Psychiatric Mental Health Nursing

Application of the Nursing Process

Psychiatric Mental Health Nursing

Application of the Nursing Process

Gertrude K. McFarland, *R.N., D.N.Sc., F.A.A.N.*
Health Scientist Administrator, Nursing Research Study Section
Division of Research Grants, National Institutes of Health, U.S. Public Health Service, Bethesda, Maryland
Formerly, Nurse Consultant, Division of Nursing, Health Resources & Services Administration, U.S. Public Health Service, Rockville, Maryland

Mary Durand Thomas, *R.N., C.S., Ph.D.*
Research Assistant Professor, Department of Psychosocial Nursing
University of Washington, Seattle, Washington

With 87 contributors from the United States and Canada

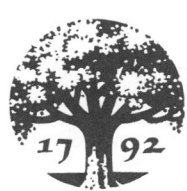 **J.B. LIPPINCOTT COMPANY**

Philadelphia   Grand Rapids   New York   St. Louis
San Francisco   London   Sydney   Tokyo

Acquiring Editor: Ellen M. Campbell
Project Editor: Dina Kamilatos
Indexer: Alexandra Weir Nickerson
Art Director: Susan Hess Blaker
Interior Design: Patti Maddaloni
Cover Art: Tom Vilot
Production Manager: Caren Erlichman
Production Coordinator: Kevin P. Johnson
Compositor: Tapsco, Inc.
Printer/Binder: The Murray Printing Company
Cover Printer: Lehigh Press

1 3 5 6 4 2

Library of Congress Cataloging-in-Publication Data

Psychiatric mental health nursing : application of the nursing process
  / [edited by] Gertrude K. McFarland, Mary Durand Thomas ; with 87
  additional contributors from the United States and Canada.
      p.   cm.
    Includes bibliographical references.
    Includes index.
    ISBN 0-397-54678-5
    1. Psychiatric nursing.   I. McFarland, Gertrude K.
  II. Thomas, Mary Durand.
    [DNLM: 1. Nursing Process.   2. Psychiatric Nursing.   WY 160 P974]
  RC440.P7373 1990
  610.73'68—dc20
  DNLM/DLC
  for Library of Congress   90–5958
                                                                      CIP

The opinions expressed herein are those of the authors and do not necessarily reflect those of the U.S. Department of Health and Human Services (National Institutes of Health, and Health Resources & Services Administration), and the Department of Veterans Affairs.

Photographs used throughout this text were chosen to illustrate or enhance the reader's understanding of specific concepts or conditions. It should not be implied that the persons pictured in these photographs have sought or received psychiatric services.

Case studies and care plans have been drawn from the clinical experiences of the authors and contributors. Names and details have been changed to maintain confidentiality.

Any procedure or practice described in this book should be applied by the health-care practitioner under appropriate supervision in accordance with professional standards of care used with regard to the unique circumstances that apply in each practice situation. Care has been taken to confirm the accuracy of information presented and to describe generally accepted practices. However, the authors, editors, and publisher cannot accept any responsibility for errors or omissions or for any consequences from application of the information in this book and make no warranty, express or implied, with respect to the contents of the book.

Every effort has been made to ensure drug selections and dosages are in accordance with current recommendations and practice. Because of ongoing research, changes in government regulations and the constant flow of information on drug therapy, reactions and interactions, the reader is cautioned to check the package insert for each drug for indications, dosages, warnings and precautions, particularly if the drug is new or infrequently used.

Consultants

Doris L. Carnevali, RN, MN

Associate Professor, Emeritus, Department of Community Health Care Systems, School of Nursing, University of Washington, Seattle, Washington

Margaret Heitkemper, PhD, RN

Associate Professor, Department of Physiological Nursing, School of Nursing, University of Washington, Seattle, Washington

James B. Lohr, MD

Chief of Inpatient Psychiatry, Veterans Administration Medical Center; Assistant Professor of Psychiatry, School of Medicine, University of California at San Diego, San Diego, California

Judith T. Maurin, RN, PhD, FAAN

Professor and Associate Dean for Academic Affairs, University of Utah, College of Nursing, Salt Lake City, Utah

Oliver Hilton Osborne, RN, PhD, FAAN

Professor, Department of Psychosocial Nursing; Adjunct Professor, Department of Anthropology, University of Washington, Seattle, Washington

Sister Callista Roy, RN, PhD, FAAN

Professor, School of Nursing, Boston College, Chestnut Hill, Massachusetts. Research Professor in Nursing, Mount St. Mary's College, Los Angeles, California

Mary Trainor, PhD, CS

Associate Professor, School of Nursing, George Mason University, Fairfax, Virginia. Nurse Psychotherapist in Private Practice, Kensington, Maryland

James E. Wilson, PharmD

Department of Psychiatry, College of Medicine; Department of Pharmacy Practice, College of Pharmacy, University of Nebraska Medical Center, Omaha, Nebraska

Contributors

Deanah I. Alexander, MSN, RN, CS

Clinical Coordinator of Psychiatric Services, Veterans Administration Medical Center, Amarillo, Texas

- *Nursing Diagnosis: Aggression (mild, moderate, severe, extreme/panic)*
- *Nursing Diagnosis: Anger*
- *Nursing Diagnosis: Altered Impulse Control*

Heather Andersen, RN, MN

Lecturer, School of Social Work; Adjunct Lecturer, Department of Community Health Care Systems, School of Nursing, University of Washington, Seattle, Washington

- *Chapter 3: Strategies for Preventing and Coping With Burnout*

Joan M. Baker, RN, CS, MS

Clinical Nurse Specialist, Psychosocial Nursing, University of Washington Medical Center; Clinical Assistant Professor, Department of Psychosocial Nursing, University of Washington, Seattle, Washington

- *Chapter 21: Clients With Anxiety Disorders*

Barbara Hyatt Baskerville, RN, BSN, MSN

Assistant Professor, Psychiatric Nursing, Division of Nursing Education, University of the District of Columbia, Washington, DC

- *Chapter 33: Milieu Therapy*

Donna R. Baughcum, RN, CS, MN

Psychiatric Nurse Clinical Specialist, McLean Counseling Associates, McLean, Virginia

- *Chapter 29: Abused Persons*

Karen A. Benson, RN, PhD

Lecturer, Pathophysiology, Seattle University, Seattle, Washington

- *Nursing Diagnosis: Emotional Lability*

Sharon L. Bernier, RN, PhD

Psychiatric Nurse Consultant and Therapist in Private Practice, Washington, DC

- *Chapter 30: Mental Health Issues and Nursing in Corrections*

Patricia A. Betrus, RN, CS, PhD

Assistant Professor, Department of Psychosocial Nursing, University of Washington, Seattle, Washington

- *Chapter 9: Neurobiology of Mental Disorders*

Joan E. Bowers, RN, EdD

Associate Professor and Chairperson, Department of Community Health, Psychiatric Mental Health and Gerontology Nursing, University of Nebraska College of Nursing, Omaha, Nebraska

- *Nursing Diagnosis: Family Coping, Potential for Growth*
- *Nursing Diagnosis: Dysfunctional Family Processes*
- *Chapter 37: Family Therapy*

Kathleen C. Buckwalter, RN, PhD

Professor, College of Nursing, University of Iowa, Iowa City, Iowa. Geropsychiatric Consultant, Abbe Center for Community Mental Health, Cedar Rapids, Iowa

- *Chapter 25: Psychosocial Needs and Care of the Elderly*
- *Chapter 47: Community Mental Health and Home Care*
- *Chapter 48: Rural Mental Health Care*

Mary T. Bush, RN, CS, MN

Staff Nurse, Emergency Department, Providence Medical Center, Seattle, Washington

- *Chapter 40: Electroconvulsive Therapy and Other Biologic Therapies*
- *Appendix IV: Laboratory Values*

Howard K. Butcher, RN, MSN

Clinical Education Specialist, Psychiatric Institute of Washington, Washington, DC

- *Chapter 4: Conceptual Frameworks for Psychiatric Mental Health Nursing Practice*
- *Chapter 12: Assessment of the Psychiatric Mental Health Client*
- *Nursing Diagnosis: Powerlessness*

Joan M. Cunningham, RN, MA

Associate Professor of Nursing, County College of Morris, Randolph, New Jersey. Clinical Specialist, Crisis Intervention Team, St. Mary's Hospital, Passaic, New Jersey

- *Chapter 35: Crisis Intervention*

Mary J. D'Amico, RN, MN

Nursing Clinical Coordinator, Royal Ottawa Psychiatric Hospital; Assistant Professor, School of Nursing, University of Ottawa, Ottawa, Ontario, Canada

- *Nursing Diagnosis: Decisional Conflict*

Verrelle M. Davis, RN, MSN

Assistant Professor, School of Nursing, Seattle University, Seattle, Washington

- *Nursing Diagnosis: Emotional Lability*

Gordon L. Dickman, MA

AASECT Certified Sex Educator, Seattle Sexual Health Center, Seattle, Washington

- *Nursing Diagnosis: Sexual Dysfunction*
- *Chapter 38: Sex Therapy*

Katie Cosper Duncan, RN, BSN

Unit Coordinator, Mental Health Unit, Scripps Memorial Hospital, La Jolla, California

- *Nursing Diagnosis: Regressed Behavior*

Carol Ann Dunphy, ARNP, MN

Nurse Practitioner, Seattle-King County Department of Public Health, AIDS Prevention Project, Seattle, Washington

- *Chapter 32: Mental Health Needs of Clients Along the Continuum of Human Immunodeficiency Virus (HIV) Infection*

Ethel Stitt Ekland, RN, MN

Geropsychiatric Clinical Nurse Specialist, Western State Hospital, Fort Steilacoom, Washington

- *Nursing Diagnosis: Hopelessness*
- *Nursing Diagnosis: Altered Perception/Cognition (confusion)*

Christina L. S. Evans, RN, CNA, MSN

Specialist, Nursing Administration in Psychiatric Nursing, Kingswood Hospital, Ferndale, Michigan. Doctoral Student, Wayne State University, Detroit, Michigan

- *Chapter 53: The Future Practice Environment and the Psychiatric Nurse Administrator*

Monique M. Farill, RN, MN

Psychiatric Clinical Nurse Specialist, Central Fulton Mental Health Center, Atlanta, Georgia

- *Nursing Diagnosis: Depression*

Britt Finley, BSN, RNC, CAC, MEd

Associate Professor, Psychiatric-Mental Health Nursing, Montana State University, College of Nursing, Missoula Extended Campus, Missoula, Montana

- *Nursing Diagnosis: Substance Abuse (alcohol)*
- *Nursing Diagnosis: Substance Abuse (drugs)*
- *Chapter 16: Clients With Psychoactive Substance Use Disorders*

Margaret I. Fitch, RN, PhD

Director of Nursing Research and Professional Development, Toronto General Division, The Toronto Hospital, Toronto, Ontario, Canada

- *Nursing Diagnosis: Defensive Coping (specify)*

Theresa S. Foley, RN, CS, PhD

Assistant Professor, Psychiatric Mental Health Nursing Graduate Program, School of Nursing, University of Michigan, Ann Arbor, Michigan

- *Nursing Diagnosis: Rape Trauma Syndrome*

Noreen Cavan Frisch, RN, PhD

Chair, Department of Nursing, Humboldt State University, Arcata, California

- *Nursing Diagnosis: Impaired Resource Management (specify)*

Elizabeth Kelchner Gerety, RN, CS, MS

Clinical Nurse Specialist, Psychiatry Consultation, Portland Veterans Affairs Medical Center, Portland, Oregon

- *Nursing Diagnosis: Grieving, Anticipatory Grieving, Dysfunctional Grieving*
- *Chapter 49: Psychiatric Consultation–Liaison Nursing*

Maryanne Godfrey, ARNP, MN

Psychotherapist in Private Practice, Everett, Washington

- *Chapter 22: Clients With Personality Disorders*

Marjory Gordon, RN, PhD, FAAN

Professor, School of Nursing, Boston College, Chestnut Hill, Massachusetts

- *Chapter 11: Nursing Process and Clinical Judgment*

Barbara Grimes, RN, MSN

Assistant Administrator for Clinical Services, Havenwick Hospital, Auburn Hills, Michigan

- *Nursing Diagnosis: Rape Trauma Syndrome*

Ruth Jalane Hagerott, RN, CS, MA

Psychiatric Nursing Director, Western State Hospital, Fort Steilacoom, Washington. Clinical Assistant Professor, Department of Psychosocial Nursing, University of Washington, Seattle, Washington

- *Nursing Diagnosis: Agitation*
- *Nursing Diagnosis: Bizarre Behavior*

Peggy Ann Hansen, ARNP, MN

Counselor and Biofeedback Therapist in Private Practice, Northwest Stress Management, Seattle, Washington

- *Chapter 34: Stress Management*

Mary Ann Hertz, RN, CS, MSN

Psychiatric Nurse, Charleston Veterans Administration Medical Center, Charleston, South Carolina

- *Nursing Diagnosis: Altered Growth and Development*

Illa Ann Hilliard, RN, CS, MSN

Director of Nursing, Eastern State Hospital, Medical Lake, Washington. Clinical Assistant Professor, Department of Psychosocial Nursing, University of Washington, Seattle, Washington

- *Nursing Diagnosis: Guilt*

Sonia D. Hinds, RN, MSN

Psychiatric Nurse Educator, District of Columbia Department of Human Services, Commission on Mental Health Services, Washington, DC

- *Chapter 26: Clients With Alzheimer's Disease*

Agnes L. Hoffman, RN, CS, PhD

Associate Professor, Department of Psychosocial Nursing, University of Washington, Seattle, Washington

- *Nursing Diagnosis: Diversional Activity Deficit*
- *Nursing Diagnosis: Loneliness*

Leta M. Holder, RN, EdD

Associate Professor of Psychiatric Mental Health Nursing, Georgia College, Milledgeville, Georgia

- *Nursing Diagnosis: Potential for Injury*
- *Nursing Diagnosis: Knowledge Deficit (specify)*

Marilyn G. Holnsteiner, BSN, MN

Charge Nurse of Women's and Eating Disorder Program, Belle Park Hospital, Houston, Texas

- *Nursing Diagnosis: Potential for Elopement*

Mary I. Huntley, RN, PhD

Associate Professor, School of Nursing, Mankato State University, Mankato, Minnesota

- *Nursing Diagnosis: Wellness-Seeking Behavior*

Robin S. Johnson, ACSW, DSW

Associate Director, Social Work Department, University of Washington Medical Center, Seattle, Washington

- *Chapter 3: Strategies for Preventing and Coping With Burnout*

Maisie Schmidt Kashka, RN, PhD

Assistant Professor, College of Nursing, Texas Woman's University, Denton, Texas

- *Nursing Diagnosis: Wellness-Seeking Behavior*

Helen Kirkpatrick, RN, MScN

Clinical Nurse Specialist, Hamilton Psychiatric Hospital, Hamilton, Ontario, Canada

- *Nursing Diagnosis: Powerlessness*

Connie B. Klopfenstein, RN, MN

Psychiatric Clinical Nurse Specialist, Transplant Team, Emory University Hospital. Formerly, Coordinator, Psychiatric Emergency Clinic, Grady Memorial Hospital, Atlanta, Georgia

- *Nursing Diagnosis: Depression*

Ann Knecht-Kirkham, RN, CS, MS

Assistant Professor of Psychiatric Nursing, Harris College of Nursing, Texas Christian University, Fort Worth, Texas

- *Chapter 43: Transactional Therapy*

Mary Kunes-Connell, RN, MSN

Assistant Professor, School of Nursing, Coordinator, Psychiatric–Mental Health Nursing, Creighton University; Clinical Specialist, AMI Saint Joseph Center for Mental Health, Omaha, Nebraska. Doctoral Student, Adult Education, University of Nebraska, Lincoln, Nebraska

- *Nursing Diagnosis: Altered Nutrition, Less than Body Requirements*
- *Chapter 14: Clients With Disorders Usually First Evident in Infancy, Childhood, and Adolescence*
- *Chapter 23: Children and Adolescents: Developmental Issues and Concerns*
- *Chapter 31: Clients With Eating Disorders*

Gail M. Lascik, RN, CS, MN

Nursing Education Coordinator, Clinical Nurse Specialist, Eastern State Hospital, Medical Lake, Washington. Clinical Assistant Professor, Department of Psychosocial Nursing, University of Washington, Seattle, Washington

- *Nursing Diagnosis: Boredom*

Suzanne Sexton Leichman, RN, CS, MA

Psychiatric Clinical Nurse Specialist, Western State Hospital, Fort Steilacoom, Washington. Clinical Instructor, Department of Psychosocial Nursing, University of Washington, Seattle, Washington

- *Nursing Diagnosis: Maturational and Situational Crisis*

Martha J. Lentz, RN, PhD

Research Assistant Professor, Department of Physiological Nursing, University of Washington, Seattle, Washington

- *Nursing Diagnosis: Sleep Pattern Disturbance*

Barbara S. Levinson, RN, MSN, CS

Director of Nursing, Belle Park Psychiatric Hospital, Houston, Texas. Doctoral Candidate in Psychiatric Mental Health Nursing, University of Texas, Austin, Texas

- *Chapter 42: Cognitive Behavioral Therapy*

Irene Daniels Lewis, RN, DNSc, FAAN

Associate Professor of Geropsychiatric Nursing, San Jose State University, Department of Nursing, San Jose, California

- *Chapter 46: The Mental Health Care Delivery System*
- *Chapter 55: Education*

Sharon A. Link, RN, MSN

Head Nurse, Clinical Nurse Specialist, Crisis Stabilization Unit, Grady Memorial Hospital, Atlanta, Georgia

- *Chapter 20: Clients With Mood Disorders*

Carolyn A. Livingston, ARNP, PhD

AASECT Certified Sex Therapist and Sex Educator, Seattle Sexual Health Center; Clinical Instructor, Department of Psychosocial Nursing, University of Washington, Seattle, Washington

- *Nursing Diagnosis: Sexual Dysfunction*
- *Chapter 38: Sex Therapy*

Melodie A. Lohr, BSN, MSN

Program Director, Mental Health Unit, Scripps Memorial Hospital, La Jolla, California

- *Nursing Diagnosis: Regressed Behavior*
- *Chapter 17: Clients With Schizophrenia*
- *Chapter 39: Psychopharmacology*

Maxine E. Loomis, RNCS, PhD, FAAN

Professor and Director, Doctoral Program, University of South Carolina, College of Nursing, Columbia, South Carolina

- *Chapter 7: Group Dynamics Theory*
- *Chapter 36: Group Therapy*

Beverly Koehler Lunsford, RN, MN

Director, Adolescent Health Programs, Community of Hope Health Services, Washington, DC

- *Chapter 28: Mental Health Needs of Homeless Persons*

Mary-Lou Martin, RN, MScN

Clinical Nurse Specialist, Hamilton Psychiatric Hospital; Assistant Clinical Professor, McMaster University, Hamilton, Ontario, Canada

- *Nursing Diagnosis: Impaired Social Interaction*

James C. McCann, RN, DNSc

Nurse Consultant, Nurse Education Practice Resources Branch, Special Projects Section, Division of Nursing, Health Resources and Services Administration, U.S. Department of Health and Human Services, Rockville, Maryland

- *Chapter 50: Impact of the Medicare Prospective Payment System on Psychiatric Care*

Joan Hanser McConnell, RN, MS

Assistant Director of Nursing, Psychiatry and Rehabilitation Services, Sacred Heart Medical Center, Spokane, Washington. Clinical Assistant Professor, Department of Psychosocial Nursing, University of Washington, Seattle, Washington

- *Nursing Diagnosis: Fear*

Gertrude K. McFarland, RN, DNSc, FAAN

Health Scientist Administrator, Nursing Research Study Section, Division of Research Grants, National Institutes of Health, U.S. Public Health Service, Bethesda, Maryland

- *Chapter 4: Conceptual Frameworks for Psychiatric Mental Health Nursing Practice*
- *Chapter 12: Assessment of the Psychiatric Mental Health Client*
- *Chapter 13: Introduction: Nursing Diagnoses in Psychiatric Mental Health Nursing*

Helen S. A. Murphy, RN, MN

Program Planner, Division of Alcohol and Substance Abuse, Department of Social and Health Services, Olympia, Washington. Clinical Instructor, Department of Psychosocial Nursing, University of Washington, Seattle, Washington. Psychiatric Instructor, South Puget Sound Community College, Olympia, Washington

- *Nursing Diagnosis: Altered Health Maintenance*

Charlotte Naschinski, RN, MS

Acting Director, Nursing Education Section, District of Columbia Commission on Mental Health Services, Washington, DC

- *Chapter 6: The Communication Process*
- *Nursing Diagnosis: Impaired Communication*
- *Chapter 24: Life Events of Adulthood and Related Mental Health Needs and Treatment*

Fe Nieves-Khouw, RN, CS, MSN

Psychiatric Unit Coordinator, District of Columbia Commission on Mental Health Services, Washington, DC

- *Chapter 41: Behavior Therapy*
- *Chapter 44: Reality Therapy*

Joan Norris, RN, PhD

Associate Professor of Psychiatric Mental Health Nursing, Associate Dean and Director of Graduate Nursing and Research, School of Nursing, Creighton University, Omaha, Nebraska

- *Chapter 15: Clients With Organic Mental Syndromes and Disorders*
- *Chapter 27: Chronically Mentally Ill Clients*

Linda-Lee O'Brien-Pallas, RN, PhD

Assistant Professor, Faculty of Nursing, University of Toronto, Toronto, Ontario, Canada

- *Nursing Diagnosis: Defensive Coping (specify)*

Annette M. O'Connor, RN, PhD

Assistant Professor, Career Investigator, Patient Decision Making Research, University of Ottawa School of Nursing, Ottawa, Ontario, Canada

- *Nursing Diagnosis: Decisional Conflict*

Frederica W. O'Connor, RN, PhD

Assistant Professor, Department of Psychosocial Nursing, University of Washington, Seattle, Washington

- *Chapter 10: Health Promotion and Disease Prevention in Psychiatric Mental Health Nursing*

Ellen Frances Olshansky, RNC, DNSc

Assistant Professor, Department of Parent and Child Nursing, University of Washington, Seattle, Washington

- *Nursing Diagnosis: Altered Parenting (actual, potential)*

Helen Palisin, RN, PhD

Independent Writer and Consultant, Seattle, Washington. Formerly, Coordinator, Psychiatric Nursing, Creighton University, Omaha, Nebraska. Postdoctoral Research Fellow and Visiting Scholar, Child Development and Mental Retardation Center, University of Washington, Seattle, Washington

- *Chapter 5: Developmental and Psychological Theories*
- *Chapter 45: Alternative Therapies*

Donna Poole, RN, CS, MSN

Hospital Consultation Liaison Nurse Specialist, Group Health Cooperative Medical Center; Clinical Instructor, Department of Psychosocial Nursing, University of Washington, Seattle, Washington

- *Nursing Diagnosis: Ineffective Individual Coping*
- *Nursing Diagnosis: Self-Care Deficit*

Gail J. Ray, RN, CS, EdD

Chairperson and Associate Professor, Department of Nursing, Gonzaga University, Spokane, Washington. Clinical Assistant Professor, Department of Psychosocial Nursing, University of Washington, Seattle, Washington. Formerly, Director of Quality Assurance and Clinical Nurse Specialist, Eastern State Hospital, Medical Lake, Washington

- *Chapter 54: Quality Assurance in Psychiatric Nursing*

Janet M. Rhode, ARNP, MN

Counselor and Biofeedback Therapist in Private Practice, Northwest Stress Management, Seattle, Washington

- *Chapter 34: Stress Management*

Susan M. Robertson, ARNP, MN

Utilization Review Analyst, Blue Cross of Washington and Alaska; Clinical Instructor, Department of Psychosocial Nursing, University of Washington, Seattle, Washington

- *Nursing Diagnosis: Self-Concept Disturbance (Personal Identity Disturbance, Self-Esteem Disturbance, Body Image Disturbance, Role Performance Disturbance)*

Eldine I. Sanger, RN, BSN

Nurse Coordinator, Psychiatric Unit, University of Washington Medical Center; Clinical Associate, Department of Psychosocial Nursing, University of Washington, Seattle, Washington

- *Nursing Diagnosis: Post-Overdose Syndrome*

Jean Scheideman, RN, CS, MA

Psychosocial Nurse, Community Psychiatric Clinic and Private Practice, Seattle. Clinical Instructor, Department of Psychosocial Nursing, University of Washington, Seattle, Washington

- *Nursing Diagnosis: Altered Perception/Cognition (delusions)*
- *Nursing Diagnosis: Suspiciousness*

Sandra C. Sellin, RN, MS

DNS Candidate, University of California, San Francisco; Associate Clinical Instructor, Psychosocial Nursing, City College of San Francisco, San Francisco, California

- *Chapter 52: Ethical Issues in Psychiatric Mental Health Nursing*

Julie K. Sengstacken, RN

Director of Staff Growth and Development, Belle Park Hospital, Houston, Texas

- *Nursing Diagnosis: Manipulation*

Billie M. Severtsen, RN, EdD

Assistant Professor, Intercollegiate Center for Nursing Education, Spokane, Washington

- *Nursing Diagnosis: Spiritual Distress*

S. Robin Shanks, RN, MSN, JD

Senior Risk Management Consultant, Corroon & Black Corporation, Nashville, Tennessee

- *Chapter 51: Legal Issues in Psychiatric Mental Health Nursing*

Lois Elaine Smith, RNC, MN

Director, Community of Hope Health Services, Washington, DC

- *Chapter 28: Mental Health Needs of Homeless Persons*

Geraldine M. Spillers, RN, MSN

Head Nurse, Affective Disorders Unit, National Institutes of Health, Clinical Center, Department of Nursing, Bethesda, Maryland

- *Nursing Diagnosis: Suicide Potential*

Katsuko Tanaka, RN, CS, MN

Staff Nurse, Addiction Treatment Center, Veterans Administration Medical Center; Clinical Assistant Professor, Department of Psychosocial Nursing, University of Washington, Seattle, Washington

- *Nursing Diagnosis: Post-Trauma Response*

Mary Durand Thomas, RN, CS, PhD

Research Assistant Professor, Department of Psychosocial Nursing, University of Washington, Seattle, Washington

- *Chapter 2: Therapeutic Relationships With Clients*
- *Chapter 8: Cultural Concepts and Psychiatric Mental Health Nursing*
- *Nursing Diagnosis: Altered Perception/Cognition (hallucinations)*

Jennifer A. Turner, RN, MSN

Director, Psychiatric Nursing, Grady Memorial Hospital, Atlanta, Georgia

- *Chapter 20: Clients With Mood Disorders*

Lillian Eleanor Wade, RN, BSN, MSN

Clinical Specialist, Psychiatric Nursing, Department of Human Services, Commission on Mental Health Services, Washington, DC

- *Chapter 26: Clients With Alzheimer's Disease*
- *Chapter 33: Milieu Therapy*

Janet Weber, RN, MSN

Instructor, Department of Nursing, Southeast Missouri State University, Cape Girardeau, Missouri

- *Nursing Diagnosis: Impaired Resource Management (specify)*

Jan Westwell, RN, MScN

Clinical Nurse Specialist, Hamilton Psychiatric Hospital; Clinical Lecturer, School of Nursing, McMaster University, Hamilton, Ontario, Canada

- *Nursing Diagnosis: Impaired Social Interaction*

Georgia Whitley, RN, EdD

Assistant Professor, Psychiatric Mental Health Nursing, School of Nursing, Northern Illinois University, Dekalb, Illinois

- *Nursing Diagnosis: Anxiety (mild, moderate, severe, extreme/panic)*
- *Nursing Diagnosis: Noncompliance (specify)*
- *Nursing Diagnosis: Ritualistic Behavior*
- *Chapter 18: Clients With Delusional (Paranoid) Disorder*
- *Chapter 19: Clients With Psychotic Disorders Not Elsewhere Classified*

Marilyn Peddicord Whitley, RN, CS, PhD

Professor, Director and Chair, Department of Nursing, Northern Montana College, Havre, Montana

- *Chapter 1: The History of Psychiatric Mental Health Nursing*

Joanne Davis Whitney, RN, MS

PhD Candidate, Department of Physiological Nursing, University of California at San Francisco, San Francisco, California

- *Nursing Diagnosis: Somatization*

Vivian Wolf-Wilets, RN, MA, PhD, FAAN

Professor, Department of Psychosocial Nursing, University of Washington, Seattle, Washington

- *Nursing Diagnosis: Altered Perception/Cognition (memory loss)*
- *Chapter 34: Stress Management*

Preface

We had a number of goals in mind when we set out to develop *Psychiatric Mental Health Nursing: Application of the Nursing Process.* The foremost of these was to focus on that unique body of knowledge that is nursing, and so we chose the nursing process as the organizing framework for presenting psychiatric mental health nursing content. The text has been designed to provide a comprehensive understanding of nursing assessment, nursing diagnosis, goal setting, nursing intervention, evaluation, and other information essential for providing quality nursing care.

This is most clearly evident in Unit II, Nursing Diagnosis and Process, which presents nursing content on more than fifty nursing diagnoses judged to be the most useful for psychiatric mental health nursing practice; these were selected from developmental work of the North American Nursing Diagnosis Association (NANDA), the American Nurses' Association (ANA) task force, and our own research. The unit begins with a chapter on the nursing process and clinical judgment by Marjory Gordon, and one on nursing assessment. Dr. Gordon, a nurse educator and leader in nursing diagnoses and clinical judgment, summarizes her chapter by reminding us that information collection and interpretation are continuous throughout the nursing process. The nursing process begins with the collection of information in order to determine if a problem exists and continues through to the evaluation of a treatment plan. When a diagnostic cue to a health problem is assessed, the diagnostic judgment process is initiated. Interpreting the diagnostic meaning of the information and the formulation of a problem using standardized terminology results in a nursing diagnosis. This diagnosis is used as a basis for the therapeutic judgments involved in care planning, implementation, and evaluation.

Chapter 13 presents major nursing diagnoses and develops each in depth—for example, aggression, anxiety, defensive coping (specify), maturational and situational crisis, depression, dysfunctional family processes, family coping, potential for growth, altered impulse control, altered perception/cognition (confusion, delusions, hallucinations, memory loss), post-trauma response, self-concept disturbance, impaired social interaction, spiritual distress, and wellness-seeking behavior. A consistent outline is followed for each diagnosis: definition and description, theory and research,

related/risk factors, defining characteristics, and nursing process and rationale. Every nursing diagnosis section also includes a case study and research highlights.

The nursing process serves as a theme in other units of the text as well. For instance, Unit III, Clients With Major Psychiatric Disorders and the Nursing Process, incorporates content on the major classes of psychiatric disorders from the DSM-III-R. Following a description of the psychiatric disorder, the text discusses assessment, treatment modalities, related nursing roles, and common nursing diagnoses. In Chapter 14, for example, Mary Kunes-Connell draws from her experience as a child psychiatric clinical nurse specialist, to examine the dynamics and behaviors associated with conduct disorders, and presents practical assessment guidelines for interviewing the child and family, along with identifying common nursing diagnoses. In Chapter 15, Joan Norris, a psychiatric mental health nurse educator and expert in working with the chronically mentally ill, specifies common nursing diagnoses associated with organic mental disorders. Britt Finley, also a psychiatric mental health nurse educator and a specialist in caring for clients with psychoactive substance use disorders, contrasts the etiological explanations of these disorders in Chapter 16, and describes treatment modalities and nursing roles.

A comprehensive and up-to-date text must also include the fundamental information essential to the provision of quality nursing care. Thus, Unit I presents the theoretical and conceptual bases for psychiatric mental health nursing. It begins with the historical perspective (Chapter 1) and continues with a chapter on therapeutic relationships with clients, in which Mary Durand Thomas discusses the importance for psychiatric nurses to be aware of their own beliefs, feelings, behaviors, and values, along with the psychiatric nurse qualities of respect, genuineness, empathy and hope (Chapter 2). Strategies for preventing and coping with burnout useful for psychiatric mental health nurses in today's high stress health care environment are presented in a creative chapter (3) by Heather Andersen and Robin Johnson. Developmental and psychological theories, the communication process, and group dynamics theory are comprehensively examined in Chapters 5, 6, and 7. Chapter 4, by Howard Butcher and Gertrude McFarland, reviews selected nursing conceptual frameworks (Peplau, Roy, Orem, King, Rogers) and examines how they fit with nursing process and nursing diagnoses in this text. Concepts essential for the mental health needs of persons from diverse cultures are included in Chapter 8. The neurobiology of mental disorders (Chapter 9) and content on health promotion and disease prevention (Chapter 10) conclude the unit.

We also wanted to be responsive to the issues and developments facing contemporary society, each of which confronts our professions with unique challenges. Thus Unit IV, Mental Health and Illness in Special Population Groups, focuses on target populations with special mental health needs, such as the chronically mentally ill, clients with Alzheimer's disease, homeless persons, abused persons, the imprisoned, clients with eating disorders, and clients along the continuum of HIV infection. The authors of these chapters describe the population group and then discuss assessment parameters, treatment modalities, related nursing roles, and common nursing diagnoses. Donna Baughcum, a psychiatric clinical nurse specialist, incorporates her wealth of experience in working with abused persons in Chapter 29. She notes that abused individuals, whether adults or children, have been robbed of power and control over their own lives and often distrust others who offer assistance; an empathetic, sensitive nurse who is knowledgeable about the complex dynamics of abuse can make all the difference in effecting a positive resolution of the trauma inflicted by the abuse. Mary Kunes-Connell notes in Chapter 31 that the psychiatric mental health nurse plays a vital role in the prevention, identification, and treatment of eating disorders such as anorexia nervosa, bulimia nervosa, and obesity. Carol Dunphy draws on her expertise as a nurse practitioner in an AIDS prevention project in Chapter 32, and identifies nursing diagnoses and describes client goals, nursing interventions, and outcome criteria for the worried well, HIV-positive asymptomatic persons, and those manifesting HIV disease.

Unit V, Specialized Psychiatric Therapies and Treatment Programs and the Nursing Process, provides state-of-the-art content and research findings in chapters on a wide variety of therapies, such as milieu therapy, stress management, crisis intervention, group therapy, family therapy, sex therapy, psychopharmacology, electroconvulsive therapy and other biological therapies, cognitive behavioral therapy, and alternative therapies. Each chapter provides a description of and rationale for the use of the therapy for clients with specific psychiatric disorders, and then discusses the role(s) that psychiatric nurses assume in such a therapy. Common nursing diagnoses among clients treated with each therapy are also identified. For example, in Chapter 36, Maxine Loomis, a psychiatric mental health nursing educator, includes a discussion of the therapeutic factors present in

therapy groups. In Chapter 37, Joan Bowers identifies assumptions that underlie the family approach in psychiatric mental health nursing, discusses selected family therapy models, describes nursing roles in relation to family therapy, and identifies common nursing diagnoses of families in family therapy. Gordon Dickman and Carolyn Livingston, sex therapists and educators, describe in Chapter 38 the various sex therapies, including medical and psychotherapeutic interventions, treatment models for various sexual disorders, nursing roles, and common nursing diagnoses for individuals in sex therapy. Melodie Lohr, a psychiatric nurse program director, provides (with consultation from James Wilson, Pharm.D.) an excellent overview of neuroleptic, antiparkinsonian, lithium, antidepressant, antianxiety, and other psychotropic medications in Chapter 39, by addressing indications for use, guidelines for administration, side effects, and nursing roles.

Finally, in addition to focusing on current developments, we wanted to address *projected* challenges and issues confronting psychiatric mental health nursing. By incorporating current theory and research, as well as content on nursing diagnoses and process, Unit VI describes the current status of and future issues for the mental health care delivery system, community mental health and home care, rural mental health care, psychiatric consultation–liaison nursing, the Medicare prospective payment system, legal issues, and ethical issues in psychiatric mental nursing. For example, drawing from her experience as a psychiatric consultation liaison nurse (PCLN), Elizabeth Gerety delineates the four major functions (clinical, administrative, research, and education) of this role, which are influenced by organizational and clinical needs, as well as the needs, goals, philosophy, and clinical expertise of PCLNs.

The text concludes with Unit VII, Status and Directions in Psychiatric Mental Health Nursing, which describes the status of the future practice environment and the nurse administrator, quality assurance in psychiatric nursing, and education as each relates to psychiatric mental health nursing. Christina Evans, herself an established psychiatric mental health nurse administrator, reviews in Chapter 53 trends that will impact on psychiatric mental health nursing care and programmatic changes that will assist psychiatric nursing administrators in keeping pace with these trends. She notes that the future practice environment will offer many challenges in the constantly changing health care environment, as well as the potential for satisfaction to psychiatric mental health nurses. To be successful in the future, psychiatric mental health nursing must begin to plan for that future.

Because we wanted the best quality content possible, we carefully selected a diverse group of professionals to serve as contributing authors to the text, based upon their unique expertise in specialties such as psychiatric mental health nursing, nursing education, nursing research, nursing theory, medical-surgical nursing, physiology, psychiatry, psychology, social work, and pharmacology. We also appointed a board of senior consultants to assist us in a rigorous peer review process for the entire manuscript. The most complete, indepth, and current content is thus ensured throughout the text.

As senior authors, we brought complementary expertise and education to this text. Gertrude K. McFarland's advanced educational preparation is in psychiatric mental health nursing science. She began her career as a psychiatric mental health nurse specialist, served as a nurse consultant in undergraduate education at the national level for many years, provided leadership to the North American nursing diagnosis movement for almost two decades, and is currently the research administrator for a nationwide research program. Mary Durand Thomas, a nurse anthropologist, has extensive background as a psychiatric mental health nursing educator. She has worked with the severely mentally ill and served as a consulting psychosocial nurse clinician for a native American tribe, and has also been actively involved in the development of nursing diagnoses.

The entire team of expert contributors and consultants helped us achieve our goal of developing a scholarly work. Relevant theory and research are incorporated throughout the text. In addition, each chapter and nursing diagnosis section features **Research Highlights** that may summarize or critique a study which is cited in or related to the content of the chapter, describe the implications of a particular research study for psychiatric mental health nursing practice, suggest areas where additional nursing research is needed, or present related research by means of a brief annotated bibliography. James McCann, previously a psychiatric nurse consultant for the Health Care Financing Administration, USPHS, chose the last option in Chapter 50, describing among other studies, "A Two Year Follow-Up of a Comparative Trial of the Cost-Effectiveness of Home and Hospital Psychiatric Treatment."

In order to demonstrate the application of theory and research to practice, we have also included clinical examples throughout the text. A **Case Study** is presented in each nursing diagnosis section. In the section on Decisional Conflict in Chapter 13, for example, Annette O'Connor, a career investigator in patient decision making and a nurse educator, describes the nurse's interview with a client, then formulates a specific nursing diagnosis, and discusses goals, nursing interventions and discharge planning. A Case Study, along with a specific **Nursing Care Plan,** is featured in each chapter where relevant; for example, in Chapter 25, Psychosocial Needs in Care of the Elderly, Kathleen Buckwalter, a psychiatric nurse

educator and psychogerontologist, describes a 78-year-old widower in the case study, followed by a specific care plan that addresses specific nursing diagnoses and such client goals as: maintain optimal level of cognitive/perceptual and affective functioning and be protected from harm.

Other useful features of the text include the following:

- **Content outlines** provide an orientation to each chapter and quick reference for the major chapter topic areas.
- **Reader objectives** are specific for each chapter.
- A **detailed table of contents** and the **index** help in quickly locating key content covered in each chapter or section of the text.
- The **application of the nursing process** and **examples of therapeutic responses to clients** are integrated throughout the text.
- **Boxed material** throughout the text provides examples, summarizes important concepts and information, or expands content discussed in the narrative; for example, Box 12-2 offers an example of a Psychiatric Nursing Assessment Guide Organized by Functional Health Patterns in Chapter 12, Assessment of the Psychiatric Mental Health Client.
- **Charts** are consistently used in each nursing diagnosis section in Chapter 13. Chart 1 summarizes the definition of the nursing diagnosis category and lists the major related factors as well as the major defining characteristics. Chart 2 summarizes the nursing process described in the narrative.
- **Tables** are used to organize detailed content clearly and logically.
- **Photographs** are used to capture emotions not as readily conveyed in words or to demonstrate special skills (for example, the photos used in Chapter 28, which so vividly express the plight of the homeless, and the Aggression section in Chapter 13, which demonstrate interventions for severe or extreme aggression).
- **Figures,** liberally used throughout the text, show content in diagram form, by providing an example of the content or expanding on the narrative (for example, a diagram of Peplau's Interpersonal Relations Conceptual Framework in Chapter 4, or Figure 52-1, the Ethical Decision Making Model).
- The **Appendices** summarize useful content: the list of currently approved NANDA nursing diagnoses and NANDA Taxonomy I Revised; the ANA Classification of Human Responses of Concern for Psychiatric Mental Health Nursing Practice; the DSM-III-R classifications; and a listing of laboratory values.
- An **Instructor's Manual** accompanies the text and provides information to aid faculty in preparing teaching/learning activities for students using the textbook. Each chapter contains an

overview, an outline of the chapter organization in the text, behavioral objectives, key terms, helpful classroom and clinical strategies, and supportive resources for students, such as current additional readings and audiovisuals. A unique feature is the listing of distributors for the audiovisual resources that are identified throughout the manual.

We as nurses encourage students and practicing nurses to continue participating in the exciting endeavor of developing psychiatric mental health nursing and the nursing process. As authors, we hope this text will serve as both a starting point and a continuing reference in that endeavor.

Gertrude K. McFarland, R.N., D.N.Sc., F.A.A.N.
Mary Durand Thomas, R.N., C.S., Ph.D.

Acknowledgments

Many individuals have contributed time and effort and expertise to the development of **Psychiatric Mental Health Nursing: Application of the Nursing Process.** A diverse group of experts in their fields served as contributing authors to selected chapters and sections. We also worked with a board of consultants who gave us invaluable assistance in the peer review process throughout the creation of the manuscript. All of these individuals are listed elsewhere in the text, along with their credentials and affiliations. We extend a sincere thank-you to each one of them.

We would also like to express special thanks to Elizabeth Gerety, Julie McKim, Patricia Sosnovec, and Mary Cowan, for their development of the Instructor's Manual that accompanies the text.

The talented professionals at J. B. Lippincott—Ellen Campbell, Diana Intenzo, Dina Kamilatos, and Nancy Mullins—have each contributed their skill and wisdom. We are most appreciative.

Supportive colleagues and friends are too numerous to mention individually, except for Dr. Lillian S. Brunner, F.A.A.N., eminent scholar and prolific Lippincott author, who had initial confidence in a fledgling author many years ago and has provided encouragement and periodic consultation ever since.

Finally, we thank our families: Al McFarland and John and Emma Ramseier; and John B. Thomas, Hugh Thomas, James M. Thomas, Evelyn Durand, and the late Walter G. Durand.

Contents in Brief

Detailed Contents

6

The Communication Process

7

Group Dynamics Theory

8

Cultural Concepts and Psychiatric Mental Health Nursing

9

Neurobiology of Mental Disorders

10

Health Promotion and Disease Prevention in Psychiatric Mental Health Nursing

15

Clients With Organic Mental Syndromes and Disorders

16

Clients With Psychoactive Substance Use Disorders

17

Clients With Schizophrenia

18

Clients With Delusional (Paranoid) Disorder

19

Clients With Psychotic Disorders Not Elsewhere Classified

20

Clients With Mood Disorders

UNIT V
Specialized Psychiatric Therapies and Treatment Programs and the Nursing Process

33
Milieu Therapy

34
Stress Management

35
Crisis Intervention

36
Group Therapy

37
Family Therapy

38
Sex Therapy

51

Legal Issues in Psychiatric Mental Health Nursing

52

Ethical Issues in Psychiatric Mental Health Nursing

UNIT VII
Status and Directions of Psychiatric Mental Health Nursing

53

The Future Practice Environment and the Psychiatric Nurse Administrator

54

Quality Assurance in Psychiatric Nursing

55

Education

Appendices

Appendix I

Appendix II

Appendix III

Appendix IV

Index

Psychiatric Mental Health Nursing

Application of the Nursing Process

Theoretical and Conceptual Bases for Psychiatric Mental Health Nursing

1

Marilyn Peddicord Whitley

The History of Psychiatric Mental Health Nursing

OBJECTIVES

After reading this chapter, the reader will be able to:

1. Describe American pre-modern treatment practices for mental illnesses
2. Describe the American evolution of the profession of psychiatric mental health nursing
3. Understand the impact of scientific, social, and legislative decisions on the treatment of the mentally ill and on psychiatric mental health nursing services
4. Identify contemporary roles of psychiatric mental health nurses
5. Understand the modern challenges associated with providing psychiatric mental health nursing care.

INTRODUCTION

Today psychiatric mental health nurses are employed in state hospitals, community mental health centers, and in general hospitals. Some nurses with advanced preparation and credentials establish independent practices. In some states, these advanced practitioners may prescribe medications and receive direct third-party payment for their services. These independent nursing roles have evolved over the last century.

EARLY TREATMENT OF THE MENTALLY ILL IN AMERICA

It is useful to review the past care given to the mentally ill in the United States as a means for understanding the development of psychiatric mental health nursing. The first hospital for the mentally ill in the United States, the Eastern Lunatic Hospital, opened in Williamsburg, Virginia in 1773. Others opened after the Revolutionary War. In America's more populated urban areas, a few mentally ill were admitted to the newly constructed general hospitals; however, mental patients constituted fewer than 10% of those hospitalized in the major general hospitals in Philadelphia and New York. These hospitals used a variety of treatment methods, the most prevalent being moral treatment strategies, the use of medications such as purgatives and emetics, and blood-letting techniques. Some hospitals also used a special tranquilizing chair, invented by Benjamin Rush, in which patients were seated, tied down, and suspended in the air for relief of agitation.[8]

During this early period, caregivers, including the few nurses available to care for the mentally ill, offered custodial care to institutionalized patients. Some nurses dispensed early forms of medication, but the care was physically oriented; no attempt was made to deal with patients' interpersonal or emotional issues.[9]

After the American Revolution, the growing belief that an individual could be changed by humanitarian treatment led to social reforms. Small private institutions that catered to the upper classes, such as the McLean Asylum in Massachusetts, began to develop at about the turn of the 19th century. Supportive moral treatment was offered to persons believed to have experienced unmanageable emotional difficulties. Some of these treatment centers reported extremely high cure rates.

The American form of moral treatment was based on principles recommended by the French psychiatrist, Phillippe Pinel (1745–1826). That is, emphasis was placed on a relationship between a few patients and a physician that was marked by good will on the part of the physician. However, even greater attention was given to a comfortable physical setting and interactive influences with others as curative agents. A family-like atmosphere in which staff members and their families associated with patients, as a matter of course, was utilized in these moral treatment environments.[3]

Under the direction of physicians, some of the early graduates of America's first schools of nursing helped provide the treatment atmosphere. Activities such as exercise, organized games, structured work, educational classes, and religious devotions were provided by these nurses.[4]

During the 19th century, America experienced an increase in urbanization, unemployment, and periodic economic depressions. These phenomena, along with the population growth that resulted from massive immigration, drew attention to America's mentally ill among the poor and eventually led to the building of very large mental institutions. By their very size, these hospitals militated against moral treatment, which eventually fell into disuse. The large institutions became even larger as social reformers, critical of the confinement of the mentally ill in jails and almshouses, exerted pressure for the confinement of additional individuals in state hospitals. It was during this time that increasing emphasis was placed on treating the mentally ill as if they had physical illnesses and were in need of scientific, rather than moral, care.[3] (See also Chapter 46.)

First Stage Psychiatric Nursing

During the latter decades of the 19th century, nursing leaders began to found schools to educate nurses in the care of the mentally ill. Linda Richards, an early nurse leader, was instrumental in forming schools for the training of nurses in hospitals for the mentally ill. She worked with a physician during the early 1880s to establish a school of nursing at McLean Asylum. Nurses graduating from this school learned the care of both the mentally and physically ill. The latter was accomplished through affiliations with general hospitals. The content of the mental illness portion of the curriculum included elements of the moral treatment approach. Because few of these nurses worked in mental institutions, however, and the working conditions required 12- to 14-hour days, six to seven days a week, the nurses in those institutions were often able to give little more than custodial care.[6]

Civil Rights and the Mentally Ill

Because of their symptoms, the mentally ill were most often indigent and suffered from multiple social, psychological, and financial problems. Family and friends often wished to have them confined to institutions out of the mainstream of society. Civil suits arose around the issue of wrongful commitment, an issue made more complex by the lack of precision in the diagnosis of mental illness. The courts found themselves in the confusing position of trying to preserve citizens' civil rights, while, at the same time, protecting the citizenry at large from the perceived dangers of the mentally ill.[3]

Classification of Mental Illnesses

A classification system that would help identify the truly mentally ill was sorely needed. Near the end of the 19th century, observation of the large cohorts of mentally ill then confined in well-established institutions in both America and Europe gave rise to such a classification of mental illnesses. Major categories of mental illness were identified, and various somatic causes of mental impairment, such as syphillis and epilepsy, were discovered. With the somatic explanations of etiology, many somatic treatments were utilized. Hydrotherapy, shock treatments (including electric shock), and several systems of suspension and spinning of patients, called centrifuge therapy, were used. Psychosurgery, especially the various forms of lobotomy, became popular. Systematic drug therapies such as insulin, narcosis, and Metrazol therapy were widely used. Psychotherapies, including Freudian psychoanalysis and its many derivatives, became popular in the second quarter of the 20th century.[8]

By the 1940s, under close physician supervision, nurses often administered hydrotherapy and insulin therapy. They also participated in the administration of electric shock treatments and continued in their attempts to maintain sanitary and safe conditions within the state hospitals.[4]

POST-WORLD WAR II

The post-World War II era brought significant and far-reaching influences on psychiatric nursing. These included changes in the practice of psychiatry, adoption of psychoactive drugs, critiques of social scientists, and federal legislation.

Changes in Psychiatric Practices

Practitioners who had experiences in treating war veterans suggested that people could be aggressively treated with drugs and psychotherapy, particularly group and milieu therapies. The English psychiatrist, Maxwell Jones, in *The Therapeutic Community*,[11] questioned current custodial methods, suggested better staff–patient relationships, and increased patient participation in therapeutic programs. Jones also suggested mechanisms for housing and treating the mentally ill, reminiscent of moral treatment, and reintroduced the concept of smaller units for treatment. (See also Chapter 33.)

Psychoactive Medications

During the 1950s, pharmacologic experimentation showed that chlorpromazine (Thorazine) contained properties that had the ability to reduce psychotic behaviors. This drug was given in experimental doses to institutionalized patients, and markedly reduced the amount of violence in state institutions. It also reduced delusions and hallucinations, and for some patients, significantly shortened their stay in state hospitals.

Social Science Research

Studies by social scientists of mental illness and its treatment offered new perspectives. Stanton and Schwartz's monograph, *The Mental Hospital*,[19] described the social structure of Chestnut Lodge Hospital in Rockville, Maryland. Alexander Leighton described the treatment of the mentally ill in a Canadian Newfoundland community in his book *My Name is Legion*.[13] Hollingshead and Redlich published an extensive research report, *Social Class and Mental Illness*,[10] which demonstrated that mental institutions served lower-class individuals at a higher rate than individuals from the middle and upper classes. Their study gave a class taint to mental institutions.

The establishment of milieu therapy and the increased use of group treatment, psychoactive drugs, and social science research changed the role of nurses in the treatment of the mentally ill. Maxwell Jones and others taught nurses to engage in group therapies. Nurses became caregivers of recognized importance within the treatment milieu, eventually managing those treatment environments. Nurses administered medications and observed their effects on patients.

Social science studies helped change the attitudes of nurses and other caregivers about the origin of the impoverished nature of the mentally ill. Although treatment facilities catering to the patient with a greater ability to pay for care still existed, the increased effectiveness of treatment techniques in public facilities made it possible for patients from all social strata to seek treatment in the same milieu. It was also during this era that psychiatric nurses began to exchange their white uniforms for street clothes, since these seemed to facilitate nurses' blending more easily into the treatment milieu. These social trends and shifting treatment modalities, along with the impact of early nurse leaders, began to shape psychiatric nursing.[7]

Early Nursing Leaders

Hildegard Peplau, in *Interpersonal Relations in Nursing*,[18] encouraged nurses to interact with patients for therapeutic purposes. Peplau used a structure for interaction that has come to be known as the *interpersonal process*. Other theorists (Ida Orlando,[17] Imogene King,[12] June Mellow,[16] Myra Levine,[14] and Joyce Travelbee[20]) offered more ideas to help guide nurses' actions. Nursing roles shifted from an emphasis on custodial care to an emphasis on the therapeutic nurse–patient relationship. Sociological and biologic theories of development and adaptation also influenced nursing practice strategies. Once interpersonal relationships were formed, psychiatric nurses tried to help patients adapt to environmental situations through the adoption of appropriate behaviors in personal and work environments.

Federal Legislation

The National Institute of Mental Health (NIMH) was created in 1949 as an outcome of the National Mental Health Act passed by Congress three years earlier. Promoted by psychiatrists close to and within NIMH, The Mental Health Study Act was passed in 1955. The results of an ensuing five-year study indicated that the existing network of American mental hospitals was inadequate to serve the needs of mentally ill Americans. In 1963, President Kennedy signed the Community Mental Health Centers Act, which divided the country into mental health catchment areas. The care of the mentally ill moved from centralized state institutions to decentralized, local community-based mental health centers operated under federal guidelines. The funds and policies for this action flowed from federal programs and were an attempt to design a more equitable distribution of treatment.

Under NIMH initiatives, caregiving for the mentally ill was opened to professions other than psychiatry: NIMH funded educational opportunities and research projects for psychiatric nursing, social work, psychology, and psychiatry. This action led to the development of interdisciplinary care techniques. Many psychologists and social workers became directors of the community mental health centers where the mentally ill came to receive drug, milieu, and group therapies. Psychiatrists often served as consultants to the interdisciplinary treatment teams, becoming only one of the team members who held clinical and administrative authority. Paraprofessionals and mental health volunteers also became a part of the treatment arena, offering their services under professional guidance to the mentally ill through participation in the treatment milieu.

THE MODERN ERA

During the 1960s and 1970s, the mentally ill were dispersed from state hospitals to community mental health centers for care. Rights to individual freedoms and treatment were guaranteed through the courts. An expanding and widely available array of drugs allowed outpatient treatment of patients who would formerly have been institutionalized. The drugs helped control hallucinations and delusions, and many mentally ill persons lived in board-and-care arrangements. Some, however, went irregularly to community mental health centers and stopped taking the drugs that had been prescribed.

Many nurses were educated by federally supported educational programs at the graduate level. Some acquired education and credentials in many therapies, including transactional analysis, behavior modifica-

tion, and rational–emotive therapy. Psychiatric nurses also became family, sex, and marital therapists, as well as child and adult psychotherapists.

The American Nurses' Association[2] (ANA) began to develop standards for practice in the early 1970s, and in 1982 an ANA special committee completed a comprehensive set of standards applicable to all settings in which psychiatric mental health nurses practice (Box 1-1).

Beginning in 1973, a group of American and Canadian nurses first met about the issue of nursing diagnosis. The group is currently organized as the North American Nursing Diagnosis Association (NANDA). The development of a taxonomy of nursing diagnoses and formulation of a process for identifying and accepting diagnoses has moved nursing in the direction of establishing its unique practice domain. (See Chapter 11 and Appendix I.)

In 1984, at a joint meeting, the Executive Committees of the Division on Psychiatric and Mental Health Nursing Practice of the American Nurses' Association and the Council of Specialists in Psychiatric/Mental Health Nursing approved a plan to establish a task force of specialists to develop a list of phenomena of concern to psychiatric–mental health nurses. That task force identified a classification system for organizing human responses to actual or potential health problems.[15] (See Appendix II.)

The New Federalism in the 1980s, and the decentralization of decision making for revenue spending, swiftly reduced the size and power of the NIMH. The agency's focus changed from one of promoting service to one of research into the etiology of mental illness. Cutbacks in federally funded treatment and housing programs for the mentally ill created new problems for state and local agencies trying to serve the mentally ill, since they were unable to regain sufficient monies through the federal block grant funds sent to their jurisdictions. Many deinstitutionalized mentally ill persons, even those who were associated with community-based treatment programs, lost essential support, such as housing. Large groups of these individuals became homeless.[21]

These policy shifts, juxtaposed with the growing numbers of people who are mentally ill, poor, and unattached to adequate living or treatment facilities, have presented new challenges to psychiatric mental health nursing. The reduction of support by NIMH in the areas of research and education will leave the nation with inadequate nursing resources for the care of the mentally ill in the future, unless political interventions are quickly instituted.[1,5]

Currently, nurses have roles in all settings in which the mentally ill receive treatment. They work in inpatient units as staff nurses, therapists, clinical nurse specialists, and unit managers. They are employed in outpatient settings as directors, as clinical supervisors, and as therapists using a variety of individual and group treatment strategies. A number of nurses prepared at the graduate level have private practices. Some use their psychiatric mental health skills to treat a variety

BOX 1–1
Standards of Psychiatric and Mental Health Nursing Practice

PROFESSIONAL PRACTICE STANDARDS

Standard I: Theory
The nurse applies appropriate theory that is scientifically sound as a basis for decisions regarding nursing practice.

Standard II: Data Collection
The nurse continuously collects data that are comprehensive, accurate, and systematic.

Standard III: Diagnosis
The nurse utilizes nursing diagnoses and standard classification of mental disorders to express conclusions supported by recorded assessment data and current scientific premises.

Standard IV: Planning
The nurse develops a nursing care plan with specific goals and interventions delineating nursing actions unique to each client's needs.

Standard V: Intervention
The nurse intervenes as guided by the nursing care plan to implement nursing actions that promote, maintain, or restore physical and mental health, prevent illness, and effect rehabilitation.

Standard V-A: Psychotherapeutic Interventions
The nurse (generalist) uses psychotherapeutic interventions to assist clients to regain or improve their previous coping abilities and to prevent further disability.

Standard V-B: Health Teaching
The nurse assists clients, families, and groups to achieve satisfying and productive patterns of living through health teaching.

Standard V-C: Self-Care Activities
The nurse uses the activities of daily living in a goal-directed way to foster adequate self-care and physical and mental well-being of clients.

Standard V-D: Somatic Therapies
The nurse uses knowledge of somatic therapies and applies related clinical skills in working with clients.

Standard V-E: Therapeutic Environment
The nurse provides structures, and maintains a therapeutic environment in collaboration with client and other health care providers.

Standard V-F: Psychotherapy
The nurse (specialist) utilizes advanced clinical expertise in individual, group, and family psychotherapy, child psychotherapy, and other treatment modalities to function as a psychotherapist and recognizes professional accountability for nursing practice.

Standard VI: Evaluation
The nurse evaluates client responses to nursing actions to revise the data base, nursing diagnoses, and nursing care plan.

PROFESSIONAL PERFORMANCE STANDARDS

Standard VII: Peer Review
The nurse participates in peer review and other means of evaluation to assure quality of nursing care provided for clients.

Standard VIII: Continuing Education
The nurse assumes responsibility for continuing education and professional development and contributes to the professional growth of others.

Standard IX: Interdisciplinary Collaboration
The nurse collaborates with interdisciplinary teams in assessing, planning, implementing, and evaluating programs and other mental health activities.

Standard X: Utilization of Community Health Systems
The nurse (specialist) participates with other members of the community in assessing, planning, implementing, and evaluating mental heath services and community systems that include the promotion of the broad continuum of primary, secondary, and tertiary prevention of mental illness.

Standard XI: Research
The nurse contributes to nursing and the mental health field through innovations in theory and practice and participation in research.

(American Nurses Association, 1982)

---

of client groups such as those suffering from substance abuse or sexual dysfunction. Others hold psychiatric liaison roles in general hospitals, offering psychiatric mental health services to the medically and surgically ill, as well as the dying. Some psychiatric mental health nurses focus on caring for children or adolescents. Others work with the elderly, and some have created roles in general hospitals and other settings in which they offer supportive mental health services to caregivers. Finally, it is important to note that there are a number of psychiatric mental health nurses who hold positions on local and national boards and in federal agencies where funding and agency policies are formulated.

Throughout American history, sympathy for publicly funded programs for those who cannot support themselves has been dependent on the size of the need and on the presence of effective advocates for those populations. Currently, psychiatric mental health nurses can use their skills in patient advocacy, serving the mentally ill by working through the political process, and keeping the needs of the mentally ill in the public view. This can be done while continuing to improve the effectiveness and efficiency of psychiatric nursing care.

SUMMARY

Treatment of the mentally ill is influenced by philosophical and cultural belief as well as by biologic and social science discoveries. Psychiatric mental health

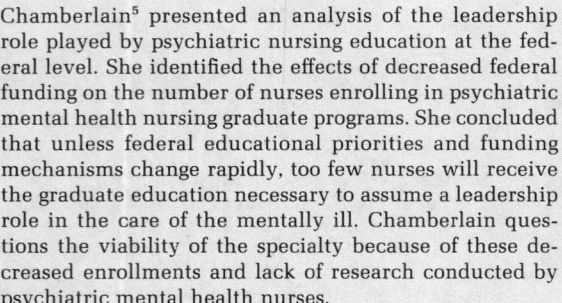

Research Highlights

Chamberlain[5] presented an analysis of the leadership role played by psychiatric nursing education at the federal level. She identified the effects of decreased federal funding on the number of nurses enrolling in psychiatric mental health nursing graduate programs. She concluded that unless federal educational priorities and funding mechanisms change rapidly, too few nurses will receive the graduate education necessary to assume a leadership role in the care of the mentally ill. Chamberlain questions the viability of the specialty because of these decreased enrollments and lack of research conducted by psychiatric mental health nurses.

Aiken[1] presented an overview of the unmet needs of the chronically mentally ill. She suggested a number of strategies for improving the delivery of services and asserted that nurses are the caregivers best suited to improve the care of the chronically mentally ill. However, she also pointed out that only a few nurses are choosing to prepare themselves to work in psychiatric mental health nursing. There is a great need to strengthen the specialty of psychiatric mental health nursing and particularly to develop a cadre of psychiatric mental health nurse researchers.

nursing has been evolving as a profession over the past 100 years, but the profession came of age only during the period after World War II. During the 1980s, shifts in federal funding priorities have caused a decrease in housing and treatment facilities for the mentally ill.

Psychiatric nurses are prepared to offer modern treatments to the mentally ill. However, adequate funding is required to support the delivery of those services. Contemporary psychiatric mental health nurses can serve as patient advocates, while continuing to improve the effectiveness and efficiency of psychiatric nursing care.

References

1. Aiken LH. Unmet needs of the chronically mentally ill: will nursing respond? Image J Nurs Sch. 1987;19:121–125.
2. American Nurses' Association. Standards of psychiatric and mental health nursing practice. Kansas City, MO: American Nurses' Association; 1982.
3. Bockoven JS. Moral treatment in American psychiatry. New York: Springer; 1963.
4. Carter FM. Psychosocial nursing. 3rd ed. New York: Macmillan; 1981.
5. Chamberlain JG. Update on psychiatric–mental health education at the federal level. Arch Psychiatr Nurs. 1987;1:132–138.
6. Deutsch A. The mentally ill in America. Garden City, NY: Doubleday, Doran & Co; 1937.
7. DeYoung C, Tower M, Glittenberg J. Out of uniform and into trouble again. Thorofare, NJ: Slack; 1983.
8. Freedman AM, Kaplan HI. Comprehensive textbook of psychiatry. Baltimore: Williams & Wilkins; 1967.
9. Goodnow M. Outline of nursing history. 6th ed. Philadelphia: WB Saunders; 1938.
10. Hollingshead A, Redlich F. Social class and mental illness. New York: John Wiley & Sons; 1958.
11. Jones M. The therapeutic community: a new treatment method in psychiatry. New York: Basic Books; 1953.
12. King IM. Nursing theory—problems and prospect. Nurs Sci. 1964;2:394–403.
13. Leighton AH. My name is legion. New York: Basic Books; 1959.
14. Levine ME. Adaptation and assessment: a rationale for nursing intervention. Am J Nurs. 1966;66:2450–2453.
15. Loomis ME, O'Toole AW, Brown MS, Pothier P, West P, Wilson HS. Development of a classification system for psychiatric/mental health nursing: individual response class. Arch Psychiatr Nurs. 1987;1:16–24.
16. Mellow J. The evolution of nursing therapy and its implications for education. 65-9538, Boston University School of Education, Health Sciences, Nursing (Dissertation), 1965.
17. Orlando IJ. The dynamic nurse–patient relationship function, process and principles. New York: GP Putnam's Sons; 1961.
18. Peplau HE. Interpersonal relations in nursing. New York: GP Putnam's Sons; 1952.
19. Stanton AH, Schwartz MS. The mental hospital. New York: Basic Books; 1954.
20. Travelbee J. Interpersonal aspects of nursing. Philadelphia: FA Davis; 1966.
21. Whitley MP, Osborne OH, Godfrey MA, Johnston K. A point prevalence study of alcoholism and mental illness among downtown migrants. Soc Sci Med. 1985;20:579–583.

2

Mary Durand Thomas

Therapeutic Relationships With Clients

OBJECTIVES

After reading this chapter, the reader will be able to:

1. *Describe the nature of therapeutic nurse–client relationships*
2. *Discuss the importance for psychiatric nurses to be aware of their own beliefs, feelings, behaviors, and values*
3. *Describe the psychiatric nursing qualities of respect, genuineness, empathy, and hope*
4. *Discuss issues in therapeutic relationships including therapeutic alliance, transference, countertransference, termination, and discharge*
5. *Identify potential goals for a one-to-one nurse–client relationship*
6. *Describe the therapeutic tasks of each phase of a nurse–client relationship*
7. *Discuss the process of supervision in psychiatric nursing.*

NATURE OF THERAPEUTIC NURSE–CLIENT RELATIONSHIPS

The nurse's therapeutic relationship with clients is an interpersonal helping process based on theory. It is *interpersonal* in that the nurse reaches out as one human being to another to enable the client to experience being listened to and having his or her personal worth affirmed. The relationship is *helping* because it is focused toward the client's care, well-being, learning, and growth. Reaching out and willingness to help, however, are not enough. To be therapeutic, a relationship with a client requires the use of *theory-based* knowledge and skills.

Therapeutic nurse–client relationships can be distinguished from social relationships. The primary purpose of a therapeutic relationship is to help the client, as compared with a social relationship, which has as its purpose mutual satisfaction or enjoyment. Of course, the nurse can find the relationship with a client a learning experience and satisfying, but that is not the primary purpose of the relationship. Other characteristics are shown in Table 2-1. In a therapeutic relationship, the focus is the client's thoughts, feelings, and behaviors, with self-disclosure by the nurse limited to that which is helpful to the client. A therapeutic relationship, although sometimes long-term, is usually planned with a specific termination that is based on goal attainment or discharge. Social relationships, on the other hand, may last a lifetime or may terminate in gradual and unplanned ways, as well as in planned ways. In spite of the unique features of the therapeutic relationship, skills, such as problem solving, learned in other relationships are often applicable.

There are inpatient and outpatient settings during which one nurse and one client talk together regularly over an extended period of time. The one-to-one nurse–client relationship is discussed later. In addition, the principles involved in therapeutic relationships are the context for other psychiatric nursing interventions, including providing physical care, structuring client activities, and encouraging interactions among clients.

SELF-AWARENESS

Because the nurse's self is central to therapeutic relationships with clients, the success of such relationships is influenced by the depth of the nurse's self-awareness. Increasing one's self-awareness requires looking inward, as well as looking realistically at the environment. Self-awareness cannot be static, but must be transformed and modified throughout life.[5] To be self-aware involves knowledge in four interconnected areas.[5]

1. The *psychological component* includes a sensitivity to one's own emotions, factors that affect those emotions, how crises are dealt with, and a knowledge of needs, motivations, and personality.
2. The *physical component* comprises awareness of bodily sensations, including reactions to stress, sexuality, body image, and physical potentials.
3. The *environmental component* involves interpersonal relationships and interaction with the natural environment.
4. The *philosophical component* includes personal history and values, the meaning given to life, and awareness of personal finiteness.

Becoming more self-aware is an ongoing process. The nurse approaching a situation that engenders strong feelings can examine why the situation and thoughts about the situation gave rise to such feelings. Personal patterns of behavior and ways of interacting with others can be reviewed for choices about what is valued in life.[30] (Box 2-1 gives an example of such an exercise.) Writing letters to oneself or keeping a journal can lead to greater awareness of what constitute significant experiences. In *The Transparent Self*, Sidney Jourard argued that self-knowledge comes through the courage of self-disclosure to another.[15] By sharing thoughts, emotions, reactions, and experiences with another, self-understanding is increased. Self-awareness is basic to being genuine with clients and to making choices consistent with personal ethical values.[20]

TABLE 2–1
Characteristics of therapeutic and social relationships

CHARACTERISTIC	THERAPEUTIC RELATIONSHIPS	SOCIAL RELATIONSHIPS
Goal	Client's well-being, growth, and learning	Mutual satisfaction
Content	Focus is on client's thoughts, feelings, and behaviors; nurse's self-disclosure based on helpfulness to client	Amount of self-disclosure more likely to be similar by both individuals; may range from openness to superficiality
Length	Time-limited; planned termination based on goal achievement or client's discharge	May last years; ending of relationship often gradual and unplanned but may be planned

---

BOX 2–1
Learning About Values from Patterns

DIRECTIONS

Which of these words describe you? Draw a circle around the seven words you feel best describe you as an individual. Then, underline the seven words you feel most accurately describe you as a professional person. (You may circle and underline the same word.)

ambitious	reserved	assertive	opinionated
concerned	generous	independent	indifferent
easily hurt	outgoing	reliable	dynamic
capable	self-controlled	fun-loving	dependent
suspicious	solitary	likable	obedient
intellectual	argumentative	unpredictable	slow to relate
compromising	thoughtful	affectionate	
logical	imaginative	self-disciplined	
moody	easily led	helpful	

HERE ARE SOME QUESTIONS TO REFLECT ON AND ANSWER:

Are you happy with your patterns? Do you like who you are?
Would you like to change? In what way? Why?
What are some alternatives?
List some goals for yourself.
What values are reflected in the patterns you have chosen?
What is the relationship between these patterns and your personal values?
Which pattern(s) is (are) negative to you? Why?
In what patterns are you aware of the most inconsistencies in attitude or behavior?
What words would you add to this list to describe yourself?
What patterns do you feel a nurse should ideally possess?

QUALITIES FOR THE PSYCHIATRIC NURSE TO BRING TO RELATIONSHIPS

There are a number of qualities that the effective psychiatric nurse brings to relationships with clients. These qualities include respect, genuineness, hope, and empathy.

Respect

Respect of the nurse for the client is consideration for the individuality and uniqueness of another person and concern for that person's welfare. It involves recognizing the client's feelings, beliefs, and experiences as being part of the client's humanness. This is especially important with psychiatric clients whose behavior may have led to their being rejected by others. Respect is communicated through active listening to what is said. It is manifested through concern for comfort, such as offering a chair or a cup of tea. The client who experiences the nurse's respect might conceptualize it as, "That nurse really cares about me as an individual."

Genuineness

The nurse's genuineness in relationships with clients means that he or she is "real." There is a congruence between what the nurse believes or feels and what is expressed. This congruence is basic to establishment of interpersonal trust. For example, the nurse would say "I'm glad to see you" to a client only if that is an expression of a sincere sentiment. Genuineness in relationships with clients is crucial because they are being asked to reveal information about themselves; it is easier to be self-disclosing with an individual who is authentic than with someone whose communications are counterfeit. To be genuine does not require that the nurse express every feeling experienced or information inappropriate to the situation, nor does it mean that the nurse interacts with the client as in a social relationship. Rather, the issue is that the information or emotions that are communicated be authentic and therapeutic.

There is some disagreement concerning how much personal information it is useful to disclose to clients. In all human relationships, an individual discloses parts of the self.[1] One way of evaluating how much self-disclosure is useful is by consideration of what might be achieved for the client.[1,31]

1. What would be accomplished by self-disclosure and what is the theoretical rationale? Some possibilities might be encouragement of emotional expression, provision of support for client goals, or discussion of problem solving.
2. What is the timing of the disclosure? Too much information about the nurse early in the relation-

ship would more likely be a reflection of the nurse's anxiety, and it could be overwhelming for the patient. At that point, information about the nurse's role in working with the client would be more useful than personal information.

3. How would the client interpret the disclosure? The client could interpret a nurse's self-disclosure accurately or could misunderstand or misinterpret its meaning.

4. What are the client's feelings about the nurse? It is when the client is not experiencing an extreme of positive or negative feelings toward the nurse that self-disclosure is more likely to be helpful and less likely to be problematic.

5. What are the nurse's feelings about the client? If they could be detrimental, it is important that the nurse use self-awareness and seek consultation or supervision to understand the basis for the feelings so that such feelings are not communicated in a punitive way.

All nurses are at times asked to disclose information that they do not wish to share. In such situations, being genuine may mean responding honestly, "It makes me uncomfortable when you ask me about my personal life."[1] Other responses for limiting inappropriate self-disclosure while remaining genuine are given in Box 2-2.

Empathy

Empathy is significant in the nurse–client relationship. It is the experience of accurately comprehending what the client is experiencing. The process is complex and involves observing the client's physical demeanor and listening to the content and the style of what is said. It is not just a cognitive understanding that is gained, but also a spontaneous, emotional awareness. *Empathy* is "a particular mode of gathering data about the internal

---

BOX 2–2
Deflection of Requests by Client for Inappropriate Self-Disclosure by Nurse

Benign curiosity: "I wonder why you ask me that."
Redirection or refocusing: "I'm wondering about your switching the subject. We were talking about . . ."
Observation of a pattern: "I notice that whenever we are talking about your wife, you ask me about myself."
Clarification: "You've asked me several times about my religion. What are you concerned about?"
Feedback and limit-setting: "I'm not really comfortable talking with you about . . ."

(Based on Auvil CA, Silver BW. Therapist self-disclosure: when is it appropriate? Perspect Psychiatr Care. 1984; 22:57–61.)

---

experiences of another" (reference 3, p 421). It requires the ability to alternate between affectively participating with the client and intellectually observing the client. "It is a sensing of the client's inner world of private personal meanings 'as if' it were the therapist's own, but without ever losing the 'as if' quality" (reference 26, p 104).

However, the nurse's experience of empathy is not of value to the client unless the empathy is meaningfully communicated. Being *empathic* is the ability to comment about the client's inner experience in such a way that the client feels understood and soothed.[3] A client who experiences the empathic communication of the nurse might conceptualize it as, "Even when I can't explain how I feel very clearly, the nurse seems to understand." Empathy is different from sympathy, for which the client's experience would more likely be: "The nurse feels sorry for me." It is also different from the nurse's projection of feelings onto the client, for which the client's experience might then be: "The nurse thinks we feel just alike."

One caveat concerning empathy is important. For a client who is concerned about separateness from others and fears that others can mind read, it is important for the nurse to communicate explicitly the behavioral clues in the client that led to the experience of empathy. For example, the nurse might say: "From what you told me about the voices you're hearing and the way you are looking from side to side, I get the feeling that you are fearful for your safety."

Hope

Hope, or what Peplau has termed "a bias of optimism" (reference 23, p 12), is an assumption that all clients have the potential for learning and change. "When people exhibit behaviors that appear to contradict this assumption, it is thought to be because they have met with repeated negative experiences and have thus lost respect for themselves, trust in their abilities, and faith in their potential" (reference 24, p 8). Even clients who are very deteriorated can be sensitive to nurses' beliefs about their potential. One very sick client, speaking of a previous hospitalization, said, "I could tell that the doctors and nurses gave up on me. They stopped sitting down to talk with me, they just gave me pills but no talk because I'm a hopeless case."

The nurse who is hopeful recognizes small changes and successes and communicates them to the client. This assists the client in seeing the self as confronting problems, rather than as being overwhelmed by them.[11] The nurse can also indicate the expectation that clients will make changes they wish to make at the time that is right for them. To be hopeful about the potential for change, does not mean that clients should be forced to change. Rather, the nurse's hope or optimism provides the client with the experience of knowing that another person believes that change is possible.

ISSUES IN THERAPEUTIC RELATIONSHIPS

Therapeutic Alliance

Therapeutic alliance is defined as the client's active collaboration with the treatment process. A client who actively participates in problem solving with a nurse and other members of the health care team, for example, would be seen to have a high level of therapeutic alliance. It is a concept that originally came out of psychoanalysis, but has now been applied to relationships with clients in other settings.[7,12] The concept is important because therapeutic alliance correlates highly with therapeutic outcomes. A client's alliance with psychosocial treatment in the hospital setting, for example, is correlated with a better condition at discharge.[7] A scale for rating therapeutic alliance is shown in Box 2-3.

Clients may have a low level of therapeutic alliance for a number of reasons.[4,17] Initially, the client may be overwhelmed by symptoms or frightened by a new environment, or be unclear about what is expected. The client may want to change, but be anxious about changing and, thus, continue to use defense mechanisms. The client may be hospitalized or in therapy because of court referral or commitment and may feel coerced or trapped. Or the client's goals and methods for achieving change may be different from those of the nurse. A client's openness to change implies recogni-

---

BOX 2-3
Six-Point Scale for Rating the Therapeutic Alliance of the Hospitalized Patient

1. Patient is actively involved in therapy—explores problems, makes realistic plans for discharge, and so forth.
2. Patient is initially passive but toward discharge becomes more active in therapy, discharge planning, and so forth.
3. Patient is passively receptive in therapy.
4. Patient is variable—at times realizes he has an emotional problem but alternates in psychotherapy between acknowledging and denying this need.
5. Patient sees no need for hospitalization and is passively waiting for discharge; is not taking part in discharge planning.
6. Patient sees no need for hospitalization and is constantly demanding discharge; sees no need for aftercare or therapy; totally denies emotional problems; actively refuses treatment.

(Adapted from Clarkin JF, Hurt SW, Crilly JL. Therapeutic alliance and hospital treatment outcome. Hosp Comm Psychiatry. 1987;38:871–875. Used with permission.)

---

tion of problems or pathology, and this, in turn, may be too painful to contemplate.

The nurse can encourage the client's alliance with the treatment process through the qualities discussed previously: respect, genuineness, empathy, and hope. In addition, assessing specific reasons for low therapeutic alliance may guide further action, such as acknowledging the client's feeling of coercion. Or anxiety might be the focus of interventions. Finally, because the client may be unclear on how to become involved in treatment, it is helpful to elicit the client's participation in setting clear goals and to help the client find behaviors that approach those goals.

Transference and Countertransference

Transference and countertransference, like therapeutic alliance, were first identified in the psychoanalyst–client relationship. Similar processes have come to be recognized as occurring in other relationships. *Transference* has been defined as the client's

> . . . experience of feelings, drives, attitudes, fantasies, and defenses toward a person in the present which do not befit that person. Rather, they are a repetition of reactions originating in regard to significant persons of early childhood, unconsciously displaced onto figures in the present (reference 13, p 155).

The nurse may be the subject of such transference. The feelings and attitudes involved in the client's transference are not appropriate to the present situation and, thus, involve distortions.[25] Transference reactions may be specific and occur within a particular relationship, such as with a particular nurse. Or there may be a more generalized transference reaction that represents a repetitive way an individual reacts in certain types of interactions, such as expecting all older women to be aggressive.[28] Transference is significant for the nurse to understand for two reasons: (1) It can be helpful in sorting out explanations for client behavior in certain relationships. Otherwise, a nurse may inaccurately explain the client's behavior as a response to something the nurse has said, rather than as a way the client is distorting the relationship. (2) As such distortions become more clearly identified, the nurse is in a better position to assist the client in examining the distortions.

Countertransference is the converse of transference in that it is the displacement onto the client of feelings, beliefs, and attitudes arising from the helping person's early childhood experiences with significant persons. The distortions implicit in countertransference can be detrimental to the nurse–client relationship. The nurse can be alerted that countertransference may be occurring if any of the following self-observations are made: (1) sexual or aggressive fantasies toward the client; (2) dreaming about the client; (3) extremes of liking or disliking for the client; (4) recurrent anxiety or guilt feelings about the client; (5) preoccupation with the client in nonclinical situations; (6) a tendency to focus on information presented by the client in only one way; and (7) defensiveness with others about interventions with the client.[28]

Countertransference is sometimes viewed in a broader sense as any strong emotional reaction to a patient. A research project that studied countertransference in this broader sense in an inpatient setting identified the following characteristic patterns of reaction to types of psychopathology from health team members:[8]

1. With clients who were highly demanding, manipulative, hostile, emotionally labile, or who sabotaged treatment, the primary countertransference response was anger.
2. Clients who were psychotically withdrawn and slow to change elicited helplessness and confusion.
3. Suicidal-depressed behavior in clients tended to evoke positive interest and protectiveness.
4. Clients who had a potential for agitation and violence invoked a variety of discipline-specific responses, with fearfulness and a lack of group cohesiveness the most common responses among nurses.[8]

It is useful for nurses to be aware of their own emotional responses to clients and to discern what it is in the situation, as well as in the way they are thinking about the situation, that leads to certain strong feelings. Supervision (discussed later) can be useful in helping the nurse to decrease the distortions inherent in countertransference.

Termination and Discharge

Groundwork for termination starts at the beginning of the relationship with the clarification of how long the relationship will continue. Even though the nurse's therapeutic relationship with a psychiatric client is expected to end when therapeutic goals are achieved or the client is discharged from the hospital, termination or discharge can evoke strong reactions in the client and often in the nurse.[6,19] The termination process reawakens feelings around past separation and loss experiences, and the experience has been termed *separation anxiety*[19] and *mourning*.[29] The client may view termination or discharge as a personal rejection and may feel hopeless or helpless. Anger may be expressed verbally or through less overt means such as missed appointments or denial of the significance of the relationship. New symptoms may appear, or former symptoms may recur.

The nurse can help the client to work through reactions to termination by encouraging discussion of the impending separation as well as the feelings that are being experienced. To assist the client in this way, it is important that nurses seek self-awareness of the meanings that a separation has for them. With this knowledge, the nurse will be more genuine with the client and more responsive to the client's experience of separation.

Preparation for hospital discharge is often made more complex by the need for the client to make multiple decisions concerning outpatient therapy, finances, and living arrangements after hospitalization.[17] Thus, an additional goal during this time is to assist the client to become involved in relationships outside the hospital environment. This may take the form of encouraging the client to take passes, to make contact with an outpatient therapist, and to initiate activities that will continue after discharge.

THE ONE-TO-ONE NURSE–CLIENT RELATIONSHIP
Goals

Psychiatric nursing has traditionally placed great emphasis on the one-to-one nurse–client relationship. This emphasis was affirmed and strengthened with the publication of Peplau's *Interpersonal Relations in Nursing*[22] in 1952.[16] In the past, such relationships often extended over lengthy hospitalizations. In the present era of short-term hospitalization, their relevance has been questioned.[21] However, one-to-one nurse–client relationships continue to be important in many inpatient and outpatient settings.

The nurse–client relationship can be directed to goals at any of a number of levels. Loomis has suggested a framework for specifying, in contractual form, which level of change is being sought in a range of inpatient and outpatient settings (Table 2-2). In a Level I, Care Contract, the goal of nursing intervention is care not cure. The client may lack the ability or motivation for

TABLE 2–2
Levels of change contracts

LEVEL AND TYPE OF CONTRACT	INTERVENTION TECHNIQUES
I. Care Contracts	Provide physical or custodial care required
	Protection from loss of functional abilities
II. Social Control Contracts	Crisis intervention
	Brief therapy
III. Relationship Contracts	Insight or redecision work
	Cognitive restructuring
	Marital, family or relationship counseling
IV. Structural Change Contracts	Script analysis
	Reparenting and redecision work

(Adapted from Loomis ME. Levels of contracting. J Psychosoc Nurs. 1985;23(3):8–14. Used with permission.)

change, and the contract may actually be with a third party such as the state or parents. The nurse provides needed physical care, assists in activities of daily living, and attempts to minimize negative outcomes. In a Level II, Social Control Contract, the client seeks help because of a developmental life change or stressor that has precipitated a life crisis. The nursing interventions are usually short-term and pragmatically directed toward solving the immediate problem. In Level III, Relationship Contracts, the focus is on the repetitive or cyclical nature of the client's relationship problems. The nurse and client work together to make the connection between the client's early life decisions and current relationships and life-style. Relationship contracts often include adjunctive couple or family counseling. Level IV, Structural Change Contracts, involve intensive, usually long-term, psychotherapy intended to affect pathologic structure as well as current relationship issues.[18] Nurses involved in Level III and Level IV contracts have master's degree preparation and sometimes specialized training in particular approaches.[18]

Phases

The nurse–client relationship, regardless of level, can be divided into three phases: orientation, working, and termination. In addition it is useful to consider the preinteraction and posttermination periods. Each of the phases gives rise to unique relationship issues and calls for accomplishment of specific tasks (Box 2-4). The phases of the nurse–client relationship actually overlap one another, especially if the time period is short.[21]

PREINTERACTION PERIOD

During the preinteraction period, the nurse knows there will be meetings with a particular client and prepares for those meetings. This preparation can take the form of reviewing assessment data collected by others about this particular client. As the nurse reviews these data, certain expectations and reactions may be evoked. The expectations and reactions may be "What if the client . . . ?" "Will I be able to respond appropriately?" "What would be an appropriate response?" It is useful for the nurse to consider possible client behaviors and appropriate interventions, both for planning purposes and as a means of anxiety reduction. If additional help is necessary, the nurse can seek help from another nurse—a preceptor, for example—or from the literature. Before the interaction, the client also has certain expectations. These expectations may be based on what has been heard from other clients in the particular setting, or they may be expectations for helping relationships in general or, perhaps for a nurse–client relationship, based on past experiences.

ORIENTATION PHASE

During the orientation phase, the nurse and the client who are strangers to each other, but each with expec-

---

BOX 2–4
Tasks of Each Phase of the Nurse–Client Relationship

PREINTERACTION
Discover what has been learned by others about the client
Assess own expectations and own reactions to knowledge about client
Give consideration to ways of handling difficult situations
If necessary, obtain assistance from supervisor, preceptor, consultant, or literature

ORIENTATION
Initiate meetings with client
Gather assessment data and identify nursing diagnoses
Discuss goals with the client
Foster a therapeutic alliance
With the client formulate a treatment contract (goals, frequency and length of sessions, length of relationship, where sessions will be held, mutual roles and responsibilities)
Consider own thoughts and feelings that occur in response to client

WORKING
Maintain the relationship
Refine nursing diagnoses and perhaps identify others
Encourage discussion of current relationships and issues that are problematic for client
Observe for patterns of behavior during session that reflect issues that are problematic for client
Identify patterns of behavior, such as lateness or unwillingness to participate, that indicate client's anxiety about the relationship
Help client to describe experiences in a concrete, specific way
Evaluate progress toward goals
Consider own thoughts and feelings that occur in response to client

TERMINATION
Acknowledge the forthcoming termination
Evaluate what has been learned during the relationship
Encourage client to participate in other relationships
Decrease the frequency and intensity of the sessions
Share own reactions to termination in a way that is appropriate to the particular client

POSTTERMINATION
Review what was helpful to client and what can be improved upon in relationships with other clients

---

tations for the other, plan goals and arrange ways in which they can work collaboratively. The nurse meets with the client and gathers additional assessment data. On the basis of the data gathered and the nurse's observation of the client, nursing diagnoses are formulated. The nurse and client clarify goals and how they will be attained. This entails developing the treatment contract including frequency, length, and place of sessions, and how termination will be decided. Mutual roles and responsibilities are defined, in part, through discussion. For example, the nurse might summarize a discussion of roles and responsibilities by saying: "Then we'll meet here in this office at one o'clock every Tuesday and Thursday for as long as you are in the hospital. You'll bring up any problems you are having with getting angry with your family or with other clients on the ward and I'll discuss them with you." As the nurse and client actually carry out these plans there is an opportunity to further clarify roles and responsibilities. The identification of goals and ways of achieving them is useful in forming the therapeutic alliance because it communicates to the client that the nurse has hope and believes that help is possible and available. The nurse's respect for the client, genuineness, and empathy also foster the formation of a therapeutic alliance. During the orientation phase, the nurse considers his or her own thoughts and feelings that occur in response to the client. Not only is this useful in increasing the nurse's self-awareness, it may indicate the type of response that the client evokes in others.

WORKING PHASE

By the working phase, the client has an increased commitment to the work of the relationship and is less guarded. This phase calls for maintenance of the therapeutic alliance as a context for pursuing the agreed-upon goals. The goals to be pursued depend upon the level of the contract. Generally, for the client and the nursing student or the beginning nurse, the goals would be at Level I, Care, or Level II, Social Control. Nursing diagnoses can be refined or new diagnoses identified as the nurse learns more about the client. The nurse encourages discussion of current relationships and issues that are problematic for the client. The client is helped to describe experiences in a concrete, specific way. Patterned ways in which the client interacts with the nurse are observed for similarities to behaviors that create problems for the client in other relationships. The client's level of anxiety about the topics discussed is continually assessed. Low levels of anxiety can enhance learning. But higher levels of anxiety can interfere with therapeutic alliance, make learning difficult, and result in behaviors, such as lateness, that interfere with progress toward goals. Throughout the working phase, the client's progress toward goals is evaluated.

TERMINATION PHASE

The termination phase may be directly related to achieving the goals defined for the nurse–client relationship. Or it may be in response to factors such as the client's discharge from the hospital or the nursing student's completion of clinical experience. The task of this phase is to bring a therapeutic end to the relationship. This is accomplished by acknowledging the forthcoming termination and by evaluating what has been learned during the relationship. The relationship is attenuated by decreasing the frequency and intensity of the sessions and by encouraging the client to increase participation in other relationships. In spite of the planned nature of the ending, reactions to termination, as discussed earlier, may be difficult for both client and nurse. The nurse encourages the client to share thoughts and feelings about the forthcoming termination. In addition, the nurse's genuine sharing of his or her reactions to termination in a way that is appropriate to a particular client can be an opportunity for new learning for the client.

POSTTERMINATION PERIOD

During the posttermination period it is useful for nurses to review their part in the relationship. An honest appraisal of what was helpful to the client and what could be improved upon can assist nurses to grow in clinical skills.

SUPERVISION

Supervision, as utilized in psychiatric mental health nursing, is the interpersonal process whereby a supervisor assists a supervisee to improve therapeutic relationships with clients.[9,10,14] In addition to improving therapeutic knowledge and skills, a related purpose of supervision is to provide support for the nurse who is receiving supervision.[2] The process consists of a series of conferences between a supervisor and one or more supervisees that focus on the supervisee(s)' clinical work with clients. To share information about what has transpired in the nurse–client relationship, the supervisee shares audiotapes, videotapes, or process recordings (transcriptions of the nurse's and client's verbal and nonverbal communication).

Topics discussed in supervision, in addition to the actual sessions with the client, could include effects of the milieu on the client and the supervisee, relevant theoretical concepts, the supervisee's "blind spots" in understanding the client, and the relationship of supervisor and supervisee. Although supervision is expected to increase the supervisee's awareness of his or her own behavior, supervision is different from therapy in that the focus is kept on the learning necessary to improve therapeutic relationships.

Both supervisor and supervisee attitudes and tasks change during the course of supervision.[9,10,14] The phases have been regarded as paralleling the nurse–client relationship in having beginning, working, and termination phases.[14] And some of the themes, such as dependency or anger, that occur between the nurse and client may be reflected in the supervisor–supervisee relationship.[14] Supervisee behaviors that contribute to optimal learning include (1) taking an active role in the learning process by presenting material from the session as clearly as possible; (2) sharing responsibility for the working relationship with the supervisor; and, probably most difficult, (3) being willing to share problems and expose vulnerabilities, strengths, and weaknesses.[14]

SUMMARY

The nurse's therapeutic relationship with clients is an interpersonal helping process based on theory. Because

Research Highlights

As an aid to increasing self-awareness, it is important to consider one's own thoughts and feelings as a new clinical situation is approached. Carole Schoffstall, a nursing faculty member, wanted to identify nursing students' concerns about working with mentally ill clients in psychiatric clinical settings.[27] Over a three-year period, she collected data from nursing students utilizing a "fantasy exercise" carried out before their psychiatric clinical experience. Each student was asked to write a specific fantasy about what it would be like to go to a psychiatric hospital and begin psychiatric nursing experience. There were common themes in the fantasies: (1) The highest percentage of students (26%) related fantasies that indicated their perception of lacking sufficient therapeutic skills, for example, "I will get a patient to start talking to me and totally misunderstand what is being said and not know how to react." (2) Some students (18%) expressed a fantasy about a unique contribution they would make during the experience, for example, "A patient who has never opened up to anyone before, will open up after I listen and show that I really care." (3) Other students (18%) wrote fantasies that indicated an expectation of personal growth, for example, "I'll come out knowing why I act like I do." (4) Twelve percent of the fantasies reflected concerns about physical danger or fear (e.g., "being strangled and/or raped"). (5) Another 12% of the fantasies indicated that students were concerned about similarities of patients to themselves (e.g., "get locked up and the staff thinks I'm a patient"). (6) On the other hand, some fantasies (10%) reflected concerns about the patients being very different (e.g., "I will meet someone considered 'insane' who is really on a super-advanced mental plane, and learn all sorts of bizarre things"). (7) Finally, a few (4%) indicated concern about the clinical experience with psychiatric patients being emotionally painful. The commonality of these "fantasies" was thought to be based on societal stereotypes of the mentally ill and of psychiatric hospitals.[27]

the nurse's self is central to therapeutic relationships, the success of such relationships is largely dependent on the depth of the nurse's self-awareness. To be effective, a psychiatric nurse brings to therapeutic relationships the qualities of respect, genuineness, empathy, and hope. Issues of concern in therapeutic relationships include therapeutic alliance, transference, countertransference, and termination. Psychiatric nursing places great emphasis on the one-to-one nurse–client relationship. Such a relationship can be directed to goals at various levels from care to structural change. The phases of the nurse–client relationship can be divided into three phases: orientation, working, and termination. Supervision is the interpersonal process whereby a supervisor assists a supervisee to improve therapeutic relationships with clients.

References

1. Auvil CA, Silver BW. Therapist self-disclosure: when is it appropriate? Perspect Psychiatr Care. 1984;22:57–61.
2. Benfer BA. Clinical supervision as a support system for the caregiver. Perspect Psychiatr Care. 1979;17:13–17.
3. Book HE. Empathy: misconceptions and misuses in psychotherapy. Am J Psychiatry. 1988;145:420–424.
4. Busch P. Therapy with the noninvolved client. J Psychsoc Nurs Ment Health Serv. 1987;25(11):21–25.
5. Campbell J. The relationship of nursing and self-awareness. ANS. 1980;2(4):15–25.
6. Campaniello JA. The process of termination. J Psychiatr Nurs. 1980;18(2):29–32.
7. Clarkin JF, Hurt SW, Crilly JL. Therapeutic alliance and hospital treatment outcome. Hosp Commun Psychiatry. 1987;38:871–875.
8. Colson DB, Allen JG, Coyne L, et al. An anatomy of counter-transference: staff reactions to difficult psychiatric hospital patients. Hosp Commun Psychiatry. 1986;37:923–928.
9. Critchley DL. Clinical supervision. In Critchley DL, Maurin JT, eds. The clinical specialist in psychiatric mental health nursing: theory, research, and practice. New York: John Wiley & Sons; 1985.
10. Critchley DL. Clinical supervision as a learning tool for the therapist in milieu settings. J Psychosoc Nurs Ment Health Serv. 1987;25(8):18–22.
11. Frank JD. Therapeutic factors in psychotherapy. Am J Psychother. 1971;25:350–361.
12. Frieswyk SH, Allen JG, Colson DB, et al. Therapeutic alliance: its place as a process and outcome variable in dynamic psychotherapy research. J Consult Clin Psychol. 1986; 54:32–38.
13. Greenson R. The technique and practice of psychoanalysis, vol 1. New York: International Universities Press; 1967.
14. Hughes CM. Supervising clinical practice in psychosocial nursing. J Psychosoc Nurs Ment Health Serv. 1985;23(2):27–32.
15. Jourard SM. The transparent self. 2nd ed. New York: Van Nostrand; 1971.
16. Lego S. The one-to-one nurse–patient relationship. Perspect Psychiatr Care. 1980;18:67–89.
17. Leibenluft E, Goldberg RL. Guidelines for short-term inpatient psychotherapy. Hosp Commun Psychiatry. 1987; 38:38–43.
18. Loomis ME. Levels of contracting. J Psychosoc Nurs Ment Health Serv. 1985;23(3):8–14.
19. Nehren J, Gilliam NR. Separation anxiety. Am J Nurs. 1965;65:109–112.
20. Nelson MJ. Authenticity: fabric of ethical nursing practice. Topics in Clinical Nursing. 1982;4(4):1–6.
21. Nix J, Dillon K. Short-term nursing therapy: a conceptual model for inpatient psychiatric care. Hosp Commun Psychiatry. 1986;37:493–496.
22. Peplau HE. Interpersonal relations in nursing: a conceptual frame of reference for psychodynamic nursing. New York: GP Putnam's Sons; 1952.

23. Peplau HE. The nurse as counselor. J Am Coll Health. 1986;35(1):11–14.

24. Purkey WW, Schmidt JJ. The inviting relationship: an expanded perspective for professional counseling. Englewood Cliffs, NJ: Prentice-Hall; 1987.

25. Rawn ML. Transference: current concepts and controversies. Psychoanal Rev. 1987;74:107–124.

26. Rogers CR, Truax CB. The therapeutic conditions antecedent to change: a theoretical view. In Rogers CR, ed. The therapeutic relationship and its impact: a study of psychotherapy with schizophrenics. Madison: University of Wisconsin Press; 1967.

27. Schoffstall C. Concerns of student nurses prior to psychiatric nursing experience: an assessment and intervention technique. J Psychosoc Nurs Ment Health Serv. 1981;19(11):11–14.

28. Schroder PJ. Recognizing transference and countertransference. J Psychosoc Nurs Ment Health Serv. 1985;23(2):21–26.

29. Schultz FK. The mourning phase of relationships. J Psychiatr Nurs. 1964;2(11):37–42.

30. Uustal DB. Values clarification in nursing: application to practice. Am J Nurs. 1978;78:2058–2063.

31. Weiner MF. Therapist disclosure: the use of self in psychotherapy. 2nd ed. Baltimore: University Park Press; 1983.

3

Heather Andersen
Robin S. Johnson

Strategies for Preventing and Coping With Burnout

OBJECTIVES

After reading this chapter, the reader will be able to:

1. *Understand the importance of self care and its role in psychiatric nursing practice*
2. *Identify the causes and symptoms of burnout*
3. *Develop a self-care plan.*

The psychiatric nurse who possesses an intact, healthy self is more effective in clinical practice than the nurse whose self is not cared for. The support and nurturing of that self is ultimately the task of the individual professional nurse. Maintenance of effective clinical practice necessitates that planning for the care of the self be started early in a nurse's work experience, with modifications made throughout the career. Although the potential for burnout is also present in other nursing environments, the chronic nature of many psychiatric illnesses, the attached stigma, and the interpersonal demands of psychiatric nursing intensify the need for supportive strategies in psychiatric nursing. To assist in developing strategies for self support, this chapter will explore how the meaning attached to work affects the work experience. Conditions that lead to burnout will be identified, and strategies to prevent those conditions will be examined. An opportunity for the learner to consider a self-care plan will be provided.

STRESS AND BURNOUT

Understanding the stresses of psychiatric nursing requires attention both to the personal disposition of the individual experiencing a life event[6,10] and to the social conditions under which these events are experienced.[2,15] A complex interplay exists between stressful life events, individual personality, and illness; and failure to recognize this fact can leave even the experienced psychiatric nurse vulnerable to burnout.

The term "burnout" was first used by Freudenberger in 1974 to explain the attitudinal and behavioral changes observed in mental health workers in "alternative" help-giving facilities such as free clinics.[4] More recently, burnout has been defined as:

> A syndrome characterized by progressive physical and emotional exhaustion involving the development of negative job attitudes and perceptions and a loss of empathetic concern for patients. It is caused by chronic emotional stress resulting from prolonged intensive involvement with people (reference 12, p 305).

A further definition draws attention to the unity of caring and caregiving that is fundamental to nursing practice:

> The separation of caregiving and caring is a good definition for the modern epidemic of "burnout." . . . It is a peculiarly modern mistake to think that caring is the cause of . . . burnout, and that the cure is to protect oneself from caring. In fact the loss of caring is the sickness. . . . Expert caring liberates and facilitates in a way that the one caring is also enriched in the process. When nurses are permitted to care for patients and families to the best of their knowledge and ability, the stresses in nursing are reduced to those legitimate to the realm of caring (reference 1, p 1074).

Cumulative involvement with clients, family, and peers, together with a work environment that includes frequent crises, excessive workload, role conflicts, and minimal control of decision making, leaves nurses especially prone to burnout. For the psychiatric nurse in clinical practice, this outcome translates into loss of concern for others. Physical and emotional exhaustion combine to leave the nurse devoid of empathy, respect, or any positive feelings for clients.[11] The nurse's relationship with fellow professionals also is adversely affected. Yet occupational stress does not inevitably cause burnout. Two psychiatric nurses in similar positions that involve high stress, such as working with the homeless mentally ill, may respond very differently: one may continue to find fulfillment in the work, whereas the other soon begins to contemplate a career move. Burnout is not the same as job stress. Rather, burnout occurs as a consequence of job stress that is repeated and unresolved.[13]

Factors Leading to Burnout

Burnout may arise from at least three primary causes: individual, organizational, and occupational (Box 3-1). Individual personality factors can contribute to lack of adequate care of the self: burnout is correlated with the traits of unassertiveness, low self-confidence, dependency, and poor personal commitment to one's work.[5,8] Furthermore, some individuals drawn to human services such as nursing often put the needs of others first and fail to recognize their own needs.

Organizational factors can also inhibit self care. For example, psychiatric nurses work closely with other health care professionals, especially psychiatrists and social workers. Six key areas of organizational stress for interdisciplinary teams are communication problems with administration, communication problems within the team, role ambiguity, conflicting goals of the clinical staff and the administration, the nature of the system or institution, and lack of institutional support for direct caregivers.[16] These factors are particularly relevant to mental health nursing.

Nursing as an occupation is inherently stressful because it involves working with people who have a physical or mental illness. Working with people in crisis can force psychiatric nurses to confront their own personal issues as well as those of clients. Various aspects of the work itself play key roles in the burnout risk to care providers, such as lack of adequate funding, rotating shift work, client and family conflicts, and low ratio of staff to clients. Exposure to suffering is inherent to all human service work, and psychiatric nurses see a great deal of it: these nurses are forced to confront the grim realities of life from a perspective few in our society experience. In addition, a nurse may be stigmatized for working with populations that are stigmatized, such as the mentally ill, the aged, and, most recently, those with AIDS.

Psychiatric nurses and other health care workers can find satisfaction in meeting the needs of those in physical, psychological, and spiritual distress. Such workers are seldom given recognition—financial, professional,

---

BOX 3–1
Factors That Inhibit Self Care

INDIVIDUAL

Low self-esteem
Workaholism
Financial problems
Compromised values
Family demands
Relocation, increased mobility
Hidden agenda
Emotional health
Conformity–submissiveness
Rigid personality
Competitiveness
Overaggressiveness; impatience
Frustration
Lack of control
Feeling of powerlessness
Low social support
Fear of success or failure
Inability to let go
Inability to set limits
Lack of attention to own needs and wants
Physical and psychological isolation

ORGANIZATIONAL

Communication problems with others in the system
Communication problems with administration
Communication problems within the team
Role ambiguity
Conflicting goals of clinical staff and administration
Role conflict
Nature of the system or institution
Lack of institutional support for direct caregivers

OCCUPATIONAL

Exposure to suffering
Lack of adequate funding
Rotating shift work
Client/family conflicts
Low ratio of staff to clients
Lack of time
Chronicity of client illness

---

or societal—for their work with those who suffer. They may be unable to acknowledge how they feel about these and other dimensions of their chosen profession. The nurse who has the skills to do so will develop strategies to identify and manage the factors that lead to burnout. On the other hand, nurses who do not develop coping skills, or those working in situations for which their existing coping skills are inadequate, may begin to show the signs of repeated unmanageable stress.

Manifestations of Burnout

Burnout can manifest itself in physical and behavioral signs and symptoms (Box 3-2). Fatigue, moodiness, irritability, insomnia or hypersomnia, and over and under eating as well as excessive alcohol consumption can indicate depression, which, in turn, can indicate burnout. Medications such as barbiturates, narcotics, tranquilizers, and even antibiotics and vitamins may be abused. Abuse of alcohol may be less easy to detect in a society where drinking is socially sanctioned as a stress-reducing "medication." Gastrointestinal disturbances, including ulcers, colitis, nausea, diarrhea, and constipation, are most likely to develop in women, including nurses, who are highly educated and hold jobs of high responsibility and low authority.[14] Cardiovascular problems, hypertension and angina, and respiratory problems evidenced by allergic flare-ups, colds, and chronic infections such as sore throats may be further symptoms of burnout.

Other signs of burnout may be directed toward clients, fellow workers, or the hospital. For example,

the psychiatric nurse may refer to clients in a detached or dehumanizing manner, label them in derogatory terms or with cliches, or make them the topic of malicious jokes or humor. Nurses may constantly complain about clients, supervisors, or fellow workers. There

---

BOX 3–2
Signs of Burnout

PHYSICAL

Fatigue
Feelings of exhaustion
Inability to recover from a cold
Feeling physically "run down"
Frequent headaches
Gastrointestinal disturbances
Weight gain or loss
Sleeplessness
Shortness of breath

BEHAVIORAL

Work harder and harder, yet accomplish less and less
Come to work late and leave early (or vice versa)
Have a vague feeling that something is wrong
Feel bored
Increase absenteeism
Feel resentful
Feel disenchanted
Feel confused
Feel guilty
Have feelings of futility
Be quick to anger
Feel instant irritation
Have a suspicious attitude about others
Feel omnipotent
Be rigid
Be unable to make decisions
Have heightened sense of responsibility for clients
Abuse alcohol, other drugs, or both

may be rigidity of behavior such as uncompromisingly "following procedure" to the exclusion of teamwork or individualized patient needs. The nurse may minimize physical closeness to the client by avoiding eye contact, spending more time with staff than with clients, or reducing the number of meetings with clients. There may be overintellectualization about situations that arouse powerful emotions as a way of denying the strength of the feelings. The nurse may surrender the capacity to care fully for the individual encountered in daily interactions.

How, then, are psychiatric nurses to permit themselves to care without losing themselves in the process; to practice responsibly and to recognize stress; to be warmed by their work, yet resist being drawn in and burned by it? The answer may lie in how the work experience is framed and in the meaning given to it.

PREVENTION OF BURNOUT

Although some symptoms of burnout may be experienced by many nurses during their careers, steps can be taken to prevent these problems. These steps must include attention to the creation of meaning, to specific strategies to manage behavior, and to the development of a plan of self care.

Creation of Meaning

The meaning given to an experience greatly affects a person's interpretation of the experience. The plight of a 22-year-old client with AIDS who has severe dementia from neurologic involvement can be viewed by a 24-year-old nurse in a variety of ways, ranging from the senseless or tragic through the anger- or anxiety-provoking to an opportunity to explore the nurse's own ideas about powerlessness and mortality. The nurse who views this client as one to be pitied may miss an opportunity to learn about the strength of the human spirit, both of the client and of the nurse.

Meaning is the interpretation given to a particular life experience by the individual undergoing that experience. It is the "why" of "He who has a why to live for can bear almost any how" (reference 3, p 121). "Meaning" can also connote a conscious awareness of the reasons for undergoing an experience. A valuable coping skill will be developed by nurses who work to understand what the suffering they witness means to them. In so doing, they may be able to transcend the self and use a formerly painful experience as a means of personal growth.

When a nurse can create meaning and assist colleagues in doing the same, then work, stress, and the self all contribute to the creation of new dimensions that develop the self and enhance work rather than detracting from it. There is no conflict between warding off the conditions under which burnout occurs and adopting a lifestyle that is positive and preventive. The professional nurse must have both a cognitive under-

standing of the conditions leading to burnout and a plan of self care that includes diversified personal and professional growth activities. These activities are not only intrinsically enriching; they also become the means to avoid the conditions under which burnout occurs. It is very important to view burnout prevention from the positive perspective of self-care promotion rather than from a focus on the fear of becoming professionally burned out.

Behavioral Strategies

Prevention of burnout can be addressed from a variety of perspectives. Good physical care is important, such as appropriate diet, rest, and exercise and the attainment of a balance between work and recreation. The psychiatric nurse who experiences symptoms of burnout requires a thoughtfully developed plan for treatment.

There are a variety of ways to begin to increase the ability as a nursing professional to take care of the self (Box 3-3). Attention needs to be given to proper nutri-

---

BOX 3–3
Strategies for Self Care

ACTING ASSERTIVELY

Requesting what one wants
Delegating responsibility or tasks if overloaded
Directing/intervening/confronting when appropriate
Offering alternatives
Seeking resources
Questioning
Expressing opinions and offering information
Setting limits
Refusal of requests that are inappropriate or dangerous to client

CULTIVATING

Offering to help
Bringing individuals together
Supporting colleagues
Educating others
Socializing

CATHARSIS

Discharging pent-up emotions
Talking things over with coworkers
Physical activity

WITHDRAWING

Leaving situation for a time-out period
Refusing to respond affect for affect
Resigning position

HUMOR (Facilitates the Four Other Major Strategies)

(Hutchinson S: Self-care and job stress. Image: Journal of Nursing Scholarship. 19(4):192–196; 1987)

TABLE 3–1
Care plan for the self

SIGNS AND SYMPTOMS	NURSING INTERVENTION	OUTCOME CRITERIA
Fatigue, weariness, overextended, "too busy," overwhelmed	Learn and incorporate a number of assertiveness skills, especially those that focus on limit setting, saying no Develop healthier lifestyle habits such as balanced diet and adequate rest and recreation	Appropriate limits set on time and energy committed to work and personal life Healthier physical self: well rested, weight and blood cholesterol within normal limits Decrease in the number of colds and flu episodes during the year
Sense of apathy, lack of a sense of meaning in one's professional worklife	Explore through readings, work with a mentor, discussions with colleagues, or in classroom settings the meaning one gives to working with those who suffer, experience loss, have catastrophic illness, etc.	Gain a deeper awareness of why one is doing this work and what internal rewards or energy it offers the helper

tion, including reducing the use of alcohol, sugars, and fats; to regular exercise; and to adequate rest and relaxation. Moreover, nurses must develop a strong network of personal and professional supporters. Above all, ways must be found to develop and strengthen as well as to draw on personal values in dealing with feelings that are aroused when struggling with conflicts in the work place and other aspects of living.

Acting assertively in professional interactions is also helpful in coping with conditions that may lead to burnout.[9] Acting assertively demonstrates knowledge of what is needed and the ability to ask for it in a manner that preserves the rights of others. In being assertive, the psychiatric nurse learns to set limits, to question rationale, and to seek appropriate resources. Assertiveness can be demonstrated by proper delegation of care, and by refusal to carry out inappropriate assignments. Assertiveness can also be demonstrated by the psychiatric mental health nurse who, in utilizing the nursing process, contributes her professional understanding of the client to the interdisciplinary conference for client care planning. Nurses who use

Research Highlights

Hare J, Pratt C, Andrews D. Predictors of burnout in professional and paraprofessional nurses working in hospitals and nursing homes. Int J Nursing Study. 1988; 25(2):105–115.

These authors surveyed 312 professional and paraprofessional nurses in 10 acute-care and long-term care facilities to determine the relations between work and personal factors and the nurses' perceptions of burnout. The questionnaire consisted of a variety of scales to assess interpersonal, intrapersonal, and situational (demographic) areas plus the Maslach burnout inventory, which measures the frequency and intensity of emotional exhaustion, depersonalization, and feelings of personal accomplishment. A stepwise multiple regression analysis indicated that the most powerful predictors of burnout or its absence were work relationships and coping strategies. That is, higher satisfaction with informal support received at work was associated with a lower frequency and intensity of emotional exhaustion. Also, the use of problem-focused coping skills was associated with a greater sense of personal accomplishment, whereas the use of emotion-focused coping (e.g., "venting" actions such as cursing, smoking, yelling, withdrawing) was related to a greater sense of burnout.

Although this study did not look specifically at nurses working in strictly psychiatric settings, the findings could still be relevant. Because institutions have the greatest control over organizational rather than personal issues, Hare and associates recommend attention to improving the quality of the work environment. On the basis of this study, it appears that attention would need to be paid to structural issues as well as to process issues in developing an organizational plan to reduce the risk of burnout among staff.[7]

Hutchinson S. Self and job stress. Image: J Nursing Scholarship. 1987;19(4):192–196.

This qualitative field research explored self-care strategies of hospital-based nurses with data derived from participant observation in four clinical areas and from indepth interviews with 20 nurses. The nurses relied on the following self-care strategies: asserting, cultivating, catharsis, and withdrawing. Humor, an additional self-care strategy, facilitated the other strategies.

The findings from this study could be most helpful to those psychiatric nurses who experience a great deal of powerlessness in their job setting. Hutchinson concludes that self-care strategies can be used to combat the problems nurses confront in their daily work. "Such strategies should ultimately provide them with a sense of control over stressful situations and relationships. Such personal power should lead to job power, thus enhancing the nurse, the person and the profession" (reference 9, p 196).

assertive strategies they have learned report that they feel better in that they know they have clearly communicated their concerns to others and have had some influence on their environments.[9]

Prevention of burnout requires careful planning and an attitude of vigilant hopefulness. The framework to begin creating a life-long care plan for the self can come from a multitude of sources, including philosophy, religion, education, family of origin, peer groups, and the belief systems that both inform and flow from these.

Development of Self-Care Plan

One of the difficulties in diagnosing burnout is that it is rarely recognized by those who are experiencing it. Early signs are subtle and often overlooked. Box 3-1 lists factors that can inhibit self care on individual, organizational, and occupational levels. These factors have been identified to assist in symptom recognition, diagnosis of burnout, and planning of treatment for the self. Developing a plan of optimal care of the self will keep the psychiatric nurse aware of the presence of those factors and experiences that reduce satisfaction in work. Table 3-1 is a sample of a self-care plan. The reader is encouraged to begin work on a personal plan of care.

SUMMARY

A psychiatric nurse may develop coping skills that will assist in avoiding the negative symptoms of stress overload and burnout. Such skills may assist in early identification of situations that potentiate stress overload. Skills also can be learned to deal assertively with work situations that create conditions leading to burnout. The psychiatric nurse who is prepared to cope with these various stressors will be able to focus the nursing process on the relationship with the client and be open to the many rewards to be gleaned from those interactions.

References

1. Benner P, Wrubel J. Caring Comes First. Am J Nursing. 1988;88:1073–1076.
2. Brown GW. Meaning, measurement and stress of life events. In: Dohrenwend BS, Dohrenwend BP (eds). Stressful Life Events: Their Nature and Effects. New York: John Wiley; 1974.
3. Frankl VE. Man's Search for Meaning: An Introduction to Logotherapy. New York: Washington Square Press; 1963.
4. Freudenberger HJ. The staff burn-out syndrome in alternative institutions. Psychother Theory Res Pract. 1975;12:73–82.
5. Gann ML. The Role of Personality Factors and Job Characteristics in Burnout: A Study of Social Workers. University of California, Berkeley: Doctoral dissertation; 1979.
6. Glass DC. Behavior Patterns, Stress and Coronary Disease. Hillsdale, NJ: Lawrence Erlbaum Associates; 1974.
7. Hare J, Pratt C, Andrews D. Predictors of burnout in professional and paraprofessional nurses working in hospitals and nursing homes. Int J Nursing Studies. 1988;25(2):105–115.
8. Heckman SJ. Effects of Work Setting, Theoretical Orientation and Personality on Psychotherapist Burnout. California School of Professional Psychology, Berkeley: Doctoral dissertation; 1980.
9. Hutchinson S. Self-care and job stress. Image: J Nursing Scholarship. 1987;19(4):192–196.
10. Lazarus R. Psychological Stress and the Coping Process. New York: McGraw-Hill; 1984.
11. Maslach C. Burnout: The Cost of Caring. Englewood Cliffs: Prentice-Hall; 1982.
12. McCarthy P. Burnout in psychiatric nursing. J Advanced Nursing. 1985;10:305–310.
13. McConnell EA. Burnout in the Nursing Profession: Coping Strategies, Causes and Costs. St Louis: CV Mosby; 1982.
14. Norris J, Kunes-Connell M, Stockard S, Ehrhart PM, Newton GR. Mental Health–Psychiatric Nursing. New York: John Wiley; 1987.
15. Phillips SL, Fischer LS. Measuring social support networks in general populations. In: Dohrenwend BS, Dohrenwend BP (eds). Stressful Life Events and Their Contexts. New Brunswick, NJ: Rutgers University Press; 1984.
16. Vachon LS. Team stress in palliative/hospice care. Hospice J. 1987;3(2):75–103.

4

Howard K. Butcher
Gertrude K. McFarland

Conceptual Frameworks for Psychiatric Mental Health Nursing Practice

OBJECTIVES

After reading this chapter, the reader will be able to:

1. *Compare and contrast Peplau's interpersonal relations conceptual framework, Orem's self-care conceptual framework, Roy's adaptation conceptual framework, King's open-system conceptual framework, and Rogers' science of unitary human beings*

2. *Discuss application of Peplau, Orem, Roy, King, and Rogers' conceptual frameworks to psychiatric mental health nursing practice.*

INTRODUCTION

The ongoing development of a distinct body of knowledge for nursing is critical. If nursing is to continue to evolve as a profession, nurses must develop, through the process of scientific inquiry, the body of knowledge specific to nursing, upon which practice is based. If psychiatric mental health nursing is to develop fully as a professional specialty, then psychiatric mental health nursing must turn to nursing science to organize and guide practice. In this chapter, developments of nursing science by Peplau,[31-38] Orem,[25-28] Roy,[1,48-54,57] King,[15,19-21] and Rogers[42-47] will be examined, utilizing human beings, environment, health, and nursing as a framework for analysis.[11,13,24]

PEPLAU'S INTERPERSONAL RELATIONS CONCEPTUAL FRAMEWORK

Hildegard Peplau's seminal book, *Interpersonal Relations in Nursing*,[31] made a major contribution to theory-based nursing practice. Peplau used knowledge derived from behavioral science, particularly from the work of Harry Stack Sullivan. Peplau views nursing as an "educative instrument, a maturing force that aims to promote forward movement of personality in the direction of creative, constructive, productive, personal and community living" (reference 31, p 16). The crux of nursing that facilitates this growth is the nurse–client relationship. The nurse–client relationship is conceptualized as moving through four overlapping phases: orientation, identification, exploitation, and resolution. As the nurse–client relationship evolves, the nurse assumes various roles, initially as a stranger, but later as a teacher, leadership, surrogate, resource person, and counsellor for significant other (Fig. 4-1).

In Peplau's model, nursing is "being able to understand one's own behavior to help others identify felt difficulties and to apply principles of human relations to the problems that arise at all levels of experience" (reference 31, p xiii). In the 1950s, Peplau's framework laid the groundwork for psychiatric nursing practice.[14] Furthermore, the concept of nurse–client relationship has become an integral component of broader nursing frameworks such as King's. Currently, there is renewed interest in Peplau's view of psychodynamic nursing, as nursing moves toward theory-based practice.

Human Beings

Peplau describes humans as living in an unstable environment and life as the process of striving toward stable equilibrium, a fixed pattern that is never reached except in death.[31] She believes that humans have the ability to learn and to develop skills for solving problems and adapting to the tensions created by their needs.

The person is a self-system, who comprises biochemical, physiological, and interpersonal characteristics and needs. The person develops through interactions with others. An individual's behavior patterns are influenced by past developmental experiences, present contextual variables, and future expectations and goals. It is the person's perception of these factors that is most significant in determining behavior.[13,37]

Anxiety is a basic concept, integral to Peplau's conceptualization of human beings. Behavioral activities are designed for the purpose of reducing anxiety generated from unmet needs and toward facilitating the emergence of higher needs. Anxiety is an energy produced when communications with others threaten the biological or psychological security of the individual. There are four stages of anxiety: mild, moderate, severe, and panic. Identifiable behavior patterns emerge from varying degrees of anxiety, such as withdrawal or somatization.[13,34] The person is viewed as an "antianxiety system" because the direction of development is toward behaviors that prevent undue anxiety.[37]

Communication with others, another basic concept, helps human beings attend to and clarify perceptions of reality and achieve a sense of understanding with another person.[31] An awareness of nonverbal and verbal communication and the symbolic meaning behind these communications must be assessed by the nurse and understood, if the nurse is to influence the client's communications in a manner that contributes to health. A person's thought patterns are assessed and modified through communication. Clear and supportive communication is integral to a person's development.

Environment

Peplau implicitly defines the *environment* in terms of "existing forces outside the organism and in the context of culture" (reference 33, p 163) from which mores, customs, and beliefs are acquired. Specifically, Peplau describes an *interpersonal environment* as consisting of

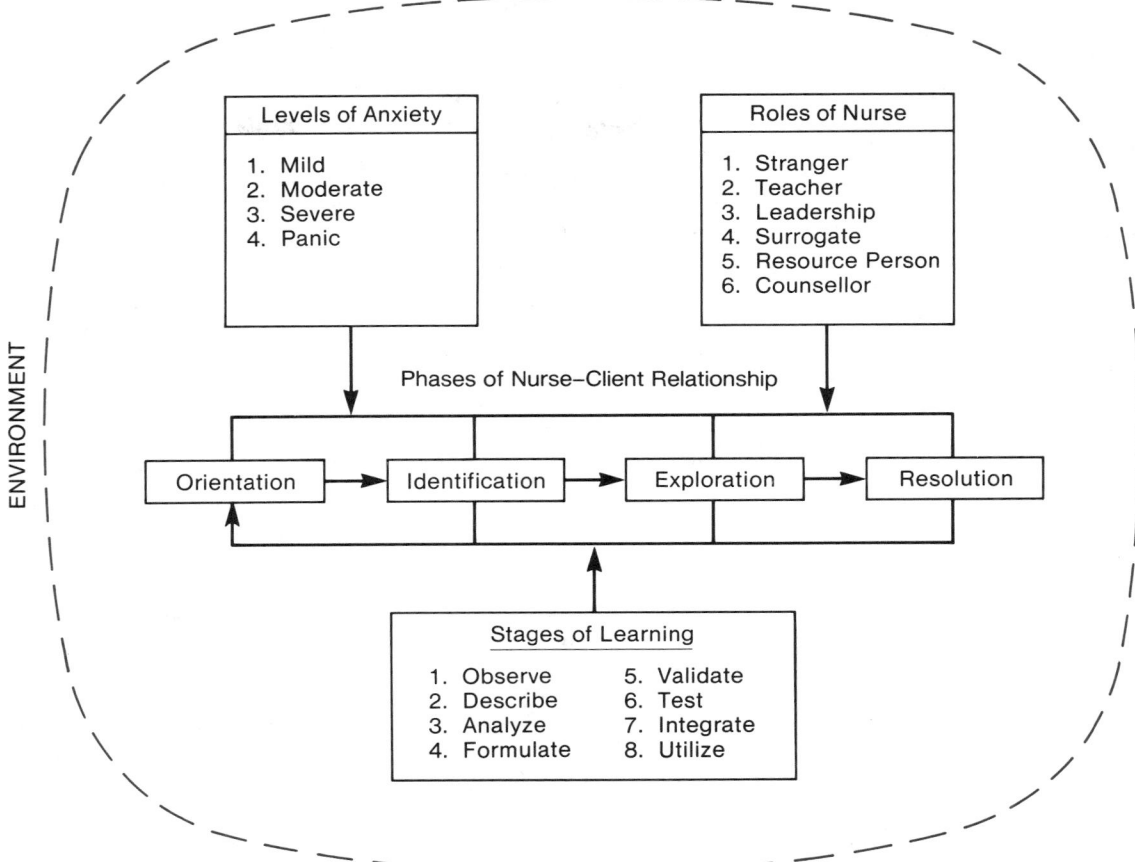

FIGURE 4–1. Peplau's[31–38] interpersonal relations conceptual framework.

interactions between person and family, child and parent, or patient and nurse as the context in which health is promoted and human goals fulfilled. The hospital's physical and social environment and the nurse–client interpersonal environment are viewed as primary responsibilities of the nurse. Environmental systems may be either illness maintaining or health promoting.[33]

Health

Health is viewed as a developmental process and is described as the "forward movement of personality and other ongoing human processes in the direction of creative, constructive, productive, personal and community living" (reference 31, p 12). Health and illness are viewed on a continuum. A person's degree of health is related to the degree of anxiety experienced and the ability to transform this anxiety into productive, asymptomatic behavior. Health-promoting behaviors are those that facilitate need satisfaction, self-awareness, and meaningful integration of each life's experiences, including illness. Thus, health is viewed primarily as a reduction of anxiety.[13]

Nursing

Peplau defined *nursing* as a "significant, therapeutic and interpersonal process."[31] The essence of nursing, according to Peplau, is the relationship between nurse and client. Nurses must first become aware of themselves, their personal needs, and their personal reactions. Nurses can then manage their own behavior and use themselves as the stimulus or therapeutic agent to assist clients to respond and modify behavior. Peplau characterizes nurses as active partners with clients, in a mutual learning experience. A client is accepted "as he/she is" rather than trying to model the person to meet the nurse's personal expectations. Also, Peplau[31,32,36,38] described the nurse as being a client-focused, nondirective listener, maintaining a nonjudgmental approach, offering unconditional warmth, and providing hope. The nurse needs to be authentic with the client by being clear and direct about the limits of a situation. The nurses's consistency and clarity are important principles. The nurse's focus is on the client and his or her problem. To be helpful to clients, nurses need to develop an understanding of clients' perceptions of themselves in the situations confronting them.

The interpersonal process is described as a participatory relationship between nurse and client, in which the nurse governs the purpose and the process, and the client controls the content. The interpersonal process is operationally defined in terms of four interlocking, distinct phases: orientation, identification, exploitation, and resolution. The identification and exploitation phases are often referred to as the *working phase*. Table 4-1 illustrates the role of nurse and client in each of the four phases. The nurse and client have changing goals and roles as they pass through each phase. Operationally, the nurse's role is a process in terms of any or all of the identified roles. In the first role of stranger, both the nurse and client are unknown to each other. The nurse should not prejudge the client. As a resource person, the nurse provides information and answers questions within the context of the larger problem. The teacher is

a combination of all the roles, and always proceeds from what the client knows and develops around his or her interest in wanting and using information.[31] The leadership role is directed toward the development of a democratic relationship. The nurse encourages active participation and a relationship of mutual cooperation in the direction of care. The surrogate role is described as being outside the client's awareness and results in the client viewing the nurse as a variety of symbolic figures. The nurse's function is to assist clients in recognizing similarities between herself and the persons recalled by the clients. The nurse then helps the clients see the difference between herself and the recalled persons. Peplau[31] believes the counselor role is of greatest importance in all nurse–client relationships. Components of the counselor role include increasing the client's awareness of conditions required for health and

TABLE 4–1
Nurse–client roles in Peplau's phases of the nurse–client relationship

| ORIENTATION PHASE | WORKING PHASE | | RESOLUTION PHASE |
	Identification	Exploitation	
CLIENT			
Seeks assistance	Participates in identifying problems	Makes full use of services	Abandons old needs
Conveys educative needs	Begins to be aware of time	Identifies new goals	Aspires to new goals
Asks questions	Responds to help	Attempts to attain new goals	Becomes independent of helping person
Tests parameters	Identifies with nurse	Rapid shifts in behavior; dependent <--> independent	Applies new problem-solving skills
Shares preconceptions and expectations of nurse because of past experience	Recognizes nurse as a person	Exploitative behavior	Maintains changes in style of communication and interaction
	Explores feelings	Realistic exploitation	Positive changes in view of self
	Fluctuates dependence, independence, and interdependence in relationship with nurse	Self-directing	Integrates illness
	Increases focal attention	Develops skills in interpersonal relationships and problem-solving	Exhibits ability to stand alone
	Changes appearance (for better or worse)	Displays changes in manner of communication (more open, flexible)	
	Understands purpose of meeting		
	Maintains continuity between sessions (process and content)		
NURSE			
Responds to emergency	Maintain separate identity	Continue assessment	Sustain relationship as long as client feels necessary
Gives parameters of meetings	Exhibit ability to edit speech or control focal attention	Meet needs as they emerge	Promote family interaction
Explains roles	Testing maneuvers decrease	Understand reason for shifts in behavior	Assist with goal setting
Gathers data	Unconditional acceptance	Initiate rehabilitative plans	Teach preventive measures
Helps client identify problem	Help express needs, feelings	Reduce anxiety	Utilize community agencies
Helps client plan use of community resources and services	Assess and adjust to needs	Identify positive factors	Teach self-care
Reduces anxiety and tension	Provide information	Help plan for total needs	Terminate nurse–client relationship
Practices nondirective listening	Provide experiences that diminish feelings of helplessness	Facilitate forward movement of personality	
Focuses client's energies	Do not allow anxiety to overwhelm patient	Deal with therapeutic impasse	
Clarifies client's preconceptions and expectations of nurse	Help client to focus on cues		
	Help client develop responses to cues		
	Use word stimuli		

(From Forchuk C, Brown B. Establishing a nurse–client relationship. J Psychosoc Nurs Ment Health Serv 1989;27(2):30–38. Used with permission.)

providing these when possible, identifying threats to health, and facilitating learning through the use of evolving interpersonal events. The nursing roles change as the nurse and client work through the phases of the relationship.

Peplau[35] described eight stages of the learning process. After the nurse identifies which learning stage the client is in, the nurse helps the client move on to the next stage. The learning stages are to observe, to describe, to analyze, to formulate, to validate, to test, to integrate, and to utilize. Each stage has specific questions[35] to help the client move on to the next stage. For example, if a person is at "observe" the nurse would ask: "What do you see, what do you hear?"

Assessment within Peplau's conceptual framework would involve assessing the client's level of anxiety and stage of learning and determining the phase of the nurse–client relationship. The nurse, when functioning in the roles of the nurse, uses therapeutic communication techniques as interventions specific to the phase of relationship and stage of learning as a means to reduce the client's level of anxiety and to increase interpersonal and problem-solving competencies. Increasing competencies lead to the forward movement of personality that Peplau defines as health.

OREM'S SELF-CARE CONCEPTUAL FRAMEWORK

Three theories are interrelated and basic to Orem's framework.[11,13,24–28] The *theory of self-care deficit* proposes that the recipients of nursing care are persons who are incapable of continuous self-care or independent care because of health-related or health-derived limitations. The *theory of self-care* is based on the premise that a relationship exists between deliberate self-care actions and the development and functioning of individuals and groups. The *theory of nursing systems* discusses therapeutic self-care requisites and the actions or systems involved in self-care; that is, "activities that individuals initiate and perform on their own behalf in maintaining life, health, and well-being."[27] Self-care is learned, deliberate behavior that people perform to meet and maintain certain specific needs (self-care requisites). At different times in each person's life, the person (self-care agent) has differing abilities or skills in performing self-care (self-care agency). Self-care agency refers to the power of individuals to engage in self-care. When a self-care need is not met, a self-care demand is present; self-care deficits exist when people are unable to meet their self-care demands. A nurse, family member, or friend (dependent-care agent) may be used in an educative or consultative relationship to help alleviate or correct the deficit. In health care facilities, nurses perform this role and help people meet their self-care requirements by (1) organizing a wholly compensatory system in which acting and doing for the client is central; (2) designing with the client a partially compensatory system, in which either the nurse or the client may have the major role; or (3) participating in a supportive–educative system in which support, guidance, provision of a developmental environment, and teaching are central components.[28]

Human Beings

In Orem's self-care model, human beings are viewed as integrated wholes, functioning biologically, symbolically, and socially.[28] Integrated human functioning includes physical, psychological, interpersonal, and social aspects. Self-care is a learned requirement for human beings to maintain health and well-being, as they have universal, developmental, and health deviation self-care requisites.

UNIVERSAL SELF-CARE REQUISITES

Universal self-care requisites (USCR) are common to all human beings and are associated with life processes and with the maintenance of the integrity of human structure and functioning. The eight universal self-care requisites include sufficient intake of air, food, and fluid; maintenance of elimination; balance between rest and activity and between solitude and social interaction; prevention of hazards; and a sense of normalcy. Many psychiatric clients are hospitalized because they are unable to meet multiple universal self-care requisites. For example, a client in a manic episode of bipolar disorder may not have eaten in three days (insufficient food–fluid intake); may be hyperactive and unable to sleep (imbalance of activity and rest); be highly intrusive and interfering with others (imbalance between solitude and social interaction); lack judgment and problem-solving ability relative to personal safety (unable to protect self from hazards); and have strong underlying feelings of poor self-concept and self-image (lack of a sense of normalcy). Examples of nursing diagnoses identified by the authors of this chapter as being related to Orem's universal self-care requisites include altered nutrition, sleep pattern disturbance, agitation, impaired social interaction, potential for injury, self-concept disturbance, and wellness-seeking behavior.

DEVELOPMENTAL SELF-CARE REQUISITES

Developmental self-care requisites (DSCR) focus on human developmental processes and events during various stages of the life cycle and on events that may adversely affect development.[11] For example, developmental stages of childhood through adulthood create specialized self-care demands that need to be met to prevent developmental disorders and to promote development in accord with the human potential. Loss of significant others, loss of possessions, and educational deprivation are some of the conditions that may adversely affect human development. The developmental history of psychiatric clients often includes traumatic experiences during key phases of the person's development. For another client, the onset of mental illness may be related to the person's difficulty in adjusting to developmental changes. Examples of nursing diagnoses, which were selected by the authors of this chapter as being related to DSCR, include maturational crisis, situational crisis, grieving, dysfunctional grieving, and altered growth and development.

HEALTH DEVIATION SELF-CARE REQUISITES

Health deviation self-care requisites (HDSCR) are associated with the self-care required in conditions of illness, injury, or disease, or may result from medical measures required to diagnose or correct the condition. The six health deviation self-care requisites are (1) seeking appropriate medical assistance for conditions of human pathology, (2) attending to the effects of human pathology, (3) carrying out medically prescribed measures effectively, (4) caring for or regulating uncomfortable or deleterious effects of prescribed medical measures, (5) accepting self in relation to a state of health in need of health care and modifying the self-concept, and (6) altering one's life-style to promote personal development while living with the effect of pathology and medical measures.[28] Defensive coping (specify), noncompliance (specify), and altered health maintenance are nursing diagnoses that were identified by the authors of this chapter as being closely related to one or more of Orem's HDSCR that are not being met.

Environment

The concept of environment is not well developed in Orem's conceptual framework. Orem does state that "requisites for self-care have their origins in human beings and their environment" (reference 28, p 36). Therapeutic self-care demands can be adversely affected by internal or external conditions. The focus of the theory of self-care is toward personal self-management in the person's environment, under stable or changing conditions. The assessment of the person's sociocultural orientation, socioeconomic conditions, health care system, and family system elements may be viewed as environmental factors that condition the person's ability to perform self-care.

Health

Orem views health as a state of wholeness and well-being. Persons are whole when they are structurally and functionally sound. Any deviation from normal structure or functioning is referred to as "an absence of health" (reference 28, p 174). When self-care is not being maintained, illness, disease, or death will occur. Self-care is a person's own personal continuous contribution to personal health and well-being. Thus, health is integral to the concept of self-care in this model. Orem's view of health is based on the concept of preventive health care. It includes the promotion and maintenance of health (primary prevention), the identification and treatment of disease (secondary prevention), and the prevention of complications (tertiary prevention). Orem also discusses the impact of values and beliefs on self-care practices. Conflicts between self-care values and other cultural values may influence the selection of unhealthy activities. Orem relates care, restoration, regulation, maintenance, recovery, and rehabilitation to the concept of health.

Nursing

The special concern of nursing, according to Orem, is "the individual's need for self-care action and the provision and management of it on a continuous basis in order to sustain life and health, recover from disease or injury, and cope with their effects" (reference 28 p 59). The nursing perspective encompasses the client's perspective of his or her own health situation and the physician's perspective of the patient's health situation. Nursing care is appropriate when the person is not able to engage in self-care or dependent care (i.e., a parent's care for a child). Nursing actions are helpful in moving the client toward responsible action in self-care or toward increasing the competence of a dependent care agent in giving care to a family member. Nursing goals and interventions are based on assessing and diagnosing the therapeutic self-care demand, self-care agency, and basic-conditioning factors.

From an action perspective, nursing is a human property that enables nurses to engage in the diagnostic, prescriptive, and regulatory operations necessary to design and produce systems of nursing care for persons with self-care or dependent care deficits associated with the health state or with the health care requirements of persons in need of care.[28] The power capabilities that enable nurses to perform these actions are developed through nurses' preparation for nursing practice, life experiences, and their motivation and enduring interests to provide nursing care to others.

NURSING AGENCY

The nurse's ability to carry out the nursing process within a self-care framework is called nursing agency. Nursing agency is developed in three areas: social (contractual role of nurse), interpersonal (therapeutic use of self), and technological (the work operations of nursing professionals). Nurses activate their nursing agency to overcome, substitute for, or compensate for health-derived or health-associated self-care deficits of persons under care.[28]

NURSING PROCESS

All self-care actions that are needed to meet self-care requisites (USCR, DSCR, and HDSCR) are referred to as the client's *therapeutic self-care demand* (TSCD). The first area of assessment is referred to as *basic-conditioning factors* (BCFs), factors that may modify all self-care requisites and power components. The factors include age, sexual features, developmental state, health state, sociocultural orientation, socioeconomical elements, health care system elements, family system elements, and pattern of living. These basic conditioning factors provide the structure for data gathering because each factor has the potential of revealing the conditioning effect of the requisites and the quality of self-care agency. The use of antecedent knowledge about human structure and function, including social functions and development, determines the conditioning effect of the BCFs on each requisite.[56] Figure 4-2 illustrates the relationship between TSCD, self-care agency, nursing agency, and self-care. The therapeutic self-care demand (TSCD) is calculated by assessing the universal, developmental, and health deviation self-care requisites relative to the basic-conditioning factors. The nurse then identifies those action demands that the client needs to perform to meet self-care requisites.[40,56]

The nurse assesses the client's self-care agency (SCA), which is the summation of the human capabilities needed for performing self-care. Self-care agency is also assessed relative to the BCFs. Ten components of self-care agency are assessed in terms of development, operability, and adequacy, to determine the client's ability to engage in deliberate self-care. The self-care agency power components include (1) attention span and vigilance, (2) control of physical energy, (3) control of body movement, (4) ability to reason, (5) motivation,

(6) decision-making skills, (7) knowledge, (8) repertoire of skills, (9) ability to order self-care actions, and (10) ability to integrate self-care actions into patterns of living.[25] Self-care agency is a key concept in psychiatric nursing. Mental illness may have a direct effect on a client's reasoning ability, decision-making ability, and control of physical energy.

Each action demand is analyzed in relation to power components in the client's self-care agency. If the self-care agency is less than the TSCD (required self-care) to meet a particular action demand, then a self-care deficit is present. The self-care deficit statement is analogous to nursing diagnosis.

According to the authors of this chapter, nursing diagnoses state the existing level of the self-care agency needed to meet current and future demands and state the relationship between the self-care action required of an individual and the ability to carry out such actions. Compatibility between nursing diagnoses and self-care deficit theory is possible by relating the human response to the limitation in self-care agency or the limiting action demand, for example, self-concept disturbance related to inadequate knowledge of how to modify the environment and life-style to maximize independence.

TYPES OF NURSING SYSTEMS

Orem[28] presents three types of nursing systems. The first type is called "wholly compensatory" and requires the nurse to do everything, or nearly everything, collaboratively with the patient. An example would be a psychiatric client on one-to-one supervision who requires total care. The second type is known as "partly compensatory." In this situation, all five helping methods may be used, with the client doing what he or she can and the nurse supplementing the activity that the client is unable to perform. The third type of system, one important for helping psychiatric patients, is the supportive–educative system. It involves guiding, teaching, and environmental support. Within this system, the nurse assists the client in decision making, behavioral control, and acquiring the needed knowledge and coping skills for the promotion of self-care.

CATEGORIES OF HELPING

The five categories of helping identified by Orem[28] include (1) acting for or doing for, (2) guiding, (3) supporting physically or psychologically, (4) providing an environment conducive to individual development, and (5) teaching. In psychiatric nursing, the therapeutic one-to-one nurse–patient relationship and the provision of psychotherapy by a qualified nurse therapist would be examples of the helping method supporting psychologically. Milieu therapy is an example of providing an environment conducive to individual development. In the production management phase of nursing systems, the nurse implements the nursing system design. On the basis of the clients' self-care deficits and the selected ways of helping, the client compensates or overcomes the self-care deficits. The nurse assists the client

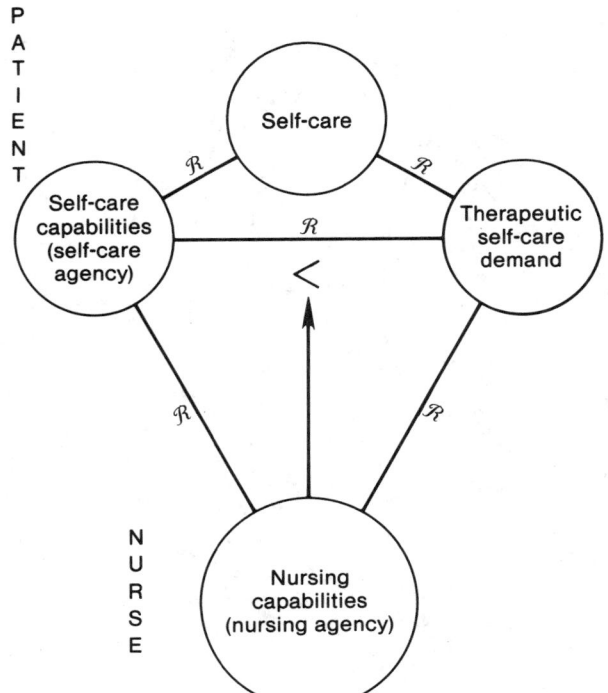

FIGURE 4–2. Self-care deficit theory. R = relationship; < = deficit relationship; current or projected. (From Orem DE. Nursing: concepts of practice, ed. 3, New York; McGraw-Hill Book Co.; 1985. Reproduced by permission of the C.V. Mosby Co., St. Louis. Used with permission.)

or family in self-care matters to achieve identified and described health-related results.

Orem's self-care conceptual framework identifies the object, goals, elements, products, and boundaries of nursing within this framework. "Self-help or self-care" is advocated. The nurse's role is in deciding how best to help each client, given his or her abilities for self-care, so that an independent level of function can be regained, the present level can be maintained, or a dignified meaningful death can be supported. This conceptual framework looks at the relationship between what a human being must do to maintain life, health, and well-being (therapeutic self-care demand), and that human being's ability to do so (self-care agency). When self-care agency is less than the therapeutic self-care demand, a self-care deficit exists. Nursing systems are then designed to help individuals deal with these deficits. When the ultimate goal of nursing is to engage clients in meeting self-care requirements for health, psychotherapeutic approaches (such as insight-ori-

ented/problem-solving therapy, behavioral therapy, psychoanalytical approaches, and interpersonal psychotherapy) are conceptualized as appropriate helping methods in providing psychological support as a means for meeting self-care requirements within this framework.

ROY'S ADAPTATION CONCEPTUAL FRAMEWORK

Roy provides a conceptual framework for nursing that views the person as an adaptive system interacting with a changing environment (Fig. 4-3). Roy's adaptation conceptual framework[1,11,13,24,48–54,57] is based on von Bertalanfy's systems theory[5] and on Helson's[17] adaptation level theory, as well as specific philosophical assumptions.[49] As a systems model, Roy's framework utilizes the concepts of input, output, control processes,

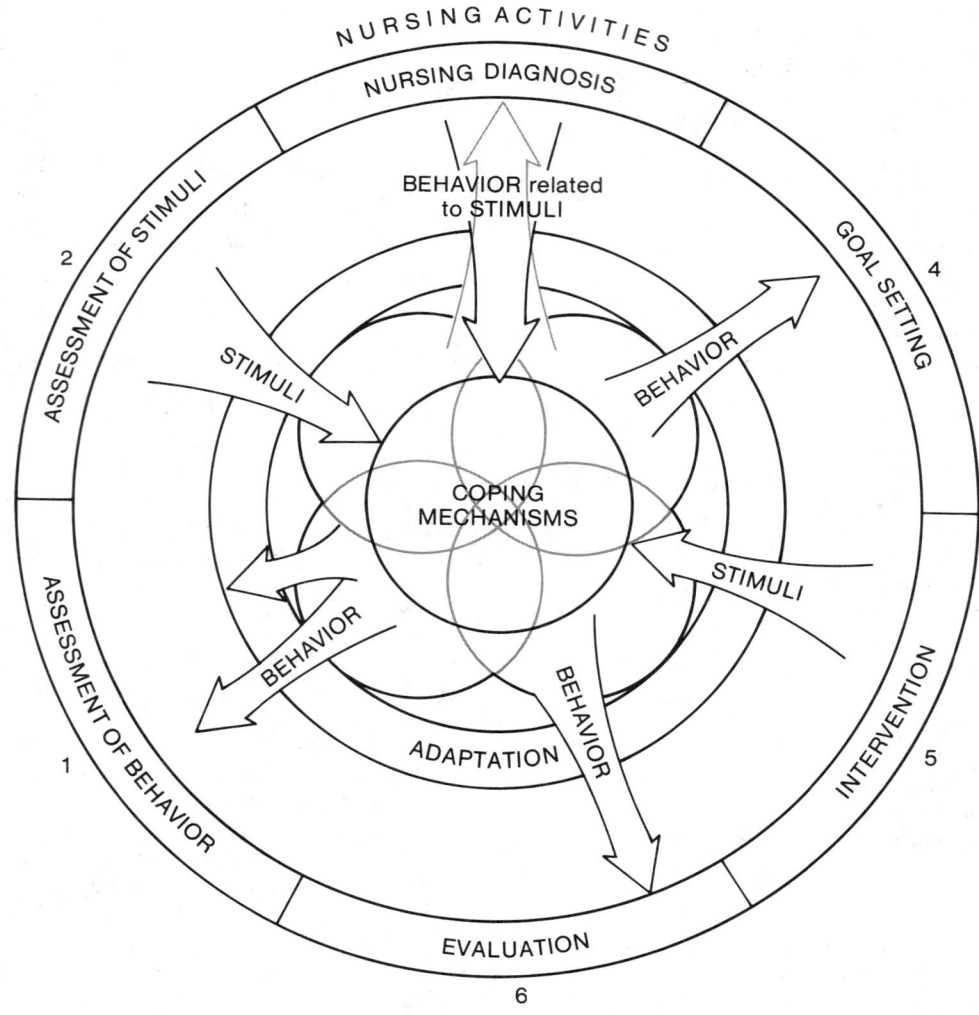

FIGURE 4–3. Roy's adaptation model. (From Andrews H, Roy C. Essentials of the Roy adaptation model. Norwalk, CT: Appleton-Century-Crofts, 1986:103. Used with permission.)

and feedback. The individual or group is affected by stimuli (input), which is then processed by both the regulator (physiologic) and cognator (psychological) control processes. A behavioral response is manifested in one of four modes of adaptation: physiological, role, self-concept, and interdependence. The response or output may be either an adaptive or ineffective response. The feedback mechanism relays information back to the system as input, and the process of adaptation continues. Roy's central concept of adaptation is integral to the concepts of human beings, environment, health, and nursing. *Adaptation* is defined as a process of promoting integrity or, more specifically, as a process of responding positively to environmental changes.[51] Adaptation, both as a process and a point in time, is a person's response to the environment that promotes his or her general goals, including survival, growth, reproduction, and mastery.[53] A given adaptation level is made up of pooled stimuli and is "a constantly changing point which represents the person's own standard or range of stimuli that he will tolerate with ordinary adaptive responses" (reference 53, p 43).

Human Beings

The Roy adaptation framework views the human being or group as an adaptive system, with coping mechanisms (control processes) manifested by the four adaptive modes. Although the focus of nursing is on the person, Roy has also stated that the model may be applied to family, organizational structures, community, or society.[50] The human being is an adaptive system that is integrated while in constant interaction with a changing environment. The systems and parts of the body can be studied separately, but in reality, they are interwoven and balanced to produce a functioning human being with inseparable biological, psychological, and social needs. Roy uses the term *coping mechanisms* to describe the control processes of the person as an adaptive system.

Roy identifies two major internal coping mechanisms: the regulator and the cognator subsystems. The regulator sybsystem receives input from the external environment and from changes in the person's internal state.[51] The regulator then processes the changes through neurochemical endocrine channels to produce responses. For example, a client experiencing the DSM-III-R diagnostic disorder, generalized anxiety disorder, with a nursing diagnosis of anxiety (severe) related to spouse's illness, may be experiencing an increase in blood pressure, hyperventilation, rapid pulse rate, muscular tension and rigidity, agitation, cold sweats, and faintness because of stimulation of the sympathetic nervous system and release of catecholamines. Excessive and prolonged anxiety increases the person's susceptibility to illness by decreasing the effectiveness of the immune system and through tissue or organ damage. Thus, the regulator subsystem describes the person's physiologic response to stress.

The second major coping mechanism, termed the cognator subsystem, encompasses complex cognitive–affective pathways of perceptual information processing, learning, judgment and emotion.[51,52] The cognator subsystem is related to the higher brain functions. Stimuli to the cognator are both external and internal in origin. Output behavior from the regulator subsystem can serve as feedback stimuli to the cognator subsystem. Perceptual–information processing includes the activity of selective attention, coding, and memory. Learning includes the activities of problem solving and decision making, whereas emotion encompasses the defense mechanisms that seek relief from anxiety and from making affective appraisals and attachments.[1] In the example of the client experiencing anxiety (severe) related to the spouse's illness, the client's perceptual capacity may be restricted, problem solving may be inefficient, insight may be limited, and the client may be using the defenses of projection, displacement, and reaction formation. Research efforts to further describe and study the interrelationships of the regulator and cognator subsystems are in progress. The interrelationships of the regulator and cognator hold the key to the concept of holism.[52] Furthermore, the person as an adaptive system is seen within the perspective of assumptions related to humanism and beliefs about the purposefulness of human existence.

The stimuli processed by the regulator and cognator control processes is manifested through coping behavior in four adaptive modes: *physiological, self-concept, role function,* and *interdependence.* The *physiological mode* focuses on five basic needs in a hierarchy (oxygenation, nutrition, elimination, activity and rest, and protection), and four regulator processes (the senses, fluid and electrolytes, neurologic function, and endocrine function).[52] Anatomy, physiology, pathophysiology, and chemistry provide the theoretical background for the physiological mode. Behavior in this mode is the manifestation of physiological activity of all the cell tissues, organs, and systems composing the human body. The underlying need of the physiological mode is physiological integrity.[1] The behavioral assessment of the physiological mode provides the nurse with an indication of how the client is managing to cope with environmental changes affecting the physiological coping mechanisms.[39,51,53] Examples of nursing diagnoses identified by the authors of this chapter as being related to Roy's physiological mode are altered nutrition and sleep pattern disturbance.

The *self-concept mode* is defined as the composite of beliefs and feelings that one holds about one's self at a given time and is formed by internal perceptions and the perception of others' reactions.[52] The physical self includes two components: body sensations and body image. The personal self is viewed as having three components: self-consistency, self ideal, and moral–ethical–spiritual self. Self-consistency is the continuity of self over time; the self-ideal is what one expects of the self and what one wants to accomplish; and the moral–ethical–spiritual self involves spiritual values and one's belief system. The five components of the self-concept model form the basis for the behavioral assessment of psychic integrity. Inherent in each component of the self-concept is one's self-esteem. Self-esteem, spiritual distress, body image disturbance, personal identity disturbance, powerlessness, and ineffective individual coping are examples of nursing diagnoses selected by the authors as associated with Roy's self-concept mode.

The third adaptive mode is *role function*. Role function emphasizes the need for social integrity. Role function also relates to the performance of duties based on given positions in society. The way a human being performs a role is dependent upon that person's interaction with others in a given situation.[53] Health and illness experiences affect a human being's role performance. Roy classifies roles into primary, secondary, and tertiary types. Role performance disturbance and altered parenting are examples of nursing diagnoses related to Roy's role function mode identified by the authors of this chapter.

Interdependence is the fourth adaptive mode and is defined as the close relationships of people that involve the willingness and ability to love, respect, and value others; and to accept and respond to love, respect, and value given by others.[51,52] The interdependence mode emphasizes the need for social integrity. The nature of the relationship one has with significant others and support systems is the basis of interdependence. To be mutually satisfying, interdependent relationships must demonstrate reciprocal, receptive, and contributive behaviors.[57] Impaired social interaction; family coping: potential for growth; dysfunctional family processes; grieving; altered parenting; sexual dysfunction; and aggression (specify), are examples of nursing diagnoses identified by the authors of this chapter as most closely related to Roy's interdependence mode.

Environment

In Roy's adaptation conceptual framework, the environment is conceived as the source stimuli affecting the person's adaptive system. The environment encompasses all the internal and external conditions, circumstances, and influences surrounding or affecting the development and behavior of the person or groups.[51] Factors in the environment that affect the human being are categorized as focal, contextual, and residual stimuli. Focal stimulus is that which immediately confronts the person in a given situation, such as loss of a loved one. When the focal stimuli fall within the person's range of adaptation, the response is adaptation; when the focal stimuli fall outside the range of the adaptive level, the person responds ineffectively.[48] Contextual stimuli are all the other stimuli present at the time that may influence a response to the focal stimuli, such as feelings of shame, which affect grieving. Residual stimuli are the beliefs, attitudes, and traits of an individual developed from the past but affecting the current response. Previous losses, unresolved grief, coping style, and culture are examples of some of the contextual and residual stimuli that may

impinge on an individual experiencing grieving related to the loss of a significant other. Assisting the client in managing contextual stimuli promotes adaptation by broadening the client's zone of adaptation.

Health

Roy[51] defines *health* as a state and process of becoming an integrated and whole person. Also, Roy[51] views health as a condition of life that involves integration of the four modes of adaptation. An individual's integration throughout life is dynamic, and it changes in accordance with the person's ability to respond positively to various environmental changes. Health is a reflection of adaptation or the interaction of the human being and environment. Adaptation is the means by which a person sustains health. Successfully coping with a wide variety of stressors is characteristic of health and adaptation. Ineffective responses do not contribute to the integrity of the human being. A lack of integration, therefore, represents a lack of health.[51]

Nursing

Nursing is defined as a "theoretical system of knowledge which prescribes a process and action related to the care of the ill or potentially ill person" (reference 50, p 4). Also, Roy[51] differentiates nursing as a science from nursing as a practice discipline. *Nursing science* is a "developing system of knowledge about persons that observes, classifies, and relates the processes by which persons positively affect their health status" (reference 50, pp 3–4). *Nursing practice* is "nursing's scientific body of knowledge used for the purpose of providing an essential service to people, that is, promoting ability to affect health positively" (reference 51, pp 3–4). The goal of nursing is to help human beings adapt to changes in their physiological needs, self concepts, role functions, and interdependent relationships during health and illness. Nursing fulfills its unique role as a facilitator of adaptation by assessing behavior in each of the four adaptive modes and intervening by managing the influencing stimuli.[51]

NURSING PROCESS

Roy[51] identifies the nursing process as including assessment of behaviors, assessment of influencing factors, nursing diagnosis, goal setting, intervention, and evaluation. Roy further describes two levels of assessment.[51] The first is behavioral assessment and involves the systematic examination of behavioral responses in each of the four adaptive modes: physiological, self-concept, role function, and interdependence. In assessing behavior in each adaptive mode, the nurse uses skills of observation, measurement, and interviewing to obtain behavioral data.[1,50,51,53] Once data are collected, the nurse judges whether the behavior is adaptive or ineffective. Does the behavior support the health of the client? The judgment is based on the comparison of the client's behavior with known norms signifying adaptation. For example, a client experiencing severe anxiety may exhibit some of the following ineffective behaviors in the physiological mode: (rest and activity) unable to relax, insomnia, muscle tension; (oxygenation) increased heart rate, respiratory rate, blood pressure, palpitations, pallor of skin; (nutrition) anorexia, dry mouth; (fluid and electrolyte balance) water retention, decreased potassium; (elimination) decreased urinary output, constipation. In the self-concept mode, verbal expressions of insecurity and inability to deal with the situation are examples of ineffective behaviors underlying anxiety. In the first-level assessment, the nurse also identifies adaptive responses that require the nurse's support. The nurse then prioritizes the ineffective behaviors.

Once all four modes are assessed, the nurse moves to the second level of assessment. For each adaptive and ineffective behavior, the nurse identifies factors (stimuli) influencing the behavior. The stimuli are classified as focal, contextual, or residual. Although the focus of first-level assessment is on the here and now, second-level assessment uses information from the past, as well as from the present. Common stimuli affecting adaptation include culture, beliefs, social and economic status, family structure, development stage, perception, knowledge skills, and illness (pathology). Behavior in one adaptive mode may function as a stimulus in another, indicating the interrelationship of modes. Roy stresses the importance of validating with the client all assumptions and inferences made concerning the identification of adaptive or ineffective behaviors and influencing stimuli.

Problem identification involves a statement of the client's adaptive or ineffective behavior and the most relevant influencing factors. The nursing diagnosis statements describe the problem and its influencing or related factors. Roy[51] describes three methods of formulating a nursing diagnosis. Two examples follow:

1. Label the cluster of behaviors within each mode along with the focal, contextual and residual stimuli; for example, in the physiologic mode, a priority may be sleep pattern disturbance related to loss of significant others, lack of social support, undeveloped coping skills, and repeated losses
2. Summarize the behaviors across the modes that are affected by the same focal, contextual, and residual stimuli (cross-moded diagnosis); for example, the problem may be best understood as anxiety related to loss of significant other, lack of social support, undeveloped coping skills, and repeated losses evidenced by lack of sleep, loss of orientation, and pacing.

Once nursing diagnoses have been identified and prioritized, goals are established through mutual agreement of the nurse and client. Each goal is stated in terms of the expected client behavioral outcome for a nursing intervention.[51] Nursing intervention involves the management of stimuli. The focal stimulus is selected for intervention whenever possible. Management of stimuli may involve altering, increasing, decreasing, removing, or maintaining stimuli. If it is not possible to manage the focal stimulus, contextual stimuli must be managed in an effort to broaden the adaptation level. The intervention with the highest probability of achieving the valued goal is selected. Options for nursing interventions are shared with the client.

The final step in the nursing process using the Roy adaptation framework is evaluation. The nurse evaluates outcomes by assessing the client's behavior relative to the preset goals. If the goals have been achieved, the interventions are considered to be effective and adaptive. This occurs when behaviors have been maintained and ineffective behaviors have been changed to adaptive. For those goals not achieved, the nurse must identify alternate approaches by assessing behavior and stimuli and continuing in an ongoing manner.[1]

Roy's emphasis on the four adaptive modes reflecting the biobehavioral nature of human beings and emphasis on nursing diagnoses provides a unique framework to guide psychiatric mental health nursing practice. The framework's emphasis on the management of stimuli provides a conceptual fit with behavioral theory and milieu therapy. The emphasis on a cognitive–emotional coping mechanism (cognator) provides a conceptual fit with cognitive theory and short-term psychotherapeutic interventions. Psychodynamic theory provides a useful theoretical base for understanding the relationship between stimuli and behaviors. Robitaille-Tremblay and her colleagues,[41] for example, have developed a psychiatric nursing assessment tool based on the Roy adaptation framework, and Schmidt[54] has applied this framework to clients diagnosed as having schizophrenia. Exploring the relationships of the philosophical assumptions to psychiatric mental health nursing care may be an area for future development.[53]

KING'S OPEN-SYSTEM CONCEPTUAL FRAMEWORK

King states that human interaction is the foundation of nursing process.[19–21] King proposed a conceptual framework for nursing and later developed the theory of goal attainment. King's open-system conceptual framework[11,13,15,19–21,24] is composed of three dynamic interacting open systems: (1) the personal systems, (2) interpersonal systems, and (3) the social systems (Fig. 4-4). King views nursing as a process that involves action, reaction, interaction, and transaction (Fig. 4-5). Through this process, nursing assists clients in meeting basic needs in performing the activities of daily living and in coping with health and illness.[19] Transaction follows when a reciprocal relationship is established by the nurse and client, and both mutually set the goals to

Human Beings

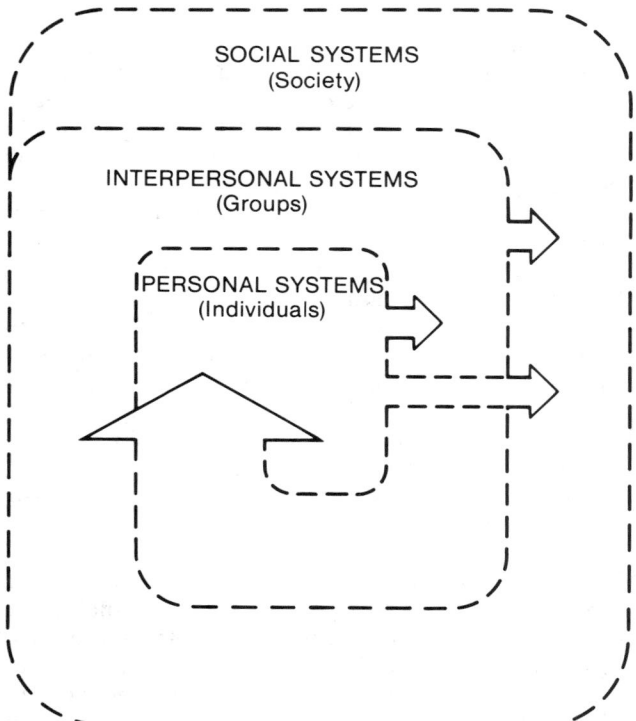

FIGURE 4–4. *King's open-system model. (From King IM. A theory for nursing. New York: John Wiley & Sons, 1981:11. Used with permission.)*

be achieved.[19] King's work builds on the tradition of Henderson,[18] Peplau,[31] and Orlando.[29] The framework's emphasis on human interaction, open systems, and goal attainment are particular features that provide a strong conceptual fit with psychiatric mental health nursing practice.

Human beings are viewed by King as open systems with permeable boundaries that allow the exchange of matter, energy, and information with the environment. Human beings are assumed to be social, sentient, rational, reacting, perceiving, controlling, purposeful, action oriented, and time oriented human beings. King[20] identifies the concepts of perception, growth and development, body image, time, and space as key concepts within the *personal system.* Altered perception–cognition, altered growth and development, body image disturbances, and impaired resource management (time) are examples of nursing diagnoses identified by the authors as most closely related to King's personal system. The *interpersonal system* is the interaction between two or more people. As the number of interacting individuals increases, the complexity of the interactions also increases. The five concepts within the interpersonal system are interaction, communication, transaction, role, and stress. Impaired communication, altered parenting, and impaired social interaction are examples of nursing diagnoses identified by the authors as most closely related to King's interpersonal system. King[20] defines a *social system* as "an organized boundary system of social roles, behaviors, and practices developed to maintain values and the mechanisms to regulate the practises and rules." Social systems describe units of analysis in society in which individuals form groups to carry on activities of daily living to maintain life and health, and, it is hoped, happiness.[19] The concepts of organization, authority, power, status and decision making are defined within the social system. King[20] suggests that the interplay of these forces influences social behavior, interactions, perceptions, and health. Powerlessness, decisional conflict, role performance disturbance, and dysfunctional family processes

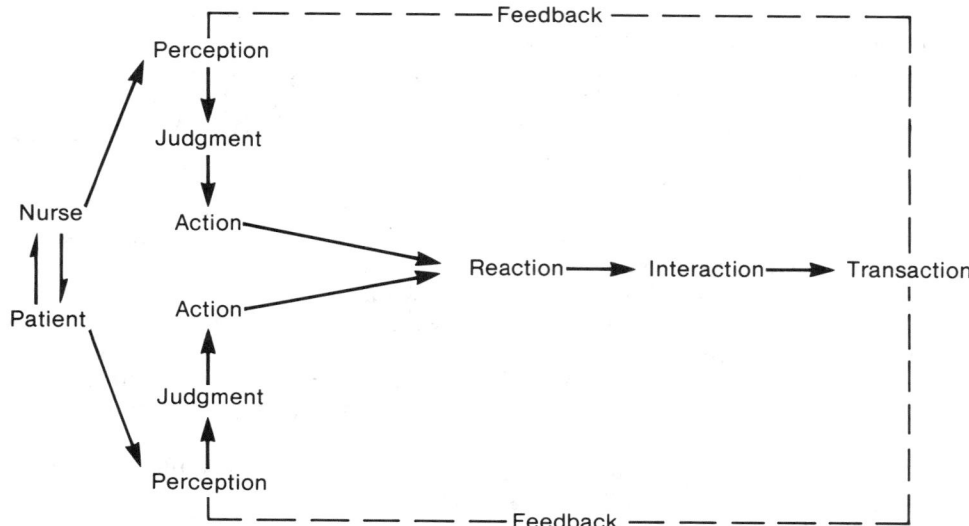

FIGURE 4–5. *King's process of human interactions. (From King IM. A theory for nursing. New York: John Wiley & Sons, 1981:145. Used with permission.)*

are examples of nursing diagnoses identified by the authors that are most closely related to King's conceptual framework.

The concepts within the personal, interpersonal, and social systems are the substantive knowledge base for nursing practice. Furthermore, disturbances in health status relate directly to the concepts. For example, a client with a DSM-III-R diagnosis of bipolar disorder, manic episode, may have a personal system characterized by altered perceptions of reality, whereby the perception of time, space, and body image are severely impaired. Underlying the grandiose delusions may be a profound sense of inadequacy and very low self-esteem. This client's interpersonal system may be characterized by the recent stressor of losing a job and the resulting loss of residence. The loss of role functioning leads to a crisis. The manic behavior serves as a defense to ward off feelings of depression. The mania severely affects this client's ability to communicate and transact effectively with his environment. Because of delusions and psychosis, the client's social system is affected. His sense of organization, authority, status, power, and ability to make decisions, all are impaired. All the concepts within King's open-system conceptual framework may be relevant to understanding a client with mental illness.

Environment

King conceptualizes the environment as an open system interacting with the personal system. In a technological world, human beings are in continuous transaction with the environment.[15] An understanding of the ways that human beings interact with the environment to maintain health is essential knowledge for nurses. King views the person as continuously adjusting to stressors in the environment, since a continuously changing environment is a potential source of stressors.

King refers to both the external and internal environment. The internal environment of human beings transforms energy to enable them to adjust to the continuous external environmental changes. The external environment includes the formal and informal organization.[20] King's view of environment also encompasses the process of human interaction. Human beings and the environment are linked together by the process of interaction. The nurse is viewed as part of the client's environment. Environment is also addressed in King's view of social systems. Cultural, social, political, and economic forces that are characteristics of a specific social system may influence life and health. Social systems influence interactions between individuals, social relationships, and the setting of rules of behavior and modes of action taken.[20] Beliefs, attitudes, values, and customs are learned within social systems. Nurses can make alterations in the environment that are conducive to promoting health. "The moving forces in nursing are embedded in the dynamics of society in which the process of change alters the environment" (reference 20, p 11). Within the social environment, nursing can focus practice on the health needs of communities through the establishment of mutually set goals and the planning of community health programs.[15]

Health

The goal of nursing is to help individuals attain, maintain, and restore their health so they can function in their social roles.[20] *Health* is defined as the "dynamic life experiences of human beings which implies the continuous adjustment to stressors in the internal and external environment through optimum use of one's resources to achieve maximum potential for daily living" (reference 20, p 5). In this conceptual framework, health is viewed as a functional state and illness as an interference with the functional state. More specifically, King defines *illness* as "a deviation from normal, that is, an imbalance in a person's biological structure or in his psychological make-up, or a conflict in a person's social relationships" (reference 20, p 5). King recognizes the influence of culture on these definitions of health and illness.

Nursing

Nursing is defined as "a process of action, reaction, and interaction whereby nurse and client share information about their perceptions in the nursing situation," and as "a process of human interactions between nurse and client whereby each perceives the other and the situation; and through communication, they set goals, explore means and agree upon the means to achieve goals" (reference 20, pp 2, 141). A nursing situation is the immediate environment, spatial or temporal reality, in which the nurse and client establish a relationship to cope with the client's health status and help the client adjust to changes in activities of daily living should the situation demand adjustment. The quality of nurse–client interactions may have either a positive or negative impact on the promotion of health.[20] Nursing is practiced through the nursing process, and it is within the interpersonal system of nurse–client relationships that the nursing process is applied. The nursing process is a dynamic, ongoing interpersonal process (rather than simply a problem-solving process) in which the nurse and client are viewed as a system, with each affecting the behavior of the other and both being affected by factors within the situation.[20] Within the traditional steps of assessment, diagnosis, planning, implementation, and evaluation, the nurse assesses the perception, reaction, and action to set mutual goals. Mutually planning the means to achieve goals is accomplished through interaction, whereas the implementation and evaluation of goals occurs through nurse–client transactions.

THEORY OF GOAL ATTAINMENT: NURSING PROCESS

The theory of goal attainment describes the nature of nurse–client interactions that lead to the achievement of health-related goals. The theory provides a guide for nurses in establishing mutual goals based on the nurse's assessment of the client's concerns, perceptions, disturbances in health, and perceived problems. King[20] believes goal attainment results in outcomes that are measurable events in nursing situations.

The major concepts in the theory of goal attainment are interaction, perception, communication, transaction, self, role, stress, growth and development, time, and space. *Interaction* is a process of perception and communication between person and person, and person and environment, represented by verbal and nonverbal behaviors. *Perception* is each person's representation of a subjective world experience. *Communication* is a process whereby information is given from one person to another either directly in face-to-face meetings or indirectly through telephone, television, or the written word. *Transaction* is defined as observable behavior of human beings interacting with their environment that leads to goal attainment (reference 20, pp 145–147). King[20] describes *self* as a personal system synonymous with the terms *I, me,* and *person.* Self is a "unified, complex whole person who perceives, thinks, desires, imagines, decides, identifies goals and selects means to achieve them" (reference 20, p 26). *Role* is a set of behaviors expected of persons occupying a position in a social system; rules that define rights and obligations in a position; a relationship with one or more individuals interacting in specific situations for a purpose. *Stress* is defined by King as a dynamic state whereby a human being interacts with the environment to maintain balance for growth, development, and performance. *Growth and development* are defined as "continuous changes in individuals at the cellular, molecular and behavioral levels of activities" (reference 20, p 148). *Time* is a sequence of events moving onward to the future, a continuous flow of events in successive order that implies change, a past, and a future. *Space* is described as that element that "exists in all directions and is the same everywhere; a physical area called territory and is defined by the behavior of individuals occupying space; such as, gestures, postures and visible boundaries erected to mark off personal space" (reference 20, p 148).

Assessment occurs during the interaction between the nurse and client.[20] The nurse enters the relationship with special knowledge and skills, whereas the client brings knowledge of self and perception of the problems that are of concern. The nurse collects information about the client's level of growth and development, view of self, perception of current health status, communication patterns, role socialization, pattern of interaction with the environment, roles and life stressors, and perceptions of time and space. Data concerning activities of daily living; exercise and recreation; medication; nutrition; cultural factors; and physical,

emotional, and spiritual needs, all are important to the assessment process.[20] The client's age, sex, medical diagnosis, socioeconomic status, and culture influence the clients' perceptions of their health needs.

King has asserted that nursing diagnoses are compatible with the theory of goal attainment.[55] *Nursing diagnosis* is defined as a statement that "identifies the disturbances, problems or concerns about which the patient seeks help" (reference 20, p 177), which is synthesized using substantive knowledge of the concepts and their relationship within the personal, interpersonal, and social systems. Diagnoses are clinical judgments derived from mutually identified problems in the conceptual areas of interaction, perception, communication, transaction, role, stress, self, time, space and growth, and development. All these concepts have great relevance to clients with psychiatric mental health problems.

The next phase of transaction includes identifying and mutually setting goals. Information is shared, and mutual goals are explored. Clients are encouraged to participate, as much as possible, in making decisions about how the goals are to be met. Nursing orders are written that indicate the plan of care to be implemented by nursing personnel. Implementation is a continuation of nurse–client transactions and occurs through purposeful therapeutic interaction. Implementation within King's framework may include a broad range of nursing actions, including health teaching, counseling, physical care, carrying out delegated medical therapy, therapeutic communication, and coordinating resources. Communication theory and interpersonal theory are useful therapeutic theories that conceptually fit with King's open-systems framework.

Evaluation involves descriptions of the outcomes identified, as goals are attained. King[20] proposed a goal-oriented nursing record system (GONR) to facilitate the documentation of both process and outcome of nurse–client transactions. King suggests the GONR may be used as a quality assurance measure in measuring effectiveness of care and goal attainment. The GONR includes a data base, problem list, goal list, plan, and format for progress notes.

ROGERS' SCIENCE OF UNITARY HUMAN BEINGS

Martha Rogers' science of unitary human beings[11,13,24,42–47] offers nursing a view that is different from those of Peplau, Orem, Roy, or King. Rogers states that an "abstract system basic to nursing's science of unitary human beings is rooted in a progressive world view coordinate with current and emerging knowledge theories" (reference 46, p 183). Rogers' concepts of energy fields, open systems, wholeness, pattern, evolving diversity, and multidimensionality are supported by modern science.[23] In her organistic simultaneity world view, the nurse and client are integral within a field of conscious awareness that is beyond space and time.

They participate together in the unfolding of increasingly conscious participation in change. Table 4-2 illustrates the differences between the traditional Cartesian–Newtonian world view and the emerging organistic world view.

Human Beings–Environment

Rogers[46] identifies unitary human beings and their environment as the central focus of nursing. She defines *unitary human beings* (human field) as an irreducible, multidimensional energy field identified by pattern and manifesting characteristics that are specific to the whole and that cannot be predicted from knowledge of the parts.[46] *Environment* (environmental field) is defined as an irreducible, multidimensional energy field identified by pattern and integral with the human field.[46]

Rogers[42–47] identifies four building blocks as central to her conceptual model: energy fields, a universe of open systems, pattern, and multidimensionality.

Energy field is the fundamental unit of the living and nonliving. Fields are irreducible, and do not have parts. Energy is dynamic and in constant motion.[46] Special relativity theory has shown that all mass is a form of energy. Quantum field theory supports the notion that the universe is a set of infinite energy fields in mutual interaction with one another. Rogers identifies two energy fields, the environmental energy field and the human energy field.[43,45] Energy fields are open continuously and are infinite. Thus, the human and environmental energy fields are integral with one another, and there is a mutual continuous simultaneous flow of energy between persons and their environment.[45,47] The person and environment are inseparable and evolve together. In open systems, causality is invalid. Equilibrium, adaptation, homeostasis, and steady-state are contradicted.[45–47] Rather, open systems are characterized by growing diversity and creativity.

Pattern gives identity to human and environmental fields.[45] One perceives "manifestations of field pattern." All pattern evolves and emerges out of the human–environmental field mutual process. Observable patterns of human behavior, personality, thought, feelings, and movement are examples of unique, individual human–environmental field patterns. Pattern is a reflection of the whole.

All reality is postulated to be multidimensional. Rogers defines multidimensionality as a nonlinear domain without spatial or temporal attributes.[47] Modern science supports the notion that there is no linear time, no past, present, or future. There is no separation in space. Space–time spreads all over in an infinite now. The relative nature of change is explicated by the concept of multidimensionality. Multidimensionality is a difficult concept to comprehend from a three-dimensional perspective. Infinite energy fields are beyond the space constraints of the physical body and beyond the time constraints of the present. Human experiences of timelessness during meditative experiences or exercise provide glimpses of the reality described by multidimensionality.[9,16,23]

The three principles of homeodynamics integrate the major concepts and describe the nature and direction of change. The principle of integrality describes the inseparability of human beings from their environment, engaged in mutual process of energy exchange. The principle of resonancy describes the continuous change from lower- to higher-frequency wave patterns in the human and environmental fields. Change toward higher frequency refers to the acceleration in the rate of change. Evolution is accelerating. The principle of resonancy also includes the notion that human beings experience their environment as a resonating wave of complex symmetry. Rhythmic patterns of wave frequencies are manifested at all levels of the universe. The principle of helicy depicts the "continuous, innovative, unpredictable, increasing diversity of human and environmental field patterns characterized by non-repeating rhythmicities" (reference 47, p 8). Change is always in the direction of greater diversity and innovation because past experiences become preserved in the space–time structure and each experience further patterns the field. *Unpredictable* refers to the noncausal nature of change and the uncertainty inherent in the universe.

Manifestations of patterning emerge out of the human–environmental field process and are continuously innovative.[44] Movement and change are always in the direction of higher frequency and greater diversity. Manifestations of field patterning include diversity, rhythms, motions; the experience of time; sleep–wake and beyond-waking states; and pragmatic,

TABLE 4–2
Comparison between the prevailing world view and Rogers' emerging world view[3,23,42–47]

PREVAILING VIEW	ROGERS' VIEW
Cell theory	Field theory
Mechanistic	Organistic
Closed system: feedback	Open system: innovation
Human: homeostatic	Human being: homeodynamic
Human: biopsycho–social–spiritual parts	Human being: unitary patterns
Causality: single, multiple	Mutual process: pattern
Reductionism	Synthesis
Parts	Wholeness
Relationships	Interconnectiveness
Human–environment: dichotomous	Human being–environment: integral
Being	Becoming, unfolding
Dynamic equilibrium	Continuous, evolving diversity
Assessment	Pattern appraisal
Nursing diagnosis	Health pattern description
Nursing intervention	Mutual patterning
Disease	Well-being, meaning
Deficits	Strengths, actualizing potentials
Structure	Rhythm
Adaptation	Transcendence

imaginative, and visionary approaches to conscious participation in change. Human–environmental field assessment is organized according to the manifestations of human–environmental field process. Figure 4-6 integrates Rogers' four concepts, principles of homeodynamics, manifestations of patterning, and the emerging Rogerian practice methodology.

Health

Health is the dynamic well-being of the individual or group. The dynamic well-being is manifested through the human–environmental field process. Health and illness are expressions of the human–environmental field in the process of unfolding.[16] Health and illness are not dichotomous, rather they are viewed equally as expressions of the life process, and the meaning of the experience of health and illness is derived from an understanding of the life process in its totality. Health encompasses disease and nondisease, and both are re-

flections of the larger whole. In this context, health is a process of unfolding potentials. Health can be further described as the active participation in the life process by choosing and executing behaviors that lead to maximum fulfillment of a person's potential.[22]

Nursing

Rogers views nursing as a learned profession that is both a science and an art. The science of nursing is an "organized body of abstract knowledge arrived at by scientific research and logical analysis," whereas the art of nursing "is the imaginative and creative use of the knowledge in human service" (reference 46, p 182). The uniqueness of nursing lies in the phenomenon of concern, and the phenomenon of concern of nursing, Rogers believes, is unitary human beings and their environment. The irreducible nature of human beings as energy fields differentiates nursing from other

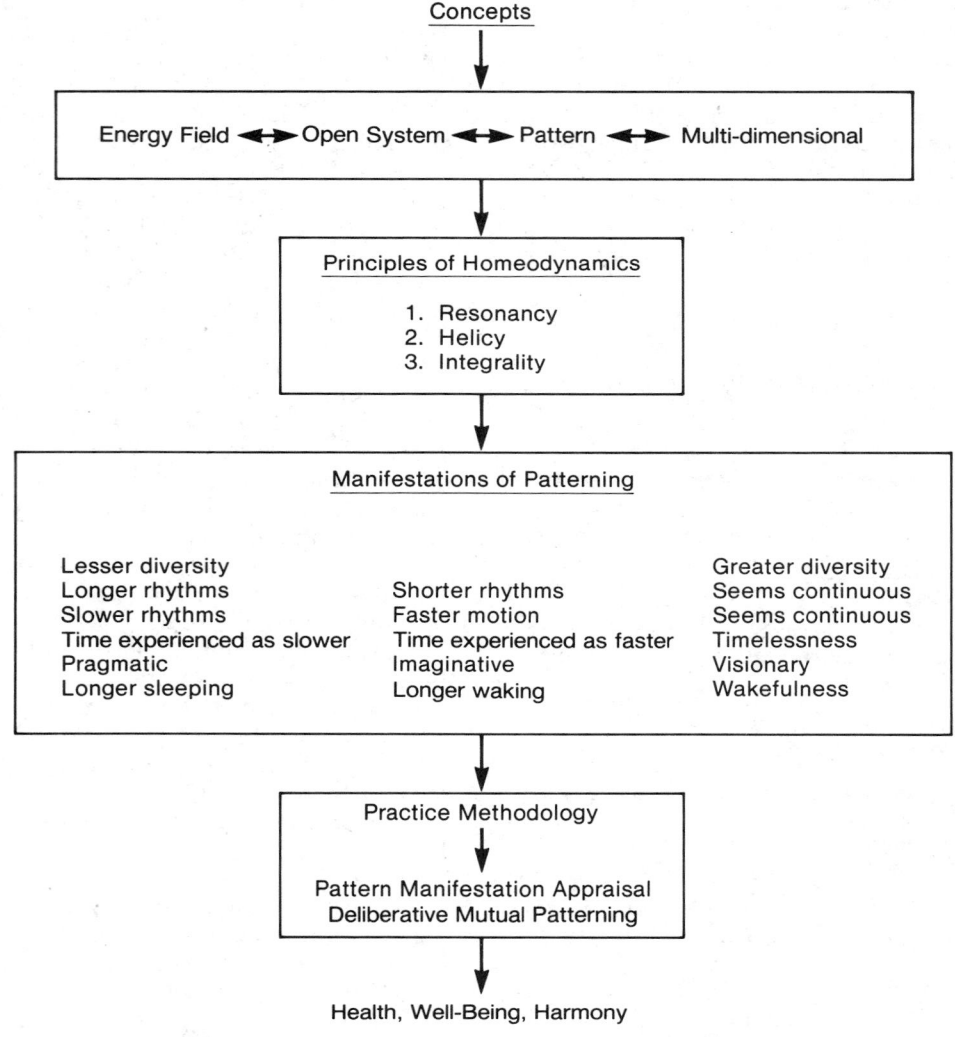

FIGURE 4–6. Rogers' science of unitary human beings.[3,42–47]

sciences.[45] The purpose of nursing is to help individuals and groups achieve maximum well-being.

Practice methodologies are evolving consistent with the philosophical beliefs inherent in Rogerian science. Nursing process and diagnosis are not consistent practice methodologies within Rogers' multidimensional view of the world. Barrett[3] has proposed a Rogerian practice methodology that is derived from the principles of homeodynamics. Barrett describes two phases: (1) pattern manifestation appraisal and (2) deliberative mutual patterning.[3] Pattern manifestation appraisal is the continuous process of identifying manifestations of the human–environmental field that is related to current health events. Deliberative mutual patterning is the continuous process whereby the nurse with the client patterns the environmental field to promote harmony to health related events. The client is integral to both the appraisal and patterning phases, which are nonlinear and not necessarily sequential.[3] All information about the human–environmental field mutual process is relevant to revealing the total pattern of the client. Data, however, are interpreted within a unitary perspective. For example, vital signs are reconceptualized as manifestations of field patterning that reflects the whole, rather than as indicators of the status and functioning of a particular organ system. Rogerian science also guides the nurse to focus on additional areas of pattern appraisal not evident in other nursing frameworks. Areas of pattern appraisal evolve from Rogers' manifestations of patterning and include the appraisal of the experience of time; sleep-wake and beyond-waking patterns; sense of rhythm; frequencies of light, color, and sound; pragmatic, imaginative, and visionary approaches to knowing participation in change; indicators of increasing diversity, faster rhythms, and creativity; sense of connectiveness to the environment; sense of wholeness and integrity; patterns of communication; and personal myth.[16,22,47] Box

---

BOX 4–2
Deliberate Mutual Patterning[23]

Guided imagery	Meditation modalities
Therapeutic touch	Color
Music	Light
Humor	Facilitating pattern recognition
Dialogue	Exploring meaning of experiences
Motion	Guided reminiscence

4-1 lists emergent health patterns that provide a focus of pattern appraisals.

Noninvasive appraisal and patterning techniques, such as therapeutic touch and guided imagery, are also relevant within the science of unitary human beings. Ference's Human Field Motion Tool,[12] Barrett's Power as Knowing Participation in Change Tool,[2] and Paletta's Temporal Experience Scales[30] are pattern appraisal tools developed specifically within this conceptual system. The use of imagery, touch, sound, light, color, motion, dialogue, humor, and meditative modalities are energy forms that can be designed creatively by the nurse to pattern the field toward harmony and well-being. Box 4-2 identifies deliberate mutual pattern strategies.

Implications for Psychiatric Nursing Practice

Practicing from a Rogerian perspective means focusing on unitary human beings as an irreducible whole, different from and more than the sum of parts. This is a generally accepted principle in nursing, but is difficult to articulate. Although other frameworks have more clearly distinct biopsychosocial–spiritual and cultural aspects, unitary human beings have no parts. Rather, the focus of practice from a Rogerian perspective is on pattern. Pattern is a reflection of the whole person–environmental mutual process. Mental health nurses focus on unitary patterns, rather than biological, social, psychological, spiritual, or cultural parts of clients. The person–environment is viewed as an inseparable unity. The simultaneous mutual process between the person and environment means that a search for causal relationships and diagnostic statements are invalid. Rather, the focus is on discovering the pattern and mutually exploring the meaning of the pattern. In addition to their health-promotion aspects, other frameworks allow diagnoses and identification of deficits, whereas the emphasis in the Rogerian conceptual system is on strengths and the health potentials of human beings. Rather than formulating nursing diagnoses, the nurse writes a pattern description or profile, which may be a single word, short phrase, profile, listing, or short narrative that captures the essence of the human–environmental mutual process.

BOX 4–1
Pattern Manifestation Appraisal[4,12,16,22,23]

The experience of time: temporal experience
Sleep–wake and beyond-waking patterns
Sense of rhythm
Frequencies of light, color, and sound
Pragmatic, visionary approaches to knowing participation in change
Indicators of increasing diversity
Faster rhythms, creativity
Sense of connectiveness to environment
Sense of wholeness and integrity
Personal myth
Power
Human field motion
Near death experiences
Multiple manifestations
Pain–comfort cycles

In terms of evaluating the person, the nurse must be aware that the experience of time is relative and unique for each individual. Time pressure underlies patterns of anxiety.[10] Psychotic experiences involve alterations in time perception. Furthermore, knowledge of a person's hopes and dreams is as relevant as their past patterns because each person is a synthesis of their past and future all at once, living in a relative present. Delusions and hallucinations are viewed as manifestations of a multidimensional reality, the meaning of which needs uncovering. Change is viewed as always being positive. Even illness may have an integrative, transformational evolutionary potential.

The nurse practicing from a Rogerian perspective views clients as equals. Nurses are environmental energy fields, integral and in mutual process with those receiving nursing care. Nurses and clients participate together in a mutual process, patterning each other in a process of change. The focus of care is toward the mobilization of health potentials, empowering the client's ability to participate knowingly in change, enabling self-healing potentials, facilitating the recognition of rhythmic patterns, and the balancing, harmonizing, and synchronizing of person–environment rhythms. The nurse uses nondirective approaches in dialogue, providing choices and options to enable clients to choose knowingly. Humanistic psychologies, psychosynthesis, transpersonal psychology, and Gestalt psychology are more compatible approaches within the Rogerian conceptual system, whereas psychoanalytic,

Research Highlights[6,7]

Pleasant guided imagery is an independent nursing intervention designed for the purpose of promoting field integrity, harmony, wholeness, and well-being. Often persons experiencing pleasant guided imagery report feelings of time standing still or timelessness; moving through space or motion; floating and weightlessness; being beyond everyday experience or transcendence; expansion outward or boundarylessness; and increased imagination. Presently there are no empirical studies investigating the subjective experience of pleasant guided imagery. Thus, there is little understanding of the subjective feelings experienced during pleasant guided imagery, and there are no theoretical interpretations of the subjective feelings that would guide future developments concerning the usefulness of pleasant guided imagery as a nursing intervention.

The purpose of the study was to conceptualize and investigate the experience of pleasant guided imagery within Martha Rogers' science of unitary human beings as a means to develop an understanding of the subjective experience of pleasant guided imagery. Rogers' science of unitary human beings emphasizes human feelings as manifestations of the environmental and human field mutual process. According to Rogers' principle of resonancy, the human and environmental fields are identified by pattern, perceived as a mosaic of waves, and manifesting continuous changes from lower- to higher-frequency wave patterns in human and environmental fields. Within Rogers' conceptual system, movement toward faster motion, timelessness, beyond waking, more diversity, and toward being visionary, can reflect a movement toward a higher wave frequency pattern. The Human Field Motion Test is a measure of the relative frequency of the wave frequency pattern of the human energy field. Because the subjective feelings reported during pleasant guided imagery seem synchronous with Rogers' manifestations of patterning, this study postulated that pleasant guided imagery is a multidimensional environmental field energy pattern, integral with the human field, with a potential to pattern the human field toward a high-frequency wave pattern. The patterning of the energy field toward a higher-frequency wave pattern accelerates unitary human development and motion toward wholeness, harmony, and health.

A pretest and posttest control group design consisting of 60 volunteer participants, who were health care employees from a large community hospital, was used to test two hypotheses derived from Rogers' principle of resonancy: (1) participants experiencing an 11-minute pleasant guided imagery tape will have significantly lower posttest scores on the Time Metaphor Test (representing a movement toward a perception of timelessness, a higher-frequency wave pattern) than participants in the control group who experienced an 11-minute educational tape; (2) participants experiencing pleasant guided imagery will have significantly higher posttest scores on the Human Field Motion Test (representing a higher-frequency wave pattern of the human energy field) compared with participants in the control group.

A repeated measures ANOVA yielded a significant Treatment X Trials interaction effect ($F = 4.358$, $df = 1,118$, $p > 0.05$) supporting hypothesis 1. Hypothesis 2 was not supported. However, participants experiencing pleasant guided imagery had higher scores on those scales on the Human Field Motion Tool, which most closely reflected Rogers' manifestations of patterning (increased imagination, more visionary, more boundaryless, and more transcendent). Given the support of hypothesis 1 and the movement toward higher human field motion on the transcendent, visionary, and boundarylessness scales on the Human Field Motion Tool, Rogers' science of unitary human beings may provide an initial tentative theoretical interpretation of the subjective feelings of motion, timelessness, boundarylessness, transcendence, and increased imagination experienced during pleasant guided imagery as a patterning of the human field toward a higher-frequency wave pattern. Within Rogers' nursing science, a higher-frequency wave pattern facilitates actualization of the human field potential and unitary human development, which facilitates transcendence beyond three-dimensional constraints, such as time and space, that impede motion toward wholeness, harmony, and well-being. Further evaluation of the Human Field Motion Tool is needed.

behavioral, and cognitive approaches are not consistent with a unitary perspective of human beings.

However, models for practice evolving from Rogerian science are emerging. For example, Barrett[4] has developed a nursing theory of power derived from Rogers' science of unitary human beings. *Power* is defined as the capacity to participate knowingly in the nature of change characterizing the continuous patterning of the human and environmental fields as manifested by awareness, choices, freedom to act intentionally, and involvement in creating changes.[4] Barrett has suggested that the power theory may be particularly useful in working with clients who have issues of hopelessness with suicidal ideation, drug and alcohol dependence, grief and loss, self-esteem issues, marital discord, career conflicts, and other major life-style changes or phase-of-life manifestations.[4]

The Power as Knowing Participation Tool is used as an initial appraisal of the client's power pattern. Teaching then begins by describing the definition of power as knowingly participating in change. Deliberate mutual patterning strategies can then be designed to increase one's awareness of choices and empower one to feel more free and involved in making desired changes in one's life. The tool can be used to evaluate the changing power-patterning profile as the client participates in nursing care.

Compton has reconceptualized drug addiction within a Rogerian perspective.[8] Drug addiction is viewed as a means to increase one's awareness of the multidimensional nature of reality. Thus, meditation, imagery, and other high-frequency, multidimensional experiences are proposed as therapies to increase field frequency without the use of drugs.[8]

SUMMARY

Nursing science includes a number of conceptual frameworks, and is the foundation of nursing practice. Conceptual frameworks are designed to guide nursing practice and are useful to the practicing psychiatric mental health nurse. Knowledge of multiple frameworks is encouraged; each framework provides a unique perspective of human beings, environment, health, and nursing. Five nurse theorists—Peplau, Orem, Roy, King, and Rogers—were described. Peplau's central theme focuses on the nurse–patient relationship. Orem's framework is based on the premise that a relationship exists between self-care deficits and deliberate self-care action, resulting in independent action. Roy's framework utilizes the concepts of input, output, control processes, and feedback in describing the notion of adaptation. King's framework is composed of three dynamic interacting open systems: personal, interpersonal, and social. Rogers' science of unitary human beings centers on human environmental fields and irreducible wholes. Each of these conceptual frameworks is useful in guiding psychiatric mental health nursing practice.

References

1. Andrews H, Roy C. Essentials of the Roy adaptation model. Norwalk, CT: Appleton-Century-Crofts; 1986.
2. Barrett EAM. An empirical investigation of Rogers' principle of helicy: the relationship of human field complexity, human field motion, and power. New York: New York University; 1983. Dissertation.
3. Barrett EAM. Using Rogers' science of unitary human beings in nursing practice. Nurs Sci Q. 1988;1(2):50–51.
4. Barrett EAM. A nursing theory of power for nursing practice: derivation from Rogers' paradigm. In: Riehl-Sisca J, ed. Conceptual models for nursing practice. 3rd ed., Norwalk, CT: Appleton & Lange; 1989.
5. von Bertalanfy L. General system theory. New York: George Braziller; 1968.
6. Butcher HK. Repatterning of time experience and human field motion during the experience of pleasant guided imagery: an experimental investigation within Rogers' science of unitary human beings. Toronto: University of Toronto; 1986. Thesis.
7. Butcher HK, Parker NJ. Guided imagery within Rogers' science of unitary human beings: an experimental study. Nurs Sci Q. 1988;1(3):103–110.
8. Compton MA. A Rogerian view of drug abuse: implications for nursing. Nurs Sci Q. 1989;2(2):98–105.
9. Cowling WR. The relationship of mystical experience, differentiation, and creativity in college students. In: Malinski VM, ed. Explorations on Martha Rogers' science of unitary human beings. Norwalk, CT: Appleton-Century-Crofts; 1986.
10. Dossy L. Space, time, and medicine. Boulder, CO: Shambhala; 1982.
11. Fawcett J. Conceptual models of nursing. 2nd ed. Philadelphia: FA Davis; 1989.
12. Ference HM. The relationship of time experience, creativity traits, differentiation and human field motion: an empirical investigation of Rogers' correlates of synergistic human development. New York: New York University; 1979. Dissertation.
13. Fitzpatrick J, Whall A. Conceptual models of nursing: analysis and applications. Bowie, MD: Brady; 1983.
14. Forchuk C, Brown B. Establishing a nurse–client relationship. J Psychosoc Nurs Ment Health Serv. 1989;27(2):30–38.
15. Gulitz EA, King IM. King's general systems model: application to curriculum development. Nurs Sci Q. 1988;1(3):128–132.
16. Hanchett ES. Nursing frameworks and community as client: bridging the gap. Norwalk, CT: Appleton & Lange; 1988.
17. Helson H. Adaptation level theory. New York: Harper & Row; 1964.
18. Henderson V. The nature of nursing: a definition and its implications for practice, research and education. New York: Macmillan; 1966.
19. King IM. Toward a theory of nursing: general concepts of human behavior. New York: John Wiley & Sons; 1971.
20. King IM. A theory for nursing: systems, concepts, process. New York: John Wiley & Sons; 1981.
21. King IM. King's general systems framework and theory. In: Riehl-Sisca J, ed. Conceptual models for nursing practice. 3rd ed. Norwalk, CT: Appleton & Lange; 1989.
22. Madrid M, Winstead-Fry P. Rogers' conceptual model. In: Winstead-Fry P, ed. Case studies in nursing theory. New York: National League for Nursing, 1986:73–102.
23. Malinski VM. Explorations on Martha Rogers' science of unitary human beings. Norwalk, CT: Appleton-Century-Crofts; 1986.

24. Marriner A. Nursing theorists and their work. St. Louis: CV Mosby; 1986.

25. Nursing Development Conference Group. Concept formalization of nursing process. 2nd ed. Boston: Little, Brown & Co; 1979.

26. Orem DE. Nursing: concepts of practice. New York: McGraw-Hill; 1971.

27. Orem DE. Nursing: concepts of practice. 2nd ed. New York: McGraw-Hill; 1980.

28. Orem DE. Nursing: concepts of practice. 3rd ed. New York: McGraw-Hill; 1985.

29. Orlando IJ. The dynamic nurse–patient relationship. New York: GP Putnam's Sons; 1961.

30. Paletta JL. The relationship of temporal experience to human time. New York: New York University; 1988. Dissertation.

31. Peplau HE. Interpersonal relations in nursing. New York: GP Putnam's Sons; 1952.

32. Peplau HE. Talking with patients. Am J Nurs. 1960;60:964–967.

33. Peplau HE. The crux of psychiatric nursing. Am J Nurs. 1962;62:50–54.

34. Peplau HE. Anxiety. In: Burd SF, Marshall MA, eds. Some clinical approaches to psychiatric nursing. London: Macmillan; 1971.

35. Peplau HE. Process and concept of learning. In: Burd SF, Marshall MA, eds. Some clinical approaches to psychiatric nursing. London: Macmillan; 1971.

36. Peplau HE. Psychiatric nursing: role of nurses and psychiatric nurses. Int Nurs Rev. 1978;25:41–47.

37. Peplau HE. The psychotherapy of Hildegard E. Peplau. Field WE, ed. New Braunfels, TX: PSF Productions; 1979.

38. Peplau HE. Nurse–patient relationships. Presented at Lakehead Psychiatric Hospital; April 27, 1984; Thunder Bay, Ontario, Canada.

39. Rambo B. Adaptation nursing: assessment and intervention. Philadelphia: WB Saunders; 1984.

40. Riehl-Sisca J. Orem's general theory of nursing: an interpretation. In: Riehl-Sisca J, ed. Conceptual models for nursing practice. 3rd ed. Norwalk, CT: Appleton & Lange; 1989.

41. Robitaille-Tremblay M. A data collection tool for the psychiatric nurse. Can Nurse. 1984;80(7):26–27.

42. Rogers ME. An introduction to the theoretical basis of nursing. Philadelphia: FA Davis; 1970.

43. Rogers ME. Nursing: a science of unitary man. In: Riehl JP, Roy C, eds. Conceptual models for nursing practice. 2nd ed. New York: Appleton-Century-Crofts; 1980:329–337.

44. Rogers ME. Science of unitary human beings: a paradigm for nursing. In: Clements IW, Roberts FB, eds. Family health: a theoretical approach to nursing care. New York: John Wiley & Sons; 1983.

45. Rogers ME. Science of unitary human beings. In: Malinksi VM, ed. Explorations on Martha Rogers' science of unitary human beings. Norwalk, CT: Appleton-Century-Crofts; 1986.

46. Rogers ME. Nursing: a science of unitary human beings. In: Riehl-Sisca J, ed. Conceptual models for nursing practice. Norwalk, CT: Appleton & Lange; 1989.

47. Rogers ME. Nursing: Science of unitary, irreducible human beings: Update 1990. In: Barrett EAM, ed. Vision of Rogers' science-based nursing. New York: National League for Nursing; 1990.

48. Roy C. Adaptation: a conceptual framework for nursing. Nurs Outlook. 1970;18(3):42–45.

49. Roy C. Explication of the philosophical assumptions of the Roy adaptation model. Nurs Sci Q. 1988;1(1):26–34.

50. Roy C. Introduction to nursing: an adaptation model. Englewood Cliffs, NJ: Prentice-Hall; 1976.

51. Roy C. Introduction to nursing; an adaptation model. 2nd ed. Englewood Cliffs, NJ: Prentice-Hall; 1984.

52. Roy C. Roy's adaptation model. In: Parse RR, ed. Nursing science: major paradigms, theories and critiques. Philadelphia: WB Saunders; 1987.

53. Roy C, Roberts SL. Theory construction in nursing: an adaptation model. Englewood Cliffs, NJ: Prentice-Hall; 1981.

54. Schmidt CS. Withdrawal behavior of schizophrenics: application to Roy's model. J Psychosoc Nurs. 1981;19(11):26–33.

55. Smith MJ. Perspectives in nursing science. Nurs Sci Q. 1988;1(2):80–85.

56. Taylor SG. Nursing theory and nursing process: Orem's theory in practice. Nurs Sci Q. 1988;1(3):111–119.

57. Tedrow M. Interdependence: theory and development. In: Roy C, ed. Introduction to nursing: an adaptive model. Englewood Cliffs, NJ: Prentice-Hall; 1984.

5

Helen Palisin

Developmental and Psychological Theories

OBJECTIVES

After reading this chapter, the reader will be able to:

1. *Identify the central psychic mechanism that is the foundation for Freud's theory*
2. *Describe the psychic structures proposed by Freud*
3. *Describe the psychosexual stages of development described by Freud*
4. *Identify the psychic structure involved in Erikson's theory of life cycles*
5. *Describe the tasks in Erikson's eight stages of development*
6. *Discuss the relation of anxiety to the self-system in Sullivan's theory*
7. *Identify the role of the self-system in the six eras of development described by Sullivan*
8. *Describe the three major stages in Piaget's theory*
9. *Describe the three central concepts in Piaget's theory of intellectual development*
10. *Describe Adler's view of how the perception of inferiority influences development*
11. *Explain the factors in Horney's theory that contribute to the development of self-image and character*
12. *Discuss the behaviorist approach to documenting developmental processes*
13. *Describe the philosophy that is central to the existentialists' position*
14. *Discuss the three modes of being-in-the-world in the existentialist philosophy*
15. *Identify Stern's domains of the development of the self*
16. *Identify the rationale for treatment with selected theories.*

INTRODUCTION

Many theories have emerged in the last century that have had a significant impact on beliefs about how humans develop. Several of these theories continue to influence thought, practice, and research, providing insights into the organization of behavior and hypotheses about the development of symptoms and behavioral disorders. The theorists to be discussed in this chapter focus on different parts of the developmental process. For instance, Freud emphasized the sexual aspect; Erikson, the societal; Sullivan, the interpersonal; Piaget, Adler, and Horney, the cognitive; Skinner, the behavioral; and the existentialists, the spiritual.

PSYCHOSEXUAL THEORY— SIGMUND FREUD

Sigmund Freud (1856–1939) started his career as a neurologist and later developed the method of *free association*. Through this technique, he became aware that there was a great deal of psychic energy that went into preventing some feelings from coming into consciousness. He identified this energy as *repression* and considered the concept to be the foundation of his theory. Over time, Freud noticed that the content being repressed was related to early sexual experiences. This observation led him to theorize that development was based on a sexual drive expressing itself as the organism matured; thus, he viewed human development in terms of psychosexual stages.[7-10]

As infants begin their existence outside the uterus, they are flooded with new stimuli and cellular excitation, electrolyte and physicochemical changes occur, energy is generated, and tensions develop. Freud believed the source of an instinct is this process of excitation within an organ.[11] In this way, the organs of the body give rise to instincts whose aims are related to the functions of those organs. These instincts and the energy associated with them fill the psychical structure Freud called the *id*.

Freud theorized that no conflict exists within the id itself—all functions exist side by side, simply fulfilling their aims. However, when the newborn has to obtain substances from the environment to survive, aims are met by initiating activity—by breathing, crying, kicking, or sucking. At this interface between internal and external reality, one portion of the id was thought to be modified and differentiated into the *ego*. Freud described the ego as an outer layer or external cortex of the id. Its function is to deal with the conflicts between the internal and external worlds and mediate between what the organism needed and what was possible. Its goal is unity and synthesis.

Freud was continually revising his theory and eventually came to believe that a sexual instinct was the principal force in development. He labeled the energy attached to it *libido*. It is the tracking of this instinct— its aims, objects, repressions, and mechanisms of defense to keep it from awareness—that is unique to Freud's theory. He identified five psychosexual or libidinal stages of development: *oral, anal, phallic, latency,* and *genital*. These stages are more easily understood if they are seen as a progression of the physical development of the newborn.

Oral Stage. It is through the structures in the oral region that the organism exchanges air, takes in nutrients, and has contact with the mother's body. Through experience, the infant learns to associate the satisfaction of its needs with that area of the body. Tension reduction occurring simultaneously with pleasurable sensations is the forerunner of the later mature sexual pattern. Freud considered these oral experiences the beginning of sexuality and also as the foundation for relations with objects and people in the environment. As growth continues, the muscles of the oral area become sophisticated, with activities such as chewing, drinking, facial expressions, and verbalizations coming under voluntary control.

Anal Stage. The sequence of maturation continues, with one area of the body maturing before the next emerges into awareness. By the end of the first year, the anal zone becomes a source of interest to both the infant and the parents. The infant develops an awareness of a full rectum and, later, control over the innate urges. Freud believed that the full bowel as a stimulating mass on a sexually sensitive mucous membrane is the forerunner of another organ that will develop later —the penis.[11] Along with the pleasurable sensations, there is the production of feces, which can be something of a "gift" to the parents and social environment or can be stubbornly withheld. In this way, the anal area and its activities become a means of interacting with the environment, much as the oral region did earlier.

Phallic (Oedipal) Stage. Eventually, the child discovers that the perineal area really has two separate zones that provide different pleasurable sensations and satisfactions. Freud believed this was the first emergence of sexuality in an observable form. This phallic stage, which begins around 2 or 3 years of age, involves the awareness of the genitals and a recognition that they are associated with different roles and relationships in the family. Freud used the Greek myth of Oedipus Rex, who married his mother, to discuss the conflicts and prohibitions the child encounters during this stage. The society's values about incestuous thoughts and behaviors are transmitted to the child via the family—primarily by the father or father surrogate. The ego has by now taken charge of mediating between bodily needs, wishes, thoughts, and reality, and Freud believed the ego's resolution of this Oedipal conflict gave rise to a third psychic structure—the *superego*. The superego contains the moral teachings and values of the family and society and ultimately becomes the conscience (Fig. 5-1).

Latency Stage. The Oedipal period is followed by the stage of latency, which occurs when the child is about 6 years old. By this time, which usually coincides with

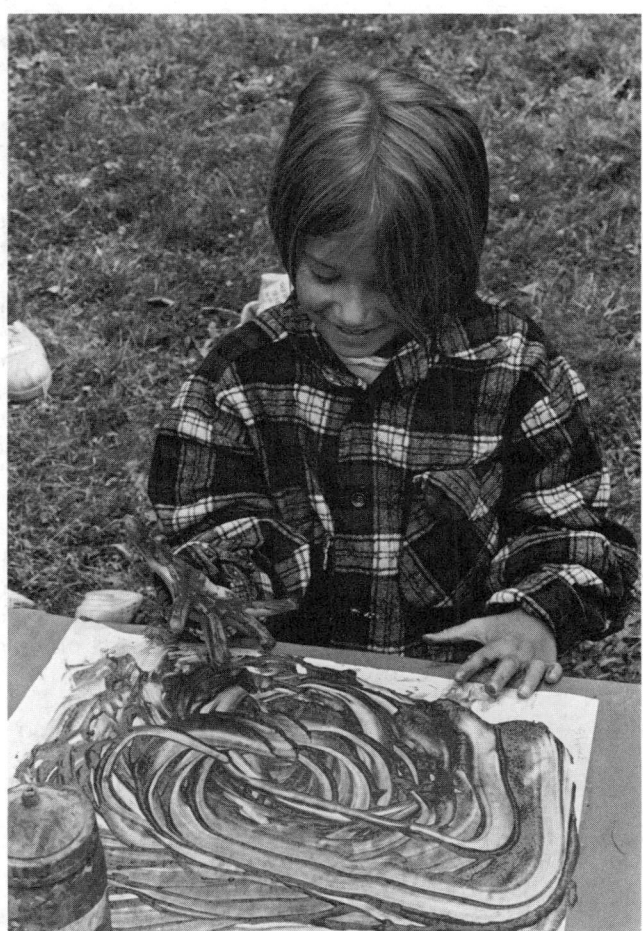

FIGURE 5–2. Art offers a creative outlet and respite from other pressure in a child's life. (Courtesy of Tony Schiro)

entry into school, the child has learned to control his or her energies and drives in socially acceptable ways. During the next several years, until the beginning of adolescence, the sexual drives of the previous period are channeled or "sublimated" into other activities such as school work and group interests. Also, the basic pattern of relating to people and objects in the environment that will characterize adult relationships is established (Fig. 5-2).

Genital Stage. Adolescence marks the beginning of the final psychosexual stage of genitality. It is the period when the sexual drive reemerges but becomes associated with fully maturing genitals and seeks its expression outside the family. One important task during this stage is for the young adult to establish psychological freedom from the parents and family. Healthy development was seen as resulting from successful integration of id, ego, and superego in dealing with the sexual drive. The ego must learn to deal with the libido of the id, the external world, and the evaluation of the superego. By the end of adolescence, the individual is transformed from a pleasure-seeking infant into a socialized adult. The sexual impulses of infancy become

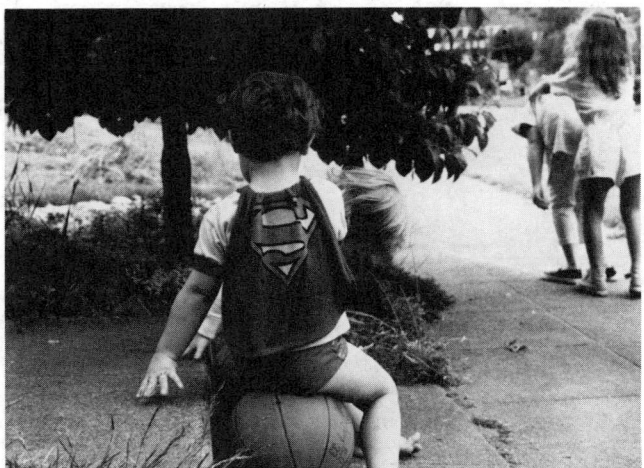

FIGURE 5–1. Unstructured play allows children to express themselves in imaginative ways. Note the preschool boy's selection of symbols associated with males in this culture. (Courtesy of Helen Palisin)

fused and synthesized with the genital impulses of the adult.

Summary. Currently, there remains controversy about the role of sexual instinct as an organizing force.[16] However, it would be a mistake to discard Freud's other contributions, such as the concept of repression; the structures of id, ego, and superego; and the technique of free association.

Perhaps Freud's greatest contribution came in emphasizing the interaction of physiological and mental activities at a time when the prevailing philosophy was a dualism of mind and body. He believed all mental and physical responses first occurred outside of awareness—in the *unconscious*. The responses are available to consciousness unless they are repressed because the content is unacceptable for some reason. When the energy attached to an instinct is barred from consciousness, it seeks discharge through other routes and may result in symptoms if its true content is not acknowledged. Therapy consists of expanding the field of consciousness to acknowledge the thoughts or feelings and to allow the energy to be associated with its original aim. This is done through free association and interpretation of dreams. Thereafter, a fully conscious decision can be made by the individual about how to respond to the information.

Whatever the fate of his theory, Freud was responsible for stimulating much interest and scientific inquiry into human development. His work influenced most of the theorists reviewed in the following sections.

LIFE CYCLE THEORY—ERIK ERIKSON

Erik Erikson (1902–   ), a child analyst, accepted Freud's theory of sexuality but seemed less certain that it and the libido were the prime organizing principle of the organism's development. His emphasis was on the ego qualities and strength that emerge from critical periods during the life cycle.[4]

Erikson believed there are crises throughout the life cycle between the individual's needs and society's expectations. The task of the ego is to resolve these crises at each stage of development. The eight stages are: *trust vs mistrust, autonomy vs shame, initiative vs guilt, industry vs inferiority, identity vs role confusion, intimacy vs isolation, generativity vs stagnation,* and *ego integrity vs despair.* Erikson cautioned that the stages are not absolute, clearly polarized achievements but rather processes that continue to unfold as development progresses.[4]

Trust–Mistrust. Trust develops from the consistency, continuity, and sameness of experiences associated with people and objects in the environment. The confidence that comes from having needs met also results in a sense of confidence about the ability to obtain what is needed. Erikson described it as a sense of being "all right" (reference 4, p 249), a sense that the world is safe and that others can be relied on. He noted that one of the cultural institutions that reinforces this idea is organized religion: in most religions, there is some ideal of a Provider who will dispense benefits, as well as a sense of faith in the efficacy of one's strivings and the kindness of the powers of the universe. In contrast, mistrust comes from a lack of conviction about the meaning of parental behavior and leads to a feeling of having been deprived or abandoned in some way (Fig. 5-3).

Autonomy–Shame. The physical growth and maturation of muscles sets the stage for two social responses—holding on and letting go. In this second stage, toddlers' feelings of autonomy about their anal activities and being able to stand on their own two feet contrasts with feeling shame or doubt about these functions and abilities. During this time, children need the experience of free choices, of testing the environment and learning about the people and objects in it and how they relate to the self. The experiencing and testing can lead to a sense of law and order as well as a sense of justice. Shame comes from a self-consciousness about one's bodily functions and doubt about one's abilities and relationships. Erikson believes that shame can lead to the extremes of compulsion neuroses or to the opposite—shamelessness. Similarly, doubts about the self or others may be expressed in paranoic fears and beliefs.

Initiative–Guilt. Erikson's third stage of initiative vs guilt corresponds to Freud's phallic phase, but Erikson added another dimension of understanding to this period. The child develops a combination of increasing interest in the environment with curiosity about the differences between the sexes. As a result, the child

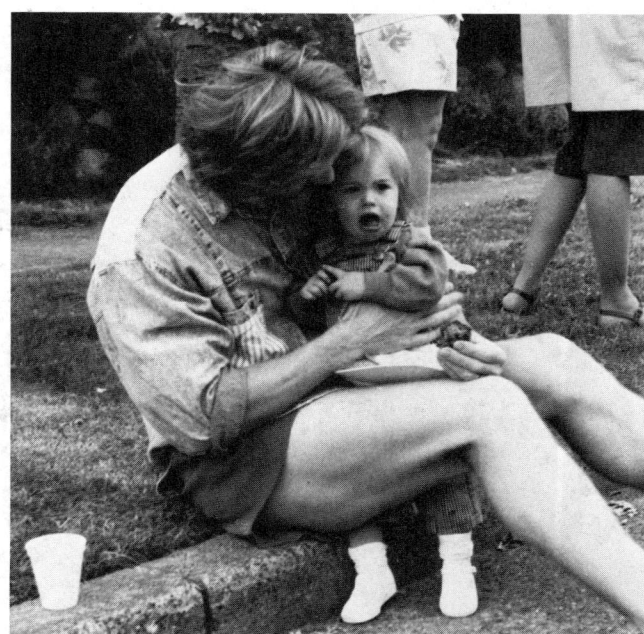

FIGURE 5–3. Trust develops when support from others in the environment is available when needed. (Courtesy of Helen Palisin)

attempts to take on the role of the parent of the same sex. The sexual behaviors of the child are merely imitation of adult behaviors and similar to earlier imitations such as eating with utensils, toileting, and speech. However, in contrast to other imitations and initiatives, the emulation of sexual roles may cause parental anxiety and responses that lead to feelings of guilt in the child.

Industry–Inferiority. The school years bring the possibility of success, of being an industrious and competent child who can function outside the family in a productive way. This age is characterized by the child's willingness to be enthusiastically involved in productive situations in the home, school, or neighborhood. Feelings of inadequacy occur if the child is unable to accomplish the tasks or to acquire the skills to do so. The possibility of being a competent worker and potential provider and of obtaining recognition for producing things is important to the child at this age. Feelings of inferiority about one's ability may lead to a reliance on work and technology in a thoughtless and conformist way. Erikson noted that in all cultures, children receive some systematic instruction in the technology of that culture, whether it is in the field, jungle, or classroom (Fig. 5-4).

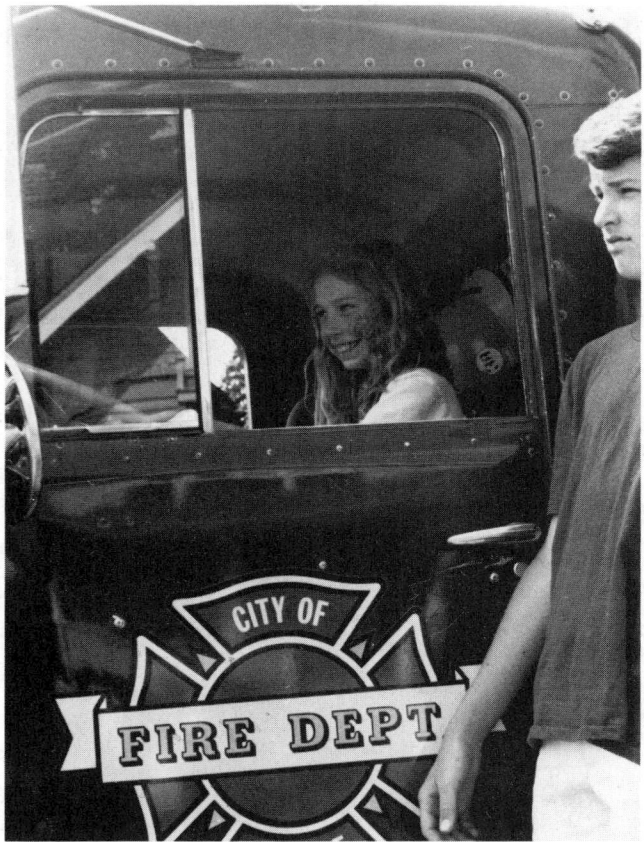

FIGURE 5–4. This 12-year-old enjoys the opportunity to imagine herself in a responsible adult role in society. (Courtesy of Helen Palisin)

Identity–Role Confusion. The fifth stage, identity vs role confusion, is the time of puberty, when the maturing person must deal with new physiology and stimuli and reevaluate roles and images. Erikson thought that a significant source of role confusion came from the concerns about the future and having an occupational identity about what one is to become. It is a time of concerns about how to connect skills, roles, and ideals with reality. Erikson noted that the long conversations typical of adolescent love are efforts to sort out one's image by filtering it through another person. There also are concerns about sexual identity and overdependence on and independence from others. The confusions of this period may be expressed through delinquency, overidentification with heroes, and the apparent simplicity found in cliques, stereotypes, and authoritarian regimes.

Intimacy–Isolation. In the young adult, both the body and ego are mature enough to seek physical intimacy with another person. Ideally, the expression of genitality of this period is in a spirit of mutual respect and emotional intimacy rather than the identity-seeking sexual strivings that precede this stage. Isolation occurs as a result of distancing oneself from close affiliations, friendships, and sexual unions, as well as avoiding such intimacies as inspirational experiences or the intuitions from the recesses of the self.[4] Erikson observed that just being in a relationship did not ensure intimacy if there was no mutuality and that isolation could be experienced even in marital relationships if respect and empathy were absent. He described such situations as isolation by mutual consent of the partners to protect themselves from facing the next critical task of the life cycle—generativity.

Generativity–Stagnation. The seventh stage, generativity vs stagnation, is the establishment and guidance of the next generation. The notion of generativity goes beyond actual childbearing to encompass being productive and creative in one's life and work. It involves an expansion of ego interests, in contrast to a sense of stagnation and personal limitations or emotional impoverishment. Generativity can also exist in religious communities or other commitments where procreation has been renounced. In these situations, generativity transcends its usual form to express itself through caring and charity for the creatures of the world.

Ego Integrity–Despair. The last stage, ego integrity vs despair, has as its foundation the preceding seven stages. Although Erikson had no clear definition for ego integrity, he described it as a transcendance of all that has gone before, integrated in a new and meaningful way. It involves love, self-acceptance, new relationships with one's parents, and a sense of dignity about one's own lifestyle. The result is an emotional integration and a sense of spirituality and world order. Despair, on the other hand, is a dissatisfaction with one's life, a fear of death, and a sense that time is too short to begin things anew (Fig. 5-5).

Summary. Erikson emphasized that each step is part of the foundation for the next one and thus is essential to it. In a similar way, the resolution at each step enlarges the area of accumulated successful experiences. The length of time allowed at any stage is determined by the culture in which the individual lives. Resolution of a stage results in a new ego quality that helps the individual integrate with the social structure of the culture. The long, slow childhood and dependence on parental figures can contribute to basic fears and anxieties whose residues persist into adulthood. When these problems are aggravated by unresolved issues of the life cycle, symptoms develop. Treatment is through the psychoanalytic techniques for adults and play therapy for children.

Erikson recognized that his stages were fairly global and lacked details about terminology and methodology —which makes research difficult. His emphasis on cultural expectations and the ego's tasks in meeting those expectations provides a useful complement to Freud's theory of sexual stages. Erikson's purpose was to offer some guidelines for comparison with physical and cognitive stages of development.

INTERPERSONAL THEORY— HARRY STACK SULLIVAN

Harry Stack Sullivan (1892–1949), originally trained in psychoanalysis, thought the principal factor in development was what the organism experienced during its interactions with the human environment.[25,26] In his view, these experiences occur in three modes: *prototaxic*, *parataxic*, and *syntaxic*. Prototaxic experiences occur at the physicochemical and sensory levels and are beyond recall. In the parataxic mode, the infant recognizes different events and generalizes from them to interpret patterns of the experiences. The syntaxic mode comes with communication through gestures or speech and permits validation of the private experiences.

Sullivan believed the child learns about itself through experiences while being cared for by another and that these experiences are the basis for the interpersonal process. He described the influence of this process in terms of eras rather than age-related stages. These eras are infancy, childhood, juvenile, preadolescence, early adolescence, and late adolescence.

Infancy Era. During infancy, interactions between needs and their satisfaction set up patterns of energy transformations. These occur in "zones" of interaction such as the oral zone and the anal zone. But infants experience their bodily needs and the emotional state of the caretaker simultaneously and eventually learn to associate the bodily satisfaction with the affect of the caretaker. This crucial linkage is the foundation for interpersonal relations, which are carried into future experiences. The learning is not the kind ordinarily associated with human cognition. Rather, it is at an associative level based on a repeated pattern of interactions.

Sullivan described tenderness and anxiety as two affective states of the caretaker that are transmitted to the infant. Tenderness brings feelings of euphoria, whereas anxiety brings disorganization. Infants respond on a primitive level to decrease anxiety and increase euphoria, much as an amoeba will retract from noxious stimuli to a more pleasurable environment. However, infants' lack of motility means they cannot escape such stimuli except through emotional withdrawal.

Sullivan hypothesized that the experience of severe anxiety is probably like being hit on the head with a two-by-four, resulting in confusion and not much information about what happened. Although severe anxiety will interfere with learning, lesser amounts are necessary for learning and the process of socialization. During toilet training, for example, mild anxiety will heighten the child's awareness about the expected activity. When tenderness from the parent is experienced

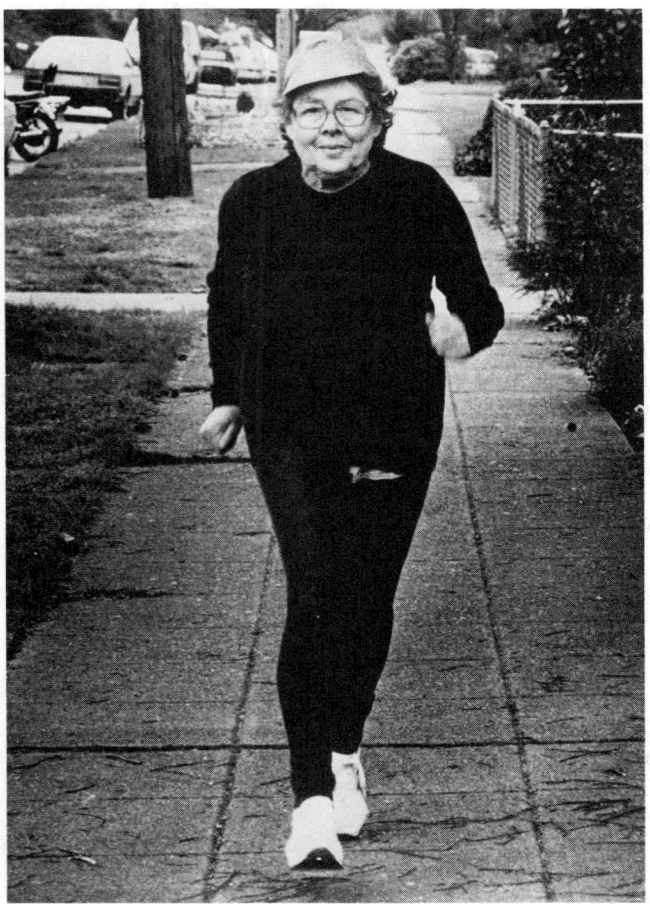

FIGURE 5–5. Full enjoyment of life reflects ego integrity in late adulthood. (Courtesy of Rick Schweinhart, Mercer Island Reporter)

along with the satisfaction of needs, learning results. In this case, the need to relieve bowel pressure will eventually be coupled with anticipation of parental approval when the fecal contents are deposited in the right place. As a consequence, it is likely to happen again, with more rewards.

This ongoing process of experiencing energy transformations in terms of tenderness and anxiety was thought to bring the development of the *self-system.* Sullivan was emphatic that his concept of self—the I, Me, My—was not based on any physicochemical structure or biologic need, was not the id, ego, or superego, but came into being as a mental representation of interpersonal experiences. As these experiences continue over time, the infant organizes around a "good-me" when satisfaction and tenderness occur, a "bad-me" when anxiety is present, and a "not-me" when intense anxiety occurs. The "not-me" is characterized by emotional withdrawal.[25]

Childhood Era. During the childhood era, early forms of speech develop. These are important because they begin to provide opportunities to the child for validating personal, subjective experiences. But language also can bring on a fusion of perceptions, with the result that distinctions in the child's experiences are lost. For example, the child will very likely have had both good and bad experiences with the mother, resulting in a mix of positive and negative feelings about her. The separate experiences will eventually belong to the concept of "mother"—a word that also carries societal messages about how one is to perceive and feel about this person. So the child could find some experience at odds with the concept. Speech is thus a two-edged sword—it provides an opportunity for sharing experiences, but the limitations of words may also reduce the complexity of the perceptions.

Sullivan believed that children are learning about punishment and pain and that these events may be accompanied by parental anxiety. In these situations, children may also learn from adults how to use words to explain and rationalize behaviors. In a childhood where there is a predominance of pain, punishment, and parental anxiety, the child learns to use words to deceive his or her true needs, feelings, and behaviors and to obscure the true self. Words are used to explain, to rationalize, and to condense complex reactions. So the tensions associated with unexpressed affective states are distributed in complicated and covert ways in an effort to minimize anxiety and to maintain the security of the self system (Fig. 5-6).

Juvenile Era. The process of maintaining security and minimizing anxiety was thought by Sullivan to continue through to the juvenile era. In this era, the child is exposed to authority figures outside the home and to the pressures of other children. During these school years, the child learns to compete, to compromise, and to modify or give up ideas. The child is under pressure from both adults and other children to behave in certain ways, to conform and not be different, and to "act

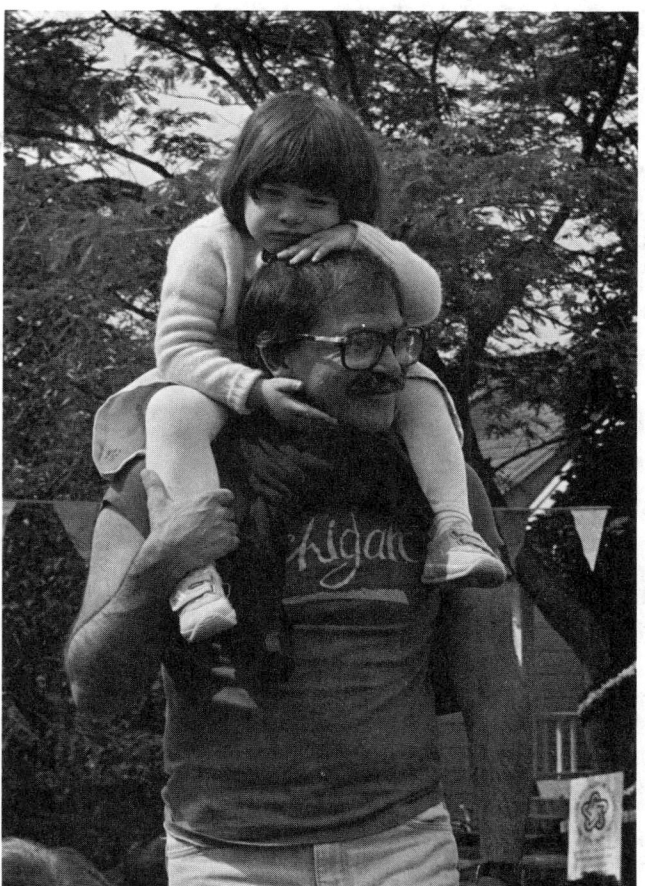

FIGURE 5–6. Security comes from freedom to express feelings and thoughts that may differ from those of others in the environment. (Courtesy of Tony Schiro)

right" (reference 25, p 233). Although this pressure aids in socialization, it can be unfortunate if the child learns to relinquish those experiences and feelings that are unimportant to others; problems arise when these really do matter, but the child suppresses them to avoid being denigrated or ignored (Fig. 5-7).

Preadolescent Era. The era of preadolescence is characterized by interest in another person of the same sex—a chum. It is the first manifestation of a capacity for adult forms of affection and love and occurs because there is ease with another person who is having similar experiences in growth and development. Because of the opportunity for closeness and validation of personal worth outside the family system, it is also a time for the child to reassess herself or himself and establish the foundations for tenderness and interpersonal intimacy. In Sullivan's view, love exists only if the satisfactions and security of the other are as important as one's own.

Early Adolescent Era. In early adolescence, there develops a true genital interest and the appearance of what Sullivan described as the *lust dynamism.* "Dynamism" refers to an enduring pattern of energy transfor-

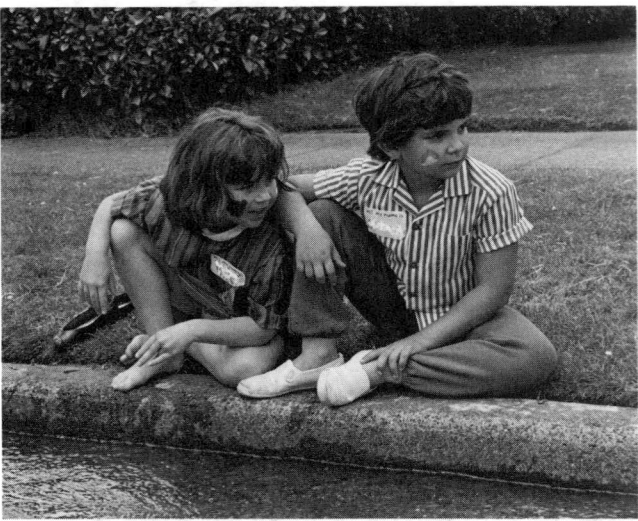

FIGURE 5–7. Experiences spontaneously shared with other children offer an opportunity for emotional satisfactions outside the family and contribute to a sense of interpersonal competence. (Courtesy of Tony Schiro)

mations. He did not think there was a relation between lust and the need for intimacy. He viewed the latter as an older need that had its beginnings as loneliness and a need for tenderness in infancy, whereas lust is a new arrival during this era attributable to the eruption of reproductive biology. He saw three needs that had to be integrated at this stage—for maintaining the security of the self-system, for intimacy, and for lustful satisfaction—as sometimes being on a collision course. Sullivan felt strongly that clinicians should not dwell on sexual problems, because these tended to disappear when problems in interpersonal relations were treated satisfactorily.

Late Adolescent Era.
In the stage of late adolescence, the aim is to become integrated into larger society, to take on responsibilities, and to be able to manage anxiety instead of being overcome by it. The need for tenderness, begun in infancy, moves the young adult to seek companionship despite the anxiety encountered in the process and can lead to a mature relationship between the self and the larger society.

Symptoms and problems in living arise when the individual cannot deal with anxiety and uses excessive avoidance of anxiety-laden situations or cannot use effective methods to deal with it. Sullivan noted that relationships from the past will unconsciously influence relationships in the present in what he called *parataxic distortion*.[25] The anxiety that originally arose from interpersonal situations can be identified and re-examined in the relationship with the therapist.

Summary.
Sullivan's theory about the mechanisms of anxiety and the self-system was based on adult patients in his psychiatric practice. He recognized that his views were not influenced by healthy people, who were not likely to become patients and thus available

for study. Sullivan's principal contribution was in adding other dimensions to Freud's formulations. It is clear that he believed the interpersonal factors in the environment and the learning associated with them had a larger influence on human development than did any physiological ones.

COGNITIVE THEORY—JEAN PIAGET, ALFRED ADLER, KAREN HORNEY

Piaget

Jean Piaget's (1896–1980) theory is based on methodical observations of his own and other children. Although there are many classifications of his stages of mental development, Piaget and his colleague Barbel Inhelder summarized them into three major ones: sensorimotor, concrete operations, and formal operations. Piaget stressed that the ages at which these develop are not absolute and that it is quite normal to have functions at different levels of maturity appearing simultaneously within one period.[13,21]

Sensorimotor Stage. The sensorimotor stage begins at birth and continues to 18 or 24 months. In the newborn period, the infant comes equipped with a few automatic reflexes that will be the basis for further development. The reflexes lead to physiological needs being rewarded, and because of these stimulus–response experiences, more complex structures and behaviors develop. For example, the infant is born with a sucking reflex and will turn toward a touch on the cheek. Over time, as this reflex is rewarded with milk and other nutrients, the infant's response becomes more mature, and he or she will approach the nipple directly and begin sucking in an organized way. The association of the reflex with feeding encourages repetition of the behavior. These repetitions become habits that are rewarded and lead to still another level of development. This feedback loop of behavior patterns turns simple structures into more complex ones.

Piaget identified two processes as being involved. The first, the internal response to stimuli, is called *assimilation*. The second is the modification of the internal structure to develop new patterns of action and is called *accommodation*. The processes are complementary and part of the organism's adaptation to its environment and its need to organize its experience. Although the organism's functioning was observed to begin at the very primitive level of recognizing and responding to cues, the process leads to increasingly mature behavior. Intellectual development was seen to result from this interaction of external events and internal factors. Piaget believed that increasingly intelligent behavior results from a balance of assimilation and accommodation.

Another important aspect of Piaget's theory is the concept of *decentration*. In the early stages of existence, the organism is in an undifferentiated state. Awareness of the environment as something separate from the self probably is minimal or nonexistent. The first interaction, the initial breath, functions at a purely physico-chemical level of response. As experience accumulates and structures become more complex, there is a point at which behavior indicates an awareness that this environment and the people and objects in it are separate from the self. This process is called decentration. These processes of assimilation, accommodation, and decentration are central concepts of Piaget's theory.

Concrete Operations. The processes continue into childhood and adolescence. The foundations of mental structures developed during the sensorimotor period will increase in complexity as the child continues to interact with and experience the environment and the objects in it. During the stage of concrete operations, the child will begin to develop mental representations of objects or people. There is an expansion of the sensorimotor, subjective self to a decentering that includes social and intellectual development. It leads from a state of relative lack of differentiation between the self and others to a state of being able to coordinate several points of view (Fig. 5-8).

Formal Operations. The beginning of the formal thought stage of development also marks the end of childhood. The mental structures laid down in the

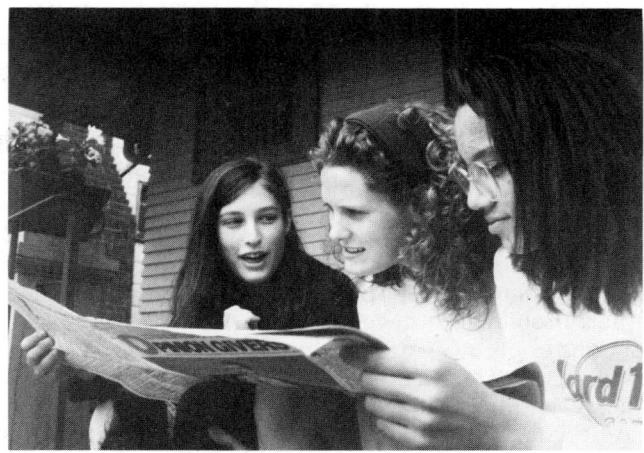

FIGURE 5–9. *Intellectual discussions often occur in the context of social activities with peers. (Courtesy of Jessica Huffine)*

sensorimotor period, then integrated and restructured during the stage of concrete operations, are once more reorganized into a new mental structure that is now able to deal with abstract thought. The preadolescent child begins to test hypotheses and theories and to reason in ways that are not dependent on concrete objects or situations.

Achievement of the stages is based on sensory experience and on how much stimuli the child can process from the environment. The organism in equilibrium can integrate the physiological, the external, and the abstract. Piaget also placed emphasis on the organism as an active participant in organizing its experience. He notes that the stroke on the newborn's cheek does not *cause* the rooting behavior—the reflex is within the infant as a response to the stimulus. This participant involvement continues throughout development and at every stage in the process of assimilating and accommodating. It is the individual who selects the response and gives personal meaning to the experience.

Piaget's theory of intellectual development has had its greatest impact in education at all levels. Although his theory is primarily viewed as cognitive, he repeatedly emphasized that sensory, emotional, and social experiences underlie all the mental operations (Fig. 5-9).

Adler and Horney

Two other theorists, Alfred Adler and Karen Horney, also emphasized the importance of cognition in development. As psychoanalysts and colleagues of Freud, they believed in unconscious processes but not that these processes were driven by sexual instincts. Both believed that problems in emotional development came from learned events originating in the environment and that perceptions, attitudes, and values about oneself arose from interpersonal experiences.

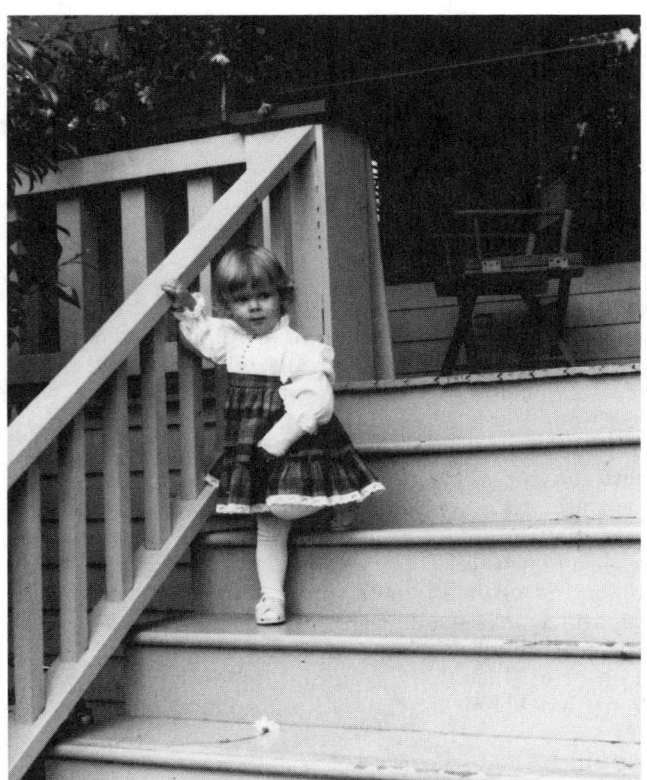

FIGURE 5–8. *Rapidly developing physical, spatial, and cognitive skills enable this toddler to investigate new challenges. Note the cast from earlier explorations. (Courtesy of Helen Palisin)*

ADLER

Alfred Adler (1870–1937) thought the physical and social dependence of infancy gave rise to a perception of inferiority. In his view, the feeling of inferiority is natural to the human situation and leads to efforts to improve one's existence. The sense of inferiority may come either from organic defects or from environmental inadequacies and results in efforts to compensate. Adler interpreted the Oedipal conflict in terms of just such a conflict about power between the child and the father. Problems in development arise when the perceptions of inferiority result in relating to the environment in hostile ways and in attempts to dominate others—an *inferiority complex*.[1,20]

Adler maintained that the child's perception of inferiority could be interpreted through the child's behavior and could also be corrected by bringing the goals of the behavior to the child's attention. For example, the child's hostility toward the parents and a need for superiority over them can be expressed through behaviors that embarrass them. In Adler's view, the situation could be remedied by helping the child identify what the behavior is accomplishing. Adler promoted his theories and methods in public lectures, educational efforts in schools, teaching in large clinics, and group sessions.[1]

HORNEY

Karen Horney (1885–1952) believed the infant has two basic response sets: those related to satisfaction and those that promote a sense of security. The need for security was evident to Horney from the efforts that went into avoiding or minimizing anxiety. This basic anxiety arises from negative attitudes and behavior toward the child, which result in isolation and a feeling of helplessness. Development unfolds under the influence of two factors—temperament and environmental influences. Thus, a critical aspect in the development of problems is the child's response to the attitudes of others. The organization of thoughts, feelings, habits, and way of perceiving events lead to the development of a *self-image* and *character*. Both could be changed through recognition, insight, and understanding. Horney promoted the technique of self-analysis albeit in conjunction with traditional approaches to therapy.[15]

Summary. All three theorists have influenced approaches to counseling and therapy. Current therapists such as Beck and Ellis acknowledge the contributions of Piaget, Adler, and Horney in influencing their own perspectives about the identification and treatment of problems in human development.[2,3]

BEHAVIORIST THEORY— JOHN WATSON, B. F. SKINNER

Watson

John Watson (1878–1958), a psychologist, argued that speculations about what is going on inside an organism's body or mind is not a very scientific approach to understanding development.[22,28] He believed the methodology used by the Russian physiologist Pavlov could be applied to humans as well. Pavlov carefully designed experiments to observe animals' external, objective behavioral responses to stimuli, with the long-range goal of documenting the properties of the nervous system. Watson thought a similar mapping could be done of human behavior. Instead of making inferences about feelings and states, Watson believed the emphasis should be on observations of external behaviors such as reflexes and habits that help the organism adjust and adapt to the environment.

Watson and his followers such as B. F. Skinner did not suggest that there are no internal capacities such as mind, consciousness, or awareness—only that the accuracy of the inferences about such structures is difficult to assess. They thought it was more useful to document the conditions under which the behaviors occur and provide the database for physiologists and biochemists to develop theories about the structures involved in human development. Their belief was that the organism will eventually reveal itself under careful and systematic observation. The foundation of this approach is that organisms tend to adapt and adjust behaviors or responses based on the rewards obtained from the environment.

Skinner

B. F. Skinner (1904–   ) noted that there are two types of responses—*respondent* and *operant*. Respondent behavior is the type associated with a reflex, such as the salivation of Pavlov's dogs, and occurs in response to an external stimulus such as food. Operant behavior occurs without an apparent external stimulus and appears to be spontaneous and voluntary, such as painting a picture or crossing a street. Both types may receive reinforcement from the environment, which will increase the probability that the behavior will be repeated. Thus, the infant or child develops and acquires new patterns of behavior through exposure to the rewards associated with earlier behaviors.[8,22,23]

Skinner emphasizes that observation of external behavior is more useful than relying on verbal reports, for there may be a difference between feelings as subjective states and reports of what one feels. He notes that words have some limitations in communicating private experience—their accuracy depends on how well the public and private events agree. The chief problem is that the words used to describe feelings have been learned through contingencies of reinforcement. Consequently, the labels attached to internal affective events have been shaped by the responses of others.

Summary. Behaviorism is basically a learning theory, and that has been one of its greatest contributions. Skinner's development of the principles of operant conditioning and schedules of reinforcement have led to the development of programmed instruction and the use of learning machines. The principles also have been used in therapeutic settings with adults and children, where the focus is on eliminating problematic behaviors or encouraging new behaviors through schedules of rewards and punishments.

EXISTENTIAL THEORY— SOREN KIERKEGAARD, ROLLO MAY, VIKTOR FRANKL, ERICH FROMM, DANIEL STERN

Kierkegaard

The acknowledged founder of modern existentialist thought is Soren Kierkegaard, a Danish philosopher of the early 19th century. He attacked the prevailing philosophical belief of dualism—that mind and body could be separated, that reality could be dichotomized into objective and subjective components, and that truth existed in some external abstract system rather than in the concrete reality of the individual's experience. Although his work was ignored in his lifetime, it eventually influenced generations of philosophers, psychologists, psychiatrists, and theologians and has been directly or indirectly responsible for the foundations of psychoanalytic, interpersonal, and cognitive theories of development.[17–19]

May

Rollo May (1909–   ) notes that the term *existence* comes from the root *ex-sistere*, which means to *stand out* or *to emerge* (reference 18, p 12). The central belief of existentialism is that the individual is not a static entity or set of mechanisms such as instincts and drives but rather is a being always in the process of becoming, emerging, existing. This belief means that humans cannot be defined in preconceived ways but are free to be whatever they wish to be. But along with this freedom come choices and decisions, which, in turn, bring responsibility for one's own existence. Responsibility involves decisions based on complete awareness of wishes, fears, and instincts and the courage that comes from acknowledging those sources of influence.

Existentialists describe three modes of existing in the world. *Umwelt* refers to relations with the biologic world; *Mitwelt* involves relationships with other humans; and *Eigenwelt* is the relationship with the self (reference 18, p 61). The three modes are always functioning simultaneously and influence each other. Loss of reality or loss of authenticity occurs if one mode is either excluded or becomes an exclusive way of relating to the world. May saw anxiety as not being able to know the world one is in and not being able to orient oneself in one's own existence. According to this theory, problems arise when one's subjective reality is not confirmed in some way and there is an attempt by others, however subtle, to deny the truth of the individual's experience.

May believes that two of the modes of being have received considerable attention by other theorists. He sees Freud's theory of the physiological aspects of behavior as *Umwelt*, whereas Sullivan's addressed the interpersonal or *Mitwelt*. However, the mode of relatedness to the self had yet to be fully explored.[18]

The existential literature focuses mainly on adult behavior, with very little about how the sense of being or the sense of self develops from infancy and through childhood. May believed that the sense of being emerges in the first 2 years of life, but he cautioned that although this is also the time of the emergence of the ego, the two should not be confused. Morris suggests that there is an *existential moment* in puberty when the person recognizes for the first time that he or she is responsible for his or her own conduct.[19] Others, such as Klein and Mahler, have developed theories about how the infant individuates after birth and separates from the mother, but their theoretical formulations are embedded within libidinal or ego development, not the self as a central organizing principle.[24] The following three theorists provide some views of what the self is and how it develops.

Fromm

Erich Fromm (1900–1980), a psychoanalyst, believed the development of the child's sense of self is influenced by the culture, family, and an inherited constitution.[12,20] As the child grows and becomes aware of separateness and an increasing ability to function independently, either respect for individuality or suppression of it may be encountered. With respect from the environment for uniqueness, the modes of existence—Umwelt, Mitwelt, and Eigenwelt—become more and more integrated and authentic. Over time, this process leads to the structure of the self and self-awareness. However, with growth, separateness, and independence comes an aloneness, which may create a feeling of helplessness and anxiety. This aloneness may be more of a problem for the child who has experienced hostility or has a poor self-image or little self-respect. The healthy child and adult will have the inner strength to continue with individuation rather than returning to a dependent state or other forms of escape.[12]

Frankl

The psychiatrist Viktor Frankl (1905–   ) believes that to freedom and responsibility, a third factor—spirituality—should be added. In his view, the spiritual side of the self or *will-to-meaning* is the dimension that adds meaning to life. He uses the Greek term *logos*, which translates to *meaning* or *spirit*, as the central concept in human functioning. This logos is not the spirituality of organized religion but a spirituality of self-awareness about choices, the factors that are influencing them, and the consequences of decisions. He emphasizes that it is not a spirituality in which specific values are inculcated into the child, but rather an awareness of the factors that are influencing the possibilities and alternatives. He thinks it is essential that parents or therapists be very clear about their own values and biases and avoid *covert* attempts to influence decisions.

In Frankl's view, neuroses do not develop from conflicts involving instincts but rather from conflicts between values and moral or spiritual problems. Such existential frustrations are not in themselves pathological, because the spiritual distress is a crisis that can lead to further growth and development. Frankl is not concerned with the salvation of the soul but with the health of the soul, believing that the healthy one that comes to grips with the meaning of its existence and takes responsibility for it will also be saved (Fig. 5-10).

Frankl believes that the aim of existence is not self-actualization but self-transcendence. He thinks that individuals who come in contact with the depth of their being—whether it is a belief in God or some other value—will also become self-actualized as a secondary benefit. Frankl developed *logotherapy*, which uses the technique of *paradoxical intention* to confront a problem or phobia directly and take the energy out of the fear and anxiety that is interfering with a meaningful existence.[5,6]

Stern

Noting that the self and its boundaries are at the heart of most philosophical inquiries, Daniel Stern has proposed a theory of how the self emerges during infancy.[24] Combining the insights of psychoanalytic theory with data from developmental psychology, he believes that infants can individuate themselves from birth and progress through increasingly complex modes of relatedness. The problem in the past has been how to get reports about the experiences from infants who are not yet able to speak. But he also recognized that speech is only one form of communication; behaviors can provide a wealth of information to observers.

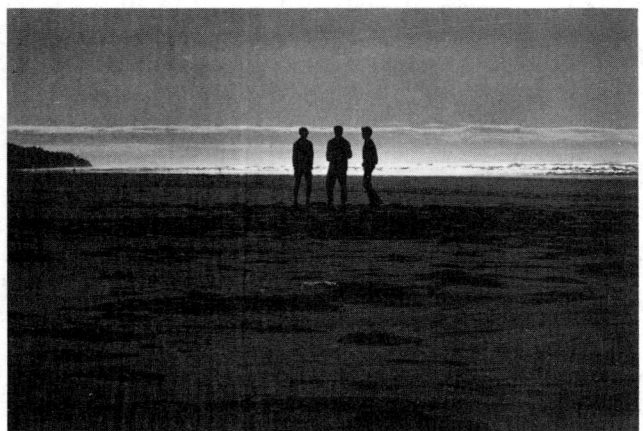

FIGURE 5-10. The search for meaning during adolescence can bring both a sense of loneliness and an opportunity for emotional and spiritual intimacy. (Courtesy of Jessica Huffine)

For example, an infant can establish independence by averting the gaze, shutting the eyes, staring past the speaker, or becoming glassy eyed.[24] These behaviors are the precursors of later self-expressive communication such as gestures, cries, babbling, and, eventually, walking away and returning to the mother.

Stern's approach is to separate knowledge about infancy into two categories—the *observed infant* and the *clinical infant*. The observed infant is the one whose behaviors and responses are seen by parents and researchers, whereas the clinical infant is the one who is reconstructed by the adult later. They are not the same entities, but there is an overlap or an area in which they interface. In Stern's view, the information provided by the clinical infant brings subjective validity to the observed infant.[24]

Findings of studies of the observed infant have led to Stern's theory about the development of the self. He believes there are four domains of the self that emerge in the first 2 years of life: the *emergent self*, which occurs from birth to 2 months, the *core self* from 2 to 6 months, a *subjective self* from 9 to 18 months, and the *verbal self*, which emerges sometime after that.[24] These four domains do not end abruptly but are integrated within the life span.

Emergent Self. Experiments reveal that newborns are able to make sensory discriminations about their environment. They are able not only to distinguish among auditory, olfactory, tactile, and visual stimuli but also can discern what is communicated verbally and what is communicated behaviorally. The transfer of information across sensory modalities convinces Stern that there is an emerging organization of learning among the infant's experiences.[24] The infant is likely to have separate, unrelated experiences that are not yet integrated—not undifferentiated, just separated by long periods of sleep, but which will become assimilated and connected and organized in time. This subjective world of organization is operating outside of awareness but eventually becomes the matrix from which subsequent activities will arise.[24]

Core Self. By the second month of life, infants seem to make a qualitative change in their interpersonal relatedness. They also appear to be more integrated in their interactions with others. This is evident from the infant's ability to share, even for a brief period, a focus of attention or feeling states. This ability will become more differentiated into a sense that the mother and self are quite separate entities. Stern argues that the first task of the infant is the "formation of self and other, and only then is the sense of merger-like experiences possible" (reference 24, p 70) (Fig. 5-11).

Subjective Self. Around 9 months of age, the infant shows evidence of sharing his or her subjective life. Without using words, the infant can effectively get the parent's attention to come share an experience. The infant also has the capacity to detect whether affective

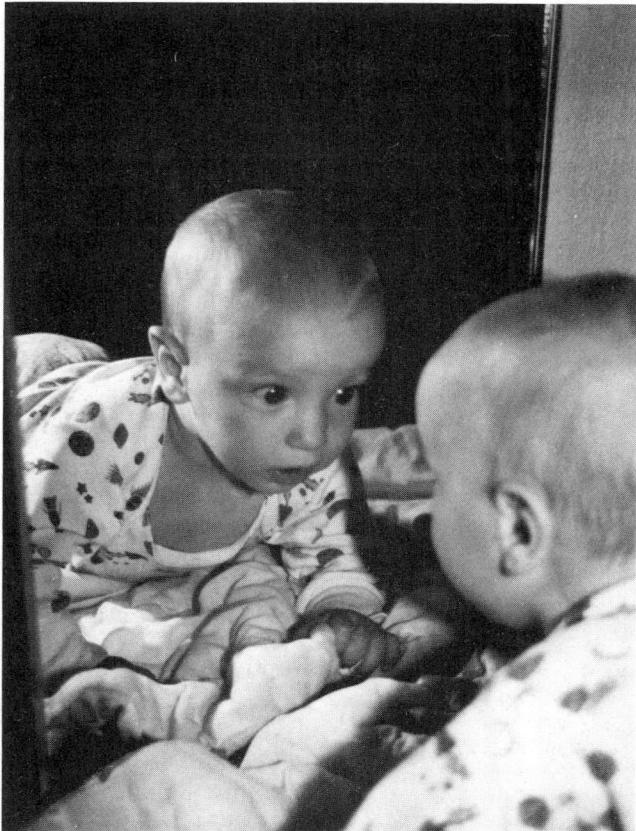

FIGURE 5–11. Discovery of the self begins early and continues throughout the life span. (Courtesy of Jessica Huffine)

feelings in others are congruent with the affective states within the self.

Verbal Self. As language emerges by 24 months, the self has a new medium of exchange. But Stern also notes that the totality of subjective experiences is only partially translated into words. Those experiences that are unarticulated can become a source of alienation. Speech is a means of using symbols at an abstract level.

But although this may be a loss, there is also a new form of relatedness, because language means a new way of communicating. Although it is abstract, it does offer an opportunity for being-with others in their personal experiences.

Stern's theory is new and has yet to be tested, but his integration of many theories, in combination with data from experimental designs and parent observations, will generate considerable attention in the future. Although Stern does not identify himself as an existentialist, his concerns with the development of the self and reliance on infant "reports" to understand the emergence of the self are consistent with that philosophy.

SUMMARY

The developmental levels for some of the theorists—Freud, Erikson, Sullivan, and Piaget—are summarized in Table 5-1. Their theories all begin with the organism at birth and the tasks to be accomplished in order to survive. All these theorists believe that the physiological substrate is an important factor in guiding the organism's experience. Each also sees the process of human development as one of increasing complexity —id to ego to superego, an ego moving through life tasks, the emergence of a self-system, and a mental structure reorganizing itself in response to new stimuli.

Developmental problems arise when the infant or child's individual needs are not recognized or permitted open expression. These needs may be instincts, ego tasks, security of the self-system, intellectual expression, or self-awareness. When consistently denied expression and emergence into awareness, they eventually express themselves through surrogate behaviors that may reduce or interfere with the realization of the individual's full potential.

At this stage, knowledge of development is much like a jigsaw puzzle. The outline is the biology of the organism, and some sections or theories are in place. There are some links among the sections, and they each have a place in the total picture.

TABLE 5–1
Stages of development according to various theorists

FREUD: PSYCHOSEXUAL STAGES	ERIKSON: LIFE CYCLE TASKS	SULLIVAN: INTERPERSONAL ERAS	PIAGET: COGNITIVE STAGES
Oral	Trust vs mistrust	Infancy	Sensorimotor
Anal	Autonomy vs shame		
Phallic	Initiative vs guilt	Childhood	Concrete operations
Latency	Industry vs inferiority	Juvenile	
	Identity vs role confusion	Preadolescence	Formal operations
Genital		Early adolescence	
		Late adolescence	
	Intimacy vs isolation		
	Generativity vs stagnation		
	Ego integrity vs despair		

Research Highlights

Thomas A, Chess S. Genesis and evolution of behavioral disorders: From infancy to early adult life. Am J Psychiatry. 1984;141:1–9.

The increasing interest in the concept of temperament in child development research is due largely to the results of the New York Longitudinal Study (NYLS) originated by Thomas & Chess.[27] They reported that temperament in infancy was related to problems in later life—a result which suggested that temperament could be used in the early identification and prevention of problems. However, subsequent examination of the study revealed serious methodological issues which make the NYLS rating scales unreliable for predicting later problems. Conse-quently, the validity of temperament as a predictor of social–emotional development has not yet been established.

From the case studies described by the authors, the most appropriate use of the concept of temperament may be in clinical situations where assessment and intervention are more important than predictions of later outcomes. The specific items of temperament scales can be used to help parents identify behaviors that are creating difficulties for them and to help provide an opportunity for problem-solving and reassurance. Rating scales can also be used by adolescents and adults to increase self-awareness and a recognition of their individuality in responding and interacting with the environment.

References

1. Ansbacher HL, Ansbacher RR, eds. The individual psychology of Alfred Adler. New York: Harper & Row; 1964.
2. Beck AT. Depression. Philadelphia: University of Pennsylvania Press; 1985.
3. Ellis A. Humanistic psychotherapy. New York: McGraw-Hill; 1973.
4. Erikson E. Childhood and society. New York: WW Norton; 1950.
5. Frankl VE. Man's search for meaning. Boston: Beacon Press; 1959, 1968.
6. Frankl VE. The doctor and the soul. New York: Vintage Books; 1986.
7. Freud S. The question of lay analysis. London: Imago Publishing; 1926, 1947.
8. Freud S. An autobiographical study. New York: WW Norton; 1952.
9. Freud S. The origins of psychoanalysis. New York: Basic Books; 1954.
10. Freud S. Collected papers. Vol. 1. New York: Basic Books; 1959.
11. Freud S. Three essays on the theory of sexuality. New York: Basic Books; 1975.
12. Fromm E. Escape from freedom. New York: Farrar & Rinehart; 1941.
13. Ginsburg A, Opper S. Piaget's theory of intellectual development. Englewood Cliffs: Prentice-Hall; 1969.
14. Hall CS, Lindzey G. Theories of personality. New York: John Wiley & Sons; 1978.
15. Horney K. Self-analysis. New York: WW Norton; 1968.
16. Masson JM. The assault on truth. New York: Farrar Strauss & Giroux; 1984.
17. May R. Existential psychotherapy. Toronto: CBC Publications; 1967.
18. May R, Angel E, Ellenberger HF, eds. Existence. New York: Touchstone Books; 1958.
19. Morris VC. Existentialism in education. New York: Harper & Row; 1966.
20. Mullahy P. Oedipus: myth and complex. New York: Grove Press; 1955.
21. Piaget J, Inhelder B. The psychology of the child. New York: Basic Books; 1969.
22. Skinner BF. About behaviorism. New York: Vintage Books; 1976.
23. Skinner BF. Whatever happened to psychology as the science of behavior? Am Psychologist. 1987;42:780–786.
24. Stern DN. The interpersonal world of the infant. New York: Basic Books; 1985.
25. Sullivan HS. The interpersonal theory of psychiatry. New York: WW Norton; 1953.
26. Sullivan HS. The psychiatric interview. New York, WW Norton; 1954.
27. Thomas A, Chess S. Genesis and evolution of behavioral disorders: From infancy to early adult life. Am J Psychiatry. 1984;141:1–9.
28. Watson JB. Psychology as the behaviorist views it. Psychological Rev. 1913;20:158–177.

6

Charlotte Naschinski

The Communication Process

OBJECTIVES

After reading this chapter, the reader will be able to:

1. *Define* communication
2. *Describe the communication process*
3. *Discuss how the factors of culture, anxiety, perception, and style affect communication*
4. *Describe therapeutic communication skills including questioning, conveying information, reflection, clarification, focusing, suggesting, feedback, silence, and listening.*

DEFINITION

Communication is a dynamic and complex process through which information and personal beliefs or attitudes about the self or the environment, as well as instructions from one person to another, are imparted. Communication is an essential component of interpersonal relationships including those between nurses and clients. Hence, it is essential for the nurse to be cognizant of the complexity of the communication process.[5] This chapter describes the components of the communication process (sender, message, receiver, feedback), factors affecting communication (culture, anxiety, perception, and communication style), and therapeutic communication skills.

COMMUNICATION PROCESS

Communication involves a series of ongoing reciprocal events. Components of the communication process include a sender of a message, the message itself, a receiver of the message, and feedback (Fig. 6-1).

Sender

The sender has a message to be shared with the receiver. The origin of the message may be internal or external sensory input (e.g., a thought or event). The sender selects words, sentences, and nonverbal cues to create the intended message, a process known as encoding. Unconscious factors influence the selection and processing of input, as well as the choice of verbal and nonverbal cues, to create the message.

Message

The *message* is the translation of thoughts, purpose, and intention into a code that is carried through a channel to the receiver.[3]

ANALOGUE AND DIGITAL COMMUNICATION

Messages may be communicated in either an analogue or digital manner.[14] In analogue communication, concepts are represented by their physical, self-explanatory likeness. The similarities may be in shape, color, or proportion to the events represented. Primitive picture writings found in Egyptian tombs are examples of analogue communication. These pictures convey messages about the person and the life of the entombed without the use of words. Analogue communication usually is nonverbal.

Digital communication is usually verbal communication in which concepts, ideas, and objects are represented by signs and symbols such as s-h-o-e for shoe. The signs and symbols are then arranged to create a syntax of language that allows versatility and abstraction. Digital communication, however, lacks adequate semantics in the field of relationships. For example, a description of feelings that exist in relationships, such as love, is very difficult using digital communication. The variety of signs or symbols making up a language must be known by a number of persons and retain the same or similar meanings across different situations.[13]

Human beings communicate both digitally and analogically, but both modes can be problematic for accurate communication. The analogic behavior of crying for example, runs the risk of being misunderstood in that crying may represent sadness, elation, surprise, or anger. However, difficulty exists in translation from the analogic to the digital mode. For example, the feelings involved in intimate relationships may be more accurately expressed by pictures, poetry, and music, than by words.

NONVERBAL COMMUNICATION

Nonverbal communication is any form of communication that does not use words. It is equally as useful and important and can even override verbal communication. For example, a client who states, "I'm feeling fine," may communicate the opposite message to an astute nurse through facial grimacing, vocal quivering, and restlessness. Nonverbal communication can be

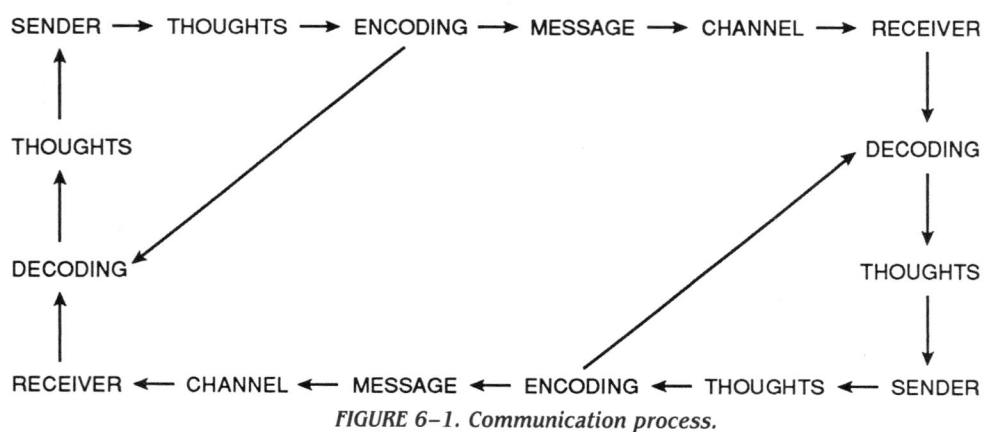

FIGURE 6-1. Communication process.

used to augment or substitute for verbal communication, convey feeling, or reflect the relationship between the sender and receiver. Concepts important to understanding nonverbal communication include kinesics, paralanguage, and proxemics.

Kinesics. Facial expression, eye contact, and gestures are included in this field of study.[4] These body movements can reflect emotion, emphasize an idea, or reflect a willingness to interact. Accurate interpretation of a person's facial expression, eye contact, and gestures is dependent, in part, on understanding that person's cultural background. For example, lack of eye contact can be interpreted as an indication of low self-esteem or embarrassment. However, when members of the Wodaabe nomads of Niger meet, they are forbidden to look directly into each other's eyes.[2] In fact, it has been stated that there is no one gesture that has the same social meaning in all societies.[4]

Paralanguage. Included in paralanguage are the vocal phenomena of voice qualifiers (pitch and range), vocal differentiators (crying and laughing), identifiers ("ah" and "un-hun"), and voice quality.[6] Personality characteristics and emotional states are inferred through paralanguage. For example, a person who speaks loudly and forcibly can be viewed as assertive and confident; whereas a person who speaks haltingly, in low tones, with little change in pitch, may be thought to be depressed.

Proxemics. Proxemics is the study of the relationship of space to social interaction including, for example, zones of intimate, personal, social, and public space.[9] How people feel about each other, the nature of the activity they are engaged in, and culture, all influence the distance employed during the interaction. For example, distance may be used as a means of conveying respect when interacting with a dignitary or as a means of protection when interacting with a feared person. Physical objects, as well as space, may be used to effect interpersonal distance.

DENOTATIVE AND CONNOTATIVE MEANINGS

Words have both denotative and connotative meanings. The denotative meaning is the one that is in most general use. Connotative meaning is an additional meaning for a word derived from past experience. Connotative meaning includes emotions, associations, and referents added to a word's denotative meaning. For example, the word *key* would be defined relatively the same by most English-speaking persons; yet the connotative meaning of this word would be different to a prisoner, a warden, and a homeowner.

CONTENT AND CONTEXT

In addition to a content level, which is usually verbal, messages have a context level that is at least partially nonverbal and indicates how a communication is to be taken. The context functions as a modifier of messages. In other words, the content is a dependent variable, whereas the context is the independent or determining variable.[1] For instance, the nurse saying matter-of-factly to the client, "You must stay in bed," both provides instruction (content) and also defines the relationship (context) of the nurse to the client as someone who has the right and responsibility to give instructions. Thus, the relationship aspect of a communication is a communication about a communication or *metacommunication*.[17]

It is through social context of communication that the subtle variations of metacommunication are learned. Accurate interpretation of metacommunication is dependent on knowledge of the social matrix in which the exchange of messages takes place.[12]

IMPOSSIBILITY OF NOT COMMUNICATING

All behavior in interactions contains a message. Action or inactivity, words or silence, all have message value. Some form of communication takes place when individuals are together whether it is intentional or unintentional, successful or unsuccessful. Even when a person purposely tries to not communicate by remaining silent, the withdrawal, facial expression, or body posture are forms of communication.[17]

The Receiver

The receiver is the recipient of the message. The receiver perceives and interprets the meaning of the communication through a process known as decoding. The receiver responds based on personal perception and interpretation, thereby providing feedback and becoming the sender.

To organize internal and external input for interpretation and response, the receiver "punctuates" the events of the interaction by organizing them into a linear sequence, with a beginning and an end. *Punctuation* is useful in that it simplifies a complex communication sequence. However, individuals in an interaction may punctuate the sequence differently. For example, a psychiatric client indicates that the reason for his elopements is that staff members do not trust him and will not grant him privileges. The staff personnel state that they do not approve privileges because the client has demonstrated his irresponsibility by eloping. In this example, the problem is that the persons involved have failed to metacommunicate about their respective patterning of the interaction.

Feedback

When the receiver responds to the sender's message, feedback has occurred. Feedback comprises the information received by the initiator of the interaction about the message generated. Feedback serves a regulatory function in communication to assure that the message sent is the message received. To be most helpful, feedback should be given clearly and tactfully, be appropriately timed, and be relevant to the persons and context. These characteristics are evident in the following example: Dr. S enters a client's room when Ms. K, the staff nurse, is providing care. Dr. S abruptly states, "I'd like a report on my clients." Ms. K replies, "I do have information I'd like to share with you. However, I am busy now. Would you be able to meet me in the nurses' station in ten minutes?" Understanding and consensus between communicators is facilitated by feedback.[12]

FACTORS AFFECTING COMMUNICATION

A number of factors can affect the whole or any one component of the communication process. Knowledge of, and attention to, these factors facilitate successful communication. The factors affecting communication to be described are culture, anxiety, perception, and communication style.

Culture

Communication is learned within a specific cultural context. Groups within a given society, such as the family, religious groups, and socioeconomic class, influence norms, values, and mores that guide behavior, including what, how, and with whom a person communicates.

Both verbal and nonverbal modes of communication can differ in meaning from one society to another. Culture is reflected in the meaning of verbal communication. A lack of comparable words can make translation from one language to another particularly difficult. Even within a given society with members speaking the same language, the meaning of a word can vary because of the existence and influence of subcultures. For example, a *poke* often refers to a person who proceeds slowly; however, in some subcultures, a *poke* is a paper bag.

Interpretation of all forms of nonverbal communication (body movements, paralanguage, and use of space) is influenced by culture. In addition, the use and interpretation of cultural artifacts influences communication. Cultural artifacts are items or substances that reflect a culture or subculture such as manner of dress, cosmetics, and jewelry. For example, the use of perfume may be interpreted in one society as an invitation for interaction, whereas, in a society that values the body's natural odors, the use of perfume would be considered offensive.

Anxiety

Anxiety also affects communication, especially the encoding and decoding of messages. Anxiety is a complex phenomenon that results in cognitive, affective, physiologic, and behavioral responses.[10] Behavioral responses may be adaptive and enable the person to cope with anxiety, or they may be inadequately adaptive, leading to continuation of, or an increase in, the anxiety level. A mild or moderate level of anxiety can result in increased motivation, learning, and productivity. For example, a client who responds to the diagnosis of diabetes mellitus with moderate anxiety is more likely to seek out and be responsive to information about and treatment for the illness than is the client who responds with severe anxiety.

Successful communication with a person experiencing anxiety is dependent on recognition of the existence of anxiety, identification of its source, and reduction of anxiety. Careful attention to verbal and nonverbal communication can reveal the presence and origin of anxiety. Consider the following statements of clients: "I don't know how my husband will treat me after my mastectomy"; "Do people always wake up after surgery?"; and "I'll never be able to drive a car with an artificial leg."

Perception

The behavior of a person is directly related to the perceptual field at the moment in which the behavior occurs.[7] To understand the intended meaning of a communication, the communicator's perception must be understood. Perception involves reception, selection, organization, and interpretation of sensory data.

The selection of, and response to, the myriad of sensory data available at any one moment is influenced by the functioning of the nervous system, past experience, needs, and emotional state of the person. Dysfunction of any part of the nervous system can result in limited or altered perception. Past experiences can bias an individual toward certain events in a stereotyped way. These biases can result in the inability to determine differences or changes in a person or a situation or the derivation of faulty conclusions about another's behavior. A nurse, for example, with the bias that all clients who abuse alcohol are immature and dependent, may fail to notice that clients with a drinking problem are able to make independent decisions.

Needs and emotional states also affect perception. Needs motivate a person to behave in a certain manner. Clues to persons' need states are found in their perceptions. For example, a picture of a family eating Thanksgiving dinner may be perceived in a variety of ways. A person with unmet physiologic needs may "see" the array of food items; whereas a person with unmet love and belonging needs may "see" close relationships among the family members. Emotional states can result in distortion or blocking of sensory input that, in turn, may result in an inability to attend and respond to stimuli. The intense emotional reactions experienced in a fire, for example, may result in a person not being able to find an exit door.

Communication Style

Successful communication is dependent on the use of a communication style in which the communicators consider self, other, and context throughout the communication process. *Self* refers to one's own feelings, perceptions, and self-worth in a given communication sequence. *Other* refers to the other person's feelings, perceptions, and self-worth in the same communication sequence. *Context* refers to both the context in which the communication takes place and the content.

CONGRUENT STYLE

The interaction of self, other, and context determines the communication style. In the *congruent style of communication*, the context as well as the needs and feelings of self and other are considered. The verbal and nonverbal behavior is in synchrony and is appropriate to the context. Self-worth is maintained and communication is effective when a congruent style is utilized.[15]

INCONGRUENT STYLES

Incongruent styles in which self, other, or context is denied include placating, blaming, superreasonable, and irrelevant.[15,16] Examples of incongruent styles can be recognized by the words spoken, the body language used, and their effect on the other.

Placating. In this style of communication, the goal is "peace at any price." The placator ignores self and assumes all responsibility for the other and the context. The placator uses self-derogatory words and displays body language suggesting submissiveness.

Blaming. Self becomes the predominant focus in the blaming style of communication. Neither feelings and needs of the other nor the context are taken into consideration. The blamer uses accusatory and hostile words and displays body language that conveys superiority.

Superreasonable. In this communication style, the context is the focus of communication, and the feelings and needs of both persons are denied. Both the verbal and nonverbal behavior of the person utilizing a superreasonable style are impersonal and devoid of feelings.

Irrelevant. The irrelevant style of communicating ignores self, other, and the context. The words spoken are unrelated to the circumstances. Feelings of self and other are avoided. The nonverbal behavior displays motion and distraction. Table 6-1 summarizes the different aspects of congruent and incongruent communication styles.

ASSERTIVE COMMUNICATION STYLE

Another way of viewing communication that considers self, other, and the context, is termed *assertive commu-*

TABLE 6–1
Incongruent and congruent communication styles[15,16]

STYLE	VERBALIZATION	BODY LANGUAGE	EFFECT	CONSIDERS: SELF Yes	No	OTHER Yes	No	CONTEXT Yes	No
INCONGRUENT									
Placating	I'm wrong My fault Forgive me	Hand wringing Head hung Eyes down Posture of supplication	Pity		X	X		X	
Blaming	You always/never Why don't you You made me	Pointed finger Leaning forward Glaring Tight muscles	Reverse blame	X			X		X
Superreasonable	Impersonal Factual Logical Monotone	Upright posture Rigid No eye contact	Coldness Hurt		X		X	X	
Irrelevant	Frequent change of subject Nonsequiturs	Laughing Jokes Gestures Looking about	Confusion Impatience Anxiety		X		X		X
CONGRUENT									
	I think I feel What are your thoughts/feelings	Eye contact Relaxed posture Gestures match words	Tension reduced Self-worth maintained	X		X		X	

nication and is differentiated from responses described as aggressive or passive.

Assertive Communication.

The assertive communicator sets goals, acts on those goals decisively, and accepts responsibility for the consequences of actions taken.[10] The person who uses assertive communication is sensitive to the feelings and rights of self and others. Statements often begin with "I" and clearly indicate the position of the person. The assertive person is gentle but firm when necessary and able to negotiate workable outcomes.

Aggressive Communication.

The aggressive communicator ignores the rights and feelings of others in an effort to control and manipulate them or the environment. Verbal messages frequently start with "you," include threats or demands, and disavow responsibility for the outcome of behavior. Nonverbal behavior is in synchrony with verbal messages and may include finger-pointing, a loud threatening tone of voice, or clenched fists.[8]

Passive Communication.

The passive communicator seeks peace and avoids conflict or confrontation. Behavior is passive and dependent, often reflecting a denial of one's own feelings and rights. Ultimately, the passive communicator experiences frustration, inadequacy, and depression.

The following example illustrates the communication patterns discussed: A staff nurse's request for leave on Christmas is denied by the head nurse. The staff nurse responding aggressively might say, "You never grant my requests. It will be your fault if my children do not enjoy Christmas because I have to work." The staff nurse utilizing passive communication states, "You are right. The needs of the patients and unit are more important than my need to be with my family." A response of an assertive nurse might be, "I understand that the unit must be adequately staffed, yet I want to be with my family on Christmas. Ms J, registered nurse who is scheduled for evening shift, has agreed to work the day shift. I will work the evening shift on Christmas."

THERAPEUTIC COMMUNICATION SKILLS

Effective use of communication skills enhances the communication process. Therapeutic communication skills help ensure that the message sent is the one received so that mutual understanding is achieved. Understanding the client's thoughts, feelings, and the meaning of those feelings helps the nurse utilize the nursing process. Communication skills are learned skills that must be incorporated into the nurse's existing interpersonal skills and be utilized appropriately to be effective. The skills selected for discussion in this chapter include questioning, conveying information,

reflection, clarification, focusing, suggesting, feedback, silence, and listening.

Questioning

Questioning is a useful communication skill to obtain information. Questioning is a direct approach and, when used to excess, serves to control the nature and range of the client's responses. When the intent is to engage the client in conversation, it is best to use open-ended questions, and when the goal is to obtain factual information, closed-ended questions are useful.

OPEN-ENDED QUESTIONS

Open-ended questions focus on the topic, but allow multiple options for response. They allow the client to clarify, elaborate, describe, or compare experiences, thoughts, and feelings. With open-ended questions, the client is allowed the freedom to structure the conversation. These questions often begin with such words as how, what, and when. Examples of open-ended questions include: "How were you feeling when . . . ?"; "What was happening that . . . ?"; "When you were . . . , what were you thinking and feeling?" Questions beginning with "why" should be used with caution. "Why" questions often place the client on the defensive and are difficult to answer. Consider the following "why" questions: "Why do you refuse your medications?"; "Why do you feel that way?"

CLOSED-ENDED QUESTIONS

Closed-ended questions are worded so that they can be answered with very few words or merely a *yes* or *no*. For the most part, these questions should be used sparingly, as they limit therapeutic exploration and lead to an interrogative tone. However, closed-ended questions are useful in obtaining factual information when a client rambles or is limited in capacity for speech. Examples of these questions include: "Were you feeling angry when your husband said that?"; "How many times have you been hospitalized?"; or "Do you feel less anxious after you take the medicine?"

Conveying Information

When using the communication technique of conveying information, the nurse supplies new or additional information. When a nurse is asked a direct information-seeking question by a client, information that is useful should be provided. However, caution should be used in imparting information in the form of advice or providing personal information.

Reflection

Reflection is conveying to the client the nurse's understanding of the client's expressed thoughts (content) or implied feelings. Through the use of this communication skill, the client is encouraged to develop or evaluate thoughts and clarify implied or incongruent feelings. In reflecting content, the nurse repeats the statement made by the client. This allows the client to hear and think about what was said and lets the client know the nurse heard and understood. For example, the client states, "My thoughts are disjointed," and the nurse responds, "Your thoughts are disjointed?" Effectiveness of this communication skill diminishes with its misuse or overuse.

Reflection of feeling is a statement of the nurse's perception of the feeling implied in a client's comments. Through the use of reflection, the client realizes the nurse is aware of his feelings and is encouraged to further elaborate on or clarify comments. Reflective statements should allow opportunity for the client to disagree or offer a different perception. For example, "You seem to be feeling depressed," rather than, "You are depressed."

Clarification

When a client is upset or experiencing disturbing emotions, verbalizations are often not clear or obvious in meaning. When this occurs, the nurse should clarify, even when it is necessary to interrupt the flow of the conversation. Clarification responses are attempts to find the meaning of a communication and are worded tentatively or in the form of a question. Examples include: "I'm not sure I understand. Tell me again about . . ."; "To whom are you referring when you say 'they'?"; When you say . . . do you mean . . . ?".

Focusing

Some clients experience difficulty focusing on one topic for any length of time as a result of anxiety or as a defense against involvement. Instead, they may speak in broad generalities, change the subject frequently, or focus on the nurse. In focusing, the nurse helps the client identify and concentrate on a specific thought or feeling. The purpose of focusing is to facilitate goal-directed communication and to focus on significant data. Focusing techniques include facilitating description of perceptions, encouraging comparisons, and sequencing events. For example, when the client stated, "Our relationship has been so helpful to me," the nurse replied, "In what way has our relationship helped you?" Persistent focusing on an anxiety-generating topic or feeling can impede or stop the communication process, however.

Suggesting

Suggesting is the presentation and exploration of alternatives. Once the client and nurse have identified a problem or task, exploration of options and choices is appropriate. The nurse assists the client to explore advantages, drawbacks, meanings, and implications of potential options through the communication skill of suggesting. The nurse must use a nondogmatic, uncoercive manner when offering suggestions such as, "Others have found . . . useful" or "Do you think that . . . would work for you?"

Feedback

The communication skill of feedback is a description of some aspect of a person's communication and its impact on another. Through feedback, the client can become aware of the impact of behavior and can modify or correct methods of communicating. Feedback is most useful when the focus is on behavior and when it is descriptive, rather than judgmental; for example, "I found it difficult to comment during the meeting due to your frequent interruptions," rather than "You sure are inconsiderate." Focus feedback on behavior related to a specific here-and-now situation. The sooner and more specific feedback is, the more useful it becomes. Feedback should also be focused on exploration of alternatives, rather than offering answers, advice, or ultimatums. What was said and done, rather than why, should be emphasized. When providing feedback, consider the ability of the recipient to receive it. Choose a time, place, and words conducive to acceptance of the feedback.

To facilitate communication, the nurse must also be able to receive feedback. The nurse, too, can modify or correct communication based on feedback. The nurse who assumes responsibility for communication requests and accepts feedback. The feedback provided should be received and evaluated objectively by the nurse.

Silence

Communicating without verbalization can be a very effective communication skill. It is, however, a skill that can be difficult to master, for verbalization between people is the expected social behavior. Some nurses find silence uncomfortable because they feel they are not doing anything for the client.

Silence, however, serves a variety of purposes. It can convey concern, interest, or acceptance of the client. Silence allows both the nurse and the client to collect thoughts and formulate responses. It can encourage the client to assume more initiative in the conversation. Silence can also provide the opportunity for nurses to evaluate the client's and their own level of anxiety, as well as the opportunity for relief from emotionally charged content.

Listening

Listening is essential for accurate assessment of the client. Listening is more than simply not speaking. It is

Research Highlights

Patterson reviewed, analyzed, and evaluated past and present models for research on nonverbal communication and made recommendations for future research.[11] The following summarizes major points of Patterson's article concerning recent and future research. Since 1976, a variety of theoretical models for nonverbal behavioral research have emerged. An earlier role for cognitive activities, such as expectancies, scripts, or affective assessments, in the communication process are stressed. Recent models have become more complex and more specific for the study of nonverbal communication. Recent empirical studies are characterized by increased sophistication, greater comprehensiveness, and close attention to mediating mechanisms directing the process of nonverbal communication.[11]

A concern of primary importance in future research on nonverbal communication is examination of factors that determine patterns of initiating interaction. What specific motivational and situational determinants underlie interaction? In addition, distinction must be made between those interactions that are guided by purposeful goals and those than are casual and spontaneous.[11]

A second emphasis needed in future research is attention to the verbal component of interaction. Historically, research has focused on verbal or nonverbal components. Research is needed that examines verbal content and nonverbal cues as a system.[11]

Future research on nonverbal exchange should extend the focus from dyadic exchanges to include larger groups. The relative simplicity of studying two-person exchanges and the predominance of dyads in social settings provide justification for studying dyads. The study of groups would allow examination of different functions of nonverbal behavior. Lastly, different methods and settings for research should be explored to extend generalizability of findings and facilitate creative approaches to addressing research questions.[11]

an active process in which the nurse gives complete attention to the content of the client's message, how the client states the message, and what feelings are being relayed by the client.

The nurse's nonverbal behavior must convey that full attention is being given to the client (e.g., body posture and eye contact should convey interest). In addition, the nurse should suspend thinking of personal experiences as well as personal judgments of the client. Listening conveys concern and respect for the client and can reinforce or encourage client verbalizations. The nurse may also encourage the client to verbalize by nonverbal gestures such as a smile or a nod of the head.

SUMMARY

Effective communication is a cornerstone upon which the nurse–client relationship is built and nursing process is implemented. Components of the communication process include sender, message, receiver, and feedback. Through encoding, the sender selects and arranges words and nonverbal cues to create a specific message. The receiver perceives, organizes, and interprets the message sent. Through responding to the message, the receiver provides feedback and becomes the sender. Feedback, a regulatory process, facilitates understanding and consensus between communicators. A number of factors affect the whole or components of the communication process (e.g., culture, anxiety, perception and communication style). Utilization of therapeutic communication skills enhances nurse–client communication. Other than when specific information is needed, questions that focus on the topic, but that allow multiple options for response, are most useful. In general, those communication techniques that encourage the client to develop or evaluate thoughts, express or clarify feelings, and enhance problem solving are most therapeutic.

References

1. Bateson G. The logical categories of learning and communication. In: Bateson G, ed. Steps to an ecology of mind. New York: Ballantine Books; 1972.
2. Beckwith C. Niger's Wodaabe: people of the taboo. Natl Geogr. 1983;164:483.
3. Berlo D. The process of communication: an introduction to theory and practice. New York: Holt, Reinhart & Winston; 1960.
4. Birdwhistell R. Kinesics and context. Philadelphia: University of Pennsylvania Press; 1970.
5. Bridge W, Clark J. Communication in nursing care. London: Wm & M Publishers; 1981.
6. Brooks W. Speech communication. 2nd ed. Dubuque, IA: William C Brown; 1971.
7. Brunner J. Beyond the information given. New York: WW Norton; 1973.
8. Clark C. Assertive skills for nurses. Wakefield, MA: Contemporary Press; 1978.
9. Hall E. The hidden dimension. New York: Doubleday & Co; 1966.
10. McFarland G, Leonard H, Morris M. Nursing leadership and management: contemporary strategies. New York: John Wiley & Sons; 1984.
11. Patterson M. Nonverbal exchange: past, present and future. J Nonverbal Behav. 1984;8:350–359.
12. Ruesch J. Disturbed communication. New York: WW Norton; 1972.
13. Ruesch J. Therapeutic communication. 2nd ed. New York: WW Norton; 1973.
14. Ruesch J. Communication and psychiatry. In: Kaplan H, Freedman A, Sadock B, eds. Comprehensive textbook of psychiatry, vol 1. Baltimore: Williams & Wilkins; 1980.
15. Satir V. Peoplemaking. Palo Alto, CA: Science & Behavior Books; 1972.
16. Satir V. Making contact. Milbrae, CA: Celestial Arts; 1976.
17. Watzlawick P, Beavin J, Jackson D. Pragmatics of human communication. New York: WW Norton; 1967.

7

Maxine E. Loomis

Group Dynamics Theory

OBJECTIVES

After reading this chapter, the reader will be able to:

1. *Identify groups that occur in health care settings*
2. *Identify goals for task, teaching/learning, and social/support groups*
3. *Discuss the impact that membership, physical arrangements, and resources have on group structure*
4. *Give examples of group contracts in the health care setting*
5. *Discuss the impact that leadership issues and interaction of members have on group process*
6. *Identify strategies for increasing group cohesiveness*
7. *Identify ways of determining group effectiveness.*

INTRODUCTION

Group membership is a natural experience in the lives of most human beings.

Consider six students who have just signed up to develop a care plan for patients with the nursing diagnosis of ineffective individual coping. These students are friends, but they have never before worked on a class project together. Now, they are aware that a portion of their grade depends on their individual contributions as well as on how creatively they can put their ideas together in the next 2 weeks.

Tomorrow afternoon, the College of Nursing faculty will consider a proposal for a new curriculum at its monthly meeting. A representative task force of faculty and students has worked for the past year to develop an innovative curriculum that reflects professional nursing practice in a rapidly changing health care environment. The task force members feel good about their process of working together and are proud of the new courses and curriculum plan they have developed. Today, however, the task force is concerned about possible faculty resistance to their new ideas. Even though there has been ample opportunity for faculty input and discussion, the task force is meeting to plan a strategy for addressing concerns that may be voiced in the formal faculty meeting.

Tonight at a Cassandra meeting, a group of radical feminist nurses will meet to provide support for each other in dealing with the patriarchal values they confront within the university and health care system. This group of nursing students and faculty has been meeting monthly for the past year to discuss issues from a feminist perspective. Support is readily available within the group, as the members are committed to eliminating horizontal violence—a process by which nurses express their frustrations with powerlessness by abusing each other. Group cohesiveness is high, and the members look forward to the meetings, where they can collaborate rather than compete with each other.

Finally, at the local community mental health center, the clinical specialist who is case manager for a multiproblem family has called a team conference of professionals from eight community agencies involved with the family. Their goal is to develop a coordinated plan for helping the alcoholic grandfather, the unemployed abusive father, his wife who works evenings as a waitress, the adolescent daughter who is on drugs and planning to quit high school and get married, and the two youngest boys who are already having difficulties at school. The nurse is pleased that the boys' teachers, the high school counselor, a social worker from the welfare agency, and the family minister and doctor have agreed to come. Now, her role as team leader is to assist the group in developing a plan that will help each of the family members and improve the family's functioning. Perhaps collectively they can arrive at a plan that will be better than what any one of them could develop individually.

These are just a few examples of the importance of groups in peoples' everyday lives. Group membership is a way of relating to other people as well as a means of accomplishing certain tasks.

Basis of the Theory of Group Dynamics

Group dynamics theory has developed from research that defines and predicts how groups of individuals and individuals within groups will behave. The theory is based on the assumption that when people are together in groups, activities occur that are more than a simple collection of individual member behaviors; i.e., the group is more than the sum of its parts. Just as a basketball team executes a fast break as a collective activity, so a group's dynamics or process is the result of collective activity. Group cohesiveness, for example, is an experience that can be described only in terms of group dynamics.

Whereas the early research on group dynamics focused primarily on the influence that groups could have on individual attitudes and behaviors, group researchers in the 1960s and 1970s devoted a great deal of attention to the impact that groups could exert on the social system and the processes of individual, group, and organizational change. The term "change agent" was introduced to describe the role of working with groups of individuals to achieve an outcome greater or better than any member could have accomplished in isolation. Problem-solving groups and administrative teams were used in a variety of work settings to build morale and accomplish tasks.

Within health care settings, groups are an important means of arriving at treatment decisions. Mental health care is often delivered by a multidisciplinary treatment team, and psychiatric mental health nurses are often responsible for functioning as team leaders and team members. It is therefore imperative that these nurses understand and utilize group dynamics theory.

The Group

A group can be defined as a collection of individuals who are to some degree interdependent,[7] the definition that is used throughout this chapter. It is important to recognize that it is the interdependence—needing each other to accomplish a task or achieve a goal—that makes these individuals a group. A number of people waiting in line in the hospital cafeteria would not be considered a group. If the people waiting in line were required to decide who got the last hamburger, they could become a group for the purpose of making that decision, or they might each individually decide to leave and eat elsewhere, in which event they would not become a group. This functional definition should assist psychiatric mental health nurses in focusing on the elements of group dynamics most important to their roles as professional nurses.

GROUP OBJECTIVES
Types of Groups

The objectives or goals of groups will differ depending on how group members answer the following questions: "Why?"; "Why should I join?"; "Why are we meeting?"; "Why was this group formed in the first place?" Groups are often considered to be a more economical means than individual sessions of accomplishing certain objectives. When information is being delivered, as in staff orientation or inservice classes, a large number of people can be reached at one time by teaching them in a group. Three major types of groups will be discussed in this section: task groups, teaching/learning groups, and social/support groups.

TASK GROUPS

Many tasks cannot be accomplished individually. Certainly, the delivery of modern health care is an excellent example of the professional interdependence and cooperation required in our society. The more complex the task, the more likely a group or multiple groups of people will be required to accomplish the objective. Individuals with unique skills and attributes are often brought together to achieve complex goals.

The primary purpose of a task-oriented group is to accomplish specific outcomes. During this process, the group places high priority on decision making and problem solving related to accomplishing the tasks. Psychiatric mental health nurses participate in numerous task groups during the course of their careers. For example, the clinical nurse specialist at the community mental health center decided to call a team conference because she was aware that each of the agencies in contact with the W family mentioned earlier had adopted a different approach in dealing with the multiple problems. The minister was being critical of the grandfather's drinking and Mr. W's abuse of his wife and children, while the high school counselor was encouraging Tanya, the adolescent daughter, to examine the role she played in provoking her father. The social worker had been encouraging Mrs. W to leave home with the children, while the psychiatric nurse was attempting to develop a family therapy contract with the entire family. It therefore became imperative that all of the mental health professionals working with the Ws meet to exchange information, formulate a shared diagnosis of the family's problem(s), and arrive at an integrated plan of care for the family and each of its members. Each professional could not help the family adequately in isolation from the others. Their task, although complex, was clear: to develop a plan for working with the W family they could all agree to implement.

TEACHING/LEARNING GROUPS

The primary goals of instructional groups are exchange of knowledge, skill acquisition, or both. The classroom setting in which there is a designated teacher and eager students is the most familiar type of teaching/learning group. Nursing students are also familiar with small group seminars and clinical discussion groups and their importance in the educational process. What makes a collection of nursing students a group is their interdependence in the learning process. A physiology lecture in which there is a one-way exchange of information does not fit the definition of a group being used in this text. However, a small group of students who decide to study together and share notes in preparation for a physiology exam becomes a small group whose dynamics or group process have a significant impact on the accomplishment of the goal of passing the test.

Many educators believe that the use of group discussions and group projects enhances the teaching/learning process. Group learning activities are based on the assumption that students learn more and retain information better when they have responsibility for teaching or sharing that information with each other. There also are certain nursing activities, such as restraining a combative patient, that require a team effort to be done safely. Because of the numerous nursing activities that require a team approach, it is important that nurses learn to work together in groups.

Consider again the group of six junior students who have just signed up to develop a care plan for patients with the nursing diagnosis of ineffective individual coping. These students, who are friends, must begin by developing a strategy for working together. They could very well begin by sharing their individual objectives for the project. Karen might want to work for an "A" on the project to pull up her grade in the course. Mark wants to spend as little time as possible on the project because of his varsity cheerleading schedule, while Helen, Grace, and Whitney are eager to learn all they can about helping patients cope with stressful life events. Tony, the designated group leader, is very competitive and intent on turning in the best class project with an eye toward future graduate study. Of course, Professor S's objective is that the students enhance each other's learning through the process of working together on the project. Thus, in teaching/learning groups, individual goals differ from group goals. This process of group learning is also important for many of the patient therapy and self-help groups that will be discussed in Chapter 36.

SOCIAL/SUPPORT GROUPS

The primary goal of most social/support groups is to meet the interpersonal and affiliation needs of group members. These groups usually gather around some common activity or topic to have fun and support each other. A social group might buy season football tickets together, form a gourmet cooking club, or play bridge together once a week. A support group might consist of a number of nurses who have returned to school to obtain a B.S.N. or M.S. degree or a group of male nurses who share the discrimination attendant on being a minority within their profession.

Social and support groups are discussed together here because both objectives often are met within the same group. Social groups that meet to have fun also provide support, which is most often seen when one of the members becomes ill or experiences some other personal or family crisis. Feminist nurses who share a common professional concern may also become friends and choose to share social time together. Social support, in general, has been found to be an important factor in predicting how people will respond to job stress,[10] illness,[9] and normal life events.[2]

Identifying Group Objectives

The objectives for any given group are a blend of the needs and goals of each individual member, the group leader's objectives, and the expectations of the system in which the small group functions. Table 7-1 contains examples of the types of member needs, leader objectives, and system expectations that can be present in various task, teaching/learning, and social/support groups.

There are several questions that will yield information regarding the objectives of a specific group.

1. What are the goals/objectives that individual members are attempting to meet in the group?
2. What are the leader's goals and objectives for the group?
3. What are the expectations of the system with respect to the group outcomes and objectives?
4. Realistically, can all leader and member objectives and system expectations be met in this group?

This last is the point at which the real work begins: it may not be possible to meet all individual objectives within the same group. Sometimes, there is a discrepancy between the task of the group (e.g., developing a new curriculum plan in the next year) and the needs of individual members (e.g., making a good impression on the dean or defining the body of nursing knowledge). At other times, a leader's agenda (e.g., doing the best group project in the class) may conflict with a member's objective (e.g., spending as little time as possible completing the project). The group and leader will

TABLE 7-1
Types of groups and objectives

TYPE OF GROUP & EXAMPLES	GROUP OBJECTIVES		EXPECTATIONS OF BROADER SYSTEM
	Member Needs	Leader Objectives	
Task	Getting the job done	Completing the task with member participation	Task achievement
Examples:			
Curriculum task force	Develop new curriculum; make sure that clinical specialty content is included	Develop new curriculum within 1 year	Produce a curriculum plan that will meet NLN criteria for accreditation
Team conference	Clarify roles in family treatment plan	Coordinate care for multiproblem family	Provide the best possible treatment for multiproblem family
Teaching/Learning	Knowledge or skill acquisition	Imparting information or teaching skills	Learning objectives will be met
Examples:			
Class project	Writing an "A" project	Doing the best group project in the class	Students will learn more by working in groups
Football team	Play well enough to get a professional contract	Inspire players to function as a team	Win the conference title
Social/Support	Have fun/receive support	Have fun together; meet needs of all members	Have fun/provide support within existing structure
Examples:			
Cassandra meeting	Give and receive support	Schedule and convene meetings	Don't change the status quo
Gourmet cooking group	Enjoy sharing good food with friends	Plan meetings; eat well	None

need to negotiate and perhaps renegotiate the group objective(s) while considering all stated needs, goals, and objectives.

Many groups function within a larger system or organization that has certain expectations of its employees, students, and members. Some systems reward creativity, whereas others value stability. A college of nursing could be administered like a strict hierarchical unit or could value the creative exchange of ideas among students and faculty at all levels of the academic enterprise. The values, norms, and expectations of the system will influence the goals and objectives of any group that functions under its auspices.

The key factor in identifying group objectives is to arrive at an understanding of the congruence or divergence among the needs of individual members, the objectives of the group leader, and the expectations of the system within which the group functions. Although arriving at agreement is not always easy, determining group objectives will help prevent future conflict, controversy, and confusion as the group attempts to move forward.

GROUP STRUCTURE

A number of considerations go into determining the group structure. The most significant of these variables are the composition of the group, the physical arrangements, and the resources available to accomplish the task. Each of these factors must be clarified before the group contract for task completion, meeting teaching/learning objectives, or social/support needs can be implemented.

Group Composition

Group composition is usually the first structural variable to be considered: someone needs to decide who the group members will be before the group can get on with its activities. As illustrated in Table 7-2, group composition will differ depending on the objectives of the group.

In a task group, the members are often selected for their ability to contribute to completion of the task. The chair of the new curriculum task force needs faculty who have a visionary approach to preparing nurses for future changes in the health care system. However, members also are needed who can design a coherent curriculum, write behavioral objectives, and solicit and integrate faculty input during the planning process.

Teaching/learning group membership is based on peoples' need to know certain content. Membership may be voluntary, as in prenatal classes, or involuntary, as in a required course in medical–surgical nursing. Whether participation in a teaching/learning group is voluntary or involuntary can make a difference in one's interest in or commitment to learning. That is one reason that within a required course, faculty often develop small group projects in which students can select projects of personal interest.

Social/support groups are usually voluntary, and participation is based on personal interest. A support group for nurses experiencing job stress can be initiated by an individual nurse and need not be organized by a hospital or agency. In this case, membership may be open to any interested nurse, and the composition of the group might vary from meeting to meeting.

The size of the group should also be based on the needs of the members and the group objectives. Five or six members is usually considered to be the smallest group that will allow for diversity of membership and the development of group interaction. However, some task groups with a clear, time-limited agenda can function well with only two, three, or four members who have expertise specific to the task. On the other hand, a group of more than 10 to 12 members usually will break into smaller subgroups because of the difficulty

TABLE 7–2
Group structure and group objectives

GROUP OBJECTIVES	GROUP COMPOSITION	PHYSICAL ARRANGEMENTS	RESOURCES
Task	Based on ability to contribute to task completion By virtue of position May represent special interests	Meetings or work sessions related to task Time-limited; based on completing task	Provided by sponsor or organization
Teaching/Learning	Membership may be voluntary (elective experience) or involuntary (required course) Based on need to know	Classroom or other structured settings Time-limited	Covered by course fee and personal
Social/Support	Usually voluntary; based on personal interest Membership may be open and changing	Structure can differ based on member preference Often open ended	Personal May solicit donations

of attending to a large number of people simultaneously. If the group objectives can be accomplished by subgroups, committees, or task forces, provision can be made for beginning with a larger group and dividing the work into smaller projects. Most teaching/learning and social/support seem to function best with eight to ten members.

Physical Arrangements

Physical arrangements for the group should be made with the size and activities of the group clearly in mind, as the space and physical environment can have a profound effect on group functioning. For example, one Cassandra group had been meeting one evening a month in various members' homes. The members looked forward to these meetings as an opportunity to share personal and professional concerns about their own experiences within a patriarchal health care system. In an attempt to schedule the meetings earlier, the group agreed to meet the following month at a quiet local restaurant. No one had anticipated the impact of background restaurant noise, a long table seating 12 people, and the interruption of attentive waiters on the usual group process. Although everyone had an excellent meal, there was no way to discuss concerns or to experience support from the entire group. The physical environment had altered the group objectives.

The previous example illustrates the profound impact of the environment. The physical environment should facilitate rather than interfere with group functioning. The furnishings, heat, light, space, sound, privacy, and geographic location of the room will affect the group process. Group leaders and members should be constantly aware of the effects of physical arrangements on the group and select or alter the environment to facilitate group functioning.

Resources

The resources available to the group will also influence its ability to meet its objectives. With task groups and teaching learning groups, the provision of necessary resources usually reflects the commitment of the sponsoring organization to the objectives of the group. All too often, a committee is charged with a task and embarks on its work only to discover that there is no secretarial or staff support available or, even worse, that the committee members are expected to do the work on their own time with no adjustment in their usual workload. If the group members are especially committed to accomplishing their objectives, they may be willing to do the work without organizational support. Over time, however, this arrangement becomes wearing, and the organization's administrators are likely to face "morale problems" and a paucity of people who are willing to volunteer for or serve on committees.

The Group Contract

The final step in planning the group structure is the group contract: an openly negotiated, clearly stated set of mutual expectations that indicates what the group members and leader(s) can expect of each other regarding their activities together.[8] The contract consists of a set of shared objectives as well as a clear understanding of the structure for arriving at mutually determined outcomes. The group must be specific about such issues as time and physical arrangements, resources, and membership responsibilities. When the members and leader(s) have a common understanding of what they can expect from each other, they have formulated a group contract. This group contract is a reference point against which the members and leader(s) can compare any changes in their commitment to working together. It also serves as a way of measuring the group's progress in achieving its objectives. The contract can be renegotiated or terminated at any time. While the contract is in effect, the contract can be used to facilitate the activities of the group.

Figure 7-1 is an illustration of the components of the group contract and the effect the contract can have on group process and outcomes.

GROUP PROCESS

Group process is a general concept that refers to all of the activities within a group during the life of that group. Group process includes what is said and done in the group, as well as how members interact with each other, the timing of those interactions, and the roles the leader and members play in relation to one another. Some group members and leaders refer to the group as if it had a life of its own that is something more than the sum of all the individual members and their interactions. At times, they will refer to "the group's level of confusion" or ask, "what does the group want to do about that?"

In fact, every group does develop a process that is unique. The specifics of this process are impossible to predict even if one knows all of the individual members apart from the group, because when they get together as a group, they affect each other in unique ways. There are, however, some general group process issues with which all groups must deal. The role and style of the leader, the roles that specific members will play, the patterns of communication, and types of power and influence that will be exerted within the group are common group process issues. The phases of group development and the presence or absence of group cohesiveness affect the functioning of all groups.

Leadership Issues

Skilled group leaders are similar to perceptive photographers. When composing a picture, photographers

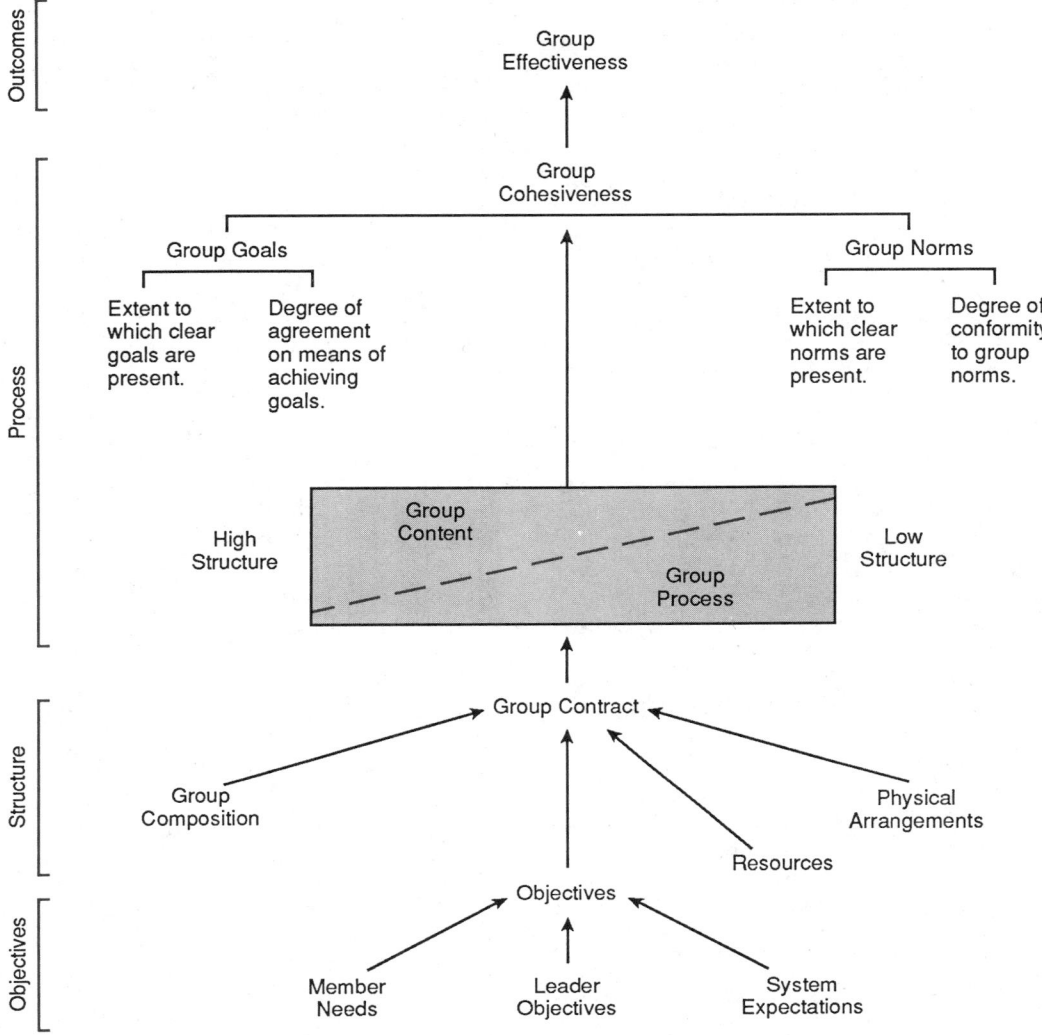

FIGURE 7–1. Model of small group dynamics.

must decide on a point of focus; i.e., what should be considered foreground and what background. The focus may be on a flower at the base of a tree, the tree surrounded by violets, or a panoramic view of the entire woods set against a Carolina blue sky. Although it is possible to be aware of the violets, the tree, the woods, and the horizon simultaneously, photographers must select a focus for each picture. This process is most quickly accomplished by using a zoom lens.

Group leaders likewise need to learn to use a zoom lens as they attempt to influence the process of a group. At times, the leader may be attending primarily to what is going on with one individual member, then focusing on how the other group members are responding to that member, and then on how the specific situation fits into the process of the group. The skilled group leader is able to attend to all levels of activity simultaneously in order to decide where and how to intervene. Whether or not the leader is attending to the

group process, there is always a process level of activity in addition to the overt content of group member interactions.

The important question is what use the leader should make of the group process. Figure 7-1 contains a box that shows the possible relationships between group content and process. Some groups, such as highly structured task groups, would be located at the far left end of the box, whereas groups in the middle would be those focusing equally on content and process. For example, the leader of a task group might be aware of the competition between two group members for the leader's praise. On the basis of this observation, the leader might decide to put each competitor in charge of a subproject related to the task, compliment the two equally for their contributions, and never even address the issue of how their competition was interfering with the group's goal. In this case, the leader has taken care of the process problem that was affecting the content-oriented group task without ever drawing the group's attention to the process issue. In this situation, the leader's knowledge of group process was useful in helping the group move more directly toward completion of its task.

Group Development Issues

Most people are concerned about entering a new situation, as the uncertainty usually causes some anticipatory thoughts and anxiety about what will occur. Will the other people like me? What will be expected of me? Can I meet the expectations? Will I get something out of it?

Assuming that most people enter a group experience with some initial uncertainty, one would expect that they will start out by being cautious in the group, to check out the leader and other members to determine whether they belong in the group. Yalom[12] has described this period of initial testing as the "in or out" period in the group's process. All of the members will be attempting to determine what their role will be in relation to the process and content of the group. Who will contribute most to the group objectives? Who will play an important role in conflict resolution? How will tasks be distributed? What does one have to do to gain recognition in this group?

Another phenomenon during the initial phase of most small groups is the development of patterns of power and influence. Yalom[12] has characterized the resolution of power and influence issues as the "top or bottom" phase in the group's process. Although there is no set time period for resolving the issues of power and influence, a group in which these issues are not clarified will experience difficulty in accomplishing its primary objective.

Regardless of how the group addresses the issues, it must find answers to the questions "who is in charge?" and "who will be influential in the group?" French and Raven[4] have identified five bases of social power that may also be applicable to health care groups: reward, coercive, legitimate, referent, and expert. *Reward* and *coercive* powers both refer to the recipient's perception of the influencing agent as being capable of rewarding or punishing them for their responses to the attempt at influence. *Legitimate* power stems from internalized values in the recipient and dictates that the influencing agent has a legitimate right to influence the recipient, who is obligated to accept this influence. *Referent* power is based on the attraction that the recipient feels for the person attempting to influence him or her: on the desire to be like, to identify with, and to be closely associated with that person. *Expert* power refers to the recipient's perception that the individual attempting to influence is better informed than the recipient on the topic under discussion.

This formulation seems clear until one realizes that what occurs in most groups is a mixture of bases of power and influence. The nurse may be the legitimate leader of a support group for high-risk pregnant women. Because the group is a voluntary outpatient experience, the nurse has no clear base of reward or coercive power. The hospital is not likely to refuse to deliver the baby if a member does not attend group sessions, nor would this be a part of the contract. The nurse may be an expert in group process, but she may never have had a baby, or at least not under high-risk conditions. She must therefore share her expert base of power and influence with other group members who can speak from their own feelings and experiences. Referent power may also be shared by the leader and several group members, depending on their interpersonal attractiveness to the group.

The third and final issue around which members demonstrate their initial concerns is developing patterns of communication. On the surface, this appears to be a matter of resolving who will talk with whom about what. Yalom[12] characterizes the underlying issue as "near or far." The resolution of the concerns regarding role, power, and influence leaves the group free to deal with just how open or closed the members will be with each other. Member openness and communication is important in all groups; it appears to be most important in social/support groups.[6]

When the group has satisfactorily dealt with these initial concerns, it is ready to enter the working phase in which group cohesiveness is the primary concern.

Group Cohesiveness

Group cohesiveness is the glue that holds groups together, helps them over rough spots, allows them to fend off outside threats, and helps the members to accomplish their objectives. Group cohesiveness can be defined as the result of all the forces that influence members to stay in the group.[3] Most people can recognize a cohesive group when they see or experience one. The members display a team spirit and feel good about one another and their group identification. They are loyal and supportive of each other and of the goals and values of the group. When there is an issue to be resolved or a task to be done, they mobilize their collective forces, decide on a method for approaching the problem, and move steadily toward resolution. Anyone who has been a member of such a cohesive group usually recalls the experience with positive feelings and may even wish to create such a group in the future. But how?

Group cohesiveness relates very directly to the goals and norms of the group (Fig. 7-1). Cohesiveness is enhanced by clear goals or objectives that all group members agree to and value. A laboratory study by Raven and Rietsema[11] indicated that the incentive value of a particular group goal for a particular person will depend, not only on the goal itself, but also on how explicitly the goal is formulated, how clear the paths are for goal attainment, and the likelihood of successful attainment of the goal. The extent to which clear goals are present and the degree of agreement as to the means of achieving those goals will greatly influence the development of group cohesiveness.

Group norms also have a significant impact on cohesiveness. Norms are the standards for behavior that is expected within the group. Group norms become the spoken and unspoken rules for acceptable behavior within the group, and group functioning is disrupted when members deviate from the norms. A deviant is someone who departs from or opposes the standards of the group. Initially, considerable effort and communication are directed to deviant members, especially if the group perceives that there is a reasonable chance of changing their opinions or behaviors. Research demonstrates that when it becomes clear that the deviants cannot or will not change, communication toward them declines markedly.[5] The group may redefine its boundaries to exclude deviant members, and they might even be asked or told to leave.

Group leaders play a significant role in the development of cohesiveness because of their influence in clarifying group norms and goals. Leaders are primarily responsible for structuring the goals and norms of the group to maximize their potential for cohesiveness. With guidance from the leader, members can arrive at agreement regarding means of achieving goals as well as expectations for the roles of each person in the group. In this way, group cohesiveness becomes an essential determinant of group effectiveness.

GROUP OUTCOMES

The primary measure of group effectiveness is its outcomes. Evaluation questions can be designed to determine group outcomes. Has the group accomplished its original objectives? Has the group accomplished other things in addition to or in place of its stated objectives? Have the needs of individual members been met? Have the system expectations been accomplished?

In a task group, the evaluation of group outcomes usually is fairly direct. Did the curriculum task force produce an innovative new curriculum within the 1-year time they were given? Did the treatment team develop and implement a collaborative treatment plan that helped the W family? Although the content objective is most often evaluated, some group leaders and members are equally concerned about process outcomes. Did all members participate in and contribute to the group task? Did they benefit as individuals from participating in the group? Did they leave feeling good about their group experience? If the task was related to a job or an outside assignment, were the system's expectations met? Was the report completed on time and of high quality?

These same criteria are important in evaluating a teaching/learning group. In addition, much emphasis is placed on whether the content was learned and retained. The instructor who structured group class projects will evaluate and grade the group's product. Student grades on the final examination and perhaps even state board examination scores might also be consid-

ered an indication of learning from the project. If the goal of a patient education class is to change behavior, then maintenance of the new behaviors would be a good test of the group's effectiveness. For example, how many members quit smoking, and was this change permanent?

Social/support group outcomes are perhaps the most difficult to determine because their objectives are often latent or not behaviorally specific. The focus of evaluation is usually on group process. What did the members like or dislike about the group? Did they feel supported by or close to the other members? Did they enjoy the group experience? In groups such as Cassandra, where the agenda can change from one meeting to the next, consistent attendance at meetings and attraction to the group can be seen as a measure of group effectiveness.

In summary, the group objectives, structure, process, and outcomes are all important factors to be considered in group dynamics. They are also important variables to be considered in developing, participating in, and evaluating group effectiveness.

SUMMARY

It is important that nurses learn the principles of group dynamics because they will work frequently with client groups and professional health team groups in most practice settings. A group is a collection of individuals who are interdependent for the completion of a task or attainment of some objective. The study of groups includes examining the objectives, structure, process, and outcomes.

Three general types of groups discussed in this chapter are task groups, teaching/learning groups, and social/support groups. Each type has unique goals or objectives the members are attempting to accomplish collectively. The purpose of a task group is to accomplish a specific outcome. The primary goals of a teaching/learning group are knowledge or skill acquisition. The primary goal of most social/support groups is to meet the interpersonal and affiliative needs of group members.

The outcome of all the planning and discussion that goes into forming a group is the group contract. This contract is an openly negotiated, clearly stated set of mutual expectations that indicate what the group members and leader(s) can expect from each other regarding their activities together. It is important to determine whether the leader and member objectives and broader system expectations can be met realistically within a specific group. The leader should consider the group composition, physical arrangements, and available resources when structuring a group.

The skilled group leader is able to attend to both content and process issues while the group is meeting. This includes an awareness of the roles of specific members, the patterns of communication, and the types of power and influence that are exerted within the group. Group cohesiveness is the most important variable affecting the process and outcomes of a group.

Research Highlights

Beeber LS, Schmitt MH. Cohesiveness in groups: a concept in search of a definition. Adv Nursing Sci. 1986; 8(2):1–11.

The authors of this well-written, thought-provoking article raise a number of important questions about the emphasis placed on group cohesiveness in the literature on nursing, group therapy, and group dynamics. They argue that the many and varied definitions of group cohesiveness have resulted in "a diffuse concept implying more than is stated in any of its definitions" (p 2). Because there is no clear conceptual definition, it has been difficult to develop clear operational definitions for conducting research on group cohesiveness. The authors strongly recommend clarification of the defining characteristics of the concept as well as nursing research to determine the clinical indicators of high cohesiveness and its consequences in therapy and support group situations.

The authors' concerns and recommendations are well founded. The ways in which health care groups accomplish their work represent a vast, uncharted territory for the clinical researcher. Much of the available research on group dynamics has been conducted by social and organizational psychologists on convenience samples of college students, workers, or business managers, and because of the difficulties of conducting research in natural settings

with actual groups, many group process studies have been conducted in laboratories with simulated group experiences. It is not clear how generalizable these findings are, because they have been few replication studies in the real world where groups function.

Regarding group cohesiveness, Loomis[7] proposed a model and an operational definition of group cohesiveness that is included in this chapter and which could be utilized in conducting clinical research. She hypothesized that the extent to which clear goals are present and the degree of agreement about the means of achieving those goals will influence the development of cohesiveness in health care groups. Further, the extent to which clear norms are present and the degree of conformity to the group norms will influence the development of cohesiveness in health care groups. The interactions among clarity and agreement regarding group goals and norms need to be explored. To what extent do these or other factors influence group cohesiveness? The multiple definitions of cohesiveness may indicate that it is a concept composed of a number of related variables that will require definition and correlational research before Loomis' hypotheses can be addressed adequately. Indeed, there is a great need for psychiatric mental health nurse researchers and clinicians to work together to expand the knowledge base for practice.

Cohesive groups are likely to be more productive and create a higher degree of member satisfaction. Group cohesiveness is enhanced by clear objectives that all members agree to and value. It is also enhanced by clear norms and member conformity to those norms. Group effectiveness is measured by the extent to which the group accomplishes its original objective(s) and is satisfied with the outcomes.

References

1. Beeber LS, Schmitt MH. Cohesiveness in groups: a concept in search of a definition. Adv Nursing Sci. 1986;8:1–11.
2. Cronenwett LR. Network structure, social support, and psychological outcomes of pregnancy. Nursing Res. 1985; 34:93–99.
3. Festinger L. Informal social communication. In: Cartwright D, Zander A, eds. Group Dynamics. New York: Harper & Row; 1968.
4. French JRP Jr, Raven B. The bases of social power. In:

Cartwright D, Zander A, eds. Group Dynamics. New York: Harper & Row; 1968.
5. Lauderdale P, Parker J, Smith–Cunnien P, Inverarity J. External threat and the definition of deviance. J Personality Social Psychology. 1984;46:1058–1068.
6. Lieberman MA, Yalom ID, Miles MB. Encounter groups: First facts. New York: Basic Books; 1972.
7. Loomis ME. Group process for nurses. St Louis: CV Mosby; 1979.
8. Loomis ME. Levels of contracting. J Psychosocial Nursing Mental Health Services. 1985;23:9–14.
9. Norbeck JS. Social support: a model for clinical research and application. Adv Nursing Sci. July. 1981;43–59.
10. Norbeck JS. Types and sources of social support for managing job stress in critical care nursing. Nursing Res. 1985;34:225–230.
11. Raven BH, Rietsema J. The effect of varied clarity of group goal and group path upon the individual and his relation to his group. Human Relations. 1957;10:29–44.
12. Yalom ID. The theory and practice of group psychotherapy. Ed 3. New York: Basic Books; 1985.

8

Mary Durand Thomas

Cultural Concepts and Psychiatric Mental Health Nursing

OBJECTIVES

After reading this chapter, the reader will be able to:
1. *Describe characteristics of culture*
2. *Explain ethnocentrism and cultural relativism*
3. *Identify areas in which cross-cultural differences may become apparent in psychiatric mental health nursing*
4. *Discuss the interaction of culture and mental illness*
5. *Describe ways of being culturally sensitive in carrying out the nursing process in psychiatric mental health nursing.*

INTRODUCTION

Interpersonal relationships are central to psychiatric mental health nursing. An important influence in interpersonal relationships is the cultural background of clients and families and the cultural background of the nurse. The concept of culture helps psychiatric mental health nurses to understand why the extended Samoan family members, who accompanied a teenage boy to the emergency room, are unwilling to leave him alone with staff on the psychiatric ward; to understand why the Korean American client, who was admitted for depression, describes stomach pain, rather than hopelessness; or to understand why the client, who is a recent arrival from South America, refuses a capsule saying it is "hot." Most important, the concept of culture helps psychiatric mental health nurses to understand that some of their own beliefs that they regard as universal may, in fact, be meaningful only within the confines of their own culture. In a pluralistic society, an understanding of the potential impact of cultural differences is especially relevant for psychiatric mental health nurses because they frequently care for individuals coming from different cultural backgrounds.

CHARACTERISTICS OF CULTURE

Culture has been defined as ". . . that complex whole which includes knowledge, belief, art, law, morals, custom, and any other capabilities and habits acquired by man as a member of society" (reference 24, p 1). Recent views of culture by anthropologists have emphasized certain characteristics of culture.

1. *Culture is learned:* Culture is not a racial or biologic feature, but is acquired through interaction with others. Culture, however, does influence how biologic needs are met. For example, an American child learns that a bed in a room alone or with a sibling is where the biologic need for sleep is met, whereas a Pacific island child learns that the culturally appropriate place to sleep is on a mat shared with other family members. Learning about where to sleep, as with other cultural learning, occurs as part of the fabric of daily life. The process of learning may be structured through formal teaching or ceremonies: but, more often, it is an informal learning process by which the ways of doing things, thinking about things, and conceptualizing the world are assimilated as a result of living in a particular society among people who share these concepts. This process of acquiring culture is termed *enculturation.*
2. *Culture involves shared meanings:* The shared assumptions and beliefs of a culture group, learned through enculturation, makes the actions of others understandable. Culture provides guidance for what behaviors are appropriate in particular situations and allows the prediction of how others will behave. That culture is shared does not mean that particular beliefs are shared by every member of the culture group. For example, among four generations of Greek immigrants in an American city, there were generational differences in knowledge about the "evil eye."[21] This illustrates how there may be generational, as well as individual, differences in maintaining cultural beliefs. It is important to recognize that there are differences among people in a culture group, and members should not be stereotyped as being alike in all ways.

   Culture is not deterministic, and individuals in any social group manifest variations in behavior. Individuals can, in fact, behave in ways considered eccentric or deviant by others within their own group. Interestingly though, definitions of what behaviors are deviant are themselves part of the cultural meanings that are shared.
3. *Culture involves symbols:* Symbols are representations of cultural ideas. Examples of culture-specific symbols include icons, other objects associated with religion, and money. But, the primary symbols for representing shared meanings are words: It is language that allows for sharing meanings and for transmitting these shared meanings to the next generation.
4. *Culture is integrated:* Saying that culture is integrated means that various domains of the culture (e.g., politics, economics, kinship) are interrelated. For example, ideas and practices relating to illness are often inseparable from the domain of religious beliefs and practices, and illnesses may be attributed to supernatural beings or to humans with special powers.[4]

ETHNOCENTRISM AND CULTURAL RELATIVISM

The belief that one's own culture is better than that of others is termed *ethnocentrism.* An ethnocentric perspective is an expected outcome of enculturation, since all individuals learn to regard their own culture—that is, the way they conceptualize the world—as "natural," "normal," and "real." Thus, beliefs from a culture that is different seem less natural, less normal, and less real. A problem with an ethnocentric perspective is that it closes off attempts to understand culturally diverse beliefs and ways of living. On the other hand, the position of *cultural relativism* holds that each culture can be evaluated only according to its own standards of right and wrong. Although this position has been criticized as being too extreme, it encourages the understanding of behavior occurring in another culture from the viewpoint of that other culture, rather than from an ethnocentric perspective. For example, a kind of skin lesion that occasionally occurs among infants on one of the Caroline Islands is attributed by islanders to the mother's anger, which manifests itself in the child's skin lesion. An ethnocentric perspective would be to say that it is "really" an infected mosquito bite. A relativistic perspective would be to understand how the islanders' concern with prevention of such lesions leads them to treat pregnant women and new mothers with special concern so that they will not be angry or unhappy.

CULTURAL DIVERSITY

There are many variations from one culture to another. The focus here will be on the kind of cultural variability that is likely to become apparent in psychiatric mental health nursing interactions with clients and families.

Health, Illness, and Treatment

Beliefs about what states are healthy or unhealthy are, to some extent, culturally based. For example, different culture groups may or may not differentiate between mental health and physical health. An individual is also influenced by culture in terms of (1) whether mood changes and physical sensations are noticed; (2) how they are evaluated and labeled as minor symptoms, serious illness, or as trivial and irrelevant; and (3) the decisions made for course of treatment.[1]

In Haitian culture, for example, fat people are thought to be healthy and happy, whereas thin people are considered to be in poor health and prone to psychological problems.[10] Symptoms that are of particular concern to Haitian Americans are pain and weakness, and, as a means of self-diagnosis, these and other symptoms are often compared with those that have been experienced by relatives. What course of treatment an individual decides upon is partially dependent upon such factors as whether the affliction is regarded as temporary and, therefore, not in need of care beyond self-medication, or whether it is a state needing specialized care. A differentiation is made between natural illnesses, called "diseases of the Lord," and supernatural illnesses, which are thought to result from a breach of agreements with voodoo spirits. If treatment beyond home remedies is necessary, either a folk healer or a medical doctor, or both, may be utilized in treating most natural illnesses. Supernatural illnesses or lingering natural illnesses are thought to be better treated by a voodoo healer through rituals to appease specific spirits.[10]

Cultural beliefs, then, enter into the choice of practitioner, as well as expectations of how the practitioner and the sick person and perhaps the sick person's family will interact. The client who comes to a mental health clinic or hospital may previously have visited a folk practitioner or may be seeing both simultaneously (Fig. 8-1). Often the two forms of treatment vary in a number of ways. In a study comparing Puerto Rican treatment by outpatient psychotherapists and spiritist healers, there were several differences in practitioner characteristics, styles of interacting, and forms of treatment.[9] Table 8-1 shows a comparison of psychotherapy and spiritism as practiced in Puerto Rico.

Food

Cultural variation in food preferences is commonly known. But this represents more than a simple difference in choice of ingredients or style of preparation. Beliefs concerning food uses and food taboos can be strong and closely linked to cultural identity. Food brought to a client can have such symbolic meanings as

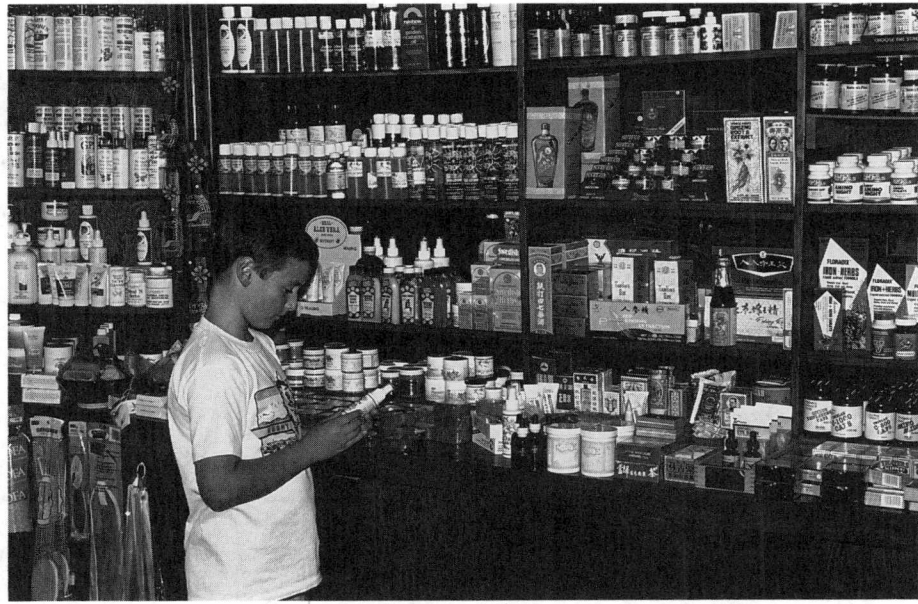

FIGURE 8–1. A client who comes to a mental health clinic or hospital may be taking herbal medicines or visiting other practitioners. (Tenzing Momo, Inc., Pike Place Market, Seattle, Washington. Courtesy of Mary Durand Thomas)

TABLE 8–1
Contrasts between psychotherapy and spiritism

ASPECT	PSYCHOTHERAPY	SPIRITISM
Diagnostic process	Screening interview	Spiritist observes patient
	Patient describes problem	Spiritist describes patient's difficulties
	Therapist listens to patient's explanations and complaints before making diagnosis	Spiritist "captures" or "receives" patient's problems into his or her body through visions
Practitioner characteristics	Therapist usually of a higher social class than patient	Spiritist usually of same social class as patient
	Therapist's role validated by education and professional status	Spiritist's role validated by special, often ecstatic, experiences
	Therapist usually viewed as authoritative, but readily cooperative and capable of misjudgment	Spiritist viewed as vehicle of divine authority, much more powerful than patient
	Therapist often a young adult man or woman (more women than men)	Spiritist usually an older woman (approximately three women to one man)
	Therapist viewed as knowledgeable, but exhibits only limited empathy	Spiritist viewed as having special knowledge of spirits and unusual empathy
	Therapist thought to be a normal, middle-class, educated person	Spiritist thought to have unusual, not normal, attributes
Treatment	Patient receives advice and/or psychotropic drugs as primary treatment as well as individual or group psychotherapy	Patient receives valuable, but not central, advice; treatment consists of personal rituals (e.g., prayers) and exorcistic rites conducted by spiritist; herbal preparations sometimes used
	Focus of therapy on adaptation and amelioration of conflict; practical solutions suggested	Changes in coping style insisted on; personal transformation of patient emphasized, possibly with goal of becoming a healer
	Therapist seldom works with family	Spiritist almost always includes near or extended family in diagnosis and treatment, at least through patient
	Therapist rarely discusses relevance of problems to general meaning of life	All treatment deals with life and cosmologic meaning

From Koss JD. Expectations and outcomes for patients given mental health care or spiritist healing in Puerto Rico. Am J Psychiatry 1987;144:56–61. Copyright 1978, The American Psychiatric Association. Reprinted with permission.

indicating caring, demonstrating interpersonal closeness, or conveying healing properties.[11]

Clients from some culture groups may classify foods according to hot and cold theory and may self-prescribe some foods on the basis of their perceptions of their condition. Foods classified as hot—which may be, but are not necessarily, hot in temperature—are used to treat illnesses classified as cold. Conversely, foods classified as cold are used to treat hot illnesses. There is variation within and between culture groups about what foods are considered hot and cold. Both indigenous and scientific medicines may also be categorized in this way.[6]

Temporal Orientations

The way in which persons conceptualize and measure time is cultural. The Western concept of time is linear wherein time is thought of as a movement from the past, through the present, toward the future, and that upward progress occurs in moving from past toward future time.[17] In contrast, some non-Westerners view time as cyclic, with the overall direction of the cycles being downward.[17] There are also cross-cultural differences concerning which time period is most emphasized. Some culture groups, for example, place greater emphasis on the present than they do the future. A community mental health center client from such a culture group, feeling better in the present, may not

keep an appointment, because concern about future relapse would be relatively unimportant. Additional examples of temporal orientation include such cultural concepts as saving time and not wasting time.

Family Relationships

The family or extended kin group of a psychiatric client may be wary of Western mental health practitioners for a number of reasons. There may be cultural beliefs concerning the untrustworthiness of anyone outside the kin group—let alone outside the culture group. Such beliefs may have been reinforced by past experiences with mental health practitioners who offered different explanations of illness. In addition, language barriers and discrimination from the dominant society may have forced the client and extended family to rely more completely on family resources. All of these factors may result in a special effort to monitor the care given their family member.

Deciding about psychiatric care, as with other kinds of decisions, may be made by family members other than the individual who is ill. In a study of psychiatric help seeking by individuals of various culture groups in Canada, it was found that Chinese families made prolonged efforts to treat a mentally disturbed individual at home before seeking outside help.[13] These efforts, which sometimes lasted as long as 20 years, involved one pragmatic trial-and-error method after another.

Because there is a range of cultural explanations for mental illness among such families, including violation of Confucian moral ethics or filial piety, imbalance of yin and yang, or breakdown of family relationships, each family member might have a different view of the most likely cause and the most appropriate treatment. Treatment methods would then become prioritized on the basis of the proponent's age, status, wisdom, sex, and ordinal position within the family. When the family's tolerance and resources were exhausted, Western medical treatment might be sought. But this was done with the family feeling that they had failed in their efforts at treatment. When the family member's illness was still problematic after discharge, the home care cycle was reactivated, with suggestions again being made and prioritized within the family.[13]

Sometimes health workers, with their own cultural beliefs in individualism, are puzzled by responsibilities clients feel toward their extended families. American Indians, for example, highly value harmonious relationships with an extensive network of kin and interact with them in numerous ways.[16] In addition, generosity and sharing are valued over personal acquisitiveness.[20]

Matheson gives an example of a highly stressed American Indian client without money to purchase gasoline to travel to a clinic appointment, but who, at the same time, is acting in a culturally appropriate way by housing a number of relatives[16] (Fig. 8-2).

Interpersonal Style of Communication

As with language differences, nonverbal communication can vary among culture groups. Direct eye contact may be interpreted in some cultures as communicating hostility or disrespect, rather than self-confidence and openness. A client's silence may indicate respect for the ideas of another, rather than lack of involvement. Differences in personal space are also culturally influenced. The distance separating two culturally different individuals who face one another may be regarded as intrusive by one and as too distant by the other.[5] It has been noted that North American nurses may be offended by Middle Eastern clients who seem to

FIGURE 8–2. American Indians highly value harmonious relationships with an extensive network of kin. (Courtesy of John Byron Thomas)

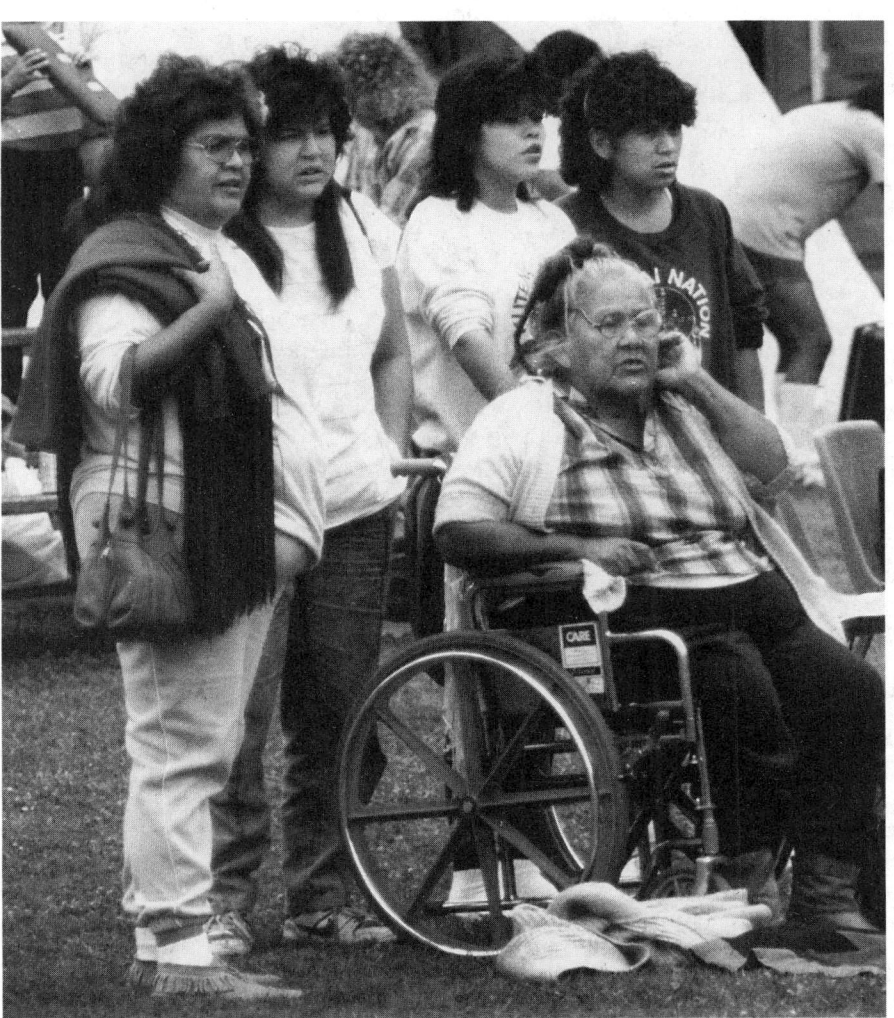

invade their privacy by standing too close and staring too intently. Conversely, the nurses, who then back away or avert their eyes, seem cold and reserved to the Middle Easterners.[14] Both the nurses and the clients are interpreting the behavior of someone with different cultural norms in terms of their own norms.

Differences in interpersonal styles of communication between black clients and non-black therapists is thought to be a partial explanation for the overdiagnosis of schizophrenia in blacks.[8] Wariness or a reluctance to express feelings to a white therapist because of past experiences may be misinterpreted as paranoia and flat affect.[8]

CULTURE AND MENTAL ILLNESS
Culture-bound Syndromes

There are episodes of deviant behavior that occur in non-Western societies that have been labeled *culture-bound syndromes*; that is, they are regarded as specific to one or a limited number of culture groups. An example is "wild man" behavior in the New Guinea Highlands.[18] There, an adult male's ability to participate in economic exchanges and to use this ability to build his personal renown is highly valued. Typically, wild man behavior occurs among young men who are politically and economically powerless to discharge a number of economic obligations such as paying back bride price. The affected man, who is said to have been bitten by a ghost or to be acting like a ghost, rushes around his community aggressively, using weapons to threaten people, stealing small objects, and destroying gardens. After a few days, he reverts to his usual behavior and claims no memory for the event. Members of his group do not blame him for the behavior, but recognize it as an indication of the need to reduce economic demands placed on him.[18]

Wild man behavior and other culture-bound syndromes typically occur in individuals who are of a particular sex or age. It has been suggested that these syndromes afflict individuals within a society who fall into relatively powerless positions because of age or sex, and who cannot live up to certain culturally valued behaviors.[15] In culture-bound syndromes, the pattern of behavior, the sanction for its occurrence, and the expected response of others all represent culturally shared meanings. Thus, the activation of such behaviors is thought to communicate to the group the problems the individual is experiencing with some cultural ideal and also prescribes the group response which, while not changing the cultural ideal, make adjustments for that individual.[15] Certain kinds of psychopathology that occur in the West—such as agoraphobia, anorexia nervosa, and kleptomania—have been analyzed as representing a similar conflict between personal predicament and public concerns.[15]

Culture-bound syndromes have also raised questions about the relevance of culture in classifications of psychiatric diseases, such as DSM-III-R, and how culture-bound syndromes ought to be considered in relation to such classifications.[7,19] Such syndromes alert psychiatric mental health practitioners to the interactive and powerful influence of culture in all psychiatric disorders.

Cultural Component in Manifestations of Illness

Even when a similar disorder occurs across cultural boundaries, the manifestations of the illness, such as the content of hallucinations and delusions, vary. For example, the client expressing concern that the FBI is communicating with him through the television set has likely had different cultural experiences than the person who believes he is in communication with tree spirits. In fact, when the psychiatric mental health nurse is unfamiliar with the range of beliefs that exist in the client's culture, there may be difficulties in distinguishing the normal experiences from the pathologic. Westermeyer suggests that hallucinations and delusions may be distinguished from cultural beliefs by the lack of agreement by other culture group members; accompanying psychological, behavioral, and social deterioration; and the presence of other psychopathologic manifestations.[25]

Cross-cultural variation has been noted in the emphasis on the physical symptoms of individuals with psychiatric disorders. For example, much higher levels of somatization have been observed in Hispanic individuals with depression or schizophrenia than in Anglos with the same diseases.[2] In another report, Korean individuals experiencing somatic symptoms characteristic of a major depressive episode (psychomotor retardation, sleep disturbances, fatigue, loss of appetite, and weight loss) considered themselves to be suffering from a physical disease characterized by an epigastric mass.[12] Culture, then, can influence the way that a psychiatric disturbance is manifested, as well as which symptoms are emphasized.

CULTURAL SENSITIVITY AND THE NURSING PROCESS

Sometimes nurses are concerned that, by recognizing cultural differences in clients, they are guilty of prejudice. However, recognizing cultural differences is part of recognizing and respecting the uniqueness of each individual. This is very different from stereotyping, which assumes that all members of a culture group are alike, an assumption that leads to dismissal of individual differences among members of the group and, in turn, to devaluing and discrimination. To recognize cultural differences without stereotyping, it is helpful to remember that culture group membership, although very important, is only one attribute of the individual. An individual, after all, comprises many attributes:

male or female, of a certain age and generation, with a unique personality and life experiences.

The psychiatric mental health nurse, to give culturally sensitive care to an individual from another culture group, can consider how culture affects the entire nursing process. As part of a general nursing assessment, the psychiatric mental health nurse collects information about the client's background such as culture group membership, religion, and language(s).[23] Given the focus of the nurse–client relationship and time constraints, the assessment may then elicit cultural information in relation to the particular client problem. Tripp-Reimer and her colleagues suggest such specific questions as: "What do you think has caused your problem?" "Why do you think it started when it did?" "What kind of treatment do you think you should receive?" "What are the chief problems your sickness has caused you?" (reference 23, p 81). After making a nursing diagnosis, cultural factors that influence interventions can be elicited with further questions such as: "What have you been doing for this problem/condition in the past and presently?" "How should a person who has this condition/problem act?" "How should one who has this condition/problem be treated by family members?" (reference 23, p 81).

In caring for culturally different clients, the psychiatric mental health nurse often intervenes as a *culture broker.* Culture brokerage involves translating, bridging, or linking the scientific health care system with clients of different cultures.[22] This can involve gaining a more comprehensive understanding of the client's perception of the disease, helping the client to understand the health care system, helping practitioners to adapt scientific methods of care into culturally appropriate ones, and to translate differing perspectives of cause, meaning, and treatment.[22]

SUMMARY

Characteristics of culture include that (1) it is learned through enculturation; (2) it involves shared meanings; (3) it involves language and other symbols; and (4) it is integrated. The belief that one's own culture is better than that of others is termed ethnocentrism. The position of cultural relativism encourages understanding behavior occurring in another culture from the viewpoint of that other culture, rather than from an ethnocentric perspective. Cross-cultural differences occur in such cultural domains as perceptions of health, illness,

Research Highlights

Ethnic minority group members have been reported to utilize mental health services less frequently than the majority group and to terminate therapy early.[3] Flaskerud, from a review of the literature, identified nine major ways in which mental health professionals have been encouraged to alter the mental health service delivery system to make it compatible with cultural expectations of Asian, Hispanic, and black American clients. These are as follows:

1. Therapists who share the culture (ethnic/racial) background of the clients
2. Therapists who share the language or language style of the clients
3. Location of the agency in the client community
4. Flexible hours and appointments
5. Provision of, or referral to, services for social, economic, legal, and medical problems
6. Use of family members in the therapy process
7. Use of a brief therapy approach
8. Use of, or referral to, clergy or to traditional healers in the treatment process
9. Involvement of consumers in determining, evaluating, and publicizing services (reference 3, pp 129–131).

Flaskerud termed these nine components a culture-compatible approach to mental health services.[3] To examine the relationship between this approach and utilization of services, she chose client records from four community mental health agencies respectively serving: principally Asian American clients; principally black American clients; principally Mexican American clients; and a mixed ethnic–racial population that was preponderantly white American. Data were collected from client records on a variety of client characteristics including whether they remained in treatment for more than four visits or whether they dropped out before that time. Interviews were held with staff and clinical directors to gather data on agency and community characteristics as a measure of the nine components of a culture-compatible approach.[3]

Flaskerud found that three components were the best predictors of dropout status: language match of therapists and clients; cultural match of therapists and clients; and agency location in the client community.[3] However, there were no significant relationships between any of the nine components of the culture-compatible approach and utilization of mental health services as measured by dropout status.[3] On the other hand, pharmacotherapy, although not originally considered a culture-compatible component, was found to be significantly related to remaining in therapy. Flaskerud noted that pharmacotherapy is congruent with the somatization of psychological disturbances and, thus, could actually be considered as a component of a culture-compatible approach.[3] She suggested that several methodologic issues may have affected the lack of significant relationships with any of the original culture-compatible components.[3] In any event, more research is needed on the important topic of making mental health services available and acceptable to culturally diverse groups.

and treatment; food; temporal orientation; family relationships; and interpersonal style of communication. The psychiatric mental health nurse, to give culturally sensitive care to an individual from another culture group, can consider how culture affects the entire nursing process. The role of culture broker involves translating, bridging, or linking the scientific health care system with the beliefs of clients of different cultures.

References

1. Angel R, Thoits P. The impact of culture on the cognitive structure of illness. Culture Med Psychiatry. 1987;11:465–494.
2. Escobar JI. Cross-cultural aspects of the somatization trait. Hosp Commun Psychiatry. 1987;38:174–180.
3. Flaskerud JH. The effects of culture-compatible intervention on the utilization of mental health services by minority clients. Commun Ment Health J. 1986;22:127–141.
4. Glick LB. Medicine as an ethnographic category: the Gimi of the New Guinea Highlands. In: Landy D, ed: Culture, disease, and healing: studies in medical anthropology. New York: Macmillan, 1977.
5. Hall E. The hidden dimension. New York: Doubleday, 1959.
6. Harwood A, ed. Ethnicity and medical care. Cambridge: Harvard University Press; 1981.
7. Hughes CC. Culture-bound or construct-bound? The syndromes and DSM-III. In: Simons RC, Hughes CC, eds: The culture-bound syndromes: folk illnesses of psychiatric and anthropological interest. Boston: D. Reidel Publishing; 1985.
8. Jones BE, Gray BA. Problems in diagnosing schizophrenia and affective disorders among blacks. Hosp Commun Psychiatry. 1986;37:61–65.
9. Koss JD. Expectations and outcomes for patients given mental health care or spiritist healing in Puerto Rico. Am J Psychiatry. 1987;144:56–61.
10. Laguerre MS. Haitian Americans. In: Harwood A, ed. Ethnicity and medical care. Cambridge: Harvard University Press; 1981.
11. Leininger MM. Transcultural eating patterns and nutrition: transcultural nursing and anthropological perspectives. Holistic Nurs Pract. 1988;3:16–25.
12. Lin KM. Hwa-Byung: A Korean culture-bound syndrome? Am J Psychiatry. 1983;140:105–107.
13. Lin TL, Lin MC. Service delivery issues in Asian–North American communities. Am J Psychiatry. 1978;135:454–456.
14. Lipson JG, Meleis AI. Culturally appropriate care: the case of immigrants. Top Clin Nurs. 1985;7(3):48–56.
15. Littlewood R, Lipsedge M. The butterfly and the serpent: culture, psychopathology and biomedicine. Culture Med Psychiatry. 1987;11:289–335.
16. Matheson L. If you are not an Indian, how do you treat an Indian? In: Lefley HP, Pedersen PB, eds. Cross-cultural training for mental health professionals. Springfield, IL: Charles C Thomas; 1986.
17. Melges FT. Time and the inner future: a temporal approach to psychiatric disorders. New York: John Wiley & Sons; 1982.
18. Newman PL. "Wild man" behavior in a New Guinea Highlands community. Am Anthropol. 1964;66:1–19.
19. Prince R, Tcheng-Laroche F. Culture-bound syndromes and international disease classifications. Culture Med Psychiatry. 1987;11:3–19.
20. Trimble JE. Value differentials and their importance in counseling American Indians. In: Pedersen PP, Draguns JG, Lonner WJ, Trimble JE, eds. Counseling across cultures, rev ed. Honolulu: University of Hawaii Press; 1981.
21. Tripp-Reimer T. Retention of a folk healing practice (matiasma) among four generations of urban Greek immigrants. Nurs Res. 1983;32:97–101.
22. Tripp-Reimer T, Brink PJ. Cultural brokerage. In: Bulechek GM, McCloskey JC, eds. Nursing interventions: treatments for nursing diagnoses. Philadelphia: WB Saunders; 1985.
23. Tripp-Reimer T, Brink PJ, Saunders JM. Cultural assessment: Content and process. Nurs Outlook. 1984;32(2):78–82.
24. Tylor EB. Primitive culture: researches into the development of mythology, philosophy, religion, language, art and customs. London: J Murray; 1871.
25. Westermeyer J. Cultural factors in clinical assessment. J Consult Clin Psychol. 1987;55:471–478.

Patricia A. Betrus

Neurobiology of Mental Disorders

CONCEPTS FROM NEUROSCIENCE
Cells of the Brain
Synaptic Transmission
Brain Structures
MOOD DISORDERS
Monoamine Theories
   Catecholamine Depletion Theory
   Catecholamine Theory
   Role of Other Neurotransmitters
   Issues with Neurotransmitter Depletion Theories
   Monoamine Depletion Theory Revised
Sleep and Circadian Theories
Biologic Markers for Affective Disorders
   Dexamethasone Suppression Test
   Thyroid-Releasing Hormone Challenge Test
THOUGHT DISORDERS
Dopamine Theory of Schizophrenia
Relationship of Cerebral Atrophy to Negative-Symptom
   Schizophrenia
ORGANIC MENTAL DISORDERS
IMPLICATIONS FOR NURSING RESEARCH AND PRACTICE

OBJECTIVES
After reading this chapter, the reader will be able to:
1. Describe the anatomic structures and biochemical processes relevant to normal brain functioning
2. Identify how alterations in brain functions can influence the development and progression of mental disorders
3. Describe the mechanisms underlying psychopharmacologic interventions for mental disorders.

INTRODUCTION

Investigation into neurobiologic bases of mental disorders is an attempt to explain in biologic terms the behavior of individuals experiencing psychiatric disorders. Scientists are investigating various physiologic and chemical processes in the brain to develop models of mental disorders. Clinicians can use this information in considering psychopharmacologic and somatic interventions with psychiatric clients. Before discussing the neurobiology of psychiatric disabilities, important concepts of basic neuroscience will be reviewed to facilitate an understanding of the complex interactions between brain processes and mental disorders.

CONCEPTS FROM NEUROSCIENCE

Cells of the Brain

The human brain is made up of billions of cells. At birth, the immature human brain contains principally glial cells and neural cells, called neurons. By approxi-

mately 12 years of age the human brain has completed its development. Neurons constitute approximately half the total volume of the brain; the second half is composed of glial or support cells. Glial cells perform several functions for the neurons of the brain, including structural support, insulating neurons from each other, supplying the chemicals neurons need to exchange messages with other neurons, storing and providing the nutrients necessary for survival of the neuron and, finally, providing a housekeeping activity by destroying and removing neurons that are injured or deteriorate from age.

Neurons, the functional cells of the brain, are the information-processing and transmitting component of the human brain (Fig. 9–1). Neurons are composed of several distinct parts. The *soma* or cell body, surrounded by a membrane, contains structures that are responsible for nutrition, transport, genetic information, and the basic proteins or enzymes necessary for the creation of transmitter substances. Attached to the soma of the neuron are *dendrites*, that look like spiny tree limbs. Messages passing from one neuron to another are transmitted to the dendrites. Dendrites are

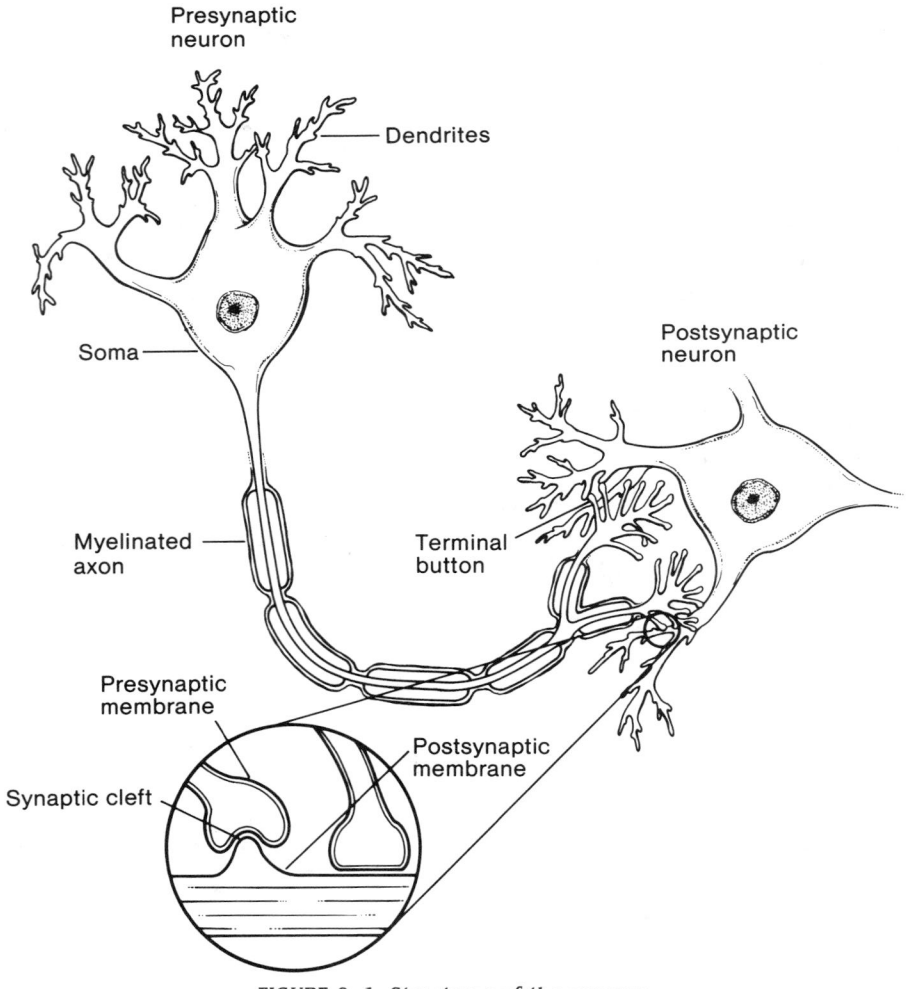

FIGURE 9–1. Structures of the synapse.

principally responsible for receiving information from other neurons.

Also attached to the soma are *axons*, long thin tubes that carry information from the soma of the neuron to little knobs at the end of the neuron called *terminal buttons*. Axons contain internal microtubules that transport chemicals to the terminal buttons. Axons also carry messages from the cell body to the terminal button, which is electrical by nature. The axon is covered by a layer, called *myelin*, that speeds the transmission of the electrical information. When a message, carried from the cell body by the axon, arrives at the terminal button, a chemical, called the *transmitter substance,* is secreted. The transmitter substance travels across a space between the terminal button and a nearby receiving neuron. The terminal button, the space between the neurons, and the receiving area of the next neuron, are collectively referred to as a *synapse*. The chemical information either excites or inhibits the receiving cell and helps determine the message that the subsequent cell will propagate.

Synaptic Transmission

Information is passed from one neuron to another in only one direction at the synapse. The membrane of the terminal button is referred to as the *presynaptic membrane,* and the membrane of the receiving neuron is called the *postsynaptic membrane.* The space between the two cells is called the *synaptic cleft.* The transmitter substance, secreted by the presynaptic cell, is synthesized by catalytic enzymes from amino acids (and choline, for acetylcholine) in the soma of the neuron. Many transmitter substances are then packaged in vesicles and travel from the soma to the terminal button through a tube system in the axon. When such a substance arrives in the terminal button, the vesicles bind with the presynaptic membrane, open up, and expel the transmitter substance into the synaptic cleft. The transmitter substance travels across the synaptic cleft and, if it is appropriate, binds with receptors on the postsynaptic membrane, thereby activating the postsynaptic cell.

There are several types of substances that can act as transmitter substances in the central nervous system

---

BOX 9–1
Synthesis Patterns of Neurotransmitters

ACETYLCHOLINE

Acetyl-CoA + Choline $\longrightarrow$ Acetylcholine
Choline acetyltransferase

DOPAMINE

Tyrosine $\longrightarrow$ L-Dopa $\longrightarrow$ Dopamine
Tyrosine hydroxylase   Dopa decarboxylase

NOREPINEPHRINE
Same path as to dopamine then:

Dopamine $\longrightarrow$ Norepinephrine
Dopamine β-hydroxylase

SEROTONIN

Tryptophan $\longrightarrow$ 5-Hydroxytryptophan $\longrightarrow$ Serotonin
Tryptophan hydroxylase   5-HPT decarboxylase

γ-AMINOBUTYRIC ACID

Glutamic acid $\longrightarrow$ γ-Aminobutyric acid
Glutamic acid decarboxylase

(CNS). The classifications and a partial list of transmitter substances are displayed in Table 9–1.

The discussion of the neural bases of mental disorders will focus principally on the transmitter substances acetylcholine (ACh), norepinephrine (NE), dopamine, serotonin, and γ-aminobutyric acid (GABA) because scientists have presented the most information pertaining to their effects in the CNS in relation to mental disorders. However, as can be seen from the partial list of transmitter substances included in Table 9-1, there are many other substances that could have as yet undiscovered roles in neural effects on mental disorders.

Important to understanding the neural role in mental disorders is an understanding of transmitter synthesis and synaptic effects in the brain. Box 9-1 outlines the synthesis patterns of the four major neural transmitters (NT).

Critical events occurring during synthesis can either increase or decrease the availability of transmitter substance. Chemicals that increase or facilitate activation at the postsynaptic membrane are called *agonists;* conversely, chemicals that decrease or block postsynaptic events are called *antagonists.* There are two processes that influence the amount of transmitter substance created during synthesis. The first event is the availability of the precursor substance in the CNS. The precursors of transmitter substances are the amino acids and choline that cross the blood–brain barrier. Increasing or decreasing dietary intake of these amino acids can change their availability in the CNS for the production of transmitter substances. The second event that can change the amount of transmitter substance is interference with the enzymes that convert the precursors to transmitters. There are specific chemicals that block the effects of synaptic enzymes; when this happens less transmitter can be produced.

There are certain chemicals (antagonists) that can

TABLE 9–1
Major categories of transmitter substances*

MONOAMINES	AMINO ACIDS	PEPTIDES
CATECHOLAMINES Norepinephrine Dopamine **INDOLAMINES** Serotonin Melatonin	Aspartic acid Taurine Glutamic acid Glycine γ-Aminobutyric acid	Substance P Endorphins Enkephalin Somatostatin Cholecystokinin Bombesin

* Acetylcholine is a transmitter substance that does not fit any of the established categories.

make the synaptic vesicle membrane "leaky." When this occurs the transmitter substance leaks out into the cytoplasm. Chemical antagonists that are contained in the cytoplasm can degrade the transmitter substance. The end result is a decrease of transmitter substance available to be released from the presynaptic cell.

Several events can change the availability of transmitter substance or its ability to bind to the postsynaptic cell. Some chemicals (agonists) speed up the release of transmitter substance from the presynaptic membrane; similarly, others (antagonists) block and slow down the release of the transmitter substance. Antagonists at the postsynaptic receptor sites can bind to the receptors (blocking them), but not cause activation of the postsynaptic membrane. Other chemicals (agonists), which are similar to the transmitter substance when present in the synaptic cleft, can bind and cause activation of the postsynaptic cell.

Finally, after the transmitter substance has left the receptor site, it remains in the synaptic cleft until it is broken down by the specific antagonists present in the synaptic cleft. Certain agonists block the effects of the degradation chemicals. This keeps the transmitter substance in the synaptic cleft where it has the ability to rebind with receptor sites. Understanding the role of agonists and antagonists is crucial to comprehension of the complex theories of mental disorders and to an understanding of how many of the psychoactive drugs work. Table 9-2 summarizes alterations in synaptic transmission.

Brain Structures

The major divisions of the brain and associated structures are presented in Table 9-3.

TABLE 9–2
Overview of alterations in synaptic transmission

PROCESS	ALTERATIONS	NET EFFECT
Precursor availability	Increase	Agonistic
	Decrease	Antagonistic
Catalytic enzymes	Chemicals that block effects of catalytic enzymes	Antagonistic
Synaptic vesicle	Chemicals increase membrane permeability	Antagonistic
Presynaptic membrane	Chemicals increase expelling of NT to cleft	Agonistic
	Chemicals slow down or block expelling of NT	Antagonistic
Receptor sites	Chemicals bind, but do not cause activation	Antagonistic
	Chemicals bind and cause activation	Agonistic
Breakdown of neurotransmitters	Chemicals that cause breakdown	Antagonistic
	Chemicals that block the breakdown process	Agonistic
Reuptake	Chemicals speed reuptake	Antagonistic
	Chemicals slow down reuptake	Agonistic

TABLE 9–3
Divisions of the brain important for psychiatric nursing

DIVISION	STRUCTURES	COMPONENTS
Telencephalon	Cerebral cortex	Frontal lobe Parietal lobe Temporal lobe Occipital lobe
	Basal ganglia	Caudate Putamen Globus pallidus
	Limbic system	Amygdala Fornix Mammillary body Hippocampus Nucleus accumbens Stria terminalis
Diencephalon	Thalamus Hypothalamus	Suprachiasmic nucleus
Mesencephalon	Tectum Tegmentum	
Metencephalon	Cerebellum Pons	Raphe nuclei Locus coeruleus Substantia nigra
Myelencephalon	Medulla oblongata	

The brain is completely surrounded by cerebral spinal fluid (CSF), allowing it to float within the skull. After transmitter substances are broken down, either the end products (metabolites) are carried into the CSF and removed from the CNS, or the end products are taken back into the presynaptic cell and reused in the synaptic synthesis process.

The information so far elaborated has been a brief review of neuroscience necessary to aid understanding of the neural events related to the mental disorders. Only information relative to understanding mental disorders has been presented. For those who desire a more detailed knowledge of neuroscience, *The Physiology of Behavior* by Carlson[12] or *The Principles of Neuroscience* by Kandal and Schwartz[36] may be consulted.

MOOD DISORDERS

Mood disorders, previously termed "affective disorders," are mental disorders in which the prominent aspect is a disturbance of affect, mood, or feelings.[33] Individuals with mood disorders also can display dysfunctions in physiologic systems such as arousal, food intake, reproduction, circadian rhythms, and pituitary regulation.

Monoamine Theories

The neurobiologic theories generated to describe depression suggest a functional deficiency in monoamines, generally a deficiency in norepinephrine or serotonin or both.[27,32] The first evidence to suggest a neurotransmitter deficiency came from the treatment of hypertension with a drug in the 1950s. Reserpine, a drug used to control hypertension, when given to non-depressive persons, produced a side effect of depression in approximately 15% of the individuals.[10,49] It was soon established that reserpine triggers the membrane of the synaptic vesicles, which carry transmitter substance to the terminal button, to become leaky. When the transmitter substance is leaked into the cellular cytoplasm, it is unprotected and can be degraded by monoamine oxidase (see Table 9-2 for effects of degradation). The end result of this process is to reduce the amount of transmitter substance available. This process occurs in both norepinephrinergic and serotoninergic neurons.

Confirmatory evidence was provided by individuals who were taking a drug called Iproniazid for tuberculosis. It was noted that some depressed tuberculosis patients experienced mood elevations when treated with Iproniazid. Iproniazid, the first monoamine oxidase inhibitor (MAOI) used for depression, was found to be effective.[22,27] Monoamine oxidase inhibitors act by increasing the amount of serotonin and norepinephrine in the brain by blocking the degradation in the synaptic cleft of these transmitters by monoamine oxidase. Thus, MAOIs act as agonists at the synapse.

Monoamine oxidase inhibitors were the first class of drugs to be used to treat depressive disorders. However, they were not effective for all depressions and have some serious side effects and adverse reactions. Soon a class of drugs, tricyclics, that have a different effect on the synapse, was discovered. The effect of tricyclic drugs is to block the reuptake of the transmitter substance into the presynaptic cell. When this occurs, the transmitter substance remains in the synaptic cleft with an increased ability to bind with the postsynaptic receptors. Thus, as with the MAOIs, the net effect is agonistic. If depression is responsive to these categories of drugs that increase the amount of transmitter substances, specifically norepinephrine and serotonin, then support is provided for the monoamine depletion theories.[1,32]

CATECHOLAMINE DEPLETION THEORY

The monoamine theory became narrowed to emphasize principally norepinephrine as the disordered system. The principal site of synthesis for norepinephrine is in the locus coeruleus, located in the midpontine region of the brain. The locus coeruleus is associated with normal functions such as sleep, arousal, and response to the environment. Dense networks of fibers arise from this structure and send projections to the hypothalamus, hippocampus, and cortical areas. Evidence to support the specific catecholamine depletion theory is related to the low norepinephrine metabolite levels found in the urine, plasma, and CSF of depressed individuals.[49,50] 3-Methoxy-4-hydroxyphenylglycol (MHPG) is the metabolite of norepinephrine that has been suggested to be at lower levels in depressed persons. Depressed persons who have low levels of MHPG

before agonistic drug treatment (with tricyclics or MAOIs) show a return to normal levels of MHPG after clinical mood states have returned to normal.[42] Persons who have low levels of MHPG respond well to treatment with desipramine; in contrast, persons who are depressed, but do not have low MHPG levels, do not respond well to treatment with desipramine. Imipramine is a drug that has potent reuptake-blocking effects.[28,42]

Further evidence in support of the catecholamine depletion theory occurs from the improvement in mood of some depressed clients for whom amphetamines are prescribed. Amphetamine is an agonist at the presynaptic membrane. The action of amphetamines is to increase the release of catecholamines from the terminal buttons and, to some extent, slow the reuptake of the transmitter substance into the presynaptic membrane. Thus, the net effect of amphetamine administration is to increase the total amount of transmitter substance available to the postsynaptic cell.

CATECHOLAMINE THEORY

The chemical L-3,4-dihydroxyphenylalanine (L-dopa) is a precursor to the synthesis of norepinephrine. It is capable of crossing the blood–brain barrier and gaining entrance into the CNS. Thus, if the catecholamine depletion theory is credible, then administration of L-dopa should relieve the symptoms of depression. However, this does not occur, even in large doses.[46]

The administration of L-dopa has been found to precipitate hypomania or mania in individuals with bipolar disorder (in which manic episodes alternate with depressive episodes). Furthermore, MHPG levels are elevated in some individuals in the manic phase of the bipolar disorder.[11] As a consequence, the catecholamine depletion theory was modified to the catecholamine theory, which states that depression is a result of reduced norepinephrine, and mania is a result of an increased level of norepinephrine. A review of evidence for the catecholamine theory raised many unanswered questions. The evidence of low norepinephrine levels could be substantiated in only a limited number of depressed individuals.[1]

ROLE OF OTHER NEUROTRANSMITTERS

A number of other neurotransmitters were investigated for their relationship to depression. However, investigation of alterations in other neurochemical transmitters confused the picture even more by presenting contradictory results.

Decreased serotonin levels were investigated as a determinant in depression. Interest in serotonin was generated because the effects of MAOIs and selected tricyclics at the serotoninergic synapses is analogous to norepinephrine.[32] The major nuclei in which serotonin is found are the nuclei raphae of the medulla. These nuclei are associated with sleep–wake cycles and, through their connections to the hypothalamus, with libido, food intake, and pituitary hormone secretion. They are located in the hindbrain at midpontine level and send projections to the hypothalamus, hippo-campus, cingulate lobe, and the septal area. Reduced levels of serotonin, as measured by its metabolite 5-hydroxyindoleacetic acid (5-HIAA), were found in the urine, plasma, and cerebral spinal fluid of some depressed individuals.[57,58] L-Tryptophan, a precursor to serotonin, can potentiate the therapeutic effects of MAOIs. 5-Hydroxytryptophan (5-HT), the immediate precursor to serotonin, has been found to exhibit antidepressant effects for selected depressed individuals. Imipramine, which is a very potent reuptake blocker for serotonin compared with norepinephrine, is effective for depressions in which serotonin levels are reduced.[6] The behavioral correlates that seem to be present with the subtypes of depression, serotoninergic or norepinephrinergic, are activation (agitated) or lethargy (retarded), respectively.

The other neurotransmitter that has some supportive evidence for its role in depression is γ-aminobutyric acid (GABA). The principal role of GABA in the CNS is inhibitory; it restrains the firing of the locus coeruleus.[5] Low levels of GABA have been found in the plasma and CSF of depressed individuals.[7,25] In preliminary studies, progabide, a GABA agonist, has been shown to have antidepressant effects.[43]

ISSUES WITH NEUROTRANSMITTER DEPLETION THEORIES

Although the foregoing picture is confusing and complex, there appears to be substantial psychopharmacologic and biochemical evidence to support neurotransmitter depletion theories. However, there are several issues involved in depletion theory to be clarified. Sachar has identified the following as critical issues:[46]

1. Most studies have evaluated changes in the concentration of monoamines by assay of their metabolites. However, it is difficult to relate brain levels of these transmitters to levels of their metabolites in the urine, plasma, or CSF. The decrease of the metabolite could result from a variety of causes, including decreased synthesis of the transmitter, decreased release, or increased degradation, or a combination of any of these factors. It is also difficult to separate the percentage contribution of brain metabolite to peripheral metabolite in urine and plasma measurements.
2. The nuclei implicated in mood disorders are in a small area of the brain. Alterations of neurochemicals in these small areas are difficult to assess from general transmitter metabolism. The studies that measure metabolites involve combined metabolites from all areas of the brain.
3. Perhaps the most serious critique of the depletion theory comes from clinical evidence. Tricyclics, which are very effective in the treatment of depressive disorders, cross the blood–brain barrier and have an *immediate* effect by blocking the reuptake of neurotransmitters. However, the clinical response to these drugs occurs from two to four weeks after treatment begins. Furthermore, tricy-

clic drugs vary in their abilities to block neurotransmitter reuptake. Because some tricyclics have a greater ability to enhance the neurotransmitters' availability to the receptors, those tricyclics should then produce greater results, yet their efficacy is approximately the same as that of others if therapeutic blood concentrations are achieved.

A final problem with the current research in mood disorders is the focus on only one transmitter substance as a causative factor. Most structures in the brain contain several types of neurons that secrete different transmitter substances. Furthermore, structures that contain primarily one type of transmitter substance have direct neural connections with other areas of the brain and influence by inhibition or excitation these secondary areas. These areas interact and integrate with each other to influence actions. The changes in secretion of one transmitter substance may have direct effects on other transmitter substances in the same brain structure or in other brain structures. For example, dopamine and acetylcholine (ACh) have an interactive effect in the substantia nigra. Changes in dopamine (either increases or decreases) subsequently produce changes in ACh levels (either increase or decrease). Given these integrative relationships, the relationship of mood disorders to brain transmitter substances may actually reflect not the changes in the identified transmitter substance, but those in a related transmitter. This can happen either in the same structure or in a structure in which the first transmitter substance has an inhibitory or excitatory effect. For these reasons, scientists have continued to search for explanations.

MONOAMINE DEPLETION THEORY REVISED

Reexamination of the biochemical processes has led scientists to speculate on a new theory for the neurobiologic basis of affective disorders. The theory originates from the awareness that antidepressants have effects on parts of the synapse other than just as reuptake blockers. Antidepressants, as well as electroconvulsive therapy, can reduce the sensitivity of β-adrenergic receptors. This reduction of receptor sensitivity has been called *down regulation*. The antidepressants produce down regulation of these postsynaptic receptors. The down regulation also reduces the activity of norepinephrine-stimulated adenylate cyclase.[46] Similarly, antidepressants can also decrease the sensitivity of specific serotonin receptors by down regulation.

An associated effect of the long-term administration of tricyclic drugs is that this administration causes a decrease in the number of presynaptic receptors. The receptors on the presynaptic membrane, called autoreceptors, normally inhibit the release of transmitters from the presynaptic cell (they function as a negative-feedback control system).[12] Thus, down regulation of the presynaptic autoreceptors would enhance synaptic function. The process of down regulation, whether it occurs in the presynaptic autoreceptors or postsynaptic receptors, takes approximately the same amount of time as is required for the therapeutic effects of antidepressants. It has been speculated that the predominant effect of tricyclics is on presynaptic receptors, and this action is responsible for their therapeutic response.

Sleep and Circadian Theories

Individuals experiencing affective disorders exhibit specific changes in the architecture of sleep. Healthy individuals spend approximately ten minutes falling asleep (sleep latency), and sleep is divided into phases of rapid-eye-movement (REM) and non-REM sleep (stages 1 to 4). When young adults fall asleep, they begin at stage 1 and progress to stage 4. The first REM period, lasting only a few minutes, usually begins in approximately 60 minutes (REM latency). The first third of the night non-REM sleep dominates, after which REM periods become more frequent and last longer, dominating the last hours of sleep. The sleep–wake (rest–activity) cycle follows the cycle of light–darkness and is controlled by a weak oscillator (biologic clock).

The sleep abnormalities exhibited in depression are prolonged sleep latency, increased wakefulness, decreased arousal thresholds, and early-morning awakenings.[18,26] Specific changes in REM sleep are shorter REM latency and REM sleep that dominates the first half of sleep, rather than the second.[24,39,41] When affective disorders are treated with tricyclics or MAOIs, the effect on sleep is to restore a normal pattern of REM sleep or to reduce the frequency and intensity of REM sleep.[35,40]

The brain contains several oscillators (biologic clocks), each of which is associated with a circadian rhythm for a specific physiologic function. The sleep–wake cycle is a weak oscillator compared with core temperature and adrenocorticotropic hormone (ACTH; the pituitary hormone that controls secretion of cortisol from the adrenal cortex) which are strong oscillators. The circadian theory of depression suggests that the oscillator for temperature, cortisol, and REM sleep (strong oscillator) is advanced compared with the sleep–wake oscillator (weak oscillator). It has been suggested that the phase advance of the strong oscillator may be a component of the pathophysiologic process in affective disorders.[59] The phase advance of the strong oscillator pulls the sleep–wake cycle (weak oscillator) so that the time of awakening is advanced, resulting in early-morning awakening.[21] This presses REM sleep forward into the first half of the night, a consistent pattern in affective disorders. Changing the phase relationship of REM sleep by phase advancing sleep (i.e., sleep onset at 5 PM and waking at 2 AM) brings the oscillators back in synchrony and produces a remission in depression.[60] Additional evidence in support of the phase-advance theory is the affect of MAOIs, which tend to delay the phase advance of circadian rhythms.[62] These theories are in their formative phase, but show great potential for the understanding of affective disorders.

Biologic Markers for Affective Disorders

The neurobiologic theories of affective disorder support a disruption of the neurotransmitters (either by blockade or receptor changes) in nuclei that are associated by direct neural links with the hypothalamus. In fact, the hypothalamus receives neural input (either direct or indirect) from almost all regions of the brain. Changes in neurotransmitter patterns in a variety of brain areas alter neurotransmitter patterns in the hypothalamus.

The hypothalamus exerts direct control of the anterior pituitary by a process known as *neuroendocrine transduction*. In this process electrical signals determine the secretion patterns of hypothalamic neurotransmitters that stimulate specialized hypothalamic cells to secrete releasing or inhibiting factors. These factors (hormones) travel by a portal system (in the blood) to determine the release patterns of anterior pituitary hormones.[29] Thus, changes in the neurotransmitters in the hypothalamus, as evident in individuals with affective disorders, should exhibit changes in the hormonal secretion patterns from the pituitary.

Alteration in cortisol production was the first disrupted hormonal pattern to be studied. It was known that acutely depressed individuals showed extremely elevated levels of circulating cortisol.

Cortisol, a glucocorticoid, is secreted by the adrenal cortex and regulated by the hypothalamic–pituitary–adrenal axis. ACTH, released from the pituitary, is the major regulator of cortisol production. The release of ACTH is controlled by corticotropin-releasing factor (CRF) from specialized neural cells in the hypothalamus. The secretion of CRF is stimulated by serotonin and acetylcholine and inhibited by norepinephrine (Box 9-2).

ACTH is secreted from the pituitary in bursts. The lowest levels of ACTH are secreted in the late evening and the highest levels occur in the early morning, just after awakening. There are eight to nine secretory bursts during the day, for a total of approximately 16 mg of cortisol released per day. Feedback loops, to the pituitary and hypothalamus, exist to regulate the release of ACTH and, subsequently, cortisol.

Individuals experiencing affective disorders evidence increased levels of cortisol as measured in the plasma, CSF, and urine.[14–17] The elevated levels of cortisol secretion were evident in both unipolar and bipolar depressives.[14,16,17] The secretion pattern is shifted, with the greatest increase occurring from 6 to 8 AM. In addition to elevated cortisol levels, individuals also had a flattened curve with loss of its normal circadian pattern.[47]

DEXAMETHASONE SUPPRESSION TEST

Dexamethasone is a synthetic glucocorticoid that exerts negative-feedback to the pituitary and hypothalamus. Dexamethasone has the effect of turning off the secretion of ACTH and, subsequently, cortisol. In nor-

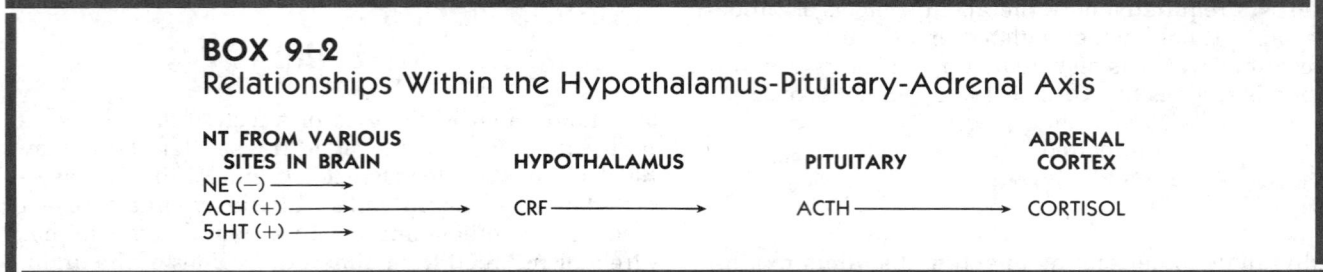

BOX 9–2
Relationships Within the Hypothalamus-Pituitary-Adrenal Axis

NT FROM VARIOUS SITES IN BRAIN	HYPOTHALAMUS	PITUITARY	ADRENAL CORTEX
NE (−) ⟶			
ACH (+) ⟶ ⟶ ⟶	CRF ⟶	ACTH ⟶	CORTISOL
5-HT (+) ⟶			

mal persons, a 1-mg dose of dexamethasone given at 11 PM reduces cortisol levels to less than 5 μg/dL for the next 24 hours. In depressives, the suppression effect of dexamethasone does not occur. The nonsuppression of cortisol is called a positive dexamethasone test. The most general pattern of nonsuppression is early escape, that is, depressed individuals suppress cortisol normally in the morning but escape from suppression later in the day.[14–17] Thus, the dexamethasone suppression test (DST) was the first biologic marker for affective disorder.

Although DST is used as a biologic marker for mood disorders, it does not identify all depressed individuals. It identifies only approximately 50% (sensitivity) of individuals with clinical diagnoses of depression.[8,48,55] Another consideration of how well a test identifies a subgroup is its specificity; that is, how well the test discriminates one type of disorder from another. The DST is highly specific for melancholia and does not exhibit nonsuppression for other diagnoses such as schizophrenia.[14,16,17]

Given that only 50% of depressed persons respond with nonsuppression, the use of DST clinically as a biologic marker is limited. A positive DST result is confirmatory of depression. However, a negative DST result does not rule out the diagnosis of major depression. Furthermore, studies suggest a positive correlation between the severity of depression with the rate of DST nonsuppression. There is also a correlation between the DST nonsuppression index and suicide risk.[19]

Finally, individuals identified as nonsuppressors, when tested before antidepressive medication treatment, return to a normal suppression pattern when the treatment is successful. Individuals who do not show the reversal effect subsequent to treatment (i.e., remain nonsuppressors) are at increased risk of timely relapse.[9,23]

THYROID-RELEASING HORMONE CHALLENGE TEST

The thyroid gland link to the CNS is known as the hypothalamic–pituitary–thyroid (HPT) axis. The hypothalamus releases thyroid-releasing hormone (TRH) from specialized neurons, which stimulate the pituitary cells to release thyroid-stimulating hormone (TSH) into the blood. The TSH, in turn, stimulates the release of thyroxine (T_4) and triiodothyronine (T_3) from the thyroid gland. Release of TRH is facilitated by dopamine and norepinephrine and is inhibited by serotonin. The levels of TSH have a circadian rhythm, with the highest levels of secretion from 4 AM to 8 AM.

The symptoms of hypothyroidism, particularly changes in weight, are evident in some individuals who are depressed. A TRH test is used to determine if the HPT axis is functioning normally. This test has been adapted as a biologic marker for depression. Individuals fast overnight and, in the morning, an indwelling catheter is put in place. Baseline levels of TSH are measured. A 500-mg bolus of synthetic TRH is infused. The TSH blood levels are measured at 15, 30, 60, and 90 minutes. The baseline level of TSH is subtracted from the subsequent level and a ΔTSH is obtained.[38] In normal persons, the ΔTSH level is 7 to 15 IU/mL. In depressives, there is a blunted response of TSH to the TRH challenge.[31,37,56] The blunted TRH challenge is 85% specific to unipolar depression, with a sensitivity of approximately 40%.[54]

Indications for clinical use of the TRH challenge test are similar to those for DST. A positive test result is confirmatory for the diagnosis of major depression, but a negative test result does not eliminate the diagnosis. However, the use of the two tests together, DST and TRH, yields an increased sensitivity of 84%.[25]

THOUGHT DISORDERS

Thought disorders are mental disorders in which the process of cognition (self-awareness, self-perception) is disrupted. Schizophrenia, the primary thought disorder, is characterized in the acute phase by loss of reality testing, profound misinterpretation of perception, or markedly aberrant beliefs. Individuals with schizophrenia may also exhibit bizarre behavior, unusual postures, mannerisms, or rigidity.

It has been suggested that there are two subtypes of schizophrenia based on the relative preponderance of symptoms and neurobiologic evidence. Positive-symptom schizophrenia (the most common form) is dominated by hallucinations, delusions, and bizarre or disorganized behavior. Individuals with a preponderance of positive symptoms tend to respond well to antipsychotic medication. The pattern of positive-symptom schizophrenia is that individuals function fairly well before their first psychotic episode and improve to pre-morbid levels of functioning after psychotic episodes.[2-4]

In contrast, negative-symptom schizophrenia is characterized by absence of functioning in a number of areas: poverty of speech, flattened affect, poor social adjustment, and impaired attention. Schizophrenia in which negative symptoms dominate responds poorly to antipsychotic medication and has a poorer prognosis.[3,4]

Dopamine Theory of Schizophrenia

The most prominent neurobiologic theory of schizophrenia is an excess secretion of dopamine in specific areas of the brain.[13,52] Evidence for this theory comes from a knowledge of the effects of neuroleptic drugs in reducing dopamine transmission. The first suggested mechanism of action is receptor blockade. Antipsychotic drugs are capable of binding to dopamine receptor sites, but do not cause activation of the postsynaptic cell. By binding to receptors, antipsychotic drugs prevent dopamine from occupying receptors and, thereby, decrease the action of endogenous dopamine. Moreover, the potency of antipsychotic drugs in binding to dopamine receptors closely approximates the relative therapeutic potency of these drugs.[52]

There are two types of dopamine receptors. One type, D1, activates adenylate cyclase (the enzyme that converts ATP to cyclic AMP) in the postsynaptic cell. This receptor has a low attraction for most antipsychotic drugs. The second type of receptor, D2, located on the postsynaptic membrane, inhibits adenylate cyclase. The D2 receptor possesses a high attraction for antipsychotic drugs. This is the site at which, it is believed, antipsychotic drugs work.[53] Dopamine synapses also possess autoreceptors on the presynaptic membranes. These autoreceptors act by inhibitory feedback to regulate dopamine transmission. Antipsychotic drugs are believed to stimulate these autoreceptors.[20]

Dopaminergic agonists (drugs that can bind at dopamine receptors and cause activation), such as L-dopa, amphetamines, and cocaine, cause a syndrome of behavior similar to schizophrenia. In fact, acute amphetamine psychosis is behaviorally similar to paranoid schizophrenia and has been used as a model for study of this disorder. Furthermore, antipsychotic medications act as antidotes for these behaviorally similar disorders.[61]

Final evidence for the dopamine excess theory is provided by a study of pituitary prolactin. Dopamine is the major transmitter inhibiting prolactin secretion by D2 receptors. If antipsychotic drugs act by reducing the transmission of dopamine, they then should also have an effect of increasing secretion of prolactin from the pituitary. This result, an increase secretion in prolactin, occurs when antipsychotic medications are given.[51]

The location of increased dopamine secretion is believed to be the mesolimbic dopaminergic system.[20] Dopamine cell bodies arise in the tegmental area and the substantia nigra. The axons project to the limbic system, specifically to the nucleus accumbens, stria terminalis, and amygdala, and in general to the cortex. Interest has focused on the nucleus accumbens because it has been postulated to act as a gate or filter for information concerned with affect and with certain types of memory projections from the hippocampus, hypothalamus, and frontal cortex.[20] Disregulation in this system could be seen as a basis for psychosis, delusions, and other thought disorders associated with schizophrenia.

Conceptually, the problems with the dopamine excess theory is that it is difficult to define the mechanisms of causation principally from the actions of antipsychotic medications.[13] It may be that the pharmacologic interventions produced the changes in interaction with the disease and shed no light on the causation at all. Finally, antipsychotic drugs are most effective in alleviating positive-symptom schizophrenia and are relatively ineffective for negative symptoms.

Relationship of Cerebral Atrophy to Negative-Symptom Schizophrenia

New technology for imaging the structural and biochemical processes occurring in the brain have generated tentative theories on negative-symptom schizophrenia. These technologies reveal an association between cerebral atrophy (or ventricular enlargement) and negative-symptom schizophrenia.[34,44,45] The theory of cerebral atrophy as a factor in the etiology of symptoms of schizophrenia is uncertain because of several contradictions. First, the finding of cerebral atrophy is not present in all individuals experiencing negative-symptom schizophrenia.[34] Second, the changes are not specific to only negative-symptom schizophrenia. Similar patterns of cerebral atrophy can occur in some individuals who are experiencing mania or Alzheimer's dementia.[34,45,46] Thus, the relationship between negative-symptom schizophrenia and cerebral atrophy warrants further research and clinical scrutiny.

Other models of schizophrenia (e.g., the endorphin model) exist; however, the evidence is sketchy, at best. As of yet, there are no established biologic markers used to confirm the diagnosis of schizophrenia.

ORGANIC MENTAL DISORDERS

Organic mental disorders as characterized by the DSM-III-R arise from damage to specific sites or areas of the brain. The damage may be caused by advanced degeneration related to aging, trauma or injury, seizures, or acute or chronic ingestion of toxic substances. In all cases, there is substantial disruption to normal neural processes. The symptoms that arise may be classified into disorders such as dementia, delirium or altered sensorium, and related processes. The specific symptoms give an indication of the areas of the brain that have been affected. In dementia, for example,

Research Highlights

Dexamethasone Testing and Mood Disorders

Research in the neurobiology of mental disorders has direct implications for the practice of psychiatric nursing. One example of research application is the seminal work of Carroll and associates.[14-17] In a series of studies Carroll related dexamethasone suppression testing to the diagnosis and treatment of depression. From an understanding of this research the practicing psychiatric nurse can alter interventions with the mood-disordered individual. The first implication for practice can be elicited from the relationship between the level of DST nonsuppression and severity of depression. These individuals exhibit severe physical disruptions (vegetative symptoms). Nutrition, sleep, and fatigue are focal problems that the nurse must develop specific interventions by which the individual can be assisted before therapeutic improvement.

The second implication for practice can be elicited from the relationship between the level of DST nonsuppression and the increased risk of suicide potential. For individuals who are hospitalized, increased precautions should be instituted. For individuals who remain in the community, precautions, such as decreasing isolation, behavioral contracts, and intense follow-ups, should be a part of the nursing care plan.

Finally, individuals who exhibit DST nonsuppression before treatment and remain as nonsuppressors after clinical improvement are at increased risk of imminent relapse. Discharge and community treatment plans must be geared to the increased possibility of relapse. Individuals, as well as the families, should be counseled about the possibility of relapse, including how to monitor for the warning signs and symptoms. Counseling about the potential of relapse will help build the trust relationship between the nurse, individual, and family. In addition, it will assist the individuals who do experience a relapse to understand that it is not their fault nor the families', thereby reducing guilt and blame within these families. The community plan should include intense professional follow-up and monitoring so that, if needed, intervention can be prompt.

Research in neurobiology has direct practice implications for the psychiatric nurse. Nurses are in the ideal position as care providers and case managers to become active participants in this research process.

---

disruption frequently occurs in the diencephalon, affecting the hippocampus and other limbic structures. The disruption may be either alterations in biochemical processes or actual lesions and structural damage.

IMPLICATIONS FOR NURSING RESEARCH AND PRACTICE

Knowledge of the neurobehavioral determinants of mental disorders is of the utmost importance for effective psychiatric mental health nursing. Basic knowledge of anatomic structures and biochemical processes are instrumental building blocks for practice. When equipped with this knowledge, nurses can be more effective in providing education to clients, their families, and the general community. Knowledge of the biologic antecedents of mental disorders often helps families and significant others in understanding therapeutic regimens required to facilitate keeping individuals in the general community. Moreover, explanations to the family of the biologic bases of mental disorders often reduce their feelings of guilt, enhancing the therapeutic interaction.

Psychopharmacologic treatment of mental disablements is a reality for most individuals. The nurse must be able to understand the mechanisms of action, biochemical alterations, and potential adverse and side effects that accompany the use of pharmacologic interventions. In addition, nurses must be able to communicate with the multidisciplinary health care team on a equal status.

SUMMARY

The knowledge of the neurobiologic bases of mental disorder is a rapidly growing field. Much of our current knowledge has been the result of research within the past decade. What is certain is that there exists a genetic predisposition for affective disorder and schizophrenia. The expression of the predisposition is in the central nervous system. Current theory suggests alteration in specific neurotransmitters. However, as knowledge of general neuroscience grows, these beliefs will be modified and expanded.

References

1. Akiskal H, McKinney W. Overview of recent research in depression. Arch Gen Psychiatry. 1975;32:285–305.
2. Andreasen N. Positive vs negative schizophrenia: a critical evaluation. Schizophr Bull. 1985;11:380–389.
3. Andreasen N. Brain imaging: applications in psychiatry. Science. 1988;239:1381–1388.
4. Andreasen N, Olsen S, Dennert J, Smith M. Ventricular enlargement in schizophrenia: relationship to positive and negative symptoms. Am J Psychiatry. 1982;139:297–302.
5. Aston-Jones G, Foote S, Bloom F. Anatomy and physiology of locus coeruleus neurons: functional implications. In: Ziegler M, Lake C, eds. Norepinephrine. Baltimore: Williams & Wilkins; 1984.
6. Baldessarini RJ. Chemotherapy in psychiatry. Cambridge: Harvard University Press; 1977.
7. Berrettini W, Nurnberger J, Hare T, Gershon E, Post R. Plasma and CSF GABA in affective illness. Br J Psychiatry. 1982;141:483–487.
8. Brown W, Johnston R, Mayfield D. The 24 hour dexametha-

sone suppression test in a clinical setting: relationship to diagnosis, symptoms and response to treatment. Am J Psychiatry. 1979;136:543–547.

9. Brown W, Shuey I. Response to dexamethasone and subtype of depression. Arch Gen Psychiatry. 1980;37:747–751.

10. Bunney WE, Davis JM. Norepinephrine in depressive reactions: a review. Arch Gen Psychiatry. 1965;13:483–494.

11. Bunney WE, Murphy D, Goodwin F, Borge G. The switch process from depression to mania: relationship to drugs which alter brain amines. Lancet. 1970;1:1022–1027.

12. Carlson N. Physiology of behavior. 3rd ed. Boston: Allyn and Bacon; 1984.

13. Carlton P, Manowitz P. Dopamine and schizophrenia: an analysis of the theory. Neurosci Biobehav Rev. 1984;8:137–151.

14. Carroll B, Curtis G, Davies B. Urinary free cortisol excretion in depression. Psychol Med. 1976;6:43–50.

15. Carroll B, Curtis C, Mendels J. Cerebrospinal fluid and plasma free cortisol concentration in depression. Psychol Med. 1976;6:235–244.

16. Carroll B, Curtis G, Mendels J. Neuroendocrine regulation in depression: I. Limbic system–adrenalcortical dysfunction. Arch Gen Psychiatry. 1976;33:1039–1044.

17. Carroll B, Curtis G, Mendels J. Neuroendocrine regulation in depression: II. Discrimination of depressed from non-depressed patients. Arch Gen Psychiatry. 1976;33:1051–1058.

18. Coble P, Foster F, Kupfer D. Electroencephalographic sleep diagnosis of primary depression. Arch Gen Psychiatry. 1976;33:1124–1127.

19. Coryell W, Schlesser M. Suicide and the dexamethasome suppression test in unipolar depression. Am J Psychiatry. 1981;138:1120–1121.

20. Creese I. Dopamine receptors explained. Trends Neurosci. 1982;5:40–43.

21. Czeisler C, Zimmermann J, Ronda J, Moore-Ede M, Weitzman E. Timing of REM sleep is coupled to the circadian rhythm of body temperature in man. Sleep. 1980;2:329–346.

22. DiMascio A, Killam K, eds. Psychopharmacology: a generation of progress. New York: Raven Press; 1978.

23. Ettigi P, Hayes P, Narasimhaehari N. D-Amphetamine response and dexamethasone suppression test as predictors of treatment outcome in unipolar depression. Biol Psychiatry. 1983;18:499–503.

24. Foster F, Kupfer D, Coble P, McPartland R. Rapid eye movement sleep density: an objective indicator in severe medical–depressive syndromes. Arch Gen Psychiatry. 1976;33:1119–1123.

25. Germer R, Hare T. CAF GABA in normal subjects and patients with depression, schizophrenia, mania and anorexia nervosa. Am J Psychiatry. 1981;138:1098–1101.

26. Gillin J, Duncan W, Pettigrew K, Frankel B, Snyder F. Successful separation of depressed, normal and insomniac subjects by EEG sleep data. Arch Gen Psychiatry. 1979;36:85–90.

27. Gold P, Goodwin F, Chrousos G. Clinical and biochemical manifestations of depression: relation to the neurobiology of stress. Part 1. N Engl J Med. 1988;319:348–353.

28. Gold P, Goodwin F, Chrousos G. Clinical and biochemical manifestations of depression. Relation to the neurobiology of stress. Part 2. N Engl J Med. 1988;319:413–420.

29. Gold M, Kronig M. Tests of the hypothalamic–pituitary–adrenal axis. In: Gold M, Pottash A, eds. Diagnostic and laboratory testing in psychiatry. New York: Plenum Medical; 1986.

30. Gold M, Pottash A, Extein I. Diagnosis of depression in the 1980s. JAMA. 1981;245:1562–1564.

31. Gold M, Pottash A, Extein I. The TRH test in the diagnosis of major and minor depression. Psychoneuroendocrinology. 1981;6:159–169.

32. Goodwin F, Bunney W. A psychobiological approach to affective illness. Psychiatr Ann. 1973;3(3):19–53.

33. Goodwin FK, Jamison KR. The natural course of manic–depressive illness. In: Post RM, Ballenger JC, eds. Neurobiology of mood disorders. Baltimore: Williams & Wilkins; 1984.

34. Grinspoon L, ed. Schizophrenia and the brain. Part II. Harvard Med School Ment Health Lett. 1988;5(1):1–3.

35. Hartmann E, Cravens J. The effects of long term administration of psychotropic drugs on human sleep. III. The effects of amitriptyline. Psychpharmacologia. 1973;33:185–202.

36. Kandal E, Schwartz J. The principles of neuroscience. New York: Elsevier/North-Holland; 1985.

37. Kirkegaard C, Bjorum N. TSH responses to TRH in endogenous depression. Lancet. 1980;1:152.

38. Kronig M, Gold M. Thyroid testing in psychiatric patients. In: Gold M, Pottash A, eds. Diagnostic and laboratory testing in psychiatry. New York: Plenum Medical; 1986.

39. Kupfer D. REM latency: a psychobiological marker for primary depressive disease. Biol Psychiatry. 1976;11:159–174.

40. Kupfer D, Bowers M. REM sleep and central monoamine oxidase inhibition. Psychopharmacologia. 1972;27:183–190.

41. Kupfer D, Foster F. Interval between onset of sleep and rapid-eye-movement sleep as an indicator of depression. Lancet. 1972;2:684–686.

42. Marano H. Depression: new knowledge, new tests and new therapy. Med World News. 1981;Jan:31–45.

43. Morselli P, Bossi L, Henry J, Zarifian E, Bartholini G. On the therapeutic action of SL 76 002, a new GABA-mimetic agent: preliminary observations in neuropsychiatric disorders. Brain Res Bull. 1980;5(suppl 2):411–414.

44. Nasrallah H, Jocoby C, Chapman S, McCalley-Whitters M. Third ventricular enlargement on CT scans in schizophrenia: association with cerebellar atrophy. Biol Psychiatry. 1985;20:443–450.

45. Nasrallah H, McCalley-Whitters M, Jacoby C. Cortical atrophy in schizophrenia and mania: a comparative CT study. J Clin Psychiatry. 1982;43:439–441.

46. Sachar E. Disorders of feeling: affective disorders. In: Kandal E, Schwartz J, eds. The principles of neuroscience. New York: Elsevier/North-Holland; 1985.

47. Sachar E, Hellman L, Roffwang H. Disrupted 24 hour patterns of cortisol secretion in psychotic depression. Arch Gen Psychiatry. 1973;28:19–24.

48. Schatzberg A, Rothschild A, Stahl J. The dexamethasone suppression test: identification of subtypes of depression. Am J Psychiatry. 1983;140:88–91.

49. Schildkraut JJ. The catecholamine hypothesis of affective disorders: a review of supporting evidence. Am J Psychiatry. 1965;122:509–522.

50. Schildkraut JJ. Current status of the catecholamine hypothesis of affective disorders. In: Lipton M, DiMascio A, Killam K, eds. Psychopharmacology: a generation of progress. New York: Raven Press; 1978.

51. Seeman P, Lee T. Antipsychotic drugs: direct correlation between clinical potency and presynaptic action on dopamine neurons. Science. 1975;188:1217–1219.

52. Seeman P, Lee T, Bird E, Tourtellotte WW. Elevation of brain neuroleptic/dopamine receptors in schizophrenia. In: Baxter C, Melnechuk T, eds. Perspectives in schizophrenia research. New York: Raven Press; 1980.

53. Snyder S. Neurotransmitters and CNS disease: schizophrenia. Lancet. 1982;2:970–974.

54. Sternbach H, Gerner R, Gwirtsman H. The thyrotropin-releasing hormone stimulation test: a review. J Clin Psychiatry. 1982;43:4–6.

55. Stokes P, Pick G, Stoll P. Pituitary–adrenal function in depressed patients: resistance to dexamethasone suppression. J Psychiatr Res. 1975;12:271–281.

56. Targum S, Sullivan A, Byrnes S. Compensatory pituitary-thyroid mechanisms in major depressive disorder. Psychiatry Res. 1982;6:85–96.

57. Traskmann L, Asberg M, Bertilsson L, Sjostrand L. Monoamine metabolites in CSF and suicidal behavior. Arch Gen Psychiatry. 1981;38:631–636.

58. Van Praag H, Korf J, Puite J. 5-Hydroxyindoleacetic acid levels in the cerebrospinal fluid of depressive patients treated with probenecid. Nature. 1970;225:1259–1560.

59. Wehr T, Goodwin F. Biological rhythms and psychiatry. In: Areiti S, Brodie HKH, eds. The American handbook of psychiatry, vol. 2. 2nd ed. New York: Basic Books; 1981.

60. Wehr T, Wirz-Justice A, Goodwin F, Duncan W, Gillin J. Phase advance of the circadian sleep–wake cycles as an antidepressant. Science. 1979;206:710–713.

61. Weinberger D, Wagner R, Wyatt R. Neuropathological studies of schizophrenia: a selected review. Schizophr Bull. 1983;9:193–212.

62. Wirz-Justice A, Groos G, Wehr T. The neuropharmacology of circadian time keeping. In: Aschoff J, Daan S, Groos G, eds. Vertebrate circadian systems: structure and physiology. Heidelberg: Springer-Verlag; 1982.

10

Frederica W. O'Connor

Health Promotion and Disease Prevention in Psychiatric Mental Health Nursing

OBJECTIVES

After reading this chapter, the reader will be able to:

1. *Distinguish between primary, secondary, and tertiary disease prevention and between health protection and health promotion*
2. *Define mental health*
3. *Cite two major themes in contemporary definitions of health*
4. *Analyze a situation involving risk for health breakdown using Kagan and Levi's model*
5. *Identify several foci for interventions to prevent or ameliorate psychosocially mediated disorders*
6. *Identify advantages and disadvantages associated with utilization of direct and indirect nursing strategies to impact others' health*
7. *Specify criteria influencing the choice of one mode or locus of intervention in preference to others*
8. *Critique a plan for health promotion or disease prevention, discussing the locus of the intervention, potential difficulties, and ethical considerations.*

DEFINITIONS AND CONCEPTS

The 1979 Surgeon General's Report, *Healthy People*,[21] provided a strong stimulus for health protection and health promotion activity in the United States. Disease prevention is commonly divided into three levels: primary, secondary, and tertiary. Primary prevention involves efforts to prevent the development of a disease or disorder in susceptible people; secondary prevention involves early diagnosis and treatment of a disease or disorder to shorten its duration, reduce discomfort, and lessen sequelae; and tertiary prevention involves interventions to limit disability and promote maximum function where disorders cannot be fully reversed.

Primary prevention is further divided into health-protecting and health-promoting interventions. Health-*protecting* interventions are defensive actions undertaken to prevent particular health problems. For example, programs to teach young people about the dangers of drug use and show them ways to resist social pressure are designed to protect health. Health-*promoting* interventions do not have a disease referent; rather, they include activities undertaken to promote or support higher levels of health. For example, interventions that raise self-esteem or enhance self-efficacy promote mental health. Both health protection and health promotion can be undertaken in the presence of disease, particularly chronic illness or disability.

Mental health is often viewed as the absence of definable psychopathology. There is little research to suggest criteria for mental health. However, several definitions are widely used. The American Psychiatric Association defines mental health as a relative, rather than an absolute, state of being. "The best indices of mental health are simultaneous success at working, loving, and creating with the capacity for mature and flexible resolution of conflicts between instincts, conscience, important other people, and reality" (reference 1, p 89). Jahoda identified six characteristics of mental health. She stated that the mentally healthy person gives evidence of positive self-attitudes, growth and self-actualization, personality integration, autonomy, reality perception, and environmental mastery.[6] Menninger defined mental health as "the adjustment of human beings to each other and to the world around them with a maximum of effectiveness and happiness" (reference 11, p 1).

These definitions refer primarily to the psychological and social dimensions of health. There is increasing evidence, however, that events in the psychological and social dimensions also interact with events and outcomes in the physical, spiritual, and intellectual dimensions.[16] For example, recent research showed that marital discord and separation or divorce is associated with significantly poorer immune function that may render a person more vulnerable to physical illness.[8] Because interpersonal events may impact physiological health, it is reasonable that psychological or social interventions may benefit health in general, not just psychosocial functioning.

The two major themes in the definitions of health that focus on the person are stability and actualization.[16] Stability-oriented definitions emphasize an individual's ability to maintain personal equilibrium and integrity and to fulfill normative expectations within society.[3,15] Actualization-oriented definitions emphasize the integration of mind, body, spirit, and environment; the expanding of consciousness; and the release of human potential.[4,13]

These definitions represent a change from earlier conceptions, where health was defined as the absence of disease. Within the last decade, there has been increasing emphasis on health as a positive state that can be purposefully strengthened and developed.[2,21] However, health is a relatively new field of study, and professional and societal understanding and application of health-promotion knowledge is only beginning.

INTERVENTIONS THAT PROMOTE HEALTH AND PREVENT ILLNESS

Health-promotion activities are often envisioned within the province of individual behavior. Health is enhanced and protected when individuals either engage in activities believed to foster resilience and well-being or avoid circumstances that increase the likelihood of disease. However, the potential range of approaches is much broader than the focus on the individual. Health promotion includes "activities directed toward increasing the level of well being and actualizing the health potential of individuals, families, communities and society" (reference 17, p 27). The World Health Organization's definition of health-promoting activities includes building healthy public policy, creating environments that support health, strengthening community actions, developing personal skills of healthy living, and reorienting health services.[20] The potential focus of health promotion and disease prevention includes not only individuals, but also families, communities, and larger societal groups.

POTENTIAL POINTS OF INTERVENTION TO PROMOTE MENTAL HEALTH

A theoretical model developed by Kagan and Levi[7,9] illustrates the interacting psychosocial variables in disease causation and therefore the levels at which preventive interventions can occur (Fig. 10-1). The initial stressor may be physical, psychological, or social, but the actual disorder occurs because of intermediary psychosocial processes. In this model, psychosocial stimuli (Fig. 10-1, box 1) interact with a person's biologic and psychological characteristics (box 2); this combination may or may not produce an emotional or other physiological response (box 3). Depending on the situation, this response gives rise to precursors of disease (box 4) or to disease (box 5). At all points, this process is promoted or impeded by interacting vari-

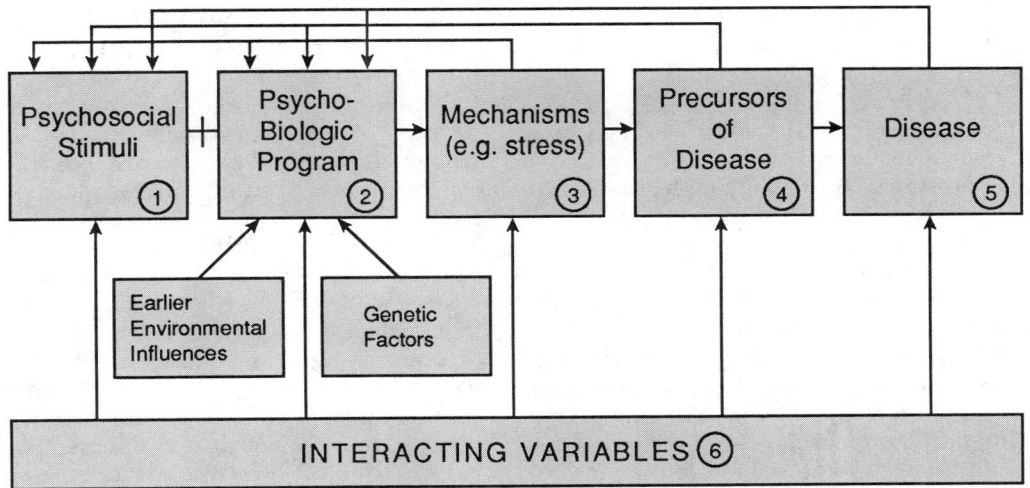

FIGURE 10–1. *Theoretical model for psychosocially mediated disease. The combined effect of psychosocial stimuli (1) and the psychobiologic program (2) determines psychological and physiological reaction mechanisms, such as stress (3) that may lead to precursors of disease (4) and to disease (5). This sequence can be promoted or counteracted by interacting variables (6), such as social support or an excessively critical interpersonal environment. The sequence is a cybernetic system with continuous feedback. (Kagan and Levi, 1975; used with permission)*

ables, such as good coping skills or the presence of a supportive person (box 6). This sequence is not a one-way process but rather constitutes part of a cybernetic system with continuous feedback among the variables. Several examples will clarify the use of these terms.

Examples of psychosocial stimuli thought to be pathogenic under certain circumstances are loss of a parent or parental neglect, domestic violence, high levels of criticism, stigmatization, changes in male–female roles, and rapid social change. These events interact with people's psychobiologic characteristics, which in this model refer to the level of constitutional vulnerability resulting from inherited characteristics and previous experiences. At special risk are the very young, the elderly, persons genetically predisposed to a particular disorder, and those already disabled in various ways. Conversely, children and adults who are biologically and psychologically healthy and resilient are more resistant to the effects of environmental stressors. When sufficiently intense and enduring events overwhelm an individual's constitutional health and strength, the result is a disease or reaction that may be a precursor of disease. Examples of high-risk behavioral or psychological reactions are suicide, anxiety, and depression. At any point along this trajectory, physical or psychosocial factors can intervene to promote or ameliorate the disease-causing process. Examples of disease-predisposing factors are low self-esteem, poor problem-solving skills, social marginality, and the lack of protective interacting variables. Ameliorating, or protective, interacting variables include mental processes such as habituation, adaptation, learning, and other coping skills; psychosocial processes such as group belonging, access to advice, availability of someone with whom to discuss difficulties; and physical factors such as good nutrition and available health services.[9]

This model demonstrates the many interconnected factors in the person–environment ecosystem. An important implication is that there are many potential points of intervention where the progression from the experience of a noxious psychosocial event or situation to the development of a mental disorder can be interrupted. For example, interventions might be directed toward reducing the incidence of high-risk psychosocial events or perhaps toward changing a person's interpretation of the events—reframing them so that an occurrence that was originally viewed as threatening comes to be seen as challenging (Fig. 10-1, box 1). Alternatively, intervention might involve providing or urging others to provide increased levels of protective interacting variables, such as being available to discuss problems, and providing extra assistance with tasks (box 6). This would be especially useful if there is no way to change the event itself. A third possibility is intervention focused on high-risk reactions (box 3). In this case, the stressful circumstances and the basic characteristics of an individual remain unchanged, but the person learns to alter physiological or psychological reactions to the stressor.[12] An example is replacing stress-related symptoms with a relaxation response.

When health promotion and disease prevention are viewed this comprehensively, not only are many points of potential intervention identified, but a whole range of possible prevention activities becomes apparent. A psychosocial nurse is likely to think first of direct care interventions, such as remaining with a very anxious client in order to reduce the person's reaction to an event or providing information to a person who has misinterpreted an event in order to reduce the stressfulness of the event. A second approach involves teaching people how better to promote mental health in themselves and in others. Examples are teaching relaxation techniques to people who experience stress so they can interrupt symptoms on their own behalf or teaching parents how to interact with their young children in ways that build self-esteem in order to strengthen the child's psychobiologic program or personality. A third approach is directed toward institutions such as businesses, schools, community agencies, or legislatures with the goal of changing legislation or organizational activities in ways that promote mental health. For example, a health professional or community member might persuade a mental health agency to organize a volunteer friendly visitor program to support older adults living independently. This program would promote health by providing an additional source of positive interacting variables. A critical care nurse might suggest the hiring of a psychosocial nurse to facilitate a support group for nurses on the unit. Citizens have lobbied for laws and policies outlawing racial or ethnic discrimination to reduce distressing psychosocial conditions and to provide circumstances that do not impede minority children's opportunities to develop healthy self-esteem. In the first example above, the nurse behaves directly in a health-promoting way with the final target of health promotion activity. In the second and third examples, the nurse teaches and persuades others, and their subsequent actions determine the mental health benefits.

CRITERIA FOR SELECTING INTERVENTIONS TO PROMOTE MENTAL HEALTH AND PREVENT PSYCHIATRIC ILLNESS

Given the many possible points and levels of intervention to promote mental health and prevent psychiatric illness, it is important to consider factors that influence the choice to intervene in particular ways. Appropriate considerations are effectiveness, cost, and the ethical implications associated with various options. This analysis entails consideration of such factors as resources and the target individual's or group's attitudes, cognitive ability, and affective state. For example, the effectiveness of teaching others how to promote their health depends on their being aware (or at least their becoming aware) of the need for changed behavior and then being willing to learn and to institute new behavior, ideally within a supportive environment. In the absence of a specific circumstance that is perceived as both threatening and alterable without too much difficulty, many people are uninterested in investing time and energy in behavioral change.[18] Lifestyle changes must be maintained to continue to exert benefits, and when people institute more healthful behaviors or lifestyles, relapse may occur because of the lack of support (a positive interacting variable) needed to maintain new behavior.[10] Nonetheless, in the course of everyday life, most people occasionally notice ways their behavior impairs their health or effectiveness and are motivated to learn and use new behavior.

However, in some situations, one-to-one approaches to helping people change their behavior are seriously limited, because one-to-one approaches do not modify the environmental forces that continually produce risk for other people. Wide-scale social problems and specific environmental hazards are best handled by broad interventions. Examples are governmental mandates for nondiscriminatory employment and housing policies and access to buildings for physically disabled persons. Interventions at the societal level are also often cost effective, because the health of many people can be affected. Some ethicists emphasize the immorality of intervening at the individual level where there is good reason to believe that interventions at the environmental level would be more effective.[5]

An illustration of an environmental approach is a research project on stress reduction conducted among San Francisco bus drivers.[19] Numerous previous studies had shown that bus drivers have a high prevalence of hypertension and diseases of the gastrointestinal and musculoskeletal systems, and it seems probable that certain aspects of their occupation increased their risk of these problems. It would be useful clinically to teach drivers about posture, healthful eating habits, and stress management. However, from an environmental perspective, and perhaps to prevent the development of these disorders altogether in new drivers, it would be more effective to identify and change those characteristics of the job itself that are associated with increased risk. An examination of the social environment of bus drivers determined that drivers are continually under the "tyranny" of a schedule that in fact cannot be met. Nevertheless, drivers are regularly reprimanded for failure to keep the unrealistic schedule. Further, there is considerable social isolation in the job. The researchers discovered that the drivers typically remain at the bus yard to wind down for as long as 3 hours after their shifts. It is late when they get home, and they often go right to bed, with minimal contact with their spouses and children. Syme[19] proposes such environmental interventions as devising realistic schedules, locating rest stops nearer central cities so drivers could have contact with other drivers during the shift if they so chose, and informing the public of the difficult circumstances faced by bus drivers. If these interventions were instituted, the prevalence of the three clinical disorders might be sharply reduced.

Many environmental changes have the advantage of protecting individuals' health without requiring purposeful change efforts that people might be unwilling or unable to make. When environments are altered, people often change voluntarily, almost automatically. The suggestion that bus drivers' rest stops be located so that the drivers would have opportunities to interact with one another during their work hours assumes that if the environment were hospitable, most drivers would elect to have contact with one another.

Pragmatic considerations often require psychosocial nurses to help people manage and grow as well as they can in environments that are less than optimal. Although individual approaches may be all that can be attempted realistically in many situations and may achieve the goal, the bus driver example illustrates that such an approach is incomplete from a public health standpoint when significant environmental stressors are present. Hence, it is important to document situations that threaten health and to inform and influence legislators and business and community leaders to implement alternative approaches when current circumstances threaten the health of community members or employees.

An important disadvantage of some legislative or other macro-level interventions directed at changing the environment is that they might reduce an individual's freedom. For example, if a law mandates student busing to achieve racial and social equality, a child may lose the option of attending the nearest school. It is important to consider the implications of proposed societal or environmental changes for individuals' opportunities to exercise personal determination.[5]

As the model in Figure 10-1 suggests, approaches to a particular (actual or potential) problem may be multilevel, and approaches that involve both individual and environmental changes undoubtedly produce some of the most beneficial and lasting improvements in health-promoting behavior.

SUMMARY

Health promotion and disease prevention are important components of the nursing role. Disease prevention is commonly divided into primary, secondary, and tertiary. Primary prevention is further divided into health protection and health promotion. Health is frequently described as a multidimensional phenomenon, but there is much interplay among the dimensions, and difficulties in one area usually impact other dimensions. Health definitions typically emphasize stability or actualization. Activities that promote health range from behavioral change in an individual to the establishment of healthy public policy and reorientation of health services.

A theoretical model developed by Kagan and Levi[7] illustrates variables involved in a psychosocially mediated disorder. A threat to health begins with an event that has potentially negative psychosocial implications. The impact depends partly on the psychological and biologic predisposition of the individual involved, and the result may be either disease or precursors of disease. The trajectory from a high-risk event to the appearance of a disorder can be greatly altered by inter-

Research Highlights

A prevention study tested the effectiveness of nurse home visits to high-risk families for 2 years following the birth of a first baby in preventing child abuse and neglect.[14] The sample consisted of first-time mothers with characteristics that predispose to infant health and development problems: mothers were younger than 19 years, single, and of low socioeconomic status. Women in the visited group received nurse visits prenatally and periodically for 2 years after the birth of the baby. The three principal nursing activities were: parent education regarding infant development, needs, and care; involvement of family members and friends in child care and support of the mother; and linking the family with other health and human services. In this high-risk population, 19% of the unvisited mothers vs 4% of the visited mothers had confirmed instances of child abuse or neglect during the 2 years. Visited mothers were observed to punish and restrict less frequently, and they provided a larger number of appropriate play materials. There were trends toward higher developmental levels in their infants. Visited mothers demonstrated less conflict with the babies and less spanking, and the babies showed better temperament. There were fewer trips to the emergency room in the first year by visited mothers. During the second year of life, visited women presented in the emergency room fewer times and with fewer accidents and poisonings than their counterparts in the comparison group. However, visited mothers reported more instances of their babies' resisting eating. The pattern of results indicates that nurse visits prevented a number of caregiving dysfunctions, including neglect and abuse, in high-risk families.

The home visits represent intervention primarily at the levels of box 1 and box 6 of Figure 10-1. It is likely that normal infant behavior was less stressful for mothers who had been taught what to expect and how to respond. The nurse visits almost certainly functioned as a supportive interacting variable as well. Further, the intervention may have strengthened mothers' sense of their own competence, enhancing their psychobiologic program for the future. Visited mothers very likely also responded to their infants in ways that promoted the babies' psychosocial development, reducing their future vulnerability to health threats. In addition, the nurses worked to increase the mothers' natural support systems and to link mothers to needed health and welfare services, so there was a defined element of increasing environmental support in this intervention. Although this primary intervention was designed explicitly to prevent child abuse and neglect, the intervention strengthened and supported general welfare and parenting skills, promoting the health of both mother and infant.

This study was a large-scale undertaking; however, similar interventions could be arranged for clients by individual nurses. In many instances, nurses are in a position to readily identify high-risk situations, individuals, or reactions. When any of these conditions is identified, nurses can locate the resources needed to support clients, explore with clients how they might change their behavior or circumstances to protect their health, and work with others to bring high-risk situations to the attention of those in a position to make changes.

acting variables, which are interpersonal, cultural, or environmental influences whose effects may either worsen or relieve the threat. There are many points in this person–environment ecosystem where intervention can affect the health outcome. Nurses can intervene directly with individuals to promote health, or they can teach and influence others, including legislators and employers. Appropriate considerations when selecting a locus for intervention are probable effectiveness, cost, and ethical concerns.

References

1. American Psychiatric Association. Psychiatric glossary. Washington, DC: American Psychiatric Press; 1984.

2. Antonovsky A. Unraveling the mystery of health. San Francisco: Jossey-Bass; 1987.

3. Aubrey L. Health as a social concept. Br J Soc. 1953;4:109–124.

4. Dunn HL. Points of attack for raising the level of wellness. J Natl Med Assoc. 1975;49:223–35.

5. Faden RR. Ethical issues in government sponsored health campaigns. Health Educ Q. 1987;14:27–37.

6. Jahoda M. Current concepts of positive mental health. New York: Basic Books; 1958.

7. Kagan A, Levi L. Health and environment—psychosocial stimuli: a review. In: Levi L, ed. Society, stress and disease. Vol. 2: Childhood and adolescence. London: Oxford University Press; 1975.

8. Kiecolt–Glaser JK, Fisher LD, Ogrocki P, Stout JC, Speicher CE, Glaser R. Marital quality, marital disruption, and immune function. Psychosom Med. 1987;49:13–34.

9. Levi L. Psychosocial factors in preventive medicine. In: US Department of Health, Education, and Welfare: Healthy people: the Surgeon General's report on health promotion and disease prevention. DHEW Publication No. 79-55071A. Washington, DC: US Government Printing Office, 1979.

10. Marlatt GA, Gordon JR. Relapse prevention. New York: Guilford; 1985.

11. Menninger KA. The Human Mind. Ed 3. New York: Alfred A Knopf; 1945.

12. Nakagawa–Kogan H, Betrus P. Self management: a nursing mode of therapeutic influence. ANS. 1984;6(4):55–73.

13. Newman M. Theory development in nursing. Philadelphia: FA Davis; 1979.

14. Olds DL, Henderson CR, Chamberlin R, Tatelbaum R. Preventing child abuse and neglect: a randomized trial of nurse home visitation. Pediatrics. 1986;78:65–78.

15. Parsons T. Definitions of health and illness in the light of American values and social structure. In: Jaco EG, ed. Patients, physicians and illness. Ed 3. New York: Free Press; 1979:120–144.

16. Pender NJ. Health and health promotion: conceptual dilemmas. In: Duffy ME, Pender NJ, eds. Conceptual issues in health promotion: report of proceedings of a Wingspread Conference. Indianapolis: Sigma Theta Tau; 1987:7–23.

17. Pender NJ. Health promotion in nursing practice. Ed 2. Norwalk, CT: Appleton–Lange; 1987.

18. Sennott–Miller L, Miller JLL. Difficulty: a neglected factor in health promotion. Nurs Res. 1987;36:268–272.

19. Syme SL. Strategies for health promotion. Prev Med. 1986;15:492–507.

20. Turner J. WHO: Charter for health promotion. Lancet. 1986;2:1407.

21. US Department of Health, Education, and Welfare: Healthy people: the Surgeon General's Report on Health Promotion and Disease Prevention, DHEW Publication No. 79-55071A. Washington, DC: US Government Printing Office, 1979.

Nursing Diagnosis and Process

11

Marjory Gordon

The Nursing Process and Clinical Judgment

OBJECTIVES

After reading this chapter, the reader will be able to:

1. *Identify nursing assessment and diagnosis as the principal components of diagnostic judgment*
2. *Discuss the development of a diagnostic taxonomy and its use in clinical reasoning and judgment*
3. *Describe the hypothesis generation and testing model used to explain diagnostic judgment*
4. *Identify care planning—goals, nursing interventions, and outcomes and evaluation—as the components of therapeutic judgment.*

The nursing process is a systematic method for organizing the delivery of psychiatric–mental health nursing and represents an application of the generic method of problem identification–problem solving to clinical care. A similar process is used by many other health care providers: psychiatrists, social workers, and clinical psychologists also identify problems within their domains of practice and assist clients in solving their problems.

The components of the nursing process are assessment, diagnosis, planning, implementation, and evaluation. These components provide both the novice and the expert with a structure for helping individuals, families, or communities to identify and modify or resolve potential and actual health problems. Clinical reasoning and judgment form the cognitive basis for each of these components.

NURSING STANDARDS AND NURSING PROCESS

The nursing process is an important dimension of practice. Standards exist for the use of each component, so that nurses may compare their practice with the professional standards prepared by the American Nurses Association Council on Psychiatric–Mental Health Nursing (see Chapter 1). The nursing process also is an integral part of the definition of professional nursing. The American Nurses Association's definition condenses the five components of nursing process into two. In their definition, *diagnosis*, the problem-identification component, refers to both assessment and diagnosis; *treatment*, the problem-solving component, refers to the planning–implementation–evaluation components:

> Nursing is the diagnosis and treatment of human responses to actual or potential health problems.[1]

Human responses are behaviors manifested by the client. These behaviors comprise the clinical data used by the nurse to make a nursing diagnosis. For example, consider the following information about a client: overwhelming sadness, frequent crying, and comments about being "not good for much." These are human responses that can be observed during assessment. A nursing diagnosis provides an understanding of these responses that is useful for the problem-solving phase of the nursing process; that is, for treatment planning.

NURSING PRACTICE AND NURSING PROCESS

In addition to providing a structure for care delivery, the nursing process is the basis for other related activities. For example, documentation on the client's chart is based on the elements of the nursing process; nurses document a client's nursing history and examination,

nursing diagnoses, treatments, and responses to treatment. Quality assurance programs use nurses' documentation of the nursing process to measure the quality of care delivery. Also, nurse staffing of units is based on factors derived from nursing process documentation. The recording of nursing process can be used as a basis for setting charges for nursing care and for establishing health statistics about the occurrence of nursing problems. For example, the nurse in private practice or in a community agency may be reimbursed for the nursing treatment of dysfunctional grieving.

In addition, some nursing leaders are interested in establishing a Nursing Minimum Data Set (NMDS), the minimum, essential information for describing nursing care delivery. This would include, for example, the NMDS that would provide a standard for describing diagnostic, intervention, outcome, and acuity data across all health care settings.[22] The NMDS is of particular value in compiling national and international health statistics. For these reasons, the accuracy of reasoning that underlies the diagnostic and therapeutic judgments within the nursing process is of great concern in maintaining high-quality care delivery in psychiatric–mental health nursing.

CONCEPTUAL FOCUS FOR NURSING PROCESS

The nursing process, thus far, has been defined only as a problem-identification–problem-solving method, not unique to nursing. The reader may be wondering what makes it nursing process, as opposed to medical process or social work process.

It is the conceptual focus and the content of reasoning that makes problem identification–problem solving a *nursing* process. The definition of professional nursing specifies a focus for the nursing process; that is, human responses to actual or potential problems. The term *human responses* refers to observable behaviors that indicate actual or potential health problems. Conceptual models that guide nursing have a holistic, biopsychosocial approach to the phenomena of concern in nursing: client–environment interaction, intervention, and health.

There is a pluralism in nursing regarding ways of thinking about these phenomena.[17] One nurse may find it useful to think about clients with affective disorders from the perspective of the adaptation conceptual model,[18] whereas another nurse may use Orem's self-care agency framework when working with these clients.[16] It is important that a *nursing* model of practice guide *nursing* process. As frameworks are used in nursing practice, it will become clear which frameworks are most useful for guiding the treatment of particular problems at various acuity levels. The concept of the client of nursing and client–environment interaction is relevant to what is assessed and is the focus for diagnosis within the nursing process. The concept of health influences goal setting and evaluation decisions;

the concept of nursing intervention used by a nurse influences decisions about care planning and treatment. Clearly, the conceptual framework a nurse employs influences all clinical judgments within the nursing process.

Clinical reasoning and judgment are critical thinking skills. They involve logical reasoning and the evaluation, analysis, and synthesis of information. *Reasoning* is a term used to describe thinking strategies; clinical judgment is the product of reasoning. On the basis of clinical reasoning and judgment, the nurse determines during assessment which client behaviors require attention. Reasoning is also required to derive meaning from behavioral information, to identify treatment outcomes that are attainable, and to select treatments that would lead to those outcomes. As implementation of a nursing care plan proceeds, clinical reasoning is applied to observations of the client's immediate responses to treatment. Outcome evaluation after a period of treatment also utilizes clinical reasoning abilities. In this chapter, the components of the nursing process will be discussed within the framework of clinical reasoning and judgment. Examples and illustrations will assist the reader in understanding how these skills are used in assessment, diagnosis, care planning, implementation, and evaluation.

CLINICAL JUDGMENT AND NURSING PROCESS

The professional practitioner uses three types of judgment within the nursing process: diagnostic, therapeutic, and ethical.[6,14] *Diagnostic judgment* is a product of information collection (assessment) and analysis; *therapeutic judgment* results in treatment decisions, including evaluative judgments about the outcomes of treatment; *ethical judgment* involves moral decisions based on philosophical principles and values. Within the nursing process, there is an ethical, or value, dimension that enters into diagnosis and treatment decisions.

Newell and Simon view judgment as an act;[15] it concludes an extended process of reasoning and involves identifying something. Judgment in any domain—diagnostic, therapeutic, or ethical—is the expression of an understanding that results from intellectual work.

The nursing process is usually presented to readers as a series of steps. This is the textbook picture; in practice, many times, the nurse does not proceed stepwise through the process. Immediately after assessment of one sign, the nurse may intervene. For example, when cues signifying immediate danger to self or others are observed, a nursing action is taken, bypassing full assessment and diagnosis.

Diagnostic Judgment and Nursing Diagnosis

Through reasoning, judgments are made about the health status of a client seeking psychiatric or mental health services. The judgments are formulated as nursing diagnoses, which then serve as a basis for treatment planning. The judgment process includes information collection and analysis and formulation of the diagnosis.

Judgment enters into the situation because each problem is defined by more than one cue. The key is to learn the critical cues for each problem; that is, the cues that are diagnostic. These will be present when the condition is present. Secondly, judgment has to be used, because cues may signify more than one problem; clinical information is ambiguous. For example, crying can mean many things. The key is to learn the diagnostic process, diagnostic reasoning, and the common problems encountered.

INFORMATION COLLECTION AND ANALYSIS

Diagnostic judgments about actual or potential health problems are not made in isolation. Information has to be collected and analyzed. The term *assessment* refers to the collection and evaluation of information. Information collection and analysis requires accuracy and efficiency. It must be accurate, because diagnostic and therapeutic judgments are based on assessment information; errors in assessment thus can lead to misdiagnosis and incorrect treatment. Efficiency is necessary because nursing assessment takes time, and time translates into health care costs. Deliberate and systematic assessments use time wisely. A second reason for emphasizing efficiency is that gathering excess, irrelevant information may strain cognitive processes and can result in diagnostic errors. Excess information collection, for example, with prolongation of an admission interview, also can tire the client.

Information collection is a component of the nursing process that is used throughout all nurse–client interactions and in all care delivery settings. As may be seen in Box 11-1, it is not confined to the admission nursing history and examination. It is used as a basis for immediate action in an emergency situation, to establish baselines, to provide information to individualize treatment, and to evaluate a client's progress. It is useful to think of assessment as a component of the nursing process that is used *whenever information is needed* for diagnostic, therapeutic, or evaluative judgments. Judgment has to be exercised in what information to collect and in how the information is to be used in reasoning and judgment.

The primary source of assessment information is the client. Significant others, such as family or household members, may provide information if the client consents or if the client is a minor or is judged not competent to provide a nursing history. Information about health patterns is gathered by interview and observation. An interview elicits the client's subjective viewpoint. It includes descriptions of life patterns, experiences, beliefs, and values. Observations of gait, posture, and speech patterns are useful to evaluate further the physical manifestations of self concept and mood states. Interactions with care providers and family or

BOX 11–1
Types of Nursing Assessment Situations

1. *Initial Assessment.* Information collection and analysis in this situation is designed to identify nursing diagnoses and client's strengths. The initial assessment is usually called the nursing history and examination. It is the most complex of the assessment situations in nursing practice because the universe of diagnostic possibilities is open. An initial health pattern review is done at admission in conjunction with a psychiatric intake interview.
2. *Problem-Focused Assessment.* Information collection and analysis is focused on the signs and symptoms of diagnoses previously identified. The focused cue search is used to evaluate daily progress toward attainment of projected outcomes.
3. *Emergency Assessment.* Information collection and analysis is quickly done in order to institute immediate life-sustaining action. An example of the need for emergency assessment is a client who is a danger to himself or others.
4. *Time-Lapse Reassessment.* Information collection and analysis of change in health status over time is done within a screening assessment and the previously identified diagnoses. This is used in clinic situations, long-term care, or other situations where a significant period of time has elapsed between nurse–client encounters.

Adapted from Gordon M. Nursing diagnosis: process and application. New York: McGraw-Hill; 1987.

companions are part of an examination of a client's responses to the immediate social environment. When the nurse's judgment dictates, physical examination is carried out. Inspection, auscultation, and palpation are used. This may be indicated if, for example, a psychiatric client is also prone to congestive heart failure or if information is needed for referral to a physician.

As may be noted from this brief description, judgment is exercised in regard to what information to collect and why the information is warranted. Screening assessment tools and other guidelines used in health care agencies can assist the beginner, but clinical judgment has to be exercised about the need to collect information beyond that specified in the tool.

As information is collected, it is simultaneously analyzed for clarity and reliability. This is a second area of judgment. For example, if the client says, "I don't know if the divorce was . . . (inaudible)," the nurse should clarify. Similarly, if the client states that his first attempt at suicide was 6 months ago and later states that he started having "jittery feelings and cut his wrists" 7 months ago, the reliability and accuracy of the judgment that these events are connected needs to be checked with the client. The product of the assessment is a database that provides the supporting data for diagnoses, information for individualizing treatment, and baseline information for the evaluation of treatment. Accurate judgments result when consideration is given to the following *during* information collection:

Is clarification or verification necessary?
Is other information needed to evaluate the data (e.g., previous baseline values)?
Is the information reliable? That is, were measures done accurately, and did I hear and observe accurately?

As information is collected during a functional assessment, inferences are made to derive meaning from the data. A general rule to follow is that inferences and transformations of observational information obtained from a client should be validated. For example, a psychiatric client who is receiving a drug that can cause

constipation may say that she has trouble moving her bowels. Does this signify constipation? Actually, it may be that the "trouble" is not constipation that is relieved by laxatives but rather is related to pain on defecation such as that produced by hemorrhoids. Thus, inferring that the client's statement "trouble moving bowels," means constipation would lead to misdiagnosis. It is important not to assume what appears to be the obvious explanation without further investigation or validation of cues that could have multiple meanings.

First-level inferences, or assumptions, can lead to misdiagnosis if not validated. Inferences represent *created* information, not information that another observer could see, hear, and validate. When inferences are used in formulating a diagnosis, it is important that their accuracy be checked with the client. It is easy for human beings to place their own subjective interpretations on assessment data. For example, what conclusion can be drawn from the following information obtained early in an admission interview:

Mrs. R is a 73-year-old widow who has come to the mental health clinic. Her husband was killed in an auto accident 1 year ago. She has been crying a lot over little things and sometimes for no reason at all. She says she has "not had any energy" for the last 2 weeks and feels "really bad." She is surprised that she is so "apathetic" about her two grandchildren and her household duties. She has not gone to her rughooking group for the last 2 months. She readily admits that she has no one particular physical problem—just a generalized feeling that she is "sick all over."

Evaluate the accuracy of the following conclusions (inferences) in turn:

1. Mrs. R's basic reason for crying is her husband's death.
2. Mrs. R is neglecting her household duties.
3. Mrs. R is exhausted and "run down" from maintaining the house by herself.
4. Mrs. R feels apathetic about her grandchildren since her husband's death.

If you selected item one, you may be considering dysfunctional grieving as a possibility. Yet item one needs to be validated: she said she was crying over "little things" and "sometimes for no reason at all;" she did not say crying over her husband's death. Did you consider item two to be a valid inference? If so, you will probably generate the diagnostic hypothesis of impaired home maintenance management* related to activity intolerance. Actually, she said she was apathetic about her household duties; you may have *inferred* that she was neglecting them. If you selected item three, you probably imagined a 73-year-old lady, perhaps with heart disease, taking care of a big house since her husband died. This view may lead to considering the diagnostic hypothesis of activity intolerance* and wondering if she could have heart failure. Yet "exhaustion" and being "run down" are not in the database, nor is a big house. If you chose item four, half of your inference would be valid: she did say she was apathetic about her grandchildren, but she did not say it was since her husband's death.

This exercise and the interpretations that have been put on this information by nurses serve to point out that caution must be observed when "creating" information from observations. Wrong interpretations can cause errors in diagnostic and therapeutic judgments.

Situations occur in which it is not possible to validate inferences. If a psychiatric client has impaired thought processes or is mute, it may be impossible to validate inferences and assumptions during assessment. In these cases, indirect information may be obtained from the family or friends of the client as well as from the client's nonverbal behavior. It may also be helpful to have another nurse validate impressions.

Too early closure on interpretations of the client's status can lead to diagnostic errors. Errors of this type can be avoided if a diagnosis is not made until critical defining characteristics of the condition are present. These are the signs and symptoms that are present when a particular condition is present. In contrast to premature closure is the failure to make a diagnosis when the necessary information is present. This second type of diagnostic error can occur when information of low reliability and validity is used in judgment;[4] this produces low levels of confidence. Both types of errors can be avoided by learning the critical characteristics of commonly encountered nursing diagnoses and recognizing that these characteristics are indicators of the condition. Inadequate assessment leading to missed cues, failure to consider alternative explanations for cues, and biased interpretations of cues can also lead to diagnostic errors.

FORMULATING THE DIAGNOSIS

As information is being collected, it is being analyzed and interpreted. Interpretations of the initial clinical data are part of the diagnostic judgment process, and the process of formulating a diagnosis begins with the first information collected. In this section, consideration will be given to diagnostic categories for labeling judgments about health problems and to diagnostic judgment. Diagnostic categories are considered first, as these are the concepts used in diagnostic reasoning and judgment.

USE OF DIAGNOSTIC CATEGORIES

In 1973, a concerted effort was begun to label the health problems that nurses diagnose and treat. Approximately every 2 years, under the auspices of the North American Nursing Diagnosis Association (NANDA), nurses from the United States and Canada have met to classify nursing diagnoses. Currently, 98 diagnoses have been entered in a taxonomy of human response patterns called "NANDA Taxonomy I, Revised," which appears in Appendix I. This is the diagnostic classification system endorsed by the American Nurses Association.

The broad human response patterns used to structure the taxonomy may be seen in Appendix I. When diagnoses are approved by the NANDA membership, they are incorporated into the Taxonomy. Classification of nursing diagnoses, or taxonomic development, is based on hierarchical placement of categories describing clinical phenomena.[10,19] General categories are at the higher levels and specific categories at the lower, more precise levels. In Taxonomy I, for example, Pattern 5, Choosing, has multiple levels, as may be seen in Box 11-2. With the current arrangement, specific clinically usable diagnoses are at the lowest, most precise levels. As an example, the diagnosis ineffective coping contains ineffective denial and defensive coping. The taxonomy is designated as number one to indicate that it requires testing, further conceptual analysis, and development.

NANDA has always encouraged all professional nurses to participate in the identification and classification of health conditions that nurses diagnose and treat. A task force of the Division on Psychiatric and Mental Health Nursing Practice of the American Nurses Association has begun to identify nursing diagnoses in their specialty practice area (See Appendix for list). It is projected that after sufficient development, diagnoses not already classified in the NANDA Taxonomy I, Revised, will be entered in the NANDA Diagnosis Review Cycle. Work is currently being done to develop the diagnoses according to the NANDA criteria for submitting a diagnosis.

Definition of a Nursing Diagnosis

There are many definitions of nursing diagnosis in the literature. Those cited by the NANDA include one process definition that is derived from a consensus study and three definitions that address what nursing diagnostic categories describe.[13] The process definition is:

> A nursing diagnosis is a clinical judgment about an individual, family, or community that is derived through

---

* Other NANDA nursing diagnosis.

BOX 11-2
Example of Taxonomic Arrangement in
NANDA Diagnostic Classification
System: Pattern 5.0, Choosing, in
NANDA Taxonomy I

5.0 CHOOSING: A human response pattern involving the
     selection of alternatives
  5.1 Altered Coping
    5.1.1 Individual Coping
      5.1.1.1 Ineffective Coping (Individual)
        5.1.1.1.1 Impaired Adjustment
        5.1.1.1.2 Defensive Coping
        5.1.1.1.3 Ineffective Denial
    5.1.2 Family Coping
      5.1.2.1 Ineffective Family Coping
        5.1.2.1.1 Ineffective Family Coping: Disabled
        5.1.2.1.2 Ineffective Family Coping: Compromised
      5.1.2.2 Family Coping: Potential for Growth
    5.1.3 (Community Coping)
  5.2 (Altered Participation)
    5.2.1 (Individual)
      5.2.1.1 Noncompliance (Specify)
      5.2.1.2 Decisional Conflict (Specify)
      5.2.1.3 Health Seeking Behaviors (Specify)
    5.2.2 (Family)
    5.2.3 (Community)

Adapted from Carroll-Johnson R. NANDA Taxonomy I. In:
Carroll-Johnson R, ed. Classification of nursing diagnoses:
proceedings of the Eighth Conference. Philadelphia: JB Lippincott; 1988.

a deliberate, systematic process of data collection and analysis. It provides the basis for prescriptions for definitive therapy for which the nurse is accountable. It is expressed concisely, and it includes the etiology of the condition when known (reference 20, p 109).

This definition offers a clear grasp of how nursing diagnosis is integrated into the nursing process. The remaining three definitions identify various foci of nursing diagnostic categories: normal variations or altered patterns of human functioning,[12] patterns of unitary man,[19] and actual or potential health problems nurses are capable of treating and licensed to treat.[8] The third definition was written when the idea of nursing diagnosis was just beginning to be implemented in nursing practice. Today, the author would suggest that "actual or potential problems" is vague and that an individual nurse uses a concept of nursing diagnosis that is consistent with the nursing model or framework that guides his or her practice.[7] For example, *ineffective adaptation* would be the conceptual definition of a nursing diagnosis when using Roy's adaptation framework. *Dysfunctional* or *potentially dysfunctional patterns* would define the focus of nursing diagnosis when using the functional health patterns framework.

The NANDA Taxonomy provides nurses with diagnostic labels for their clinical judgments. This permits communication of thoughts to others and improves continuity of care. Having a standardized nomencla-

ture also facilitates documentation, provides a focus for health statistics and quality assurance, and provides a basis for cost analysis and for reimbursement for nursing care.

Future efforts in classification need to address a number of issues. One is the concept of nursing diagnosis. What is included and excluded as a nursing diagnosis? This question has both professional and legal aspects. For example, medical diagnoses are not viewed as nursing diagnoses. From a nursing perspective, they are collaborative problems in the interdependent domain of practice. Nurses, however, are independently responsible for the nursing diagnoses that co-occur with these conditions. Nevertheless the nursing literature does not reflect consensus on this and other issues related to the concept of nursing diagnosis.[5,11]

The psychiatric nurse's professional responsibility to the consumer is continually to improve diagnostic skills. In the next section, the focus will be on these skills and on how diagnostic judgments are made.

Diagnostic Judgment

When something is not immediately perceptible, signs have to be used for its identification. Persons learn that a large snarling, growling dog signifies aggression and possible harm. This is an example of learning the meaning of cues. The same process is used in diagnostic judgment: professionals learn that certain clinical signs or symptoms are defining characteristics that signify a health problem. The sign or symptom is known as a cue to the problem. If a cue is nearly always present when a problem is present and absent when the problem is absent, it is called a diagnostic cue. In very simple terms, the response to one or more diagnostic cues during assessment is:

What are the most likely explanations for the data being observed? (hypothesis generation)
Which nursing diagnosis is the best explanation for the observed behaviors? (hypothesis testing)

The following assessment data contain diagnostic cues that signify a health problem (nursing diagnosis). Select diagnostic cues from the assessment data and identify the most likely hypotheses that require further assessment:

Mrs. K is a 30-year-old who visits the mental health clinic in her town at the urging of her family and her principal in the grammar school in which she teaches 6th grade. She is married and has four children between 2 and 8 years of age. About 6 months ago, Mrs. K's father was discharged from the hospital after treatment for a broken hip and came to live with Mrs. K and her family. Since he moved in, she has felt very irritable and nervous. The principal in her school has reported that she is extremely hard on the children in her class. In the last 3 or 4 months, she has had episodes of dry mouth and sweaty palms nearly every day.

The initial assessment data reveal four important diagnostic cues: irritability, nervousness, dry mouth, and sweaty palms. To the experienced clinician, these cues are some of the classic signs of anxiety. Even so, with any diagnosis, other hypotheses likely to explain the cues should be considered. The current contextual information is that Mrs. K works, has a family with young children, and has had her father living with her for about 6 months. Further assessment would be done to see if the cues are explained by anxiety or if irritability and nervousness might be a cue to something other than anxiety. Ineffective individual coping with her situation and responsibilities is one diagnostic explanation for the cues that should be considered. At this point in the assessment, thinking is directed toward hypothesis generation, which provides a pool, or set, of diagnostic hypotheses to explain the initial cues. Early in the diagnostic judgment process, hypotheses may be very broad, such as "emotional problem," or early cues might point to specific diagnoses, such as anxiety. As assessment progresses, the diagnostic hypothesis is refined.

Likely diagnostic hypotheses are tested by further assessment to determine if signs and symptoms of the conditions are present. The focused search is for characteristics that have to be present if the condition is present; that is, the critical defining characteristics. Cue recognition, diagnostic hypothesis generation, and hypothesis testing depend on knowledge of the critical characteristics of each common nursing diagnosis.

Accurate diagnoses also depend on knowledge of cues that differentiate between nursing diagnoses. Consider the example of differentiating the diagnostic hypotheses of anxiety and fear. In this case, differential cues are collected to determine if the nervousness is focused on something specific (fear) or if it is diffuse (anxiety). Diagnostic inaccuracies can result if differential characteristics are not known, and these inaccuracies can influence treatment. Ineffective treatment and prolongation of the client's problems can result from incorrect nursing diagnoses.

When the client's problem is formulated, further questions and observations may be needed to identify the factor(s) contributing to the problem. These factors are the link between diagnosis and treatment. If the main factors contributing to the existence and maintenance of a problem can be identified, then treatment can be focused, and the condition can be alleviated or resolved. Otherwise, treatment is symptomatic or palliative. Many of the nursing diagnoses encountered in psychiatric–mental health nursing, such as body image disturbance, self-esteem disturbance, and depression, have complex related factors. In addition, the underlying cause of a problem may be masked by other contributing factors and revealed only as treatment progresses.

THERAPEUTIC JUDGMENT AND NURSING INTERVENTION

Therapeutic judgment underlies the planning, implementation, and evaluation of nursing intervention. As with the previous components of the nursing process, there is lack of agreement on names; terms such as *nursing intervention, nursing action, nursing therapy,* and *nursing treatment* are in current use. Judgments in the therapeutic domain of clinical reasoning are exceedingly important. These judgments can directly affect the client's welfare because in this phase of the nursing process, actions are taken or suggested to the client. Conditional logic provides a framework for therapeutic reasoning; this type of logical reasoning is represented in an "If–then" proposition:

If A, B, and C are done, then X will occur

Assume that A, B, and C are a set of therapeutic actions that will be instituted by the nurse, the client, or both. The prediction is that if A, B, and C are done, then the outcome will be X. The condition, X, is a measurable behavior(s) that indicates the condition identified by the nursing diagnosis is modified or resolved. For example, an outcome might be that a client can maintain employment for 1 year. These ideas should be kept in mind as the planning, implementation, and evaluation phases of nursing intervention are discussed.

Nursing Intervention

The definition of *nursing intervention* proposed by Bulechek and McCloskey is as follows:

> A nursing intervention is an autonomous action based on a scientific rationale that is executed to benefit the client in a predicted way; the action is related to the nursing diagnosis and the stated goals (reference 2, p 8).

This definition describes autonomous actions; that is, interventions within the province of nursing. It does not include medical orders, such as assisting the client to carry out drug therapy. The focus is on treatments nurses prescribe for nursing diagnoses, such as relaxation therapy, diversional activities, social skills training, or participation in a therapeutic milieu.

Note that this definition states that actions are based on a scientific rationale. At present, the theoretical basis for diagnosis-specific interventions is based more on clinical wisdom than on research findings, as there have been insufficient clinical studies of most nursing diagnoses to provide a rationale for interventions. Each professional has a responsibility for identifying the diagnosis-specific interventions that maximize the client's health potential. With such data from practicing nurses, knowledge for practice can be generated. For example, consider 100 adult patients with a particular diagnosis. Research findings from a study of these patients' case records may reveal that 95% or more will reach the desired health outcome, X, when A, B, and C interventions are done. Then it is concluded that interventions A, B, and C, have a high probability of leading to the specified outcomes. This is how knowledge can be generated from the psychiatric nurse's clear specification and documentation of interventions and outcomes.

At this time, the theoretical basis for most nursing diagnosis-based interventions is not research based but rather a logical rationale for how the intervention will "benefit in a predicted way." The definition above also points to another important consideration in the ethics of practice. It states that ". . . actions are executed to benefit the client. . . ." The ethical mandate to any professional is "to do no harm."

The definition also states that an action is related to the nursing diagnosis and goal or projected outcome. As will become clear when care planning is discussed below, nursing diagnoses provide the focus for selecting interventions to resolve the problem. Projected health outcomes describe behaviors indicating this resolution.

Care Planning

After the problem and etiologic factors are specified in the diagnostic statement, the outcomes are projected by the client and nurse, and interventions are identified that will help the client reach the projected outcomes. A health outcome is a concise statement describing an observation. Outcomes specify the behaviors that will be present when the problem is resolved. For example, if a client with advanced Alzheimer's disease has developed a pressure ulcer over a bony prominence, the nurse may reason that if pressure is relieved, the area kept dry, and nutrition maintained, the outcome will be intact skin.

The problem is used as a focus for stating outcomes; the contributing factors (reasons for the problem) usually provide an indication of the length of time it will take for outcomes to be reached. For example, treatment outcomes for knowledge deficit (medication regimen) could be achieved more quickly than could helping a client to raise his self-esteem to a functional level.

Implementation of the Plan

With a well-designed nursing care plan, nursing actions are goal directed. During implementation of the nursing care plan, information is collected and analyzed to determine if interventions are influencing progress toward the projected outcome. Interactions with the client during implementation of nursing care also provide an opportunity to validate further the nursing diagnoses and the projected outcomes that have been identified.

Evaluation of Outcomes

Outcomes provide a focus for evaluating progress toward resolution of a problem identified by a nursing

Research Highlights

As discussed in this chapter, clinical judgment is an important part of all phases of the nursing process. Research on reasoning and judgment skills in the health professions suggests that human beings are capable of adapting their cognitive strategies to the requirements of the task. Beyond the generic behaviors of diagnosticians, there is no single strategy used by all accurate decision makers. Clearly, when microcomponents are studied, there are many pathways to an accurate diagnosis.

Generic components of strategies have been identified. These include the use of divergent and convergent thinking, inductive and deductive reasoning, and intuitive, nonanalytical reasoning. Accuracy in diagnosis seems to depend on clinical knowledge and the use of a strategy consistent with task variables.[4] For example, in a complex task involving large amounts of information, predictive hypothesis testing using divergent thinking process is a useful strategy to control errors. Memory requirements in the task are reduced quickly if information can be obtained to predict the likely possibilities from the universe of possibilities early in the diagnostic task.[9] This strategy narrows the diagnostic task and reduces the information that has to be processed in short-term memory. Ciafrani's studies supported this finding.[3] Controlling the amount of information, thus avoiding overload, seems to be important in reducing errors.

The work of Tanner and her associates suggests that the models developed in studies of physicians' and clinical psychologists' reasoning also can be used to describe nurses' clinical reasoning and judgment in the area of nursing diagnosis.[21,23] Claims that clinicians use early hypothesis generation and hypothesis-directed cue search in their practice are based on the assumption that research tasks are high-fidelity reproductions of clinical conditions. Clearly, subjects are able to accomplish the behaviors described in the models in study settings. More research is needed to establish whether clinicians' behaviors are valid representations of their reasoning in clinical practice or merely induced by the laboratory setting.

Much interesting work is beginning in the area of clinical nursing judgment. In a 5-year project, Gordon and Murphy developed instruments to measure the effect of teaching on baccalaureate staff nurses' clinical reasoning and judgment.[14] Overall findings suggested that four 3-hour classes on a professional model for practice, diagnostic categories, and the diagnostic process, combined with selected exercises, increased diagnostic skills. Research is needed to identify the effect of particular learning experiences within the global approach used in this project. This would enable students to focus on activities that most significantly influence learning.

diagnosis. Evaluative judgments answer the question, "How is the problem responding to the nursing intervention?" Outcomes are the criteria used to determine progress toward problem resolution. For example, if self-esteem disturbance was the problem, and a critical characteristic is self-negating verbalizations, then a reasonable outcome of care would be self-affirming verbalizations. This outcome would be one criterion for judging progress toward resolution of self-esteem disturbance, and the evaluation would be done by assessing self-verbalizations. If outcomes are not attained, it may be that the interventions are not effective, the time to outcome attainment has been underestimated, or the problem, contributing factors, or both have not been specified correctly.

SUMMARY

Information collection and interpretation are continuous throughout the nursing process. The process begins with information collection for purposes of determining if a problem exists and continues to the evaluation of a treatment plan. If a diagnostic cue to a health problem is assessed, the diagnostic judgment process is initiated. Interpreting the diagnostic meaning of the information and formulation of a problem using approved terminology results in a nursing diagnosis. The diagnosis is used as a basis for therapeutic judgments involved in care planning, implementation, and evaluation.

References

1. American Nurses Association. Nursing: A social policy statement. Kansas City: American Nurses Association; 1980.
2. Bulechek G, McCloskey J. Nursing intervention: treatments for nursing diagnoses. Philadelphia: WB Saunders; 1985.
2a. Carroll-Johnson R. NANDA Taxonomy I. In: Carroll-Johnson R, ed. Classification of Nursing Diagnoses: Proceedings of the Eighth Conference. Philadelphia: JB Lippincott; 1988.
3. Ciafrani K. The influence of amounts and relevance of data on identifying health problems. In: Kim MJ, McFarland G, McLane A, eds. Classification of nursing diagnoses: proceedings of the Fifth Conference. St Louis: CV Mosby; 1984.
4. Elstein A, Schulman L, Sprafka S. Medical problem solving: an analysis of clinical reasoning. Cambridge: Harvard University Press; 1978.
5. Gordon M. Issues in nursing diagnosis. In: McLane A, ed. Classification of nursing diagnoses: proceedings of the Seventh Conference. St Louis: CV Mosby; 1987.
6. Gordon M. The nurse as thinking practitioner. In: Hannah K, Reimer R, Mills W, Letourneau S, eds. Clinical judgment and decision making. New York: John Wiley & Sons; 1987.
7. Gordon M. Nursing diagnosis: process and application. New York: McGraw-Hill; 1987.
8. Gordon M. Nursing diagnosis and the diagnostic process. Am J Nursing. 1976;76:1298–1300.
9. Gordon M. Predictive hypothesis testing. Nursing Res. 1980;29:39–45.
10. Kritek P. Report of group work on taxonomies. In: Kim MJ, McFarland G, McLane A, eds. Classification of nursing diagnoses: proceedings of the Fifth Conference. St Louis: CV Mosby; 1984.
11. Kim MJ. Diagnostic: The dilemma of physiological problems: without collaboration, what's left? Am J Nursing. 1985; 85:281–284.
12. McLane A, ed. A taxonomy of nursing diagnoses: toward a science of nursing. Milwaukee Professional Nurse. 1979; 20:33.
13. McLane A. Classification of nursing diagnoses: proceedings of the Seventh Conference. St Louis: CV Mosby; 1988.
14. Murphy C, Gordon M. Integrated model of clinical judgment. Boston College, Chestnut Hill, MA; unpublished manuscript, 1985.
15. Newell A, Simon H. Human problem solving. Englewood Cliffs, NJ: Prentice-Hall; 1972.
16. Orem D. Nursing: concepts of practice. New York: McGraw-Hill; 1980.
17. Riehl J, Roy C Sr. Conceptual models for nursing practice. Ed 2. Norwalk, CT: Appleton-Century-Crofts; 1980.
18. Roy C. Essentials of the Roy adaptation model. Norwalk, CT: Appleton-Century-Crofts; 1986.
19. Roy C. Theoretical framework for classification of nursing diagnosis. In: Kim MJ and Moritz D, eds. Classification of nursing diagnoses: proceedings of the Third and Fourth Conferences. New York: McGraw-Hill; 1982.
20. Shoemaker J. Essential features of nursing diagnosis. In: Kim MJ, McFarland GK, McLane AM, eds. Classification of nursing diagnoses: proceedings of the Fifth Conference. St Louis: CV Mosby; 1984.
21. Tanner CA, Padrick KP, Westfall U, Putzier D. Diagnostic reasoning strategies of nurses and nursing students. Nursing Res. 1987;36:358–363.
22. Werley HH, Lang NM. Identification of the nursing minimum data set. New York: Springer; 1988.
23. Westfall UE, Tanner C, Putzier D, Padrick KP. Activating clinical inferences: component of diagnostic reasoning in nursing. In: Kim MJ, McFarland G, McLane A, eds. Classification of nursing diagnoses: proceedings of the Fifth Conference. St Louis: CV Mosby; 1986.

12

Gertrude K. McFarland
Howard K. Butcher

Assessment of the Psychiatric Mental Health Client

OBJECTIVES
After reading this chapter, the reader will be able to:
1. Discuss the principles for conducting a nursing
   assessment of a psychiatric client
2. Describe the components of the mental status
   examination
3. Cite examples of specific psychological tests and
   discuss the rationale for these tests
4. Discuss the influence of organizational factors,
   client characteristics, and mental health team
   characteristics on the development of a psychiatric
   mental nursing assessment guide
5. Describe strategies for conducting a focused
   assessment and formulating a nursing diagnosis
6. Describe a psychiatric nursing assessment that is
   organized by functional health patterns.

INTRODUCTION

This chapter will describe (1) principles for conducting a nursing assessment of a psychiatric client; (2) developing a psychiatric mental health nursing assessment guide; (3) strategies for conducting a focused assessment and formulating a nursing diagnosis; (4) components of the mental status examination; and (5) aspects of psychological testing.

PRINCIPLES FOR CONDUCTING A NURSING ASSESSMENT OF THE PSYCHIATRIC CLIENT

Setting Priorities

Setting priorities during the assessment phase of the nursing process is as important in the evaluation of the psychiatric client as it is for clients with other health problems. The psychiatric mental health nurse must quickly assess whether or not the client is experiencing a psychiatric emergency, such as suicidal gestures and thoughts or assaultive impulses, that may require immediate intervention. General overall physical health must also be assessed to determine if any physical emergencies exist. This is especially important with the increase in the incidence of drug and alcohol abuse and potential withdrawal reactions. Psychiatric mental health nursing assessment guides can be developed so that collecting such information is given priority in the data collection process.

The Environment

The environment in which the psychiatric mental health nurse conducts the initial interview is an important variable, because the environment can influence whether or not a constructive and useful interview is conducted. A quiet, uninterrupted setting, where the client can talk openly with the nurse in privacy is generally helpful, since intrusion of privacy can be experienced as dehumanizing. Chapter 33, *Milieu Therapy*, discusses strategies for developing a therapeutic milieu, some of which can be adapted in the development of an environment conducive for conducting the initial interview.

Establishing an Interpersonal Relationship

The initial contact with a psychiatric client is important in developing trust and in establishing a therapeutic relationship. Chapter 2, *Therapeutic Relationships With Clients*, and Chapter 6, *The Communication Process*, provide essential knowledge for developing a relationship that is therapeutic. Client characteristics, such as level of fatigue, attention span, thought processes, and level of physical wellness, are important considerations in determining the pace of the initial interview, as well as how much of the database is actually collected during the initial interview session. The conveyance of empathy, unconditional positive regard, and caring can set the stage for a constructive and positive interview experience for the client and for the ability to collect the needed database.

DEVELOPING A GENERAL PSYCHIATRIC MENTAL HEALTH NURSING ASSESSMENT GUIDE

Organizational factors, client characteristics, and mental health team characteristics are essential considerations when developing a general assessment guide for clients in a particular psychiatric setting or practice.

Organizational Factors

Professional practice standards and the mission, philosophy, goals, and policies of a health care organization influence, to an extent, the type of clients admitted and the treatment interventions usually provided. A nursing department espousing a particular conceptual nursing framework as a basis for clinical practice is another important organizational consideration. Chapter 4, *Conceptual Frameworks for Psychiatric Mental Health Nursing Practice*, provides examples of how nursing conceptual frameworks guide psychiatric mental health nursing practice and how nursing diagnoses fit within a particular nursing framework. The nursing conceptual framework espoused is useful in organizing the data to be collected and in structuring the assessment guide. Gordon's Functional Health Patterns (Box 12-1) can also serve as a clinically practical way of structuring and organizing the assessment guide. Gordon's 11 functional health patterns represent a holistic nursing perspective, as "all human beings have in common certain functional patterns that contribute to their health, quality of life and achievement of human potential. These common patterns are the focus of nursing assessment" (reference 6, p 92). Data collection for each of the 11 functional health patterns can be useful in developing initial or working nursing diagnoses, as well as the health assets and health potential of the client that may be useful in developing a meaningful plan of care. Standardization of the data to be collected initially need not interfere with the psychiatric mental health nurse's interpretation of the data based upon the philosophy and conceptual framework that the nurse is using. Box 12-2 provides an example of a general psychiatric nursing assessment guide using the functional health patterns as an organizing framework.

BOX 12–1
Typology of 11 Functional Health Patterns[6]

Health Perception–Health-Management Pattern: Describes client's perceived pattern and well-being and how health is managed

Nutritional–Metabolic Pattern: Describes pattern of food and fluid consumption relative to metabolic need and pattern indicators of local nutrient supply

Elimination Pattern: Describes patterns of excretory function (bowel, bladder, and skin)

Activity–Exercise Pattern: Describes pattern of exercise, activity, leisure, and recreation

Cognitive–Perceptual Pattern: Describes sensory perceptual and cognitive pattern (mental status, pain comfort, sensory modes)

Sleep–Rest Pattern: Describes patterns of sleep, rest, and relaxation

Self-Perception–Self-Concept Pattern: Describes self-concept and perception of self (e.g., body comfort, body image, feeling state)

Role–Relationship Pattern: Describes pattern of role engagements and relationships

Sexuality–Reproductive Pattern: Describes client's patterns of satisfaction and dissatisfaction with sexuality pattern

Coping–Stress Tolerance Pattern: Describes general coping pattern and effectiveness of the pattern in terms of stress tolerance

Value–Belief Pattern: Describes the pattern of values (including spiritual) or goals that guide choices or decisions

Client Characteristics

Development of a general assessment guide is influenced also by the developmental characteristics of the psychiatric client population on a specific unit (i.e., child and adolescent, adult, or geropsychiatric units). Hospital or nursing units focusing on specific psychiatric conditions, such as eating disorders, substance abuse disorders, affective disorders, or schizophrenia, may consider collecting more specific assessment data with relevant functional health patterns for the specific client populations served.

Mental Health Team Characteristics

Psychiatric mental health nurses need to conduct a comprehensive nursing assessment, hence, the importance of developing a comprehensive assessment guide. How the nursing database is integrated into the total psychiatric database depends on the unique characteristics of the health team members, their backgrounds, experience, roles, and the ability of psychiatric mental health nurses to articulate their roles and negotiate with other team members. Collection of duplicate information from a client should be avoided. For example, a psychiatric clinical nurse specialist may be responsible for collecting most of the initial database on a client that will be useful to both psychiatric mental health nurses and other team members. On the other hand, if, for example, detailed information on the family and social history has already been collected by the social worker, the psychiatric mental health nurse can use this data and interpret it from a nursing perspective.

STRATEGIES FOR CONDUCTING A FOCUSED ASSESSMENT AND FORMULATING A NURSING DIAGNOSIS

The psychiatric nursing assessment guide provides an overall means by which the nurse can assess the client and formulate initial or working nursing diagnoses. Four aspects are involved in the diagnostic process: collecting information, interpreting information, clustering information, and naming a cluster or problem.[6] As data is collected, cues need to be clarified and verified. The cues are interpreted by assigning meaning to each one to determine what it signifies. Hypotheses about nursing diagnoses are generated. Cues are related and clustered as they are collected. The cluster of data identifying a problem can be named by using the list of nursing diagnoses. Although the psychiatric nursing assessment guide can be used to identify possible nursing diagnoses, a focused assessment should then be completed. Each nursing diagnosis section contains an assessment section that further validates and clarifies the cluster of cues or the defining characteristics and identifies possible related factors necessary to formulate a specific nursing diagnosis. (See examples in each nursing diagnosis section for specific nursing diagnoses.)

COMPONENTS OF THE MENTAL STATUS EXAMINATION

The *Mental Status Examination* evaluates client functioning in the here and now. However, a client's mental status may change over time. Common aspects of the mental status examination include: attitude, manner, and behavior; mental content; sensorium; emotional tone; and insight (see Box 12-3 for further expansion). The Mini Mental Status Examination (Box 12-4) is a shortened version of the more comprehensive mental status examination. Aspects of this examination can readily be incorporated into a psychiatric nursing assessment guide, particularly one organized by functional health patterns (see Box 12-2 for example).

ASPECTS OF PSYCHOLOGICAL TESTING[11]

Standardized psychological testing has become an integral component of a comprehensive assessment of the

BOX 12-2
Psychiatric Nursing Assessment Guide Organized by Functional Health Patterns[6,10,11]

General Information
Name   Address/Phone
Age   Allergies

Pattern assessment (assess not only complaints, limitations, and problems but also what is being done to alleviate the problem or problems, as well as positive health practices and previous coping skills).

1. HEALTH PERCEPTION–HEALTH MANAGEMENT PATTERN

Physical or psychiatric emergency?
Risk factors
    Suicidal behavior
    Self-destructive behavior
    Aggressive behavior
    Elopement potential
    Other risk factors for injury
Perception of own health state? Chief complaint?
Past psychiatric history?
Previous illness or surgery?
Current illness?
Past and current health seeking behaviors?
Current treatments? On any prescription medications?
Adherence to therapeutic recommendations?
Motivation?
Prevention practices?
General appearance

2. NUTRITIONAL AND METABOLIC PATTERN

Weight? Loss or gain?
Nutritional status? Diet?
Fluid intake?
Drug and alcohol consumption?
Ability to swallow?
Breastfeeding (if applicable)?
Skin, tissue, or mucous membrane integrity?
Dentures?
Body temperature?

3. ELIMINATION PATTERN

Bowel elimination?
Urinary elimination?

4. ACTIVITY–EXERCISE PATTERN

Physical mobility?
Motor activity pattern?
Fatigue level?
Self-care ability? Level of independent functioning?
Growth and development (in relation to age group norms)?
Recreation and leisure activities?
Home maintenance?
Daily activity pattern?
Respirations?
Shortness of breath?
Coughing?
Cyanosis?
Pulse (rate, rhythm, peripheral pulses)?
Blood pressure?
Edema?
Extremities (cold, cyanosis)?

5. SLEEP–REST PATTERN

Sleep habits? Feel rested?
Rest habits?
Methods to promote sleep and relaxation?

6. COGNITIVE–PERCEPTUAL PATTERN

Ability to see, feel, taste, touch, smell?
Special aids?
Orientation?
Level of consciousness?
Pain? Discomfort? How are these managed?
Hallucinations? Delusions?
Obsessions? Phobias?
Memory?
Judgment?
Ability to concentrate?
Decision-making ability?
Education?
General fund of knowledge?
Abstraction ability?
Insight?

7. SELF-PERCEPTION–SELF-CONCEPT PATTERN

Any perceived threat or danger to self or others?
Apprehension? Tension?
Affect/mood? Anxious? Depressed?
Mood change? Lability?
Energy level?
Assertiveness?
Perceived control over situations?
Self-worth? Self-esteem?
Body image? Personal identity?

8. ROLE RELATIONSHIP PATTERN

Significant loss? Grieving?
Ability to perform roles? Occupation?
Marital status?
Communication pattern (nonverbal and verbal)?
Social support system?
Family structure and system?
Parenting practices and problems?
Interpersonal interactions?

9. SEXUALITY AND REPRODUCTION PATTERN

Sexuality pattern? Satisfaction? Dysfunctions?
History of sexual abuse?
Menstrual history?
Contraceptives (use or problems)?

10. COPING–STRESS TOLERANCE PATTERN

Current stressors? Life challenges?
Recent major life changes?
Response and adjustment to trauma?
Defense mechanisms?
Coping strategies?
Resources available to cope with stressors?
Potential for family growth during stress?

11. VALUE–BELIEF PATTERN

Ethnic cultural background?
Overall life belief and values?
Religious affiliation and importance of religion?
Useful religious practices? Which ones are desired while in hospital?
Desire for chaplain visit?

NURSING FORMULATION

1. Strengths and weaknesses
2. Nursing diagnosis(es)

BOX 12–3
Mental Status Examination[16]

ASPECTS OF THE EXAMINATION

1. Attitude, manner, and behavior
   a. Appearance, dress, facial expression, activity, posture, and demeanor are noted.
   b. Disturbances include deviations of degree of activity, mannerisms, distortions of motility, and uncooperativeness.
2. Mental content
   a. This consists of the thoughts, concerns, and trends that are uppermost in the client's mind.
   b. Disturbances of content include delusions, hallucinations, obsessions, and phobias.
3. Sensorium and intellect
   a. The degree of the client's awareness and the level of his or her functioning are noted.
   b. Disturbances of orientation, memory, retention, attention, information, and judgment can be elicited with standardized questions and test materials.
4. Stream of thought
   a. This includes the quantitative and qualitative aspects of the client's verbal communication.
   b. Disturbances include over- and underproductivity, disconnectedness, unintelligibility, and incoherence.
5. Emotional tone
   a. This includes the client's report of subjective feelings (mood or affect) and the examiner's observations of facial expression, posture, and attitude.
   b. Disturbances include both quantitative deviations (elation, depression, apathy) and incongruence (disagreement among the client's subjective report, behavior, and mental content).
6. Insight
   This means the degree to which the patient can appreciate the nature of his or her condition and the need for treatment.

(From Clarence J. Rowe, M.D., An Outline of Psychiatry, 9th ed. Copyright © 1989. Wm. C. Brown Publishers, Dubuque, Iowa. All Rights Reserved. Reprinted by permission.)

---

mental health of a client. Psychological testing is done for the purpose of testing intelligence, personality, neuropsychologic functioning, and for diagnosis.

Intelligence Testing

The purpose of intelligence testing is to assess cognitive and intellectual abilities. The *Wechsler Adult Intelligence Scale* (WAIS-R)[18] is the most widely used standardized test of general intelligence. The test, usually administered by a psychologist, measures verbal, nonverbal, and perceptual motor abilities.

Personality Testing

The purpose of personality testing is to assess personality functioning and psychodynamics. There are several commonly administered tests:

- The *Minnesota Multiphasic Personality Inventory*[1] (MMPI) is a 567 true/false questionnaire designed to measure major aspects of personality related to hypomania, paranoia, hypochondriasis, hysteria, psychopathic deviation, psychasthenia, schizophrenia, masculinity and femininity, and depression.
- The *Thematic Apperception Test* (TAT)[15] is a projective test consisting of a series of 30 pictures. A number of these pictures are presented to the client with instructions that a story be constructed or created about the picture. Interpretation of the client's responses identifies various needs and psychological conflicts.
- The *Rorschach Test*[3] is also a projective test, and consists of a set of ten inkblots. The patient is asked what he or she sees in the inkblot, what it looks like, and what it suggests. Personality style and structure, cognitive style, emotional controls, and the ability to perceive reality are examined.
- In the *Draw a Person Test* (DAP),[9] the client is asked to draw one or more persons and possibly a tree, the family, or an animal. The clinician may also question the patient about the meaning of the drawing. This test is used as a projective test for personality analysis and screening for organic brain damage.
- The *Bender–Gestalt Test*[14] involves presenting the client with cards, one at a time, and asking the client to copy the geometric designs of each of them. The test is used to detect organic abnormality and is also employed as a projective technique to assess personality functioning.
- In the *Sentence Completion Test* (SCT)[8] the client is presented with 75 to 100 sentence stems that he or she is asked to complete with the first response that comes to mind. The test taps much conscious data and can identify the patient's preoccupations, concerns, fears, and goals.
- The *Millon Clinical Multiaxial Inventory*[12] (MCMI-2) is a 175 true/false questionnaire that assesses both Axis I clinical syndromes (anxiety, depression, psychotic thinking) as well as Axis II personality disorders such as narcissistic, hystrionic, and passive–aggressive personality disorders.
- The *Luria-Nebraska Neuropsychological Battery*[5] consists of 16 scales to help identify neuropsychological functioning, whereas the *Halstead-Reitan Neuropsychology Battery* uses several different tests to measure concept formation and tactile and motor functions related to neuropsychological dysfunction.

Structured Interviews

The *Schedule for Affective Disorders and Schizophrenia* (SADS)[2,17] is a detailed interview guide that provides a description of the current episode of illness, as well as the client's level of psychopathology and functioning during the week before the evaluation. The interview consists of eight scales: depressive mood and ideation,

BOX 12–4
Mini Mental State Examination[4]

Patient _____

Examiner _____

Date _____

MAXIMUM SCORE	SCORE	
		ORIENTATION
5	( )	What is the (year) (season) (date) (day) (month)?
5	( )	Where are we: (state) (county) (town) (hospital) (floor)?
		REGISTRATION
3	( )	Name 3 objects: 1 second to say each. Then ask the patient all 3 after you have said them. Give 1 point for each correct answer. Then repeat them until he learns all 3. Count trials and record. Trials _____
		ATTENTION AND CALCULATION
5	( )	Serial 7s. 1 point for each correct. Stop after 5 answers. Alternatively spell "world" backwards.
		RECALL
3	( )	Ask for the 3 objects repeated above. Give 1 point for each correct.
		LANGUAGE

9	( )	Name a pencil, and watch (2 points)
		Repeat the following "No ifs, ands, or buts." (1 point)
		Follow a 3-stage command:
		   "Take a paper in your right hand, fold it in half, and put it on the floor" (3 points)
		Read and obey the following:
		   Close your eyes (1 point)
		   Write a sentence (1 point)
		   Copy design (1 point)
		Total score
		ASSESS level of consciousness along a continuum

Alert	Drowsy	Stupor	Coma

INSTRUCTIONS FOR ADMINISTRATION OF "MINI-MENTAL STATE" EXAMINATION

Orientation
1. Ask for the date. Then ask specifically for part omitted (e.g., "Can you also tell me what season it is?") One point for each correct.
2. Ask in turn "Can you tell me the name of this hospital?" (town, county, etc.). One point for each correct.

Registration
Ask the patient if you may test his memory. Then say the names of 3 unrelated objects, clearly and slowly, about 1 second for each. After having said all 3, ask him to repeat them. This first repetition determines his score (0–3), but keep saying them until he can repeat all 3, up to 6 trials. If he does not eventually learn all 3, recall cannot be meaningfully tested.

Attention and Calculation
Ask the patient to begin with 100 and count backwards by 7. Stop after 5 subtractions (93, 86, 79, 72, 65). Score the total number of correct answers.
If the patient cannot or will not perform this task, ask him to spell the word "world" backwards. The score is the number of letters in correct order (e.g., dlrow = 5, dlorw = 3).

Recall
Ask the patient if he can recall the 3 words you previously asked him to remember. Score 0–3.

Language
Naming: Show the patient a wrist watch and ask him what it is. Repeat for pencil. Score 0–2.
Repetition: Ask the patient to repeat the sentence after you. Allow only one trial. Score 0 or 1.
3-Stage command: Give the patient a piece of plain blank paper and repeat the command. Score 1 point for each part correctly executed.
Reading: On a blank piece of paper print the sentence "Close your eyes," in letters large enough for the patient to see clearly. Ask him to read it and do what it says. Score 1 point only if he actually closes his eyes.
Writing: Give the patient a blank piece of paper and ask him to write a sentence for you. Do not dictate a sentence, it is to be written spontaneously. It must contain a subject and verb and be sensible. Correct grammar and punctuation are not necessary.
Copying: On a clean piece of paper, draw intersecting pentagons, each side about 1 in., and ask him to copy it exactly as it is. All 10 angles must be present and 2 must intersect to score 1 point. Tremor and rotation are ignored.
Estimate the patient's level of sensorium along a continuum, from alert on the left to coma on the right.

Research Highlights

Nursing research can be useful in building a scientific knowledge base about the comprehensive psychiatric mental health nursing assessment of clients. Included among priority areas for nursing research are

- Development of the validity and reliability of psychiatric mental health assessment tools
- Determination of the usefulness of psychiatric nursing assessment guides in assisting psychiatric mental health nurses in formulating initial nursing diagnoses

- Determination of the influence of aspects of the environment on the quality of the initial interview
- Evaluation of the influence of caring on the establishment of a constructive interpersonal relationship during the initial nursing assessment
- Identification of client satisfaction with the assessment process
- Comparison of various combinations of team member roles in the assessment process

endogenous features, depressive-associated features, suicidal ideation and behavior, anxiety, manic syndrome, delusions–hallucinations, and formal thought disorder. The interview guide is used to increase the reliability of diagnostic judgments. In some clinical settings, skilled psychiatric mental health nurses administer this test.

The *Brief Psychiatric Rating Scale* (BPRS)[13] is a broad, highly efficient, rapid evaluation scale yielding a comprehensive description of major symptom characteristics. The scale has been used to evaluate patient change in psychoactive drug research; examination and evaluation of psychiatric diagnosis; to describe, measure, and classify psychiatric clients and their psychopathology; and to develop clinical prediction models for treatment response expectations.

Nurses need to collaborate with the psychologist to review the test assessments and to incorporate these findings into the overall treatment plan.

SUMMARY

The environment, nature of interpersonal relationships, and health care needs must all be considered in conducting a nursing assessment of a psychiatric client. Organizational factors, client characteristics, and mental health team characteristics are important considerations in developing a mental health nursing assessment guide. After an overall assessment is conducted, a focused assessment will be useful in formulating more specific nursing diagnoses. Finally, psychiatric mental health nurses must work collaboratively with other mental health team members in collecting a comprehensive database that will be useful in developing the treatment plan.

References

1. Dahlstrom WG, Welsh GS, Dahlstrom LE. An MMPI handbook, vol. 2. Research application. Minneapolis: University of Minnesota Press; 1975.

2. Endicott J, Spitzer RL. A diagnostic interview: The schedule for affective disorders and schizophrenia. Arch Gen Psychiatry. 1978;35:837–844.

3. Exner JE. The Rorschach: A comprehensive system, vol. 1. Basic foundations, 2nd ed. New York: Wiley; 1986.

4. Folstein JF, Folstein SE, McHugh PR. Mini-mental state: a practical method for grading the cognitive state of patients for the clinician. Oxford: Pergamon Press; 1975.

5. Golden CJ, Purisch AD, Hammeke TA. The Luria-Nebraska neuropsychological battery, Forms I & II manual. Los Angeles: Western Psychological Services; 1985.

6. Gordon M. Nursing diagnoses: process and application, 2nd ed. New York: McGraw Hill Book Company; 1987.

7. Hamilton Psychiatric Hospital. Health pattern assessment. Nursing Department: Hamilton, Ontario, Canada; 1989.

8. Loevinger J, Wessler R, Redmore C. Loevinger's Washington University sentence completion test of ego development. Measuring ego development, vol. 2. San Francisco: Jossey-Bass; 1970.

9. Machover K. Personality projection in drawing of the human figure. Springfield, Ill: Thomas; 1949.

10. McFarland G. Nursing Diagnosis: The critical link in the nursing process. In McFarland G, McFarlane E. Nursing diagnosis and intervention: planning for patient care. St. Louis: CV Mosby; 1989.

11. McFarland G, Wasli E. Nursing diagnosis in psychiatric/mental health nursing. Philadelphia: JB Lippincott; 1986.

12. Millon T. Manual for the MCMI-II. Minneapolis: National Computer Systems; 1987.

13. Overall JE. The brief psychiatric rating scale in psychopharmacology research. Psychometric Laboratory Reports, No. 29. Galveston: University of Texas; 1972.

14. Pascal G, Suttell BJ. Bender Gestalt test. New York: Grune & Stratton; 1951.

15. Rosenwald A. The thematic apperception test. In Rubin A, ed. Projective techniques in personality assessment. New York: Springer; 1968.

16. Rowe CJ. An outline of psychiatry, 9th ed. Dubuque, Iowa: Brown Publishing; 1989.

17. Spitzer RL, Endicott J. Schedule for affective disorder and schizophrenia. Biometrics Research. New York: State Development of Mental Hygiene; 1975.

18. Wechsler D. Manual for the Wechsler adult intelligence scale-revised. New York: Psychological Corporation; 1981.

13

Nursing Diagnoses

AGGRESSION (MILD, MODERATE, SEVERE, EXTREME/
    VIOLENCE)
AGITATION
ANGER
ANXIETY (MILD, MODERATE, SEVERE, EXTREME/PANIC)
BIZARRE BEHAVIOR
BOREDOM
COMMUNICATION, IMPAIRED
COPING, FAMILY, POTENTIAL FOR GROWTH
COPING, INEFFECTIVE INDIVIDUAL
CRISIS, MATURATIONAL AND SITUATIONAL
DECISIONAL CONFLICT
DEFENSIVE COPING (SPECIFY)
DEPRESSION
DIVERSIONAL ACTIVITY DEFICIT
ELOPEMENT, POTENTIAL FOR
EMOTIONAL LABILITY
FAMILY PROCESSES, DYSFUNCTIONAL
FEAR
GRIEVING, ANTICIPATORY GRIEVING, DYSFUNCTIONAL
    GRIEVING
GROWTH AND DEVELOPMENT, ALTERED
GUILT
HEALTH MAINTENANCE, ALTERED
HOPELESSNESS
IMPULSE CONTROL, ALTERED
INJURY, POTENTIAL FOR
KNOWLEDGE DEFICIT (SPECIFY)
LONELINESS

MANIPULATION
NONCOMPLIANCE (SPECIFY)
NUTRITION, ALTERED, LESS THAN BODY REQUIREMENTS
PARENTING, ALTERED (ACTUAL, POTENTIAL)
PERCEPTION/COGNITION, ALTERED (CONFUSION,
    DELUSIONS, HALLUCINATIONS, MEMORY LOSS)
POST OVERDOSE SYNDROME
POST TRAUMA RESPONSE
POWERLESSNESS
RAPE TRAUMA SYNDROME
REGRESSED BEHAVIOR
RESOURCE MANAGEMENT, IMPAIRED (SPECIFY)
RITUALISTIC BEHAVIOR
SELF-CARE DEFICIT
SELF-CONCEPT DISTURBANCE (PERSONAL IDENTITY
    DISTURBANCE, SELF-ESTEEM DISTURBANCE, BODY
    IMAGE DISTURBANCE, ROLE PERFORMANCE
    DISTURBANCE)
SEXUAL DYSFUNCTION
SLEEP PATTERN DISTURBANCE
SOCIAL INTERACTION, IMPAIRED
SOMATIZATION
SPIRITUAL DISTRESS
SUBSTANCE ABUSE (ALCOHOL)
SUBSTANCE ABUSE (DRUGS)
SUICIDE POTENTIAL
SUSPICIOUSNESS
WELLNESS-SEEKING BEHAVIOR

INTRODUCTION: NURSING DIAGNOSES IN PSYCHIATRIC MENTAL HEALTH NURSING
State of the Art
Organization of Chapter
Future Directions

NURSING DIAGNOSIS SECTIONS
Each nursing diagnosis section is organized according to the following outline:
DEFINITION AND DESCRIPTION
THEORY AND RESEARCH
RELATED/RISK FACTORS
DEFINING CHARACTERISTICS
NURSING PROCESS AND RATIONALE
Assessment
Nursing Diagnosis
Client Goals and Nursing Interventions
Evaluation
CASE STUDY
RESEARCH HIGHLIGHTS
SUMMARY
REFERENCES

OBJECTIVES

After reading this chapter, the reader will be able to:

1. *Define and describe each nursing diagnosis category presented in the chapter*
2. *Discuss relevant theories and/or research studies for each nursing diagnosis category presented in the chapter*
3. *Identify related factors or risk factors for each nursing diagnosis category presented in the chapter*
4. *Identify defining characteristics for each nursing diagnosis category presented in the chapter*
5. *Specify focused assessment criteria for each nursing diagnosis category presented in the chapter*
6. *Formulate two examples of client–specific nursing diagnoses for each nursing diagnosis category presented in the chapter*
7. *Discuss appropriate client goals and nursing interventions for each nursing diagnosis category presented in the chapter*
8. *Examine outcome criteria for each nursing diagnosis category, indicating attainment of the identified client goals*
9. *Assess a client; formulate a specific nursing diagnosis or diagnoses; identify client goals; select and implement, as possible, appropriate nursing interventions; and evaluate outcomes of care*
10. *Identify one research question for each nursing diagnosis category presented in the chapter.*

NURSING DIAGNOSES IN PSYCHIATRIC MENTAL HEALTH NURSING PRACTICE

State of the Art

The North American Nursing Diagnosis Association (NANDA) "is organized to develop, refine and promote a taxonomy of nursing diagnostic terminology of general use to professional nurses" (reference 11, p 1). (See also Chapters 1 and 11.) NANDA has identified 98 nursing diagnoses to date, which appear in the NANDA's Taxonomy I, Revised. (See Appendix I.) As has been mentioned, NANDA's work is sanctioned by the American Nurses' Association. Although much progress has been made since 1973, the nursing diagnoses, as developed by NANDA, are incomplete for psychiatric mental health nursing practice. "At its February 1984 meeting, the Executive Committee of the Division on Psychiatric and Mental Health Nursing Practice of the American Nurses' Association (ANA) authorized support for identification of the phenomena of concern for psychiatric mental health (PMH) nursing practice" (reference 3, p 16). Loomis et al[3] present a listing of subpatterns and human responses in the perceptual/cognitive and socio/behavioral human response patterns. Based upon this developmental work, and on their combined expertise as educators, researchers, and clinicians, McFarland[1,2,4–10,16] and Thomas[12–15,17] selected a list of over 50 nursing diagnosis categories judged to be most useful for psychiatric mental health nursing practice. Definitions were developed for each nursing diagnosis consistent with common usage. In this chapter, each of these major nursing diagnoses are presented and developed in-depth, according to a consistent outline, by psychiatric mental health nurse experts.

Organization of Chapter

The first subsection of each nursing diagnosis section —*Definition and Description*—presents a clear definition of each nursing diagnosis category, differentiating this category from other categories. Meaning is further enhanced by a thorough literature review of relevant theory and research in the subsection *Theory and Research*.

The *Related Factors* identify the most common (although not exhaustive) internal or external factors that contribute to the development, existence, and/or maintenance of a client's health problem. Related factors are included in a nursing diagnostic statement, making it more specific and thus more useful in providing directions for the selection of nursing interventions. *Risk Factors* are identified for potential nursing diagnosis categories.

Defining Characteristics are the most common cluster of both subjective and objective signs and symptoms present in a client with a nursing diagnosis. Although much of the work on defining characteristics, as well as on related factors, is based on clinical observation and group consensus, available research is incorporated within the discussions presented. Chart 1 in each section summarizes the definition, related/risk factors, and defining characteristics.

The nursing process is then thoroughly addressed. Focused assessment criteria are presented for each nursing diagnosis category, followed by examples of how the nursing diagnosis category can be made more specific. A discussion of major client goals and relevant nursing interventions, including rationale, is followed by specification of outcome criteria as a means of determining whether client goals have been met. Chart 2 in each section summarizes the nursing process. Both charts can be useful in care planning. Each nursing diagnosis section also includes a *Case Study* and *Research Highlights*.

Future Directions

While state of the art information is presented in each section, the development of nursing diagnoses and a taxonomy is an evolving and an ever-changing process. Continuous clinical nursing research is needed to validate the nursing diagnoses identified to date and to continue to identify additional ones where gaps in the taxonomy remain for psychiatric mental health practice. Each psychiatric mental health nurse is invited and encouraged to observe clinically the usefulness of the nursing diagnosis categories presented, to engage in research as much as possible, and to provide feedback through professional channels in order to continue to build on the current knowledge base.

Gertrude K. McFarland

References

1. Kim M, McFarland G, McLane A, eds. Classification of nursing diagnoses: Proceedings of the Fifth National Conference. St. Louis: CV Mosby Co; 1984.
2. Kim M, McFarland G, McLane A. Pocket guide to nursing diagnoses. 3rd ed. St. Louis: CV Mosby Co; 1989.
3. Loomis M, O'Toole A, Brown M, Pothier P, West P, Wilson H. Development of a classification system for psychiatric/mental health nursing: individual response class. Arch Psychiatric Nursing. 1987;1.
4. McFarland G, McFarlane E. Nursing diagnoses and interventions: Planning for patient care. St. Louis: CV Mosby Co; 1989.
5. McFarland G, Naschinski C. Anticipatory & dysfunctional grieving and inappropriate aggression: A descriptive study. In: Hurley M, ed. Classification of nursing diagnoses: Proceedings of the Sixth conference. St. Louis: CV Mosby Co; 1986.
6. McFarland G, Naschinski C. Impaired communication: A descriptive study. Nurs Clin North Am. 1985;20:775–785.
7. McFarland G, von Schilling K. Eltern und ihre Trauer bei

Tod, lebensbedrohlicher Erkrankung oder Behinderung ihres Kindes. Notwendige Kenntnisse und Hilfsmoglichkeiten. Der Kinderarzt. 1985;33:1517–1522.

8. McFarland G, Wasli E. Care of the adult psychiatric patient. In: Brunner L, Suddarth D. Lippincott manual for nursing practice. 3rd ed. Philadelphia: JB Lippincott Co; 1982.

9. McFarland G, Wasli W. Nursing diagnoses and process in psychiatric mental health nursing. Philadelphia: JB Lippincott Co; 1986.

10. Meldman M, McFarland G, Johnson E. The problem oriented psychiatric index and treatment plans. St. Louis: CV Mosby Co; 1976.

11. North American Nursing Diagnosis Association. Bylaws of the North American Nursing Diagnosis Association. St. Louis: North American Nursing Diagnosis Association; 1986.

12. Sanger E, Thomas MD, Whitney J. A guide for nursing assessment of the psychiatric inpatient. Arch Psychiatric Nursing. 1988;2.

13. Thomas MD, Coombs R. Nursing diagnosis: Process and decision. In: LaMonica E, ed. The humanistic nursing process. Monterey: Wadsworth Health Sciences; 1985.

14. Thomas MD, Sanger E, Whitney J. Nursing diagnosis of depression: Clinical identification on an inpatient unit. J Psychosoc Nurs and Ment Health Serv. 1986;24:6–12.

15. Thomas MD, Sanger E, Wolf-Wilets V, Whitney JD. Nursing diagnosis of patients with manic and thought disorders. Arch Psychiatric Nursing. 1988;2(6):339–344.

16. Thompson J, McFarland G, Hirsch J, Tucker S, Bowers A. Mosby's manual of clinical nursing. 2nd ed. St. Louis: CV Mosby Co; 1989.

17. Whitney JD, Sanger E, Thomas MD, Wolf-Wilets V. A validation study of the nursing diagnosis "somatization." Arch Psychiatric Nursing. 1988;2(6):345–349.

AGGRESSION

(MILD, MODERATE, SEVERE, EXTREME/VIOLENCE)

Deanah I. Alexander

DEFINITION AND DESCRIPTION

Aggression is a forceful, inappropriate, nonadaptive verbal or physical action designed to pursue personal interests. It may result from such feelings or emotional states as anger, anxiety, tension, guilt, frustration, or hostility. Behaviors can be classified into categories of disturbing behaviors, behaviors endangering self, and behaviors endangering others.

The levels of aggression are mild, moderate, severe, and extreme/violence. *Mild aggression* is characterized by actions that convey displeasure or tension, such as sarcasm, verbal responses that are slightly derogatory (e.g., name calling), facial expressions such as grimacing or sticking out the tongue, and hand movements that have sexual connotations. *Moderately aggressive* actions are more forthright in conveying displeasure, anger, or hostility. Some examples are slamming doors, throwing objects not at a target, verbal degradation (e.g., personal insults), and verbal harrassment (e.g., nagging). Many actions fit under either mild or moderate, depending on their intensity and duration. Severe and extreme aggression are best described as the far end of the continuum in destructive behaviors.[2] *Severe aggression* may include the above-described behaviors in increased forcefulness. The presence of a target in physical aggression occurs in these two levels. Threats of physical violence also are part of this stage of aggression. *Extreme aggression/violence* is linked with the physical acting out of anger, frustration, tension, or hostility. The verbal and facial descriptors may or may not be present during the act of violence depending on the amount of guilt and suppression/repression used. A threat of physical harm that is carried out is an example of aggression that has moved from severe to extreme. Extreme aggression includes a loss of control over one's behavior.

THEORY AND RESEARCH

Studies of aggression have been limited primarily to clients with a diagnosis of mental illness or to clients receiving care in long-term care settings. The majority of these studies have focused on physically aggressive behavior that would endanger the client or another person.[6] Long-term care settings have a high incidence of residents with diagnoses of both organic brain syndrome and aggressive behavior.[8,12] These clients' aggression seems to stem from disorganization and frustration felt in a loosely structured milieu and thus differs from aggression seen in psychiatric clients, who may suffer from paranoid delusions or hallucinations and are prone to be violent in response to fixed false beliefs or to the receiving of messages to harm self or others. Clients with longer stays and less control over situational activities have a higher incidence of aggressive behavior.[12]

Violent behavior and aggression are thought to be underreported in psychiatric settings.[2,7] Professional denial of the unwanted behavior has been recognized and likened to the denial of battering in families. The types of aggression that are most likely to be reported are self-injurious behaviors or behaviors that injure other clients rather than aggression aimed at staff. In dealing with extreme aggression/violence, the most frequent intervention is restraint, chemical or physical. Verbal intervention is used as an adjunct.

Numerous studies state that the prediction of future violence in the criminally insane ranges from 30% to 95%.[10] In the mentally ill population, clients with schizophrenia have been considered the most dangerous group, but their rate of violent behavior is low; i.e., 5 in 10,000.[10]

Neurobiologic research on aggressive behavior has identified several neurotransmitters that may be responsible for the increase or decrease in aggression. An increase in acetylcholine and dopamine appears to enhance aggression in mammals. Norepinephrine effects are variable: studies have shown both enhancement and inhibition.[3] Dopamine antagonists are the basis of antipsychotic medications, which accounts for their effect. Serotonin and gamma-aminobutyric acid (GABA) appear to inhibit aggression in animals and humans. Benzodiazepines enhance GABA activity, thus reducing aggression, although there is evidence that in humans, the chronic use of low-dose benzodiazepines may increase aggressive behavior.[3]

The extent to which aggression is a learned behavior is not yet resolved. However, because aggression is made up of a wide range of behaviors, it appears that there is also multiple causation.[4,5,11]

RELATED FACTORS

Outbursts of aggression or rage occur in the following diagnostic categories: alcohol idiosyncratic intoxication, alcohol intoxication, amphetamine intoxication, antisocial personality disorder, borderline personality disorder, cocaine intoxication, dementia, inhalant intoxication, intermittent explosive disorder, late luteal-phase dysphoric disorder, mental retardation, multi-infarct dementia, nicotine withdrawal, oppositional defiant disorder, organic personality disorder, posttraumatic stress disorder, primary degenerative dementia of the Alzheimer type, and sedative, hypnotic, or anxiolytic intoxication.[1]

Although DSM-III-R does not list aggression per se as occurring in the psychotic disorders such as schizophrenia and bipolar disorder, the diagnostic criteria include behaviors that fit within the definition of aggression. Aggression may occur in response to hallucinations such as hearing voices that give direction to hurt self or another. This aggression is more likely to be of the severe or extreme type. An individual experiencing a manic state may evidence all of the types of aggression. The use of sarcasm and biting humor as well as derogatory comments are common responses to a feeling of low self-esteem and fear of loss of control. The mild and moderate types of aggression can easily be recognized in individuals who have not been classified as mentally ill. These responses to feelings of anger, frustration, and guilt often are condoned by society. The person who has deep-rooted anger and sublimates this with sarcasm or a "dry" sense of humor may be admired, and thus rewarded, for self control.

Aggression that endangers others may be in the form of physical acting out seen in the severe and extreme types. These behaviors may be common in males from disadvantaged populations.[10] Those with poor access to resources and those living in a high stress environment are more prone to violence. A previous episode of violence increases the person's probability of repeating the action unless there has been external intervention. Childhood experience with aggression in the family setting is also a factor. Children who have seen aggression may learn that behavioral response. Adults who are aggressive but do not recall any childhood experience may have blocked an experience, which may surface with intensive psychotherapy.

The various types of toxicities and organic brain disorders in which aggression occurs point to alteration of neurologic function as a related factor. The elderly seem to be more prone to experience multiple physiologic factors that can lead to aggression. In addition, sensory impairment, physical discomfort, communication problems, and environmental overstimulation or understimulation can contribute to the development of aggression.[9] Another related factor in severe and extreme aggression is the availability of weapons, victims, and a substance that alters self-control, such as drugs or alcohol.

DEFINING CHARACTERISTICS

Behaviors that indicate impending or mild aggression are those indicating anxiety, anger, hostility, or guilt.

Verbal signs are sarcasm, raised or quavering voice tone and pitch, rapid or hesitant speech, derogatory comments, and threats. Physical signs such as pacing, tightened lips, narrowed eyes, reddened face, and fast or irregular breathing often indicate impending aggression. Prodomal signs may include disturbed thought process or perception, anger disproportionate to an event, fatigue, hypersensitivity to stimuli, and misinterpretation of stimuli.

The client who expresses fear of self or others has the potential of losing control. The event or events that could result in actual loss of control are unique to each person. For example, a person who remains in control in a structured environment may quickly decompensate as changes occur.

Physical signs of aggression are pacing; muscle tension; sharp, quickened movements; and striking or throwing objects. The observation of overcontrolled behavior indicates mild aggression that may escalate to various degrees. The overly controlled person is one who may be consciously trying to keep aggression under control or using reaction formation.

Physical activity in aggression ranges from purposeless movement to physical assault. The throwing of an object in anger provides a temporary release of energy. The child who falls to the floor in a temper tantrum while kicking and beating the air is providing an example of aggressive movement that indicates an intense emotion being discharged.

The nurse should be alert to the possibility of aggressiveness in clients with suspiciousness and inability to trust. The suspiciousness may be in the form of delusions of persecution or generalized paranoia. Suspiciousness, along with a high degree of disorganization, often is evident in toxic or organic states.

The use of humor as an outlet for mild or moderate aggression has been described since the time of Freud. The sarcastic wit of one person to vent frustration or anger toward the butt of the joke is a repression of aggression. By including a third person as the audience, the first receives validation of an acceptable release of aggression.

Mild and moderate aggression may be expressed sexually through hand gestures or sexually related derogatory phrases. Graffiti is another form of mild aggression that is often coupled with sexual expression. Seductiveness may be used as mild to moderate aggression when the intention is to tease. Severe and extreme sexual aggression is observed in sadism, masochism, and rape. The self-mutilating acts such as cutting that are observed in the client with borderline personality disorder are certainly self-aggressive (Chart 1).

NURSING PROCESS AND RATIONALE

Assessment

The nurse who assesses situations in terms of the potential for aggression but conveys an expectation that

CHART 1
Aggression: Definition, Related Factors, and Defining Characteristics

DEFINITION

Aggression is a forceful, inappropriate, nonadaptive verbal or physical action designed to pursue self-interests. It may result from such feelings or emotional states as anger, anxiety, tension, guilt, or hostility, which, in turn, result from a variety of precipitating factors. The levels of aggression are mild, moderate, severe, and extreme/violence.

RELATED FACTORS

Intoxication
Antisocial personality disorder
Borderline personality disorder
Intermittent explosive disorder
Late luteal-phase dysphoric disorder
Mental retardation
Organic mental disorders
Schizophrenia
Bipolar disorder
Anger
Hallucinations
Delusions of persecution
Frustration
Cultural factors
Interpersonal conflict
Availability of weapons
Blocked personal goals
Sensory impairment

DEFINING CHARACTERISTICS

Sarcasm
Verbal or physical threats
Change in voice tone
Degrading comments
Pacing
Throwing or striking objects or people
Suspiciousness
Suicidal ideation
Homicidal ideation
Self-mutilation
Invasion of personal space
Increase in agitation/irritability
Disturbed thought process/perception
Misinterpretation of stimuli
Anger disproportionate to event

Nursing Diagnosis

Formulation of a nursing diagnosis of aggressive behavior follows assessment of the client and the situation. Moderate aggression related to frustration would be the diagnosis in the case of a client who becomes angry and responds by throwing objects, slamming doors, and yelling. A client who is sarcastic and uses biting humor may be displaying mild aggression related to feelings of inferiority.

Client Goals and Nursing Interventions

The primary goal in nursing intervention with the aggressive client is to direct the expression of the emotion in a socially acceptable manner. The client who is using mild aggressive forms may need little intervention if this behavior is not disruptive to the client or those around him or her. Clients who primarily use moderate aggression will benefit from psychotherapy, individual or group, to find the underlying emotion. The client who has aggression as a response to confusion, as in organic brain syndrome, generally will respond positively to a set routine, which will lessen overstimulation and provide something consistent on which the client can depend. Allowing these individuals to participate actively in their care will decrease their frustration. The neurologically impaired client will benefit from frequent reorientation to time, place, person, etc. The client is best approached in a calm, firm manner using a moderate voice tone to increase the feeling of security. Giving simple directions rather than asking questions helps decrease aggression. Use of touch as a therapeutic intervention can aid in reorientation and in decreasing frustration in some clients. An example is holding the hand of a person while giving a simple direction such as "come and sit with me on the couch." However, to clients with suspiciousness or neurologic impairment, touch may be a trigger that precipitates physical aggression.

Teaching problem-solving techniques and assertiveness are appropriate interventions for clients who are cognitively clear; i.e., not confused. The teaching must be done while the client is either not aggressive or in a mild stage. Teaching problem solving by breaking it into steps lessens the amount of overload a client feels at learning new behavior (Box 13-1).

The expression of severe and extreme aggression frequently calls for external control in order to protect the client and others. The long-term goals are to maintain the client's dignity and to reinforce self-esteem. It is the nurse's responsibility to be familiar with the seclusion and restraint policies of the institution, as well as with the legal implications.

Chemical restraint is the use of medication to calm or sedate the client. These medications may be ordered PRN, dependent on the behavior exhibited. In the client who appears to be escalating toward severe/ex-

aggression will not occur increases the self-control of clients. Client verbalizations of fear of loss of control or of feelings of wanting to harm others should be heeded. History taking will include a review of aggressive thoughts and actions toward others and self and of past problem-solving methods. Observation of the general mood and actions of the client may give subtle clues of increasing aggression. Physical signs to watch for are rapid gait, abrupt or constant movements, narrowed eyes, and quavering voice. These are signs of mild to moderate aggression and may precede a more intense level of aggression.

BOX 13–1
Problem-Solving Steps

1. Stop before acting.
2. State the problem.
3. Identify alternative solutions.
4. Evaluate the alternatives individually by considering their positive and negative features.
5. Choose one alternative and plan to carry it out.
6. Determine the resources needed to carry out the plan.
7. Set a specific time to try the alternative behavior.
8. If the chosen alternative does not work, go back to Step 1.

treme aggression, the use of PRN medication may prevent violence.

Other interventions include modification of the environment, such as eliminating a source of noise, removing others from the surroundings, or moving to a place where the client is not overwhelmed by sensory input. A clearly stated expectation of control of aggressive impulses will reassure the client. Verbal statements that the staff will provide external control to prevent harm reassures the client that he or she is safe and that the client and others will remain in control. The fear of losing control and the unknown consequences of being out of control can lead to panic reactions in clients already under stress. The nurse's statement that control will be maintained must be delivered as a reassurance rather than as a threat.

The nurse should be aware of the territoriality of the client and be wary of initiating touch with a client who may misinterpret physical contact. The client should be given freedom to move about in a defined area unless physical restraint is a probable action. It also is best to keep an escape open for both the client and the nurse. The client who feels trapped is more likely to lash out in violence, and the nurse should not take on a hero role if there is not sufficient back-up for physical restraint.

PHYSICAL RESTRAINT

Physical restraint should be used as a last resort and never as a punishment. Informing a client of seclusion and restraint use should not be a threat but a sharing of information. When the decision is made to restrain the client, the intervention team should act as a unit. This team is a trained response group for intervention in severe, extreme aggression. Safe intervention using physical restraint requires a minimum of four team members. One person is the preappointed leader, who gives the direction for action. Often, having the intervention team visible will provide an incentive for the client to maintain self-control. The team should act quickly in removing the client to a safe environment and applying restraints. While the team is in action, the leader should talk calmly to the client, explaining what is taking place. All team members should be aware of their own emotions and should guard against responding with anger.

Team members should maintain awareness of the strength of their hand grip. It is necessary to grip the resistive client firmly; however, as the client calms, or as control is gained, the grip can be loosened so as to not injure the client. The team also should be aware of the interactions among themselves. Humor is common as a tension release but is inappropriate while the client is being transported or restrained. The use of small talk or talking about the client is likewise inappropriate. Other safety measures for staff include the removal of their jewelry, eyeglasses, name tags, and any ornaments that may cause harm or be used as a weapon.

The basic hold used in restraint or transporting a client is called the basket hold (Fig. 13-1). This hold is accomplished by crossing the client's arms in front with the staff member holding the client's wrists. The staff member is in back of the client in the completed basket hold. From this position, the staff member can ease the client down to the floor if necessary.

Transporting a client may involve walking with support or a carry. This is accomplished by having a staff member on each side supporting the client's arms at the elbow and above the wrist. The staff members must adjust their strides to each other and to the client so he or she is not dragged. If the client is very resistive, it may be necessary to walk the client backward in order to have better control (Fig. 13-2). The possibility that the client will fall to the floor while walking backward should be kept in mind. If a client falls or is eased down to the floor, the staff should attempt to cushion the impact, with special attention to preventing injury to the head.

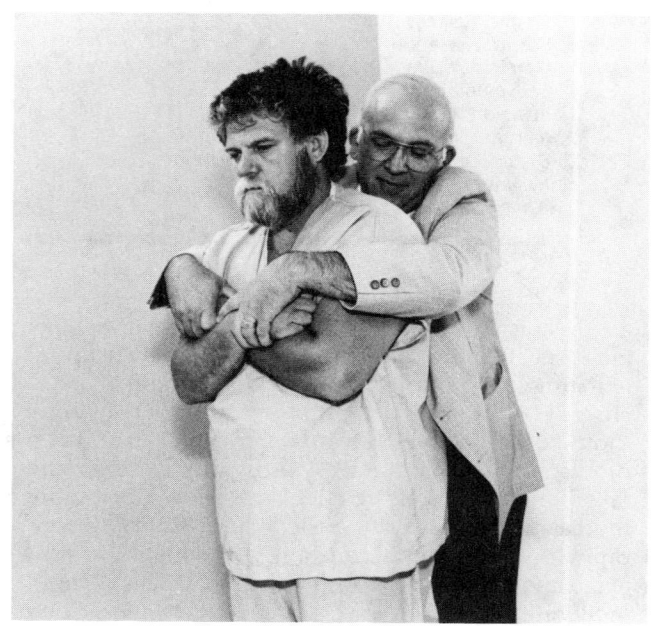

FIGURE 13–1. Basket hold.

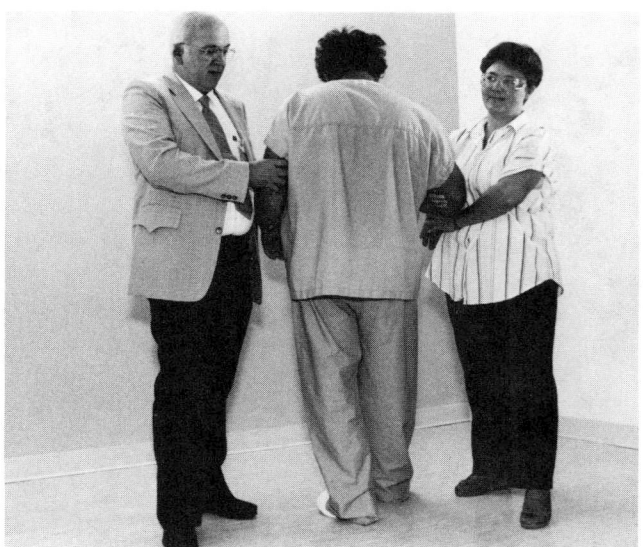

FIGURE 13–2. Walking a client backward.

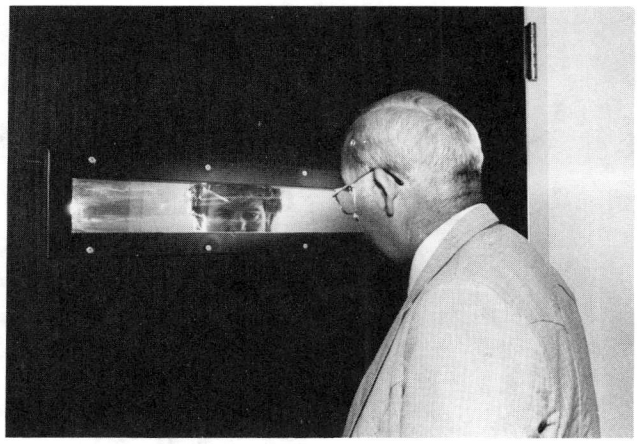

FIGURE 13–4. Visual check of seclusion room.

check the seclusion room visually before entering (Fig. 13-4).

Among those clients with extreme aggression are those who pull the hair of another. Quick intervention is required to prevent or lessen the harm. In Figure

If it is necessary to carry a client, there must be adequate staffpower, usually between three and five staff members. The client's head and shoulders are supported by one or two staff, either with a basket hold or as in the walk. Hip support usually involves the most weight and may require one or two staff. One person usually is sufficient to carry the feet. If too many staff members attempt to help, there is an increased risk of injury.

The use of physical restraint is pictured in Figure 13-3. The client is in full restraint and secured with locking leather restraints around the wrists, ankles, and waist. A client restrained on his back must be observed continually because of the danger of aspiration. If a client must be restrained for more than short periods of time, it is preferable to place him on the abdomen or side. Any time a client is restrained, the nurse must make frequent visual checks, at least every 15 minutes, and provide continuous monitoring of the client's status. For those clients who are placed in a seclusion room, an additional safety measure is to

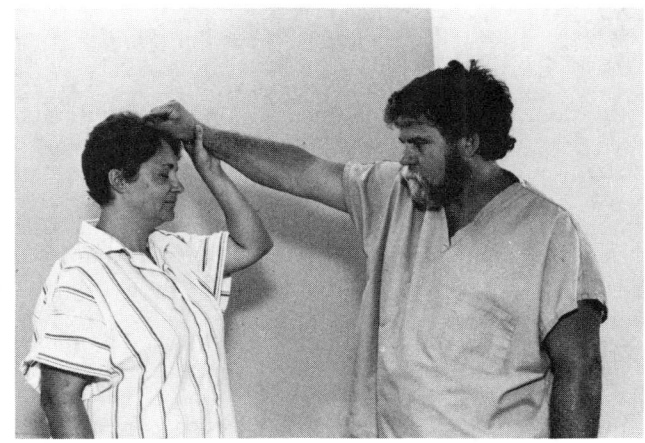

FIGURE 13–5. Breaking a hair pull.

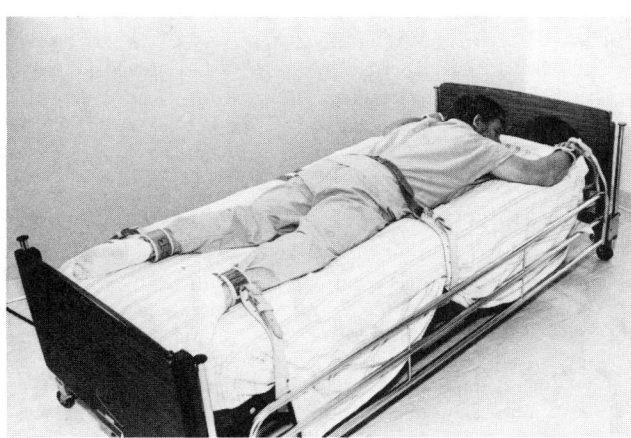

FIGURE 13–3. Client in full restraint.

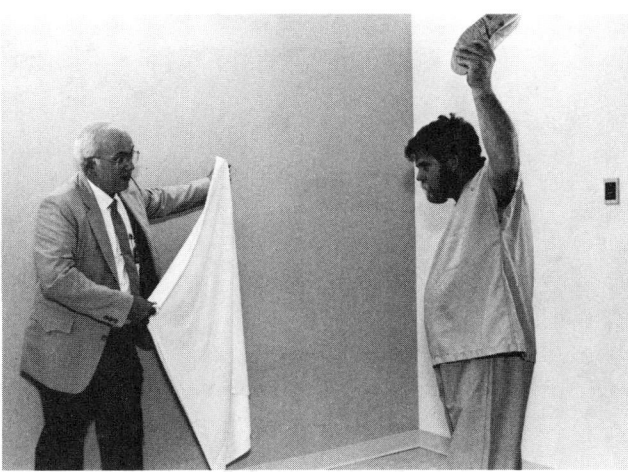

FIGURE 13–6. Client threatens with object.

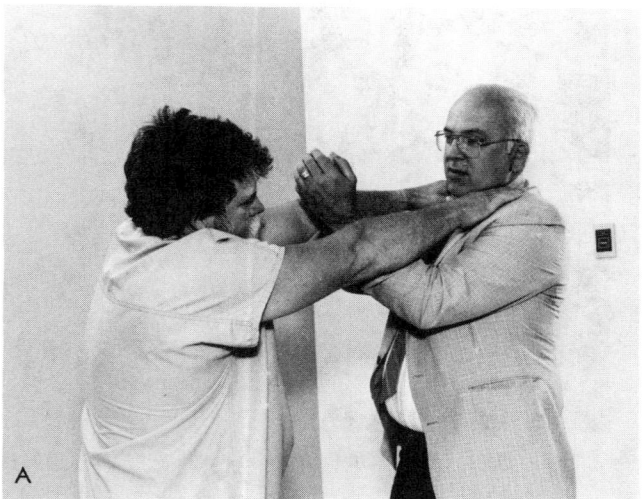
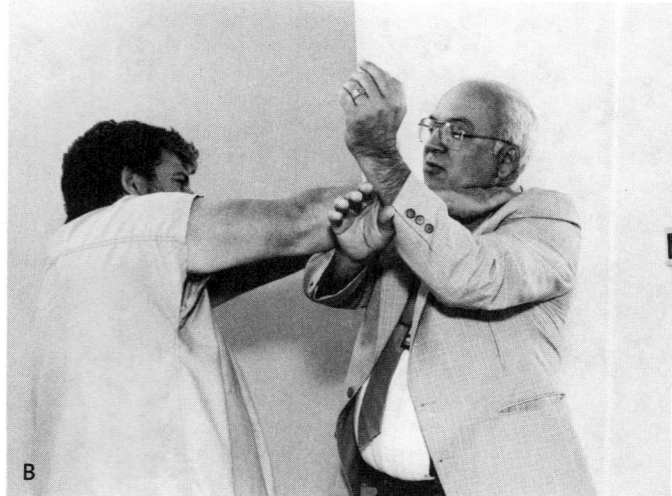

FIGURE 13–7. Breaking a front choke hold.

13-5, the nurse is shown breaking a hair pull by raising her hand quickly to catch the client's arm at the wrist. When this is done quickly, there is automatic release of the hair. The nurse can proceed from this to a basket hold by grasping the client's wrist and stepping around to the back of the client.

A common aggressive response is to throw or threaten to throw an object. The nurse should stand slightly to the side rather than directly in front of the client and have a broad base to allow for quick avoidance movement. The client will watch where he intends to throw the object, and the nurse should observe the client for eye movements. By having a weapon, the client feels control and often will hesitate actually to throw it. Depending on the lethality of the object, the nurse will need to decide if the client can be managed by the intervention team. Two common intervention techniques are to throw a small towel to distract or to precipitate the throwing of the weapon or to throw a sheet over the client to allow staff time to act (Fig. 13-6).

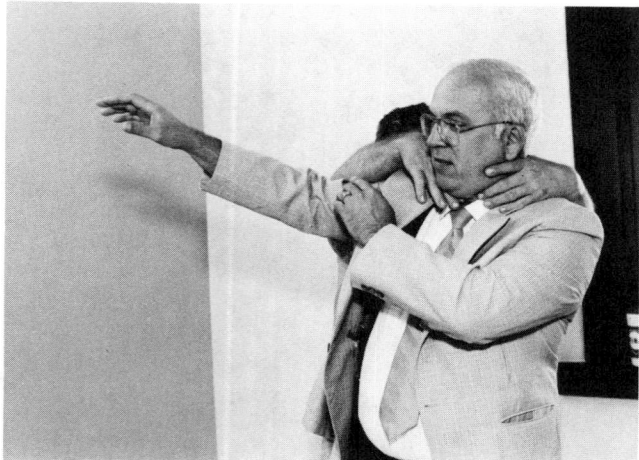

FIGURE 13–8. Breaking a rear choke hold.

If the client is excessively aggressive, wetting the sheet will cause it to stick and thus further hamper the client's movements. If a sheet is thrown, client safety must be assessed; the client should not be left tangled in the sheet.

When the client attempts to choke the nurse (known as a choke hold) from either the front or the back, a quick twist from the nurse with one arm held up can break this hold (Figs. 13-7 and 13-8).

In any intervention with the severely/extremely aggressive client, the nurse must know his or her strengths and limitations. It is important to realize that a single nurse cannot and should not attempt to handle every aggressive response. Practice in the use of restraining holds and team response is essential in providing safe and effective control of severe and extreme aggression.

Evaluation

The degree to which nursing interventions have been effective can be measured by outcome criteria. For the nursing diagnosis of aggression, these criteria would include the extent to which the patient is able to express emotions with appropriate words, to remain calm, to refrain from threatening or harming self or others, to utilize the steps of problem solving, and to express needs appropriately (Chart 2).

CASE STUDY

A 34-year-old woman was hospitalized with dysthymia and borderline personality disorder. She had been brought to the hospital by her family after she threatened them verbally and attempted to harm herself by falling down stairs and walking in front of cars. She repeatedly stated that she was a "bad person" and became hostile and aggressive when nurses attempted to reflect her feelings. She refused to participate in any therapies and socialized only with confused geriatric clients on the unit. As her hospitalization

CHART 2
Aggression: Summary of the Nursing Process

NURSING INTERVENTIONS	OUTCOME CRITERIA

CLIENT GOAL: EXPRESS EMOTION IN ACCEPTABLE MANNER
Provide physical outlet
Encourage verbal expression of feelings
Create a safe, protective environment
Give positive feedback for acceptable behavior
Set firm limits politely

Does not harm/threaten self or others
Expresses emotions appropriately

CLIENT GOAL: FEEL MORE IN CONTROL OF SITUATIONS
Assist in problem-solving process
Allow client to make decisions as appropriate
Teach assertiveness skills
Give positive feedback
Comply with reasonable requests
Contract for desired behaviors

Expresses needs appropriately
Utilizes steps in problem solving

CLIENT GOAL: NOT HARM OTHERS
State expectation of no severe or extreme aggression
Clear environment of bystanders
Use physical restraint if necessary
Administer medication in collaboration with physician
Use seclusion procedures as appropriate
Explain rationale for seclusion/restraint

Is calm
Does not harm others

---

progressed, she became more reclusive to her room and more aggressive to any staff members she encountered. The client had repeated episodes of banging her head on the wall of her room until she was bleeding. Staff who attempted to intervene were met with moderate to severe aggression. She would scream obscenities, throw objects (but not at staff), and run toward staff in a threatening manner.

A major nursing diagnosis was severe aggression related to negative feelings about self. The goal was for the client to interact verbally with staff without severe aggression toward self or them. A contract was made with the client for one shift at a time that she would not harm others or herself in order to give her an increased feeling of control over her

situation and her actions. During her periods of nonaggression, the staff would talk with her about nonthreatening subjects and topics that interested her. On several occasions, the client did not honor the contract and was found beating her head against the wall. At these times, a staff member would physically hold her with a hug while reassuring her that staff would not allow her to harm herself or others. The client initially responded stiffly to the physical touch but later would respond with a hug of her own. She agreed to attend therapies and eventually did go to assertiveness training and occupational therapy. After her hospitalization, the client was referred to outpatient group therapy, where she continued to gain insights into her own behavior.

Research Highlights

A significant number of nursing home residents have mental disorders or behavioral problems. The impact is compounded by the increase in the numbers of elderly who reside in long-term care facilities. In a sample of clients of a large nursing home, 26% had active aggression, 26% had verbal aggression, and 14% were self-destructive.[8]

A study of aggressive behavior in long-term care was conducted by Winger, Schirm, and Stewart in units of a Veterans Administration Hospital.[12] The researchers attempted to identify the characteristics of individuals who exhibit aggression and the relation of the length of stay, health status, dependency, and perceived control over situations of daily living. A sample of 101 clients was

chosen from nursing home and intermediate-care units, and the behaviors of the subjects were rated according to an inventory with three primary categories: (1) disturbing behaviors; (2) behaviors endangering self; and (3) behaviors endangering others. The three primary categories included a total of 23 behaviors. Ninety-one per cent of the nursing home clients demonstrated aggressive behaviors as did 66% of the intermediate-care group. The trends that were apparent in these data were that aggressive clients had longer lengths of stay, had lower mental status scores, and had less control over situational activities. Another observation was that nursing home staff tended to perceive the aggression in the elderly as not serious.

SUMMARY

Aggression, classified in four types—mild, moderate, severe, and extreme—is a behavioral response to various emotions and other factors. The response is based on a variety of factors such as environment, developmental tasks, use of defense mechanisms, and experiences. The behaviors that make up aggression range from angry affect to violence toward self or others. Nursing actions directed toward intervention focus on safety needs as well as on meeting the emotional needs of the individual. The use of physical restraints as part of nursing intervention was outlined. Research suggests that individuals who perceive control of their situation are less likely to be aggressive.

References

1. American Psychiatric Association. Diagnostic and Statistical Manual of Mental Disorders. Ed 3, revised. Washington, DC: American Psychiatric Association; 1987.
2. Brizer DA, Convit A, Krakowski M, Volavka J. A rating scale for reporting violence on psychiatric wards. Hosp Community Psychiatry. 1987;38(7):769.
3. Eichelman B. Neurochemical bases of aggressive behavior. Psychiatr Ann. 1987;17(6):371.
4. Fawcett J, ed. Dynamics of Violence. Chicago: American Medical Association; 1972.
5. Felthous AR, Kellert SR. Childhood cruelty to animals and later aggression against people: a review. Am J Psychiatry. 1987;144:710.
6. Green RG, Donnerstein EI, eds. Aggression: theoretical and empirical reviews. Vols 1 and 2. New York: Academic Press; 1983.
7. Lion J. Training for battle: thoughts on managing aggressive patients. Hosp Community Psychiatry. 1987;38(8):882.
8. Silver JM, Yudofsky SC. Aggressive behavior in patients with neuropsychiatric disorders. Psychiatr Ann. 1987; 17(6):367.
9. Struble LM, Sivertsen L. Agitation behaviors in confused elderly patients. J Gerontol Nurs. 1987;13(11):40.
10. Talley S, King MC. Psychiatric emergencies: nursing assessment and intervention. New York: Macmillan; 1984.
11. Valzelli L. Psychobiology of aggression and violence, New York: Raven Press; 1981.
12. Winger J, Schirm V, Stewart D. Aggressive behavior in long-term care. J Psychosoc Nurs. 1987;25(4):28.

AGITATION

Ruth Jalane Hagerott

DEFINITION AND DESCRIPTION

Agitation is behavior that is excited, tense, with rapidly fluctuating levels of physical activity. It is manifested by pacing, purposeless, potentially injurious movements; loud and rapid speech; tense facial expression; cursing; wringing hands; jittery, nervous movements of the face or extremities; perspiration; short attention span; distractibility; or angry verbal or physical outbursts.

THEORY AND RESEARCH

Agitation has been explained by psychodynamic theory,[3] interpersonal theory, social learning theory,[15] and the concept of frustration.[9,11] Multiple etiologies may have a direct or indirect bearing on the manifestation of the observed excitement and increased physical activity. The accurate identification of the cause can be a critical factor in long-term intervention (e.g., paradoxical drug reaction, metabolic disorders). The reaction to stressful events or relationships may be particularly important, and dramatic changes in behavior are commonly observed when a person or event intrudes on the delicate balance of an already disturbed client.[2] Some research on agitation is directed toward the identification and management of the underlying cause,[19] such as untoward response to psychotropic medications[23] or other responses to disruptions in the patient's physiologic–neurologic homeostasis.[6,18] Other studies focus on prevention of violence, whatever the cause of the agitation.[13,20]

RELATED FACTORS

Agitation can occur in psychiatric disorders, such as schizophrenia, bipolar disorder, major depression,[14] delirium, and dementia.[1,21] It often occurs when psychotic symptoms increase, such as in manic agitation.[17] Agitation is commonly referred to in describing the acutely disturbed psychotic or nonpsychotic patient. It is a nursing diagnosis that is frequently associated with psychiatric emergencies. These emergencies can range from a highly assaultive or self-destructive outburst owing to the increase in voices experienced by the schizophrenic; to the paranoia of the demented client; to the thwarting of a grandiose manic patient; to a client who is experiencing a toxic reaction to drugs (as in akathisia[5]), amphetamines, caffeine,[1] or alcohol;[12] or to physical conditions, such as temporal lobe epilepsy[10] or infarcts of the right hemisphere.[18]

Agitation has been observed in otherwise normal individuals when exposed to a crisis situation (e.g., war, natural disasters, bereavement) in which they often experience extreme fear, isolation, and sleep deprivation.[16]

DEFINING CHARACTERISTICS

The most common defining characteristic associated with agitation is an increase in motor activity.[21] Pacing, frequent changing of clothes, and disrobing are manifestations of heightened level of activity. The affect associated with agitation may be a tense, worried, or angry expression. The frequency and timbre of vocalizations may increase, including nervous laughter or crying, or the client may appear fearful and withdrawn. Demands for attention from staff members or other clients may take an obtrusive tone, and lack of attention may precipitate an outburst. Irritability, coupled with a loud demeanor, elicits negative responses in others that then lead to an increased level of frustration and agitation in the client, which may result in striking out or other aggressive behavior.[22,24]

Increases in perspiration, respiration, pulse, and blood pressure may be observed in the agitated person. Decreased interest in, or ability to, sleep and refusal of food and drink are also commonly associated with agitation.[21] Psychotic clients experiencing agitation may not be able to describe their experiences, or they may say "my mind is racing," "my chest is pounding," or "I can't sit still" (Chart 1).

NURSING PROCESS AND RATIONALE

Assessment

Agitation may be manifested initially by subtle and less apparent clues, with an increasing number and intensity of behaviors as the client's discomfort escalates (see Levels of Agitation in Chart 1). Early awareness of changes in the client's behavior, followed by assessment of the underlying cause, are key in an effective assessment process.

As the agitation increases, so does the level of physi-

CHART 1
Agitation: Definition, Related Factors, and Defining Characteristics

DEFINITION

Agitation is behavior that appears excited or tense, with rapidly fluctuating levels of physical activity.

RELATED FACTORS

Noise
Crowded environment
Lack of privacy
Agitation of others
Lack of direction and control
Threats by others
Unstructured and unpredictable ward milieu
Staff coercion
Level of tension on ward
Isolation
Level of stability and cognitive functioning
Fluctuation of moods
Poor impulse control
Internal conflicts
Anger
Frustration
Psychiatric disorders, e.g. schizophrenia, bipolar disorder, personality disorder, organic mental disorders
Disturbed neurochemical balance
Learned response to stress
Alcohol or drug abuse or withdrawal
Previous history of expressing agitation through violence
Epilepsy
Drug reaction (akathisia)
Interpersonal conflicts
Crisis
Sleep deprivation

DEFINING CHARACTERISTICS

Levels of Agitation	Behaviors
FIRST	Feeling of tension Increase in physical activity Increase in normal volume and rate of speech Mild perspiration Slight tremors Anxious affect Facial musculature tense
SECOND	Increase in cognitive arousal Acceleration of activity Sense of growing tension Clenching of fists and hands Further increase in rate and volume of speech Demanding Verbal assaults or threats Hypervigilance
THIRD	Frenetic activity Pacing, crying, shouting Cursing Heavy perspiration Sense of impending loss of control and potential violence

cal activity. There is a sense of escalating tension and irritability in response. Often a heightened startle reflex is noted. Verbal response often becomes loud, hostile, or abusive, or a combination of such. Assaultive or self-destructive acts often result if the agitation is allowed to escalate. It is important that the nurse be observant and know the individual's special behavioral manifestations, such as increasingly loud laughter, frequent trips to the water fountain or bathroom, sudden requests to leave the ward, an anxious facial expression, and urgency in the voice. Otherwise the client's behavior may be overlooked until the behavior is unmanageable.

Nursing Diagnosis

Based upon client data, a more specific nursing diagnosis can be formulated; for example, agitation related to manic episode;[24] agitation related to confusion;[21] or agitation related to pharmacologic toxicity.[1]

Client Goals and Nursing Interventions

The client goals of recognizing and developing self-management skills regarding agitation can be a major accomplishment. The nurse assists the client by endeavoring, in a mutual effort, to identify precipitating factors, modifying the manner in which the client and staff members generally respond to the agitation and being available to support the client in utilizing the newly learned methods. In those psychiatric clients who have a unique pattern of escalating tension, it is crucial for effective and timely intervention that the nurse utilize keen observational skills. When the nurse understands what the client is experiencing, nursing interventions can occur early. Clients will manifest less agitation once psychotic symptoms are under control.[15] Clients with schizophrenia, for example, often report that their increased activity is the result of command hallucinations that are extremely irritating and frightening. Clients experiencing extreme agitation may have little ability to help themselves. Therefore, protection of the client and prevention of further escalation is the responsibility of those assessing and treating the client. Once the agitation is under control and the client protected from the results of destructive behavior either to self or others, the client goal is to describe the internal process that led to the growing tension and agitation. Secondly, the client should be assisted in identifying ways that this distress can be communicated early to those who can assist in managing the tension and resulting behavior. The provision of support and acceptance of the client, while at the same time setting appropriate limits, will assist the nurse and client to build a foundation for further, more extensive, interaction and mutual care planning.

Current research indicates that how members of the staff respond to the agitated client is clearly an issue in the management of the highly problematic population. Countertransference and responding anger and frustration on the part of staff members often prevent effective intervention at the early stages and may blur the staff's ability to accurately assess the underlying cause of the behavior and also lead to division within the staff, which further complicates the management of this behavior.[8]

After resolution of the crisis, the nurse needs to consider the following sequence of interventions:

1. Careful evaluation of the circumstances under which this behavior occurs and how it might endanger the client or others.
2. A comprehensive plan for how to prevent recurrence of these crises.
3. An alternative plan to intervene if the agitation does recur, including requests for medication as needed (prn) or removal from a stimulating environment so that escalation will be limited by prompt psychopharmacologic and environmental intervention.
4. Role-modeling support and clarity in communicating that the nurse is readily available to assist the client in controlling the agitation.
5. Careful ongoing observation and listening for additional clues to precipitating factors in the internal or external environment of the client.
6. Communication among all staff members about the anticipated warning signs and expectations for interventions.
7. Evaluation of consistency of approach among staff members.
8. Education and practice with the client about how to identify the warning signs of escalating agitation and how to communicate these signs to the nurse to facilitate early intervention
9. Education of family members about client distress and how they can assist with management. Do a comparative evaluation of instances for which the agitation was successfully managed with the times when more extreme measures were required.
10. Modification of approach as required, including requests for medication reevaluation, change of staff or room assignment, or communication with family.

A discharge summary to another agency would include a description of the precipitating factors, the patient's agitated behavior, and the expected response from presently utilized interventions.

Evaluation

If the client continues to experience increasing episodes of agitation, then there needs to be further evaluation of the underlying cause and further intervention

---

CHART 2
Agitation: Summary of the Nursing Process

NURSING INTERVENTIONS	OUTCOME CRITERIA
CLIENT GOAL: EXPERIENCE DECREASED AGITATION	
Assess level of and cause of agitation	Experiences decreased episodes of agitation
Decrease level of stimuli	
Identify own feelings toward client so that interventions are not based on anger, punitive measures	
Communicate in a calm, quiet, slow manner, offering support and limits where appropriate	
Administer medications as required to control excitement or underlying condition (e.g., epilepsy)	
Protect from self-harm or harm to others	
CLIENT GOAL: IDENTIFY FEELINGS AND THOUGHTS PRIOR TO AGITATION	
Provide opportunity for client to communicate personal experience	Communicates feelings before escalation of agitation
Establish a plan with the client to include how he or she can communicate feelings of agitation. Provide timely intervention (e.g., sitting with the client, removing the client from a stimulating environment, psychopharmacologic interventions)	Participates in plan and verbalizes understanding of same
Assess the interventions for effectiveness through observation of behavior and verbal feedback from client regarding his or her experience (calm, agitated)	Verbalizes a need for nursing interventions
CLIENT GOAL: UTILIZE PHYSICAL OUTLETS AND PROPER DIET	
Establish regular exercise regimen	Exercises regularly
Support client efforts to control agitation by providing opportunities for walking	Understands the need for adequate exercise, diet, rest, quiet, and space and practices same
Provide adequate space and quiet	
Monitor diet for ingestion of excessive sugar and caffeine	When feeling agitated, maintains low-sugar, caffeine-free diet and requests a quiet space and time
Assess client response to exercise and availability of quiet and space compared with need for psychopharmacologic intervention	

planned and implemented. If change is noted, such as the need for more frequent PRNs or quiet time, then, again, the underlying cause needs to be evaluated. Possible changes in the environment, such as absence of a favorite nurse or the admission of another client who becomes antagonistic, might be factors causing the client to experience more anxiety and lessen the ability to utilize control over the agitation. There could be a subtle change in the client's health status or diet that might contribute to the increased agitation. If the nurse makes assumptions that nothing significant has changed and that the client is "not cooperating with treatment," this could be critical in terms of lost valuable time and misdirected intervention (Chart 2).

CASE STUDY

Bob R was a 35-year-old, 250-lb man who had been admitted to a Veterans Administration Hospital 15 years earlier after a short six-month period in the service. He had been discharged from the hospital for brief periods, only to be readmitted because of his periods of extreme agitation and violence. His verbal skills were severely limited, and his primary focus of conversation was that he would someday be a "truck driver" and would leave the hospital forever. His childlike behavior and gentleness could explode into severe agitation when he was confronted by other clients regarding his incessant chatter about trucks or when prevented by staff personnel from leaving the ward for a walk at any time of the day or night. Once his agitation escalated to crisis proportions, he was placed in sheet restraint, often for as long as 24 hours, where he would rave and thrash until he became exhausted or the medication would take effect. After these episodes, there would be periods, sometimes as long as a month, when he was quiet and relatively subdued. He was diagnosed with chronic schizophrenia, and his prognosis was extremely poor. A keen observation, made by the nurse one day while watching Bob, uncovered a subtle clue that the man might be experiencing a seizure. This led to a neurologic evaluation, and the diagnosis of temporal lobe epilepsy. Bob was seen hovering by the wall with a vacant expression on his face and a slight twitch in his left facial muscles. When the nurse requested that he describe his experience, he vividly described his feeling as one of "having my brain stretched." The nursing diagnosis for this client was agitation related to schizophrenia and temporal lobe epilepsy. The goal of the nursing interventions was to elicit Bob's cooperation in controlling the agitation before it escalated to dangerous proportions.

Once the neurologic evaluation was completed, Bob was placed on regular doses of phenytoin (Dilantin) and was educated to know that if he experienced those "strange feelings," he was to approach the nurse and request additional medication. He had a PRN order for diazepam (Valium), 25 mg, to offset the ensuing postseizure agitation. He was also told, and all staff members were informed, that if he felt the need to leave the ward and walk, he would be allowed to do so. He understood these instructions and was cooperative in following through. The extreme agitated incidents were almost entirely obliterated, except when staff failed to follow through on the agreed upon plan. He was allowed to roam the grounds of the hospital and was eventually discharged to a less restrictive environment. He was retained on phenytoin (Dilantin) and PRN diazepam (Valium) up to the day of discharge. At the time of discharge, his diazepam use had decreased.

SUMMARY

With agitation and the potential for further escalation, it is critical to observe, assess, and intervene quickly and appropriately. The immediate identification and assessment of the client's mental status and timely short-term intervention are paramount to maintaining the safety of the client and others. It is imperative that nurses consider multiple related factors when assessing the agitated client. Provision of safety and security are key to the successful management of agitation. It is essential that rapport and communication be established to better identify the long-term effective interventions required to address the underlying cause and to develop a plan that will assist the patient in managing the disruptive experience of agitation.

Research Highlights

In the management of agitated clients who are commonly seen by the internist or emergency room physician, effective drug management has been researched. Haloperidol (Haldol), chlorpromazine (Thorazine), perphenazine (Trilafon), and thiothixene (Navane) have been utilized.[6] The immediate danger to clients and staff is considered in the psychopharmacologic intervention of agitated behavior. Often, the desired short-term effect is the focus until a psychiatric diagnosis has been formulated.[25] Three classes of medication are generally considered to be beneficial for short-term effect on agitation and excitement: antipsychotics for schizophrenia and mania; antianxiety for the anxious, agitated client (although these have been found to aggravate violence in some clients in whom there is central nervous system disease or sedatives in use); and sedative medications. Intermediate-acting barbiturates, such as sodium amytal, have been advocated because there is less danger of respiratory depression.[20]

References

1. American Psychiatric Association. Diagnostic and statistical manual of mental disorders. 3rd ed, revised. Washington, DC: American Psychiatric Association; 1987.
2. Arieti S, ed. American handbook of psychiatry, vol. 3, Adult clinical psychiatry. New York: Basic Books; 1974.
3. Bleuler M. The schizophrenic disorders. New Haven: Yale University Press; 1978.
4. Boettcher EG. Preventing violent behavior: an integrated theoretical model for nursing. Perspect Psychiatr Care. 1983;21:54–58.
5. Braude WM, Barnes TRE, Gore SM. Clinical characteristics of akathisia: a systematic investigation of acute psychiatric inpatient admissions. Br J Psychiatry. 1983;143:139–150.
6. Cavanaugh SV. Psychiatric emergencies. Med Clin North Am. 1986;70:1185–1202.
7. Clark JB, Queener SF, Karb VB. Drugs: pocket nurse guide. St Louis: CV Mosby; 1986.
8. Colson DB, Allen JG, Coyne L, Dexter N, Jehl N, Mayer CA, Spohn H. An anatomy of countertransference: staff reactions to difficult psychiatric hospital patients. Hosp Commun Psychiatry. 1986;37:923–928.
9. Dollard J, et al. Frustration and aggression. New Haven: Yale University Press; 1939.
10. Gorton JG, Partridge R, eds. Practice and management of psychiatric emergency care. St Louis: CV Mosby; 1982.
11. Izard CE. Human emotions. New York: Plenum Press; 1977.
12. Jessor R, Graves TD, Hanson RC, et al. Society, personality and deviant behavior. Huntington, NY: Kreiger Publishing; 1975.
13. Jones MK. Patient violence: report of 200 incidents. J Psychosoc Nurs. 1985;23(Jun):12–17.
14. Kaplan HI, Sadock BJ, eds. Comprehensive textbook of psychiatry/IV, vol. 1. 4th ed. Baltimore: Williams & Wilkins; 1985.
15. Kerr TA, Snaith RP, eds. Contemporary issues in schizophrenia. Royal College of Psychiatrists, Washington, DC: American Psychiatric Press; 1986.
16. Kutash IL, Schlesinger LB, et al. Handbook on stress and anxiety. San Francisco: Jossey-Bass; 1980.
17. Model JG, Lenox RH, Weiner S. Inpatient clinical trial of lorazepam for the management of manic agitation. J Clin Psychopharmacol. 1985;5:109–113.
18. Price BH, Mesulam M. Psychiatric manifestations of right hemisphere infarctions. J Nerv Ment Disorders. 1985;173:610–614.
19. Risse SC, Barnes R. Pharmacologic treatment of agitation associated with dementia. J Am Geriat Soc. 1986;34:368–376.
20. Roth LH, ed. Clinical treatment of the violent person. Rockville, MD: US Department of Public Health & Human Services, MIMH, Publication no (ADM) 85-1425; 1985.
21. Struble LM, Sivertsen L. Agitation: behaviors in confused elderly patients. J Gerontol Nurs. 1987;13:(11):40–44.
22. Tanke ED, Yesavage JA. Characteristics of assaultive patients who do and do not provide visible cues of potential violence. Am J Psychiatry. 1985;142:1409–1413.
23. Van Putten T. The many faces of akathisia. Compr Psychiatry. 1975;16(1):43–47.
24. Yesavage JA. Bipolar illness: correlates of dangerous inpatient behaviour. Br J Psychiatry. 1983;143:554–557.
25. Young GP. The agitated patient in the emergency department. Emerg Med Clin North Am. 1987;5:765–781.

ANGER

Deanah I. Alexander

DEFINITION AND DESCRIPTION

Anger is an emotional state of intense displeasure and frustration. Subjectively, anger includes sentiments from animosity to rage; from slight irritation to explosive hostility. Most often, anger is seen as a source of energy that is discharged on other persons, objects, or self. Anger can be sublimated to discharge energy in a positive direction, such as by taking action on a disputed issue, or in a negative direction, leading to aggression.

THEORY AND RESEARCH

The word anger evokes pictures in a person's mind that often are based on experiences from childhood on. The child who is angry may hold his (or her) breath, pout, or have a temper tantrum. As he grows, he may mimic the release of anger he has seen in adults. This is an example of modeling, the behavior manifested to a child by significant adults being taken on by the child. An example is the child who, seeing his parents yell or hit in anger, demonstrates the same behaviors in his anger.[6]

Anger often leads to action to release the intense associated feeling. These actions may passively harm another or the angry person himself. The more forthright expression of anger is linked with aggression, which is described under the nursing diagnosis entitled Aggression.

The emotions of anger and anxiety frequently go hand in hand, but anger is often a more comfortable feeling. With anger, there is a corresponding feeling of power: others can be pushed away and therefore kept at a safe distance from threatening emotions.[8] Anger results when the motor response is directed at the real or perceived source of threat, whereas anxiety occurs when the motor response is undirected or aimed toward avoidance.[7] The concept of anxiety is described more extensively under the nursing diagnosis entitled Anxiety.

Anger in the clinical setting has been classified into dimensions such as justified, unjustified, normative, maladaptive, and suppression. Biaggio[4] further suggests that these dimensions be assessed initially to plan effective intervention with psychotherapy. Use of the self-report to elicit the client's perceptions of the incident is suggested. Observation of the angry response may not always be possible. The domains of treatment are described as behavioral, cognitive, physiological, and affective.

Anger has been identified as a stage of grieving that comes in response to the loss over which one has no control. The "in control" person may display symptoms of sublimated anger such as use of sarcastic humor or a passive–aggressive nature in which anger is indirectly discharged.

RELATED FACTORS

Disproportionate anger is a major symptom in psychiatric disorders such as borderline personality disorder, late luteal-phase dysphoric disorder, nicotine withdrawal, and oppositional defiant disorder.[1] Anger often is present in other disorders that have an element of grieving (depression) or fear of loss of control (post-traumatic stress disorder).

Cultural expectations affect one's ability to acknowledge anger as well as the action taken in response to the feeling. Differences in culture also dictate in which situations anger is an acceptable response. A child raised in a society that denies one's right to be angry may very well respond covertly by developing somatic symptoms such as headache, gastrointestinal disturbance including diarrhea or constipation, jaw tensing, or skin disturbance including dermatitis or flushing. The adult response to anger includes the aforementioned and may result in other physiologic changes.

The object of the anger is influential in the response elicited and may determine whether the emotion is labeled "appropriate." The more global the object, the more acceptance the person is likely to receive in support of the anger. For example, the individual who is angry at the injustices of the world is more likely to receive support (may in fact become a leader in undoing those injustices) than one who singles out a responsible person upon which to vent the anger.

Past use of defense mechanisms will influence whether the anger is acknowledged or denied and also how the accompanying energy is spent. If an individual has found that openly expressing anger meets with positive results, then the behavior is reinforced. The environment in which the anger is provoked also will influence the emotional and behavioral response. The angry person is likely to keep anger in check and release it at a safe time or toward a person who is considered safe or at least less of a threat, even if that release is inappropriate and misdirected.

Violent acts, such as rape, murder, and battery, incorporate anger in both the victim and the aggressor.

Anger rapes are common among reported rapes.[5] In such cases, the rapist uses the violent act to discharge the energy created by pent-up anger. Survivors of rape report anger as a common feeling in the recovery process. This response may be dealt with by internalizing the anger, causing guilt and depression, or by externalizing the anger, leading to acting out behavior to punish society or self for the crime. A further discussion is included in the section on rape trauma syndrome in this chapter.

DEFINING CHARACTERISTICS

Anger's most characteristic component is its intensity. The cluster of behaviors that identify anger include frowning; gritting the teeth; raising, drawing together, or lowering the eyebrows; pacing, clenching the hands; and facial flushing. There is an accompanying feeling of intense distress and an urge to act to negate that distress.[3] Individually these behaviors do not signify that the person is angry.

Voice changes also can characterize anger. Voice tone may be lowered and words spoken between clenched teeth, or the tone may rise to a yell or shout. Often, the person delivers speech in short, clipped phrases. The whole characteristic of speech is either that of trying to keep control or that of having lost control.

Anger carries with it a great amount of energy that can spur the angry person to action, destructive or constructive, or drain the individual of desire to interact with the world. The depressed individual might respond to anger by withdrawing in an attempt to keep control over the pent-up anger.

Although the term "anger" often has a negative connotation, the behavioral response to it can be constructive. The individual who takes action to release the energy of anger may clean the house, organize a project, or do the opposite of what precipitated the anger. For example, the student who fails a test may become angry at the result and direct energy toward studying for the next examination (Chart 1).

NURSING PROCESS AND RATIONALE

Assessment

Assessment data will include the appropriateness of the anger, its effect on daily living, and the time frame. Observation of the behavioral signs described under Defining Characteristics is important. A useful method in identifying the presence and type of anger is taking a history from the individual and significant others to pinpoint the angry behaviors. Information should be gathered from a client who is angry and significant others in separate interviews. For example, the nurse might ask the spouse if he or she notices any behavior that predictably accompanies the client's anger, such as aversion to certain foods, decline in normal sociali-

---

CHART 1
Anger: Definition, Related Factors, and Defining Characteristics

DEFINITION

Anger is an emotional state of intense displeasure and frustration. Subjectively, anger includes sentiments from animosity to rage; from slight irritation to explosive hostility.

RELATED FACTORS

Borderline personality disorder
Late luteal-phase dysphoric disorder
Nicotine withdrawal
Oppositional defiant disorder
Depression
Post-traumatic stress disorder
Cultural factors
Developmental factors
Perception of situation as unjust
Perception of threat or affront
Social factors

DEFINING CHARACTERISTICS

Intense distress
Frowning
Gritting of teeth
Pacing
Eyebrow displacement; e.g., raised, lowered, knitted
Clenched fists
Increased energy
Fatigue
Withdrawal
Change in tone of voice
Flushed face
Emotional overcontrol

---

zation, complaints of body aches, or denial of the feeling of anger.

Some clients are uncomfortable with the word "anger," although they can describe themselves as upset or irritable. These clients may believe that to be angry is bad or that one will be punished for being angry. In such a case, it is more effective to use the client's word until the client can believe that it is acceptable to be angry.

Nursing Diagnosis

An example of a specific situation when a nursing diagnosis of anger could be made is when a client expresses frustration with a marital relationship and demonstrates sarcasm, withdrawal from social interactions, and temper outbursts. The client may not be readily aware of being angry but acknowledges the frustration felt in regard to the relationship. A nursing diagnosis of anger related to marital relationship is appropriate in this case.

Client Goals and Nursing Interventions

The long-term goal in helping persons with anger is for them to have appropriate responses to the feeling. Short-term goals include recognizing the symptoms of anger in oneself and acknowledging the feeling.

Behavioral treatment, such as assertiveness training or social skills training, is appropriate for clients who typically use inappropriate or ineffective responses, including those with justified anger. In assertiveness, the person is required to role play and practice new responses to situations. Social skills training also requires role playing and focuses more on bodily responses such as eye contact, posture, and facial mannerisms. Cognitive treatment, focusing on education and information, is helpful for persons using suppression or having unrealistic expectations of themselves or others that lead to anger.

Physiological treatment, such as relaxation training, is aimed at reducing the physiological response that is especially intense or of long standing. Counterconditioning such as humor can be used to modify angry responses and is particularly useful for a client with chronic anger.

Persons who lose control when angry often do not recognize the feeling that precedes the loss of control. Instead, they perceive themselves as going from a calm state to rage with no forewarning. Helping the client describe the feeling and the intensity often lessens the impact of the feeling and the fear of loss of control. It also is important to give recognition to a justifiable anger and help the client with problem solving so he or she can select an appropriate action. For example, "I sense your anger at _____; what will happen if you decide to _____?" The blanks can be filled with the situation that elicited the anger and the client's proposed response to the situation.

The use of physical activity in channeling anger expression provides a sense of control over the intense feeling and disperses energy. Activity of large muscles may result in more satisfactory use of the energy that accompanies anger. Examples of such activities are walking, jogging, hammering, dancing, calisthenics, volleyball, softball, and archery. Activities that can also utilize a substitute image of the target may increase the client's awareness of the anger and allow for its release in an acceptable form. The client who participates in archery might visualize the subject of the anger as the target. An important caution for this intervention is assessing whether the client has enough control to visualize only without taking action with a weapon against the object of the anger. It also is important to assess potential guilt, in which case this intervention should be used with care.

Use of an "anger box" that permits physical release of the tension of anger and encourages the use of imagery to facilitate the resolution of anger may be helpful. Such a box is made of wood and has an opening into which the client throws clay pigeons. The opening has a backing on which a picture or a target can be placed. The advantages of using clay pigeons are that the cost is minimal and the weapon potential is low. Moreover, the noise made by the breaking of the clay can be very satisfying and calming to the angry person.

Nurses frequently are the target of displaced anger from clients and their significant others.[2] Intervening with an angry client calls for the nurse first to recognize her or his own response. A nurse who responds by becoming defensive or angry may create further complications rather than help resolve the problem. The nurse must recognize the nature and dynamics of the client's anger in order to respond as a professional: two angry persons interacting cannot resolve the feeling until one at least partially discharges the anger. This discharge may be by physical aggression (inappropriate or appropriate) or by one person becoming the listener and taking a submissive role in verbal aggression. The modeling of assertive techniques sets the stage for future learning. The person who can deal assertively with anger has an increased feeling of control over the emotion rather than a feeling of being controlled by it. If a source of the anger external to the relationship can be identified, the nurse is less likely to feel threatened, and the client receives more support.

Limit setting is necessary in some cases where the client is physically or verbally aggressive or with children who lack self-control. With external limits set, the angry person can have a sense of relief that someone is in control, because loss of control is feared. Children often ask for the external control through behavioral clues such as repeating inappropriate actions in a testing manner to see where the limit is and who will set it. A child may also respond to anger by clinging or becoming more dependent. This is an internalized response that can be dealt with by gentle limit setting. In working with children, it is most important to talk about the behavior as inappropriate and to emphasize that the child is still valued for himself or herself.

Evaluation

The subjective measurement of the lessened frustration felt by the client is imperative in evaluation. Other criteria for evaluation are a reduction in anger-related disruption in relationships and daily living activities. The positive use of anger is another measurement of the success of therapeutic intervention (Chart 2).

CASE STUDY

Charles J, a 37-year-old Caucasian man, was hospitalized involuntarily after he set fire to his friend's house. The admitting diagnoses were major depression and borderline personality disorder. He had a history of minor conflicts with the law, primarily fighting and public nuisance. Over the preceding 2 weeks, he reported feeling increasingly despondent and that life was futile at times. In the personal history, he revealed that he had worked at menial jobs, which he had trouble keeping because he would get into

---

CHART 2
Anger: Summary of the Nursing Process

NURSING INTERVENTIONS	OUTCOME CRITERIA
CLIENT GOAL: IDENTIFY FEELINGS OF ANGER IN SELF	
Have client keep diary of feelings of anger	Recognizes anger before losing control
Acknowledge client's feelings and experience	Takes responsibility for own emotions
Validate justification of anger without taking sides	Acknowledges that some anger is justified
CLIENT GOAL: USE CONSTRUCTIVE RELEASE OF ENERGY OF ANGER	
Teach assertive techniques	Decrease in impulsive release of anger
Encourage physical activity using large muscles	Increased feelings of self-worth
Facilitate verbal expression of anger to appropriate source	Demonstrates internal control over behavior
	Harnesses energy generated by anger in nondestructive manner
CLIENT GOAL: IDENTIFY COGNITIONS THAT LEAD TO FEELINGS OF ANGER	
Assist client to identify thoughts that precede feelings of anger	Takes responsibility for emotional response
Assist client to examine responses to situations where anger was experienced	
Teach positive self-talk	

---

fights with coworkers. After losing his last job as a dishwasher, he moved in with a friend, and it was this friend's house he set afire. He denied having hallucinations, delusions, or illusions. Past mental health treatment had been in an outpatient clinic with individual psychotherapy. Charles described the recent event as happening "out of the blue. I came home and my clothes were laying around the house. I thought maybe he wanted me to move. I guess I got mad." Physically, Charles was intimidating; he wore dark sunglasses most of the time, dressed in black or dark colors, was 6'6", and weighed approximately 280 pounds. When he interacted with others, he was soft-spoken and was most comfortable with frail geriatric clients. He was cooperative with his regimen of occupational therapy and individual psychotherapy but was reluctant to attend group therapy because he was afraid he would get mad at someone.

The staff made the nursing diagnosis of anger related to threat and altered impulse control. In planning care for Charles, the goal for him was to learn to identify his feelings before he lost control and acted on impulse. He started attending an assertiveness class, and staff used the class exercises to point out his intimidating appearance. As he started to change his appearance by not wearing his sunglasses indoors and by removing his dark stocking cap, staff gave him positive feedback. Trust continued to build, and

his primary therapist asked him to keep a log of his feelings. Nurses then became more confronting to test his awareness of his emotions and his behavior. When he appeared to be getting angry, they asked him what he was feeling and helped him put a name on his feelings. Charles progressed to the point of not acting out his anger and was discharged to the partial hospitalization program. He became more comfortable with group therapy through the use of confrontation and support and benefited from role-playing situations. Charles was encouraged to walk as a physical release for his tension and anger, and he reported that this was helpful. The prognosis was considered good for Charles if he continued in the partial hospitalization program.

SUMMARY

Anger as a nursing diagnosis can be applied to many clients. Anger is defined as an emotional state of intense displeasure. The related factors include selected mental disorders, cultural or developmental factors, or perception of threat or of a situation as unjust. For the implementation to be most successful, the client must

Research Highlights

A survey of mentally retarded adults in a mental health clinic revealed that 30% had self-control problems.[3] A study of the effectiveness of anger management training for this population was conducted. Individuals participating were mildly or moderately retarded and were treated in a group format. The interventions were relaxation training, self-instructions, problem solving, and an anger management program consisting of all three interventions. Utilizing self-reports, videotaping, and supervision ratings, the investigators found similar increases in self-control in all the groups.[3] The significance of the research is its demonstration that mentally retarded individuals can benefit from anger management training.

be a participant in the diagnosis and treatment. Goals of decreasing the discomfort felt with anger and making constructive use of the energy released are important in working with clients experiencing anger.

References

1. American Psychiatric Association. Diagnostic and Statistical Manual of Mental Disorders. Ed 3, revised. Washington, DC: American Psychiatric Association; 1987.
2. Antai-Otong D. When your patient is angry. Nursing. 88 1988;18(2):45.
3. Benson B, Rice CJ, Miranti SV. Effects of anger management training with mentally retarded adults in group treatment. J Consult Clin Psychol. 1986;54:728-9.
4. Biaggio MK. Clinical dimensions of anger management. Am J Psychother. 1987;41:417-27.
5. Foley T. The client who has been raped. In: Lego S, ed. The american handbook of psychiatric nursing. Philadelphia: JB Lippincott; 1984.
6. Hayes SC, Rincover A, Volosin D. Variables influencing the acquisition and maintenance of aggressive behavior: modeling versus sensory reinforcement. J Abnorm Psychol. 1980;89:254-62.
7. Rothenberg A. On anger. Am J Psychiatry 1971;128:454-60.
8. Sullivan HS. The psychiatric interview. New York: WW Norton; 1954.

ANXIETY

(MILD, MODERATE, SEVERE, EXTREME/PANIC)

Georgia Whitley

DEFINITION AND DESCRIPTION

Nursing practice in the 20th century has been impacted by a society existing at a time described as the Age of Anxiety. A large proportion of clients treated by nurses in a variety of settings exhibit characteristics of anxiety, especially in mental health settings. Whether the client's anxiety is a presenting problem or is related to therapeutic regimens or lack of knowledge, it is important for the nurse to assist the client in identifying and managing the anxiety.

Anxiety is defined as a vague, uneasy feeling, the source of which is often nonspecific or unknown to the individual. This often nonspecific or unknown origin differentiates anxiety from the nursing diagnosis *fear*, in which the feeling of dread is related to an identifiable source the person can validate. Four levels of anxiety have been identified: mild, moderate, severe, and extreme/panic. Differentiation of these levels assists the nurse in assessing, diagnosing, and establishing goals and interventions specific to the individual responses of the client. Defining characteristics (signs and symptoms) have been identified and occur in various degrees depending on the level of anxiety experienced. Perceptual abilities, information processing, and problem-solving skills are affected in proportion to an individual's level of anxiety.

Experiences that provoke anxiety begin in infancy. Anxiety is a part of everyday life and provides a self-protective mechanism: it occurs when self-esteem, identity, or personhood are threatened. Responses to anxiety range from adaptive, constructive actions such as learning, problem solving, goal setting, and skill acquisition to maladaptive, disturbed coping behaviors such as inability to make decisions, conflict, repetitive behavior, and rigidity of responses.

THEORY AND RESEARCH

Four prominent theories of human behavior and their consequent conceptualizations of anxiety have influenced the development and use of the concept of anxiety within the framework of nursing. Psychoanalytic theory describes anxiety as the result of neurotic fixations at earlier stages of development. In this view,

the occurrence and persistence of anxiety disproportionate to the real situation is labeled *neurotic anxiety*. Behaviorists describe anxiety as a learned or habitual response to stimuli that contain no actual threat. This anxiety response has been reinforced and so will recur in the future. Interpersonal theorists state that anxiety is first conveyed by the mother to the infant, with the child, and later the adult, experiencing anxiety in relation to perceived approval or disapproval of actions. Biologic theories of anxiety incorporate genetic, biochemical, and pharmacologic bases in their conceptualization of anxiety. Scientists have related neuroregulators, endorphins, and specific brain receptors for benzodiazepines to the generation and regulation of anxiety.

The need to define and separate anxiety as a state from anxiety as a trait was identified by Spielberger.[21] State anxiety is precipitated by a stressful life situation over which the individual may feel lack of or diminished control. *Trait anxiety* refers to the amount of anxiety that a person usually experiences, with some individuals having an overall greater proneness to experience anxiety than do others. These two types of anxiety can be measured by the State–Trait Anxiety Inventory developed by Spielberger, Gorsch, and Lushem.[22]

A classic work on anxiety by Peplau, a leader in psychiatric and mental health nursing, has influenced subsequent nursing treatment.[19] In this report, sources of anxiety are defined as threats to the security of the person such as threats to biologic integrity, values, behavior patterns, and views of self. Peplau describes mild, moderate, severe, and panic levels of anxiety. In mild or moderate anxiety, capabilities are increased, whereas in extreme or panic levels of anxiety, capabilities are overworked or paralyzed. Mild anxiety increases observational capacity, so that the person is aware and alert and perceives connections between elements of situations. The perceptual field is somewhat narrowed in moderate anxiety, attention being fixed on the situation of concern with little attention to the periphery. In mild and moderate anxiety, learning can take place, as the individual is able to observe and formulate meanings and relations as well as to validate with others and use the learning product. In severe anxiety, on the other hand, attention is directed to scattered details, and learning is greatly diminished

145

because the person begins to seek means for reducing the discomfort caused by the anxiety. At the panic level, the individual is unable to attend to external events and is controlled by the severe internal distress being experienced.

Nurses have debated whether anxiety should be considered a diagnostic category or whether it is more appropriately a defining characteristic for ineffective coping and knowledge deficit or a precursor to fear. Anxiety was deleted by the North American Nursing Diagnosis Association as a nursing diagnosis for 2 years but was reinstated after several studies suggested that anxiety is prevalent and widely distributed in nursing practice, that it is amenable to nursing interventions, and that nurses do distinguish between fear and anxiety.[5,10,25] Seven studies of nursing diagnosis have revealed that the diagnosis anxiety is one of the most common, with ranks ranging from third through eighth in frequency of occurrence.[6,9–11,13,17,18] Validation studies related to the nursing diagnosis anxiety have contributed to nursing knowledge of this phenomenon.

RELATED FACTORS

The definition of the nursing diagnosis anxiety indicates that the source or related factors for anxiety are often nonspecific or unknown to the individual. The use of defense mechanisms such as suppression, repression, and denial may make information regarding the causative factors unavailable to the client at a conscious level. Through assessment procedures and analysis of assessment data, nurses and other health professionals may identify related factors for anxiety. If specific causative factors are not apparent, the nurse may document that the related factors are unknown at this point, continue to collect data, and attempt to identify related factors at a future time. The identification of specific related factors will assist in the selection of nursing interventions appropriate for the treatment of anxiety for a given etiology.

Threat to self-concept is a related factor that assumes the most prominent position in the literature and with nurses in the identification of causes of anxiety in clients.[24] This related factor is very broad and includes real or anticipated disapproval from a significant person, expectations of the individual that are not fulfilled, and needs for self-esteem and respect that are not met.[19] Self-concept may also be related to failure or success, needs for prestige and recognition, and physical possessions.

Unmet needs is a related factor that is ranked high by nurses and includes a broad spectrum of human needs.[24] These needs include physiologic, safety, belonging and love, self-esteem, self-actualization, and aesthetic.[14]

Situational and maturational crises encompass an extensive spectrum of human events. Situational crises occur when unanticipated events threaten a person's biologic, social, or psychological integrity,[1] e.g., loss of or change in a job. Maturational or developmental crises are successive events that occur normally in each individual's life during periods of physical and psychosocial role transitions such as adolescence.

Sets of socially expected behavior patterns related to the individual's functioning within various groups are called roles. *Threats to or changes in role functioning* may cause anxiety. Factors that may threaten role functioning include situations that precipitate incompatible role behaviors, incongruent cultural and self expectations of role behaviors, incompatibility of various roles, lack of knowledge of specific role expectations, lack of clarity in role definitions, and inconsistent responses to role behaviors by significant others. Changing or unclear sex roles in contemporary society frequently are a cause of role conflict and disturbance. Threats to or changes in role functioning frequently involve conflicts between dependent and independent functioning. Developmentally, these difficulties arise most prominently in the transitions from adolescence to young adulthood and from middle to older adulthood. Constraints of illness, hospitalization, and disability may cause role changes secondary to dependency and independence issues.

A threat to or change in health status may precipitate anxiety. These threats or changes may be related to physical and psychological illnesses or disabilities, to medical treatment and iatrogenic effects, to alterations in access to health care services, and to changes in living situations. The person may lack adequate knowledge regarding signs and symptoms related to health status or may be overwhelmed by knowledge and lack the defense of denial. In addition, physical and psychological changes related to aging predispose the individual to alteration in health status.

Threats to or changes in interaction patterns may be a related factor in client anxiety. Interaction patterns may be disrupted by physical or emotional separation from family, friends, job, home, or physical environment. Also, inability of the individual to interact because of physical or psychological disorders may threaten or disrupt patterns of interaction; e.g., a spouse who begins hallucinating or loses short-term memory changes interaction patterns, leading to anxiety in the other spouse.

Threats to or changes in the environment have been identified as a causative factor in the development of anxiety. Environmental factors include unsafe neighborhoods as evidenced by high crime rates, change of residence, natural disasters, nuclear threat, and health hazards caused by environmental pollution.

The *socioeconomic status* of the individual may be influenced by a variety of factors, including changes in employment status, the assumption of additional financial responsibilities, and health problems necessiting continuing care. Any of these situations may generate anxiety within the person or persons experiencing the changes or threats.

Conflicts about essential values and goals in life may elicit anxiety. The most common type of conflict is the double approach–avoidance, when the person can see both desirable and undesirable aspects of both alternatives.[7] An example is the individual who must choose between living with maladaptive coping patterns or taking the risk of seeking therapy. A second kind of conflict, avoidance–avoidance, is one in which the person must choose between two undesirable goals. A third kind of conflict, approach–avoidance, occurs when the individual wishes simultaneously to obtain and to avoid a goal. An example is the client who wishes to express feelings yet is fearful of doing so. A fourth conflict is approach–approach, in which two equally desirable goals are perceived, with attainment of only one being possible.

Contagion is an important characteristic of anxiety: it can be transmitted from person to person. Anxiety as a contagious phenomenon may also be communicated within families and groups. Parents who have high anxiety levels may transfer that anxiety to their children. In addition, families can experience unique anxiety levels and anxiety-provoking issues that are typically expressed by individual family members in specific behaviors.

Tillich described anxiety as being central to survival and as a result of the individual's awareness of possible nonbeing.[23] The balance between survival and death is addressed by the crux of anxiety, preservation of the self. Thus, both awareness of possible nonbeing in a theoretical context and the threat of more immediate death brought on by a terminal illness are etiologically related to anxiety.

DEFINING CHARACTERISTICS

The cluster of signs and symptoms observed in persons with the nursing diagnosis anxiety may be categorized into physiological, psychological, and cognitive indicators. These categories are chosen because of their utility in nursing assessment and intervention in relation to anxiety. As previously discussed, anxiety occurs at various levels of intensity, and the defining characteristics will be present according to the level of anxiety experienced (Table 13-1). For example, apprehension has been identified as a defining characteristic of anxiety. An individual might be experiencing mild, moderate, severe, or extreme apprehension, depending on the level of anxiety, mild through panic.

The autonomic nervous system mediates the *physiological* responses associated with anxiety. These responses are of two types: the sympathetic response activates body processes and the parasympathetic conserves body responses. In anxiety, the sympathetic reaction usually dominates, and the body is prepared for a "fight or flight" response. When the sympathetic branch is activated, the adrenal glands are stimulated to release epinephrine, causing blood to be channeled from the gastrointestinal tract to the heart, muscles, and central nervous system. The existing parasympathetic response also results in observable physiological reactions. The physiological responses, when associated with mild or moderate anxiety, will heighten the individual's capabilities, whereas the physiological responses associated with severe or panic levels will limit, overwork, and immobilize capabilities to function. High levels of anxiety affect coordination and responsiveness, causing the individual to be clumsy or accident prone. Because the physiological responses to anxiety are mediated through the autonomic nervous system, the body achieves the internal adjustments without conscious or voluntary actions by the individual.

Clients often describe the *psychological* manifestations of anxiety with expressions such as "nervous," "uptight," or "tense." The person may appear to be jumpy and worried with the expectation that something negative will happen. These phrases and behaviors express the apprehension and overalert state of the

TABLE 13–1
Features of the levels of anxiety: mild, moderate, severe, extreme/panic

	PHYSIOLOGICAL	PSYCHOLOGICAL/BEHAVIORAL	COGNITIVE
Mild	Slight sympathetic arousal with slight increase in pulse, breathing rate, and blood pressure	Behaviors and feelings generally positive	Alert, aware; perceives connections between elements of situations
Moderate	Sympathetic nervous system activation with muscular tension, perspiration, dilation of pupils, peripheral vasoconstriction, further increase in pulse, breathing rate and blood pressure	Feelings of tension, apprehension, helplessness, and concern	Perceptual field is somewhat narrowed; attention is fixed on situation of concern; little attention to peripheral events
Severe	Fight or flight responses: generalized sympathetic nervous system response	Increasingly negative feelings including inadequacy, wariness, and distress	Attention is directed to scattered details; learning capacity is greatly diminished
Extreme/panic	Continued physiological arousal with possible eventual parasympathetic nervous system response	Emotionally overwhelmed; may regress to primitive coping behaviors	Unable to attend to external events; responds to severe internal distress

individual. Higher levels of anxiety are experienced as uncomfortable and unpleasant, and the individual will attempt to avoid the anxiety, sometimes with extreme behaviors. Anxiety is often seen in combination with depression and hostility. These emotions may function in a reciprocal fashion, with one generating or reinforcing another.

Cognitive functioning may be enhanced or diminished by anxiety, depending on the level of anxiety experienced by the individual. In mild anxiety, sensory input is heightened, whereas in moderate anxiety, some of the sensory acuity is lost. At a severe level of anxiety, sensory input is further limited and is also distorted, so that processing occurs in a scattered, disorganized mode. In panic, perceptions are grossly distorted, and the individual has difficulty distinguishing reality from unreality. Concentration, learning, and problem solving are also enhanced by mild and moderate anxiety. The severe levels of anxiety cause difficulties with concentration and in understanding relations between and among the foci of learning. At the panic level, the ability to concentrate, learn, and solve problems is virtually nonexistent (Chart 1).

NURSING PROCESS AND RATIONALE
Assessment

Assessment for anxiety not only determines whether this nursing diagnosis is appropriate but also identifies

---

CHART 1
Anxiety: Definition, Related Factors, and Defining Characteristics

DEFINITION

Anxiety is a vague uneasy feeling, the source of which often is nonspecific or unknown to the individual.

RELATED FACTORS

Threat to self-concept
Unmet needs
Situational crisis
Maturational crisis
Threat to or change in role functioning
Threat to or change in health status
Threat to or change in interaction patterns
Threat to or change in environment
Threat to or change in socioeconomic status
Unconscious conflict about essential values/goals of life
Interpersonal transmission/contagion
Awareness of death

DEFINING CHARACTERISTICS
Physiological

Increased pulse	Decreased pulse
Increased blood pressure	Decreased blood pressure
Increased breathing rate	Faintness and fainting
Flushed face	Abdominal pain
Breathing difficulties	Nausea
Heightened reflexes	Diarrhea
Twitching	Urinary urgency
Trembling	Urinary frequency
Tremors	
Restlessness	
Extraneous movements	
Insomnia	
Weakness	
Pupil dilation	
Anorexia	
Dry mouth	
Increased perspiration	
Facial tension	
Voice quivering	

Psychological/Behavioral

Increased tension	Jittery
Apprehension	Poor eye contact
Worried	Glancing about
Distressed	Feelings of inadequacy
Focus on self	Rattled
Uncertainty	Increased helplessness
Fearful	Increased wariness
Scared	Expressed concerns regarding change in life events
Fear of unspecified consequences	

Cognitive

Difficulty concentrating
Diminished learning ability
Diminished ability to solve problems
Blocking of thoughts
Reduced or scattered perceptual field
Forgetfulness
Impaired attention
Diminished productivity
Preoccupation
Confusion

the level of anxiety manifested by the patient as well as the particular manifestations of anxiety and their effect on the individual's daily life. In addition to relating the assessment to defining characteristics, one should conduct a focused assessment for stressors or threats related to the etiologies of anxiety.

Four behavioral patterns are commonly used to cope with anxiety. An adaptive, growth-producing coping behavior is that of problem solving and using anxiety to learn positive, adaptive behaviors. Three other patterns—withdrawal and avoidance, acting out, and somatization—are maladaptive coping behaviors because they do not help the person deal with the anxiety, only avoid it at the expense of reality perception and growth. *Withdrawal and avoidance* involve retreating from and evading anxiety-provoking experiences. In *acting out* behaviors, the individual discharges the tension and feelings through aggressive behaviors. When the person uses *somatization* to deal with anxiety, the anxiety is converted into physical symptoms and given visceral or physiological expression. During the assessment process, the nurse will observe the nature of these responses to anxiety. Throughout the nursing process, the nurse continues to re-evaluate the patient's anxiety level. Persons who experience severe anxiety and use maladaptive coping patterns may have difficulties that fall into the category of anxiety disorders as listed in the DSM-III-R[3] (see Chapter 21).

Nursing Diagnosis

Arriving at a nursing diagnosis of anxiety for a particular client will involve, not only assessment for the presence of defining characteristics and possible related factors, but subsequently the designation of the level of anxiety and, whenever possible, the duration. The diagnostic process will include assessing the impact of the manifestations of anxiety in the individual client on the management of daily living; e.g., working, parenting, eating, sleeping, and relating with others. An example of a nursing diagnosis is severe anxiety related to threat to self-concept.

Client Goals and Nursing Interventions

Once the nursing diagnosis has been established, the nurse is ready to delineate client goals related to managing or functioning in the presence of the level of anxiety exhibited. It would be inappropriate and unrealistic to think that anyone can be totally free from anxiety. Rather, the ultimate goal is to help the person identify and tolerate mild or moderate anxiety and to use it constructively.

If the assessment reveals that the client's anxiety is at the severe or panic level, the immediate goal is to assist the person to reduce the level of anxiety. Nursing interactions with the client will be directed toward providing reassurance and comfort through a calm, accepting, nondemanding approach. The physical environment needs to be comfortable and nonstimulating. A staff member may need to stay with the client. During this time, a trusting relationship can be established between the nurse and the client. To facilitate the development of trust, empathy, and unconditional positive regard for the client should be communicated by the nurse.

When the client's anxiety has decreased, analysis and discussion of the feelings of anxiety and the surrounding situations can be initiated. The client must first be able to recognize the presence of anxiety, then to identify anxiety-provoking situations. Discussion of the client's response to anxiety eventually will assist in: (1) evaluating whether these responses are maladaptive and (2) problem solving regarding adaptive responses. The client is encouraged to express feelings and is given positive feedback during symptom-free intervals. Secondary gains derived from maladaptive behaviors are reduced, and alternative interests in the external environment are encouraged. Volunteer work, new interests, hobbies, helping others, and gradual participation in social activities are encouraged during this phase of treatment.

A final client goal is to initiate health teaching and referrals regarding constructive methods of handling anxiety. Health teaching related to constructive handling of anxiety offers varied and interesting choices that the nurse and client can explore and adapt to individual needs. Relaxation training is an option frequently presented in nursing literature.[5,16] A common technique is progressive muscular relaxation (PMR). Initially, the client systematically tenses and relaxes gross muscle groups while attending to the differences in sensation during contraction and relaxation. The goal of PMR is for the client to identify tension and to use PMR to reduce it.

Exercise provides a method for preventing or reducing anxiety and stress. Assessment of the client before an exercise should include a health history, physical examination, and laboratory tests as indicated. If appropriate for the client, a repetitive endurance exercise that uses large muscle groups is recommended. Examples are brisk walking, running, jogging, cycling (stationary or rolling), skipping rope, climbing stairs, dancing, and skiing. Activities may be modified for individual factors such as disability or advanced age. The process of individualizing the regime for the client is the principal strategy for both initiation and maintenance of the program. Data about daily patterns and preferences, experiences, health beliefs, resources, and social supports are utilized to increase client readiness and to individualize the program.[2] Planning with the client should include goals and mutual expectations. Contracting with clients is effective and is enhanced by follow-up visits to monitor the success of the plan.

After exploring the client's musical preferences, the nurse and client can select music appropriate to facilitate relaxation and to decrease anxiety. Portable tape cassette players with headphones are an effective means of providing accessibility and privacy for the client listening to music.

Nursing interventions for clients with anxiety can be varied and individual. In addition to the initial interventions aimed at decreasing anxiety and later interventions to help the client develop insight, nurses can provide health teaching aimed at helping the client learn constructive methods of coping with anxiety. It is hoped that these health-promotion activities will assist clients to gain self-management skills and a sense of environmental mastery.

Evaluation

The final step in the nursing process, evaluation, is set in motion by establishing outcome criteria that reflect the client's goals and measure the extent to which they were achieved and thus whether the anxiety was modified or diminished. For the client goals regarding anxiety discussed previously, the outcome criteria would include a statement about the reduction or elimination of the defining characteristics indicative of anxiety. In addition, outcome measures of recognition of anxiety, problem solving about adaptive vs maladaptive coping behaviors, and the use of mild or moderate anxiety for

personal growth would be included. Data that indicate whether the client has learned about and is utilizing strategies to prevent anxiety from reaching harmful levels will be collected to measure outcomes in this area. Evaluation of interventions may include use of anxiety scales or inventories in addition to the subjective and objective observations of the nurse and client (Chart 2).

CASE STUDY

Jason K, an 18-year-old single Hispanic man, is a freshman at a large state university. During an interview with a nurse at the university health service, he states that his grades are low and that he is unable to study because of poor concentration. He reports that he sits with his books and notes and tries to study but cannot remember what he has been reading. He reports that he feels restless and gets up to pace about his dormitory room frequently when trying to study. As he talks with the nurse, his posture is tense and rigid, with many extraneous movements of the hands, feet, and legs, and his voice quivers occasionally. He describes difficulty getting to sleep and states that he sleeps only 2 to 3 hours before awakening. His reason for coming to the health service is to obtain relief for the distress and fatigue, which he describes as increasing with each day. Jason relates his current condition to the stress of his studies and to

CHART 2
Anxiety: Summary of the Nursing Process

NURSING INTERVENTIONS	OUTCOME CRITERIA
CLIENT GOAL: EXPERIENCE REDUCED LEVEL OF ANXIETY Assess level of anxiety: mild, moderate, severe, panic Talk with and reassure client in a calm, supportive, nondemanding manner Communicate in short, concise sentences Provide a quiet, nonstimulating, and safe milieu Consult with physician regarding pharmacologic therapy if indicated	Defining characteristics of anxiety are reduced or eliminated
CLIENT GOAL: RECOGNIZE THE PRESENCE OF ANXIETY IN SELF Help the client identify anxiety by asking, "are you uncomfortable now?" Give feedback to the client regarding behaviors that indicate anxiety Encourage client to discuss perception of and feelings about anxiety	Recognizes presence of anxiety
CLIENT GOAL: EXPLORE PREDISPOSING AND PRECIPITATING FACTORS IN ANXIETY Discuss ways of predicting anxiety Encourage client to recall and analyze instances of anxiety in detail	Explores factors that predispose to or precipitate anxiety
CLIENT GOAL: DEVELOP ADAPTIVE COPING STRATEGIES AND RESPONSES Assist the client in identifying adaptive solutions and methods to deal with anxiety Teach problem-solving process and practice with client Practice use of positive coping behaviors through discussion and role playing Encourage social activities, new interests, hobbies	Utilizes constructive coping strategies
CLIENT GOAL: INTEGRATE HEALTH-PROMOTING, ANXIETY-REDUCING ACTIVITIES INTO LIFESTYLE Assist client to utilize mild or moderate anxiety for positive growth Teach progressive muscular relaxation Practice assertive communication skills Talk over concerns with appropriate persons Practice using music for relaxation Participate in physical activities: sports, walking, jogging, biking, swimming	Uses selected health-promoting, anxiety-reducing activities

being away from his extended family. He feels that he needs outside help because his attempts at studying more, going to bed early, and talking with the resident advisor on his floor in the dormitory have not seemed to help. No particular sports or exercise programs are patterned into Jason's life.

Jason states that he feels tired and tense most of the time and relates this to his interrupted and inadequate sleep pattern. He usually goes to bed between 11 and 12 P.M. but does not fall asleep for about 2 hours. He then awakens in 2 to 3 hours and sleeps again for 1 to 2 hours. He is usually up before 6 each morning. He relates that he feels tense and jittery and is unable to relax or even to be attentive when watching television and misses talking with his Hispanic friends. Jason describes recent difficulties with concentration and short-term memory and states that he is distract-

Research Highlights

Annotated Bibliography

Aukamp V. Knowledge deficit and anxiety as nursing diagnoses in the third trimester of pregnancy: an exploratory study to identify the defining characteristics and contributing factors. [Doctoral dissertation]. Austin, Texas: The University of Texas, 1986.

Aukamp's study addressed the defining characteristics and contributing factors for anxiety and the amount of nurse–pregnant women agreement about the defining characteristics and contributing factors. The researcher collected data from nurses and patients and used both qualitative and quantitative methods. Both groups verbalized feelings of anxiety and apprehension. Nurses and pregnant women also agreed that threat to or any change in health status and fear of the unknown were contributing factors in anxiety.

Burke SO. A developmental perspective on the nursing diagnoses fear and anxiety. Nurs Papers 2:59, 1982.

Burke provides a descriptive review of what developmental theorists, researchers, and experts on the nursing of children can offer in the clarification of the relation between fear and anxiety. Clinical uses of the diagnoses fear and anxiety and the differences are discussed, and nursing interventions for each are outlined.

Fadden T, Fehring RJ, Rossi EK. Clinical validation of the diagnosis anxiety: In: McLane AM, ed. Classification of nursing diagnoses: proceedings of the Seventh Conference. St Louis, CV Mosby, 1987.

Fadden and associates provide a clinical validation study of the defining characteristics of anxiety. These researchers concluded that most of the defining characteristics were observed and validated by the clinical specialists. However, significant content diagnostic validity levels were not reached.

Jones PE, Jakob DF. Anxiety revisited from a practice perspective. In: Kim MJ, McFarland GK, McLane AM, eds. Classification of nursing diagnoses: proceedings of the Fifth National Conference. St Louis, CV Mosby, 1984.

The findings suggest that anxiety is prevalent and widely distributed in nursing practice settings and that the reported contributing factors are amenable to nursing interventions. The authors point out that apparent ambiguities in the terms "anxiety" and "fear" indicate the need for further investigation.

Kim MJ, Seritella RA, Gulanik M, et al. Clinical validation of cardiovascular nursing diagnoses. In: Kim MJ, McFarland GK, McLane AM, eds. Classification of nursing diagnoses: proceedings of the Fifth National Conference. St Louis, CV Mosby, 1984.

Kim and coworkers attempted clinical validation of nursing diagnoses in cardiovascular patients, in whom anxiety was the eighth most frequent diagnosis. The defining characteristics most frequently listed by the nurses were psychosocial indicators of stress (anxious, tense, restless, tranquilizer use, hyperalertness, nervous mannerisms, hyperkinetic, questioning, and depressed) and concern about life events (illness, future, family, finances, job). The authors suggest the need for further validation, because the frequency of occurrence was not large enough for meaningful interpretations.

Metzger KL, Hiltunen EF. Diagnostic content validation of ten frequently reported nursing diagnoses. In: McLane AM, ed. Classification of nursing diagnoses: proceedings of the Seventh National Conference. St Louis, CV Mosby, 1987.

Metzger and Hiltunen attempted to obtain validity estimates on selected nursing diagnoses, including anxiety. Critical cues identified for anxiety were anxious, apprehension, increased tension, worried, fear of specific consequences, and distressed. Findings indicated a need for further refinement.

Whitley G. Validation of the nursing diagnosis anxiety: a nurse consensus survey [Doctoral dissertation]. DeKalb: Northern Illinois University, 1986.

This consensus survey included input from 312 nurses who delineated four defining characteristics of anxiety as critical and 24 as acceptable and rejected one. Twenty-three nurses made spontaneous comments regarding the desirability of building levels into the nursing diagnosis anxiety.

Yokum CJ. The differentiation of fear and anxiety. In: Kim MJ, McFarland GK, McLane AM, eds. Classification of nursing diagnoses: proceedings of the Fifth National Conference. St Louis, CV Mosby, 1984.

Work on the differentiation of fear and anxiety led to the conclusion that distinct differences exist. Anxiety is defined, and sympathetic and parasympathetic responses, behavioral indicators, and subjective experiences are delineated. Anxiety reduction is discussed.

able and restless. Examination reveals blood pressure 134/88 mm Hg; pulse 92 per minute and strong, regular; breathing rate 26 per minute. Severe anxiety was the nursing diagnosis. An important initial goal was the experience of a reduced level of anxiety. The nurse collaborated with the physician, and pharmacologic therapy was initiated. A series of nursing counseling sessions was planned in which Jason was assisted in identifying the source of his anxiety, and adaptive methods and solutions for dealing with anxiety were explored. One mutually agreed on intervention called for Jason to be become involved in the Spanish Club on campus.

SUMMARY

Anxiety is a vague uneasy feeling, the source of which is often nonspecific or unknown to the individual. Anxiety occurs throughout the life cycle, birth through old age, and is interpersonally contagious. The work of Peplau, a leader in psychiatric and mental health nursing, was discussed. Four levels of anxiety were described in relation to nursing care: mild, moderate, severe, and panic. Two frequently occurring related factors in anxiety are threat to self-concept and unmet needs. Defining characteristics of anxiety occur in the physiological, psychological, and cognitive realms. The goals of nursing assessment of the client for anxiety include determining whether this diagnosis is appropriate, determining the level of anxiety manifested by the individual, and observing for stressors that indicate the etiology of the anxiety. The ultimate therapeutic goal for individuals with anxiety is to identify and tolerate mild or moderate anxiety and to use it in a constructive manner. If assessment reveals that anxiety is at a severe or panic level, the immediate goal is to assist the client in reducing the level of anxiety. Evaluation encompasses whether the client's anxiety has been modified or diminished, whether the client recognizes the presence of anxiety and is able to use problem solving in relation to adaptive/maladaptive coping behaviors, and whether mild or moderate anxiety can now be used for personal growth.

References

1. Aguilera DC, Messick JM. Crisis intervention: theory and methodology. Ed 5. St Louis: CV Mosby; 1986.
2. Allan JD. Exercise program. In: Bulecheck GM, McCloskey JC, eds. Nursing interventions: treatments for nursing diagnoses. Philadelphia, WB Saunders; 1985.
3. American Psychiatric Association. Diagnostic and Statistical Manual of Mental Disorders III-Revised. Washington, DC: American Psychiatric Association; 1987.
4. Bulechek GM, McCloskey JC, eds. Nursing interventions: treatments for nursing diagnoses. Philadelphia: WB Saunders; 1985.
5. Burke SO. A developmental perspective on the nursing diagnoses fear and anxiety. Nurs Papers. 1982;2:59–64.
6. Castles MR. Interrater agreement in the use of nursing diagnosis. In: Kim MJ, Moritz DA, eds. Classification of nursing diagnoses: proceedings of the Third and Fourth National Conferences. New York: McGraw-Hill; 1982.
7. Dollard J, Miller H. Personality and psychotherapy. New York: McGraw-Hill; 1950.
8. Horrocks J, Jackson D. Self and role: a theory of self-process and role behavior. Boston: Houghton Mifflin; 1972.
9. Jones PE. The revision of nursing diagnosis terms. In: Kim MJ, Moritz DA, eds. Classification of nursing diagnoses: proceedings of the Third and Fourth National Conferences. New York: McGraw-Hill; 1982.
10. Jones PE, Jakob DF. Anxiety revisited from a practice perspective. In: Kim MJ, McFarland GK, McLane AM, eds. Classification of nursing diagnoses: proceedings of the Fifth National Conference. St Louis, CV Mosby; 1984.
11. Kim MJ, Amorosa K, Gulanick M, et al. Clinical validation of nursing diagnoses. In: Kim MJ, Moritz DA, eds. Classification of nursing diagnoses: proceedings of the Third and Fourth National Conference. New York: McGraw-Hill; 1982.
12. Kim MJ, McFarland GK, McLane AM, eds. Classification of nursing diagnoses: proceedings of the Fifth National Conference. St Louis, CV Mosby; 1984.
13. Kim MJ, Seritella KA, Gulanick M, et al. Clinical validation of cardiovascular nursing diagnoses. In: Kim MJ, McFarland GK, McLane AM, eds. Classification of nursing diagnoses: proceedings of the Fifth National Conference. St Louis, CV Mosby; 1984.
14. Maslow AH. Motivation and Personality. Ed 2. New York: Harper & Row; 1970.
15. McFarland GK, Bates TI. Nursing care plan: anxiety. In: Kim MJ, McFarland GK, McLane AM. Pocket guide to nursing diagnoses. Ed 3. St Louis, CV Mosby; 1989.
16. McFarland G, Wasli E. Nursing diagnoses and process in psychiatric mental health nursing. Philadelphia: JB Lippincott; 1986.
17. McKeehan KM, Gordon M. Utilization of accepted diagnoses. In: Kim MJ, Moritz DA, eds. Classification of nursing diagnoses: proceedings of the Third and Fourth National Conferences. New York: McGraw-Hill; 1982.
18. Metzger KL, Hiltunen EF. Diagnostic content validation of ten frequently reported nursing diagnoses. In: McLane AM, ed. Classification of nursing diagnoses: proceedings of the Seventh Conference. St Louis, CV Mosby; 1987.
19. Peplau H. A working definition of anxiety. In: Burd S, Marshall M, eds. Some clinical approaches to psychiatric nursing. New York: Macmillan; 1963.
20. Scandrett S, Uecker S. Relaxation training. In: Bulecheck GM, McCloskey JC, eds. Nursing interventions: treatments for nursing diagnoses. Philadelphia: WB Saunders; 1985.
21. Spielberger CD. Conceptual and methodologic issues in anxiety research. In: Anxiety: current trends in theory and research. New York: Academic Press; 1972.
22. Spielberger CD, Gorsuch RL, Lushem RE. Manual for the State–Trait Anxiety Inventory. Palo Alto: Consulting Psychologist Press; 1970.
23. Tillich P. The courage to be. New Haven: Yale University Press; 1952.
24. Whitley G. Validation of the nursing diagnosis anxiety: a nurse consensus survey [Doctoral dissertation]. DeKalb: Northern Illinois University; 1986.
25. Yokum CJ. The differentiation of fear and anxiety. In: Kim MJ, McFarland GK, McLane AM, eds. Classification of nursing diagnoses: proceedings of the Fifth National Conference. St Louis, CV Mosby; 1984.

BIZARRE BEHAVIOR

Ruth Jalane Hagerott

DEFINITION AND DESCRIPTION

Behavior that appears odd, socially unacceptable, undesirable, distracting, and grotesque is termed *bizarre*. It is manifested by odd and inappropriate dress; mannerisms, such as posturing, repetitive gestures, grotesque facial grimaces; incomprehensible verbalizations; incongruent affect; weird laughter; and symptoms of severe regression, such as assuming a fetal position or defecating or urinating without regard for normal convention.

THEORY AND RESEARCH

Bizarre behavior is commonly referred to in describing psychosis and occurs in a number of psychiatric illnesses. It is one of the major causes for the distress the general public demonstrates toward the mentally ill, and one that, other than violence toward self and others, can draw immediate attention to the person's problem.

Bizarre behavior is often the result of regression as part of the phenomenological picture of schizophrenia or mania.[4,8,9] Whether the individual is mute, immobile and curled in a fetal position, or gleefully smearing feces, bizarre behavior demonstrates an inability or unwillingness to communicate on an adult level.[8,9]

It has been hypothesized that the bizarre behaviors that occur in schizophrenia are attempts by the individual to not communicate;[6,14] that is, a way of avoiding communication is to speak in unintelligible terms or to behave in unpredictable or unconventional ways. Although bizarre behavior does allow the individual to avoid the expression of specific problematic thoughts or feelings, it simultaneously is very much a means of communicating the state of that person. Thus, bizarre behavior is the client's substitute for coherent speech and appropriate behavior, but it also serves as a window through which the receiver of the message may understand the disturbed sender.[14] It can, however, prove a difficult barrier in client–therapist interaction and make prediction of prognostic outcome difficult.[6]

RELATED FACTORS

Bizarre behavior can occur in psychiatric conditions such as schizophrenia, bipolar disorder, delirium, dementia, and psychoactive substance-use disorders.[2] It often occurs together with hallucinations and delusions.

Bizarre behavior has been observed in conjunction with toxic psychosis as an effect of cocaine, phencyclidine (PCP), diphenhydramine (benadryl), or alcohol use.[12,13,15,16] It has been observed in conjunction with temporal lobe epilepsy, systemic infections, metabolic disorders (e.g., hypoglycemia[11]), trauma, neoplasms, postoperative states,[2] and with minor disruptions in physiologic status, such as constipation.

Bizarre behavior has been observed in otherwise normal persons who are exposed to protracted periods of isolation, sensory deprivation, and sleep deprivation, or who experience a grief reaction. Sensory loss or impairment may also contribute to what observers perceive as bizarre behavior. Grief reactions may lead to bizarre behaviors that are perceived as acceptable within certain time limitations.[2]

Cultural factors can influence the nature, frequency, and interpretation of bizarre behavior. What might be acceptable in one context may not be in another. Varying degrees of bizarre or dysfunctional behavior will be tolerated, but eventually, if the behavior is seen as maladaptive or inadequate for survival, the individual member will be isolated, deserted, treated, or incarcerated.[5]

DEFINING CHARACTERISTICS

Certain behaviors have typically been identified as bizarre. Grooming and style of dress are often the most apparent signs of a disruption in mental processes and communication style. An example might be a woman who applies makeup, exaggerating her eyes, mouth, and eyebrows to the extent that she resembles a clown. This may demonstrate the need to outline features that are otherwise unclear or fragmented, according to reports of distortion in perception experienced by schizophrenics or those clients under the influence of drugs (LSD).[6,7] Clients with schizophrenia, who do not see their features in the appropriate places, may mark on their faces where they perceive their eyes should be or outline them so they are more obvious.

The clothing may not match in color or style and is inappropriate to the occasion or weather. Clients have been observed dressed in shorts and no shoes in a cold, driving rain or, by contrast, bundled in a heavy coat on a day when the temperature is near 100°F. They may wear outer garments that are inappropriate to the location or weather, such as hats or gloves, for delusional concerns that they would otherwise turn to stone or have their brains fall out (Fig. 13–9).

Peculiar posturing, body carriage, or movements have also been noted. The client who crouches beneath a sink with limbs outstretched in a manner that reminds one of a wounded bird might be communicating unwillingness to participate in an expected activity. Although temporarily removed from location or prevented from continuing the posturing, the client will return to the preferred location and former position.[8]

The same client may communicate verbally in monosyllables or sentences absent of referents for noun phrases [e.g., "(You) wear brights; (I) wear Sundays."] In the former example, the client was attempting to indicate approval or pleasure with bright colors or, in the case of "Sundays," formal dress, but could not do so in complete sentences. They may also mumble incomprehensible, nonsensical phrases or suddenly shout obscenities without apparent provocation.[1]

The ingestion of inedible objects is one of the more dangerous manifestations of the client demonstrating bizarre behavior. Clients have been known to swallow objects such as nails, pins, needles, or coat hangers, and substances such as bleach, lye, or ammonia, and masticate on curtains, sheets, their own clothing and body parts. Clients may do these things without cognizance of the consequences of their behavior, but, rather, as an extreme manifestation of their inability to communicate otherwise.

All of the aforementioned behaviors are considered to be manifestations of an underlying cognitive deficit and inability to communicate appropriately, which includes a vivid portrayal of disrupted self-image,[6] regardless of the multifaceted etiologic factors[3,10] (Chart 1).

NURSING PROCESS AND RATIONALE

Assessment

Bizarre behavior may be manifested initially in subtle ways, such as minor changes in grooming and dressing, verbalizations that are less understandable, peculiarities in gestures or posture, ritualistic behavior that increases in frequency to the point of interfering with a client's functioning. Withdrawal and changes in eating and sleeping behavior may accompany an increase in bizarre behavior. Illness or physical problems, such as diarrhea, constipation, flu, may be enough to upset the client's homeostasis and increase the incidents of strange behavior formerly under control or not previously noted. Noting subtle changes in the level of stress in the client's internal and external environment early in its onset and assessing the underlying cause are paramount to effective intervention. Because the behavior reflects the inner world of the client, it is imperative that the client's perception of what others interpret as bizarre be explored to whatever extent possible. Often the decrease in bizarre behavior is an indication that the overall condition of the client is improving (for example, one client who removed his dentures requested their return once the psychotic symptoms, such as delusions and hallucinations, began to abate).

Nursing Diagnosis

When delineating the nursing diagnosis of bizarre behavior, a specific phrase, such as bizarre behavior related to schizophrenia or bizarre behavior related to pharmacologic toxicity is added. In so doing, the nurse will be better prepared to plan care that is based on an

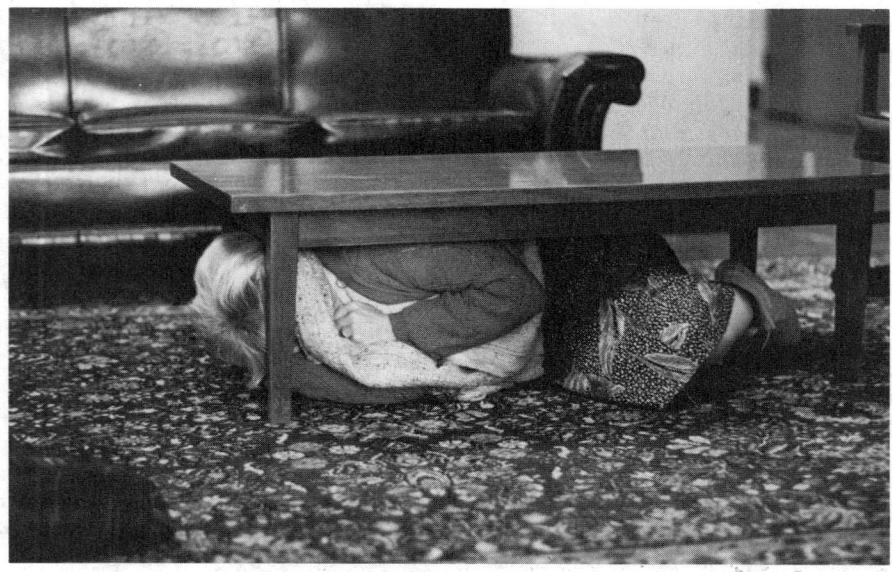

FIGURE 13–9. Clients may manifest bizarre behavior in body posturing and in clothing. (Courtesy of Lindsey Ekland)

CHART 1
Bizarre Behavior: Definition, Related Factors, and Defining Characteristics

DEFINITION

Bizarre behavior is behavior that appears odd, socially unacceptable, undesirable, distracting, and grotesque.

RELATED FACTORS

PSYCHIATRIC AND OTHER DISORDERS
Schizophrenia
Mood disorders
Psychoactive substance use
Toxic conditions such as thyrotoxicosis, uremia, hypoglycemia, water intoxication
Delirium or dementia
Neoplasm
Alzheimer's disease
Epilepsy (especially temporal lobe)
Tourette's disorder

TRAUMA
Head injuries
Surgical procedures

STRESSFUL LIFE EXPERIENCES
Loss
Sleep deprivation
Disasters/war
Mass hysteria
Starvation
Loss of body part or function (amputation, paralysis)

DEFINING CHARACTERISTICS

INABILITY TO COMMUNICATE APPROPRIATELY

Grunts	Rituals
Howls	Posturing
Guttural sounds	Aimless or stereotyped
Screams	movements
Snorts	

REGRESSIVE MANIFESTATIONS
Poor judgment
Inappropriate grooming and dress
Self-neglect
Self-abuse

IMPAIRED SOCIAL RELATIONS
Withdrawal
Isolation
Aggression
Hyperactivity

awareness of the underlying problem that manifests in bizarre behavior.

Client Goals and Nursing Interventions

Dangerous consequences can result from bizarre behavior, either in terms of danger to self, as the result of poor judgment, or danger from others, as a result of the annoyance of other disturbed clients. Thus, an initial goal is modification of behavior such that it is more adaptive and such that the ideas, feelings, or experiences the client is attempting to communicate are accomplished in a more appropriate manner and without harm to self or others.

Noting the client's behavior and providing protection from the untoward consequences are the first obligation of the nurse. Once these measures have been addressed, the nurse then utilizes support and acceptance so that the client will experience enough confidence to communicate thoughts and feelings, and then the nurse can, it is hoped, reach the healthy parts of the client and build upon them.

After careful assessment and establishment of rapport, the nurse considers the following sequence of intervention:

1. Protection by monitoring proper clothing, diet, and hygiene, and prevention of harm to the client or to others from impulsive or aggravating behavior that may precipitate aggression or reprisal on the part of other clients.

2. Clear communication that includes reality orientation and consistent role-modeling. Prescribe specifically the words and messages that are understood by the client.

3. Consistent active listening to ascertain the nuances in the client's seemingly bizarre and "nonsensical" verbalizations or behaviors, to be perceptive to the grains of truth or understanding of the client's message [e.g., if the client refers to an object that seems totally unrealistic (like reindeer under the couch), rather than dismissing the client's reference, explore it further].

4. Clarification of the nurse's understanding with the client or others who might know him or her better and strive to reach beyond the barriers created by the psychotic process and behavior. In the client record, provide a glossary of terms and meanings this client has so that all personnel can understand the client's communication.

5. Development of a plan to provide substitute behaviors that the client can utilize. Prescribe the specific behaviors, scripts, attitudes that all personnel are to adopt in interacting with the client.

6. Work with the client and other team members to identify those behaviors that will provide small increments of success. Prescribe the specific positive-feedback behaviors that the client finds rewarding and the circumstances under which they are to be used.

7. Once the client has been educated about the substitute behavior and what to expect in terms of the staff's response and support, consistency in nursing responses communicates a clear message to the client. To do otherwise would be confusing and nontherapeutic for the client. Therefore, specific caregiver behaviors are clearly outlined in the treatment plan.

8. When addressing bizarre behavior, the nurse needs

to retain an acceptance and sense of humor when communicating with the client. Often clients will resort to strange maneuvers to get attention, which (even if most of their thought processes are disrupted) does not necessarily indicate that they are totally unaware that their behavior is peculiar. A sense of timing in the use of humor or a clear indication of doubt that they need to resort to this style of communication is learned by knowing the individual client and utilizing a great deal of discretion.

9. Provide opportunities for clients to participate in a group in which they not only will be accepted, but in which they will also be able to try more appropriate means of communication. Then, when clients receive feedback that communication is unclear or strange, they will be more able to accept this and attempt to do otherwise.

The client goals of decreasing bizarre behavior, learning alternate behaviors, and increasing the ability to recognize when he or she is resorting to that style of communication can be a major accomplishment. The nurse would, initially, prescribe gentle reminders to the client that new ways to communicate needs have been learned. Later in the course of interaction, the nursing orders will change to prescribe the occasions, timing, and behavior to be used in setting firm limits. The treatment is intended to increase the likelihood that the client will not regress, but will continue to work at more appropriate communication. For example, when a client appears, obviously unwashed, with a dirty shirt and no shoes, requesting to go to breakfast, the nursing order can be to indicate, calmly and in a nonjudgmental tone, that the client needs to dress appropriately for the meal, and once that is done, he may then go to breakfast. When he regresses in his dressing, repeat the instructions clearly and neutrally, if he does not respond to the initial ones. Remark warmly on how much better he looks, *after* he has changed his clothes and washed. This kind of reminder may have to occur more than once, but it is clearly stated each time that this is an expectation, and nothing else will be adequate. Usually, the client will comply. At that time, the client goal of taking responsibility for self (even in a limited way) needs to be acknowledged.

Evaluation

If the client becomes agitated or increasingly bizarre when a simple limit is imposed, then there needs to be further evaluation of the underlying cause, and more tailored interventions (e.g., medication, quiet time) may be required. Possible change of environment, such as absence of a favorite nurse, the admission of an aggressive individual who teases or otherwise antagonizes the client, may be factors leading the client to resort to less effective means of communicating needs or frustrations. If the nurse operates on the assumption that nothing has changed, other than the client in question, and does not consider factors in the external as

well as the internal environment of this person, valuable time may be lost and intervention may be misdirected.

Discharge planning for these clients includes a description of the alternate behaviors and communications they have learned so that these then can be reinforced by the family or receiving agency, commonly a group home and mental health clinic. This kind of information often is omitted, because the main focus is on types and dosages of medication. Unfortunately, the omission of what the client has learned and how to help the client retain and continue to use new, effective behaviors is a serious oversight. Nursing has a key role in ensuring that the elements of client education go out of the present environment and into the future with the client (Chart 2).

CASE STUDY

Vera R was a 30-year-old woman who had been in and out of the mental hospital for over ten years. She never wore a dress, always baggy men's trousers and suspenders, and often did not wear shoes, even in cold rain. She wore a large Stetson hat and carried a large stack of books. She muttered to herself, contorted her face to the point that she appeared deformed, and repeatedly insisted that she was Charles Lindbergh, Clark Gable, Gary Cooper, or some other heroic male figure. Her favorite was Charles Lindbergh. She would rarely admit that her name was Vera, nor would she demonstrate by dress or manner that she identified herself as a woman. She did not become agitated, nor was she self-destructive, other than her lack of attention to the weather, which endangered her health because of exposure. She was isolated and seldom communicated anything coherently. She had no friends among the other clients because, even to them, she was so odd and unreachable that they no longer made any efforts to be friendly. Eating, sleeping, making her daily trips to the library, and muttering to herself were the manifestations of her existence. In her mind, she was a world-famous flyer, Rhett Butler in *Gone With the Wind,* the weathered cowboy who conquered the West, or other male figures who were prominent in the daily news, such as astronauts or political candidates, but never did she acknowledge being a woman.

The primary nursing diagnosis was bizarre behavior related to chronic schizophrenia. The goals were to enable her to communicate her needs verbally, to dress appropriately, and to identify herself as Vera R. Nursing interventions were based on the premise that she was reachable, if one were gentle and consistent in reaching out to her. Rapport had to be developed by merely sitting beside her or, if she were willing, walking with her to the library.

Over an extended period, Vera R was treated with medication and milieu therapy in a state mental hospital. She was included in all the regular ward meetings and was a member of her designated group who shared information and feedback with the staff leader and client participants. Her grooming and dress were monitored so that she did not develop upper respiratory or skin infections from neglect or exposure. She was encouraged to wear clothing appropriate to the weather and occasion and was assigned to a female student who role-modeled female dress and behavior to reinforce some degree of social control and cultural expectations. She responded relatively well to the assigned

CHART 2
Bizarre Behavior: Summary of the Nursing Process

NURSING INTERVENTIONS	OUTCOME CRITERIA
CLIENT GOAL: INCREASE APPROPRIATE COMMUNICATION, DECREASE RELIANCE ON BIZARRE BEHAVIOR	
Assess for predisposing conditions of problem	Communicates thoughts in understandable manner
Establish rapport	
Communicate clearly, using concise, simple statements	Resorts to regression and inappropriate communication less frequently
Maintain consistency in own words and actions	
Clarify client's meaning after careful listening or observation	Demonstrates decreased anxiety during communication process
Orient to reality without discounting patient's response or interpretations	
Accept client's regression as part of process—do not respond judgmentally	
Structure opportunities for client to practice reality-oriented communication and interactions with staff, other clients, and family (e.g., conditions of a visit off the unit would be that client engages in a reality-oriented conversation five minutes daily and participates in activity without resorting to bizarre behavior)	
CLIENT GOAL: DECREASE BIZARRE BEHAVIOR	
Protect from acts of self-harm or neglect	Dresses appropriately for weather and occasion
Role-model appropriate behavior; provide clear feedback if behavior is bizarre or inappropriate	Demonstrates understanding of limits and expectations
Set consistent limits; define expectations and rewards	
Give neuroleptic medication as required to control psychotic symptoms and monitor; assess their effectiveness	Reports decrease in psychotic symptoms
Assess to identify location, intensity, and predisposing conditions. If there appears to be no physical basis for this behavior, provide feedback and assist client to control behavior	Does not resort to bizarre contortions, clothes, and such, to communicate needs

student and would, on designated days when the student was present, wear a dress. The remainder of the time, however, she persisted in wearing masculine attire that was consistent with her delusional system. Her general grooming and choice of outerwear appropriate to the weather continued to be an ongoing area of need. Her delusions were fixed, and although on rare occasions, she would respond to "Vera," she was persistent in her beliefs that she was a masculine figure of fame and influence and would correct treatment staff members when they called her by name,

insisting that she was Charles Lindbergh. She was not a hazard to society or herself and was eventually discharged to an extended care facility where her lack of self-care could be monitored, and she could be safeguarded from developing health problems as a result of self-neglect and poor judgment. Her bizarre manner of dressing and her distorted self-image were addressed in the treatment plan that was forwarded to the mental health center and that also included strategies and interventions that had proved effective in the hospital environment.

Research Highlights

Crucial to the study of psychiatric illnesses is the identification of the range of behaviors that are to be included by a particular diagnostic category. It is, for example, important to be clear about what is indicated when the term *schizophrenia* is used. Such clarity is basic to gaining more understanding about etiology and course of illness, as well as about appropriate treatments. At times, schizophrenia has been broadly defined, including a wider range of behaviors; at other times, it has been more narrowly defined. One problem in this definitional process is that no single symptom is always indicative of the presence of schizophrenia.[3]

In recent years, one approach to defining schizophrenia as well as subtypes has been through the study of clustering of signs and symptoms, especially positive and negative symptoms. Positive symptoms represent a distortion of normal behavior and include bizarre behavior, as well as hallucinations and delusions. Negative symptoms, on the other hand, represent a loss of function and include such behaviors as affective flattening and poverty of speech.[3] Research is being conducted to learn if subtyping that is based on positive and negative symptoms has any predictive validity for the course of illness and the treatment response. In addition, brain imaging is being used to identify whether or not particular phenomenologically based subtypes can be linked with particular biologic defects.[3]

SUMMARY

Bizarre behavior, which includes distorted verbal communications, can occur in psychiatric and nonpsychiatric conditions. Distorted communication and regressed behavior have been linked to schizophrenia, as well as other related factors. The assessment by the nurse and other treatment staff members for the etiology of the bizarre behavior clearly influences the nursing interventions and is subject to modification based on additional information. Recognition on the part of the nurse that bizarre behavior can be the manifestation of either psychological or physiologic factors is inherent in a complete assessment. Basic interventions to protect and establish communication with the client are paramount to the success of interventions required to address the underlying cause and to continue to help the client develop and utilize more effective behaviors. The nurse needs to remember that such clients are suffering individuals who need help to reach beyond the prison of their thought disorder long enough to contact others and receive a response that helps them continue to move away from the bizarre to the normal.

References

1. Allen HA, Allen DS. Positive symptoms and organization within and between ideas in schizophrenic subtypes. Psychol Med. 1985;15:71–80.
2. American Psychiatric Association. Diagnostic and statistical manual of mental disorders. 3rd ed, revised. Washington, DC: American Psychiatric Association; 1987.
3. Andreason NC. The diagnosis of schizophrenia. Schizophr Bull. 1987;13:9–22.
4. Bleuler M (Clemens S, trans). The schizophrenic disorders: long term patient and family studies. New Haven: Yale University Press; 1978.
5. Foulks E, et al. Current perspectives in cultural psychiatry. New York: Spectrum Publications; 1977.
6. Johnson DR. Representation of the internal world in catatonic schizophrenia. Psychiatry. 1984;47:299–314.
7. Jones J, Dougherty J, Cannon L. Diphenhydramine-induced toxic psychosis. Am J Emerg Med. 1986;4:369–371.
8. Kaplan HI, Sadock BJ, eds. Comprehensive textbook of psychiatry, 4th ed. Baltimore: Williams & Wilkins; 1983.
9. Keefe RS et al. Characteristics of very poor outcome schizophrenia. Am J Psychiatry. 1987;144:889–895.
10. Lanin-Kettering I, Harrow M. The thought behind the words: a view of schizophrenic speech and thinking disorders. Schizophr Bull. 1985;11:1–15.
11. Malouf R, Brust JC. Hypoglycemia: causes, neurological manifestations and outcome. Ann Neurol. 1985;17:421–430.
12. Merigian KS, Roberts JR. Cocaine intoxication: hyperpyrexia, rhabdomyolysis and acute renal failure. J Toxicol Clin Toxicol. 1987;25:135–148.
13. Schwartz RH, Einhorn A. PCP intoxication in seven young children. Pediatr Emerg Care. 1986;2:238–241.
14. Watzlawick P, Beavin JH, Jackson DD. Pragmatics of human communication: a study of interactional patterns, pathologies, and paradoxes. New York: WW Norton; 1967.
15. Wetli CV, Fishbain DA. Cocaine-induced psychosis and sudden death in recreational cocaine users. J Foren Sci. 1985;30:873–880.
16. Whitley MP, Osborne OH, Godfrey MA, Johnston K. A point prevalence study of alcoholism and mental illness among downtown migrants. Soc Sci Med. 1985;20:579–583.

BOREDOM

Gail M. Lascik

DEFINITION AND DESCRIPTION

Boredom is an emotional state of dampened energy related to the person's perception of being involved in pursuits or surroundings that are tedious, monotonous, and lacking in interest. It is the unpleasant experience of being trapped or caught in a situation or relationship that the person believes must be endured, temporarily or permanently. The individual may feel obligated, powerless, or fearful to change the situation. The result is boredom.

Boredom is not only the inability to find something that satisfies; it is the inability to find satisfaction in what is being done and the inability to find stimulation and meaning internally.[9] Being bored is having nothing to do at a certain time . . . having something to do but not wanting to do it . . . or being tired of the same old thing, being "bored to tears," "bored to death," or "bored stiff." Boredom is different from depression in that the bored person does not have the extensive feelings of guilt, unworthiness, sinfulness, hopelessness, failure, and self-blame characteristic of depression. Anger is much closer to consciousness in boredom than in depression, and the bored person does not feel suicidal.[5]

THEORY AND RESEARCH

The person with borderline personality disorder who has chronic feelings of emptiness or boredom; the adolescent who has nothing to do and no one to do it with; the workaholic who has reduced life to uninspired and mechanical routines; the hospitalized client who paces the halls and chain smokes; the student who sits staring off into space; the assembly line worker who gets hurt; the elderly client who continually pushes the call bell; all may be examples of individuals suffering from boredom.

The causes of boredom can be considered from several different theoretical viewpoints, including psychophysiological, psychodynamic, behavioral, cognitive, and existential. From a *psychophysiological approach,* boredom is seen as a consequence of inattention. Developmentally, there must be a degree of cortical maturation before the person has the capacity to be attentive. Altered EEGs and decreased reaction time are among the physiological variables associated with feelings of boredom.[8] Sensory deficits that limit the individual's ability to perceive or process external stimulation may also contribute to boredom.

The *psychodynamic view* states that boredom results from conflicting internal forces and is secondary to repression of forbidden instincts. Because of the repressed impulses, the individual has an impoverished fantasy life, limits sensory input, and utilizes a nonsymbolic communicative style that is simple and concrete and has few metaphors or verbal images.[4,11] A therapist may become bored in response to a client's resistance or in response to the therapist's own unacceptable feelings toward the client.[6]

Behavioral theorists hypothesize that boredom results from sensory deprivation or lack of stimuli in the environment. When there is too much predictability and too little novelty in the situation, relationship, or environment, the person will experience boredom.[3]

Cognitive theory posits that sensory monotony alone is not a sufficient condition for the occurrence of boredom. Rather, the individual's subjective perception of the event as lacking meaning or stimulation is the critical factor. Being bored is a state in which there is little cognitive activity, which gives rise to a feeling of subjective monotony and a high degree of frustration.[7]

Existential theorists believe that boredom results from existential frustration. In this view, feelings of meaninglessness and boredom are intricately interwoven with nonproductive use of leisure time and disengagement from others. The person is cynical, lacks direction, and questions the point of most of life's activities. Without a sense of life purpose, belief in the importance of relationships, dedication to a cause, or pursuit of creative activities, feelings of pervasive blandness and boredom result. Modern man's dilemma is that one is not told by instinct what one *must* do or any longer by tradition what one *should* do, nor does one know what one *wants* to do.[12]

Researchers have suggested that boredom results in lowered output, decreased job performance, and increased accidents; increased turnover or dropout rates; increased truancy and acting out behavior in school children; increased usage of alcohol, drugs, and food; extramarital affairs and divorce; acts of aggression and violence; decreased morale; and poorer mental health.[2,3,5,7] Boredom affects all individuals regardless of sex, race, age, creed, intelligence, status, or occupation. The nurse as well as the client can experience feelings of boredom.

RELATED FACTORS

Boredom may be a temporary or momentary experience or so persistent and pervasive that it seems to be a permanent part of the person's life. Boredom may involve a deficit in stimulation, a deficit in meaning, or deficits in both stimulation and meaning.[9] Types and examples of boredom are summarized in Table 13-2.

Boredom occurs in a number of psychiatric conditions, especially borderline, histrionic, and narcissistic personality disorders and psychoactive substance-use disorders. Many of the problems these clients have with attention-seeking behavior, risk-taking behavior, and the use of alcohol and drugs are attempts to avoid the emptiness or boredom they experience.[1,4]

The hospitalized client is particularly vulnerable to boredom. The physical environment may be drab and visually unstimulating. There often is too much free time with limited diversional activities. The person may be socially inept, withdrawn, or isolated. Those recuperating from a lengthy illness or who have been immobilized for extended periods often have inadequate stimulation or insufficient variety of stimulation.

Elderly clients with losses of vision, hearing, taste, and mobility have handicaps that limit the variety and amount of their sensory input. Hearing aids with dead batteries or which stay in the drawer, broken or lost glasses, bland and unappetizing food, and sitting alone in an immobile geri-chair or wheelchair do little to break the monotony and thus may lead to boredom.

Age, interests, and life satisfaction affect a person's perception of what is meaningful or stimulating. The success of an individual's coping mechanisms will influence feelings of boredom.[7] Feeling caught or trapped in a situation or relationship provides the basis for the development of boredom. Individuals who are confined to a bed or hospital area, restricted in their choices and in the variety of foods, activities, and social interactions are captives in a situation intended to be beneficial. Being captive may also involve the individual's perception of role requirements or expectations, such as the married couple who do the same thing the same way and repeat the same script day after day.

TABLE 13-2
Boredom: types, deficits, and examples

TYPE AND DEFICITS	EXAMPLES
APATHETIC BOREDOM REPRESENTING DEFICIT IN STIMULATION[9]	
Repetitive tasks Too low expectation with little challenge Gap between intellectual level and either task at hand or other people Interlude between two activities Sensory deprivation Lack of stimuli (environmental, interpersonal)	Hospitalized client confined to bed with drab walls, limited food selections, and extended periods of unstructured time Elderly client who has visual and hearing losses; loss of mobility
ANXIOUS BOREDOM REPRESENTING DEFICIT IN MEANING[9]	
Disliked tasks Existential meaninglessness Unrealistic expectations	Client stays involved in activities or job but does so reluctantly because client dislikes or does not believe in some of the things he or she has to do Client frustrated over excessive expectations—"why try?"
DEPRESSIVE BOREDOM REPRESENTING DEFICIT IN STIMULATION AND MEANING[9]	
Relationships that have become routinized Isolation or lack of relationships Overly predictable lifestyle Fearful of taking risks, so "play it safe" Lack of creativity and decreased fantasy life	Institutionalized elderly who see no hope in anything changing, so they vegetate Person who avoids relationships because others are frightening or "dangerous"

DEFINING CHARACTERISTICS

Signs that may indicate the presence of boredom can be separated into emotional, behavioral, and cognitive indicators. *Emotional indicators* are uninvolvement, lack of concentration, absence of motivation, feelings of emptiness, and absence of excitement or enthusiasm for what is happening. The client is caught between not feeling good about what is being done but not wanting to do anything else that would feel better. The client may feel frustrated and retreat into angry retaliatory silence or may engage in excessive questioning, challenging, or confrontation.[5,11]

Behavioral indicators include undirected agitation, which usually is repetitive and not goal directed (i.e., "nervous" activities). These are habitual behaviors with high rates of repetition such as eating, smoking, and drinking. Bored individuals may writhe as if in agony or merely fiddle, fidget, jitter; wander about aimlessly; yawn and stretch; run their hands through their hair or rub their heads; scratch themselves; peer about distractedly; or doodle.[5,11]

Cognitive indicators include mental confusion and uncertainty about what is occurring and what can be done to correct it.[5] There is a decrease in cognitive activity, including decreased attentiveness and problem solving. Daydreams or fantasies may occur. The person may ruminate on how boring the situation is.[5,7,11]

The most common characteristic of boredom is the loss of a sense of personal meaning, whether in relation to a particular experience or encounter or to an entire life situation. A bored condition is intensified when it is deep enough to trigger fear. Fear is connected with boredom because of the fear of being bored coupled with the fear of change, the very remedy boredom requires. It constitutes an emotional double bind, fear of what is happening and fear of doing anything creative about it[9] (Chart 1).

NURSING PROCESS AND RATIONALE

Assessment

When assessing boredom, it is important to consider the individual's behaviors, thoughts, and feelings as well as the values and belief systems. What environmental factors affect the individual? What is the client's perception of what is happening? Recognition

---

CHART 1
Boredom: Definition, Related Factors, and Defining Characteristics

DEFINITION
Boredom is an emotional state of dampened energy related to one's perception of being involved in pursuits or surroundings that are tedious, monotonous, and lacking in interest.

RELATED FACTORS
Borderline personality disorder
Narcissistic personality disorder
Histrionic personality disorder
Psychoactive substance-use disorder
Deficit in stimulation
　Repetitive tasks
　Low expectations
　Sensory deprivation
　Lack of environmental or interpersonal stimuli
Deficit in meaning
　Disliked tasks, unrealistic expectations, existential meaninglessness
Deficit in stimulation and meaning
　Isolation, overly predictable lifestyle, lack of creativity and decreased fantasy life
Fear of taking risks
Institutionalization/confinement
Social withdrawal
Impairments in vision, hearing, mobility
Internal conflicts
Existential conflicts

DEFINING CHARACTERISTICS
Lack of motivation
Decreased attention span/inattentiveness
Repetitive oral activities—eating, smoking, drinking
Fidgeting, restlessness
Disinterest or uninvolvement
Dullness in facial expression
Mental confusion
Decreased cognitive activity
Doodling
Daydreaming
Yawning/stretching
Frustration
Lack of goals
Identifies self as bored
Routinized relationships

---

of the overt and covert cues that indicate that boredom is a problem is important for early intervention.

A client who abuses alcohol or drugs, has frequent changes in jobs, drops out of school, has been involved in several accidents, sits staring off into space, chain smoking, restlessly paces the hall complaining there is nothing to do, or is confined to a gerichair for most of the day may be suffering from boredom. A client may be able to identify the feeling of boredom or may need assistance to recognize and label that feeling as such.

There are several tools to measure the presence and severity of boredom. Leckart developed a 36-item Boredom Survey to assess the presence of boredom and a Need for Stimulation Scale to measure the amount of stimulation needed to maintain a comfortable level of arousal.[5] Savitz and Friedman identified six diagnostic interview questions that differentiate boredom (too much predictability) from confusion (too little predictability).[10] Frick's Boredom Confusion Adaptation Scale differentiates boredom, confusion, and adaptation in school children through a series of 33 "like me"–"unlike me" questions.[3] Farmer and Sundberg developed a 28-item self-report Boredom Proneness Scale to measure the tendency to experiencing boredom.[2] Crumbaugh and Maholick published a 20-item questionnaire to measure Purpose in Life.[12]

The physical environment may contribute to the development of boredom. Analysis of the amount of stimulation available and the diversity and meaningfulness of the stimulation is critical. What environmental factors can be controlled or changed? What must be worked around? Can music, pictures, radio, television, or structured activity periods be used to break the monotony?

Exploration of the emotional, behavioral, and cognitive aspects of boredom include: What is the client feeling (besides bored)? What is the client doing while feeling it? What is the client thinking about at the time? What is the overall focus and direction of the person's life? Is the client reaching beyond the self, beyond the humdrum daily routine of staying alive? What is the client's belief system; quality of interpersonal relationships; long-range hopes and goals; creative interests and pursuits? Identification of the amount and diversity of stimulation, the sense of life purpose, the quality of relationships, and current coping skills will guide the nurse in making appropriate interventions.

Nursing Diagnosis

Examples of specific nursing diagnoses that can be formulated include boredom related to sensory deprivation, boredom related to low expectations, and boredom related to existential conflicts.

Client Goals and Nursing Interventions

Client goals focus on altering the amount and variety of stimulation, increasing productive use of leisure time, expanding social interactions, and enhancing a sense of meaningfulness. Cognitive interventions may include having clients keep a Boredom Journal; i.e., to write their definitions of boredom, describe themselves when bored, identify illogical thought patterns and payoffs, describe how they experience curiosity, assess the intimacy level in their relationships, and write a prescription for changing their boredom.[9] It is helpful for the nurse to assist the client to identify what is boring; when, where, and with whom boredom occurs; what routines reinforce the boredom; and feeling states associated with the boredom.[5] Cognitive interventions are based on the premise that boredom may arise out of irrational beliefs such as, "I am not able to do anything athletic." When the client is able to replace such beliefs with positive self-talk, behavior and feelings of boredom may change.

Behavioral interventions focus on overcoming inertia and activating the client to do something different. Can a task be dropped or done differently or less often? The person can be encouraged to try doing something that seems out of character for someone of comparable age, intelligence, or social sophistication. The client can be assisted in prioritizing problems, making a plan of attack with simple behavioral goals, and putting the plan into action.[5]

Affective interventions focus on increasing the per-

son's awareness of feelings of boredom and the associated feelings of frustration and anger. The nurse explores with the client constructive ways of handling anger, because avoidance of confrontation in relationships can lead to feelings of boredom, since those involved are afraid to keep changing and growing.[5,9]

Other techniques include watching what others do to reduce boredom and trying new approaches; reframing the situation by looking at it from a new perspective; using imagination or fantasy (What would you be doing if . . . you never went to college . . . never met your spouse . . . could change your identity . . . had a different job?) By improving interpersonal relationships, it is possible to develop curiosity and concern for others and thus to reduce boredom. Boredom increases when one is a distant spectator rather than an active participant in life.[9,12]

Evaluation

The extent to which nursing interventions have been effective can be evaluated by considering the ways in which the client has altered the amount and variety of stimuli in everyday living and whether the client indicates an increased sense of control and meaningfulness in daily activities. Further indicators are the extent to

CHART 2
Boredom: Summary of the Nursing Process

NURSING INTERVENTIONS	OUTCOME CRITERIA
CLIENT GOAL: ALTER AMOUNT AND VARIETY OF STIMULI Assess typical day or problematic areas Explore creative responses to problems/boring tasks Encourage to develop meaningful rewards (short and long term) Discuss ways to alter schedule/work routine/environment	Identifies repetitive or boring aspects of daily schedule Increases amount of novelty during day Completes tasks with minimal interruptions Alters environment to reduce incidents of boredom
CLIENT GOAL: INCREASE PRODUCTIVE USE OF LEISURE TIME Discuss constructive options for use of leisure time Provide opportunities to learn new leisure skills Encourage participation in recreational activities Promote activities at which client can succeed Structure environment so that amount of free time is reduced	Lists interests and sets priorities Minimizes thrill-seeking activities that are potentially harmful Schedules varied and productive leisure-time activities
CLIENT GOAL: INCREASE RANGE OF SOCIAL INTERACTION Explore social network and quality of interpersonal relationships Assist to identify fears and risks in current relationships Teach social skills/communication skills Role play interpersonal situations to practice confrontation/assertiveness skills	Develops a positive social network Initiates contact with others when feeling bored Increases assertiveness skills
CLIENT GOAL: DEVELOP SENSE OF MEANINGFULNESS Explore values and belief systems Encourage to develop and incorporate meaningful rewards into life Provide opportunities to make decisions about life Assist client to reframe situation	Develops future goals for self Reduces feelings of entrapment Reframes repetitive tasks to focus on purpose Increases sense of control over life/situations/relationships

Research Highlights

Savitz and Friedman developed a procedural tool to determine whether clients were bored, confused, or in an adaptive state.[10] This study was based on the theoretical framework that individuals seek optimally predictable situations and was designed to test interview questions to determine if there was too much predictability (boredom) or too little predictability (confusion) in the client's life. Fifty outpatient clients from a family practice clinic were used to select the specific questions to be used and the scoring method. Twenty-nine additional outpatients were selected for further study of the scoring responses and to test the reliability and validity of the instrument.

Six interview questions discriminated between bored, confused, and adaptive responses. Subjects subsequently met with a therapist who assisted bored clients to add novelty and variability to their lives and confused clients to simplify, organize, and regulate their lives. At the end of the 4-week treatment period, the interview schedule was readministered. Of the six subjects identified as confused on the pretest, five changed to adaptive on the retest; of the 10 who were bored, 9 changed to adaptive at the end of the treatment period.

which the client's range of social interactions and productive use of leisure time have increased (Chart 2).

CASE STUDY

Frank J, a 26-year-old manufacturer, sought counseling after his wife threatened to divorce him. He complained that he had a boring existence and that his relationship with his wife was dull and unexciting. He knew his use of marijuana had increased over the past year but believed it helped him reduce the stress of his job and marriage. His primary nursing diagnosis was boredom related to ritualized interaction patterns and to lack of stimuli at work. Initially, his feelings of frustration and entrapment at work and at home were explored. He identified the lack of stimuli and variety in his job and relationships and his sense of frustration in not changing. Exploration of ways to alter his routines, increase leisure time activities with his wife, improve communication skills, and explore the risks and benefits involved in change significantly improved his sense of power and control over his life. His fears of "causing trouble" by being assertive and direct with his needs were becoming a self-fulfilling prophecy. Boredom was reduced by labeling it, focusing on the significance of his work, and varying his routines both at work and at home.

SUMMARY

Boredom is an emotional and cognitive state that results from lack of variety or stimulation, lack of meaningfulness, or a combination of sensory deficit and meaninglessness. After diagnosis and assessment of boredom, interventions focus on reducing social isolation or withdrawal, developing a sense of life purpose, increasing creativity in problem solving, increasing meaningful environmental stimuli, and taking action to vary routines.

References

1. American Psychiatric Association. Diagnostic and Statistical Manual of Mental Disorders. Ed 3, revised. Washington, DC: American Psychiatric Association; 1987.
2. Farmer R, Sundberg N. Boredom proneness—the development and correlates of a new scale. J Personality Assess. 1986;50(1):4–17.
3. Frick S. Diagnosing boredom, confusion, and adaptation in school children. J School Health. 1985;55(7):254–257.
4. Kulick E. On countertransference boredom. Bull Menninger Clin. 1985;49(2):95–112.
5. Leckart B, Weinberger LG. Up from boredom, down from fear. New York: Richard Marek Publishers; 1980.
6. Morrant JCA. Boredom in psychiatric practice. Can J Psychiatry. 1984;29:431–434.
7. Perkin RE, Hill AB. Cognitive and affective aspects of boredom. Br J Psychol. 1985;76(pt 2):221–234.
8. Pibram KH. Language of the brain. Englewood Cliffs: Prentice-Hall; 1971.
9. Rediger GL. Lord, don't let me be bored. Philadelphia: Westminster Press; 1986.
10. Savitz J, Friedman M. Diagnosing boredom and confusion. Nurs Res. 1981;30(1):16–19.
11. Taylor G. Psychotherapy with the boring patient. Can J Psychiatry. 1984;29:217–222.
12. Yalom I. Existential psychotherapy. New York: Basic Books; 1980.

COMMUNICATION, IMPAIRED

Charlotte Naschinski

DEFINITION AND DESCRIPTION

Communication is an essential component of interpersonal relationships. It is the primary means by which a person influences or is influenced by another person. *Communication* is a complex continuous process including both verbal and nonverbal behavior.

The components of the communication process are sender, message, receiver, and feedback. The *sender* formulates a *message* for transmission to a *receiver*. Words and actions are selected by the sender to facilitate accurate interpretation of the meaning of the message by the receiver. However, many variables may affect the receiver's ability to accurately receive and interpret the meaning of the message. *Feedback* occurs when the receiver responds to the sender's message. It provides information to the original sender concerning how the message was understood and allows correction when necessary.

Communication can be ineffective at a given point. However, for a nursing diagnosis of impaired communication to be valid, a pattern of faulty or ineffective communication must exist. Definitions of *impaired communication* include a state in which an individual experiences a decreased or absent ability to use or understand language and nonverbal behavior in human interaction,[4] and a communication pattern in which the receiver often arrives at a meaning that differs from that intended by the sender.[5]

THEORY AND RESEARCH

The following discussion highlights communication theories described in Chapter 6. Watzlawick and associates[9] note that it is impossible to not communicate. Human beings communicate both digitally and analogically, and every communication has a content and a relationship aspect such that the latter classifies the former and is, therefore, a metacommunication. Understanding metacommunicative statements requires knowledge of the culture and consideration of the communicator's self-definition.

Ruesch[7,8] describes two basic systems of codification of a message: analogue and digital. He further describes four possibilities for the correspondence of the information between communicators.[7] Feedback can facilitate understanding. The goal reached when feedback is successful is a sense of gratification or satisfaction with communication.

Other authors have described specific aspects of nonverbal behavior that have enhanced understanding of the communication process. The role of body movement in communication was described by Birdwhistell.[1] The relationship of space to social interaction was described by Hall.[2]

Research in communication has primarily focused on specific verbal or nonverbal aspects in dyadic exchanges. Concerns for future research include examination of factors that determine patterns of initiating interaction, verbal content and nonverbal cues as a system, and communication in groups.[6]

RELATED FACTORS

Many variables affect communication. When variables consistently provide a negative influence on communication, a pattern of impaired communication can result. Related factors include developmental stage, physical condition, stress, perception, culture, and communication style and skills. Several of these factors are described in more detail in Chapter 6.

Developmental Stage

Communication, like other human functions, is mastered through learning a series of progressive tasks over time. Each age period contains challenges for development that can immediately or subsequently affect the ability to communicate.[7] Assessment of a person's communication ability requires knowledge of the salient features of their current age level and their developmental history.

Physical Condition

Physical condition may directly or indirectly affect the ability to communicate. Any interference with reception or processing of sensory input and the generation of output directly affects communication. Examples of such conditions include trauma, infections, neoplasms, metabolic disturbances, and vascular problems involving the sensory organs, nerve fibers, or central nervous system. The conditions may be pathophysiologic, or they may be situationally imposed such as endotracheal intubation, tracheostomy, or medications. An indirect relationship may exist between a physical condition and communication. For example, a person may withdraw from communication because of pain or embarrassment related to a physical condition.

Stress

Excessive stress can result in impaired communication and mental or physical dysfunction. The affective or emotional responses to stress many include anxiety, anger, or depression. These emotional responses can further impede communication. Severe anxiety lowers cognitive functioning, narrows the perceptual field, and limits decision-making skills. Overt expression of intense anger can result in negative consequences. Depression can result in lack of vitality, withdrawal from interaction with others, and a decrease in verbalization, even to the point of muteness.

Perception

Behavior, including communication, is directly related to a person's perception. Effective communication is dependent on accurate perception of self, other, and the context. Nervous system dysfunction, biases, poor self-concept, needs, and emotions can limit perception and result in impaired communication.

Culture

Communication is learned within a given cultural context. Culture is reflected in the meaning of verbal communication and the interpretation of nonverbal communication. Lack of understanding and consideration of cultural differences can lead to impaired communication.

Communication Style and Skills

Communication is enhanced by a style of communicating that considers self, other, and the context, such as the congruent and assertive styles. In addition, the use of communication skills that encourage development and evaluation of thoughts, expression or clarification of feelings, and problem-solving results in effective communication. Their absence contributes to impaired communication.

DEFINING CHARACTERISTICS

Identification of the defining characteristics of impaired communication is, in part, dependent upon understanding the characteristics of successful communication that include the ability to receive, process, and transmit messages; focus attention on appropriate stimuli; select and organize words that describe the intended meaning; use synchronized verbal and nonver-

bal communication; send a message that is complete, well-timed, and appropriate to the context; provide feedback that is relevant, clearly stated, and appropriately timed; listen actively; and receive gratification from communication.[3] Absence of these characteristics may indicate impaired communication (Chart 1).

NURSING PROCESS AND RATIONALE

Assessment

Through interview and observation, the nurse gathers data about the client's patterns of communication: Is the client able to perceive and attend to appropriate

---

CHART 1
Impaired Communication:
Definition, Related Factors, and
Defining Characteristics

DEFINITION

Impaired communication is a state in which an individual experiences a decreased or absent ability to use or understand language and nonverbal behavior in human interaction.

RELATED FACTORS

Physical condition or state
Psychologic or emotional state
Developmental or age-related factors
Severe stress
Severe anxiety
Extreme anger
Severe depression
Significant impairment of perception
Inadequate self-concept
Cultural difference
Faulty communication style or skills

DEFINING CHARACTERISTICS[3–5]

Unable to speak dominant language
Does not or cannot speak
Speech impediments
Disorientation
Verbosity or laconism
Inappropriate selection or organization of words
Unable to focus on appropriate stimuli
Inconsistent verbal and nonverbal messages
Inconsistent nonverbal messages
Ill-timed or inappropriate messages in relation to
    context
Absent, irrelevant, or inappropriate feedback
Inadequate listening skills
Lack of gratification
False perception
Reluctance or inability to express feelings
Unrestrained or inappropriate emotional expression
Incongruent or nonassertive communication style
Ineffective communication skills

stimuli? Does the client transmit messages that are understood, complete, well-timed, and appropriate to the context? Does the client select and organize words that describe the intended meaning? Does the client use consistent verbal and nonverbal communication? Is the client able to listen and both send and receive feedback? With whom does the client most frequently and most comfortably communicate? About what does the client most frequently communicate? Does the client describe self as very, sometimes, or seldom verbal? In what circumstances does the client feel comfortable expressing thoughts and feelings? Are there any barriers that hinder or limit the client's ability to communicate? Does the client experience gratification from communication? How does the client express feelings and emotions? What is the client's communication style and repertoire of communication skills?

The data gathered from the client can be validated and augmented by obtaining data about the client's ability to communicate from the client's significant others, nurse peers, and other members of the health care team. All assessment data gathered are analyzed for the presence of defining characteristics that support a pattern of impaired communication.

CHART 2
Impaired Communication: Summary of the Nursing Process[3–5]

NURSING INTERVENTIONS	OUTCOME CRITERIA
CLIENT GOAL: ATTEND TO APPROPRIATE STIMULI	
Assess for inattention or hypervigilance to stimuli	Responds to relevant stimuli
Assess for disorientation	Demonstrates full orientation
Assess for imaginary or false perception	Perceives stimuli accurately
Reduce or increase environmental stimuli	Experiences resolution of physical
Teach the client to focus on relevant stimuli	problems that interfere with
Focus full attention on client	communication to the extent possible
Orient to time, place, and person	
Correct faulty perception	
Assist in resolution of physical problems interfering with communication	
CLIENT GOAL: SEND CONCISE, CLEAR MESSAGES	
Assess for amount, selection, and organization of words	Uses appropriate numbers of words
Assess for the presence of speech impediments	Selects and organizes words in a manner
Assess for style of and skills in communication	appropriate to the receiver and context
Assess client's ability to express feelings	Experiences to the extent possible resolution of speech impediments
Demonstrate and teach facilitative communication styles and skills	Expresses feelings appropriately
Teach and support client's expression of feelings	Uses effective communication style and
Teach use of other than verbal means of communication	skills
CLIENT GOAL: EMPLOY CONGRUENT VERBAL AND NONVERBAL COMMUNICATION	
Assess the match of verbal to nonverbal communication	Uses appropriate amount and balance of
Assess the consistency of nonverbal communication	verbal and nonverbal communication
Validate with the client meaning of nonverbal communication	Demonstrates congruent verbal and
Assist client to evaluate use and effect of verbal and nonverbal communication	nonverbal communication
Point out discrepancies in verbal and nonverbal communication	
Demonstrate congruent verbal and nonverbal communication	
CLIENT GOAL: SEND AND RECEIVE FEEDBACK	
Assess the frequency and nature of feedback sent	Demonstrates effective listening skills
Assess client's response to feedback provided	Provides relevant and appropriate
Assess client's listening skills	feedback
Provide relevant and appropriate feedback to client	Asks for feedback
Request feedback from client	Responds appropriately to negative and
Support client's efforts to provide and utilize feedback	positive feedback
Teach, demonstrate, and encourage use of effective listening skills	Uses feedback to correct and modify communication
CLIENT GOAL: EXPERIENCE GRATIFICATION FROM COMMUNICATION	
Assess client's feelings resulting from communication	Provides and receives confirming
Assess client's self-esteem	responses
Provide confirming responses to client	Reports self-regard
Support client's use of confirming responses	Expresses satisfaction from communication
Support or increase client's self-esteem	

Nursing Diagnosis

To proceed from the diagnostic category of impaired communication to a more specific nursing diagnosis, assessment data must be obtained or reviewed for related factors. Is there a physical condition or developmental problem that inhibits the client's ability to communicate? Is the client experiencing feelings or emotions that interfere with effective communication? How accurate is the client's perception of self, others, and the environment? Is the client's cultural background different from the current cultural context? Are the client's communication style and skills ineffective or inadequate? An example of a specific nursing diagnosis is impaired communication related to cultural differences.

Client Goals and Nursing Interventions

The overall goal for any client experiencing impaired communication is reduction or resolution of this impairment. Subgoals reflect the specific components of the communication process that are impaired: able to receive and attend to sensory input; able to transmit messages; able to use verbal and nonverbal communication, send and receive feedback, and experience gratification.

Specific interventions are selected that address the related factor(s) and meet the subgoal. Because communication is a learned behavior, a primary mode for nursing intervention is teaching. The nurse may role-model or directly teach the client desired communication behaviors. At times, the nurse may manipulate the environment to promote communication (e.g., reduce environmental stimuli, provide privacy, or provide pad and pencil or pictures as alternative methods for communicating). Referrals to other care providers may be necessary when a physical condition or cultural difference exists that the nurse is unable to address.

Evaluation

In the evaluation step of the nursing process, the nurse observes for specific client behaviors indicative of reduction in or resolution of impaired communication; more specifically, those behaviors that reflect the attainment of the identified subgoals (Chart 2).

CASE STUDY

Ann B, a 36-year-old office manager, was admitted to a psychiatric unit with a diagnosis of bipolar disorder, manic. Her appearance was disheveled: her clothing was mismatched and only partially fastened, her makeup appeared hastily applied and incomplete. Ann was in almost constant motion, beginning but seldom completing any activity, including meals. She sought out interactions, but often left abruptly. Her conversation reflected rapid, incomplete, and sometimes unrelated thoughts. She seemed to attend and respond to a number of internal and external stimuli simultaneously and did not take the time to receive feedback or listen. She expressed frustration over unmet needs and unsuccessful communication. Her physical health had been good, although the potential existed for problems related to her hyperactivity (e.g., insomnia, inadequate nutrition, exhaustion). She had been started on a therapeutic regimen of lithium carbonate (Lithane) to control manic symptoms.

Among the actual nursing diagnoses that were identified for Ann was impaired communication related to hyperactive behavior. One identified goal was for Ann to attend to appropriate stimuli. Care was taken to reduce environmental stimuli such as noise and the number of activities. The length of interaction with her was limited according to her tolerance level. She was given assistance in focusing on relevant stimuli; faulty perceptions were corrected in a nonjudgmental way.

A second goal was for Ann to communicate thoughts and feelings concisely and clearly, using congruent verbal and nonverbal communication. Initially, questions or comments were stated in a manner requiring only short responses from Ann. She was assisted in examining the effects of her communication on others. Discrepancies in verbal and nonverbal communication and inconsistencies in nonverbal communication were pointed out to her. Role-playing and demonstrations were used to teach her how to synchronize verbal and nonverbal communication.

A final goal was for Ann to effectively send and receive feedback. When appropriate, she was encouraged to send and request feedback in conversation with others. Ann was also taught effective listening skills, and encouraged to listen to others. She was given positive feedback for her own attempts and for her success in receiving and providing feedback.

SUMMARY

Communication is a complex, continuous process including both verbal and nonverbal behavior. A number of variables can affect the communication process, for example, developmental stage, stress, and perception. When a client experiences an absent or decreased abil-

Research Highlights

Research in communication has primarily focused on specific verbal or nonverbal aspects in dyadic exchanges. Concerns for future research include examination of factors that determine patterns of initiating interaction, verbal content, and nonverbal cues as a system, and communication in groups.[6]

ity to use or understand language, the nursing diagnosis of impaired communication should be considered.

References

1. Birdwhistell R. Kinesics and context. Philadelphia: University of Pennsylvania Press; 1970.
2. Hall E. The hidden dimension. New York: Doubleday & Co; 1966.
3. Kim M, McFarland G, McLane A. Pocket guide to nursing diagnoses. 3rd ed. St Louis: CV Mosby; 1989.
4. McFarland G, Naschinski C. Communication. In Thompson J, McFarland G, Hirsch J, Tucker S, Bowers A. Clinical nursing. St Louis: CV Mosby; 1986.
5. McFarland G, Wasli E. Nursing diagnoses and process in psychiatric mental health nursing. Philadelphia: JB Lippincott; 1986.
6. Patterson M. Nonverbal exchange: past, present and future. J Nonverbal Behav. 1984;8:350–359.
7. Ruesch J. Disturbed communication. New York: WW Norton; 1972.
8. Ruesch J. Therapeutic communication, 2nd ed. New York: WW Norton; 1973.
9. Watzlawick P, Beavin J, Jackson D. Pragmatics of human communication. New York: WW Norton; 1967.

COPING, FAMILY, POTENTIAL FOR GROWTH

Joan E. Bowers

DEFINITION AND DESCRIPTION

Family coping, potential for growth is defined as the effective management of adaptive tasks by the family members who are involved with the client's health challenge. The family members are now exhibiting the desire and readiness for enhanced health and growth for self and in relation to the client. The members' basic needs are being sufficiently gratified, and other adaptive tasks are effectively addressed so that these self-actualizing goals may emerge.[22]

THEORY AND RESEARCH

Although family is variously defined in the literature, for purposes of this chapter Terkelsen's[33] definition will be used: *A family is a small social system made up of individuals related to each other by reason of strong reciprocal affections and loyalties and comprises a permanent household (or cluster of households) that persists over years and decades.*[33]

The healthy family manifests characteristics that fall into three general areas. First, the healthy family has clear boundaries that are sufficiently open to allow members access to communication and support from the extended family, members of the social support network, and the community within which it functions. In addition, boundaries are present within the family such that the individual members or groupings of members have access to each other for support and communication. However, this boundary must also allow the members freedom from intrusion appropriate to the developmental level to promote individuation and autonomy. A second area is the ability of the family to meet the requirements of society, including the protection and nurturing of the younger generation, as well as the provision of a safe haven in which members' needs may be met. The third area encompasses those characteristics that facilitate the family's ability to meet the situational demands that confront it on a continuing basis. Included here are the family members' sense of attachment and commitment to each other and to the health of the family unit. The ability to adapt to varying circumstances, whether arising from external demands or from the developmental

demands within the family, is another important component. Communication process within the family, including decision making and power allocation and enactment, are also in this category.

Families will vary considerably in their ability to cope with demands from the environment. An inclusive dimension that describes families who cope well in the face of these demands is *hardiness*,[25] defined as the basic strength that families call upon to manage the hardships and difficulties of transitions and crises.

The Family as a System

Concepts from general system theory (GST) provide a framework for viewing the family as a unified whole rather than a collection of individuals operating in concert. The theory, developed by von Bertalanffy,[6,36] a biologist, was generalized to explain social systems in general, and, later, was used to analyze family as a type of social system. The concept of boundary, for example, has been applied to the family as a system. Boundaries are those markers that indicate what and who are contained within the family system as compared with what and who are outside of the system. Boundaries also include the rules that govern who participates in each subsystem within the family.[27]

The family as a system has a history and a trajectory. It functions within a community and optimally maintains connections to various other social systems, such as church, school, employment, neighborhood, and social groups. These connections are a critical resource for the family in the face of crisis. For example, social support has been found to mediate the effects of crisis,[15] to influence the exercise of discipline in a family with a developmentally delayed member,[3] and to influence the outcomes of pregnancy for both the mother[29] and the newborn infant.[23]

Ideally, the family functions as a major source of attachment and socialization for its members. Three major concepts that describe family are cohesion, adaptability, and communication.[30,37]

COHESION

Cohesion refers to the amount of closeness experienced by the family members. The degree of cohesion within and among family members is highly correlated with developmental stage. For example, the parent–infant dyad is in a highly cohesive or enmeshed relationship. Information flows very freely across the boundary between these two family members. The parent is highly attentive to signals and cues from the child; the reverse is true as well. This behavior is highly adaptive for the survival of the infant. As the child matures and begins to develop autonomy and is concurrently at less risk for mortality, the boundary between the parent(s) and the child becomes less permeable. Information flows less freely within the parent–child dyad. Parents feel more comfortable in leaving the child with a caretaker for a time. The child learns that the parent(s) will return and so can be content with a caretaker to substitute for the parent(s). This pattern evolves to adolescence, when the young person, with help from the parents, draws ever more rigidly the boundary between self and the parent. Were the parent to resist or not facilitate this process, the young person would be at risk for difficulty in resolving the tasks of adolescence that include emancipation and moving on to become invested in peer relationships and a career trajectory. With the onset of maturity, this boundary is ideally renegotiated to one of relatively more permeability than was true during the offspring's adolescence. There may be some gender differences in this renegotiation process, with mothers and daughters experiencing this to a greater degree than other potential parent–adult offspring dyads.

The other extreme of this family pattern, known as disengagement, can occur as well. If the parent is burdened by his or her own problems and cares, distancing from the child may occur. In some instances, when one parent is enmeshed with a child, the other parent may become disengaged and distanced from the family. This can be seen particularly when a child is handicapped by either a physical or a developmental problem. The process of disengagement may occur between spouses, as in the case of a childless couple who pursue their own career interests and grow further apart, or between any two members or groups within the family who find themselves diverging in interests, values, or affective involvements.

ADAPTABILITY

The second major factor of family functioning to be considered is *adaptability,* defined as the ability of the family system to change and to develop new rules in the face of emerging demands either from externally (e.g., job change) or internally triggered events (e.g., child's development). The rigid family would have difficulty in bending rules for special occasions or in developing different rules as the child is able to assume more responsibility. The chaotic family has few if any rules, and the members behave more like totally autonomous individuals than like members of a family community. The effects of rigidity may also be seen in the elderly couple who have lived most of their lives with traditional gender-based role assignment. Death

or divorce may leave one or both members lacking in some basic survival skills, such as home management (cooking, laundry) for the man or financial management for the woman.

COMMUNICATION

Finally, the communication process within the family and between the family and the community contributes to healthy family functioning. Communication serves two major purposes—a content message and a message that defines the relationship.[38] Both choice of language and various nonverbal factors convey the relationship-defining message. For example, the parent may say to the child, "Get off that chair immediately." The content message is a clear command to behave in a particular fashion. The relationship message tells the listener that the speaker is in a position of authority in relationship to the child. More than this though, communication within the family, to be healthy or functional, must be direct and open. The message should convey what the speaker intends to convey, and it should not be so veiled that the person being addressed is left to question what is meant by the sender of the message.

Role Theory

Roles assumed by family members are predicated on position, age, gender to some extent, and function within the system. Roles within the family are elaborated over time and lead to reciprocal expectations about role enactment.[17] In the event of illness in a member, role functions may have to be assumed by the other members of the family for brief or prolonged periods. For example, attention to mechanical functioning of household equipment may have been the responsibility of the oldest daughter. In the event that she is incapacitated by illness, another member may need to attend to this family responsibility (or services of a maintenance person may need to be purchased, possibly stressing the family budget).

When roles are temporarily redistributed within the family, members may experience role overload. The transition engendered by the health crisis demands reorganization within the family system and brings stress to the system, regardless of the extent or the duration of the need. In the event of chronic illness through which a member is incapacitated and unable to continue in certain aspects of role functioning, the role loss may result in depression and resentment. Other issues involved in dealing with this loss may surface around autonomy, control, authority, and gender identity.[16]

Developmental Theory

Assessment of family functioning in the face of an illness crisis must be placed in the context of the developmental stage and the inherent tasks with which the family is dealing. Duvall's[9] model of family development has been used extensively in analyzing the stages and tasks of healthy family functioning. Duvall defines *family development* as the ongoing process that includes meeting the needs of the individual members, as well as the demands of the larger social system. The consequences of this process are the progressive differentiation and transformation of the system, analogous to the consequences of development for the individual person.

A number of models have been developed that offer explanations of this process.[7-9] Aldous and D'Antonio[1] discussed four family system characteristics that are affected as the family moves through each developmental stage: (1) family interdependence; (2) selective boundary maintenance; (3) adaptability to and initiation of change; and (4) family task performance. A brief summary of the eight stages as proposed by Duvall and adapted from Wright and Leahey[39] and Friedman[12] follows.

STAGE 1: MARRIAGE

Marriage, the joining of families, is at least a two-generational phenomenon and, even though the couple are adult and emancipated (in most instances), the marriage brings together their two families in a new relationship. The tasks of this stage include:

1. Establishment of couple identity including the negotiation of issues between them as individuals, such as daily-living patterns, employment decisions, and the use of space and time.
2. Realignment of relationships with their respective families to include the spouse or partner.
3. Decisions about parenthood including the when and, in some instances, the how of parenthood need to be negotiated by the couple.

STAGE 2: FAMILIES WITH INFANTS

Stage 2 begins with the birth of the first child and continues until that child is beyond infancy, usually around age three. Tasks for this stage are focused on:

1. Integration of the infant into the family.
2. Accommodation of new parenting and grandparenting roles.
3. Maintenance of the marital relationship.

STAGE 3: FAMILIES WITH PRESCHOOLERS

Stage 3 includes the period from when the eldest child reaches age three until that child enters school. This is a time of high stress in young families because of child-rearing demands, low financial resources, and heavy commitment of the parent(s) to career development. Two major tasks for this stage include:

1. Socialization of the child(ren): Both parents have critical roles to play in this process.

2. Parent and child adaptation to separation: In preparation for entry into school, the child needs gradual experiences in interacting with peers and adults other than family members.

STAGE 4: FAMILIES WITH SCHOOL CHILDREN

The entry of the oldest child into school marks the beginning of this stage for the family. During this stage, the family becomes more and more involved with community activities and attachments. The family boundary begins to open up to allow for both the temporary absences of the members as well as the entry of outsiders such as schoolmates for short periods. This stage encompasses the following tasks:

1. Development of child's peer relationships: The sibling subsystem in the family provides the paradigm for the development of peer relationships.[26]
2. Parent accommodation to outside influences on their child(ren). Congruence of the parents' values with the school and community at large form the basis for this task.

STAGE 5: FAMILIES WITH TEENAGE CHILD(REN)

Stage 5 begins when the oldest child in the family reaches teen age. It is notoriously a time of tensions and upheavals in the family. This stage, because of the multiple changes in the individual child and the consequent demands on the family, frequently heralds a developmental crisis for the family. Like other crises, this can imply both danger and opportunity for the system. The tasks to be accomplished in this stage include:

1. Negotiation of increasing autonomy for the adolescent: This stage introduces a major demand on the family system for adaptability in developing new rules and in renegotiating roles.
2. Refocus on midlife, marital, and career issues.
3. Beginning focus on concerns for the older generation.

STAGE 6: FAMILIES AS LAUNCHING CENTERS

Stage 6 is characterized by the first child leaving home. It ends when the last child has exited from the parental home. Strains during this stage may occur because the parents are assessing their own achievements and may be moving in different directions as they each progress toward self-development. The opportunity to renegotiate an enhanced marital relationship is also inherent in this stage. The tasks of this stage include:

1. Development and consolidation of independent identities for parents and their young adult offspring.
2. Renegotiation of the marital relationship: Although family living and women's roles have evolved over the past two decades, the departure of the children

from the family home still brings a need for shifts in role allocation.

STAGE 7: FAMILIES IN THE MIDDLE YEARS

The last child's departure from the parents' home signals the onset of this stage in the family trajectory. It ends with retirement or the death of one of the spouses. This is a time of freedom from the burdens of parenting. It may bring continuing and even heavier financial burdens as the couple try to provide assistance both to their children, who may be struggling with their early family development, and to the members of the older generation, who may be in need of support. The major tasks of this stage that confront families include:

1. Sustaining satisfying and meaningful relationships with aging parents and with children.
2. Strengthening the marital relationship: This task may be made more difficult because of the increased focus on this relationship secondary to the absence of offspring in the home and the career plateau that the individuals may be facing in their jobs.
3. Dealing with the disabilities and the death of the older generation.

STAGE 8: FAMILIES IN RETIREMENT AND OLD AGE

Stage 8, the last stage of the family life cycle, is begun with retirement of one or both of the couple members. It continues through the death of one spouse and ends with the death of the second spouse. Adaptation during this stage is heavily influenced by the adequacy of financial resources and the members' health status. Society's devaluation of the aged and the many losses common to aging make this period of life problematic.[12] This stage confronts the family with the following tasks:

1. Maintaining both individual functioning and the marital relationship, including sexual gratification while adapting to the aging process.
2. Shifting from a work role to eventual full retirement: This shift has implications for economic functioning and for social roles of both members of the couple.
3. Adjusting to loss through death of one's spouse, siblings, and peers. Loss of the spouse is especially problematic for men, many of whom die within a year after the death of the wife.
4. Continuing to maintain connections with family members despite the tendency for the older person to gradually disengage from social relationships.

Another variation in this model occurs when the couple separate, divorce and eventually remarry. Tables 13-3 and 13-4 outline the phases of these stages along with the developmental tasks that face these families.

Family Stress Theory

McCubbin and Patterson's double ABC-X model (an adaptation of Hill's model;[19]) explains the family's re-

TABLE 13–3

Dislocations of the family life cycle requiring additional steps to restabilize and proceed developmentally

PHASE	EMOTIONAL PROCESS OF TRANSITION PREREQUISITE ATTITUDE	DEVELOPMENTAL ISSUES
DIVORCE		
The decision to divorce	Acceptance of inability to resolve marital tensions sufficiently to continue relationship	Acceptance of one's own part in the failure of the marriage
Planning the break-up of the system	Supporting viable arrangements for all parts of the system	Working cooperatively on problems of custody, visitation, finances
		Dealing with extended family about the divorce
Separation	Willingness to continue cooperative coparental relationship	Mourning loss of intact family
	Work on resolution of attachment to spouse	Restructuring marital and parent-child relationships; adaptation to living apart
		Realignment of relationships with extended family; staying connected with spouse's extended family
The divorce	More work on emotional divorce: overcoming hurt, anger, guilt, etc.	Mourning loss of intact family; giving up fantasies of reunion
		Retrieval of hopes, dreams, expectations from the marriage
		Staying connected with extended families
POST DIVORCE FAMILY		
Single-parent family	Willingness to maintain parental contact with ex-spouse and support contact of children with ex-spouse and his family	Making flexible visitation arrangements with exspouse and his family
		Rebuilding own social network
Single-parent (noncustodial)	Willingness to maintain parental contact with ex-spouse and support custodial parent's relationship with children	Finding ways to continue effective parenting relationship with children
		Rebuilding own social network

(From Carter EA, McGoldrick M. The family life cycle: a framework for family therapy. New York: Gardner Press; 1980:18.)

TABLE 13–4
Remarried family formation: a developmental outline*

STEPS	PREREQUISITE ATTITUDE	DEVELOPMENTAL ISSUES
Entering the new relationship	Recovery from loss of first marriage (adequate "emotional divorce")	Recommitment to marriage and to forming a family with readiness to deal with the complexity and ambiguity
Conceptualizing and planning new marriage and family	Accepting one's own fears and those of new spouse and children about remarriage and forming a step-family	Work on openness in the new relationships to avoid pseudomutuality
	Accepting need for time and patience for adjustment to complexity and ambiguity of Multiple new roles	Plan for maintenance of cooperative coparental relationships with exspouses
	Boundaries: space, time, membership, and authority	Plan to help children deal with fears, loyalty conflicts, and membership in two systems
	Affective issues: guilt, loyalty conflicts, desire for mutuality, unresolvable past hurts	Realignment of relationships with extended family to include new spouse and children
		Plan maintenance of connections for children with extended family of ex-spouse(s)
Remarriage and reconstitution of family	Final resolution of attachment to previous spouse and ideal of "intact" family	Restructuring family boundaries to allow for inclusion of new spouse–stepparent
	Acceptance of a different model of family with permeable boundaries	Realignment of relationships throughout subsystems to permit interweaving of several systems
		Making room for relationships of all children with biologic (noncustodial) parents, grandparents, and other extended family
		Sharing memories and histories to enhance stepfamily integration

(From Carter EA, McGoldrick M. The family life cycle: a framework for family therapy. New York: Gardner Press; 1980:19)
* Variation on a developmental schema presented by Ransom et al (1979).

sponse to crisis.[24] The model proposes that in the precrisis period, the stressor interacts with the family's perception of the stressor (how they evaluate it) and the existing family resources (both psychosocial and tangible assets) to create family attempts to cope with the crisis fallout. The adaptation factors during this phase include (1) family's existing and newly developing resources, (2) their perception of the crisis, the pileup of stressors, and their resources, and (3) their coping strategies. Together these factors account for or predict the outcome of the crisis events. These authors hypothesize that the outcome ranges from "bonadaptation," in which the family is stronger and more resourceful secondary to the crisis; through "adaptation," in which the family may suffer some minor to major deficits as a consequence of the crisis; to "maladaptation," in which the family is seriously disrupted with negative consequences for the system and for the individuals. The value of this model for the health care professional is the opportunity it provides to examine the many factors that influence the family's coping with health issues and predicaments over time. Figure 13-10 illustrates the model and the relationship among the factors on a longitudinal time dimension.

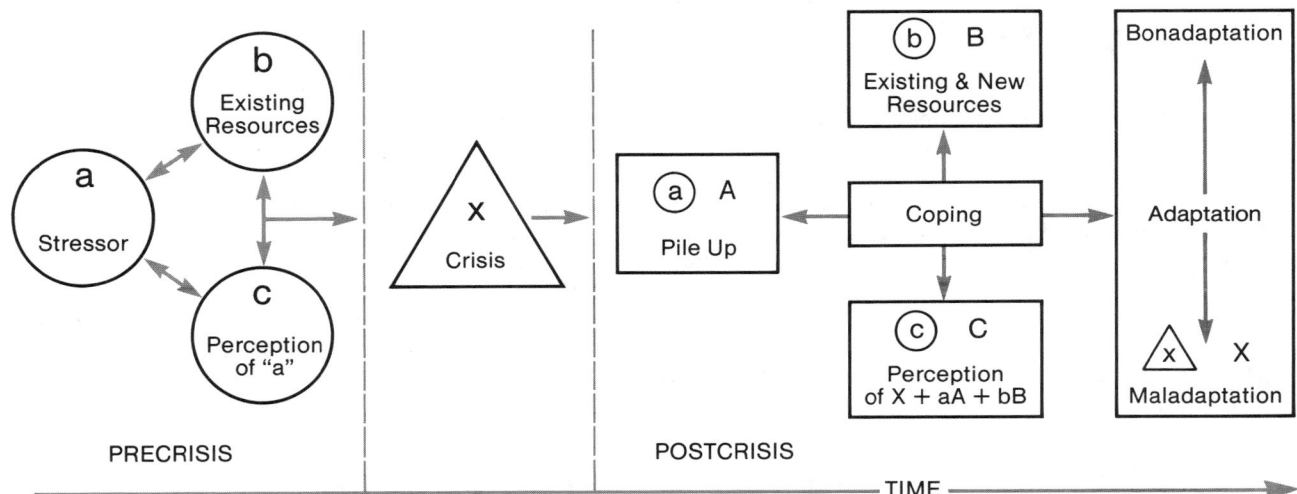

FIGURE 13–10. Double ABC-X model. (From McCubbin HI, Cauble AE, Patterson JM. Family stress, coping, and social support. Springfield, IL: Charles C Thomas, 1982:46)

RELATED FACTORS

Family coping in response to the member's health challenge will vary along several dimensions. First, the age and relationship of the primary client to the family will influence the coping responses of the family. The middle-aged family may be particularly vulnerable when their aging parents begin to require assistance and their adult children are also in need of assistance. Couples in this circumstance may be at risk for experiencing overload in the event of a member's health problem.

The nature of the onset of the illness event, that is, whether it was sudden and unpredicted or gradual and anticipated, will seriously affect the family's coping response. Both the nature of the health challenge (for example, whether it is a physical or a psychiatric challenge) and its severity will affect the family's ability to cope and to grow from the experience. This factor is complex in that it contains several different aspects. If a major physical illness for which there is a reliable treatment has been diagnosed in a member, the challenge to the family's coping resources will be quite different from that in which the illness is severe and the availability of effective treatment strategies is uncertain or not yet accessible. Mishel,[28] in a series of research investigations, has explored the effect of uncertainty on the individual's and the family's coping strategies in the case of life-threatening illness. In a terminal illness, regardless of the etiology, the family's coping tasks will again be different from those in the situation in which the member is expected to survive with few if any residual effects after medical or surgical treatment.

Another factor that can influence the family's coping response to the health challenge is that of other situational or transitional crises that may be impinging on the family concurrently. A parent's health crisis around the time that the youngest child is getting ready to leave for college could temporarily overwhelm the family. As noted earlier, the middle-aged family may experience multiple demands concurrently from both the older and the younger generations in their family.

Other preexisting factors that will influence family coping response are the family dynamics. The nature of the boundaries[26] between members within the family and between the family and the community or extended family will influence their ability to seek and to use available support as a means of coping with a member's health challenge. The openness of the communication process in the family[31] and the family's history of conflict patterns and conflict resolution are other forces that influence coping responses. The family's earlier experiences in dealing effectively with health challenges also contribute to current coping processes.[24]

In the event of psychiatric disorder in the member, the social stigma that continues to be attached to mental illness is shared by the family of the disabled member as well. The consequences of the illness and of the stigma may tax the family's coping resources to the point that recovery and potential for growth may be delayed at best or blocked at worst. Adaptation in these families is further hampered because the affected member's behavior may be socially unacceptable and, therefore, may lead to the withdrawal from the family of its community support systems. In a study designed to investigate the quality of life experienced by caregivers of persons with schizophrenia, Seymour and Dawson[32] found that families reported a much higher overall quality of life when the disturbed member was in the hospital, rather than in the community or at home. A similar situation may be experienced by the family caregiver of a member with Alzheimer's disease. In this instance, the affected member's loss of social interaction skills may be an embarrassment to family and friends. In the early stages, these members of the family's network may reduce contact with the family because of this embarrassment. In later stages, if the affected member is volatile or violent, there may be a further withdrawal of the family from social contact as well.

DEFINING CHARACTERISTICS

For the family's potential for growth to emerge, certain processes will already have been accomplished. First, the member with the health problem will either have recovered or stabilized sufficiently so that the family is experiencing a sense of balance. The basic needs of all of the involved family members will have been met in a timely fashion. For example, provisions for meeting the physical and emotional needs of the family's school age children will have been made. Adults who have been spending large amounts of time at the hospital and in dealing with the client's needs will have been able to meet their own needs for sustenance, rest, and emotional comfort as well. The adolescent members of the family will have had physical and emotional needs met and will have been delegated family-focused responsibilities that they are capable of meeting.

Assessment of the family's readiness to learn from the illness experience involves both observations of interactions among and between the family members and the client as well as self-reports by the family about their readiness for new experiences. First, family members will talk either among themselves or with the health professionals about their reevaluation of goals, values, priorities, or relationships. For instance, after the mother's recovery from an acute depression that required a brief hospitalization, she and her husband decide that they will not pursue the purchase of a second home, but will use their accumulated savings to hire a part-time housekeeper for a year.

Another way in which the family demonstrates readiness to engage in growth occurs when one or more members begin to discuss changes in life-style that are related to a family member's health problem. The middle-aged couple who seek out information about exercise and dietary changes after the husband's experience with severe anxiety attacks related to his job stresses offers an example of this indicator. Another example is provided by the parents of teenagers who, as a consequence of the health problems with which they have been dealing, have had to expect more responsibility from the children. When the response from the teenagers is negative, the parents inquire of the health professional about counseling resources to help them deal more effectively with the developmental changes facing their family (Chart 1).

NURSING PROCESS AND RATIONALE
Assessment

The assessment of a family for purposes of determining the level of coping can be conducted through various modes. The nurse may observe a shift in the behavior of the family members that indicates a readiness to engage in more self-fulfilling behaviors than had been possible while the primary client was in an acute state. The family members may be asked to report on their readiness either through direct questions about need fulfillment or through the use of a standardized assessment tool. And finally, the family may be asked to come together to participate in an assessment process in which both the verbal responses to structured or unstructured questions, and observations of the interaction process will form the data for the health professional's diagnosis and intervention with the family.

The nurse will be interested in gathering information about:

1. The family and household composition.
2. The family's perception of their current functioning.
3. The family's developmental stage and how well the members are meeting the tasks as a group and individually.

The nurse also gathers information about the family's functioning through observations for:

1. Indications of appropriate attachments between and among members, such as verbal and nonverbal expressions of concern for members.
2. Evidence of clear boundaries both within the family and between the family and the community, and the absence (or presence) of destructive coalitions within the family. For example, do the parents work together in setting reasonable limits for the children?
3. Signs of clear and open communication, including (a) members speak for themselves, (b) questions and comments are direct and say what they mean, (c) nonverbal communication is consistent with the verbal message, (d) members are free to express a range of emotions.
4. Evidence that family members enact roles that are appropriate and feasible given the family needs and the individual's capabilities.
5. Indications that appropriate controls are exercised fairly and consistently in the family.
6. Information about the beliefs and goals that influence the family, including family myths[11] that may serve either to enhance or block the health professional's efforts to work with the family. An example might be the parents of an adopted child who are afraid to set appropriate limits because they think the child might then not love them.
7. Sociocultural and ethnic factors that might play a role in determining the family's current functioning. The system of support and reciprocity may be particularly important, for example, to an African-American family whose extended family members are currently sharing their house at the expense of family privacy.

CHART 1
Family Coping, Potential for Growth: Definition, Related Factors, and Defining Characteristics

DEFINITION

Family coping, potential for growth is the effective management of adaptive tasks by family members who are involved with the client's health challenge. The family members are now exhibiting the desire and readiness for enhanced health and growth for self and in relation to the client.

RELATED FACTORS

Family developmental stage
Client's role in the family
Available family resources
    Financial status
    Educational background of members
    Social support
Nature of the health challenge
    Physical illness vs psychiatric illness
    Chronic vs acute problem
    Availability of effective treatment
    Treatable vs terminal illness
Family functioning including communication patterns, conflict resolution patterns, flexibility
Family's prior experiences with health challenges
Other concurrent demands on family resources

DEFINING CHARACTERISTICS

Member with health problem either recovered or stabilized (this may include those families in whom the member with the health problem is dying)
Family experiences a return to sense of balance
Indicators that basic needs for all family members are met in a timely fashion
Family members indicate through verbal and nonverbal behaviors the readiness to learn, to engage in new behaviors

8. Family financial resources and the educational levels of family members.

This last information may be obtained from the client's clinic or hospital record. For adults who have little education, the nurse will have formed some impression of the person's intellectual functioning as well.

Nursing Diagnosis

The diagnostic category, family coping, potential for growth, is used by the nurse for families who are in process of coping effectively with a health crisis or issue. For example, the parents of a teenager who has been suspended from school decide that efforts to deal with the behaviors leading up to this episode have been ineffectual and, without outside help, their child is headed for serious trouble. They make a counseling appointment at the local mental health clinic at which they are assessed by a nurse who does screening for the family intervention unit. She finds them to be a family who demonstrate concern and an ability to be flexible, and her assessment is that they will profit from a brief intervention that will serve to get them on track in helping their adolescent to be more responsible in school. A more specific nursing diagnosis for this family might be family coping, potential for growth related to family dissatisfaction with current family functioning and the 14-year-old son's expulsion from school.

Client Goals and Nursing Interventions

When the family is coping effectively and indicates through various behaviors a potential for further growth, the nurse will observe a willingness of the family members to learn from the current experience such as the member's health challenge. Goals for the family might include helping the parents to function more closely as a team in defining and enforcing expectations and limits for their child(ren). If the parents have had difficulty in adapting to the challenges presented by their child's push for greater autonomy, they may need help from the nurse in developing a negotiation process for rules and limits.

A second family goal might be for the family to develop strategies for dealing with the behavior of the children other than the referral child (that is, the child who presented symptoms that brought the family to the attention of the health professional). A family that is demonstrating a potential for growth will quickly see opportunities for transfer of learning from the counseling session to other situations in their life at home. Other families may need some coaching to see the similarities in their children's behavior or to recognize the

ways in which they are inconsistent in setting limits for all of their children. A similar situation may occur in the family with an adult offspring with a chronic mental illness; here, the family may need assistance in determining appropriate and effective limit setting for intrusive behaviors.

Parents may need to increase their knowledge about normal growth and development to enhance their parenting effectiveness. They may be offered appropriate reading suggestions for this purpose or they may be referred to a community resource, such as the local YWCA or their church, for classes in parenting. A support group of parents with similar issues also may be an appropriate referral. Finally, parents may need to be encouraged to take time for themselves as a couple, both to increase their satisfaction with their marriage and to work out some of the issues that will help them function as a team in the face of the various demands that children place on them.

The older family may need help in identifying goals that relate to the return of emancipated adult offspring after a job loss or the dissolution of a marriage. These parents may need help in drawing up a contract with the returned offspring, such that their privacy and autonomy are maintained *and* their expectation that the arrangement is temporary is clearly communicated. Cultural differences in the experience of parental responsibility for adult children should be investigated; these may be different from the nurse's expectations.

This same older couple may be faced with helping their parents to adapt to diminishing ability to live alone and possibly with supplementing their parents' fixed income. Families with responsibility for a senile or demented member may demonstrate a critical need for help in accessing some form of respite for themselves, to function effectively and meet their own health and psychosocial needs.

Evaluation

Family behavioral changes, such as those noted, will generally result in problem resolution. The family will report a change in their child's behavior (and attitude) at home, and on checking with the school, the change should be evident there as well. The parents will report the ways in which they have assessed their own behavior and that of their other children and the efforts they have made to be more consistent in limit setting and in dealing appropriately with issues based on the child(ren)'s level of maturity. An indication that suggested reading material has been sampled and found helpful in furthering growth in the family will also be forthcoming. Or alternatively, parents may have enrolled in a class or joined a support group in the community. In addition the couple will offer indication that they have begun nurturing their own relationship more carefully by taking time for themselves away from the children (Chart 2).

CHART 2
Family Coping, Potential for Growth: Summary of the Nursing Process

NURSING INTERVENTIONS	OUTCOME CRITERIA
PARENT GOAL: FUNCTION MORE CLOSELY AS A TEAM IN DEFINING AND ENFORCING EXPECTATIONS AND LIMITS FOR THEIR CHILDREN	
Assist the parents to develop a negotiation process for rules and limits	Parents report having come to agreement on certain expectations
Encourage parents to take time for themselves as a couple	
PARENT GOAL: DEVELOP STRATEGIES FOR DEALING WITH THE BEHAVIOR OF CHILDREN OTHER THAN THE REFERRAL CHILD	
Assist the parents to discuss ways in which they may transfer learning from the strategies they have learned to use in their relationships with the referral child to their relationships with their other children	Parents identify ways learning can be transferred
	Parents report the usefulness of strategies in relationships with their other children
PARENT GOAL: INCREASE THEIR KNOWLEDGE ABOUT NORMAL GROWTH AND DEVELOPMENT	
Suggest appropriate references for reading	Parents describe increased knowledge about normal growth and development
Suggest community resources such as parenting classes	

CASE STUDY

The J family consists of Ron, 47, Gladys, 44, and their four children, Claudia, 23, Bernard, 20, James, 19, and Peter, 17. Ron is employed in the construction industry and Gladys is a full-time homemaker. Claudia is a filing clerk for the utility company, a job she began part-time while still in high school. She continues to live at home with her parents. Bernard is a junior at the state university and lives on campus about 200 miles away. He visits only at major holidays and school breaks. James is a freshman at the local community college and lives at home, as does Peter who is a senior in high school. James' parents were unprepared for his behavior on an early winter weekend when he refused to come from his room and by Sunday morning was screaming and threatening to do harm to them and to himself. The police were called and he was admitted to a psychiatric inpatient service for a 72-hour observation period. Because a clear history of drug use could not be obtained, his provisional diagnosis was phencyclidine (PCP) intoxication.[2] His parents were asked to return the next day for a family assessment.

The Js were anxious and eager to be seen as cooperative. However, they had little information to offer about their son's behavior and activities since he started classes at the community college. They validated James' comments about the amount of conflict at home and, after some probing, Ron admitted that he has a bad temper and frequently beat up on his sons when they were younger. The staff had determined that the basis for James' violent episodes was indeed the use of PCP.

James remained on this unit for three weeks. His behavior steadily improved, but he continued to have outbursts, and a more extended treatment period was recommended. His parents began to attend a support group at the hospital. They found that these parents who were also dealing with their children's behavior disorders were able to provide many helpful ideas and suggestions for how the Js thought about and responded to James, their other children, and their concerned neighbors and friends.

When James was discharged from the drug treatment program at the state hospital, the J family was prepared for his return. The parents had revised some of their own ideas about their expectations for and from their children. For example, James was encouraged to return to school. He was also told that he was welcome to continue living at home, but that his welcome would be contingent on his being a responsible member of the family group. In the event that he decided to leave school, a new set of plans would be drawn up by the parents. Ron and Gladys were very clear in letting him know that, as an adult, he would be expected to conform to their limits or he would have to move out on his own. They also were very clear in their resolve to deal with all of their children fairly and in a manner that would clearly communicate to them these new expectations for their continued welcome in their parents' home. Claudia began to think about moving out on her own. Ron was adamantly against this, but Gladys was willing to consider it, and so the three talked together about the pros and cons of such a move. The Js' other sons were pleased to have the benefit of less focus on themselves while Claudia worked on her negotiations. They were both doing well in school and responded easily to their parents' changing expectations. They were glad to see James recovering from his problems and were supportive of his return home and to school.

SUMMARY

Important concepts from general systems theory and family systems theory include the concepts boundary, cohesion, adaptability, and communication. Developmental theory concepts include the notion of stage of development and tasks (for the family and its members) associated with that stage. Family stress theory concepts include coping, perception, resources, maladaptation, and bonadaptation.[24] Related factors that might influence the family's coping response were discussed. Some examples of these were the differential effects of

Research Highlights

The major constructs that contribute to understanding family dysfunctional behavior in general are drawn from family systems, development, stress, and communication theories. A significant thread of psychiatric research on families has focused on the construct "expressed emotion" (EE). Expressed emotion has been described as the most thoroughly researched psychosocial variable in recent years.[21] This research originally developed from the effort to understand factors that predicted rehospitalization of persons with a diagnosis of schizophrenia.[4] Brown and his group conducted their research in Britain, and several similar research foci were subsequently developed at various sites in the United States.[10,14,20]

The Camberwell Family Interview[5] has been used extensively in these studies. It is described as a reliable, systematic assessment method for measuring the components of EE. These components include the family's criticism, hostility, dissatisfaction, warmth, overinvolvement, and positive remarks toward the schizophrenic member. The more recent studies have primarily focused on criticism, hostility, and overinvolvement; these variables have been found to correlate significantly with clinical relapse.[21]

An extension of this research explored the interaction effect of neuroleptic medication and EE. This study found that medication-noncompliant clients who came from families deemed high in EE had very high relapse rates. Medication-compliant clients from families with low EE, on the other hand, had low relapse rates.[35] Several crucial questions that are unanswered by this line of research were proposed by Kanter and his colleagues[21] and will be summarized briefly. The first question is whether high EE actually *causes* relapse. A controversy exists over whether the level of EE speaks to the family's effect on the client, or the reverse. Furthermore, only relapse of positive symptoms of schizophrenia, primarily in young male patients, has been successfully predicted. A second question raised by these authors is for the clinical validity of a global EE rating. Rather than this global rating, they suggest that the several variables (criticism, hostility, emotional overinvolvement) that seem closely related to relapse should be investigated independently of each other, rather than as pieces of a unified construct. The third question asks about the clinical significance of EE ratings. Here, Kanter and his colleagues deem that the EE scales conceal subjective judgments about the families ". . . behind the objective veneer of complex scientific methodology" (reference 21, p 377). This issue of scapegoating the families of persons with schizophrenia has been raised by other professionals[34] and also by mental health advocacy groups. Finally, a major concern about any research on schizophrenia has to do with the need for prospective study of families at risk. Even more important, is the need for research that investigates successful family coping in the presence of schizophrenia in a member.[21]

On a positive note, the research on EE has generated a number of intervention programs for families with a schizophrenic member.[10,18,20] The more successful of these psychoeducational approaches educates families about the causes, phenomena, and treatment of schizophrenia. This is followed by more personalized work around particular problems in coping with the affected member's behaviors and symptoms.[21]

a member's illness on the family, depending on the roles fulfilled by that member; the nature of the onset of the illness event; the available treatment and the prognosis for the member's health problem; and the effects of stigma and uncertainty on the family. Client goals included helping parents function more effectively as a team; helping the family develop strategies for dealing with the behaviors of other than the referral child; and meeting the educational needs of the family, including normal growth and development, as well as knowledge about treatments and medications. Expressed emotion and the components of this construct —criticism, hostility, and overinvolvement—were also discussed.

References

1. Aldous J, D'Antonio W. Families and religions. Beverly Hills: Sage Publishers; 1983.
2. American Psychiatric Association. Diagnostic and statistical manual of mental disorders. 3rd ed, revised. Washington, DC: American Psychiatric Association; 1987.
3. Brandt PA. Stress-buffering effects of social support on maternal discipline. Nurs Res. 1984;33:229–234.
4. Brown GW, Carstairs GM, Topping G. Post hospital adjustment of chronic mental patients. Lancet. 1958;2:685–689.
5. Brown GW, Rutter M. The measurement of family activities and relationships: a methodological study. Hum Relations. 1966;19:241.
6. Buckley W, ed. Modern systems research for the behavioral scientist. Chicago: Aldine Publishing; 1968.
7. Carter EA, McGoldrick M, eds. The family life cycle: a framework for family therapy. New York: Gardner Press; 1980.
8. Combrinck-Graham L. A developmental model for family systems. Fam Process. 1985;24:139–150.
9. Duvall EM. Marriage and family relationships. 5th ed. Philadelphia: JB Lippincott; 1977.
10. Falloon IRH, Boyd JL, McGill CW. Family care of schizophrenia: a problem-solving approach to the treatment of mental illness. New York: Guilford Press; 1984.
11. Ferreira A. Psychosis and family myth. Am J Psychother. 1967;21:186–197.
12. Friedman MM. Family nursing: theory and assessment. 2nd ed. Norwalk, CT: Appleton-Century-Crofts; 1986.
13. Goffman E. Stigma: notes on the management of a spoiled identity. Englewood Cliffs, NJ: Prentice Hall; 1963.
14. Goldstein MJ, Doane JA. Family factors in the onset, course and treatment of schizophrenic disorders: an update on current research. J Nerv Ment Dis. 1982;170:692–700.
15. Gottlieb BH. Social support and the study of personal relationships. J Soc Pers Relation. 1985;2:351.
16. Gray-Price H, Szczesny S. Crisis intervention with families

of cancer patients: a developmental approach. Top Clin Nurs. 1985;7:58–70.

17. Hardy ME, Conway ME. Role theory: perspectives for health professionals. New York: Appleton-Century-Crofts; 1978.
18. Heinrichs DW, Carpenter WT. The coordination of family therapy with other treatment modalities for schizophrenia. In McFarlane WR, ed. Family therapy in schizophrenia. New York: Guilford Press; 1983.
19. Hill R. Families under stress. New York: Harper & Row; 1949.
20. Hogarty GE, Anderson CM, Reiss DJ. Family psychoeducation, social skills, training, and maintenance chemotherapy in the aftercare treatment of schizophrenia. Arch Gen Psychiatry. 1986;43:633–642.
21. Kanter J, Lamb HR, Loeper C. Expressed emotion in families: a critical review. Hosp Commun Psychiatry. 1987;38:374–380.
22. Kim MJ, McFarland GK, McLane AM. Pocket guide to nursing diagnoses. 3rd ed. St Louis: CV Mosby; 1989.
23. Kirgis CA, Woolsey DB, Sullivan JJ. Predicting infant APGAR scores. Nurs Res. 1977;26:439–442.
24. McCubbin HI, Patterson JM. Family adaptation to crises. In McCubbin HI, Cauble AE, Patterson JM, eds. Family stress, coping, and social support. Springfield, IL: Charles C Thomas; 1982.
25. McCubbin MA, McCubbin HI, Thompson AI. Family hardiness index. In McCubbin HI, Thompson AI, eds. Family assessment inventories for research and practice. Madison: University of Wisconsin–Madison; 1987.
26. Minuchin S. Families and family therapy. Cambridge: Harvard University Press; 1974.
27. Minuchin S, Rosman BL, Baker L. Psychosomatic families:

anorexia nervosa in context. Cambridge: Harvard University Press; 1978.
28. Mishel MH. Uncertainty in illness. Image: J Nurs Scholarship. 1988;20:225–232.
29. Nuckolls KB, Cassel J, Kaplan BH. Psychosocial assets, life crisis and the prognosis of pregnancy. Am J Epidemiol. 1972;95:431–441.
30. Olson DH, Russell CS, Sprenkle DH. Circumplex model VI: theoretical update. Fam Process. 1983;22:69–83.
31. Satir V. Conjoint family therapy, revised ed. Palo Alto: Science and Behavior Books; 1967.
32. Seymour RJ, Dawson NJ. The schizophrenic at home. J Psychosoc Nurs. 1986;26:28–30.
33. Terkelsen KG. Toward a theory of the family life cycle. In Carter EA, McGoldrick M, eds. The family life cycle: a framework for family therapy. New York: Gardner Press; 1980.
34. Terkelsen KG. Schizophrenia and the family, II: adverse effects of family therapy. Fam Process. 1983;22:191–200.
35. Vaughn CE, Leff JP. The influence of family and social factors on the course of psychiatric illness: a comparison of schizophrenic and depressed neurotic patients. Br J Psychiatry. 1976;129:125–137.
36. von Bertalanffy L. General system theory. New York: George Braziller; 1968.
37. Walsh F, ed. Normal family processes. New York: Guilford Press; 1982.
38. Watzlawick P, Beavin JH, Jackson DD. Pragmatics of human communication. New York: WW Norton; 1967.
39. Wright LM, Leahey M. Nurses and families: a guide to family assessment and intervention. Philadelphia: FA Davis; 1984.
40. Wright LM, Leahey M, eds. Families and chronic illness. Springhouse, PA: Springhouse Corp; 1987.

COPING, INEFFECTIVE INDIVIDUAL

Donna Poole

DEFINITION AND DESCRIPTION

Ineffective individual coping is defined as the impairment of adaptive behaviors and problem-solving abilities of a person in meeting life's demands and roles.[10] People tend to experience problems in daily living when familiar coping strategies are no longer effective. Often the individual is facing a life situation with inadequate preparation or without experience. As tensions and conflicts mount, the individual's daily functioning is likely to become impaired. The severity of the ineffective coping is related to the type, duration, and intensity of the stressor; the perception or interpretation of the stressor; and the coping strategies employed.[5] For example, denial can be a useful coping strategy initially in the face of an overwhelming situation; however, when denial interferes with needed problem solving, it is no longer a useful method.

Coping consists of a set of behaviors and cognitive processes through which the individual manages the internal and external demands of daily living.[6] Generally, coping is a process that individuals engage in daily without much thought. When coping is effective, anxiety remains at a manageable level, and physical and mental illness can be prevented.[13] Coping activities take a wide variety of forms, including all the diverse behaviors that people engage in to meet actual or anticipated challenges.[1]

THEORY AND RESEARCH

Stressors

There are many causes for the phenomenon of ineffective individual coping.[13] However, most theorists and researchers agree that ineffective individual coping usually is a response to a stressor. Selye defines stress as the rate of wear and tear on the body and defines a stressor as that which produces stress. Selye views stress as a positive life force and distinguishes between negative stress (distress) and positive stress (eustress).[12] However, few other theorists make this distinction.

According to Lazarus and Folkman, stressors can generally be placed into three categories: major changes, often cataclysmic and affecting large numbers of persons; major changes affecting one or a few persons; and daily hassles.[6] Major changes affecting large numbers of persons are usually treated as universally stressful. Examples include natural disasters and mass homicide. The actual event may be long, as in a war, or over quickly, as in a tornado. However, the length of the event does not predict the amount of stress generated: the physical and psychological aftermath of even a brief disaster can be extended over a long time, whereas individuals may adjust to extended periods of exposure to a stressor.

The number of persons affected does not alter the power of stressors to disturb. Events outside an individual's ability to control frequently lead to problems with ineffective coping. Examples include the death of a loved one, a life-threatening or incapacitating illness, or being laid off from work. Major life changes such as divorce may be so threatening that ineffective individual coping is the result. Some theorists contend that any major life change, positive or negative, can be a stressor.[6]

Events that arise out of everyday living are less dramatic than cataclysmic events, but they may be even more important in adaptation and health.[6] An argument with a partner, a car that won't start, or a dog knocking over the trash can produce irritations and distress that may precipitate ineffective individual coping.

Perceptions

Difficulties arise when the great variations in human response to universal stressors are overlooked.[6] The ability to cope with the demands of life is more related to the individual's response to stressors than to the stressor itself. Because illness is largely a subjective experience, clients with similar conditions who face some of the same stressors may have significantly different ways of coping, resulting in very different outcomes in response to similar events.[2] Thus, unusual or extremely difficult stressors do not necessarily lead to ineffective coping. If the client has the resources and skills to deal with the demands presented, coping is likely regardless of the stressor.[3] The client's belief in his or her own ability to handle the stressor is often just as important as the ability itself to the successful resolution of a stressful situation.[7]

In order to evaluate how and why stress affects people differently, several factors must be examined. Lazarus and Folkman identify two critical processes in this evaluation: cognitive appraisal and coping.[6] They define cognitive appraisal as an evaluative process that determines why and to what extent a particular transaction or series of transactions is stressful to an individual. In other words, it is how and what the individual is thinking about the event that makes it uniquely stressful for him or her. Coping is defined as the process through which the individual manages the demands that are perceived as stressful and the emotions they generate. Aguilera and Messick support these two factors, which they call perception of the event and coping mechanisms.[1] They add a third evaluative factor: situational support. By evaluating these three "balancing factors," it is possible to evaluate how the same stressful event may affect individuals differently.

Coping Skills

Leventhal and Nerenz describe coping as the planning, selecting, and executing of responses to a stimulus.[7] Coping is based on the individual's interpretation of the stimuli and may be a response either to the objective features, to the emotional reaction, or to both. For example, a person with an upset stomach may respond to the objective feature by taking an antacid, whereas the same individual who suspects an ulcer may respond to the fear and anxiety by making an appointment with a physician.

The effectiveness of coping skills is dependent on a number of other factors, such as self-esteem, self-efficacy, role models, and social support.[7] Positive factors, such as high self-esteem or successful role models, are more likely to lead to effective coping skills. Negative factors, such as the inability to solve problems and the absence of social supports, are more likely to lead to ineffective individual coping.

RELATED FACTORS
Stressors

The nursing diagnosis of ineffective individual coping is associated with most of the major psychiatric disorders. Any stressful situation or any condition that predisposes an individual to personal vulnerability has the potential to precipitate ineffective coping. Common stressors include maturational or situational crises, multiple life changes, inadequate support systems, or work overload, including too many deadlines. As previously stated, it cannot be assumed that a stressor will always produce ineffective coping.

Perceptions

The individual can be thought of as a regulatory system that strives to reach specifiable goals.[7] When an individual's goals are unrealistically high, the potential for ineffective individual coping is increased. Unmet expectations and unrealistic perceptions often precipitate ineffective individual coping.

Coping Skills

Lifestyle or personal habits often predispose an individual to ineffective coping. People who fail to take vacations or who do not take the time or do not have the ability to relax are at risk for ineffective individual coping. An individual's physical stamina may influence the ability to cope effectively. Therefore, other potential risk factors include poor nutrition and little or no exercise.

Coping methods that are inappropriate or inadequate for the situation may also lead to ineffective individual coping. For example, physical violence is an inappropriate response to a threat to one's self-esteem. On the other hand, failure to defend oneself from a physical threat may likewise have dire consequences.

DEFINING CHARACTERISTICS

Defining characteristics are clues to the presence of ineffective individual coping, and they offer supporting evidence in the formulation of the diagnosis. The most obvious sign of ineffective individual coping is the client's verbal report of the inability to cope. In a society where self-reliance is valued, clients often demonstrate an inability to ask for help. During periods of great stress, anxiety or other emotional states may interfere with a client's problem-solving ability. Clients may verbalize an inability to meet role expectations or to meet their basic needs. The client may express a pessimistic viewpoint or may refuse or reject help when help would obviously be useful. However, often, it is nurses' observations of a client's behavior, rather than the client's verbalizations, that are the first clue to ineffective individual coping.

Changes in a client's usual behavioral pattern may be an indication of ineffective individual coping; e.g., changes in usual patterns of social participation or in usual communication patterns. Individuals who have frequent illnesses or accidents may be manifesting their ineffective coping in somatic ways.

Individuals who are not coping effectively may engage in behaviors that are not socially acceptable or that annoy and irritate others. Examples are destructive behaviors toward the self, others, or property; verbal manipulation; excessive dependency on others; nonproductive lifestyles; self-absorption; and avoidance behaviors.

Everyone needs and uses defense mechanisms; however, when used excessively or inappropriately, these mechanisms cease to be useful coping strategies. For example, it often is useful to suppress anger to allow for a "cooling off" period. However, repeated attempts to suppress anger without issue confrontation and problem solving may later result in an explosive outburst (Chart 1).

CHART 1
Ineffective Individual Coping: Definition, Related Factors, and Defining Characteristics

DEFINITION

Ineffective individual coping is the impairment of adaptive behaviors and problem-solving abilities of a person in meeting life's demands and roles.

RELATED FACTORS

Personal vulnerability
Maturational crises
Situational crises
Multiple life changes
No vacations
Inadequate relaxation
Inadequate support systems
Little or no exercise
Poor nutrition
Unmet expectations
Work overload
Too many deadlines
Unrealistic perceptions
Inadequate coping method

DEFINING CHARACTERISTICS

Verbalization of inabilty to cope
Inability to ask for help
Inability to solve problems
Inability to meet role expectations
Inability to meet basic needs
Alteration in societal participation
Destructive behavior toward self or others
Inappropriate use of defense mechanisms
Change in usual communication patterns
Verbal manipulation
High illness rate
High rate of accidents
Expressions of pessimism
Refusal or rejection of help
Overdependence on others
Nonproductive lifestyle
Self-absorption
Avoidance behavior

NURSING PROCESS AND RATIONALE

Assessment

The first step in assessing for ineffective individual coping is to determine the client's perception of the event or situation, because that perception generally determines the reaction. In addition, the client's history of managing stressful situations should be assessed by asking the client to recall stressful life events and tell how they were managed. The client also should be asked to evaluate past life situations for the effectiveness of coping. These reports provide valuable information about the client's coping pattern and stress tolerance pattern.[4] Assessment questions include:

1. Are you tense a lot of the time? What helps? Do you use any medication, drugs, or alcohol to help you cope with your tension?
2. Who's most helpful to you in talking things over? Is this person available to you now?
3. Have there been any big changes in your life in the last year or two?
4. When (if) you have big problems (any problems) in your life, how do you handle them?
5. Most of the time, is this (are these) way(s) successful in managing your problem?[4]

It often is useful to explore with the client the cause to which he or she attributes the present situation. Some clients will blame themselves; others will seek to place blame on external causes. Blaming oneself does not necessarily result in poor coping skills, nor is attributing blame to an external cause associated with more effective coping. The process of attributing blame affects individuals differently. Is the client's attribution of blame perpetuating the crisis and limiting his or her coping skills? Has the client considered other attributions less damaging to self-esteem? Attributions that are more helpful to the client may result in the growth of coping skills and in a positive resolution.[11]

Nursing Diagnosis

Once assessment data have been gathered, the nurse begins to form a judgment on the meaning of the data. A nursing diagnosis of ineffective individual coping is made specific to the individual; i.e., ineffective individual coping related to personal vulnerability and unrealistic expectations. The diagnosis of ineffective individual coping is not appropriate when describing excess food or alcohol intake, noncompliance, or uncooperative behavior unless the client has a perception of life stress and the inability to solve problems also is present.[4] It is usually good practice to validate the nursing diagnosis with a client. The nurse's relationship with a client is ideally one of a partnership, requiring the problem and the goal to be agreed on.

Client Goals and Nursing Interventions

When an individual is facing a stressful situation and is struggling to make sense out of an event, nursing intervention can play a crucial role in facilitating movement toward a positive resolution. Individuals under stress are generally more susceptible to suggestion and more willing to accept help.[1,11]

Interventions occur throughout the nursing process; they are not limited to the intervention phase. For example, during the assessment phase, the goal is to encourage the client to verbalize feelings and opinions related to his or her emotional state. The nurse must engage in several interventions in order to accomplish this goal. First, it is the responsibility of the nurse to create an atmosphere of trust and caring. The nurse can do this by demonstrating consistency and trustworthiness. The client also must feel that the nurse is accessible. Because individuals who are experiencing ineffective coping often are unable to assert themselves, it often is necessary to be a strong advocate for these clients. It is not uncommon for individuals who are coping ineffectively to engage in inappropriate behaviors that may necessitate limit setting by the nurse.

Other nursing interventions are directed toward the goal of assisting the client to recognize and verbalize his or her own coping patterns and the subsequent consequences of behaviors. To begin to reaffirm or develop coping behaviors, it is important for clients to recognize their own personal strengths, skills, and resources. The nurse should listen carefully as the client speaks, paying close attention to behavioral cues such as facial expressions, gestures, eye contact, tone and intensity of voice, and body positioning. It is then possible to reflect the nurse's observations to the client for his or her consideration.

Because clients with ineffective coping have limited problem-solving abilities, it is not uncommon for them to experience suicidal or homicidal ideation. It is therefore important to determine the risk of a client's in-

flicting self-harm or harm to others and to intervene appropriately. Assisting the client to identify potential solutions to current problems is a most useful intervention with these clients as well as with others.

Once clients have identified effective coping patterns, the next step is for them to begin to practice and use their new-found skills and behaviors. Often, it is useful to teach the client the problem-solving process. The nurse can provide a safe environment for practicing new behaviors. It often is helpful to assist the client to identify existing and potential support systems and external resources that will reinforce the development of new coping skills. Clients often need assistance in identifying alternatives to fulfill unmet needs. Finally, clients need to be assisted to set achievable goals. Unrealistically high goals lead to a sense of failure and ineffectiveness, whereas easily achievable goals do not offer a challenge or a sense of accomplishment.

Evaluation

Finally, no intervention for this nursing diagnosis is complete without planning to prevent further problems. Has the client's plan to cope with the most recent

---

CHART 2
Ineffective Individual Coping: Summary of the Nursing Process

NURSING INTERVENTIONS	OUTCOME CRITERIA
CLIENT GOAL: IDENTIFY RESPONSE TO STRESSFUL EVENT(S) Assess behaviors and related factors Provide an atmosphere of trust and caring Communicate accessibility to the client Be an advocate in stressful situations Set limits on inappropriate behavior Encourage verbalization of feelings, perceptions, and fears	Verbalizes feelings and beliefs related to stressful event(s)
CLIENT GOAL: IDENTIFY EFFECTIVE AND INEFFECTIVE COPING PATTERNS Assess client's coping patterns by listening carefully as client speaks and observing nonverbal communication Determine risk of client's inflicting self-harm and intervene appropriately Assist to identify strengths, values, and resources Assist to identify past coping methods Assist to identify current problems and potential solutions	Identifies own coping pattern and the consequences of that behavior Describes own strengths, skills, and resources Verbalizes hope and potential solutions to the current problem
CLIENT GOAL: UTILIZE EFFECTIVE COPING MECHANISMS Assist to develop strategies based on strengths and experience: Teach problem-solving techniques Provide a safe environment for exploring new behaviors Assist to identify available support systems and resources Explore alternatives to fulfill unmet needs Assist to set achievable goals	Makes decisions Requests support from others Practices new coping skills Takes action to change troublesome situations in personal environment Reports needs are adequately met
CLIENT GOAL: ENGAGE IN PLANNING TO PREVENT FURTHER EPISODES OF INEFFECTIVE INDIVIDUAL COPING Assist to evaluate current lifestyle and stressors that can be modified to enhance coping Refer for continued therapy or counseling if needed	States new skills and abilities developed Describes how similar situations will be handled in the future Accepts recommendation for further therapy or counseling if needed

stressor produced the expected results? Are there predictable stressful events the client is likely to encounter? Has the client resumed his or her previous level of functioning? Is it possible for the client to assume a higher level of functioning than prior to the stressful event? For example, a client who is proud of the way in which he or she handled a difficult, stressful situation may experience an increase in self-esteem and self-confidence. Clients who come through stressful situations at a lower level of functioning, or clients who were not functioning well prior to the stressor, may require continued psychotherapy or counseling. Clients with high levels of functioning may also desire counseling for personal growth and development (Chart 2).

CASE STUDY

Eleanor R, a 17-year-old woman, was hospitalized after a visit to a local hospital emergency room. In the ER, she was crying uncontrollably and complained of not being able to cope with her life any more: "I don't know what's going to happen to me if I don't get some help." She had been sent to the ER via ambulance by her mother, who remained at home. Recent stressors included being expelled from high school in her senior year for failure to attend ("I can't get out of bed in the morning"), being unable to locate her

father, receiving a reprimand at work, needing extensive automobile repairs, having financial difficulties, and a recent argument with her boyfriend. Her "final blow" came when she called her counselor at his home and was reprimanded for doing so.

Eleanor gave a history of being required to help support the family starting from age 9, when she took a paper route. She currently lives with her mother and a younger sibling. The mother expressed verbal support but was too overwhelmed with her own low-paying job and her own night school classes to be of much actual support. The family members expressed love for each other, but admitted they often fought. The client expressed feeling overwhelmed by her current responsibilities and fear of assuming further adult responsibilities, such as living on her own and completely supporting herself.

A major nursing diagnosis was ineffective individual coping related to inadequate support systems. Verbalization of inability to cope and difficulty meeting basic needs were defining characteristics supportive of this nursing diagnosis. Eleanor was encouraged to identify her responses to stressful events and to plan new coping strategies through one-to-one interactions with her primary nurse. She also participated in social skills and assertiveness groups. The hospital liaison to the community school system was called in for a consultation. A family conference was held by the nurse family specialist to assess family interactions and to provide support for all family members.

One week later, at discharge, Eleanor was able to state how she might have handled the same situation differently

Research Highlights

Some researchers believe there are an insufficient number of nursing diagnoses for psychiatric mental health clients and that some of the diagnoses, such as ineffective individual coping, are not specific enough to guide individualized nursing care.[13] Another group of researchers developing a classification system for psychiatric mental health nursing did not include ineffective individual coping in their classification system.[8]

Vincent surveyed psychiatric mental health clinical nurse specialists to determine what signs and symptoms they observed when formulating a diagnosis of ineffective individual coping.[14] In this validation study, the inability to solve problems was the only one of the three NANDA-accepted critical defining characteristics to be nearly always present (identified 83% of the time by clinical nurse specialists). Verbalizing of the inability to cope was seen as nearly always present by only 66%, whereas the verbalization of inability to ask for help was seen as nearly always present by only 23%. The most frequent defining characteristics listed were not on the NANDA list: anxiety was reported to be nearly always present by 94% and reported life stress was reported to be nearly always present by 89%. These results suggest that the list of defining characteristics is not yet complete and that the critical defining characteristics need further refinement. Further validation studies are required before forming any definite conclusions.

McFarland and Naschinski surveyed 45 psychiatric nurse experts in one facility on the clarity and usefulness of current NANDA diagnoses for psychiatric mental

health nursing.[9] None of the nursing diagnosis labels accepted by NANDA was viewed as clear in meaning by 90% or more of the respondents. Among NANDA-accepted nursing diagnostic labels, ineffective individual coping ranked fourth in clarity and was perceived as clear by 87% of the respondents, following diversional activity deficit, anticipatory grieving, and rape trauma syndrome (89% each). Other nursing diagnosis labels identified by psychiatric nurse experts as being more clear than ineffective individual coping have not yet been approved by NANDA. These were: depressive mood (94%), threatened or attempted suicide (93%), suspiciousness (93%), hyperactive behavior (91%), regressive behavior (91%), and substance misuse (90%). The results of this study suggest there still are diagnoses to be identified within psychiatric mental health nursing. The distinction between accepted and proposed nursing diagnoses must be further explored and clarified. Ineffective individual coping is similar in description to several of the proposed diagnoses. Therefore, it is incumbent on the nurse clinician to ensure that life stress and the inability to solve problems are present before making the diagnosis of ineffective individual coping. As stated previously, it also is useful to validate the diagnosis with the client.

There is no need to be alarmed or confused by the apparent lack of agreement and the contradictions among experts on the nursing diagnosis ineffective individual coping. Further research will refine and clarify the diagnostic categories, the defining characteristics, and the related factors.

and was able to say how she intends to handle similar situations in the future. Although many of the same stressors remained at discharge, she expressed confidence in her ability to seek help from appropriate resources and to tolerate her own internal stress. Discharge planning involved referral to an agency that provided individual counseling and limited family therapy sessions. Eleanor had visited her therapist once before discharge and expressed confidence in the discharge plan. All family members verbalized satisfaction at the course of the hospitalization.

SUMMARY

Ineffective individual coping is the impairment of adaptive behaviors and problem-solving abilities of a person in meeting life's demands and roles. Poor coping can occur in persons with psychiatric conditions or under a variety of other circumstances. Generally, ineffective individual coping is associated with a life stress for which the person is inadequately prepared or has no experience to draw on in responding. After assessment, nursing interventions are directed toward mobilizing current coping mechanisms and practicing newly learned coping skills. After the stressful event and the return to normal functioning, emphasis is placed on planning to prevent future episodes of ineffective individual coping.

References

1. Aguilera DC, Messick JM. Crisis intervention: theory and methodology. St Louis, CV Mosby; 1986.
2. Burckhardt CS. Coping strategies of the chronically ill. Nurs Clin North Am. 1987;22(3):543–550.
3. Carnevali DL. Nursing care planning: diagnosis and management. Philadelphia, JB Lippincott; 1983.
4. Gordon M. Nursing diagnosis: process and application. San Francisco: McGraw-Hill; 1987.
5. Hagerty BK. Psychiatric–mental health assessment. St Louis: CV Mosby; 1984.
6. Lazarus RS, Folkman S. Stress: appraisal and coping. New York: Springer Publishing; 1984.
7. Leventhal H, Nerenz DR. A model for stress research with some implications for the control of stress disorders. In: Meichenbaum D, Jaremko ME, eds. Stress reduction and prevention. New York: Plenum Press; 1983.
8. Loomis ME, O'Toole AW, Brown MS, Pothier P, West P, Wilson HS. Development of a classification system for psychiatric/mental health nursing: individual response class. Arch Psychiatr Nurs. 1987;1(1):16–24.
9. McFarland GK, Naschinski CE. Validation and identification of nursing diagnoses labels for psychiatric mental health nursing practice. In: McLane AM, ed. Classification of nursing diagnoses: proceedings of the Seventh Conference. St Louis, CV Mosby; 1987.
10. McLane AM (ed). Classification of nursing diagnoses: proceedings of the Seventh Conference. St Louis: CV Mosby; 1987.
11. Peterson LC. Attribution theory and its application in crisis intervention. Perspect Psychiatr Care. 1984;22(4):133–136.
12. Selye H. Stress without distress. New York: Lippincott and Crowell; 1974.
13. Thomas MD, Sanger E, Whitney JD. Nursing diagnosis of depression. J Psychosoc Nurs Ment Health Serv. 1986; 24(8):6–12.
14. Vincent KG. The validation of a nursing diagnosis: a nurse consensus survey. Nurs Clin North Am. 1985;20(4):631–640.

CRISIS, MATURATIONAL AND SITUATIONAL

Suzanne Sexton Leichman

DEFINITION AND DESCRIPTION

A crisis occurs when an individual experiences events that are perceived as threatening and for which coping skills are inadequate. There are two kinds of crises: maturational and situational. A *maturational crisis* occurs with normal change and growth. Also known as developmental crises,[6] maturational crises occur during significant transition periods of personality development, such as adolescence, young adulthood, marriage, parenthood, or retirement. A *situational crisis* may occur because of a single event, or a series of events, which together overwhelm the person's ability to cope. Events leading to a crisis are not necessarily negative; many changes in a short period may overtax the ability to cope, even if the changes are positive. What one person perceives as threatening and a crisis may be seen by another as a growth challenge. When events are perceived as threatening, and personal resources are not adequate for successful coping, a crisis may result.

THEORY AND RESEARCH

Crises occur when a person's equilibrium is disturbed by a hazardous event or a change in role that the person perceives to be a threat or a loss.[4] The crisis is a turning point. It is a period during which customary coping skills are insufficient. Disorganization and anxiety develop as the person struggles to cope.

Caplan[4] describes four characteristic phases of a crisis. In phase 1, tension rises as the usual problem-solving techniques are tried. In phase 2, the individual experiences a lack of success in coping, and the tension and discomfort increase. In phase 3, the individual feels pressured to use all energy reserves to resolve the situation. This may mean trying previously unused coping skills or seeking help from others; also, the person may try to approach the problem by trial and error, redefine the problem to make it more manageable, or give up certain goals that begin to seem unattainable. If the problem situation continues, or cannot be satisfactorily resolved, phase 4 occurs in which the tension and anxiety build to a crescendo, and major disorganization occurs.[4]

Every crisis presents an opportunity for disorganization or growth.[4] If the person becomes overwhelmed with anxiety and all attempts at coping fail, the result may be a decrease in functioning during the crisis, and the person may never be able to achieve the former level of functioning.[8] If new coping skills are learned and the person receives support from significant others, including health care professionals, functioning may be at the same or a higher level after the crisis.[1,4]

A person is more open to suggestions in crisis than at other times.[5] The feelings of helplessness motivate the individual to accept help and learn new ways of coping. This presents an opportunity for emotional growth as a result of successful learning.[4,5] Therefore, long-standing problems may be resolved during a crisis. How the person manages in a crisis influences future capacity to cope with problems.[3]

Distinctions should be made between maturational and situational crises. Maturational crises occur during transition states from one developmental stage to another. The developmental stages have been described by Erikson, among other developmental psychologists[6] (see Chapter 5). Each state presents unique stressors and challenges toward growth called developmental tasks. Achievement in each stage relies on tasks mastered in previous stages. Psychosocial development proceeds by critical steps or turning points "between progress and regression, integration and retardation" (reference 6, p 271). The turning points are the major transition states in development:

Prenatal to infancy
Infancy to childhood
Childhood to puberty and adolescence
Adolescence to adulthood
Maturity to middle age
Middle age to old age
Old age to death (reference 8, pp 38,39)

The transition states are critical periods during which "natural changes in roles, body image and attitudes toward oneself and the world create internal turmoil and restlessness" (reference 8, p 39). Maturational crises usually evolve over an extended period, and they frequently require that one make characterologic changes.[1] Because maturational crises follow developmental stages, they are considered part of normal development. Additionally, they can be anticipated, making it possible to prepare for them.

However, not everyone experiences crises during transitional states. With personal resources and support from others, the turning points can be periods of challenge and growth. Successful mastery requires expenditure of energy and nurturance from others.[8] Maturational crises occur when one does not have the social supports and personal resources to cope with the anxiety during transition states.

Situational crises occur as a result of unexpected, traumatic events, such as a house fire or a death; they cannot be anticipated, nor can a person prepare for them. When situational events occur during a developmental transition period, the individual may be stressed beyond the ability to cope (e.g., an adolescent diagnosed as being diabetic, a young father losing his job shortly after his baby is born, or an elderly couple having to move to lower-income housing when they retire). In each instance, a significant situational event is experienced during a transitional period, and the latter is exacerbated by the former. The person may have coped with the trials of the transition period until the situational event.

RELATED FACTORS

Individuals, families, or communities may experience situational crises after many events. Natural disasters, such as fires, floods, hurricanes, or earthquakes, increase vulnerability to crisis. Economic and political events also stress people's coping abilities. These may include a stock market crash, the closing of the major industrial plant in a small community, changes in government, or consequences of war. Also at high risk for crisis are those who have suffered from rape, robbery, burglary, kidnapping, or hostage-taking. All of these may receive public attention.

However, events that do not receive media attention are also causes for situational crises. The event that triggers a crisis need only be significant to the individual involved, for example, an automobile accident, which may require auto repairs, insurance claims, reporting to the state motor vehicle bureau, and finding other ways to get around. The loss of a job can precipitate a crisis, particularly if the loss represents a threat to the person's competency and self-esteem. A promotion might also constitute a crisis situation if the person is not prepared to accept the additional responsibility, extra hours, or increased pressures and stress.

"The potential for a crisis state exists within every human by virtue of living and experiencing life" (reference 3, p 17). Some people have a greater risk of experiencing a crisis because they (1) have a high probability of exposure to stressful events, (2) have inadequate social supports, (3) lack coping skills, or (4) have a poor history of handling stress.[3]

Factors Affecting Crisis Outcome

The outcome of a crisis results primarily from three balancing factors: perception of the event, coping mechanisms, and social supports.[1,3,5] The single most important balancing factor is the *perception of events as a threat*. An individual in crisis manifests one of two primary patterns. In one, the person acknowledges events as threatening and asks for help in coping. Here, the individual is aware of what is being experienced, but feels powerless to effect a change. In the second pattern, the individual presents somatic problems or anxiety surrounding, but not directly referring to, a significant event. Here, the individual is unaware of not coping and describes anxiety manifestations.

The second balancing factor is *coping mechanisms*. A crisis is a highly stressful period in which the individual believes that, despite the use of all available resources, the crisis has not been managed. Successful coping mechanisms contribute to restoring equilibrium by reducing anxiety and giving the person a sense of control. The more varied the number of ways of handling situations, the greater the potential for crisis management. People with few or fixed ways of coping have fewer resources on which to rely. Hence, past patterns of crisis management influence the ability to cope with the current crisis.

Social support is another balancing factor in a crisis. In the struggle to resolve the crisis, a person is susceptible to the influences of others. The norms and behaviors of those in the individual's environment affect the perception of events and define acceptable ways of coping. The way a situation is defined is, in part, culturally based.[4] Cultural prescriptions influence how an individual or family will be supported while in crisis. The pain and discomfort experienced motivate one to accept help from others. Likewise, the person in crisis affects the family or group of which he or she is a member.[4] An individual in crisis may also be expressing a disturbance or disequilibrium within the family.[9]

DEFINING CHARACTERISTICS

Defining characteristics of crisis may include signs and symptoms of severe to extreme anxiety; insomnia or hypersomnia; fatigue or loss of energy; inability to perform activities of daily living (ADL); feelings of worthlessness or helplessness; diminished ability to think or concentrate; disorganization; and diminished functioning and depression (Fig. 13-11). In addition, a client in crisis commonly experiences a variety of physical symptoms.

Anxiety is a major dynamic in a crisis and is viewed as the most common psychological response to a stressor.[10] Anxiety, as an uncomfortable sensation, motivates the individual to avoid or escape the perceived hazardous situation. It affects problem solving, learning, and communicating by distorting perceptions and

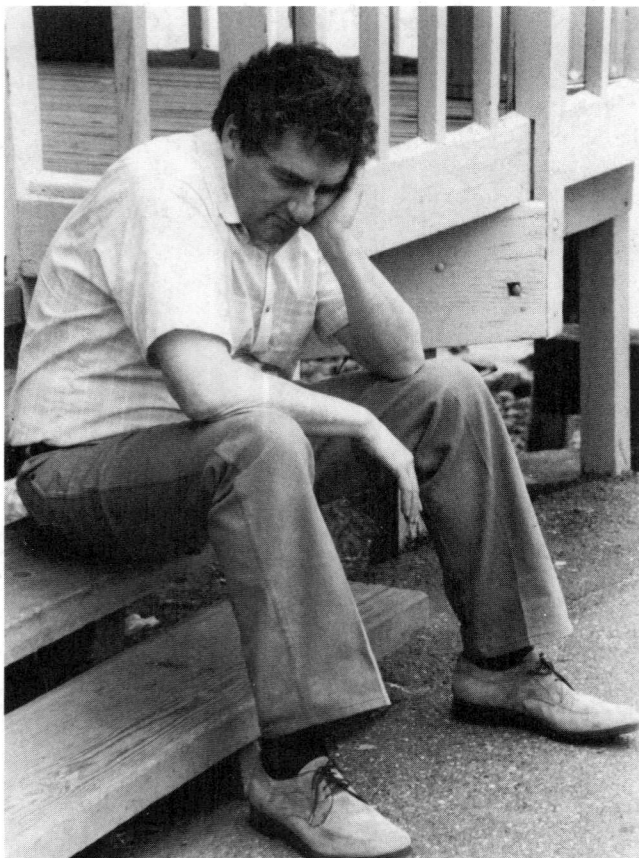

FIGURE 13–11. Persons undergoing situational crisis may experience fatigue, loss of energy, inability to perform ADL, feelings of worthlessness, disorganization, diminished functioning, and depression. (Courtesy of Suzanne Sexton Leichman)

altering the capacity to process information from the environment.[7] In a crisis, anxiety increases, even though the individual attempts to reduce it.

Therefore, clients in crisis may complain of not being able to do anything right, or feelings of powerlessness or guilt. They may blame themselves or others. They may express anger about what has happened to them and have difficulty problem solving or utilizing resources effectively (Chart 1).

NURSING PROCESS AND RATIONALE

Assessment

The first area to be assessed is the anxiety level. Next, the psychiatric mental health nurse assesses the client's perception of what has occurred by encouraging the client to talk about the events leading to the present situation and noting whether the client's description is clear or vague and confusing. How the client handled previous crises is also assessed. Data are collected on the client's strengths and weaknesses according to the five dimensions: physical, psychological,

cultural, social, and spiritual. From this assessment the coping skills and social supports that will help in dealing with the crisis are determined. It is also important to identify such physical symptoms of depression or anxiety as changes in sleeping, eating, or elimination patterns, or recent changes in weight.

Nursing Diagnoses

Examples of specific nursing diagnoses include maturational crisis related to first-time parenthood; situational crisis related to house fire resulting in loss of housing and personal belongings; and maturational and situational crises related to adolescent identity issues, homesickness during first quarter at college, and concern about failing courses and losing an athletic scholarship.

CHART 1
Maturational and Situational Crisis: Definition, Related Factors, and Defining Characteristics

DEFINITION

A crisis occurs when an individual experiences events that are perceived as threatening and for which coping skills are inadequate. Maturational crises occur during periods of developmental change. Situational crises occur because traumatic events overwhelm the person's ability to cope.

RELATED FACTORS

Maturational stage: adolescence, parenthood, retirement
Situational events: house fire, loss of a job, divorce
Perception of events
Coping mechanisms
Social supports

DEFINING CHARACTERISTICS

Signs and symptoms of severe to extreme anxiety
Insomnia or hypersomnia
Fatigue or loss of energy
Inability to perform activities of daily living
Feelings of worthlessness and helplessness
Diminished ability to think or concentrate
Disorganization
Diminished functioning
Depression
Physical symptoms
Feelings of powerlessness
Guilt
Self-blame
Blaming others
Anger
Inability to problem solve
Inability to use coping resources effectively

Client Goals and Nursing Interventions

The first goal in intervening with a client in crisis is to reduce anxiety, because a high anxiety level will interfere with the ability to concentrate and solve problems. Structuring interactions, including specifying time, place, and frequency of sessions, helps the client know what to expect. In the structured sessions, the psychiatric mental health nurse focuses on anxiety reduction so that the client will be more comfortable in telling the story. Active listening is particularly important. The demeanor of the nurse is one of concern and caring. Other interventions might include teaching the client to deep-breathe and relax, having a cup of tea, or finding a quiet, private place to talk. Reducing anxiety helps the client to regain a sense of control amid the chaos experienced.

Sometimes, the nurse encounters people in crisis in the course of other activities. For example, a nurse asks a man about his wife, who is being treated for a sarcoma with aggressive chemotherapy. He responds with a discussion of how he himself is doing. The nurse's treatment of his situational crisis is to listen so that he can put into words for the first time his crisis and his response.

The second goal is for the client to develop a realistic perception of the situation. The client is encouraged to tell the story in order. The nurse assists the client to clearly describe sequential events by asking who, what, when, and where questions as needed. This clarifies what has happened and helps to develop a more realistic perspective.

The third goal is to assist the client to develop adequate coping skills. The psychiatric mental health nurse and the client discuss past coping mechanisms and identify those that were more successful. The nurse then helps the client to explore new coping skills and to use them in role-playing. The nurse also teaches problem solving and how to anticipate situations, plan scripts or behaviors, and consider possible outcomes. This enables the client to cope with changes without feeling overwhelmed.

The fourth goal is to develop adequate social supports. The psychiatric mental health nurse encourages the client to identify possible support persons (family, neighbors, friends) who could be supportive and might help if asked. Role-play may be utilized to help the client anticipate conversations with others. For example, a client is anxious about spending a weekend at his mother's house. The nurse has the client describe an anticipated conversation with his mother; the client plays himself and the nurse plays the mother. Another technique is to reverse the roles so that the client plays the mother and the nurse plays the client.

The fifth goal is for the client to take action toward resolving the defined problem(s). The client is encouraged to take responsibility for resolving the crisis by acting upon a problem-solving option. To increase confidence and the chances of success, the client then rehearses the situation with the nurse.

The final goal is to enable the client to evaluate actions that have been taken. To accomplish this, the client is assisted in identifying desired outcomes. When a client is fearful of succeeding, the nurse may give the client permission to succeed. The nurse also encourages the client to reevaluate actions taken and teaches how to choose another option if the one tried does not work.

Evaluation

Crisis resolution may take up to a year. The nurse may not have contact with the person throughout the recovery process, which complicates evaluation. However, evaluation may take place at any time by evaluating the client's current level of functioning and comparing it with the precrisis level of functioning. The psychiatric mental health nurse may evaluate the client's ability to perform the outcome criteria: Is the client able to identify strengths? Has the client tried a new coping skill? Has the client identified people to whom he or she can turn for help? Additionally, the nurse can simply ask the client, "What have you learned?" (Chart 2).

CASE STUDY

Lynne, a 28-year-old mother of three (ages 10 months, 3 years, and 5½ years) was admitted to a small rural hospital complaining that she was depressed and could no longer function. At the time of admission, she was distraught and very tearful. She was withdrawn and responded minimally to routine questions, but said that she was so upset when her husband of eight years told her that he wanted a divorce that she put their children in the car and drove 130 miles to her sister's home. Her sister offered to take care of her children and convinced her to come to the hospital. This was her first psychiatric hospitalization. Her admission nursing diagnoses were situational crisis related to possible divorce and ineffective individual coping. Her DSM-III-R diagnosis was adjustment disorder with depressed mood.[2]

At first, Lynne was fearful of being in the hospital and would not interact with other patients. She chose to stay in her room with the door closed and the lights dimmed. Through brief, hourly, goal-directed conversations with her nurse during the first day, she gradually organized her thoughts. She described her feelings of hurt that her husband did not want to live with her, and of panic because she would have to raise her children alone. Unaware of where she had been and what she had done during the 24 hours before her hospitalization, she feared that she was "losing her mind." However, the more she described her situation, the clearer her thinking became. She then described her relationship with her husband. They had met in college and dated for six months before getting married; Lynne had dropped out of school to work so that her husband could finish his degree. She intended to resume her education when her husband graduated, but became pregnant with their first child and then moved when her husband accepted a job in another town. Lynne had mixed feelings about it

CHART 2
Maturational and Situational Crisis: Summary of the Nursing Process

NURSING INTERVENTIONS	OUTCOME CRITERIA
CLIENT GOAL: EXPERIENCE REDUCED ANXIETY Assess client's anxiety level Structure interactions, including time, place, frequency Focus on reducing anxiety Encourage client to describe feelings	Reports a decrease in anxiety Describes feelings experienced during crisis
CLIENT GOAL: DEVELOP REALISTIC PERCEPTION OF THE SITUATION Encourage client to tell the story in a step-by-step fashion Encourage clear description of sequential events	Describes events associated with the crisis
CLIENT GOAL: DEVELOP ADEQUATE COPING SKILLS Assess client's strengths: physical, psychological, cultural, social, spiritual Have the client state ways of coping in the past. What has worked? What has been tried with this crisis? What helped? What didn't? Explore new ways of coping to expand client's repertoire Teach problem solving Explore options Try out skills in role-playing. Teach client to anticipate outcomes, "What if . . . ?"	Identifies strengths Demonstrates new coping skills
CLIENT GOAL: DEVELOP ADEQUATE SOCIAL SUPPORTS Have client identify social supports (family, neighbors, friends, caseworkers, etc.) Have client role-play anticipated conversations with others	Identifies people who would help by name
CLIENT GOAL: TAKE ACTION TOWARD RESOLVING THE PROBLEM(S) Encourage client to take responsibility for resolving crisis by acting upon a problem-solving option To increase confidence have client rehearse the situation first	Rehearses an option for action Reports taking action on an option
CLIENT GOAL: EVALUATE ACTIONS Teach client how to evaluate actions taken. What was done? What was the desired outcome? How will client know if actions were successful? For people who are afraid to succeed, give permission to succeed	Reports evaluation of actions Reports selection of another option or problem to work on

because it meant leaving family and friends and increased the likelihood that she would not be able to finish her education. She stated that she was satisfied with their marriage, but admitted to having more arguments with her husband in the past four months. She added that she continually felt depressed and tired during the month before she was admitted and was discouraged enough to consider going to a counselor, but lacked the energy to do so.

Her psychiatric mental health nurse guided her through problem-solving steps, exploring possible options and weighing pros and cons. Lynne identified new ways to cope with the problem such as seeking a counselor to help her and her husband talk about their problems. She was encouraged to identify her own strengths and to acknowledge areas for which she could allow herself to ask help from others. She also identified specific people with whom she would feel comfortable in asking for help. Her sister was supportive, but lived too far away to help with day-to-day difficulties; however, she felt comfortable in sharing and discussing her problems with two close friends; she also identified a neighbor who would care for her children.

On the third day of her hospitalization, Lynne called her husband on her own initiative and asked him to come to the hospital to discuss their situation. The following day, she and her husband met with the physician and the psychiatric mental health nurse. In the sessions, Lynne told her husband that she did not want a divorce and asked him to join in couples therapy. Her husband said that he had been abrupt in asking for a divorce, and he agreed that they needed help. The nurse pointed out that they had both reacted impulsively and needed to learn how to talk about their thoughts and feelings before acting. Lynne's husband described feeling apprehensive that she might run away again. Lynne apologized for her behavior and told him some of the new ways of coping she had learned. The psychiatrist cautioned Lynne to follow through carefully with the plans, because of the seriousness of her situation at hospitalization. Lynne and her husband agreed to attend couples therapy with a private psychiatrist in their home town, focusing on developing open communication so that they could resolve their problems. After this session, Lynne was discharged.

SUMMARY

A crisis occurs when an individual experiences events perceived as threatening and for which coping skills are inadequate. Disorganization and anxiety develop as

Research Highlights

Tomlinson PS. Spousal differences in marital satisfaction during transition to parenthood. Nurs Res. 1987;36: 239–243.

The purpose of this study was "to determine if child-bearing had a significant impact on the marital relationship and to determine whether sex role attitudes, marital equity, father involvement and infant temperament influenced marital adjustment in new parents" (reference 11, p 239). Couples with a first pregnancy were included if the delivery and the baby were healthy. The sample consisted of 96 couples who completed both pre- and posttest questionnaires. Pretests were mailed one to two weeks after recruitment, and posttests were completed around the baby's 12th week. To control for joint responses, couples were asked to answer the questionnaires independently.

Significant findings suggested that the marital relationship before the birth had a strong influence on the marital adjustment during early parenthood.[11] Postbirth marital satisfaction was found to be significantly lower than pre-birth for both partners. It was also found that equal roles between husband and wife contributed to postbirth marital satisfaction. Sex role attitudes contributed minimally to the postbirth marital satisfaction. Traditional sex roles contributed negatively to the postbirth marital satisfaction for the women, but not for the men. Postbirth marital satisfaction for fathers was more positively influenced by marital equality than was that of the mothers. Infant temperament had little effect on postbirth marital satisfaction. The researchers attributed this to the young age of the infants. In general, the impact of parenthood on marriage was not severe for most of the couples.

The study describes factors that influence perception of changes during transition to parenthood. The factors described could be significant in identifying someone with a diagnosis of maturational crisis due to adjustment to parenthood. For example, a client experiencing problems in adjusting to parenthood might complain of dissatisfaction in the marital relationship or disturbance in roles.

the person struggles to cope. There are two kinds of crises: maturational, which occurs during developmental changes, and situational, which develops after a hazardous event. Goals for intervention include assisting the client to develop a realistic perception of the situation, adequate coping skills, and social supports. The outcome of a crisis may result in the individual functioning at a lower, at the same, or at a higher level than before the crisis. Every crisis presents the threat of disorganization or the challenge for growth. This is a valuable opportunity for the psychiatric nurse to effect change.

References

1. Aguilera DC, Messick JM. Crisis intervention: theory and methodology. 5th ed. St Louis: CV Mosby; 1986.
2. American Psychiatric Association. Diagnostic and statistical manual of mental disorders. 3rd ed, revised. Washington, DC: American Psychiatric Association; 1987.
3. Brownell MJ. The concept of crisis: its utility for nursing. Adv Nurs Sci. 1984;6(July):10–21.
4. Caplan G. Principles of preventive psychiatry. New York: Basic Books; 1964.
5. Dixon SL. Working with people in crisis: theory and practice. St Louis: CV Mosby; 1979.
6. Erikson EH. Childhood and society. New York: WW Norton; 1963.
7. Hagerty BK. Psychiatric-mental health assessment. St Louis: CV Mosby; 1984.
8. Hoff LA. People in crisis: understanding and helping. 2nd ed. Menlo Park, CA: Addison-Wesley Publishing; 1984.
9. Langsley DG, Kaplan DM. The treatment of families in crisis. New York: Grune & Stratton; 1968.
10. Lowery B. Stress research: some theoretical and methodological issues. Image: J Nurs Scholarship. 1987;19:42–46.
11. Tomlinson PS. Spousal differences in marital satisfaction during transition to parenthood. Nurs Res. 1987;36:239–243.

DECISIONAL CONFLICT

Annette M. O'Connor and Mary J. D'Amico

DEFINITION AND DESCRIPTION

Clients in primary, secondary, and tertiary psychiatric-care settings, like most people, often are faced with a need to make decisions or choose between alternative actions. Do I take the medication or not? Should I live at home or go out on my own? ECT or not? Which job opportunities should I pursue? Do I continue with this relationship? Which psychiatrist should I choose? Suicide or not? Families of clients have complementary decisions to make. Should I take my sister to the psychiatric emergency unit? Should I agree to take my son home after discharge from the inpatient psychiatric hospital? Do I consent to have my child receive this psychiatric treatment?

Decision making, according to Orem, is the first phase of deliberative self-care:

> Persons who can produce effective self-care have knowledge of themselves and of environmental conditions. They have also affirmed the appropriate thing to do under the circumstances. Before they could affirm the appropriate thing to do, they had to gain antecedent knowledge of the courses of action open to them and the effectiveness and desirability of these courses of action. Effective producers of self-care bring the first phase of self-care to closure by making a decision about the actions they will take and those they will avoid (reference 19, p 79).

Models for judging the effectiveness and desirability of alternative courses of action have been developed by economists and psychologists.[8] Although theorists disagree about the way individuals make or ought to make judgments and decisions, many agree that *expectations* and *values* are essential inputs.[21] Expectations and values correspond to Orem's concepts of effectiveness and desirability. Expectations are beliefs or subjective judgments about the likelihood of the consequences or outcomes of a course of action. Values or utilities are preferences for or the relative desirability of those outcomes. Values are preferences under conditions of certainty; utilities are preferences under uncertain or risky conditions and incorporate a person's attitude toward risk as well as desirability.

Generally, individuals are more likely to choose an alternative that makes desirable outcomes likely and undesirable outcomes unlikely; conversely, individuals are less likely to choose a course of action that makes undesirable outcomes likely or desirable outcomes unlikely. Unfortunately, many important decisions are likely to produce both desirable and undesirable outcomes. Moreover, the desirable outcomes may be divided among the alternatives. For example, Psychiatrist A is most knowledgeable, but Psychiatrist B has better interpersonal skills. Therefore, no single alternative will satisfy all objectives, and every alternative poses a risk of undesirable outcomes. These difficult decisions have been referred to as choice dilemmas[6] or conflicted decisions.[25] They are characterized by difficulty in identifying good alternatives, risk and uncertainty of outcomes, high stakes in terms of potential gains and losses, and the need to make value tradeoffs in selecting a course of action.[13] Janis and Mann describe decisional conflict as "the simultaneous opposing tendencies within the individual to accept and reject a given course of action" (reference 11, p 46).

In summary, decisional conflict (specify) is a state of uncertainty about course of action to be taken when choice among competing actions involves risk, loss, regret, or challenge to personal values. The "specify" component of the nursing diagnosis refers to the focus of the conflict; for example, choices regarding health, family relationships, career, finances, or other life events.

THEORY AND RESEARCH

The majority of decision-making research has focused on healthy individuals making everyday decisions[21] or on health professionals making clinical decisions.[2,5,29] The theoretical perspectives used differ widely, as discussed in the review of decision making and judgment theories by Hammond and associates,[8] and conclusions from these studies may not be generalizable to a client's health decisions, because judgments and decision processes differ with the type of decision being made.[21] Moreover, concurrent medical and psychiatric problems, emotional distress, and the added social influence of health professionals may make the problems clients experience in making decisions unique.

Little research has been conducted in clinical practice to examine the prevalence of decisional conflict experienced by clients in psychiatric or other clinical settings. The variation in responses to decisional conflict described by Janis and Mann[11] has received minimal attention. Hiltunen's[10] phenomenologic study with five clients in a home health setting supported the eti-

192

ology of loss and the symptoms of vacillation, stress, self-focusing, and diminished self-concept. Studies of life–death decisions made jointly by clients and clinicians or families demonstrated the difficulty these groups had in making decisions and the potential influence of expectations and values.[3,22] Basic work in methods of eliciting decisions from clients has been conducted by Llewellyn–Thomas, Holmes, O'Connor, Yoshida, and their coworkers[9,15–18,34] (O'Connor A, unpublished data). These investigators are extending their research to descriptive and prescriptive studies of clients' actual health decisions.

Buchanan, D'Amico, O'Connor, and Blenkarn are examining clients' decisions about suicide. Preliminary unpublished data revealed that individuals who seriously considered suicide and those who did not differed in their expectations and utilities for the outcomes of the decision alternatives. Compared with hospitalized clients who did not consider suicide, clients who seriously considered suicide had: (1) a higher expectation of dying if they were to attempt suicide; (2) a lower utility/value for their current functional state; and (3) a higher utility/value for death. These promising preliminary data need to be replicated with a prospective design and groups of clients in inpatient, outpatient, and emergency psychiatric settings before substantive conclusions can be drawn. The impact of therapeutic interventions such as cognitive therapy or decision therapy on changing expectations, utilities, suicide intentions, and behavior also need to be evaluated.

In summary, nursing studies of client decision making and decisional conflict are in the early stages of development. With better understanding of prevalence and etiology of the diagnosis, decisional conflict will evolve from a conceptual definition that is empirically validated in other contexts to a diagnosis that is scientifically grounded in health contexts.

RELATED FACTORS

Although responses to a difficult decision differ according to the perceived level of risk and the perceived magnitude of the loss and regret, other clinical, personal, and environmental factors exacerbate the perceived difficulty. Psychiatric disorders have a significant impact on the person's ability to make decisions. For example, cognitive functioning may be impaired by schizophrenia, mood disorders, or organic brain disease. Severe or extreme anxiety, which diminishes a person's ability to think clearly,[11] may make even simple decisions difficult. The psychiatric problem not only influences the degree of difficulty clients have with decisions but also creates new difficult decisions for the client. With new information about their state of health, clients usually have to consider how they are going to respond to the diagnosis and treatment or lifestyle advice given.

Inexperience with decision making or lack of information may contribute to the unclear or unrealistic perceptions about courses of action and their consequences, thereby magnifying the conflict. Hesitation in making a decision may also be influenced by a person's lack of the knowledge or skill needed to implement the decision once it is made. Social factors also influence the conflict experienced. The client may lack the requisite social support to implement the decision. Alternatively, the support network may interfere with the decision-making process by imposing views on the client. Health professionals can contribute to the difficulty by imposing their values and belief systems or by assuming control over decision making.

DEFINING CHARACTERISTICS

Clients experiencing a choice dilemma may demonstrate symptoms of hesitation, vacillation, or feelings of uncertainty about the course of action to take. They may express concern about the undesirable consequences of the choice facing them and question their personal values in their deliberation. Delayed decision making is a common response to difficult decision making. The client may be self-focused and manifest physiological signs of distress such as increased muscle tension and heart rate and restlessness. For some decisions, autonomic indicators of stress increase as subjects move toward a decision and gradually return to the resting state after the decision is made.[11]

Subjectively, clients may express feelings of distress. Responses differ according to the degree of conflict inherent in the decision. A low degree of conflict may be attractive and stimulating; a moderate degree may produce defensiveness, whereas a high degree may bring about hypervigilance and panic.[25] The intensity of stress symptoms depends in part on the perceived magnitude of the losses anticipated from whatever choice is made and the magnitude of anticipated regret over the positive aspects of the rejected options (Chart 1).

NURSING PROCESS AND RATIONALE
Assessment

Several guides have been developed to assess the qualitative nature of decisional conflict, including Janis and Mann's decisional balance sheet[11] and Pender's values clarification exercise.[20] The dimensions assessed include the client's personal goals, the perceived alternatives and their consequences, expectations, and values. These data are used by clinicians and clients to judge the source of the conflict; the clarity, comprehensiveness, and appropriateness of alternatives; the clarity and realism of the expectations; and the clarity of values and implicit tradeoffs. The comprehensiveness of data collection and the need for other contextual data will depend on the clinical context and time constraints. Some important parameters are:

CHART 1
Decisional Conflict: Definition, Related Factors, and Defining Characteristics

DEFINITION

Decisional conflict (specify) is a state of uncertainty about the course of action to be taken when choice among competing
  actions involves risk, loss, regret, or challenge to personal values (specify focus of the conflict; for example, choices
  regarding health, family relationships, career, finances, or other life events).

RELATED FACTORS

Interference with decision making
Lack of experience with decision making
Support system deficit
Lack of information about alternatives or their consequences
Unclear alternatives, expectations, and values while attempting decision making
Unrealistic alternatives or expectations
Threat to values
Lack of knowledge or skills to implement the decision made
Impaired cognitive functioning
Anxiety

DEFINING CHARACTERISTICS

Verbalization of feelings of distress related to uncertainty about choices
Verbalization of undesired consequences of alternative actions being considered
Vacillation between alternative choices
Delayed decision making
Questioning personal values and beliefs while attempting decision making
Self-focusing
Physical signs of distress or tension (increased muscle tension, restlessness, increased heart rate, etc.)

1. **Appearance.** Briefly note the client's apparent age, sex, race, and appearance and overt signs of distress or composure.
2. **Client's Perception of Problem.** Ask the client to describe the problem from his/her point of view. Validate impressions.
3. **Factors Contributing to Difficult Decision Making.** Ask the client to identify factors that may be making the decision difficult. As appropriate to the context, probe with questions regarding personal and environmental factors (knowledge, experience, support system, other social influences, personal resources) that are helping or hindering the decision making.
4. **Personal Goals and Perceived Alternatives.** What are the goals the client wishes to achieve? What, in the client's view, are the alternatives?
5. **Expectations.** From the client's point of view, what outcomes are possible with each alternative? How likely are these outcomes?
6. **Values/Utilities.** How desirable and undesirable are these outcomes? Ask client to rank order. Which outcome is the best, the next best, the worst?
7. **Resources to Implement Decisions.** Are there perceived difficulties implementing the alternatives? Does the client have the knowledge, motivation, and resources to implement the alternatives?

Quantitative approaches to eliciting expectations and values also have been developed,[6,14] and some have been tested for reliability, validity, and suitability for clinical practice[9,15–18] (O'Connor A, unpublished data). Many studies have illustrated the difficulties encountered in eliciting expectations and values.[7,12,30,31] Individuals' expectations or judgments about the likelihood of events do not always correspond with reality. People often tend to ignore what is known about the likelihood of event and base their expectations on the ease with which instances can be brought to mind (the availability bias) or on how similar an event is to the major characteristics of the population or process from which it is generated (the representativeness bias). Thus, clients will consider the hazards of taking recreational drugs to be less likely than the probabilities reported in the literature if they have never witnessed others experience these effects or if they consider themselves to be different from others.

Methodologic problems also exist when eliciting values.[7,12,27,30] Values are difficult to obtain for outcomes that are unfamiliar, complex, or not directly experienced. Dramatic preference reversals have occurred depending on whether the outcomes are framed positively or negatively, on whether risks involve gains or losses, on how much regret was expected, and on the reference point from which the person was stating a preference.[12,30] These problems make it difficult to get consistent answers about preferences. Slovic and associates[27] have stated that in value elicitation, "there may be no substitute for an interactive elicitation procedure, one that employs multiple methods and acknowledges the elicitor's role in helping the respondent to create and enunciate values.'' The need for quantitative assessment of expectations or values will depend on the need for refined judgments of probability and value tradeoffs and on the acceptability to clinicians and clients.

Nursing Diagnosis

The data collection is completed and the nursing diagnosis of decisional conflict is formulated when the following have been clarified and validated with the client: (1) the client is uncertain about which alternative to choose; (2) the choice that has to be made is identified; (3) the factors that make the decision difficult are noted; and (4) the contributory factors that are amenable to nursing interventions are identified. For example, if parents are having difficulty because of their anxiety in deciding whether to agree to medicate their child for attention deficit disorder, the nursing diagnosis would be decisional conflict (about medicating their child) related to extreme anxiety. If the parents are unsure about what to decide because they are unaware of treatment alternatives and the likely outcomes, the diagnosis would be decisional conflict (about medicating their child) related to knowledge deficit about alternatives and consequences. If the parents are aware of alternatives but have unrealistic expectations about the outcomes of various choices, the contributory factor would be unrealistic expectations rather than knowledge deficit.

Client Goals and Nursing Interventions

The expected outcome of decisional conflict intervention is that the client will make an effective decision. The difficulty in judging effectiveness is that there is no criterion for judging the correctness of a decision, because the decision is based, in part, on the opinions and preferences of the individual.[21] Some theorists have imposed a mathematical or logical structure on the decision that defines the consistency of a set of responses.[21] For example, expected utility theory provides a set of rules for combining expectations and utilities to determine the alternative with the highest expected value. Unfortunately, there is poor correspondence between decisions using mathematical models and intuitive decisions.[30]

Despite the difficulty in establishing criteria for effective decision making, some outcomes need to be specified to guide action. These criteria are based on the following assumptions:

■ People who have a clear understanding of the nature of the conflict make better decisions;
■ Informed decisions are better than uninformed decisions unless the client needs denial as a defense;
■ Decisions that are consistent with personal values are better than those that are inconsistent;

■ Decisions that are congruent with subsequent behavior are better than those that are not congruent.

Therefore, effective decisions will be defined as those that are informed, consistent with values, and congruent with behavior. An informed decision is one in which clients: (1) are aware of relevant alternatives and their outcomes; (2) have clarified expectations of outcomes that are reasonably aligned with reality; and (3) are aware of the nature of the conflict in the decision. Decisions are consistent with personal values when clients acknowledge the implicit tradeoffs that are made, select alternatives consistent with the priority ordering of preferences, and express satisfaction that they are clear about the alternative they need to choose and are convinced it is the best choice under the circumstances and at the time. The last criterion for an effective decision is that it is implemented (congruent with behavior). The client may change the decision later but at least attempts to implement the choice made.

Once client goals have been mutually established, interventions are selected to achieve those goals. Decision therapy is the process of assisting individuals to make effective decisions. Possible approaches range from unstructured counseling to the use of structured decision aids and are based on different theoretical perspectives on how decisions are or ought to be made.[1,8,14,21,33] An organized approach to examining the decision problem is useful in clarifying the individual's perception of the decision and the elements that make the decision difficult:[13,21]

1. Structure the problem by exploring personal objectives and corresponding attributes and generating proposed alternatives.
2. Assess the possible impact of the alternatives by determining the magnitude and likelihood of the possible outcomes (expectations). Compare client expectations with available knowledge.
3. Identify the client's preferences or values/utilities for the outcomes of each alternative. Identify value tradeoffs implicit in the decision.
4. Compare the alternatives and evaluate to determine the optimum preference.
5. Plan decision implementation and strategies for dealing with the consequences of the decision.

Part of this process begins in the assessment phase: data generated from the assessment represent a first approximation of the decision problem. It is subsequently revised by a two-way interaction where clinician and client fill gaps, clarify, and share expertise. Rothert and Talarczyk[23] outline the roles and expertise of the clinician and client when making decisions about following treatment regimens. For example, clinicians can provide information about the options available, the risk/probability of various outcomes, and the health care resources required and available. Client's expertise includes preferences or values and available personal, social, and economic resources. Control over who guides and who is involved (e.g., significant others) in the deliberation process should be dependent on the client's preference. For example, Degner and Aquino Russell[3] have found that clients can be classified into one of three profiles of preference for control: those who want to keep, share, or give away control for decision making. Depending on preferences, the client may guide the deliberation with clinician input on the scientific facts (for "keepers"), the guidance may be started by the clinician with input and final decision by the client (for "sharers"), or the clinician may adopt an advisory role with informed consent given by the client (for "givers away").

The specific interventions used in decision therapy depend on the data provided by the client in the first approximation of the decision problem and on the clinician's and client's judgment about how clear, complete, salient, accurate, and parsimonious the first approximation is. Goals, alternatives, or outcomes that are too narrow or incomplete are expanded. Options or outcomes that are too numerous are reduced to appropriate alternatives and salient outcomes. For areas in which information is lacking, the clinician or client provides the data or searches from an appropriate source. Unrealistic expectations are realigned with research data or conventional wisdom. Values are clarified using qualitative[8,18] or quantitative[14,16,28] methods.

Once clients have identified the appropriate alternatives, realistic expectations, and value tradeoffs, they are in a better position to make an informed decision consistent with their values. Following selection, the next step is to act on the decision. Orem refers to the operational phase of the decision as the second phase of self-care:

> The choice made sets the goal for phase two because it specifies what action will be taken. The questions raised by the self-care agent now include: How can I proceed in relation to my choice? What must I do? What resources do I need? Do I have them? Can I perform all actions correctly. . . . Will other duties interfere? How will I know I am proceeding correctly? What rules will I follow? How will I know I am getting . . . results. . . . Who can help me if I need help? (reference 19, p 81).

Some questions will be considered prior to choice, but rarely are all operational details planned. For the decision implementation phase, personal and environmental resources are evaluated. When deficits occur, the clinician may assist the client to acquire the necessary self-help skills and to mobilize the external resources as required.

The effectiveness of decision therapy or decision aids has had little evaluation. In a review of evaluated studies, Pitz and Sachs[21] concluded that some positive benefits have been found such as clarifying the problem, generating more alternatives through goal-oriented approaches, and recognizing the best action. One trial[26] of decision therapy to assist parents to reduce the ambivalence about medication for hyperactive children was not any more effective in reducing ambivalence than an information session between clinician and parent.

However, it was effective in making parents more aware of the importance of deliberating about their decision. Clearly, there is a need for more trials of decision therapies.

Evaluation

The outcomes of nursing intervention can be measured by the extent to which the client:

Identifies appropriate alternatives;
Expresses realistic expectations about the outcomes of alternatives;
Indicates the relative importance of each outcome;
Acknowledges the uncertainty and implicit tradeoffs inherent in the decision;
Selects a course of action consistent with expectations and values;
Acquires/uses knowledge and skills to implement the course of action;
Expresses satisfaction at having made the best decision under the circumstances.

Depending on clinician and client preferences, quantitative scales can be used to complement the qualitative evaluation of decision therapy[26] (O'Connor A, unpublished data).

A summary of the nursing process for the decisional conflict diagnosis is presented in Chart 2. The overall goal is for the client to make a decision that is informed, consistent with values and expectations, and congruent with behavior. Decision therapy is the nursing intervention and can involve exploring goals and alternatives, realigning expectations, clarifying values, facilitating alternative selection, and teaching or reinforcing self-help skills to implement the decision.

CASE STUDY

Brian D is a 21-year-old who has recently been admitted for the third time with the diagnosis of schizophrenia. Brian's previous discharge occurred 1 month ago. He stayed in a group home and functioned well until 2 weeks ago, when he stopped taking neuroleptic medications because of side effects. Over the next 2 weeks, he started hearing voices, which he described as God telling him to get people together to try to "save" them. He left the group home, ate little, was unkempt, and slept on the street. He roamed buses, telling people that he had come again to save them. Initially, he would leave a bus when requested to do so, but eventually, he refused to leave a bus, and he threatened the passengers who did not listen to him. The police were called, and he arrived handcuffed in the emergency department. After a few days of antipsychotic medication in the hospital, the voices and threatening behavior subsided. The primary nurse began to discuss plans for discharge with him. At that time, Brian expressed extreme ambivalence toward taking his medication once he went back to the group home. Excerpts from the interview include:

1. **Appearance.** 21-year-old Caucasian man well groomed and in no apparent distress.

> **CHART 2**
> **Decisional Conflict: Summary of the Nursing Process**
>
> | **NURSING INTERVENTIONS** | **OUTCOME CRITERIA** |
> |---|---|
> | **CLIENT GOAL: BE INFORMED ABOUT ALTERNATIVES AND CONSEQUENCES OF DECISION** | |
> | Clarify goals, alternatives, outcomes | Identifies appropriate alternatives |
> | Review other known alternatives and outcomes | Expresses realistic expectations |
> | Reduce to appropriate alternatives and salient outcomes | Identifies source of conflict |
> | Clarify expectations | |
> | Realign unrealistic expectations with reality | |
> | **CLIENT GOAL: UNDERSTAND THE VALUE TRADEOFFS IMPLICIT IN DECISION** | |
> | Clarify desirability of possible outcomes | Prioritizes outcomes |
> | Clarify priority of outcomes | Identifies implicit tradeoffs in making decision |
> | Explore implicit value tradeoffs in making a decision | |
> | **CLIENT GOAL: SELECT ALTERNATIVE CONSISTENT WITH EXPECTATIONS AND VALUES** | |
> | Facilitate alternative selection | Selects alternative most likely to achieve most important outcomes |
> | **CLIENT GOAL: IMPLEMENT DECISION** | |
> | Teach and reinforce self-help skills in order to implement decision | Acquires/uses skills to implement decision |
> | Explore strategies to deal with the consequences of the decision | |

2. **Client's Perception of Problem.**

   CLIENT: "I *hate* those medications. I feel so bad when I'm on them. But I also hate the voices. I get so scared and no one wants to be around me when they come."

   NURSE [validates]: "You don't know whether you should take the medication or not; you're finding it hard to decide."

   CLIENT: "Yes, that's it."

3. **Factors Contributing to Difficult Decision Making.**

   NURSE: "It is a hard decision to make. If you agree, we can discuss the things that make it hard for you to decide. Do you think that would be ok?"

   CLIENT: "OK."

4. **Goals and Perceived Alternatives.** After discussion, the client indicates that what he wants out of life is to be free of the voices and to feel physically well (free of side effects) so that he can get back with his family and function normally in a job and with his friends. The alternatives facing him are to take the medication or not.

5. **Expectations.**

   NURSE: "Let's begin by talking about what you think the advantages and disadvantages of taking and not taking medication are. If you took the medications, what would be the pluses and minuses of that choice?"

   CLIENT: "When I take the medications the voices go away, I'm not as scared, but then the side effects come back even on the lower doses. . . . I feel bad. . .dizzy . . . my neck gets stiff and I can't swallow . . . my mouth gets dry . . . I don't feel like myself."

   NURSE: "So taking the medication makes the voices go away and you're less scared, but it also makes you feel bad from the side effects."

   CLIENT: "Yeah."

   NURSE: "Have I left anything out?"

   CLIENT: "No."

   NURSE: "If you didn't take the medication, what would be the pluses and minuses of that choice?"

   CLIENT: "I wouldn't have the side effects so I would feel all right that way . . . the voices might come back and scare me . . . and my family and friends wouldn't want anything to do with me. But maybe it won't happen this time. God will take care of me, and it won't be as bad."

   NURSE: "So from your point of view, not taking the medication means no side effects but the voices may come back and people you care about avoid you . . . or the voices may not come back because God will take care of you."

   CLIENT: "Yes."

   NURSE: "Any other points about not taking medication?"

   CLIENT: "No."

6. **Values/Utilities.**

   NURSE: "I guess there are two kinds of feeling bad you experience: feeling bad from the side effects and feeling bad from the voices and your friends' and family's avoidance. Do you know which one is worse for you: the side effects or the voices and being avoided?"

   CLIENT: "I don't know. I hate both of them."

   The decision appears to involve making tradeoffs between dysfunction from side effects and dysfunction from hearing voices. Eliciting priorities or tradeoffs is deferred until expectations are realigned with reality.

   NURSE: "I've listed the pluses and minuses of the decision you have to make. Maybe we can look these over together. We can review what you can realistically expect from selecting each alternative and explore how important each of these advantages and disadvantages is to you. Then maybe the best decision for you will be clearer to you."

The decision facing Brian caused conflict because he stood to lose whatever alternative he chose. The decision was made more difficult by his unclear preferences about the importance of dysfunction of side effects vs dysfunction from hearing voices. His expectations about the consequences of not taking the medication were unrealistic because of magical thinking ("God will take care of me"). The specific nursing diagnosis that was formulated was decisional conflict (about taking medications) related to unclear preferences concerning side effects vs voices and unrealistic expectations concerning ability to manage without medications.

The first client goal to be formulated was that Brian would have realistic expectations about decision alternatives. The primary nurse's initial intervention to meet this goal was to reaffirm the appropriateness of the alternatives Brian had identified and his realistic expectations of what would happen if he took the medication. Next, the nurse realigned Brian's expectation that God would take care of him if he did not take the medication. For example, the nurse asked him if God had taken care of him when he stopped his medication before. Eventually, Brian was able to verbalize realistic expectations concerning the consequences of not taking the medication.

The second client goal was that Brian would select an alternative consistent with his values. The intervention was to clarify Brian's priority of outcomes (dys-

Research Highlights

Few studies have examined the diagnosis of decisional conflict or evaluated decision therapies to deal with it. Slimmer and Brown[26] evaluated decision therapy with parents in the process of deciding to medicate their children for attention deficit disorder–hyperactivity prior to entry in a clinical trial. One of the study objectives was to determine whether decision therapy increased parents' positive attitudes toward the decision. A pretest–post-test experimental design was used in which parents were randomized to receive decision therapy using Janis and Mann's[11] decisional balance sheet or a control conference in which the parents were given information about the medication but were not given guidance in making a decision. The 1-hour decision therapy session used Janis and Mann's six-step hierarchical process,[11] in which parents initially discuss the alternatives available to them and finally rank order their decision alternatives. Semantic differential scales were used as pretest and post-test instruments to assess parental attitudes toward stimulant drug administration. Positive attitudes were measured along three dimensions: (1) personal assurance that the decision is the best possible one at this time (evaluative dimension); (2) expectations for positive consequences of the decision (activity dimension); and (3) belief that the decision is relevant and worth deliberation (potency dimension). Decision therapy was found to increase positive beliefs that the decision is relevant and worth deliberating but had no impact on personal assurance and expectations. The investigators concluded that the intervention has the potential of making parents aware of their ambivalence and of the need to deliberate but does not necessarily get them to engage in the actual decision.

This study is an important beginning to the evaluation of decision therapy. It should be replicated in a variety of decision contexts with the following improvements in design to rule out possible biases that may have influenced the results:

1. Evaluation of therapy should take place in a treatment setting to rule out the effect of parents about to be entered in a drug trial.

2. The preference for control over decision making and ambivalence or degree of decisional conflict should be assessed before intervention, and subjects should be stratified according to these factors. Analyses should be conducted to test the relative impact of therapy on each subgroup.

3. The sample size should be increased. There were as few as four subjects per cell, and therefore the power to detect important differences may have been too low. As a corollary, an important difference in scores should be designated a priori.

4. The instruments need validity testing and reliability testing for repeated measurement. Other scaling methods should be tried. Other variables can be measured: perceived clarity of the uncertainty, tradeoffs, alternatives and conflict, and perceived clarity of the action the client believes should be taken.

5. The length and type of decision therapy should be tested (e.g., one vs multiple sessions; therapies that use different strategies to realign expectations, explore implicit tradeoffs, or plan to deal with the consequences of decisions).

More basic studies also are needed to understand the manifestations and etiology of difficult health decisions and to evaluate possible therapies. Potential research questions that can be posed include:

- How frequently do clients select various decision alternatives?
- To what extent do expectations, values, and other factors discriminate between, predict, and explain clients' selection of different alternatives?
- What proportion of clients experience conflict in making the decision?
- What factors predict and explain the decisional conflict?
- How efficacious are decision therapies in promoting effective decision making?

function from medication vs dysfunction from disease) and to clarify the value tradeoffs implicit in the decision. Brian realized the decision involved making tradeoffs between the severity of side effects and the severity of disease symptoms. After careful reflection, he came to the conclusion that the side effects of treatment were worse than the symptoms of his disease. He admitted that he may change his priorities once he starts experiencing symptoms of the disease again.

The final client goal was for Brian to plan decision implementation. He planned to cut down on his medication while in the hospital in case he changed his mind. The primary nurse also assisted Brian to explore strategies for dealing with the consequences of his decision once he was discharged from the hospital.

SUMMARY

Decisional conflict is a state of uncertainty about a course of action to be taken when choices among alternatives involve risk, loss, regret, or challenge to personal life values. The magnitude of the conflict experienced can be influenced by impaired cognitive functioning, emotional distress, social interference, or social support deficit. Unclear alternatives, expectations, or values or unrealistic expectations may enhance vacillation or hesitation in making a decision. Diagnostic assessment involves finding out from the client what makes the decision difficult. The client's personal goals are elicited, as well as the perceived alternatives, expectations, values, and resources to implement the alternatives. From these data, the nature of the conflict and contributing factors are specified in a diagnostic statement. The overall goal is that the client select and implement a course of action that is consistent with expectations and values. Decision therapy is then tailored to the particular contributing factors. Therapeutic strategies may include exploring alternatives, realigning expectations, clarifying values, and facilitating selection of an alternative. Plans are made to deal with the consequences of the decision. Decisional conflict is a recent addition to the taxonomy of nursing diagnoses and requires scientific investigation to understand better the prevalence of the problem, the factors that explain and predict the problem, and the efficacy of interventions designed to promote effective decision making.

References

1. Beach LR, Wise JA. Decision emergence: a Lewinian perspective. Acta Psychol. 1980;45:343–356.
2. Benner P, Tanner C. How expert nurses use intuition. Am J Nurs. 1987;87:23–31.
3. Degner LF, Aquino Russell C. Preferences for treatment control among adults with cancer. Res Nurs Health. 1988;11:367–374.
4. Degner LF, Beaton J. Life–death decisions in health care. Washington DC: Hemisphere Publications; 1987;34–85; 144–54.
5. Dowie J, Ellstein A, eds. Professional judgment. New York: Cambridge University Press; 1988.
6. Fischer G. Utility models for multiple objective decisions: do they accurately represent human preferences? Decis Sci. 1979;10:451–479.
7. Fischhoff B, Slovic P, Lichtenstein S. Knowing what you want: measuring labile values. In: Wallsten TS, ed. Cognitive processes in choice and decision behaviour. Hillsdale, New Jersey: Laurence Erlbaum; 1980.
8. Hammond KR, McClelland GH, Mumpower J. Human judgment and decision making. New York: Praeger Publishing; 1980.
9. Holmes MM, Rothert ML, Rovner DR, Elstein AS, Hoppe RB, Metheny WA. Comparison of physicians vs. premenopausal women in importance ascribed to potential outcomes of estrogen replacement therapy [Abstract]. Clin Res. 1984; 32:648.
10. Hiltunen E. Decisional conflict: a phenomenological description from the points of view of the nurse and client. In: McLane A, ed. Classification of nursing diagnoses: proceedings of the Seventh Conference. St Louis, CV Mosby; 1987.
11. Janis IL, Mann L. Decision making. New York: The Free Press; 1977.
12. Kahneman D, Tversky A. The psychology of preferences. Science. 1982;246:160–171.
13. Keeney RL. Decision analysis: an overview. Operations Res. 1982;30:803–838.
14. Keeney RL, Raiffa H. Decisions with multiple objectives: preferences and value tradeoffs. Toronto: John Wiley & Sons; 1976:369–70; 506.
15. Llewellyn–Thomas HA, Sutherland HJ, Tibshirani R, Ciampi A, Till JE, Boyd NF. The measurement of patients' values in medicine. In: Dowie J, Ellstein A, eds. Professional judgment: a reader in clinical decision making. New York: Cambridge University Press; 1988:395–408.
16. Llewellyn–Thomas HA, Sutherland HJ. Procedures for value assessment. In: Cahoon MC, ed. Recent advances in nursing: research methodology. Edinburgh: Churchill Livingstone; 1987:169–85.
17. O'Connor A. Effects of framing and level of probability on patient's preferences for cancer chemotherapy. J Clin Epidemiol. 1989;42:119–126.
18. O'Connor A, Boyd NF, Tritchler DL, Kriukov Y, Sutherland H, Till J. Eliciting preferences for alternative cancer drug treatments: the influence of framing, medium, and rater variables. Med Decis Making. 1985;5:453–463.
19. Orem DE. Nursing: concepts of practice. Ed 2. Toronto: McGraw-Hill; 1980.
20. Pender NJ. Health promotion in nursing practice. Ed 2. Norwalk, Connecticut: Appleton & Lange; 1987:159–83.
21. Pitz GF, Sachs NJ. Judgment and decision: theory and application. Ann Rev Psychol. 1984;35:139–163.
22. Rostain A. Deciding to forgo life-sustaining treatment in the intensive care nursery: a sociologic account. Persp Biol Med. 1986;30:117–134.
23. Rothert ML, Talarczyk GJ. Patient compliance and the decision-making process of clinicians and patients. J Compliance Health Care. 1987;2:55–71.
24. Schoemaker PJH. The expected utility model: its variants, purposes, evidence, and limitations. In: Paelinck JHP, Vossen PH, eds. The quest for optimality. New York: Gower Publishing; 1984:70–111.
25. Sjoberg L. To smoke or not to smoke: conflict or lack of differentiation? In: Humphreys P, Svenson O, Vari A, eds. Analyzing and aiding decision processes. New York: North-Holland; 1983.
26. Slimmer LW, Brown RT. Parents' decision making process in

medication administration for control of hyperactivity. J Sch Health. 1985;55:221–225.

27. Slovic P, Fischhoff B, Lichtenstein S. Response mode, framing, and information-processing effects in risk assessment. In: Hogarth R, ed. New directions for methodology of social and behavioural science: Question framing and response consistency. San Francisco: Jossey-Bass; 1982.

28. Sox HC, Blatt MA, Higgins MC, Marton KI. Medical decision making. Boston: Butterworths; 1988.

29. Tanner C. Research on clinical judgement. In: Holzemer W, ed. Review of research in nursing education. Thorofare, New Jersey, Slack; 1983:2–31.

30. Tversky A, Kahneman D. The framing of decisions and the psychology of choice. Science. 1981;211:453–458.

31. Tversky A, Kahneman D. Judgment under uncertainty: heuristics and bias. In: Kahneman D, Slovic P, Tversky A, eds. Judgment under uncertainty: heuristics and biases. New York: Cambridge University Press; 1982.

32. Weinstein MC, Fineberg HV. Clinical decision analysis. Toronto: WB Saunders; 1980.

33. Wilson CZ, Alexis M. Basic frameworks for decisions. In: Koontz H, O'Donnell C, eds. Management: a book of readings. Ed 3. Toronto: McGraw-Hill; 1972.

34. Yoshida M, Kalnins I. Children's health decision making: making the healthiest choice possible. Proceedings of the 12th World Conference on Health Education, Dublin, Ireland; 1986:131.

DEFENSIVE COPING

(SPECIFY)

Margaret I. Fitch and Linda-Lee O'Brien-Pallas

DEFINITION AND DESCRIPTION

Defensive coping refers to the overuse of defense mechanisms to protect the individual against feelings of anxiety, threat or frustration. *Defense mechanisms* are mental processes, usually occurring unconsciously, that serve as an armor for the individual's sense of self.[12,14,15,29] All defense mechanisms include some degree of self-deception and distortion of reality and, at times, may seem irrational.

It is not the use of the defense mechanisms per se, but rather the type, frequency, and rigidity of their use that may be problematic. The mechanisms are integral to both normal and abnormal behavior—operating in everyone at times. They become pathologic when they cause the individual to lose contact with reality. In less extreme situations, they may contribute to inability to problem solve effectively, to ineffectiveness in learning new coping behaviors, or to ineffectiveness in carrying out normal roles and responsibilities.

THEORY AND RESEARCH

Observation of the process of coping has shown that individuals differ in their response to stress. Coping strategies are selected to serve two fundamental purposes: managing or altering the problem (event) perceived to be causing the distress and regulating the emotional response to the problem.[18] The former are called *problem-focused coping* and the latter are called *emotion-focused coping*. The five main coping modes identified by Cohen and Lazarus include information-seeking, direct action, inhibition of action, intrapsychic processes, and turning to others for support.[11] These modes may well serve purposes of both problem solving and emotion regulation. Currently, little is known about which particular individual will select which particular strategy or combination of strategies in any given situation. Individuals may select the same strategies for a variety of different situations and yet may select different strategies for the same situation at different times.[13,17,27] Persons tend to perceive events and behave in ways that reinforce their self-concept and self-esteem.[24,28] An event appraised as harmful or frustrating to the self will evoke defensive-coping strategies to protect what is important to the individual and defend against a painful experience.

Defense mechanisms that are enacted to defend or protect against anxiety and reduce distress involve some degree of self-deception and distortion of reality. They may be classified as *escape techniques* or *compromise techniques*.[12] The former enable an individual to escape or avoid the situation that generates anxiety, whereas the latter involve changing the situation in some way. Escape techniques include repression, denial, fantasy, and regression. Compromise techniques include, among others, rationalization, projection, sublimation, and displacement (Table 13-5).

Defense mechanisms are employed by everyone at one time or another to deal with life's events. Although the mechanisms can appear irrational, they can serve useful purposes for the individual using them. During crises that would overwhelm or disable, the use of defense mechanisms assists in gaining time to gather strength, maturity, and knowledge to manage the situation realistically and constructively.[16] The literature abounds with descriptions of how individuals use defense mechanisms (including fantasy, projection, denial) to deal with life's events.[7,8,19,20,25] Crisis literature particularly underscores defense mechanisms as vital in helping individuals deal with such events as severe burns, quadriplegia, the death of a child, or the diagnosis of cancer.[10,16,21,23]

Although defense mechanisms may be helpful in protecting the individual from overwhelming, unpleasant feelings (particularly on a short-term basis), they can close the cognitive field to further input. They may not allow further cognitive appraisal as new information that could reduce the sense of threat attributed to the event becomes available. The use of these mechanisms can be described as inappropriate when the emotional response (1) prevents seeking and cooperating with treatment for illness, (2) interferes with everyday functioning, (3) evokes behaviors that cause more pain and distress than the event itself, or (4) evokes responses that appear as conventional psychiatric symptoms.

Defense mechanisms were first described by Sigmund Freud in 1894.[14] He identified defenses as major means of managing instinct and affect, as unconscious, as discrete from one another, as reversible and adaptive, as well as pathologic. After World War II, as nor-

TABLE 13–5
Defense mechanisms: types, definition, and examples

TYPE	DEFINITION	EXAMPLE
Compensation	An individual makes up for a felt lack in one area by emphasizing strengths in another	A student who feels devoid of athletic ability becomes an outstanding member of the debating team
Denial	Failure to acknowledge the reality of an anxiety-producing situation	A woman ignores behavior changes in her husband that would indicate to others that he is having an affair
Displacement	Shifting of feelings from an emotionally charged person or object to a substitute, less threatening, person or object	A nurse becomes angry with a second nurse for not helping her; later, the second nurse berates a family member for asking too many questions
Dissociation	Temporary but drastic modification of character or sense of personal identity to avoid emotional distress	A soldier, fearful of leading his patrol into enemy territory and not wanting to acknowledge cowardice, becomes unable to remember where he is
Fantasy	Symbolic wish fulfillment with nonrational thought	A young boy, unable to protect his mother from his father's abuse, daydreams of singlehandedly killing a herd of wild animals that surround his home, thereby saving the family
Identification	Internalizing the characteristics of an idealized person	A young woman has high regard for her aunt and chooses to become a nurse just like her
Intellectualization	Reasoning or logic is used in an attempt to avoid confrontation with an objectionable impulse or affect	A man deals with intellectual formulations about the nature of death and the thoughts of various philosophers and scientists on the subject rather than the personally relevant feelings about his father's recent death
Introjection	Taking on another person's ego and becoming like that other person	A young child incorporates the personality of an adult and actually behaves like one
Isolation	Splitting of affect from the rest of a person's thinking	When a man who had been angry with his father (yet also loved him) hears of his father's death, he acknowledges the death, but deals with it in a mechanical way—he prevents himself from having feelings about the event
Projection	False attribution of the person's own undesirable feelings, thoughts, and impulses to others	A client states that a coworker does not like her, as a projection of her own dislike for the coworker
Rationalization	Finding logical or acceptable, but incorrect, reasons or excuses for behavior that is unacceptable to one's self-image	A college student who has low grades because of careless study habits rationalizes that he could have good grades if he had different instructors
Reaction formation	Substitution of behavior, thoughts and feelings diametrically opposed to unacceptable ones	A man who finds his sexual impulses unacceptable adopts puritanical beliefs and totally devotes himself to fighting pornography
Regression	Return to an earlier, more comfortable level of development	A child upset by the arrival of a new sibling may return to thumb-sucking or bed-wetting
Repression	Involuntary exclusion from consciousness of those ideas, feelings, and situations that are unacceptable to the self	After a painful interpersonal experience, the individual involved cannot recall his part in the interaction
Sublimation	Establishment of a secondary goal that an individual can satisfy in place of a primary goal that is socially unacceptable or physically impossible	A teenager with strong aggressive tendencies gains social acceptance through sports
Suppression	Voluntary exclusion from level of thought of those feelings and situations that produce discomfort and some anxiety	A student with a poor report card "forgets" to give it to his parents for their signature
Undoing	A person symbolically acts out in reverse something unacceptable that has already been done	A man, raised to believe sex is immoral and dirty, relieves his sexual desires from time to time by masturbating; afterward, feeling tremendous guilt, he tries to undo the way he has fouled his hands (by touching his genitals) and develops a compulsion to wash his hands over and over

mal populations were studied, the need for a hierarchy of defense mechanisms and relative psychopathology emerged. Many defenses were being described, but a common nomenclature or classification system did not exist.[6] Defenses were effective in "repressing" conflict and in "denying" stress, but the individual defenses differed in the diagnoses associated with their use and the implications for long-term biopsychosocial adaptation.

A major contribution to classifying defenses was made by Vaillant, who hypothesized a four-level hier-archy of defenses. His 30-year study of psychologically healthy men[33] illustrated that these men tended to progress through the ego function levels during the course of their lifetimes. His 12-year follow-up of heroin addicts[32] suggests patients tend to recover sequentially through these levels.

The first, most disturbed, level includes the "narcissistic" or "psychotic" mechanisms of denial of external reality, delusional projection, and distortion. These can be found in dreams, in young children, and in psychosis; the psychotic defenses rarely respond to simple psychological intervention. The second level is characterized by immature mechanisms, such as schizoid fantasy, projection, passive–aggressive behaviors, and acting out. Immature defenses externalize responsibility and allow individuals with personality disorders to refuse help. These mechanisms rarely respond to verbal interpretation, but rather, require supportive confrontation and alteration (rendering the individual less angry or lonely). The third level includes mechanisms of intellectualization, repression, reaction formation, displacement, and dissociation. These defenses are common to the psychopathology of everyday life, and they manifest themselves clinically as phobias, obsessions, compulsions, and somatization. Usually, they create more problems for the individual experiencing them than for others and are responsive to interpretation. The fourth, most healthy level comprises "mature" mechanisms: sublimation, altruism, suppression, anticipation, and humor. Although they still distort reality and alter feelings and relationships, they do so with "grace and flexibility." Empirical evidence has shown that people who deploy these mechanisms are happier and enjoy better mental health and more gratifying personal relationships than do individuals who use immature defense mechanisms.[2,5,15,33]

With the tendency of ego psychological models to describe hierarchical approaches to coping and defense, some processes are automatically considered superior to others.[14,22] The idea exists that a person has coped with the situation and met the demands successfully or a person has defended and coped ineffectively. According to Lazarus and Folkman, this hierarchical assumption should be abandoned and, instead, the effectiveness of strategies should be considered for each person individually.[18]

> No one strategy is considered inherently better than another. The goodness (efficacy, appropriateness) of a strategy is determined only by its effects in the long term (reference 18, p 134).

Confronting life's events, whether anticipated or unexpected, may well evoke the use of defensive mechanisms to protect against anxiety and reduce emotional pressures. When individuals are uncertain about possessing the abilities to cope with a particular event, they may experience a growing sense of threat, harm, or fear. Defensive mechanisms can provide avenues for escaping the reality of the event or altering the event in some way. Issues may arise when the use of these defense mechanisms is exaggerated or extreme and interferes with required problem solving and everyday functioning.

RELATED FACTORS

Whether or not an event is appraised as anxiety generating or threatening is a function of both environmental and personal factors. Regardless of whether the event is real, anticipated, or imagined, or the appraisal is realistic or unrealistic, the coping behaviors are based on the meaning assigned to the event by the individual. Events that occur suddenly or that are perceived to be unpredictable, uncontrollable, or ambiguous present a greater sense of threat than do those without these characteristics. If the event impinges upon ideas or goals that are important to the individual, the appraisal of threat will be heightened. Any event that demands loss or change may evoke feelings of threat or anxiety. Feelings of loss may accompany the predictable transitions in life (e.g., adolescence, marriage, birth of a child, retirement, dying) as well as the unpredictable events (e.g., birth defect, suicide of a family member, traffic accident, job loss). In particular, illness may elicit feelings of vulnerability and threat.

The individual's level of knowledge, skills, and abilities for any particular event will influence feelings of threat. An appraisal of harm or threat is assigned when an individual believes that his or her coping resources are not sufficient to meet demands created by a particular situation. If a similar situation occurred in the past, the previous experience will provide the frame of reference regarding the ability to manage it. Evidence is also accumulating that an individual's social support (sense of being cared for) has an influence on feelings of distress.[1,3,4] The capabilities to deal with uncertainty, to maintain motivation, to cope, and to maintain an emotional balance are also considered important personal factors.[10] In general, ego strength and increased self-esteem reduce vulnerability to stress.[18]

More specifically, Bond and associates[5] used factor analysis to demonstrate empirically a positive relationship between adaptive (mature) defenses and maturity in ego development. Vaillant and associates[30] provided evidence that defensive style (a cluster of defense mechanisms evidenced in an individual across a range of specific acts) is an enduring and important facet of personality development, although specific defenses may be used more-or-less frequently during times of crises and different stages of psychosocial development. In the growth of the adolescent toward adulthood, defensive styles mature. However, fatigue, alcohol, organic brain disease, and certain mental illnesses will shift an individual's defenses toward less mature styles. Childhood environment, sex, culture, and social class do not seem to influence the development of mature defenses. Although further work is needed, Vaillant suggests the significant variation in the development and use of mature defense mechanisms likely depends on person–situation interactions. Preliminary work points out the importance of social support in affecting the maturity of individuals and vice versa.[26,33]

According to Bond and Vaillant,[6] linking defenses with specific illnesses can create confusion. They suggest defenses should refer to a style of dealing with conflict and stress, whereas diagnosis (illness) should refer to a constellation of symptoms and signs. If the examination of defenses were separate from the issue of diagnosis (illness), they maintain, that would allow much more precision to be awarded to the fluctuations in a person's style as that individual deals with a particular stress, at a particular point in time, under particular circumstances, and with a particular level of psychosocial development. As an individual's circumstances change, changes may become evident in the use of different defense mechanisms. The work by Bond and Vaillant[6] suggests that defense style and diagnosis may be two independent dimensions. Within a psychiatric patient sample, no DSM-III diagnosis was associated with the use of any particular number or type of defense style, except for those with affective disorders. The patients with affective disorders resembled the control group in their responses. The study provides support for the notion that people with the same diagnosis can use very different defense styles. On the other hand, Vaillant and Drake[31] found that two thirds of a sample of 74 men with personality disorders primarily used immature mechanisms. Projection, fantasy, and hypochondriasis were particularly common in the most severely psychosocially impaired men. Conversely, altruism and suppression were rarely identified in these men.

DEFINING CHARACTERISTICS

The nursing diagnosis of defensive coping applies to the individual who overuses the mental mechanisms of defense to protect against anxiety. In general, ineffective coping may be evidenced by ineffective problem-solving abilities and impairment of adaptive behaviors.[9] Individuals may express feelings of not being able to cope with the current situation, but many may not be able to ask for help. Obvious problems may be denied to reduce the anxiety associated with acknowledging their presence. Individuals may use grandiose behaviors or project fears and responsibilities to others. In an attempt to control anxiety, they may uncharacteristically overuse food, cigarettes, drugs, or alcohol. Furthermore, they may express feelings of inability to meet role expectations, or even their basic needs.

More particularly, individuals may delay seeking assistance for obvious problems, to the detriment of either health or well-being. Problems or issues that are identified by others are not perceived as having personal relevance, or their impact is minimized. Individuals can hold a distorted view of themselves, their abilities, and their role(s) in specific situations. There may be evidence of a high need for social approval, but discomfort with intimacy and self-disclosure. There may be an inability to acknowledge personal failures or having certain thoughts, feelings, and impulses. There is evidence of difficulty in testing reality and difficulty in establishing and maintaining personal relationships. In therapeutic environments, lack of participation in therapy, lack of follow through, and self-neglect have been reported.

Additionally, each defense mechanism has its own unique set of defining characteristics. As an example, individuals with life-threatening illness (e.g., cancer) may deny the knowledge or meaning of the illness and delay seeking medical attention. The clients may not perceive the personal relevance of any symptoms or any danger. They may use home remedies to relieve the discomfort and minimize what symptoms they have. The source of the discomfort may be attributed to an organ other than the one involved with cancer. These individuals do not admit the impact of the disease in their life or admit fear of death or of invalidism. They make dismissive gestures when speaking of distressing events, or change the topic. They displace the fear of the impact of their conditions and display inappropriate affect.

In contrast, individuals attempting to protect against a negative self-image may project a falsely positive image. They may deny obvious weaknesses or problems and project blame and responsibility for problems on to others. They are hypersensitive to slight criticism and rationalize any failures. They project a heightened sense of their capabilities (grandiosity) and may display a superior attitude toward others. They may engage in hostile laughter and ridicule others and have difficulty maintaining relationships (Chart 1).

NURSING PROCESS AND RATIONALE
Assessment

The first step in assessing an individual's use of defensive strategies is to gather data on the environment–person interaction. Are the behavioral, cognitive, and emotional strategies accomplishing what the individual wants without undue harm to self or others?

The data collected for clinical assessment will depend, in large measure, upon the context of the situation. Important areas for data collection are listed below, and may take several interviews to complete. Ultimately the goal of assessment is to determine if the individual's coping resources fit with the demands of the event and whether the person's desired goals are met. The key aspect of the assessment is understanding the meaning assigned to the event by the individual and the purpose served by the defensive coping strategies. The environment must be supportive and nonjudgmental for the data to emerge successfully.

AREAS TO BE ASSESSED

The Nature of the Situation (Event)
- Determine the specific event at issue
- Assess the event for its unexpectedness, predictability, controllability, duration
- Assess the potential for harm or threat (especially to functional self-esteem)
- Determine the demands created by the event

The Individual
- Appearance: briefly note apparent age, sex, ease of deportment, and overt signs of distress or composure
- Perception of the event: ask the individual to explain in his or her own words the perception of the

CHART 1
Defensive Coping: Definition, Related Factors, and Defining Characteristics

DEFINITION
Defensive coping is the overuse of mental mechanisms as a defense against the emotional discomfort of anxiety.

RELATED FACTORS
Demands of an event on individual exceed the individual's coping resources
Unexpected loss of person, object, functional capacity, or expected life span
Lack of ego strength or ego development
Threat to values and goals
Previous stressful experiences with similar events
Mood disorders or other psychoses
Exacerbation of existing health problem
Emergence of a new health problem
Accumulation of stressful life events
Unavailable social support

DEFINING CHARACTERISTICS
Distortion of reality or sense of self/abilities
Inability to ask for help
Inability to problem solve effectively
Denial of obvious problems or of personal relevance of problems
Delay in seeking help for obvious problems
Projection of fears or responsibilities to others
Rationalization of personal failures
Grandiosity or heightened sense of abilities
Inability to meet usual role expectations or basic needs
Dramatic increase in use of drugs, alcohol, food, cigarettes
Difficulty in testing reality
Inability to establish close relationships
Lack of participation in therapy and follow-through
Inappropriate affect

situation as it is experienced, and the "assigned" meaning to the event (e.g., How much discomfort is felt? How much harm or threat?)

- Coping resources: ask the individual to describe the ability to manage this type of situation; what are seen as important goals or objectives; what he or she did in the past when there was a feeling of discomfort
- Self-concept: ask the individual to describe sense of self (e.g., How do you feel about yourself? What can you do? What do you want to achieve?)

The Context of the Interaction
- Determine individual's past experiences with similar events (Has this type of event happened before? What did the individual do?)
- Determine social supports in existence (supportive, tangible)

- Assess the individual's ability to deal with uncertainty, motivation to cope, usual coping patterns, knowledge, and abilities
- Identify what other events are occurring at the same time
- Identify if there is a discrepancy between self-ideal and perceived self in the current situation

Coping Strategies and Outcome
- Identify the emotional, behavioral, and cognitive responses to the event and what purpose they serve for the individual (problem solving, emotion controlling)
- Assess if the desired outcomes are achieved (Is the client feeling more comfortable?)
- Assess the skills possessed by the client
- Assess the communication patterns and their effectiveness
- Assess the effectiveness of interactions with others

Having identified if the use of defensive coping strategies is effective, it is valuable to study the particular use the individual has for defense mechanisms. What does the individual gain from the use of defense mechanisms? The nurse's subsequent clinical judgment reflects whether there is inappropriate use or overuse of defense mechanisms. Care must be taken to ensure that the nurse's judgment incorporates what purpose the defense serves for the individual. The client's use of specific defenses may not be personally desirable to the nurse, but they may serve a useful purpose to the client. If the mechanisms are serving a desired purpose for the client, careful consideration precedes any intervention to alter the use of the defense mechanisms. Any attempt to interfere with the client's use of defense mechanisms will undoubtedly cause the individual to experience increased tension and anxiety.

Nursing Diagnosis

The diagnostic category, defensive coping, can be made more specific for a particular client by including the type(s) of defense mechanisms in use and the related factors. An example would be: defensive coping (intellectualization) related to accumulation of stressful life events.

Client Goals and Nursing Interventions

Defense mechanisms are used to regain or maintain a sense of balance or well-being in the face of threat or actual harm. In particular, a person wants to feel a reduction in anxiety and a movement toward a desired goal without undue cost. The major issue is the lack of criteria for describing effective use of defense mechanisms. Effectiveness in their use will be different for different individuals.[18] In part, effectiveness is defined on the basis of personal opinion and preferences of the individual, but this must be balanced against any harm that might occur to self or others. In each situation, the efficacy (appropriateness) of the defensive strategies must be evaluated for the person concerned within the particular situation. In one situation, it may be very important for the individual to maintain a stance of denial and avoidance, whereas in another, that same strategy creates additional difficulties for the individual or for others.

For the client with defensive coping, the nurse plans interventions with two goals in mind. The first goal is to avoid increasing feelings of anxiety or threat for the client unnecessarily. The second goal is to be alert for indications that there is a readiness on the part of the client to decrease the use of defense mechanisms and to utilize that readiness to assist the individual to move in the desired direction.

Fundamentally, nursing interventions are based on a clear understanding of why the client is exhibiting particular behaviors. In general, interventions can be directed toward reducing the sense of harm or stress and the related emotions, where this is possible, and increasing the perception of strength in coping resources.[9] The nurse needs to be a careful observer and assessor as well as an active listener and supporter. Initially, in light of overwhelming threat, the individual will strive to protect the self-concept (image, integrity). Nursing interventions focus on preserving the person's integrity and, at the same time, deal with the behavior the client is using (e.g., denial, intellectualization). The nurse must seek to reduce the stressful aspects of a situation and to gently correct any misconceptions.

When the client exhibits readiness to move away from the closed cognitive stance of defensive coping, the nurse adjusts to the client's pace. The process of helping with and supporting adaptation involves exploring realistic interpretations of the events together. The nurse needs to understand what makes the event threatening from the client's perspective, and what is required to meet the demands of the situation. The abilities possessed by the person also need to be identified. In turn, the nurse may need to help the client acquire new knowledge and skills and to aid the client in maintaining a reasonable emotional balance during the transition period. Specific help may be necessary to assist the client in designing clearly defined, mutually agreeable goals; in identifying specific strategies to accomplish the goals; in facilitating the individual's ability to recognize and challenge distortions in thinking. Appropriate links with other health professionals and community agencies may need to be arranged and those with significant others maintained or strengthened.

If an individual continues to need particular defenses to manage the distress being experienced, the nurse needs to think very carefully about the type of interventions that are most appropriate. In certain instances, interventions aimed toward "facing the truth" could leave a previously "defended" person defense-less and, perhaps, do more harm than good. In addition, it has been suggested that "well-defended" individuals are not susceptible to intervention, and the most appropriate approach is one of support and patience—dealing with the areas one can. This can create a dilemma for health professionals when, in their opinion, the defensive stance retards the person's ability to deal with real threats that are amenable to resolution. On the other hand, in some situations, interventions are best geared toward confronting the defensive position.

Evaluation

The nurse will need to use both observation of, and interaction with, the individual to evaluate the extent to which nursing interventions have had the desired effect. The desired effect is defined in the context of the particular situation and the desired outcome identified by the individual involved. Evaluation involves separating one's own personal or professional notion of "effective" outcomes from those the individual may hold as "effective" outcomes.

In general, nursing interventions can be evaluated by observing whether the client's anxiety level has decreased, whether there has been a decrease in the frequency and rigidity of defense mechanisms, and whether the nature of the client's involvement with others has changed. In addition, the effectiveness of the client's problem solving and ability to meet usual role obligations can be evaluated (Chart 2).

CASE STUDY

Jane, a thirty-year-old wife and mother of two children, recently had a mastectomy (for a Stage II tumor) and received adjuvant chemotherapy on an outpatient basis at a nearby clinic. She has been referred to the psychiatric program at the same clinic because of drastic behavior changes. In the six weeks since she returned home after surgery, she has denied that she has had any cancer. She maintains that receiving chemotherapy is just a safeguard to prevent cancer. She shows no interest in caring for her children and spends much of her available time and energy shopping for new clothes. Given their limited funds, Jane's husband is concerned about her many charge card purchases.

Jane, who did not smoke or drink alcohol before surgery, is now smoking two packages of cigarettes a day, and Jane's husband says he can often smell alcohol on her breath when he comes home from work. When first seen by the nurse at the psychiatric clinic, Jane was composed but appeared very anxious; she smoked frequently throughout their first session and continued to deny that she had had cancer, even in view of her recent surgery and the chemotherapy she was receiving. After two sessions with Jane, the nursing diagnosis was formulated of denial of cancer related to threat to self of recent mastectomy. The chosen approach to Jane was to maintain her in her protected stance as long as was necessary and to meet with Jane twice weekly to provide supportive therapy, allowing Jane to proceed at her own pace. After four sessions, Jane was

> **CHART 2**
> **Defensive Coping: Summary of the Nursing Process**
>
> **NURSING INTERVENTIONS**   **OUTCOME CRITERIA**
>
> **CLIENT GOAL: EXPERIENCE PROTECTION TO THE SELF AGAINST THREAT AND ANXIETY**
> Support the individual's personhood, uniqueness and right to be   Experiences decreased anxiety or distress
>   involved in decision-making
> Seek to understand the individual's perspective of the situation (i.e.,   Uses immature defense mechanisms less
>   what is stressful, what is harmful or threatening, what evokes   frequently
>   feelings of conflict)
> Clarify in a gentle manner any misconceptions the client may have
> When possible, make the client's social milieu more predictable and
>   supportive
> When possible, reduce the stressful aspects of the situation (i.e.,
>   physical discomfort, visitors, rest, demands on client)
> Assist client to deal with emotions
> Encourage the maintenance of social networks and the expression of
>   feelings
> If required, confront any behaviors that are harmful to others
> Tailor interventions to match client's defense style (i.e., provide work
>   that can be viewed as helpful to individual who uses self-
>   sacrificing behaviors; provide creative arts for the individual who
>   uses sublimation and suppression)
>
> **CLIENT GOAL: DECREASE THE INAPPROPRIATE USE OF DEFENSE MECHANISMS**
> Assist the individual to explore the nature and characteristics of the   Expresses a realistic appraisal of the
>   situation, its demands, feelings involved, the coping resources   situation, its demands, and the coping
>   required, and identify when discrepancies exist between   resources available
>   expectations and reality   Verbalizes a sense of personal integrity and
> Assist the individual to identify desired goals   movement toward desired goals
> When possible, reduce the stressful aspects of the event and enhance   Decreases the frequency of use of immature
>   the individual's coping abilities through: defense mechanisms and instead uses
>   more mature coping behaviors
>   Setting concrete, realistic goals with the individual   Uses effective problem solving
>   Identifying specific strategies to achieve the goals   Meets usual role expectations (personal and
>   Setting realistic time frames for reaching the goals   work) or the role expectations of
>   Reviewing capabilities and learning from past experiences (especially   current situation
>   what is helpful in reducing emotional discomfort)
>   Exploring patterns in thinking (especially negative thoughts) and the
>   use of defensive behaviors
>   Teaching the necessary knowledge and skills (especially for adaptive-
>   coping strategies)
>   Acknowledging accomplishments toward desired goals
>   Maintaining social networks
>   Encouraging the expression of fears and concerns

able to acknowledge that the surgery was very stressful for her and that she had not been behaving "normally" lately. By the sixth session, Jane was able to acknowledge that she had, in fact, had a breast removed because of cancer, but that the cancer was contained. Once Jane had moved to the stage of acknowledging her disease, the nurse encouraged Jane to explore the meaning of cancer and a mastectomy in her life. She assisted Jane to acknowledge her overuse of certain defensive behaviors and move to more appropriate coping strategies.

Jane finished her course of chemotherapy, but she continues to see the nurse at the clinic for supportive care. She is able to talk about the fact that she lost her mother to cancer when she was only 13. Jane's behavior is back to normal, and she is able to see the link between her recent behavior, her own surgery and chemotherapy, and her mother's death.

In case Jane's cancer were to recur, the nurse would want to consider the potential for defensive coping related to behavioral patterns with initial diagnosis and surgery.

SUMMARY

Individuals vary in their responses to life events. The explanation for this variation lies in the arena of cognitive appraisal. Individuals judge events in relation to the potential for harm or threat and their own coping resources in relation to managing the demands of events. Distress or anxiety arise when individuals perceive that they do not have the required resources to manage the events. One way of coping is through the use of defense mechanisms. These mental mechanisms serve as protection through escape from reality or alteration of the situation in some way. It is not their use per

Research Highlights

That defense mechanisms are used by a wide variety of individuals can be seen in recent studies. Viney and Westbrook identified strategy preferences and associated emotional reactions in three studies of chronically ill patients.[34] These were inpatients who suffered from a variety of conditions that would last six months or that had caused a permanent disability; the patients were between 18 and 65 years of age. A self-appraisal of coping technique was used whereby patients ranked six clusters of coping strategies in order of 1, most likely to use, to 6, least likely to use in relation to dealing with their illnesses. Patients preferred optimism–fatalism strategies (expecting the best or the worst regardless of reality), whereas nonpatients preferred action-oriented and interpersonal coping strategies. Coronary patients selected fewer escape strategies (e.g., denial, avoidance) than other chronically ill patients. Action strategies tended to be associated with psychological reactions such as little uncertainty and helplessness. The preferences for escape strategies were linked with patterns such as much anxiety and indirectly expressed anger while in the hospital and considerable helplessness and little sociability at home. These data may be useful in designing interventions to help patients cope with their illnesses.

Bond and associates[5] designed a self-administered questionnaire that would indicate a person's perception of his or her habitual defense style. It was tested in a sample of 98 psychiatric patients and 111 nonpatients. Factor analyses for each group separately, or the entire combined group, revealed the presence of four defense clusters. Defense style 1 consisted of apparent derivatives of defense mechanisms viewed as immature (i.e., withdrawal, regression, acting out). Defense style 2 consisted of apparent derivatives of omnipotence, splitting, and primitive idealization. Defense style 3 consisted of apparent derivatives of reaction formation and pseudoaltruism. Defense style 4 consisted of apparent derivatives of suppression, sublimation, and humor. High ego strength scores and mature ego development scores correlated positively with defense style 4. Bond also reported that 60% of the patients used defense style 1 in conjunction with other styles, whereas only 11% of the nonpatients used it in conjunction with other styles. In contrast, 48% of the patients used style 4 in conjunction with other styles, whereas 90% of the nonpatients did so.

se that creates concerns, but rather, the type, frequency, and rigidity of their use. Assessment needs to focus on the usefulness of the mechanisms to an individual. Interventions are directed toward the goal of reducing the sense of distress and increasing the perception of strength in coping resources.

References

1. Baider L, DeNour AK. Couples' reactions and adjustments to mastectomy. Int J Psychiatry Med. 1984;14:265–270.
2. Battista JR. Empirical test of Vaillant's hierarchy of ego functions. Am J Psychiatry. 1982;139:356–357.
3. Bishop DS, et al. Stroke, morale, family functioning, health status and functional capacity. Arch Phys Med Rehabil. 1986;67:84–87.
4. Block AR, Bayers SL. The spouse's adjustment to chronic pain behavior: cognitive and emotional factors. Soc Sci Med. 1984;19:1313–1317.
5. Bond M, Gardner ST, Christian J, Sigal JJ. Empirical study of self rated defense styles. Arch Gen Psychiatry. 1983;40:333–338.
6. Bond MP, Vaillant JS. An empirical study of the relationship between diagnosis and defense style. Arch Gen Psychiatry. 1986;43:285–288.
7. Cassileth BR, et al. Psychological status in chronic illness. N Engl J Med. 1984;311:506–511.
8. Cassileth BR, et al. Psychological analysis of cancer patients and their next of kin. Cancer. 1985;55:72–76.
9. Clark S. Nursing diagnosis: ineffective coping. Part I. A theoretical framework; Part II. Planning care. Heart Lung. 1987;16:670–674.
10. Coelho GV, Hamburg DA, Adams JE. Coping and adaptation. New York: Basic Books; 1974.
11. Cohen F, Lazarus RS. Active coping processes, coping dispositions and recovery from surgery. Psychosom Med. 1973;35:375–389.
12. Coleman J. Psychology and effective behaviour. Glenville: Scott, Foresman & Company; 1969.
13. Folkman S, Lazarus RS. An analysis of coping in a middle-aged community sample. J Health Soc Behav. 1980;21:219–239.
14. Freud A. The ego and the mechanisms of defense. New York: International Universities Press; 1946.
15. Haan N. Coping and defending: processes of self environment organization. New York: Academic Press; 1977.
16. Hoff LA. People in crisis: understanding and helping. Toronto: Addison-Wesley; 1978.
17. Ilfield FW. Coping styles in Chicago adults: description. J Hum Stress. 1980;6:2–10.
18. Lazarus RS, Folkman S. Stress, appraisal and coping. New York: Springer Publishing; 1984.
19. Lipowski ZJ. Psychosocial aspects of disease. Ann Intern Med. 1969;71:1197–1206.
20. Mages NL, Mendelsohn GA. Effects of cancer on patients' lives: a peronological approach. In Stone GC, Cohen F, Adler NE, eds. Health psychology. San Francisco: Jossey-Bass; 1979.
21. Mechanic D. Some modes of adaption: defense. In Monat A, Lazarus RS, eds. Stress and coping: an anthology. New York: Columbia Press; 1977.
22. Menninger K. Regulatory devices of the ego under major stress. Int J Psychoanal. 1954;35:412–420.
23. Moos RH, Tsu VD. The crisis of physical illness: an overview. In Moos R, ed. Coping with physical illness. New York: Plenum Press; 1977.

24. Norris J, Kunes-Connell M. Self esteem. Nurs Clin North Am. 1985;20:745–761.

25. Northhouse L. The impact of cancer on the family: an overview. Int J Psychiatry Med. 1984;14:215–242.

26. Nuckolls KB, Cassel J, Kaplan BH. Psychological assets, life crises and the prognosis of pregnancy. Am J Epidemiology. 1972;95:431–441.

27. Pearlin LI, Schoolar C. The structure of coping. J Health Soc. Behav 1978;19:2–21.

28. Reasoner RW. Self esteem through the life span. Fam Commun Health. 1983;6(Aug):11–28.

29. Saxon DF, Haring PW. Care of patients with emotional problems. St. Louis: CV Mosby; 1979.

30. Vaillant GE, Bond M, Vaillant CO. An empirically validated hierarchy of defense mechanisms. Arch Gen Psychiatry. 1986;43:786–794.

31. Vaillant GE, Drake RE. Maturity of ego defenses in relation to DSM-III Axis II personality disorder. Arch Gen Psychiatry. 1985;42:597–601.

32. Vaillant GE. A 12-year follow-up of New York narcotic addicts, IV: Some characteristics and determinants of abstinence. Am J Psychiatry. 1966;123:573–584.

33. Vaillant GE. Adaptation to life. Boston: Little Brown & Co; 1977.

34. Viney LL, Westbrook MT. Coping with chronic illness: strategy preferences, changes in preferences and associated emotional reactions. J Chron Dis. 1984;37:489–502.

DEPRESSION

Monique M. Farill and Connie B. Klopfenstein

DEFINITION AND DESCRIPTION

The nursing diagnosis of *depression* refers to an emotional state manifested by sadness, discouragement, self-depreciation, and, at times, inability to act for self that is found in all age groups and ranges from mild to severe. Depression can be a transient mood fluctuation in response to stress, a symptom associated with a number of mental and physical disorders, and a clinical syndrome encompassing a multitude of symptoms. When psychological, physiologic, and interpersonal functioning is significantly affected as a result of depression, it can be considered a mental health problem.

THEORY AND RESEARCH

Several explanations contribute to the understanding of depression. Included in these are psychophysiologic, sleep, genetic, behavioral, psychoanalytical, and interpersonal models of depression. The psychophysiology of depression, as well as the role of this psychophysiology as a determinant of depression, is yet to be fully understood.[24] Alterations in levels of central nervous system neurotransmitters, including norepinephrine, dopamine, and serotonin, in areas that regulate appetite, sleep, and emotional processes, occur in those with severe depression. Norepinephrine and serotonin levels have been found to be decreased in certain depressions.[32] Cholinergic hyperactivity in major depression has been noted.[32] Siever and Davis have attempted to integrate neurotransmitter theories. They view depression as an interrelated failure of the regulation of neurotransmitter systems.[31] Neuroendocrine system regulation is influenced by neurotransmitters and their receptors. An imbalance in either system can affect all parts of both systems. Involved in neuroendocrine dysfunction are the hypothalamic–pituitary–adrenal system (HPA) and the hypothalamic–pituitary–thyroid system (HPT).[28]

Electroencephalograph (EEG)-recorded sleep disturbances in major depression include prolonged rapid eye movement (REM), increased REM activity with sleep, shortened REM sleep latency (the number of minutes of stage 2 sleep before the onset of the first REM period), reduced deep sleep (stage 3 or 4 of sleep), and disturbances in continuity of sleep.[32] Circadian biologic rhythm (24-hour cycle) disturbances have been linked to depression as frequently found in individuals who have irregular sleep schedules because of travel or shift work, or who experience sleep deprivation, as in the puerperium.[6,27]

Depressive illness tends to be familial. There is a 50% to 70% risk of developing a major depressive disorder with two parents who have bipolar affective illness, and a 25% risk with one parent who has a bipolar affective illness.[25] The prevalence of depression in children of depressed parents is greater than in those of parents without a history of depression.[35]

Behavioral models of depression are based on social learning theory. A cyclic pattern is proposed in which stress disrupts involvement with others, with reduction in the amount and quality of positive reinforcement. This leads to an increase in negative self-evaluation and outlook on the future, which in turn develops into dysphoria, withdrawal, and further negative reinforcement.[21] The cognitive theory of depression is based on the premise that cognition, "the process of acquiring knowledge and forming beliefs, is a primary determinant of mood and behavior" (reference 36, p 1119). Depressed people learn to view themselves, the world, and the future negatively, which leads to a sense of low self-worth and feelings of rejection, alienation, dependency, helplessness, and hopelessness. This fosters avoidance, increased dependency, withdrawal, and possible suicide.[36] Learned helplessness theory is based on the result of repeated exposure to adverse conditions beyond an individual's control. This is translated into the belief that nothing is controllable. In the event of stress, a helplessness stance is adopted leading to depression.[26]

Psychoanalytic explanations of depression postulate that loss, a real or perceived withdrawal of affection in childhood, is a crucial predeterminant of depression in all age groups. Early concepts proposed by Freud and Abraham include the role of ambivalence toward the lost love object, identification with the lost object, and subsequent anger turned inward. This pattern is thought to be reactivated in relationships with others. Later theories emphasize unrealistic expectations of self and others and loss of self-esteem as essential antecedents to depression. Progression from a usual dysphoric reaction in experiencing loss, followed by a loss of state of well-being that reaches clinical proportions, is viewed as a failure to work through the loss.[3]

Interpersonal theory emphasizes the importance of social bonds to human functioning. An individual's adaptive responses to the psychosocial environment are determined by early developmental experiences in forming attachment bonds. When early attachment bonds have been impaired or disrupted, the individual is subsequently vulnerable to increased interpersonal and social problems leading to depression.[29]

RELATED FACTORS

Depression is related to many factors including psychiatric and medical conditions, drugs, psychosocial stressors, gender, and age. Depression occurs in mood disorders, other psychotic disorders, organic mental disorders, adjustment disorders, psychoactive substance use disorders, and anxiety disorders.[2,9] Individuals with personality disorders, especially those with obsessive–compulsive, dependent, avoidant, and borderline personality disorders, are susceptible to depression.[2]

Any illness impinging on cerebral functioning and impairing blood flow to the brain can produce depression. Box 13-2 lists medical conditions that are associated with or can lead to depression.[8] The psychological stressors caused by physiologic dysfunctions can also result in depression. For instance, a debilitating disease can severely restrict usual life-style, resulting in depression. Conversely, physiologic dysfunctions such as gastrointestinal disturbances and chronic pain can be manifestations of depression.[8,17]

Drug-induced depressions are seen in psychiatric and non-psychiatric settings. Box 13-3 lists drugs associated with depression.[7,8,19,20,33] The elderly are particularly susceptible to depression from the many medications prescribed for them.[33] Although drug-induced depression is reversible when the drug is discontinued, this is not always a feasible alternative. Increased use of illegal drugs, such as cocaine and cannabis, has increased the occurrence of depression in adolescents.

Psychosocial stressors, including acute stressful events, chronic daily stressors, and social role stress or conflict, can contribute to depression. Examples of these are death of a spouse, urban living, chronic unemployment, and role change of women.[11,12,18,34] The Social Readjustment Rating Scale, developed by Holmes and Rahe, although not specific to depression, gives an indication of the range of stressors that can affect the well-being of an individual.[18] Environmental and personal resources, an individual's sense of mastery of the environment, interpersonal skills, and personality traits work in concert with psychosocial stressors as possible determinants of depression.[4] For instance, dependency and obsessional traits in an older person experiencing role changes, loss of family members, and diminished environmental resources can result in depression.[1,5]

Depression is more common in women than in men. This is not merely a measure of increased help-seeking behavior in women. Possible explanations are psychobiologic considerations, learned helplessness, sex role conflicts, lack of social supports when unemployed and involved in the care of small children, empty nest syndrome, and lack of an intimate relationship.[1,12] For men, depression increases with age. This is associated

with change in role status after retirement.[14] A trend is occurring with a narrowing of rates of depression in the two sexes.[34]

BOX 13–2
Physiological Dysfunctions Associated With or Leading to Depression[7,8,17,19]

HORMONAL

Adrenal Cortex Dysfunctions
Insufficiency (Addison's disease)
Hyperadrenalism (Cushing's syndrome)

Thyroid Dysfunction
Hypothyroidism
Hyperthyroidism

Parathyroid Dysfunctions
Hypoparathyroidism
Hyperparathyroidism
Hypoglycemia
Hyperglycemia (hyperosmolar nonketotic coma in the elderly)
Diabetes mellitus
Premenstrual tension

NEUROLOGIC
Multiple sclerosis
Huntington's chorea
Alzheimer's disease
Dementia: senile, presenile
Normal-pressure hydrocephalus
Wernicke–Korsakoff syndrome
Head injury: subdural hematoma
Myasthenia gravis
Parkinson's disease
Migraine headaches
Cerebral arteriosclerosis
Creutzfeldt–Jakob disease
Seizure disorder: temporal lobe

METABOLIC
Liver failure
Porphyria
Uremia

NUTRITIONAL

Eating Disorders
Obesity
Anorexia
Bulimia
Iron deficiency anemia
Alcoholism
Pernicious anemia

INFECTIOUS
Influenza
Hepatitis
Viral pneumonias
Encephalitis
Subacute or chronic meningitis
Fungal infections
Infectious mononucleosis
Neurosyphilis
Tuberculosis
Occult infections

NEOPLASTIC
Lymphoma
Intracranial tumors
Carcinoma: pancreatic

CARDIOVASCULAR
Cerebral ischemia
Sinus arrhythmias
Myocardial infarction
Congestive heart failure
Angina

COLLAGEN VASCULAR
Rheumatoid arthritis
Systemic lupus erythematosus

BOX 13–3
Drugs Associated With or Leading to Depression

PSYCHOTROPICS
Benzodiazepines
Amphetamines (upon withdrawal)
Phenothiazines
Barbiturates

ANTIHYPERTENSIVES
Propranolol
Reserpine
Clonidine
Hydralazine
Methyldopa
Nifedipine

ANTINEOPLASTIC
Vincristine sulfate

ANTI-INFLAMMATORIES AND ANALGESICS
Phenylbutazone
Indomethacin
Phenacetin
Corticosteroids

ANTIPARKINSONIAN
Levodopa

ANTIGLAUCOMA
Carbonic anhydrase inhibitors

CARDIOVASCULAR
Digitalis
Metoprolol
Procainamide
Atenolol

HORMONES
Estrogen
Progesterone

ANTISEIZURE
Carbamazepine

(Modified from Flomenbaum NE, et al. Treatment of depression in the physically ill. Emerg Med. 1984;17(Jan):8.)

DEFINING CHARACTERISTICS

Depression may be exhibited in a variety of ways, with the most common characteristics in appearance being sad downcast facial expression, poor eye contact, stooped posture, neglect of personal hygiene and dress, and frequent crying. Anxiety is frequently associated with depression and may be a premorbid personality trait or a symptom unique to the present situation. Overwhelming feelings of hopelessness, despair, dissatisfaction, confusion, emptiness, personal devaluation, guilt, and low self-confidence are almost always present. These may culminate in suicidal ideation and plans. Depressed clients may self-isolate and show apathy and anhedonia in general. Psychomotor retardation as well as psychomotor agitation may be noticeable. Hallucinations or delusions of a self-deprecatory nature are common in depression of a psychotic degree.

Depressive symptoms in children and adolescents are similar to adult depressive symptoms.[30] In the elderly, depression mimics the symptoms of dementia (disorientation and impairment of memory and of intellect).[10]

Family and friends of depressed clients may describe strained interpersonal relationships caused by irritability and hostility.[2,13,15,23] All of these defining characteristics are interrelated. The level of dysfunction is dependent on the number and severity of these characteristics (Chart 1).

NURSING PROCESS AND RATIONALE
Assessment

Because of their self-isolation, apathy, anhedonia, and poor eye contact, assessment of depressed clients through interviewing can be difficult. The nurse needs to be aware of, and responsive to, both verbal and nonverbal cues of clients. It is essential to gather information about previous episodes, medical history, family patterns, precipitating factors, and present symptomatology (including suicidal thoughts) as soon as possible. The family may be useful as a source of information. Depression inventories or scales can also be used to assist in assessing the presence or severity of the depression. The Beck Depression Inventory (BDI) and the Zung Self-Rating Depression Scale (SDS) are just two of many scales available for this purpose.[36] Because the mental status can be affected by depression, a

---

CHART 1
Depression: Definition, Related Factors, and Defining Characteristics

DEFINITION
Depression is an emotional state manifested by sadness, discouragement, self-depreciation and, at times, inability to act for self.

RELATED FACTORS
Mood disorders
Other psychotic disorders
Organic mental disorders
Psychoactive substance use disorders
Adjustment disorders
Anxiety disorders
Drug-induced depression
Personality disorders
Medical conditions
Psychosocial stressors

DEFINING CHARACTERISTICS
Despair
Guilt
Apathy
Anger
Sleep disturbances
Changes in activity level
Decreased interaction with others
Low self-esteem
Hopelessness
Anxiety
Anhedonia
Withdrawal
Appetite changes
Poor eye contact
Frequent crying
Suicidal ideation

CHART 2
Depression: Summary of the Nursing Process

NURSING INTERVENTIONS	OUTCOME CRITERIA

CLIENT GOAL: EXPERIENCE IMPROVEMENT IN PHYSIOLOGIC FUNCTIONING

Assess sleep pattern	
Arrange for individualized bedtime schedules based on client's usual routine	Reports return of "normal" sleep schedule
Discourage daytime sleeping	Reports feeling rested following sleep
Encourage daytime activity	Demonstrates increased energy level
Decrease caffeine intake	Reports decreased agitation
Teach relaxation techniques	
Encourage regular sleep schedule	
Assess level of activity	
Assist in self-care as needed	Makes decisions about self-care
Recommend a variety of activities for participation	Verbalizes increased interest in participation in activities
Explore client's perception of activities available	Demonstrates increased level of self confidence in participating in activities
Gradually increase participation in number and level of complexity of activities	Demonstrates decreased level of psychomotor retardation
	Participates in self-care
Assess nutritional intake	
Observe eating pattern	Reports a normalization of food intake
Monitor weight	Demonstrates less variation in weight and acceptable weight for sex and age
Offer nutritional snacks between meals	
Determine favorite foods and include in daily intake as often as possible	
Assess other physiologic changes	
Maintain elimination	Reports regular bowel and bladder elimination
Assess alteration in libido	Reports return of libido to predepressed state
Monitor menstrual cycle, if appropriate	Reports regular menstrual cycle, if appropriate
Monitor vital signs	Verbalizes fewer psychosomatic symptoms related to depression
Investigate physical complaints	

CLIENT GOAL: EXPERIENCE INCREASED SENSE OF WELL-BEING

Assess level and severity of depression	
Perform MSE as appropriate	Verbalizes awareness of early depressive characteristics in self, whom to contact, and when to seek professional help when discharged
Administer self-rating scales of depression as appropriate	
Observe non-verbal and behavioral communication	
Assess suicide potential by determining thoughts, intent, or plan	
Facilitate expression of feelings	
Initiate frequent, short contacts with client	Verbalizes thoughts and feelings more appropriately
Use nonjudgmental, supportive approach (i.e., reflection and validation of feelings)	Initiates interaction with nurse
Discuss diagnosis and accompanying symptoms	Verbalizes understanding of symptoms and diagnosis
	Verbally participates in decisions regarding treatment
	Reports decreased feelings of helplessness and hopelessness
	Reports decreased number and frequency of depressive characteristics
	Verbalizes knowledge of alternative choices to suicide
	Reports increased interest in former activities
Assist in improvement of self-esteem	
Assist in setting and achieving small goals	Makes positive statements about self
Question negative self-statements made by client	Plans realistic goals for self
Teach to change negative self-statements to positive ones	Reports increased self-confidence and self-esteem
Allow uninterrupted time for client	Gives self-credit for progress and accomplishments
Administer prescribed medication	
Teach client about medication	Verbalizes purpose and desired effects of medication
Assess for desired effect	Verbalizes prescribed dosage and when to take medication
Assess for adverse effects	Verbalizes symptoms of adverse reactions to medications and knows the action to take
Monitor vital signs	

(continued)

CHART 2 (*continued*)
Depression: Summary of the Nursing Process

NURSING INTERVENTIONS	OUTCOME CRITERIA
CLIENT GOAL: MAINTAIN OR IMPROVE CURRENT INTERPERSONAL RELATIONSHIPS	
Assess present interpersonal relationships	
Determine extent of withdrawal from others	Initiates interactions with others
Identify person with whom client can interact	Interacts with others appropriately
Set limits on behavior destructive to IPR	Actively seeks out others for social group activities
Encourage interaction with others	Expresses anger or hostility appropriately
Assess family relationships	
Identify family members who are supportive	Initiates interactions with family members
Identify family members who are nonsupportive	Verbalizes thoughts and feelings to family members appropriately
Set limits on behavior of client and family members destructive to family relationships	Explores situations that create disharmony
Teach family about diagnosis and symptoms of client	
Teach client about behavior of family that creates additional impairment for client	
Encourage family activities if they contribute to the well-being of the client	
Assess role functioning	
Determine different roles client plays in life (spouse, parent, child, sibling, employee, etc.)	Identifies own roles in relationships with others
Encourage adoption of new role behaviors through role-playing	Verbalizes any conflicts in connection with these roles
	Participates in role obligations appropriately

mental status examination by the nurse is necessary on a daily basis.

Nursing Diagnosis

The diagnostic category of depression is made more specific for a client by including related factors. An example would be depression related to substance abuse.

Client Goals and Nursing Interventions

The goals for the client and nursing intervention can be addressed within three major categories: improvement in physiologic, psychological, and interpersonal functioning. Specific interventions for addressing problems in these three areas are suggested in Chart 2.[12,13,15,19,20,22,23,29]

To achieve any measure of success with a depressed client, the nurse will need to establish a positive supportive relationship with the person as quickly as possible. Many depressed clients feel they do not deserve the nurse's time and so will make excuses or behave in such a way to discourage positive interaction. Sleep disturbances, appetite changes, and inactivity are some of the more troublesome characteristics that the nurse will need to address in the physiologic category. Improvement in the client's feeling of well-being needs to be a focus of each interaction, no matter how brief and for what specific purpose. For example, even when advising the client of meal time or medication, the nurse needs to interact in a way that conveys respect and value for that person as a unique human being.

The nurse needs to always be alert for changes in suicide potential. If the client makes statements like "There's nothing left for me," "I'm finished," or "I'm tired of trying," a further assessment of current suicidal ideation and plan is indicated.[13,23]

Assisting the client to establish or maintain a therapeutic relationship with the nurse can serve as a model for relationships with peers and family.

Some depressed clients may be placed on antidepressant medications. Therefore, it is important for the nurse to clearly understand and be able to explain adverse effects of the medication.[8,16,32] Orthostatic hypotension is more common early in treatment with tricyclic antidepressants. The client's blood pressure is checked lying and standing before the first dose. If the systolic pressure decreases more than 15 mm Hg standing, the person is likely to experience a decrease of more than twice that with the medication.[15]

Evaluation

Nursing interventions can be evaluated for their effectiveness by observing whether the client has shown an improvement in sleep pattern, posture, eye contact, appetite, activity level, positive self-statements, along with increased interest in planning for the future and satisfying interactions with others (see Chart 2).

Research Highlights

On the basis of previous evidence that cognitive therapy with nonelderly depressed clients can be more effective than pharmacotherapy, Chaisson and associates,[5] in their two-part exploratory pilot study (1) determined whether or not mental health professionals from a variety of disciplines could develop mastery levels as cognitive therapists and (2) evaluated the effects of cognitive therapy by these therapists on elderly clients. The samples for this study consisted of 12 mental health professional trainees, six of whom had a bachelor's degree in nursing, and 33 elderly clients divided in four groups. The knowledge of trainees was measured by the cognitive therapy scale at the end of a ten-week, 20-hour, training program in cognitive skills and again at the end of the six-week therapy group. Eight of the 12 mental health professionals met the criteria for selection as cognitive therapists.

The Beck Depression Inventory (BDI) and Zung Self-Rating Depression Scale (SDS) rated levels of depression in elderly subjects before and after the six-week cognitive therapy group. The level of depression in all clients before testing ranged from mild to severe according to the BDI and SDS ratings. None of the elderly clients were delusional, hallucinating, or suicidal.

A significant positive correlation was found between the cognitive therapy skills level of the eight therapists and the decrease in depression of elderly group members. Although depression of group members decreased, the change was not significant. However, the researchers suggested that a longer-term group would likely have led to greater decreases in depression of group members.[5]

CASE STUDY

Ms P, a 34-year-old woman, was hospitalized in a short-term observation and evaluation psychiatric unit with a DSM-III-R diagnosis on Axis II of borderline personality disorder. Ms P had a long-term history of mental health problems including frequent changes in employment, unstable relationships, and frequent short-term mood shifts often accompanied by suicidal ideation. As a child, Ms P had experienced many losses: the death of her mother when she was five years old, the lack of emotional support from a father whom she perceived as very critical, and relocation to several different family members who cared for her in the absence of her father.

The precipitating stressors leading to this hospitalization were a change of employment supervisors in the past month and a reportedly negative performance evaluation by this new supervisor three days before admission.

At the time of admission, Ms P experienced intensive feelings of depression and hopelessness in her ability to maintain employment or care for herself. She had made a suicidal gesture by cutting her wrists, and she expressed active suicidal ideation. She reported a decrease in appetite, early morning awakening, and extreme fatigue. Ms P noted that at work she had become very withdrawn, feeling unable to perform her duties.

A major nursing diagnosis was depression. Other nursing diagnoses were suicide potential, hopelessness, impaired social interaction, sleep pattern disturbance, and role performance disturbance.

Goals of this hospitalization were improved physiologic functioning; increased sense of well-being to be evaluated by client's exhibiting no suicidal behavior, verbalizing alternative choices to suicide, and expressing hope for the future; and improved interpersonal relationships to be measured by active participation in communicating with clients and nursing staff and by developing communication skills for a more effective working relationship with Ms P's supervisor.

Initially, suicide precautions were taken. Ms P was encouraged to participate in unit activities. Expression of feelings was facilitated by the nurse through frequent interaction with the client. Ms P was, in exploration with the nurse, able to identify the relationship between her depressed and hopeless feelings and the performance evaluation. In reviewing the sequence of the performance evaluation, she realized that she had made several cognitive errors. Through role-playing with the nurse, Ms P was able to explore different ways of interacting with her supervisor. Discharge planning included involvement in a community peer support group and outpatient follow-up at the community mental health center.

SUMMARY

Psychophysiologic, sleep, genetic, behavioral, psychoanalytic, and interpersonal explanations of depression have been discussed. Related factors for the nursing diagnosis of depression include psychiatric and medical conditions, drugs, psychosocial stressors, gender, and age. Defining characteristics encompass impairment of physiologic, psychological, and interpersonal functioning. Evaluations of the effectiveness of nursing interventions in the three areas of functioning include improvement in sleep, appetite, and activity level; positive self-statements and increased interest in planning for the future; and improved quality of interactions with others.

References

1. Akiskal HS, Tashjian R. Affective disorders: II. Recent advances in laboratory and pathogenic approaches. Hosp Commun Psychiatry. 1983;34:822–830.
2. American Psychiatric Association. Diagnostic and statistical manual of mental disorders. 3rd ed, revised. Washington DC: American Psychiatric Association; 1987.
3. Bemporad JR. Long-term analytic treatment of depression. In Beckham EE, Leber WR, eds. Handbook of depression: treat-

ment, assessment and research. Homewood, IL: Dorsey; 1985.

4. Billings AG, Moos RH. Psychosocial stressors, coping, and depression. In Beckham EE, Leber WR, eds. Handbook of depression: treatment, assessment and research. Homewood IL: Dorsey; 1985.

5. Chaisson M, Butler L, Yost E, Allender J. Treating the depressed elderly. J Psychosoc Nurs Ment Health Serv. 1984;22(May):25–30.

6. Erranti JE. Sleep deprivation or postpartum blues? Top Clin Nurs. 1985;6:9–18.

7. Field WE. Physical causes of depression. J Psychosoc Nurs. 1985;23(Oct):7–11.

8. Flomenbaum NE, Freedman AM, Levy NB, Simpson GM, Talley J. Treatment of depression in the physically ill: multidisciplinary viewpoints in a roundtable discussion. Emerg Med. 1984;17:2–20.

9. Fogelson DL, Bystritsky A, Sussman N. Interrelationships between major depression and anxiety disorders: clinical relevance. Psychiatr Ann. 1988;18:158–167.

10. Fopma-Loy J. Depression and dementia: differential diagnosis. J Psychosoc Nurs. 1986;24(Feb):27–29.

11. Friedman ML. Families of unemployed workers: need for nursing intervention and prevention. Arch Psychiatr Nurs. 1987;1:81–89.

12. Glazebrook CK, Munjas BA. Sex roles and depression. J Psychosoc Nurs. 1986;24(Dec):9–12.

13. Goldwyn RM. Educating the patient and family about depression. Med Clin North Am. 1988;72:887–895.

14. Gordon VC, Ledray LE. Depression in women: the challenge of treatment and prevention. J Psychosoc Nurs. 1985;23 (Jan):26–34.

15. Hackett TP, Cassem MH. Massachussets General Hospital handbook of general hospital psychiatry. 2nd ed. Littleton MA: PSG Publishing; 1987.

16. Hayes PE, Kristoff CA. Adverse reactions to five new antidepressants. Clin Pharm. 1986;5:471–479.

17. Holland JC, Korzun AH, Tross S, et al. Comparative psychological disturbances in patients with pancreatic and gastric cancer. Am J Psychiatry. 1986;143:982–986.

18. Holmes T, Rahe R. Social readjustment rating scale. J Psychosom Res. 1976;11:213–218.

19. Jenike MA. Depressed in the ER. Emerg Med. 1984; 17(Mar):102–120.

20. Lazarus LW, Davis JM, Dysken MW. Geriatric depression: a guide to successful therapy. Geriatrics. 1985;40(Jun):43–51.

21. Lewinsohn PM, Hoberman HM, Teri L, Hautzinger M. An integrative theory of depression. In Reiss S, Bootzin R, eds. Theoretical issues in behavior therapy. New York: Academic Press; 1985.

22. Manderino MA, Bzdek VM. Mobilizing depressed clients. J Psychosoc Nurs Ment Health Serv. 1986;24(May):23–28.

23. Maurer FA. Acute depression: treatment and nursing strategies for this affective disorder. Nurs Clin North Am. 1986;21:413–427.

24. Mendlewicz J. Depressive disorders: epidemiology and heredity. In Beckham EE, Leber WR, eds. Handbook of depression: treatment, assessment, research. Homewood, IL: Dorsey; 1985.

25. Mendlewicz J. Genetic research in depressive disorders. In Beckham EE, Leber WR, eds. Handbook of depression: treatment, assessment, and research. Homewood, IL: Dorsey; 1985.

26. Peterson C, Seligmen MEP. The learned helplessness model of depression: current status of theory and research. In Beckham EE, Leber WR, eds. Handbook of depression: treatment, assessment, and research. Homewood, IL: Dorsey; 1985.

27. Plumlee AA. Biological rhythms and affective illness. J Psychosoc Nurs Ment Health Serv. 1986;24(Mar):12–17.

28. Rothschild AJ. Biology of depression. Med Clin North Am. 1988;72:765–790.

29. Rounsaville BJ, Klerman GL, Weissman MM, Chevron ES. Short-term interpersonal psychotherapy (IPT) for depression. In Beckham EE, Leber WR, eds. Handbook of depression: treatment, assessment, and research. Homewood, IL: Dorsey; 1985.

30. Ryan ND, Puig-Antich J, Ambrosine P, et al. The clinical picture of major depression in children and adolescents: Arch Gen Psychiatry. 1987;44:854–861.

31. Siever LJ, Davis KL. Overview; toward a dysregulation hypothesis of depression. Am J Psychiatry. 1985;142:1017–1031.

32. Thase ME, Frank E, Kupfer DJ. Biological processes in major depression. In Beckham EE, Leber WR, eds. Handbook of depression: treatment, assessment, and research. Homewood, IL: Dorsey; 1985.

33. Todd B. Depression and antidepressants. Geriat Nurs. 1987;8(Jul/Aug):302.

34. Tsuang MT, Tohen M, Murphy JM. Psychiatric epidemiology. In Nichole AM, ed. The new Harvard guide to psychiatry. Cambridge: Belknap; 1988.

35. Weissman MM, Gammon D, John K, Merikangas KR, Prusoff BA, Sholomskas D. Children of depressed parents: increased psychopathology and early onset of major depression. Arch Gen Psychiatry. 1987;44:847–853.

36. Wright JH, Beck AT. Cognitive therapy and depression: theory and practice. Hosp Commun Psychiatry. 1983;34: 1119–1126.

DIVERSIONAL ACTIVITY DEFICIT

Agnes L. Hoffman

DEFINITION AND DESCRIPTION

The nursing diagnosis of *diversional activity deficit* has been defined as the state in which an individual experiences a decreased stimulation from or interest or engagement in recreational or leisure activities.[24] Defining characteristics of this diagnosis include a wish for "something to do," self-report of "boredom," or reference to environmental constraints (e.g., hospital setting, prison, "homebound" status, or a combination thereof).

Recreational or leisure activities are defined and described from both objective and subjective perspectives. Objective approaches typically use some type of residual time definition (i.e., leisure is seen as nonwork time) combined with an activity-type definition in which certain activities (e.g., arts, crafts, music, sports) are defined a priori as *leisure*.[10,12] The objective approach to defining leisure activity fails to take into account the participant's perceptions, values, attitudes, and meanings associated with activities. Any one activity can be experienced as leisure by one person, but as work by another. Presumably, a busy homemaker preparing dinner for her family does not have the same subjective experience as a person preparing a gourmet dinner for friends on a holiday. The objective approach to defining leisure in terms of activities leads to certain systematic biases relative to the work–free time dichotomy.[21] For example, for the unemployed, the excess of free time or "time on one's hands" may not translate into more satisfying leisure activity. Instead, the "forced leisure" time may become an antecedent to diversional activity deficit. Excessive free time may also be experienced by those whose activities are compromised because of mental or physical disability or frailty, as in the elderly.[3,25,36]

A subjective definition of leisure was proposed by a number of researchers in the field.[18,29,33] *Leisure behavior* is defined as engagement in activities that are perceived by a participant as recreational, relaxing, or stimulating. Leisure experience is characterized by anticipation and recollection of activity engagement and opportunity for recreational and personal growth.[19,22] A significant issue of the subjective perspective is the position that leisure activity is not so much what people do as how they do it and what it means to them.[23]

THEORY AND RESEARCH
Optimal Arousal Theory

The concept of stimulation has emerged as central to understanding recreational and leisure activities.[7,11,35] The amount of stimulation that is comfortable to a given individual has been referred to as the *optimal stimulation level*. When too much stimulation occurs, a person experiences sensory overload and loss of control; at the other extreme, lack of sufficient stimulation leads to lethargy and boredom. Boredom is a frequent complaint of individuals experiencing actual or perceived leisure deficits.[8,30]

Optimal arousal theory of leisure addresses the conditions or factors that facilitate or impede the human tendency to engage in leisure behaviors. Engagement in leisure behavior is to meet a need for an optimal amount of change, novelty, variety, and arousal.[19] If satisfaction with leisure activities–pursuits drops below optimal level, the probability increases that the person will experience leisure deficit (i.e., chronic inadequacy or dissatisfaction with leisure experience), which can adversely affect mental and physical health.[35]

Need Satisfaction

Literature reviewed by Tinsley and Tinsley[35] suggests that psychological needs at all five levels of Maslow's[27] hierarchy may be satisfied by participation in leisure activities. Their model of causal effects of leisure experience proposes that satisfaction of a person's psychological needs through leisure activity has a salutary effect on mental health, physical health, and satisfaction with life, which, in turn, have a salutary effect on personal growth.

Personal interviews with individuals in retirement (n = 300) were based on Maslow's hierarchical need theory to determine the relationship between recreational activities and levels of life satisfaction.[31] A stronger need for love and association than self-esteem or self-actualization was found for this population. The observed hierarchy could be due to rewarding outcomes associated with affiliation in retirement.

Symbolic Interaction

A symbolic interactionist perspective postulates that an individual's reality is based upon personal perception and interpretation of actions and events.[28] The meaning of a significant symbol, such as leisure, has its origins in interaction and is defined and changed by individuals within a society, or subgroup, through the process of communication. Thus, meanings are derived from subjective interpretations of the social context.

A symbolic interactionist framework was used to interview 60 married couples about their leisure experiences.[33] The dimensions of leisure experiences included (1) free choice of activity, (2) motivation to engage in an activity, and (3) outcomes of enjoyment and relaxation from activity engagement.

Self-expression was a critical factor in distinguishing between "anomic free time" and "engaging leisure" activities in an analysis of 695 "real-life situations" recorded by 18 subjects.[32] Subjective qualities (e.g., pleasure and self-realization) were also critical characteristics of the consequences of leisure in an analysis of subjects' (n = 140) self-report essays of leisure experiences.[16]

RELATED FACTORS

Diversional activity deficit is attributed to individual characteristics, environmental contexts, and the interaction between persons and their environment. Individual characteristics may include a belief in the "work ethic" and excessive absorption in work-related activity leading to inadequate participation in recreational activities that provide leisure outcomes. An inadequate socialization toward leisure and inadequate leisure education may compromise capabilities to engage in recreational activities. Social skill deficits may hinder engagement in leisure activities requiring effective interaction with others.

Intrapersonal and interpersonal factors, as well as energy level and motivation associated with depression and schizophrenia, can adversely influence engagement in and outcomes from diversional activity participation.[9,30] Various chronic health conditions (e.g., arthritis, emphysema, dementia), as well as certain physical disabilities (e.g., spinal cord injury, back injury), may preclude involvement in selected or preferred diversional activities and, thus, contribute to leisure deficit.[36]

Environmental contexts may also preclude engagement in selected recreational activities. For example, institutional environments, such as "total institutions" (e.g., nursing homes, state mental hospitals, prisons),[15] may deprive the individual access to diversional activities and to use of leisure opportunities. Health conditions that impose a "homebound" status also limit access to activities.

Related factors also may involve interaction between the individual and environment.[1] Although a given en-

vironment may offer access to an array of diversional activities, the individual may choose not to participate in the activities for various reasons. For example, choice and motivation may be lacking, or the activities may not be experienced as enjoyable or relaxing.[19,33] Leisure resources may be incompatible with recreational preferences or with capabilities.

DEFINING CHARACTERISTICS

Defining characteristics of diversional activity deficit involve descriptions of the use of time as unsatisfying or as not sufficiently stimulating or relaxing. An individual may express different leisure preferences, voice concern about lack of access to leisure resources, or complain of a restricted environment.

Other responses to leisure deficit may include apathy, disinterest, and decreased motivation to participate in leisure activity. The experience of boredom is a typical subjective response (Chart 1).

CHART 1
Diversional Activity Deficit: Definition, Related Factors, and Defining Characteristics

DEFINITION
A state in which an individual experiences a decreased stimulation from or interest or engagement in recreational or leisure activities.[24]

RELATED FACTORS
Individual Factors

Leisure socialization deficits
Social skill deficits
Lack of motivation–energy
Work ethic orientation
Health status–disability
Depression
Schizophrenia
Physical illness

Social Factors

Inadequate social–personal resources
Sociocultural norms, roles
Inadequate physical resources, finances
Restricted environmental settings
Recent relocation
Lack of recreational resources
Altered social network

DEFINING CHARACTERISTICS

Expression of dissatisfaction with leisure time
Descriptions of leisure as not sufficiently stimulating or relaxing
Complaints of boredom
Apathy
Disinterest
Inactivity

NURSING PROCESS AND RATIONALE

Assessment

Assessment of the client's diversional activity deficits involves identification of current and past leisure interests, skills, and amount and style of activity participation. A comprehensive assessment includes eliciting critical leisure activity information (e.g., values, preferences, life-style, social network) such as that outlined in a tool developed by Ferguson.[13]

1. Readiness for activity participation
2. Preferred type of activity participation
3. Leisure behavior patterns and history
4. Personal leisure values
5. Interpersonal resources for leisure involvement
6. Strengths or assets for leisure involvement
7. Life-style adjustments needed for healthy leisure function
8. Available leisure support systems or resources in the community
9. Economic factors influencing leisure access and involvement
10. Leisure-related problems

The identification of leisure-related problems is important for individual program planning. Examples of problems that affect leisure participation and performance include too much free time, not enough free time, the need to adjust life-style because of injury, the use of free time in a harmful or self-destructive way, and shyness that inhibits participation in group activi-

ties.[13] Situational factors that require modifications in leisure activity can include age, gender, medication effects, injury, relocation, and confinement.[2,4,6] Environmental factors that hinder or preclude access to recreational resources are important to include in the assessment protocol.

Nursing Diagnosis

Examples of specific nursing diagnoses include diversional activity deficit related to the life transition of retirement and relocation, or diversional activity deficit related to hospital confinement and illness.

Client Goals and Nursing Interventions

A thorough assessment of the client's leisure needs and activity enables planning a prescriptive program, with the client assuming responsibility for choice of diversional activities.[17,34] The client is assisted in identifying activities of interest, any barriers interfering with participation in leisure activities, and how such barriers can be overcome. Environmental factors and the client's preferences are major considerations in formulating activity plans. The client's perception of particular recreational activities and the resources required can be ascertained. The prescriptive program is designed to reduce diversional activity deficits, meet recreational needs, and support the client's total treatment plan. After selecting an activity and participating in it,

---

CHART 2
Diversional Activity Deficit: Summary of the Nursing Process

NURSING INTERVENTIONS	OUTCOME CRITERIA
CLIENT GOAL: IDENTIFY FACTORS THAT INTERFERE WITH PARTICIPATING IN ENJOYABLE LEISURE ACTIVITIES	
Engage the client in comprehensive assessment of leisure activities	Describes typical pattern of recreational activity
Assist the client to identify what interferes with participation	Identifies factors currently interfering with diversional activities
CLIENT GOAL: IDENTIFY ONE OR MORE LEISURE ACTIVITIES THAT CAN BE ADAPTED TO CURRENT STATUS AND RESOURCES	
Ascertain client's perceptions and interest in particular recreational activities	Plans for one or more activities that are feasible in terms of requirements and resources
Maintain emphasis on client's choice of activities for participation	
Assist the client to explore resources required for selected activity and means to obtain them	
CLIENT GOAL: EXPRESS RELAXATION, ENJOYMENT AND/OR STIMULATION FROM INVOLVEMENT IN ACTIVITY SELECTED	
Support client's engagement in activity selected	Expresses satisfaction with the activity (or the modified activity) as having met a need for relaxation, enjoyment, or stimulation
Assist client to evaluate experiences and make whatever modifications are needed	

Research Highlights

Iso-Ahola and Mobily[20] conducted a field study in which they investigated recreational involvement among 149 patients with psychiatric disorders and 63 patients with cancer who were in inpatient settings. The significant main effect of the type of illness indicated that patients who had diagnoses of different forms of depression did not differ from one another in the frequency of their participation in recreational activities, but the participation frequency of patients with cancer was about ten times less than that of other patients. The patients with cancer were hypothesized to be experiencing severe "reactive" depression, which resulted in responses of social withdrawal as well as reduced participation in leisure and recreational activities. The finding that psychiatric patients participated only about three times and patients with cancer about 0.3 times per week in the planned activities was interpreted as indicants of a lack of interest in the activities offered them in the hospital environment. Given these findings, the investigators suggested that program evaluation of leisure activity offerings be conducted.

Although the findings of this study provide information about the level of activity participation of selected patients in one hospital setting and is useful in program planning, it does not address more qualitative indices of participation. For example, neither the subjects' preferences for activity participation nor the outcomes experienced from participation were examined. These factors, along with other individual characteristics, such as discomfort and pain associated with illness and energy level, may have contributed substantially to the finding by these investigators of low activity participation rates.

---

the client can be assisted in evaluating the experience and on making whatever modifications are necessary.

Implementation of the plan requires careful attention to the client's leisure literacy and competence. Leisure education and counseling[5,14,26] may be prerequisite to the client's engagement in diversional activities that can bring about the outcomes of leisure satisfaction and relaxation. In one study, residents in psychiatric transitional facilities were provided leisure education to increase their independent leisure functioning. This new challenge led to enhanced community adjustment and increased the quality of life for residents in the facility.[9]

Evaluation

The expected outcomes for effective implementation of the plan prescribed to reduce diversional activity deficits include the client's engagement in diversional activities that are freely chosen, satisfying, and relaxing or stimulating. Such engagement in leisure activities would be expected to provide opportunities for enhanced well-being and personal growth (Chart 2).

CASE STUDY

Martha, aged 67, was admitted to an inpatient psychogeriatric unit with a psychiatric diagnosis of adjustment disorder with depressed mood. Recent life events included the death of her husband one year earlier and subsequent relocation to a congregate housing facility for retired persons arranged by her only child, Harry. Harry reported that his mother was "very dependent" upon his father, who died suddenly of a heart attack. Because she was unable to manage an "independent" life-style, the son sold their home and helped her move to her present residence. Harry noted that his mother had "not adjusted well" to her new location and the activity director reported that she had not attended any activities offered to residents. Martha claimed the activities are not of interest to her; she missed the type of recreation she and her husband had together, as well as activities associated with their home such as gardening and shopping trips with neighborhood friends.

One of the nursing diagnoses formulated was diversional activity deficit related to depression, recent relocation, and altered social network. The nursing care plan to address her diversional activity deficit diagnosis included (1) conduct comprehensive assessment of leisure activity based on the protocol by Ferguson;[13] (2) involve Martha in formulation of a prescriptive plan of leisure activities that are meaningful and enjoyable to her; and (3) monitor activity engagement and reduction of diversional activity deficit, improved affective status, and reduction of social isolation with improved social network changes.

After discharge from the inpatient setting, Martha's progress was slow, but incremental, during the first year. With continued support and encouragement from her son and the activity director, as well as continuation in the day-care program, Martha's activity involvement increased. She reported leisure activity satisfaction and an increased sense of well-being, as well as new acquaintances in her retirement residence community.

References

1. Barris R. Activity: The interface between person and environment. Phys Occup Ther Geriat. 1987;5(2):39–49.
2. Bialeschki MD, Henderson K. Leisure in the common world of women. Leisure Stud. 1986;5:299–308.
3. Burrus-Bammel LL, Bammel G. Leisure and recreation. In: Birren JE, Schaie KW, eds. Handbook of the psychology of aging. 2nd ed. New York: Van Nostrand; 1985.
4. Chambers DA. The constraints of work and domestic schedules on women's leisure. Leisure Stud. 1986;5:309–325.
5. Chinn KA, Joswiak KF. Leisure education and counseling. Ther Recreat J. 1981;15:4–7.
6. Crepeau EL. Activity programming for the elderly. Boston: Little, Brown & Co; 1986.
7. Csikzentmihaly M. Beyond boredom and anxiety. San Francisco: Jossey-Bass; 1975.

8. DeChenne TK. Boredom as a clinical issue. Psychotherapy. 1988;25:71–81.
9. Dunn JK. Leisure education: meeting the challenge of increasing independence of residents in psychiatric transitional facilities. Ther Recreat J. 1981;15:16–23.
10. Edington RR, Compton PM, Hanson CJ. Recreation and leisure programming: a guide for the professional. Philadelphia: WB Saunders; 1980.
11. Ellis GD, Witt PA, Aguilar T. Facilitating "flow" through therapeutic recreation services. Ther Recreat J. 1983;17:6–14.
12. Farrell P, Lundigren HM. The process of recreational programming. New York: John Wiley & Sons; 1978.
13. Ferguson DD. Assessment interviewing techniques: a useful tool in developing individual program plans. Ther Recreat J. 1983;17:16–21.
14. Fine AH, Feldis D, Lehrer BE. Therapeutic recreation and programming for autistic children. Ther Recreat J. 1982;16:6–11.
15. Goffman E. Asylums. New York: Anchor; 1961.
16. Gunter BG. The leisure experience: selected properties. J Leisure Res. 1987;19:115–130.
17. Hoffman MD. Recreation therapy: a prescriptive approach. Ther Recreat J. 1981;15:16–21.
18. Iso-Ahola SE. Basic dimensions of definitions of leisure. J Leisure Res. 1979;15:15–26.
19. Iso-Ahola SE. A theory of substitutability of leisure behavior. Leisure Sci. 1986;8:367–389.
20. Iso-Ahola SE, Mobily KE. Depression and recreation involvement. Ther Recreat J. 1982;16:48–53.
21. Kabanoff B. Work and nonwork: a review of models, methods, and findings. Psychol Bull. 1980;88:60–77.
22. Kaplan M. Leisure: lifestyle and lifespan. Philadelphia: WB Saunders; 1979.
23. Kelly JR. Leisure in later life: roles and identities. In: Osgood NJ, ed. Life and work: retirement, leisure, recreation, and the elderly. New York: Praeger; 1982.
24. Kim MJ, McFarland GK, McLane AM. Pocket guide to nursing diagnosis. 3rd ed. St Louis: CV Mosby; 1989.
25. Lawton MP. Activities and leisure. Annu Rev Gerontol Geriatr. 1985;5:127–164.
26. Li RK. Activity therapy and leisure counseling for the schizophrenic population. Ther Recreat J. 1981;15:44–49.
27. Maslow AH. Motivation and personality. 2nd ed. New York: Harper & Row; 1970.
28. Mead GH. Mind, self, and society. Chicago: University of Chicago Press; 1934.
29. Neulinger J. The psychology of leisure. Springfield, IL: Charles C Thomas; 1981.
30. Patrick GD. Clinical treatment of boredom. Ther Recreat J. 1982;16:7–12.
31. Romsa G, Bondy P, Blenman M. Modeling retirees' life satisfaction levels: the role of recreational, life cycle and socio-environmental elements. J Leisure Res. 1985;17:29–39.
32. Samdahl DM. A symbolic interactionist model of leisure: theory and empirical support. Leisure Sci. 1988;10:27–39.
33. Shaw SM. Gender and leisure: inequality in the distribution of leisure time. J Leisure Res. 1985;17:266–282.
34. Rubenfield MG. Diversional activity, deficit: theory and etiology. In: Thompson JM, McFarland GK, Hirsch JE, Tucker SM, Bowers AC. Clinical nursing. St Louis: CV Mosby; 1986.
35. Tinsley HE, Tinsley DJ. A theory of the attributes, benefits, and causes of leisure experience. Leisure Sci. 1986;8:1–45.
36. Voeltz LM, Wuerch BB. A comprehensive approach to leisure education and leisure counseling for the severely handicapped person. Ther Recreat J. 1981;15:24–35.

ELOPEMENT, POTENTIAL FOR

Marilyn G. Holnsteiner

DEFINITION AND DESCRIPTION

Elopement has been defined as "the unauthorized departure of a voluntary or involuntary client from hospital grounds, regardless of whether the client returned to the psychiatric unit or was discharged."[10] *Potential for elopement* is the existing possibility that a psychiatric client will leave the hospital or residential treatment facility against therapeutic advice. This diagnosis does not negate a voluntary client's right to rationally elect to terminate treatment. Elopements can occur with clients of any age and from many locations (e.g., from care areas, from hospital grounds, from passes, and from hospital-sponsored outings).

THEORY AND RESEARCH

Studies of elopement have attempted to distinguish those who elope from those who do not and to identify stressors involved with elopements. The population studied most often has been adolescents, ages 15 to 19, because the largest number of elopements occur in this age group.[1] In predicting elopers versus nonelopers, demographic data, personality factors, and diagnostic labels have been considered.[1] Males elope more often than females; singles more often than married clients; and Caucasians more often than other races. Also, elopements occur more often in the summer months.[1] Males with a prior history of home or school truancy had a 65% probability of eloping from a facility; whereas females had a 62% probability of eloping. Those female adolescents who eloped and were returned to the facility had greater than 80% probability of subsequent elopements.[5]

RISK FACTORS

Elopements can either be planned or occur impulsively. Risk factors are present in any age group and can trigger either planned or impulsive elopements. Potential for elopement occurs in various psychiatric conditions. Psychiatric diagnoses of elopers vary and have included clients with depression, borderline personality disorders, psychoactive substance use disorders, and, occasionally, schizophrenia and acute organic mental disorders.[1,9] Clients with diagnoses of major depression and borderline personality disorder were more likely to elope if they manifested rage toward authority figures, rebelliousness, and antisocial behaviors, in contrast with those clients with the same diagnoses who manifested helplessness and withdrawal behaviors.[3] A comparison of female adolescent psychiatric inpatients who eloped and those who did not elope, using the Minnesota Multiphasic Personality Inventory, identified lack of verbal skills, problems with interpersonal relationships, impulsive behavior, and problems with authority figures as four personality traits associated with elopement.[4] In addition, feelings of anger, boredom, homesickness, depression, and fear have been identified by elopers as psychological reasons for their planning to elope. Suicidal clients have been known to plan elopements so that they can attempt suicide outside the hospital. Hallucinations and delusional thoughts can lead to a sudden elopement by psychotic clients.

Potential stressors associated with elopements have centered around the psychotherapeutic relationship,[2,11] family dynamics,[6,12] and the social functioning of the hospital unit.[7,8] Various phases in the psychotherapeutic relationship can trigger elopement plans in a client, for example, resistance to psychiatric treatment at the beginning, need to demonstrate independence and individuation or fear of closeness during the middle and later phases, and fears of abandonment during therapist's absences and during the termination phase.[2]

In the early phase of the psychotherapeutic relationship, fear of opening up to an authority figure can result in complete resistance to treatment of any kind. In the working phase of the relationship, the client experiences increased anxiety as feelings are shared and he or she begins caring for the therapist and the relationship. Clients experiencing changes within themselves during therapy, or experiencing intense feelings that they have previously kept buried, may resort to old familiar patterns of coping (i.e., running away).[8] Absences by the therapist, such as illness or vacations, cause fears of abandonment and can result in elopement. Clients preparing for upcoming discharge or those in the termination phase of the relationship will sometimes demonstrate their independence and individuation by leaving.[2]

Family dynamics also have played a major role in causing elopements and potential elopements. Conflicts over family values, disciplinary practices, and communication problems, coupled with a strong need for independence and individuation, have resulted in elopement. Changes in the structure of the family, such as a divorce, a new stepparent's assumption of more responsibility and authority in the family, births, or deaths of members, can lead to elopements.[12] Often, a perceived sense of responsibility for keeping the family together, protecting one family member from another, or bringing to attention unwanted facts about the family will lead to a client's planning of an elopement.[8] In addition, family members or a girlfriend or boyfriend may be pressuring the client to leave the hospital by writing letters or by criticizing the treatment or treatment team.

Some clients recreate their family dynamics on the unit, and when they perceive staff members as being judgmental, controlling, punitive, and unable to give support, they plan elopements to free themselves of constraints.[6] Differences between the staff's and the client's perception of the need for hospitalization also have been stressors.[7] Admissions under duress result in many elopements, especially within the first three weeks of hospitalization. Elopements can be in response to the social functioning of the psychiatric unit;[8] intrastaff conflicts; changes with program, staff, or other clients; crisis situations occurring on the unit, such as physical violence between clients; and peer or family pressures.

Difficulties in school, such as failing classes or grades, truancy, and social pressures, can result in elopements. Those clients, regardless of age, who have developmental issues centering around dependence–independence, individuation and the resultant separation anxiety, and fear of intimacy can become potential elopers.

On admission the best indicator of potential for elopement is a previous history of running away from home or a detention center. A prototype of the client who potentially elopes describes an action-prone, peer-dependent client.[3] This client, regardless of age, is distrustful and uses rebellion and rage to bolster self-esteem. When dependency on authority figures arouses intense anxiety, any kind of relationship with authority figures may be rejected. These clients have difficulty accepting criticism from authority figures and the normal restrictions and behavioral limits imposed by these figures. They turn to friends and peers on the unit for approval and permission. Their peers become objects of love or objects of ambivalence as dependency needs tend to be denied or repressed. They proclaim hospitalization as inappropriate because they believe that they have no problems and are capable of living on their own.

The content of hallucinations or delusional thoughts may lead a client to suddenly bolt toward a door or break a window to escape a perceived danger and, thus, pose a high elopement risk.

DEFINING CHARACTERISTICS

On a psychiatric unit, certain behaviors may indicate elopement plans. Clients who previously have been resistive to treatment and to staff, and who suddenly change their attitude and want to be included in the upcoming outing plans or want a weekend pass to take care of business, represent potential risks of eloping. Peers may be observed whispering to each other or talking in groups and, when a staff member approaches, the clients become quiet or disperse. Clients may ask questions about the number of staff members working, location and time of outings, which keys open which doors, which doors are locked or unlocked. On locked units, clients will watch the doors closely as people go in and out, and they may periodically test doors to see if they are closed properly. Others watch where staff members keep their keys. On unlocked units, clients may be observed watching staff members routine in making rounds, learning which slips are necessary to leave on a pass, or they may be found by other staff members exploring the hospital grounds or courtyards, and appear anxious when discovered. Clients may pack up all their clothes and hide them in the laundry basket or closet, or take them all home on pass, knowing they will not be returning. Some clients hide objects they find on the unit such as razors, keys, paper clips, plastic knives, or equipment from workmen to use either as tools to aid in opening screens or doors or to use as a weapon against staff in an elopement attempt. Sometimes, relatives or friends are included in the elopement plan, and there are reports of unauthorized individuals being seen on the hospital grounds and around units. Clients may also say goodbyes to peers and some staff when going out on a pass as though they will not be back (Chart 1).

NURSING PROCESS AND RATIONALE
Assessment

The first step in assessing for elopement potential is to ask during the admission process whether the client has ever run away from home or school, or has been placed in a detention center for truancy or running away. In addition, the nurse assesses how impulsive the client is, current coping mechanisms, and his or her mode of interacting with family, friends, and authority figures. When exploring coping mechanisms, ask the client how anger, sadness, and anxiety are usually expressed. Assess whether the client uses alcohol or drugs, sexual experimentation, running away, or self-mutilation as a means of coping. Ask questions geared toward gaining the client's understanding of the reasons for being hospitalized as well as related feelings. Note whether the client is on voluntary or involuntary status.

Behavior such as checking doors or windows, standing by unit doors, whispering with peers, asking questions about the time and location of the outing, or how many staff members are working would be observed.

When a client is on elopement precautions, the elopement risk is assessed every shift and communicated in shift reports and in documentation. The treatment team evaluates daily whether or not the client is

CHART 1
Potential for Elopement: Definition, Risk Factors, and Defining Characteristics

DEFINITION

The potential for elopement is the existing possibility that a client will leave the hospital or residential treatment facility against therapeutic advice.

RISK FACTORS

Chemical abuse
Conflict with authority figures
Rebelliousness
Antisocial behavior
Lacks verbal skills
Poor interpersonal skills
Impulsiveness
Hallucinations
Delusional ideations
Psychotherapeutic relationship
Family difficulties
Social functioning of unit
Fears about intimacy
Stressful environmental factors
Loneliness
Loss of significant other
Peer pressure
Situational crisis
Unmet needs

Incongruent values–role expectations
Intrastaff conflicts
Not confiding in adults
Anxiety
Internal conflicts
Poor coping skills
School difficulties
Developmental factors
History of runaway behavior
Peer-dependent
Acts out feelings
Rejects adult relationship
Inability to accept criticism
Denial of problems
Disregard for social norms, rules
Feelings of meaninglessness

DEFINING CHARACTERISTICS

Unable to accept normal restrictions and behavioral limits by adults
Overly aggressive toward staff
Ambivalence toward hospitalization
Rage over being controlled
Asking questions about doors, keys, rounds
Asking questions about outings, number of staff
Saving objects for tools or weapons
Testing limits
Testing doors
Whispering with peers
Packing clothes
Expresses desire to leave

tial problem of running away when faced with various types of stresses during hospitalization; for example, potential for elopement related to anxieties over being hospitalized, potential for elopement related to family pressures to leave the hospital, potential for elopement related to anxiety over staff changes, or potential for elopement related to anxiety over therapist's absence.

Client Goals and Nursing Interventions

If upon admission or later on during hospitalization, the client is assessed as presenting an elopement risk, the client is placed on elopement precautions. The frequency of observations (every 30 minutes, every 15 minutes, or 1:1 status) will depend on the degree of risk the client presents (i.e., presence of plan, ideations, suspicious behavior). The precautions also include supervising the client when attending off-unit activities, or they may require that the client remain on the unit. On open units, clients are observed for showing an exceptional interest in learning staff times for making rounds and where pass slips are kept. Such behaviors are communicated to all staff members so that those clients exhibiting suspicious behavior can be observed more closely, and the times for performing nursing rounds can be made less predictable. The client is encouraged to tell staff members when experiencing increased anxiety, overwhelming feelings, and an urge to run. It is crucial at the early stages of treatment to let the client know that the nurse is available to talk and is willing to listen. Helping the client to identify ways that hospitalization can be utilized and, thus, accept the need to be in the hospital, accept the treatment program and activities, and accept staff's help is a crucial goal to meet if early elopements are to be prevented.

It is important for clients to become oriented to unit rules and regulations and to have the functioning of the unit explained by other clients (unit leaders preferably). By assignment of the same nurse daily to each shift to care for this client, the client can develop a close relationship with someone in authority and learn to work through conflicts. The unit system needs to allow for individualized treatment plans, but provide controls. The client is helped to make the connection between behaviors and actions and resultant consequences (positive and negative).

Because control is often a central issue and the client may be trying to achieve independence and individuation, nurses need to allow the client to have as much say in unit government, community meetings, treatment goals and plans, and unit activities as possible. The client needs to feel that opinions and feelings are heard and taken into consideration by staff members. It is important to help the client develop self-confidence and self-esteem by pointing out assets and accomplishments. It is also important to help the client identify the areas in life over which there is little or no control.

When clients lack verbal skills, they sometimes act out feelings by breaking rules, drinking, taking drugs,

to continue on elopement precautions and the frequency of observations. Before hospital outings or passes, the client's recent stressors are assessed, as are abilities to cope.

Nursing Diagnosis

Potential for elopement is identified as a nursing diagnosis when the client's history or current behaviors, or both, indicate a high risk of an elopement occurring. This diagnosis may be used at various times in the treatment process, and it addresses the client's poten-

sexual acting-out behavior, self-destructive behavior, as well as by running away. A goal is to increase verbal skills during hospitalization. The nurse can teach these clients how to identify feelings (anger, sadness, hurt, anxiety, and the like) and how to express those feelings, rather than act them out. Role-playing is an excellent way to understand another's point of view and to learn healthier approaches to problems.

Along with teaching expression of feelings, nurses can assist the client in identifying current coping methods and can teach alternative coping skills. A goal during hospitalization is to try new coping methods, such as seeking out staff to talk, when feelings of running away surface. This is a long-term project that will carry over into discharge planning. Assertiveness-training skills can also be taught as a way of helping the client to get needs met.

It is important for the nurse to recognize situations that cause high or escalating stress for the client so that close observations for potential elopement can be initiated. During such periods, the client may resort to old coping patterns and may need to have a safe place provided where anger can be physically expressed, such as a gym with a punching bag or a quiet room with a mattress to hit. Others may need protective measures to guard against self-mutilative behaviors. Clients on an unlocked unit who pose an imminent threat of eloping, may be dressed in hospital gowns to facilitate early recognition by other hospital employees that precautions are being followed and to stop the client if seen. Some clients will not be able to tolerate an open unit and may require transfer to a locked unit or facility.

Because these clients often have dependency issues and fear of abandonment, it is very important that changes on the unit (e.g., new staff coming, staff members leaving or going on vacation, client discharges, changes in the treatment program) be dealt with openly and the clients allowed time to ventilate feelings and adjust to the changes.

Before hospital outings or the client leaving on pass, if the nurse assesses the client as presenting too high a risk of elopement, the treatment team is consulted and the client is watched closely. If while on an outing, the client exhibits behaviors that the nurse assesses to pose an elopement risk, the nurse will initiate closer interactions and physical contact with the client, have clients buddy up with one another, or return the client to the unit. If the client elopes during an outing, the safety of the whole group is addressed before attempting to deal with the client. The hospital is called to assist in notifying the physician, next of kin, and legal authorities, as deemed necessary by the client's legal status and age.

Those clients who are psychotic and experiencing hallucinations and delusions and who pose an elopement risk need to be medicated and supervised closely until stabilized on medications. The priority goals with such clients are to protect from harm and to decrease psychotic behavior.

When clients elope from the hospital, the legal status, age of the client, and assessment of whether the client poses a danger to self or others determine who the nurse notifies about the elopement. Upon return to the hospital, it is important to assess the client physically for any harm that may have occurred during the elopement and to assess the mental status of the client and notify the physician of findings. Explore with the client what the elopement accomplished and the reasons for the elopement, rather than responding punitively. Some clients who return after an elopement verbalize improved communication with staff members, increased understanding of their problems or treatment, and view it as having a positive outcome. Other clients may continue to actively resist treatment and plan future elopements.

Evaluation

A primary part of evaluating whether or not the goals and interventions worked with a client posing an elopement risk is noting if the client actually eloped. If the client was successful in eloping, the treatment team needs to analyze the behaviors that occurred before the elopement, the stressors, and what steps might have been taken to prevent the elopement. If no elopement attempts occurred, the treatment team looks at what interventions worked. Has teaching been effective? How is the client responding to the nurse–client relationship? Has the client begun expressing feelings verbally rather than through destructive behaviors? Does the client acknowledge a need for treatment and an understanding of treatment goals? Has the client begun to try new coping skills such as seeking out staff members or peers when feeling increased anxiety or the need to run? In evaluating the client's progress or lack of progress, the treatment team looks at changes in behavior, verbalizations by the client, and observations by the staff (Chart 2).

CASE STUDY

A 15-year-old single girl, who looks older than her stated age, was admitted with the psychiatric diagnosis of major depression and borderline personality disorder. The client was hospitalized by her parents because they were unable to control her impulsive, self-destructive behaviors which included chemical abuse of alcohol and marijuana, frequent runaway attempts, and chronic truancy from school. The client's parents had divorced when she was five and she had been shuffled back and forth between them ever since. The client described her life as unhappy and her parents and authority figures as angry, rejecting, and ridiculing. Psychological testing indicated an individual who was nonconforming and resentful of authority, who had marked problems with impulse control, one who acted out in asocial ways, was distrustful of other people, and avoided close relationships. Family relationships were very conflicted and a major source of her distress. Testing also revealed extreme concern about abandonment by significant people in her life and showed evidence of ineffective coping skills (e.g., drug abuse, sexual promiscuity, running away).

Nursing diagnoses identified were (1) potential for elopement related to previous runaway behavior, chronic

CHART 2
Potential for Elopement: Summary of the Nursing Process

NURSING INTERVENTIONS	OUTCOME CRITERIA
CLIENT GOAL: REFRAIN FROM RUNNING AWAY FROM THE HOSPITAL	
Upon admission, assess the elopement risk	No elopements during hospitalization
Assess the client's understanding of need for hospitalization and feelings about being hospitalized	
Enlist aid of other clients to orient client to unit rules and regulations	
During hospital stay, place client on elopement precautions whenever risk is present	
Assign same nurse to work with client each day	
Set up 10 to 15 minute talks daily	
Assess elopement risk every shift while on precautions; note if plan, ideations, or suspicious behavior is present	
Report risk potential to all staff by shift report and documentation	
Evaluate daily with treatment team whether or not elopement precautions should be continued	
CLIENT GOAL: ACKNOWLEDGE NEED FOR HOSPITALIZATION	
Explore with client ways to constructively utilize hospitalization	Verbalizes need for hospitalization
Explain rationale for groups, activities, community meetings	Exhibits decreased anxiety and anger over unit rules, groups, activities
Provide opportunities for client to voice opinions and assist in decision-making process with unit government, treatment plan and goals, unit activities	
CLIENT GOAL: LEARN AND DEMONSTRATE INCREASED VERBAL SKILLS WITH REGARD TO EXPRESSION OF FEELINGS	
Teach client to recognize and identify feelings and connect them with events of the day	Identifies feelings and connects them with events
Teach client various ways to verbalize these feelings directly to others (i.e., role-playing, assertiveness training exercises)	Increased verbalization of feelings to peers, family, staff
Help client identify behaviors and their resultant consequences	
Help client to identify ways to handle fears of closeness and concerns about dependency	
CLIENT GOAL: LEARN AND BEGIN TO TRY OUT NEW COPING SKILLS DURING HOSPITALIZATION	
Help client to identify current coping methods and teach new coping skills	Identifies alternative coping skills to try in different situations
Encourage client to seek out staff to talk whenever he/she feels like running away, harming self, drinking	Tries out new coping skills (i.e., seeks out staff when feels like running, asks for gym or quiet room)
Recognize situations that cause high stress and warning signs	No elopements during periods of high stress or change
During stressful periods, provide safe place for client to express anger and/or institute protective measures to prevent harming self or others	
During periods of change with staff, clients, or unit, provide time for client to verbalize feelings about the change and adjust to the change	
If client elopes, notify the physician, legal guardian, or legal authority per elopement policy and procedure	
When client returns to the hospital, explore with client reasons for elopement and feelings surrounding elopement	

lack of consistent family support, and concern about abandonment; (2) depression; and (3) dysfunctional family processes. The first diagnosis was later refined and changed to: elopement related to feelings about intimacy and about increased sharing of feelings with family.

Initially elopement precautions were taken to protect the client from running away and causing harm to herself. The same staff member worked with her throughout the hospitalization; thus, she was able to develop a relationship slowly with an adult and also had consistency with limit setting. She was oriented to the unit by fellow clients to help her adjust to the system. She tested rules and became sexually involved with male peers through the first few months, but seemed to slowly respond to the consistent limit setting and finally accepted the need for hospitaliza-

tion. Staff members worked to teach her increased verbal skills, which she began to utilize more and more in family and group sessions. Staff members also worked with her to identify her current coping methods and explore alternative approaches. She also worked on her drug abuse problem through A.A. and N.A. meetings. Under periods of high stress with her family, she tended to resort to severe limit testing and highly provocative sexual behavior, and eventually she eloped from an A.A. meeting. Upon returning to the hospital, she identified as reasons for eloping, heightened emotions over increased sharing of feelings in family sessions and what she perceived as rejection from her father. She then continued to work at expressing feelings more openly with her family. However, one month later she eloped from her room through a screen she had unlocked

Research Highlights

Elopement from the perspective of clients who eloped was researched.[7] This study was designed to help nurses gain a greater understanding of how psychiatric clients view their own elopements (i.e., the reasons for eloping and the experiences during the elopements) to prevent future elopements. Clients interviewed upon their return to the hospital shared their perception of the event and feelings that led up to the elopement. Although the sample size was small (*n* = 7), the findings suggest areas for further investigation. A theme of meaninglessness was found to be an integral component in how clients explained their elopement. Clients did not see the need for hospitalization, except as a place to stay. They denied having any problems. They saw the treatment program and activities as something to do, or as infantilizing punishment. Decisions were made for them and about them, but they saw little reason or meaning for these decisions. They could not see the connection between treatment programs and meeting a higher level of functioning. They experienced nurses as having limited impact on their level of functioning. Instead, they viewed them as intermediaries to contact doctors, or as functionaries providing concrete services such as giving out cigarettes and organizing activities. They considered nurses as too busy, lacking in caring and warmth, and lacking knowledge or influence to make changes. These clients' expectations of nurses, however, when they came into the hospital were that they were trained staff who would talk to them and elicit their problems.

The implications of this study are threefold. First, the psychiatric nurses need to gain an understanding of the client's reality (beliefs, expectations, roles about health care, psychiatry, nurses, hospital) to anticipate problems that may occur during hospitalization and negotiate shared perception with the client. Unless treatment can be made understandable to clients, they may see little value in hospitalization and seek situations that they hope will have meaning and worth to them by eloping. Second, psychiatric nurses and other treatment team members need to understand clearly the rationale for their groups, meetings, and activities on the unit and discuss these openly so that clients can be helped to understand their importance and utilize them more fully. In addition, clients can be encouraged to give feedback and suggestions on programs. Especially important in meeting the needs of these clients is evaluating treatment programs for any activities that tend to infantilize clients and giving consideration to what alternative approaches are available. Third, psychiatric nurses must be able to objectively evaluate personal communication styles and those of peers to help clients feel that their care has priority and that nurses are available to talk to and teach them.

---

using a piece of metal. Again she returned to the hospital. She identified intense feelings about commitment and intimacy as leading to her elopement, and continued to work on learning new ways to handle stress and feelings. Discharge planning involved assisting in placement in a halfway house, because of the resistance to treatment by both her parents and their spouses, and a plan for outpatient follow-up at a community mental health center. Prognosis remained guarded for future elopements from treatment.

SUMMARY

Elopements from hospitals or residential treatment centers can occur in any age group, but they are seen primarily with adolescents and young adults described as action-prone and peer-dependent. Reasons for eloping center around family conflicts, changes in the social functioning of the psychiatric unit, or the psychotherapeutic relationship. Following assessment and diagnosis, nursing interventions are directed toward helping the client recognize and accept the need for hospitalization, and teaching the client increased verbal and coping skills, assisting the client to identify and try alternative coping skills in different situations, and protecting the client during periods of high stress when maladaptive coping patterns may return.

References

1. Altman H, Brown M, Sletten, I. And . . . silently steal away, a study of elopers. Dis Nerv Syst. 1972;33(1):52–58.
2. Benalcazar B. Study of fifteen runaway patients. Adolescence. 1982;17(67):553–566.
3. Goodrich W, Fullerton C. Which borderline patients in residential treatment will run away. Resident Group Care Treat. 1984;2(3):3–14.
4. Grayson C. Minnesota Multiphasic Personality Inventory differences between female adolescent psychiatric inpatient elopers and nonelopers. Diss Abstr Intern. 1984;44(7-B):2243.
5. Howard R, Haynes J, Atkinson D. Factors associated with juvenile detention truancy. Adolescence. 1986;21(82):357–364.
6. Loeb R, Burke T, Boglarsky C. A large-scale comparison of perspectives on parenting between teenage runaways and nonrunaways. Adolescence. 1986;21(84):921–930.
7. McIndoe K. Elope: why psychiatric patients go AWOL. J Psychosoc Nurs Ment Health Serv. 1986;24(1):16–20.
8. McNaught T, McKamy L. Elopement of adolescents: dynamics in the treatment process. Hosp Community Psychiatry. 1978;29(5):303–305.
9. Miller D, Stone M, Beck N, Fraps C, Shekim W. Predicting AWOL discharge at community mental health center: a "split-half" validation. Am J Psychiatry. 1983;140:479–482.
10. Molnar G, Keitner L, Swindall L. Medicolegal problems of elopement from psychiatric units. J Forensic Sci. 1985;30(1):44–49.
11. Rinsley D. Principles of therapeutic milieu with children. In Sholevar GP, Benson RM, Blindor BJ, eds. Emotional disorders in children and adolescents: medical and psychological approaches to treatment. New York: SP Medical and Scientific Books; 1980.
12. Steinberg L. Single parents, stepparents, and the susceptibility of adolescents to antisocial peer pressure. Child Dev. 1987;58:269–275.

EMOTIONAL LABILITY

Verrelle M. Davis and Karen A. Benson

DEFINITION AND DESCRIPTION

Emotional lability is a condition in which an individual's emotions show a ready tendency to change. Emotions are subjective experiences of feelings and the accompanying physiological changes. They may be identified in a client by assessment of physiological changes and observation of characteristic body language and of verbal and behavioral expression. Emotions are regarded as labile when they change abruptly, repeatedly, and unpredictably.

THEORY AND RESEARCH
Neurotransmitter Levels

Mood imbalances may be related to increases or decreases in one or more of the neurotransmitter systems, including norepinephrine, serotonin, dopamine, and acetylcholine.[15] Parkinson's disease is an example of a disorder in which levels of dopamine are altered. The mood changes seen in parkinsonism are associated with changes in dopamine levels in the brain, especially the substantia nigra and the pathways to the caudate and putamen. The depression seen with this illness is associated with decreased dopamine levels, whereas paranoid psychosis, perhaps with anger and fear, is more often associated with drugs used to treat parkinsonism, because these drugs elevate levels of dopamine.[13] Imbalances of various neurotransmitters occur in bipolar disorder, an illness involving emotional lability.

Disruption of Neural Tracts

Disruption of neural tracts also can result in changes in emotional response. The effects of this disruption depend on the function of the affected tracts. Causes of disruption include tumors, direct or hypoxic injury, and disorders that destroy the myelin covering of the nerve.

The limbic system is a relatively "old" part of the brain and forms the most medial edge of the cerebrum. It includes some structures that lie beneath the cortex and surround the basal ganglia and is thought to be associated with emotion and affect. Projections travel to the brainstem and spinal cord and to the motor areas of the cortex (through hypothalamic projections) and association areas (direct projections). Damage to the limbic frontal cortex may cause behavioral disturbances. This sometimes occurs if demyelination from multiple sclerosis affects this area of the brain and often results in labile emotions. Psychosurgery, if it involves one of the two major connections between the frontal lobe and the limbic–subcortical structures, produces a dissociation between verbalization and the observed response, a lack of inhibition, and accentuation of premorbid personality traits.[20] The area of pathology may determine which mood is the dominant one: for example, if demyelination affects primarily the right side of the brain, laughter will be the dominant emotion, whereas left-brain pathology may result in crying. Dementia with emotional lability has been reported following multi-infarct injury to the subcortical area.[7]

Temporal Lobe Changes

Pathology of the temporal lobes may be associated with changes in mood and behavior. The temporal lobe, located to the side of and below the frontal lobe, contains the auditory receptive areas and has connections to most other parts of the brain, including the amygdala (anterior part of the temporal lobe), which mediates input from the temporal lobe to other brain centers. These connections undergo changes in transmembrane (electrochemical) potential that bring them close to threshold. When the threshold for action potential is lowered, such as occurs in a seizure disorder when the stimulation is repeated consistently, the temporal lobe–amygdalar connections are facilitated. This may allow sensory input access to discharge centers for autonomic arousal that would not be allowed under ordinary conditions. This change can result in a lowered threshold for seizures or in diffuse behavioral instability.[16] The mood lability seen in rabies is probably associated in some way with damage to the medial temporal lobes, as the characteristic small (Negri) bodies formed in nerve cells in the brain in this disease are found in this area.[14]

Hormone Levels

Changes in endorphin levels accompanying variations in estrogen and progesterone levels may be responsible for some rapid mood cycling in women.[15] Other hormones also seem to be related to labile emotions.

Although Kuevi and coworkers[11] did not find changes in peripheral hormone levels in their 44 postpartum patients, they did find that those who had "postpartum blues" had lower levels of peripheral catecholamines (norepinephrine and epinephrine) during the times they were depressed.

RELATED FACTORS

Emotional lability can occur in a number of DSM-III-R[1] conditions: bipolar disorder; cyclothymic disorder; borderline personality disorder; histrionic personality disorder; organic personality syndrome; and alcohol, sedative, hypnotic, or anxiolytic intoxication. It can also occur in eating disorders, late luteal-phase dysphoric disorder, multiple sclerosis, and epilepsy.

Drugs may have mood changes as a side effect. For example, rapid mood cycling is positively correlated with administration of exogenous steroids, particularly when the regimen is alternate-day corticosteroid therapy.[17,19] Weddington and Banner[22] reported one case in which metoclopramide, a dopamine antagonist that stimulates gastric emptying through release of acetylcholine and sensitization of gastric smooth muscle to stimulation, caused dysphoria, insomnia, racing thoughts, and labile affect in a patient being treated for hiccups. This drug also increases serum prolactin, which could be responsible for the changes in mood. Levy and Remick,[12] in a discussion of possible etiologic factors for clients' experiencing very frequent or "rapid cycling" mood disorders, included as possible causes rapid and frequent medication changes, drug noncompliance or erratic adherence, or changes induced by a tricyclic antidepressant.

Lability of mood associated with other central nervous system (CNS) dysfunction may not be easy to quantify or relate to a specific cause. For example, patients placed on extracorporeal circulation during open-heart surgery report intellectual disturbance and lability of mood for several months after surgery. The degree of disturbance is positively correlated with time on the pump, the length of time the perfusion pressure was below 50 mm Hg, and the pCO_2 during the extracorporeal circulation period. This correlation implies insidious hypoxic lesions of the brain.[6]

Emotional lability has also been reported in disorders in which the direct area of pathology has not been defined. Alcoholism, particularly in the elderly, may involve emotional lability along with confusion, depression, and other symptoms.[2] In senile dementia, there is a positive correlation between affective "incontinency" (loss of control of emotional expression), lability of affect, and cerebellar atrophy.[9]

Although some of the pathology associated with particular changes in affect has been described, the identification of emotions depends also on other factors. For example, the emotional expression on the face depends on the correct functioning of connections from the frontal cortex to the brainstem nuclei and from the brainstem to the facial muscles controlling expression.

The self-description of emotions depends on intact cortical functions and speech functions. Alertness is elicited by stimulation from an intact reticular activating system and is required to some degree for awareness of stimuli. Alteration in activity related to affect also involves many neural tracts.

Circadian rhythm research is finding evidence of a relation between the circadian system and mood. Two subtypes of mood disorders are cyclic: rapid-cycling manic depressive illness and seasonal affective disorder. Some of the classic symptoms of depression seem to indicate rhythm disturbances—diurnal variation, early morning awakening, and alterations in sleep–wake patterns. Temporal isolation experiments, where all external time cues that alter biologic rhythms are removed, have lessened depressive symptoms and altered mood.[18]

Psychosocial factors, including beliefs about what constitutes socially accepted emotional expressions and role expectations, influence to some degree how feelings will be manifested. In addition, an overstimulating environment may increase emotional lability.[3] The excess stimulation may come from being with too many people, especially over a period of time, from being in an unfamiliar environment, from too much noise, from arguments or conflict, or from the emotional expressions of others.[4] Hooley[10] reported an association between high expressed emotion levels in clients' spouses and unexpressive behavior in clients. Environmental overstimulation can be a particular problem for a client who is prone to emotional lability (e.g., bipolar disorder) and who also has some cognitive deficits that impair judgment about optimal stimulation.

DEFINING CHARACTERISTICS

Abruptly vacillating mood shifts are characteristic of emotional lability. The client alternates between emotional expressions such as laughing and crying; social intrusiveness changing to withdrawal; and hostility, anger, irritability, or sarcasm oscillating with docility. Because of this changeability of the emotions, the client may express concerns about being unpredictable and out of control. On the other hand, the client may be unaware of the inappropriateness of his or her emotional expressions and their effect on other people (Chart 1).

NURSING PROCESS AND RATIONALE

Assessment

Emotional responses are learned within environmental situations that reflect cultural norms for appropriateness and acceptability of expression. When abruptly changing and alternating emotions are displayed in a

CHART 1
Emotional Lability: Definition, Related Factors, and Defining Characteristics

DEFINITION

Emotional lability is a condition in which an individual's emotions show a ready tendency to change. Emotions are regarded as labile when they change abruptly, repeatedly, and unpredictably.

RELATED FACTORS

Physiological imbalances
    Neurotransmitters
    Pharmacological agents
    Hormone levels
    Metabolic disturbances
Pathological stressors
    Tumors
    Trauma
    Hypoxic injury
    Inflammation
    Surgery
    Alcohol
Degenerative conditions
    Multi-infarct dementia
    Parkinson's disease
    Multiple sclerosis
    Cerebellar atrophy
    Neurologic alterations
Sociopsychological stressors
    Grieving
    Perceived stress
    Anticipated or actual threats to security
    Interval conflict with values, goals
    Transference reactions
    Over-responding to feelings
DSM-III-R disorders
    Bipolar disorder
    Cyclothymia
    Eating disorders
    Histrionic personality disorder
    Borderline personality disorder
    Organic mood syndrome
    Schizoaffective disorder

DEFINING CHARACTERISTICS

Alternating, abrupt, unpredictable mood shifts
Euphoria or elation alternating with sadness
Laughter alternating with crying
Anxiety or agitation alternating with tranquility
Hostility, anger, irritability, or sarcasm alternating
    with docility
Concerns about being unpredictable or lack of
    awareness of emotional expressions

Nursing Diagnosis

An example of a nursing diagnosis that might be made relevant to a particular client is emotional lability related to histrionic personality disorder and stress of hospitalization.

Client Goals and Nursing Interventions

Use of medication is an important intervention in nursing management of clients with emotional lability. Major categories of medications that alter states of consciousness, result in quiescence, and reduce motor activity and anxiety are neuroleptics, anxiolytics, antidepressants, antimanics, and sedative–hypnotics, which may be used alone or in combination. Teaching about the drugs being used, their expected actions, and their possible side effects can help the client understand the importance of the medication in maintaining some feeling of control.[21] In turn, the client who has more control may be more likely to be compliant with the medication regimen.[5]

In order to assist the client to feel safe, the nurse maintains a consistent relationship based on caring, concern, and a sense of hopefulness that the client will feel more secure in the environment. Management of the environment is necessary to decrease stimulation and to develop structure, routine, and consistent limits. Physiological and psychological stressors are reduced to the extent feasible. The client's feelings of control can be enhanced by clear guidelines of appropriate behavior, available choices, and a sense of predictability from others and the environment. Environmental management is also important for other clients, who may be made anxious by the unpredictability of the client experiencing emotional lability. It is important that these other clients know that the nurses are aware of the problem and that they will act to control the situation.

To encourage the client who is cognitively able to develop an increased awareness of changing emotions and their personal and social consequences, the nurse provides opportunities for the client to examine patterns of behavior and any unsatisfactory consequences. By encouraging the client to be with others in noncompetitive activities and by exploring the client's interpersonal involvement in various situations, the nurse becomes active in a collaborative process that assists the client in gaining self-awareness of relationships with others, thus decreasing potentially negative responses. The client is encouraged to assume responsibility for behavioral expression and actions, to modify beliefs that are not reality based, and to discuss feelings rather than act on them.

In making plans with a client whose emotional lability may continue, the nurse explores with the client the resources available to alleviate stressors, meet needs, decrease problems for others that may be related to emotional expression, learn about the relation of cognition and feelings, and learn alternative ways of

manner beyond established social norms, assessment is called for. This assessment includes identifying etiologic factors that may be responsible for the emotional lability as well as ways in which the environment may be contributing to an intensification of the lability. In addition, assessment is made of the client's ability to recognize the effect of behavior on others.

expressing feelings. A treatment plan may include teaching about medications that help to maintain emotional balance and homeostasis, the need for professional assistance, and practices to ensure a healthy lifestyle.

Evaluation

The effectiveness of nursing care can be evaluated by the extent to which there is a decrease in the frequency and intensity of emotional expression. Other outcome measures include acceptance of verbal and environmental limits, appropriate participation in interactions with others, appropriate expressions of emotions, and identification of alternative ways of handling emotions (Chart 2).

CASE STUDY

Kathy G, 28 years old and married, was considered a healthy, well-adjusted person until about 4 years ago. At that time, she lost her job as an executive secretary and began overeating during the day to alleviate her feelings of failure and sadness and to calm herself when she felt anxious and agitated. Mood swings became a problem, and there was marital discord, which intensified after the birth of twin boys 2 years ago. She felt increasingly over-

whelmed with the care of the boys, especially when they became toddlers. In the months prior to hospitalization, her husband frequently confronted her, freely expressing his anger and irritation with her inability to "get hold of herself" and care for the twins. Kathy was usually mute after these verbal attacks but seemed to obtain some relief and satisfaction from binge eating. She decreased her social contacts out of concern that she might suddenly burst into tears or become giddy with laughter or both. On admission to the hospital, she expressed that she felt "out of control" with her feelings, her marriage, her ability to mother the boys, and her eating. She was unable to concentrate on one topic or sit for more than a few minutes, flayed her arms as she talked in a loud voice, and had sudden swings in mood.

Her DSM-III-R diagnosis was bipolar disorder, mild, and her primary nursing diagnosis was emotional lability (anxiety, irritability, sadness, and withdrawal) related to bipolar disorder. Client goals were to regain a sense of self-control, to develop coping skills, and to maintain medication and treatment programs. Nursing interventions included administering and monitoring the action and dosage of lithium and developing a relationship based on a consistent caring, dependability, and hopefulness that she could gain more self-control and remain on medication. Initially, a nonstimulating environment was provided until Kathy could tolerate group activities. With the setting of clear limits on her loud behavior, pointing out the effects of her behavior on others, and examining alternative coping mechanisms; e.g., identifying increasing feelings of anxiety as she became more agitated, going to a quieter place, taking deep breaths, and, finally, examining her thoughts prior to feeling anxious, Kathy

---

CHART 2
Emotional Lability: Summary of the Nursing Process

NURSING INTERVENTIONS	OUTCOME CRITERIA
CLIENT GOAL: FEEL SAFE IN ENVIRONMENT AND MORE IN CONTROL	
Maintain consistent client–nurse relationship based on caring and concern	Increases time spent in groups
Provide quiet, low-stimulation environment	Appears more relaxed
Set clear limits, behavioral expectations	Responds to verbal and environmental limits
Reinforce client's positive coping skills	Decreases frequency and intensity of emotional expression
Develop awareness of own feelings and reactions concerning self-control	Accepts positive reinforcement
Positively reinforce client for utilizing successful alternative emotional or behavioral expression	
Provide structured schedule of activities	
Administer specific medications to maintain homeostasis	
CLIENT GOAL: BECOME AWARE OF CHANGING EMOTIONS AND THEIR PERSONAL AND SOCIAL CONSEQUENCES	
Assist client to examine patterns of behavior resulting in unsatisfactory consequences	Stops self prior to invading rights of others
Model, role play, rehearse social interactions	Participates appropriately with others
Provide opportunities for noncompetitive activities with others	Demonstrates appropriate expression of emotions
Assist client to modify beliefs that are not reality based	Identifies thoughts that lead to exaggerated expressions
Encourage client to reward self for successes in new skill development	Verbalizes successes experienced utilizing alternative coping skills
CLIENT GOAL: MAKE REALISTIC PLANS	
Plan with client ways of alleviating stressors and finding available resources	Identifies factors that result in increased emotional lability
Support medication program, need for professional assistance, healthy lifestyle practices	Identifies approaches to decreasing etiologic stressors
Encourage client in planning realistic goals	Identifies alternative ways of handling emotions

Research Highlights

Studying a general sample of undergraduates unselected for bulimia, researchers have found a positive relation between depression and bulimia. In a sample of undergraduate women, Greenberg and Harvey[8] found that coexistent high levels of depression and dietary restraint were a better indicator of binge eating than was either variable alone. Other investigators have reported that both impulsivity and substance abuse are associated with bulimia and disorders involving an elevated mood. However, the interaction of depression and dietary restraint did not always predict the severity of binge eating.

The study by Greenberg and Harvey[8] attempted to identify other variables that could enhance predictions of the severity of binge eating. They assessed depressive, elated, and labile cyclic mood disturbances with binge eating. The subject sample of 73 undergraduates unselected for bulimia completed four instruments; the Long Form Beck Depression Inventory, Restraint Questionnaire, Binge Scale, and General Behavior Inventory. The results replicated earlier findings that the interaction of dietary restraint and depression was a significant predictor of binge eating. In addition, this study found that lability of affect, particularly the shifts between elated and depressed mood, is an even better predictor of the severity of binge eating. Lastly, the researchers suggested that biphasic mood variation has a causal role in binge eating that earlier had been attributed to depression.

began to feel she did have alternative coping skills and was not a victim of her emotions.

By the time of discharge, Kathy had developed an awareness of her binge eating and alcohol consumption as a relief from her overwhelming feelings of powerlessness and hopelessness. She identified alternative strategies for living with her mood disorder by learning about the need to take lithium consistently, becoming involved in group and couple counseling, and beginning an exercise and nutrition program. She began to acknowledge her likable qualities and abilities and to develop relationships with others. In addition, she identified some of the related stressors in living with her family while trying to carry out multiple role responsibilities. She began to relate being emotionally labile to feelings of being overwhelmed and to utilize alternative coping behaviors for feelings of anxiety. A continuing goal was to regain and maintain more consistently satisfying relationships based on an appraisal of her strengths and limitations. She had difficulty accepting the potential for relapses. This led to some episodes of discontinuing medication, rehospitalization, and periodic cycles of depression.

SUMMARY

Labile emotions are associated with feelings and behaviors evidenced by mood fluctuations. Related factors include neurologic, hormonal, chemical, environmental, traumatic, and pathological stressors and psychosocial–cultural influences that interrelate to create an imbalance in homeostasis. Defining characteristics consist of behaviors and moods that indicate variable and changing emotional expressions. The nursing process involves a thorough assessment of the relation of past and present stressors and imbalances the client may be reacting to, the safety and control issues, the client's awareness of the impact of emotional expression on self and others, and the ability to alter behavior when emotional expressions are greater in amount and frequency than is usually appropriate. Priority nursing interventions are to consider the safety issues for the client's and others' well-being. The client's abilities to make behavioral changes are identified within a context of realistic assessment of cognitive and physiological norms. Evaluation of client emotional expression, behavior, ability to be in control, and related factors is continuous.

References

1. American Psychiatric Association. Diagnostic and Statistical Manual of Mental Disorders. 3rd ed. Revised. Washington, DC: American Psychiatric Association; 1987.
2. Bienenfield D. Alcoholism in the elderly. Am Family Physician. 1987;36:163–169.
3. Brenners DK, Harris B, Weston PS. Managing manic behavior. Am J Nurs. May, 1987;87:620–623.
4. Brown G. Interview: expressed emotion and life events in schizophrenia and depression. J Psychosoc Nurs. 1986; 24(7):31–33.
5. Dracup K, Meleis A. Compliance: an interactionist approach. Nurs Res. 1982;31(1)31–36.
6. Elsass P, Henriksen L. Acute cerebral dysfunction after open-heart surgery. Scand J Thor Cardiovasc Surg. 1984;18(2):161–165.
7. Erkinjuntti T. Types of multi-infarct dementia. Acta Neurol Scand. 1987;75(6):391–399.
8. Greenberg BB, Harvey PD. Affective lability versus depression as determinants of binge eating. Addict Behav. 1987;12(4):357–361.
9. Gutzman H, Kulal K. Emotion control and cerebellar atrophy in senile dementia. Arch Geront Geriatr. 1987;6(1):61–71.
10. Hooley J. Expressed emotion and depression: interactions between patients and high- versus low-expressed-emotion spouses. J Ab Psychol. 1986;95(3):237–246.
11. Keuvi V, Carson R, Dixson A. Plasma amine and hormone changes in "post-partum blues." Clin Endocrin. 1983; 19(1):39–46.
12. Levy JM, Remick RA. Clinical aspects and treatment of rapid cycling mood disorders. Can J Psychiatry. 1986;31(5):436–441.
13. Mayeux R. Emotional changes associated with basal ganglia disorders. In: Heilman K, Satz P, eds. Neuropsychology of Human Emotion. New York: Guilford Press; 1983.
14. Mueller J. Neuroanatomic correlates of emotion. In: Temoshok L, Van Dyke C, Zigans L, eds. Emotions in Health and

Illness: Theoretical and Research Foundations. New York: Grune & Stratton; 1983.

15. Price W, DiMarzio L. Premenstrual tension syndrome in rapid-cycling bipolar affective disorder. J Clin Psychiatry. 1986:47:415–417.

16. Pritchard P. Personality and emotional complications of epilepsy. In: Heilman K, Satz P, eds. Neuropsychology of Human Emotion. New York: Guilford Press; 1983.

17. Reus V. Diagnosis and treatment in endocrinology from Cushing's syndrome to disorders of mood. In: Van Dyke C, Temoshok L, Zigans L, eds. Emotions in Health and Illness: Applications to Clinical Practice. New York: Grune and Stratton; 1984.

18. Ryan L, Montgomery A, Meyers S. Impact of circadian rhythm research on approaches to affective illness. Arch Psych Nurs. 1987;1(4):236–240.

19. Sharfstein S, Sack D, Fauci A. Relationship between alternate day corticosteroid therapy and behavioral abnormalities. JAMA. 1982;248(22):2987–2989.

20. Stuss D, Bendon D. Emotional concomitants of psychosurgery. In: Heilman K, Satz P, eds. Neuropsychology of Human Emotion. New York: Guilford Press; 1983.

21. Wartman S, Morlock L, Malitz F, Palm E. Patient understanding and satisfaction as predictors of compliance. Med Care. 1981;21(9):886–891.

22. Weddington W, Banner A. Organic affective syndrome associated with metoclopramide: case report. J Clin Psychiatry. 1986;47(4):208–209.

FAMILY PROCESSES, DYSFUNCTIONAL

Joan E. Bowers

DEFINITION AND DESCRIPTION

Dysfunctional family processes is a state in which the survival or developmental needs of one or more members of a family that usually functions effectively are not being met.[14] Each family manifests its dysfunction in a variety of ways related either to difficulty in coping with the usual daily stressors or as a result of crisis secondary to situational or developmental demands (see nursing diagnosis entitled Family Coping, Potential for Growth). An example of a family engaged in dysfunctional process related to situational factors would be parents who are engaged in marital conflict because of reduced role flexibility and whose 8-year-old child is setting fires in the neighborhood. This family may come to the attention of the nurse or the mental health professional because of the behavioral disturbance in the child, and the assessment process would lead the psychiatric mental health nurse to recognize that this behavioral disturbance is a symptom of underlying marital conflict and secondary ineffectual limit setting these parents enact with their child.

THEORY AND RESEARCH

The theories that have been developed to explain dysfunctional processes in families can be seen on a continuum from behavioral models[25] to cybernetics theory[9] to communication theory[30] to general systems theory[20] to the more psychodynamic models such as those of Bowen and Ackerman.[13] All of these theories share a perspective of the family as a system; that is, an entity composed of persons in interaction in a continuing relationship.[3] Although the terminology and emphases may differ, various commonalities regarding the goals and functions of the family are shared by these models.

Dimensions of Family Health

Barnhill[1] presented a synthesis of the family literature and proposed eight basic dimensions that distinguish healthy from dysfunctional families (Box 13-4).

Expressed Emotion

The construct of expressed emotion was developed from observations that clients with a diagnosis of schizophrenia were more likely to relapse when they spent extended amounts of time (35 or more hours per week) with family member(s) who were critical of the client's social behaviors and competence. More recent efforts to replicate the early studies on expressed emotion determined that continued maintenance on neuroleptic medications ameliorated the effect of both of these variables (extended time spent with family and family's criticism of the client) on the client's continued avoidance of relapse, rehospitalization, or both. Further research has examined the effects of expressed emotion on relapse of clients with depression.[19,34] For groups with either neurotic or bipolar depression, significant relations were found between expressed emotion and the relapse rate. The research has extended further to examine expressed emotion and maintenance of persons with senile dementia of the Alzheimer's type.[24] Here, the results were negative; that is, expressed emotion does not seem to be related to outcomes for these clients and their families (see nursing diagnosis entitled Family Coping, Potential for Growth).

Family Paradigm Model

Three major constructs that describe family functioning, known as the Family Paradigm,[28] are: *configuration*, the family's belief that the environment is one they are able to master; *coordination*, the family's sense that the environment functions similarly for all its members; and *closure*, the family's view of the environment as a source of new and changing experience. These constructs differentiate successful families from those with a chronically disturbed member.

Strategic Family Therapy Model

Haley[9] has proposed that the occurrence of a serious psychiatric disturbance in a young person is a symptom of dysfunctional processes within the family. The Stra-

---

BOX 13–4
Dimensions of Family Health

1. Individuation *v* enmeshment
2. Mutuality *v* isolation
3. Flexibility *v* rigidity
4. Stability *v* disorganization
5. Clear *v* unclear or distorted perceptions
6. Clear *v* unclear roles or role conflict
7. Role reciprocity *v* unclear or conflictual roles
8. Clear *v* diffuse or breached generation boundaries

From Barnhill L. Healthy family systems. Family Coordinator. 1979; 28:94.

---

tegic Family Therapy approach is focused on empowering the parents to structure their world so as to help the young person to leave home.[9]

In summary, a number of theories about family functioning and dysfunctional processes have been advanced. Primarily, these theories view the family as a system, and they share many concepts. Some, like that of Reiss,[27] are heavily grounded in empirical research. Others, such as Haley's,[9] were developed primarily from extensive interaction with families who have sought help in dealing with a member's symptomatic behaviors.

RELATED FACTORS

The family's response to either a situational or a developmental challenge is mediated by a variety of factors. The *developmental stage* of the family and the success with which it has traversed the preceding stages provides background for coping with the current issues. Earlier challenges that have confronted the family can have either a negative or a positive influence on the response to the contemporary events.

The *coping strategies* the family has learned and used successfully can be very important resources in meeting the demands of the current crisis. On the other hand, if the family has recently been bombarded with demands, members may be feeling overwhelmed or depleted in the face of the new demands of the current crisis.

Some families have developed sufficient "stress resistance"[8] from earlier experiences with developmental and situational challenges that they will continue to cope at a high level even in the face of what would appear to be an overwhelming burden. A related concept used in understanding family response to stressors is that of *hardiness*,[17] which is conceptualized as a family resource and includes the internal strengths and durability of the family unit. These families are characterized as having a sense of control over the outcomes of life events and hardships. Further, they view change as beneficial and growth-producing, and they take an active rather than a passive approach to managing stressful situations.

The family's *precrisis relational patterns* may contribute to the difficulties they experience in facing a major demand. For example, the parents may have *rigidly defined role patterns* that help them to maintain their marital relationship, in the absence of a satisfying interpersonal component of the marriage. Having to deal with a crisis could very easily undo this delicate balance, such that the family may be torn apart by what appears to the observer to be a normal developmental challenge.

Another important variable is *cultural background*. The meaning the family gives to a crisis may be quite different from that the psychiatric mental health nurse would expect under the circumstances. In order to account for these differences, Olson and his colleagues[23] developed an assessment tool that asks families to report on various family characteristics as they are now. A second set of the same items asks how satisfied members are with these areas of family functioning. The family instrument of Roberts and Feetham[29] has a similar format.

Additionally, the nature of the challenge or crisis may impose a special burden on the family and result in dysfunctional coping patterns. For example, a traditional family in which a member has broken the law and been apprehended may be so overwhelmed by the inherent loss of face that the members are unable to cope with even very minor demands following the arrest.

The nature of a health challenge will influence the family's response. For example, the primary client's age and role functioning within the family may have a significant influence on the family's ability to manage the health challenge effectively. Thus, the incapacitation of the primary breadwinner by a life-threatening illness probably will evoke a different response from the family than the diagnosis of a chronic but not life-threatening disorder in the family's school-age child. Also, the family that has to cope with a member's illness for which there is effective treatment with certain outcomes will have fewer problems on the average than the family whose member is found to have AIDS, a disorder for which there is currently no cure, with inevitable death. The *uncertainty*[21] that attaches to the course and outcome of some health problems may also adversely affect the family's ability to manage the stressor effectively.

In summary, the family that is operating in a dysfunctional mode may be coping with a variety of factors such as *excessive internal* or *external demands*, inadequate *coping strategies*, or the *uncertainty* or *stigma* attached to the event, to name a few. When dysfunctional family process is observed, a thorough *family assessment* is in order.

DEFINING CHARACTERISTICS

The family that is manifesting dysfunctional process may demonstrate difficulty in meeting or inability to meet the needs of its members in one or more of the following domains: physical, emotional, spiritual, and cognitive.

The family's internal processes may provide clues to the difficulties it is experiencing. Some of these elements include inability to engage in effective problem solving, lack of respect between the parents for each other's parenting styles, and rigidity in function and roles between and among family members. Inappropriate boundary maintenance within the family, that is, between members of a dyad or between members of different generations, can be an important clue that the family is not functioning well. A lack of connectedness to the community may be a symptom of family dysfunction. For example, the family with rigid boundaries between itself and the community may be one in which the members are constrained to keep secrets about such behaviors as family violence or sexual abuse. On the other hand, the family with very loose boundaries between itself and the external environment allows too much opportunity for coming and going and therefore may convey too little sense of belongingness to its members, particularly the dependent children. A family in which one or both of the parents are incapacitated through drug abuse may demonstrate this symptom of inadequate boundaries and connectedness. For example, the parents' drug use may make them unavailable to the dependent children and thus unable to meet the children's needs adequately and consistently.

Additionally, the family in which there is little emphasis on the development of autonomy for its members may be demonstrating that it is having difficulty that would profit from intervention by a health professional. An example of this is the family in which the oldest child, who is now reaching adolescence, is still expected to obey curfew rules appropriate at an earlier age.

Another way in which a family may give evidence of dysfunction is through the inability to deal constructively with a traumatic event. An example is the family that becomes disorganized through lack of communication or the experience of guilt in relation to a child's serious illness. The failure to accomplish current or past developmental tasks is also symptomatic of a dysfunctional family. The young married couple who fail to set appropriate boundaries between themselves as a new family unit and their respective families of origin is a case in point (Chart 1).

NURSING PROCESS AND RATIONALE

Assessment

Evidence that the family is operating in a dysfunctional mode should signal the need for an assessment of the family as a unit. If one of the members is acutely disturbed, the nurse may need to decide whether to include that member in the initial assessment. A skilled clinician will more likely wish to include the disturbed member in order to get a complete picture of the family

---

CHART 1
Dysfunctional Family Processes: Definition, Related Factors, and Defining Characteristics

DEFINITION

A family displaying dysfunctional process is one in which one or more member(s)' survival or developmental needs are not being met.

RELATED FACTORS

Family developmental stage, including successful achievement of earlier developmental tasks
Learned coping/management strategies
Previous stressors
Concurrent stressors (pile-up of stressors)
Family hardiness, family stress inoculation
Family functioning, including role patterns, communication patterns, cohesion, flexibility, conflict resolution patterns
Cultural variables, including stigma attached to the challenge confronting the family
Concurrent demands on family resources

DEFINING CHARACTERISTICS

Physical needs not met (food, clothing, shelter, security)
Psychosocial needs not met (respect, affirmation, social support, autonomy)
Spiritual needs not met
Cognitive needs not met (intellectual stimulation, learning opportunities, validation of perceptions)
Poor problem-solving skills
Rigid role function/assignment
Boundary issues relative to family developmental stage
Unclear or inconsistent communication
Unmet developmental tasks (individual or family)
Family system at risk of disintegration

---

process that affects and is affected by that member's functioning. In this assessment process, the family members will be asked to respond to a variety of questions about the family and its individual members. Both the family's verbal responses and observations of the members' interactions will provide data for the health professional's diagnosis and interventions. Additionally, the family members may be asked to complete one or more standardized instruments about themselves and about the family.[6,18,22,23]

In conducting the assessment of the family, the psychiatric mental health nurse will focus on:

1. Family and household composition.
2. Members' perceptions of the family's current functioning, including their definition of the problem facing them, the strategies they've used for dealing with similar problems in the past, their satisfaction with those outcomes, and their resources for dealing with the current problem.

3. The family's developmental stage, including how well it is meeting tasks both as a group and as individuals.

Other observations that the nurse makes about family interaction will add to this information base:

4. Indications of clear boundaries and the absence (or presence) of destructive coalitions within the family. Destructive coalitions are frequently cross-generational; for example, a father-daughter pair who criticizes the mother's lack of limit setting with a mentally retarded son.

5. Evidence of appropriate attachments between and among the family members, such as listening patiently.

6. Illustrations of clear and open communication, such as nonverbal communication that is congruent with the spoken message.

7. Signs that the members' roles are appropriate and feasible given the individual's abilities and the needs manifested by the family.

8. Evidence that appropriate controls are used fairly and consistently in the family, such as the observation that all of the children are expected to be quiet while an adult is speaking.

9. Illustrations of the goals and beliefs that may influence the family and that may block the health professional's efforts to work with the family toward change.

10. Indicators of the family members' intellectual functioning and educational levels, as well as their financial resources.

11. Manifestations of the ways in which the member's behavioral symptom influences one or more members in the family (the reverse of this would also be important).

Many of these indicators will not be important if they appear in isolation; rather, the nurse will be interested in observing family *patterns* of interaction, such as those described in the Case Study, that support the dysfunctional process.

Nursing Diagnoses

The nursing diagnostic category—dysfunctional family process—may be made more specific for a particular family. For example, the diagnosis might be dysfunctional family process related to many concurrent stressors and problematic coping strategies.

Client Goals and Nursing Interventions

The goals the family initially identifies may focus on the individual member's symptoms or problem behaviors. In conducting the family assessment, the nurse may wish to help the family to explore the relation between the presenting problem and family *system* functioning.[31,32] The psychiatric mental health nurse specialist may choose an assessment approach that has been proposed[26,34,36] for helping the family both to focus on system properties and to begin to discover its own ability to heal itself. For example, reflexive questions are characterized by a general curiosity about the possible connectedness of events that include the problem.[34] Future-oriented questions ask the family to speculate and thus provide the members with an opportunity to introduce new ideas into the problem-solving process.[26] Several examples of such questions appear in Box 13-5.

Barnhill's[1] dimensions of family health may be used as the basis for proposing goals when the family is found to be operating in a dysfunctional mode (see Box 13-4).

1. Goals can include the development of greater autonomy counterbalanced by appropriate levels of closeness for all family members. In the case of unhealthy coalitions, the reestablishment of appropriate hierarchical boundaries might provide another family goal (see item 8).

2. In families where one or more members have become disengaged, a goal of increased affective connections among members may be an appropriate goal.

3. Increased flexibility in the allocation and enactment of roles within the family may be an important goal in rigid systems. Families may need to develop more flexibility in the rules and regulations that govern members' behavior. Boundaries between the family and the larger community may need to be made more flexible in order for the family to have access to important feedback and other forms of social support.

BOX 13–5
Examples of Interventive Questioning

REFLEXIVE QUESTIONS

The clients are required to reflect on their situation in order to provide an answer.[34] For example, a family with a depressed member might be asked, ''Who worries the most about (the depressed member)?'' ''Who worries next most?'' ''When Dad is worrying about (the depressed member), how does he let you know this?'' ''When Dad is worrying, what do the rest of you do?''

FUTURE QUESTIONS

The family is asked to consider how the pattern of their relationships will continue in the future.[26] For example, the family with an anorexic daughter might be asked how much longer they think it will be before the girl will give up her bulimia. When the daughter is asked the same question, she answers, ''Probably next year when I move out.''[36]

4. Families in which there is little predictability or structure may need help in developing patterns that are easily managed and that contribute to members' sense of stability. Budgeting of finances, meal planning, and consistent behavioral expectations for children and adults are a few of the organizational elements that might be goals for nursing intervention with a dysfunctional family.

5. The goals for the family regarding perceptions might focus on improving communication skills. Subgoals might include that all members speak for themselves, that questions and comments be direct, saying what they mean, that nonverbal communication be consistent with the verbal message, and that members be free to express a range of emotions.

6. Family members should know what is expected of them in each of the particular roles that is assigned or assumed. These roles should be feasible for the members to enact.

7. An example of role conflict would be a situation in which the mother must be gainfully employed to provide an adequate family income but receives no relief in her family caretaking role. This family might elect the goal of increasing role reciprocity around caretaking needs.

8. Breached generational boundaries are generally an indication of a moderate to severe dysfunction in the family system. Father–daughter incest is an example of breached generational boundaries.[10] In families with a diagnosis of drug dependency in a member, that member is frequently found to be in an enmeshed relationship (or cross-generational coalition) with a parent or other involved adult family member.[15]

Outcome criteria for a family intervention should include two foci. First, the presenting symptom should be used to propose changes in functioning that would signify positive outcomes from the intervention. Some early reports of family therapy outcomes have been criticized because the measures of individual functioning in the symptomatic member were not included in the research report.[16] The cessation of symptoms or other behavior changes for the individual thus should be specified as part of the outcome criteria. The other major focus could be developed by using the Barnhill schema (see Box 13-4) for determining family goals and family level outcome criteria (Chart 2).

CASE STUDY

The R family was assessed by a psychiatric staff nurse on an inpatient unit to be operating at a dysfunctional level at the time the 13-year-old daughter, Kim, was hospitalized for a transient psychotic episode. On the basis of this assessment, the Rs were referred for family therapy with a psychiatric mental health clinical nurse specialist, to which they readily agreed. The family had experienced serious difficulties for the last 8 months, ever since the 10-year-old, Nancy, was hospitalized in acute distress with insulin-dependent diabetes. Ken, 38, employed as a maintenance engineer for a large firm, had left the family for several months because he could not handle the stress and demands. His wife, Maribelle, 35, conducted a daycare center in their home to supplement the family income. The other family members included twin boys, Danny and David, age 6. Kim was described by her parents as very bright but at risk for failing in school because she had refused to attend classes following her 2-week hospitalization.

A significant family issue was the stress brought on by Nancy's brittle diabetes. At the time the family was seen, Nancy had developed peripheral neuropathy in her upper extremities and had difficulty administering her own insulin. In addition, she would permit only her mother to administer the medication. Nancy and her mother thus shared a very special relationship, which was also demonstrated by the extreme concern that Ms. R felt about Nancy. This was a serious issue for Kim, who felt deprived and jealous of the attention showered on Nancy. Mr. R, once again back in the

CHART 2
Dysfunctional Family Processes: Summary of the Nursing Process

NURSING INTERVENTIONS	OUTCOME CRITERIA
PARENT GOAL: FACILITATE CHILDREN'S PSYCHOSOCIAL DEVELOPMENT BY HOLDING THEM RESPONSIBLE FOR BEHAVIOR AT HOME AND IN SCHOOL	
Assist parents to develop negotiation skills regarding rules and limits	Parents report satisfaction with change in children's behavior and attitude
Encourage parents to use contracts for desired behavior changes	
PARENT GOAL: RENEGOTIATE BOUNDARIES BETWEEN PARENTS AND CHILDREN WITHIN THE FAMILY	
Encourage parents to spend time with each of the children as individuals and to take time for themselves as a couple	Parents report more sharing of responsibility for tasks related to care of children
	Parents and children report increased levels of satisfaction with relationships
PARENT GOAL: INCREASE KNOWLEDGE ABOUT NORMAL GROWTH AND DEVELOPMENT	
Suggest appropriate references for reading	Parents describe increased knowledge about normal growth and development
Suggest community resources such as parenting classes	

Research Highlights

Thompson and Doll[33] studied 125 family caregivers to determine the extent of the burden related to having a family member with a serious psychiatric illness return to the home after hospital discharge. Instruments used included an index of family members' embarrassment[7] and the Incomplete Sentence Blank.[30] The authors reported that fully 73% of the respondents were adversely affected in one or more ways by the presence of their member in the home. Seventy-four per cent of these participants were deemed to be coping with chronic feelings of being overloaded. The three principal findings were: (1) families of discharged psychiatric patients have been placed in an emotionally demanding situation in which they report feeling burdened; (2) this experience of emotional burden is reported by families regardless of the relationship to the member patient (parent versus spouse), social class, or race; and (3) the family's experience of burden needs to be separated into subjective and objective components to facilitate a clearer understanding of the phenomenon.

Cook[4,5] studied caretaking of former psychiatric patients from a feminist perspective. Mothers in this study reported higher levels of worry, anxiety, depression, and emotional drain than fathers.

home, also appeared to be suffering from the change in focus within the family secondary to his younger daughter's illness. The two boys seemed to be functioning well, although they were both more reserved and shy than might be expected of children their age. The psychiatric mental health clinical nurse specialist made a nursing diagnosis of dysfunctional family process related to concurrent demands on family resources and, secondarily, to the family's problematic coping strategies. Several individual-level nursing diagnoses were also determined to be applicable. Kim was given a nursing diagnosis of situational low self-esteem with resulting behaviors of moderate aggression and altered impulse control. Nancy received a nursing diagnosis of self-care deficit related to management of her diabetes regimen.

The family was seen for a total of ten sessions over a period of 3 months by the clinical nurse specialist. The therapy goals focused on helping the parents to empower Kim by holding her responsible for her behavior at home and in school. This goal was counterbalanced by a second one of having Ms. R reestablish appropriate boundaries between herself and Nancy, thus allowing the mother to provide more attention to her other children. The marital relationship was not addressed directly. Attention was paid indirectly first by focusing on the need to have Mr. R learn to administer insulin to Nancy, thus drawing him back into the family circle. Second, the parents worked together to determine and implement limits for Kim and the other children. The couple thus shared more responsibility for their children's welfare and began to demonstrate increased togetherness in their marital relationship as well.

At the time of termination, Kim was attending classes at an alternative school. She was pleased with this arrangement and had learned to use the bus system, a requirement that initially paralyzed her. Several months later, at Christmas time, Ms. R wrote to the clinical nurse specialist that although life was never perfect, the family was doing well. She enclosed Kim's school photograph, showing an attractive, shy, but smiling teenager.

SUMMARY

Concepts that facilitate an understanding of dysfunctional family process include those from role theory such as role flexibility, role conflict, and role reciprocity. Both situational and developmental demands influence family functioning. Other family concepts include boundary, hierarchy, limit setting, coalition, interaction patterns, and individuation. The concepts of stigma and uncertainty assist in understanding family response to demands. Barnhill's model of family functioning[1] includes the concepts of autonomy, enmeshment, mutuality, isolation, flexibility, rigidity, and clear perceptions. Research on family interaction patterns by Reiss and Oliveri[28] provides the concepts of configuration, coordination, and closure.

The degree of hardiness[17] or stress inoculation[8] that the family has developed may explain differences across families in coping with similar stressors. Cultural factors need to be understood by the health professional who conducts the family assessment and intervention. Caregiver burden[4,5,7,33] also influences the family's level of functioning in dealing with a member with a chronic mental illness.

References

1. Barnhill L. Healthy family systems. Family Coordinator. 1979;28:94–100.
2. Brown GW, Carstairs GM, Topping G. Post hospital adjustment of chronic mental patients. Lancet. 1958;2:685–689.
3. Buckley W, ed. Modern Systems Research for the Behavioral Scientist. Chicago, IL: Aldine Publishing; 1968.
4. Cook JA, Pickett S. Feelings of burden and criticalness among parents residing with chronically mentally ill offspring. J Appl Soc Sci. 1987–88;12:79–107.
5. Cook JA. Who "mothers" the chronically mentally ill? Fam Relations. 1988;37:42–49.
6. Epstein NB, Baldwin LM, Bishop DS. The McMaster Family Assessment Device. J Marital Fam Ther. 1983;9:171–180.
7. Freeman H, Simmons O. Feelings of stigma among relatives of former mental patients. Soc Prob. 1961;8:312–321.
8. Garmezy N, Rutter M, eds. Stress, Coping and Development in Children. New York: McGraw-Hill; 1983.
9. Haley J. Leaving Home: The Therapy of Disturbed Young People. New York: McGraw-Hill; 1980.
10. Herman JL. Father–Daughter Incest. Cambridge, MA: Harvard University Press; 1981.
11. Hoffman L. Foundations of Family Therapy: A Conceptual Framework for Systems Change. New York: Basic Books; 1981.

12. Holman AL. Family Assessment: Tools for Understanding and Intervention. Beverly Hills, CA: Sage; 1983.

13. Jones SL. Family Therapy: A Comparison of Approaches. Bowie, Maryland: Robert J Brady Co; 1980.

14. Kim MJ, McFarland GK, McLane AM. Pocket Guide to Nursing Diagnoses. 3rd ed. St. Louis: CV Mosby; 1989.

15. Madanes C, Dukes J, Harbin H. Family ties of heroin addicts. Arch Gen Psychiatry. 1980;37:889–894.

16. Masten A. Family therapy as a treatment for children: A critical review of outcome research. Fam Process. 1979;18:323–335.

17. McCubbin M, McCubbin HI, Thompson AI. FHI: Family Hardiness Index. In: McCubbin HI, Thompson AI, eds. Family Assessment Inventories for Research and Practice. Madison, WI: University of Wisconsin-Madison; 1987.

18. McCubbin HI, Thompson AI, eds. Family Assessment Inventories for Research and Practice. Madison, WI: University of Wisconsin-Madison; 1987.

19. Miklowitz DJ, Goldstein MJ, Nuechterlein KH, Snyder KS, Mintz J. Family factors and the course of bipolar affective disorder. Arch Gen Psychiatry. 1988;45:225–231.

20. Minuchin S. Families and Family Therapy. Cambridge, MA: Harvard University Press; 1978.

21. Mishel MH. Uncertainty in illness. Image: Journal of Nursing Scholarship, 1988;20:225–232.

22. Moos RH, Moos BS. A typology of social environments. Fam Process, 1976;15:357–371.

23. Olson DH, Portner J, Lavee Y. Family adaptability and cohesion scales (FACES III). St. Paul, Minnesota: University of Minnesota Press; 1985.

24. Orford J, O'Reilly P, Goonatilleke A. Expressed emotion and perceived family interaction in the key relatives of elderly patients with dementia. Psychol Med. 1987;17:963–970.

25. Patterson GR. Living with Children: New Methods for Parents and Teachers, rev ed. Champaign, IL: Research Press; 1976.

26. Penn P. Feed-forward: Future questions, future maps. Fam Process. 1985;24:299–310.

27. Reiss D. Varieties of consensual experience III: Contrasts between families of normals, delinquents and schizophrenics. J Nerv Ment Dis. 1971;152:73–95.

28. Reiss D, Oliveri ME. Family paradigm and family coping: A proposal for linking the family's intrinsic adaptive capacities to its responses to stress. Fam Relations. 1980;29:431–444.

29. Roberts CS, Feetham S. Assessing family functioning across three areas of relationships. Nurs Res. 1982;31:231–235.

30. Rotter J, Williams B. The incomplete sentence test as a method of studying personality. J Consult Psychol. 1947;11:43–48.

31. Satir V. Conjoint Family Therapy, rev ed. Palo Alto, CA: Science and Behavior Books; 1967.

32. Smoyak S. Introducing families to family therapy. In: Smoyak S, ed. The Psychiatric Nurse as a Family Therapist. New York: John Wiley; 1975.

33. Thompson EH, Doll W. The burden of families coping with the mentally ill: An invisible crisis. Fam Relations. 1982;31:379–388.

34. Tomm K. Interventive interviewing. I: Strategizing as a fourth guideline for the therapist. Fam Process. 1987;26:3–13.

35. Vaughn C, Leff JP. The influence of family and social factors on the course of psychiatric illness: A comparison of schizophrenic and depressed neurotic patients. Br J Psychiatry. 1976;129:125–137.

36. Wright LM, Leahey M. Families and psychosocial problems: Assumptions, assessment and intervention. In: Leahey M, Wright LM, eds. Families and Psychosocial Problems. Springhouse, PA: Springhouse Corporation; 1987.

FEAR

Joan Hanser McConnell

DEFINITION AND DESCRIPTION

Fear is a feeling of dread related to an identifiable source that can be validated. Its primary difference from *anxiety* is that the source of fear can be identified, whereas, in anxiety, the source is nonspecific or unknown to the individual. Fear concentrates on a specific danger, whereas anxiety frequently occurs as vague feelings of dread or uneasiness.[18] Because fear and anxiety can occur simultaneously, careful assessment as well as thoughtful planning are necessary for nursing interventions to be effective.

THEORY AND RESEARCH

Fear has a definite and important role in normal childhood development. It is a mechanism for successfully coping with dangers, such as traffic or thin lake ice. The avoidance behavior exhibited in response to these fears keeps the child safe.[3,15] Avoidance behavior in response to fear continues to play a protective adaptive role in adults as well as in children. Avoiding a speeding car by jumping out of the way is a lifesaving response to fear. This same avoidance reaction to fear, however, can be problematic, such as when treatment of illness is avoided because of lack of knowledge and the resulting fear of pain or death.[14,18]

Correlations between childhood fears and adult fears have been clearly identified.[2–4,7] The age of onset of fear and its duration and intensity are variables that are important in determining whether or not it will persist into adulthood.[3] Coping strategies related to fears are also understood in relationship to development.[10,15] As normal children grow to adulthood, the repertoire of cognitive, behavioral, and emotional skills and responses also grow and develop. Children traumatized by fears frequently demonstrate developmental difficulties as they mature. As adults they may manifest maladaptive coping skills in relation to fear. Some research indicates that a genetic control factor is involved in fear from infancy onward.[9] Fear can complicate psychiatric disorders and the treatment of clients who experience them.[6,11,12,14]

RELATED FACTORS

Fear can occur in clients across the age span. Separation from significant others can elicit fear in children or adults during hospitalization. Knowledge deficits of disease processes and treatment regimens can cause fears that complicate recovery.[16] Side effects of medications or potential impairments, such as movement disorders, may interfere with compliance in the long-term treatment of some mental disorders. Increased knowledge may also increase fear. Clients who become aggressive or out of control during a psychotic episode fear the occurrence of such behavior in the future.

Victims of physical and sexual abuse are fearful of pain, bodily harm, or even death at the hands of the abuser. Abused children frequently express the fear of separation from families if the abuse is reported. Many battered women report fear of loneliness or their own abilities to survive as reasons for remaining in abusive situations.

Fear can occur in psychiatric clients because of problems in appraising the situation accurately and because of problems in coping with the sources of fear. Hallucinations and delusions, such as voices telling a person to harm himself or the fixed idea that there is a plot of murder, can be very frightening. Cognitive losses experienced by clients with dementias leave them without the ability to utilize coping strategies that may have been effective in the past when managing fear. Clients with a new diagnosis of Alzheimer's disease often fear the debilitating losses that are to come. Many psychiatric clients are fearful about how others may react when they are told of recent hospitalizations. Fear of loss of jobs, income, and family support are often verbalized by clients.

Fears related to death and dying are common in clients facing terminal illnesses. Isolation, sensory impairments, and loneliness are feared by the elderly experiencing losses of family and friends as they near the end of life. Hospitalization often exacerbates these fears as a very real loss of control over many aspects of daily living becomes a reality.

DEFINING CHARACTERISTICS

Clients expressing fear describe the situations in a variety of ways. Descriptions can be graphic and highlight the emotions experienced: "I was frozen with fear;" "It scared me to death;" "There was nothing I could do to stop him from hitting me." Clients experiencing perceptual distortions, illusions, or hallucinations, may react with fear to these distortions. The client suffering from Alzheimer's disease who is unable to recognize and interpret objects may fear common objects in the environment.[1] Increased alertness, tension, and concentration on danger are also found in descriptions of fearful situations.

Physiologic manifestations of fear that may be observed include increased heart and respiratory rates, pupil dilation, diaphoresis, and increased muscle tension. Children frequently cry if the stimulus for the fear is especially terrifying, as when experiencing painful procedures or experiencing nightmares. Involuntary urination or defecation can occur in children or adults when fear is experienced.

"Fight-or-flight" responses result in aggression toward the feared object or withdrawal from the situation.[12] The fight-or-flight responses may be maladaptive, or they may be effective mechanisms for coping with fear. Clients fearful of change risk maintaining lives complicated by painful emotional situations. The client fears the change necessary to make life bearable so "flees" or avoids the situation by leaving the hospital or by cancelling therapy appointments. Maladaptive fight responses in reaction to the fear may include behavioral disturbances, such as temper tantrums or consistent oppositional behavior. Facing fears and learning effective methods for dealing with feared persons or situations illustrate effective fight response.[11,13] The battered wife who leaves her spouse utilizes the flight response effectively (Chart 1).

NURSING PROCESS AND RATIONALE

Assessment

A comprehensive assessment of the client who may be experiencing fear involves observing for physiologic, emotional, and behavioral changes. Factors including age, developmental level, and environment, influence how the nurse obtains assessment data. Careful direct questioning of clients who appear frightened can assist them in describing their fear. Statements such as, "tell me what's frightening you" or "you seem frightened, tell me about that," encourage descriptions of the source of the fear and its experience by the client. Directed play techniques using props, such as dolls and stuffed animals, assist young children to describe their fears.[8] Withdrawn or aggressive behaviors are often present as a response to fear and complicate the assessment process.

Previous coping methods and strategies for dealing with fears that have worked in the past for the client are assessed. In addition to observing patterns of coping, questions such as—"Have you experienced similar fears before?" "What helped you overcome them?" "Has anything like this happened to you in the past?" "What made it better?"—all assist in gathering assessment data from the client.

Nursing Diagnosis

Examples of nursing diagnoses for the client who is fearful may include fear related to separation from sig-

---

CHART 1
Fear: Definition, Related Factors, and Defining Characteristics

DEFINITION

Fear is a feeling of dread related to an identifiable source that can be validated. Fear is differentiated from anxiety primarily in that the source of fear is related to an identifiable source, whereas, in anxiety, the source is nonspecific or unknown to the individual.

RELATED FACTORS

Loss of control
Pain
Death
Separation
Loneliness–isolation
Knowledge deficit
Knowledge of threats posed by an approaching
    experience
Bodily harm
Environmental stimuli (i.e., physical threats, abuse)
Sensory impairment
Language barrier
Hallucinations
Delusions

DEFINING CHARACTERISTICS

Fright
Apprehension
Increased tension
Terror
Alertness
Fight (aggression)
Flight (withdrawal)
Concentration on danger
Sympathetic stimulation
    Increased heart rate
    Increased respiratory rate
    Pupil dilation
    Increased muscle tension
    Diaphoresis
Impulsiveness
Focus on "it, out there"
Attempts to destroy source of fear

---

nificant other, fear related to loss of control, or fear related to bodily harm.

Client Goals and Nursing Interventions

The goals for the client experiencing fear are (1) to reduce or eliminate the fear, (2) to control fear by use of effective coping strategies, and (3) to manage daily life in the presence of fear. Nursing interventions are aimed at assisting the client to identify and describe the fears, remove the source of the fear, or assist the client to do so, and provide information when the fear is related to a knowledge deficit. Fears experienced by hospitalized psychiatric patients are often related to loss of control or separation from family members. Providing information about daily routines, unit rules, expectations of clients, and encouraging contact with significant others, reduce or eliminate many fears. Young children may exhibit extreme fear when hospitalized. Provision of a safe, secure environment and of consistent nursing care, as well as information geared to their developmental level, serves to reduce fears of abandonment or bodily harm. Contextual play situations provide an extremely effective method of dealing with fears of young children.[8]

Effective client teaching significantly decreases fears associated with medical, surgical, and psychiatric treatment.[5,13,17] Interventions aimed at increasing coping skills and problem-solving abilities also are helpful to fearful clients. Identifying specific strategies and role-playing them with clients provides opportunities to master skills that may be utilized in fearful situations. Providing information before a difficult or painful procedure may be contraindicated in clients with dementias. Information about an upcoming diagnostic test can communicate, on an emotional level, that something distressing is coming up.[1] Because of the cognitive impairments associated with these illnesses, the client may be unable to understand or remember the information. Providing information would cause or increase fear, rather than decreasing it. The nurse can help the client to access resources for care after discharge and establish a supportive community network. Behavioral, cognitive, and interpersonal approaches, all can be effectively utilized by the nurse to assist clients in reducing, eliminating, or managing fear.

Evaluation

The most important outcome for clients is the absence or reduction of fear. The ability to use successful coping skills when faced with fear will reduce the characteristics associated with the feared situation (Chart 2).

CASE STUDY

Jason, a nine-year-old boy, was hospitalized with a diagnosis of conduct disorder. Although it was his first psychiatric hospitalization, he had a long history of impulsivity, aggressiveness toward peers, and nightmares. His family history included drug and alcohol abuse and prostitution, and he had suffered physical abuse and neglect. He had run away from home several times and had been placed in foster care. On admission, Jason refused to have blood drawn for diagnostic tests and became physically aggressive towards staff when this procedure was attempted. The physical aggression persisted and was accompanied by crying, screaming, and verbal threats toward any staff who approached him. One nursing diagnosis formulated was fear of bodily harm. Other nursing diagnoses included ineffective individual coping and aggression. Safety and limits were provided for the child within the structure of the inpatient setting. Attempts to draw blood were not made for a few days. Nights were particularly difficult because the child's nightmares increased in intensity, and he verbalized being frightened of being harmed in the dark. Staff stayed with Jason until he fell asleep, and a night light was provided. His verbalizations about his fears increased, especially with his primary nurse. Four days after admission he allowed staff to draw blood. In the children's discussion group he was able to talk about his fears of needles and

---

CHART 2
Fear: Summary of the Nursing Process

NURSING INTERVENTIONS

CLIENT GOAL: REDUCE OR ELIMINATE THE FEAR
Assist client to describe source of fear
If possible, remove the source of fear or assist the client to do so

Assist client to accurately perceive the environment
Provide information regarding illness, treatment expectations, and environment
Provide a safe environment

CLIENT GOAL: CONTROL FEAR BY USE OF EFFECTIVE COPING STRATEGIES
Assist client to develop new coping skills
Teach problem-solving skills
Identify and role-play with client strategies to use in fearful situations
Assist client to regain control by distraction, teaching relaxation techniques, leaving the feared situation

CLIENT GOAL: MANAGE DAILY LIFE IN THE PRESENCE OF FEAR
Teach relaxation techniques
Arrange for follow up outpatient care

Assist client to identify and access community resources
Provide information to caregivers to assist client in managing fears

OUTCOME CRITERIA

Describes the fear
Removes the source of fear or alters perception of fear
Becomes knowledgeable about illness and treatment

Increases sense of safety and security

Lists and/or demonstrates effective coping skills and strategies for fear reduction

Demonstrates relaxation techniques
Maintains contact with supportive community resources
Lists community resources
Develops network of helpful, knowledgeable caregivers

Research Highlights

The study of normal fear in children has been suggested as useful in the understanding of healthy fear development, as well as in determining those fears that represent problematic reactions. As a part of this effort and to gather baseline information on typical coping mechanisms of children in relation to specific fears, Sipes and his colleagues studied 2728 ninth grade students in public schools in the Rocky Mountain region of the United States.[15] The students were instructed to write an essay in response to the questions: "Most of us as children were afraid of something—the dark, dogs, or being alone. What caused you the greatest fright when you were young? Show, by example, how you reacted to the fear. What has helped you to overcome or conquer the fear?" The results of the study determined that there are five relatively common childhood fears that accounted for almost 70% of those fears listed by the children. These fears included fear of the dark, people, spooks, being alone, and animals.

No single fear was reported with enough frequency to be assumed a fear common to most children. Of greatest interest in this report of fears are the changes that have occurred when compared with earlier similar studies. Children's fears seem to be changing, most likely in response to society and to changes in family structure. More fears associated with separation and abandonment were reported than in the earlier studies. Coping strategies listed by the children in this study were similar to those found in earlier studies. Seventy-seven percent of the coping strategies used to overcome fears were believed to be the result of growing up or of repeated or prolonged exposure to the feared event. One finding related to gender was that boys were significantly more likely to deal with fear by attacking or destroying the feared object, whereas girls turned to other people, escaped, or used other strategies to "take control" of the situation.

blood and said that "next time" he would not hurt anyone but might "yell some." A primary focus of his continued hospitalization became assisting him to overcome his fears and gain control of his behavior related to them.

SUMMARY

Fear is a feeling of dread related to an identifiable source that can be validated. The fight-or-flight reactions that occur in response to fear may be maladaptive, or they may be effective mechanisms for coping with fear. The goals for the client experiencing fear are to reduce or eliminate the fear, to control fear by the use of effective coping strategies, and to manage daily life in the presence of fear.

References

1. Beck C, Heacock P. Nursing interventions for patients with Alzheimer's disease. Nurs Clin North Am. 1988;23:95–124.
2. Erikson E. Childhood and society. New York: Norton; 1963.
3. Ferrari M. Fears and phobias in childhood: some clinical and developmental considerations. Child Psychiatry Hum Dev. 1986;17:75–87.
4. Fischer M, Rolf J, Hasozi JE, Cummings L. Follow-up of a preschool epidemiological sample: cross age continuities and prediction of later adjustment with internalizing and externalizing dimensions of behavior. Child Dev. 1984;55:137–150.
5. Foa EB, Kozak MJ. Emotional processing of fear: exposure to corrective information. Psychol Bull. 1986;99:20–35.
6. Franklin JA. The changing nature of agoraphobic fear. Br J Clin Psychol. 1987;26(Pt 2):127–133.
7. Harris SL, Ferrari M. Developmental factors in child behavior therapy. Behav Ther. 1983;14:54–72.
8. Lentz KA. The expressed fears of young children. Child Psychiatry Hum Dev. 1985;16:3–13.
9. Marks IM. Genetics of fear and anxiety disorders. Br J Psychol. 1986;149:406–418.
10. Mooney KC, Graziano AM, Katz JN. A factor analytic investigation of childrens' nighttime fear and coping responses. J Genet Psychol. 1985;146:205–215.
11. Moores A. Facing the fear. Nurs Times. 1987;83(27):44–46.
12. Moores A. Frightened of fear. Nurs Times. 1987;83(13):34–38.
13. Moss R. Overcoming fear. AORN. 1986;43:1107.
14. Pipes RB, Schwarz R, Crouch P. Measuring client fears. J Consult Clin Psychol. 1985;53:933–934.
15. Sipes G, Rardin M, Fitzgerald B. Adolescent recall of childhood fears and coping strategies. Psychol Rep. 1985;57:1215–1223.
16. Thompson D. Coronary fears. Nurs Times. 1987;83(24):68.
17. Wright LK. Life threatening illness. J Psychosoc Nurs. 1985;23(9):7–11.
18. Yocum CJ. The differentiation of fear and anxiety. In: Kim MJ, McFarland GK, McLane AM eds. Classification of nursing diagnosis: proceedings of the fifth national conference. St. Louis: CV Mosby; 1984.

GRIEVING, ANTICIPATORY GRIEVING, DYSFUNCTIONAL GRIEVING

Elizabeth Kelchner Gerety

GRIEVING

DEFINITION AND DESCRIPTION

Grieving is a psychobiologic response of suffering that follows the actual or perceived loss of an object that is of value. Valued objects are significant others, parts or functions of the body, roles, relationships, personal possessions, status, and patterns and conditions of living. Grieving begins as early as infancy when there is a separation from the mother figure or the loss of a significant other.[2] It continues throughout the life span, whenever an individual is faced with the loss of something that is meaningful and valuable. Grieving is a universal phenomenon characterized by both internal processes and observable reactions. It encompasses a wide range of complex, and sometimes bewildering, thoughts, feelings, physical and emotional reactions, and behaviors that surround the experience of loss and its expected resolution. It is a stressful, subjective experience that is influenced by the current meaning or value of the lost object as well as by past successes or failures associated with the loss.[3,6,14,21,24,36] The Diagnostic and Statistical Manual of Mental Disorders (DSM-III-R) uses the category, Uncomplicated Bereavement, when an individual experiences normal grieving after the death of a significant other.[1]

THEORY AND RESEARCH

There is no one comprehensive theory that explains the classification and management of normal grief.[3] Lindemann's classic study in 1944, described acute grief as a syndrome with a remarkably uniform course and characteristic symptoms.[19] Researchers and clinicians who have continued to systematically study the experience of grief since that time agree that there are many factors that influence grief responses, the process of mourning, and the length of time that it takes to complete grief work.[26] Individual responses to loss are affected by previous experiences with loss and other variables, such as the age and support system of the person facing the loss; cultural, ethnic, and religious backgrounds; physical and mental health, and whether the loss was sudden or anticipated.[2,6,8,24]

Despite the fact that grief and mourning do not progress in a linear fashion, they are generally described as occurring in a sequence of phases, clusters of reactions, or stages that change over time.[2,6,16,26] During the initial period after a significant loss, somatic distress and physical sensations, which may be transitory or continue over a period, commonly occur. Adaptive denial, which protects from overwhelming stress of the loss, is manifested by blunting and blocking out painful aspects, as well as initial overt acceptance of the loss. Anger and aggression may be directed toward the people or circumstances that the person believes are responsible for the loss. Feelings of pain, anguish, acute sadness, weeping, and despair are concomitant with developing awareness of the loss, which begins within a few hours or a few days after the loss occurs. Successful mourning is dependent upon the individual's being able to tolerate the intense emotions that occur during this particular time.

Activities that initiate the recovery process lead to restitution, the work of mourning. For example, a new amputee agrees to be fitted for a prosthesis and diligently participates in his rehabilitation program.[8] Much of the grief work during this time is intrapsychic, as the individual struggles to cope with the painful void left by the loss. Successful mourning is similar to successful wound healing. Both processes need an orderly sequence and an interval of time that cannot be compressed. Attempts to interfere with this orderly sequence and necessary time frame may lead to pathologic consequences. Just as preexisting factors influence the ultimate outcome of wound healing, they also affect the ultimate outcome of mourning.[6] Resolution of the grief experience, with a redefinition of oneself and one's situation, occurs when the individual is able to reflect on both the positive and negative aspects associated with the loss[2] (Fig. 13-12).

Children's grieving is influenced by age, developmental stage, grieving responses of parents, the availability of supportive others, and the significance of the loss.[24] Confusion and misunderstanding sometimes occur when the assumption is made that children's grieving patterns are similar to the ways in which adults grieve. Although there are some similarities between adults' and children's responses to loss, there are specific differences in the manner in which children acknowledge a significant loss and in the manifestation and duration of their grief. Children may attempt to cope with feelings of loss through play activities and

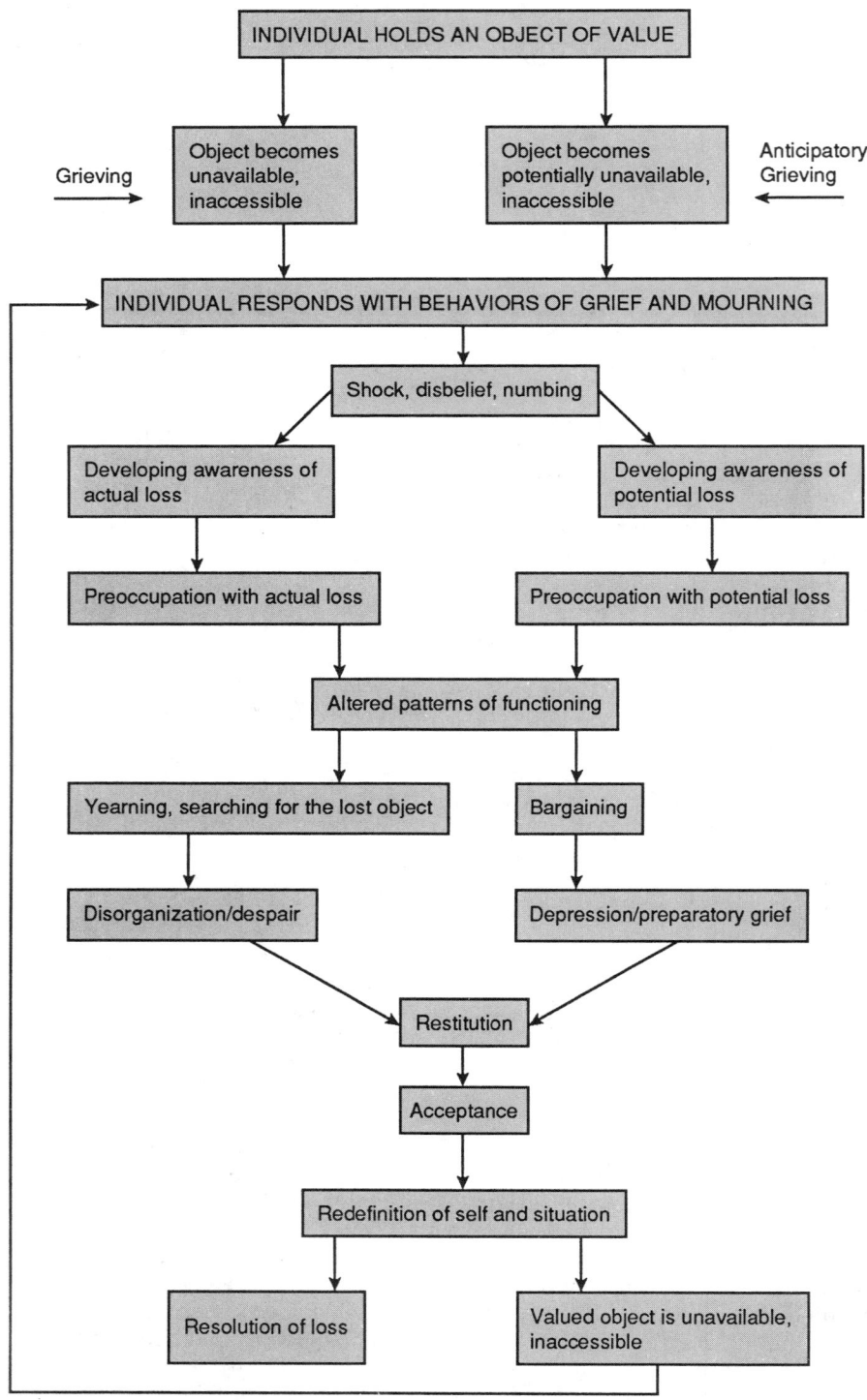

FIGURE 13-12. Operational description of grieving and anticipatory grieving.

games that are a reenactment or a variation of the loss. Some losses evoke frightening and painful feelings that can be endured for only brief periods. Children are more likely to express grief through angry outbursts or misbehavior, as opposed to expressions of overt sadness.[26] The grief and mourning of children is a controversial research issue because of disagreement among researchers in the area of cognitive development and interpretation of behaviors. It is difficult to define differences between adolescent and adult reactions to death. There is a lack of research on the adolescent's concept of death.[14]

RELATED FACTORS

The loss of a significant other is the most common loss that evokes intense grieving. Sometimes the person who is deemed to be significant is a nonintimate other, such as a celebrity or leader of a country. People may grieve as deeply over the loss of meaningful possessions as they do over the loss of a significant other.[2,31] The loss of a pet can be important. Loss is experienced when an individual's home is burglarized or destroyed during a natural disaster. The theft of a motor vehicle is a loss that can be difficult to resolve. Developmental losses can result in grieving. Aging, with a loss of health, stamina, and autonomy, represents a loss of self that is mourned. The loss of body parts, caused by traumatic injury or through surgery, and the loss of body image, contribute to grief reactions. The loss of important resources, such as a familiar environment, because of retirement or promotion, the loss of ideals, or the loss of one's country may foster grieving reactions.

DEFINING CHARACTERISTICS

Normal, uncomplicated grief is a subjective experience in which an individual acknowledges or "owns" a loss.[31] Somatic distress or physical sensations are common during normal grieving. Although clinical observations and research studies show an association between grief after the death of a significant other and an increase in medical problems and mortality, the psychobiology of grief has not been investigated in depth or in detail. Current studies demonstrate a correlation between grief and activation of the adrenocortical and adrenal medullary and sympathetic nervous systems; however, it has not been determined if the correlations are causally related.[13] There are sexual differences in expressions of suffering and distress in Western culture.[3] Sighing and crying occur more frequently among women. Women talk more openly about their symptoms than men. Many men are socialized to conceal their feelings of grief from others, including those closest to them.[14,20] The grieving person may experience intense feelings that are not pathologic.[36] For example, Mary M., whose husband died from a heart attack, recalls being furious with him for leaving her so abruptly. "How could he do this to me! I was so angry at him that I shook him when he was lying in the casket. The funeral director had to rearrange him afterward." There may be intense yearning for the lost object or a sense of relief after an anticipated loss actually occurs.[2,36]

Cognitive manifestations of normal grieving include the initial inability to directly face a sudden loss, difficulty in thought organization and concentration, and hallucinatory experiences.[36] Amputees, or women who have had mastectomies, frequently experience a form of kinesthetic and tactile hallucinations when they feel postoperative phantom limb pain and other sensations in the area of the amputation. People who have been widowed may experience a sense of presence of the dead person, as well as auditory, visual, or tactile hallucinations.[29] Sally Z, a young widow whose husband died from cancer, described feeling comforted when, "I know John visited me the weekend after he died. I saw a shadow on the edge of the bed, and I saw the water bed move on his side. I know he was there." Absentmindedness and a decreased interest in external events, outward attire, and usual social activities are behavioral characteristics of normal grieving. Symbolic searching for the lost object or person, which may continue for several months or, sometimes, years, may include visiting places that are reminders of the lost object or person. The grieving person may treasure or carry around, objects that are associated with the loss[2,3] (Chart 1).

CHART 1
Grieving: Definition, Related Factors, and Defining Characteristics

DEFINITION

Grieving is a psychobiological response of suffering that follows the actual or perceived loss of an object that is of value.

RELATED FACTORS[6,31]

Loss of significant person
Loss of meaningful possessions
Loss of part of the self
Loss of other important resources

DEFINING CHARACTERISTICS[2,3,19,36]

Somatic distress, physical sensations (e.g., difficulty breathing, tightness in the throat, slight sense of unreality, depersonalization, feelings of weakness)
Altered feelings (e.g., sadness, anger, numbness, guilt, loneliness)
Cognitive changes (e.g., disbelief, confusion, preoccupation with the loss)
Behavioral changes (e.g., decreased appetite, sleep disturbances, dreams of the lost object, social withdrawal)

NURSING PROCESS AND RATIONALE

Assessment

Assessment for behaviors associated with normal grieving is a necessary component for developing nursing strategies to assist the person to be strengthened and to grow during the grieving process.[21] Individual defense mechanisms and cultural norms may cause psychological pain to be expressed through physical complaints and somatic distress. Assess for the possibility of grief-related depression in the elderly, to avoid the misdiagnosis of an organic dysfunction.[26] Determine the phase or stage of grieving. Recognize that phases or stages are not delineated by specific entry or exit criteria, and they do not necessarily occur in a sequential order. There may be a shifting back and forth, as well as an overlapping, of phases as each person copes in his or her own unique way.[31]

Nursing Diagnosis

The nursing diagnosis of normal grieving is based on the client's recognition of having experienced a significant loss and on the nurse's identification of responses that are indicative of normal grieving. An example nursing diagnosis is grieving related to the loss of familiar environment, social position, and forced retirement.

Client Goals and Nursing Interventions

The initial goal for the individual experiencing shock and disbelief is to accept the reality of the loss. Encourage description about the loss by asking questions such as, "When did it happen?"; "How did you learn about it?"; "Where were you when you heard?"[36] Try to provide privacy when conveying news of a sudden, unexpected, or traumatic death. Prepare the client, and significant others who may be present, for what they can expect when they see the body of their loved one. When parents choose to see their stillborn baby, let them know that the infant will be cold and discolored. Be sure to explain the presence of abnormalities or maceration.[35] A second goal of grief work for the person who has had a significant loss is to experience the pain of grieving.[36] Sometimes, nurses feel very helpless when grieving clients express intense feelings of anger, hostility, or sadness. Try to avoid personalization of negative and hypercritical behaviors, and do try to encourage discussion of feelings of frustration and sadness. A third goal for the grieving person is to adjust to an environment in which the lost object or significant other is missing. Evaluate the need for a mental health clinic referral for short-term grief therapy (Fig. 13-13). Consider referrals to special groups, such as Reach for Recovery for the woman who has had breast surgery, or an ostomy group for the client who has had bowel sur-

gery. Other groups such as Parents Without Partners, Widow to Widow, Compassionate Friends, and Candlelighters assist family members who have lost a spouse or a child. Pet support groups provide an opportunity to discuss common feelings of loss and to explore ways in which to cope with the loss of an animal that held a very special place.

Evaluation

Resolution of denial and subsequent demonstration of acceptance of the loss, are outcomes that indicate that the goal of accepting the reality of the loss has been achieved. The nature and subjective meaning of the loss influence the length of time for acceptance of its reality. The resolution of anger and the acknowledgement of recognition of painful thoughts and feelings indicate that the client has met the goal of experiencing the pain of grief. The use of adaptive-coping skills and the initiation and maintaining of a constructive lifestyle signify adjustment to an environment in which the lost object or other is missing (Chart 2).

CASE STUDY

Nurses initially felt intimidated and helpless when Jim R, a 51-year-old married landscape architect, lashed out at them for what he perceived to be inconsistencies in his dressing changes and therapy schedules after his below-the-knee amputation for chronic osteomyelitis. His primary nurse diagnosed Mr. R as experiencing grieving related to the loss of his leg. Jim R manifested intense feelings of anger and hostility that were directed toward his caregivers. Expected outcomes for Mr. R were for him to be able to overtly acknowledge his feelings of loss and to participate in ongoing recommended treatments and plans for rehabilitation. Nurses used nondefensive responses as they encouraged him to talk about specific examples of dressing change and

continued on page 250

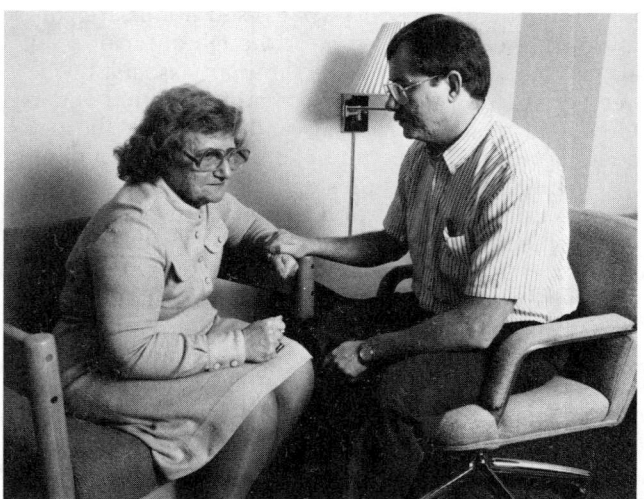

FIGURE 13–13. *Psychiatric clinical nurse specialist provides grief therapy for recently widowed woman. (Courtesy of M. Moody/VAMC Portland, OR)*

CHART 2
Grieving: Summary of the Nursing Process[20,24,26,35,36]

NURSING INTERVENTIONS

CLIENT GOAL: ACCEPT REALITY OF THE LOSS
Encourage verbalization about the loss (e.g., "when did it happen?")
Provide privacy for conveying news of the loss
Permit visual and tactile contact with the deceased, when appropriate
Offer support in dealing with bewilderment
Acknowledge similarity of others' responses to loss
Correct misinformation about the loss
Recognize–respect impact of customs on grieving process
Encourage client to seek help from others
Permit a reasonable period for denial
Point out reality in a nonthreatening manner
Encourage discussion of past or present memories of lost object or person

CLIENT GOAL: EXPERIENCE THE PAIN OF GRIEF
Encourage verbalization of thoughts and feelings
Assess for possible suicidal intent
Facilitate constructive expression of anger
Allow for variations in expressions of grief
Convey assurance that feelings of guilt are a part of normal grieving
Allow reminiscing about loss

CLIENT GOAL: ADJUST TO ENVIRONMENT IN WHICH THE LOST OBJECT OR SIGNIFICANT OTHER IS MISSING
Evaluate impact of loss on family system
Encourage social interaction
Consider referral to special support groups
Encourage and teach good health habits
Assist in development of constructive coping styles

OUTCOME CRITERIA

Experiences resolution of denial
Demonstrates acceptance of the loss

Experiences resolution of anger
Acknowledges recognition of painful thoughts and feelings

Uses adaptive coping skills
Initiates and maintains a constructive life style

Research Highlights (Grieving)

Infertility, the inability to conceive or to continue a pregnancy, can result in grieving that is related to the loss of self-concept and self-worth, powerlessness, and a sense of failure. A study was conducted to examine the effectiveness of a structured group fertility-counseling program on the frequency of grief reported by couples who were undergoing infertility evaluation or treatment.[20] A questionnaire that focused on feelings of anger, frustration, loss of control, self-concept, and the marital and sexual relationship, was administered at the first and final sessions. Responses from the first questionnaires were used to obtain information on pretreatment grief, self-concept, marital and sexual satisfaction, and to develop group goals. Analysis of pre- and posttest scores of subcategories of grief showed significant sexual differences and suggested that the group counseling had positive effects for women, who reported a higher prevalence of grief than men in all of the categories in both pre- and posttests. Posttests showed a decrease in intensity of grief for the women; the intensity of grief remained essentially the same for the men. Women reported a significant improvement in self-concept; men reported minimal changes in this area. Group counseling appeared to have no effect on the marital and sexual relationship of the couples.

In another study, research that compared the grief of amputees and widows showed that the initial grief of these two groups was comparable in intensity; however, postamputation grief was more persistent and unchanged after one year.[8] Examination of referrals of acute amputees to an interdisciplinary psychiatric consultation service identified normal grieving in 45 of the 86 amputees. The three highest ranking symptoms were despondency, anxiety, and insomnia. Analysis of postamputation grieving showed that there is no single appropriate response to expect from this population. Previous experiences with loss influenced their postamputation grief. Clients with preoperative preparation had less complicated grief reactions. Effective counseling interventions included (1) allowing a gradual assimilation of information during adaptive denial, (2) answering questions honestly with only as much detail as asked for by the client, (3) allowing ventilation of anger, (4) exploring coping mechanisms and support systems. Psychiatric consultation interventions and recommendations for the acute amputees in this study population contributed to more effective pain management and improved client–caregiver relationships. A comparison of data with amputees who had no psychiatric consultation showed a somewhat shorter stay in the critical-care unit and shorter duration of hospitalization for the amputees who received a mental health consultation.

schedule problems. The primary nurse worked with other members of his treatment team to minimize inconsistencies in his overall plan of care. These interventions facilitated constructive expression of his frustration and anger and served to decrease the feelings of helplessness and vulnerability that both the client and nurses were experiencing during Mr. R's initial postoperative recovery. He moved beyond the ventilation and displacement of anger and began to discuss the painful feelings and uncertainties he was experiencing as a result of the amputation. His criticisms of staff decreased, and he began to seek information about rehabilitation activities that would lead to resuming his work as a landscape architect.

SUMMARY

The subjective meaning of a significant loss influences the manifestation and duration of grieving. The resolution of previously felt strong emotions to an important loss occurs as emotional bonds are untied and readjustments to the environment are made. New relationships and interests are established. The individual gradually reenters an active life-style and interacts with the external world in gratifying ways that no longer focus on the loss.[24,31]

ANTICIPATORY GRIEVING

DEFINITION AND DESCRIPTION

Anticipatory grieving is a psychobiologic response to a potential loss. It is an adaptive mechanism that can assist a person to begin to integrate the factual and symbolic aspects of a potential loss in preparation for letting go of the valued object.[9,25,27,31,36]

THEORY AND RESEARCH

The term *anticipatory grieving* was initially used during World War II to describe a syndrome that was observed in many military families who were separated from their loved ones and experienced all of the phases of grief because of the severe threat of the potential death of a loved one.[19] Although anticipatory grieving can serve as a protection from the impact of a sudden loss, it can also be a disadvantage when significant others reinvest in new relationships before the actual occurrence of the loss of a loved one. For example, the "missing" loved one may return, or the seriously ill person may recover or go into a remission.

Kubler-Ross's work, which describes stages, or coping mechanisms of people who are dying, provides a useful framework for examining some of the similarities and differences between grieving and anticipatory grieving related to death, as well as to other important losses. These coping mechanisms are denial and isolation, anger, bargaining, depression, and acceptance. Successful anticipatory grieving is not dependent upon a sequential progression through, or an experiencing of, each of these stages.[16] Denial, "No, not me, it can't be true," serves as a buffer and a temporary defense, which allows for mobilization of less extreme defenses. Anger, characterized by feelings of rage, envy, and resentment, is frequently accompanied by the person asking out loud or inwardly, "Why me?" Bargaining maneuvers, attempts to postpone the inevitability of a loss related to death, are usually made with God and shared with a member of the clergy, instead of with loved ones. Bargaining attempts to forestall a loss not associated with death, are more likely to be discussed with others. Depression, the preparatory grief for the final separation from the significant other or object, occurs as the result of an *impending* and not a past loss. Acceptance, which is not to be confused with giving up or feeling hopeless, follows the mourning of an impending loss.

The restitution and resolution in anticipatory grieving differs from grieving after an actual loss.[3,24] During anticipatory grieving, there can always be a degree of hope that something will happen to prevent the actual loss from occurring. In grieving there is nothing that can be done to change the extent of the loss. Grief decreases with the passage of time; anticipatory grief may increase in intensity as the actuality of the loss becomes imminent. The anticipatory grieving of the terminally ill person leads to a "definite end point"—death. The person who is grieving after an actual loss can prolong the grieving experience. Grieving includes experiencing reestablishment. There is no reestablishment for the terminally ill person who is experiencing anticipatory grieving; instead, there may be a realization or resolution of one's impending death (see Fig. 13-12).

RELATED FACTORS

Experiences and events that contribute to or precipitate anticipatory grieving are similar to those that result in grieving. However, in anticipatory grieving there is the *perceived potential* of a significant loss.

DEFINING CHARACTERISTICS

Reactions to a potential loss are similar, in many respects, to the reactions after an actual loss. One of the hallmarks of anticipatory grieving, however, is the roller-coaster effect that sometimes inhibits the grieving process because of the awareness that the anticipated loss has not actually occurred.[31] The social context of the individual may reinforce denial when people are encouraged to be optimistic and to seek nontraditional or experimental alternatives for coping with an impending loss. The anger during anticipation of the loss of a significant other is sometimes directed toward that person, who is perceived to be deserting the individual who is grieving. Ambivalence is more characteristic in anticipatory grieving than in normal grieving. The individual may be torn between impatience for the loss to be over and the hope that the loss will not occur. Allthough the actual occurrence of the loss reactivates the grieving process, it may also bring a sense of relief and be anticlimactic[24] (Chart 3).

NURSING PROCESS AND RATIONALE

Assessment

Observe for behaviors that are indicative of grieving. Assess the subjective meaning of the experience of loss, the individual's personality, the appropriateness or inappropriateness of perceptions of the anticipated loss, and the social reality in which the potential loss is occurring. Find out what the client knows or imagines about the potential loss.[27,31] The physician requested a psychiatric consultation for evaluation of Tim L's denial of the need for surgery to have his gangrenous toe amputated. Mr. L, an elderly gentleman with a mild

---

CHART 3
Anticipatory Grieving: Definition, Related Factors, and Defining Characteristics

DEFINITION

Anticipatory grieving is a psychobiologic response to a potential loss.

RELATED FACTORS[6,15,25]

Perceived potential death of self
Perceived potential loss of:
  Significant other
  Health, body parts, or body image
  Meaningful possessions
  Other important resources

DEFINING CHARACTERISTICS[15,24,36]

Cognitive changes (e.g., shock, disbelief, lack of interest or difficulty in follow through with routine activities, sense of unreality, realization of impending loss)
Behavioral changes (e.g., expression of distress, altered sleep and communication patterns, self accusation of negligence, withdrawal and emotional distance from others)
Altered feelings (e.g., anger, irritability, guilt, sorrow, loneliness, ambivalence, hope that loss will be averted)
Somatic symptoms (e.g., emptiness in stomach, exhaustion, decreased appetite)

---

dementia, was adamant in his refusal, as he cited numerous reasons for avoiding surgery. Further assessment by his primary nurse revealed that this was Mr. L's first hospitalization, and his refusal to agree was based on his unawareness that the amputation would be preceded by an anesthetic.

Nursing Diagnosis

The diagnosis of anticipatory grieving is based on an assessment that the person facing a potential significant loss is experiencing behaviors indicative of grief and mourning before the actual occurrence of the loss. An example nursing diagnosis is anticipatory grieving related to potential loss of breast from mastectomy.

Client Goals and Nursing Interventions

Encourage the identification of past coping strengths for dealing with the present anticipated loss. Assure clients and their families that acute grief symptoms are not indicative of "craziness," and that it is normal to experience intense and chaotic thoughts and feelings.[14] Recognize the importance of adaptive denial to protect the client from the full emotional impact of an anticipated loss.[7,16] Sara W, who had had a modified radical mastectomy, was completing chemotherapy, when she learned that a mammogram showed a suspicious area in her remaining breast. She was aware that others might think that she was minimizing the seriousness of the situation because of her matter-of-fact manner after she was told of the report. She recognized, however, her need to wall off, to isolate, the full potential emotional impact of the tentative findings at that particular time, until she obtained more factual information.

Interventions for potential maladaptive denial of life-threatening or terminal illness could include suggesting that the client and significant others discuss the impact of their lives on each other and to explore what their contributions to future generations will be.[4] Future imaging without having to deal directly with the threat of death can be accomplished by encouraging the client and family to imagine what the lives of their descendants will be like. The groundwork is laid for moving beyond denial by dealing with mortality in a more general and less-threatening manner.

Offering hope for coping with an impending loss enables the client to talk about the loss and to explore constructive ways with which to deal with it.[22] Try to incorporate personal observations of the client and family as well as observations from other client–family interactions that allow hope for the client's ability to cope with the loss. During terminal illness, hope may be directed toward small, immediate goals, instead of long-term ones.

Interventions which encourage reminiscence about

an anticipated loss and discussion about the possible positive aspects of the loss, in addition to the negative aspects, help to reduce the feeling of loss. When Ken T could no longer maintain the family home after his wife's death, he benefited from interventions that helped him to recall the pleasant memories he would always have, as he selected the items to take to his small apartment at the retirement center. He was able to smile at the thought of someone shoveling the snow from the long driveway. The ability to make informed decisions is an important goal for constructive anticipatory grieving. It may be necessary for the nurse to repeat information that contains emotionally charged content. Assure the client and family that it is quite normal to be unable to remember and to have difficulty understanding information the first time that it is explained. Do not give more information than they are able to assimilate.[8]

During terminal illness, participation of constructive anticipatory grief work includes the client and family making informed decisions about final arrangements. On the basis of an assessment of behaviors indicative of anticipatory grieving and the client or family's overall identification of the need for information, consider initiating questions such as: "Have you thought about the kind of service you would like after you die?"; "Have you thought about whether you want to be buried or do you wish to be cremated?"; "Have you and your family talked about . . . ?" Many families want to discuss these topics and need permission from a health professional to initiate this content.

Recognize that the pattern of past relationships between the client and significant others will be similar to the way they relate to each other in the context of a potential loss.[22] Dan P was admitted to the cardiac intensive care unit to rule out a myocardial infarction. Nurses in the unit were somewhat critical of and concerned about Mrs. P's pattern of extremely brief visits, which were consistently followed by her abruptly leaving her husband and crying in the family waiting room. As they talked with Mrs. P about their concerns, they learned that Mr. P had never been able to tolerate any member of his family crying in front of him and that it would add to Mr. P's stress if Mrs. P was to cry at his bedside instead of leaving immediately when she recognized she was on the verge of tears.

Emphasize the importance of family members paying attention to their self-care needs for rest and activity. Bob K, who had terminal cancer, expected his wife to spend all of her free time after work and on her days off, at his bedside. Mrs. K became resentful of his demands, but she felt guilty about taking time away from her husband to resume her exercise program. A nursing intervention that encouraged her to pay attention to her needs for leisure activity and time away from her husband, led to Mrs. K's experiencing less tension, improved sleep, and a substantial increase in tolerance for her husband's demands.

Facilitate ongoing communication between the client and significant others by recognizing that they may differ in the phases of grieving that they are experiencing.[22] Although Joe W accepted that he was termi-

nally ill, Mrs. W remained in a state of anger as she refused to openly acknowledge that her husband was dying. Nursing interventions for Mrs. W included nondefensive responses to her harsh criticisms of the staff and the hospital and conveying to her how much it meant to her husband to have her be able to visit with him and help with his personal care. Mr. and Mrs. W maintained ongoing communication with each other, even though they remained at different stages in their grieving process, until the time of his death.

During terminal illness, promote the client and significant others to maintain constructive interpersonal relationships with each other by encouraging them to think and to talk about who they want to be present at the time of death. Assist them to recognize that a request or choice for absence at the time of death is not to be equated with a lack of love or caring.[22] This goal was accomplished with Mr. and Mrs. A. Mrs. A talked with her husband's primary nurse about the last evening she spent in the hospice unit before her husband died. "I kissed him good night. I knew that was the last time I would see him alive. Even though he didn't tell me, I know that he knew he would die that night. I also knew that he loved me, but he didn't want me to see him die."

Evaluation

Participation in constructive anticipatory grief work, the overall client goal, is facilitated by the ability to verbalize thoughts and feelings about the anticipated loss. People who are unaccustomed to talking about their thoughts and feelings may have difficulty discussing their reactions to a potential loss and, thus, be at a greater risk for experiencing dysfunctional grieving. The ability to make informed decisions related to an impending loss is indicative of participation in constructive anticipatory grief work. An essential outcome for the goal of participation in successful anticipatory grief work is for the client to be able to maintain constructive interpersonal relationships with others. Participation in constructive anticipatory grief work in terminal illness is evident when the client's family members are able to maintain interpersonal contact with the client by continuing to talk with and to touch their loved one, even though the person may not be able to respond. Mrs. C comforted herself, as well as her teenage daughter who was comatose and dying, as she stroked her daughter's forehead and whispered softly, "Go to sleep, sweet lady. Pretty soon you will see Jesus" (Chart 4).

CASE STUDY

Hank J, a 34-year-old married man, who was diagnosed with a moderately fast growing astrocytoma, planned to return to his employment in an auto body shop when he completed his series of radiation therapy. "I'm going to miss me," he observed before an unexpected setback, when he had a severe myocardial infarction near the completion of his radiation treatments. He expressed concerns for his wife, ten-year-old daughter, and eight-year-old son. He

CHART 4
Anticipatory Grieving: Summary of the Nursing Process[6,16,22,25,34]

NURSING INTERVENTIONS	OUTCOME CRITERIA
CLIENT GOAL: PARTICIPATE IN CONSTRUCTIVE ANTICIPATORY GRIEF WORK	
Find out what is known or imagined about the potential loss	Verbalizes thoughts and feelings about the anticipated loss
Encourage discussion of fears and concerns	
Recognize influence of past experiences with loss	
Avoid premature disruption of denial during period of shock and disbelief	
Avoid reinforcement of denial	
Avoid defensive responses to negative criticisms and convey recognition of client's concerns	
Offer hope for coping with loss	
Encourage discussion of positive and negative aspects of potential loss	
Find out what client–significant others understand about current situation	Makes informed decisions in relation to the anticipated loss
Promote identification of information needs	
Facilitate opportunities to obtain information from health providers	
Provide information in words that are easily understood	
Facilitate exploration of options	
On basis of individual assessment, provide family with ongoing information of client's status and plan of care	
Facilitate communication between client and significant others	Maintains constructive interpersonal relationships
Encourage use of support from others	
Encourage family to maintain self-care needs	

emphasized the need for ongoing direct information, "so I can mobilize what is inside of me"; and he identified the need for information on what to expect in the future, "What kind of reactions will I have as I get sicker?" Mr. J recognized that his sense of humor helped him to cope with daily frustrations. Both Mr. and Mrs. J worried about the financial implications of his cancer and cardiac diagnosis. Mrs. J experienced increased stress from assuming the major responsibility for running the house during her husband's hospitalization and radiation treatments. She reported that their son was having trouble keeping up with his school work and that he was getting into frequent fights with classmates. One day she confided, "I guess I've been so busy preparing for Hank's dying that I am forgetting he is still living." Mr. J and

Research Highlights (Anticipatory Grieving)

Hampe's investigation of the needs of families during anticipatory grieving identified a total of eight needs of grieving spouses: (1) to be able to visit any hour of the day or night for as long a time as deemed necessary; (2) to be able to help with the physical care of the spouse; (3) to have professionals respond with prompt acknowledgement and competency to the client's physical and emotional needs; (4) to be kept informed by nurses and physicians of the spouse's daily progress and general condition, such as diagnosis, complications, and current treatment plans; (5) to be informed of the nearness of death; (6) to be able to verbalize and to ventilate thoughts and feelings about anxieties, the client's care, or problems in general; (7) to have comfort and support from family members; (8) to have the health-care providers show friendliness and concern to the spouse.[11]

Dracup and Breu used Hampe's research findings to meet the needs of grieving spouses of critically ill clients in a coronary care setting.[5] A standardized plan of care with specific nursing interventions for meeting the needs of families of critically ill clients was developed. Hampe's interview tools were used to conduct interviews with clients whose spouses were admitted to a cardiac care unit because of serious cardiovascular disease and a poor prognosis. One-half of the spouses received consistent nursing interventions using the standardized plan of care that also incorporated information from an analysis of the interview data which identified the family member's needs, according to Hampe's categorizations. The other one-half of the group received nursing interventions according to the standardized plan of care. A comparison of responses of family members in the two groups indicated that the needs of family members in the experimental group were met with a greater consistency and completeness than the needs of the family members in the control group. Although the researchers were unable to determine the specific nursing interventions that effected the change, they assumed that the standardized plan of care that incorporated Hampe's research findings of the needs of grieving spouses made the difference.

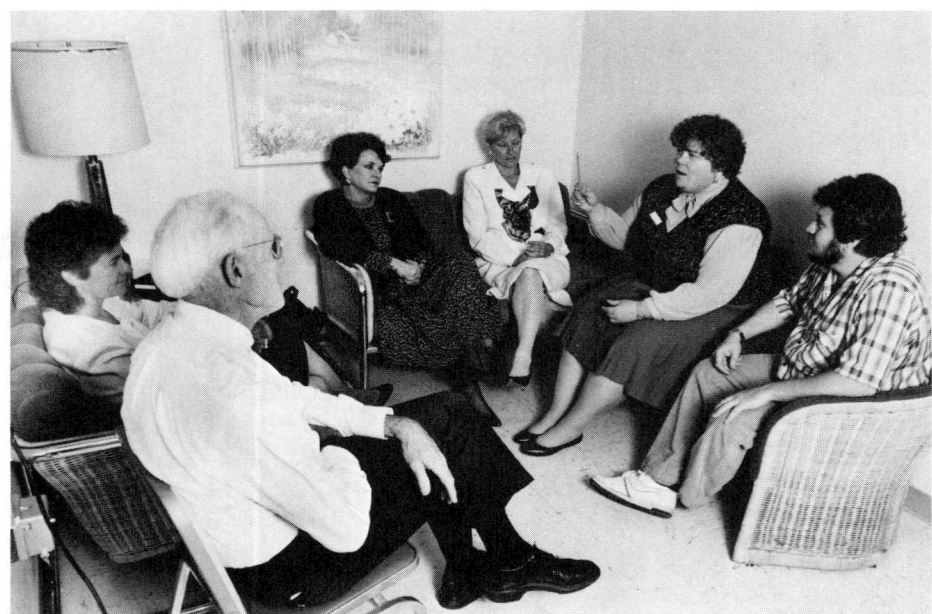

FIGURE 13–14. A nurse leads an encouragement group for families of terminally ill clients. (Courtesy of M. Moody/VAMC Portland, OR)

his family were experiencing anticipatory grieving related to impending death of self and the potential loss of a significant other. After the myocardial infarction, Mr. J also experienced normal grieving, related to loss of health and loss of employment.

Because the client and his wife were accustomed to openly discussing family problems and issues together, they were extremely responsive to nursing interventions that promoted verbalization of their thoughts and feelings about the actual and anticipated losses they were facing. Nursing interventions directed toward their making informed decisions included describing what they could expect as Mr. J's tumor progressed, referring them to the social worker and social security representative for assistance with financial issues, and encouraging them to contact an attorney to discuss legal issues. They were also referred to a weekly cancer support group for clients and families. Outcomes indicative of their making informed decisions included the making of individual wills and establishing guardianship for their children in the event that both parents died before the children became adults. The client and his wife also talked about his desire to be cremated. He agreed to his wife's request that his ashes be buried and identified with a grave marker, so that their children would have a

place to go to remember their father after his death. Mr. and Mrs. J were encouraged to talk with their son's teachers and school counselor. They were provided with information about a Child in Crisis group for children who anticipated or were experiencing the loss of a loved one. Both children attended this group, and the son's difficulties at school were resolved after a few weeks. Mr. and Mrs. J's past patterns of talking openly with each other, and their ongoing use of support from their family, friends, and church community, enabled them to maintain constructive interpersonal relationships as they lived with the knowledge of Mr. J's fatal illness (Fig. 13-14).

SUMMARY

Anticipatory grieving is a normal and expected process for coping with the potential loss of a significant object. Nursing interventions are based on an individual client assessment. The overall goal for people who are experiencing anticipatory grieving is to participate in constructive grief work.[22,24,25,34]

DYSFUNCTIONAL GRIEVING

DEFINITION AND DESCRIPTION

Dysfunctional grieving is a state in which the grieving process is abnormally delayed, prolonged, or exaggerated, or a combination thereof. The intensity of a loss is so overwhelming for some individuals, that they resort to maladaptive behaviors or remain stuck in an interminable state of grief. Descriptions of dysfunctional

grieving include the inhibition, suppression, or absence of the grief process, as well as the exaggeration, distortion, or prolonging of certain symptoms or behaviors in excess of cultural expectations.[12,17,18,31] The DSM-III-R diagnosis, major depression, may be made when an individual experiences marked preoccupation with worthlessness, prolonged and significant functional impairment, and marked psychomotor retardation after a major loss.[1,3]

THEORY AND RESEARCH

Lindemann used the phrase, *morbid grief reactions*, to discuss delayed and distorted reactions to loss that he believed were distortions of normal grief. He viewed pathologic grief as a single entity, with syndromes that were related to repressed unconscious ambivalent drives, and he believed that the absence of grief during a significant loss increased the potential for future disabling disturbances.[18,19] Rynearson disagreed with Lindemann and other theorists who describe normal grief as occurring in predictable, successive stages and pathologic grief as representing a denial or an arrest of these stages. He argued that, because there are insufficient data from longitudinal studies to validate a model in which grief occurs in discrete stages, it is premature to cite denial or arrest of the grieving process as the basis for pathologic grief. He developed a propositional revised typology of pathologic grief:

(1) *Dependent grief syndrome* links clinging or over-reliant attachment to responses of immediate pining and chronic grief. (2) *Unexpected loss syndrome* links unexpected loss to responses of immediate disbelief, avoidance, and anxiety leading to chronic anxious withdrawal. (3) *Conflicted grief syndrome* links conflicted ambivalent attachment to minimal immediate response, but delayed responses of anxiety and pining.[30]

According to psychoanalytic theorists, the inability to freely recognize the *meaning* of the loss, even though there is recognition that a significant loss has occurred, increases the likelihood of dysfunctional grieving.[3]

RELATED FACTORS

Dysfunctional grieving may occur after a person experiences some of the same perceived or actual losses that contribute to grieving or anticipatory grieving; for example, losses associated with biopsychosocial well-being, meaningful possessions, and role changes. Dysfunctional grieving is usually associated with the loss of an immediate family member. In children and adolescents, it is almost always related to the loss of a parent or a parent substitute. Certain personalities are prone to dysfunctional grieving: people whose relationships are characterized by anxious attachments and ambivalence; clinging and overly dependent individuals who have a strong need to engage in compulsive caregiving; and individuals who go to great lengths to emphasize their emotional self-sufficiency and independence.[2] Circumstantial factors, such as uncertainty of the loss and multiple losses associated with natural disasters or accidents, may contribute to dysfunctional grieving.[17,36] The reluctance and inability of an individual's social support system to acknowledge and help the individual cope with a loss contributes to unresolved grieving. Social negation of a loss, the socially unacceptable and unspeakable loss, as well as social isolation can prevent the resolution of a loss. People may not be able to openly mourn an abortion, a death from suicide, or the death of an illicit lover. Chronic fatal illness leads to dysfunctional grieving when a person is unable to use adaptive-coping skills to maintain a constructive life-style in the face of ongoing losses associated with illness. Secondary gains to maintain grieving beyond what is seen as a reasonable period, such as reluctance to give up the tragic role of "suffering well" and increased attentiveness from and protection by others, may prevent a person from having to accept the reality of a loss or to reinvest energy in other relationships.[31] The absence of anticipatory grieving or a thwarted grieving response contributes to dysfunctional grieving. People who do not allow time for personal grieving and delay their own mourning because of the need to maintain the morale of others, are at risk for experiencing dysfunctional grieving.[15,19,25]

DEFINING CHARACTERISTICS

Dysfunctional grieving is characterized by the intensification of many of the same emotional reactions and feelings that are present in normal grieving. Pollock identifies three possible outcomes that are characteristic of dysfunctional grieving after a significant loss: an arrest of the mourning liberation process at a particular stage of the loss experience; fixation points, such as anniversary reactions without arrested mourning; and pathologic mourning processes, such as severe despondency and depression, suicide, homicide, serious somatazations, with no liberation from mourning the loss.[28]

Prolonged episodes of panic, hostility toward oneself, and deflated, low self-esteem after a significant loss, are indicators of dysfunctional grieving.[12,25] Other manifestations include unabated specific searching behaviors for the lost person or lost object, as well as aimless searching behavior. The searching may recur on specific anniversary dates of the loss.[17] An increase in smoking and alcohol consumption may signal the presence of dysfunctional grieving. Developmental regression, aggression and hostility to others, and an ongoing drop in academic performance may be behavioral manifestations of dysfunctional grieving in children and adolescents.[26]

Cognitive manifestations of dysfunctional grieving after a death include prolonged alteration in concentration and suicidal ideation as a means of rejoining the dead person. A pattern of increased illness in an individual who has been previously healthy may be a somatic manifestation. The client may complain of physical distress under the upper half of the sternum, with the feeling that something is "stuck" inside.[2,17,25,26,36] "The criteria that most clearly distinguish healthy forms of defensive process from pathological ones [in dysfunctional grieving] are the length of time during which they persist and the extent to which they influence . . . mental functioning or come to dominate it completely"[2] (Chart 5).

CHART 5
Dysfunctional Grieving: Definition, Related Factors, and Defining Characteristics

DEFINITION

Dysfunctional grieving is a state in which the grieving process is abnormally delayed, prolonged, or exaggerated.

RELATED FACTORS[15,17,25,36]

Perceived or actual loss of significant other, self, or meaningful possessions
Inadequate social supports
Multiple, overlapping losses
Lack of resolution of previous loss or losses
History of complicated grief reactions
Uncertainty of loss
Prolonged, stressful anticipated loss

DEFINING CHARACTERISTICS[2,12,15,17,22]

Cognitive changes (e.g., perception of loss occurring "yesterday," as opposed to months and years; prolonged or excessive denial; suicidal ideation)
Behavioral changes (e.g., difficulty maintaining social relations, excessive reliving of past experiences, decreased participation in religious or ritualistic activities, refusal to follow prescribed therapies)
Altered feelings (e.g., delayed, distorted, excessive emotional reactions; prolonged depression)
Somatic (e.g., persistent physical complaints, choking sensation and breathing attacks, symptoms representing identification with the person who died)

NURSING PROCESS AND RATIONALE

Assessment

Dysfunctional grieving is sometimes difficult to diagnose because of the similarity of behaviors with those that occur during normal grieving.[21,28] A loss history, that includes deaths and other losses, helps to validate the presence of dysfunctional grieving.[36] Try to obtain information about the social and psychological circumstances surrounding the loss. Was the loss sudden, from an accident or suicide, or did it evolve over a period of time, such as with a lingering illness? Observe for behaviors that are indicative of unresolved feelings of anger and guilt in connection with the loss. What was the individual's developmental stage at the time of the loss?[2] Consideration should be given to the client's cultural background when assessing for dysfunctional grieving, because there may be cultural variations in manifestations of normal grieving.

Nursing Diagnosis

The diagnosis of dysfunctional grieving is based on assessment data that indicate that the client is stuck in a particular phase of grieving or is experiencing prolonged, extended, or excessively intense responses to a loss. The diagnosis includes the extent to which these responses interfere with the individual's adaptation to an environment without the lost object, for example, dysfunctional grieving related to a lack of resolution of previous loss of family members through death and divorce, and prolonged, stressful anticipated death of husband from chronic illness.

Client Goals and Nursing Interventions

The overall client goal is to resolve dysfunctional grieving. Assist clients to progress through the phase in which they are stuck.[17,23,25] Adults, adolescents, and children may benefit from interventions that encourage them to use storytelling, to draw pictures, keep a journal, or talk into a tape recorder to identify and to discuss unresolved losses.[14] A family chart, such as a genogram, which structurally diagrams family names, births, deaths, marriages, and divorces over three to four generations, can provide factual information that may lead to the identification of unresolved losses.[10] A loss history, through a five-generational genogram, enabled a nursing home resident to begin to talk about unresolved losses related to death and divorce. Consider a referral for further evaluation by a mental health professional for clients who experience suicidal ideation with intent. Participation in recommended therapies is an outcome for the person whose unresolved grieving, usually denial, interferes with compliance with a recommended regimen. Find out the client's expectations for recovery and encourage discussion of present and anticipated problems related to management of daily living with the loss. Observe for responses by the caregivers that may reinforce maladaptive denial by the client. Discourage the use of medication or alcohol to minimize feelings of loss. Emphasize that grieving for a significant loss does not signify weakness and inability to deal with a painful situation. Assisting the client to redefine the relationship with the lost person or object, contributes to the resolution of ambivalence as well as acknowledgment of an increase in positive feelings about the significant other or the object which was lost[36] (Fig. 13-15).

Although physical symptoms and complaints may be indicative of masked grief, physical disease must be ruled out before assuming that somatic complaints are indicative of dysfunctional grieving.[36] Severe and ongoing physical complaints and problems may necessitate a referral for brief psychotherapy. Teach the client that relaxation techniques, exercise, yoga, meditation, imagery, and good nutrition can help to prevent and to overcome problems with physical and emotional health while working through the grieving process.[14]

Verbalization of increased feelings of self-esteem is a goal for clients who have lived with socially unspeakable losses and losses that are perceived as stigmatizing. Convey unconditional positive regard to help them in their recovery from losses that have had a profound impact on self-esteem.[17] Prompt responses to expressions of physical concerns and needs conveys recognition of individual worth and self-esteem to clients experiencing dysfunctional grieving related to chronic physical illness or disability.[32]

Recognize the influence of family dynamics on the client's ability to resume or develop constructive relationships after a loss in which there is dysfunctional grieving, and evaluate the need for a referral for family therapy.[23,36] Clients who experience dysfunctional grieving as the result of an amputation or disfiguring surgical intervention may be very hesitant to socialize with old friends or to initiate new social contacts. Role-playing can be an effective technique for encouraging dysfunctionally grieving widows and widowers to try

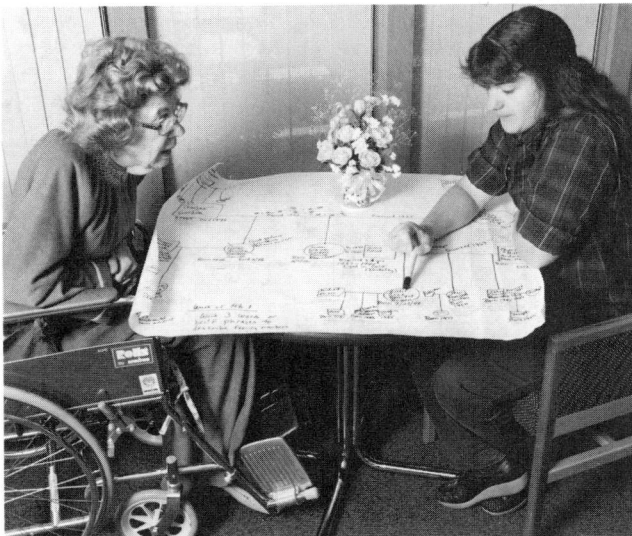

FIGURE 13–15. The primary nurse uses a genogram to help her geriatric client identify and discuss unresolved losses. (Courtesy of M. Moody/VAMC Portland, OR)

out and to practice social skills in which they previously participated as a couple. Consider referral to a support group to promote participation in constructive social relationships. Although self-help groups are beneficial for coping with many kinds of losses, they are contraindicated for people who are experiencing dysfunctional grieving.[30]

Evaluation

Observe for behaviors that demonstrate that the client is engaged in normal grieving and is not continuing to experience prolonged or excessive emotional reactions. Participation in recommended therapies is an outcome for clients whose unresolved grieving has interfered with compliance with a recommended regimen. Acknowledgment of an increase in positive feelings about the lost person or object indicates a lessening or absence of ambivalence. Evaluate for a decrease in physical symptoms and complaints in clients who initially sought medical treatment for unrecognized, unresolved grief. Verbalization of increased self-esteem indicates resolution of dysfunctional grieving for people who have experienced socially unacceptable and stigmatizing losses. Evaluate the client's ability to resume or develop constructive social relationships[23,36] (Chart 6).

CASE STUDY

Max M, a 55-year-old, divorced, insulin-dependent man, was admitted to a surgical unit for evaluation of chronic osteomyelitis in his left foot. During his admission intake, he informed his primary nurse that he was considering suicide if he had to have an amputation. He told her about a psychiatric admission three years previously for treatment of depression after his only daughter was killed in a boating accident and that he had continued to have recurrent suicidal ideation since that admission. Mr. M said that he had recently moved to a new community without notifying his community mental health therapist of his new address. His osteomyelitis caused him to be laid off from his custodial position. The primary nurse's initial nursing diagnosis was dysfunctional grieving related to unresolved past losses, recent losses of health and occupation, and potential surgical interventions. Initial client goals were (1) no suicide attempt or self-harm during hospitalization; (2) verbalizing thoughts and feelings related to his past, present, and anticipated losses; (3) participating in recommended treatment interventions. The primary nurse also initiated a referral to the psychiatric consultation–liaison clinical nurse specialist to evaluate the client and to make recommendations for his nursing management. Mr. M informed the clinical nurse specialist that he had no intent of attempting suicide while he was in the hospital and that his suicidal plan had consistently been to walk into the ocean until he would eventually drown. He was very agreeable to signing a release of information to contact his community mental health therapist to schedule an appointment for Mr. M immediately after his discharge from the surgical unit. The clinical nurse specialist concurred with the current plan of nursing care and recommended additional interventions: establishing a ''No Self-

CHART 6
Dysfunctional Grieving: Summary of the Nursing Process[17,23,25,30,32,36]

NURSING INTERVENTION	OUTCOME CRITERIA
CLIENT GOAL: RESOLVE DYSFUNCTIONAL GRIEVING	
Avoid imposing a predetermined time table for grief work	Engages in normal grief work
Provide opportunity for discussion of experiences that preceded loss	Participates in recommended therapies
Monitor for suicidal intent	Demonstrates absence of abnormal, prolonged, and excessive emotional reactions
Evaluate the impact of denial of participation in therapies	
Use a gradual approach to present and explore increasing facts about the loss	
Postpone nonessential teaching for adaptation to loss until there is a decrease in denial	
Legitimize feelings of anger and aggression as common responses to loss	
Acknowledge the universal need for normal grieving	
Encourage discussion of feelings of ambivalence	Acknowledges increase in positive feelings about lost significant other or object
Help client recognize that angry feelings do not obliterate positive feelings	
Help client recognize that it is not necessary to have physical symptoms to have contact with a health provider	Reports abatement of somatic symptoms
Encourage use of relaxation techniques and exercise	
Evaluate need for referral for brief psychotherapy	
Convey unconditional positive regard to client	Verbalizes increased feeling of self esteem
Encourage recognition of past as well as current strengths in coping with loss	
Teach client to identify and deal with stigmatizing behavior from others	
Support structured attempts to try new coping strategies and plan for feedback regarding their effectiveness	
Promote relearning of previous social skills	Resumes or develops constructive social relationships
Consider role-playing for development of social skills and relationships	
Encourage cultivation of new relationships	

Harm Contract'' for the duration of his admission, providing time for him to talk about his thoughts and feelings about past and present losses, and providing opportunities for him to talk about experiences that preceded his current loss of well-being. Mr. M was greatly relieved to learn that it was necessary to amputate only his fifth toe and not his entire foot. He complied with, and participated in, all recommended treatments and interventions. He was discharged after an uneventful recovery from his surgery, and he planned to keep his mental health clinic appointment.

Research Highlights (Dysfunctional Grieving)

Vachon, a psychiatric nurse and sociologist, conducted research to explore unresolved grief in people with cancer who were referred to her for psychotherapy.[33] She hypothesized that people with a history of unresolved grief who have a diagnosis of cancer are at an increased risk for experiencing distress, which necessitates their seeking or being referred for therapy. Her literature review of pathologic grief and related research into possible connections between cancer, loss, or stressful life events, revealed minimal investigation of the significance of unresolved losses in people who have a diagnosis of cancer. Her content analysis of all available cancer referrals showed that 76% of the group had previous grief experiences and 60% of the total group had experienced unresolved grief from previous losses. Vachon did not find a significant correlation between unresolved grief and variables of sex, type of cancer, referral source, significant problems during childhood, or a history of previous mental health problems. She recommended that the education of cancer clinicians include assessment of unresolved grief in people with cancer to provide referrals for helping them to identify this grief as a potential source of their current distress. She further recommended that completion of the tasks of mourning for previous losses be considered an individual choice, because the exploration of unresolved grief may be too threatening for some clients.[33]

SUMMARY

Dysfunctional grieving, a state in which the grieving process is abnormally delayed, prolonged, or exaggerated, represents a distortion of normal grieving. It is essential that nurses recognize behaviors that are indicative of dysfunctional grieving so that appropriate nursing interventions can be planned for the client to resolve this state of grieving and to engage in grieving.

References

1. American Psychiatric Association. Diagnostic and statistical manual of mental disorders. 3rd ed, revised. Washington, DC: American Psychiatric Association; 1987.
2. Bowlby J. Loss: sadness and depression—attachment and loss, vol 3. New York: Basic Books; 1980.
3. Carr AC. Grief, mourning, and bereavement. In: Kaplan HI, Sadock BJ, eds. Comprehensive textbook of psychiatry, vol 2. 4th ed. Baltimore: Williams and Wilkins; 1985.
4. Collison C, Miller S. Using images of the future in grief work. Image. 1987;19:9–11.
5. Dracup KA, Breu CS. Using nursing research findings to meet the needs of grieving spouses. Nurs Res. 1978;27:212–216.
6. Engel GL. Psychological development in health and disease, Philadelphia: WB Saunders; 1968.
7. Engel GL. Grief and grieving. Am J Nurs 1964;64(9):93–98.
8. Frierson RL, Lippmann SB. Psychiatric consultation for acute amputees. Psychosomatics. 1987;28:183–189.
9. Fulton R, Gottesman D. Anticipatory grief: a psychosocial concept reconsidered. Br J Psychiatry. 1980;137:45–54.
10. Guerin PJ, Pendagast EG. Evaluation of family system and genogram. In: Guerin PJ, ed. Family therapy theory and practice. New York: Gardner Press; 1976.
11. Hampe SO. Needs of the grieving spouse in a hospital setting. Nurs Res. 1975;24:113–120.
12. Horowitz MJ, Wilner N, Marmar C, Krupnick J. Pathological grief and the activation of latent self-images. Am J Psychiatry. 1980;137:1157–1162.
13. Irwin M, Daniels M, Weiner H. Immune and neuroendocrine changes during bereavement. Psychiatr Clin North Am. 1987;10:449–465.
14. Johnson SE. After a child dies: counseling bereaved families. New York: Springer; 1987.
15. Kim MJ, McFarland GK, McLane AM. Pocket guide to nursing diagnoses. 3rd ed. St Louis: CV Mosby; 1989.
16. Kubler-Ross E. On death and dying. New York: Macmillan; 1969.
17. Lazare A. Unresolved grief. In: Lazare A ed. Outpatient psychiatry diagnosis and treatment. Baltimore: Williams & Wilkins; 1979.
18. Lindemann E. Beyond grief: studies in crisis intervention. New York: Aronson; 1979.
19. Lindemann E. Symptomatology and management of acute grief. Am J Psychiatry. 1944;101:141–148.
20. Lukse MP. The effect of group counseling on the frequency of grief reported by infertile couples. JOGNN. 1985;14(suppl):67s–70s.
21. Martocchio BC. Grief and bereavement: healing through hurt. Nurs Clin North Am. 1985;20:327–341.
22. McFarland GK, Gerety EH. Grieving, anticipatory. In: Kim MJ, McFarland GK, McLane AM. Pocket guide to nursing diagnoses. 3rd ed. St. Louis: CV Mosby; 1989.
23. McFarland GK, Gerety EH. Grieving, dysfunctional. In: Kim MJ, McFarland GK, McLane AM. Pocket guide to nursing diagnoses. 3rd ed. St. Louis: CV Mosby; 1989.
24. McFarland GK, Wasli EL. Coping–stress–tolerance: grieving, anticipatory; grieving, dysfunctional. In: Thompson J, McFarland GK, Hirsch J, Tucker S, Bowers A. Clinical nursing. St. Louis: CV Mosby; 1986.
25. McFarland GK, Wasli EL. Nursing diagnoses and process in psychiatric mental health nursing. Philadelphia: JB Lippincott; 1986.
26. Osterweis M, Solomon F, Green M, eds. Bereavement: reactions, consequences, and care. Washington, DC: National Academy Press; 1984.
27. Parkes CM, Weiss RS. Recovery from bereavement. New York: Basic Books; 1983.
28. Pollock GH. The mourning-liberation process in health and disease. Psychiatr Clin North Am. 1987;10:345–354.
29. Rees WD. The bereaved and their hallucinations. In: Schoenberg B, Gerber I, Wiener A, Kutscher AH, Peretz D, Carr AC, eds. Bereavement: its psychosocial aspects. New York: Columbia University Press; 1975.
30. Rynearson EK. Psychotherapy of pathologic grief, revisions and limitations. Psychiatr Clin North Am. 1987;10:487–499.
31. Stephenson JS. Death, grief, and mourning: individual and social realities. New York: Macmillan; 1985.
32. Stewart T, Shields CR. Grief in chronic illness: assessment and management. Arch Phys Med Rehabil. 1985;66:447–450.
33. Vachon MLS. Unresolved grief in persons with cancer referred for psychotherapy. Psychiatr Clin North Am. 1987;10:467–486.
34. Welch D. Anticipatory grief reactions in family members of adult patients. Issues Ment Health Nurs. 1982;4:149–158.
35. Whitaker CM. Death before birth. Am J Nurs. 1986;86:157–158.
36. Worden WJ. Grief counseling and grief therapy. New York: Springer; 1982.

GROWTH AND DEVELOPMENT, ALTERED

Mary Ann Hertz

DEFINITION AND DESCRIPTION

Altered growth and development is the state in which an individual demonstrates deviations in norms from his or her age group. Growth and development is seen as a process, a progressive movement along a normally predictable continuum throughout life. Deviations from normal in childhood and adolescence (0–18 yrs) are multicausal and minor to major in terms of influence on clinically relevant developmental patterns.

This section will focus on altered growth and development of children and adolescents. Psychiatric mental health nurses build upon their knowledge of normal growth and developmental needs when they utilize the nursing process in the development of a case plan for emotionally disturbed children and adolescents. Attention to age-appropriate developmental needs and identification of the child's strengths and achievements are crucial to a complete assessment and the consequent care plan. Psychiatric mental health nurses have a responsibility to provide knowledgeable information to care providers across many systems. To do this and to promote optimal care, the nurse must understand the needs of children, patterns of their growth and development (physical, psychological, social, and intellectual), and the dynamics of behavior and of interpersonal relationships.

The following brief vignettes are examples of the range of problems that may come to the attention of a psychiatric mental health nurse.

Sandie W, aged three years, has made no attempt to communicate verbally. She resists her parents attempts to comfort her, hold her, or play with her. Her mother appears depressed and anxious.

John S, aged seven years, is not able to concentrate on any activity for more than two to three minutes. His first-grade teacher complains that she cannot contain him in the classroom. He talks constantly and disrupts the classroom activities. His parents and his teacher have noticed that John has no friends. Neighborhood children now avoid him because of his explosive and aggressive behavior.

Paul P, 12 years old, was placed in his first foster home at the age of two as a result of a court determination that he was abused and neglected. His mother was 16 when he was born. He is the son of an alcohol-involved father who sexually and physically abused him over a period of five years. Over the years, he has been placed in 13 foster homes. He is now being evaluated for a long-term group home placement. His case worker describes his behavior as alternating from seductive, immature clinging to violent and vengeful outbursts. Most of the foster home placements failed as a result of his unpredictable mood swings and impulsive aggressive behavior.

THEORY AND RESEARCH

Current understanding of normal development is derived from a wide range of research, literature, and clinical studies. For the most part, the varied aspects of normal child development have been explored by various disciplines and different approaches within disciplines, for example, developmental psychology, psychoanalysis, psychology, and the neurosciences.[2,9,13]

Until recently, explanatory research into deviations from normal development utilized two major theoretical frameworks. Anna Freud, Sigmund Freud, Erikson, and Piaget contributed to the theoretical frameworks sometimes labeled the *organismic–structural approach and universal stages*.[6] The other major theoretical framework is the *mechanistic–functional approach and individual differences theory*.[2] The organismic–structural approach postulates that all growth is evolving toward its species-specific adult form. The theory requires that a determination of an end point (e.g., old age) be made in advance. In contrast, the mechanistic-functional approaches and individual differences theory postulates that development is caused and variably shaped by environmental factors.[6] Today, scholars and clinicians are attempting to incorporate the advantages of both organismic and mechanistic approaches. Studies of children who deviate pathologically from the norm provide evidence that emotional, biologic, and motivational influences are important factors contributing to relative maturity and progression through developmental sequences.[1,2,8,9]

Greenspan's research, focusing on the mother–child dyad, is an example of work motivated by a need to create an integrated developmental theory, interweaving research data and theoretical propositions that combine organismic–structural and mechanistic–functional theories. The purpose of his continuing research and scholarly writings is to provide clinicians identifiable landmarks for assessment, intervention, and evaluation. Greenspan's *developmental structuralist* approach examines how individuals organize experience at each stage of development. His longitudinal action research provides detailed examples of adaptive and maladapted states and behaviors and descriptions of growth-promoting and growth-inhibiting environments.[10]

The presence or absence of genetic susceptibility and biologic factors in altered growth and development continues to be a rich area of research for the neuroscientists. Research in the neurosciences implicate lesions in the reticular, brain stem, and vestibular areas in autism. The lesions, if they exist, account for abnormal processing of sensory input or motor output. Other research explores the theory that children with autism fail to develop hemispheric specialization.[4] Biochemical researchers have found higher levels of serotonin in peripheral blood of children with autism than in normal controls, and 5-hydroxy-N,N-dimethyltryptamine (bufotenine) in the urine of autistic patients and their families, but not in controls, thus implicating genetic influences.[12]

Sociocultural and psychological factors are evident in continuing research that tests the concepts of Bowlby, Kanner, M. Klein, and others. Attachment and loss behaviors of children diagnosed in the *Diagnostic and Statistical Manual of Mental Disorders, 3rd ed, revised* (DSM-III-R) category of developmental disorders were studied by Shapiro et al., to determine if they responded differently than normal children.[16] They found no statistical difference between the groups in relation to ability to demonstrate reaction to loss and strange situations. Most demonstrated reactions expected of normal children. Affective display of distress on separation tended to correlate with security of attachment although it did not reach statistical significance.[16] The role of attachment–relationship history in victim behavior and victimizer behavior of preschool children was studied by Troy and Sroufe, who postulated that childhood relationship behavior is predictive of adult relationship behavior.[17] Their findings documented the impact of early relationships on later social functioning in that children with histories of rebuff, rejection, and poor attachment behaviors demonstrated either anxious–avoidant or anxious–resistant relationship patterns. Children with secure attachment (predictable, consistent, growth-fostering) relationship history were associated with nonvictimization. This study suggests that children raised in parent–child exploitive relationships become victims of their history, an important dynamic in generational child abuse. The research cited was intended to be illustrative of multifactorial influences on normal growth and development. The individual's capacity to organize experience

at certain levels of development sets the stage for positive growth or negative results, as in altered growth and development.

RELATED FACTORS

Significant alterations in growth and development are the hallmark factors in all the Developmental Disorder class of the DSM-III-R, for example: autistic disorder, academic skills disorder, language and speech disorders, motor skills disorders, and attention-deficit hyperactivity disorder.

Alterations in growth and development are best understood when related factors are identified and assessed. Within the framework of childhood and adolescence, biopsychosocial responses to genetic, sociocultural, and psychological assaults influence vulnerability and adaptational ability throughout the crucial formative years. Building on Greenspan's interactional model, it is not difficult to see that if a child is subjected to noxious psychological elements in the environment, is born with biologic deficits, and experiences a myriad of sociocultural handicaps, he or she is at high risk. Three major forces, biologic, sociocultural, and psychological, interact in combination with the individual's learned or inborn adaptational responses. The biologic or organic factor is a consequence of hereditary, congenital, and postnatal environmental influences. Sociocultural factors are the environmental context of the individuals development and the psychological forces derive from interactions with caretakers, especially during infancy and early childhood.

DEFINING CHARACTERISTICS

Physical manifestations associated with genetic abnormalities are the most obvious signs of deviation from normal growth and development. Down's syndrome, obvious from birth, is a case in point. However, when the developing fetus is subject to assault as a result of varied factors, such as poor maternal nutrition, alcohol ingestion, cigarette smoking, or certain infections, the result is not always obvious until the child is past the neonatal stage. Early detection of signs and symptoms of deviations from normal requires that nurses who see children continue to do careful assessments, particularly when, by history, they have knowledge of risks presented by the mother's health habits.

Individual patients will present unique combinations of signs and symptoms. For example, a child or adolescent with attention deficit disorder may have a high or normal IQ, but have a learning disability, speech disorder, and a poor self-image. Clinical evidence of depression is often seen in children who are aware of, or are reminded of, their differences. Some children and adolescents will withdraw, whereas others cover their depression with aggressive acting-out behavior.

Defining characteristics, at minimum, include those

behaviors most readily accessible to the observer. Other characteristics are more subtle and come to light only over time, for example, the less severe signs and symptoms of a developmental receptive language disorder, such as difficulty in understanding only certain types of words, or an inability to comprehend long or complex statements. The list of defining characteristics included in Chart 1 is not intended to be all-inclusive. Consideration of the following functional areas will guide the clinician in identifying characteristics unique in each case: (1) physical and neurologic integrity of the individual; (2) range, depth, and stability of emotions and affect; (3) anxieties and fears; (4) ability to engage in and maintain relationships with family,

---

CHART 1
Altered Growth and Development: Definition, Related Factors, and Defining Characteristics

DEFINITION

The state in which an individual demonstrates deviations in norms from his or her age group.

RELATED FACTORS

Prenatal and perinatal insults
Potentially noxious sociocultural and psychological environment

Stage of Development	Biologic Factors	Sociocultural Factors	Psychological Factors

Prenatal
Perinatal
Neonatal
Infancy
	Prenatal and Perinatal factors
	Endocrine
	Infectious
	Toxic
	Metabolic
	Genetic
	Length of gestation
	Neurochemical
	Neurophysiologic
	Neuroanatomic
		Family stability
		Single-parent
		Age of mother
		Age of father
		Socioeconomic status
		Values
		Child-rearing experiences of parents
		Presence or absence of problems related to
		  Membership in minority group
		  Access to health care
		  Support of general welfare
		  Education of parents
			Adaptional pattern of biologic parents
			Intelligence of parents/ caretakers
			Emotional development of parents/caretakers
			Ability of parent to bond to infant

Childhood and Adolescence	All of the above *plus*
	Ingestion of toxic elements
	Diseases or trauma affecting bodily integrity
		All of the above *plus*
		Housing: urban vs rural
		Racial influences
		Child-rearing patterns, beliefs and practices of caretakers
		Education of parents/ caretakers
		Educational opportunities afforded child
			All of the above *plus* the child's
			Experience of attachment or loss
			Resolution of developmental tasks consequent to
			  Interactions with mother and father
			  Role of father
			  IQ
			  Object relations in family

DEFINING CHARACTERISTICS

Absence of speech at expected age
Abnormal speech patterns
Unable to or impaired ability to perform daily living skills normal for age and developmental level
Impersonal treatment of others
Abnormal social play, solitary or disruptive
Impaired ability to make peer friendships
Absence of ability to engage in creative play
Specific academic skill deficit (e.g., reading, expressive writing, arithmetic)
Easily distracted, short attention span
Inattentive
Excessive talking
Excessive restlessness

peers, and other adults; and (5) ability to communicate his or her concerns in age appropriate ways through play or verbally[11] (see Chart 1).

NURSING PROCESS AND RATIONALE
Assessment

Assessment for deviations from normal growth and development requires that the psychiatric mental health nurse be comfortable with families who are greatly stressed and distressed. Regardless of the fact that some parents may possess prior knowledge that their child will be abnormal, perhaps as a result of amniocentesis, the reality of the child's condition and their plight cannot be fathomed until after the fact. Living with a child who is obviously different precipitates a kind of psychic pain that may at times seem unbearable. In the effort to survive, each parent's coping skills and defense mechanisms are severely tested. It is not unusual to hear parents deny or diminish the importance of significantly deviant behaviors or even visible evidence of physiological defects and, at the same time, express fear, horror, or anxiety about only one aspect of their child's behavior. It often happens that only one parent, generally the mother, has expressed concern to the pediatrician or family physician that all is not well. Lamentable though it may be, many parents are told to "wait and see, maybe the child will grow out of it." It is tragic because early intervention can ameliorate behavioral complications.

Signs and symptoms of deviations from normal growth and development typically appear in clusters. For example, reported or observed delay in accomplishing developmental tasks or in reaching developmental milestones is often accompanied by evidence of low self-esteem in school-aged children.

Families who present themselves at diagnostic clinics seeking answers to their questions and hoping for help from professionals often come in a state of fear and anxiety mixed with hope. At a diagnostic clinic for multiple-handicapped children, some parents may state that they hope the child's behavior will be attributed to a hereditary defect, chemical reaction to food, or birth trauma caused by a clumsy obstetrician. Their greatest fear is that they will be labeled "bad parents," who have caused their child's abnormality. Consequently, when eliciting a comprehensive description of the problem and family history that includes data about the parents and their families of origin, it is wise to plan for several interviews. The nurse can anticipate the family's need for a nonthreatening interview environment by providing a relaxed and private setting for the interviews. This will set the stage for reducing the family's anxiety and for fostering trust. The temptation to give the family quick, commonsense advice is quite strong given their sometimes intense expression of need. However, any advice at this stage will almost certainly influence the quality and quantity of information communicated to nurses by the family.

It is useful to come to the assessment with an interview schedule that includes items that relate to biologic and neurologic, sociocultural, and psychological factors to solicit needed diagnostic data. Open-ended, nonthreatening questions that require behavioral answers elicit more information. "You just told me that Johnny is hyperactive. Would you describe his behavior for me so I may get an accurate picture of what you mean by hyperactive?"; or "What does (did) he do exactly?" Many parents respond to questions about their child's behavior with affective statements of their own feelings in response to the behavior. In contrast, if the child is asked to describe his or her problems, the response is more likely to be an accurate description, such as "I have trouble sitting still"; or "I hit kids and they don't like me." Perhaps it is because the child hears his "sins" told to him over and over. Adults who are frustrated and worried tend to verbally assault children repeatedly with the "badness" of their actions in the mistaken belief that "they," the children, will correct the behavior once they have been told.

To make an effective assessment, it is useful for the nurse to:

1. Utilize a comprehensive interview guide that elicits biologic, sociocultural, and psychological data, and the parent–child perception of the problem
2. Schedule time for more than one interview
3. Provide a private, relaxed environment for the interviews
4. Use open-ended questions as often as possible
5. Listen rather than talk
6. Observe family interactions, verbal and nonverbal
7. Observe for defining characteristics of the deviation
8. Record data in behavioral descriptive terms.

Nursing Diagnosis

An example of a nursing diagnosis is altered growth and development related to parental substance abuse and inadequate caretaking, or altered growth and development related to nervous system abnormality.

Client Goals and Nursing Interventions

When the etiology of the developmental disorders is multifactorial, ranging from hereditary genetic aberrations, to noxious environmental influences, early nursing intervention strategies should address the problems that have a quality of immediacy to the client and the family. This is a technique that is effective in managing the feelings of being overwhelmed on the part of the family and sometimes the helpers. The psychiatric mental health nurse can guide the family by helping them identify two or three problems with which they would like immediate assistance. Poor impulse control is often cited as most troublesome to the child and to all who deal with him or her. An attempt should be made to identify a specific circumstance, for example, evening meals, an occasion with a beginning and an end point. The intervention will be a behavioral prescription that gives the parties involved concrete direction and can be evaluated for outcome (e.g., improved table behavior).

Evaluation

Working with complex problems in a complex system such as a family requires patience, persistence, and ingenuity on the part of the nurse. Developing outcome criteria that will be useful to the client, the family, and the nurse is as important as all the preceding steps. For the family, the criteria serve as indicators of their success or need to reevaluate the planned interventions. Behaviors can be counted and timed during the assessment phase, then incorporated as baseline data. Parents, caretakers, and even the clients themselves, if old enough, can track improvement or lack of improvement on a very simple counting evaluation tool. Younger children respond very positively to visual, concrete representations of their progress, especially if simple rewards are built into the goals, such as stars or special treats. The family needs to be advised that when a behavioral program is initiated, it is not unusual to see an increase in the undesirable behavior for a time before the behavior begins to decrease. Warning of this phenomenon beforehand will often prevent discouragement and feelings of frustration (Chart 2).

CASE STUDY

Allen B, a 16-year-old mentally retarded (IQ 64) boy, was admitted to the adolescent psychiatric unit on an emergency basis. He was accompanied by his social service case worker who related that Allen's parents were no longer willing to keep him in their home because he had sexually molested a younger sibling and, when confronted, threatened to harm them or take his own life. He has been in counseling at the local community mental health center off and on since the age of ten. The mental health center records revealed multiple family problems, including an unaccepting stepmother and unstable employment of his father, with frequent family moves in and out of state. The father was known to have rejected the fact of his son's mental disability and refused all specialized services for Allen.

Allen's behavior on the ward was described by staff as follows: loud, explosive, and rapid speech; intruding into the space of other patients and staff; frequent, sudden body contact with female staff and patients; short attention span (about three to five minutes); inability to control explosive behavior during recreation with peers; boasting about knowledge and skills he did not possess. A positive feature noticed by staff was his obvious need to be liked and noticed and his unique and often appropriately timed sense of humor. The primary nursing diagnosis was altered growth and development related to moderate mental retardation. Other nursing diagnoses were: impaired communication; altered impulse control related to attention deficit; personal identity disturbance related to lack of adequate parental role model; and impaired social interaction related to knowledge and skill deficits in social interaction and control of sexual impulses.

An individualized care plan was developed for Allen that took into account his intellecual capacities and developmental level of function (generally about nine to ten years of age). The care plan featured a consistent structured daily routine that incorporated developmentally-appropriate activities, as well as special time-limited tasks he was able to accomplish. Allen's reward schedule differed from the other clients' because he was not able to sustain positive

---

CHART 2
Altered Growth and Development: Summary of the Nursing Process

NURSING INTERVENTIONS	OUTCOME CRITERIA
CLIENT GOAL: EXPERIENCE ABILITY TO COMPLETE A TASK	
Assess need for medication	Demonstrates ability to complete a task without intervening
Assess attention span	activity
Assess response to external stimuli	
Provide low-stimulus environment	
Acknowledge child's frustration	
Provide task with few and simple steps; teach steps of task	
CLIENT GOAL: GAIN POSITIVE RECOGNITION FROM ADULT	
Teach caretakers technique of immediate positive-feedback as reinforcement for expected behaviors	Parents/caretakers increase positive behaviors
Teach caretakers about the purpose and methods of planned ignoring	Parents/caretakers experience constructive parenting
	Demonstrates decreased negative behavior
	Verbalizes positive statements about self

Research Highlights

Brandt reported on a study designed to obtain information on social support and negative life events and their influence on maternal caregiving of mothers with developmentally delayed children.[3] The subjects of this descriptive study were 91 mothers of children ages six months to three years old with developmental disabilities. Most of the subjects were white, married, full-time homemakers who had completed high school. The children in the study had a median of 2.5 disabilities. The method of study was a self-administered questionnaire, completed by the respondents anonymously and returned by mail. Forty percent responded. The measure of social support was obtained utilizing the Personal Resource Questionnaire by Brandt and Weiner. Impact of life events was measured by the Life Experiences Survey, a tool of established reliability and validity. The study was important in that multiple variables were examined, thereby making it consistent with clinical nursing experience. In terms of social support the following significant findings were reported: Fewer resources were available to employed mothers than to mothers who were homemakers, mothers between the ages of 19 and 28 years, and mothers who were divorced, separated, or never married. Satisfaction with help received differed with the type of problem situation. When the need was for information or help in emergencies and child care, a greater percentage of mothers reported satisfaction. If the mother needed emotional support and affirmation in an interpersonal context, most were only somewhat satisfied or dissatisfied with the help received. Perceived support, the third variable examined, was moderately rated overall. However, a significant difference was found between mothers with income of 19,999 dollars or less and mothers with incomes of 20,000 dollars or more. The lower-income group perceived their support to be less than the higher-income group. The number of resources and perceived support were positively related, as were the number of resources and average satisfaction during problem situations.

Analysis of the Life Experience Survey revealed that there was some difference in negative life events among groups of mothers. If the children had three or more disabilities, the mothers obtained higher scores on negative life events.

Although the results of this study cannot be generalized because of the low return rate and the absence of a random sample, the results are consistent with other research findings that mothers and, in many instances, the family's support network, may find adaptive abilities stressed to the limit when a child is developmentally disabled. Greenspan's work illustrates the influence of maladaptive parental response on growth promotion or growth inhibition for children.[10] Nursing research that continues to explore the influence of an individual's or group's ecological system on adaptional response to life stresses and crisis situations will continue to be relevant to nurse practitioners, especially when the findings can be utilized to develop and implement nursing intervention strategies.

behaviors for more than one day or sometimes, one eight-hour shift. It was clear he needed more immediate awards. Rewards were as simple as 15 minutes alone with a staff person of his choice to engage in an activity of his choice. Within two months, Allen's intrusive behavior disappeared completely. He was able to accept waiting for attention and to make his needs known in a more appropriate manner. He was discharged to a therapeutic foster home operated by a male, single foster parent. The community mental health center assigned a staff case manager to the foster home providing as-needed support and direction to the foster parent.

SUMMARY

The etiology of alterations in growth and development may be multifactorial for any one person. Explanations for deviations from normal include the classic work of Sigmund Freud and other psychoanalytic theorists, behavioral theorists, environmental theorists, the more recent work of neuroscientists, and the theories that combine biologic, environmental, and psychological theory with clinical observation of adaptation and coping. Upon completion of assessment, nursing interventions are developed in collaboration with the family and the child toward amelioration of problem behav-

iors that interfere with the child's reaching a maximum potential.

References

1. Bender BG, Linden MG, Robinson A. Environment and developmental risk in children with sex chromosomes abnormalities. J Am Acad Child Adolesc Psychiatry. 1987;26:499–503.
2. Block J. Assimilation, accommodation, and the dynamics of personality development. Child Dev. 1982;53:291–295.
3. Brandt PA. Social support and negative life events of mothers with developmentally delayed children. In: Raff B, Carroll P, eds. Social support and families of vulnerable children, vol 20, no. 5. Birth Defects Foundation; 1984.
4. Campbell M, Rosenbloom A, Perry R, et al. Computerized axial tomography in young autistic children. Am J Psychiatry. 1982;139:510.
5. Cantwell DP. The hyperactive child: diagnosis, management and current research. New York: Spectrum; 1975.
6. Fischer KW, Silvern L. Stages and individual differences in cognitive development. Annu Rev Psychol. 1985;36:613–648.
7. Fish B, Ritvo ER. Psychosis of childhood. In: Noshpitz JD, ed. Basic handbook of child psychiatry, vol 2. New York: Basic Books; 1979.
8. Galler JR, Ramsey F. A follow-up study of the influence of

early malnutrition on development: delayed development of conservation (Piaget). J Am Acad Child Adolesc Psychiatry. 1987;26:23–27.

9. Goldstein HS. Cognitive development in low attentive, hyperactive, and aggressive 6 through 11-year-old children. J Am Acad Child Adolesc Psychiatry. 1987;26:214–218.

10. Greenspan SI. Normal child development. In: Kaplan H, Sadock B, eds. Comprehensive textbook of psychiatry/IV; vol 2. Baltimore: Williams & Wilkins; 1985.

11. Greenspan SI: Psychopathology and adaptation in infancy and early childhood. New York; International Universities Press; 1981.

12. Neurobiological research in autism. (Special Issue). J Autism Dev Disord. 1982;12:103–205.

13. Powell ML. Assessment and management of developmental changes and problems in children, 2nd ed. St. Louis: CV Mosby; 1981.

14. Rheingold HL. Development as the aquisition of familiarity. Annu Rev Psychol. 1985;36:1–17.

15. Rutter M, Schopler E, eds. Autism: a reappraisal of concepts and treatment. New York: Plenum Press; 1978.

16. Shapiro T, Sherman M, Colamari G, Koch D. Attachment in autism and other developmental disorders. J Am Acad Child Adolesc Psychiatry. 1987;26:480–484.

17. Troy M, Sroufe LA. Victimization among preschoolers: role of attachment relationship history. J Am Acad Child Adolesc Psychiatry. 1987;26:166–172.

GUILT

Illa Ann Hilliard

DEFINITION AND DESCRIPTION

Guilt is an emotional and interactional response to a perceived or actual failure to meet expectations of self, others, or a Supreme Being. It runs a progressive course (Fig. 13-16). It is initiated by the awareness of expectations, followed by acts of omission or commission that violate those expectations and, in turn, is accompanied by conscious or unconscious guilt responses. The outcome of a guilt episode may be negative and characterized by decreased self-esteem, destructive thoughts, or immobilization, such as inability to make decisions, or it may be positive, wherein there is growth, change, forgiveness, and reparation.

Traditional guilt is frequently defined as a mode of interaction manifested by poor self-concept, a sense of wrongdoing, anxiety and discomfort, sadness, and the fear of punishment. It is usually associated with offending others—frequently parents—or with going against social mores.[13,17,18] Existential guilt expands this definition to include the failure of an individual to respond to the self, be responsible for oneself, or develop one's potential. The individual transgresses against self in making choices that lead away from being authentic. At the core of existential guilt is failure to accept the responsibility for one's life and actions—responsibility reflected through choices.[3,18] Guilt is generally viewed as something to be avoided; however, without it, there would be chaos and a lack of social order.

THEORY AND RESEARCH
Theoretical Perspectives

A number of theories have emerged to explain the phenomenon of guilt. Although separated for discussion, several theories have implications in the assessment and treatment of an individual experiencing guilt.

Freud. Freud theorized that guilt emerges in the Oedipal stage of development and symbolizes a conflict between the superego (internalized standard of behavior, judge) and the id (pleasure drive). When experienced, guilt brings into awareness the need to make a conscious choice regarding acceptable behavior. If the superego is too harsh, it can lead to unreasonable guilt and loss of self-esteem or self-imposed punishment. If the superego is too lenient or nonexistent, a person has no internalized standard of behavior. The superego is founded on the internalized values of parents and, thus, is experienced similarly to the child's reaction to parents in their authority roles.[7]

Erikson. Building upon Freud's theory is Erikson's developmental framework. Erikson viewed the preschool period (three to six years of age) as a developmental crisis in which initiative is primary. If initiative is thwarted to the extent that anger and antagonism become overwhelming, guilt becomes dominant and can hinder or negatively influence the individual's self-concept. This can have a lasting influence on a person's belief about his or her ability to influence others or the environment and creates feelings of helplessness.[6]

Rank. Rank considered the role of the will in relation to guilt. He saw the need for parental influence to assist children in channeling aggressive impulses, but he warned not to squelch or suppress them to the point where "willing" by the child is perceived as bad or wrong. Excessive guilt is theorized to cause some individuals to reach the point of not being able to feel or to "will."[18]

Sullivan. Sullivan theorized that guilt occurs when individuals consciously violate their personal ideal systems or moral codes. Sullivan viewed guilt as a form of anxiety. When an individual's defense mechanisms are activated to a degree that removes the guilt from conscious awareness, crazy guilt results. In other words, unconscious acting-out occurs because guilt is not worked through on a conscious level. Sullivan speculated that the process of rationalizing is used to avoid the anxiety. If this is a dominant pattern, the individual fails to develop a conscience and frequently violates social norms by manipulating and using others for personal gain.[16]

Berne. Berne, in his transactional analysis theory, placed the emphasis on communication between the parents and child and the subsequent internalized message that continues with the individual. Three ego states—parent, child, and adult—are identified. Guilt is activated when the parental messages of "shoulds" and "shouldn'ts" come into conflict with the child ego state of feelings and spontaneous behavior. Berne viewed guilt as a type of self-punishment or response to a parental program. The adult ego state mediates to bring guilt into compliance with reality and to provide balance.[2]

267

Piaget and Kohlberg. Piaget and Kohlberg's moral development theory identified a series of sequential stages in which the cognitive framework for guilt progresses from preconventional, to conventional, to postconventional thinking. Preconventionally, the concern is with the effect or consequences of behavior—particularly in terms of punishment or avoidance of punishment. In conventional thinking, the focus is on approval by others or compliance with rules, order, or authority. The mature or postconventional stage of moral thinking is characterized by consideration for others' rights, claiming of personal values, and flexibility in making judgments. In this last stage, guilt is present when one transgresses against self or others.[9]

Ellis. Ellis placed primary focus on thinking and the messages the individual sends to self. He posited that inner thoughts are the dominant factor influencing a person's feelings, guilt, and behavior. He stressed the need to examine the activating event, the belief or thoughts stimulated, the emotional consequences, and the disputing beliefs or reframing necessary to relieve guilt.[4,5]

Yalom. Yalom conceptualized existential guilt as going beyond traditional guilt. It arises from transgressions against self that trap a person into not developing his or her potential. Existential guilt is a powerful force that can block decision making and cause the person to sacrifice living life fully. Closely linked to decision making is the responsibility an individual takes for his or her own life: past, present, and future. An individual's affirmation results from values chosen, behaviors reflective of self, and congruence between knowing and experiencing. Recognizing personal contributions to the past and responsibility for the present and future can be a difficult and painful experience. Unsuccessful resolution can lead to loneliness and fear. Decisions and feelings must be claimed for resolution of existential guilt to be realized.[18]

Jung. Jung viewed existential guilt as a result of resistance to individuation and betrayal to humanity. His view of responsibility includes being responsive to the world as well as to oneself.[3]

Research Perspectives. Guilt has been researched from a number of perspectives. Several findings with implications for nursing have emerged. Excessive guilt can interfere with recovery or lead to serious health consequences. In a study of burn clients, controlling for burn severity and time since admission, it was found that clients who blamed themselves for burn injury experienced more pain and depression and demonstrated poorer compliance with nursing activities.[10]

Patterns of guilt may vary as illustrated by a study comparing guilt feelings in concentration camp survivors and controls. Although there were no significant differences between the survivor and control groups, there were differences between men and women. Women expressed significantly more guilt than men about behaviors contrary to moral or ethical principles.[12]

Guilt, which can interfere with the normal process of grieving, can be reduced by timely interventions. For example, in a study of bereaved parents of dying children, parents who were involved in a long-preparation group were able to resolve some of the guilt feelings, whereas parents who were involved in a short-preparation group made significantly more statements indicating guilt at the end of the study period.[8]

Finally, guilt can be a significant issue to be dealt with, even though it may not be the primary symptom or presenting problem. In a study of a group of subjects with a diagnosis of major depression, it was found that individuals with excessive guilt predictively had fam-

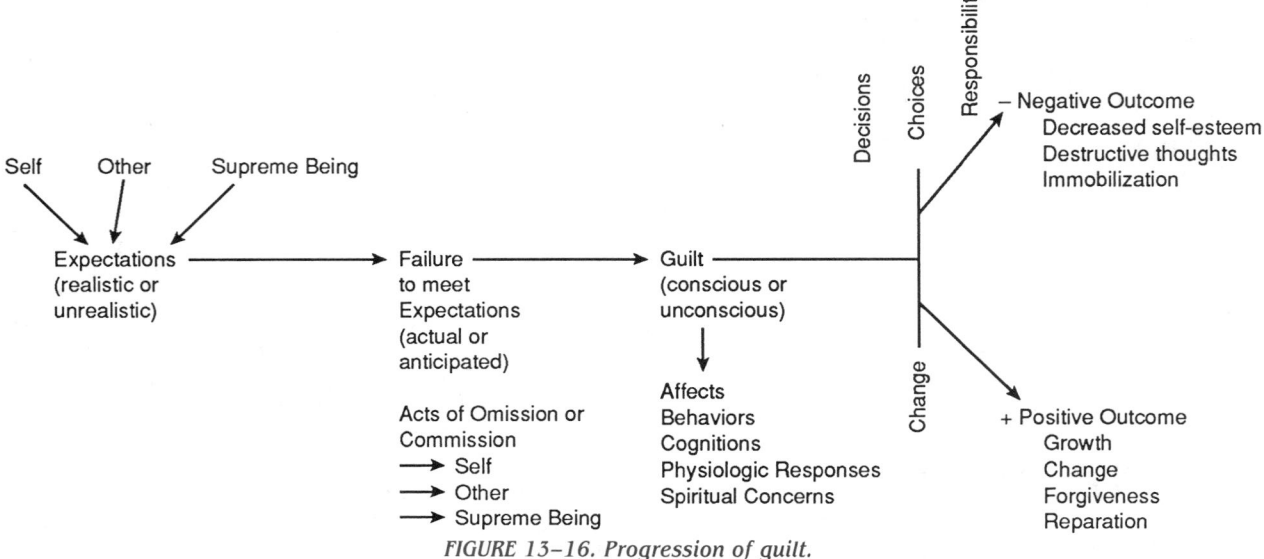

FIGURE 13–16. Progression of guilt.

ily members with significant depression. One of the two most discriminating predictors for familial depression was excessive guilt.[11]

RELATED FACTORS

Guilt can be experienced in a number of life situations including acts against one's self, crisis situations in which expectations are not met, or as a feature of psychiatric conditions. Acts against the self include actions that violate known health rules or increase health risks: smoking, obesity, substance abuse, lack of or excessive exercise. Other acts against self are failing to behave according to personal beliefs and values, suppressing desires or needs to meet others' expectations and avoid conflict, and choosing to avoid risks or new experiences to avoid the anxiety of the unknown. Crisis situations frequently associated with guilt include birth of a handicapped child, contracting a serious and chronic or terminal illness (e.g., genital herpes, AIDS), involvement in a serious accident, or realizing one is going to have to care for a chronically ill spouse or significant other. Psychiatric disorders in which guilt frequently is a characteristic include anorexia nervosa, bulimia nervosa, depressive episodes, posttraumatic stress disorder, and alcohol abuse.[1] Clients are viewed as experiencing irrational guilt when their guilt emanates from imagined situations or from minor transgressions that are perceived as very powerful.

Regardless of the cause of the guilt, its meaning can be appreciated only if viewed within a cultural context. From this context expectations are established. Societal or subcultural norms and values can play a crucial role in the guilt experienced by the nurse or the client. For example, a nurse may initiate resuscitation procedures for a 96-year-old man in a nursing home, but feel guilty for obeying the rules, rather than honoring the client's wish to die and protecting his right to choose death with peace and dignity. In another situation, a client may choose a life-style unacceptable to a family or church group. These groups may disenfranchise the individual because the norms are broken and, yet, the individual may still wish to belong. It is also within a cultural context that forgiveness and reparation can have a healing effect.

DEFINING CHARACTERISTICS

Defining characteristics of guilt include behaviors, affects, cognitions, physiological responses, and spiritual concerns. The pattern of response may be typical of an individual; however, not all individuals exhibit the same cues or patterns. Moreover, the clustering of responses may vary depending on the area of focus related to guilt.

Two examples illustrate variations in presenting symptomatology. One client may identify feelings of failure as the primary problem. These feelings may be accompanied by addictive behaviors; cognitions of justifying, ruminating, and utilizing many "shoulds"; physiologic signs of dry mouth and tachycardia; and spiritual struggles involving a sense of needing to be punished, lack of self-forgiveness, and wishes to undo. Another client may seek assistance for a pattern of behaviors accompanied by feelings of anxiety, helplessness, and depression; obsessive thoughts of self-blame; and spiritual issues of inconsistencies in his value system, discrepancies and conflicts between his beliefs and behaviors, and preoccupation with sinfulness (Chart 1).

NURSING PROCESS AND RATIONALE
Assessment

The nurse observes client behaviors and listens for statements that indicate a belief that certain actions are wrong or bad, or for the presence of an "I am bad" self-concept. Examples of such statements are: "Oh! I shouldn't have done that." "If only he hadn't been there." "I never should have said that." "I always mess up." "I never do anything right." "If only I had lived differently." The underlying themes in guilt frequently include failure of the individual's actions to meet expectations or standards set from self, others, or Supreme Being. Within this context, patterns of symptoms are identified from the characteristics outlined in Chart 1.

Assessment and diagnosis establish the foundation to ensure accuracy of the nursing interventions. The nurse needs to determine if the individual is struggling with developmental factors relating to autonomy or initiative. Sequentially, autonomy issues are associated with shame and initiative issues with guilt. Although related, shame differs from guilt.[14] Shame frequently is experienced by the client despite others' differing views. For many persons shame is more difficult to talk about than guilt. Guilt is more frequently associated with actions, whereas shame is often connected with body image and a failure of self. Therefore, self-consciousness is escalated to a greater degree with shame than with guilt. The big factor for discriminating the two is that issues around autonomy are usually associated with shame and issues around initiative are associated with guilt. Frequently, there is overlap, and it may be very difficult to differentiate the diagnosis.

Nursing Diagnosis

Clearly focused nursing diagnoses provide direction for nursing care. The nursing diagnosis of guilt can be formulated specifically for a particular client. Examples of diagnoses include guilt related to failure to prevent parents' divorce; guilt related to having an abortion; guilt related to parenting failures; guilt related to unrealistic expectations of self; guilt related to assuming unrealistic responsibility for others; and guilt related to significant life choices.

CHART 1
Guilt: Definition, Related Factors, and Defining Characteristics

DEFINITION

Guilt is an emotional and interactional response to a perceived or actual failure to meet expectations of self, others, or a Supreme Being. It runs a progressive course initiated by the awareness of expectations, followed by acts of omission or commission that violate those expectations, in turn, accompanied by conscious or unconscious guilt responses.

RELATED FACTORS

Psychoactive substance use disorders
Crisis situations
Eating disorders
Depressive episodes
Post-traumatic stress disorder
Alcoholism
Violation of personal values
Existential dilemmas
Violation of socially accepted behaviors

DEFINING CHARACTERISTICS
Affects (feelings)

Anxiety
Fear
Pain
Helplessness
Anger
Anguish
Depression
Remorse
Burdened
Unworthiness
Vague discomfort
Embarrassment
Sadness
Despair
Ashamed
Failure
Isolation
Conflict (sexual)
Excess responsibility

Cognitions (thoughts)

Self-blame
Projection
Denial
Ruminating
Justifying
Preoccupied (short attention span)
Tunnel vision
Selective inattention
Obsessive thoughts
"Shoulds"/"shouldn'ts"

Behaviors

Arguing
Social isolation (avoidance)
Punitive actions toward self or others
Repetition of guilt-producing behavior
Use of drugs or alcohol
Overeating or undereating
Overworking
Compulsive exercising
Avoiding eye contact
Fidgeting
Crying
Accidents

Physiologic Signs

Tachycardia
Palpitations
Dry mouth
Sweaty palms
Loss of appetite
Nausea
Fainting
Hyperventilation
Diarrhea
Urinary frequency and urgency
"Butterflies"
General adaptation syndrome

Spiritual Concerns

Violation of moral order
Inconsistency with value system
Sense of needing punishment
Discrepancies and conflicts between beliefs and behaviors
Lack of self-forgiveness
Anger toward Supreme Being or representatives
Questions meaning of suffering
Unable to forgive or be forgiven
Preoccupation with spiritual issues
Withdrawal from religious ties
Questions own meaning of life, death, belief system
Wishing to undo
Looking for punishment from Supreme Being
Preoccupation with sinfulness
Inability to experience pleasure

Client Goals and Nursing Interventions

Regardless of the specific goals and interventions, the process for intervening follows a common course. Initially, the client may or may not be aware of experiencing guilt. The nurse may ask direct questions regarding guilt, beginning with what the client presents as the primary problem or need. "When you don't meet your expectations or those of others, do you feel guilty?" "If you don't work 60 hours a week, do you feel guilty?" "I notice you keep saying 'I should . . .'; do you feel guilty when you are saying this?" "I notice you keep identifying conflicts in your choices as you talk about your beliefs; are these situations connected with a sense of guilt?" If the individual is aware of and claims the guilt, the nurse can proceed with helping the client work through the guilt. If the client is unaware of experiencing guilt, efforts are directed toward assisting the client to identify the comments, feelings, physical symptoms, and behaviors related to guilt and to claim the response. It is often useful to establish a historical perspective by having the client recall and describe a situation in which guilt was experienced. The nurse guides the client to include description of all dimensions. "What happened prior to experiencing your sense of guilt?" "What were some of your thoughts, feelings?" "How did your body react when you experienced guilt in that situation?" "Do you see any similarities between what happened then and what is happening now?" Frequently the client will make connections because most persons have patterns of experiencing and coping with guilt. It is essential that the client be able to identify and claim the guilt feeling because resolution will be blocked or hindered without this process.

The second step is to relate guilt feelings with mechanisms that offer relief. Directly asking the client what relieves guilt feelings is frequently helpful. Sometimes the client needs assistance in focusing on specific behaviors used to combat guilt and determining how constructive these behaviors are. Examples of such behaviors are drinking; overworking; compulsive exercising; entertaining thoughts that lead to justifying, projecting, anger, sadness; constantly apologizing; or setting spiritual priorities such as praying, singing, or going to confession.

When the client is able to identify some means of providing relief for guilt, the next step is to explore in detail the situation or situations that precede the guilt feelings. At this point a specific situation may be explored or specific thoughts, behaviors, or experiences occurring just before the feelings may need to be described in detail. The nurse may need to guide the exploration by inquiring into specific areas. "What were your expectations?" "What were you saying to yourself?" or "What was your 'self-talk'?" "What messages did you receive from others?" "Did you feel you should do or feel anything?" "What feelings did you experience: failure, despair, burdened, helpless, conflict?"

"What physical discomfort or symptoms have you been experiencing: loss of appetite, butterflies, nausea?" The client is encouraged to describe in as much detail as possible any experience immediately preceding the guilt feelings.

Once the guilt is recognized and labeled, the client analyzes the connections that led to feeling guilt. "What happened when the guilt was felt?" "Then, what followed after the initial guilt?" For many clients, seeing the connections and understanding the feelings within a context is enough to precipitate the relinquishment of the guilt. For some clients, additional explanations about cause are necessary, and other similar situations need to be thoroughly explored.

Finally, new options for coping are explored and tried. These may include thought-stopping techniques, revising self-talk scripts, making decisions and assuming responsibility for self, practicing assertiveness, and initiating or restructuring of relationships. For some clients, self-help books are of assistance (e.g., references 2, 3, 4, 5, and 7). These are particularly helpful if the client uses a lot of negative self-talk or shoulds.

If the foregoing steps are taken and the nurse identifies that the guilt is long-standing, developmental in origin, part of very low self-esteem, unresponsive to the interventions just described, or a continuing destructive factor for the client, psychotherapy is an option to consider.

Evaluation

Evaluation is an ongoing process for the client and nurse. During the work on reducing the guilt, feelings may be more intense for a short period, or a great sense of relief may be experienced. The ongoing evaluation monitors progress and guides the establishment of effective coping strategies. Outcome criteria are individualized and depend upon the needs of the client (Chart 2). The positive or negative outcome of the guilt episode depends on the coping skills of the individual, the therapeutic intervention, and the individual's choices.

CASE STUDY

Nancy, a medical technician, is a 32-year-old single mother of a daughter aged four. She initiated therapy after an abortion. She wanted the baby, but Bill, her live-in partner of six months and father of the baby, did not. Nancy also remembered how difficult it had been when she decided to have her daughter and not marry.

Nancy perceived herself as independent, responsible, and doing what was expected of her by others. She looked at situations as right or wrong, successful or unsuccessful. If a situation was ambiguous she made completion in her thoughts to reduce anxiety, rather than talking with the other individual involved. She always placed the blame on herself when things did not work out. Nancy spent much time apologizing to others and trying to make everything "right" to gain approval and acceptance. She thought that

---

CHART 2
Guilt: Summary of the Nursing Process

NURSING INTERVENTIONS	OUTCOME CRITERIA
CLIENT GOAL: ESTABLISH NEW MEANS OF COPING WITH GUILT	
Assist client to identify negative self-talk	Identifies negative self-talk contributing to guilt when it begins
Assist client to identify situations triggering negative self-talk	
Teach thought-stopping techniques	Uses thought-stopping technique
Assist client to revise self-talk script	Uses revised self-talk script
Assist client to evaluate results of changes in self-talk	Reports decrease in guilt
CLIENT GOAL: DEFINE AND CHOOSE REALISTIC EXPECTATIONS FOR SELF	
Assist client to identify expectations to which he or she responds	Discriminates sources and impact of expectations
Assist client to explore source of expectations: self, others, Supreme Being	
Assist client to differentiate areas he or she controls (i.e., realistic–unrealistic)	Identifies areas of control or lack of control
Assist client to identify impact of attempts to respond to unrealistic expectations	
Assist client to establish realistic expectations	Chooses realistic expectations for self
CLIENT GOAL: CHANGE REPEATED BEHAVIORS LEADING TO GUILT	
Assist the client to identify guilt-producing behaviors	Describes actions leading to guilt
Assist client to list positive and negative outcomes or rewards of behaviors	Claims responsibility for positive and negative outcomes of behavior
Explore with the client options for alternate behaviors	Selects option creating less guilt
Discuss with client results of new approaches	

---

whatever she started needed to be completed. In trying to meet her own and others' expectations, she often experienced feelings of anger, anxiety, guilt, and self-doubt. Positive feelings increased momentarily when she helped someone.

These characteristics were apparent in her relationships, as several incidents with Bill illustrate: After agreeing to pay half the abortion expenses, Bill spent his money on a hunting rifle. Nancy expressed her anger, then felt guilty about making Bill angry. When Bill refused to be involved sexually for two months after she asked him to use protective measures because she was unable to use birth control pills, Nancy felt responsible for pushing him away. Although Nancy asked Bill to move out because the relationship was filled with conflict and he was not paying his share as agreed, she invited him to move back when he had a death in the family. She felt guilty for not being with him at his time of need.

In her relationships with her parents, she always tried to please. When her parents divorced when she was eight, the children were separated. She and her oldest sister lived with her father, whereas the three younger children lived with her mother. She learned not to express her feelings because these were met with anger by her stepmother. The dominant message she received from her mother was "be perfect." Her role with her father was his defender.

Research Highlights

Pagel and associates conducted a longitudinal study of caregivers of spouses with Alzheimer's disease.[15] A two-wave assessment of caregivers, using interviews and a battery of psychological tests, was completed with subjects selected from referrals to the project by a variety of care providers in a large metropolitan area. The researchers found that guilt was the significant factor in the degree of depression experienced. Those who blamed themselves (i.e., felt guilty and responsible) for their spouses' uncontrollable behavior experienced more depression at follow-up than was predicted from their initial interview level of depression. Those who did not blame themselves were not depressed. Depression scores for spouse caregivers of home and institutionalized clients did not differ. Finally, the objective aspects of the spouse's disability did not account for the degree of stress caused by the situation.[15]

These findings support those of other studies that excessive guilt can lead to serious health consequences, interfere with normal grieving, and be a significant issue for nursing care, even though it is not the presenting issue. They underscore the need for nurses to consider the possibility of guilt as a dynamic in many situations with clients and their families. In addition, the need to ascertain the clients' perceptions and experiences, as well as the objective facts of a situation, is imperative.

With her daughter, Nancy set expectations but often failed to follow through. She feared she was expecting her daughter to be perfect, just as her mother did.

In working with Nancy, the guilt could be approached from several perspectives. Possible nursing diagnoses were guilt related to having an abortion; guilt related to conflictual relationship with Bill—over child, sexual withdrawal, finances; guilt related to failure as parent—not following with discipline; guilt related to unrealistic expectations of self; guilt related to perceived failure with parents—not being a "perfect child," preventing the divorce. The therapist in collaboration with Nancy chose to focus on guilt related to unrealistic expectations of self. This focus was selected because it was the crux of Nancy's presenting problems and permeated her life dilemmas. As therapy progressed, Nancy became more aware of her historical pattern of incorporating others' expectations as her own. She was able to accept how unreachable many of these expectations were. Slowly, she began to select her own expectations and make realistic choices that she claimed as her own. During the early part of this change, Nancy's anxiety and guilt escalated as she felt she was being disloyal and would be abandoned. With the continuing process of freely choosing to meet her own expectations, the guilt decreased, her self-talk became more positive, and her behaviors were less stressful. Her tolerance increased for aloneness, although she has not yet reached the point of celebration of her own worth and being. Therapy continues.

SUMMARY

Guilt, a human response that may be experienced by the nurse or client, may be constructive or destructive. Increasing knowledge about guilt can lead to effective nursing interventions and assist the client in establishing positive styles of coping with guilt.

References

1. American Psychiatric Association. Diagnostic and statistical manual of mental disorders. 3rd ed, revised. Washington, DC: American Psychiatric Association; 1987.
2. Briggs DC. Celebrate your self. Garden City: Doubleday; 1977.
3. Brooke R. Jung and the phenomenology of guilt. Anal Psychol. 1985;30:165–184.
4. Burns D. Feeling good: the new mood therapy. New York: New American Library; 1980.
5. Ellis A, Harper R. A guide to rational living. Englewood Cliffs, NJ: Prentice–Hall; 1971.
6. Erikson EH. Childhood and society. 2nd ed. New York: WW Norton; 1964.
7. Freeman L, Strean HS. Guilt: letting go. New York: John Wiley & Sons; 1986.
8. Johnson S. Counseling families experiencing guilt. Dimens Crit Care Nurs. 1984;3:238–244.
9. Kessler S, Kessler H, Ward P. Psychological aspects of genetic counseling III. Management of guilt and shame. Am J Med Genet. 1984;17:673–697.
10. Kiecolt–Glaser JK, Williams DA. Self-blame, compliance, and distress among burn patients. J Pers Soc Psychol. 1987;53:187–193.
11. Leckman JF, Caruso KA, Prusoff BA, Weissman MM, Merikangas KR, Pauls DL. Appetite disturbance and excessive guilt in major depression. Arch Gen Psychiatry. 1984;41:839–844.
12. Lobel TE, Kav-Venaki S, Yahia M. Guilt feelings and locus control of concentration camp survivors. Int J Soc Psychiatry. 1985;31:170–175.
13. McFarland G, Wasli E. Nursing diagnosis and process in psychiatric mental health nursing. Philadelphia: JB Lippincott; 1986.
14. O'Toole AW. The phenomenon of shame: Part 2. Arch Psychiatr Nurs. 1987;1:308–317.
15. Pagel MD, Becker J, Coppel DB. Loss of control, self-blame, and depression: an investigation of spouse caregivers of Alzheimer's disease patients. J Abnorm Psychol. 1985;94:169–182.
16. Sullivan H. The interpersonal theory of psychiatry. New York: WW Norton; 1953.
17. van Wormer K. Guilt feelings in the spouse of the terminally ill. Home Health Nurs. 1985;3(5):21–25.
18. Yalom ID. Existential psychotherapy. New York: Basic Books; 1980.

HEALTH MAINTENANCE, ALTERED

Helen S. A. Murphy

DEFINITION AND DESCRIPTION

Altered health maintenance is a person's inability to identify, manage, or seek out help to maintain health.[5] The focus here will be on the difficulty that many psychiatric clients have in maintaining their physical health.

THEORY AND RESEARCH

Psychiatric clients are at risk for the occurrence of medical illnesses. In a multisite study of the utilization of medical facilities, clients with psychiatric diagnoses visited medical practitioners one and one-half to two times more frequently than clients without such diagnoses.[4] Conversely, a high rate of medical illness has been observed in both inpatient and outpatient psychiatric populations and in clients with various psychiatric diagnoses.[1,3,6,7] The medical disorders may be unrelated but co-occurring or in some cases, for example, cardiac decompensation or iron deficiency anemia may be involved in the etiology or exacerbation of the psychiatric symptoms.[3,6] Of 100 patients admitted to an inpatient unit in one study, 46 had previously unrecognized medical illnesses that were specifically related to psychiatric symptomatology, and an additional 34 had coexisting medical illnesses requiring treatment.[3]

Mortality among psychiatric clients is higher than for the general population.[2,8] In an extensive follow-up of 500 psychiatric outpatients, mortality was nearly twice that of a demographically similar nonpsychiatric population.[8] As might be expected, deaths occurring from suicide, homicide, and other unnatural causes partially accounted for this high mortality. However, nearly two-thirds of the deaths were from medical illnesses, including cardiovascular disease, cerebrovascular disease, malignant neoplasms, and other diseases.[8]

RELATED FACTORS

A number of interacting related factors are involved in altered maintenance of physical health by psychiatric clients. Because of decreased energy and motivation, altered cognitive abilities, and impaired judgment, psychiatric clients may ignore their own health care or be inconsistent in following suggested treatment regimens.[7] Promotion of health and prevention of disease may be impaired by inadequate or inaccurate informa-

tion. Clients may become malnourished or dehydrated, placing them at further risk for various diseases.[3] Symptoms of confusion, depression, agitation, assaultiveness, and delusions may mask underlying medical disorders.[1] Psychiatric clients may lack the social and communication skills necessary to obtain the help they need.[7] Negative feelings may be aroused in health-care workers leading to less than optimal care.[1] Clients may be unable or unwilling to communicate pain or discomfort. In one study (see Research Highlights), for example, clients with schizophrenia expressed no discomfort when suffering from life-threatening illnesses.[9] Finally, inadequate resources (money, housing, transportation) may pose problems for psychiatric clients in maintaining their health and in obtaining medical care.

DEFINING CHARACTERISTICS

Altered health maintenance may be manifested in a number of ways. The client may be missing dentures, may have glasses in need of repair, or be without a needed hearing aid. There may be indicators of malnourishment or dehydration, obvious physical signs of disease such as an elevated temperature or blood pressure or skin lesions. Or there may be less obvious symptoms such as generalized weakness.[1] In addition, there may be edema, bruises, or other signs of injury. The client may be unaware of these problems or may misinterpret their meaning (Chart 1).

NURSING PROCESS AND RATIONALE
Assessment

Manifestation of physical illness or injury in a psychiatric client may be very subtle, necessitating good physical assessment and behavioral observation. For some clients, information about physical problems can be elicited with careful questioning. Vital signs and laboratory test results may indicate problems. It is also helpful to gather information from family members, significant others, previous medical records, or health-care professionals who have knowledge of the client's previous history. When a client is suffering from delusions or hallucinations, listening to the content may provide information about concerns that the client is unable to express more directly. For example, the client may make statements like, "Jane needs to go to

274

CHART 1
Altered Health Maintenance: Definition, Related Factors, and Defining Characteristics

DEFINITION

Altered health maintenance is an individual's inability to identify, manage, or seek help to maintain health.

RELATED FACTORS

Decreased energy and motivation
Altered cognitive abilities
Impaired judgment
Malnourishment
Dehydration
Psychiatric symptoms masking underlying disorder
Poor communication skills
Inadequate resources

DEFINING CHARACTERISTICS

Missing dentures
Missing or damaged eyeglasses
Absence of needed hearing aid
Manifestations of malnourishment
Manifestations of dehydration
Physical signs of disease
Generalized weakness
Physical signs of injury
Hypothermia

the hospital;" or "There's blood on my arm, nurse. Wipe it off." This type of statement could indicate internal pain or suffering being experienced by the client.

Nursing Diagnosis

An example of a nursing diagnosis for a client is alteration in health maintenance related to impaired judgment and inadequate financial resources.

Client Goals and Nursing Interventions

The first goal is to assist clients in reducing current physical impairments. Steps are taken to correct any immediate problems such as malnourishment or dehydration. Consultations are sought from other health-care providers, or assistance is given to the client in making contacts with proper caregivers. Arrangements may be made, for example, for a client to have a dental check up or to have glasses repaired. The client is provided with information about available health care and, if necessary, assisted in contacting agencies for follow-up.

A second goal is to help the client establish behavior patterns that maintain physical health. The nurse works with the client toward the removal or reduction of cognitive deficits, removal of stressors, teaching positive adaptation skills, and providing support. The nurse encourages the client to report significant or continuing signs or symptoms of illness or any significant change in emotional status. The nurse discusses with the client the need for medication that reduces symptoms of psychosis which may lead to behavior that causes alterations in health status.

A third goal is increasing the use of support systems. It is important to encourage involvement of the family or significant others in the care and treatment of the client. They may be able to recognize early signs of illness ignored by the client. Family members and significant others can also provide cultural or other information to health-care workers. This, in turn, would allow for adaptation of health-care regimens to make compliance more likely. The nurse provides education to the family and the client about what community resources are available to aid in health maintenance, when the client should seek health care (e.g., when signs and symptoms do not abate and there is an apparent threat to health), and how to contact resources such as hospitals, clinics, or mental health centers for assistance.

Evaluation

The effectiveness of nursing interventions can be evaluated by the extent to which the client demonstrates a decrease in physical impairments, an increase in behavior patterns that contribute to health maintenance, and an increase in support system involvement (Chart 2).

CASE STUDY

John is a 30-year-old, single man who had been an inpatient in a psychiatric hospital for two years with a diagnosis of schizophrenia, chronic undifferentiated type. He was discharged three months ago with a one-month supply of neuroleptic medication and a referral for follow-up care at a community mental health-care center located close to his group home. John did not take his prescribed medications or keep appointments with his counselor at the mental health center. His judgment and insight became grossly impaired, and he saw no need to eat or drink or wear protective clothing while out-of-doors. John was found wandering on the street and received immediate treatment for dehydration and exposure in a general hospital. Upon resolution of the acute crisis, John was brought to a psychiatric facility where he received a nursing diagnosis of altered health maintenance related to impaired judgment. Nursing goals were formulated to assist the client with self-care and improved judgment through assisting the client in recognizing the signs and symptoms of alterations in health, what community resources are available and how to contact them, and the importance of support systems.

CHART 2
Altered Health Maintenance: Summary of the Nursing Process

NURSING INTERVENTIONS	OUTCOME CRITERIA
CLIENT GOAL: DECREASE PHYSICAL IMPAIRMENT(S)	
Assess the client's health care needs	Demonstrates a decrease in physical symptoms
Take necessary steps to correct any problems such as malnutrition or dehydration	
Assist client toward the removal or reduction of cognitive deficits and removal of stressors	
Teach positive adaptation skills	
Assist client in the acquisition of necessary appliances to improve sensory perceptions (e.g., corrective lenses, hearing aid, dentures, crutches, or cane)	Obtains needed corrective appliances
Provide emotional support	
Seek consultations with other health care providers as necessary	
Provide client with information about available health care and, if necessary, assist in making contacts	
CLIENT GOAL: ESTABLISH BEHAVIOR PATTERNS THAT CONTRIBUTE TO HEALTH MAINTENANCE	
Assess behaviors that contribute to alterations in health	Demonstrates ability to recognize health threats
Work with client to remove or reduce cognitive deficits and stressors	
Discuss with client the need for medication that reduces symptoms of psychosis	Identifies reasons for medications
Encourage the client to report significant or continuing signs or symptoms of illness or any significant change in emotional status	Reports any significant or continuing symptoms
FAMILY GOAL: HAVE SUPPORT SYSTEMS AVAILABLE	
Encourage family members or significant others to provide cultural information to health care workers	Family or significant other displays understanding of altered health states
Encourage family to assist in early recognition of altered health states	
Discuss with family or significant others when the client should seek health care assistance	
Communicate to the client and family what community resources are available to aid in health maintenance and how to contact resources such as clinics or mental health centers for assistance	Client or significant other identifies available health care resources

Research Highlights

Talbott and Linn conducted a study of the responses of chronic schizophrenic clients to serious medical illnesses.[9] A total of 30 nurses and doctors responsible for the medical, surgical, and nursing care of chronic mental patients in seven New York State hospitals were interviewed. In addition, the medical records for those patients were reviewed. Several themes emerged from the interviews and medical record review. The most pervasive finding was that many psychotic clients, particularly those with a diagnosis in which severe pain would be expected, such as myocardial infarction, verbalized no discomfort. Other conditions that clients tolerated without complaint included major fractures, third-degree burns over large portions of the body, perforated peptic ulcers, childbirth, occlusions of peripheral arteries with gangrenous extremities, incarcerated hernias with gangrenous bowel changes, and a variety of malignancies with or without metastases. Most were diagnosed by the astute observation of the staff of such behavior as limping after a leg fracture, alterations in mood or emotional state in a patient who previously exhibited destructive and assaultive behavior, but who sat quietly in a chair after perforation of a peptic ulcer. A second major finding in this study was that clients who were self-mutilating demonstrated no evidence of pain or discomfort. Examples involved incidence of self-inflicted burns with matches, cigarettes, or against radiators; self-inflicted cuts and hacking with glass or sharp metal objects to the point of suicide; banging of extremities; and opening of wounds of surgical incisions with bare hands. A third finding was that chronic schizophrenic clients were able to tolerate foul-smelling lesions on their own person without evidence of concern. Finally, there was widespread evidence that these clients were unable or unwilling to tolerate medical care, plaster casts, sutures, surgical dressings, traction, intubation, immobilization, and bed rest.[9]

SUMMARY

Chronic psychiatric clients are at high risk for physical illness and mortality because of several factors: (1) underutilization of health care services because of decreased energy and motivation, inadequate or inaccurate information regarding health practices, psychotic symptomatology, or inadequate resources; (2) nonresponsiveness to painful stimuli; (3) an inability or unwillingness to tolerate medical care. These factors make it imperative for nurses to be cognizant of significant changes in clinical findings or in a client's behavioral changes that may indicate alterations in health status. Client goals are focused on the reduction of present physical impairments, establishing behavioral patterns that maintain health, and the utilization of support systems.

References

1. Bunce DFM, Jones R, Badger LW, Jones SE. Medical illness in psychiatric patients: barriers to diagnosis and treatment. South Med J. 1982;75:941–944.

2. Eastwood MR, Stiasny S, Meier HMR, Woogh CM. Mental illness and mortality. Compr Psychiatry. 1982;23:377–385.

3. Hall RC, Gardner ER, Stickney SK, Lecann AF, Popkin MK. Physical illness manifesting as psychiatric disease, II. Analysis of a state hospital inpatient population. Arch Gen Psychiatry. 1980;37:989–995.

4. Hankin JR, Steinwachs DM, Regier DA, Burns BJ, Goldberg ID, Hoeper EW. Use of general medical care services by persons with mental disorders. Arch Gen Psychiatry. 1982;39:225–231.

5. Kim M, McFarland G, McLane A. Pocket guide to nursing diagnosis, 3rd ed. St. Louis: CV Mosby; 1989.

6. Koranyi EK. Physical health and illness in a psychiatric outpatient department population. Can Psychiatric Assoc J. 1972;17:SS109–SS116.

7. Lima BR, Pai S. Concurrent medical and psychiatric disorders among schizophrenic and neurotic outpatients. Community Mental Health J. 1987;23:30–39.

8. Martin RL, Cloninger R, Guze SB, Clayton PJ. Mortality in a follow-up of 500 psychiatric outpatients, I. total mortality, and II. cause-specific mortality. Arch Gen Psychiatry. 1985;42:47–54; 58–66.

9. Talbott J, Linn L. Reactions of schizophrenics to life-threatening disease. Psychiatr Q. 1978;50:218–227.

HOPELESSNESS

DEFINITION AND DESCRIPTION

Hopelessness is a state in which individuals see limited or no desirable alternatives or personal choices available, and they are unable to mobilize energy on their own behalf.

THEORY AND RESEARCH

Hope can be conceptualized as having two spheres: generalized and particularized.[8] *Generalized hope* is broad in scope and not attached to a particular object. *Particularized hope* identifies and asserts what a hopeful person perceives as most important to have occur. Particularized hope may be concrete or intangible; it may be stated in definite or implied terms. Particularized hope is a hope for something valued to be attained or expanded, for an event to occur; generalized hope is to just have a hopeful attitude. Generalized and particularized hope can be structured according to six dimensions: the *affective* dimension, feelings of confidence or uncertainty about the outcome; the *cognitive* dimension, the process of wishing, imagining, wondering, perceiving, thinking, remembering, learning, generalizing, interpreting, and judging; the *behavioral* dimension, the action orientation of the individual; the *affiliative* dimension, the sense of relatedness; the *temporal* dimension, the experience of past, present, and future time; and the *contextual* dimension, life situations that surround the hopeless person.

Hopelessness has been clearly linked to suicide potential.[1,2] When hopelessness is defined as negative expectations, it is a "stronger indication of suicidal intent than is depression itself" (reference 2, p 1148). Clients with chronic schizophrenia are more likely to commit suicide when hopelessness develops with depression. The bleakness of a future living with a chronic mental illness can lead to expressions of hopelessness.[7]

RELATED FACTORS

There are many conditions associated with chronic or terminal illness that lead to hopelessness. These conditions are prolonged activity restrictions and attendant isolation; a failing or deteriorating physiologic condition; prolonged pain, discomfort, and weakness; impaired functional ability; prolonged treatments; prolonged diagnostic studies that yield no results; dependence on equipment for monitoring or life support for prolonged periods; new and unexpected signs or symptoms of previous disease process; repeated hospitalizations; and transfer to a different ward or hospital leading to the perception of finality.[9,13] Additional conditions that can result in hopelessness are long-term stress, isolation, abandonment, and a lost belief in transcendent values or God. Hopelessness may co-occur with powerlessness or depression and a lessened will to live.[9,12,13] Hopelessness may develop when dread of impending death, loss of friends or family through death or estrangement, failure of ambitions for the future, or stigma associated with illness are experienced.

DEFINING CHARACTERISTICS

Five observable behaviors are associated with the presence of hopelessness: (1) inability to reach a desired goal as defined by the individual; (2) negative future expectations in that the individual believes that the future has nothing good or positive to give; (3) perceived loss of control such that the individual feels helpless to influence future outcomes; (4) passivity by which the individual accepts the futility of planning to meet goals; (5) emotional negativism in which the individual expresses emotional responses of despair, despondency, or desperation.[6]

Individuals who experience hopelessness give verbal cues of the perception that the situation seems impossible with no solutions. Expressions of feelings of emptiness, pessimism, and being overwhelmed prevail. Such expressions as, "I might as well give up because nothing I do matters," indicate a state of hopelessness. "I've never been lucky so why should I get a break now"; and "I know I'll never get what I want so why try"; or "It's all too much for me to think about," would also be indications of hopelessness in the client.[13]

The hopeless client lacks initiative, is passive, demonstrates decreased affect, is apathetic, and does not participate in care planning. Even though the hopeless client does not participate in care, it is usually not actively resisted. Instead the individual may passively and unenthusiastically allow care to be given. The client may passively accompany the nurse to a ward meeting, but is unlikely to participate. There may be shrugging in response to a question. Other indications might be increased sleep, decreased appetite, decreased verbalizations, turning away from the speaker, and decreased response to stimuli. There is a sense of loss or deprivation, lack of interest or ambition, a sense of impossibility, and expressions of helplessness[4,5] (Chart 1).

CHART 1
Hopelessness: Definition, Related Factors, and Defining Characteristics

DEFINITION

Hopelessness is a state in which individuals see limited or no desirable alternatives or personal choices available and are unable to mobilize energy on their own behalf.

RELATED FACTORS

Chronic or terminal illness
Prolonged activity restrictions creating isolation
Failing or deteriorating physiologic condition
Prolonged pain, discomfort, weakness
Impaired functional abilities
Prolonged treatments
Prolonged diagnostic studies that yield no results
Prolonged dependence on equipment
New and unexpected signs or symptoms of previous disease process
Repeated hospitalizations
Transfer to a ward or hospital leading to perception of finality
Long-term stress
Isolation
Abandonment
Lost belief in transcendent values or God
Sense of having little or no power
Lessened will to live
Dread of impending death
Loss of friends or family through death or estrangement
Failure of ambitions for future
Stigma associated with illness

DEFINING CHARACTERISTICS

Expresses inability to reach a desired goal
Negative future expectations
Expresses feelings of loss of control to influence future outcomes
Responses of despair, despondency, or desperation
Verbal cues that situation is perceived as impossible with no solutions
Expresses lessened will to live
Expresses dread of impending death
Expresses feelings of emptiness or pessimism
Expresses feelings of being overwhelmed
Lack of initiative
Passivity
Decreased affect
Decreased appetite
Shrugging in response to other's attempts at communication
Increased sleep
Decreased verbalization
Turning away from speaker
Decreased response to stimuli
Lack of interest or ambition
Expressions of helplessness

NURSING PROCESS AND RATIONALE

Assessment

The nursing assessment consists of listening to and observing the client. The nurse listens for themes of hopelessness, pessimism, emptiness, and being overwhelmed. The nurse observes for behaviors indicative of hopelessness such as passivity and unresponsiveness.[10] Some cues are muted or subliminal. Thus, an awareness of the nurse's own feelings of hopelessness when interacting with a client may be an indication of the client's hopelessness and should alert the nurse to assess the client for hopelessness.

Beck's Hopelessness Scale[3] is a set of 20 statements that are marked true or false by the client. One statement, for example, is "I just don't get the breaks, and there's no reason to believe I will in the future" (reference 3, p 862). With a diagnosis of hopelessness, there is the need to assess further for suicide potential.

Nursing Diagnosis

Examples of specific nursing diagnoses of hopelessness that can be formulated include: hopelessness related to prolonged activity restriction; hopelessness related to failing vision; and hopelessness related to inability to return to living with family of origin.

Client Goals and Nursing Interventions

To increase the client's participation in the plan of care, the nurse sets expectations consonant with the client's abilities. Facilitation of the expression of the client's wants and choices promotes a sense of options and control the client no longer sees. The client is encouraged to gradually increase the number of decisions made each day. Positive feedback is given when the client participates or shows improvement in appearance.[11,13]

The nurse plans to increase the client's optimism about the present by focusing on the moment and what is possible. Statements made by the nurse express realistic hope for the client. It is important that nurses do not deny what the client is experiencing or ignore areas that are problematic (e.g., pain, stigma, isolation); rather, clients are helped to reframe their situation in positive terms. If appropriate, negative statements can be identified and then realistic positive statements substituted. The nurse helps the client distinguish between the possible and the impossible so that the client does not waste time on what cannot be achieved. Strengths of the client are emphasized, not weaknesses. The nurse helps the client to set workable daily goals and to monitor specific responses for signs of progress.

By informing the client what to expect and what not to expect, optimism is promoted.[13]

To increase the client's positive expectations of the future, the nurse directs the client's thinking to problems that can be resolved and assists in the development of feasible goals for the next few days or weeks. Statements by the nurse, such as, "In a few days you will be sitting in the chair," and "I'll see you tomorrow," direct the client toward the future.

The family or other significant persons can be supportive. The family needs to know the client goals. By discussing the client's plans, the family can join in realistic support for the client. Also encouraging the family to express love and need for the client with words and actions promotes client well-being. The nurse can demonstrate touch and closeness as acceptable behaviors for client care.[13]

Evaluation

Outcome criteria used to evaluate the effectiveness of the nursing interventions for hopelessness include the following: (1) The client begins to participate in care planning and implementation; (2) the client expresses interest in the happenings of the moment or the day; (3) the client is able to plan for the future; and (4) family members are able to participate in a positive manner with touch and words expressing their need for the client (Chart 2).

CASE STUDY

Jenny T was admitted to the intensive care unit with recurring fevers. She had been experiencing symptoms of pain and fatigue for four years and had not been able to work for eight months. "I'll never get better," and "What's the use" were frequent comments. The medical diagnosis on admission was fever of unknown origin. Among the nursing diagnoses identified was hopelessness related to prolonged undiagnosed illness and multiple diagnostic procedures.

When assessing resources, the nurse determined that Jenny had a supportive husband and son and that former coworkers were still interested in her as a friend and coworker. Jenny was too fatigued to have visitors, but the nurse mentioned the names of family members and friends while giving care. "Jim phoned, he hopes you are better today, he sends his love." "Mary called, she is interested in visiting you soon. She said you were an important member of her staff."

Jenny had difficulty recognizing improvements day after day. The nurse spoke gently to Jenny, "You may not be able to tell any improvement today, but I can tell that your fever is less." And another time she said, "You sat up for five minutes this morning and seven minutes this time. Next time will be a little longer."

With antibiotics and reassuring care, Jenny gradually improved enough to be transferred from intensive care. Jenny began phoning family and friends and started taking an interest in her son's activities. She was discharged with a diagnosis of systemic lupus erythematosus. Jenny was able to make plans to rest at home while keeping in contact with her work situation. Jenny would state, "I know I am not going to get better for a while, it takes time for the medications to work."

CHART 2
Hopelessness: Summary of the Nursing Process

NURSING INTERVENTIONS	OUTCOME CRITERIA
CLIENT GOAL: PARTICIPATE IN PLAN OF CARE	
Respect client as a competent person	Makes suggestions
Facilitate expression of choices	Participates in care
Gradually increase number of decisions made each day	
Compliment on increased participation or improved appearance	
CLIENT GOAL: EVIDENCE OPTIMISM ABOUT THE PRESENT	
Assist the client to look at the moment	Expresses interest in the moment
Express hope for the client	
Assist with positive statements	
Emphasize strengths not weakness without denying reality of the situation or the client's feelings	
Work toward realistic daily goals	
Teach the client to monitor specific symptoms for signs of progress	
Inform what to expect and what not to expect	
CLIENT GOAL: DEVELOP POSITIVE EXPECTATIONS OF THE FUTURE	
Direct thinking to problems that can be resolved	Expresses plans for the foreseeable future
Develop realistic goals for the next few days	
FAMILY GOAL: GIVE SUPPORT TO CLIENT	
Discuss the client goals with family	Family interacts with client in supportive manner
Encourage family to express need for the client	
Model supportive interactions with acceptable behaviors	

Research Highlights

Beck and associates investigated whether hopelessness, depression, and suicidal ideation would predict eventual suicide in patients who were hospitalized with suicidal ideation.[3] The sample included 207 subjects, admitted to a psychiatric inpatient ward and considered suicidal, but who had not made a recent suicide attempt. Ninety-six of the subjects were male and 111 were female; the ages ranged from 17 to 65 years. The Beck Hopelessness Scale was used to assess hopelessness. The subjects were also assessed for depression and suicidal ideation. The subjects were followed for five years after admission, or until the time of their deaths. Of the 207 subjects, 34 died from all causes. Fourteen of the 34 were judged to have committed suicide. The Hopelessness Scale was significantly related to eventual suicide. A cutoff of 9 on the Hopelessness Scale was found to clearly separate the suicidal noncompleters from the completers. Only one of the suicide completers had obtained a score of 9 or less whereas 13 had a score of 10 or more. For the noncompleters, 76 had a score of more than 9 and 78 had a score of less than 9.

The results support the idea that presence of hopelessness increases the probability of future suicide among clients who are thinking of suicide. The severity of depression did not significantly differentiate between those with suicidal ideation who committed suicide and those who did not.

Hopelessness is a state in which individuals see limited or no desirable alternatives or personal choices available and are unable to mobilize energy on their own behalf. Behaviors associated with hopelessness include (1) the inability to reach a desired goal as defined by the individual, (2) negative future expectations, (3) a perceived loss of control with resultant feelings of helplessness, (4) passivity and acceptance of futility of planning to meet goals, (5) emotional negativism. The nurse seeks to help the client find some realistic areas for control, for quality of life, and satisfaction within the reality of the client's situation.

References

1. Beck AT, Steer RA, Kovacs M, et al. Hopelessness and eventual suicide: a 10-year prospective study of patients hospitalized with suicidal ideation. Am J Psychiatry. 1985;142:559–563.
2. Beck AT, Kovacs M, Weissman A. Hopelessness and suicidal behavior: an overview. JAMA. 1975;234:1146–1149.
3. Beck AT, Weissman A, Lester D, et al. The measurement of pessimism: the hopelessness scale. J Consult Clin Psychol. 1974;42:861–865.
4. Beyea SC, Peters DD. Hopelessness and its defining characteristics. In: McLane AM, ed. Classification of nursing diagnoses: proceedings of the seventh conference. St Louis: CV Mosby; 1987.
5. Bruss CR. Nursing diagnosis of hopelessness. J Psychosoc Nurs Ment Health Serv. 1988;26:28–31.
6. Campbell L. Hopelessness: a concept analysis. J Psychosoc Nurs Ment Health Serv. 1987;25:18–22.
7. Drake RE, Cotton PG. Depression, hopelessness and suicide in chronic schizophrenia. Br J Psychiatry. 1986;148:554–558.
8. Dufault SP, Martocchio BC. Hope: its spheres and dimensions. Nurs Clin North Am. 1985;20:379–391.
9. McLane AM, ed. Classification of nursing diagnoses: proceedings of the seventh conference. St Louis: CV Mosby; 1987.
10. Miller JF. Inspiring hope. Am J Nurs. 1985;85:22–25.
11. Schneider JM. Hopelessness and helplessness. J Psychosoc Nurs Ment Health Serv. 1980;19:12–21.
12. Smith DY. Guided imagination as an intervention in hopelessness. J Psychosoc Nurs Ment Health Serv. 1982;20:29–32.
13. Weber JR. Hopelessness. In: Carpenito LJ, ed. Nursing diagnosis: application to clinical practice. 2nd ed. Philadelphia: JB Lippincott; 1987.

IMPULSE CONTROL, ALTERED

Deanah I. Alexander

DEFINITION AND DESCRIPTION

Altered impulse control is a mode of interacting manifested by acts performed with little or no regard for their consequences.[8] Frequently, an action is taken impulsively to gratify an immediate desire of the individual. Such action is self-satisfying but may also be destructive to the person or others. Impulsive acts are a temporary release and so require repetition for short-term relief of uncomfortable emotions.

Impulse control disorders are often confused with compulsion disorders, such as obsessive compulsive disorder. In impulse control disorders, a building of tension occurs before the impulsive action, and there is an element of gratification *during* the action that is not found in a compulsion.[4] In both compulsive and impulsive behavior, guilt, anxiety, and remorse may follow the release behavior.

THEORY AND RESEARCH

The origins of altered impulse control can be reviewed by looking at psychoanalytic, psychosocial, and biologic explanations. According to psychoanalytic theory, emotional maturation results in learning to tolerate frustration and to delay gratification or to find alternatives.[2] Poor impulse control or gratification of a desire of the moment is seen as an ego dysfunction because of the lack of control or the socially unacceptable release of the impulse. The psychosocial theory of impulse control stresses early life events that influence a person's ability to delay gratification and to find appropriate releases.[5] The biologic explanations of altered impulse control have correlated brain lesions with persistent violence, linked certain hormones with aggressive behavior, and linked temporal epilepsy with violent behavior.[7,11] A possible connection between poor impulse control and a deficiency in the serotonin system has been investigated.[7] Hypoglycemia has also been identified as a concomitant of altered impulse control.[7]

RELATED FACTORS

Descriptions of altered impulse control have focused on spontaneous and explosive patterns, but altered impulse control is also related to behaviors such as promiscuity. The occurrence of altered impulse control is most frequently documented in impulse control disorders; e.g., intermittent explosive disorder, kleptomania, pathological gambling, pyromania, and trichotillomania (pulling out of one's own hair). Altered impulse control also occurs in personality disorders, obsessive compulsive disorder, psychoactive substance use disorders, and eating disorders. Paraphilias are also considered alterations of impulse control because of the recurrent sexual urge.[1,3,7,11]

It has been suggested that a multi-impulsive personality disorder exists in which there are overlapping types of impulsive behaviors, such as concurrent alcohol abuse and opiate addiction.[7] The eating disorders of bulimia nervosa and anorexia nervosa may be associated with alcohol abuse or addiction, and clients may recall similar feelings of being out of control.

Uncontrolled outbursts of rage are a manifestation of altered impulse control sometimes correlated with epilepsy.[9] One study found that 94% of clients with uncontrolled rage outburst had evidence of brain dysfunction.[9] Other physiological disturbances related to altered impulse control are head injury, mental retardation, and delirium.[11]

Exposure to family violence and dysfunctional relationships may lead to the development of altered impulse control. Clients with such backgrounds have a higher incidence of dysfunctional coping in many areas of their lives.[5] The client's ego strength is also related to the formation of altered impulse control. If the ego functions are blurred, the client will have a more difficult time tolerating frustration and anxiety.

DEFINING CHARACTERISTICS

The client who has altered impulse control usually has disturbances in several areas of behavior, emotions, and relations with others. The overall picture is of inability to delay gratification and a lack of concern for immediate consequences. The disorder affects the client's interactions with family and possibly with the legal system. Although the client experiences gratification during the impulsive action, it is not unusual for there to be guilt or remorse after the fact. The family interaction may contribute to these feelings if the client has shamed the family, become involved in legal proceedings, or acted against significant others.

The client who has altered impulse control and explosive behavior is likely to have amnesia for all or part of the explosive event, whereas the victim is likely to remember the events in detail. The combination of the amnesia and resulting guilt and embarrassment may lead to denial by the client that there is something wrong. The use of rationalization and projection is common in clients with altered impulse control. Clients who have neurologic deficits or mental retardation may respond blandly after an impulsive event and be quite confused over others' responses to them.

The client who has a diagnosis of a personality disorder, such as borderline personality disorder, will demonstrate impulsive acts that may or may not be explosive. This client may act out aggressively because of boredom or in search of thrills. The action may be directed at self, as with self-mutilation, or at another person or an animal. The impulsiveness may also take the form of law breaking such as shoplifting, robbery, or destroying property.

Other examples of altered impulse control are fire setting and sexual promiscuity. The fire setting may be a retaliation or may be a search for excitement. Sexual promiscuity temporarily reinforces the self-esteem of the person but may also include elements of using or punishing the partner as well as of self-punishment. Often, clients with altered impulse control have self-messages of lack of willpower and low self-esteem.

Thus, clients with altered impulse control differ greatly in the specific behaviors manifested. However, the common features are the difficulties in thinking through consequences and delaying gratification. Impulsive behavior is most likely to occur when frustration or anxiety is experienced and to be accompanied by desire for immediate tension relief regardless of the consequences (Chart 1).

NURSING PROCESS AND RATIONALE

Assessment

Assessment of altered impulse control must begin with determining the patterns of impulsive behavior. The client may be an unreliable historian for a number of reasons, so a client history should be supplemented by information from responsible others or from legal documentation, such as police records. The impulsive client is likely to use rationalization and may also be manipulative, thus requiring skillful interviewing techniques.

Once assessment data have been gathered, it is necessary to determine who is seeking treatment for the behavior. Impulsive behavior often affects others, who seek treatment for the impulsive client. The impulsive client is most amenable to treatment during a crisis, such as the alcoholic client following a binge or a blackout. Pending legal involvement may also prompt treatment, such as a court order requiring treatment as a condition of probation.

Nursing Diagnosis

An example of a specific nursing diagnosis is altered impulse control related to frustration with interper-

---

CHART 1
Altered Impulse Control: Definition, Related Factors, and Defining Characteristics

DEFINITION

Altered impulse control is a mode of interacting manifested by acts performed with little or no regard for the consequences. An act of impulsiveness is often done on the spur of the moment in order to gratify a need of the individual. The action is self-satisfying but may also be destructive to the person or others. The impulsive acts are a temporary release and so require repetition for short-term relief of uncomfortable emotions.

RELATED FACTORS

Impulse control disorders
    Intermittent explosive disorder
    Kleptomania
    Pathological gambling
    Pyromania
Personality disorders
Obsessive compulsive disorder
Psychoactive substance use disorders
Promiscuity
Eating disorders
Paraphilias
Altered serotonin levels
Head injury
Mental retardation
Childhood exposure to dysfunctional family
Poor ego strength
Epilepsy

DEFINING CHARACTERISTICS

Difficulty in problem solving
Difficulty in thinking through consequences
Difficulty in delaying gratification
Low frustration tolerance
Overuse of rationalization and projection
Experiences pleasure during impulsive behavior
Boredom
Poor historian

---

sonal relationships. This diagnosis would be appropriate for a client who has a pattern of responding to frustration in relationships by immediately walking out on others.

Client Goals and Nursing Interventions

Increasing the client's ability to solve problems and to think through consequences can expand the range of behavioral responses. The client who impulsively slams a door or tells someone to "get lost" will benefit from consideration of alternative actions that express emotions but do not infringe on others' rights. It is most effective if assistance with problem solving occurs over a long period of time, because learned responses are the target of change. Accepting clients' angry feelings while stressing the need to change the behaviors occurring in response to the feelings allows the client to retain a positive feeling about self. Teaching assertiveness skills gives the client control in choosing a response to emotions. Client teaching should include the fact that relapses will occur and advice on how to handle them rather than being defeated by them. A diary to record the feelings that precede and accompany impulsive actions may be used to identify false or self-damaging beliefs as well as to identify patterns of behavioral response.[10] Limit setting for behavior is helpful in defining what is appropriate and what is not.

Planning care for the impulsive client requires a consistent treatment format involving the client and significant others. Peer support groups, such as Alcoholics Anonymous and others with a similar base, are useful in treatment and for continuing support. Nursing care should be based on genuine concern and honesty with the client. Education about the behavior helps with insight and is a starting point for raising the self-esteem of these clients.

Nursing care may also include the administration of medications such as lithium, propranolol, or carbamazepine for the control of outbursts of rage and anticonvulsants for those with neurologic imbalance.[9] Disulfiram (Antabuse) may be prescribed in alcohol addiction as a deterrent to drinking. Informed consent and medication teaching concerning the adverse actions, side effects, and actions is imperative with all clients and may help with medication compliance. Medications such as lithium and anticonvulsants usually are given as long-term therapy, and this must be stressed to the client and significant others.

Evaluation

The evaluation focuses on the client's ability to solve problems and delay gratification. The client who is learning techniques of self-control will benefit from a supportive relationship that gives positive feedback for appropriate behavior. Consistency of approach should be reviewed, because the treatment is likely to be long term. Safety concerns should also be evaluated if the client has had behavior that endangered either self or others (Chart 2).

CASE STUDY

A 20-year-old woman, Georgia B, was treated in the outpatient clinic for a complaint of anxiety and impulsive acts. Georgia's entrance into therapy was at the insistence of her boyfriend, who expressed concern at her self-destructive behavior of cutting her arms when "her mood was down." Georgia said she realized that these behaviors were not normal, but she was not overly concerned because she did not feel suicidal and said she cut herself because she didn't know what else to do when she was frustrated. Her injuries had become progressively more severe; the cuts were deeper, requiring sutures, and several became infected. The couple's relationship was described by both as being "worth working on," although her boyfriend admitted being frightened by Georgia's unusual behavior. Her diagnosis was borderline personality disorder. A nursing diagnosis of altered impulse control related to interpersonal anxiety was formulated in treatment planning.

Georgia and her boyfriend were seen individually initially and then as a couple for counseling. The goal of treatment for Georgia was to identify the feelings that preceded her cutting episodes and to deal with these feelings in a more appropriate manner. The goals for Georgia's boyfriend included dealing with his frustration toward Georgia and allowing him to analyze how her behavior affected him. During the individual therapy, Georgia was able to identify her feelings of boredom and her need to control prior to cutting. She was also able to identify the potential serious consequences of her behavior. Her boyfriend realized that he gave secondary gain to her when she had hurt herself. Together, they improved their communication skills, and anxiety was decreased for both persons.

SUMMARY

Altered impulse control is a nursing diagnosis that can be identified in clients with psychiatric disorders such

---

CHART 2
Altered Impulse Control: Summary of the Nursing Process

NURSING INTERVENTIONS	OUTCOME CRITERIA
CLIENT GOAL: INCREASE ABILITY TO SOLVE PROBLEMS AND THINK THROUGH CONSEQUENCES OF BEHAVIOR	
Set limits on inappropriate behavior	Demonstrates increased ability to solve problems
Assist client to consider:	Decrease in impulsive behavior
Situations and emotions that lead to impulsive behavior	
Consequences of impulsive behavior	
Alternative behaviors and their consequences	
Contract with client for appropriate behaviors	
Teach assertiveness skills	
Maintain consistency in interactions with client	

Research Highlights

The value of contracts for changing behaviors has recently been documented in clients with borderline personality disorder who demonstrate impulsive self-destructive and aggressive acts. O'Brien, Caldwell, and Transeau[10] tested a written treatment contract that identified the problem behavior, goal(s), a target date, and the responsibilities of the client and the nurse. The subjects were newly admitted (within 72 hours) and demonstrated impulsivity or unpredictability in at least two areas that were self-damaging. At the conclusion of the study, clients who had functioned under the written treatment contract showed a decrease in self-destructive behaviors. The investigators concluded that the contract and the process of making it helped strengthen communication with the client with borderline personality disorder and helped in making behavioral changes.

as fire setting, chemical abuse, borderline personality disorder, and organic brain disorders. The common defining characteristic of altered impulse control is the lack of regard for consequences. The behavioral pattern must be assessed to determine the most effective nursing intervention(s). Interventions that are useful are assistance in problem solving, contracting, having the client keep a diary of feelings and response, or assertiveness training. The primary goal is for the client to learn to think through consequences and delay gratification, thus controlling behavior that often causes problems for the client.

References

1. American Psychiatric Association. Diagnostic and Statistical Manual of Mental Disorders. 3rd ed, rev. Washington, DC: American Psychiatric Association; 1987.
2. Booth GK. Disorders of Impulse Control. In: HH Goldman (ed): Rev Gen Psychiatry. 2nd ed. Norwalk, Connecticut: Appleton and Lange; 1988.
3. Hamilton JD, Decker N, Rumbaut RD. The manipulative patient. Am J Psychother. 1986;40(2).
4. Hoogduin K. On the diagnosis of obsessive-compulsive disorder. Am J Psychother. 1986;40(1).
5. Kaplan HI, Sadock BJ. eds. Comprehensive Textbook of Psychiatry. 4th ed, Vol 4. Baltimore, MD: Williams & Wilkins; 1985.
6. Kellner R. Personality Disorders. Psychother Psychosom. 1986;46:58–66.
7. Lacy JH, Evans CDH. The impulsivist. Br J Addict. 1986;81:641–649.
8. McFarland GK, Wasli EL. Nursing Diagnosis and Process in Psychiatric Mental Health Nursing. Philadelphia: JB Lippincott; 1986.
9. Mattes JA. Psychopharmacology of temper outbursts. J Nerv Ment Dis. 1986;174(8):464–470.
10. O'Brien P, Caldwell C, Transeau G. Destroyers: Written treatment contracts can help cure self destructive behaviors of the borderline patient. J Psychosoc Nurs. 1985;23(4):19–23.
11. Roy A, Virkkunen M, Guthrie S, Linnoila M. Indices of serotonin and glucose metabolism in violent offenders, arsonists, and alcoholics. Ann NY Acad Sci. 1986;487:202–220.
12. Wishnie HA, Nevis–Oleson J. eds. Working with the Impulsive Person. New York: Plenum Press; 1979.
13. Woodcock JH. A neuropsychiatric approach to impulse disorders. Psychiatr Clin North Am. 1986;9:341–352.

INJURY, POTENTIAL FOR

Leta M. Holder

DEFINITION AND DESCRIPTION

Potential for injury is defined as a state in which an individual is at risk of injury as a result of interaction among human factors (host), energy sources (agents), and physical–sociocultural factors (environment).

THEORY AND RESEARCH

During the past decade there has been an increased emphasis on identifying the factors that precipitate injuries. Thompson classified these factors in three categories: human, energy sources, and physical–sociocultural environment.[18]

Human factors refer to internal variables that are inherent characteristics related specifically to the client. Age, physical or psychological condition, intellectual ability, growth and development, habits, cultural values, and stress are examples of these factors.

Energy sources that can produce injury include agents classified as mechanical–gravitational (vehicle accidents, firearms); radiant (sunburns); thermal (heat exhaustion, burns); chemical (poisons); electrical (electrical shock); and lack of oxidation (drowning, suffocation).

Environmental factors can be subdivided into two major categories, physical and sociocultural. Physical factors include mechanical devices and unsafe conditions such as slippery floors, furniture with sharp edges, inadequate light, matches, smoking in bed, gas leaks, and availability of illicit drugs. Sociocultural factors include lack of safety education, negligence or abuse, lack of supervision, and family crisis situations. These lists are examples and not inclusive of all environmental factors.[18]

RISK FACTORS

Human Factors

Specific human risk factors predisposing the psychiatric client to potential for injury include confusion, disorientation, hallucinations, or delusions. The client's mental status may prevent him or her from adequately assessing the environment. The client may lose the ability to interpret the here and now and require self-protection.

There are numerous ways that psychiatric clients can potentially or actually harm themselves. Self-mutilation, ingestion of toxic substances, and noncompliance with treatment regimens may occur. The client who bangs his head against the wall in response to a hallucination, ingests a poisonous substance because of misinterpretation, or refuses to comply with necessary treatments because of delusional thinking is at risk for injury. Falls that occur because the client has an unsteady gait from medications or because the client is in an agitated state and unable to adequately assess the environment are additional examples.

Researchers have found that falls account for most client injuries.[5] Studies have noted that the client's mental status is a primary risk factor in falls. Swartzbeck and Milligan noted that in 44% of all patient falls, the client's mental status was recorded as being disoriented or confused.[17] In a later study, Swartzbeck reported that over 50% of the patients involved in falls had a problem with mentation. She recommended that clients with problems involving communication, wandering, combative, or otherwise inappropriate behaviors, be considered at high risk for potential of injury.[16]

Other human risk factors include neurologic conditions that affect the client's ability to process information and interpret reality, thereby increasing vulnerability to injury. Diseases recognized as causing impaired thinking and responding include Huntington's disease, Alzheimer's disease, head trauma, Korsakoff's syndrome, and organic mental syndrome. These diseases can also cause problems with mobility, which can lead to falls.

Substance abuse is another area in which the potential for injury is a major consideration. The client who is intoxicated may be unpredictable. In such a condition, the client can exhibit impaired judgment, poor perception, hallucinations, and behavioral changes that include hyperexcitability and aggressive or assaultive behavior. These clients can harm themselves in a number of ways. Automobile accidents, falls, and cigarette burns are most frequently reported.[9,14] Barile notes that clients who are acutely intoxicated represent a physical threat to themselves because of their impulsive behavior and unsteady motor skills.[1]

An additional area of current research is the client's potential for injury related to tardive dyskinesia. Tardive dyskinesia is a neurologic condition that is manifested by involuntary, repetitive movements of the face, extremities, and trunk. It is associated with the use of neuroleptic medications and can be irreversible.

Clients experiencing these symptoms are predisposed to falls. Whall and associates found that 30% of all psychiatric clients experienced tardive dyskinesia.[19] In another study by Munetz and Roth, it was found that many clients have such a strong desire to avoid psychosis that they want to maintain their medication regimen regardless of the possibility that they might develop this side effect.[11] They noticed that although clients are willing to listen to information about tardive dyskinesia, their fear of becoming psychotic and their trust in the clinician's judgment are frequently the deciding factors in whether they will take the prescribed medications.[11] Clients taking neuroleptic medications need to be assessed for signs of tardive dyskinesia, and clients with tardive dyskinesia need to be identified as at risk for injury.

Other side effects produced by various medications have been linked to patient injury, particularly falls. Clients taking either psychotropic, sedative, hypnotic, tranquilizer, or antidepressant drugs can develop orthostatic hypotension secondary to the neuroleptic medication.[3,11] A client who rises quickly from a lying or sitting position can become dizzy and fall. One additional potentially dangerous complication of neuroleptic treatment is the neuroleptic malignant syndrome. Symptoms include muscular rigidity and akinesia followed by hyperthermia. Potential for injury is a major concern because the accompanying muscular rigidity may increase the risk of falls.[10]

Suicide ideation in a depressed client is another example of a human risk factor. Clients with severe depression may harm themselves in an aborted attempt at suicide. Although suicide is one of the leading causes of death in the United States it is estimated that there are eight to ten attempts for every completed suicide.[18]

Other psychiatric clients who should be recognized as at risk for potential for injury are those with borderline personality disorder. These individuals usually present a history of self-mutilation behavior. It is generally agreed that this behavior is either impulsive and in response to tension or is manipulative.[12,15] These clients, on occasion, may attempt suicide, and any threat should be taken seriously. Usually, however, they are more likely to respond to their anxiety with acts of self-mutilation. An example was reported in a case study by Curtis.[2] A client was admitted to a hospital after self-inoculation of contaminated material. During hospitalization this self-mutilation behavior continued as the client deliberately tampered with intravenous lines to prolong the illness.[2]

The violent or aggressive client should also be considered as at risk for injury. This individual may harm himself or other clients in the immediate environment. Also, these clients may be harmed by others as they try to protect themselves.

Psychomotor deficits are frequently identified as factors in accidents. An unsteady balance or gait is a major contributor to falls. If the client stumbles, it is more difficult to reestablish his balance. Also, decreased reaction time can lead to injury because the client is unable to respond quickly to the safety hazard.

Cognitive and emotional difficulties are prime factors to be considered with the psychiatric client. The client may lack the ability or the motivation to prevent accidents. If the client is experiencing a high level of anxiety then he may be unable to focus on anything but his immediate self. Hazardous factors in the environment will be ignored.

Additional internal human risk factors listed by Kim, McFarland, and McLane are as follows: "weakness, poor vision, balancing difficulties, reduced temperature and/or tactile sensation, reduced large or small muscle coordination, reduced hand-eye coordination, . . . cognitive or emotional difficulties, and history of previous trauma."[8] Seizure disorders, hearing impairment, and lack of judgment about safety hazards are additional host factors that can lead to injury.

Energy Factors

Energy sources can also be risk factors and predispose the psychiatric client to injury. Photosensitivity is a common side effect of the phenothiazines.[13] The potential for motor vehicle accidents is increased by the use of psychotropic medication. Poisoning, electrical shock, and drownings are still other sources of possible injury.

Physical Environmental Factors

Selected physical environmental risk factors identified in the environment of psychiatric clients can include slippery floors, unanchored rugs, unlighted rooms, litter or liquid spills on floor or stairways, obstructed passageways, unsupervised bathing, unsupervised cigarette smoking, struggling within bed restraints, and smoking in bed.[8] Changes in the environment, cluttered rooms, and loud noise levels should also be considered as factors that can predispose the client to accidents.

Sociocultural Environmental Factors

Sociocultural environmental factors include lack of safety education, fatalistic attitudes about accidents, neglect or abusive child rearing, lack of resources, and family stress.[18] Lack of family and client motivation is still another factor that should be considered (Chart 1).

NURSING PROCESS AND RATIONALE

Assessment

Direct observation, examination, and client interviews can yield data that will indicate whether or not the psychiatric client is at risk. The nurse needs to consider

CHART 1
Potential for Injury: Definition and Risk Factors

DEFINITION

Potential for injury is a state in which an individual is at risk of injury as a result of interaction among human factors (host), energy sources (agents), and physical–sociocultural factors (environment).

RISK FACTORS
Human Factors (internal)

Adverse reaction to psychotropic medications

SENSORY DEFICITS	PSYCHOMOTOR DEFICITS
Impaired vision	Weakness
Hearing loss	Unsteady gait
Decreased tactile sensation	Poor muscle coordination
Decreased smell sensation	Seizures
Decreased taste	

EMOTIONAL DISORDER	COGNITIVE DEFICITS
Anxiety	Lack of motivation
Confusion	Lack of ability
Disorientation	
Hallucinations	
Delusions	
Depression	
Aggressiveness	

Energy Factors

Overexposure to sun
Driving while intoxicated
Poisoning
Electrical shock

Physical–sociocultural (Environmental Factors)

PHYSICAL

Slippery floors, i.e., rugs, spills, wax
Unlighted rooms
Clutter
Unsupervised bathing and feeding
Loud noise level

SOCIOCULTURAL

Financial problems
Lack of knowledge
Lack of resources
Family stress

injury, the nurse assesses human factors, energy sources, and both the physical and sociocultural environment. That is, the presence of the specific risk factors previously discussed should be assessed in each category. Of particular importance is to assess for unsteady gait, poor eyesight, confusion, physical disabilities, neurologic problems, communication problems, negative attitudes, changes in the environment, unsafe footwear, drugs and alcohol, and a history of previous falls.[5]

Nursing Diagnosis

If a diagnosis of potential for injury is made, the diagnosis must be specific and indicate the specific risk factors present. For example, a client admitted with a medical diagnosis of Alzheimer's disease exhibiting signs and symptoms of unsteady gait, confusion, and disorientation may be given a nursing diagnosis of potential for injury related to unsteady gait, confusion, and disorientation.

Client Goals and Nursing Interventions

Once the nursing diagnosis is made, the nurse then identifies specific goals and objectives focused on providing for the safety of the client. These objectives are patient oriented and are related to the specific risk factors identified. Examples include the following: client will be oriented to time, person, and place; or client will encounter safe environment. The overall goal should be that the client will experience no injury.

The nursing care plan includes nursing interventions aimed at patient and family education. The client needs to be aware of risk factors and should be taught techniques that can reduce the chance of injury. The family can reinforce patient teaching, and family participation helps them feel needed and involved. This can help in preparing the family for the client's return home.

The primary focus is on providing for the safety of the client. Assistance with any activity the client is unable to perform alone is important. Injuries can be decreased by frequent observations of clients identified as being at risk. Assigning these clients in a room close to the nursing station makes observation easier. Informing all staff of the need for observation and providing needed assistance are other important factors. In addition, some hospitals have implemented risk management programs in which clients at risk are identified by a coding system marking patients' armbands, room, bed tags, and chart. This serves as a reminder to all staff that the client needs additional assistance.[3,5,7]

If the client is confined to bed, side rails should be used cautiously because confused and disoriented clients may attempt to climb over the rails and fall. Posey jacket restraint can be considered.

the degree of impairment before diagnosing the client as at risk for injury. Many clients can successfully adapt to their limitations. Several authors suggest that more than one limitation or risk factor should be present before the client is diagnosed as being at risk.[2,3]

When assessing psychiatric clients for potential for

Another area to be addressed is the effect of the medications. Hypnotics, tranquilizers, and psychotropic drugs often produce drowsiness and orthostatic hypotension. Orthostatic hypotension can be controlled by teaching the client to rise slowly from a sitting or lying position. Medication such as laxatives and diuretics can indirectly cause injury if the client, experiencing mobility problems, tries to hurry to the bathroom; therefore, frequent reminders to call for assistance and prompt response may be necessary. Client teaching is a necessity when the client is capable of learning. There are some instances, however, in which the only protection for the client is one-to-one observation. One-to-one observation is usually limited to those situations in which the potential for injury is imminent. The client that is actively suicidal is a prime example of one that must be assigned one-to-one observation.

The second major area to be addressed in the nursing care plan is the client's environment. The environment needs to be as safe as possible and yet aesthetically pleasing and homelike. Loose rugs are avoided and any spills are cleaned up immediately. The lighting is adequate with night-lights left on if the client is prone to wander. If the client is at risk of harming self or others, then seclusion may be indicated. Kendrick and Wilber note that when in seclusion the room should be securely fixed with nonbreakable windows.[7] All furniture is removed and a mattress and flame-retardant blankets provided for the client's comfort. Close observation of this client is important.[7]

Evaluation

A daily assessment of the effectiveness of the nursing interventions for the prevention of injury is critical. Assessment of any changes in the client's condition or environment that warrants revisions in the plan of care is necessary. A review of the objectives to determine if they are being met is an effective method of evaluation (Chart 2).

CHART 2
Summary of the Nursing Process: Potential for Injury

NURSING INTERVENTIONS	OUTCOME CRITERIA
RELATED TO HUMAN FACTORS	
Client Goal: Not Injure Self	
Frequent observations	Injury prevented
Assist with ambulation	
Assist with activities of daily living as needed	
Provide reality orientation as needed	
Provide patient and family education	
RELATED TO ENERGY FACTORS	
Client Goal: Not Injure Self	
Encourage wearing of long-sleeved shirt and hat when exposed to sunlight	Injury prevented
Supervised use of equipment	
Provide reinforcement of safety tips as needed	
RELATED TO PHYSICAL AND SOCIOCULTURAL FACTORS	
Client Goal: Encounter Safe Environment	
Apply jacket restraints as needed	Injury prevented
Remove unnecessary furniture	
Place call light within reach	
Supervise bathing and eating as needed	
Provide family education	
Encourage family attendance in support groups	

CASE STUDY

Mr. B, a 42-year-old man, was admitted with a diagnosis of schizophrenia paranoid type. His social history indicated that he was married and the father of two sons. He had a degree in chemical engineering and was employed at one of the local industries. His psychiatric history revealed that this was his third admission in five years. His last admission was 14 months ago. His wife stated that he had done well until he stopped taking his medication. She noted that he had gradually become suspicious and hostile.

The client's physical appearance was unkempt. He acknowledged that he was hearing voices, and accused other clients of being from the KGB. Such accusations made other clients defensive and angry, feelings that were intensified by the client's agitated behavior, to the point that the other clients threatened to hit him.

Mr. B's nursing care plan included a nursing diagnosis of potential for injury related to alterations in thought process and agitation. A second nursing diagnosis was noncompliance (medications).

Concern was expressed by the nursing staff that he would injure himself, or that another client would injure him in self-defense. It was determined that seclusion and sedation were the only safe alternatives. Care was taken to reassure him that he was safe. Frequent assessments of his physical and emotional status were made, and, within hours, he was able to control his behavior and return to his room.

In the days that followed, careful observation was necessary to be sure that he was ingesting his medication. Once his condition stabilized, he was assigned to a medication group. As he complied with his medication regimen, a steady improvement was noted.

SUMMARY

Risk factors are those elements that can predispose the client to injury. They can be classified as human factors, energy sources, and physical–sociocultural factors. Human factors include internal defects, impaired

Research Highlights

Tardive dyskinesia is a neurologic condition producing involuntary movements caused by long-term neuroleptic drug use. It is considered a major problem because of its prevalence, resistance to treatment, and disabling nature. This condition can predispose the client to injury because of the abnormal movements of the extremities and trunk. Signs and symptoms of tardive dyskinesia include lateral knee movement, foot tapping, heel dropping, foot squirming, inversion and eversion of foot.

There is some controversy concerning the reversibility of tardive dyskinesia.[4,6] Some authorities believe that early detection and discontinuation of the medication may be effective. Whall and associates have reported on a feasibility study focused upon the development of a valid and reliable screening method.[19] The setting for their study was four aftercare homes. Sixty subjects from 26 to 74 years of age were included. The raters were trained in a 12-hour training program in the use of an Abnormal Involuntary Movement Scale tool. Results of the study indicated that this method of screening was reliable. The nurse raters maintained an 80% agreement level with earlier experts that used the tool in a laboratory setting. Thirty percent of the population studied showed symptoms of tardive dyskinesia.[19] This was similar to earlier studies by Jeste and Wyatt who reported an overall prevalence of 26% in clients on long-term treatment with neuroleptics.[6]

sensory input, as well as psychomotor deficits that lead to problems with mobility. Cognitive deficits that decrease ability and motivation are also included. Finally, emotional disorders with accompanying high levels of anxiety and distorted thinking deter the client in assessing his environment for hazards. This may lead to behavior that is injury provoking. Energy sources that are hazardous to the client's safety include overexposure to the sun (photosensitivity), driving while intoxicated, poisoning, and electrical shock. Physical and sociocultural factors refers to those factors found in the environment. Slippery floors, poor lighting, and cluttered rooms and passageways are common examples. Unsupervised bathing and feeding can be hazardous conditions associated with the psychiatric client who is out of contact with reality. Sociocultural factors include lack of financial resources to repair, replace, or purchase needed items. Family stress is another factor, as well as their lack of knowledge due to cultural mores and poverty.

Nursing care for clients at risk should be focused on patient and family education. Families need to be involved so that they may reinforce the teaching and prepare for the client's return home. A major focus for client safety is the environment. In many situations adaptations are necessary to safeguard the client.

References

1. Barile L. The client who is addicted to alcohol. In: Lego S, ed. The American handbook of psychiatric nursing. Philadelphia: JB Lippincott; 1984.
2. Curtis J. When patients harm themselves. Hasting Cent Rep. 1984;14(Apr):22–23.
3. Fife DD, Solomon P, Stanton M. A risk/falls program: code orange for success. Nurse Manage. 1984;15(Nov):50–53.
4. Gardos G, Cole JO. Overview: public health issues in tardive dyskinesia. Am J Psychiatry. 1980;137:776–781.
5. Innes EM, Turman WG. Evaluation of patient falls. QRB. 1983;(Feb):30–35.
6. Jeste DV, Wyatt RJ. Understanding and treating tardive dyskinesia. New York: Guilford Press; 1982.
7. Kendrick DW, Wilber G. Seclusion: organizing safe and effective care. J Psychosoc Nurs. 1986;24(Nov):26–28.
8. Kim MJ, McFarland GK, McLane AM. Pocket guide to nursing diagnoses, 3rd ed. St Louis: CV Mosby; 1989.
9. Lewin-Pitz L. Violence. AD Nurse 1986;18(Sep/Oct):18–25.
10. Masters JC, Spitler R. Neuroleptic malignant syndrome. J Psychosocial Nurs. 1986;24(Sep):11–16.
11. Munetz MR, Roth LH. Informing patients about tardive dyskinesia. Arch Gen Psychiatry. 1985;42:866–871.
12. Silver D. Psychodynamics and psychotherapeutic management of the self-destructive character disorder patient. Psychiatr Clin North Am. 1985;8:2.
13. Skidmore-Roth L. Medication cards for clinical use. Englewood Cliffs, NJ: Prentice–Hall; 1986.
14. Smith MC. The client who is abusing toxic substances other than alcohol. In: Lego S, eds. The American handbook of psychiatric nursing. Philadelphia: JB Lippincott; 1984.
15. Smith MC, Lego S. The client who has a borderline personality disorder. In: Lego S, ed. The American handbook of psychiatric nursing. Philadelphia: JB Lippincott; 1984.
16. Swartzbeck EM. The problem of falls in the elderly. Nurse Manage. 1983;14(Dec):34–38.
17. Swartzbeck EM, Milligan WL. A comparative study of hospital incidents. Nurse Manage. 1982;13(Jan):39–43.
18. Thompson J. Potential for injury. In: Thompson JM, McFarland GK, Hirsch JE, Tucker SM, Bowers AC. Clinical nursing. St Louis: CV Mosby; 1986.
19. Whall AL, Engle V, Edwards A, Bobel L, Haberland C. Development of a screening program for tardive dyskinesia feasibility issues. Nurs Res. 1983;32(May/Jun):151–155.

KNOWLEDGE DEFICIT
(SPECIFY)

Leta M. Holder

DEFINITION AND DESCRIPTION

Knowledge deficit is defined as lack of information or skills that would assist the client in managing a health problem or a potential health problem. The parameters of this diagnosis extend from the organically disabled client to the individual who lacks the needed information for maintaining adequate health care because of the newness of the situation. Therefore, when this diagnosis is used, the specific type of knowledge deficit must be included with the related factor(s) when known, for example: knowledge deficit (medications) related to lack of exposure to information.

THEORY AND RESEARCH

Currently, educational interventions are a common part of mental health services.[2,9,16,18] Before the early 1960s, this was not always true.[7] Redman postulates that the delay in the development of client teaching in psychiatric–mental health nursing was due to the assumption that psychiatric clients would be unable to comprehend or use the information.[9] It is now recognized that in addition to information concerning health care issues, the psychiatric client needs skill training focused on the development of social relationships and coping strategies.[7,16,17]

There is also an increased emphasis on family involvement. Research supports the inclusion of families in the plan of care, so that both the family and client can work together to implement short- and long-term goals. A recent study by Johnson noted that families are asking mental health professionals for help.[2] Support groups offering information about specific diagnoses and family coping strategies have proved effective.[2,16]

Another method of family involvement was addressed in a study by Williams and associates.[18] Families with children admitted to an inpatient unit were expected to participate in a family program focused on stress management and behavior management. The family members were asked to come to the inpatient unit to observe and work with their child under the supervision of the staff. Two-thirds of the families surveyed noted their satisfaction with this program.[18]

RELATED FACTORS

Numerous factors impinge on the psychiatric client's knowledge base, and each must be considered. Physical disorders causing knowledge deficits are those disorders that impair cognitive abilities. Cognitive functioning can become impaired at any age. Wacht noted that 15% of all newborns are at risk for mental disability because of prenatal or birth injury.[15] Whitman and associates note that 10% of all infants born to adolescent mothers will demonstrate developmental delays.[17] They estimate that this is approximately three times higher than for the population as a whole. In addition, there are congenital defects that cause mental impairment. Down's syndrome and hydrocephalus are two primary examples. Brain damage resulting from trauma, infections, or neoplasms also produces cognitive disabilities. Several other causative factors of intellectual impairment are generally associated with middle- to old-age. These include degenerative disorders, such as Alzheimer's disease, Parkinson's disease, and multiple sclerosis.

The more complex the learning task, the greater the limitation cognitive disability places on the client. Cognitive processes that may be affected include interest, attention span, perception, abstraction, and generalization. Consequently, the learning styles of these clients usually are on a lower level than their chronological age would indicate.

Sociocultural factors that influence knowledge deficit are many. A primary example is lack of exposure. This can be due to not having opportunities because of economic hardship, cultural mores, or simply not having experiences of a similar nature. Neglect is another factor. It is estimated that 2% of all children are subject to neglect in their lifetime.[3] Neglect can lead to social deprivation, which, in turn, leads to developmental deficits and cognitive delays.[19] Inner-city children have been identified as a high-risk population for deficits in health-care information because of poverty, powerlessness, and deprivation.[4] In addition, cultural beliefs that do not place a high value on Western medical care, customs that limit cross-ethnic involvement, and language barriers can restrict an individual's exposure to health-care information. The drastically reduced length of hospital stay is implicated in clients' and their families' increased need for information. Clients are going home with greater health-care needs than ever before. The client and family are expected to adhere to complicated medical regimens for which they often have no past knowledge base on which to build.[10]

Emotional disorders that are manifested by hallucinations, delusions, confusion, disorientation, depression, mania, or anxiety predispose the client to knowledge deficit. The client who is not thinking clearly has difficulty processing information. Clients who exhibit delusional thinking may intertwine their delusions with the information being given. An example is the client with paranoid schizophrenia who believes that the staff is trying to teach him to harm himself with medications. Clients who are confused and disoriented have limited recall, and the client exhibiting signs of mania has a short attention span. The client with depression has retarded psychomotor and cognitive response. Finally, the client with a high level of anxiety has either a narrowed or scattered attention focus. Carey notes that if the client is not motivated to learn and change behavior, then no amount of client teaching will be effective.[1] Lack of motivation is not uncommon in the psychiatric population.

DEFINING CHARACTERISTICS

Behaviors that indicate knowledge deficit are numerous. Clients who do not adhere to medical regimens, who exhibit inappropriate or exaggerated behaviors, or who use elaborate defense mechanisms, all may be exhibiting knowledge deficit. It is not unusual for a client to use these mechanisms to protect self-esteem. Another behavior that may indicate knowledge deficit is the client's inability to demonstrate a procedure or perform a health-care skill, even though the content has been taught.

The client may not possess the information needed to comply with the prescribed medical regimen. If the client lacks relevant skills, then acting-out inappropriately or using exaggerated coping mechanisms is common. Denial, withdrawal, rationalization, or projection are among the defense mechanisms frequently used to avoid acknowledgment of a learning need.

Other indications of knowledge deficit are statements and questions asked by the client. The client may verbalize a need for knowledge, request more information, or show that there is a problem by verbalizing incorrect information. An adequate assessment of all communication is necessary to identify statements and questions that indicated a knowledge deficit (Chart 1).

NURSING PROCESS AND RATIONALE

Assessment

Rankin and Duffy have identified four areas that must be assessed:[8] information needed by the client and family, attitudes, skills, and factors in the client's environment that may pose barriers to the performance of the desired behavior. Stanton adds to this list the need to consider the learning state and readiness of the clients.[12] She notes that personal characteristics, prior experiences, sociocultural group, religious group, prev-

---

CHART 1
Knowledge Deficit: Definition, Related Factors, and Defining Characteristics

DEFINITION

Knowledge deficit is lack of information or skills that would assist the client in managing a health problem or potential health problem.

RELATED FACTORS

Intoxication
Genetic disorders
Degenerative disorders
Disorders that interfere with cognition
Developmental stage
Impaired intellectual capacity
Low attention span
Lack of readiness to learn
Mental disorders
Poor self-concept
Poor motivation
Lack of exposure to information
Cultural mores
Sensory deprivation
Unfamiliarity with information
Suspiciousness
Emotional state (e.g., level of anxiety)

DEFINING CHARACTERISTICS

Verbalization of lack of information
Request for information
Inaccurate follow-through of instructions
Inappropriate or exaggerated health behavior
Statements of misconception
Inadequate performance of skills
Exaggerated use of defense mechanisms

---

alent life needs, stage of illness, intellectual capacity, and developmental stages are also factors to be assessed. When dealing with a psychiatric client, mental status, communication level, attention span, perception, and the ability to think abstractly need to be considered. Next, the client's level of anxiety and readiness to learn is determined. Learning can take place when the client is experiencing mild levels of anxiety, but learning does not occur when the client's level of anxiety is at a severe or extreme panic stage.

Nursing Diagnosis

After the pertinent data have been collected, categorized, and sorted, decisions can be made about educational needs. These educational needs are based on identifiable problems and can be formulated as a nursing diagnosis. An example might be: knowledge deficit related to lack of exposure to information about the psychobiology and treatment of depression.

Client Goals and Nursing Interventions

Identification of client goals is the next step in the process. The client, family, and the treatment team need to work together to develop these goals. If all have a clear understanding of what is expected, learning will be easier to achieve. Once these goals are delineated, the nurse and client can set priorities. It is not unusual for clients to have multiple learning needs; yet all of these needs cannot be addressed simultaneously. The client should be an active participant in deciding which is the most important. Once the priorities have been identified, the nurse is ready to consider content and what information is needed by the client. Generally, clients need information that will assist them in making realistic choices, as well as information that teaches new skills, coping mechanisms, and specifics about the mental disorder and treatment regimen.[11]

Libraries (hospital or local colleges) contain a wealth of available resources, including textbooks, nursing journals, and other documents. There are a number of agencies that will provide teaching pamphlets (Box 13-6). Care must be taken, however, in using prepared teaching pamphlets. Researchers have noted that most pamphlets are developed for a higher reading level than the average for the population.[13,14]

Once the content has been identified, the next step is to determine teaching strategies. The learning needs

---

BOX 13-6
Sources for Client Education Information

PROFESSIONAL ORGANIZATIONS

American Association of Sex Educators, Counselors, and Therapists
Suite 304
5010 Wisconsin Avenue, N.W.
D.C. 20016

American Nurses Association, Inc.
2420 Pershing Rd.
Kansas City, Missouri 64108

American Psychiatric Association
1700 18th Street, N.W.
Washington, D.C. 20009

American Hospital Association
840 North Lake Shore Drive
Chicago, Illinois 60611

National Council on Aging Washington
1828 L Street, N.W.
Suite 504
Washington, D.C. 20036

VOLUNTARY AND NONPROFIT ORGANIZATIONS

Al-Anon (Family Group Headquarters, Inc)
200 Park Avenue South
Room 1602
New York, New York 10003

American Council on Alcohol Problems
119 Constitution Avenue, N.E.
Washington, D.C. 20002

Council of Guilds for Infant Survival
1629 K Street, N.W.
Washington, D.C. 20006

Mental Health Materials Center
419 Park Avenue South
New York, New York 10016

National Association for Retarded Citizens
2709 Avenue East
Arlington, Texas 76011

The Public Television Library
475 L'Enfant Plaza, S.W.
Washington, D.C. 20024

Alcoholics Anonymous World Services, Inc.
468 Park Avenue South
New York, New York 10017

Child Study Association of America
9 East 89th Street
New York, New York 10028

Epilepsy Foundation of America
1828 L Street, N.W.
Washington, D.C. 20036

National Association for Mental Health
1800 North Kent Street
Arlington, Virginia 22209

National Council on Alcoholism
733 3rd Avenue
New York, New York 10017

Sex Information and Education Council of United States
84 5th Avenue, Suite 407
Hempsted, New York 10011

GOVERNMENTAL SOURCES

National Clearinghouse for Alcohol Information
P.O. Box 2345
Rockville, Maryland 20857

National Clearinghouse for Mental Health Information
22400 Rockville Pike
Rockville, Maryland 20857

National Clearinghouse for Drug Abuse Information
5600 Fishers Lane
Room 10A-J3
Rockville, Maryland 20857

OTHER

Family Communications, Inc
4802 5th Avenue
Pittsburgh, Pennsylvania 15213

United States Pharmacopeial Convention, Inc.
Publication Department
12601 Twinbrook Parkway
Rockville, Maryland 20852

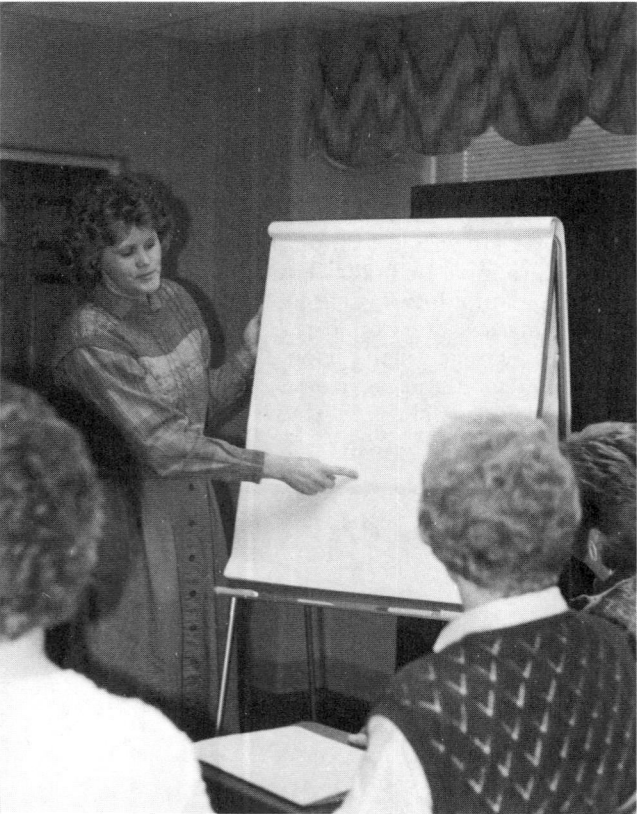

FIGURE 13–17. Client-teaching sessions are an essential nursing intervention.

and learning style of the client must be coordinated with appropriate teaching strategies and available resources. It is generally accepted that learning takes place within three major domains: cognitive, affective, and psychomotor. The approach taken by the nurse, the selection of teaching strategies, and the method of evaluation are influenced by the category of learning involved.

After the teaching plan has been developed, the next step is implementation. First a climate is created that is conducive to learning. This means that the psychiatric client should be both physically comfortable and emotionally ready to begin. The session should be conducted in an environment that is free from noise and distractions. In some instances, privacy may be needed. The atmosphere needs to be one of trust, and the client is encouraged to interact and ask questions. Timing is particularly crucial in informal or spontaneous teaching situations. When the client or family asks for information, these opportunities should be capitalized upon. If the nurse cannot stop and give an impromptu teaching session, then the groundwork for a later session should be laid.[8,9,11] A statement such as, "Let's talk about this when you finish group," will show the nurse's interest and concern (Fig. 13-17).

The nurse strives to actively involve the client once the teaching session has begun. Client teaching is not doing something *to* a client, but working *with* a client.

One mechanism for involving the client is to elicit feedback throughout the session. Plewes advises that feedback be given immediately at the comprehension level of the learner and that praise be incorporated.[6]

Evaluation

No teaching project is complete until an evaluation has been conducted. If the client-teaching process has not been successful, then revisions can be made. When working with any client, the nurse understands that learning of information may not be sufficient to motivate the individual to make behavioral changes. This is particularly true when working with a psychiatric client. The stress level may be too high to permit follow-through with the learned activity, or the attention span and communication level may be so impeded that it is a deterrent to transferring the knowledge to practice. This is not an indication, however, that the client or nurse has failed. It is simply an indication that the teaching may need to be revised. Rorden has identified seven steps in teaching and includes evaluation.[11] They are as follows:

1. Confirm knowledge base and motivation
2. Get the learner's attention
3. Clarify objectives
4. Present content of lesson and get feedback
5. Provide an example
6. Reinforce learning
7. Summarize and evaluate learning[11] (Chart 2).

CASE STUDY

Mrs. Angela M, a 48-year-old Italian woman, was hospitalized with a psychiatric diagnosis of bipolar disorder, depressed type. This was the fifth admission in a ten-year span. On admission, the client exhibited sad affect, psychomotor retardation, decreased energy, poor appetite, sleep disturbance, and difficulty in concentrating. When interviewed, the client verbalized feelings of worthlessness and suicide ideation. Over the years, several antidepressant medications had been used by the client, but with minimal results. Before this admission, the client had been taking doxepin, one of the tricyclics. After a review of her history, the physician prescribed phenelzine, a monoamine oxidase (MAO) inhibitor.

A total of three nursing diagnoses were used to structure this client's nursing care: suicide potential related to depression; self-care deficit related to psychomotor retardation, decreased energy, and difficulty in concentrating; and knowledge deficit (medications) related to lack of exposure to information. Therefore, precautions were initiated and maintained until the staff was able to determine that the client was no longer actively suicidal. The client was encouraged to perform self-care activities, but assistance was necessary during the first ten days. As the client's personal hygiene improved, there was a marked increase in her self-esteem. As the client improved she was involved in a one-to-one medication teaching session and later she was assigned to group medication classes. The focus of these classes was on self-medication administration, medication

---

CHART 2
Knowledge Deficit: Summary of the Nursing Process*

NURSING INTERVENTION	OUTCOME CRITERIA
CLIENT GOAL: INCREASE KNOWLEDGE ABOUT MAO INHIBITORS Encourage attendance in medication group Reinforce information on drug action, timing of expected effects, and adverse reactions	Verbalizes correct information about MAO inhibitors Reports symptoms if adverse reactions experienced
CLIENT GOAL: SELF-ADMINISTER MEDICATIONS Give instructions on name of drug, dosage and schedule Monitor self-administration of medication	Administers medications accurately
CLIENT GOAL: INCREASE KNOWLEDGE ABOUT DIETARY/MEDICATION RESTRICTIONS Give information on dietary–medication restrictions Provide list of foods and drugs that must be avoided Be sensitive to client's cultural preferences in foods	Lists foods and drugs that must be avoided Adheres to diet and medication restrictions

* The summary is limited to knowledge deficit (medications–MAOs).

Research Highlights

Plum conducted a qualitative study of what factors were helpful and harmful to recovery from a major mental illness by analyzing autobiographic accounts of psychiatric clients.[7] There were 34 articles published in professional journals from 1856 to 1985. Twenty of these articles met the criteria for inclusion in the study. Review of the early articles (1856–1940) indicated a theme of spiritual and metaphysical treatment regimens. Beginning in 1959, the articles began to indicate patient teaching as a major beneficial prescription. The need for staff to provide information and methods for coping with the information were common themes in most accounts. Plum noted that there must be a focus upon skill-training for developing and sustaining social relationships and coping with information and stress relations. The advice to professionals from recent accounts was "establish trust and explain everything."[7] What better source is there for determining the needs of clients than clients themselves?

---

dosage, recognition of adverse reactions, and dietary restrictions. Learning about dietary restrictions was particularly difficult for Angela because she enjoyed preparing large meals of combination foods (e.g., pizza, lasagna, macaroni and cheese, eggplant parmigiana) for her family and friends. Discharge planning was included. The client was prepared to administer and monitor her own medication. An appointment for follow-up through the outpatient clinic of a community health center was made for her before discharge.

SUMMARY

Knowledge deficit (specify) is defined as lack of information or skills that would assist the client in managing a health problem or a potential health problem. Problems causing knowledge deficit can be psychological, physiologic, or social. The nursing care plan for these clients takes into consideration assessment of learning styles as well as learning needs. Client-teaching strategies must be appropriate to the content area as well as the learning styles of the client.

References

1. Carey RL. Compliance and related nursing actions. Nurse Forum. 1984;21:157–161.
2. Johnson SW. Mutual expectations. J Psychosoc Nurs. 1986;24(Oct):35–36.
3. Kauffman CK, Neill MJ, Thomas JN. The abusive parent. In: Johnson SH, ed. Nursing assessment and strategies for the family at risk. Philadelphia: JB Lippincott; 1986.
4. Marchant R. Caring for hospitalized inner-city children. Pediatr Nurs. 1985;2:129–131.
5. Munetz MR, Roth LH. Informing patients about tardive dyskinesia. Arch Gen Psychiatry. 1985;42:866–871.
6. Plewes CRB. Helping nurses become better patient educators. Can Nurse. 1984;10(4):41–42.
7. Plum KC. How patients view recovery: what helps, what hinders. Arch Psychiatr Nurs. 1987;1:285–293.
8. Rankin SH, Duffy KL. Patient education: issues, principles and guidelines. Philadelphia: JB Lippincott; 1983.
9. Redman BK. The process of patient education. 7th ed. St. Louis: CV Mosby; 1988.
10. Roncoli M, Whitney F. The limits of medicine spell opportunities for nursing. Nurs Health Care. 1986;7(Dec):45–49.
11. Rorden JW. Nurses as health teachers. Philadelphia: WB Saunders; 1987.

12. Stanton MP. Teaching patients: some basic lessons for nurse educators. Nurse Manage. 1985;10:59–62.

13. Streiff LD. Can clients understand our instructions? Image. 1986;18(2):48–52.

14. Vivian AS, Robertson EJ. Readability of patient education materials. Clin Ther. 1980;3:129–136.

15. Wacht MA. The mentally disabled child. In: Johnson SH, ed. Nursing the family at risk. Philadelphia: JB Lippincott; 1986:40–56.

16. Walsh J. Psychoeducational program evaluation. J Psychol Nurs. 1987;25(Mar):3.

17. Whitman TL, Barrowski JG, Schellenbach CJ, Nath PC. Predicting and understanding developmental delay of children of adolescent mother: a multidimensional approach. Am J Ment Defic. 1987;92:40–56.

18. Williams PD, Elder JH, Griggs C. The effects of family training and support on child behavior and parent satisfaction. Arch Psychiatr Nurs. 1987;1:89–97.

19. Yeates KO, MacPhee D, Campbell FA, Ramey CT. Maternal IQ and home environment as determinants of early childhood intellectual competency: A developmental analysis. Dev Psychol. 1983;19:731–739.

LONELINESS

Agnes L. Hoffman

DEFINITION AND DESCRIPTION

Loneliness, an affective state important to psychosocial well-being, is a complex problem that knows no limits of class, ethnicity, or age.[1,5] Its complexity is highlighted by such diverse experiences as those portrayed by a poet, a religious hermit, a homeless orphan, a widow, a first-term college student, or a person alienated from society. Loneliness is widespread, unpleasant, and can have life-threatening consequences. It has been linked to alcohol dependence, depression, suicide, physical illness, as well as the strength of social interactions.

Loneliness, when considered from a subjective perspective, has been defined as an emotional state of feeling empty, abandoned, and alone. It is "the unpleasant experience that occurs when a person's network of social relationships is deficient either qualitatively or quantitatively" (reference 11, p 31). Often confused with loneliness are the concepts of aloneness, solitude, and social isolation. Being alone, experiencing solitude, or social isolation is not equivalent to the experience of loneliness. Rather, loneliness results from deficiencies in an individual's social relationships that are experienced as distressing.

THEORY AND RESEARCH

Theoretical approaches vary in how the nature of social deficits experienced by lonely individuals are explained. The cause of the experience may be attributed to the person, the environment, developmental influences, or contemporary occurrences. Five major explanatory viewpoints on loneliness, which are not mutually exclusive, can be delineated. They are psychodynamic, learning, phenomenologic, cognitive, and interactional perspectives.

Psychodynamic Perspective

The psychodynamic formulation of loneliness postulates an inherent, universal human need for intimacy[14] that is present from infancy throughout life[4] and has roots in developmental, interpersonal antecedents.[17] Without intimacy, psychological stability falters and deteriorates and developmental tasks are compromised.

Research findings have demonstrated the critical importance of child–parent relationships and the experience of loneliness.[2,3,6,13] In a manner similar to the infant who sees the mother as part of the self, the lonely person distorts others as part of the self and is unable to view self as separate from the environment. When alone, then, the lonely person feels incomplete. But loneliness is a desperate experience that is unbearable and must be defended against.[9] Underlying the use of defenses to cope with loneliness is despair, which results in a state of detachment. The person counteracts the need for closeness with an urge for independence and detachment from others.[17]

Learning Perspective

Loneliness approached from a learning perspective proposes that affected persons experience insufficient social reinforcement.[18] Social relations are viewed as a special class of reinforcement. The reinforcement history of the person's social relations becomes a standard or criterion for assessing current social relations. For example, a person may experience positive outcomes after confiding in a friend and learn to expect social reinforcement following similar interpersonal involvement. A relocation that results in physical separation from current friendships may then be an antecedent of feelings of loneliness. However, given a positive reinforcement history relative to friendships, the individual would be expected to pursue opportunities to establish new friends and alleviate feelings of loneliness.

Phenomenologic Perspective

A phenomenologic perspective postulates that humans are ultimately alone and that loneliness is an essential condition of existence. The issue for phenomenologists is not how to prevent, avoid, or alleviate loneliness, but how to live with loneliness. Moustakis emphasizes the importance of distinguishing between loneliness anxiety and true loneliness.[7,8] Loneliness anxiety is a system of defense mechanisms that distracts people from dealing with critical life questions and that motivates them continually to seek activity with others. In contrast, true loneliness stems from the reality of being alone and of facing life's ultimate experiences (e.g., birth, death, change, tragedy) alone. From Moustakis' viewpoint, true loneliness can be a creative force, which, albeit painful at times, can be a productive, creative experience.

Cognitive Perspective

Cognitive approaches emphasize an individual's perception and evaluation of social relations. In other words, it is what the person thinks about social relationships that is important. If social relationships are evaluated as unsatisfactory, loneliness results.

In articulating the role of cognition in conceptualizing loneliness, Peplau and colleagues draw on attribution theory.[10] The causes attributed to the experience of loneliness can be of crucial importance in determining explanations of why relationships have failed and what options are available to alleviate suboptimal social relations. It is proposed that the most problematic attributions are those that attribute causes of relevant events to internal, stable, or uncontrollable factors. For example, an individual regards his problem with social relationships as owing to his appearance and shyness, which he believes he cannot change.

Interactionist Perspective

The interactionist viewpoint emphasizes that loneliness is not solely a function of personality factors, nor of situational factors, but it is a product of their combined interactive effects.[15,16] The interplay between situations and personal characteristics as joint determinants of loneliness needs study to predict which people will experience loneliness under what kinds of conditions or situations.

Study of widowed and recently separated individuals led to postulation of loneliness as a "normal" reaction involving two types of loneliness, with different antecedents and affective responses. One, emotional loneliness, results from the absence of a close, intimate attachment, such as a lover or spouse, and is accompanied by affective responses akin to separation anxiety. The second, social loneliness, is a response to the absence of meaningful friendships or a sense of community and is accompanied by experiences of boredom and feelings of being socially marginal.[15,16]

RELATED FACTORS

Loneliness may be experienced as a response to a change in either actual social relations or in the individual's needs or desires for relationships. For example, change may involve ending a close relationship through death or divorce, physical separations from loved ones, or a decreased satisfaction with current relationships. Existential loneliness may occur in relation to major life events, such as the birth of a child.

A variety of personal and situational factors may increase a person's vulnerability to experience social deficits. Personal factors may include developmental experiences that led to difficulty forming intimate relationships. Characteristics such as shyness or introversion may present barriers to initiating or maintaining social relations. Situational factors, such as those surrounding widowhood, may reduce opportunities for interactions with married friends and may require special efforts to establish social relations compatible with single-life status.

Loneliness can occur in a number of psychiatric conditions in which interpersonal relationships are typically disturbed. The conditions include schizophrenia, major depression, delusional disorder, early phase of dementia, and substance use disorders. In addition, loneliness can occur in chronic or terminal illness with treatments such as radiation or isolation, aging with increased risk of illness and decreased mobility, and loss of relationships through death.

DEFINING CHARACTERISTICS

Defining characteristics of loneliness are complicated by the fact that loneliness is not a unitary phenomenon, but a subjective experience, unique to the affected person. Manifestations of loneliness differ in duration and have been categorized as chronic, situational, or transient.[18] *Chronic loneliness* involves long-term deficits in the individual's ability to relate to others effectively. *Situational loneliness* is relatively short-term and results from a major disruption of the person's pattern of social relationships. *Transient loneliness* refers to the occasional feelings of loneliness that most people experience from time to time.

Variations in defining characteristics include specific affective, cognitive, and behavioral manifestations. An investigation of affect associated with loneliness showed four clusters of feelings identified by subjects ($n = 3500$) as loneliness: desperation, depression, impatient boredom (which included anger), and self-deprecation.[12]

Cognitive patterns of loneliness are influenced by expectations and interpretations of social situations. Personal accounts or explanations of events may reveal cognitive distortions and invalid assumptions used to interpret social situations. When loneliness persists over time, individuals tend to blame themselves for their social failures, which may increase the risk of depression and decrease efforts to improve their social relationships. A tendency to focus excessively on self and internal experiences produces vigilant attention. That is, they may be anxious in social settings and oversensitive to minimal social cues, resulting in a "tendency to misinterpret or exaggerate the hostile or affectionate intent of others."[16] Such misinterpretations may result in negative evaluations of other persons and a tendency to devalue new acquaintances.

Behaviors manifesting loneliness include self-preoccupation, avoidance of social interaction, engagement in many solitary activities (e.g., watching television, reading, fantasizing), and may involve use or abuse of alcohol or psychoactive drugs (Chart 1).

CHART 1
Loneliness: Definition, Related Factors, and Defining Characteristics

DEFINITION

Loneliness is an emotional state of feeling empty, abandoned, and alone. It is the "unpleasant experience that occurs when a person's network of social relationships is deficient either qualitatively or quantitatively" (reference 11, p 31).

RELATED FACTORS
Ontologic

Existential situations
Creativity

Personal Characteristics

Introversion–shyness
Cognitive distortions
Social skill deficits

Environmental Influences

Separation or death of a significant person
Constricted social network (e.g., being "homebound")
Relocation
Suboptimal social opportunities
Employment changes

Psychiatric Conditions

Schizophrenia
Depression
Delusional disorder
Substance use disorders
Dementia, early phase

Personal–Environmental Interaction

Chronic or terminal illness or treatments such as radiation or isolation
Aging with an increased risk of illness and decreased mobility and loss of relationships through death

DEFINING CHARACTERISTICS
Affective Patterns

Emptiness
Alienation
Depression
Desperation

Cognitive Patterns

Self-blame
Cognitive distortion
Invalid assumptions
Negative self or other evaluation
Vigilant attention

Behavior Patterns

Identifies self as lonely
Solitary activities
Social withdrawal
Self preoccupation
Substance abuse

NURSING PROCESS AND RATIONALE
Assessment

When a client uses the self-description, "I feel lonely," the unique and intended subjective meaning needs to be determined through systematic questioning. The meaning of loneliness varies and different standards are applied when loneliness is identified. For example, one client may be experiencing shyness or inadequate interpersonal skills to initiate or maintain adequate social contacts, another may feel lonely because of relocation and geographic separation from family and friends.

The foregoing defining characteristics of loneliness point to important areas of assessment for the person who experiences loneliness. These include the client's history of loneliness (i.e., chronic pattern or situational response), affective (e.g., emptiness, sadness, anger), cognitive (e.g., beliefs about the causes of loneliness, cognitive distortions, negativity), and behavioral manifestations (e.g., avoidance of social interaction, solitary activities).

Nursing Diagnosis

Examples of nursing diagnoses of loneliness may include loneliness related to recent death of spouse and reduced social contact with married friends; loneliness related to increased social isolation, illness, and "homebound" status; loneliness related to relocation and geographic separation from friends and relatives.

Client Goals and Nursing Interventions

Depending on the factors related to loneliness for a particular client, goals may include that the client (1) experience reduced problematic cognitions or expectations for interpersonal relationships that are unrealistic or unlikely to be met; (2) experience decreased behaviors that are barriers to satisfying interpersonal relationships; (3) experience increased satisfaction in interpersonal relationships that are available; and (4) be able to live with existential loneliness.

To decrease cognitive barriers to satisfying interpersonal relationships, it is important that the individual experience a nonthreatening relationship with a trusted individual. Such a relationship serves as a corrective experience in learning that interpersonal relationships can be satisfying. It provides the opportunity for discussing the painful feelings of loneliness and for clarifying and examining cognitive distortions and invalid assumptions that the client is making about interpersonal relationships. Reduction of unrealistic expectations for interpersonal relationships is important for the person experiencing a serious mismatch between desires for social contact and social opportunities as, for example, a man in a nursing home who expects his adult daughter who is married and working outside the home to spend every day with him. A client can be assisted in considering whether there are some tasks or some activities that can be enjoyably done alone. For some clients, surrogate relationships with pets, TV personalities, or radio talk show hosts may be helpful.

The client may need assistance in changing behaviors that serve as barriers to satisfying relationships, for example, learning ways to initiate relationships. For the client manifesting particular problems in interpersonal relationships, a group targeted to the particular problem may be appropriate. For example, a client may benefit from a social skills training group, an assertiveness training group, or a group focused on overcoming shyness.

To experience increased satisfaction in the interpersonal relationships that are available, the nurse can assist in identifying individuals within the client's existing social network and enjoyable activities that could be shared with these individuals. The client can also be assisted in discussing ways of extending a social network, such as by participation in a group based on a particular interest. If there are relationships available that the person does not find satisfying, the basis for the dissatisfaction can be examined.

Learning to live with existential loneliness may be a goal for a client. For an individual who has faced aloneness in relation to a major life crisis, talking about the experience with a nurse may be a growth experience.

Evaluation

The criteria by which outcomes can be evaluated include the client's being able to discuss the painful feelings of loneliness, having realistic expectations about available interpersonal relationships, and being able to enjoy activities alone. It would be expected that the client for whom problematic behavior interfered with forming relationships would show a reduction in such behavior. For the client with limited relationships, there would be an expectation of either an increased number of relationships or more interactions with those individuals already in relationship (Chart 2).

CASE STUDY

Mona, age 72, has lived in a low-income retirement home in the Northwest for the past two years. Although her husband's death was four years ago, Mona admits that she still "misses" him and feels his "passing" was untimely and "unfair." She attributes the causes of her present loneliness to her status as a widow, lack of opportunities for male companionship, and boredom with the other residents of the home except for one companion, Dorothy. During the past three weeks Dorothy has been visiting her daughter in California, partly to determine possible relocation there. Mona missed what she described as their "daily walks," trips to the library, and watching "favorite TV programs" together.

Recently Mona has voluntarily shared comments to the home receptionist, such as "What's the use of going on?"; "What's left in life for me?"; "Is Dorothy ever coming

CHART 2
Loneliness: Summary of the Nursing Process

NURSING INTERVENTIONS	OUTCOME CRITERIA
CLIENT GOAL: EXPERIENCE REDUCED PROBLEMATIC COGNITIONS OR UNREALISTIC EXPECTATIONS CONCERNING INTERPERSONAL RELATIONSHIPS	
Provide supportive relationship	Discusses painful feelings of loneliness
Encourage discussion of beliefs and expectations for relationships, situational influences on relationships, and activities that can be done alone	Expectations and cognitions are congruent with personal situation.
	Engages in enjoyable activities alone or with pet
CLIENT GOAL: EXPERIENCE DECREASED BEHAVIORS THAT ARE BARRIERS TO SATISFYING INTERPERSONAL RELATIONSHIPS	
Discuss and role-play new behaviors to substitute for those that are problematic	Examines interaction between self and significant others
Encourage participation in relevant group	Reduction in behaviors that are barriers to satisfying interpersonal relationships
CLIENT GOAL: EXPERIENCE INCREASED SATISFACTION IN INTERPERSONAL RELATIONSHIPS THAT ARE AVAILABLE	
Discuss with client ways of enhancing present social network, extending numbers of relationships, and making relationships more enjoyable	Increases effective use of existing interpersonal network
	Structures time and activities with others
	Extends interpersonal network
	Expresses increased satisfaction with interpersonal relationships
CLIENT GOAL: BE ABLE TO LIVE WITH EXISTENTIAL LONELINESS	
Provide relationship in which client's experience can be discussed	Discusses experience of existential loneliness

Research Highlights

A phenomenologic investigative method was used by Rubenstein and Shaver to study subjective features of loneliness.[12] In the early phases of their research, they listened carefully to individual accounts of the experience of loneliness and analyzed open-ended questionnaires (n = 3500) that addressed feelings associated with loneliness, reasons for, and reactions to, loneliness. Factor analysis of the findings showed feelings to include desperation, depression, impatient boredom, and self-depreciation; reasons for being lonely as alienation, being unattached, being alone, forced isolation, and dislocation; and responses to loneliness as sad passivity (e.g., cry, sleep, do nothing), active solitude (e.g., study or work, read, work on hobby), spending money, and social contact (e.g., visit or call a friend).

From the foregoing findings the texture and complexity of loneliness can be sensed, but its structure and dynamics remain unclear. Because informants were respondents to newspaper announcements, their reports of loneliness may differ from clients in clinical settings.

back?" The new activity director reported that during the past two weeks Mona had seldom been seen out of her room, except at meal times, and had attended none of the group activities sponsored by the home.

Nursing assessment data included Mona's history of loneliness since her husband's death and subsequent movement from her "beloved" birthplace, decreased interest in her daughter's weekly visit or in her grandchildren, "who have a life of their own now," dissatisfaction with other residents and activities at the retirement home. Her current behavior included taking walks by herself "now that Dorothy was gone" and spending her time "in my room mostly, not doing much of anything, not having much energy for things." Her strengths included self-disclosure, positive view of self, a pleasant appearance, and willingness to deal with issues concerning her present life situation.

The nursing diagnosis was loneliness related to widowhood, lack of opportunities for male companionship, boredom with other residents, and recent separation from a close friend. Lack of interaction with other residents and lack of involvement in activities at the retirement home also contributed to Mona's experience of loneliness and social isolation.

Goals for Mona included (1) expansion of social relationships with residents in the retirement home and (2) development of an activity plan for engagement in selected leisure activities. The clinical specialist made plans with Mona to meet on a weekly basis to discuss her concerns, expectations, and activities, and to set goals pertaining to use of time and social interactions with residents and relatives. Mona responded well to weekly sessions which were continued for 12 weeks. Her affect improved, although she still saddens when speaking of her husband and of Dorothy. She has increased her participation in activities and her interaction with two new residents, one of whom shares her daily walks.

SUMMARY

Loneliness is an emotional state of feeling empty, abandoned, and alone. Major explanatory viewpoints on loneliness are psychodynamic, learning, phenomenologic, cognitive, and interactional perspectives. The cause of the experience may be attributed to the person, the environment, developmental influences, or contemporary occurrences. Loneliness may be chronic, situational, or transient, and has affective, cognitive, and behavioral manifestations. When the client uses the self-description of loneliness, the nurse assesses for the client's subjective meaning, identifies factors related to the loneliness, and tailors goals and interventions to the specific client experience of loneliness.

References

1. Butler R. Why survive? Being old in America. New York: Harper & Row; 1975.
2. Bowlby J. Attachment. New York: Basic Books; 1969.
3. Bowlby J. Separation. New York: Basic Books; 1973.
4. Fromm–Reichmann F. Loneliness. Psychiatry. 1959;22:1–15.
5. Gordon S. Lonely in America. New York: Simon & Schuster; 1976.
6. Harlow HF, Harlow M. The affectional systems. In: Shrier B, Harlow H, Stollnitz M, eds. Behavior of non-human primates, vol 2. Orlando, FL: Academic Press; 1945.
7. Moustakas CE. Loneliness. Englewood Cliffs, NJ: Prentice–Hall; 1961.
8. Moustakas CE. Loneliness and love. Englewood Cliffs, NJ: Prentice–Hall; 1972.
9. Peplau HE. Loneliness. Am J Nurs. 1955;55:1476–1481.
10. Peplau LA, Miceli M, Morash B. Loneliness and self-evaluation. In: Peplau LA, Perlman D, eds. Loneliness: a sourcebook of current theory, research, and therapy. New York: John Wiley & Sons; 1982.
11. Perlman D, Peplau LA. Toward a social psychology loneliness. In: Gilmour RG, Duck S, eds. Personal relationships in disorder. London: Academic Press; 1981.
12. Rubenstein C, Shaver P. The experience of loneliness. In: Peplau LA, Perlman D, eds. Loneliness: a sourcebook of theory, research, and therapy. New York: John Wiley & Sons; 1982.
13. Spitz RA. Hospitalism. In: Psychoanalytic study of the child, vol 1. New York: International Universities Press; 1945.
14. Sullivan HS. The interpersonal theory of psychiatry. New York: Norton; 1953.
15. Weiss RS. Issues in the study of loneliness. In: Peplau LA, Perlman D, eds. Loneliness: a sourcebook for theory, research, and therapy. New York: John Wiley & Sons; 1982.
16. Weiss RS. Loneliness: the experience of emotional and social isolation. Cambridge, MA: MIT Press; 1973.
17. Welt SR. The developmental roots of loneliness. Arch Psychiatr Nurs 1987;1:25–32.
18. Young JE. Loneliness, depression, and cognitive therapy: theory and application. In: Peplau LA, Perlman D, eds. Loneliness: a sourcebook of theory, research, and therapy. New York: John Wiley & Sons; 1982.

MANIPULATION

Julie K. Sengstacken

DEFINITION AND DESCRIPTION

Manipulation is a mode of interaction that results in an attempt to control others, without regard for their personal feelings, rights, or goals. The behavior is used to fulfill the individual's desires and needs or to avoid discomfort, change, or growth. Manipulation should be considered a destructive behavioral pattern when it creates difficulties in interpersonal relations or undermines the treatment progress of the client or other clients within the therapeutic milieu.

Manipulation may involve the use of aggressiveness, cleverness, and deception to influence others toward the gratification of unmet needs within the person who is manipulative. The object of manipulation is assumed to be reluctant to contribute such satisfaction and, thus, must be maneuvered in some manner, by the person manipulating, into an activity that satisfies needs. In essence, the purpose of manipulation is to change a frustrating object into a gratifying object or to force the environment into compliance with the desires of the person who is manipulating.[6]

THEORY AND RESEARCH

Using a psychoanalytic model, manipulation can be described as a response to an internal crisis within the person who manipulates and that is resistant to usual coping mechanisms and defenses. When usual methods of coping fail to reduce anxiety, it is thought that the ego grants the id permission to have gratification at the expense of others, and manipulation ensues.[4] Neo-Freudians believe manipulation occurs in response to a person's need to appear flawless so as to obtain love.[5] Because this is an unobtainable goal, manipulation occurs as a means to achieve power over others.

Learning theorists focus on positively and negatively reinforcing experiences that mold behavior.[5] Manipulative efforts that elicit the desired response invite repetition.

Fredrick Perls, the father of gestalt therapy, describes manipulation as a conflict between self-support and environmental support.[5] The person who manipulates, lacking self-trust, believes he should entrust others. However, entrusting others is also difficult, which leads to manipulation. Gestalt theory holds that the behavior is secondary to distrust.

The existential perspective focuses on the risk surrounding individuals in everyday existence and the resulting sense of powerlessness in facing existential situations.[5] Manipulation is believed to be used to gain a sense of control over life or to combat powerlessness.

RELATED FACTORS

Manipulation may be seen in a myriad of psychiatric diagnoses (e.g., psychoactive substance abuse disorders, borderline personality disorder, eating disorders). In these mental disorders, manipulation becomes destructive, interrupting relationships or personal growth and, thus, becomes a nursing concern. Many factors singly, or in combination, may be used to explain manipulation. Investigating the stressors behind the behavior is important in the nursing process, because interventions will be directed toward these related factors.

Learned behavior may be seen as a stressor if the individual uses manipulation to reduce stress to the exclusion of more adaptive coping responses. Ineffective role-modeling for problem-solving skills and processing feelings may limit the behavioral repertoire and, thereby, perpetuate manipulation. When ego dystonic feelings, such as powerlessness, fear, hostility, inadequacy, and anxiety arise, the client may become so overwhelmed that he or she manipulates to gain an increased sense of control over feelings. In effect, the client attempts to control undesirable feelings through the control of others by manipulation.

The environment may also present stressors. Many clients with conflicts related to structure and authority manipulate in an effort to increase personal power. Hospitalization frequently places clients in a submissive, dependent role with little understanding of the treatment program offered. Highly rigid environments, or those with excessive conflict, may result in attempts to bring control by manipulation. An environmental evaluation should always coincide with client assessment for manipulation.

Another area to be addressed is the nurse–client relationship. Clients who manipulate often have difficulty trusting and developing intimate relationships in which feelings, needs, and desires can be discussed. When a nurse is perceived by the client as authoritarian, rigid, aloof, or distant, the client may mistrust, feel inadequate or hostile, which may set into action a manipulative response.

Manipulative behavior is seen in a variety of psychiatric diagnoses, particularly in the following personality disorders: antisocial personality disorder, border-line personality disorder, histrionic personality disorder, narcissistic personality disorder, avoidant personality disorder, and passive–aggressive personality disorder. It may, in fact, present as a dominant feature in these conditions. Psychiatric disorders in which manipulation is also seen are factitious disorder and malingering, as both are characterized by intentionally feigned symptoms.

DEFINING CHARACTERISTICS

Certain behaviors may indicate the presence of manipulation. For example, power struggles, defying authority, demanding or bargaining behavior, threats, and procrastination, all may be defining characteristics of manipulation. Other behavioral cues can include helplessness, tears, frequent requests, and repeated attempts to gain pity or sympathy.

The manipulative individual is often described as ingratiating and oversolicitous. The client may seem self-centered and may use the weaknesses of others against them, thereby alienating others. Often feelings of vulnerability within the nurse are the first clues that the client is manipulating.

Finally, clients who manipulate have a disturbed manner of relating to others in that they fear intimacy. Because they lack trust, empathy, and a sense of relatedness, relationships they form may be short-lived and opportunistic. Frequently, those around them feel as if they have been used. Manipulation may serve to reduce anxiety and, hence, increases the probability of repeated use in future coping. Therefore, it is essential to identify manipulative patterns so that appropriate nursing action can be taken (Chart 1).

NURSING PROCESS AND RATIONALE

Assessment

Manipulative has become a derogatory label, too often applied to the client who presents as uncooperative, hostile, overly dependent, demanding, or otherwise hard to handle.[2] In assessing for manipulation, it is imperative that the nurse avoids labeling as a means to deal with his or her own negative feelings. Where manipulation does exist, the guidelines that follow may be useful in the development of effective nursing assessment.

A first step is self-assessment or the examination of the nurse's own response to a particular behavior. Often, unresolved issues in the health-care provider manifest in responses that may serve to perpetuate manipulative behavior in the client. Consider the nurse with low self-esteem. Attempts by the client to manipulate with flattery may decrease her objectivity and elicit rescuing behavior, particularly if the client suggests that she is "the only one who understands." Likewise, a nurse who fears anger may fail to set appro-

---

CHART 1
Manipulation: Definition, Related Factors, and Defining Characteristics

DEFINITION

Manipulation is a mode of interaction that results in the control of others, without regard for their feelings, rights, or goals. Manipulation is utilized to fulfill desires or needs or to avoid discomfort, change, or personal growth.

RELATED FACTORS

Feelings of fear
Feelings of powerlessness
Feelings of hostility
Developmental factors
Conflict with authority
Inability to tolerate intimacy
Unidentified, unmet social needs
Blocked needs or desires
Problematic nurse–client relationship
Learned behavior
Conflicted milieu
Unmet dependency needs
Feelings of anxiety
Rigid environment
Self-esteem factors

DEFINING CHARACTERISTICS

Lack of empathy toward others
Develops opportunistic relationships
Ability to sway others
Attempts to get special treatment
Lack of relatedness to others
Lack of trust in relationships
Difficulties in accepting controls or limits
Behavior directed toward meeting own needs often violating others' rights
Disturbed communication patterns
Demanding and threatening behavior
Disregarding rules or routines
Ingratiating or oversolicitous
Uses weaknesses against others
Elicits negative feelings in others
Attempts to gain recognition
Bargaining behavior
Tearfulness
Procrastination
Dishonesty
Self-centeredness
Cons others for personal profit
Impersonal use of others
Critical of others
Distorted beliefs
Identity problems
Defies authority
Frequent requests
Helpless behavior
Power struggles
Lacks insight
Exploits others
Lacks regard for the truth
Intimidating others
Flattery
Use of aliases

priate limits or confront a client who manipulates and who has a history of violence. In both cases, the response, or lack of response, by the nurse permits continued manipulation by the client. Clearly, self-awareness on the part of the care provider is an essential element in dealing with manipulation.

In addition to self-assessment, nursing personnel may derive useful information from the feedback of the multidisciplinary treatment team. Team meetings are especially valuable when working with the manipulative client because varying degrees of objectivity represented within the team allows quicker identification of manipulative behavior. In this same setting, support is available for the staff member who serves as the object of manipulation.

Nursing Diagnosis

A nursing diagnosis of manipulation should be considered when the behavior has created difficulty in the client's interpersonal relationships or within the therapeutic milieu. An example of a specific nursing diagnoses is manipulation related to conflict with authority.

CLIENT GOALS AND NURSING INTERVENTIONS

The management of manipulative behavior involves development of a trusting relationship between the client and the nurse. Because those clients who manipulate generally have difficulty with trust, it is important to incorporate specific interventions into the nursing care plan designed to augment the development of trust. These interventions may include a kind, but firm, approach with open honest communication. Allow sufficient time for gradual evolution of the relationship, meeting regularly with the client to discuss what need manipulation is meeting, and to confront the manipulative behavior itself. All staff members should set uniform limits to facilitate consistency and provide models for trust. Often, clients who manipulate deal with feelings of insecurity by attempting to control others, which serves to render the environment more predictable and, thus, more secure. Therapeutic limit-setting increases the level of security by "providing temporary and artificial ego boundaries."[1] The development of trust takes time, and efforts toward this end may be facilitated by a predictable environment and supportive, but firm, staff members.

Another area to be addressed relative to manipulation is the client's coping mechanisms. Maladaptive coping mechanisms must be replaced with healthy ones to help the client deal with stress and anxiety. Assist the client in identifying existing strengths and encourage the use of talents in socially accepted activities. Promote assertive behavior and the use of relaxation techniques as alternatives to manipulation. Other coping strategies, such as communication skills, leisure activities, and seeking support from others, may also be helpful and should be modeled and encouraged by staff. To decrease manipulative behavior, the client must incorporate alternative methods of coping into the repertoire of behaviors.

The use of manipulation is often secondary to feelings of powerlessness, and it is important to identify and address this issue in the nursing care plan. Allow the client to make decisions wherever possible to impart a sense of control over surroundings. One way to deal with powerlessness is by involving the client in his or her own treatment plan. Identification of client expectations for treatment encourages both a sense of responsibility for one's health and a regained sense of autonomy for the patient.

Evaluation

As a final step in the nursing process, ongoing evaluation of treatment must take place. Monitor nursing interventions and treatment progress by asking the following questions:

1. Are consistent limits present?
2. Are all members of the treatment team familiar with the care plan?
3. Are feelings among the staff toward the patient (anger, pity) preventing therapeutic treatment?
4. How are feelings towards the patient coped with?
5. Have the signs and symptoms of manipulation been reduced?

By using this approach the client is outfitted with new tools and alternative behaviors to manipulation, thereby improving the prognosis (Chart 2).

CASE STUDY

A 14-year-old girl, Debbie, was hospitalized by her mother after being unmanageable at home and was given the psychiatric diagnosis of conduct disorder. Debbie's father and mother were legally separated. The mother refused to let the daughter live with the father, and a trial of living with the grandparents did not work out because of Debbie's disobedience.

Debbie was angry about being admitted to a psychiatric hospital, and as soon as her mother left, she attempted to run away. Once back on the unit, Debbie telephoned her mother reporting that the staff had struck her and she should come and get her. The mother spoke to the psychiatrist and the nursing staff who explained what had happened. The mother refused the daughter's request to go home. Debbie then telephoned her father suggesting that the mother and psychiatrist would allow her to live with him and that he should come and get her. When the father sought to verify this, he was told the truth.

Debbie refused to take part in the treatment program and frequently threatened to run away. She called a friend asking her to bring in marijuana, hoping that infraction of rules would result in her discharge. Debbie's appearance and be-

Chart 2
Manipulation: Summary of the Nursing Process

NURSING INTERVENTIONS

CLIENT GOAL: DEMONSTRATE DECREASED USE OF MANIPULATION
Identify client attempts to manipulate staff
Assist client in recognizing unhealthy coping mechanisms
Assist client in identifying strengths
Encourage use of talents in socially accepted activities
Encourage use of assertive behaviors within the milieu
Assist client to learn relaxation techniques
Assist client in identification of alternative methods of coping
Use kind, but firm, approach
Provide consistent limits with reasonable expectations
Give positive feedback for healthy coping behavior
Encourage leisure activities, participation in unit functions and
  therapeutic milieu to expose client to new coping methods and
  provide environment to "try out" new skills

CLIENT GOAL: IDENTIFY AND DISCUSS FEELINGS
Assign consistent staff member to facilitate trust and therapeutic
  relationship
Encourage open and honest communication by use of confrontation
  of deceptive communication patterns and positive role-
  modeling
Define acceptable behaviors and confront manipulation each time it
  occurs
Assist client in discussing feelings and offer feedback to help gain
  insight
Encourage active involvement in treatment planning to increase
  sense of autonomy and responsibility for self

OUTCOME CRITERIA

Identifies manipulative behaviors and
  demonstrate new coping methods

Demonstrates effective communication patterns

havior had quite an impact upon the milieu. She emphasized her sexual attractiveness, acting seductively and causing jealous quarrels among her male peers. She tried to elicit pity and sympathy whenever possible. She managed to divide the staff and then set up arguments between her "allies and adversaries."

Debbie displayed numerous characteristics of manipulation, including disturbed communication patterns, dishonesty, and difficulty in accepting limits. A nursing diagnosis of manipulation related to self-esteem issues was made.

During a team meeting, the staff discussed their frustration with Debbie's behavior. Staff members recognized that it was common for manipulative clients to evoke negative feelings in others, and it was decided that regular team meetings would serve as a forum to increase communication, plan appropriate treatment, and discuss feelings. A consistent staff member was assigned to Debbie to aid in the development of a trusting relationship. Staff used a kind, but firm, approach and confronted Debbie's manipulative behavior each time it occurred. A more predictable environment was established by setting limits on her behav-

Research Highlights

Walt and Gillis designed a study to determine to what extent nurse's attitudes about mental illness affected the treatment of clients.[7] A sample size of 162 (58 registered nurses; 104 mental health workers) was used. Ellsworth's modification of the Opinions About Mental Illness Scale was used to measure staff behavior as seen by clients,[7] with staff falling into one of the following categories:

1. Authoritarianism: emphasized restrictive control and firm measures. Seen by clients as inconsiderate, domineering, and rigid people who were unable to be trusted, related to, or understood.

2. Protective Benevolence: comfortable, but superficial and detached relationships. Stresses "homey" atmosphere and physical comfort. Seen by clients as being aloof, distant, and reluctant to be involved.

3. Accountability: emphasis on client participation in treatment and personal interaction is stressed. Seen by clients as warm, sensitive, and understanding.

Considering research results, one might speculate that the authoritarian and protective benevolent staff types may be targeted by clients who manipulate.

ior and assisting Debbie in structuring her time. As trust developed, Debbie began talking about her feelings. She shared with staff that her father had "touched" her and that when she told her mother of the incident, her mother had "kicked him out." She discussed her feelings of shame and guilt over both the incident and the break-up of her parents' marriage.

Through the use of the therapeutic milieu, a trusting relationship, consistent limits, and opportunities to explore feelings, Debbie began to gain awareness of her manipulative behavior. When Debbie was discharged from the inpatient setting, discharge plans included continued outpatient therapy for both herself and her mother.

SUMMARY

Manipulation is an interpersonal process used to control others. Often the motivation behind the behavior involves feelings of lack of power and lack of trust. The nurse's most valuable means of responding therapeutically is through self-awareness and the skillful use of the nursing process. Although manipulative attempts by the client are frustrating, the nurse who remembers the client's needs for trust, security, and control will provide a positive learning experience for a challenging client.

References

1. American Psychiatric Association. Diagnostic and statistical manual of Mental Disorders. 3rd ed, revised. Washington, DC: American Psychiatric Association; 1987.
2. Chitty K, Maynard C. Managing manipulation. J Psychosoc Nurs. 1986;24:6.
3. McMorrow ME. The manipulative patient. Am J Nurs. 1981;June.
4. Rutter M. Developmental psychiatry. Washington, DC: American Psychiatric Press; 1980.
5. Shostrom E. Man the manipulator. Nashville, New York: Abingdon Press; 1967.
6. St Clair H. Manipulation. Compr Psychiatry. 1966;7:4.
7. Walt AP, Gillis LS. Factors that influence nurses' attitudes toward psychiatric patients. J Clin Psychiatry. 1979;35:2.

NONCOMPLIANCE

(SPECIFY)

Georgia Whitley

DEFINITION AND DESCRIPTION

Health-care providers have focused much attention upon the area of client compliance during recent decades. With the acceptance of noncompliance as a nursing diagnosis, the attention to this topic was joined by controversy. Questions arose on the possible negative and passive connotations of this diagnosis, and the issue continues to be debated. The role of the client is perceived to be that of a partner in all aspects of care, to the extent that the client wishes to be and is able to be.

Noncompliance is defined as a person's informed decision not to adhere to, or participate in, a therapeutic recommendation.[8] The nursing diagnosis, noncompliance, is listed with the word *specify* following it in parentheses, which means that the nurse is to specify the particular therapeutic recommendation that the client is not following. Client compliance is extremely important in psychiatric–mental health nursing because of the complications that may result from the presence of a chronic mental illness that is not treated in an optimal manner. The magnitude of the problem of compliance with health-care regimens is illustrated by the existence of deviation from prescribed regimens by one-third to one-half of all persons treated.[6] Challenges to providers are not only to increase patient compliance, informed decision making, and participation, but also to identify factors that predict compliance, to develop methods for measuring compliance, and to develop more acceptable treatments.

THEORY AND RESEARCH

The first model to be studied in an attempt to predict noncompliance was the medical model.[4,9] Variables such as medical diagnosis, type of treatment, seriousness of illness, resultant pain and disability, and duration of treatment were studied. This model has not proved to consistently or accurately predict noncompliance.[4,9] A variation of the medical model was the attempt to predict noncompliance based upon the perceptions of health-care workers. This model also has not been a consistent or accurate predictor of noncompliance.[4,9]

In contrast, the *health belief model* provided a theoretical base for dealing with readiness to take health action.[13] Developed in the early 1950s, this model purports that health action is related to (1) belief that one is susceptible to a specific disease, (2) belief that the disease would have serious effects upon one's life, (3) awareness of actions to be taken and belief that these actions would reduce or eliminate the disease, and (4) belief that the threat of taking action is not as great as the threat itself.[13] Components of the model include individual perceptions, modifying factors, and variables that affect the likelihood of taking action. Although a statistically significant relationship has been demonstrated between individual components and compliance, the model cannot predict compliance.

Studies of demographic and sociological characteristics, including educational level, marital status, mental status, age, sex, race, religion, and socioeconomic level, have produced contradictory results. Variables that have become generally acceptable as having a significant relationship to compliance are age and mental status.[5,9] Specifically, the very young, the elderly, and persons who have the diagnosis of paranoid schizophrenia can be identified as being at risk for noncompliance with health-care protocols.[9]

Three studies can be cited from nursing literature that address the nursing diagnosis noncompliance.[1,10,15] In a study of nursing diagnoses used in psychiatric mental health nursing, noncompliance was one of four NANDA diagnoses found to be most unclear in meaning.[10] Furthermore, noncompliance was one of the five NANDA labels that was rated as moderately to very useful for psychiatric mental health nursing by only 70% to 79% of the respondents. In this study, several respondents commented on the negative aspects of labeling a patient as noncompliant. In another study describing how the diagnosis noncompliance is used in clinical practice, 52% of the respondents did report using this diagnosis.[1] Of those using the diagnosis, a consensus definition did not emerge. Respondents who did not use the diagnosis indicated that they considered it a value-laden label, that it did not address the real problem of the client, or that they felt that noncompliance denoted a lack of mutual decision making. A third study of noncompliance, descriptive in nature, revealed that the defining characteristics and etiologies as presented in the study were present in clients.[15] Each etiology was linked with specific defining characteristics. Defining characteristics from both the

NANDA listing and from the health belief model were selected with a high degree of frequency.

Noncompliance with treatment protocols by persons with the diagnosis of schizophrenia is predictably greater than with most other client groups, which signals a special need for assessment and appropriate interventions by nurses working with these clients. A review of the literature indicates that little research has focused on factors that affect compliance among individuals with schizophrenia.[2] Educational programs for persons with schizophrenia are common, but many have not been evaluated. A framework for research has been derived from operational conditioning concepts and applied to medication adherence by clients with schizophrenia.[3] Although this framework does not provide an explanation of all aspects of compliance or noncompliance, it does provide a framework that accounts for the factors correlated with compliance in prior studies. Factors correlated with compliance can be grouped into four areas: personal factors, therapy factors, helper and milieu factors, and multiple factors (acceptance of role, support of family, perception of physician, perception of illness, attitude toward treatment milieu).[2] An experimental study involving newly discharged clients with affective disorders showed a statistically significant difference between compliance in a control group and a directive-patient education group.[17] These findings imply that patient education did have an effect upon compliance and support incorporation of these programs in psychiatric mental health nursing to increase compliance.

RELATED FACTORS

The NANDA definition of noncompliance, a person's informed decision not to adhere to a therapeutic recommendation, must be interpreted when establishing related factors for noncompliance. This definition is being expanded because choices, not always informed, are made by an individual at many levels, including a range of consciously made decisions through unconscious choices, the dynamics of which the individual is not aware. An example of the unconscious forces at work in decision making is the client who uses denial in relation to a health problem. The threat of illness is so great that the person denies that it is there and, thus, does not participate in the treatment. Other issues that must be confronted when dealing with the related factors in noncompliance are the skills and abilities of the client to comply. Examples of factors included in this category are visual or hearing deficits and inability to read or write.

Factors identified by NANDA as contributing to noncompliance are divided into two major categories. The first is the client value system with three subcategories: health beliefs, cultural influences, and spiritual values. The second is client and provider relationships with no subcategorization. The work of Ryan on related factors for noncompliance provides more specific differentiation of these factors.[14-16]

Inadequate knowledge is a frequently identified cause for noncompliance. However, research in compliance has demonstrated that adequate knowledge alone does not yield compliance; thus, this may or may not be a final related factor. An example of inadequate knowledge owing to not having been given information is the client who says, "No one ever told me about the side effects of this medication." An example of ignoring information is the client who says, "The nurse talked about what would happen during my treatment, but I figured what I didn't know wouldn't hurt me so I told her I didn't want to hear about it." Inaccurate information may be due to inaccuracies of teaching, old information, or distortions by the client. *Alterations in thought processes* that lead to noncompliance can occur, for example, in clients with psychiatric problems such as schizophrenia, bipolar disorders, substance abuse, paranoid disorders, and organic mental syndromes and disorders.

Deficits that impair the client's *ability to read or write*, such as physical problems, psychological difficulties, or educational deficiencies, may lead to noncompliance. *Visual or hearing difficulties* may interfere with the client's ability to read directions for prescribed medications.

Clients may be *inadequately motivated* to comply because of disbelief in the seriousness of an illness or belief that one is not susceptible to the illness. Another reason for inadequate motivation is that the client finds the illness less problematic than the treatment. An example is the client who has schizophrenia and chooses to live with the resultant behaviors, rather than take psychotropic drugs indefinitely.

Denial is a coping mechanism frequently used by persons in an attempt to deal with changes in health status. The use of denial may mean denying the presence of a problem, or the need for or effectiveness of treatment protocols. *Anxiety* is another frequent response to threats to one's health. Anxiety may cause one to use denial to cope, or it may cause distortion of information and mismanagement of treatment. *Fear* may be expressed about the outcome of the illness or the effects of the treatment and may also lead to noncompliance. *Anger* and *depression* may occur separately or in tandem and interfere with the individual's perceptions of the health situation and protocols and, thus, also interfere with compliance.

Health beliefs, cultural influences, and spiritual beliefs may precipitate *conflicts in value systems* that lead to noncompliant health behaviors. Values may also involve giving priority to another role responsibility rather than that of client role. Thus, the value and belief systems of clients serve as related factors in noncompliance with health care regimens. Another related factor is the belief that the therapy is necessary and helpful, but the client is unable to maintain the behavior required to implement the therapy because of *addictive and habitual behaviors* such as smoking, alcohol or drug abuse, and overeating.

The social support system of the client is defined as the client's relationships with others and with the environment including significant others, job, church, community, and material resources.[14] *Inadequate social support* may occur because family members are not taught about regimens and why they are important and, thus, may not offer the assistance or encouragement that would help the client comply. Inadequate community support may also contribute to noncompliance. *Inadequate resources* such as lack of financial resources, equipment, facilities, or transportation are barriers that may lead to noncompliance. *Deficits in the health-care system* such as relationships between the client and caregivers, adequacy of the health-care system, and the complexity of a regimen are factors that, if ineffectual, lead to noncompliance.[14] Additionally, past negative experiences with health care may adversely affect adherence. If a treatment is not effecting improvement, or if the patient is decompensating, the patient may become noncompliant.

DEFINING CHARACTERISTICS

The defining characteristics observed in clients with the nursing diagnosis noncompliance include behavior indicative of failure to adhere to a therapeutic recommendation by direct observation or statements by patient or significant other, indications from objective tests, evidence of development of complications, evidence of exacerbation of symptoms, failure to keep appointments, failure to progress, and inability to set or attain mutual goals.[7] The last defining characteristic is especially important in psychiatric nursing because it implies the mutually active relationship between nurse and client in establishing treatment parameters (Chart 1).

NURSING PROCESS AND RATIONALE

Assessment

A thorough assessment is vital when the nurse suspects noncompliance, because many times this diagnosis is ruled out during the assessment process. The nurse needs to pay special attention to the differentiation of knowledge deficit, decisional conflict, and noncompliance, and to the ways in which the three diagnoses can articulate with one another. Proper diagnosis and identification of related factors are essential, for this directs the psychiatric mental health nurse to appropriate interventions.

Data gathering will first be directed toward seeking out any behavior indicative of failure to adhere and will be collected through direct observation or by statements by the client or significant others. Objective tests, including physiologic measures and detection of markers, provide compliance data to the nurse. An example of these would be determinations of the serum lithium levels in blood samples drawn for the client with a diagnosis of bipolar disorder who is maintained on lithium therapy. Although many factors influence

---

CHART 1
Noncompliance: Definition, Related Factors, and Defining Characteristics[8,11,14]

DEFINITION

Noncompliance is the individual's informed decision not to adhere to a therapeutic recommendation.

RELATED FACTORS

Alteration in Cognition

Inadequate knowledge
Alterations in thought processes
Inability to read or write
Sensory deficits

Alteration in Perception

Inadequate motivation
Alterations in affective state: denial, depression, anger, fear, anxiety
Conflict in value system: health beliefs, cultural influences, spiritual values
Belief in therapy but unable to change behavior

Inadequacies in Social System

Inadequate social support
Inadequate resources

Deficits in Health-Care System

Complexity of regimen
System inadequacy
Nontherapeutic relationship with health-care professional
Past negative experiences
No improvement or decompensation with treatment

DEFINING CHARACTERISTICS

Behavior indicative of failure to adhere to a therapeutic recommendation by direct observation or statements by patient or significant others
Indications from objective tests (physiologic measures, detection of markers)
Evidence of development of complications
Evidence of exacerbation of symptoms
Failure to keep appointments
Failure to progress
Inability to set or attain mutual goals

---

blood lithium levels, very low levels or absence of lithium in the blood would certainly suggest noncompliance.

Other assessment determinations include return of symptoms, development of complications, and failure to progress as expected. If the client is not keeping follow-up appointments, the nurse may suspect nonadherence and may contact the client or significant other by telephone or a home visit. Additionally, other health-care personnel or other agencies may need to be alerted and asked to assist in evaluating what is happening with this client. Setting and working toward mutual goals has been identified as a desired process between nurse and client. When this process breaks down, the nurse needs to assess for noncompliance on the part of the client.

Nursing Diagnosis

Identification of specific related factor(s) of the client's noncompliance is a critical step in the nursing process for the selection of specific nursing interventions that will assist the client to comply with appropriate health-care measures. For example, a client who misses clinic appointments is found to be motivated to attend, but is unable to get to the clinic after a family member who had provided transportation moved away. Noncompliance (with clinic appointments) related to the transportation problem is an example of a nursing diagnosis.

Client Goals and Nursing Interventions

Once the assessment data is available and the nursing diagnosis has been established, the nurse is ready to delineate appropriate goals with the client. Goals will be relevant to the specified noncompliance and the particular related factor(s) for this client. General goals for clients who are noncompliant are presented in the summary of the nursing process (Chart 2). The nurse can further develop and specify these general goals according to individual assessment data. In general, client goals are to:

- Identify an appropriate health regimen
- Explore feelings regarding the health regimen
- Acquire necessary knowledge and skill to perform health behaviors
- Modify life-style to promote health behaviors
- Maintain positive relationships with caregivers and agencies
- Practice specific health behaviors consistently.

Nursing interventions will be grounded in the concept of joint decision making between the client and caregivers. The expression of feelings about the health regimens will be encouraged throughout the process. Principles of health teaching are utilized, with special emphasis upon tailoring the program to meet individual needs. Research has demonstrated that simple instructions for the treatment regimen, simple instructions on prescription containers, written and verbal explanations of the treatment regimen, and packaging of medication are related to increased compliance.[2] Significant others need to be included in health teaching so that they understand the therapy and can be encouraged to support health-seeking behaviors, as well as to help the client eliminate barriers to such behaviors.

After the establishment of clear, specific protocols, the client needs to be given the opportunity to practice the protocols and modify the regimen, life-style, and environmental factors as necessary. A structured system that provides cues and positive feedback for carrying out the regimen must be established to maintain compliance. A systematic schedule of follow-up visits needs to be established, as well as articulation with appropriate agencies and self-help groups. Specific agency and group contacts must be initiated and followed through so that the relationships are established.

The nurse must remain cognizant of the fact that it is the client's prerogative to adopt health maintaining behaviors or not to do so. Caregivers help to provide the most positive structure for the client, taking into consideration specific guidelines, individuality, client decision making, family–social support, and the team of health professionals and agencies. However, it is the client who decides whether or not the value of compliance exceeds the payoffs of noncompliance.

Evaluation

Outcome criteria that reflect client goals are used to measure the extent to which the goals are achieved. General outcome statements that articulate with general client goals are presented in Chart 2. More specific measures are utilized in individual client situations. For example, if the client has been noncompliant (in taking psychotropic medication) related to denial of illness, the nursing interventions will be aimed at dealing with the client's denial of illness as well as establishing an appropriate medication regimen. An outcome measure that can be observed is whether or not the client continues to verbally deny the illness. An objective measurable outcome criterion would be blood or urine levels of the psychotropic medication. Other measures would include pill-counts, self-monitoring records, patient reporting, and reporting by significant others. Measurement of compliance is complex and inexact at this point, thus, multiple checks assist in more accurate measures (see Chart 2).

CASE STUDY

Jim B, a 20-year-old single man, was a sophomore at a small, private college when he became unable to concentrate and his grades dropped. His roommates described his behavior as bizarre. He talked to himself and had grandiose delusions about being a center on the college basketball team. He withdrew from classes and went home to live with his parents and younger brother. When the bizarre behavior continued, he was hospitalized on the psychiatric unit of the local hospital. He stayed there for several weeks and responded well to medication, group therapy, and therapeutic activities. Upon discharge he was to be maintained on his medications and to have frequent appointments for follow-up at the local mental health center. During the first months after discharge, Jim did well and was able to work part time at a nearby sporting goods store. Recently, however, Jim

CHART 2
Noncompliance: Summary of the Nursing Process[8,11,14]

NURSING INTERVENTIONS	OUTCOME CRITERIA
CLIENT GOAL: IDENTIFY APPROPRIATE HEALTH-RELATED BEHAVIORS Discuss alternative approaches with client Encourage client to select from appropriate choices those which are most personally desirable Discuss the relationship between emotional needs and compliance	Identifies specific health-related behaviors
CLIENT GOAL: PERFORM SPECIFIC HEALTH-RELATED BEHAVIORS CONSISTENTLY Implement patient teaching relevant to specific behaviors Simplify protocols and instructions Provide opportunities for supervised practice Discuss response to regimen with client and modify as needed Incorporate significant others into regimen as appropriate Establish cues and positive reinforcement for carrying out protocols Refer and articulate with other agencies and other health-care personnel as indicated	Performs specific health behaviors
CLIENT GOAL: MODIFY LIFE-STYLE TO ACCOMMODATE AND PROMOTE IDENTIFIED HEALTH-RELATED BEHAVIORS Refer client and significant others to self-help and community groups if available Assist client to analyze current patterns of behavior and social interactions to determine influence upon health regimen Plan and implement necessary changes with client Plan daily activities so that health behaviors are structured and cues, reminders, and positive reinforcers are provided Set up self-monitoring record-keeping system and provide for periodic review of progress	Modifies life-style and accommodates health regimens
CLIENT GOAL: MAINTAIN A PRODUCTIVE RELATIONSHIP WITH CAREGIVERS AND HEALTH AGENCIES Provide regularly scheduled visits to monitor progress and give positive support Provide a means of making contact if the client is discouraged or needs support Clarify agency services and roles of caregivers Promote client autonomy and self-expression Modify relationships and simplify regimens as appropriate to meet individual needs	Maintains relationships with caregivers and agency that support positive behaviors

has again been unable to concentrate, has been talking about himself in grandiose terms, and is unable to function in his job. When Jim and his mother appeared for his clinic appointment, his mother reported that Jim had not been taking his medication. Jim states that he no longer needs medication. Jim has always been slender and lost 10 pounds during the acute phase of his illness. When he is agitated and pacing, he does not attend to his nutritional needs. One of Jim's nursing diagnoses is noncompliance (medications). One of the goals is to determine the related factors for Jim's refusal to take his medications. An appropriate plan of nursing care will then be developed based upon these findings.

SUMMARY

Noncompliance is a person's informed decision not to adhere to a therapeutic recommendation. The definition of noncompliance is based on the assumption that the client role is one of partnership with caregivers to the extent feasible. Noncompliance is a frequent problem for psychiatric–mental health clients.

Etiological factors were presented using four general categories as developed by Ryan[14] with specific etiologies grouped under the general categories. The importance of comprehensive assessment to ascertain the cause was emphasized because of the importance of this in determining effective nursing interventions. Defining characteristics developed by NANDA were presented. The characteristic that describes behavior indicative of failure to adhere has been identified as critical. Emphasis upon assessment is especially important when considering this diagnosis because noncompliance may occur as a defining characteristic of another nursing diagnosis. Client goals were identified for the diagnosis of noncompliance. Mutuality of goal setting and selection of interventions was emphasized. Use of principles of health teaching was included in nursing interventions for noncompliance. Simplicity of regimen, involvement of significant others, a systematic schedule, and appropriate referrals, all need to be built into the plan of care. Evaluation is based upon the extent to which client goals were achieved. Evaluation of compliance is complex and requires all data possible, including objective tests and measurements, as well as subjective data from the client, significant others, health professionals, and referral groups.

Research Highlights

The following are some of the nursing research problems related to noncompliance that merit further study:[1,2,7]

1. Determine the usefulness and acceptability of the term noncompliance as a nursing diagnosis
2. Arrive at a consensus nursing definition of noncompliance
3. Conduct validation studies of the proposed defining characteristics of noncompliance
4. Conduct validation studies of the proposed related factors of noncompliance
5. Determine the influence of having clients involved in planning treatment protocols. Target groups for this study should be those clients who are known to have a high rate of nonadherence
6. Develop instruments to aid in identifying gaps in information that may relate to noncompliance
7. Compare the effectiveness of individual teaching, group teaching, and inclusion of a significant other in the teaching process
8. Develop an instrument to evaluate the presence of risk related to noncompliance and a particular individual's likelihood of noncompliance
9. Compare factors identified by the client, physician, nurse, and family as significant in the noncompliance of specific clients to determine differences in perception
10. Evaluate educational programs using pre- and post-testing of treatment and control groups to determine the role of the program in effecting client compliance
11. Conduct descriptive studies of nursing process with noncompliant clients, with a focus on interventions and outcomes to build a body of knowledge regarding this process.

References

1. Breunig KA, Brukwitzki G, Schulte J, Crane L, Schroeder PM, Lutze J. Noncompliance as a nursing diagnosis: current use in clinical practice. In: Hurley ME, ed. Classification of nursing diagnoses: proceedings of the sixth conference. St. Louis: CV Mosby; 1986.
2. Davidhizar RE. Compliance by persons with schizophrenia: a research issue for the nurse. Issues Ment Health Nurs. 1982;4:233–255.
3. Davidhizar RE. The schizophrenic client's reinforcement and punishment for medication adherence. Issues Ment Health Nurs. 1984;6:173–187.
4. Haynes RB. Determinants of compliance, the disease and the mechanics of treatment. In: Hayes RB, Taylor DW, Sackett HD, eds. Compliance in health care. Baltimore: Johns Hopkins University Press; 1979.
5. Haynes B. Improvement of medication compliance in uncontrolled hypertension. Lancet. 1979;2:1265–1269.
6. Haynes RB, Taylor DW, Sachett DL, eds. Compliance in health care. Baltimore: Johns Hopkins University Press; 1979.
7. Kim MJ, McFarland GK, McLane AM, eds. Classification of nursing diagnoses: proceedings of the fifth national conference. St. Louis: CV Mosby; 1984.
8. Kim MJ, McFarland GK, McLane AM. Pocket guide to nursing diagnoses. 3rd ed. St. Louis: CV Mosby; 1989.
9. Marston MV. Compliance with medical regimes: a review of the literature. Nurs Res. 1970;19:312–316.
10. McFarland GK, Naschinski CE. Validation and identification of nursing diagnoses labels for psychiatric mental health nursing practice. In: McLane AM, ed. Classification of nursing diagnoses: proceedings of the seventh conference. St. Louis: CV Mosby; 1987.
11. McFarland GK, Wasli EL. Nursing diagnoses and process in psychiatric mental health nursing. Philadelphia: JB Lippincott; 1986.
12. McLane AM, ed. Classification of nursing diagnoses: proceedings of the seventh national conference. St. Louis: CV Mosby; 1987.
13. Rosenstock JM. What research in motivation suggests for public health. Am J Public Health. 1960;50:295–301.
14. Ryan P. Noncompliance. In: Thompson JM, McFarland GK, Hirsch JE, Tucker SM, Bowers AC. Clinical nursing. St. Louis: CV Mosby; 1986.
15. Ryan P, Falco SM. A pilot study to validate the etiologies and defining characteristics of the nursing diagnosis of noncompliance. Nurs Clin North Am. 1985;20:685–695.
16. Ryan P, Falco SM. The nursing diagnosis of noncompliance: a pilot study. In: Hurley ME, ed. Classification of nursing diagnoses: proceedings of the sixth conference. St. Louis: CV Mosby; 1986.
17. Youssef FA. Compliance with therapeutic regimes: a follow-up study for patients with affective disorders. J Adv Nurs. 1983;8:513–517.

NUTRITION, ALTERED, LESS THAN BODY REQUIREMENTS

Mary Kunes-Connell

DEFINITION AND DESCRIPTION

As a nursing diagnosis, *altered nutrition, less than body requirements* is defined as "a state in which an individual experiences an intake of nutrients insufficient to meet metabolic needs."[13] This definition emphasizes an inadequate nutrient intake in addition to a decrease in caloric intake as requisites for determining that an individual has an altered nutritional intake. Despite the fact that this diagnosis can be a sequela to a number of emotional states, psychiatric illnesses, and therapies, as well as the inability of many psychiatric clients to meet their own self-care needs, surprisingly little has been documented regarding specific nutritional concerns confronting psychiatric clients. More psychiatric nursing attention should be paid to some very important aspects of nutritional care, including: (1) an understanding of the interplay between emotional status, psychiatric treatment, and nutritional intake; (2) assessment of nutritional status on admission, during hospitalization, and at the time of discharge; (3) incorporation of a nutritional assessment into an individualized treatment plan promoting an optimal nutritional status; (4) monitoring and analysis of the nutritional content of the client's food choices; and (5) nutritional discharge planning.

THEORY AND RESEARCH

Adequate nutrition implies a caloric intake designed to maintain a weight appropriate to a person's sex, height, and body frame in addition to nutrients sufficient for maintaining a healthy lifestyle.[8] Shaw and Cronin[8] have provided an extensive summary of recommendations from the various nutritional and medical organizations. These guidelines are meant to provide a foundation for planning and preparing meals to meet the standards of adequate nutrition. It is not enough for an individual to have the knowledge of essential nutrients and their Recommended Daily Allowance (RDA); the individual also must have the financial and environmental resources to purchase and prepare food. Furthermore, the individual must have the cognitive and physical abilities to plan meals appropriately as well as the motivation to do so.[4] Finally, an individual must have an understanding of factors that might affect the absorption of nutrients.[4-6,8,23]

Recent research conducted by Ryan and Rao[24] indicates that the psychiatric hospitals under study were able to provide clients access to meals planned in accordance with the United States Recommended Daily Allowances. Nevertheless, despite adequate planning on the part of nutritionists in psychiatric settings, many psychiatric clients continue to exhibit altered nutritional status, with many displaying inadequate nutritional intake.[4,6,19,23,24] As Ryan and Rao[24] point out, it does not suffice for a hospital staff to provide nutritionally sound meals; additional efforts are needed to educate clients regarding the impact of their disorder and treatments on their nutritional status as well as to provide adequate assistance with activities of daily living —e.g., feeding—as needed.

RELATED FACTORS

Inadequate nutritional intake may be the result of a number of diverse personal and extrapersonal factors. The factors related to alteration in nutrition, less than body requirements, include biologic, emotional, cognitive, and sociocultural factors.[4,11,15,24]

Numerous psychiatric and emotional disorders have profound physiological effects on the body. Alcoholism and substance abuse can suppress the appetite, leading to a decrease in food intake.[4] In addition, excessive alcohol intake impairs liver and pancreatic functioning and often results in gastric inflammation. Therefore, many nutrients taken in by the alcohol abuser are malabsorbed; vitamin B complex, magnesium, zinc, folic acid, and vitamin K are just a few examples. Over the long term, the lack of these nutrients can result in a variety of neurologic, cardiovascular, and dermatologic problems.[4,6,9]

A disorder receiving increasing attention is that of self-induced water intoxication. Effects of neuroleptics and excessive dopamine release, for example in schizophrenia, on hypothalamic functioning are only two of the many reasons psychiatric clients may be at risk for water intoxication.[12,21] Water intoxication has resulted in the well-known psychiatric effect of psychotic behavior. However, there is an increasing body of evidence that the psychological effects are secondary to a physiological alteration in the serum electrolyte sodium. Illowsky and Kirch[12] discuss the growing belief that hyponatremia is the principal cause for the psychiatric, as well as the gastrointestinal, elimination, and neurologic complications. These authors point out that not all clients with polydipsia will develop water intoxication or hyponatremia, as most clients will be able to conserve sodium through the eventual suppression of antidiuretic hormone (ADH). However, Illowsky and Kirch summarize a number of studies indicating that ADH is not suppressed in some clients in whom water intoxication and hyponatremia result.

Stress and anxiety play a significant role in decreasing the psychiatric client's ability to meet optimal nutritional needs. From a physiological standpoint, severe anxiety increases the release of epinephrine and norepinephrine. These hormones shunt blood from the digestive organs to the muscles, heart, and brain. Second, and more importantly, during stress, the body prepares itself for "fight or flight." The body's response to stress is to fuel itself for this response.[5] The body increases its release of glucocorticoids as well as growth hormone. Glucocorticoids increase glucose production, while growth hormone decreases the effectiveness of insulin in glucose metabolism.[5] The decreased blood flow, along with the increased glucose production, creates a state of anorexia whereby the individual has a decreased intake of essential nutrients.[5,25]

Psychotropic medications frequently play a contributory role in inadequate nutritional intake.[16,20,23] They do not directly decrease nutritional intake; rather, the side effects (e.g., dry mouth) may make it difficult to meet nutritional requirements. Other side effects that hinder the client's ability to maintain a positive nutritional intake are glossitis, abnormal jaw and tongue movements, nausea, vomiting, diarrhea, and abdominal pain. The difficulties that can be created include chewing problems, swallowing problems, gastric and intestinal distress, and absorption problems. Table 13-6 lists common side effects of psychotropic medications that could, if undetected or untreated, have a negative impact on the psychiatric client's nutritional status.

Schizophrenia, dysthymia, depressive episodes, and psychoactive substance use disorders can produce anergia and decreased motivation. These conditions thus tend to diminish the client's initiative and ultimate capacity to meet nutritional needs.[1,4,10,17,22,25] A client with a manic episode or schizophrenia, on the other hand, may be so agitated that time is not taken to eat. Suspiciousness and delusions can create serious disruptions in an individual's attempt to meet nutritional needs; for example, the client may believe that people are poisoning the food or drinks.

Interestingly, the need for psychological and emotional comfort may create a set of circumstances leading to an inadequate nutritional intake. It is hypothesized that an infant's need for nurturance, in a situation where this nurturance is not given, may be accomplished by using food in a "refeeding" process. Refeeding occurs when an infant partially digests the food, regurgitates it, and reswallows it. Mayes and associates[18] analyzed 66 cases of infants and children with rumination disorder. These authors discovered that this self-induced disorder occurs not only in infants, but also in mentally retarded children. Infant rumination may be the result of faulty parent–child relations, whereas rumination in mentally retarded children is thought to be the result of the need for continued self-stimulation. Both types of rumination result in nutritional deficits.[18]

TABLE 13–6
Effects of psychotropic medications that may affect nutritional status[16,19,20]

DRUG CLASSIFICATION	DRY MOUTH	CHEWING PROBLEMS	SWALLOWING PROBLEMS	UNPLEASANT TASTE
ANTIPSYCHOTICS	X	X (Tardive dyskinesia: buccolinguo-masticatory triad)	(Laryngospasm/ bronchospasm)	X
TRICYCLIC ANTIDEPRESSANTS	X	X (Glossitis)		X
MONOAMINE OXIDASE INHIBITORS	X			
BICYCLIC ANTIDEPRESSANTS	X			X
CHOLINERGIC BLOCKING AGENTS	X			
ANTIANXIETY AGENTS	X	X (Swollen tongue)	X (Bronchospasm)	X
LITHIUM CARBONATE	X			X
CARBAMAZEPINE	X	X (Glossitis)		

Organic impairment caused by organic mental disorders, alcohol or other drug use, or mental retardation often results in the inability to make decisions about self-care. This lack of judgment can lead to a client's neglect of basic human needs. The lack of judgment may be reflected in inappropriate selection or preparation of meals. The memory impairment associated with some of these disorders may cause the client to "forget" to eat, even after frequent reminders.[1,22]

Sociocultural factors impact an individual's perception of his or her physical self. Larocca[15] discusses the profound influence of the media on the prevalence of eating disorders. "Thin is in" would appear to be the motto of the 1980s and has led to individuals of average weight distorting their body image to the point of developing an eating disorder.

Of growing concern in the mental health field is the increasing number of mentally ill persons who are homeless and destitute. For these individuals, social isolation, inadequate financial resources, and lack of food storage and preparation facilities contribute to the potential for inadequate nutrition.[4]

DEFINING CHARACTERISTICS

The defining characteristics for altered nutrition, less than body requirements are complex, because the manifestations tend to reflect the severity and duration of the diagnosis, as well as the specific nutrients involved. The more severe the nutritional deficit and the longer its duration, the more apparent and serious will be the defining characteristics.[26] Also, the nature of the defining characteristics will depend on the specific nutrient deficiency. For example, a client with a vitamin B12 deficiency will demonstrate confusion, dementia, pallor, loss of appetite, diarrhea, and tingling of the extremities, among other signs. A client with protein deficiency would manifest edema, muscle wasting, and changes in hair texture and skin color.[6,26]

Despite the specificity of the defining characteristics for certain nutrients, there also are manifestations associated with an overall decrease in intake that should alert the psychiatric mental health nurse to potential problems. These defining characteristics include[15,26] general physiological changes (decreased metabolic rate, decreased body temperature, lethargy, fatigue, weakness, weight loss); cognitive changes (decreased attention span, decreased concentration, confusion, delirium); cardiovascular changes (lower blood pressure, lower pulse rate, changes in cell counts); emotional changes (irritability, apathy, depression, amotivation, anergia); integumentary changes (changes in color or texture of hair, skin, nails; oral/mucous membrane breakdown); and fluid and electrolyte changes (alterations in serum fluid and electrolytes) (Chart 1).

NURSING PROCESS AND RATIONALE
Assessment

It is important for the psychiatric mental health nurse to assess nutritional status and intake generally in order to determine the need for further evaluation. This general nutritional screening includes: (1) client diagnosis; (2) weight; (3) general factors influencing eating habits such as meal patterns (times, preparations, amounts), likes and dislikes, allergies, sociocultural variables, special diets; and (4) physical, medical,

NAUSEA	VOMITING	CONSTIPATION/ DIARRHEA	GASTRIC DISTRESS	ANOREXIA
		X		X (Possible)
X	X	X	X	X
X	X	X	X	X
X	X	X		X
X	X	X	X	
		X		X (Possible)
X	X	X	X	X
X	X	X	X	

CHART 1
Altered Nutrition, Less than Body Requirements: Definition, Related Factors, and Defining Characteristics

DEFINITION

A state in which an individual experiences an intake of nutrients insufficient to meet metabolic needs.[13]

RELATED FACTORS

Side effects of psychotropic medications
   Dry mouth
   Mouth sores
   Nausea
   Vomiting
   Chewing problems (impaired jaw and tongue movements)
   Bronchospasms
   Anorexia
   Unpleasant taste
   Constipation
   Diarrhea
   Gastric distress
Anergia
Decreased motivation
Agitation
Anxiety
Depression
Grieving
Cognitive factors
   Suspiciousness
   Hallucinations
   Delusions
   Lack of judgment
Sociocultural factors
   Media ideal of thinness
   Homelessness

DEFINING CHARACTERISTICS

General physiological changes
   Decreased metabolic rate
   Decreased body temperature
   Lethargy
   Fatigue
   Weakness
   Weight loss
Cardiovascular changes
   Hypertension
   Lowered pulse rate
Changes in skin, hair, mucosa
Alteration in body fluid and electrolyte balance
Cognitive changes
   Decreased concentration
   Confusion
   Delirium
Emotional changes
   Irritability
   Apathy
   Depression
   Anergia

emotional, and cognitive factors affecting the attainment, preparation, or actual intake of nutrients.[3,14,15,21] Figure 13-18 presents a nutritional screening guide to detect potential problems that might negatively affect the client's nutritional status.

Should the psychiatric mental health nurse suspect altered nutrition, a more thorough assessment should be undertaken. Risk factors that indicate a need for further assessment include recent significant weight loss or gain, numerous somatic complaints involving the gastrointestinal system, potential or known food–drug interactions, and suspected or known eating disorders. A more thorough assessment, outlined in Figure 13-19, focuses on weight and exercise history, drug history, significant laboratory values, stress responses, body image perceptions, and diagnoses and treatments that disrupt hand to mouth coordination, chewing, or swallowing. In addition, this form includes a 24-hour recall and nutrient analysis.[3]

Nursing Diagnosis

Because any number of clients with different diagnoses, different treatment regimens, and different social and economic status can experience altered nutrition, it is important for the nurse to identify those related factors precipitating the nursing diagnoses. The related factors (e.g., anergia, paranoid ideations, chewing and swallowing difficulties associated with medication) dictate the individualized plan of care necessary to promote a long-term change in nutritional status. Therefore, a depressed client and a schizophrenic client may both experience an altered nutritional status, less than body requirements. However, the plans of care may be quite different depending on the related factors; e.g., (1) altered nutrition, less than body requirements related to amotivation and a decreased energy level (for the depressed client) and (2) altered nutrition less than body requirements related to internalized paranoid voices stating that the food is poisoned (for the client with schizophrenia).

Client Goals and Nursing Interventions

Should the assessment validate the nursing diagnosis altered nutrition, less than body requirements, general goals would include decreasing or alleviating the factors contributing to the client's compromised nutritional status, and providing a diet with the necessary nutrients in a form that the client will accept and be able to ingest to maintain a healthy nutritional status.

The goal related to decreasing or alleviating the factors contributing to inadequate intake presents a great challenge to the psychiatric nurse. Because the related factors are unique to each client, intervention strate-

(Text continued on page 320)

Saint Joseph Center for Mental Health

Nutritional Screening Form

ADDRESSOGRAPH | Diet Order | CMH-0492 Rev. 11/86

Admitting Diagnosis _____

Height _____ Weight _____ Ideal Body Weight _____

Recent WEIGHT LOSS (Yes/No) AMOUNT _____ Recent WEIGHT GAIN (Yes/No) AMOUNT _____

	YES	NO	COMMENTS
Chewing Problems			
Swallowing Problems			
Nausea/Vomiting			
Therapeutic Diet			
Adherence			
Previous Instruction			

Food Likes and Dislikes _____

Ethnic or Religious Food Preferences _____

Food Allergies or Intolerances _____

Food Cravings _____

Dexterity, Visual, Auditory, Dental, Mobility	Physical Considerations _____
Sore Throat, Enlarged Salivary Glands	Medical Considerations _____
Self-Esteem, Self-Image, Depression, Loneliness, Stress, Anxiety, Boredom, Self-Control	Emotional & Psychological Considerations _____
Ability to Make Food Choices, Etc.	Assessment _____

PLAN: _____

Name _____ Title _____ Date _____

FIGURE 13-18. Nutritional screening form. (Used with permission of AMI Saint Joseph Center for Mental Health)

Saint Joseph Center for Mental Health

Nutritional Assessment Form

ADDRESSOGRAPH   CMH/D-0493   Rev. 9/85

Substance abuse medications presenting problems	Admitting History _____ Diagnosis _____ _____
Patient's perceptions of body size & shape; hunger, satiety; food intake, activity level	Subjective _____ _____ _____
Coping mechanisms, socioeconomic, family occupation, relationships	Psychological, Social & Emotional Factors _____ _____

Weight History

    Admission Weight_____

    Current Weight_____

    Usual Weight_____

    Ideal Body Weight_____

    % Weight Change_____

    Time Frame_____

Height _____

Scale History

    How often _____

    When_____

    Notes _____

    _____

Weight Loss or Gain Methods Tried_____

_____

Exercise History

    Current, regular, physical activity_____

_____

    Frequency _____ Duration _____

Comments _____

	Lab Data	Normal Values	Behaviors Affecting Food Intake or Nutrient Status	
Hematocrit	_____	_____	___ Gagging	___ Binging
Hemoglobin	_____	_____	___ Rumination	___ Purging
Others	_____	_____	___ Regurgitation	___ Fasting
_____	_____	_____	___ Self-Induced Vomiting	___ Other (specify)
			___ _____	___ _____
			Comments_____	
			_____	

FIGURE 13–19. Nutritional assessment form. (Used with permission of AMI Saint Joseph Center for Mental Health)

Continued

Diet History

24-Hour Diet Recall -- _____ Home

_____ Hospital

Supplements -- _____ Self-Prescribed

_____ Physician Ordered

Kind and Amount

_____

_____

_____

_____

Nutrient Total/24 Hour -- RDA

Calories _____   _____

Protein (gm)_____   _____

Other _____   _____

_____   _____

_____   _____

Assessment Summary_____

_____

_____

_____

_____

_____

_____

_____

_____

_____

_____

Plan _____

_____

_____

_____

_____

_____

_____

_____

_____

Name _____ Title_____ Date_____

FIGURE 13–19 Continued.

CHART 2
Altered Nutrition, Less than Body Requirements: Summary of the Nursing Process

NURSING INTERVENTIONS	OUTCOME CRITERIA

NURSING DIAGNOSIS: ALTERED NUTRITION, LESS THAN BODY REQUIREMENTS, RELATED TO DECREASED MOTIVATION

CLIENT GOAL: DEMONSTRATE AN INCREASED ENERGY LEVEL IN ORDER TO ADEQUATELY MEET OWN ADL'S, INCLUDING NUTRITIONAL NEEDS

Provide high-calorie, easy-to-eat foods Use a cognitive approach to improve motivation 　Invite client to attend meals with staff members 　If client refuses, discuss reasons for refusal 　Objectively review each reason with client in light of its ability to produce self-enhancing versus self-defeating behaviors for the client 　Encourage client to go to meals, then re-evaluate how client feels rather than making a judgment about how client feels Do not reinforce the client's passivity by decreasing the expectations of the client—continue to place supportive but firm expectations to complete ADLs; i.e., eating. Do not force to attend meals by comments as "if you don't eat, we will have to tube feed you" Avoid cliches and false reassurances when trying to encourage client to attend meals; e.g., "dinner will make you feel better" Give positive "strokes" for any attendance at meals Do not give positive reinforcement for comments such as: "I can't eat" or "I don't have any energy" or "It won't help anyway" Develop a schedule of low-impact aerobic-type exercise (i.e. walking) for 20 minutes/day 　Point out how exercise can increase motivation and increase appetite 　Use walking time as 1:1 relationship time and/or socialization time	Attends each meal with peers or staff members Voices having increased energy to meet nutritional needs Verbalizes the connection between levels of motivation and ensuing behaviors

NURSING DIAGNOSIS: ALTERED NUTRITION, LESS THAN BODY REQUIREMENTS, RELATED TO ANXIETY

CLIENT GOAL: DEMONSTRATE A REDUCED LEVEL OF ANXIETY

Provide finger foods or other easy-to-eat foods Discuss connection between feelings of anxiety and somatic complaints e.g., loss of appetite, upset stomach Discuss anxiety-producing events with client Explore alternatives to present methods of handling stressors Use meal time as a socialization time—avoid a discussion of client's problems and issues Choose a relaxing atmosphere in which to attend meals—if possible, avoid meals on the unit Assist client to decrease stress around meal times	Maintains nutritional intake Verbalizes a connection between anxiety and physical symptoms Verbalizes ways to cope with stressors

NURSING DIAGNOSIS: ALTERED NUTRITION, LESS THAN BODY REQUIREMENTS, RELATED TO LOSS OF APPETITE

CLIENT GOAL: ATTAIN/MAINTAIN BODY WEIGHT WITHIN NORMAL LIMITS FOR HEIGHT AND AGE GROUP

Monitor weight weekly Monitor caloric intake Refer to nutritionist to determine appropriate daily caloric intake based on age, lifestyle, and activity level Collaborate with physician to provide a daily vitamin/mineral supplement If client cannot tolerate three regular meals, work out a schedule of smaller, more frequent meals with high nutritional content	Attains a weight range appropriate for height and age Consumes appropriate caloric intake (as determined by nutritionist) on a daily basis Laboratory values remain within normal limits

(Continued)

gies must be individualized. Chart 2 summarizes possible nursing interventions for the related factors anergia, anxiety, cognitive impairment or lack of judgment, and psychotropic medication side effects.

The means necessary to assist the client to achieve adequate nutrients may be as simple as removing distractions, providing a vitamin supplement, and offering finger foods to those who cannot sit still, or as complex as providing, in collaboration with the physician, intravenous or tube feedings. The methods used correlate

CHART 2 (*continued*)
Altered Nutrition, Less than Body Requirements: Summary of the Nursing Process

NURSING INTERVENTIONS	OUTCOME CRITERIA

NURSING DIAGNOSIS: ALTERED NUTRITION, LESS THAN BODY REQUIREMENTS, RELATED TO PSYCHOTROPIC MEDICATION SIDE EFFECTS

CLIENT GOAL: MAINTAIN APPROPRIATE NUTRITIONAL INTAKE DESPITE MEDICATION SIDE EFFECTS

Initiate medication teaching to discuss normal side effects and steps that can be taken by client to prevent or alleviate side effects:	Demonstrates minimal side effects of medication Maintains appropriate caloric intake despite side effects of medication
Dry mouth	
Educate client re:	
Drinking 6–8 glasses (8 oz.) of fluid/day	
Rinsing mouth daily with mild mouthwash	
Chewing sugarless gum or sucking on sugarless hard candy when experiencing dry mouth	
Avoiding acidic foods; e.g., tomatoes, if developing mouth sores	
Monitor closely for dry mouth/mouth sores	
Nausea/vomiting/gastric distress	
Educate client re:	
Taking medications with meals	
Avoiding spicy foods	
Monitor clients with these symptoms; if symptoms continue, collaborate with physician to alter dosage	
Monitor symptoms and discuss with physician	
Constipation	
Provide high-fiber diet	
Encourage intake of 6–8 glasses (8 oz.) of fluids/day	
Encourage daily exercise (walking)	
Monitor intake and output	
Monitor bowel sounds for paralytic ileus	

NURSING DIAGNOSIS: ALTERED NUTRITION, LESS THAN BODY REQUIREMENTS, RELATED TO COGNITIVE IMPAIRMENTS

CLIENT GOAL: MAINTAIN AN APPROPRIATE NUTRITIONAL INTAKE DESPITE COGNITIVE IMPAIRMENT

Assessment level of ADL impairment due to cognitive impairment	Demonstrates no weight loss
Based on client's level of judgment, staff may have to provide direct assistance in the client's selections of appropriate food and actual eating process	
If hallucinations or delusions are paranoid in nature:	Complies with medication regime
Allow the client the opportunity to choose own foods from a buffet	
Provide foods that the client can open; i.e., milk carton instead of glass of milk	
Collaborate with physician on the administration of a medication that will decrease anxiety and control hallucinations or delusions	
On discharge, refer the client to a home meal program; i.e., Meals on Wheels, if the client cannot meet own nutritional needs	

directly with the severity of the nutritional difficulties. They may include:

Daily monitoring of client's nutritional intake and output;

Referral to a nutritionist for the purpose of developing a dietary plan suitable to the client's physical status, lifestyle, age, height, and present weight;

Incorporation of the client's likes and dislikes and sociocultural and religious eating preferences when setting up a dietary plan;

Collaboration with the physician and nutritionist to provide a daily vitamin and mineral supplement, as well as a dietary plan;

Weekly or daily weighings;

Monitoring serum electrolyte values.

Evaluation

Evaluation of the client's status is based on the client's ability to ingest a diet that is adequate in nutrients for the client's height, weight, age, physical status, and lifestyle. Second, evaluation is based on the alleviation of factors contributing to the client's compromised nutritional status (Chart 2).

CASE STUDY

Kathleen, a 20-year-old woman, was admitted to a local psychiatric facility on the advice of her family. Kathleen's parents stated that she had appeared "paranoid" and suspicious of her family since breaking up with her boyfriend of 2 years. Kathleen accused the family of turning her boyfriend against her, whereas the parents stated that they liked the young man. Furthermore, they noticed that Kathleen refused to go out with her friends because she believed that these friends no longer liked her. In addition to manifesting these behaviors, Kathleen had lost 20 pounds over the last 2 months. When weight loss was explored with Kathleen, she became angry and stated that she "knows that people are trying to get her." Kathleen had also manifested poor sleeping, decreased concentration in school, and poor follow-through with work assignments. Her admitting diagnosis was schizophreniform disorder.

During the course of hospitalization, Kathleen was noted to be experiencing auditory hallucinations. She heard voices telling her that her friends were jealous of her and trying to kill her by poisoning her food. As a result, Kathleen refused to eat, leading to a further weight loss of 3 pounds during the first week of hospitalization. One of the nursing diagnoses identified was altered nutrition, less than body requirements, related to hallucinations. During the first week of hospitalization, Kathleen was given chlorpromazine 100 mg four times daily. While on this medication, she complained of a number of side effects, including dry mouth. Nursing interventions focused on reassuring Kathleen that an environnment would be provided that would keep her safe. This included thorough explanations of all medications and a discussion of the fact that these medications could help rid her of the disturbing voices and thoughts. Furthermore, the staff allowed Kathleen freedom in choosing foods that she could open or unwrap herself. Evaluation of Kathleen's status involved a daily monitoring of caloric intake along with a weekly weighing. To supplement Kathleen's inadequate nutrient intake, the nurses in collaboration with the physician supplemented her intake with daily vitamins and minerals.

A one-to-one relationship with a consistent primary nurse was established with the goal of exploring the connections between Kathleen's feelings of anxiety over her break-up with her boyfriend and her thought patterns and behaviors. Her primary nurse focused on ways Kathleen could control her thoughts and find alternative ways to deal with stress. Finally, medication teaching was implemented on ways to alleviate the annoying side effects of dry mouth.

Kathleen did demonstrate improvement in the ability to control her own thoughts and understand that these thoughts had no basis in reality. She was able to reality test her family's reactions to her former boyfriend and to find alternative ways to cope with her grieving. She was compliant on medications and reported a decrease in the side effects after 2 to 3 weeks. Finally, over a 4-week period, Kathleen gained 7 of the 23 pounds that she had lost. She was able to eat three well-balanced meals plus one snack per day.

SUMMARY

With the exception of eating disorders, little is mentioned in the literature regarding the altered nutritional intake of the psychiatric client. However, the manifestations of an inadequate intake could become a serious sequela to many psychiatric disorders and treatments. The psychiatric mental health nurse can play a key role in both detection and intervention for the client experiencing alteration in nutrition, less than body requirements. The psychiatric mental health nurse must be aware of the dynamic interplay between emotions, cognitive status, and eating behaviors, as well as the physiological effects of psychotropic medications on nutritional intake.

Research Highlights

A number of concerns surface when evaluating the nutritional needs and requirements for the hospitalized psychiatric client. Two questions that arise are: (1) are the menus nutritionally sound? and (2) if hospitals provide nutritionally sound meals, do psychiatric clients choose a well-balanced diet? Ryan and Rao[24] conducted a study of the nutritional content of the menus in a state-operated versus a privately operated psychiatric facility in order to analyze the nutritional and caloric content of the daily menus. Using a t-test analysis, a comparison of the mean nutrient composition of each hospital's menus was conducted. The results indicated that: (1) the overall content of each menu averaged between 2300 and 2400 calories per day; (2) the percentage of fat was slightly high for both hospital menus in comparison with the RDA requirements; and (3) the overall vitamin and mineral content of each daily menu was adequate as judged by the RDA standards. These findings present no real surprise in that most hospitals employ nutritional staff capable of planning an array of well-balanced meals. However, despite this finding, the researchers noted that many psychiatric clients, although gaining weight, did not take in appropriate nutrients. This study addresses the fact that planning well-balanced meals is only one step in providing adequate nutritional care for the psychiatric client. Issues such as previous eating habits, motivation level, cognitive functioning, lifestyle, psychiatric disorder, and treatment have a tremendous impact on the client's ability to meet nutritional requirements.

References

1. American Psychiatric Association. Diagnostic and Statistical Manual of Mental Disorders. 3rd ed, rev. Washington, DC: American Psychiatric Association; 1987.
2. AMI Saint Joseph Center for Mental Health, Nutritional Screening Form. Omaha, NE: 1988.
3. AMI Saint Joseph Center for Mental Health, Nutritional Assessment Form. Omaha, NE: 1988.
4. Arego DE, Koch S. Malnutrition in the rehabilitation setting. Nutrition Today. 1988;22(4):28–32.
5. Berdanier CD. The many faces of stress. Nutrition Today. 1987;20(2):12–17.
6. Carney MWP, Ravindram A, Rinsler MG, Williams DG. Thiamine, riboflavin, pyridoxine deficiency in psychiatric in-patients. Br J Psychiatry. 1988;141:271–272.
7. Cash T, Winstead B, Jana L. The great American shape-up. Psychology Today. 1986;20:30–37.
8. Cronin FJ, Shaw AM. Summary of dietary recommendations for healthy Americans. Nutrition Today. 1988;22(6):26–33.
9. Drews TR. The 350 Second Diseases/Disorders to Alcoholism. South Plainfield, NJ: Bridge Publishing; 1985.
10. Hancock L. Schizophrenia in primary care. Nurse Practitioner. 1987;12(1):8–19.
11. Hsu G. The treatment of anorexia nervosa. Am J Psychiatry. 1986;143:573–581.
12. Illowsky BP, Kirch DG. Polydipsia and hyponatremia in psychiatric patients. Am J Psychiatry. 1988;145:675–683.
13. Kim MJ, McFarland GK, McLane AM. Pocket Guide to Nursing Diagnosis. 3rd ed. St. Louis: CV Mosby Co; 1989.
14. Kunes–Connell M. Adolescent disorders. In: Norris J, Kunes–Connell M, Stockard S, Ehrhart P, Newton G. Mental Health–Psychiatric Nursing: A Continuum of Care. New York: John Wiley and Sons; 1987.
15. Larocca FE. Eating Disorders: Effective Care and Treatment. St. Louis: Ishiyaku Euroamerica; 1986.
16. Loebl S, Spratto GR. The Nurse's Drug Handbook. 4th ed. New York: John Wiley and Sons; 1986.
17. Manderino MA, Bzdek VM. Mobilizing depressed clients. J Psychosoc Nurs Ment Health Serv. 1986;24(5):23–28.
18. Mayes SD, Humphrey FJ, Handford HA, Mitchell JF. Rumination disorder: Differential diagnosis. J Am Acad Child Adolesc Psychiatry. 1988;27:300–302.
19. Monaghan M. Fluoxetine's anorexic effects. Psychiatric Pharmacy Newsletter. Omaha, Creighton School of Pharmacy 1988;1(4):2.
20. Pagliaro AM, Pagliro LA. Pharmacologic Aspects of Nursing. St. Louis: CV Mosby; 1986.
21. Prim RG. Water intoxication and psychosis syndrome: Clinical cautions. J Psychosoc Nurs Ment Health Serv. 1988;26(11):16–18.
22. Pyke J, Page J. Long term care for the chronic schizophrenic patient. Canadian Nurse. 1982;78:37–44.
23. Roe DA. Dimensions of risk assessment for drug and nutrient interactions. Nutrition Today. 1987;20(6):20–24.
24. Ryan C, Rao L. Nutrition and the psychiatric patient. Psychiatric Hospital. 1987;18(4):163–166.
25. Thompson EA. Anxiety: A mental health vital sign. In: Longo DC, Williams RA. Clinical Practice in Psychosocial Nursing: Assessment and Intervention. 2nd ed. Norwalk, Conn: Appleton-Century-Crofts; 1986.
26. Thorn GW, Adams RD, Brunwald E, Isselbacher KJ, Petersdorf RG. Principles of Internal Medicine. 8th ed. New York: McGraw-Hill; 1977.

PARENTING, ALTERED
(ACTUAL, POTENTIAL)

Ellen Frances Olshansky

DEFINITION AND DESCRIPTION

Parenting requires caring, protecting, and nurturing to provide an environment that fosters development of a child's physical, cognitive, and emotional competencies.[2] *Altered parenting* is defined as a condition in which a nurturing person's ability to create and maintain a constructive environment that promotes optimum growth and development of another person is altered or at risk.[26] The distinction between actual and potential parenting alterations is important. *Potential* parenting alterations refers to those conditions making a person at risk for such problems, whereas *actual* parenting alterations refers to those conditions under which a person is currently experiencing such problems.

The factors influencing such alteration or risk may occur during the prenatal, as well as the child-rearing, period.[23] Parental role attainment may, in itself, pose certain risks to the process of parenting, for this transition represents a major developmental stage and crisis period to those confronted with it.[6,7,20,29,35,38] The condition of altered parenting, both actual and potential, involves not only the parent, or nurturing figure, but the infant or child being nurtured. This interactional approach highlights the importance of understanding the diagnosis of altered parenting within a family context. Early identification of this diagnosis and appropriate interventions are important in prevention of later mental health problems in both the child and the adult.

THEORY AND RESEARCH

Current research studies cite theoretical explanations for the occurrence of parenting alterations that can be clustered into several categories. Several of them examine parent–infant attachment and interaction.[3,12,18] Some investigators focus on the attainment of the maternal role[33,36] and, more recently, on the paternal role,[17,25,30] on social support,[17,34] on knowledge deficits or unrealistic expectations,[32,39] and on physiologic and emotional conditions in parent or infant.[24] Each of these research categories will be discussed in turn.

Parent–infant attachment is a concept that has been studied extensively in the past several years. Klaus and Kennell,[27] Ainsworth,[1] and Bowlby[9,10] conducted initial classic work in attachment, followed by more current research by Barnard,[3] Curry,[18] and Mercer,[31–33] who have conducted nursing research in this area. Parent–infant attachment has been studied to better understand alterations in parenting as a result of impaired parent–infant attachment. The consistent finding is that, over time, a reciprocal relationship must occur in which the parents respond appropriately to their infant's cues and provide care and nurture growth and development according to those cues. In response to this nurturing and caring by the parents, the infant continues to give them appropriate cues. An impairment in this reciprocal relationship is one explanation for why parenting alterations occur. It is important to point out, however, that parent–infant attachment is culturally influenced, and there may be differences in how parents and infants demonstrate attachment based on their cultural backgrounds.

Parental role attainment is a process that occurs over time, sometimes beginning even before conception with planning for pregnancy. As a woman begins to attain the maternal role, she is also becoming attached to her new fetus/baby. Cranley[16] has developed a tool to measure maternal attachment during pregnancy, and has used a modified version of that tool to develop a measure of paternal–fetal attachment.[40] Mercer,[33] following Rubin's[36] classic work, studied the attainment of the maternal role extensively. In her large study of mothers grouped according to age, Mercer found that a pattern of attainment of the maternal role existed with a peak in role attainment behaviors at four months postpartum and a decline at eight months. Feelings of role incompetency surfaced at eight months when, it is suggested, the infant's developmental behaviors become much more challenging for the mothers.

Recently, fathers have also been studied, although much more research is needed in this area. Cronenwett and Kunst–Wilson[17] examined transition to the paternal role. May[30] studied expectant fathers' involvement in pregnancy, and Jordan[25] is studying first-time fathers' experience of pregnancy and parenthood, finding that fathers often desperately want more involvement in the pregnancy process. Less than optimal attainment of the maternal or paternal role may be an explanation for the occurrence of alterations in parenting, although, again, as with attachment behaviors, there are cultural variations in what is considered to be "optimal."

Cronenwett and Kunst–Wilson[17] conducted a study on the influence of social support and stress on the transition to fatherhood. Norbeck and Tilden[34] have done much work in the area of social support as it relates to mothering. The lack of social support has been identified as an important variable in actual or potential parenting alterations.

Knowledge deficits or unrealistic expectations on the part of parents present another major area of study related to parenting alterations. Mothers' perceptions of their infants' capabilities were examined[39] and correlated with actual performance on the part of the infants. The major finding was that infants often did not perform to their highest potential because mothers were not always aware that their infants were so capable and, therefore, did not expect as much from them. It is important to highlight that this sample was composed of mothers who believed, antenatally, their infants were capable of much less than they actually were able to do. This raises the question of whether or not mothers with unrealistically high expectations of their infants will create "super" infants, but evidence seems to be that this is not so. Mercer[32] examined postpartum mothers' views of themselves, comparing ideal with real views and related this to parenting. She found that postpartum women must go through a process of "grief work" in which they reconcile their actual baby with their fantasy baby, as well as reconcile their postpartum body with their fantasy body. Mercer believes that the process of reconciling these antenatal fantasies is key in allowing the woman to view herself as the mother of her infant.

Extensive research has been conducted on the impact of physiologic defects in children on parenting. Mercer[31] studied parents of children with defects. Less work has been done on the influence of physical defects in one or both parents on their parenting behaviors. Infants and children with emotional difficulties, too, have been studied to determine the influence such difficulties have on parenting behaviors. Recent work has revealed that mothers who are depressed may have difficulties in parenting.

To summarize, there are many reasons that parenting alterations may occur. Some major reasons are impaired parental–infant attachment and interaction, difficulty in attaining the parental role, inadequate social support, unrealistic expectations on the part of the parents or the children regarding one another, and physiologic or emotional problems in infant or parent. These factors are usually interrelated.

RELATED FACTORS

Related factors for actual altered parenting or risk factors for potential altered parenting may arise from the presence of a high-risk child, or the presence of a high-risk parent, or a high-risk condition in both child and parent.[24] Box 13-7 lists several of these high-risk conditions in both parent and child.

Many infant or child factors are related to alterations in parenting. For example, an unwanted child or a child of an undesired sex may contribute to difficulties in parenting behavior, as parents may have difficulty or resent parenting their unwanted child. Abnormalities in the child may also contribute to alterations in parenting. A child with a physical or mental handicap, or a terminally ill child can pose difficulties to parents, and a child with severe behavioral problems may be an important factor in parenting alterations.

Many parent characteristics are also related to alterations in parenting. For example, a parent who is an adolescent or is single may encounter greater risk for difficulty in parenting. A parent who is an alcoholic or drug addict, too, is at risk for difficulties in parenting. Emotionally disturbed or abusive persons, as well as physically ill or disabled persons, are at risk for alterations in parenting. Recently, questions have been raised about the issue of balancing career and family, with potentially competing demands from parenting and career responsibilities. However, it would be inaccurate to categorize this issue as contributing to alterations in parenting, as more and more individuals and couples are successfully, although often not without difficulty, doing this.

In addition to the factors in both infant or child and parent, situational factors may exist that can contribute to parenting alterations. These factors include physical separation from the nuclear family, or from the extended family, and difficulties in relationships, particu-

---

BOX 13–7
Risk Factors for Potential Alterations in Parenting

CONDITIONS IN INFANT OR CHILD

Pregnancy at risk for infant mortality, neonatal mortality, postneonatal mortality
Preterm infant or low-birth-weight infant
Physically or mentally handicapped child
Failure-to-thrive child
Hyperactive child
Terminally ill child

CONDITIONS IN PARENT(S)

Abusing or battering parent
Alcoholic parent
Addicted parent
Adolescent parent
Single parent
Emotionally disturbed parent
Terminally ill parent
Sensory defects (e.g., vision)
Chronic illness

(Adapted from Johnson SH. High risk parenting: nursing assessment and strategies for the family at risk, 2nd ed. Philadelphia: JB Lippincott, 1986.)

larly the marital relationship. Relationship problems include marital discord, divorce, separation, which may lead to lack of support between or from significant others. The presence of stepparents, live-in lovers, and relocation[15] may be other risk factors for parenting alterations. Other changes in the family unit may contribute to parenting alterations as well. Such changes include the addition of a new child to a family with children, possibly posing a threat to the already existing child(ren) and posing challenges to parents. Having a relative move into the household can also create a stressful situation for the family and, particularly, for parents.

Other situational factors related to alterations in parenting, or those that can be risk factors related to potential alterations in parenting, include economic problems such as unemployment and lack of resources. Also, lack of knowledge and limited cognitive functioning pose problems for parents. Situations, such as multiple births or a high-risk pregnancy, may lead to alterations in parenting.

A number of risk factors can be identified for potential alterations in parenting. Such risk factors include parental history of ineffective relationships with one's own parents and a history of abusive relationship with one's own parents. A history of ineffective relationships with one's own parents may also contribute to lack of available role models or ineffective role models for parenting. Unrealistic expectations on the part of the parents and the child may contribute to parenting difficulties. For example, the parents may have unrealistic expectations of a child, or of themselves in terms of parenting. They may also have unrealistic expectations of their spouses or partners. The child may have unrealistic expectations of his or her parent(s).

DEFINING CHARACTERISTICS

Several behaviors on the part of parents are defining characteristics of altered parenting. In addition, some behaviors may be manifestations of potential altered parenting. Three critical defining characteristics of actual parenting alterations are lack of attention to the needs of the infant or child; inappropriate caretaking behaviors related to feeding, toilet training, and providing sleep and rest; and a parental history of abuse or abandonment by the parent's own caretaker.[26]

In addition, many other behaviors heighten the nurse's concern that difficulties in parenting may occur or are already occurring. Such characteristics are lack of parental attachment behaviors, indicated by inappropriate visual, tactile, or auditory stimulation; identification of negative characteristics of an infant or child; and negative attachment of meanings to characteristics of the infant or child.[15,26] Such negative attachment of meanings can be manifested in the parents verbalizing their disappointment in the child's gender or physical characteristics, as well as verbalizing resentment toward the child. Additional behaviors that are strong indicators of parenting alterations are parent's verbalization of disgust at the child's bodily func-

tions, failure to comply with health care appointments for the child as well as the self, and utilizing multiple caretakers, without having one or two persons (e.g., the parents) as primary caretakers for the child. Inappropriate discipline practices or frequent accidents or illnesses on the part of the child may indicate problems with parenting and potential child abuse. Likewise, a lag in the child's growth and development may be indicative of problems. If the parent verbalizes role inadequacy or compulsively seeks role approval from others, this could potentially reflect difficulties with parenting.

The aforementioned characteristics are indicators of potential parenting alterations. It is essential to note that a nursing diagnosis of altered parenting based on one or two of those characteristics would not be valid. Of particular importance, here, is the characteristic of verbalizing disappointment or resentment toward the child. A certain amount of verbalized disappointment may be healthy, because it may be evidence that parents are grieving the loss of their fantasy child, as mentioned by Mercer,[32] to be able to move on to attach to their real child. Thus, it is important to assess these defining characteristics in the larger context. However, their occurrence would alert the nurse to seek other indicators that would confirm or refute the diagnosis of altered parenting.

Certain defining characteristics, though, are considered indicative of actual alterations in parenting: abandonment of the child, a runaway child, verbalization by the parents that they cannot control the child, and evidence of physical and psychological trauma.[26]

Chart 1 summarizes the related factors, as well as the defining characteristics of alterations in parenting as a nursing diagnosis.

NURSING PROCESS AND RATIONALE

Assessment

The nursing process is continuous and ongoing, for, as mentioned previously, it is difficult to make a diagnosis based on one or two isolated instances. A pattern of behavior must be identified before making an actual diagnosis. A potential diagnosis may be made if more definitive data are necessary to establish an actual diagnosis.

To assess any indications of alterations in parenting, the nurse must be alert to many factors. These factors can be categorized according to context variables and person variables.[2] The nurse might ask the following questions in relation to the context variables, which are adapted from Barnard[2] (the words "parent" and "she" are used interchangeably here, as much of this research is directed at mothers):

1. How old is the parent? If the parent is under age 18, it is likely that she is single, less educated, smokes, has limited prenatal care, has less social

CHART 1
Altered Parenting (Actual): Definition, Related Factors, and Defining Characteristics[15,26]

DEFINITION

Condition in which the nurturing person's (parent's) ability to create and maintain a constructive environment that promotes optimum growth and development of another person (infant, child) is altered.

RELATED FACTORS

Factors Related to the Infant or Child

Unwanted child
Child of undesired sex
Physical or mental abnormalities in child
Child with severe behavioral problems
Unrealistic expectations on part of infant or child

Factors Related to the Parent(s)

Adolescent parent
Single parent
Alcoholic parent
Drug-addicted parent
Abusive parent
Emotionally disturbed parent
Physically ill or disabled parent
Parental history of ineffective relationships
Unrealistic expectations on part of parent(s)
Lack of knowledge, skills, and limited cognitive functioning

Factors Related to Situational Conditions

Physical separation from nuclear family or from extended family
Difficulties in relationship(s), particularly marital

Presence of stepparent, live-in lovers
Relocation
Addition of new child to a family with children
Having a relative move into household
Economic problems (unemployment, lack of resources)

Other Factors

Multiple births
High-risk pregnancy

DEFINING CHARACTERISTICS

Lack of attention to the needs of the infant or child
Inappropriate caretaking behaviors (related to feeding, toilet training, providing sleep and rest)
Parental history of abuse or abandonment by own parent(s)
Lack of parental attachment behaviors (inappropriate visual, tactile, or auditory stimulation; negative identification of characteristics of infant or child; negative attachment of meanings to characteristics of infant or child)
Parents' verbalization of disgust at child's bodily functions
Failure of parents to comply with health-care appointments for child and self
Utilizing multiple caretakers without having one or two designated primary caretakers
Inconsistent and inappropriate discipline practices
Frequent accidents or illnesses on part of child
Lag in child's growth and development
Verbalization by parent of role inadequacy and compulsively seeking approval from others

---

support, greater life stress, lower socioeconomic status, children with behavioral and learning problems, poor parent–child interaction, when compared with a parent over 18.

2. What is the parent's educational level? If she has less than a high school education, she likely provides less stimulation to her child, has less social support, has less than realistic developmental expectations of her child when compared with a high school graduate.

3. What is the parent's ethnic background? If she is a disadvantaged minority, she has fewer resources available to her.

4. What is the parent's marital status? If she has no spouse or partner, she may be socially isolated.

5. What is the parent's financial status? If she is at the poverty level, she may have less social support, poorer prenatal care, and increased incidence of preterm birth.

6. Does the parent have other children, and if so, how closely spaced are they to one another? A parent with more than one child is likely to devote less attention to subsequent children, may be more depressed, and may expose the child to more noise and television.

7. Does the parent have access to transportation and to a telephone? Limited transportation or lack of a telephone predispose the parent to social isolation, depression, and more abusive relationships with the child(ren).

8. Has the parent been in situations in which she or he was abused or neglected? Prior abuse or neglect predisposes the parent to be less sensitive to cues from the child and less positive in her or his interaction with the child.

9. Has the parent experienced frequent life changes? Frequent changes are associated with less social competence.

10. Are there chronic family problems? Chronic family problems can lead to poorer child outcomes.

11. How many moves has the parent made? More than three moves per year predisposes the parent to social isolation and poorer developmental outcomes in the child.

The nurse might ask the following questions in relation to the person variables:[2]

1. If the parent is in a relationship with a spouse or partner, how stable is this relationship? Lack of stability in personal relationships is associated with less life and parenting satisfaction.
2. What is the general health of the parent? Poor parental health is associated with smoking and drug use and abuse; and frequent illnesses make the parent less available to the child and more depressed, leading to poorer family relations.
3. What was the birth weight of the child? A child who was born at a lower-than-average weight has a greater chance of having neurologic impairment, developmental problems, and is more susceptible to a poor environment.
4. What was the general health status of the child at birth? Poor infant health negatively influences parents' expectations of the child and interferes with the child's developmental process.

In addition to making an assessment based on the previous questions, the use of Gordon's[23] functional categories for nursing diagnoses is an effective way of systematically assessing the parent(s) and child(ren). The use of certain instruments is very helpful also, such as the NCAST Feeding and Teaching Scales,[4,5] HOME,[13,14] Feetham Family Functioning Survey,[21,22] and the Personal Resource Questionnaire.[11] Table 13-7 summarizes these instruments.

Nursing Diagnoses

If problems exist, a thorough assessment will reveal several relevant nursing diagnoses. Examples of some are altered parenting related to mother's use of alcohol or drugs, being single, being an adolescent, and having unrealistic expectations for a child who may or may not have multiple abnormalities. Many related factors may occur simultaneously, such as altered parenting related to being an adolescent, as well as to being single, and to having less than a high school education.

Client Goals and Interventions

The goals for the client involve easing situations that contribute to altered parenting. Various interventions may be appropriate. Interventions are often categorized according to giving information and monitoring, supporting, referring, and giving therapy for specific diagnoses. For example, information may be very appropriate on parenting skills and infant behavior, on childbirth, on planning for a new family member and preparing other children, and on what supports are available to the family. Support may be necessary regarding changing roles in the family secondary to parenting, seeking appropriate support, and clarifying one's ideas and beliefs about parenting. Referral may be necessary for marital or family counseling, social service, and child abuse or neglect. Specific therapy would be chosen depending upon the specific related factors and defining characteristics. For example, in the case study that follows it can be seen that specific therapy would center around increasing parents' time, such that social support could be sought, as well as encouraging father's involvement with the infants.

Evaluation

Evaluation of the interventions described would include noting increased involvement by the parent who was not previously involved in child care, as well as the ability of both parents to seek and use social support. Fewer complaints by the parents and evidence of more satisfying interactions with their infants will also indicate effectiveness of interventions. Verbalization by one or both parents that they are enjoying caring for and nurturing their infant is further evidence of effectiveness of interventions (Chart 2).

TABLE 13-7
Summary of selected instruments for assessment of parenting

INSTRUMENT	ASSESSMENT
Feetham Family Functioning Survey	Allows systematic assessment of relationships within families that influence or are influenced by the way the family functions[22]
Home Observation for Measurement of the Environment (HOME)	Measures specific aspects of the family's home environment that influences emotional development of child from birth through six years of age[14]
Nursing Child Assessment Feeding Scale (NCAFS)	Measures maternal–infant interaction while mother feeds her infant[4]
Nursing Child Assessment Teaching Scale (NCATS)	Measures maternal–infant interaction while mother teaches a particular task to her infant[5]
Personal Resource Questionnaire	Measures supportive resources available to person(s)[11]

CASE STUDY*

The following case study describes a family with twin babies during the first six months of the babies' lives.

Sue and Tim are twins born vaginally at 29 weeks. Sue experienced respiratory distress, requiring mechanical ventilation and oxygen for three weeks, and was discharged at five weeks. Tim also experienced respiratory distress at birth and required mechanical ventilation and oxygen for five weeks. In addition, he had a grade II intracranial hemor-

* Presented with permission from Deborah Padgett, R.N., M.N., a clinician in the Nursing Systems Towards Effective Parenting of Prematures (NSTEP-P) Project, developed by NCAST.

CHART 2
Altered Parenting: Summary of the Nursing Process

NURSING INTERVENTIONS	OUTCOME CRITERIA
CLIENT GOAL: IMPROVE PARENTING SKILLS Assess clients' level of knowledge Assess and monitor clients' skill level Support and encourage clients in trying new tasks or skills Refer when necessary (e.g., to parent support group)	Reports feeling confident in tasks and skills of parenting Demonstrates improved abilities
CLIENT GOAL: IMPROVE PARENT–INFANT INTERACTION Assess interaction that occurs between parent(s) and infant(s) Support parents in their efforts Reassure parents Teach parents about infant cues Refer when necessary (as above)	Parents and infants demonstrate ability to respond to one another's cues Parents verbalize understanding of infant cues
FAMILY GOAL: INCREASE SOCIAL SUPPORT Assess and monitor support that is available Teach parents ways to improve time management such that it is possible to seek social support Inform parents about resources available for support Refer parents to appropriate supportive resources (as above)	Parents demonstrate and verbalize ability to seek support Parents demonstrate ability to be more efficient with their time to enable them to seek out supportive resources

rhage and a surgically corrected patent ductus arteriosus. He was discharged at six weeks.

The mother works full time as a laboratory technician on the 3 P.M. to 11 P.M. shift, and the father is a full-time student. The family's social support is limited. The mother is the primary caretaker of the twins. The father assists with caretaking, but his priority is his studies. The infants cried a great deal during their first two months of life, and the mother said it was difficult for her to console them because of her fatigue. The father stated it was difficult for him to console them because of his lack of knowledge about this and his need to study. The Feetham Family Functioning Survey indicated that the mother was frustrated with the lack of time for spouse and children and disagreements with her husband over parenting approaches. Measurement by the Personal Resource Questionnaire revealed that the family lacked adequate social support.

The family's environment consists of a two-bedroom apartment, with a small, fenced yard; the family owns a small dog. The Home Observation for Measurement of the Environment (HOME) revealed a score of 40 out of 45 points, with missed points because of not taking the infants out (e.g., to the grocery store) and the mother's lack of knowledge about developmentally stimulating toys and activities.

This case study revealed adequate data for a diagnosis of

Research Highlights

In studying parenting, it is essential that a diagnosis is not made based on a one-time occurrence, or on a one-time visit to a health-care provider. Patterns over time must be noted to accurately arrive at a diagnosis. Mercer's study[33] is an excellent example of identifying patterns over time. Her longitudinal study utilized four instruments to measure maternal role attainment at one month, four months, eight months, and twelve months postpartum. Three groups of women were studied according to age: 15- to 19-year olds, 20- to 29-year olds, and 30- to 42-year olds. The measures were: feelings about the baby (FAB),[28] gratification in the mothering role (GRAT),[37] maternal behaviors rated by the interviewer (MABE),[8] and ways of handling irritating child behaviors (WHIB).[20] The results of this study indicated certain patterns, but a positive linear increase in role attainment behaviors over the year was not noted. Instead, a peak in these behaviors (demonstrating feelings of love for the baby, gratification in the maternal role, observed maternal behavior, and self-reported ways of handling irritating child behaviors) was noted at four months, and then declined at eight months.

This is very important information, as parenting must be assessed as an ongoing interaction over time, and not as a one-sided approach on the part of the parents. Mercer's study suggests that the infants' developmental behaviors at eight months may pose a greater challenge to parenting and, thus, whereas certain parenting behaviors may decline at this time, these behavioral changes may be a normal response to the normal behavioral changes occurring in the babies. Thus, this study has important significance for nursing diagnosis, highlighting the need to assess the interaction between parents and their infants or children, taking into consideration the behavior of all participants in the interaction.

potential alterations in parenting. The father may appropriately be diagnosed with altered parenting related to decreased involvement in child care, knowledge and skill deficits in infant care, and priority for demands of schoolwork. The mother may appropriately be diagnosed with altered parenting related to the need to balance attention to each twin and to overtaxed time demands related to overload of work, home, and child care responsibilities. Possible interventions would include giving information on child care with attention to such things as appropriate toys to provide the infants that are developmentally stimulating, how to manage time to pursue social support, and how to effectively "juggle" attention between both infants. Support is necessary in regard to listening to the difficulties of giving attention "fairly" to both infants, the mother's difficulty in working full time and caring for the infants, the stresses in the marital relationship, and the lack of social support. Counseling, in the form of referral, may be necessary for the couple in dealing with some of the stressed aspects of their relationship. Specific groups, such as a new parents' group, new mothers' group, or a parents of twins group, may assist the family.

SUMMARY

Altered parenting occurs when the person(s) designated as parent is unable to meet the needs of the infant or child in an optimum manner. Current research reveals several categories of theoretical explanations for the occurrence of parenting alterations. These are disturbances in parent–infant attachment and interaction; difficulties in attainment of the parental role; lack of social support; knowledge deficits; and physiologic and emotional conditions in the parent or in the infant or child. Several defining characteristics and related factors contribute to a diagnosis of alterations in parenting. Such a diagnosis can be made accurately only over time, because patterns in behavior must be evident. Nursing interventions emphasize assessment of parenting behaviors, monitoring, giving information, supporting, referring when necessary, and giving therapy for specific diagnoses.

References

1. Ainsworth M. The development of infant–mother attachment. In: Caldwell BE, Riccuitu H, eds. Review of child development research. 3rd ed. Chicago: University of Chicago Press; 1973.
2. Barnard KB. Nursing process and diagnosis class notes, 1986.
3. Barnard KB. Nursing child assessment learning resource manual. Seattle: NCAST Publications; 1985.
4. Barnard KB. Nursing child assessment feeding scales (NCAFS). Seattle: NCAST Publications; 1979.
5. Barnard KB. Nursing child assessment teaching scales (NCATS). Seattle: NCAST Publications; 1979.
6. Belsky J. Transition to parenthood. Med Aspects Hum Sex. 1986;20:56–59.
7. Benedek T. Parenthood during the lifecycle. In: Anthony EJ,

8. Benedek T, eds. Parenthood: its psychology and psychopathology. Boston: Little, Brown, and Co; 1970.
9. Blank M. Some maternal influences on infants' rates of sensorimotor development. J Am Acad Child Psychiatry. 1964;3:668–687.
10. Bowlby J. Nature of a child's tie to his mother. Int J Psychoanal. 1958;39:350–373.
11. Bowlby J. Attachment and loss, vol 1. New York: Basic Books; 1969.
12. Brandt P, Weinert C. The PRQ: a social support measure. Nurs Res. 1981;30:277–288.
13. Brazelton TB, Koslowski B, Main M. Origins of reciprocity: the early mother–infant interaction. In: Lewis M, Rosenbloom LE, eds. Effect of the infant on its caregiver. New York: John Wiley & Sons; 1974.
14. Caldwell BM. Home observation of the environment inventory. Seattle: NCAST Publications; 1978.
15. Calloway SJ. Home observation of the environment. In: Humenick S, ed. Analysis of current assessment strategies in the health care of young children and childbearing families. Norwalk, CT: Appleton–Century–Crofts; 1982.
16. Carpenito LJ. Nursing diagnosis: application to clinical practice. Philadelphia: JB Lippincott; 1983.
17. Cranley MS. Development of a tool for the measurement of maternal attachment during pregnancy. Nurs Res. 1981;30:281–284.
18. Cronenwett LR, Kunst–Wilson W. Stress, social support, and the transition to fatherhood. Nurs Res. 1981;30:1966–201.
19. Curry MA. Maternal attachment behavior and the mother's self-concept: the effect of early skin-to-skin contact. Nurs Res. 1982;31:73–78.
20. Disbrow MA, Doerr HO, Caulfield C. Measuring the components of potential for child abuse and neglect. J Child Abuse Neglect Int J. 1977;1:279–296.
21. Dyer ED. Parenthood as crisis: a restudy. In: Parad HJ, ed. Crisis intervention: selected readings. New York: Family Service Association of America; 1965.
22. Feetham SL. The relationship of family functioning to infant, parent, and family environment outcomes in the first 18 months following the birth of an infant with myelodysplasia. [Doctoral Dissertation No. 80-20697], Michigan State University, 1980.
23. Feetham SL, Humenick SS. The Feetham family functioning survey. In: Humencik S, ed. Analysis of current assessment strategies in the health care of young children and childbearing families. Norwalk, CT: Appleton–Century–Crofts; 1982.
24. Gordon M. Nursing diagnosis: process and application. 2nd ed. New York: McGraw–Hill; 1985.
25. Johnson SH. Nursing assessment and strategies for the family at risk: high risk parenting. 2nd ed. Philadelphia: JB Lippincott; 1986.
26. Jordan PL. The experience and caring needs of expectant and new first time fathers. New Investigator Award Grant through the Division of Nursing, 1987.
27. Kim MJ, McFarland GK, McLane AM. Pocket guide to nursing diagnoses. 3rd ed. St. Louis: CV Mosby; 1989.
28. Klaus MH, Kennell JH. Maternal–infant bonding. St. Louis: CV Mosby; 1976.
29. Leifer M. Psychological changes accompanying pregnancy and motherhood. Genet Psychol Monogr. 1977;95:55–96.
30. LeMasters EE. Parenthood as crisis. In: Parad HJ, ed. Crisis intervention: selected readings. New York: Family Service Association of America; 1965.
31. May KA. Three phases in the development of father involvement in pregnancy. Nurs Res. 1982;31:337–342.

31. Mercer RT. Mothers' responses to their infants with defects. Nurs Res. 1974;23:133–137.

32. Mercer RT. The nurse and maternal tasks of early postpartum. MCN. 1981;6:341–345.

33. Mercer RT. The process of maternal role attainment over the first year. Nurs Res. 1985;34:198–204.

34. Norbeck JS, Tilden VP. Life stress, social support, and emotional disequilibrium in complications of pregnancy: a multivariate study. J Health Soc Behav. 1983;24:30–46.

35. Rossi AS. Transition to parenthood. J Marriage Fam. 1968;30:26–29.

36. Rubin R. Attainment of the maternal role, part I: processes. Nurs Res. 1967;16:237–245.

37. Russell CS. Transition to parenthood: problems and gratifications. J Marriage Fam. 1974;36:294–301.

38. Shereshefsky PM, Yarrow LJ. Psychological aspects of first pregnancy and early postnatal adaptation. New York: Raven Press; 1974.

39. Snyder C, Eyres S, Barnard K. New findings about mothers' antenatal expectations and their relationship to infant development. MCN. 1979;4:354–357.

40. Weaver RH, Cranley MS. An exploration of paternal–fetal attachment behavior. Nurs Res. 1983;32:68–72.

PERCEPTION/COGNITION, ALTERED

(CONFUSION, DELUSIONS, HALLUCINATIONS, MEMORY LOSS)

CONFUSION

Ethel Stitt Ekland

DEFINITION AND DESCRIPTION

Confusion is a condition in which clear and orderly thought is lacking, and distinctions among concepts, events, and people are indistinct. The client with confusion is unable to give a clear description of events and must rely on others to interpret happenings.[19] Confusion commonly concerns time, location, who is present, or what is transpiring but rarely the client's own identity. Various degrees of mental impairment with demonstrated deficits in memory, concentration, attention, orientation, comprehension, compliance, mood stability, and interpretation of the environment can be present.[15]

THEORY AND RESEARCH

Organic Causes

Cholinergic deficiency is the explanation for the confusion noted in a number of pathophysiological states. This deficiency is thought to occur because infection or fluid imbalance interferes with cerebral oxidative metabolism, resulting in a reduction in acetylcholine synthesis. Similarly, anticholinergic agents such as atropine and scopolamine can precipitate confusion. The fact that physostigmine salicylate, a cholinesterase inhibitor, has been used to reverse confusion lends weight to the explanation. Acute vascular lesions or other injuries to the brain may result in confusion.[12]

Rapid onset of confusion usually indicates a reversible physical cause such as infection or side effects of medication. With removal of the physical cause, such confusion disappears.[11] In contrast, global confusion with insidious onset is often indicative of irreversible dementia.[20] There can be overlap in the causes of confusion, or one cause can be superimposed on another.

For example, the confusion of delirium can occur in a person with irreversible dementia.

Stressors

Confusion can appear or be intensified in stressful situations. Stressors elevate the level of plasma cortisol, thus affecting attention and information processing.[12] This stress reaction narrows attention, such that peripheral cues are not attended to whereas central cues receive greater attention.[13] Individuals who already have difficulty giving attention have even greater difficulty paying attention to pertinent stimuli under additional stress.

Extremes of Sensory Input

Too much sensory input leading to confusion may come from internal sensations or from outside the person. Whether from internal or external sources, the person is overwhelmed by trying to process and organize unpredictable stimuli and becomes confused. All persons are thought to have a "pertinence" filter that refines incoming information. In normal persons, any new stimulation gets through for 2 seconds and then is filtered for 2 seconds so that the individual is not aware of the stimulus. Individuals who are especially vulnerable to overload do not filter out the nonpertinent stimuli, so that there is constant input. The intensity and unpredictability of the sensory input leads to the confusion.[18]

Insufficient sensory input can also cause confusion, because the person does not have enough information to understand the environment. Visual and auditory cues are used by most individuals to orient themselves to place and current happenings.[7] A decrease in sensory input may arise from hearing or vision problems or from other sensory deficits resulting from injury or changes with age. Alternatively, the person may not process incoming sensations, or the external environment may not give enough cues to orient the individuals, such as when someone is alone in a quiet, colorless room.

RELATED FACTORS

Conditions that can lead to confusion include metabolic diseases, endocrine diseases, fluid and electrolyte imbalance, oxygen deprivation, and brain injury. Stressors, especially change in environment or loss of a significant person, can precipitate confusion. Such stressors can be especially potent if they represent more sensory input than the individual can handle.

Too little sensory input can occur during social isolation or times of decreased environmental cues or from sensory organ decline. Social isolation may be voluntary or may be the result of few visitors, few familiar objects, and caretakers who spend little time with the individual.[14] Decreased environmental cues can occur in the dark, with decreased light, or when immobility limits the observable surroundings. As the sensory functions of hearing, vision, touch, taste, and smell decrease, the individual has difficulty perceiving the environment. With the misperception of the environment come misidentifications or illusions.[4,12]

Confusion can occur in a number of psychiatric conditions. It is especially probable in organic mental disorders or psychoactive substance use disorders.

Although confusion may occur at any age, acute confusion is more common in the very young and the elderly, as these age groups have a narrower range for optimal brain function and less tolerance of drug effects.[7,16] In addition, the elderly have more medical problems that increase the probability of alterations in cerebral metabolism, creating a more vulnerable brain environment. Irreversible confusion is most common in the elderly, for the elderly are more likely to experience some type of brain deficit. The likelihood of having a dementia-related diagnosis and the resultant confusion increases with age. However, confusion should not be considered an expected finding in the elderly. Any confusion or increase in the amount of confusion in a person of any age needs to be investigated.

DEFINING CHARACTERISTICS

Confused individuals exhibit a wide range of behavior. They may not know the correct time, date, month, year, or location; who is present; or what is transpiring. Not knowing the time or date could, of course, be temporary because of lack of access to a calendar or watch. Therefore, giving an incorrect month or year are more indicative of confusion. Confusion is also indicated by an individual insisting on any incorrect information, such as wrong time or location or misidentifying people, even when appropriate information has been given.

A number of behaviors seen in confusion are attempts to explain or order the world. For example, a client may assume that items that have been misplaced and cannot be found have been stolen and may accuse others of theft. Conversely, items may be taken from others because they are believed by the confused person to be his or her possessions. The confused person may go to the wrong room or use another's bed. He or she may walk about looking for someone or something or feeling compelled to carry out a task.

Not understanding what has transpired, the confused client may misinterpret the situation. There may be constant interruptions with repeated requests for information previously given. Other people's motives may be suspect. For example, a nurse who is giving medication may be accused of attempted poisoning, or the nurse assisting with physical care may be regarded as assaultive. Thus, the individual may scream, become agitated, or strike out. Behavior indicating anxiety, fear, or rage may occur—all in response to the environment as perceived by the confused client.

The confused person is distractible and has difficulty focusing attention. Other defining characteristics are hyperalert or hypoalert behavior, inability to follow instructions, talkativeness, mute behavior, or incoherent speech. The degree of difficulty can fluctuate throughout the day. Confusion, especially with restlessness and wandering, that increases with the fading light of evening is called *sundown syndrome*[5] (Chart 1).

NURSING PROCESS AND RATIONALE
Assessment

From the first interaction with the client, the nurse has an opportunity to assess for confusion. The nurse makes a quick assessment of the client's mental status with every contact. The assessment includes:

How does the client respond to the nurse's presence?
Does the client know his/her own name?
Does the client know where he/she is and what is transpiring?
Is the behavior typical for this client?

On the basis of client behavior during each interaction, the nurse can determine whether there is a change and whether further assessment for confusion is needed.

A careful history obtained from family and a review of already obtained data are part of the assessment of confusion. When did the confusion start? What events preceded the confusion? What areas of memory are affected? When is the confusion most apparent? A review of current medications, noting polypharmacy or the use of any anticholinergic drugs, may identify difficulties with cerebral metabolism. The history is reviewed for use of over-the-counter medications, street

CHART 1
Confusion: Definition, Related Factors, and Defining Characteristics

DEFINITION
Confusion is a condition in which clear and orderly thought is lacking and distinctions among concepts, events, and people are indistinct.

RELATED FACTORS
Metabolic diseases
Endocrine diseases
Fluid and electrolyte imbalance
Oxygen deprivation
Brain injury
Change in environment
Loss
Stress
Too much sensory input
Too little sensory input
Immobility
Hearing or vision deficits
Organic mental disorders
Psychoactive substance use disorders

DEFINING CHARACTERISTICS
Disorientation to time
Disorientation to location
Disorientation to who is present
Disorientation to what is transpiring
Disorientation to person
Misinterpretations
Constant interruptions
Accusations
Screaming
Distractibility
Inability to focus attention
Talkativeness
Mute behavior
Incoherent speech
Restlessness
Wandering
Manifestations of sundown syndrome
Symptoms of emotional response to confusion; e.g., anxiety, fear, rage

a Mini-Mental State examination, or a Set Test[6,9] (see Chapter 12). In evaluating the results, the sensory status, education, and cultural background of the client must be ascertained, because these may affect performance on the test. After the initial Mini-Mental State is recorded, subsequent Mini-Mental State examinations can be conducted and the results compared with the initial evaluation if there is a question of a change in the client's condition.

In addition to the Mini-Mental State, the Set Test is a useful tool for ascertaining the amount of confusion, its probable cause, and the prognosis.[9] This test requires no equipment and minimal practice. The nurse sequentially asks the client to name fruits, cities, animals, and colors. One point is given for each correct item. Each item is counted only once, up to 10 items in each category. There is no deduction for repeated items. There is no time limit, but the test is terminated if the client shows any sign of frustration. The maximum score of the Set Test is 40. A score under 15 closely corresponds to measures indicating dementia. A score over 25 is expected of those who are not demented. Scores between 15 and 25 are inconclusive. If the person seems confused but can easily name 30 to 40 items, the prognosis is markedly better than for the person with a low score, as a higher score means memory is intact and can be used when the nurse is planning and giving care.

Nursing Diagnosis

The diagnosis of confusion can be made more specific for an individual client. Examples include: confusion related to dementia, confusion related to dehydration, or confusion related to immobility and decreased sensory input.

Client Goals and Nursing Interventions

In order to prevent confusion, the nurse acts to ameliorate its various causes. For example, fluids are given to the client whose confusion is secondary to dehydration. The nurse can decrease stress in the client by giving clear explanations and simple instructions and by decreasing the number of changes the client must experience. Also, to decrease confusion, the nurse can assess the amount of stimulation each client might be receiving and alter the environment therapeutically.

To help the client understand the environment, the nurse plans care to include visual and verbal cues. The nurse can assist the client in keeping a calendar or log of events and visitors. Wall calendars, large clocks, large-lettered door signs, and reality orientation boards all give visual cues to the client. Family and friends are encouraged to bring in familiar possessions. The nurse then asks the client about the meaning of the objects. When communicating with the client, the time of day

drugs, or alcohol. Even if the onset of confusion is gradual, the cause must be sought.

Observation of behavior is especially important because confused clients may be verbally uncommunicative.[2,10] The appearance of the client, facial expression, body posture, and the amount of eye contact can be noted. The activity typical for the client at various times of the day is important. For example, a client who usually watches television after dinner is found walking the halls and unsure where he is. Observations charted over time give added depth to the assessment of the client, because signs of confusion are often subtle.

If indicated, a nurse can assess confusion more precisely through the use of a Mental Status examination,

and current activity are mentioned: for example, "Good evening, Mr. Jones. Now that you have finished eating your supper, you can watch the Wednesday evening television programs."[8]

The nurse increases the client's sense of control by giving the client as much self-determination as possible. Explanations of where the client is and what is transpiring are necessary for all confused clients and are especially important after sudden hospitalization. Simple, direct instructions decrease stress and increase a sense of control. The client benefits from simple explanations because it is reassuring that there is an explanation, even if that explanation is not understood or remembered. If the client has preferences for time of day for a bath or for which clothes to wear, these preferences are supported as much as possible. However, the client should not be required to make decisions, because this can be stressful. To further the sense of control, the client may be allowed to wander in a safe area.

For the confused client who insists on carrying out particular actions, it is useful for the nurse to respond to the implicit feelings or needs. For example, the nurse talking with a confused woman who says she must go home to take care of her children can recognize the client's loneliness and concern about her children and can acknowledge that she is a caring mother. A confused man who goes about "supervising" ward activities can be commended for wanting everything to run smoothly. The intent is to help the client feel safe and listened to and connected with someone.[17]

In order to increase the client's sense of security, the nurse modifies the environment and nurse–client interactions. The nurse communicates what is happening at the moment and limits the number of changes the client must experience. Changes in room, roommates, and mealtimes can be upsetting for the client. Even changing the location of the bed within a room should be avoided. If the client is immobile, the nurse can check for sources of stimulation. How much can the client see? From what angle does the client view the world? Can he/she see activity but not participate? Quiet scenes are helpful to the client, but watching others and not participating is distressing and adds to the confusion experienced.[3] After assessing for potential sources of illusions, the nurse provides a night light, removes or adjusts mirrors, and ties down moving curtains. The nurse explains sounds in the room and tells the client he or she is in the hospital and will be helped.

In order to provide for safety and the maintenance of basic physical health, the nurse assesses the environment and plans appropriate monitoring or alteration, depending on client behaviors. Unsafe objects (toiletries, electrical appliances, cigarettes, matches, medications) may need to be removed. The client's participation in basic activities (eating, bathing, eliminating, smoking, and wandering) is monitored as necessary and guided to ensure the client's physical health is maintained.

The nurse shares information with the family about the client's confusion and the resulting behavior. The family is helped to discover how they can orient the client, such as by stating their names and including the client's name and the current place or activity. To assist the family in discovering ways to increase the client's sense of security and control, the nurse encourages the family to bring in pictures and the client's personal belongings.

Evaluation

It would be expected that the client would be less agitated and that wandering would decrease with successful intervention. Other outcome criteria include the client's knowing own location and what the current activities are; being able to find own room; participating in daily routines in a safe manner; maintaining weight, elimination, and hygiene; and being able to interact at least minimally with others. It would be expected that the family and the client would be more comfortable together and that the client would be less confused when the family is present (Chart 2).

CASE STUDY

Matthew B was found by the police mute and disheveled in the middle of a downtown street. On admission, he was unable to give any history and seemed not to know the nurses who had cared for him during his two previous hospitalizations. Assessment involved observations of nonverbal behavior and review of records from his previous admissions. In addition, his parents and his brother were contacted, but they said they had seen little of him since he was discharged 6 months earlier. He had been living in a hotel room downtown and, when last seen 3 weeks earlier, he had seemed "mixed up." The community mental health clinic where Matthew was to have received follow-up care said he had come once but never returned. His admission psychiatric diagnoses were chronic undifferentiated schizophrenia and dementia associated with alcoholism. Initial nursing diagnoses were confusion related to long-term alcohol abuse and self-care deficit (bathing, hygiene) related to dementia.

To ensure his safety, Matthew was monitored to make sure he ate well and bathed and that he did not burn himself while smoking or wander away from the hospital. Matthew was also monitored for any symptoms of withdrawal from alcohol in case he had resumed his pattern of drinking. To decrease the confusion, the same staff members cared for Matthew consistently, and simple explanations of ward routine and what was occurring were given to him. Matthew's name was written in large letters on the door to his room to remind him where he could find his bed and his belongings.

Gradually, he began to speak in short phrases that were appropriate to the circumstances. He was generally oriented to the immediate situation and to his location and was able to maintain self-care with minimal direction. He was able to leave the ward and return safely. However, because of the dementia, he was unable to care for himself in an independent living situation. His family wanted to maintain involvement but were not able to have him live with them. Therefore, discharge planning involved arranging for him to live in a group home near his family.

CHART 2
Confusion: Summary of the Nursing Process

NURSING INTERVENTIONS	OUTCOME CRITERIA
CLIENT GOAL: MANIFEST DECREASED CONFUSION Give clear, simple explanations Decrease the number of changes in the environment Offer fluids frequently if dehydrated Maintain consistent staff	Demonstrates increased orientation Demonstrates decreased agitation and restlessness
CLIENT GOAL: UNDERSTAND THE ENVIRONMENT Describe what is occurring Provide cues: clock, calendar, newspaper, familiar objects If necessary, post signs for client's room and bathroom	Finds own room Knows day and current activity
CLIENT GOAL: DEMONSTRATE INCREASED SENSE OF CONTROL Give client as much control as possible Explain routines and procedures Allow to wander within safe limits Respond to the need presented in the behavior	Engages in own care as much as possible Is comfortable with limits and routines
CLIENT GOAL: EXHIBIT INCREASED SENSE OF SECURITY Communicate what is happening at the moment Limit the number of changes the client must experience Assess for illusions Consider a night light Explain sounds in environment Tell client he/she is being assisted by nursing staff who care about his or her well being	Manifests relaxed movements and facial expression Begins to relate to others with simple conversation
CLIENT GOAL: MAINTAIN BASIC PHYSICAL HEALTH Institute monitoring as necessary: eating, bathing, elimination, smoking, wandering	Maintains weight, elimination, hygiene Does not endanger self

FAMILY GOAL: GAIN UNDERSTANDING OF CLIENT'S BEHAVIOR AND WAYS TO ASSIST
Explain client's behavior to family
Assist family with discovering ways they can orient client,
    reduce stress, and increase client's sense of security and
    control
	Family and client are comfortable together
	Client exhibits less confusion when family is present

Research Highlights

Recognizing that nurse–client interactions are important in the care of the confused client, Armstrong–Esther and Browne[1] designed a study to determine if there is a difference in the frequency and quality of interaction between nurses and confused clients and nurses and lucid clients. Twenty-three clients, rated as either "never confused" or "almost always confused" by the nurse in charge, were selected for observation. The Clinton Assessment Procedure for the Elderly Information/Orientation Subsection was applied to divide the subjects into groups of ten lucid, six slightly confused, and seven confused. The researchers recorded activity levels, to include interactions based on a rating scale, for each subject every 15 seconds over 40 minutes in one morning. Interactions were defined as a verbal statement or question initiated by the nurse or by the patient. Each interaction included a response, rated appropriate or inappropriate.[1]

The researchers found that nursing staff interacted an average of 25 times in 40 minutes with lucid subjects compared with 11 times in 40 minutes with the confused subjects. For both groups, the staff initiated interactions more frequently than they responded to the subjects. Confused subjects initiated fewer interactions than lucid subjects and were less responsive to nurses' interactions than lucid subjects.[1]

These findings serve as a particular reminder to the nurse to increase the number of interactions with confused clients, because decreased sensory input can increase confusion. Such interactions are aimed at promoting independence and encouraging the client to participate in the conversation. The pattern of frequent interactions needs to be maintained by the nurse even if the confused person seldom responds, for the intent is to change the sensory input to the client through interaction.

SUMMARY

Confusion is a condition in which clear and orderly thought is lacking and distinctions among concepts, events, and people are indistinct. Confusion can occur from organic causes, stressors, or extremes in sensory input. Confused individuals may not know the correct time, date, month, year, or location; who is present; or what is transpiring. A number of behaviors seen in confusion are the client's attempts to explain or order the world. If the nurse believes a more extensive assessment for confusion is necessary, a Mental Status examination, a Mini-Mental State examination, or a Set Test may be given. When a nursing diagnosis of confusion is made, interventions are directed toward the goals of assisting the client to manifest decreased confusion, to understand the environment, to demonstrate an increased sense of control and an increased sense of security, and to maintain physical health. In addition, the family is assisted to gain an understanding of the client's behavior and ways they can assist.

References

1. Armstrong–Esther CA, Browne KD. The influence of elderly patients' mental impairment on nurse–patient interaction. J Adv Nurs. 1986;11:379–387.
2. Badcock KA. Early assessment of cognitive impairment in the elderly. Australian Family Physician. 1986;15:129–133.
3. Bartol MA. Reaching the patient. Geriatr Nurs. 1983;4:234–236.
4. Campbell EB, Williams MA, Mlynarczyk SM. After the fall —confusion. Am J Nurs. 1986;86:151–153.
5. Evans LK. Sundown syndrome in institutionalized elderly. J Am Geriatr Soc. 1987;35:101–108.
6. Folstein MF, Folstein SE, McHugh, PR. "Mini-Mental State." Journal of Psychiatry Research. 1975;12:189–198.
7. Gomez GE, Gomez EA. Delirium. Geriatr Nurs. 1987;8:330–332.
8. Hahn K. Using 24-hour reality orientation. J Gerontological Nursing. 1980;6:130–135.
9. Hays A. The Set Test to screen mental status quickly. Geriatr Nurs. 1984;5:96–97.
10. Hays AM, Borger F. A test in time. Am J Nurs. 1985;85:1107–1111.
11. Henderson ML. Altered presentations. Am J Nurs. 1985;85:1104–1106.
12. Lipowski ZJ. Delirium (acute confusional states). JAMA. 1987;258:1789–1792.
13. Mandler G. Stress and thought processes. In: Goldberger L, Breznitz S. editors. Handbook of Stress: Theoretical and Clinical Aspects. New York: Free Press; 1982.
14. Montgomery C. What you can do for the confused elderly. Nursing. 1987;17:54–56.
15. Nagley SJ. Predicting and preventing confusion in your patients. J Gerontological Nursing. 1986;12(8):27–31.
16. National Institutes of Health. Differential diagnosis of dementing diseases. JAMA. 1987;258:3411–3416.
17. Rader J, Doan J, Schwab SM. How to decrease wandering: A form of agenda behavior. Geriatr Nurs. 1985;6:196–199.
18. Sands S, Ratey JJ. The concept of noise. Psychiatry. 1986;49:290–297.
19. Savitz J, Friedman MI. Diagnosing boredom and confusion. Nurs Res. 1981;30:16–20.
20. Wolanin MO. Confusion: recognition and remedy. Scope of the problem and its diagnosis. Geriatr Nurs. 1983;4:227–230.

DELUSIONS

Jean Scheideman

DEFINITION AND DESCRIPTION

A *delusion* is a false, fixed belief held tightly in place by the person's need for that belief. It is not consistent with the person's sociocultural background and not open to change, challenge, or argument. A delusion is a substitute belief, as "it is the enforcement of certainty instead of the acceptance of uncertainty."[11] It arises from the fear of critical thinking and defends against the unknown, thus rendering the person more able to cope with the anxiety found in dealing with daily life. Delusions tend to resist the bombardment of reality testing, common sense, and societal pressures. Sometimes, they seem to recede in intensity and degree of influence only to reemerge when the person experiences increased anxiety caused by situational or developmental crises.

THEORY AND RESEARCH

Understanding the psychotic experience is difficult for the client and conveying the reality of it to another is even more so. Delusions have been likened to dreams that persist after sleep is over. One sequence for their formation has been postulated by a researcher who attempted to grasp the world of the psychotic through personal interviews.[3] First, there is overwhelming anxiety followed by an altered experience of self and the world. Second, this phenomenon presses the person to make sense of the experience despite realistic evidence to the contrary. Third, a certain relief, comfort, and even elation is experienced with the delusional idea. It is as though a whole new level of awareness is open. Things become crystal clear: the answer has been given.

In Britain, qualities found in delusional experience were examined in a group of 55 clients considered to be delusional.[5] Of the total sample, 35 clients were considered to have schizophrenia, whereas the rest had other psychiatric disorders. In this study it was found that nearly all delusions are held with conviction. In addition, some are preoccupying, others not; some are dismissible, others not; and many are worrisome and associated with unhappiness.

As many as 20% to 30% of clients hospitalized for

major depression experience delusions.[12] This type of depression is much more likely when the first episode occurs at age 60 or older.[12] The content of the delusions remains stable in all depressive episodes and tends to contain themes of paranoia, impending disaster, and guilt.[10] Furthermore, clients with a major depressive illness who show delusional thinking tend to have more agitation and retardation as well as less favorable outcomes of their illness than those without delusions.[10]

One study of clients with delusional depression showed a high rate of relapse (86.5%), with the majority of the relapses occurring within the first year after discharge.[1] The recurrence commonly occurred a few months after the client became totally medication-free or shortly after the neuroleptic was decreased or stopped but while the client was still receiving an antidepressant or lithium.

In looking at clients with depression who were suicidal, it was found that although delusional persons had carried out more suicide attempts in the past, at the time of hospital admission, they were assessed to be less suicidal than nondelusional persons.[20] The level of their anxiety was decreased by their delusional thinking as they attempted to establish contact with others. Therefore, they received more directed therapist reaction whereas suicidal persons were in a noncommunicative stance and less open to therapeutic intervention.

RELATED FACTORS

Delusions are commonly seen in mental illnesses such as schizophrenia, affective disorders, and paranoid disorders. They may also occur in organic illnesses caused by acute infections, metabolic disturbances, systemic illness, and substance intoxication.[2]

Elderly persons whose discriminatory capacities have been reduced by brain damage may show delusional thinking. An 85-year-old woman living in low-cost housing complained to the manager that someone was breaking into her apartment at night and stealing her things. When the manager sprinkled flour around her door to demonstrate that no footprints appeared, she changed her complaint to one of someone scaling the outside wall and coming in through her window.

Underlying most delusions is a basic low level of self-esteem that requires a delusion to keep the fragile self-system intact. Delusions of being married to a rock star or being the recipient of a large estate may help the person ward off the anxiety caused by poverty, rejection, guilt, and hopelessness.

Peplau wrote that "loneliness is the result of early life experiences in which remoteness, indifference, and emptiness were the principal themes that characterized the child's relationships with others. Because it is an unbearable experience, loneliness is always hidden, disguised, defended against, and expressed in other forms."[14] One of these forms may be the development of delusions. The child who is frequently left to personal resources for amusement, who spends hours alone waiting for the return of absent parents, or who, because of physical defects, is avoided by peers may come to need delusions for comfort and a sense of inclusion in the world. Without an opportunity to check out beliefs against those of others, delusional thinking may take hold.

The role of consensual validation has been set forth in the writings of Sullivan.[18] He believed that something akin to love is first seen in the chum relationship of preadolescence. Moreover, with the establishment of this relationship comes a great increase in the consensual validation of symbols and of information about life, which discourages the formation of delusional thinking.

In a study of elderly clients, it was found that 54% of persons with delusions of persecution have impaired social resources compared to 13% of persons who were not delusional.[8] In another study that looked at delusional clients being admitted to the hospital for the first time, two-thirds of these persons met friends less than once per week, and their social support had decreased even more when they were interviewed 2 years later.[7]

DEFINING CHARACTERISTICS

Behaviors that appear odd or incongruent with the client's realistic needs may signal delusional thinking. For example, the man who gives his only coat away in the dead of winter may be expecting imminent change, whether through wealth to buy another coat or death in which he will need none. Secrecy often surrounds delusions, for they may represent the only comfortable place in a world perceived as dangerous. Some clients seem alert and well-grounded in their thinking until one specific area of their experience is addressed. One client, who usually interacted well, became irate with another client when the latter spoke of Germany. He believed his father was Hitler, and the subject triggered a tirade of derogatory remarks to the unsuspecting person.

Clients with a history of delusions and years of involvement with treatment in and out of the hospital sometimes talk about their delusions in the past tense. Countless caregivers have perhaps chipped away the tenacious grip of a delusion when a client says to his new therapist, "You probably read all about UFOs and spaceships in my chart," thereby bringing up delusional material in a more open-to-exploration way.

Delusions have been categorized in several ways, as illustrated in Table 13-8. Rosenthal and McGuinness give a useful breakdown.[16] *Persecutory delusions* may result when a person feels victimized, believing that a hostile force is on the lookout for him or her. Agencies currently visible in the media, such as the FBI or CIA, are often cast as the force. Information heard on the radio or TV is commonly mixed with delusional thinking to create private messages for the client. Delusions may include persons in the immediate environment, with one therapist regarded as bad whereas another is accepted as good. *Negative delusions* are found in per-

TABLE 13-8
Types of delusions, definitions, and examples

TYPE	DEFINITION	EXAMPLE
Persecutory[16]	False belief that hostile forces are "out to get" the person	Person may believe that the CIA has a file on him
Negative	False belief that unworthiness has led to pain	Person may believe that the devil is in her body
Grandiose	False belief that the person is famous or important	Person may believe he is Jesus Christ
Sexual	False belief about sexuality	Person may believe that she got pregnant from kissing
Religious	False belief about matters of religion	Person may believe that she committed unforgivable sins
Somatic or hypochondriacal	False belief about the body and how it functions	Person may believe that he smells bad because his body is rotting inside
Nihilistic[13]	False belief that nothing exists	Person may believe that she is already dead
Reference	False belief that an event outside the person is referring to that person	Person may believe he caused an airplane crash by having an unclean thought at the same time
Infidelity	False belief that a partner is unfaithful	Person may believe that his wife is having an affair with his doctor
Impending death[19]	False belief that one's own death is imminent	Person may ask to be taken to the cemetery

sons who are profoundly depressed. Their hopelessness is expressed in endless repetitions of how unworthy they are: "I shouldn't be here. I should be dead" are themes that run through the stream of talk. *Grandiose delusions* tend to be better received by others, because they are more often absurd or colorful. The person who speaks of his million dollar shipping business may be the butt of cajoling listeners who encourage escalation to ever more expansive tales of future plans.

Sexual delusions occur in persons whose sexual development has been distorted by loneliness, misinformation, or strict religious practices. One young woman believed so adamantly that she was a boy that she found a surgeon to remove her breasts. In a study comparing delusional disorders in men and women, it was found that women have more frequent erotic and heterosexual delusions with affective symptoms, whereas men have more delusions with a homosexual theme.[17] Furthermore, episodes of erotomania, delusions involving the sense of being loved and sexually pursued by a man, are commonly precipitated by marital stress and the existence of a prepsychotic depression.

Delusions that are difficult to understand may also be expressed. Some clients believe they have a radio implanted in the head or have the ability to communicate with spacemen. Others focus on somatic concerns about their bodies, such as saying they are dying of cancer, being eaten by worms, or having their flesh turn into liquid. *Parasitosis* is the delusion that the skin harbors lice, worms, maggots, fungi, or bacteria.[15] The client, most often a woman in late middle age, usually first goes to a dermatologist for treatment of this condition as a skin disorder. She may even bring tiny shavings of her skin as proof of her condition.

Delusional experience has also been measured in five different dimensions.[9] They are:

1. Conviction—the degree to which the belief is held;
2. Extension—the degree to which the belief involves various areas of the client's life;
3. Bizarreness—the degree to which the belief is grotesque or fantastic;
4. Disorganization—the degree of confusion; and
5. Pressure—the degree of preoccupation and concern.

These dimensions were found to be independent, suggesting that delusions are indeed a multidimensional phenomenon (Chart 1).

NURSING PROCESS AND RATIONALE
Assessment

Assessment of delusional thinking can best be made by a slow, gentle, deliberate approach that allows the reluctant client time to build trust in the nurse. A question couched in a kind, quizzical manner may be productive in revealing a delusional system. On the other hand, some clients are only too eager to declare their delusions for all to hear, and reaching a diagnosis with them is no problem. (Occasionally, however, the person has indeed had dealings with law enforcement agencies or knows a famous person and is telling the historical truth. Conferences with family or friends may help to separate the real from the delusional in these cases.)

Clients with chronic mental illness tend to anticipate another's response to their delusions and so will share only as much as they feel comfortable doing. They may dismiss their delusions by replying, "I used to think that crazy stuff." They may express doubt: "I know something is wrong but I'm not sure what it is." Or they may blatantly declare, "that woman is pretending to be my mother but she is not." One client eloquently expressed his feelings by stating, "It's as if everyone has a key to the lock on the trunk but me. I don't know what's happening."

In order to make a nursing diagnosis, it is necessary to

CHART 1
Delusions: Definition, Related Factors, and Defining Characteristics

DEFINITION

A delusion is a false, fixed belief held tightly in place by the person's need for that belief. It is not consistent with one's sociocultural background and not open to change, challenge, or argument.

RELATED FACTORS

Schizophrenia
Affective disorders
Paranoid disorders
Acute infections
Metabolic disturbances
Systemic illness
Substance intoxication
Primary degenerative dementia
Low self-esteem
Loneliness
Lack of interpersonal relationships
Anxiety

DEFINING CHARACTERISTICS

Incongruent behavior
Sense of secrecy
Inability to concentrate
Preoccupation
Tense, inflexible manner
Misinterpretation of actions in the environment
Anxiety
Disorganized speech
Expression of delusional beliefs

Nursing Diagnosis

The nursing diagnosis can be stated more specifically for the client. Two examples are: somatic delusions related to substance ingestion and persecutory delusions related to schizophrenia.

Client Goals and Nursing Interventions

The overall goal for nursing intervention with delusional clients is to increase the self-esteem of the person and reduce anxiety so as to render the delusions less necessary. As the nurse listens to the client, an attempt is made to understand the need being expressed by the symbolic language. The person who receives praise and attention for cooking a meal in a day treatment center is less likely to need the delusion of being a corporate executive at that moment. Whatever can be done to make the here-and-now more worthwhile and palatable addresses the problem of delusional thinking.

If the delusions are related to organic causes such as metabolic disturbances or substance intoxication, it is necessary to eliminate the causative agent if at all possible. Staying with a client, remaining calm, and decreasing sensory stimuli are all ways in which anxiety can be lowered during the course of the delusional episode. These clients may be reassured by acknowledging the cause and its temporary nature.

Once the diagnosis is made, the client's communication needs to be directed to more realistic areas of concern. Too often, delusions amuse clients and staff alike, in which case the person is rewarded for talking "crazy" rather than for sharing realistic information about life experiences, which the client may feel to be humdrum. Sometimes, it is helpful if the nurse acknowledges the plausible parts of the delusion while injecting doubt into parts that seem bizarre or fantastic. Because delusional clients are often frightened, their need for space and boundaries must also be considered. Allowing them time to settle in to a new environment is important. They may remain isolated at first, even closing their eyes to prevent intrusion by others. They may require more personal space. One client chose to eat at a separate table when first admitted to the hospital, even leaving the room when another client sat down at the same table.

When the flow of delusional talk cannot be quelled, it may be useful to teach the person when and with whom to share this kind of talk. There is value in a long-term therapeutic relationship with delusional clients. Here, they may receive continuing positive reinforcement for healthy behaviors that lead to a gradual increase in self-esteem. Eventually, they may slowly begin to get in touch with the feelings that prompted the formation of the delusions in the first place as the nurse gently and consistently comments on

verify information gathered from the client, family or friends, and the referral source when possible. Some delusions are so specific to one area of experience that they are difficult to detect unless that subject is brought up. One client spoke about the "mech" in his head only after several days of polite conversation with the nurse. Other times, the delusion is so extensive and the client so preoccupied that the diagnosis is evident.

If the delusions are related to the use of substances such as amphetamines or hallucinogenic drugs such as cannabis, it is imperative to gather an accurate drug history. Persons suffering from acute infections or metabolic disturbances may also show delusional thinking. One client with organic brain syndrome as a result of chronic alcoholism had absurd delusions about his wife's infidelity.

Whether the problem has an evident biochemical cause or not, the person who is delusional appears tense and unable to concentrate and may misinterpret the actions of others. This behavior tends to arouse a sense of uneasiness in the nurse and alerts her or him to the possibility of delusional thinking.

the process and feeling of the interaction rather than the content.

Evaluation

Evaluation is a continuous process that ties into all the other aspects of clients' lives. A decrease in symptoms of depression, paranoia, or anxiety may be used in evaluating a loosening of the grip of delusional thought. Close observation and assessment of early signs that led to delusions in the past are essential in preventing their recurrence. Along with medication, the person needs an approach that addresses the full range of his or her psychosocial needs (Chart 2).

CASE STUDY

Sue was a 24-year-old woman with delusions of persecution, sexual delusions, and delusions that were difficult to understand. Underlying these delusions was a sense of unworthiness attributable to her inability to care for her daughter. A user of both cocaine and marijuana, she lost her job as a dietary aide and presented herself to the emergency room with stories of being followed, spied on, and robbed. Information from other sources suggested delusional thinking. She was admitted to the hospital several times with a nursing diagnosis of delusions related to substance intoxication. Interventions were directed at listening

for the feelings she expressed, such as fear and anger, while providing her with a sense of safety in the hospital milieu. She was given low doses of antipsychotic medication without much change in her mental status except for a decrease in anxiety, which probably was attributable primarily to her removal from the environment.

Losing custody of her daughter prompted new delusional thinking such as the conviction that she was pregnant. When confronted with the results of a negative pregnancy test, she replied, "well, wouldn't you want to be surprised?" and left the hospital to buy a layette. Although given follow-up appointments at the mental health center, she did not keep them and returned instead through the emergency room to the inpatient unit. There, she told staff that she was the mother of triplets and that her other daughters were being taken care of in a luxurious fashion by their father.

Sue was considered to have atypical psychosis and continued to have firmly entrenched delusions. She did not seem to recognize or accept her illness and was unwilling to be seen on a regular basis at the mental health center. The nurse working in community outreach at the mental health center contacted Sue to let her know of the continuing availability of help should Sue wish to make use of it in the future.

SUMMARY

Delusions, which are false, fixed beliefs, occur in organic disorders and mental illnesses. They tend to re-

CHART 2
Delusions: Summary of the Nursing Process

NURSING INTERVENTIONS	OUTCOME CRITERIA
CLIENT GOAL: FEEL LESS ANXIOUS Assess level of anxiety Provide an environment that protects client from too much stress Interact frequently using brief neutral subjects for conversation Allow client adequate physical and emotional space, not crowding the client or intruding on privacy	Demonstrates decreased level of anxiety Remains in area where interactions with others may occur
CLIENT GOAL: FEEL SENSE OF SELF-WORTH Listen to the client Indicate desire to understand Assist client to meet needs expressed by the delusion Offer positive feedback	Demonstrates greater appreciation for self, as in meeting hygiene needs Verbalizes more positive statements about self
CLIENT GOAL: EXPERIENCE LESS PREOCCUPATION WITH DELUSIONAL THOUGHT Assess for possibility of harm to self or others Refocus client on realistic issues in the here-and-now Reflect the feeling expressed by the delusion; e.g., "it must be lonesome for you there"	Does not harm self or others Communicates with others about realistic issues Exhibits nonverbal cues that are congruent with situational events
CLIENT GOAL: INCREASE KNOWLEDGE ABOUT DELUSIONS Discuss with client with whom to share delusions Accept client's limitations when delusions remain Teach family how to deal with client's delusions Teach medication management	Exhibits more success when interacting with others in the community Follows recommended medication regimen
CLIENT GOAL: ENGAGE IN PRODUCTIVE ACTIVITIES Provide time structure within client's level of functioning Direct client to activities that are socially acceptable and rewarding	Demonstrates engagement in activities that are socially acceptable and rewarding

Research Highlights

James M. Glass, professor of government and politics at the University of Maryland, demonstrated how political theory can be enriched by studying the internal world of people with delusional thinking.[6] He chose as his site for field work Sheppard and Enoch Pratt Hospital. To gather data, Glass worked in the role of participant–observer over a period of 6 years in which his position as an outsider to patient care enabled him to be the recipient of what clients called their "secrets." Dialogues with individuals lasted anywhere from 3 to 24 months. Glass believed that although delusions have been largely ignored by political philosophers, they contain social as well as intrapsychic events and may be integral to the culture's experience of itself. For example, in the delusional concepts of power appear images of domination, command, force, and control rather than those of sharing and cooperation. Thus, delusional imagery often centers on important political relations, such as victim/victimizer, slave/master, and controlled/controller. Moreover, delusions exert as much power over the self as any external tyranny. In this sense, the person with delusions is a classic victim, whose self creates its own victimizer. The distortion is a defense against the forces of reality but also represents a commitment to life. As one ex-client said to Glass, "if I ever become psychotic again and tell you delusional ideas, don't tell me I'm wrong or even interesting. Just say that you and I hold different views about things and my views are all right to hold" (reference 6, p 18).

sist reality testing and to occupy a central place in the person's thinking, serving as a defense against the anxiety experienced in the real world. As Campbell stated: "Delusions, like fever, are to be looked on as part of nature's attempt at cure, an endeavor to neutralize some disturbing factor, to compensate for some handicap, to reconstruct a working contact with group, which will satisfy special needs" (reference 4, p 9). Therefore, the primary focus of nursing interventions is to increase the person's sense of self-esteem. This may be accomplished by providing positive reinforcement for worthwhile activities in the here-and-now, as well as by assisting the client to meet those needs expressed by the delusion.

References

1. Aronson TA, Shukla S, Gujavarty K, Hoff A, DiBuono M, Khan E. Relapse in delusional depression: A retrospective study of the course of treatment. Compr Psychiatry. 1988;29(1):12–21.
2. Barile L. The client who is delusional. In: Lego S, ed. The American Handbook of Psychiatric Nursing. Philadelphia: J.B. Lippincott; 1984.
3. Bowers MB, Jr. Retreat from Sanity. New York: Human Sciences Press; 1974.
4. Campbell CM. Delusion and Belief. Cambridge: Harvard University Press; 1926.
5. Garety PA, Hemsley DR. Characteristics of delusional experience. Eur Arch Psychiatry Neurol Sci. 1987;236:294–298.
6. Glass JM. Delusion: Internal Dimensions of Political Life. Chicago: University of Chicago Press; 1985.
7. Jorgensen P. Social course and outcome of delusional psychosis. Acta Psychiatr Scand. 1987;75:629–634.
8. Jorgensen P, Munk–Jorgensen P. Patients with delusions in a community psychiatric service: A follow-up study. Acta Psychiatr Scand. 1986;73:191–195.
9. Kendler KS, Glazer WM, Morgenstern H. Dimensions of delusional experience. Am J Psychiatry. 1983;140:466–469.
10. Lykouras E, Malliaras D, Christodoulou GN, Moussas G, Christodoulou D, Tzonou A. Delusional depression: Phenomenology and response to treatment. Psychopathology. 1986;19(4),157–164.
11. Meerloo AM. Delusion and mass delusion. Nervous and Mental Disease Monographs. 1949;79.
12. Meyers BS. Late-life depression and delusions. Hosp Community Psychiatry. 1987;38:573–574.
13. Mullahy P. Psychoanalysis and Interpersonal Psychiatry: The Contributions of Harry Stack Sullivan. New York: Science House; 1970.
14. Peplau HE. Loneliness. Am J Nurs. 1955;55:1476–1481.
15. Renvoize EB, Kent J, Klar HM. Delusional infestation and dementia: A case report. Br J Psychiatry. 1987;150:403–405.
16. Rosenthal TT, McGuinness TM. Dealing with delusional patients: Discovering the distorted truth. Issues in Mental Health Nursing. 1986;8:143–154.
17. Rudden M, Sweeney J, Frances A, Gilmore M. A comparison of delusional disorders in women and men. Am J Psychiatry. 1983;140:1575–1578.
18. Sullivan HS. The Interpersonal Theory of Psychiatry. New York: WW Norton; 1953.
19. Weisman AD. On Dying and Denying. New York: Behavioral Publications; 1972.
20. Wolfersdorf M, Keller F, Steiner B, Hole G. Delusional depression and suicide. Acta Psychiatr Scand. 1987;76:359–363.

HALLUCINATIONS

Mary Durand Thomas

DEFINITION AND DESCRIPTION

A *hallucination* is a sensory perception in the absence of a corresponding stimulus. Hallucinations differ from illusions in that an illusion is a misinterpretation of a real stimulus, whereas an external stimulus is absent in a hallucination.

Although hallucinations are often thought to be manifested primarily through voices and other auditory phenomena, hallucinations can occur through any of the senses. A client may experience tastes, smells, visions, or somatic sensations (Table 13-9). Most clients who experience hallucinations do so through more than one of their senses.[10] When a client has some insight into the unreality of the sensory perception, the experience is sometimes termed a "pseudohallucination."

THEORY AND RESEARCH

A number of theories have been proposed to explain hallucinatory experiences. These theories tend to fall into one of three categories: the psychophysiological, the psychodynamic, and the interpersonal.

An example from the psychophysiological category is the dissociation–disinhibition theory, which posits that when higher cognitive functions are disrupted because of fatigue, toxicity, or disease, there is a failure to inhibit the lower cognitive functions, which results in the activation of hallucinations.[3] Another approach, based on the similarity of dreams and hallucinations, hypothesizes that brain activity associated with REM (rapid eye motion) sleep may emerge in a waking state as hallucinations secondary to the failure of a screening mechanism that normally functions during waking and most non-REM sleep stages.[3,9] The perceptual release theory suggests that, although the brain selectively excludes from consciousness the majority of impulses that are regarded as irrelevant, a certain level of sensory input is essential for this censorship mechanism to function properly.[3,24] Thus, during periods in which sensory input is disturbed or absent, memory traces are released into consciousness and experienced as hallucinations. A biochemical etiology is suggested by the occurrence of hallucinations as an adverse effect of certain medications. Levels of neurotransmitters, especially dopamine and serotonin, have been implicated.[3,9,19]

According to the psychodynamic view, hallucinations represent the intrusion of preconscious and unconscious material into consciousness as a response to psychological conflicts and unmet needs.[3,16] For example, the horrible image of a monster might be considered a projection of aggressive impulses, and voices calling the client obscene names might be interpreted as representing sexual impulses or guilt. The content of a hallucination is therefore considered to be significant in understanding a client's repressed and projected impulses, wishes, and fears.

The interpersonal explanation of auditory hallucinations posits their development over time.[8] The person is thought to experience high anxiety in a situation of great stress. The person then thinks of a supportive individual and how this individual could be helpful, which results in relief of anxiety. As such situations recur and relief of anxiety through reverie is experienced repeatedly, the person becomes concerned about being able to recall the reveries at will. The reverie becomes hallucinatory with increased withdrawal and inappropriate behavior. A cyclic process is thus initiated in which the person is embarrassed about inappropriate behavior, which results in increased anxiety,

TABLE 13–9
Types of hallucinations, definitions, and examples

TYPE	DEFINITION	EXAMPLE
Auditory	Perception of sounds or voices in absence of corresponding stimuli	Person hears unintelligible conversation, name being called, or voices commenting on behavior
Visual	Perception of colors, patterns, people, scenes, or other images in absence of stimuli	Person may see flashes of light, zigzag lines, recognizable people, or monsters
Olfactory	Perception of odors in absence of stimuli	Person may smell smoke, feces, or other generally unpleasant odors
Gustatory	Perception of tastes in absence of stimuli	Person may experience bitter taste or what is believed to be poison
Tactile	Perception of touch in the absence of stimuli	Person may experience insects crawling on the skin or the genitals being touched
Kinesthetic	Perception of movement of body parts that are not actually moving[3]	Person believes head is nodding when it is not
Cenesthetic	Perception of visceral sensations that are not perceived under physiologic conditions[3]	Person reports experiencing the flow of blood through blood vessels
Negative	Failure to perceive objects or people that are present[3,15]	Person reports that a chair is empty when there is actually a person sitting in it

leading to more withdrawal and hallucinations. The escalation leads eventually to a state where the client has virtually no interpersonal contacts and accepts hallucinations as a central part of life.

The psychophysiological, psychodynamic, and interpersonal explanations are not necessarily mutually exclusive. Multiple etiologic factors may be involved.

RELATED FACTORS

Hallucinations occur in a number of psychiatric conditions: schizophrenia, bipolar disorder, major depression, other psychoses, delirium, dementia, and conditions associated with the use or withdrawal of alcohol or other substances.[2] Hallucinations often accompany delusions, which are fixed, false beliefs.

Hallucinations may occur in epilepsy and other neurologic disorders as well as in delirium resulting from such diverse conditions as systemic infections, metabolic disorders, or postoperative states. Hallucinations can be experienced as a side effect of a variety of medications, including antidepressants, anticholinergic agents, antihypertensives, anti-inflammatory agents, and antibiotics.[3] Hallucinogenic drugs may induce later flashback hallucinations similar to those experienced at the time the drug was first used. There is a tendency for repeated use of hallucinogens to increase the probability of flashback experiences.[15]

Hallucinations can occur in otherwise normal individuals who are exposed to protracted periods of isolation, sensory deprivation, and sleep deprivation or who experience a loss.[3] Blindness, hearing loss, or speech problems can also give rise to hallucinations.[5,6,12] A study of hostage victims showed that those subjected to isolation, in combination with the stress of threatened death, experienced a progression of visual hallucinations from simple geometric forms to complex memory images.[22] Grief reactions may include auditory or visual hallucinations of the deceased. For example, among 46 widows, 28 (61%) reported hallucinatory experiences of the deceased spouse.[21]

Cultural factors can influence the nature and frequency of hallucinations. The content of hallucinations is based on an individual's experience and therefore varies from one cultural group to another. In addition, the hallucinatory experience involves different senses across cultures. The relatively higher occurrence of visual hallucinations in individuals from primitive societies has been related to social patterns of learning by doing in contrast to Western societies, where learning through words receives greater emphasis and where there is a correspondingly higher occurrence of auditory hallucinations.[1] The overall frequency of hallucinations can also vary across cultures. For example, among schizophrenic clients admitted to a hospital in Kenya, hallucinations were more common in the African, West Indian, and Asian groups than in the English groups.[20]

The extent to which hallucinations are culturally defined as symptomatic of mental illness and therefore negatively regarded can influence the willingness of individuals to admit their occurrence. Individuals in some societies view the hallucinatory experience not negatively but rather as a way of being in touch with the supernatural. In such societies, hallucinations may be sought through the use of hallucinogens, fasting, sensory deprivation, and other techniques.[13]

Certain types of hallucinations have been associated with particular conditions. For example, tactile hallucinations of insects crawling on the skin may occur during cocaine and amphetamine intoxication. Visual and tactile hallucinations of small animals crawling on the body may occur during alcohol withdrawal.[3,23] In a group of clients being treated for a variety of psychoses, clients who localized their voices on the right side were significantly more depressed than those who heard voices on the left or whose voices were not localized.[11] Visual hallucinations induced by drugs are more readily seen in darkened surroundings or with the eyes closed, whereas those that occur in schizophrenia do not change whether the eyes are opened or closed.[3] Auditory hallucinations in which a voice keeps up a commentary on the client's behavior or thoughts or in which two or more voices converse are characteristic of schizophrenia but may occur in other psychoses.[10]

DEFINING CHARACTERISTICS

Certain behaviors may indicate the presence of hallucinations. For example, a client who is preoccupied or who appears to be listening or watching something may be focusing on a hallucinatory experience. Because attention is elsewhere, the client may be unable to follow a conversation or may misinterpret what is said. The client may make lip movements during a hallucination or may laugh or react in some other way that may be consistent with the content of the hallucination but is inappropriate to the actual social context. Because an auditory hallucination may include commands such as "grimace three times before you eat a bite of food," the client may behave in a bizarre manner. Command hallucinations can also dictate more dangerous behavior involving harm to self or others.

A client may report the hallucinations being experienced, or the client may want to be alone or be hesitant to talk about hallucinating. The latter might occur because acknowledging hallucinations has in the past led to the client being criticized, ridiculed, or stigmatized as "crazy" or because the client is confused by the experience or fearful of the consequences of telling, because "the voices say not to tell." When the voices make accusations of shameful behavior, the client may feel humiliated and unable to share the terrible accusations.

Because a hallucination is experienced as real, the client may refer to the individuals seen or heard as "they" or "them" and assume the nurse knows the referent. A client who experiences a gustatory hallucination may avoid eating, and a client may brush away the crawling insects experienced in a tactile hallucination (Chart 1).

NURSING PROCESS AND RATIONALE

Assessment

The first step in assessing for hallucinations is to be alert for their occurrence. As noted above, they can occur in a wide variety of conditions. A client may be

---

CHART 1
Hallucinations: Definition, Related Factors, and Defining Characteristics

DEFINITION

A hallucination is a sensory perception that occurs in the absence of a corresponding stimulus. Hallucinations differ from illusions in that an illusion is a misinterpretation of a real stimulus, whereas an external stimulus is absent in a hallucination.

RELATED FACTORS

Schizophrenia
Mood disorders
Other psychoses
Epilepsy
Other neurologic disorders
Delirium
Dementia
Alcohol use or withdrawal
Drug use or withdrawal
May accompany delusions
Sensory deprivation
Isolation
Sleep deprivation
Loss of significant other
Cultural factors
Stress
Anxiety
Unmet needs
Internal conflicts

DEFINING CHARACTERISTICS

Preoccupied
Does not follow conversation
Listening in absence of obvious stimulus
Watchful in absence of obvious stimulus
Moving lips
Laughing inappropriately
Bizarre behavior
Dangerous behavior
Isolating behavior
Verbal references to "they" and "them"
Verbal report of hallucinations
Fear
Anxiety

---

asked directly such questions as: "Do you sometimes hear sounds or see things that other people don't hear or see?" or "Some clients are troubled by hearing voices or seeing visions. Has that been a problem for you?" In addition, if a client exhibits some of the signs and symptoms mentioned above—particularly listening or watching while seeming to be fearful—the nurse can inquire into the source of the distress. For example: "You seem very frightened. Can you tell me what you are experiencing right now?"

Once the client has acknowledged the presence of hallucinations (although it is unusual for a client to term the experience "hallucinations"), it is useful to learn more about:

The content of the hallucinations, especially the presence of command hallucinations and whether the client has ever put commands into action. "What are the voices like that you hear?" "Do the voices ever direct you to do something?" "Have you ever acted a certain way because of what you thought the voices wanted?" "Do the voices ever tell you to harm yourself?"

The meaning to the client and the client's feelings about them. "Is it frightening when you hear the voices?"

The context in which they occur and the precipitating stressors. "Are there times that you are more troubled by the voices?" "What was happening with you this morning before you started hearing the voices?"

The ways in which the hallucinations interfere with daily life. "How do the voices affect your daily living?" "Are there things you are not able to do because of the voices?"

The occurrence of hallucinations in other sensory modalities. "You mentioned hearing voices that others do not hear. Do you ever see (smell, taste) things that others don't?"

Nursing Diagnosis

The diagnostic category of hallucinations can be made more specific for a particular patient by including the type(s) of hallucination as well as related factors. An example would be hallucinations (tactile) related to ingestion of amphetamines.

Client Goals and Nursing Interventions

Because the client who is hallucinating is anxious or fearful, discussing the hallucinations may be difficult. It is important that the nurse acknowledge the client's experience without increasing the client's anxiety by forcing revelations or by attempting to reason the client out of hallucinations. In addition, focusing on hallucinations by talking about them may increase their occurrence. Therefore, after early assessment of a client's hallucinations, it is not necessary, and indeed can be counterproductive, to focus extensively on their content.

In addition to acknowledging the client's experience and feelings, the nurse can also assist the client to feel safe by increasing the structure of the environment and by communicating with simple, concrete words. The client will also benefit from a decrease in anxiety-producing situations such as having to make a decision or being required to participate in large group activities. The client whose hallucinations are biochemically based (as from an adverse reaction to a medication) can be reassured that this is a temporary reaction.

There is some risk that a client will act on a command hallucination, even though there is evidence that many clients ignore such commands.[14] Therefore, a nurse should take steps to avert risk of harm to the client or others implied by the commands.

The frequency and intensity of the hallucinations can be reduced by gently engaging the client's attention elsewhere. For example, the client may be encouraged to participate with the nurse in a simple activity. Not only does this distract the client from the hallucination, it entails experiencing a real interaction with a real person, which can be beneficial for a client who is prone to isolating behavior. The nurse who knows the contexts in which the client is most bothered by hallucinations (e.g., at bedtime) can give the client additional support at those times. Also, neuroleptic medications, which are usually prescribed initially on a regular and as necessary basis, are given to reduce psychotic symptoms, including hallucinatory behavior.

The nurse can assist the client in learning ways of handling anxiety and other emotions. It is useful for the client to learn that feelings can be shared and explored verbally. For example, the client who remembers the acute phase of illness may feel embarrassed or remorseful about behavior during that time, so working through these feelings can be beneficial. In addition, the content of the hallucinations may indicate conflicts and unmet needs. If there appears to be a theme such as guilt or dependency in the content of the hallucinations, the nurse can be alert to discussion of such issues as they are reflected in the client's daily life.

For some clients, auditory hallucinations persist and interfere with daily life after the acute phase of illness is over. Some clients have benefited from increased external stimuli such as listening to a radio or watching television.[7,17,18] Clients with persistent hallucinations may be taught *voice dismissal:* the client is encouraged to say in a loud, clear voice: "Go away and leave me alone." This should be practiced in the nurse's presence until it is done successfully. Emphasis may be added by having the client pound the table. The client can be instructed to hum instead when in a public place. This latter method will draw less attention but is not as effective as verbal dismissal.[8] Voice dismissal helps clients achieve a sense of control over hallucina-

tions. In addition, use of speech organs interrupts the subvocalized speech involved in the hallucinatory process[4] (see Research Highlights).

Other health teaching is also important with clients for whom hallucinations are a problem. As mentioned above, the nurse helps the client to learn other ways of handling anxiety by expressing feelings and becoming involved with real people. The nurse can discuss with the client the need for prescribed medications, ways of handling side effects, and the importance of not discontinuing the medications independently. It is particularly important to discuss with the client the significance of a recurrence or increased frequency and intensity of hallucinations as symptomatic of illness and the need to seek therapeutic assistance. If the client remembers hallucinating, there may be less embarrassment or remorse if it is discussed as a symptom of illness.

Evaluation

Nursing interventions may be evaluated by observing whether the client's anxiety level has decreased, whether there has been a decrease in the frequency and intensity of hallucinations, and the extent of the client's involvement in interactions with others. In addition, the client's knowledgeability about hallucinations and the need to seek treatment for recurrences can be evaluated (Chart 2).

CASE STUDY

A 53-year-old man was hospitalized with chronic undifferentiated schizophrenia. His psychiatric history spanned more than 30 years, with multiple hospitalizations interspersed with both independent and supervised living arrangements. Most recently, he had been in a single room in a hotel for transients, where he had little contact with others. He came to the emergency room because he was fearful that he would "involuntarily or voluntarily kill myself." He was experiencing auditory hallucinations, which at times included commands such as "jump out the window." The client was concerned that this would come to pass, and thus he would "involuntarily" commit suicide. On the other hand, he was so weary of the voices continually commenting on his actions and generally being a dominant feature in his life that he sometimes considered "voluntary" suicide. A major nursing diagnosis was hallucinations (auditory) related to isolation and schizophrenia. Another nursing diagnosis was suicide potential related to command hallucinations and discouragement about illness.

Initially, suicide precautions were taken, and the client was helped to feel more secure in the hospital. Gradually, he was encouraged to discuss his feelings and become involved in ward activities. He participated in a medication teaching group, where he was able to identify the purpose, side effects, and schedule for his neuroleptic medication. The hallucinations diminished significantly after he was regulated on medication but did not entirely cease. The client was helped to use voice dismissal and received some benefit. He felt that the voices had abated to a point where there was minimal interference in his life. Discharge planning involved assisting in placement in a group home and a plan

CHART 2
Hallucinations: Summary of the Nursing Process

NURSING INTERVENTIONS	OUTCOME CRITERIA
CLIENT GOAL: FEEL MORE SECURE	
Assess for occurrence of hallucinations	Reports hallucinations when they occur
Assess client's level of anxiety	Demonstrates decreased anxiety
Acknowledge client's feelings and experience	
Increase structure of environment	
Communicate with simple, concrete words	
CLIENT GOAL: REFRAIN FROM BEHAVIOR HARMFUL TO SELF OR OTHERS	
Assess content of command hallucinations	Does not harm self or others
Institute measures to protect client as well as others	
CLIENT GOAL: EXPERIENCE DECREASED HALLUCINATIONS AND LESS DISRUPTIVENESS FROM THEM	
Interrupt the hallucinations and engage the client's attention elsewhere	Reports that the hallucinations have decreased in frequency and intensity
Increase involvement with real people in real situations	Interacts with real people instead of focusing on hallucinations
Control situational factors that may increase the hallucinations	
Give neuroleptic medications and monitor their effectiveness	
CLIENT GOAL: INCREASE KNOWLEDGE ABOUT HALLUCINATIONS	
For persistent hallucinations, teach voice dismissal	Reports decrease in hallucinations
Teach that hallucinations can be a symptom of illness	Feels less remorse or embarrassment in remembering hallucinations
Teach regarding the need to seek treatment should the hallucinations increase or recur	Verbalizes plan to seek further treatment if necessary
Teach purpose, side effects, and schedule of medication	Verbalizes understanding of purpose, side effects, and schedule of medication

for outpatient follow-up at a community mental health center.

SUMMARY

Hallucinations, which include sensory perceptions through any of the senses, can occur in many psychiatric and nonpsychiatric conditions. They have been explained through psychophysiological, psychodynamic, and interpersonal theories. Following assessment and diagnosis, nursing interventions are directed toward increasing the client's feelings of safety and security, protection of the client and others, decreasing the hallucinations and their disruptiveness, and increasing the client's knowledge about this problem.

Research Highlights

The observation has been made that auditory hallucinations are accompanied by subvocalized speech (inaudible articulations of speech organs). Such subvocalizations could either be a mimicking of the hallucinated voice or be involved in generating the voice. Bick and Kinsbourne designed an experiment to discover more about this phenomenon.[4] They reasoned that if the subvocalizations were mimicking an auditory hallucination that occurred independently, then interference with speech organs should make no difference in the occurrence of hallucinations, whereas if subvocalized speech were involved in generating the hallucinated voice, then interference with speech organs should interrupt the hallucinatory process.

Eighteen inpatients with schizophrenia who were experiencing hallucinations were selected. In a randomly sequenced order, the subjects were asked to close their eyes tight, open their mouths wide, and make fists and squeeze tightly for 1 full minute. After each of these tasks, each subject was asked whether the voices got worse, stayed the same, or went away. The task of mouth opening, which precluded subvocalizations, abolished hallucinations significantly more often than did the control tasks of eye squeezing and fist clenching. Bick and Kinsbourne concluded that the following sequence occurs: the client subvocalizes, listens to his or her own covert speech, and then attributes it to another. A secondary finding of this experiment was that even clients who had experienced the hallucinations as very upsetting appeared indifferent to the possibility of having a mechanism for controlling the hallucinations. The authors suggest that this may indicate that hallucinations, even when extremely unpleasant, are serving some adaptive function for the client.[4]

Similarly, Field, in his study of hallucinations and voice dismissal, found that many clients were initially reluctant to carry out the dismissal process.[8] However, he established that a significant number of clients went on to learn and use the technique and experienced relief from hallucinations.

References

1. Al-Issa I. Sociocultural factors in hallucinations. Int J Soc Psychiatry. 1978;24:167–176.
2. American Psychiatric Association. Diagnostic and Statistical Manual of Mental Disorders, ed 3, rev. Washington, DC: American Psychiatric Association; 1987.
3. Asaad G, Shapiro B. Hallucinations: Theoretical and clinical overview. Am J Psychiatry. 1986;143:1088–1097.
4. Bick PA, Kinsbourne M. Auditory hallucinations and subvocal speech in schizophrenic patients. Am J Psychiatry. 1987;144:222–225.
5. Critchley EMR, Denmark JC, Warren F, Wilson KA. Hallucinatory experiences of prelingually profoundly deaf schizophrenics. Br J Psychiatry. 1981;138:30–32.
6. Cummings JL, Miller BL. Visual hallucinations: Clinical occurrence and use in differential diagnosis. West J Med. 1987;146:46–51.
7. Feder R. Auditory hallucinations treated by radio headphones. Am J Psychiatry. 1982;139:1188–1190.
8. Field WE. Hearing voices. J Psychosoc Nurs Ment Health Serv. 1985;23(1):9–14.
9. Fishman LG. Dreams, hallucinogenic drug states, and schizophrenia: A psychological and biological comparison. Schizophr Bull. 1983;9:73–94.
10. Goodwin DW, Alderson P, Rosenthal R. Clinical significance of hallucinations in psychiatric disorders. Arch Gen Psychiatry. 1971;24:76–80.
11. Gruber LN, Mangat BS, Abou-Taleb H. Laterality of auditory hallucinations in psychiatric patients. Am J Psychiatry. 1984;141:586–587.
12. Hammeke TA, McQuillen MP, Cohen BA. Musical hallucinations associated with acquired deafness. J Neurol Neurosurg Psychiatry. 1983;46:570–572.
13. Harner MJ. Hallucinogens and Shamanism. New York: Oxford University Press; 1973.
14. Hellerstein D, Frosch W, Koenigsberg HW. The clinical significance of command hallucinations. Am J Psychiatry. 1987;144:219–221.
15. Horowitz MJ. Image Formation and Psychotherapy. New York: Jason Aronson; 1983.
16. Kolb LC, Brodie HKH. Modern Clinical Psychiatry. Philadelphia: W.B. Saunders; 1982.
17. Magen J. Increasing external stimuli to ameliorate hallucinations. Am J Psychiatry. 1983;140:269–270.
18. Mallya AR, Shen WW. Radio in the treatment of auditory hallucinations. Am J Psychiatry. 1983;140:1264–1265.
19. Nausieda PA, Tanner CM, Klawans HL. Serotonergically active agents in levodopa-induced psychiatric toxicity reactions. Adv Neurol. 1983;37:23–32.
20. Ndetei DM, Vdher A. A comparative cross-cultural study of the frequencies of hallucination in schizophrenia. Acta Psychiatr Scand. 1984;70:545–549.
21. Olson PR, Suddeth JA, Peterson PJ, Egelhoff C. Hallucinations of widowhood. J Am Geriatr Soc. 1985;33:543–547.
22. Siegel FK. Hostage hallucinations: Visual imagery induced by isolation and life-threatening stress. J Nerv Ment Dis. 1984;172:264–272.
23. Webster M. Differential diagnosis. In: Lego S, ed. The American Handbook of Psychiatric Nursing. Philadelphia: J.B. Lippincott; 1984.
24. West LJ. A clinical and theoretical overview of hallucinatory phenomena. In: Siegel RK, West LJ, eds. Hallucinations: Behavior, Experience, and Theory. New York: John Wiley; 1975.

MEMORY LOSS

Vivian Wolf-Wilets

DEFINITION AND DESCRIPTION

Memory depends on an active system that is used to: (1) perceive or sense an event, sensation, or phenomenon; (2) modify, code, or hold that input long enough so that the brain can use that information immediately; or (3) store what was perceived in a form that can be retrieved at some future time. *Memory loss* can follow a disruption of any part of this process. Thus, perception of sensory input can be disrupted, such that the incoming perceptions will be absent or modified. Also, the brain may lose its ability to hold, recognize, or code information so that it can be used or stored. Finally, the structure and functioning of the brain can be changed so that information is not permanently stored, or if the information is stored, the individual may not be able to retrieve it. Remembering to do something at a certain time without prompting is an additionally complex task sometimes lost by clients with memory disturbances.

Memory is different from what is usually called the intelligence quotient (IQ). Most intelligence tests require judgment and reasoning, not just the ability to learn, retain, or recall sensations, events, or phenomena. It is possible for clients to have normal IQ scores but abnormally low memory scores. The reverse also occurs; some retarded individuals have an excellent or even outstanding memory but cannot judge or reason well.

Normal individuals may forget information very rapidly. How rapidly will depend on many factors such as how meaningful the information was when first presented, how long and how often the person thinks about the material, and the types of things the person does after learning the material. Similar material may interfere with the ability to recall information previously learned.

If some problems of forgetting are normal, then when is a client said to have altered memory? Table 13-10 presents some of the specific types of memory loss. These categories could be made even more specific. For example, one could have loss of visual or semantic short-term memory.

THEORY AND RESEARCH

There are a number of theories about how memory functions. Two widely accepted but contrasting theories will be presented here.

TABLE 13–10
Types of memory loss, definitions, and examples

TYPE	DEFINITION AND EXAMPLE
Recent	Cannot remember events that happened recently (in the last day, weeks, or months), e.g., is unable to remember having gone out to dinner 2 days ago
Remote	Cannot remember things from several years ago; e.g., does not remember the name of the college graduated from 15 years ago
Anterograde	Cannot remember events that happened after an incident or event; e.g., cannot remember things that happened after a car accident
Retrograde	Cannot remember events that happened before an incident or event; e.g., cannot remember the plays before a sports injury
Immediate	Cannot give back information just presented, such as repeating three words just presented
Short-term	Cannot retain information presented within the last 5 minutes; e.g., cannot remember three objects presented 5 minutes earlier[2]
Long-term	Cannot recognize or recall information presented in the past; e.g., cannot recall age or what holiday client celebrated last month
Forgetfulness	Does not remember to do things without prompting; e.g., forgets to take medication half the time
Selective memory	Remembers some things well but not other things; e.g., remembers interaction with persons but cannot remember mathematical skills
Amnesia	Loss of both short- and long-term memory;[2] e.g., cannot remember anything, including name
Transitory global amnesia	Abrupt onset of inability to form new memories for more than 15 minutes but less than 48 hours with preservation of consciousness and higher functions. A lasting amnesia for most of the episode, with possible retrograde amnesia and no overt motor seizures;[37] e.g., cannot remember what happened for a 24-hour period even though alert
Fugue state	Sudden temporary alteration(s) in the normally integrated functions of consciousness, identity, or motor behavior with an inability to recall one's past;[2] e.g., a law student who failed the bar examination is found in another state unable to recall own name or home town
Hypnotic state	Loss of memory for events or actions after receiving a hypnotic suggestion not to remember; e.g., cannot remember the hypnotist suggested client would scratch own head when a bell rings but does it anyway
Psychoactive substances	Loss or modification of memory after taking medications or exposure to chemicals having a psychogenic effect; e.g., cannot remember what happened the night before after having several drinks
Procedural	Loss of ability to carry out learned procedures; e.g., bicycle riding. This type of memory may be retained after declarative memory loss
Declarative	The loss of the ability to describe things in a statement; e.g., unable to describe a picture shown
Prospective	"The loss of the ability to remember to perform future actions; e.g., remembering to keep an appointment, to return a phone call, or to take medications" (reference 36, pp 75–76)
Benign senile forgetfulness	Forgetting that occurs in older adults and may not seriously interfere with normal functioning; e.g. "the older person may forget parts of an experience and may recall the forgotten parts later" (reference 50, p 61)
Prosopagnosia	Inability to recognize the faces of persons the client usually knows; e.g., cannot recognize spouse or daughter[25]
Anomia	Inability to name objects

Theory of Short-Term Long-Term Memory

This theory is based on a model proposed by Atkinson and Shiffrin.[5] In this view, information from the world comes into the brain from the sense organs. The information then proceeds to a sensory register, where patterns are recognized by comparing what is coming in with what is already known and stored in long-term memory. Pattern recognition can occur so quickly that it seems automatic; e.g., 95% accuracy in a fraction of a second (reference 3, pp 44–47). This type of knowing has been termed *top down*, because material is already known and in long-term memory, as shown by the arrow connecting long-term memory with pattern recognition (Fig. 13-20). When material is unknown and it is necessary to work out the meaning of the situation or the identity of objects in the environment, knowing is termed *bottom up*, and short-term memory, with or without long-term memory, is needed. There is debate about whether patterns are recognized by templates, prototypes, gestalts, or features of the phenomena or all of these means.[3,29] The context of the presentation helps provide clues for recognition. Clue recognition requires long-term memory.

Information will go on from the sensory register to immediate memory. Immediate memory is present when an individual can repeat a phrase just given or tell the name of a picture just seen. In order for this to occur, material has to have been recognized and modified by the individual's brain in such a way that the material can be given back. This may be a very complex process. For example, if an individual reads material and is asked to repeat that information orally, the brain has had to recognize visual symbols, change these to auditory symbols, and then use the nerves and muscles of speech to produce the correct sounds.

Short-term memory is the working memory where information is held for solving problems. There is a limited amount of space in short-term memory; it is estimated that only about five to nine pieces of data can be held at one time.[5] If problem solving is also being carried out, then there may even be less space available

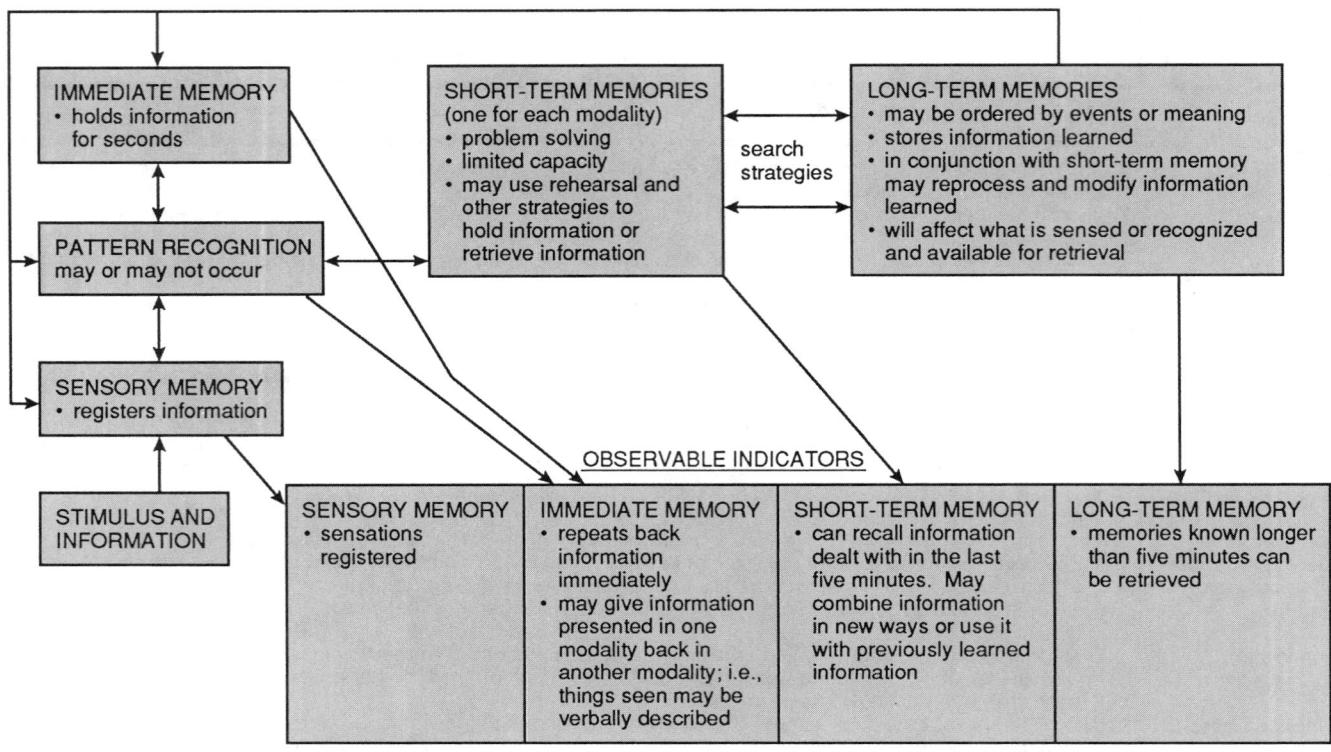

FIGURE 13–20. Interactional components of short-term and long-term memory and their observable indicators.

for information. There are strategies that are used to hold information in memory and thereby increase the amount of information that can be held. Grouping information, termed *chunking*, or repeating information, called *rehearsal*, may be done to keep information in short-term memory. Some of the information from long-term memory may be organized in what is called *schemas*, a sequence of expected events. Schemas help reduce the complexity that short-term memory must deal with and thereby aid problem solving (reference 3, p 130). When a cluster of cues in a situation enters short-term memory, they may result in retrieval of a concept label; then material related to that concept will be brought up from long-term memory. For example, if a nurse hears that a new client with schizophrenia has been admitted, this cue may retrieve material from long-term memory related to schizophrenia. Things that are associated in memory are retrieved by what has been termed "associative memory." For example, associated with the concept of schizophrenia might be the potential for such nursing diagnoses as delusions or hallucinations.

Information in long-term memory can be ordered in hierarchies of propositions that aid recall (reference 3, pp 118–123). For example, the proposition, "all drugs can have side effects; therefore the nurse should check clients for side effects if they are on drugs," can be a stimulus for a good ongoing assessment based on the memory retrieval of these hierarchially related propositions.

The manner in which material is held in short-term memory would appear to be primarily acoustic (how do the words sound). However, semantics (meaning) and syntax (how things are structured) in a sentence and a language are also used.

It is thought that while materials are in short-term memory, some of the material is going into long-term memory. If the materials are rehearsed and are at the center of attention, it is more likely that the material can be recalled easily, especially if the material has been dealt with recently. If the material is not at the center of attention and is not of importance, the material may still have been coded into long-term memory, but the trace may be so weak that it will be shown to be there only by recognition tasks or by the faster rate at which material could be relearned.

Memory is now thought to be encoded by numerous synaptic connections where learning modifies the probability of an increase or decrease of the excitation or inhibition of connected neurons. Parallel neural pathways may be involved simultaneously. For example, an individual has 100 billion neurons, and millions of these may be involved in solving a mathematics problem (reference 3, p 9). The number of brain synapses increases until age 2 years and then slowly decreases over time.[16] The metabolic rate of a child's brain, age 2 to 4, is twice that of adult.[16] Information in short-term memory may be like a fragile electrical trace while long-term memory may result in structural changes.[16]

There is still controversy about whether material encoded in long-term memory is ever lost completely. One explanation of memory loss is that material could still be present in long-term memory but might be weakened by decay over time. Alternatively, a memory may either be completely gone after a time or may take so long to retrieve that it is useless. Material in long-term memory may be stored in terms of meaning, and the material in memory may, over time, be recoded or modified in relation to meaning. For example, stories told to subjects taking memory tests may be reproduced with a minimal amount of distortion in relation to their personal view or culture if they are tested immediately, but if tested weeks or months later, subjects may reproduce the story with even more cultural or personal distortion in relation to what is meaningful to them.[8] Material in long-term memory may be remembered around episodes or events termed "episodic memory." Memories of this type may be stimulated by helping the client center attention on the place, time, or other features of the event. Using relaxation techniques in combination with centering on episodes has increased recall.[32] In general, pictures are remembered by individuals more readily than acoustic or written material. However, this can vary widely. With some individuals, these preferences may involve a whole cognitive style of learning.

Levels of Processing Theory

An alternative theory of memory is called the "levels of processing theory."[13,14,29,33] As the name implies, levels of coding are a significant feature of this theory. Stimuli are processed at different levels, namely, the *physical*, *acoustic*, and *semantic*. The semantic is thought to be the deepest level. These levels are processing variants: there are no separate structures hypothesized, as in the short-term theory. One of the basic assumptions of this theory is that deeper processing leads to a better memory. Some of the later research has indicated that this depends on the type of test given.[14]

The three levels have some resemblance to the three parts of the short-term, long-term memory theory in that sensory memory deals with physical stimuli, whereas material in short-term memory is thought usually to be held acoustically and long-term memory to be organized semantically.

RELATED FACTORS

Memory loss can occur in any condition that disrupts brain functions associated with memory. These conditions are numerous, and major causes will be mentioned.

Strokes,[46] brain tumors,[15,43] head trauma, and diseases such as Alzheimer's[38,41] and Huntington's[38] and Korsakoff's syndrome[38] account for a large percentage of the cases of memory loss. Memory loss can also be found after epileptic seizures,[18,40] cardiac arrests,[45] or exposure to toxic chemicals in the environment.

Memory loss can be secondary to prescribed treatments. Some clients who have had electroconvulsive therapy[44] complain not only of temporary memory loss but also of some permanent memory loss. Memory loss may be secondary to the drugs prescribed for the client, for example, diazepam.[22] Other commonly prescribed drugs that may impair memory are alpha methyldopa, digitalis preparations, lithium carbonate, monoamine oxidase inhibitors, tricyclic antidepressants, beta blockers, and benzodiazepines (alprazolam, triazolam, clonazepam, and lorazepam), which can produce amnesic effects[17] (Table 13-11).

Any infectious agent that destroys or modifies brain tissue as, for example, in meningitis may cause memory loss. Secondary infections are common in AIDS clients, and these may invade the brain. Syphilis and tuberculosis may affect any part of the body. Psychological states can also cause memory loss, such as dissociative personality states.[1,34] In clients with multiple personalities, some of the personalities may not be aware of the other personalities. In fugue states, clients who otherwise appear normal may be unable to remember their identity.[28] Persons under extreme stress or in states of depression or grief may find that they are blocking, not able to remember what happened. Hypnosis is a psychological state where temporary or permanent memory loss can be suggested by the hypnotist.[7,49] Some research on clients with chronic schizophrenia suggested that poor memory in these clients may be familial.[12]

Elderly persons may remember material they learned earlier in life, but their ability to learn new information may be reduced. Persons who keep mentally active are more apt to perform well in later life.[35] It should be noted, however, that extensive memory loss is not normal in aging. Medication dosages may need to be modified as persons get older, as excretion rates may change, and serum levels may increase. Larson and associates noted in the elderly, "the drugs most frequently associated with memory loss or other symptoms of dementia are sedative hypnotics, other psychotropic drugs, cimetidine (Tagamet), and antihypertensive agents. Any drug with anticholinergic effects can impair cognitive function. Even high doses of aspirin have been associated with memory loss in the elderly. Antihypertensives and pain medications are a particularly troublesome pairing, but almost any combination has the potential to cause memory difficulties in a susceptible patient" (reference 30, p 57). Other causes of memory loss in the elderly that are frequently reversible are hypothyroidism, depression, and central nervous system lesions.[30]

DEFINING CHARACTERISTICS

The behaviors that indicate memory loss will be related to the part of memory affected and the cause of the memory loss (see Fig. 13-20).

If there is sensory memory loss, the individual may not be able to recognize visual information, sensations,

TABLE 13–11
Drugs that can affect memory

DRUG AND BIOCHEMICAL EFFECT THOUGHT TO REDUCE MEMORY	PART OF MEMORY AFFECTED AND SYMPTOMS
Alcohol (inhibits serotonin uptake) (reference 42, p 15)	Severe anterograde amnesia (reference 42, p 14)
	Retrograde amnesia (may vary)
	Confabulation
	Alcoholic blackout (reference 42, p 14)
Cannabis (marijuana) (inhibits acetylcholine) (reference 42, p 15)	Fragmentation of attention and thought (reference 42, p 15)
	Immediate memory spared (reference 42, p 15)
	Short-term memory reduced (reference 42, p 15)
	Loosening of associations in long-term memory (reference 42, p 15)
D-Lysergic acid diethylamide (LSD) (serotonin release blocked (reference 42, p 15) or neurons destroyed)	Attention disrupted (small doses)
	Immediate memory spared
	Short-term memory greatly impaired
	Long-term memory abnormal with flashbacks (reference 42, p 15)
Benzodiazepines	
Diazepam, triazolam, alprazolam, clonazepam, lorazepam	Short-term memory impaired (reference 42, p 13)
	Can cause amnesic effects[17]
Lorazepam	Short-term memory deficit (reference 42, p 13)
Flurazepam (Dalmane)	May reduce alertness for up to 50 hours
Anesthetic agents: halothane	Can cause short-term memory loss in some individuals for up to 24 hours or greater after surgery[47]
Lithium carbonate (reduces norepinephrine and dopamine activity; used for bipolar depression)	Cognitive slowing (reference 27, pp 1467–1468)
	Decreased ability to concentrate
	Impaired long-term memory retrieval (reference 27, pp 1467–1468)
Antidepressants	
Amitriptyline (may be secondary to anticholinergic effects)	Reduced immediate memory (reference 27, p 1468)
	Decreased paired associate learning (reference 27, p 1468)
	Reduced performance on Porteus Maze and Trail Making Test (reference 27, p 1468)
	Impaired free recall and recall after semantic cues (reference 27, p 1468)
Nortriptyline	Impaired recall of digit span backwards (reference 27, p 1468)
Neuroleptics (antipsychotic medications)	Little or no change reported (reference 27, p 1469)
	The sedation may reduce performance and memory capabilities (reference 42, p 14)
Psychostimulants	
Amphetamines or cocaine	Do not affect memory directly[42]
	May increase vigilance and quickness (reference 27, p 1469)
Methylphenidate	In low doses, may improve learning
	In high doses, may impair memory, probably secondary to disrupted attention (reference 42, p 1470)

sounds, or speech. If this occurs, it must be determined whether the client is not perceiving the material or whether the brain is not able to encode the material so that it can be repeated immediately (immediate memory).

If short-term memory is modified, the client may not be able to hold information in memory to work on problems and may not be able to use any strategies to keep more information in memory. This may be evidenced by an inability to learn new information or to solve simple problems. The client may be able to recognize objects but may have a dazed look when asked to solve a problem. Clients are sometimes able to repeat short statements immediately (immediate memory) but do not remember them 5 minutes later (short-term memory). The client may appear uncooperative. An

example of the loss of short-term memory is the client who is being taught self-medication but does not repeat the schedule and names of the drugs after 5 minutes. A client may give an emotional response if unable to solve a problem or remember. Some clients appear depressed or stare vacantly, whereas others make an angry outburst or start crying. Some clients say they can't remember, whereas others hide the lapse by saying, "I'm just not going to tell you." This latter answer may be a cover-up, leaving the nurse to figure out another means to sort out motivation from a memory problem. Joseph points out that confabulations "on the basis of clinical observation and a review of a number of studies . . . frequently are associated with cerebral damage that involves the right hemisphere notably the frontal (often bilaterally) and parietal lobes areas intimately involved with attention, information regulation, and integration" (reference 26, p 507). For example, confabulation is found in clients who use alcohol heavily and may have Korsakoff's syndrome.

Sometimes, after individuals return to their jobs following motor vehicle accidents, coworkers complain about their not acting or following through on decisions discussed. When long-term memory is intact, short-term memory loss may not be detected. Short-term anterograde memory loss with failure to consolidate information into long-term memory or the formation of weak traces is frequently seen. These individuals might be able to repeat information immediately (immediate memory) but do not remember information 5 minutes later (short-term memory), nor remember what was discussed 24 hours later (long-term memory).

If the client has a problem with long-term memory, material learned previously will not be remembered. This loss of memory may be partial or complete. Family members might complain that they discussed important information such as financial arrangements, vacation plans, or a will with the client, then 1 week later, the client does not remember anything about it. In contrast, forgetfulness or selective memory loss might be indicated by the wife telling the nurse that, "George remembers a lot of things, but he tends to forget to take his medication on time and other things on a time schedule, so I have to remind him." The ability to remember future events, such as when to take a medication, is sometimes called prospective memory. Some authors see forgetfulness as a retrieval problem, that individuals cannot remember what they knew. The distinction seems to be before or after an event: can the client remember something coming in the future (prospectively) or can something which already has occurred be remembered?

Clients with severe Alzheimer's disease may not recognize family members and ongoing conversation.[24] Memory loss can also be so severe that the client may be at risk of serious injury or death from wandering off care units into traffic or snowstorms (Chart 1).

NURSING PROCESS AND RATIONALE

Assessment

Table 13-12 presents a summary of some of the major differences in the way memory functions can be assessed. Simple pattern recognition can be tested by drawing a cross, an apple, and a man and asking the patient to identify the figures. When testing memory, it is useful to distinguish between declarative memory and procedural memory. Declarative memory is related to the client's knowledge of propositions such as episodes or word references. In contrast, procedural memory is a test of the ability to carry out procedures.[9] For example, a client may not be able to remember events but might remember how to ride a bicycle, get out of bed, or trace a star when shown how to do it.[42]

Asking individuals to repeat information or to read

CHART 1
Memory Loss: Definition, Related Factors, and Defining Characteristics

DEFINITION

Memory loss is the inability to sense, recognize, hold, modify, code, or retrieve information or procedures. The types of memory loss differ considerably, as seen in Table 13–10.

RELATED FACTORS

Alcoholism
Strokes
Brain tumors
Alzheimer's disease
Huntington's disease
Cardiac arrest
Exposure to toxic environmental chemicals or anesthesia
Electroconvulsive therapy
Prescribed drugs such as beta blockers or benzodiazepines
Opiate and cannabis use
Dissociative personality states, fugue states
Hypnotic state
Brain infections
Aging, in combination with other factors
Stress
Dementia
Stimulus deprivation over time
Depression and grieving
Endocrine disorders such as hypothyroidism
Severe electrolyte imbalances and severe anemia

DEFINING CHARACTERISTICS

Unable to recognize information, persons, or patterns presented
Unable to repeat information or procedures just given
Unable to repeat information or procedures presented 5 minutes ago
Unable to recall information or procedures known longer than 5 minutes ago
Unable to carry out a sequence of tasks
Does not remember to do things without prompting
Cannot figure out how to summarize or condense information
May appear angry, confused, depressed, and incoherent
May lie or confabulate
May acknowledge memory loss

---

material is a test of immediate memory. A question such as "what is your name?" is a test of long-term memory. To test short-term memory, new information must be given, and it should be tested soon afterward; e.g., presenting three objects and asking the patient 5 minutes later what those objects were.

Tests for long-term memory involve asking clients something previously known such as "what is your current address?" Questions that will get at recent versus remote memory should be built into the assess-

TABLE 13–12
Nursing assessment of memory functions

	RIGHT HEMISPHERE	LEFT HEMISPHERE
MEMORY		
Immediate recall	Figure span	Digit span
		Letter span
		A-test (circle as after 45–60 seconds)
Recent memory (learning)	Orientation to self	Name
	Orientation to place (visual)	Address
	Orientation to person (visual)	
		Orientation to time
		Orientation to place (verbal identification of place)
		Orientation to person (verbal identification)
	Figures at 5 minutes	Names of objects at 5 minutes
	Drawings at 5 minutes that cannot have easy verbal labels placed on them	Babcock sentence
Retrieval	Recognition of photographs of the past	List of presidents
	Recognition of places visited in the past	Major events
	Recognition of music from the past	Fund of information (events, state capitals)
	Recognition of objects from the past	Personal history
		Medical history
Executive functions	Ability to perform sequenced activities such as dressing and bathing	Ability to carry out a series of verbal requests
		Ability to carry out a series of written requests
Cognitive functions		Mathematical calculations
		Right–left orientation
		Abstraction ability (proverbs, similarities/differences)
	Interpretation	
	Judgment	
	Insight	
BEHAVIOR		
MOOD		
APPEARANCE		

From Boss BJ, Barbara BJ. Memory impairments: Forgetfulness versus amnesia. J Neurosci Nurs. 1988;20(3):156. Used with permission.

ment. The birth date of the client and an address is usually on the driver's license; such data sources provide the possibility of verification if there is uncertainty as to accuracy of answers and the potential for fabrication. Relatives and friends may be sources of information about the client—possibly the only source that will help clarify the client's status. For example, in transitory global amnesia, the client's relatives may be the only individuals who will know how long the client has been unable to remember or whether the memory loss was preceded by any event that would rule out this diagnosis.

A number of articles present examples of memory tests. Gillis gives examples of five tests to measure cognitive dysfunction. They are the face–hand test, the misplaced objects tests, the brief mental status questionnaire, the Mini-Mental Status test, and the FROMAJE test.[20] The article by Larson and associates contains the Mini-Mental Status examination developed by Folstein.[30] Whyte presents a more theoretical article on the evaluation of the hierarchy of cognitive activity.[48] Mateer and coworkers present a new memory questionnaire in their article and the results of that questionnaire when it was used to test both brain-injured subjects with coma and controls.[36] The Set Test can differentiate memory deficits associated with dementia and depression.[23]

Once memory loss is established, only part of the nursing diagnostic work is done. The implications these defects have for client care need to be determined.[6] What activities of daily living are affected by these problems? Will the client remember to go to the bathroom? Do measures need to be taken to prevent wandering off the unit? Does the family need instruction on how to compensate for the client's forgetfulness? Will the client with alcoholism have to be driven home because short-term memory and reaction time are blocked by alcohol? Does the client with a brain tumor have to be helped to eat because he or she cannot remember how? Client care needs to be coordinated with the client and the family, physician, occupational therapist, speech therapist, physical therapist, clinical psychologist, social worker, and other members of the health team. Can the team discuss the client's prognosis so that consistent and accurate expectations are conveyed to the family? Can a home visit be done, especially if the client lives alone, so that an accurate on-site analysis can be made to determine what problems, if any, are still being encountered?

Nursing Diagnosis

Examples of specific nursing diagnoses include: memory loss related to alcoholism; memory loss (short-term) related to electroconvulsive therapy; and memory loss (short-term) related to depression.

Client Goals and Nursing Interventions

Because memory loss can occur in so many forms and so many conditions, the goals for nursing care may differ. Usually, the goals will involve: (1) compensating for the memory loss to ensure the client's safety and well-being; (2) observation of the client's performance to determine if there are any changes over time in the memory status; (3) coordination with other health personnel and significant others to assist the client in recovering memory; and (4) working with the family, friends, and community to provide the best care if compensation for memory loss is needed or for retraining the individual or modifying the environment.

The emphasis in interventions is on trying to help the client use the skills that remain in order to help the client regain or make progress on the areas lost. The individual may need a lot of encouragement, and the nurse must be careful not to present too much material or tire the client too much. Supportive behaviors such as acceptance, patience, and interactions to reduce anxiety are crucial.[10] If material is lost in relation to more than one sensory modality, then each of these modalities must be considered when assisting the client to learn. Learning new material in more than one modality is more taxing than learning new material in just one modality. However, cross-modality learning may be reinforcing. Gillis describes how an information-processing model and integrative therapy was used to teach independent self-care to older adults.[20] When working with a client who is recovering short-term memory capacity, the tasks should be simple at first in view of the limited capacity of short-term memory, recognizing that any problem solving will take more of that space. The client should be tested for and taught rehearsal, chunking, and the use of mnemonics.

Because material in memory may be organized by meaning, schemas, and propositions, this should be used in client teaching as much as possible. For example, can the problem of the client remembering to take medications be converted into a schema of steps? Environmental supports may be used as, for example, a daily pill box and a wristwatch with an alarm that rings when the medication is to be taken.

Long-term memories can be lost or be unable to be retrieved if it is not used. Reminiscence therapy is structured to try to help clients recall the past as a way of keeping mentally active and to help counteract the lack of personal identity that can occur in a long-term care setting.[11]

Environmental supports such as props, hints, reminders, a daily schedule book, or diary may all be useful aids for many types of memory loss.[10] Glisky and Schacter describe how practice drills, mnemonic strategies, and external aids can be used for remediation of organic memory disorder. Ways to work with clients for the acquisition of domain-specific knowledge are described.[21]

Pleasant events have been used as a type of therapy to overcome depression. Engaging in pleasant events has also been helpful in improving memory generally. The limbic centers of the brain that control emotion are some of the same structures that are central to the laying down of new memories. These centers are the hippocampus, the amygdala, the hypothalamus, and the thalamus. Stimulation of these brain centers by pleasant activities may modify the brain biochemistry directly, and the pleasant events may also increase general metabolism, appetite, and alertness.

Finally, two techniques, frequently taught to normal subjects as a means of helping them remember, may be useful to clients as well as health care workers. The first technique is called the PQ4R method.[3] It has been found that subjects remember better when learning material, if they first *preview* the material, looking over what it is that they will learn or read. As they preview the material, they should raise *questions* about it, such as what specific terms mean and convert subtitles into questions. Next, they *read* the materials carefully and *reflect* on the meaning (the first two Rs). Finally, they *recite* the information, then try to summarize and state what has been learned (*review*). The second technique is called the method of loci. In this method, a list of things to remember is associated with a well-known path or route.

Evaluation

When evaluating the outcomes of the nursing interventions, the nurse focuses on the particular areas in which deficits were previously noted. Nursing care interventions carried out will be evaluated to determine how effective they have been over time. In the case of memory loss, outcome criteria may have to be revised depending on the changing state of the client, as, for example, with some progressive degenerative brain conditions (Chart 2).

CHART 2
Memory Loss: Summary of the Nursing Process

NURSING INTERVENTIONS	OUTCOME CRITERIA
CLIENT GOAL: MAINTAIN PHYSICAL AND PSYCHOLOGICAL WELL-BEING	
Assess impact of memory loss on activities, such as forgetting to eat or forgetting the location of the bathroom	Maintains daily self-care
Assist the client with ADLs as necessary	Remains safe from harm
Assess the client's environment for risks such as wandering secondary to memory loss	
Make environmental changes to avert danger	
Assess the client's emotional response to memory loss; e.g. anxiety, anger, depression	Is less disturbed about situation
Acknowledge the client's feelings	
CLIENT GOAL: EXPERIENCE IMPROVEMENT IN MEMORY	
Assess type of memory loss and related factors	Has improved memory
Direct interventions to any related factors; e.g., stress, that can be influenced	
CLIENT GOAL: COMPENSATE FOR CONTINUING MEMORY DEFICITS	
Support family in discussing their concerns and feelings regarding relative's memory loss	Family identifies ways to compensate for client's memory loss
Teach client and family means to compensate for memory deficits; e.g.: Pill box with times and days indicated Calendars Lists Keeping items in same place	Client functions at the highest level possible given continuing memory deficits

CASE STUDY

Mr. Robert C, a 60-year-old man, was admitted to the psychiatric unit. He had been isolated since the death of his wife 2 years ago. Information gathered on admission indicated that he lived alone, was anemic, and sometimes forgot to shop for, prepare, and eat food. He was taking both diazepam and triazolam. His daughter encouraged him to come into the hospital because of weight loss and memory deficits. Mr. C's nursing diagnoses at the time of admission included altered nutrition, less than body requirements, due to forgetfulness; and memory loss due to lack of social stimulation and to benzodiazepines and anemia.

Mr. C remained in the hospital 10 days. During that time, all medications were tapered and then discontinued. Attention was directed toward improving Mr. C's nutritional intake. He was encouraged to participate in groups on the ward. His memory slowly improved, and he became more active with the other clients on the unit. He continued to see a psychosocial nurse counselor after being discharged. One year after discharge, he took a part-time position as a desk clerk and had expanded his social network.

SUMMARY

Memory loss is the inability to sense, recognize, hold, modify, code, or retrieve information or procedures. Major theories of memory include short-term long-term memory theory and levels of processing theory. Memory loss can occur in any condition that disrupts the brain functions associated with memory. The behaviors associated with memory loss vary with the part of memory affected and the cause of the memory loss. Nursing interventions are directed toward ensuring safety and well-being, improving memory, and assisting the family in compensating for continuing deficits.

Research Highlights

There are continuing searches for drugs that will improve memory. Most of these studies show limited, if any, improvement. One nursing study looked at improving memory in clients with dementia using lecithin and physostigmine. The pilot study on nine clients showed some improvement of clients on a tool designed to measure activities of daily living orientation, communication, and behavior.[4] Physostigmine also improved memory disturbances secondary to electroconvulsive therapy (ECT) in a study of 17 schizophrenic and depressed patients.[31] Galizia provides a review of drug studies used to improve memory or enhance recall in the elderly. She concludes, "positive results have been observed with cholinergic drugs, acetylcholine precursors, and the newer category of cerebral metabolic enhancers and nootropic agents" (reference 19, p 784).

References

1. American Psychiatric Association. Descriptions of psychoactive substance use disorders. In: Diagnostic and Statistical Manual of Mental Disorders, ed 3. rev. Washington, DC: American Psychiatric Association; pp 173–185. 1987.
2. American Psychiatric Association. Quick Reference to the Diagnostic Criteria from DSM-III-R. Washington, DC: American Psychiatric Association; 1987.
3. Anderson JR. Cognitive Psychology and Its Implications. New York: WH Freeman; 1985.
4. Antoline M, Holland C, Scruggs B. Measuring improvement in patients with dementia. Geriatric Nursing. July/August, pp 185–189: 1986.
5. Atkinson RC, Shiffrin RM. Human memory: A proposed system and its control processes. In: Spence KW, Spence JT, eds. The Psychology of Learning and Motivation. vol 2. New York: Academic Press; 1968.
6. Baas L. Memory error. Nurs Clin North Am. 1985;20:731–743.
7. Bartis S, Zamansky H. Dissociation in post hypnotic amnesia: Knowing without knowing. Am J Clin Hypn. 1986;29(2):103–108.
8. Bartlett FC. Remembering: A Study in Experimental and Social Psychology. Cambridge: Cambridge University Press; 1932.
9. Boss B. The neuroanatomical and neurophysiological basis of learning. J Neurosci Nurs. 1986;18(5):256–264.
10. Boss BJ. Memory impairments: Forgetfulness versus amnesia. J Neurosci Nurs. 1988;80(3):151–158.
11. Burnside I. Reminiscence and other therapeutic modalities. In: Nursing and the Aged: A Self-Care Approach. New York: McGraw-Hill; pp 645–686; 1988.
12. Chezan S, Bennet J, Guttman R. Familial correlation of memory function in schizophrenia. Psychopathology. 1986;19:165–169.
13. Craik FIM, Lockhart RS. Levels of processing: A framework for memory research. J Verbal Learning Verbal Behavior. 1972;11:671–684.
14. Craik FIM, Tulving E. Depth of processing and the retention of words in episodic memory. J Exper Psychology (General). 1975;104:268–294.
15. Cullum C, Bigler E. Late effects of hematoma on brain morphology and memory in closed head injury. Int J Neurosci. 1985;28:279–283.
16. Digital Discovery Series. The Infinite Voyage. Pittsburgh: WQED; 1988.
17. Edwards S. Ohio Medi Scene. Ohio State Med J. 1987, January, 17–19.
18. Eich E. Epilepsy and state specific memory. Acta Neurol Scand. 1986;74(suppl 109):15–21.
19. Galizia V. Pharmacotherapy of memory loss in the geriatric patient. Drug Intell Clin Pharm. 1984;18:784–790.
20. Gillis D. Patients suffering from memory loss can be taught self-care. Geriatr Nurs. September/October, pp 257–261; 1986.
21. Glisky E. Remediation of organic memory disorders: Current status and future prospects. J Head Trauma Rehabil. 1986;1(3):54–63.
22. Goldstein M. Valium: The miracle pill. This World. February 1988;28, 17–18.
23. Hays A. The Set Test to screen mental status quickly. Geriatr Nurs. 1984;5:96–97.
24. Heston LL, White JA. Dementia: A Practical Guide to Alzheimer's Disease and Related Illness. New York: WH Freeman; 1983.
25. Jacome D. Case report: Subcortical prosopagnosis and anosognosia. Am J Med Sci. 1986;292:386–388.
26. Joseph R. Confabulation and delusional denial: Frontal lobe and lateralized influences. J Clin Psychol. 1986;42:507–520.
27. Judd L, Squire L, Butters N, Salmon D, Paller K. Effects of psychotropic drugs on cognition in animals. In: H. Meltzer, ed. Psychopharmacology: The Third Generation of Progress. New York: Raven Press; pp 1467–1468; 1987.
28. Keller R. Amnesia or fugue state: A diagnostic dilemma. Dev Behav Ped. 1986;7:131–132.
29. Klatzky RL. Human Memory: Structure and Processes. New York: WH Freeman; 1980.
30. Larson E, Larue A, Wyma D. Memory loss: Is it reversible? Patient Care. 1987;April 30, 54–66.
31. Levin Y, Elizur A, Korczyn A. Physostigmine improves ECT-induced memory disturbances. Neurology. 1987;37:871–875.
32. Levy R. A method for the recovery of mishap-related events lost to amnesia. Aviat Space Environ Med. March, 1987;257–259.
33. Lockhart RS, Craik FIM, Jacoby L. Depth of processing recognition and recall. In: Brown J (ed). Recall and Recognition. New York: John Wiley; 1976.
34. Markowitz J, Viederman M. A case report of dissociative pseudodementia. Gen Hosp Psychiatry. 1986;8:87–90.
35. Markson E. Gender roles and memory loss in old age: An exploration of linkages. Int J Aging Hum Dev. 1985–86;22(3):205–214.
36. Mateer C, Sohlberg M, Crenian J. Focus on clinical research: Perceptions of memory function in individuals with closed head injury. J Head Trauma Rehab. 1987;2(3):74–84.
37. Miller JW, Peterson RC, Metter EJ, Millikan CH, Yanagihara T. Transient global amnesia: Clinical characteristics and prognosis. Neurology. 1987;37:733–737.
38. Moss M, Albert M, Butters N, Payne M. Differential patterns of memory loss among patients with Alzheimer's disease, Huntington's disease, and alcoholic Korsakoff's syndrome. Arch Neurol. 1986;43:239–246.
39. Ozuna J. Alterations in mentation: Nursing assessment and intervention. J Neurosurg Nurs. 1985;17(1):66–70.
40. Pedersen B, Dam M. Memory disturbances in epileptic patients. Acta Neurolog Scand. 1986;74(suppl 109):11–14.
41. Pomara N, Stanley M. The cholinergic hypothesis of memory dysfunction in Alzheimer's disease: Revisited. Psychopharmacology Bull. 1986;22(1):110–118.
42. Riley N, Gordon W. Memory for Health Professionals. Stanford, California: Conference materials, Institute for Cortex Research and Development; 1988.
43. Salazar A, Grofman J, Vance S, Weingartner H, Dillon J, Ludlow C. Consciousness and amnesia after penetrating head injury: Neurology and anatomy. Neurology. 1986;36:178–187.
44. Squire L, Zouzounis J. ECT and memory: Brief pulse versus sine wave. Am J Psychiatry. 1986;143:596–601.
45. Volpe B, Holtzman J, Hirst W. Further characterization of patients with amnesia after cardiac arrest: Preserved recognition memory. Neurology. 1986;36:408–411.
46. Waxman S, Ricourte G, Tucker S. Thalamic hemorrhage with neglect and memory disorder. J Neurolog Sci. 1986;75:105–112.
47. White MJ, Wolf–Wilets V. Memory loss following halothane anesthesia. AORNA J. 1977;26:1053–1064.
48. Whyte J. Outcome evaluation in the remediation of attention and memory deficits. J Trauma Rehab. 1986;1(3):64–71.
49. Wilson L, Kihlstrom J. Subjective and categorical organization of recall during posthypnotic amnesia. J Abnormal Psychology. 1986;95:264–273.
50. Zegeer L. Forgetfulness: A related or Alzheimer's disease? J Neurosci Nurs. 1987;19(2):61–62.

POST-OVERDOSE SYNDROME

Eldine I. Sanger

DEFINITION AND DESCRIPTION

Post-overdose syndrome is a cluster of thoughts, feelings, and behaviors that occurs shortly after a serious suicide attempt by overdose. After a client is treated for the immediate effects of the overdose in the intensive care unit, medical unit, or emergency room, a pattern of responses emerges that includes both the physiologic effects of the toxic overdose and of sleep deprivation, as well as psychological effects. These psychological effects include pressured speech, racing thoughts, and a flooding of feelings.

THEORY AND RESEARCH

Post-overdose syndrome was identified during a study of depressed clients.[20] Components of the syndrome include the toxic effects of the drug overdose, effects of sleep deprivation, and psychological effects of the serious suicide attempt in the immediate period after the attempt. Prescription drugs, nonprescription drugs, and drugs of abuse are all commonly used for overdose. Mixed-drug overdose is nearly as common as single-drug overdose and can be particularly dangerous because of the additive effects related to central nervous system depression.[4,5,17] The most commonly used drugs or substances for overdose are alcohol, tricyclic antidepressants, and benzodiazepines[18] (Box 13-8).

Delayed or Persistent Toxic Effects

Complications of overdose include the specific pharmacologic effects of the particular drug(s) ingested and the nonspecific consequences of coma. The life-threatening effects of the overdose are treated in the emergency department or intensive care unit. The delayed or persistent toxic effects that may be present, or appear after the person is medically stable, are the first component of post-overdose syndrome. For example, hypotension subsequent to overdose with central nervous system depressant drugs may persist, even after restoration of normal cardiac activity, and can be due to hypovolemia.[17] Aftereffects of lithium carbonate overdose can include sodium and water loss for days or weeks following lithium intoxication.[8] Tricyclic antidepressants can be particularly dangerous because of the risk of delayed cardiac arrhythmias, which have been reported as late as six days post-ingestion.[8,13]

Clinical relapse, in which clinical deterioration follows a period of improvement, has been reported for a variety of psychotropic drugs. Manifestations include deterioration of neurologic, hemodynamic, and respiratory status.[17] Drugs that have anticholinergic properties (tricyclics, antihistamines, antipsychotics, and many over-the-counter medications) are responsible for many acute toxic effects and also some of the most commonly reported lingering aftereffects: blurred vision and hypotension.[8,23]

Sleep Deprivation

A second component of post-overdose syndrome is sleep deprivation. Disturbed sleep is a prodromal symptom of many mental illnesses; it is likely that a sleep pattern disturbance exists in clients before an overdose because of the association of insomnia with anxiety, depression, alcoholism, severe stress, post-traumatic stress disorder, and other psychiatric conditions.[22] Sleep deprivation is intensified by a combination of such events as initial treatment of the acute phase of the overdose by lavage; toxic effects of the drug ingested (e.g., agitation caused by anticholinergic effects); environmental noise, such as machines in intensive care units; or treatment regimes, such as restraints that interfere with sleep.[16] Signs of sleep deprivation include subjective reports of sleepiness and fatigue, decreased concentration, mood deterioration, and hyperirritability.[1,7,16] A one-night loss of sleep can result in mood deterioration and sleepiness. Two nights or more of sleep loss result in decreased psychomotor performance and decreased sense of well-being. Recovery from sleep deprivation is usually completed in two to three nights.[16]

Psychological Sequelae

Psychological sequelae occur in the period immediately after a serious suicide attempt, and compose the third component of post-overdose syndrome. A major finding in a study of 25 nonpsychotic clients who had made a suicide attempt by drug overdose was the eagerness of the subjects, including those who still wished they had not survived, to talk about their suicidal crisis.[15] Common feelings reported after the overdose included anger (at both self and others) and relief

---

BOX 13–8
Post-overdose Syndrome: Drugs Commonly Used for Overdose

PRESCRIPTION DRUGS
Benzodiazepines
Tricyclic antidepressants
Neuroleptics
Barbiturates
Monoamine oxidase inhibitors
Narcotic analgesics
Lithium carbonate

NONPRESCRIPTION DRUGS
Salicylates
Acetaminophen

DRUGS OF ABUSE
Alcohol
Cocaine

MIXED-DRUG OVERDOSE COMBINATIONS
Tricyclic antidepressants and phenothiazines
Alcohol and benzodiapines

---

or happiness when they realized they would survive. Positive and negative feelings were intertwined.[15]

The literature on post-traumatic stress disorder describes several phases that may occur after a serious life event. The immediate response may include alarm, accompanied by fear; this is described as inward or outward "crying out." The intrusive phase is a cluster of signs and symptoms that include: feelings of being pressured, confused, or disorganized when thinking about themes related to the event; sleep disturbance; emotional "attacks" or "pangs" of affect related to the event; and intrusive and repetitive thoughts, emotions, and behaviors. The denial phase includes emotional numbness, sleep disturbance, and withdrawal.[9,10] The client experiencing post-overdose syndrome is also experiencing a reaction to a serious life event and has many of the same feelings and symptoms as those described in the intrusive phase.

RELATED FACTORS

Post-overdose syndrome is time-limited and related to a serious or life-threatening overdose. Related factors for suicide attempts by drug overdose are considered because that is, by definition, part of the syndrome. Related factors for attempts at suicide by overdose include the co-occurrence of major depression with another disorder, such as alcoholism, prior or current psychiatric treatment, a high (70%) history of regular alcohol use, and a previous suicide attempt (57%).[6,18] Hopelessness has been found to correlate highly with suicide intent.[3] Demographic characteristics of drug overdose clients include: a female/male ratio of 2:1; the highest incidence occurring in young adults, espe-

cially aged 20 to 24 years; and an increased frequency in single persons who have never been married or in those separated or divorced.[4]

Studies that have focused on the purpose or reasons for taking overdoses can assist in directing treatment and intervention. Three key themes emerged relevant to the purpose served by the suicide attempt in a study of 25 nonpsychotic subjects who ingested an overdose: a clear statement of the wish to die; ambivalence toward living or dying; and a view of the attempt as a way to change their lives or influence significant others.[15] Four groups of reasons were found for taking overdoses: suicidal intent; help-seeking; self-referring; and direction at a significant person.[2]

DEFINING CHARACTERISTICS

Post-overdose syndrome is of limited duration, which is dependent on the decrease in toxic effects of overdose drug(s), improvement in sleep pattern, and resolution of the acute-phase psychological reactions. Indications of the lingering effects of toxicity include alterations in fluid balance and vital signs, particularly hypotension. The client may report blurred vision, lightheadedness, dizziness, and fatigue. Decreased concentration, sleepiness, mood deterioration, and hyperirritability are signs of sleep deprivation. A flooding of feelings is observable in speaking with the client. The feelings can include guilt for making the attempt, powerlessness, and hopelessness. There is a vulnerability about how the person presents himself or herself. Repeated descriptions of the suicide attempt may be made in a detached manner, almost as if this had not happened to the client. Speech may be pressured, and racing thoughts may be reported. Reexperiencing the actual attempt is most likely to occur soon after the overdose and is related to both the need to review and piece together the recent attempt and the current vulnerability and intensity of feelings.

Among persons who made less serious attempts by overdose, the most frequently occurring defining characteristics dealt with coordination, energy levels, and the behavioral effects of neurologic suppression from the drugs ingested.[19]

The nursing diagnoses, sleep pattern disturbance and post-trauma response, both have defining characteristics that overlap with those of post-overdose syndrome. Differences between these diagnoses and post-overdose syndrome are based on the time-limited nature of post-overdose syndrome and the self-destructive focus of the trauma (Chart 1).

NURSING PROCESS AND RATIONALE

Assessment

The nurse assesses clients who are in the recovery period from a serious overdose for post-overdose syn-

Chart 1
Post-overdose Syndrome: Definition, Related Factors, and Defining Characteristics

DEFINITION

Post-overdose syndrome is a cluster of thoughts, feelings, and behaviors that occurs shortly after a severe suicide attempt by overdose. The syndrome includes the physiologic effects of the toxic overdose and sleep deprivation as well as psychological effects.

RELATED FACTORS

Suicide attempt by ingestion of drugs
Factors related to suicide attempt by ingestion of drugs
   Depression co-occurring with another disorder
   Alcohol abuse
   History of psychiatric treatment
   Prior suicide attempts
   Hopelessness
   Demographic factors
      Female
      Age 20 to 24 years
      Single, separated, or divorced

DEFINING CHARACTERISTICS

Blurred vision
Hypotension
Alteration in fluid balance
Decreased concentration
Mood deterioration
Hyperirritability
Sleepiness
Appears vulnerable
Repeated, detached description of suicide attempt
Pressured speech
Racing thoughts
Flooding of feelings: guilt, hopelessness, powerlessness

drome by observing if the defining characteristics are present. All clients who make an attempt at suicide by overdose may not experience the syndrome. Some clients move rapidly to the denial phase and do not experience the thoughts and feelings associated with the syndrome. Others are psychotic and may experience apathy and indifference.[23] A conference with family members or significant others early in the hospitalization can provide more data and support. A thorough assessment of the client and family or significant others, as well as of the current stressors and living situation, is important for understanding the family and social support system.

Nursing Diagnosis

A diagnosis of post-overdose syndrome can be made specific for a client as, for example, post-overdose syn-

drome related to ingestion of imiprimine following the break-up of a long-time relationship with a female friend.

Client Goals and Nursing Interventions

The diagnosis of post-overdose syndrome almost always co-occurs with suicidal potential. This necessitates frequent observation and contracting with the client to discuss any suicidal ideation as a means of assuring client safety.[14]

In assisting the client to regain normal physiologic functioning after a toxic overdose, it is important to use basic nursing skills of observation to monitor vital signs, and to maintain fluid balance. Hypotension, dizziness, lightheadedness, unsteady gait, and a "spacey" feeling are related to toxicity. As mentioned earlier, clinical relapse can occur after the client appears to be medically stable; therefore, the nurse must continue to observe for change. Monitoring postural changes in blood pressure can assist in prevention of falls. The client may need to be taught to change positions slowly or arise from bed only if a nurse is present. A client who has been intubated during treatment for overdose may ask why a sore throat is present; an explanation of the cause and use of throat lozenges will provide some relief. An explanation that blurred vision is a common and transitory toxic effect of many drugs may also be reassuring.

The nurse can help the client experience relief in intensity of feelings and a decrease in anxiety. After a severe suicide attempt, many clients do express relief at being alive and a wish to live.[21,24] One study found that all clients who survived a suicide attempt wished to live at the time of discharge.[2] The eagerness of clients to talk about their suicidal crisis is documented in the literature and is a rationale for support and encouragement from the nurse for a full discussion of the attempt.[15] Interventions at this time include active listening and support for expression of any feelings, reviewing the details of the attempt with the client, assisting the client in organizing information, and reassuring the client that the current intensity of feelings is a typical process after a crisis. Other general measures during this short period include permitting dependency, reducing external demands and stimulus levels, and promoting rest.

Family members may give additional information about the recent suicide attempt; they also bring their own feelings of guilt or anger.[11] Supportive contact with the family or significant others can be supplemented by a family conference with the family therapy team; a later conference or conferences can focus on interventions with the family and discharge planning.

Sleep deprivation is another problem faced by clients; the nurse can assist in improving the sleep pattern when the client reports extreme fatigue and exhaustion. Promotion of rest by a variety of nonchemical means is important, because hypnotics are not the treatment of choice after drug overdoses. Other measures include avoidance of caffeinated beverages, relaxation techniques or exercises with soft music; comfort measures such as warm milk, light snacks, massage, decreased environmental noise; and encouragement of expression of concerns when the client is unable to sleep.[12]

Evaluation

Resolution of post-overdose syndrome is indicated by an improved sleep pattern; however, the client may still experience some disturbed sleep that could be related to an underlying diagnosis such as major depression. Physiologic functioning should be close to normal; some toxic effects may persist, such as blurred vision, but the client may experience decreased anxiety about this it teaching has been effective. The client reports a subjective decrease in intensity of feelings and is able to function more independently. The client and family (or significant others) are able to work toward discharge planning (Chart 2).

CASE STUDY

Grace, a 60-year-old woman, was admitted to the psychiatric unit after treatment at her local general hospital for a serious overdose that resulted in a coma. After impulsively taking an undetermined amount of antidepressants and antianxiety medications, she called her son and was then rushed to the hospital.

The client's psychiatric diagnosis was major depression, and she related feeling depressed intermittently for the past 20 years. Treatment had been by her family physician and had included a number of antidepressants and antianxiety medications. Since her husband's death of a heart attack 18 months ago, Grace described herself as socially isolated, rarely seeing friends, not wanting to bother her son, and spending most of her time reading and watching television. She had no other living relatives.

When she arrived on the psychiatric unit she was agitated, and her speech was rapid and loud. She said, "I just can't take it anymore," and told of feeling depressed and exhausted from sleep loss. She described her impulsive suicidal attempt repeatedly in an almost detached manner—as if she could not believe she had done it. She said she was glad she had not succeeded, because it would cause her son grief. She said she could not stop thinking about the attempt, and that her thoughts were going very fast. Her vulnerability in this acute crisis manifested itself by a flooding of feelings of guilt, hopelessness, and powerlessness. Physical symptoms included extreme fatigue, unsteady gait, dizziness, and hypotension.

CHART 2
Post-overdose Syndrome: Summary of the Nursing Process

NURSING INTERVENTIONS	OUTCOME CRITERIA
CLIENT GOAL: RETURN TO NORMAL PHYSIOLOGIC FUNCTIONING AS TOXIC EFFECTS DIMINISH	
Monitor vital signs, especially postural blood pressure and pulse	Stable vital signs
Maintain fluid balance	Stable fluid/electrolyte balance
Teach changing positions slowly; assist when up if gait unsteady	Steady gait
	Diminished dizziness and blurred vision
Teach about expected toxic effects of overdose	Experiences decreased anxiety about expected toxic effects
CLIENT GOAL: EXPERIENCE IMPROVED SLEEP PATTERN AND DECREASED FATIGUE	
Avoid hypnotics	Demonstrates increased intervals of sleep
Promote sleep by nonchemical interventions such as relaxation techniques, comfort measures	Reports feeling rested
Encourage expression of feelings if unable to sleep	
CLIENT GOAL: EXPERIENCE RELIEF IN INTENSITY OF FEELINGS FOLLOWING OVERDOSE	
Provide frequent contacts for supportive listening and encouragement for discussion of feelings and events surrounding attempt	Reports subjective decrease in intensity of feelings
Reassure patient that intensity of feelings is typical	Demonstrates decreased need to review events of suicide attempt
Support brief period of dependency	
Reduce external demands and stimulus level	
Gather data and provide support during family conference and other contacts	Client and family able to work with staff to make discharge plans

Research Highlights

An extensive study of 40 clients interviewed on an intensive care unit after they had attempted suicide related diagnostic groups to feelings and reactions following the attempt.[23] Clients who had a diagnosis of neuroses experienced feelings of shame, a sense of relief at having survived, guilt, fear, and feelings of inferiority. Those persons who had a substance abuse diagnosis experienced anger more strongly than the other groups, and in addition had feelings of shame, guilt, ambivalence, and fear. Those with psychosis or prepsychosis experienced pronounced indifference and apathy, with no clear expressions of guilt or anxiety. Clients from this last group answered questions with delay and did not seek out staff contact. Once conscious, most patients wondered how they behaved while in an unconscious or half-awake condition, and if their drug overdose had side effects. An important finding was that significant others did not receive support from hospital staff, despite their need for psychological help.

Immediate nursing diagnoses included post-overdose syndrome related to ingestion of antidepressant and antianxiety medications following chronic depression, death of husband, and social isolation; suicide potential related to chronic depression and grief. Nursing interventions related to post-overdose syndrome included monitoring vital signs and fluid balance, measures to prevent falls, and teaching about the typical side effects of overdoses. Nonchemical interventions to promote sleep, such as comfort measures, relaxation techniques, and decreased stimulation, were utilized. Grace's son visited frequently and psychiatric nursing staff gathered information from him and provided support. The nurses made frequent contacts with Grace to encourage discussion of feelings and the actual events of the suicide attempt. Grace was reassured that the intensity of feelings she experienced was typical. After Grace recovered from the effects of the drug toxicity and sleep deprivation, she was able to identify goals and to plan for the immediate future. A family conference was held with her son, and discharge planning included increasing support systems. The client wished to continue seeing her long-time family physician for follow-up. After a two-week stay in the hospital, Grace was ready to return home, although somewhat anxious about it.

SUMMARY

Post-overdose syndrome is a cluster of thoughts, feelings, and behaviors that occurs shortly after a serious suicide attempt by overdose. The syndrome includes toxic effects of the drugs ingested, sleep deprivation, and psychological sequelae. Client goals include to return to normal physiologic functioning as toxic effects diminish; to experience improved sleep pattern and decreased fatigue; and to experience relief in intensity of feelings.

References

1. Association of Sleep Disorders Centers. Diagnostic classification of sleep and arousal disorders. Sleep. 1979;2:1–136.
2. Bancroft J, Hawton K. Why people take overdoses: a study of psychiatrists' judgements. Br J Med Psychol. 1983;56:197–204.
3. Beck AT, Steen RA, Kovacs M, et al. Hopelessness and eventual suicide: a 10-year prospective study of patients hospitalized with suicidal ideation. Am J Psychiatry. 1985;142:559–563.
4. Bouknight RR. Suicide attempt by drug overdose. Am Fam Physician. 1986;33:4.
5. Bryson PD. Comprehensive review in toxicology. Rockville, MD: Aspen Systems Corporation; 1986.
6. Clayton PJ. Suicide. Psychiatric Clin North Am. 1985; 8(2):203–204.
7. Degan R, Niedermeyer E (eds). Epilepsy, sleep and sleep deprivation. New York: Elsevier Science Publishers; 1984.
8. Haddad LM, Winchester JF. Clinical management of poisoning and drug overdose. Philadelphia: WB Saunders; 1983.
9. Horowitz MJ. Stress response syndromes, 2nd ed. London: Jason Aronson; 1986.
10. Horowitz MJ. Stress response syndromes: a review of post-traumatic and adjustment disorders. Hosp Commun Psychiatry. 1986;37:3:241–249.
11. James D, Hawton K. Overdoses: explanations and attitudes in self-poisoners and significant others. Br J Psychiatry. 1985;146:481–485.
12. Kim MJ, McFarland GK, McLane AM. Pocket guide to nursing diagnoses. 3rd ed. St Louis: CV Mosby; 1989.
13. Klein D, Gittelman R, Quitkin F, Rifkin A. Diagnosis and drug treatment of psychiatric disorders: adults and children. Baltimore: William & Wilkins; 1980.
14. McFarland G, Wasli E. Nursing diagnosis and process in psychiatric mental health nursing. Philadelphia: JB Lippincott; 1986.
15. Pallikkathayil L, McBride AB. Suicide attempts. J Psychosoc Nurs. 1986;24(8):13–18.
16. Riley TL, ed. Clinical aspects of sleep and sleep disturbance. Boston: Butterworth Publishers; 1985.
17. Shader RI, ed. Manual of psychiatric therapeutics. Boston: Little, Brown & Company; 1986.
18. Stern TA, Mulley AG, Thibault GE. Life-threatening drug overdose. JAMA. 1984;251(15):1983–1985.
19. Taylor JE. Clinical validation of nursing diagnoses and defining characteristics for overdose patients. Houston: University of Texas Health Science Center at Houston; 1985. Thesis.
20. Thomas MD, Sanger E, Whitney JD. Nursing diagnosis of depression: clinical identification on an inpatient unit. J Psychosoc Nurs Ment Health Serv. 1986;24(8):6–12.
21. Varadaraj R, Mendonca JD, Rauchenberg PM. Motives and intent: a comparison of views of overdose patients and their key relatives/friends. Can J Psychiatry. 1986;31:621–624.
22. Williams RL, Karacan I. Recent developments in the diagnosis and treatment of sleep disorders. Hosp Commun Psychiatry. 1985;36:951–957.
23. Wolk-Wasserman D. The intensive care unit and the suicide attempt patient. Acta Psychiatr Scand. 1985;71:581–595.
24. Wright N, Adam KS. Changing motivation in severely suicidal patients. Can Med Assoc J. 1986;135:1361–1363.

POST-TRAUMA RESPONSE

Katsuko Tanaka

DEFINITION AND DESCRIPTION

Post-trauma response is the state of an individual experiencing a sustained painful response to an unexpected extraordinary life event(s). A traumatic event may be of human or of natural origin. Normally, such an event is so overwhelming that a person cannot deal with or assimilate the experience in the usual way.

THEORY AND RESEARCH

Responses to trauma have been observed in various disaster studies such as Vietnam War combat, rape, car accident, Nazi concentration camps, the Hiroshima atomic bomb, the Buffalo Creek dam collapse, lightning strikes, the Mount St. Helens volcanic eruption, Hurricane Agnes, and the Mississippi Valley flood.[2,3,6,8,12–16,18] In spite of these very different settings, markedly consistent human responses to a traumatic event have been noted. One of the common responses is reliving the traumatic event through cognitive, affective, or sensory–motor activities (e.g., intrusive thoughts, painful emotion, or startle response). Other common responses include reduced psychic and emotional functioning (e.g., impaired memory or feeling of numbness), and an altered adaptation pattern and lifestyle (e.g., sleep disturbances, social withdrawal, or chronic anxiety) (Fig. 13-21).

Human responses to a traumatic event can be conceptualized as occurring in five stages. They are outcry, numbing, intrusion, working-through, and completion.[10] The initial response to a traumatic event is *outcry*, an alarm reaction accompanied by strong emotion, most often fear. The person may call out a warning such as "Watch out!" or shout for help, "Oh, God!" The person is quickly assessing the implications of the event and making use of all resources to survive the immediate life-threatening situation. The person may feel helpless and vulnerable or may experience the horror of death. Reactions include immobilization, panic, confusion, misdirected rage, sudden episodes of giving up, or psychotic breakdown.

Numbing is a powerful coping method used to reduce the psychological and emotional impact. Focus of attention may be narrowed, and the individual may be less attentive to new stimuli and may perseverate in a robotlike manner. The person may disavow or have a distorted perception of the traumatic event. There may be complaints of being "numb" or "dead in life." Various somatic stress responses, such as bowel symptoms, fatigue, headache, and muscle pain, may be seen. Maladaptive avoidance may include social withdrawal, alcohol or drug abuse, or fugue states.

However, in an effort to master the experience, *intrusion* of the traumatic event may erupt into conscious awareness. The person may show excessive alertness, vigilance, or startle reactions in such behavior as constantly scanning the environment for threatening cues or suddenly assuming a defensive position. Excess verbalization of the trauma or preoccupation with a search for the lost person or situation may be noted. The person may complain of flashbacks or nightmares. Waves of intense emotion with fear of losing impulse control may be felt. In overwhelming intrusion, the person may become exhausted, regress to despair, or lose the ability to function socially. These numbing and intrusion reactions fluctuate in a manner that is unique to each individual. In the struggle to master the traumatic experience, various maladaptive life-styles may be seen.

Gradually, the individual undergoes a *working-through* phase by developing a broader and more realistic view of the event and the aftermath. Failure to cope at this stage may result in chronic anxiety, depression, or multiple psychosomatic reactions. Finally, in the *completion* phase, the traumatic experience is integrated into a new sense of self and the world consistent with basic beliefs and values. Failure to achieve an integration of the trauma may cause an inability to be creative or to love, or a distortion of character.

RELATED FACTORS

Post-trauma response (PTR) results from exposure to a traumatic event. However, not everybody develops PTR or has the same degree of symptomatology. Considerable research has been conducted to find related factors that cause certain individuals to be more vulnerable than others. It is generally agreed that development of PTR involves complex interaction of many factors.[23] In existing studies, several related factors have been identified, such as personal vulnerability, severity of trauma, and post-trauma context.

Certain personal characteristics may increase susceptibility to developing PTR. Childhood trauma, adolescent developmental problems, or preexisting mental illness may bring about adverse effects in a person confronted by a traumatic event. Also, the person's coping

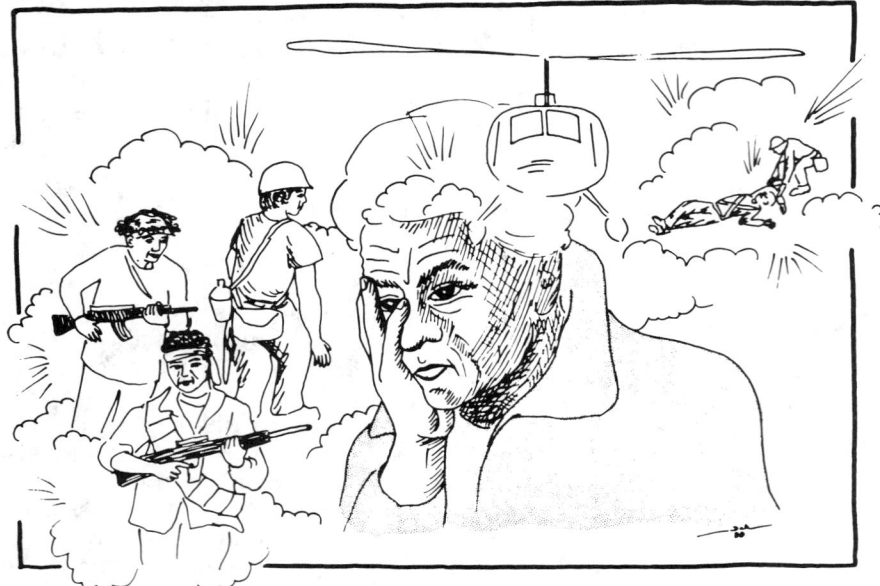

FIGURE 13–21. *Reexperiencing of the traumatic event is one of the defining characteristics of post-trauma response. (Courtesy Medical Media, Veterans Administration Medical Center, Seattle, Washington)*

resources may influence the effectiveness achieved in dealing with the trauma. If the person has adequate strength and resources, then the effect of trauma may be reduced. However, in severe trauma, personal factors may be less influential.

Severity of trauma involves both the nature and extent of trauma exposure.[7,17] Each traumatic event is unique. With the Hiroshima atomic bomb, initial impact was a sudden and dramatic shift from normal existence to an overwhelming encounter with grotesque destruction and death.[12] In addition, there was a prolonged period of continuous threat from radiation sickness and death, loss of loved ones, and genetic impairment of future generations. Rape trauma is a forced, violent sexual penetration or other sexual victimization against the victim's will and without the victim's consent[9] (see Rape Trauma Syndrome in this chapter). Genital injuries, acquired immune deficiency syndrome, venereal disease, or pregnancy may result. Also, the trauma may be prolonged by such stressors as making a decision on whether or not to press charges; identifying the assailant; facing the nature of publicity; and dealing with the responses of family, friends, and society.

Prolonged, intense, and repeated encounter with trauma tends to increase the adverse effects of PTR.[7,19] It involves a complex interaction of environmental conditions and a person's subjective experiences which include the degree of warning, threat to life, exposure to the grotesque, loss, bereavement, displacement, and moral conflict about the role of the survivor. Therefore, the individual's perception of the experience influences the PTR process. For example, when a person views the trauma as an act of fate with no one to be blamed, and not as a result of malicious intention, then the outcome of PTR may be less severe.

Post-trauma context may influence the person's working-through process of the traumatic experience. A disruptive recovery environment, in which breakdown of the family and community structures brought about a negative impact on the PTR process, was seen among the victims of Nazi concentration camps.[5] After liberation from the camp, many of the survivors had to face harsh reality such as confirmation of the death of their family members, relatives, and friends; and the destruction of their homes and communities. Many of them had to start all over again in a strange country as immigrants. These factors resulted in the loss of their support network. It is important to have social support as well as social acceptance when the survivors reenter society because these tend to bring about a favorable outcome.[3,20] Additional stresses, such as loss of a significant person or financial problems, may intensify the symptoms of PTR.

DEFINING CHARACTERISTICS

Three categories of defining characteristics of PTR have been identified: reexperience of the traumatic event, which may be identified in cognitive, affective, or sensory motor activities; psychic–emotional numbness; and altered life-style.[21] Reexperience of the trauma may be seen in various defining characteristics. For example, a client may report nightmares about the traumatic event or a feeling of guilt about surviving while others did not. Excessive verbalization of the event or search for dead persons may be observed. Overwhelming emotions, anger, or rage may be noted. Accompanied by anxiety or fear, a fight-or-flight response such as hyperalertness or a startle reaction may be observed. The client may be watchful or on guard, even when there is no reason to be, and may be jumpy or easily startled by sudden noises. The client may report fear of repetition of the experience, death, or loss of bodily control. Reexperience of trauma may be frightening and the patient may perceive the experience as "becoming crazy" and may hesitate to admit it.

Psychic–emotional numbness may be used to reduce the impact of reliving the trauma. A client may have trouble recalling some important parts of the traumatic event and may complain about feeling numb or distant from others and the rest of the world. Stereotyped behavior may be seen. For instance, a homemaker who survived an auto accident may engage in her routine task of cleaning the kitchen and go through the motions, but she feels disconnected. Indifference to surroundings, staring off into space, or flat affect may be observed.

As a client struggles with reenactment or a numbing response, various altered adaptation patterns and lifestyles may be evident. The client may report irritability, rapid mood changes, lack of impulse control, or trouble sleeping. Perception of self and the world may be changed. The client may have a negative self-concept and a loss of faith in people and the world. Self-destructive behavior, such as alcohol or drug abuse, reckless driving, fights, or illegal activities, may be observed. Deterioration in personal care, with depression and suicidal ideation, may be noted. Avoidance of activities that triggered the trauma or a development of phobia may be evident. For example, an assault victim who was beaten severely in a park at night may avoid going to parks, or may not be able to leave the house at night, or may be socially withdrawn. Failure to control recurrent intrusive traumatic experience may lead to a state of chronic anxiety. Maladaptive coping demonstrated by somatic preoccupation may be present (Chart 1).

NURSING PROCESS AND RATIONALE

Assessment

The nurse needs to determine if a prospective client has a history of trauma exposure through several sources: direct interviews and observation of the patient; information from significant others or other health professionals; or past and present medical records or other pertinent resources. During an interview, one may frame a question in the following manner: "Sometimes things happen to people that are very stressful, things that do not happen to most people and so are upsetting, like major earthquakes or floods, very serious accidents or fires, physical assault or rape, seeing other people killed or dead, being in war or combat, or some other types of disaster. During your life, have any of these kinds of things happened to you?"

If the patient has a positive history of trauma, then one may look for PTR symptoms by making statements such as the following: "When people undergo such a stressful situation, it is quite common that they may feel different about themselves. I wonder if you are experiencing some changes in yourself, the way you think, feel, or act since the stressful experience?" De-

---

CHART 1
Post-trauma Response: Definition, Related Factors, and Defining Characteristics

DEFINITION

Post-trauma response is the state of an individual experiencing a sustained painful response to an unexpected extraordinary life event(s).

RELATED FACTORS
Natural Origin Traumatic Events

Lightning-strike
Earthquakes
Volcanic eruptions
Floods

Human Origin Traumatic Events

Assault
Rape
Airplane crashes
Industrial accidents
War

Other Influential Factors

Personal vulnerability
Severity of trauma
Post-trauma context including social support

DEFINING CHARACTERISTICS
Reexperience of traumatic event

Flashbacks, nightmares, repetitive dreams, intrusive thoughts
Excessive verbalization of the traumatic events
Survival guilt, self-blame, shame, sadness, helplessness
Painful emotion, anger, rage
Anxiety, fear, panic
Hyperalertness, hypervigilance, startle reaction

Psychic–Emotional Numbness

Impaired memory or interpretation of reality, confusion, amnesia
Constricted affect, verbalization of feeling numb or alienated
Reduced functional level

Altered Life-Style

Emotional lability, lack of impulse control, irritability
Sleep disturbances
Difficulty with concentration
Chronic anxiety
Negative self-concept
Loss of faith, meaninglessness, sense of foreshortened future
Self-destructiveness (e.g., alcohol or drug abuse, reckless driving, suicide contemplation, fights, illegal activities)
Thrill-seeking activities
Difficulty with interpersonal relationships
Social withdrawal
Avoidance of situations or activities that arouse recollection of the trauma
Submissiveness, passiveness, dependency
Multiple physiologic symptoms: pains, fatigue, gastrointestinal disturbance
Deterioration in personal care
Chronic depression

fining characteristics of reliving trauma and numbing responses may be sought by asking such questions as, "Does a stressful experience keep coming back to you in some way?" "Do you dream about it or wake up with nightmares?" "Do you feel guilty about surviving?" or "Do you have trouble concentrating?" To assess altered life-style, look for readjustment difficulties or general life-style changes by inquiring: "Do you have trouble sleeping?" or "Do you feel life holds no meaning?"

It is important to be aware that talking about a traumatic event may be distressing and anxiety provoking, or it may increase PTR symptoms. Tactful intervention may be necessary if the patient becomes too anxious, including stopping the interview and providing proper support. The purpose of obtaining a history is to substantiate evidence of trauma and not explore details that are more appropriate to a therapy session. After the interview, it may be helpful to provide a brief supportive discussion about feelings the patient experienced during the interview.

Nursing Diagnosis

After the assessment, the nurse establishes a specific nursing diagnosis according to the kind of trauma and the defining characteristics; for example: post-trauma response related to assault. The family of a client with post-trauma response may be affected by the incident and the client's problems and may, for example, not understand the impact of the event on the client. A possible diagnosis may be: dysfunctional family processes related to disbelief and lack of understanding about the client's adjustment process.

Client Goals and Nursing Interventions

When the diagnosis, PTR, is made, the nurse may intervene to reduce extremes of reenactment or numbing responses by providing a safe, therapeutic environment. Reliving the trauma may be frightening to the client. Staying with the client and offering support during an episode of high anxiety may be required. Experience of anger or rage may lead to impulsive acting-out behavior. It may be necessary to set limits, to encourage ventilation of feelings, and to redirect excess energy into physical activities such as walking, jogging, or working out in a gym. It is important to reassure the client that these feelings and symptoms are often experienced by individuals who have undergone such a traumatic event. It is also reassuring for the client to be educated about other aspects of PTR. A numbing response, for example, may be used to cushion the impact of emotion evoked by reliving the experience. The client may not pay too much attention to what is happening or may have trouble remembering things. It may be necessary to orient the client to current activities and surroundings (Fig. 13-22).

When the defining characteristics of reexperiencing trauma and numbing responses are reduced, the nurse may assist the client to begin the working-through process. Through talking, the client may be able to put the pieces together to reconstruct what had occurred in a broader perspective and to validate the reality of personal involvement. It is important to encourage appropriate expression of feelings. Survival guilt or guilt about the behavior required for survival may be dealt with by reinterpreting personal motives more in the

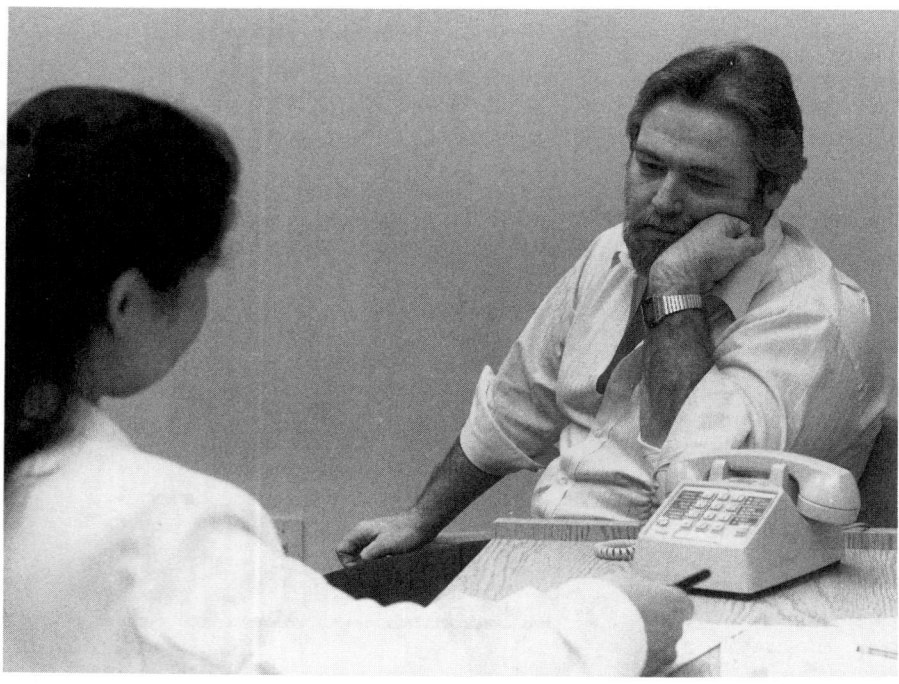

FIGURE 13–22. Through discussion, the client experiencing post-trauma response is assisted in putting what has occurred into a broader perspective. (Courtesy Medical Media, Veterans Administration Medical Center, Seattle, Washington)

direction of situational demands away from "evil" intentions. Caution must be used not to smooth over or minimize guilt feelings. A discussion of values or moral conflicts may be included in the context of the client's cultural and religious values. Changes that the client had to make after the traumatic event may also need to be addressed.

Dealing with a post-trauma victim is a difficult task, as one must confront one's mortality and value system. Therefore, nurses need to explore their own feelings engendered by the traumas they identify before attempting to intervene effectively. A nonjudgmental attitude and warm acceptance will promote therapeutic relationships. When helping trauma victims, it is important to allow the individuals to work at their own pace. Also, it is important to assist the client to find more effective strategies for managing responses and requirements of daily living while experiencing PTR. Helping the client gain new coping skills is essential. To promote the therapeutic process of PTR, it is imperative for the client to identify support resources, particularly support groups, and to make connection with them. To strengthen the client's family support, the nurse needs to assist the family members by encouraging them to ventilate feelings, helping them to understand what is happening to the client, and providing counseling sessions or referral to appropriate community resources. Building support is crucial, because social support tends to reduce PTR (see Research Highlights).

Evaluation

To evaluate the effectiveness of the intervention, the nurse assesses the client's level of self-control, the progress of trauma work, the effectiveness in meeting the daily-living requirements, and the development of support and resources. Various behavioral cues may indicate the expected outcome. For example: the client may demonstrate reduced anxiety and greater self-control by appropriately attending to the external stimuli and may verbalize feelings and needs, talk about the traumatic experience and express feelings appropriately, make adjustment to daily-living requirements with PTR process, and demonstrate new coping skills and verbalize where to find support and resources and how to utilize them (Chart 2).

CHART 2
Post-trauma Response: Summary of the Nursing Process

NURSING INTERVENTIONS	OUTCOME CRITERIA
CLIENT GOAL: FEEL MORE SELF-CONTROL	
Assess client's level of PTR	Verbalizes feelings and needs
Assess client's level of anxiety and self-control	Demonstrates reduced anxiety
Stay with client and support during high anxiety	Demonstrates self-control
Set limits for acting-out behavior	
CLIENT GOAL: GAIN A BROADER PERSPECTIVE ABOUT THE EVENT AND ITS AFTERMATH	
Provide a safe, structured setting where client can begin trauma work	Talks about the traumatic event and aftermath in realistic terms
Assist client to understand what had happened in broader perspective and validate personal involvement	Verbalizes understanding of PTR process
Teach PTR process	
CLIENT GOAL: EXPRESS FEELINGS	
Assist client to express feelings	Expresses feelings appropriately
Allow client to do the trauma work at own pace	
CLIENT GOAL: FIND ACCEPTABLE, MORE EFFECTIVE STRATEGIES FOR MANAGING RESOURCES AND REQUIREMENTS OF DAILY LIVING WHILE EXPERIENCING PTR	
Explore with client the areas of functioning in daily living most affected by PTR	Identifies responses that interfere with the patterns and requirements of daily living
Help client to discover and plan behavior, scripts, and patterns in daily living to accommodate to or compensate for PTR	Explores and tests feasible options for participating in daily living during PTR
	Reports outcomes of attempted strategies and revises or retains as appropriate
CLIENT GOAL: INCREASE SUPPORTS AND RESOURCES	
Assist client to identify current and potential support persons	Verbalizes names of support persons
Assist client to identify own strengths	Identifies ways of finding additional supportive individuals
Teach new coping skills	Demonstrates new coping skills
Link client with various community resources	Identifies ways of finding resources
	Identifies resources for continuing trauma work

Research Highlights

Research indicates that social support acts as a buffer to the impact of exposure to a traumatic experience.[4] Social support is defined as coping assistance, or the active participation of significant others in an individual's stress management.[22] Such support includes (1) instrumental support (e.g., actions, materials) to change or manage the stressful situation; (2) socioemotional aid (e.g., love, caring, sympathy, esteem, belonging) to reduce the negative feelings that accompany stress exposure; and (3) informational aid (advice, feedback, facts, or knowledge relating to current distress) to alter the perception of stress.

Stretch demonstrated a positive relationship between social support and attenuation of PTSD by surveying 238 Vietnam veterans.[20] The survey asked about support they received while in Vietnam, such as frequency of socialization, feelings of closeness and being understood in the unit, as well as support received from friends and families back in the States. Also, the survey tabulated social sup-

port the veterans received during the first year back from Vietnam by asking about experience with other people's reactions and attitudes, as well as the frequency of their encountering any negative or hostile events because of their involvement in the war. Other questions concerned the occurrence of six PTSD symptoms (i.e., intrusive memory of the Vietnam war trauma, insomnia with nightmares, inability to express feelings, problems in concentration, feelings of numbness, and survival guilt).[1] The study compared the support received and the occurrence of PTSD. Positive social interaction during the first year back from Vietnam moderated PTSD symptoms, whereas negative social interactions exacerbated the symptoms. The study concluded that social support received during the first year back from Vietnam appears to have greater influence on PTSD symptomatology than does combat experience itself.

CASE STUDY

A 38-year-old single male auto mechanic was hospitalized with an initial psychiatric diagnosis of major depression, with suicidal ideation and possible post-traumatic stress disorder (PTSD). A few weeks before, his "only friend" had died of cancer. Since then, he had become increasingly depressed, anxious, and suicidal. He complained of having sleep disturbances with recurrent nightmares and flashbacks of his Vietnam War experience. He had been confined to his apartment for the last few days and acknowledged suicidal rumination. He was brought to the hospital by his employer, who stopped by to see him when he failed to show up at work. There had been no previous psychiatric hospitalization. However, since his return from Vietnam, he had sought psychiatric help for depression and anxiety, with little apparent positive result. Further assessment confirmed that he had intensive combat experience, including witnessing the deaths of several close buddies. He commented that he didn't deserve to be alive when others weren't. After making the nursing diagnoses, suicide potential and sleep pattern disturbance, the nurse first ensured against self-harm and disturbed sleep by providing a safe therapeutic environment. The nursing diagnosis of post-trauma response related to Vietnam experience and loss of support was made as the nurse recognized his unresolved war trauma. With encouragement, he began sharing his war experiences, losses, and associated feelings with the nurse. Gradually, the client's nightmares and flashbacks became more manageable, and he was able to sleep without medication. Discharge planning was aimed at providing resources and developing a personal support system. His employer was involved in his treatment and became one of his support persons. While in the hospital, he made a friend of another Vietnam veteran. He planned to start attending church every week to make more friends. He was referred to the Veterans' Center where he could continue his trauma work through individual and group therapy. His prognosis is good, as long as he utilizes his support network and continues his trauma work which may take many years to complete. He is able to return to his community and his job.

SUMMARY

Post-trauma response may develop after an exposure to a traumatic event. Trauma victims may present themselves to a health-care facility with various symptoms of PTR such as reexperiencing the traumatic event, psychic–emotional numbness, or altered life-style. The process of PTR is discussed by using Horowitz's conceptual model.[10] After obtaining a positive history of trauma exposure, the severity of PTR is assessed. Initial nursing intervention for the nursing diagnosis of PTR is aimed toward reducing PTR symptoms by assuring a safe, therapeutic environment. Assistance for trauma work, through structured individual or supportive group therapy, is important. Further, intervention to increase support resources is also crucial.

References

1. American Psychiatric Association. Diagnostic and statistical manual of mental disorders. 3rd ed, revised. Washington, DC: American Psychiatric Association; 1987.
2. Burgess AW, Holmstrom LL. Rape trauma syndrome. Am J Psychiatry. 1974;131:981–986.
3. Card J. Epidemiology of PTSD in a national cohort of Vietnam veterans. J Clin Psychol. 1987;43:6–17.
4. Catherall DR. The support system and amelioration of PTSD in Vietnam veterans. Psychotherapy. 1986;23:472–482.
5. Chodoff P. The German concentration camp as a psychological stress. Arch Gen Psychiatry. 1970;22:78–87.
6. Dollinger SJ. Lightning-strike disaster among children. Br J Med Psychol. 1985;58:375–383.
7. Foy DW, Carroll EM, Donahoe CP. Etiological factors in the development of PTSD in clinical samples of Vietnam combat veterans. J Clin Psychol. 1987;43:17–27.
8. Gleser GC, Green BL, Winget C. Prolonged psychosocial effects of disaster. A study of Buffalo Creek. New York: Academic Press; 1981.

9.   Holmstrom LL, Burgess AW. Development of diagnostic categories. Am J Nurs. 1975;75:1288–1291.

10. Horowitz MJ. Stress–response syndromes: a review of post-traumatic and adjustment disorders. Hosp Commun Psychiatry. 1986;37:241–248.

11. Lazarus R, Folkman S. Stress, appraisal and coping. New York: Springer; 1984.

12. Lifton RJ. Death in life: survivors of Hiroshima. New York: Vintage Books; 1969.

13. Logue JN, Melick ME, Struening EL. A study of health and mental health status following a major natural disaster. Res Commun Ment Health. 1981;2:217–274.

14. McDaniel E, McClelland P. Post-traumatic stress disorder. Pract Ther. 1986;34:180–189.

15. Niederland WG. Survivor syndrome: further observations and dimensions. J Am Psychoanal Assoc. 1981;29:413–416.

16. Powell BJ, Penick EC. Psychological distress following a natural disaster: a one-year follow-up of 98 flood victims. J Commun Psychol. 1983;11:269–276.

17. Scurfield RM. Post-trauma stress assessment and treatment: overview and formulations. In: Figley CR, ed. Trauma and its wake. New York: Brunner/Mazel; 1985.

18. Shore JH, Tatum EL, Vollmer WM. The Mount St. Helens stress response syndrome. In: Shore JH, ed. Disaster stress studies: new methods and findings. Washington, DC: American Psychiatric Press; 1986.

19. Solkoff N, Gray P, Keill S. Which Vietnam veterans develop posttraumatic stress disorders? J Clin Psychol. 1986;42:687–698.

20. Stretch RH. Incidence and etiology of post-traumatic stress disorder among active duty army personnel. J Appl Soc Psychol. 1986;16:464–481.

21. Tanaka K. Development of a tool for assessing posttrauma response. Arch Psychiatr Nurs. 1988;2(6):350–356.

22. Thoits PA. Social support as coping assistance. J Consult Clin Psychol. 1986;54:416–423.

23. Wilson JP, Smith WK, Johnson SK. A comparative analysis of post-traumatic stress syndrome among individuals exposed to different stressor events. In: Figley CR, ed. Trauma and its wake. New York: Brunner/Mazel; 1985.

POWERLESSNESS

Howard K. Butcher and Helen Kirkpatrick

DEFINITION AND DESCRIPTION

Powerlessness is the perception that one's own actions will not significantly affect an outcome (i.e., a perceived lack of control over a current situation or immediate happening). Power is felt in relation to other people or objects, and is experienced when a person has the ability and freedom to feel and reason. The purpose, meaning, and goal of power operations in interpersonal relations concern nurses who wish to function therapeutically with clients.[22] If power is not experienced by the client, the feeling of powerlessness results, which can be a significant determinant of client behavior.[6] The concept of powerlessness is relevant for nursing because power and powerlessness are important aspects of the recovery process.[22]

Powerlessness is a potential problem when physical strength, psychological stamina, self-concept, energy, knowledge, motivation, or belief systems are compromised.[5] An overwhelming sense of powerlessness may occur when a client experiences a lack of control over, or lack of knowledge related to, illness, hospitalization, or treatment. Powerlessness may offer an explanation for the apathetic client who acquires little knowledge concerning health-care management. The experience of powerlessness has been associated with depression, aggression, and paranoia, and it may be a factor leading to a life-style of substance abuse, violence, and dependency.

THEORY AND RESEARCH

Power is always interpersonal, in contrast with strength, which is personal.[14] Five kinds of power may exist in the same person at different times, some of which are constructive and some destructive. (1) *Exploitative power* is the simplest and most destructive and always presupposes violence or a threat of violence; (2) *manipulative power* is power *over* another person; (3) *competitive power* is power *against* another and can be destructive or constructive; (4) *nutrient power* is power *for* the other, such as normal parental care, teaching; and (5) *integrative power* is power *with* the other person, that is, power that strengthens another's power. The goal for human development is to learn to use the various kinds of power in ways that are adequate to a given situation.[14]

Five phases of power exist as potentialities in every human being's life: power to be, self-affirmation, self-assertion, aggression, and violence. When power to be, self-affirmation, and self-assertion are blocked over a period, aggression tends to develop, and when aggressive tendencies are denied to an individual, the toll may be a "zombie-like deadening of consciousness, neurosis, psychosis, or violence" (reference 14, pp 42, 43). Violence is largely physical because the other phases, which involve reason or persuasion, have been blocked. Powerlessness, which leads to apathy, is the source of violence, and making people powerless promotes violence, rather than its control. The more personal name for powerlessness is helplessness or weakness.[14]

Powerlessness has been described as one of five alternative meanings of alienation, along with meaninglessness, normlessness, isolation, and self-estrangement.[28] Seeman[28] emphasized the individual's subjective perception of powerlessness and described it as the belief by the individual that his or her own behavior could not determine outcomes. With this understanding of powerlessness, Seeman and Evans[29] studied white, male patients hospitalized for tuberculosis and concluded that patients high in powerlessness were less knowledgeable about relevant health matters than a matched sample low in powerlessness.

Powerlessness has been linked to paranoia. Individuals who are paranoid frequently place all power and control outside themselves. Paranoia has been viewed as the expression of powerlessness whereby the individual seeks to gain mastery through the paranoid delusional system.[1] Related DSM-III-R disorders include schizophrenia, paranoid type; delusional (paranoid) disorders; and paranoid personality disorder. The individual uses paranoid beliefs to assign order, understanding, and meaning to events and occurrences over which no control is felt. Paranoia has also been linked to social positions that are characterized by powerlessness and by the threat of victimization and exploitation.[19]

Locus of control is directly related to powerlessness.[26] Persons with an internal locus of control tend to perceive that events are contingent on their own behavior, whereas those with an external locus of control tend to perceive that events are contingent on external forces such as fate, luck, or powerful people.[26] The difference between powerlessness and locus of control, according to Miller and Oertel[18] is that powerlessness is situationally determined, whereas locus of control is a fairly stable personality trait, although it is subject to some change.

Stephenson describes two kinds of powerlessness: trait and situational.[30] Trait powerlessness refers to a person's general affect, attitude, and life-style. Situational powerlessness refers to the lack of control thrust upon a coping or empowered person for a specific circumstance or series of events. Thus, it is not clear whether trait powerlessness and external locus of control are the same or different phenomena.

Loss of control and lack of knowledge are both potential causes of powerlessness.[25] Loss of control may include loss over oneself, behavior, and environment. Lack of knowledge refers to insufficient knowledge about one's illness and the impact on one's sense of self, one's family, and one's future. For example, John, a 23-year-old, was seen in a community mental health clinic. He had been recently discharged from his first hospitalization with bipolar disorder (manic). John expressed feelings of not being able to control his activities of daily living. He lacked knowledge concerning possible signs of recurrence of the illness, such as two nights without sleep and hyperactivity. He questioned whether or not he could ever return to work. The diagnosis of powerlessness related to lack of knowledge was made. The community mental health nurse assisted John to increase his understanding of bipolar disorders, including the signs and symptoms of possible recurrence. They mutually identified means to increase John's sense of control over his daily activities.

RELATED FACTORS

Powerlessness occurs in many psychiatric conditions. Being hospitalized for a mental illness or labeled with a particular psychiatric diagnosis may result in a stigma that is accompanied by feelings of powerlessness and embarrassment. Loss of reality orientation, inability to maintain self-care, difficulty in interpersonal relationships and roles, inability to maintain a positive self-concept, all of which are experienced by those who are mentally ill, can contribute to feelings of loss of control.

Society expects that sick individuals will desire and work to get well as soon as possible.[20] However, the hospital environment encourages patients to be passive.[24,25] Beginning with admission to a hospital, individuals lose many opportunities to make personal choices. The choice of doctor may or may not be one made by individuals, but choice of nurse(s) is generally out of their control, decided by the needs of the institution. The individual often has little or no control over choice of roommate, scheduling of activities, type of personal information requested during history taking, what is recorded in the chart, and who has access to it. Clients who are admitted involuntarily are often presumed to be incapable of exercising their decision-making power. Chemical or physical restraint may further reinforce loss of decision-making and control.

The importance of personal control in the hospital setting has been described by Kritek[8] when she became a patient. She felt "increasingly unable to make judgments without distortion" and was "forced to relinquish personal views, knowledge and expertise" (reference 8, p 29). Factors contributing to her feeling of powerlessness focused on the health-care system, its demands, and her feared inadequacies in meeting these demands.

When powerlessness is not contained, hopelessness can result.[24] In a description of her 20-year battle with schizophrenia, Leete[9] vividly recounts experiences with the health-care system. She chronicles power struggles over food, regulation of time and activities, and withdrawal by health-care professionals. "The more I was ostracized and punished, the angrier I became and the more I rebelled. Slowly, however, my desperation turned to resignation and hopelessness" (reference 9, p. 487). On the other hand, Leete credits her survival in one hospital to help from friends on the unit and daily individual sessions with staff.

Information and knowledge are sources of power. Physicians and nurses may provide minimal information or withhold it, even when it is solicited.[8] Withholding information or providing inappropriate information removes or inhibits control by the patient. If only highly technical explanations are provided, the recipient is still without usable knowledge.[24] The feeling of powerlessness "that is connected with putting oneself in the hands of a doctor or a nurse is reinforced when the patient cannot find out what his real worries are" (reference 21, p 67).

The side effects of psychotropic medications, such as extrapyramidial symptoms, may contribute to physiologic loss of control, which, in turn, may lead to anxieties over threatened physical integrity. A lack of knowledge about the medication, side effects, one's condition, and treatment may lead to increased feelings of powerlessness.

Life-style factors also may contribute to feelings of powerlessness. Clients who are deprived economically, socially, and educationally are the most likely to feel they lack power and control. Both hopelessness and powerlessness have been found to be associated with the subcultures of poverty.[19] Victims of poverty and oppression are caught up in a cycle of powerlessness in which the larger social systems fail to provide the needed resources.

Victims of abuse, who often lose their sense of trust, safety, and security, become psychologically paralyzed and often remain passive. Battered children and incest victims are exposed to repeated threatening experiences that can be devastating and emotionally disturbing experiences, the impact of which extends well beyond the immediate episode.[4] Adults who have been victims of abuse may feel inadequate and inferior, have low self-esteem, tend to be socially isolated, and feel powerless.

Developmental theorists[5,13,31] assert that those individuals whose psychosocial development is characterized by unmet needs, unresolved conflicts, and unmastered tasks may experience dysfunctional patterns, weak ego identity, and a negative self-concept in adulthood. Failure in meeting developmental tasks can contribute to feelings of dependency, insecurity, low self-esteem, and a life-style of helplessness.

The life-style of helplessness involves a personality trait of external locus of control. An individual with a generalized low expectancy of control in life may feel even more powerless in a situation of illness.[2] However, a person with an internal locus of control experiences more intense feelings of powerlessness when dealing with an illness than one with an external locus of control.

A person may misinterpret the causation of events, and attribute the cause as being outside of his or her control. This sense of powerlessness may be decreased by clarifying the actual controlling influences.[2]

DEFINING CHARACTERISTICS

Defining characteristics for powerlessness are cited in the nursing literature.[7,10,16,27,32] Issues of powerlessness and a feeling of low control may underlie suspicious-

ness, depression, and aggressive behavior. Powerlessness is associated with withdrawal, passivity, submissiveness, apathy, and isolation in some clients; in others powerlessness may be associated with increasing frustration, agitation, anxiety, aggression, acting-out behavior, and violence.

The loss of control imposed by illness and hospitalization compromises one's sense of independence and control and, as a result, the client may experience anger toward others. When the expression of anger is blocked on a verbal level, individuals often turn to a physical level of acting-out. Other manifestations of powerlessness are behaviors that reflect a lack of involvement or interest in decision-making about one's health care. The client may be unable to set goals, refuse to engage in activities of daily living, or appear disinterested in health-care and treatment measures. Clients experiencing powerlessness may lack the moti-

---

CHART 1
Powerlessness: Definition, Related Factors, and Defining Characteristics

DEFINITION

Powerlessness is the perception that one's own actions will not significantly affect an outcome.

RELATED FACTORS
Health-Care Environment

Hospitalization
Lack of privacy
Altered personal territory or space
Removal of personal possessions
Loss of autonomy
Social displacement
Social isolation
Physical restrictions within hospital

Interpersonal Interaction

Lack of individualization
Lack of participation in decision making
Lack of appropriate explanation by caregivers
Excessive surveillance
Misuse of rewards
Misuse of authority
Misuse of punishment
Actual or potential loss of significant other

Illness-Related

Threat to physical integrity
Altered state of wellness
Diagnosis of acute or chronic illness
Progressive physical or mental deterioration
Loss of control over body or mental ability
Lack of knowledge about illness or treatment
Interference in role functioning
Inability to perform self-care or activities of daily living
Side effects from medications
Involuntary hospitalizations
Involuntary treatment or restraint
Stigma of mental illness

Life-Style of Helplessness

Delay or distortion in accomplishing developmental tasks
Developmental changes
Lack of well-developed personal identity
External locus of control
Repeated interpersonal failures
Repeated threatening experiences
Living in abusive relationships
Extremely hostile environment
Unsupportive social environment
Lack of available social resources
Insufficient finances
Oppression

DEFINING CHARACTERISTICS

Expressions of having no control or influence over situation or outcome
Expressions of having no control over self-care
Expressions of despair, hopelessness, helplessness
Nonparticipation in care or decision making
Expressions of dissatisfaction and frustration over inability to perform previous tasks or activities
Does not monitor progress
Reluctance to express true feelings, fear of alienation from caregivers
Inability to seek information about care
Dependence on others
Depression over physical–psychological deterioration
Expressions of apathy
Suspiciousness of others
Aggressive behavior toward self or others
Violent behavior
Noncompliant behavior
Expressions of resignation
Expressions of passivity
Withdrawal
Fatalism
Aimlessness
Anxiety
Restlessness

vation to acquire new knowledge, and ask few questions concerning their illness and care, even after health teaching. Expressions of guilt, unworthiness, helplessness, hopelessness, and despair may reflect feelings of low control and powerlessness (Chart 1).

NURSING PROCESS AND RATIONALE

Assessment

Nurses assess for powerlessness by observing client behavior and exploring the possible meaning underlying the behavior. Behavior exhibited by persons experiencing powerlessness may range from passivity or apathy to aggression and violence. The nurse may observe a client who is withdrawn, isolated, and submissive and consider the diagnosis of powerlessness. On the other hand, the nurse might also consider a diagnosis of powerlessness when observing a client who is agitated and is potentially violent. In observing behavior, the nurse may note a pattern of statements reflecting feelings of low control. Statements such as "There is nothing I can do," "What can I do?" and "What do I know?" suggest feelings of powerlessness. There may be verbal expression of doubt that one's actions will

Patient Behaviors	Nurse Rating of Behaviors			
	1 Never	2 Occasionally	3 Frequently	4 Always
VERBAL RESPONSE				
Verbal expressions of lack of control over what is happening				
Verbal expressions of doubt that self-care measures can affect outcome				
Verbal expressions of giving up				
Verbal expressions of fatalism				
EMOTIONAL RESPONSE				
Withdrawal				
Pessimism				
Undifferentiated anger				
Diminished patient-initiated interaction				
Submissiveness				
PARTICIPATION IN ACTIVITIES OF DAILY LIVING				
Nonparticipation in daily personal hygiene				
Noninterest in treatments				
Refusal to take food or fluids				
Inability to set goals				
Lack of decision making when opportunities are provided				
Dependency on others for activities of daily living				
INVOLVEMENT IN LEARNING ABOUT CARE RESPONSIBILITIES				
Lack of questioning concerning illness				
Low level of knowledge of illness after being given information				
Lack of knowledge related to treatment				
Lack of motivation to learn				

FIGURE 13–23. Powerlessness behavioral assessment tool. (With permission from: Miller JF, Oertel CB. In: Miller JF, ed. Coping with chronic illness: overcoming powerlessness. Philadelphia: FA Davis; 1983)

affect an outcome or there may be expression of wanting to give up.

The Powerlessness Behavior Assessment Tool[18] (Fig. 13-23), contains four categories of behavioral assessment data. Each behavior is rated on a four-point scale indicating the frequency of the behavior. On this tool nurses should be alerted to the potential of a nursing diagnosis of powerlessness if the client's scores on individual items are 3 or more. Specific nursing interventions to alleviate powerlessness are needed for a cumulative score of 57 or more.[18]

Nursing Diagnosis

Although client behavior may suggest a diagnosis of powerlessness, a nurse makes the actual diagnosis by assessing both subjective and objective data. Because powerlessness is a subjective state, it is useful to validate inferences connected with clients' feelings of powerlessness with them. Examples of nursing diagnoses might include (1) powerlessness related to lack of knowledge about illness, treatment, and involuntary hospitalization; (2) powerlessness related to loss of control over body functioning; and (3) powerlessness related to an unsupportive social environment.

Client Goals and Nursing Interventions

The overall goals for clients are an increase in knowledge or an increase in control, or both. Nursing intervention strategies are empowerment strategies. Empowerment means recognizing clients as equal partners in their care. Empowerment entails sharing knowledge and skills with clients and enabling them to exercise autonomy in choosing options.[12]

Intervention may be directed toward barriers in the environment that limit the client's control or toward assisting clients with decision-making. In modifying the environment, one may simply remove barriers to client control, or the environment may be enhanced or modified to facilitate the client's active participation in care. Removal of barriers may include changes in bathing schedules, control over bedroom area, or provision of a staff member who speaks the client's language. Modification to the environment necessitates creativity on the part of the nurse. Preventive measures can be focused on individualizing hospital environments and including clients in planning their care.

Efforts directed toward the client are most usefully implemented by consistent staffing, which provides some stability and support for the individual. Encouraging verbalization of feelings enables clients to feel they have been heard. Clients can be encouraged to assume responsibility for their own self-care, goal setting, scheduling of activities, and independent decisions. An individualized approach to client teaching builds on the individual's uniqueness and helps in set-

ting realistic goals. Although client education will not necessarily result in compliance with treatment programs, clients cannot comply unless they know and understand the regimen they are to follow. Nurses can assist clients in differentiating situations that can be changed from those that cannot. If the goals are short-term, behavioral, and realistic, the person can progress more easily. Accomplishment of goals is a sign of progress, a positive hope-mobilizing force. Therefore, setting simple, realistic goals helps provide hope for clients. Help clients identify areas that they can control and provide positive feedback for empowering behaviors.

Behavior modification can be used to provide the client with a sense of control. Properly used, it places the responsibility with the patient, rather than with the health-care personnel. This technique is especially helpful for clients who know what action needs to be taken, but do not seem able to alter behaviors to comply with the new demands.[23] For example, behavioral techniques have been used as an empowerment strategy in the treatment of powerlessness in obese women.[17]

Evaluation

Outcome criteria indicating that the client experiences an increased ability to control activities and outcomes and maintains a sense of personal control include: (1) Verbalizations indicating that the client feels in control of situations; (2) Engagement in decision-making and problem-solving; and (3) Verbalizations indicating an increased sense of self-esteem and personal power (Chart 2).

CASE STUDY

Melodie T, 29 years old, was transferred to a tertiary care hospital after several months on a general hospital psychiatric unit. Melodie became depressed following the birth of her first child and had not responded to therapy. She was actively suicidal. The DSM-III-R diagnosis was major depression, single episode.

Melodie and her husband had been married eight years before the birth of their child, seven months ago. Both reported it had been a happy marriage. Because of the length of her illness and poor response, Melodie's husband felt increasingly hopeless. He indicated that he was thinking of "giving up" on his wife, since his primary responsibility was now caring for his daughter. Because of the potential for suicide, Melodie had not been able to leave the hospital for home visits, and she had not developed parenting skills or a relationship with the baby. The developing family bond was between Melodie's husband, John, and the baby, with Melodie increasingly excluded. John was reluctant to bring the baby in to visit, stating that the lack of privacy from other clients made it an unacceptable environment for the baby. Visiting areas were open to all patients, and patients frequently approached and wanted to touch the baby. Melodie expressed frustration and helplessness over her inability to influence her outcome, in that she was not able to form a

CHART 2
Powerlessness: Summary of the Nursing Process

NURSING INTERVENTIONS	OUTCOME CRITERIA

CLIENT GOAL: EXPERIENCE INCREASED ABILITY TO CONTROL ACTIVITIES AND OUTCOMES

Modify the Environment Preserve privacy: increase territorial rights Minimize rules and regulations Decrease surveillance of client unless essential for safety Encourage independent behavior and self-responsibility Individualize ward routine as much as possible Structure opportunities in which client can succeed Encourage client to manipulate surroundings to organize own room as desired Encourage client to create a personal and pleasant environment Provide opportunity for the client and family to participate in care Provide for engagement in meaningful activities Be sensitive to events that may induce powerlessness (unfamiliar environment, language, uncertainty of health or illness treatment)	Verbalizes feelings of being in control of situations and outcomes
Increase Decision-Making by Means of the Following Discuss daily plan of activities and allow the client to make as many decisions as possible about it Respect and support the client's decision Encourage sense of partnership with the health-care team Engage client in decision making whenever possible (selection of roommate, ADL/treatment, schedule, wearing apparel) Involve clients by having them determine what aspect of care they are ready to learn and when they want to learn it Help client differentiate those situations that can be changed from those that cannot Mutually set goals that are short-term, behavioral, practical, and attainable Shift emphasis from what client cannot do to what client can do Help client identify strengths and potential coping mechanisms, improvements in condition, and mastery over health-care situations	Exhibits decision making and is involved in making choices concerning own care Engages in problem-solving behaviors Sets goals and tries alternative behaviors to increase sense of control and power
Facilitate Verbalizations of Feelings Provide consistent staffing—identify a primary nurse Be an active listener by allowing the person to verbalize concerns and feelings Encourage client's expression of feelings and views before providing or modifying information Assist client in identifying areas of powerlessness	Verbalizes increased sense of power and control
Use Behavior Modification Help client choose positive reinforcements for slight improvements in behavior patterns Teach self-monitoring (record keeping)	
Increase the Health Team's and Significant Others' Sensitivity to Imposed Powerlessness Be alert for signs of parental attitudes Refrain from labeling client Sensitize family members to the importance of their reactions Help family members devise means of permitting patient control Involve family members and significant others in plan of care Help caregivers be less directive and overprotective	
CLIENT GOAL: INCREASE KNOWLEDGE Anticipate questions and offer information Reinforce client's right to ask questions Provide specific time (10–15 minutes) per shift that the client knows can be used to ask questions or discuss issues as desired Explain modifications of treatment program Provide relevant literature and audiovisual material based on readiness of client Provide health care teaching on issues relevant to the person's illness, health treatments, and results Teach assertiveness skills Keep the client informed about progress Teach client to solve problems and try out alternative coping	Asks appropriate questions and shows increased knowledge concerning care and treatment

(continued)

CHART 2 (*continued*)
Powerlessness: Summary of the Nursing Process

NURSING INTERVENTIONS	OUTCOME CRITERIA
Consider locus of control (internal versus external). (Those with internal locus of control may benefit from one-to-one approach and provision of information; may also need to validate mood state because they may not readily disclose anxiety. Those with external locus of control often benefit from small group approach to teaching.)	

CLIENT GOAL: MAINTAIN A SENSE OF PERSONAL CONTROL

Employ Wellness Strategies Refer to support group as needed Facilitate continuity of significant roles (return to work, family involvement, leisure activities) Help the client find alternative roles, interests, and use of talents, as needed Alleviate physical discomfort that diminishes energy reserve Assist client to plan energy-depleting tasks so that support systems are available Involve significant others—sensitizing them to the importance of their reactions and helping them devise means of permitting patient control	Integrates therapeutic regimen into life-style

bond with her daughter or to develop parenting skills. She expressed concern over whether or not she was even competent to look after the baby. Melodie also felt that she was losing her husband with whom she had had a positive relationship. The powerlessness felt by Melodie not only increased her depression, but also lessened her ability to deal with it. A nursing diagnosis was formulated of powerlessness related to social displacement (hospitalization), lack of knowledge (parenting), potential loss of significant others (husband and new baby), and lack of privacy (open visiting areas). Another nursing diagnosis was suicide potential. Goals for the first diagnosis were to increase ability to participate in family and to increase knowledge and competency in parenting.

It was agreed with Melodie and her husband that the two of them needed some time together with the baby to become accustomed to one another. Therefore, the audiovisual room was booked for one hour three times a week, to be used as a playroom. This allowed privacy from other clients and a more "normal" family setting than the open visiting areas on the ward. John brought in their daughter's favorite toys so she would be comfortable and begin to be comfortable with Melodie. Because both parents were very nervous, it was agreed that, initially, the nurse would view the visits through the one-way mirror. The presence of the nurse, although unseen, provided support for both parents and allowed postvisit discussions with Melodie. In these discussions, Melodie was encouraged to verbalize her feelings and was given support and suggestions in approaching her daughter. As these visits progressed, the family bond began to be established, which provided hope for both Melodie and her husband. Within two months of the visits being initiated, Melodie was discharged from the hospital with her husband and daughter, with follow-up by a Public Health Nurse who arranged participation for Melodie and her daughter in a parenting skills group.

Research Highlights

In a study on the clarity of the meaning and degree of usefulness of nursing diagnoses specific to psychiatric–mental health nursing, McFarland and Naschinski[11] studied 66 nurses with advanced preparation in psychiatric–mental health nursing. Of these, 86.7% considered that powerlessness had clarity of meaning; 64.5% rated powerlessness as 4 or 5 on a five-point Likert scale (5 being very useful).

Validation of the proposed defining characteristics and related factors would lead to more accurate assessment of those most at risk for powerlessness. Additional assessment tools for powerlessness need to be developed. The validity and reliability of the Miller and Oertel Powerlessness Behavioral Assessment Tool[18] needs to be established. Research clarifying the relationship of situational powerlessness and locus of control would further refine the definition of these terms. Potential research questions include: Are powerlessness and learned helplessness the same or different phenomena? Does a person with a life-style of helplessness experience situational powerlessness to a greater or lesser degree than otherwise empowered individuals? What is the relationship of powerlessness to low self-esteem and hopelessness? Are trait powerlessness and external locus of control the same or different phenomena?

Epidemiologic studies of the frequency of powerlessness as a nursing diagnosis in the psychiatric–mental health client population are needed to further establish the usefulness of this diagnosis. Nurse researchers could explore clients' perceptions concerning the effectiveness of the empowerment strategies in reducing powerlessness.

SUMMARY

Powerlessness may be experienced with any psychiatric condition. Potential related factors include health care environment, interpersonal interaction, illness-related and life-style of helplessness. Empowerment strategies are directed toward enabling an individual to have control of a situation, to increase knowledge, and to promote a sense of well-being.

References

1. Aaranson LS. Paranoia as a behavior of alienation. Perspect Psychiatr Care. 1977;15:1.

2. Abramson LY, Seligman MEP, Teasdale JD. Learned helplessness in humans: critique and reformation. J Abnorm Psychol. 1978;87:1.

3. Block DW. Alienation. In: Carlson CE, Blackwell B, eds. Behavioral concepts and nursing intervention. Philadelphia: JB Lippincott; 1978.

4. deYoung M. Incest victims and offenders: myths and realities. J Psychosoc Nurs Ment Health Serv. 1987;19:10.

5. Erikson EH. Childhood and society. New York: WW Norton & Co, 1983.

6. Johnson DE. Powerlessness: a significant determinant in patient behavior? J Nurs Ed. 1967;6:2.

7. Kim MJ, McFarland GK, McLane AM. Pocket guide to nursing diagnoses. 3rd ed. St Louis: CV Mosby; 1989.

8. Kritek PB. Patient power and powerlessness. Supervisor Nurse. 1981;(Jun), 26–34.

9. Leete E. The treatment of schizophrenia: a patient's perspective. Hosp Commun Psychiatry. 1987;38:5.

10. McFarland G, Wasli E. Nursing diagnoses and process in psychiatric mental health nursing. Philadelphia: JB Lippincott; 1986.

11. McFarland GK, Naschinski CE. Validation and identification of nursing diagnoses labels for psychiatric mental health nursing practice. In: McLane AM, ed. Classification of nursing diagnoses: proceedings of the seventh conference. St Louis: CV Mosby; 1987.

12. Malinski VM. Nursing practice within the science of unitary human beings. In: Malinski VM, ed. Explorations on Martha Rogers' science of unitary human beings. Norwalk, CT: Appleton–Century–Crofts; 1986.

13. Mahler M. The psychological birth of the human infant: symbiosis and individuation. New York: Buser Books; 1975.

14. May R. Power and innocence: a search for the sources of violence. New York: WW Norton & Co; 1972.

15. Miller JF. Concept development of powerlessness: a nursing diagnosis. In: Miller JF, ed. Coping with chronic illness: overcoming powerlessness. Philadelphia: FA Davis; 1983.

16. Miller JF. Development and validation of a diagnostic label: powerlessness. In: Kim MJ, McFarland GK, McLane AM, eds. Classification of nursing diagnosis: proceedings of the fifth national conference. St. Louis: CV Mosby; 1984.

17. Miller JF. Middescent obese women: overcoming powerlessness. In: Miller JF, ed. Coping with chronic illness: overcoming powerlessness. Philadelphia: FA Davis; 1983.

18. Miller JF, Oertel CB. Powerlessness in the elderly: preventing hopelessness. In: Miller JF, ed. Coping with chronic illness: overcoming powerlessness. Philadelphia: FA Davis; 1983.

19. Mirowsky J, Ross CE. Paranoia and the structure of powerlessness. Am Sociol Rev. 1983;48:2.

20. Parsons T. The social system. New York: Free Press; 1951.

21. Peplau H. Interpersonal relations in nursing. New York: GP Putnam's Sons; 1952.

22. Peplau H. Themes in nursing situations. Am J Nurs. 1953; 53:10.

23. Pfister-Minogue K. Enabling strategies. In: Miller JF, ed. Coping with chronic illness: overcoming powerlessness. Philadelphia: FA Davis; 1984.

24. Roberts SL. Behavior concepts and the critically ill patient. Norwalk, CT: Appleton–Century–Crofts; 1986.

25. Roberts SL. Behavioral concepts and nursing throughout the life span. Englewood Cliffs, NJ: Prentice–Hall; 1978.

26. Rotter JB. Generalized expectancies for internal versus external control reinforcement. Psychol Monogr Gen Appl. 1966;80:1.

27. Roy C Sr. Powerlessness. In: Roy C Sr, ed. Introduction to nursing: an adaptation model. Englewood Cliffs, NJ: Prentice–Hall; 1984.

28. Seeman M. On the meaning of alienation. Am Sociol Rev. 1959;24:6.

29. Seeman M, Evans J. Alienation and learning in a hospital setting. Am Sociol Rev. 1962;27:772–783.

30. Stephenson C. Powerlessness and chronic illness: implications for nursing. Balgor Nurs Ed. 1979;1:1.

31. Sullivan HS. In: Perry HS, ed. Interpersonal theory of psychiatry. New York: WW Norton & Co; 1953.

32. Thompson JM, McFarland GK, Hirsch JE, Tucker SM, Bowers AC. Clinical nursing. St Louis: CV Mosby; 1987.

RAPE TRAUMA SYNDROME

Barbara Grimes and Theresa S. Foley

DEFINITION AND DESCRIPTION

Rape trauma syndrome is a term that is used to describe the results of forced, violent sexual penetration or other forms of sexual victimization against the victim's will and consent. The trauma that develops from this attack or attempted attack includes an acute phase of disorganization of the victim's life-style and a long-term process of reorganization of life-style.[13] The syndrome was first recognized by Burgess and Holmstrom in 1974 to define the response pattern that was seen in women who came to an emergency room for treatment of rape.[2] Since that time, clinicians and researchers have recognized that other types of sexual victimization, in addition to forced violent sexual penetration, also produce the symptoms of rape trauma syndrome. Any type of unwanted sexual contact can trigger the development of symptoms. Sexual assaults can be categorized according to the situation of their occurrence. They are either stranger rape, date or acquaintance rape, marital rape, incest, or rape by a health-care provider. Although stranger rape (rape by a person with whom the victim had no prior relationship) is most commonly thought of in rape situations, it is actually the least common in occurrence. In only 12% of reported rapes was the perpetrator a stranger.[18]

Date or acquaintance rape is defined as unwanted sexual contact by someone who is known to the victim. The offender usually gains the confidence of the victim through some type of social contact before the attack. This type of rape occurs quite frequently. In a survey of 35 college campuses, 52% of 7000 women interviewed reported having experienced sexual victimization. The survey also revealed that 51% of college-aged men admitted that they would rape a woman if they knew they would not be caught and punished.[14]

Marital rape is defined as unwanted sexual contact by someone who is in a cohabiting relation with the victim. This is also a fairly common form of rape. In a 1980 survey, 14% of the women surveyed reported having been raped by their husbands. This figure is a conservative estimate because this survey did not include women who have experienced forced anal or oral intercourse, women who submitted out of a sense of duty or helplessness, or women who were unable to recognize or acknowledge their husbands' behaviors as abusive.[17]

Incest is defined as sexual contact by a member of the victim's family. Several recent surveys report that approximately 28% of females and 18% of males experience some type of unwanted sexual contact with a family member before the age of 18. Most of these assaults go unreported, leaving the child victims to deal with the effects of the assault on their own.[5]

Rape by a health-care provider is defined as sexual contact with anyone in any of the helping professions from whom the victim sought assistance or services. This is the most recently identified situational category of sexual assaults. In fact, as recently as 1971, it was claimed by some therapists that sex between a patient and therapist could be helpful.[20] Currently, it is considered to be unethical or malpractice. Masters and Johnson state that sexual contact between a patient and therapist should be considered rape rather than malpractice and that it should be regarded as a criminal offense whether the contact was initiated by the patient or the therapist.[15] In 15 states it is identified as criminal sexual assault. Despite the clear sanctions against it, sexual contacts between clients and helping professionals continue to occur. In one survey, approximately 25% of psychiatrists and psychologists reported sexual contact with their patients.[16]

THEORY AND RESEARCH

Before the 1960s, rape was considered a crime of passion. Rapists were thought of as victims of uncontrollable sexual impulses. The inability to control the impulses was attributed to one or more of the following: (1) the rape was motivated by uncontrollable sexual frustration that developed in response to a sexually inadequate or unresponsive wife; (2) the rape was motivated by some type of sexual deviation, such as that which would develop from being raised by a rejecting or seductive mother; or (3) the rape was motivated by contact with a particularly provocative and seductive woman. During the 1960s, rape came to be considered a crime of violence. Rapes were recognized as motivated by a desire to exercise power over a victim, a desire to vent rage, hatred, and contempt upon a victim, or a desire to inflict sadistic aggression upon a victim.[10]

The current theory is that rape is an act of sexualized violence.[8] In other words, dominating and humiliating a person through sexual assault involves both violence and sexuality. The act of rape is an attempt to violate, degrade, and humiliate another human being by invading their most intimate and personal individuality. It is believed that the incidence of rape may be partially attributed to the cultural valuing of traits such as power, aggression, dominance, and mastery, and the association of these traits with masculine sexuality.[1,19,21]

RELATED FACTORS

Because of lack of accurate information, many people are unaware that the prevalence of sexual assault is as high as 48% for females and 28% for males.[18] If health care professionals are unaware of the long-term effects of rape, victims who seek assistance may receive little or no follow-up beyond crisis intervention. Chronic rape trauma symptoms may develop that are not recognized or are misdiagnosed.

Because of belief in rape myths, victims can experience an increase in feelings of shame, guilt, loss of self-esteem, and fear of being disbelieved about the rape. The victim may be afraid to report the crime or seek the support of others. When rape myths are accepted by the victim's family and friends, health-care providers, members of the legal system, and members of society, the result can be blaming the victim, providing inadequate support and intervention to the victim, failure to punish the rapist, and failure to prevent the crime from being repeated. Consequently, the rape trauma syndrome can be exacerbated, and the recovery process can be interrupted or delayed. Table 13-13 lists common rape myths and the facts that dispel the myths.

In addition to belief in rape myths, there are a variety of other factors that influence the development of rape trauma syndrome and the process of recovery. These factors include the victim's coping style, level of self-esteem, type of social support available, developmental stage at the time of the assault, additional life stressors,

psychiatric history, additional history of victimization, and the type of assault.[3,8,12]

The following is a case example: Jane, a 16-year-old high school junior, was raped when a boy she met at a school dance offered her a ride home. She has an alcoholic father who has been abusive to his wife and children. Jane has a history of low self-esteem, few friends, and has never learned healthy coping skills. She is likely to blame herself, not report the rape, become more withdrawn, develop rape-related fears which may generalize, and attempt to deal with the rape by utilizing maladaptive coping skills such as denial and the use of alcohol or drugs. Consequently, she will develop rape trauma syndrome, which will become chronic without intervention. The symptoms will interfere with her mastery of the developmental tasks of adolescence and prevent her from successfully moving into the developmental stage of young adulthood.

DEFINING CHARACTERISTICS
Acute Phase

The initial phase may last from days to weeks. During this phase, some victims may present in an emergency room or clinic with obvious physical injuries that are consistent with a history of rape. During the physical examination, there may be evidence of genital trauma with the presence of spermatozoa. However, other victims may have less obvious physical symptoms. Penetration may not have occurred. As sexual dysfunction has been reported by 43% of convicted rapists[11], there may be no spermatozoa. The victim may have minimal signs of genital trauma if she submitted to the rapist out

TABLE 13–13
Rape Trauma Syndrome

RAPE MYTHS	FACTS
Rape is provoked by the victim. Victims are responsible for the rape. All women really want to be raped.	About 80% of rapes are planned in advance by the rapist. The victim is usually threatened with death or bodily harm if she resists. The Federal Crime Commission found only 4% of rapes involved "precipitative" behavior, which they reported as only a slight gesture.
Only young attractive women get raped. Only "bad girls" or promiscuous women get raped.	Rapists choose victims without regard for age, race, or socioeconomic status. Reported victim ages range from 6 months to 93 years.
Men cannot be raped by women.	There are no statistics available on the incidence of rape of males by females. In clinical practice, the authors have interviewed males who report experiences with females that meet the definition of rape. The male victims do not identify themselves as having been raped, despite experiencing the symptoms of rape trauma syndrome.
Most women are raped by strangers, when they are out alone at night or in unsafe places.	Only 12% of reported rapes are perpetrated by strangers. One-half of all rapes occur in a residence. One-third to one-half occur in the victim's residence.
Rapists are perverts or men with unsatisfied sex drives, are sick or insane. The primary motive for rape is sexual.	Rapists generally exhibit normal behavior, are usually sexually active with spouse or partner, and have a normal sex drive. Their personalities are generally within normal limits other than having a greater than average tendency toward aggression and violence.

(Modified from Foley TS, Grimes B. In: Stuart G, Sundeen S, eds. Principles and practice of psychiatric nursing. St Louis. CV Mosby, 1987.)

of fear for her life. If the victim waits several days or weeks before seeking treatment, there may be minimal or no acute physical signs of trauma remaining.

In addition to physical signs of the attack, victims may have a variety of physical and psychological responses to the rape. The rape trauma and the accompanying symptoms are so significant that the client may meet the criteria for diagnosis of post-traumatic stress disorder.[1] The physical symptoms can include nausea, vomiting, anorexia, skeletomuscular pain from tension, headaches, genitourinary disorders, rashes, or other forms of somatization.

The psychological symptoms of rape can present in a variety of ways. The manner of response can be influenced by such factors as the victim's usual style of expression, previous experience with traumatic events, coping style, and the support available. Some victims behave in a very emotional manner. They can express anxiety, anger, guilt, fear, hostility, or restlessness. They may be hyperalert, hypervigilant, and have an exaggerated startle response. They may cry, laugh, shake, talk rapidly and continuously, or have difficulty talking. Male victims often express their anger and fear in the form of physical aggression. They may destroy property or become assaultive to people with whom they have contact.[7,9]

Other victims may present in a very different manner, appearing very calm and in control. They may appear to be coping with the trauma very well. Nurses should not be misled into concluding that these victims have not been traumatized by the attack. This response is similar to the calm that sometimes occurs from shock and denial after the death of a loved one.

Other victims may present with a mixture of the styles, alternately appearing very emotional or very calm and controlled. The manner of response can be consistent with their usual behavior or completely atypical of them.

Latent Phase

Following the acute phase is a latent phase that can last from weeks to years. Victims frequently display a type of outward adjustment as they resume their usual life-style. They engage in behaviors that appear as if they are putting the rape behind them and getting on with their lives. In an attempt to distance themselves from reminders, they may make major changes such as new jobs, new place of residence, or new relationships.[3] During this phase, victims avoid talking about the rape and generally deny the need for counseling. Despite the victims' denial, the rape trauma continues to affect their lives. Symptoms, which are frequently attributed to some other cause, can include depression, sleep disturbances, eating disorders, flashbacks, anxiety disorders, phobias, sexual dysfunction, inability to concentrate, short attention span, and exacerbation of previous physical or psychiatric disorders. If symptoms continue for more than six months, victims would have a diagnosis of chronic rape trauma syndrome. In addi-

tion to the other symptoms, they may develop a chronic victim response, similar to learned helplessness. They may become involved in a series of abusive relationships. They may lose their ability to discriminate between safe and unsafe situations and, consequently, become a target for further physical or sexual assaults. They may become substance abusers in an attempt to cope with the fear, anxiety, and depression. Because these responses are generally not recognized as consequences of rape trauma syndrome, the diagnoses for many rape trauma victims are personality disorder, substance abuse disorder, major depression, or schizophrenia, without treatment for the underlying source of the symptoms.

Integration Phase

The final phase of integration can occur months to years after the assault. Victims recognize the symptoms as being rape related and begin to view themselves as survivors of a traumatic experience. They resolve their feelings of depression, anger, fear, and guilt and begin to develop healthy patterns of behavior and thinking to replace the dysfunctional patterns they may have developed after the assault.

Some victims never reach the phase of integration. They continue to avoid dealing with the rape and, as a result, continue to experience symptoms. For some victims, a precipitating event exacerbates the symptoms to such a degree that they cannot be ignored. Events such as another acute trauma, the birth of a child, the anniversary date of the rape, or some symbolic trigger may be the impetus for seeking treatment. There are numbers of victims whose denial is so strong that they do not remember the rape. The memory sometimes returns when the victim feels strong enough to deal with it, in response to a precipitating event, or during therapy for other issues. It is not unusual for victims to report unremembered rape histories during regression hypnosis, for example (Chart 1).

NURSING PROCESS AND RATIONALE
Preencounter Preparation

Nurses, like others, may believe in rape myths. Education about the scientific basis of rape response can help to dispel the myths. Nurses must examine their own emotions concerning rape, because they can be a biasing factor in assessment, diagnosis, and treatment. With the high prevalence of rape, it is to be expected that some nurses will have been victims of rape. Subsequent professional encounters with other rape victims can create intense anxiety for a nurse who has not resolved her own rape trauma. Even without a history of rape, the feelings of vulnerability and anger that can be stimulated when dealing with a rape victim can be very difficult to tolerate. Sensitivity to the difficulties of providing nursing care to rape victims and the need

CHART 1
Rape Trauma Syndrome: Definition, Related Factors, and Defining Characteristics

DEFINITION

Rape trauma syndrome describes the results of forced, violent sexual penetration or other forms of sexual victimization against the victim's will and consent. The trauma that develops from this attack or attempted attack includes an acute phase of disorganization of life-style and a long-term process of reorganization of life-style.

RELATED FACTORS

Coping style
Level of self-esteem
Social support system
Developmental stage at the time of the assault
Experience with additional life stressors
Previous psychiatric history
Type of assault
Additional history of victimization

DEFINING CHARACTERISTICS
Acute Phase

Somatic responses
　Symptoms of physical trauma
　Gastrointestinal disorders
　Skeletomuscular pain from tension
　Headaches
　Genitourinary disorders
　Dermatologic disorders
　Sexual dysfunction
Psychological responses
　Manifestations of post-traumatic stress disorder
　Denial

Shock
Fear, episodes of panic, or anxiety attacks
Guilt
Anger
Depression
Shame
Loss of self-esteem
Sleep disturbance
Eating disorders
Inability to concentrate
Short attention span
Loss of ability to trust others

Latent Phase

Somatic and psychological responses listed above (may be chronic continuation from acute phase or may be delayed onset)
Chronic or delayed onset post-traumatic stress disorder
Chronic victim response resulting in subsequent victimizations
Development of maladaptive coping patterns
Substance abuse
Self-destructive behaviors
Avoidance of reminders of the rape
Denial of symptomatic responses

Integration Phase

Recognition of symptoms as being rape related
Willingness to enter into treatment
Resolution of rape-related symptoms
Participation in activities designed to educate the public about issues of rape and to provide assistance to other victims of rape

---

for ongoing systems of support for nurses who treat rape victims is an important element of professional practice.

Nurses in any specialty area may have contact with rape victims. Knowledgeable nurses may recognize chronic rape trauma symptoms in an obstetric patient, for example, who has anxiety and depression after the birth of an infant and is exhibiting signs of detachment. Psychiatric nurses who include a victimization assessment and are alert for rape trauma symptoms can identify victims who have not previously disclosed the rape history.

Assessment

ACUTE PHASE

The nursing assessment of the recent victim of rape includes obtaining a history of the rape, assessing for physical symptoms including tests for sexually transmitted diseases and urinary tract infections, psychological symptoms, level of knowledge about rape issues, belief in rape myths, previous history of victimization,

usual coping style, and available support system. Nurses in emergency centers, offices, or clinics need to be familiar with their particular state laws on sex crimes and the procedure for obtaining evidence for the legal process. Box 13-9, a summary of the rape examination, is an example of the collection of evidence necessary for the legal process. The examination can be a painful and traumatic experience. Without supportive nursing care, the victim may perceive the examination as revictimization, resulting in a compounded rape trauma response.

LATENT PHASE

The nursing assessment for victims with chronic rape trauma syndrome includes the same data obtained from acute victims, with the exception of the physical examination. In addition, data are gathered on the victims' developmental stage at the time of the rape, subsequent history of victimization, history of changes in support system, coping style, life-style, and spiritual life since the rape.

BOX 13–9
Summary of Rape Examination

Describe appearance of patient's clothing. Report if patient changed clothing between the assault and the examination. Itemize the clothing from the assault, tag it separately, and place it in containers for evidence.
Describe appearance of patient. Describe presence of trauma to entire body, including location, exact appearance, size, and possible source of trauma (e.g., from teeth, cigarette, or other)
Itemize photos or x-rays
Describe external perineal or genitopelvic trauma
Describe internal trauma. Obtain gonococcal culture and Pap smear.
Describe any discharge.
Obtain whole blood samples for a VDRL, and compare blood and enzyme groups if an assailant is identified.
Obtain saliva specimen for same comparison.
Pull 12 head hairs from various regions of the victim's scalp for comparison.
Pull 6 to 8 strands of pubic hair from the victims pubic area.
Collect any fibers or foreign matter found on the victim's body that may have come from the scene or the assailant (i.e., plant material, dried secretions, fabric fibers, or the like)
Comb through head hairs. Collect any loose hairs for comparison. They may contain hairs from the assailant.
Comb through and collect pubic hairs for the same reason.
Obtain swabs and smears from oral, rectal, and vaginal areas.

(Summarized from the Michigan State Police Sexual Assault Evidence Collection Kit.)

Nursing Diagnosis

An example of this nursing diagnosis, made more specific for a particular client, is rape trauma syndrome, (latent phase) related to sexual assault one year ago and multiple subsequent stressors.

Client Goals and Nursing Interventions

Nursing interventions for physical symptoms of recent victims with rape trauma syndrome focus upon the goals of reducing discomfort and minimizing the possibility of the development of chronic sequelae. The victim should have instructions outlining the symptoms of a urinary tract infection or sexually transmitted diseases that may develop and the need for follow-up testing, including pregnancy testing if indicated. The use of cool compresses or ice packs in areas of bruising and edema will provide some relief initially for soft-tissue trauma. Changing to the use of heat or alternating between the use of heat and cold is recommended after 24 to 48 hours. The use of prescribed analgesics can be encouraged, particularly if the level of discomfort interferes with the victim's ability to relax or sleep. Relaxation techniques can be utilized to decrease muscle tension, facilitate sleep, and decrease symptoms of anxiety. Gastrointestinal symptoms can be reduced

with dietary measures, such as small meals of easily digestible foods.

Interventions for the psychological symptoms of recent rape victims with rape trauma syndrome or victims with chronic rape trauma syndrome who are in a crisis state should be done using a crisis model. For those victims who are unable to cope with the trauma, crisis intervention will help them to return to their previous or an improved level of functioning. Crisis intervention with rape victims deals only with thoughts and behaviors that are directly rape related. It includes offering support and reassurance that the victim is a worthwhile person, encouraging expression of feelings, helping the victim see the rape experience realistically by refuting rape myths and providing accurate information on rape issues, incorporating the use of previous coping skills or assisting the victim to develop new ones, helping the victim regain a sense of control by encouraging decision making, and assisting the victim to identify and utilize her support system.

For victims with chronic rape trauma syndrome or recent victims who are not in crisis, a less directive, more exploratory therapeutic approach would be indicated. Use of the crisis model in noncrisis situations would communicate a sense of inadequacy to the victim and could result in a decrease in feelings of mastery and level of self-esteem. For the noncrisis client, the issues to be dealt with will be the same, but the process of dealing with the issues can include an exploration of conflicts and previous life events as they relate to the rape issues. An important goal of nursing intervention with all victims is to reestablish or enhance the victim's sense of mastery over self and the environment.

There are a variety of additional interventions that have been used by nurses and other health-care workers in the treatment of rape trauma victims. These include cognitive restructuring, relaxation techniques, assertiveness training, family therapy, spiritual counseling, and group therapy.

Evaluation

The effectiveness of nursing interventions can be evaluated by the extent to which the client (1) views the circumstances of the rape in reality-based terms, (2) recognizes that certain feelings and behaviors are related to the rape, (3) recognizes the need for resolution of the rape trauma, (4) remains involved or becomes reinvolved with family and significant others, (5) assumes at least preassault levels of functioning, and (6) develops and uses healthy coping mechanisms (Chart 2).

CASE STUDY

Lois, a 26-year-old woman, was referred to the health department with the nursing diagnosis of altered parenting. She had delivered her first child three months previously. In the hospital the nursing staff noted that Lois had problems adjusting to the birth. Her appetite was poor, she cried often, and did not sleep well. In addition, she showed little interest in caring for herself or her newborn infant.

During the course of several home visits, Lois revealed

CHART 2
Rape Trauma Syndrome: Summary of the Nursing Process

NURSING INTERVENTIONS	OUTCOME CRITERIA
CLIENT GOAL: OBTAIN A MORE ACCURATE UNDERSTANDING OF THE CIRCUMSTANCES OF THE RAPE AND THE RELATIONSHIP OF SUBSEQUENT FEELINGS AND BEHAVIORS	
Assess the client's belief in rape myths Educate about rape facts Teach the client about defining characteristics of rape trauma syndrome Assist the client to relate what is being experienced with the defining characteristics	Views the circumstances of the rape in reality-based terms Recognizes that certain feelings and behaviors are related to the rape Recognizes the need for treatment
CLIENT GOAL: BE ABLE TO DISCUSS THE RAPE AND VERBALIZE FEELINGS ASSOCIATED WITH IT	
Encourage the client to discuss the rape and to verbalize feelings Acquaint the client with other victims to provide an opportunity to share/offer mutual support	Is interested in resolving the rape trauma syndrome
CLIENT GOAL: UTILIZE FAMILY AND SIGNIFICANT OTHERS TO ASSIST IN RESOLVING THE RAPE TRAUMA SYNDROME	
Encourage the client to discuss the experience and feelings with family and significant others Include family and significant others in therapy as indicated Provide education about rape myths and characteristics of rape trauma syndrome to family and significant others Encourage family and significant others to express their feelings	Calls upon family and friends for assistance in resolving rape trauma syndrome The family and significant others assist the client
CLIENT GOAL: RESOLVE PHYSICAL AND PSYCHOSOCIAL MANIFESTATIONS OF RAPE TRAUMA SYNDROME	
Provide nursing care for the physical manifestations of rape trauma syndrome Utilize education, support, reassurance, and interventions such as cognitive restructuring, desensitization, stress management, assertiveness training, and spiritual counseling as indicated	Assumes preassault levels of functioning and possibly achieves a higher level of functioning
CLIENT GOAL: RECOGNIZE INEFFECTIVE COPING PATTERNS AND SUBSTITUTE HEALTHY COPING PATTERNS	
Assist the client to identify the consequences of ineffective coping patterns and develop alternatives Refer the client to appropriate resources such as substance abuse programs, family therapy, or vocational rehabilitation	Utilizes healthy coping mechanisms to resolve the rape trauma syndrome Applies these coping mechanisms to additional life situations

that she was still having trouble sleeping, would frequently have nightmares about being mutilated, felt depressed often, and had trouble concentrating. She also reported that her anxiety attacks were increasing in frequency and intensity. Initially the public health nurse thought the symptoms were related to Lois's perception of the birth process as being traumatic and to her difficulty adjusting to her new role. During the next few visits, when the symptoms did not improve, she gathered more data. She specifically asked about Lois's previous history of trauma and victimization. Lois tearfully revealed that she had been raped by a date during her senior year in college. She did not report the rape and tried to block the memory, behaving as if nothing had happened. Her fear when being near the vicinity of the rape site increased to anxiety attacks whenever she had to go on campus. She left college right after graduation, rather than beginning graduate school as she had planned.

The public health nurse made a diagnosis of unresolved rape trauma syndrome reactivated by parturition. She referred her to a psychiatric clinical nurse specialist who was experienced in the treatment of rape trauma syndrome. The psychiatric clinical nurse specialist's interventions included helping Lois to see that she was not responsible for the rape just because she had agreed to the date. The nurse helped her to see that the present symptoms were rape related, and encouraged Lois to express feelings about the rape, the assailant, and self. With the use of cognitive restructuring, Lois learned to minimize her self-depreciating beliefs and to decrease her feelings of depression. The use of relaxation techniques helped to improve her sleep and to control the anxiety attacks. She was able to tell her husband about the rape and ask him to join her in therapy sessions. After several months of individual and couples therapy, she joined a support group with other victims of rape. The group helped Lois to identify behaviors that were chronic victim responses, increase her assertiveness skills, decrease her sense of isolation, and expand her support system. She joined a support group for mothers with infants and began to think about reapplying to graduate school.

SUMMARY

Rape trauma syndrome is a term that is used to describe the results of forced, violent sexual penetration

Research Highlights

Currently, studies that examine the long-term effects of rape are the focus of funding by the National Institute of Mental Health.[6] As with many other disorders that produce long-term effects, clinicians and researchers are beginning to examine the possibility of prevention. Previously, prevention meant teaching women how to minimize their chances of being raped. The acceptance of the theory that rape is a consequence of a socialization process that fosters sex role stereotyping and condones violence and sexual aggression toward more vulnerable individuals suggests the possibility that another area of prevention may warrant consideration. Changing the socialization process that promotes the imbalance of power between men and women and the acceptance of violent and aggressive male sexuality may decrease the prevalence of rape.

The concept is addressed in a paper by Swift who pointed out that prevention programs that teach techniques to avoid rape can reduce the risk for the individual who learns the techniques.[21] However, the prevalence of rape is not affected. Rapists are reported merely to shift their focus from less-susceptible potential victims to more-susceptible potential victims. She states that epidemiologic studies show that the highest predictor of rape victimization in a society is the status of the females in that society. The highest predictor for assaultive behavior in males is membership in a culture that condones interpersonal violence and denigrates women's roles.

The significance of the socialization process in the problem of rape was also supported in a 1981 study by Sanday. Cultures were classified as rape-free, intermediate, or rape-prone. The rape-prone cultures are characterized by male dominance, a high level of interpersonal violence, and sexual segregation.[19] A 1980 study by Burt reports that in rape-prone cultures there is a high degree of sex role stereotyping and acceptance of rape myths.[4] Further research is required in this area. The results thus far, however, suggest that preventive strategies aimed at decreasing sex role stereotyping and eliminating the acceptability of violent and aggressive expressions of sexuality may be the most effective treatment strategy for the problem of rape.

---

or other forms of sexual victimization against the victim's will and consent. The trauma that develops from this attack, or attempted attack, includes an acute phase or disorganization of the victim's life-style and a long-term process of reorganization of life-style. There are a number of factors that influence the development of rape trauma syndrome and the process of recovery including belief in rape myths, the victim's coping style, level of self-esteem, type of social support available, developmental stage at time of the assault, additional life stressors, psychiatric history, additional history of victimization, and the type of assault.

References

1. American Psychiatric Association. Diagnostic and statistical manual of mental disorders. 3rd ed, revised. Washington, DC: American Psychiatric Association; 1987.
2. Burgess AW, Holmstrom LL. Rape trauma syndrome. Am J Psychiatry. 1974;131:981–986.
3. Burgess AW, Holmstrom LL. Rape: crisis and recovery. Bowie, MD: Robert J Brady; 1978.
4. Burt M. Cultural myths and supports for rape. J Pers Soc Psychol. 1980;38:217–230.
5. Finkelhor D. Child sexual abuse: new theory and research. New York: Free Press; 1984.
6. Foley TS. Personal communication, 1987.
7. Foley TS, Davies MA. Rape: nursing care of victims. St Louis: CV Mosby; 1983.
8. Foley TS, Grimes B. Nursing intervention with sexual assault and rape victims. In Stuart G, Sundeen S, eds. Principles and practice of psychiatric nursing. St Louis: CV Mosby; 1987.
9. Goyer PF, Eddleman HC. Same-sex rape of nonincarcerated men. Am J Psychiatry. 1984;141:576–579.
10. Groth AN, Birnbaum HJ. Men who rape: the psychology of the offender. New York: Plenum Press; 1979.
11. Groth AN, Burgess AW. Sexual dysfunction during rape. N Engl J Med. 1977;14:764–766.
12. Kilpatrick DG, Veronen LJ, Resnick PA. Assessment of the aftermath of rape: changing patterns of fear. J Behav Assess. 1979;1:133–148.
13. Kim M, McFarland G. Pocket guide to nursing diagnosis. 3rd ed. St Louis: CV Mosby; 1989.
14. Koss M. National survey of intergender relationships. Preliminary results of NIMH grant funding survey of date/acquaintance rape on college/university campuses. Kent State University Department of Psychology. Kent, Ohio in collaboration with Ms. Foundation for Education and Communication, Inc., New York, 1985.
15. Masters M, Johnson V. Principles of the new sex therapy. Am J Psychiatry. 1976;133:548–554.
16. Pope K. Research and laws regarding therapist-patient sexual involvement: implications for therapists. Am J Psychother. 1986;15:564–571.
17. Russell D. Rape in marriage. New York: Macmillan; 1982.
18. Russell D. Sexual exploitation: rape, child sexual abuse, and sexual harassment. Beverly Hills: Sage Publications; 1984.
19. Sanday P. The socio-cultural context of a rape: a cross cultural study. J Soc Iss. 1981;37:5–27.
20. Shephard M. The love treatment: sexual intimacy between patients and psychotherapists. New York: Wyden; 1971.
21. Swift C. The prevention of rape. In: Burgess A, ed. Rape and sexual assault: a research handbook. New York: Garland Publishing; 1985.

REGRESSED BEHAVIOR

Katie Cosper Duncan and Melodie A. Lohr

DEFINITION AND DESCRIPTION

Regression is an unconscious defense mechanism consisting of a partial or complete return to earlier patterns of behavior. Persons are said to "behave as a child or as an infant." Not all regression is undesirable, however, and in many cases, regression serves an important and useful role.[1,11] Will[19] describes the following seven uses of regression, many of which may be quite helpful:

1. Under stress, regressed behavior may provide reassurance by uncomplicating interpersonal interactions and relieving the burden from high-level defense mechanisms.
2. With regression, attention is taken off immediate and pressing events and circumstances and placed instead on ideas and feelings from the past that have not necessarily been integrated into the personality.
3. Regressive behavior may allow the client to communicate early life events that cannot be communicated adequately with speech.
4. While regressed, a client can observe with some distance how people react to each other and to himself or herself without having to react like a mature adult.
5. Regression can be a form of remembering or escaping in time to more primitive, and perhaps more satisfying, ways of relating to others.
6. Problem solving can occur, and certain matters that otherwise would have no obvious solutions may be clarified during regressed conditions.
7. Regressed behavior can change the environment, and the person can often obtain information that would otherwise be denied.

Regression can thus be seen to have many positive aspects and, indeed, in psychoanalysis, there are often phases in which regression is desired.[9,14] Regression can, of course, be seen in everyday life in adults without gross psychopathology, and some theorists have proposed that in order to fall in love, or to be creative, or to have full emotional enjoyment of art, music, sex, and other experiences, some relaxation of ego controls is necessary. Sometimes, this response has been termed regression in the service of the ego.[13] The emotional wealth one has derived from past fulfilling relationships and experiences allows one to enjoy the happiness experienced in present situations and with others through internalized object relations.[10]

THEORY AND RESEARCH

Regression is a response that occurs when a person deals with anxiety through behaviors at a level more characteristic of and appropriate for an earlier age.[2]

Regression is often marked during adolescence, and there are a number of psychoanalytic theories that describe what is happening during this period.[5,15] There is a progressive emergence of libidinal and aggressive drives, which demand a restructuring of ego mechanisms. This restructuring is achieved by first loosening existing ego mechanisms. The theory of object relations can assist in understanding regression in adolescence. Margaret Mahler,[15] in her theory of object relations, has noted that there are several phases of separation–individuation through which the child must pass and that these are accompanied by progressively more advanced levels of symbolization. Accordingly, a period of undifferentiated object relations is followed by the phases of differentiation, practicing, and rapprochement. Inherent in every step of independent functioning is a minimal threat of object loss. During adolescence, there is a partial regression to the undifferentiated phase of ego development, after which a restructuring can take place as the adolescent moves from functioning as a child to functioning as an adult.

A form of regression that is somewhat different from the other forms discussed in this chapter should also be mentioned. Regression can occur in clients who are highly hypnotizable or who are given sedative-hypnotic interviews such as with sodium amobarbital. In such subjects, the regression may consist of an actual reliving of an event, in contrast to other forms of regression described, in which there is behavior more appropriate to an earlier stage of life. This phenomenon is sometimes called "hypnotic regression" and has been used in psychotherapy as well as in criminal investigations. Its value in the latter is not clear, as the memories of individuals undergoing hypnotic regression are often inaccurate and tainted by the desires of the subject and the examiner.[6]

RELATED FACTORS

Under certain circumstances and in certain conditions, regressed behavior occurs normally and should be accepted and worked with as coping behavior. However, regressed behavior can also be counterproductive, problematic, or actually pathological. Regressive behavior occurs basically in two contexts: in medical illness or psychosocial stress or as a component of certain psychiatric illnesses.

Stress-Related Regressed Behavior

In older children who are under stress, regression may be seen as a resumption of earlier behavior patterns such as bedwetting (enuresis) or bed soiling (encopresis), baby talk, or, in severe cases, crawling instead of walking. Such regressed behavior is often seen in children suffering from medical illnesses.[6,7,17] Sometimes, regressed behavior is mistakenly thought to represent mental retardation, when in fact, no such impairment exists, and the child's behavior is a short-term reaction to some other problem, such as school phobia or the birth of a new sibling, or the result of a more serious problem such as sexual abuse.[4]

Regressed behaviors are sometimes irritating to the medical and nursing staff in the hospital. Regressed clients are often demanding, hostile, and angry on the one hand, yet dependent and overly accepting on the other.[8] Staff members can become angry at these clients, yet be afraid to confront them directly, and this often exacerbates the regression.[3]

Regressed Behavior in Psychiatric Illness

The classic example of a psychiatric condition in which regressed behavior is often (although not invariably) a feature is schizophrenia.[7] Regression in clients with schizophrenia can take many forms, and there is often profound dependency, hostility, mutism, negativism, and other characteristics reminiscent of a much earlier period of development. Schizophrenic symptomatology has been proposed to be related to disturbances in the preoedipal phases of development, in which the separation–individuation issues are in a critical developmental period. It is not clear whether the regressed behavior of schizophrenic clients is a psychological response of the client to the stresses of psychosis, or whether regression is simply a component of the illness for some clients, perhaps with a biologic basis. It is possible that both psychological and biologic factors are important in the etiology of regression in schizophrenia.[11]

Although many psychiatric conditions are associated with some regression, there are several conditions apart from schizophrenia in which severe regression is most likely to be seen. These include severe depressions, personality disorders (especially borderline, histrionic, dependent, and passive aggressive), and severe anxiety disorders (including agoraphobia and panic disorders).

DEFINING CHARACTERISTICS

The basic characteristics of regressed behavior involve a return to patterns of behavior that were more appropriate at an earlier age. Of course, what constitutes regression is to a large extent dependent on the level of psychological development of the person. Mentally retarded persons may exhibit behaviors characteristic of a child, but such persons may not have achieved adult relationships and behaviors; thus, their behavior is not regressed; rather, it is undeveloped or immature. The term "regression" implies a loss of age-appropriate functioning previously developed in an individual. On the other hand, in very high-functioning persons, subtle changes in behavior involving increased dependence, anger, or other features, even though such behavior might be normal for other persons, may represent regression. Therefore, whether or not behavior is regressed is dependent on the baseline emotional and cognitive development of the person.[10]

In general, however, significantly regressed behavior is readily recognizable. It is apparent as increased helplessness, increased demanding behavior, aggressiveness or hostility, refusal to take responsibility for self or personal actions, and difficulty making decisions. When more severe, there may be childlike talk and behavior, conceptualization of the world or parts of it as "all good" or "all bad," and magical thinking. When it is very severe, patients may soil themselves, refuse to get out of bed, or become mute[10] (Chart 1).

NURSING PROCESS AND RATIONALE

Assessment

When assessing for regressed behavior, it is especially important to obtain information on the previous level of functioning, as this will be helpful in identifying changes in behavior that may be indicative of regression. The scope of regressive behaviors being utilized is identified, and an attempt is made to understand what these behaviors mean to the client.[16] A useful question to keep in mind is, "What is this person trying to communicate with this behavior?" Often, this information leads not only to greater understanding and empathy for the client, but also to better ways of dealing with the behavior.[19] Family and significant others are a valuable source of information, particularly regarding the client's overall support network.[2] Data needs to be collected to determine whether the regressed behavior is harmful to the client or to others (detrimental regression) or whether it is not harmful and temporarily protects the client's ego.

Nursing Diagnosis

On the basis of a thorough client assessment and, where appropriate, a family assessment, a more specific

CHART 1
Regressed Behavior: Definition, Related Factors, and Defining Characteristics

DEFINITION

Regression is an unconscious defense mechanism of a partial or complete return to earlier patterns of behavior. Regression can occur as a normal and healthy coping behavior, or it can be maladaptive and counterproductive

RELATED FACTORS

Medical illness; e.g., myocardial infarction
Family stress; e.g., divorce, abuse
Psychiatric illness; e.g., schizophrenia, severe anxiety disorders

DEFINING CHARACTERISTICS

Return to patterns of behavior that were more appropriate at an earlier age, such as

Aggression, hostility
Increased helplessness
Distractibility
Urinary or bowel incontinence
Rocking, sleeping in fetal position
Masturbating, exposing self
Refusal to get out of bed
Mutism
Destructive behavior

---

nursing diagnosis can be formulated for clients manifesting regressed behavior. An example is regressed behavior related to the stress of hospitalization.

Client Goals and Nursing Interventions

When regression is mild and apparently adaptive for the client, the nurse should be supportive and try to understand the basis of the regressed behavior. In such instances, the behavior should not be confronted directly, as the behavior itself often represents an attempt to avoid such confrontation, and directly challenging it may cause more severe regression. For example, the nurse might accept the dependency expressed by the client and help the client to deal with the precipitating stress without actually confronting the regression.[2,19]

Thus, not all regressed behavior should be challenged, as there are beneficial aspects to regression. Sometimes, regression should be accepted insofar as it helps the client deal with severe crises. In dealing with the regressed client, the nurse should constantly be aware whether nursing interventions are designed to deal with the client's problem, or if the nurse is intervening to allay his or her own anxiety about the regressed behavior.[19]

For those conditions in which regression is more severe and is detrimental to the client, one approach is the development of a behavior modification program that encourages greater independence and autonomous

---

CHART 2
Regressed Behavior: Summary of the Nursing Process

NURSING INTERVENTIONS	OUTCOME CRITERIA
CLIENT GOAL: HAVE NO FURTHER INCREASE IN REGRESSIVE BEHAVIORS	
Establish daily activities	Experiences increased structure in environment
Accept dependency expressed by the client without confronting dependency needs	Regressive dependency needs are reduced
Set limits on regressed behaviors that infringe on the rights of others or are a danger to the client's well-being or safety	Recognizes rights of others
Assist in grooming activities if necessary	Meets basic needs
Give positive feedback for even small accomplishments, independent functioning, and appropriate decision making	Experiences satisfaction from positive reinforcement for positive accomplishments
CLIENT GOAL: IDENTIFY THE PRECIPITATING STRESSOR AND EXPAND COPING STRATEGIES	
Establish rapport through empathic, trustworthy, supportive approach	Deals with emotions in a healthier way
Assist client in recognizing and expressing feelings such as anxiety, sadness, and anger related to the precipitating stressor	
Explore alternative coping strategies and reinforce coping mechanisms the client has used effectively in the past	Expands coping skills

Research Highlights

A study was conducted of suicidal adolescent girls to determine if there is a correlation between suicidal behavior and borderline personality traits and to examine separation anxiety.[17] Forty adolescent girls who had attempted suicide were given the Hansburg Separation Anxiety Test and Gunderson's Diagnostic Interview for Borderline Disorder. The results of this research, although with a limited sample, suggest that a suicide gesture in adolescence is a borderline phenomenon that has roots in the separation–individuation phase of development. The resulting separation anxiety and subsequent abandonment depression the adolescent experiences is relieved by suicide gestures as a regressive attempt to return to an earlier symbiotic state where the adolescent had experienced safety.

Because nurses often have the most contact with clients, it is important for nurses to assess clients for regressed behavior and be aware of the potential seriousness of some regressive manifestations.

functioning. Clients should be rewarded for independent functioning and appropriate decision making.[19] For example, clients may be given tokens for making their beds, combing their hair, or accomplishing other behaviors.

Evaluation

The purpose of the evaluation is to determine the degree to which the behavioral goals have been met. The client, other treatment team members, family, and significant others should be included in collecting data. Objective data gathered during the evaluation of the client with regressed behavior can then be utilized to implement new or revised intervention strategies or possibly to define more realistic goals or time frames, if needed[2] (Chart 2).

CASE STUDY

Debbie A is a 28-year-old woman with a diagnosis of chronic paranoid schizophrenia. For 4 years, Debbie lived in a chronic care facility, requiring several acute hospitalizations during that time for her mental illness. Eventual closure of this facility necessitated a transfer of Debbie into a new residential program. With Debbie's routine and surroundings disrupted, and with the absence of familiar staff and residents, she began exhibiting regressed behavior. She began isolating herself from the staff and other residents by staying in bed and eventually refusing to communicate verbally. Debbie's grooming and hygiene rapidly declined. Ultimately, a return of auditory hallucinations and paranoid delusions necessitated hospitalization on an acute-care mental health unit. Debbie was assigned a nursing case manager who, after a thorough assessment, formulated as one of her nursing diagnoses: regressed behavior related to stress of residential move and loss of familiar persons.

Debbie's case manager initiated a treatment plan utilizing behavior modification theory and interventions. In establishing a therapeutic rapport with Debbie, the case manager was supportive and accepting, giving clear and consistent messages and expectations. Short, frequent interactions were initiated, and the case manager set limits with Debbie in a supportive fashion. Initially, Debbie was expected to be out of her room for meals, of which she was to eat at least half. Supervision and encouragement were provided in grooming and hygiene practices. Scheduling of program activities and groups was structured, and limits were placed on the amount of time she could spend in her room. Each day, the daily goals were increased slightly. The case manager gave explanations of what was happening, and she was available to the client for questions and concerns. Positive feedback was given for even small self-care accomplishments.

Debbie was hospitalized for 3 weeks, during which time she showed improvement, with a lessening of defining characteristics of regressed behavior. She established a regular eating pattern, resumed independent self-care and neat grooming, and had a marked reduction in psychotic symptoms. During the last week of Debbie's hospitalization, a nurse from her new residential program came to visit her daily to begin establishment of rapport and to facilitate a smooth transition from the hospital back into the chronic care facility.

SUMMARY

Regression is an unconscious defense mechanism consisting of a partial or complete return to earlier patterns of behavior. Regression is frequently a normal part of development or a normal reaction to stress; however, there are a number of mental illnesses in which regression is a characteristic feature, including schizophrenia, severe depression, personality disorders (especially borderline, histrionic, dependent, and passive aggressive), and severe anxiety disorders (including agoraphobia and panic disorders). It is important when designing nursing interventions to decide when it is important to support the client and not challenge the regressed behavior and when the behavior should be directly challenged and an attempt made to modify it.

References

1. Balint M. The Basic Fault: Therapeutic Aspects of Regression. London: Tavistock Publications; 1968.
2. Brunner LS, Suddarth DS. The Lippincott Manual of Nursing Practice. Philadelphia: JB Lippincott; 1982.

3. Cassem NH, Hackett TP. The setting of intensive care. In: Hackett TP, Cassem NH, eds. Massachusetts General Hospital Handbook of General Hospital Psychiatry. St. Louis: CV Mosby; 1978.

4. Cooper A, Frances A, Sacks M. Psychiatry, Vol 1: The Personality Disorders and Neuroses. Philadelphia: JB Lippincott; 1968.

5. Engel GL. Psychological Development in Health and Disease. Philadelphia: WB Saunders; 1962.

6. Freud A. The role of bodily illness in the child. Psychoanal Study Child. 1969.

7. Grace HK, Layton J, Camilleri D. Mental Health Nursing: A Socio-Psychological Approach. Iowa: Wm C Brown; 1977.

8. Hackett TP. Disruptive states. In: Hackett TP, Cassem NH, ed. Massachusetts General Hospital Handbook of General Hospital Psychiatry. St. Louis: CV Mosby; 1978.

9. Houpt J, Brodie HK. Psychiatry, Vol 3: Consultation–Liaison Psychiatry and Behavioral Medicine. Philadelphia: JB Lippincott; 1968.

10. Kernberg O. Borderline Conditions and Pathological Narcissism. New York: Jason Aronson; 1975.

11. Kety SS. The concept of schizophrenia. In: Alpert M, ed. Controversies in Schizophrenia. New York: Guilford Press; 1985.

12. Lewin K. Regression, retrogression, and development. In: Carwright D, ed. Field Theory and Social Science. New York: Harper & Row; 1951.

13. MacKinnon RA. Psychiatric history and mental status examination. In: Kaplan HI, Freedman AM, Sadock BJ, eds. Comprehensive Textbook of Psychiatry. 3rd ed. Baltimore: Williams & Wilkins; 1980.

14. MacKinnon RA, Michels R. The Psychiatric Interview in Clinical Practice. Philadelphia: WB Saunders; 1971.

15. Mahler MS. On the first three subphases of the separation–individuation process. Int J Psychoanal. 1972;53:333.

16. McFarland G, Wasli E. Nursing Diagnoses and Process in Psychiatric Mental Health Nursing. Philadelphia: JB Lippincott; 1986.

17. Prugh DG, Staub E, Sands H, Kirschbaum R, Lenihan E. A study of the emotional reactions of children and families to hospitalization and illness. Am J Orthopsychiatry 1953;23:70.

18. Wade NL. Suicide as a resolution of separation–individuation among adolescent girls. Adolescence 1978;22:169–177.

19. Will OA Jr. Schizophrenia: Psychological treatment. In: Kaplan HI, Freedman AM, Sadock BJ eds. Comprehensive Textbook of Psychiatry. 3rd ed. Baltimore: Williams & Wilkins; 1980.

RESOURCE MANAGEMENT, IMPAIRED

(SPECIFY)

Noreen Cavan Frisch and Janet Weber

DEFINITION AND DESCRIPTION

The nursing diagnosis of *impaired resource management (specify)* refers to the client's inability to obtain, structure, or manage resources such as time, housing, or finances. The diagnosis of impaired resource management is made when the client indicates that he or she perceives the management of resources to be difficult and chooses to make a change with assistance from the nurse. This nursing diagnosis focuses on a wide range of client activities dealing with day-to-day living and goal attainment and is used when the client's principal difficulty is inability to obtain resources or to organize them for optimal efficiency.

A nurse may be called on to assist clients with many types of resource management. For example, a young mother may seek help in managing household finances to permit purchase of nutritional foods at reasonable cost. A client family may turn to a community nurse for information on comfortable rental housing in a child-oriented apartment complex. In both of these cases, the diagnosis provides the nurse with a framework within which to plan interventions and evaluate care directed at improving the client's use of resources. The use of this nursing diagnosis indicates that numerous activities aimed at improving resource management are legitimately within nursing's domain. For purposes of this section, however, the discussion of the diagnosis will focus on one resource, that of time, because assessment and management of time is an area of great importance to client care that has received relatively little attention.

THEORY AND RESEARCH

The concept of time has been viewed both objectively and subjectively.[12] *Objective time* refers to time as observed in the world. It is public or collective time and is measured by clocks, calendars or other instruments or is documented by natural cycles of lunar, solar, or seasonal movement. Culture influences how objective time is viewed. A sociologist who spent 2 years observ-ing the work and practice of health professionals in a large medical center documented *hospital time* as being measured in shifts, rotations, weekends, and pay period cycles.[18] Such cycles have meaning to those initiated into hospital culture (specifically nurses, interns, and residents) but may have little meaning to clients. Measurement of objective time is influenced by culture and social norms in other ways as well. Many individuals do not refer to clocks or calendars unless a work environment requires them to do so. It is commonly reported that persons on vacation cannot name the day of the week, or the hour.[2] Also, certain groups, for example, the homeless, may not think in terms of days and hours, because this measure has no relevance in their lives. Similarly, persons who live in a climate with no seasonal variation may not think in terms of winter and summer. However, when there is agreement on a time unit, objective time can be measured by several observers. These measures of objective time document the passage of time from the past and present to the future.

Subjective time refers to the individual's experience of time. It is individual and personal. A nurse scholar researching the subject over several years reported that subjective time has four dimensions of experience:[12] *perspective*—one's ability to order life events in terms of past, present, and future; *tempo*—the recognition of time passing at an identified speed; *meaning*—what time signifies for an individual; and *finality*—a sense of movement toward one's death.

A number of factors influence the experience or perception of subjective time. For example, time was perceived as passing more slowly than objective time for subjects who were tired, confined to bed, or in a quiet environment.[13–15,17] Likewise, in older institutionalized subjects, time was perceived as moving more slowly than clock time when activity on the ward increased.[7] Other investigations have suggested that amount of movement is directly related to time estimation.[9,10] Certain personality types experience time as moving quickly. For example, clients with Type A behaviors experience time as rushing, moving very quickly.[1] Other investigators have attempted to show that the elderly have a high perceived duration of time; i.e., that they overestimate passage of time when compared with clock time.[8,16] Results are inconclusive but suggest that this may be so. Individuals in a state of shock—for example, undergoing post-traumatic stress or bereavement—report loss of time perspective and speak of time as "standing still."[2]

RELATED FACTORS

Several factors related to impaired resource management (time) contribute to difficulties with time management. A very common situation is one where the client has an external locus of control and often fails to take measures to manage or organize anything in his or her environment. This client may experience impaired time management because he or she does not make decisions or set limits and therefore permits the environment to dictate what happens. Others who have a need to please will commit to certain activities without a sense of priority, resulting in "not enough time" to accomplish even the basic tasks of daily living. Also, clients who have a passive relationship with others and their environment may lack the initiative to achieve their goals. Those who lack social supports may not have time to perform all of their duties because the demand on their time is very great. Others, who tend to be overachievers in a competitive environment, find that they cannot keep up because their goals were not realistic at the outset. Individuals in both of these cases often fall into an unhealthy lifestyle of missed meals and lack of sleep, which then contributes to an inability to perform tasks efficiently.

The client may not be bound by the same measure of objective time units as the nurse, or the client may have a different subjective experience of time than the nurse. In these situations, validation of the client's view and cultural norms is essential. Such a client may ask for help if he or she identifies discomfort with the sense of time moving too slowly or too quickly.

An understanding of time requires cognitive skills to put the present in perspective and to understand one's life as having a history and a future. Psychiatric clients with disorientation and impaired cognition thus will be unable to manage time because they cannot perceive and understand time. These clients should be treated for the underlying thought process disorder first, while the nursing role with regard to time may be to structure time for the client until he or she is able to do so. Likewise, other psychiatric conditions will, by their nature, disrupt the client's regular time management patterns. An example is the client with an obsessive-compulsive disorder who cannot manage his or her day because the compulsions interfere.

DEFINING CHARACTERISTICS

One defining characteristic of this diagnosis is the client's statement of dissatisfaction with his or her own time management. This statement may come in many

forms, of which the following are examples: "I just don't have enough time in a day; I need help." "I don't know what to do with my days; they go so slowly." "I'm not able to reach my goals; something always gets in my way and I can't complete required tasks." Other defining characteristics include observations or reports that the client is not accomplishing activities of daily living or is not accomplishing activities appropriate to role demands. Examples of objective data include disorganization, poor priority setting, lack of initiative to perform activities or solve problems, and nonconstructive problem solving, whereas subjective data include client reports of boredom, disorganization, nervousness, preoccupation with worrying, and feelings of exhaustion.

Associated nursing diagnoses should be considered to ensure that the nurse is addressing the client holistically. Common nursing diagnoses that could apply in a client who is experiencing impaired resource management (specify) include sleep pattern disturbance, diversional activity deficit, self-concept disturbance, anxiety, altered perception/cognition, noncompliance, grieving, and depression (Chart 1).

CHART 1
Impaired Resource Management (Time): Definition, Related Factors, and Defining Characteristics

DEFINITION

The condition where the client is unable to structure or manage time to accomplish daily tasks.

RELATED FACTORS

Inability to plan and manage personal activities
External locus of control
Lack of social support
Unrealistic time demands; i.e., client assumes responsibilities for more activities than can be handled
Discrepancy between subjective experience of time and objective time (associated with aging, pain, bedrest, fatigue, noise, activity)
Loss of time perspective (associated with impaired cognition)
Loss of sense of tempo (associated with bereavement or shock)
Loss of sense of meaning for time (associated with depression, hopelessness, or spiritual distress)
Obsessions and compulsions

DEFINING CHARACTERISTICS

Statement that client is not satisfied with own time management
Not accomplishing activities of daily living
Not accomplishing tasks appropriate to client's social roles

NURSING PROCESS AND RATIONALE
Assessment

The nurse should assess for this diagnosis in situations where the client must adjust to a new environment or to a new social role. A new environment may be a hospital or nursing home unit. Here, the time tempo or time perspective may demand a change in and reordering of the client's internal time. A new role may be that of a first-time parent, that of a graduate student for someone who is fully employed, or that of a widow who has just lost her husband as a primary support system. In any of these examples, the individual will have new and increased demands made on his or her time and may benefit from assistance in establishing or reordering priorities to take in the increased time demands.

Nursing assessment involves a thorough investigation of how the client manages time. Past patterns of time management and the client's level of satisfaction with those patterns should be explored. A daily time log kept by the client for 3 to 4 days could be helpful. Such a log can be set up in columns to indicate how time is spent every 30 minutes. Events are recorded as they happen. This type of log will assist the client and nurse to become aware of how time actually is spent. The information gained can be used to identify useful time periods, time wasters, and interruptions. This log will also provide baseline data for the nurse and client to evaluate outcomes of planned interventions later.

In addition, an assessment of the client's perception of time is necessary to understand his or her concerns with time. Does the client perceive time to be moving rapidly or slowly at any points of the day? Does the client perceive that others in the environment take too long to achieve goals, reach their point, and conclude interactions? Do others waste the client's time, or help the client's time to pass in an enriching or stimulating way? Does the client have too few or too many activities to accomplish in a day? How does the client feel things can improve? Assisting the client to answer these questions will promote a better understanding of the reasons for and ways of changing current behaviors.

Nursing Diagnosis

An example of a specific diagnostic statement for a client who does not set priorities and has never developed a pattern of taking control of his environment would be impaired resource management (time) related to inability to plan and manage personal activities.

Client Goals and Nursing Interventions

Client goals and nursing interventions are aimed at assisting the client to acquire knowledge and thus de-velop time management skills. Although time itself cannot be manipulated, an individual can be taught management in relation to time.[6] The nurse must assess what specific objectives the client needs to achieve in order to feel satisfied with day-to-day activities and personal, social, and work roles. This can be determined by asking the client, "Where are you now?" and "Where do you want to be by the end of this month? . . . by the end of this year?" Assessment of values and priorities set by the client is essential before proceeding with a plan of time management. Perhaps the client has not been able to set priorities. This problem would direct nursing actions toward teaching priority setting by asking the client to list objectives and assign a level of priority and urgency to each of these. Table 13-14 illustrates a framework for deciding if any particular objective is one that necessitates immediate time and attention, or whether activities related to a given goal can (and should) wait until later.

Once priorities are set, activities to achieve each goal and the related objectives are defined, with the amount of time required for each activity. Activities that can be done simultaneously in order to save time are reviewed, along with those that must be done separately.

Using the support of others may also assist the client to manage better. Social support has been described as an exchange of resources intended to enhance mutual well-being and to promote the existence and availability of people on whom one can rely for assistance, encouragement, acceptance, and caring.[4] Social support increases productivity by increasing motivation and is related to successful problem solving and persistence with frustrating and challenging tasks.

The nurse may also teach the client other methods of managing time effectively. Referring to the "related to" clause in the diagnostic statement will help the nurse to individualize interventions.[3] For example, developing better decision-making skills and assertiveness training may be indicated for the client who has an external locus of control. Assertiveness training is based on principles of behavior modification and oper-

TABLE 13–14
Means of evaluating time demands

	IMPORTANT	NOT IMPORTANT
URGENT	1	3
NOT URGENT	2	4

Box 1 = Crisis
Box 2 = Take care in time or may be a crisis
Box 3 = Monitor carefully; will often attract attention, yet not important (example: phone call)
Box 4 = Time waster

Copyright 1988 by the Time Management Center, Inc., St. Louis, 1590 Woodlake Drive, Suite 111, Chesterfield, MO. Used with permission.

ates by shaping behavior techniques that are situation specific.[11] The client with unrealistic time demands can be taught to set more appropriate goals and to develop delegation skills.[5] Reduction of time wasters, implementation of efficient scheduling, and proper utilization of community resources can all assist the client to develop better time-management skills.

The pace of activities in the environment can be discussed with the client and modified for the individual who has a discrepancy between subjective and objective experiences of time. For any client in an institutional setting, the nurse has responsibility to manage the client's environment to aid in the perception that time is passing at a comfortable rate. For clients experiencing fatigue, the nurse may take measures to promote adequate rest. For clients confined to bed, the nurse may take measures to promote stimulating or enriching activities. For clients who have a basic personality orientation that time is rushing or moving very quickly, relaxation techniques may be helpful.

Evaluation

The extent to which nursing interventions have been effective is evaluated by the success of the client in carrying out those activities identified to achieve high-priority objectives. A successful plan of care is measured by the client's statement of satisfaction with current activities, roles, and accomplishments (Chart 2).

CASE STUDY

Beth L, a slightly obese, 64-year-old widow, presented at the community mental health clinic for help with feelings of being overwhelmed, and for her concerns that she was not managing her life well. Her weight was 130 pounds and her height 5 feet 2 inches. She had been living by herself for the past 6 years. She had a low to adequate income, worked outside the home as a receptionist in a nearby hotel, and owned a home that was not paid for. Beth reported that she

had been told by her medical doctor that she had an elevated serum cholesterol level, and that, despite her attempts to maintain a low-cholesterol diet, her serum level had not decreased over a 6-month period. While talking with the nurse, she began to cry and said: "I just can't find time to learn about my new prescribed diet, work, and take care of my house too! I've had to have several home repairs. When I work two nights a week, I need to sleep in the day. It's impossible to have enough time to schedule health appointments for myself. I am trying to do home repairs in order to sell the house when I retire. The furnace is broken and the house needs several other repairs before it can be sold. I can't seem to work in time for someone to repair it. I only wish I had all these things done and they never seem to get accomplished. I am also planning for retirement and have a lot of paper work to do in order to apply for low-rent housing, medical insurance, and Social Security. There is so much I don't understand, and I don't know who to ask for answers." Beth's health history revealed that she had never had a Pap smear, and, although she wore glasses, her last eye examination was 10 years ago. One nursing diagnosis formulated was impaired resource management (time) related to difficulties in planning daily activities.

With Beth's permission, the nurse scheduled a home visit to discuss her concern about not accomplishing necessary tasks. The nurse asked Beth to keep a log of her activities for the following week. Beth did so, and the time log revealed a considerable amount of time spent sitting in a chair in front of a living room window waiting for the next event. For example, Beth sat from 9 to 10 p.m. each evening waiting for the time to go to work. When someone was coming to her house, she was ready 1 to 2 hours ahead of time and sat with nothing to do. Several activities had not been carried out only because she scheduled only one activity per day.

The nurse assisted Beth in developing a list of all the activities she wished to accomplish. The nurse helped her then identify the urgency and importance of each of these in order to establish priorities. The nurse guided Beth to assert herself with others and to take control of her day-to-day life. Thus, Beth planned a calendar of daily and weekly activities with the nurse's help. Beth stated that she functioned best in the mornings, so her daily calendar scheduled critical activities early in the day. In addition, the nurse referred Beth to a local assertiveness training workshop for women.

CHART 2
Impaired Resource Management (Time): Summary of the Nursing Process

NURSING INTERVENTIONS	OUTCOME CRITERIA
CLIENT GOAL: GAIN BETTER UNDERSTANDING OF OWN USE OF TIME AND OWN PERCEPTION OF TIME	
Assess for client's perception of time and level of satisfaction with time management	Identifies objectives and priorities
Assess client's objectives and priorities	Keeps daily time log for 4 days
Instruct client to keep daily time log	
CLIENT GOAL: DEMONSTRATE BEHAVIORS THAT INDICATE EFFICIENT TIME MANAGEMENT	
Assist client with developing chart to determine urgency and, for important tasks, calendar to accomplish these	Expresses feeling organized
Teach client problem-solving and delegation of skills	Begins to use effective problem-solving skills
Assist client to identify and utilize support systems and community resources	Expresses satisfaction with ADLs
Refer client to assertiveness training class if needed	Takes initiative to act on matters and make decisions

Research Highlights

The following research provides nursing with a basis for assisting the client with time management.[13-15] Three studies completed by Smith focused on the seeming duration of time in relation to activity, change, and processing environmental information. The first study showed significant changes in perceived duration of a 40-second interval and the auditory environment, in that time was perceived to pass more slowly in a quiet environment than in an environment with continuous audiotaped stories. The second replication of the study did not confirm this finding; however, it demonstrated that tiredness was significantly related to the experience of time dragging. The third and final replication of the study confirmed the finding of the second study.

This research leads the nurse to assess the client's perception of the speed of time passage and its rhythm in relation to the client's environment. An awareness of the significance of the environment to the client's perception of time is a prerequisite to planning nursing interventions directed toward assisting the client to feel comfortable with his or her experience of time passing.

The nurse evaluated Beth's progress 1 month later. Beth had kept her daily–weekly calendar and had scheduled all activities herself. Beth reported that she enjoyed the assertiveness class. She had visited the dietitian and had scheduled a Pap smear and an eye examination for the next 2 months. Her furnace was to be repaired at the end of August in time for winter. Much paperwork remained on her kitchen table. The nurse then referred her to a local community agency to assist with her questions regarding Social Security, Medicare, and housing. The nurse encouraged Beth to schedule 1 hour of paperwork each morning followed by an activity that Beth enjoyed.

At that point, Beth stated she felt much better about her life and her ability to manage her own affairs. She had received positive reinforcement from being able to see her accomplishments and seemed able to use a daily–weekly calendar to handle future events. The nurse concluded that the plan of care was working and agreed to visit Beth in another month to assess progress and prepare for termination of the nurse's interventions.

SUMMARY

The nursing diagnosis of impaired resource management (specify) refers to the client's inability to obtain, structure, or manage resources such as time, housing, or finances. The more specific nursing diagnosis of impaired resource management (time) refers to a situation where a client is unable to structure or organize time so as to meet goals required for social, occupational, or personal roles. The client may not be able to manage time for several reasons. For example, the client may have an external locus of control and be unable to take measures to manage or organize anything in his or her environment. Also, the client may lack needed social supports or take on too many activities to be able to meet all obligations. Research indicates that clients may be dissatisfied with time management when they perceive that time is passing either much too slowly or much too rapidly. Conditions such as bedrest, fatigue, noise, activity, aging, and impaired cognition contribute to changes in the individual's perception of time passing. The nurse must assess for the presence of the diagnosis by interview, with attention to the client's subjective report of having difficulty managing time. Nursing interventions are individualized based on those factors related to the client's concerns. Evaluation of a plan of care is based on the client's subjective assessment of comfort with his or her use of time.

References

1. Burnam MA, Pennekaker JW, Glass DC. Time consciousness, achievement striving and the Type A coronary prone behavior pattern. J Abn Psychol. 1975;84:76–79.
2. Hazen H. The Limbo People: A Study of the Constitution of the Time Universe among the Aged. Boston: Routledge and Kegan Paul; 1980.
3. Kim MJ, McFarland GK, McLane AM. Pocket Guide to Nursing Diagnoses. 3rd ed. St. Louis: CV Mosby; 1989.
4. Johnson DW, Johnson FP. Joining Together: Group Theory and Group Skills. 3rd ed. Englewood Cliffs, New Jersey: Prentice Hall; 1987.
5. Koontz H, O'Donnell CO, Weirich H. Essentials of Management. 4th ed. New York: McGraw-Hill Book Company; 1986.
6. Lyles RI, Joiner C. Supervision in Health Care Organizations. New York: Wiley Medical; 1986.
7. Mellilo KD. Informal activity involvement and perceived rate of time passage for an older institutionalized population. J Gerontological Nurs. 1980;7:392–397.
8. Newman MA. Time as an index of expanding consciousness with age. Nurs Res. 1982;31:290–293.
9. Newman MA. Movement tempo and the experience of time. Nurs Res. 1976;25:273–279.
10. Newman MA, Gaudiano JK. Depression as an explanation for decreased subjective time in the elderly. Nurs Res. 1984;33:137–139.
11. Rawnsley MM. The six A's of assertiveness. In: Hein EC, Nicholson MJ, eds. Contemporary Leadership and Behavior: Selected Readings. 2nd ed. Boston: Little, Brown, and Company; 1986.
12. Sanders SA. Development of a tool to measure subjective time experience. Nurs Res. 1986;35:178–182.
13. Smith MJ. Changes in judgment of duration with different patterns of auditory information for individuals confined to bed. Nurs Res. 1975;24:93–98.
14. Smith MJ. Duration experience for bed-confined subjects: A replication and refinement. Nurs Res. 1979;28:139–144.
15. Smith MJ. Temporal experience and bed rest: Replication and refinement. Nurs Res. 1984;33:298–302.
16. Strumpf NE. Probing the temporal world of the elderly. Int J Nurs Stud. 1987;24:201–214.
17. Tompkins ES. Effect of restricted mobility and dominance on perceived duration. Nurs Res. 1980;29:333–338.
18. Zerubavel E. Patterns of Time in Hospital Life. Chicago: The University of Chicago Press; 1979.

RITUALISTIC BEHAVIOR

Georgia Whitley

DEFINITION AND DESCRIPTION

Ritualistic behavior is defined as an act, sequence of actions, a thought, or sequence of thoughts repeatedly performed in an attempt to manage anxiety. Obsessive thoughts that are unwanted, but cannot be excluded voluntarily from consciousness, typically center around religion, sex, orderliness, aggression, or dirt and germs. Compulsions are urges, which cannot easily be resisted, to perform an act. They generally relate to excessive cleaning and repetitive checking of inanimate objects. The ritualistic thoughts or acts serve to control anxiety, but do so only momentarily; thus, they must be repeated as anxiety recurs. Ritualistic behaviors may become so prominent that they interfere with the individual's employment, schoolwork, social interchanges, interpersonal relationships, and other activities of daily living. The individual who carries out ritualistic behavior often recognizes it as irrational, but is unable to stop. According to psychoanalytic theory such individuals are characterized as having great need to control not only themselves, but also other persons as well as their surroundings. It is thought that this need for control is related to their need to contain their own aggressive or sexual impulses. Ritualistic behaviors temporarily reduce the anxiety generated by these impulses. Distinguishing between behavioral traits that are helpful in achieving goals or accomplishing work, when used in moderation, and ritualistic behaviors that are fixed and nonproductive is essential. Cleanliness, precision, punctuality, perseverance, and caution are traits that can lead to productive behaviors when applied appropriately, as opposed to the problematic nature of ritualistic behaviors.

THEORY AND RESEARCH

Ritualistic behaviors are related to a fixation at, or a regression to, the anal stage of psychosexual development according to Freud.[3] These fixations and regressions are defenses that have become rigid, and they are repeated for the temporary relief of anxiety or feeling of control that they provide. This second stage of development is defined by Erikson as autonomy versus shame and doubt.[2] To give up excreta at the request of parents is to be "good" and brings parental approval. To retain them will stimulate rejection and criticism and is

equated with being "bad." Overemphasis of traits such as cleanliness, precision, punctuality, and caution can contribute to the development of ritualistic behaviors.

The self-system, according to Sullivan, seeks to avoid anxiety, increase self-esteem, and provide security. Rigidity and ritualistic behaviors can result from three security operations used by the self-system: selective inattention, false personifications, and sublimation.[6] When using selective inattention, the individual does not attend to what is said or what happens and, thus, screens out anxiety-producing stimuli. False personification involves projecting one's own self-system onto others through labeling and prejudging. By using sublimation, the individual substitutes an acceptable behavior for a desired, but unacceptable, behavior and, thereby, only partially satisfies the particular need.

Learning theorists view ritualistic behaviors as responses that the individual learns and repeats because of reinforcement of the response.[1] The ritual relieves anxiety or provides a feeling of control, however temporary. In this model, anxiety-inducing situations become paired with other stimuli. For example, unacceptable sexual or "dirty" thoughts become paired with dirty hands and precipitate anxiety that is relieved temporarily by handwashing. To regain the feeling of control or anxiety reduction produced by the ritual, it is repeated.

Ritualistic behavior has also been explained as having an organic basis. This explanation has received support from the occurrence of ritualistic behavior in families in whom there was no evidence of imitation; that is, when parent and child had differing rituals. In addition, antidepressant medications have been effective in some cases.[5]

Because etiologies vary for each theoretical model, treatment strategies are different depending upon which theoretical framework is espoused. For example, the psychoanalytic theory of causality—that ritualistic behaviors are a result of unconscious conflicts that occurred during the second developmental phase—leads to a treatment modality consisting of analysis of these childhood experiences. The cognitive–behavioral theorist, on the other hand, focuses on feelings that are predominantly conscious, treats for a much shorter period, and focuses on the client's statements about the problem. Several behavioral management strategies have been developed recently, including thought-switching, thought-stopping, flooding, distraction, and desensitization.

RELATED FACTORS

The definition of the nursing diagnosis ritualistic behavior indicates that this phenomenon occurs as an attempt to manage anxiety. Thus, the most pervasive related factor in the generation of ritualistic behavior is anxiety, a broad etiologic category. Nursing interventions will be most effective if more specific related factors are identified. The psychoanalytic view of the etiology indicates that the person has a developmental stage fixation or a regression to the anal phase. This view relates the regression or fixation to conflict between the superego and the id that may lead to unacceptable feelings about the self. The individual feels incapable of coping with life's demands, anxiety rises, and ritualistic behavior occurs as a temporary release to decrease anxiety momentarily and to give a feeling of control. The behavioral view of the relationship between ritualistic behavior and anxiety is that the individual has selected, learned, and chosen to repeat behaviors to allay anxiety. The ritualistic behavior relieves anxiety and becomes a reinforcer even though the relief is temporary. The DSM-III-R condition in which ritualistic behavior is most common is obsessive-compulsive disorder.

DEFINING CHARACTERISTICS

The cluster of defining characteristics that are observed in clients with the nursing diagnosis of anxiety are also observed in clients with the nursing diagnosis of ritualistic behavior because anxiety frequently occurs as an etiologic factor leading to ritualistic behaviors (see nursing diagnosis entitled Anxiety). The existence of repetitive acts or thoughts and the inability to control these acts or thoughts distinguishes the nursing diagnosis of ritualistic behavior from the nursing diagnosis of anxiety. In addition, clients with ritualistic behavior will demonstrate personality traits of inflexibility, expression of overabundance of detail, and low expression of feeling. The ritualistic behaviors interfere with the person's normal functioning by limiting the ability to perform activities of daily living, job responsibilities, and other activities (Chart 1).

NURSING PROCESS AND RATIONALE

Assessment

The presence of repetitive acts or thoughts that interfere with the individual's usual or normal functioning are strong indicators that focused assessment in relation to this diagnosis is essential. Data concerning the rituals may be received from the client, family members, or friends. In addition, the nurse may be able to observe the ritualistic behavior. Physical indicators, such as red, cracked, bleeding hands, may provide important diagnostic clues. Because anxiety is present in the person who exhibits ritualistic behavior, a focused

---

Chart 1
Ritualistic Behavior: Definition, Related Factors, and Defining Characteristics[4]

DEFINITION

Ritualistic behavior is an act, sequence of actions, a thought, or sequence of thoughts repeatedly performed in an attempt to manage anxiety.

RELATED FACTORS

Anxiety
Developmental stage fixation
Regression to an earlier developmental stage
Id, ego, superego conflict
Unacceptable feelings about self
Learned way of feeling control
Organic factors
Obsessive-compulsive disorder

DEFINING CHARACTERISTICS

Repetitive act or thought that is uncontrollable
Interference of rituals with job, family, or social interactions, and with activities of daily living
Manifestations of anxiety
Inflexibility
Constriction of emotional responsivity

---

assessment for anxiety is also appropriate for this individual. Situations that increase the person's need to perform the rituals need to be identified during the assessment and data collection phase.

Nursing Diagnosis

In formulating the nursing diagnosis, ritualistic behavior related to anxiety and unacceptable feelings about self, the nurse will note that defining characteristics for both anxiety and ritualistic behavior are present. The client who manifests anxiety and who engages in handwashing rituals when confronted by unacceptable feelings about self exemplifies this nursing diagnosis. In this example, the nursing diagnosis might be ritualistic behavior (handwashing) related to anxiety arising from conflictual and unacceptable feelings about self.

Client Goals and Nursing Interventions

Because of the anxiety that accompanies ritualistic behavior, the nurse may find that the first priority in working with the client is to assist the client to reduce the anxiety level. Goals and interventions appropriate for dealing with anxiety are addressed, including the administration of medications when appropriate. While assisting the client to deal with anxiety, the nurse will also help the client become more comfortable talking about ritualistic behavior. Many clients, recognizing the irrationality of the rituals, are embarrassed and attempt to maintain secrecy.[5] The client must be allowed to perform the ritual in the most discreet manner possible. Preventing performance of ritualistic behaviors or drawing attention to them will increase the client's level of anxiety and increase the need to perform the rituals. Health-care workers, family members, or significant others may need assistance in dealing with their responses to the client's ritualistic behaviors. As the client's anxiety level decreases, the nurse can encourage exploration of rituals as a way to handle anxiety and assist the client to identify factors that seem to increase or decrease the ritualistic behaviors. The client can be encouraged to say what is meant directly and opportunities can be provided for expression of feelings. As the client is able to increase the range of behaviors, anxiety is diminished, and the expanded activities serve as a new focus of attention away from the rituals. Health-care workers need to be consistent when working with clients with ritualistic behaviors.

Several behavioral techniques have been found to be helpful to clients in managing undesired repetitive thoughts or behaviors. In *thought-stopping*, the client allows the unwanted thought then commands the self to "stop." Relaxation is practiced concurrently with the "stop" command and the process is repeated until the undesired thought is stopped. A variation of this process is *thought-switching* which involves changing to an acceptable thought after stopping the obsessive thought. *Flooding* may be helpful for clients whose rituals are triggered by particular situations. In flooding, the client is repeatedly exposed to the precipitating factor in combination with a relaxation technique until the client no longer responds to the situation with anxiety and subsequent ritualistic behavior.

If ritualistic behaviors are causing physical problems for the client, the nurse will need to plan appropriate interventions to promote the physical well-being of the individual. For example, the nurse can provide a mild, lotion-added soap for the person who is carrying out compulsive handwashing and also provide medicated cream to promote healing and prevent infection.

The nurse can assist the client in making a schedule of daily activities. Included in the schedule is time for the client to complete rituals in a private, non–attention-gaining manner. The nurse needs to support the client goal of developing and testing new activities. Rewards for such positive behaviors should be offered the client. These clients usually have not learned to enjoy relaxation and pleasurable activities; therefore, the nurse needs to not only encourage these activities, but also educate clients about their importance in a healthful life-style. As the client expands positive activities, it is hoped that ways of dealing with anxiety will also be practiced and the need for rituals will decrease. These clients do not typically follow an even course of progress; they may regress when trying new behavioral patterns. Nurse and client must not become discouraged. The nurse must reassess and keep offering encouragement to the client to keep trying. It is not usually realistic to think that the client will be able to be free of ritualistic behaviors. The goals are to help the client learn to deal with anxiety; to diminish the rituals, or to find ways to engage in them with the least disruption to daily functioning; and engage in activities of daily living, social and family interactions, and job situations to the maximum degree possible for this client.

Health education is important so that the client is equipped to implement more healthful patterns of living. The client may select from a variety of methods of dealing with anxiety, including relaxation exercises, physical activities, music for relaxation, and identification of a person for talking with about concerns. Social activities, interests, and hobbies need to be scheduled on a regular basis. These activities should be simple and low-demand so that the client is not overwhelmed by them. Normal activities are planned, with time for rituals, as necessary. Persons with ritualistic behaviors tend to be intelligent and to need structure; therefore, practice in using problem-solving techniques may be helpful and acceptable to them.

Antianxiety medications, especially benzodiazepines, may be prescribed to reduce anxiety in clients with obsessive thoughts or ritualistic behaviors. Their use is appropriate during acute periods; however, other anxiety management techniques are preferable when possible. Antidepressant medications may be prescribed for depressed clients with obsessive-compulsive behaviors.

Evaluation

Outcome criteria that measure whether or not client goals were achieved set the evaluation process in motion. Criteria for client goals bearing on ritualistic behavior include the reduction or elimination of anxiety. Additional outcome criteria include whether or not the client is able to recognize and discuss ritualistic behaviors and identify factors that precipitate these behaviors. Because clients may not be able to eliminate ritualistic behaviors altogether, outcome criteria focus on achieving management that will minimize the client's focus on rituals and allow a focus on other activities. Data that indicate whether or not the client is using health-promoting strategies and is coping with the consequences of ritualistic behavior will be collected to measure outcomes in these areas (Chart 2).

CASE STUDY

Betty, a 41-year-old, married woman is a homemaker, wife, and mother. During the interview with the nurse, she states that she has become obsessed with performing cleaning rituals. These include repetitive handwashing, dishwashing, cleaning her house and, recently, going to church on Saturday to clean the pew that she and her husband will occupy on Sunday. She reports feeling very tense and wanting to stop the excessive cleaning, but being unable to do so. Her husband, Tony, insisted that his wife see their family doctor

Chart 2
Ritualistic Behavior: Summary of the Nursing Process[4]

NURSING INTERVENTIONS	OUTCOME CRITERIA
CLIENT GOAL: EXPERIENCE A REDUCED LEVEL OF ANXIETY	
Assess level of anxiety: mild, moderate, severe, panic Talk with and reassure client in a calm, supportive, nondemanding manner Communicate in short, concise sentences Provide a quiet, nonstimulating, and safe milieu Consult with physician concerning pharmacologic therapy if indicated	Experiences reduced or minimal defining characteristics of anxiety
CLIENT GOAL: DISCUSS RITUALISTIC BEHAVIORS AND CONTRIBUTING FACTORS	
Encourage client to discuss repetitive thoughts or acts Provide information about the role of rituals in everyday life Assist client to identify anxiety-provoking situations and responses to them Observe for negative responses to client by staff and initiate positive interventions	Recognizes ritualistic behaviors Identifies contributing factors
CLIENT GOAL: ENGAGE IN STRATEGIES FOR MANAGEMENT OF RITUALISTIC BEHAVIOR	
Allow client to perform ritual in most discreet manner possible Do not remark in a negative way about rituals or interfere with them	Performs rituals in a manner that minimizes them and allows for other positive behaviors
CLIENT GOAL: EXPRESS FEELINGS DIRECTLY	
Provide opportunities for direct expression of feelings Plan a daily schedule with client Encourage maximum input from client Encourage selection of activities, hobbies, and leisure time in gradual increments Discuss the role of leisure in a healthy life-style Positively reinforce healthy behaviors Be consistent and prompt in all interactions with client	Discusses feelings and expresses them directly Engages in normal activities and allows time for rituals as necessary
CLIENT GOAL: PRACTICE WAYS OF DEALING WITH ANXIETY AND ITS CONSEQUENCES	
Teach client thought-stopping and thought-switching techniques and practice these with client when appropriate situations occur or through role-playing Discuss responses to ritualistic behavior by others and how client handles those responses Focus on behaviors that decrease need for rituals and allow for greater participation in positive life-style Minimize focus on rituals Encourage the client to utilize mild or moderate anxiety for growth Teach progressive muscular relaxation Practice assertive communication skills Encourage client to talk over concerns with staff, family member, or friend Assist client to use music for relaxation Encourage client to choose a physical activity and participate in it: sports, walking, jogging, biking, swimming	Selects and uses health-promoting strategies

when she began going to church to clean their pew. He reports that he and Betty were spending more time together since their two children had left home for college, and conflicts between himself and his wife had increased. Her family physician diagnosed Betty's difficulty as obsessive-compulsive disorder, and referred her to a psychiatric nurse therapist in the local community mental health clinic.

Betty described herself to the psychiatric nurse therapist as always being a neat person who kept herself and her home in a very orderly manner, but this was not a problem until recently. She is not sure why she cannot stop cleaning now but states that she needs help to handle this problem. Betty describes feeling tired frequently and attributes this to the continuous cleaning and to ongoing arguments with

her husband. She usually retires around 10:30 P.M., but may not fall asleep until midnight. She awakens between 5 and 6 A.M. She states that the pressures of her rituals make it difficult for her to relax. She has difficulty concentrating and is distracted by pressures to clean constantly. Now she feels that her life is out of control and that other people view her behavior as very odd. The nurse identified ritualistic behavior related to overwhelming anxiety and relationship problems with husband as a priority nursing diagnosis for this client. To engage in strategies to manage ritualistic behavior and to experience a reduced level of anxiety were two goals that the psychiatric nurse therapist mutually determined with Betty. Betty was encouraged to express her feelings. A number of strategies were discussed with Betty

Research Highlights

The following are some of the nursing research problems related to ritualistic behavior that merit further study:

1. Determine the usefulness of the term ritualistic behavior as a nursing diagnosis
2. Arrive at a consensus nursing definition of ritualistic behavior
3. Conduct validation studies of the proposed defining characteristics of ritualistic behavior
4. Conduct validation studies of the proposed related factors of ritualistic behaviors
5. Conduct descriptive studies of nursing process with ritualistic clients, with a focus on interventions and outcomes to build a body of nursing knowledge about this process

to reduce her anxiety. Although Betty continued to engage in some of her cleaning rituals, the pressure to clean lessened as her anxiety level decreased, as she engaged in progressive muscle relaxation sessions, began to take her favorite dog for walks, began to identify anxiety-provoking situations, and gain insight about the reasons for her anxiety. Betty and her husband were then also referred to couples therapy.

SUMMARY

Ritualistic behavior is defined as an act, sequence of actions, thought, or sequence of thoughts repeatedly performed in an attempt to manage anxiety. Psychoanalytic theorists relate ritualistic behaviors to regression to, or fixation at, the second stage of psychosexual development for relief of anxiety. Learning theorists view ritualistic behaviors as learned responses that are repeated because of reinforcement of the response. The ritualistic behavior provides only temporary relief of anxiety. The most pervasive etiologic factor in the generation of ritualistic behavior is anxiety. Defining characteristics of ritualistic behaviors include repetitive acts or thoughts that are perceived as uncontrollable, interference of rituals with normal functioning, manifestations of anxiety, inflexibility, and constriction of emotional responsivity.

Client goals include reduction of anxiety, recognition

of ritualistic behaviors and contributing factors, implementation of strategies for the management of ritualistic behavior, direct expression of feelings, and the utilization of health-promoting strategies. The client must be allowed to perform rituals in the most discreet manner possible. Interference with rituals will increase anxiety and ritualistic behaviors. Simple, low-demand social activities and hobbies are important so that the client learns to pursue pleasurable acts and to enjoy them. Clients may not be able to eliminate ritualistic behavior, but progress consists of managing it so that the client is able to participate in normal activities and to enjoy some leisure in daily living.

References

1. Corsini R. Current psychotherapies, 3rd ed. Itaska, IL: Peacock Publishing; 1984.
2. Erikson E. Childhood and society, 2nd ed. New York: WW Norton & Co; 1963.
3. Freud S. A general introduction to psychoanalysis. Garden City, NY. Garden City Publishing; 1943.
4. McFarland G, Wasli E. Nursing diagnoses and process in psychiatric mental health nursing. Philadelphia: JB Lippincott; 1986.
5. Rapoport JL. The boy who couldn't stop washing: the experience and treatment of obsessive-compulsive disorder. New York: EP Dutton; 1989.
6. Sullivan HS. The interpersonal theory of psychiatry. New York: Norton; 1953.

SELF-CARE DEFICIT

Donna Poole

DEFINITION AND DESCRIPTION

Self-care deficit is the inability of an individual to complete activities of daily living without some assistance or without complete care. It is a state in which the individual experiences an impaired ability to perform or complete bathing or hygiene activities for the self; to perform or complete dressing and grooming activities for the self; to perform or complete feeding activities for the self; or to perform or complete toileting activities for the self. If assessment data suggest that the client performs all but one of the self-care activities, then a subcategory is used, e.g., self-care deficit (dressing and grooming) related to depression. If the client is unable to perform in all categories without some form of assistance, then the more comprehensive diagnosis would be appropriate (e.g., self-care deficit related to loss of memory). The North American Nursing Diagnosis Association (NANDA) suggests a code for functional level classification[8] (Table 13-15).

THEORY AND RESEARCH

Cultural values and beliefs have a great impact on how self-care deficits are perceived by the individual who experiences the deficit, as well as by family members and caregivers. Values and beliefs also have a significant influence on health-related behaviors, or the lack thereof.[5] In American society, there is a high value placed on independence and the ability to care for oneself. When caring for individuals with chronic illnesses, assisting the person to participate is as important for the nurse as assuring adherence to a regimen of exercise, diet, or medication. Needless to say, creating unnecessary dependence of clients upon the caregiver is paternal and coercive, and does not reflect a caring approach to client management.[7]

A major concern when caring for a psychiatric population is identifying those clients who are physically able to care for themselves but because of psychiatric disturbances do not do so. This is a particularly acute problem with clients who cannot communicate in a clear way. Examples are a severely paranoid client who will only eat white foods, such as mashed potatoes and marshmallows, because they are the only "pure" foods, or an emaciated anorexic client who will only eat a lettuce leaf because she is "fat." The person's ability to care for self is an aspect of autonomy, and interventions to provide care may be seen as interfering with this autonomy. However, what happens when the principle of autonomy comes into conflict with the principle of beneficence? When conceptualizing the self-care problems of this severely ill population, the body of literature related to the care and feeding of severely demented clients may help to put the conflict into perspective. If a client is psychotic or irrational, the ability to make autonomous decisions accordingly decreases. When possible, decisions made by caregivers on behalf of the client, should reflect the wishes of the client during well times.[1] Making the decision to step in and care for a client against his protest is rarely easy for the nurse and requires careful deliberation. The nurse must continually assess the client's judgment and ability to make decisions for himself or herself. It is often helpful to develop objective procedures for allowing the right to refuse treatment; however, procedures must deal humanely and sensitively with the clinical realities of individual cases.[5]

RELATED FACTORS

Self-care deficit may occur in a variety of physiologic and psychological disturbances. Psychiatric disturbances most frequently associated with self-care deficit are mood disorders, schizophrenia, organic mental disorders, and other psychotic disorders. However, self-care deficit can be associated with any psychiatric disorder.

Mood disorders may involve a depressive or a manic episode. Depressed clients tend to think and move slowly. They often forget, or do not seem to have the energy, to attend to activities of daily living (ADL). It is very common for depressed clients to experience a loss of appetite, which interferes with self-feeding. Manic clients are often much too agitated or otherwise involved in activity to take time out to attend to their ADLs or to eat. On the other hand, some depressed and manic clients will eat excessively.

Clients with schizophrenia experience delusions, hallucinations, or other disturbances in the form of thought. These experiences are distracting and frequently frightening for the client. People with psychotic symptoms often appear to be so absorbed in these internal processes that attention to self-care appears to have a low priority.

Clients with organic mental disorders often have all types of self-care deficits. In addition to difficulties

Table 13-15
Types of Self-Care Deficits, Definitions, and Examples

TYPE	DEFINITION	EXAMPLES
Feeding	The inability to bring food from a receptacle to the mouth.	Person hears voices telling her the food is poison.
Bathing/hygiene	Inability to wash body or body parts; inability to obtain or get to water source; inability to regulate water temperature or flow.	Person is profoundly depressed, he lies on the couch all day without bathing. When asked, he reports he has no energy and bathing seems like an overwhelming task.
Dressing/grooming	Impaired ability to put on or take off necessary items of clothing; impaired ability to obtain or replace articles of clothing; impaired ability to fasten clothing; inability to maintain appearance at a satisfactory level.	Person is experiencing manic episode of a bipolar illness. His behavior is grandiose and inappropriate. He frequently stands nude in the doorway of his hospital room or lies nude on his bed with the door open.
Toileting	A state in which the individual experiences an impaired ability to perform or complete toileting activities for him/herself.	Person is severely psychotic. She often is so absorbed with her hallucinations that she does not notice the urge to void and becomes incontinent.

SUGGESTED CODE FOR FUNCTIONAL LEVEL CLASSIFICATION
0 = Completely independent
1 = Requires use of equipment or device
2 = Requires help from another person for assistance, supervision, or teaching
3 = Requires help from another person and equipment device
4 = Dependent, does not participate in activity

(From McLane A, ed. Classification of nursing diagnoses. Proceedings of the seventh conference. St Louis: CV Mosby, 1987:497, 499–500.)

with ADLs, it is very common to have toileting deficits. In the later stages of degenerative dementia, feeding problems are very common and present a challenge for nursing.[1,2]

Other factors not associated specifically with psychiatric disorders may result in a self-care deficit. These factors may be physical, such as neuromuscular or musculoskeletal impairments, and any condition that produces an intolerance to activity, or decreases strength and endurance. Emotional and psychological factors—for example, depression, anxiety, and perceptual or cognitive impairments—may also result in self-care deficits. Pain and discomfort have physiologic and psychological components and may also contribute to self-care deficits.

DEFINING CHARACTERISTICS

With many nursing diagnoses the nurse is dependent upon the client's subjective data to formulate a nursing diagnosis. This is less true when observing for the diagnosis of self-care deficit.

With the diagnosis, self-feeding deficit, the client presents certain clear objective data. For example: Has the client lost weight? Does the client have a change in postural blood pressures and pulses, and does the client have an elevated temperature (all signs of dehydration)? Does the client have a fluid and electrolyte imbalance? If the client is hospitalized or visited in the home, the nurse has the opportunity to observe eating behaviors: Is the client able to handle the physical mechanics of feeding himself or herself? Does the client

forget to eat or have a loss of appetite? Does the client have thoughts or behaviors that interfere with eating? Clients with bathing or hygiene deficits or dressing or grooming deficits, are readily identifiable through simple observation. However, the observation should be of a *pattern* and not an isolated incident. The client with a toileting deficit may also be readily identifiable, particularly if he or she has been incontinent. Some severely debilitated psychiatric clients will walk around seemingly oblivious to their urine or stool incontinence (Chart 1).

NURSING PROCESS AND RATIONALE
Assessment

Although there are many areas of overlap in the scope of practice of health-care professionals, the area of practice dealing with self-care deficits is almost exclusively within the realm of nursing.[11] The primary skill required for the assessment of self-care deficits is observation. A single defining characteristic alone is not sufficient to make this diagnosis; rather, a pattern of behaviors should be observed.

Nursing Diagnosis

It is important for the clinician to be as specific as possible when diagnosing self-care deficit. Clients with severe impairments may have generalized deficits that include all types of self-care problems. For example,

CHART 1
Self-Care Deficit: Definition, Related Factors, and Defining Characteristics

DEFINITION

A state in which the individual experiences an impaired ability to perform or complete feeding activities for self; to perform or complete bathing and hygiene activities for self; to perform or complete dressing and grooming activities for self; or an impaired ability to perform or complete toileting activities for self.

RELATED FACTORS

Intolerance to activity, decreased strength and endurance
Pain or discomfort
Perceptual or cognitive impairment
Neuromuscular impairment
Musculoskeletal impairment
Depression
Anxiety
Psychiatric disorders

TYPE	DEFINING CHARACTERISTICS

Feeding	Unable or unwilling to:
	  Cut food
	  Bring food to mouth
	  Swallow

Bathing/
  hygiene
	Unable or unwilling to:
	  Wash body or body parts
	  Obtain a water source
	  Regulate temperature or water
	    flow
	  Use soap
	  Use deodorant

Dressing/
  grooming
	Unable or unwilling to:
	  Put on or take off necessary items
	    of clothing
	  Obtain or replace articles of
	    clothing
	  Fasten clothing
	  Maintain appearance at a
	    satisfactory level

Toileting	Unable or unwilling to:
	  Get to toilet or commode
	  Sit on or rise from toilet or
	    commode
	  Manipulate clothing for toileting
	  Carry out proper toilet hygiene
	  Flush toilet or empty commode

severely demented clients may require assistance or complete care in feeding, bathing and hygiene, dressing and grooming, and toileting. A sample diagnostic statement may be self-care deficit (functional level 2) related to progressive dementia (Table 13-15).

Other clients require nursing assistance with only one type of self-care deficit. For example, a paranoid client who has no difficulty eating or toileting, and who is always neatly dressed and groomed may refuse to bathe because of his delusional belief that the shower is actually a gas chamber. A possible diagnosis would be self-care deficit (bathing/hygiene) related to delusional beliefs about shower.

On occasion the clinician must distinguish between two similar, possibly related, nursing diagnoses. For example, how does one determine whether or not to make a diagnosis of self-care deficit, feeding or alteration in nutrition, less than body requirements? The distinction is most often made at the level of treatment or that at which the greatest emphasis is being placed with interventions. For example, if the client is dangerously emaciated from anorexia, the emphasis must be on nutrition. However, later on in treatment, once the danger has passed, the emphasis may be on the client's ability to care for self.

Client Goals and Nursing Interventions

The main goals for a client with self-care deficit include the following:[4,12]

- Perform self-care activities to extent possible
- Overcome barriers to effective self-care
- Have increased sense of responsibility for self-care.

PERFORM SELF-CARE ACTIVITIES TO EXTENT POSSIBLE

The client is often physically able to engage in effective self-care, but requires motivation or encouragement to do so. Clients with self-care deficits often lack the self-esteem to take pride in self-care activities. Encouragement may be all that is needed to stimulate and enhance self-care behaviors in many psychiatric clients. Clients can be helped to improve self-esteem by assisting them to set small, measurable, attainable goals that lead to a sense of accomplishment. Clients may need direct help, supervision, or instruction to reduce frustration and avoid discouragement. It may also be necessary for the nurse to act as a client advocate to increase sensitivity of others to the effects of their actions on the client.

OVERCOME BARRIERS TO SELF-CARE

Difficulty with communication is a frequent barrier to self-care. Clients unable to care for themselves, and unable to communicate their needs and desires about self-care activities, are dependent upon the nurse for creativity and sensitivity. Clients may give out subtle cues that at first seem meaningless or merely reactive. For example, psychotic clients may speak in symbolic ways that have meaning to themselves alone. When nurses have repeated interactions with clients, sensitive nurses may perceive cues, interpret the cues, and respond to the client in a manner that the client is able to understand.[2] Nurses can also use touch as a means of communication with clients, whether the clients have communication problems or not. For example, the nurse can use a firm, yet gentle touch when taking a blood pressure to communicate a strong positive feeling about the client and to establish a sense of caring and concern.[7]

Lack of knowledge can also be a barrier to self-care. Many times clients have the skills to take care of themselves, but they lack the knowledge to know how to be self-care-taking. One of the most important roles of the nurse is in health-care teaching. Research has demonstrated the value of health-care education with clients. In one such study of psychiatric clients with affective disorders, client education resulted in a statistically significant difference in medication compliance and, subsequently, fewer inpatient stays.[13]

In discussing barriers to self-care, the nurse must also consider the environment. Many times the most important thing a nurse can do is to establish an environment that is conducive to change and growth. Helpless, dependent, apathetic, or angry people have demonstrated the ability to grow, to mature, and to become self-sufficient in an environment that promotes health-seeking behavior, that promotes action toward positive goals, and that provides reinforcement for these behaviors.[3] Nurses must also maintain an awareness that the rational agreements or contracts of the psychiatric client may reflect only part of his or her total motivation. To help clients become self-care agents, psychiatric nurses must work toward enabling clients to confront their own opposition to treatment.[10]

HAVE INCREASED SENSE OF RESPONSIBILITY FOR SELF-CARE

As with all nursing interventions, whenever possible, clients should be included in health-care planning. Particularly when dealing with a self-care deficit, with the ultimate goal of independence, it is often useful to validate the nursing diagosis with the client. Plan the care with him or her and validate conclusions. Discuss daily routines with the client; allow him or her a voice in scheduling activities. Consult with the client in making choices about his or her treatment; do not plan activities without his or her knowledge. Evaluate outcomes of care with the client.

Psychiatric clients, as well as most people, are more likely to engage in appropriate self-care activities if they are involved in creating and deciding the course of action around their care plan.

Evaluation

With the diagnosis, self-care deficit, evaluation is most often accomplished by observation. In addition to observation, a client report is a useful adjunct to the evaluation process. Evaluation must be individualized, as various clients have vastly different abilities and rehabilitation potentials. Outcome criteria include the client's ability to identify factors that limit self-care activities. If the client is unable to perform self-care activities without assistance, can areas for which assis-

CHART 2
Self-Care Deficit: Summary of the Nursing Process

NURSING INTERVENTIONS	OUTCOME CRITERIA
CLIENT GOAL: PERFORM SELF-CARE ACTIVITIES TO THE EXTENT POSSIBLE	
Encourage or allow the client to do as much as possible for self	Performs self-care activities without assistance when physically able to do so
Provide specific, appropriate praise and encouragement	Identifies where assistance is needed
Observe for evidence of readiness to increase amount of self-care	Identifies factors limiting self-care abilities
Assist client to set measurable, attainable goals	Sets measurable, attainable goals for improving self-care
Provide help, supervision, and teaching as necessary	
CLIENT GOAL: OVERCOME BARRIERS TO EFFECTIVE SELF-CARE	
Assess for communication barriers to self-care	Communicates needs and desires about self-care activities
Use nonverbal communication as well as verbal communication when appropriate	Learns new concepts, skills, or behaviors necessary to develop or improve self-care activities
Assess for lack of knowledge about self-care	
When the client has physical limitations, explore the use of assistive devices	
Establish an environment that is conducive to change and growth	
CLIENT GOAL: HAVE INCREASED SENSE OF RESPONSIBILITY FOR SELF-CARE	
Validate self-care deficit with the client	Acknowledges the existence of self-care deficit
Assess strengths and challenges with the client	Identifies own strengths and challenges
Plan care with the client	Participates in all aspects of own care when able
Discuss daily routines, encouraging client to participate in scheduling activities	
Evaluate outcomes of care with client	

tance is needed be identified? Is the client interested in own care? Does the client ask questions, share own values, and help to prioritize care? Does the client set reasonable goals for self with reasonable time for completion? (Chart 2).

CASE STUDY

A 27-year-old man was hospitalized with chronic schizophrenia, acute exacerbation, and a secondary medical diagnosis of alcohol abuse. He reported a psychiatric history dating back six years to when he took "too much angel dust." He acknowledged hearing disturbing voices, but reported he had stopped taking his neuroleptic medication because it was causing "red spots inside of me." He had been trying to control his psychotic symptoms before admission through alcohol use.

On the unit the client often refused to get out of bed in the morning in time to attend community meeting. He usually wore a pair of jeans with holes in them, a flannel shirt without buttons, and a dirty undershirt. His jeans hung low on his hips, and his shirt did not reach the top of his pants, exposing part of his lower abdomen and the top of his pubic hair. He was most often barefoot. His mother had brought him other clothes that he refused to wear. In the evening, he would walk about the ward in hospital pajamas, loosely tied, without a bathrobe. He wore a beard and long hair, which was usually uncombed. He did shower daily without direction from others, but would only wash and wear clean clothes when asked to do so. When asked by nursing staff to pull up his pants or put on a robe, he usually complied but in a complaining manner. Items of clothing that he was not currently wearing were usually thrown around his room on the floor or under the bed.

A major nursing diagnosis was self-care deficit (dressing/grooming) related to lack of desire–motivation. Another nursing diagnosis was alteration in thought processes related to psychotic illness. As the client was treated with neuroleptic medication, the alteration in thought processes began to resolve, but there was no change in the self-care deficit (dressing/grooming).

The client's primary nurse made an appointment with the client and they sat down to discuss resolving this problem. The client reported that he did not care how he looked and, furthermore, he did not like the frequent reminders about his appearance from nursing staff. The primary nurse reported that she did not like her role in having to constantly remind him either. The client was able to agree that his appearance was sometimes a problem for him in being accepted by other people. After much discussion, it was agreed that the nurse would not offer reminders about his appearance, but that the client could not use his off-unit privileges unless he was neatly dressed and groomed and his living area was picked up. Following this, there were several days in which the client chose to stay in bed rather than dress appropriately and clean up his living area. However, as his discharge date drew nearer he was more often able to use his off-ward privileges, which he enjoyed.

Discharge-planning involved referral to a dual diagnosis program (psychiatry and substance abuse) and placement on a long-acting intramuscular neuroleptic that needed to be administered only once every two weeks. Dressing and grooming was somewhat improved, but remained an occasional problem.

SUMMARY

Self-care deficit can be diagnosed alone when the client has a generalized inability to care for himself or herself, or the diagnosis can specify deficits in feeding, bathing and hygiene, dressing and grooming, or toileting. Further specification of the diagnosis, self-care deficit, can be obtained by using the suggested code for functional level classification. Self-care deficit can be found in any psychiatric disorder, but it is most common in mood disorders, schizophrenia, and organic mental disorders. After assessment, nursing interventions are

Research Highlights

Research into nursing diagnosis reveals that self-care deficit tends to be among the ten most frequently reported nursing diagnoses. Metzger and Hiltman conducted a study to obtain validity estimates on selected nursing diagnoses.[9] They looked at the ten NANDA diagnoses most frequently reported in literature reviews from 1980 to 1984. There were only three nursing diagnoses with diagnostic content validity (DCV) scores higher than self-care deficit. For self-care deficit (bathing/hygiene) the critical cue "inability to wash body or body parts" had the highest DCV score for any critical cue studied.

Harris and others studied the nursing diagnoses in a visiting nurse population of 541 clients.[6] The focus of their study was to determine the cost of treating various nursing diagnoses. Self-care deficit was the second most frequently reported nursing diagnosis in this study. Although self-care deficit was fourth among the five nursing diagnoses requiring the most visits, it was also tenth in the ten least expensive nursing diagnoses. Whereas the average number of visits required for self-care deficit was 11 (highest being 17), the average cost per visit (112 dollars) for self-care deficit was about one-quarter the highest cost per visit (451 dollars). Total nursing costs were calculated by dividing the agency rate of 45 dollars per visit by the time spent on each diagnosis.

Self-care deficit is clearly one of the most frequently reported nursing diagnoses. This is probably related to the fact that this diagnosis is almost entirely within the scope of nursing practice and has very little overlap with the scope of practice in other health-care professions. For example, within the case study cited, the only reference made by the physician to this problem was to note in the admission and discharge summaries that the client was "disheveled." Other probable reasons for the frequency of formulating this diagnosis in client care is the relative ease in collecting data to support the diagnosis, the fact that the diagnosis can usually be made by observation, and the multiple causative factors.

directed toward assisting the client to meet personal goals for independence and in assisting the client to overcome opposition to treatment.

References

1. Akerlund BM, Norberg A. An ethical analysis of double bind conflicts as experienced by care workers feeding severely demented patients. Int J Nurs Stud. 1985;22(3):207–16.

2. Athlin E, Norberg A. Caregivers' attitudes to and interpretations of the behaviour of severely demented patients during feeding in a patient assignment care system. Int J Nurs Stud. 1987;24(2):145–153.

3. Bevvino CA, Burns B, Lewis MH, Allen JK. Planned change: an innovative nursing rehabilitation model. Perspect Psychiatr Care. 1984;22(4):149–158.

4. Connelly CE. Self-care and the chronically ill patient. Nurs Clin North Am. 1987;22(3):621–629.

5. Davidhizar R. Beliefs and values of the client with chronic mental illness regarding treatment. Issues Ment Health Nurs. 1984;6(3–4):261–273.

6. Harris MD, Peters DA, Smith JA, Yuan J. Tracking the cost of home care. AJN. 1987;87(11):1500–1502.

7. Larkin J. Factor's influencing one's ability to adapt to chronic illness. Nurs Clin North Am. 1987;22(3):535–542.

8. McLane A, ed. Classification of nursing diagnoses. Proceedings of the seventh conference. St Louis: CV Mosby; 1987:497, 499–500.

9. Metzger KL, Hiltunen EF. Diagnostic content validation of frequently reported nursing diagnoses. In: McLane A, ed. Classification of nursing diagnoses. Proceedings of the seventh conference. St Louis: CV Mosby; 1987.

10. Moscovitz AO. Orem's theory as applied to psychiatric nursing. Perspect Psychiatr Care. 1984;22(1):36–38.

11. Stokes G, Keen I. Developing self-care skills and reducing institutionalized behaviour in a long-stay psychiatric population: the role of the nurse in behaviour modification. J Adv Nurs. 1987;12(1):35–48.

12. Tilden VP, Weinert C. Social support and the chronically ill individual. Nurs Clin North Am. 1987;22(3):613–620.

13. Youssef FA. Compliance with therapeutic regimens: a follow-up study for patients with affective disorders. J Adv Nurs. 1983;8(6):513–517.

SELF-CONCEPT DISTURBANCE

(PERSONAL IDENTITY DISTURBANCE, SELF-ESTEEM DISTURBANCE, BODY IMAGE DISTURBANCE, ROLE PERFORMANCE DISTURBANCE)

Susan M. Robertson

Self-concept is the view of self, which changes dynamically throughout life. It is the foundation of personality and a filter through which perceptions are admitted into awareness. It is heavily influenced by life experiences, both expected life-stage developmental tasks and the unique stressors and trauma individual to each person's life.

Self-concept disturbance occurs when a former level of self-concept integration is challenged by life events and coping resources are inadequate to the task of reintegration. Disturbance can also result when developmental tasks are not completed or are completed with inadequate result. Self-concept disturbance will be discussed in terms of four distinct subdiagnoses: personal identity disturbance, self-esteem disturbance (both situational and chronic), body image disturbance, and role performance disturbance. These self-concept disturbances can occur simultaneously and may overlap.

PERSONAL IDENTITY DISTURBANCE

DEFINITION AND DESCRIPTION

Personal identity disturbance manifests itself in a variety of ways, all indicating confusion or inconsistency in the core self-view. Confusion may occur in identification of values, goals, beliefs, or sexual orientation. The diagnosis is applicable along a range of severity, including paranoia, grandiosity, and severe psychosis. Other individuals are less impaired but show difficulty in goal setting and mastery of developmentally appropriate tasks.

THEORY AND RESEARCH

Central to the formation of personal identity is movement from knowledge of self as doer ("I do") to self as owner of intrinsic qualities ("I do well, I am, I experience"). Thus, the self becomes differentiated from others, objects in the environment, and task mastery.[4] Early tasks in the sequence of self-concept formation are: (1) individuation, the development of a sense of self apart from others, and (2) internalization, the development of "consistent yet dynamic sets of guidelines and rules" for the self (reference 4, p 748). When these basic tasks have not been satisfactorily completed, stable personal identity is not likely to develop.

Psychodynamic theorists refer to the complete dependency of the vulnerable human infant on the parental caretaker as "symbiosis."[8] Only gradually does the infant "come to recognize an external reality—a 'not I'—that extends beyond his self-boundaries and that is first represented by the mother" (reference 1, p 29). Difficulties arise when the infant experiences loss of the mother, neglect, or inconsistent mothering during the symbiotic stage, because lack of the mother is experienced as an actual loss of self by the infant. Adult relationships of the person who has experienced deficits in nurturance during early life are fraught with difficulties.[1,6] There is a longing for, yet fear of, true intimacy with others. Depending on the extent of the damage experienced during the separation–individuation phase of early life, the individual may seek to form very intense relationships in which efforts are made to reexperience fusion. At the same time that it is pursued, this search for fusion can be frightening, as it implies a loss of self through absorption into another. The latter may be perceived as terrifying destruction of the self.[1] Fear of abandonment can be stimulated when, inevitably, the other person is unable to satisfy the escalating needs for closeness expressed by the client with personality disorder. Thus, this client repeatedly attempts to locate a person who will be able to meet his or her intense needs, only to be disappointed yet again when the other person fails to respond as desired.

Cognitive theorists view the self as a composite of

self-schemata. Self-schemata are "cognitive generalizations about the self, derived from past experience, that organize and guide the processing of self-related information contained in the individual's social experience" (reference 9, p 1495). Personal identity consists in part of social roles but also of "clusters of characteristics and enactments not associated with any particular social position or relationship" (reference 5, p 268). These clusters then form identities, which serve as blueprints for behavior in a particular situation.[5] If these identities are limited in range or poorly organized, the individual is at risk for schizophrenia. Onset and relapse of schizophrenic illness appears to occur when "all of the prominent identities are so profoundly challenged in [the individual's] living circumstances that these identities and their enactments are, for practical purposes, negated" (reference 5, p 270).

RELATED FACTORS

Both psychodynamic and cognitive theorists agree that social relations play an important role in identity formation. Psychodynamic theory suggests that inconsistent caregiving, abuse, or neglect during early life will result in persistent identity disturbance. Cognitive theory postulates that self-schemata change dynamically throughout life and are influenced significantly by interpersonal roles, themselves subject to change and flux.

Other factors that predispose to identity disturbance are chaotic or nonsupportive social environments. These may impair or preclude development of stable, well-articulated self-schemata. Disturbance in personal identity may be related to psychiatric disorders such as borderline personality disorder, identity disorder, schizophrenia, schizophreniform disorder, and mood disorders.[2] For clients with borderline personality disorder, perceived abandonment by others may engender severe anxiety and in some cases transient psychotic episodes, as these clients have not been able to complete the tasks of individuation and internalization. The client with schizophrenia may never have developed adequate identity resources and thus is highly sensitive to episodes of stress and to small environmental changes. Psychosis may result when the client is able to select only from pathological or deficient contacts with which to identify and in addition lacks the ability to create a healthier identity.[6]

DEFINING CHARACTERISTICS

Personal identity disturbance manifests itself along a continuum from mild to severe impairment in social and occupational functioning and in the degree of uncertainty about a variety of issues and choices in life. The individual suffering from this form of self-concept deficit may demonstrate relatively stable dysfunction or may function well except during episodes of stress. Typical manifestations of personal identity disturbance include confusion about values and long-term goals; inability to form stable, long-term relationships; and instability of relationships. The person may also find it difficult to make decisions independently and may be uncertain about any number of important life choices, e.g., ethical values, religious beliefs, career goals, choice of friends, and personal behavior.

In instances of severe psychopathology, dramatic behaviors are often seen when identity structure is threatened. A client with schizophrenia can experience psychotic decompensation in response to very small environmental changes because the identity is diffusely organized and unable to integrate the change. During psychosis, other people and even inanimate objects may be included within the ego boundary; e.g., the individual describes being able to think other people's thoughts.

Persons with personality disorders show other severe behavioral and affective manifestations of personal identity disturbance. For example, they often display dramatic and contradictory shifts of emotions and loyalties. Instability of long-term interpersonal relationships and difficulty setting and following through on long-term goals are also seen. There is "splitting," or the tendency for the client to respond very differently to one person than to another, thus creating conflicting impressions among others.[10] Besides splitting, the client uses other defenses such as projection, in which the client's feelings are attributed to others. Thus, the client who may be irritable about the nurse's request for compliance with hospital rules may state, "you're angry at me" to the nurse when in fact the client is experiencing his or her own anger (Chart 1).

NURSING PROCESS AND RATIONALE
Assessment

The core self-concept is assessed by a clinical interview in which inquiries are directed to the client's current view of self and characteristic interpersonal functioning. The client may be asked to describe personal attributes, both positive and negative. Social functioning is assessed by description of the quality and quantity of the client's available social support, as well as by direct observation of the client's social interactions. The client may be asked about any wished for changes in self or in significant relationships. Discussion of major life issues such as career and friendships can allow assessment of degree of certainty or uncertainty about beliefs and values as well as decision-making skills.

Nursing Diagnosis

The specific nursing diagnosis might be, for example, personal identity disturbance related to borderline per-

---

CHART 1
Personal Identity Disturbance: Definition, Related Factors, and Defining Characteristics

DEFINITION

Personal identity disturbance is an impairment in the ability to maintain a stable self-view and values in the face of environmental stressors. The diagnosis is present along a continuum of impairment and involves emotional distress accompanying uncertainty about life's major choices. All severe stressors, including physical illness, present challenges to core self-concept, which may result in personal identity disturbance.

RELATED FACTORS

Disruption of accustomed employment, housing, or other lifestyle-related activity
Emotional, physical, or sexual abuse
Inconsistent nurturing or neglect in early life
Schizophrenia
Borderline personality disorder
Identity disorder

DEFINING CHARACTERISTICS

Confusion about values, long-term goals
Instability in personal relationships
Prominent use of psychologically less-mature defense mechanisms such as projection
Difficulty making decisions independently
Dramatic affective response to minimal changes when identity structure is threatened
Inclusion of other people or inanimate objects within the ego boundary
Severe emotional distress and uncertainty about major choices in life

---

sonality disorder, personal identity disturbance related to disruption in employment and housing, or personal identity disturbance related to inconsistent nurturing.

Client Goals and Nursing Interventions

Personal identity disturbance may call for swift crisis intervention to protect the client. Psychotic decompensation requires that intensive structure be provided, as the client may be flooded with stimuli, including frightening feelings and thoughts. Anxiolytics and neuroleptic medication can be helpful in reducing intensity and duration of psychotic process. Self-inflicted injury is always a possibility and may be lethal or nonlethal. Clients with borderline personality disorder may self-mutilate in the form of superficial lacerations on the arms or legs when distressed. Clients with identity disorder can experience suicidal ideation when under stress. Nursing care involves inquiries as

to the presence of active suicidal ideation and assessment of the potential risk (i.e., is detailed planning for suicide present, and are the means to commit suicide available?).

For the nonpsychotic client, cognitive therapy can be used to facilitate the tasks of individuation and internalization. Building on the information gathered during the assessment interview, the psychiatric mental health nurse works with the client to strengthen and develop personal definition of the self-concept ("who I am"). The client may be given therapeutic assignments that foster articulation of personal values and self-directed behavior.

The individual with personality disorder presents special challenges because of the severity of the identity disturbance. This client may present requests for care in a highly anxious fashion and may be unable to tolerate delays in meeting these needs. He or she may resent the care given to more severely ill individuals who are receiving a great deal of staff attention. In a similar vein, the client may present with frequent urgent problems, the importance of which is minimized as soon as resolution is achieved. The principal task of the nurse working with this client is to balance empathy and confrontation. It is easy to get into all or nothing positions with these clients: to wish to rescue them when they are needy, to avoid them when they are angry and critical of the caretaker. It is most helpful to be consistently caring, yet clear about the limits on the extent of acting out behavior that can be tolerated within the treatment setting. The successful nurse–client relationship, then, is one in which consistent responses occur and in which the client perceives caring as well as limit setting.

Structural change and adaptational change are opposite treatment models used in the treatment of personality disorders.[7] It is important for treatment staff to use uniformity of treatment models. One model (the adaptational approach) encourages use of adaptational skills and supports the patient's defensive structures rather than exploring transference. The structural approach, by contrast, stresses transference and allows the patient to regress to experience deep-seated emotions. The latter approach is generally best accomplished in a long-term outpatient therapy or hospitalization over several months in a program modeled on the therapeutic community in which regressive behavior can be processed therapeutically.

Evaluation

Individuals with a nursing diagnosis of personal identity disturbance demonstrate improvement by a variety of indicators. For example, there is some resolution of the pronounced confusion about values and goals. The individual displays a more flexible affect and is able to use more mature defense mechanisms such as humor in order to cope. Ability to cope under continued stress also improves (Chart 2).

CHART 2
Personal Identity Disturbance: Summary of the Nursing Process

NURSING INTERVENTIONS	OUTCOME CRITERIA
CLIENT GOAL: DEVELOP RECOGNITION OF SELF VS NONSELF	
Assist client to express and process emotions	Describes attributes of self
Assess current level of self-awareness and style of interpersonal relating	Makes decisions showing increasing reliance on self
Provide low-stimulation environment if client is having difficulty processing stimuli	
Encourage self-acknowledgment of behavioral competencies	
Assist client to develop social and interactional skills	
CLIENT GOAL: TAKE ACTIONS THAT ARE CONSISTENT WITH BELIEFS	
Assist client to clarify personal values	Describes own beliefs and values
Reinforce initiative for goal-setting and purposefully directed behavior	Refers to self as initiator of planning and action
CLIENT GOAL: DEVELOP A CONSISTENT PERSONAL IDENTITY IN WHICH KEY SELF-ATTRIBUTES PERSIST IN THE FACE OF CHANGE	
Help client regroup and redefine competencies and self-worth under conditions of illness or stress	Responds to personal/environmental change without decompensation and loss of identity
Assist client in developing decision-making skills	Describes own identity based on personal meaning, distinct from situational values

CASE STUDY

Janet, a 22-year-old woman, was hospitalized for depression and suicidal and homicidal ideation. Janet was the youngest of three children. Her father was physically abusive and had left the family when Janet was less than a year old. Janet's stepfather used cocaine and was physically abusive to his wife and stepdaughters when using drugs. Janet had been sexually molested when 10 years old by an older brother. Family decision making was chaotic, and chronic anger was a feature of family life. In summary, Janet's early life experience included a number of events that can engender identity disturbance: physical and sexual abuse, paternal substance abuse (which tends to promote inconsistency and instability of family members' roles), and being parented by a mother who was herself physically and emotionally abused and thus unable to provide a consistent and nurturing environment during Janet's childhood.

At age 18, Janet met and became sexually active with a married man who lived with her for several months, but who, even after his divorce, demonstrated limited capacity for emotional closeness. The man terminated the relationship several weeks prior to Janet's hospitalization. On hospital admission, Janet reported a 20-pound weight loss in 2 months, dysphoria, sleep disturbance, suicidal ideation, and homicidal ideation directed toward her ex-boyfriend, whom she thought about obsessively.

Janet used profane language in describing significant males in her life—stepfather and boyfriend. Her affect was very intense and angry, and she frequently used abusive language toward staff. She was impulsive, and her behavior was often contradictory. She described episodes of reckless driving as well as scrupulous daily exercise and consumption of health food. She described casual sexual encounters concomitant with obsessive longing for more emotional closeness with her ex-boyfriend. She vacillated between valuing an anorexic, almost preadolescent, body size and a sexually provocative appearance. She expressed inability to identify any long-term goals except to get "revenge" on her ex-boyfriend for abandoning her. She was also unable to cite any long-term career or life goals.

Research Highlights

An individual's ethnicity can be important in the establishment of personal identity. Constantino, Malgady, and Rogler identified Puerto Rican adolescents as one group at high risk for development of mental disorder because of stressors associated with minority status, bilingualism, and cultural conflicts.[3] They designed an intervention study in which 21 Puerto Rican adolescents, sometimes with their mothers, participated in small groups. Puerto Rican heroes and heroines were presented in a modeling therapy, which was evaluated by summarizing therapists' progress reports and by participants' self-reports. After participation in the small groups, the adolescents demonstrated increased self-disclosure and self-confidence, increased pride in being Puerto Rican, and improved coping methods. In addition, they reported enjoyment in learning about famous Puerto Ricans and about their culture.[3]

The nursing diagnosis formulated was personal identity disturbance related to emotional and physical abuse and borderline personality disorder. One nurse addressed Janet's questions regarding treatment plan and "rules" and also met with her daily for one-to-one work. This personal time was for Janet to utilize in expressing needs and feelings. The nurse assisted in structuring the time by limiting the amount spent complaining about others. Janet was refocused to look at choices and decision-making abilities she herself possessed relative to difficult situations in her life. Values clarification work was done to help Janet articulate needs and how she could realistically expect others to meet these in her life at the present time. Family of origin issues also were explored, with the nurse validating Janet's anger and sense of loss regarding lack of caregiving in her childhood. Grief work about absence of family warmth and nurturance was begun.

SUMMARY

Personal identity disturbance is manifested in a variety of forms, including severe psychopathology and personality disorders. Nursing interventions include provision of environmental structure for the psychotic person and a series of graduated tasks at self-recognition and values clarification for clients who are cognitively intact.

References

1. Alder G. Borderline Psychopathology and its Treatment. New York: Jason Aronson; 1985.
2. American Psychiatric Association. Diagnostic and Statistical Manual of Mental Disorders. 3rd ed, rev. Washington, DC: American Psychiatric Association; 1987.
3. Constantino G, Malgady, RG, Rogler LH. Folk hero modeling therapy for Puerto Rican adolescents. J Adolesc. 1988; 11:155–165.
4. Dunn R. Issues of self-concept deficit in psychotherapy. Psychotherapy. 1985;22(4):747–751.
5. Gara M, Rosenburg B, Cohen B. Personal identity and the schizophrenic process: an integration. Psychiatry. 1987; 50:267–279.
6. Garcia Badaracco J. Identification and its vicissitudes in the psychoses: The importance of the concept of the 'maddening object.' Int J Psychoanal. 1986;67:136–145.
7. Gordon C, Beresin E. Conflicting treatment models for the inpatient management of borderline patients. Ann J Psychiatry. 1983;140(8):979–983.
8. Mahler M. On Human Symbiosis and the Vicissitudes of Individuation. New York: Institutional Universities Press; 1968.
9. Markus H, Moreland R, Smith J. Role of the self-concept in the perception of others. J Pers Soc Psychol. 1985;49(6): 1494–1512.
10. Masterson J. Psychotherapy of the Borderline Adult. New York: Brunner/Mazel; 1976.

SELF-ESTEEM DISTURBANCE

DEFINITION AND DESCRIPTION

Self-esteem disturbance can be conceptualized as negative feelings about self, including diminished self-confidence and self-worth. It may be *situational* (in response to a loss or traumatic change in life circumstances) or *chronic* (long-standing negative self-evaluation).[6] Self-esteem disturbance may be expressed directly or indirectly through behaviors such as failure to take care of self or follow up on health care needs.

THEORY AND RESEARCH

Self-esteem is a product of self-evaluation processes, with both cognitive and affective components.[2] It is composed, in part, of reflected appraisals—"the perceived respect, love and approval . . . of people close to us" (reference 3, p 128). Reflected appraisals have well-documented influence on the developing self-concept of children[3] and of adults.[3,13] Other elements of self-esteem include social expectations and perceptions of personal competence.[13]

Social expectations are learned beginning in childhood and achieve their maximum importance in the adult years. For example, career and work become a significant part of adult self-concept. Developmental tasks throughout the lifespan may present challenges that, in a given individual, threaten self-esteem. Lastly, the perception of personal competence which also begins to develop early, continues to have an integral role in self-esteem throughout life. Chronic low self-esteem is a possible outcome if the individual has not had environmental support for development of a sense of the self as competent.

Links between self-esteem and physical and mental health are well documented.[1,2] In some cases, low self-esteem is antecedent to health problems; in other cases, it is an outcome of health problems. The relation of self-esteem and health will be discussed further in the research highlights section.

RELATED FACTORS

Physical or mental illness and dysfunctional family systems can contribute to low self-esteem. In clinical depression, low self-esteem appears to be triggered by stressful life events.[2] Physical ill health is also correlated with diminished self-esteem.[1] In dysfunctional families, parents may themselves lack healthy self-esteem and so be unable to convey this quality to their children. If parents convey indifference or repeated negative feedback, the child's self-esteem is damaged.[9] Other damage to self-esteem occurs when the family is unable to provide genuine autonomy for the child, and inadequate problem-solving does not permit resolution of developmental crises.[12] Children experiencing these problems will not develop positive reflected appraisals or experience personal competence at mastering their environment.

A variety of traumatic experiences has been conceptualized as contributing to self-esteem disturbances. These experiences include physical and sexual abuse, war, natural disasters, accidents, or hostage experiences. Any of these experiences may challenge the perception of personal competence in relation to mastery of the environment. The original defenses used by adult or child victims of physical or sexual abuse may contribute to later psychopathology.[10] Originally developed as survival strategies, these defenses include denial of the abuse, altering the affective responses to the abuse, and changing the meanings of the abuse.[10] In other words, the child may distort feelings or beliefs about the abuse in order to survive within the family. A key element is the type and quality of responsiveness from the victim's support network when abuse is disclosed. The family's ability to believe, support, and provide safety for the child once abuse is disclosed may be the most influential factor in reducing the impact of the abuse.[4,7] When parents or other significant figures fail to provide emotional support, the victim must accommodate to the social system in which he or she lives.[8]

In severe instances of abuse or neglect in early life, multiple personality syndrome may develop.[11] This disorder may derive from spontaneous dissociative or "out-of-body" experiences during severe emotional and physical trauma such as assault or rape. Less severe reactions to incest may include long-term difficulty forming friendships and persistent feelings of low self-worth and inferiority.[5] Whatever the nature of the trauma, the key variable in the avoidance of long-term self-esteem impairment may be validation of the experience as the victim sees it, with exploration of the meanings of the experience for the victim.

DEFINING CHARACTERISTICS

Clients with self-esteem disturbance display negative self-assessment. They frequently have difficulty accepting positive feedback because it does not coincide with their self-view. They also tend to minimize their own strengths and abilities and may have inflexible, unreasonably high standards for themselves. The latter may be accompanied by preoccupation with real or imagined failure, and self-destructive behavior may be a sequela when high standards are not met. Hopelessness or uselessness is frequently communicated.

Indirect expression of self-esteem disturbance may be seen in the individual who has sustained emotional and physical trauma and who has not had available, or been able to use, appropriate support. This person will display a variety of cognitive and behavioral characteristics indicative of chronic low self-esteem ranging from expressions of shame or guilt to relatively subtle indicators such as ambivalence and lack of follow-through. The latter may be characteristic of adult children of alcoholics; these individuals are otherwise relatively well-functioning persons who have learned to distort their feelings in response to an always-changing reality within the family and who are more comfortable making decisions in response to crises than proactively. Clients with chronic self-esteem disturbance may express feelings of inadequacy and helplessness, as well as self-criticism. They may display failure to care for self, limited trust of others, self-defeating ideations and behavior, and excessive worrying and fearfulness. Clients with situational self-esteem disturbance exhibit similar defining characteristics, but they are of shorter duration and are situationally related (Chart 1).

CHART 1
Self-Esteem Disturbance: Definition, Related Factors, and Defining Characteristics

DEFINITION

Self-esteem disturbance is negative self-appraisal, with resultant diminished self-confidence and self-worth. Low self-esteem can be situational or chronic and may be expressed directly or indirectly by such means as failure to care for self.

RELATED FACTORS

Mental illness
Physical illness
Dysfunctional family system
Repeated negative experiences (including physical, emotional, sexual abuse)
Repression or denial of trauma
Absence of at least one consistently available individual, especially after trauma

DEFINING CHARACTERISTICS

Self-criticism
Negative expectations regarding outcome of own enterprises
Excessive worrying or fearfulness
Feelings of inadequacy or helplessness
Self-defeating ideations and behavior
Failure to care for self
Lack of follow-through
Limited ability to trust
Inability to accept positive reinforcement
Self-destructive behavior
Ambivalence
Unreasonable, inflexible standards for self
Minimization of own real strengths and abilities
Preoccupation with real or imagined failure
Expressions of shame or guilt
Verbalizations of inadequacies, lack of self-worth

NURSING PROCESS AND RATIONALE

Assessment

Systematic assessment for self-esteem disturbance should be begun whenever related factors are known or suspected to be present. Often, the client will verbalize negative self-appraisal, shame, or guilt directly. In many instances of chronic low self-esteem, however, it will be necessary to ask specific questions in order to obtain an understanding of the client's self-esteem.

This is particularly important in cases of physical or sexual abuse, exposure to any severe trauma (especially if prolonged), and where an individual has grown up in a severely dysfunctional family in which consistent nurturance was not available. Under these circumstances, the client may be blocking out the painful memories and may provide only subtle or disguised cues to the presence of the problem. Further, defense mechanisms for surviving in an abusive situation may have required the client to distort the situation and see the abuser as a good and loving parent or spouse. Thus, data provided may unavoidably be distorted.

Nursing Diagnosis

The nursing diagnosis of self-esteem disturbance may be made more specific for a particular client as, for example, situational self-esteem disturbance related to divorce or chronic self-esteem disturbance related to dysfunctional family system.

Client Goals and Nursing Interventions

Initial nursing activity with the client with self-esteem disturbance will focus on demonstrating caring while avoiding agreement with the client's excessively negative world view and self-view. This needs to be sensitively done so that the client can perceive that the nurse, although not agreeing with his or her beliefs, does not discount them. It also is very important to assist the client to recognize personal strengths and the positive aspects of self. These assets can reinforce the client's self-worth during times of stress and illness. Nonverbal demonstrations of the nurse's valuing of the client are also important; i.e., voice tone and body language. Praise can be effective, if sensitively used, in enhancing self-esteem.

When there is long-term contact with the client with self-esteem disturbance, the nurse works with the client to develop incremental goals for bolstering a sense of achievement and mastery. With clients with chronic self-esteem disturbance, the challenge is mutually to establish small goals that allow for the possibility of success. In hospital or day treatment settings, it is also important to facilitate constructive social interaction so that clients may expand their ability to trust where needed and to obtain necessary support from others. Support groups and process-oriented psychotherapy groups are powerful tools that can be used to enhance self-esteem. In short-term care settings, the nurse may not have sufficient contact with the client to become a significant source of positive reflected appraisals. If so, facilitation of contact with family and others important to the client may provide the needed positive feedback for self-esteem enhancement.

In working with abused clients, it is important not to pronounce judgment on the client's expressed beliefs and feelings. The client must become fully aware of his or her feelings in order to recover. This includes the experiencing of anger and directing it toward its appropriate focus so that the client can begin to understand the real effects of the traumatic experience. This must be done in a safe and controlled way, again, usually

---

CHART 2
Self-Esteem: Summary of the Nursing Process

NURSING INTERVENTIONS	OUTCOME CRITERIA
CLIENT GOAL: BE ABLE TO CARE FOR SELF Assist client with ADL care if needed Obtain client input in care planning Mutually establish small goals that allow for possibility of success with severely impaired individuals	Demonstrates initiative in self-care activities, including participation in outpatient therapy Communicates own wants and needs to others in an assertive way
CLIENT GOAL: EXPRESS MORE POSITIVE BELIEFS ABOUT SELF AND OWN COMPETENCIES Acknowledge client's feelings Assist client to recognize own strengths as well as perceived deficits	Displays full range of affect Sets and achieves meaningful goals Communicates valuing of own opinion and beliefs
CLIENT GOAL: BE ABLE TO TRUST WITHIN SELECTED RELATIONSHIPS Be alert to subtle cues indicating self-esteem deficits Anticipate low trust level and proceed with relationship at a pace sensitive to client's comfort level Assist client to clarify feelings about any abuse that has occurred	Verbalizes thoughts and feelings spontaneously Actively participates in group, individual, and family therapy

Research Highlights

Self-esteem and physical and mental health are linked, according to many studies.[1-3,9] Low self-esteem may be either antecedent to, or result from, health problems. That is, a person with low self-esteem may be predisposed to physical and mental ill health, or the health problems may lead to lowered self-esteem. A survey by Antonucci and Jackson included self-report measures of health, self-esteem, and sociodemographic variables.[1] They found that self-esteem scores were significantly higher for individuals reporting no health problems than for those who did. In other words, those who reported having health problems also had significantly lower self-esteem. This correlation was stronger for women than for men. There was also a relation between the reported severity of health problems and levels of self-esteem, with more serious health problems associated with lower levels of self-esteem. The researchers also asked subjects about physical disabilities, because such impairments might be reflected in measures of health. Indeed, physical disability was associated with even lower levels of self-esteem. The researchers, in discussing these findings, raised the question whether the degree of functional incapacity is the most important element in the relation of both health problems and physical disabilities to self-esteem.

within the context of a long-term or intensive psychotherapeutic relationship. Anger may be repressed because it is seen as so destructive by the client. There is some evidence that whereas male abuse victims tend to direct their anger outwardly, abused female patients direct their anger internally and become self-destructive.[10]

Evaluation

The client who has an increase in positive self-esteem communicates a greater valuing of personal beliefs and expresses wants and needs in a more assertive way. The client shows an increasing ability to initiate and maintain self-care activities, including participation in follow-up care when indicated (Chart 2).

CASE STUDY

John, a 15-year-old, was admitted to the hospital for treatment of depression. Although an intellectually gifted adolescent, his grades were failing. John was slight in build and sensitive about his appearance. He had few friends and frequently made self-disparaging remarks about his appearance, family, and life prospects. He was the elder of two children. His mother worked in a clerical capacity, and his father was a jazz musician who was moody and had also had one hospitalization for treatment of depression. The family had frequent financial crises because of its inconsistent income. Both parents were somewhat unavailable emotionally for their children, so John had welcomed the overtures made by an older man who was an acquaintance of his father. Prior to John's hospitalization, the man had invited John to his home under the guise of building a model boat together and had forced anal intercourse on him.

In the hospital, John was socially withdrawn and formed attachments to peers more slowly than did other teenage patients. Although the rape was obviously a key issue, there was evidence of difficulties with family and peer relations as well as school achievement before the sexual assault. John was deeply embarrassed about the assault and especially sensitive to discussion of it with women. John's primary nursing diagnosis was self-esteem disturbance related to dysfunctional family situation and recent rape. Nurses intervened in John's impaired self-esteem by developing consistent, caring relationships with him and by gently challenging his negative beliefs about himself. A male nurse and another male staff member were identified as the appropriate individuals for discussing the assault with John.

Gradually, John became more comfortable with staff, and evidenced some positive increments in self-respect and an increasing ability to be goal directed. During John's hospital stay, the family participated in family therapy sessions. In one session, the father disclosed his own hospitalization and treatment for depression to his son, and this sharing of intimate information was later reported by John to have been highly significant in his being able to feel closer to his father.

SUMMARY

Self-esteem disturbance refers to negative self-appraisal with accompanying low self-confidence and sense of self-worth. Self-esteem disturbance may be situational or chronic. Related factors include physical or mental illness, dysfunctional family system, and repeated negative experiences (including sexual, physical, or emotional abuse). Nursing interventions with clients with self-esteem disturbance are designed to improve the client's self-esteem. The nurse demonstrates caring but does not agree with the patient's excessively negative world view and cognitive distortions.

References

1. Antonucci TC, Jackson J. Physical health and self-esteem. Fam and Comm Health. 1983;6:1–9.
2. Becker J. Vulnerable self-esteem as a predisposing factor in depressive disorders. In: R. Depue, ed. The Psychobiology of the Depressive Disorders. New York: Academic Press; 1979.
3. Bell Meisenhelder J. Self-esteem: A closer look at clinical interventions. Int J Nurs Stud. 1985;22(2):127–135.
4. Brom E, Berliner L, Ramon R. Child Sexual Abuse Investigation: A Curriculum for Training Law Enforcement Officers in Washington State. Criminal Justice Training Com-

mission, Victims of Sexual Assault Programs, Bureau of Children's Services. Department of Social and Health Services, State of Washington; Seattle: Harborview Sexual Assault Center. 1983:12–24.

5. Brunngraber L. Father–daughter incest: Immediate and long-term effects of social abuse. ANS. 1986;8(4)15–35.

6. Carroll-Johnson RM. Classification of Nursing Diagnoses: Proceedings of the Eighth Conference. Philadelphia: JB Lippincott; 1989.

7. Gold E. Long-term effects of sexual victimization in childhood: An attributional approach. J Consult Clin Psychol. 1986;54(4):471–475.

8. Miller A. Thou Shalt Not be Aware: Society's Betrayal of the Child. New York: Farrar Straus Giroux; 1984.

9. Reasoner R. Enhancement of self-esteem in children and adolescents. Fam and Comm Health. 1983;6:51–64.

10. Reiker P, Carmen E. The victim to patient process: The disconfirmation and transformation of abuse. Am J Orthopsychiatry. 1986;56(3):360–370.

11. Spiegel D. Multiple personality as a post-traumatic stress disorder. Psychiatr Clin North Am. 1984;7(1):101–110.

12. Stanwyck D. Self-esteem through the life span. Fam and Comm Health. 1983;6:11–28.

13. Taft L. Self-esteem in later life: A nursing perspective. ANS. 1985;8(1):77–84.

BODY IMAGE DISTURBANCE

DEFINITION AND DESCRIPTION

Body image disturbance is defined as disruption in the way one perceives one's body. Body image disturbance can result from a variety of events; e.g., perceived or actual changes resulting from growth and aging, trauma, or loss of a body part or function. In each case, the fundamental view of self is altered by the change in physical self. These changes represent loss of a former level of integration and may occasion the need to mourn what has been lost.

THEORY AND RESEARCH

Body image is an integrated collection of visual, auditory, tactile, and proprioceptive data. Proprioception refers to "the continuous but unconscious sensory flow from the movable parts of [the] body (muscles, tendons, joints), by which their position and tone and motion are continually monitored and adjusted"(reference 11, p 43). This information combines with affective and cognitive processes to form a gestalt that is the body image. Body image may come to include external objects such as clothing or prostheses. Conversely, nerve damage may cause perceptual loss of "ownership" of a limb or body part as, for example, when the person with hemiplegia after a stroke ignores one half of the body.[11]

Body image and self-concept are closely linked because sensory input is such an integral part of interpersonal contact in infancy and childhood. As behavior and appearance are commented on by others from early life on, physical appearance is reinforced as an important part of the developing self-concept; i.e., "Who am I?"[2] Body image can thus be conceptualized as having two components: a physical component, which consists of an actual body feature or movement, and a psychological part, which develops from cognitions and feelings attached to the physical component.[12] Physical appearance is used to create for others an impression of the person as a totality (including personality and cognitive attributes). The chosen impression may be congruent with a fully integrated, genuine self, or it may reflect projection of a desired fantasy self.[12]

Aging may cause changes in body image in some individuals, as reflected by figure drawings lacking in proportion and integration.[4,6] An important determinant of the perception of aging appears to be the state of physical health and feedback from others that the individual is old; healthy older adults do not consistently report more body dissatisfaction than younger persons.[4]

RELATED FACTORS

Because the body is the vehicle by which thoughts and feelings are shared with others, normal developmental changes or debilitating injury challenge the integration of the sense of self. In normal growth and development, particularly during adolescence, sociocultural standards and interpersonal feedback heavily influence body image and, by extension, self-concept. Mutilating surgery, such as mastectomy for breast cancer, challenges the integration of the body image,[3,5,7] as does other corrective surgery and use of prostheses.[2] Hemiplegia, as produced by stroke or other neurologic deficits, produces changes in body image—actual lack of recognition of a body part or function (depersonalization of body part).[11]

Delusional beliefs about the body and its functions are often present during psychosis. A psychotic individual may perceive his or her appearance and perceptual–motor abilities to be drastically different than they are. Depressed persons negatively distort their body image, whereas other clients may distort their body image in a positive or enhancing manner.[8] The eating disorders[1] are examples of psychiatric conditions in which body image disturbance may be stimulated by maturational changes interacting with a complex variety of social, cognitive, and biological stressors. The majority of clients with eating disorders reveal by history some struggles with negative perception of the bodily changes of adolescence.[8] Girls, in particular, are apt to compare themselves with peers or with individuals representing the culturally sanctioned standards of physical attractiveness.

Intensive care patients face special challenges to body image integrity. Physical immobility may cause deficits in feedback information, and life support machinery may be perceived in a distorted, even psychotic, manner.[10]

DEFINING CHARACTERISTICS

Body image disturbance can be suspected when change or trauma has altered body structure or function. The affected body part may be concealed or deliberately exposed. Individuals may be afraid to look at a damaged body part and indeed may refuse to do so. Inability to accept change in body structure or function can also occur; i.e., an aging individual who persists in an unsafe level of strenuous physical activity that was possible earlier.

A psychotic person may demonstrate body image disturbance by expressing that his or her body and another person's are the same or that the body and inanimate objects are linked. Changes in social functioning often occur when body image disturbance is present. The individual may become preoccupied with negative feelings about the body, feel hopeless, and fear rejection by others. Grieving for loss or change may be needed (Chart 1).

NURSING PROCESS AND RATIONALE

Assessment

Body image disturbance should be assessed whenever serious physical illness and selected psychiatric illnesses are present. Operations for head and neck carcinoma, breast cancer, and creation of abdominal stoma are particularly noted to cause body image distortions.[5] It is important to observe behavior, as well as to note the client's verbalizations about his or her body. Refusal to look at or touch body parts and concealment or overexposure of body parts may indicate body image disturbance. Fear of rejection by others is important to assess because of the significance of the feedback from others in the development of body image.

Nursing Diagnosis

The nursing diagnosis of body image disturbance may be made more specific for a particular client as, for example, body image disturbance related to the changes of aging or body image disturbance related to the cognitive distortions of schizophrenia.

CHART 1
Body Image Disturbance: Definition, Related Factors, and Defining Characteristics

DEFINITION

Body image disturbance is a disruption of self-concept resulting from a change in the body or the way the body is viewed. Normal growth and aging, sociocultural standards, and trauma can all contribute to body image distortion.

RELATED FACTORS

Developmental changes (maturation, aging)
Sociocultural standards
Negative interpersonal feedback
Mutilative surgery or injury
Neurologic deficits
Psychoses and other psychiatric illnesses
Dependence on machine for life support
Actual change in body structure or function

DEFINING CHARACTERISTICS

Refusal to look at or touch body part
Concealment or overexposure of body part
Inability to accept change in body structure or function
Reduced frequency of social contact
Negative feeling about body
Preoccupation with loss of body part or function
Expressed feelings of hopelessness
Expressed fear of rejection by others
Depersonalization of body part
Refusal to verify actual change
Extension of body boundary to incorporate environmental objects

---

Client Goals and Nursing Interventions

Goals for a client with body image disturbance would include assisting the individual to experience increased self-acceptance, to grieve for changes or loss, and to participate in self-care activities.

The nurse's role with a client who has suffered body trauma is significant, as the client's body image is influenced by the reactions of others in the environment. Thus, nursing interventions that convey acceptance of the person as he or she is become important to healthy body image reintegration in cases of surgical body transformation such as creation of an abdominal stoma.[5] Involvement in social activity may need to be adjusted to the client's social sensitivity about body alteration. Using the rapport established within the nurse–client relationship, the nurse supports expression of distress, sadness, or anger as part of the grieving process for change or loss of body structure or function.

In cases of psychiatric illness (e.g., schizophrenia,

eating disorders), gentle refutation of inaccurate body image can be effective. It may be necessary to develop small, incremental goals for self-care and grooming and hygiene, especially if the client is severely depressed. This requires careful initial assessment of the client's capability for self-motivated participation.

Nursing intervention also includes bolstering the client's use of available social support and augmenting support resources where indicated. It may be important to make families feel comfortable and welcome in the treatment setting. The client and family alike may benefit from support group participation. When families are dysfunctional or too stressed by the client's illness to be supportive, a referral to a psychiatric clinical nurse specialist or other qualified family therapist is indicated. More functional family members can be included to good effect in self-care health teaching that is being made available to the client.

Evaluation

Clients will demonstrate improvement in body image by utilizing available social support and by participating in self-care activities in a manner consistent with self-acceptance of bodily changes. If illness or dysfunction is present, the client is able to grieve for the former level of body integration—a necessary process before changed body image can be integrated into the self-concept (Chart 2).

CASE STUDY

Carolyn was a 32-year-old woman with breast cancer. She was a married housewife with two children and a high school education. Premorbidly, Carolyn valued her appearance and took pride in her figure and appearance. She was frightened on learning her physician's diagnosis and did not ask any questions about treatment choices when the surgeon recommended total mastectomy.

After surgery, Carolyn was withdrawn and occasionally tearful. She displayed great reluctance to have professional staff view the operative site and refused to look at it herself. She showed anxiety before her husband's visits to the hospital and tearfulness after he left. After one such occasion, she spontaneously said to her nurse, "How can I be a woman any more?" Her husband appeared to wish to offer affection and support, but Carolyn rebuffed his efforts. It was noted by the staff that he, too, seemed anxious after several hospital visits. A nursing diagnosis formulated was body image disturbance related to disfiguring surgery.

Carolyn's primary nurse acknowledged the difficulty of viewing such a dramatic change in her body as a breast removal. She helped Carolyn with bathing and performed wound care and asked her for permission to arrange a "Reach to Recovery" volunteer visit. The nurse also anticipated the need for grieving, and when Carolyn questioned her femininity, her nurse was prepared to elicit more information about the meaning of the surgery for Carolyn, and about her fears. Carolyn's nurse responded both on a factual level and on an emotionally empathic level. In response to the couple's anxiety about the surgery, the nurse made efforts to include the husband in health teaching. She also discussed Carolyn's case with the psychiatric clinical nurse specialist, who agreed to see Carolyn and evaluate the need for family therapy.

CHART 2
Body Image Disturbance: Summary of the Nursing Process

NURSING INTERVENTIONS	OUTCOME CRITERIA
CLIENT GOAL: EXPERIENCE INCREASED SELF-ACCEPTANCE Express acceptance of the client as a person as is Explore for presence of cognitive distortions (irrational fears) and work with client over time to challenge these	Spontaneously verbalizes feelings and issues to nurse and others Recognizes negative beliefs and develops affirmations to replace them Participates in social activities without hiding or exposing affected body part(s)
CLIENT GOAL: ENGAGE IN NORMAL GRIEVING FOR CHANGE OR LOSS Accept client's distress as healthy and necessary to healing Be available to hear expression of feelings	Expresses feelings of sadness, loss, or anger where appropriate
CLIENT GOAL: PARTICIPATE IN SELF-CARE ACTIVITIES Assess client's present capability for self-motivated participation Work with client to develop mutually agreed on progress toward self-care	Views the affected body part(s) Performs hygiene and health care activities pertinent to body alteration Selects healthy lifestyle activities (exercises regularly, maintains normal weight)

Research Highlights

Breast surgery for cancer is widely noted to cause depression and various degrees of body image distortion.[3,5,7] Sexual dysfunction occurs for some women after surgery; this and other sequelae of the operation are thought to be related to premorbid psychological integration and functioning.[3,5] That is, possession of highly polarized gender role definition and highly "feminine" identification correlates with increased risk of sexual dysfunction after breast surgery.[3]

Lasry and colleagues[7] studied psychological adjustment (including body image) in women who had received one of three types of intervention for breast cancer: total mastectomy, lumpectomy, and lumpectomy plus radiation. They used a body image index that asked the women to report on satisfaction with body and breast appearance, attractiveness of self according to others, fear of not being sexually attractive, attractiveness change attributable to the operation, and several other items. Body image was more negatively affected by more extensive surgery. Radiation therapy had no significant reported effect on body image, although it did correlate with increased levels of depression compared with the lumpectomy-only group. The researchers concluded that body image is significantly better in clients with lumpectomies. They recommended that psychosocial sequelae should be given greater consideration by surgeons treating breast cancer.[7]

SUMMARY

Body image is an integral component of the self-concept. It is comprised of multisensory physical impressions and the integrated feedback from others and incorporated social normative standards. Damage to the body, illness, and even normal growth and development threaten the integration of body image.

Nursing care for persons suffering body image disturbance involves assessment of the client's perception of the change in body function or structure. Often, grief work needs to be facilitated. The responses of others in the client's social network also need to be assessed because of the importance of their feedback to the client's body image. Nursing interventions for the client suffering from body image distortion include acceptance of the client's present feelings and beliefs about his or her body and incremental increases in self-care and social activity. Supportive challenges to any cognitive distortions are also an appropriate nursing intervention.

References

1. American Psychiatric Association. Diagnostic and Statistical Manual of Mental Disorders. 3rd ed, rev. Washington, DC: American Psychiatric Association; 1987.
2. Bauman S. Physical aspects of the self: A review of some aspects of body image development in childhood. Psychiat Clin North Am. 1981;4(3):455–470.
3. Derogatis L. The unique impact of breast and gynecologic cancers on body image and sexual identity in women: A reassessment. In: Vaeth R, ed. Body Image, Self-Esteem and Sexuality in Cancer Patients. 2nd ed. Basel: Karger S; 1986.
4. Fisher S. Development and Structure of the Body Image. vol. 1. Hillsdale, New Jersey: Lawrence Erlbaum Associates; 1986.
5. Gillies DA. Body image changes following illness and injury. J Enterostomal Therapy. 1984;11(5):186–189.
6. Janelli LM. Body image in older adults: A review of the literature. Rehabilitation Nursing. 1986;11(4):6–8.
7. Lasry JC, Margolese RG, Poisson R, et al: Depression and body image following mastectomy and lumpectomy. Journal of Chronic Diseases. 1987;40(6):529–534.
8. Leon G, Lucas A, Colligan R, Ferdinande R, Kamp J. Sexual, body-image and personality attitudes in anorexia nervosa. J Abnorm Child Psychol. 1985;13(2):245–258.
9. Noles S, Cash T, Winstead B. Body image, physical attractiveness and depression. J Consult Clin Psychol. 1985; 53(1):88–94.
10. Platzer H. Body image 2: Helping patients cope with changes—a problem for nurses. Intensive Care Nurs 1987;3(3):125–132.
11. Sacks O. The Man Who Mistook His Wife for a Hat. New York: Harper and Row; 1987.
12. van der Velde C. Body images of one's self and others: Developmental and clinical significance. Am J Psychiat. 1985; 142(5):525–537.

ROLE PERFORMANCE DISTURBANCE

DEFINITION AND DESCRIPTION

Role performance disturbance as a self-concept disturbance refers to impaired role functioning that can occur as a result of illness, aging or death of partner, lack of social and interpersonal skills required for competent role performance, discrepancy between intrapersonal and societal role expectations, absence of role models, and interpersonal role disputes. Other causes of role performance disturbance include loss of employment, cross-cultural differences in role definition, and societal changes in role definition. Role changes in and of themselves are not negative; rather, it is the context of the changes and the psychological make-up of the person confronting the change that will determine whether role alteration will result in role impairment.

THEORY AND RESEARCH

The sense of self is greatly influenced by the reactions and responses of others throughout life. Relationships with others are typically organized into roles. An individual most often holds multiple roles simultaneously; i.e., spouse, parent, employee, supervisor. The perception of role competency then becomes a key determinant of the sense of self, as roles reflect both the appraisal of others and the individual's sense of competence within the environment.

Failure of a person's main interpersonal relation has been set forward as a typical cause of severe depression.[1] Marital failure poses the loss of a reciprocal role around which much of the self-concept has been organized. The depressed person may wish to deny the loss of the role or to ignore aspects of the previously held role that were not healthy. Depression can also occur if the individual can recognize the loss of the role but is unable to take the next steps—reorganizing and acting on new patterns of interpersonal relationships. Occupational roles are also closely linked with self-esteem and self-concept in the adult. Work and family roles, if positive, appear to offer a reciprocal buffering effect from life stress. Job stress negatively affects family functioning.[5] Significant variables in role performance include: (1) the importance of the relationship of the other person(s) with whom the role is enacted; (2) the beliefs that the individuals have about interactive roles; and (3) feelings related to role enactment.[3]

RELATED FACTORS

Loss is a significant related factor for role performance disturbance. Death of spouse, divorce, and loss of job challenge the integrity of the self-concept. Changes secondary to illness or aging may impact role performance significantly even if they do not cause actual role loss. The adaptation necessitated by these changes is stressful, particularly in the absence of adequate social support.

Interpersonal role conflict is another important related factor in role performance disturbance. Conflict occurs when an individual and significant other(s) have nonreciprocal expectations about their relationship.[7] If this is prolonged and the perception of the conflict as irreconcilable is also present, role performance disturbance can result.

Intrapersonal deficits result when role modeling has been absent or inadequate. Low self-esteem may lead to not learning or to lack of utilization of social skills.

Resultant intrapersonal deficits may predispose the individual to social isolation or lack of satisfaction with available relationships.[7]

Additional related factors for role performance disturbance include developmental lags in skills of social competence, changes in sex-role definitions, lack of clarity in role definition, cross-cultural differences, and role ambiguity. Substance abuse can also result in profound role performance disturbance, as nonimpaired spouses tend to take over role-related tasks of impaired partners.[6]

DEFINING CHARACTERISTICS

Role performance disturbance is often characterized by expressed dissatisfaction with the role or the ability to perform it. Conflict between simultaneously held roles may be present. Denial and avoidance of the role may occur, as when a spouse abandons a family or a person abruptly terminates a job. Role disputes are often described openly as conflictual, but failure to describe a significant relationship or idealized descriptions of relationships are also cues to interpersonal role conflict.[7]

Impaired role transition is a type of role performance disturbance that occurs when individuals encounter difficulty in trying to cope with losses and other life changes.[7] Dysfunctional grief is an example of impaired role transition.[2] Lund and coworkers[4] found a number of early bereavement indicators of poor coping at 2 years: feelings of wanting to die, confusion, aloneness, and behaviors of excessive crying, not keeping busy, and taking sleeping pills or tranquillizers. Low self-esteem prior to bereavement was correlated with dysfunctional grief 2 years after bereavement.

Role strain is a term used to describe the individual's response to stress associated with a role.[9] Stressors may include ambiguity of the role, the individual being either incompetent or overqualified for the role, and conflict between several roles held by one individual. Tension, anxiety, hostility, and depression can result when role stressors are present to a pronounced degree. The individual may ultimately decide to leave the role in order to reduce stress. Job burnout is an example of role performance disturbance that results from severe role strain (Chart 1).

NURSING PROCESS AND RATIONALE

Assessment

The role of client, especially in inpatient settings, tends to disrupt functioning in other roles and necessitates role transition. Careful data collection regarding the client's social and family roles and their disruption are important.

The meaning of the role change for the client is assessed both by the client's account and by observation of his or her behavior and interactions with others. Loss

CHART 1
Role Performance Disturbance: Definition, Related Factors, and Defining Characteristics

DEFINITION

Role performance disturbance refers to impaired role functioning, which can occur as a result of illness, lack of social and interpersonal skills required for competent role performance, role stressors, absence of role models, and other factors.

RELATED FACTORS

Interpersonal role conflict
Inadequate or unavailable role models
Loss of significant relationship
Changes in sex-role definitions
Role ambiguity
Change in physical capability to perform role secondary to illness or aging
Lack of clarity in role definition or understanding of role
Substance abuse
Social skills deficits
Cross-cultural differences
Low self-esteem
Conflict between simultaneously held roles

DEFINING CHARACTERISTICS

Expressed dissatisfaction with role or ability to perform role
Denial or avoidance of role
Impaired role transition
Role strain
Deterioration of usual patterns of responsibility in role enactment
Dysfunctional grief
Job burnout

---

of role may present such a severe threat to the individual that verbal description of it may not be possible or adequate. The person may not be able to articulate feelings, much less begin to reorganize behavior around the change or loss. Assessment of meaning for the client is, therefore, a continuing process. Anticipatory negative cognitions about self and personal efficacy as well as anxiety can accompany role transitions. Feelings of helplessness and the belief that worth to others has been made negligible is seen with loss. It is important to assess for underlying stressful role transitions or role impairments in instances of suicidal ideation or attempt and exacerbation of depression or substance abuse and other addictive disorders. Many psychiatric illnesses recur when previous levels of integration and the position of self within the individual's social matrix have been challenged.

Nursing Diagnosis

The nursing diagnosis of role performance disturbance can be made more specific for a particular client as, for example, role performance disturbance related to inadequate role models or role performance disturbance related to substance abuse.

Client Goals and Nursing Interventions

Exploration of the personal meaning of role change is an important first client goal. Expression of feelings and concerns are encouraged, with guidance from the nurse as to how the change affects values and self-worth appraisal. Need for grief work is indicated when significant loss has occurred.

A second client goal follows closely from the first; i.e., perception of self-worth in spite of inability to perform a role. Nursing intervention involves assisting the client to identify other valuable aspects of self-concept, which may be overlooked when the client is absorbed with loss or stressful role transition. The client may find use of affirmations helpful during a period of stressful coping with role change. Involvement of family and friends is also to be encouraged because of the documented benefits of social support.[4,5,7,8]

After activities toward the first two goals are in progress, the nurse can work with the client to facilitate progress toward resolution of stressful role transition or loss. Strategies that may ease role change include full utilization of available social support, development of a broader base of social support, interaction with appropriate role models, and remedial work on social skills deficits. The nurse may work directly with the client to develop these strategies or may facilitate referrals to appropriate psychotherapeutic or rehabilitative resources.

Evaluation

Resolution of role performance disturbance may occur gradually, because affect and grieving are often involved. The client who is recovering from role performance disturbance will show increasing ability to value self, will maintain relationships with significant others, and will be able to express satisfaction with new or redefined role performance (Chart 2).

CASE STUDY

Gerald was a 60-year-old man who was hospitalized for severe depression. He was agitated, had difficulty sleeping, and experienced much mood lability and frequent spells of crying. Two years before hospital admission, Gerald's wife of 35 years had died in an auto accident. She had been his most frequent companion, and he had maintained few friendships throughout his adult life. Gerald's work performance had suffered since his bereavement, and 1 month

CHART 2
Role Performance Disturbance: Summary of the Nursing Process

NURSING INTERVENTIONS	OUTCOME CRITERIA
CLIENT GOAL: EXPLORE PERSONAL MEANING OF ROLE CHANGE	
Encourage expression of feelings and concerns about current role functioning	Verbalizes feelings and thoughts about role change
Elicit meanings of role change through exploration with client	
Facilitate grieving process where appropriate	
CLIENT GOAL: BE ABLE TO PERCEIVE PERSONAL WORTH IN SPITE OF INABILITY TO PERFORM ROLE	
Help client identify other valuable aspects of self	Verbalizes and behaviorally demonstrates self-worth
Teach use of affirmations where appropriate	
Include family/friends in support efforts	Initiates and maintains contact with significant others
Refer for family therapy where appropriate	
CLIENT GOAL: PROGRESS TOWARD RESOLUTION OF CHANGE IN OR LOSS OF ROLE	
Facilitate exploration of values and interests	Expresses satisfaction with new or redefined role performance
Help client identify strategies that will ease role change	Plans for and implements other satisfying roles
Obtain vocational, rehabilitation or other referral as indicated	Seeks out appropriate role models
CLIENT GOAL: UTILIZE AVAILABLE SUPPORT AND COMMUNITY RESOURCES	
Assess family and support network's ability to respond to client's needs	Interacts with family and significant others in an appropriate way
Make referral for support group, family therapy, or rehabilitative services if indicated	Verbalizes awareness of available rehabilitative and psychotherapeutic resources
Include family in health teaching	

prior to hospitalization, he had been urged to take early retirement. Dysfunctional grieving and loss of the spouse role had compounded Gerald's difficulty with the retirement role transition. Since his wife's death, Gerald had withdrawn even more from social contact with others. Retirement appeared to exacerbate his depression and anxiety secondary to progressive loss of daily structure. The concern of his family over his distraught appearance, rapid weight loss, and "irrational" behavior led to the initial psychiatric consultation and subsequent hospitalization. His nursing diagnoses included role performance disturbance related to role transitions and dysfunctional grieving.

Gerald's nurse carefully elicited the meanings of the role loss for him. From this information and behavioral observations, three issues that needed to be addressed in his plan of care were identified. These were: (1) loss of familiar daily structure; (2) lack of experience in forming and maintaining relationships with others; and (3) self-criticism about his performance as worker and husband. It became evident that Gerald was underutilizing available social support, and the nurse facilitated several care conferences in which contact with family and friends was fostered.

Interventions to facilitate smoother role transitions in both work and social situations involved individual therapy as well as consultation with Gerald's support network. These interventions were aimed toward assisting him to identify and utilize new sources of support and to practice the social skills required of an unpartnered person. Individual therapy focused on his irrational fears of being alone and his hypercritical self-evaluation.

Research Highlights

Retirement and death of spouse have been observed to cause deleterious effects on social functioning. Decline in income or health have been proposed as factors in the changes in functioning when these role losses occur. Changes in income or health alone, however, do not seem to account for all of the variance in functioning after retirement and death of a spouse. Wan and Odell studied the relation between five predictor variables and formal and informal social participation of older men.[8] The predictor variables were prior level of participation (frequency of interaction with kin and social or professional memberships), socioeconomic status, retirement status, widowerhood status, kin network size, and deteriorative life change (declines in health, economic well-being, and life satisfaction and other negative changes). They found that "participatory lifestyle developed in the preretirement stage has more influence on social participation than major role losses and other deteriorative changes experienced in old age" (reference 8, p 190).

The effects of significant role loss, then, seem to be mediated by complex interactions among a number of important variables. Wan and Odell concluded that men may benefit from increased social participation with family and friends and through organizational memberships at all stages of life.

SUMMARY

The perception of role competence is a key determinant of the sense of self, as roles reflect the appraisal of others and the individual's mastery of the environment. Potential for role performance disturbance exists when external and internal events combine to make role performance less satisfactory or possible for the individual. Whether role performance disturbance actually develops depends on the context of the change and the psychological make-up of the individual.

References

1. Arieti S, Bemporad J. Severe and Mild Depression. New York: Basic Books; 1978.
2. Hartz, G. Adult grief and its interface with mood disorder: Proposal of a new diagnosis of complicated bereavement. Compr Psychiatry. 1986;27(1):60–64.
3. Klerman G, Weissman M. Interpersonal psychotherapy: Theory and research. In: Rush A, ed. Short-Term Psychotherapies for Depression. New York: Guilford Press; 1982.
4. Lund D, Dimond M, Caserta M, et al. Identifying elderly with coping difficulties after two years of bereavement. Omega. 1985–86;16(3):213–224.
5. Moos R, Moos B. Adaption and the quality of life in work and family settings. Journal of Community Psychology. 1983; 11:158–170.
6. Moos R, Moos B. The process of recovery from alcoholism: Comparing functioning in families of alcoholics and matched control families. J Stud Alcohol. 1984;45(2):111–118.
7. Rounsaville B, Chevron E. Interpersonal psychotherapy: Clinical applications. In: Rush A, ed. Short-Term Psychotherapies for Depression. New York: Guilford Press; 1982.
8. Wan T, Odell B. Major role losses and social participation of older males. Res Aging. 1983;5(2):173–196.
9. Ward C. The meaning of role strain. ANS. 1986;8(2):39–49.

SEXUAL DYSFUNCTION

Gordon L. Dickman and Carolyn A. Livingston

DEFINITION AND DESCRIPTION

Sexuality and sexual behavior cover a wide range of attitudes, beliefs, and activities in our society. A definition of sexual dysfunction must be broad enough to reflect this diversity.[2] It must reflect the subjective nature of sexual experience and avoid establishing an artificial norm or standard against which all sexual behaviors are measured when trying to determine whether or not they are dysfunctional.

Sexual dysfunction is defined as a state in which an individual experiences a change in sexual function that is viewed by the individual as unsatisfying, unrewarding, or inadequate.[10] This does not imply that an individual may infringe on the rights of others. Sexual function should be given the broadest possible definition to include changes in sexual beliefs and feelings, as well as changes in bodily functions. In this way, changes in sexual desire can be included along with changes in bodily function in the definition of sexual dysfunction. Sexual dysfunction can occur when being sexual alone or with a partner. It can happen to heterosexual, homosexual, bisexual, transvestite, and transsexual, younger, middle-aged, and older people. It can happen across the cultural spectrum. In short, it can happen to people, no matter what their sexual preference, life-style, or life stage may be.

Clients experiencing sexual dysfunction may try to compare their sexual behavior with some preconceived standard of normal. However, there simply is no one standard of sexual normalcy against which to measure sexual dysfunction.[2] Diversity of behavior, diversity of beliefs, and diversity of subjective experience seem to be inherent in human sexuality. When sexuality is viewed in this light, the definition of sexual dysfunction, as defined here, begins to make sense. This is a client-centered definition. Given all of the factors that can be considered in determining sexual dysfunction, the client's view is central to the consideration, as long as there is no infringement upon the rights of others.

THEORY AND RESEARCH

There is seldom one single cause for unrewarding, unsatisfying, or inadequate sexual experiences, because sexuality involves every aspect of a client's life. Sexuality has physiologic, sociologic, psychological, and spiritual components. In other words, sexual thoughts, feelings, or acts happen in the context of bodily functions; immediate and past social environments; a sexual mind-set; and feelings of connectedness with self, others, or a Higher Power.

Biomedical changes in body functions can be a source of sexual dysfunction. Disease processes, such as diabetes,[6] atherosclerosis, other blood vessel diseases, Parkinson's disease and epilepsy, chronic obstructive pulmonary disease,[14,15] and diseases of the genital area, affect the nerves, muscles, hormones, and blood supply necessary for sexual functioning. Changes in hormone levels can affect sexual desire. Physical trauma, such as spinal cord injuries and radical surgery in the pelvic area, can dramatically impair sexual functioning. One of the most overlooked physical factors contributing to sexual dysfunction are medications, particularly antihypertensives, anticholenergics, α- and β-adrenergic blocking agents, some monoamine oxidase (MAO) antidepressants, and neuroleptics.[4] Alcohol, narcotics, and sedative–hypnotic drugs likewise depress sexual functioning.[4,16] Physical causes of sexual dysfunction generate feelings related to self-worth and competency.[3] Physical and psychological explanations may go hand in hand.

A *psychoanalytic* interpretation of sexual dysfunction places the origins of the dysfunction in the unconscious past. The dysfunction is viewed as a result of internal conflicts resulting from unresolved, historical issues of which the patient is not aware. Present sexual behavior triggers defensive responses as feelings about these repressed historical events are churned up. Awareness or insight is achieved by analyzing, over time, the patient's sexual feelings and beliefs.[7]

When viewed from the *behaviorist* viewpoint, sexual dysfunction is the result of lack of information and of skills deficits. A person experiencing a sexual dysfunction has not learned successful behaviors or is missing crucial information about sexual functioning, or has learned unhelpful behaviors and information. Sexual fears and anxieties are allayed by new learning or by relearning. Desensitization exercises encourage the client to take small specific steps toward a desired sexual feeling and behavior and to learn to tolerate and ultimately extinguish negative, interfering feelings and behaviors.[1]

Cognitive and *interactional* explanations of sexual dysfunction look at a client's interpersonal interactions, as well as the client's beliefs and attitudes about sexual behavior. The dysfunctional behavior is not viewed in isolation, but as part of the client's whole life scheme. It views the client as part of work, family, social, and environmental systems. This cognitive–interactional approach acknowledges the client's ability to come to an understanding of troubling sexual issues. The client begins to make decisions around sexuality that lead to sexual health.[5]

Finally, sexual dysfunction can be viewed from a *spiritual* standpoint. Here, the dysfunction arises from a loss of connection with what the client defines as a spiritual community or Higher Power. A client will talk about having ignored or moved away from important spiritual beliefs or connections. These connections may be with the self, with significant others, or with the Higher Power. The sexual dysfunction generates feelings of guilt, loss of grace, loneliness, or of having sinned.[5]

RELATED FACTORS

Sexual attitudes arise from cultural traditions and practices, religious teachings, one's own set of personal sexual beliefs, and legislated codes of conduct. There are differences in sexual values from person to person, community to community, and region to region. There are differences between socioeconomic groups. There are differences between generations. Changes in the social roles of women and men, changes in ethnic and minority status, and changes in social temperament have a dramatic impact on how individuals feel about their sexual behavior. The faster these changes occur, as is happening in contemporary society, the less time individuals have to integrate these changes into their sexual belief system. Thus, dissonance in personal sexual values should be considered an important feature in sexual dysfunction.

Fear and anxiety can be powerful "off" switches to sexual behavior. Sexual fears and anxiety feed on real or imagined differences in physical or psychological power, feelings of vulnerability, feelings of personal attractiveness, and feelings of desirability. Sexual anxiety can result from previous sexual failures, such as in men who experience the inability to obtain an erection or who ejaculate too quickly, or in women who lack the ability to be orgasmic. With each new sexual opportunity, the fear of failure may set the scene for another perceived or real inability to function sexually.[16] Recent or past sexual abuse accounts for much sexual fear.

Sexual dysfunctions can occur in an atmosphere in which sexual knowledge and skills are minimal or lacking. Misinformation can exaggerate a dysfunction. Attending school and learning from trained educators is a normalizing experience resulting in shared social experiences, information, and skills. But, until recently, sex education has not been generally provided, resulting in enormous deficits in sexual knowledge and skills on the part of most people. What people have learned they have learned from peers, from the entertainment media, and from experience that is, for the most part, trial-and-error learning.

The presence or absence of effective social skills influences the course of a sexual dysfunction. There are always other people involved, directly or indirectly, in a sexual experience, and their rights and feelings need to be considered. People bring with them into any sexual scene the beliefs and even fantasy images of other people. This is true, even when masturbating alone. Sex partners have needs, wants, and interests that are somehow communicated to one another and to some degree met during the sexual experience. This interaction presumes the presence of social skills necessary to communicate and negotiate around these sexual needs. Like sexual information, sexual communication is not a subject people are carefully taught. Finding an appropriate partner, arranging for privacy, conveying sexual likes and dislikes, and asking for what one wants are very difficult for most people. If one is elderly, chronically ill, or otherwise socially disenfranchized, the social process of meeting one's sexual needs is doubly hard.

A sexual life-style other than heterosexual may or may not be an issue in a patient's sexual dysfunction.[16] Even though the Kinsey reports of the 1940s and 1950s showed that humans live a wide variety of sexual life-styles and exhibit a wide range of sexual behaviors, the social bias of our society remains heterosexual.[8,9] Sexual dysfunctions may occur in behaviors or life-styles that do not conform to heterosexual bias, more as a result of society's intolerance of the behaviors, than in the behaviors themselves.

DEFINING CHARACTERISTICS

Lack of sexual desire is perhaps the most common sexual dysfunction people experience.[7] Transient loss of desire caused by stress, fatigue, or illness is not identified as a sexual dysfunction. Dysfunctional lack of desire is chronic and interferes with the client's sense of well-being. There are persons who have little or no sexual desire and for whom this is not a problem.

Female sexual dysfunctions include primary and secondary orgasmic dysfunction, vaginismus, and dyspareunia.[11,13] *Primary orgasmic dysfunction* is diagnosed in women who have never had orgasms. They are described as preorgasmic. *Secondary orgasmic dysfunction* describes the female who has been orgasmic in the past but, for some reason, is not currently orgasmic. *Vaginismus* is the involuntary constriction of the outer third of the vagina. This can be so severe that vaginal penetration is impossible. *Dyspareunia* means painful penetration. Penetration is sometimes possible, but it is painful to the point that the sexual experience is no longer tolerable.

Male sexual dysfunctions include primary and secondary erectile dysfunction, premature ejaculation, and inhibited ejaculation.[17] *Primary erectile dysfunction* means the inability to sustain an erection sufficient for masturbation, vaginal, or anal penetration. *Secondary erectile dysfunction* means the inability to achieve or maintain an erection sufficient for penetration in at least 25% of his sexual experiences. Most men experience transitory erectile failure at some time in their lives, and this is not significant, unless it is chronic. Dysfunctions of ejaculatory competency are characterized by premature or inhibited ejaculation. In *premature ejaculation* the man regularly ejaculates sooner than he desires. In *inhibited ejaculation* he is not able to ejaculate during penetration.

Aging women and men may experience sexual dysfunctions related to changes in the body as well as societal expectations. Aging women may experience less vaginal lubrication and a thinning of the vaginal walls, leading to painful intercourse. Aging men usually need more time to achieve an erection, ejaculation is less forceful, and the intensity of the desire to ejaculate may be less. Both aging women and men suffer from negative cultural attitudes toward their sexuality, which may reduce sexual desire or increase sexual frustration. Loss of mobility, loss of independence, and lack of available sexual partners also contribute to sexual dysfunctions among older persons.

Foremost among feelings and behaviors that can indicate the presence of a sexual dysfunction is the difficulty or inability of the client to talk about the dysfunction. Most clients are afraid and embarassed to talk about the details of their sexual behavior. This is particularly true for clients who experience sexual dysfunction. Sex role conflicts, particularly for women, become even more important to sexual functioning as both women and men try to balance their job, family, social, and personal needs. Differences people experience in sexual attitudes, sexual appetites, and sexual behaviors that do not get addressed during the formative stage of a relationship may be a clue to the presence of dissatisfying or inadequate sexual functioning. Any life change, such as change in body or body functioning, should not be overlooked when trying to capture the central characteristics of a sexual dysfunction.

A sexual dysfunction may also be reflected in a client's behavior in social and relational contexts. There may be a marked change in interest in others; isolating behaviors or conflict; or an urgent need for attention and confirmation from significant others. Clients who are dissatisfied with their sexual functioning may test out their desirability in ways that leave them feeling even worse about themselves than before (Chart 1).

NURSING PROCESS AND RATIONALE

Assessment

It is crucial to the assessment of a sexual dysfunction that the client believes that issues of sexual health can be openly discussed in the clinical setting. An open, tolerant environment is one in which the client feels free to reveal feelings of sexual pain, frustration, or inadequacy that will be heard and responded to with compassion. Listening, language, and labels are the key ingredients of an open, tolerant environment.[1] The

---

> **CHART 1**
> **Sexual Dysfunction: Definition, Related Factors, and Defining Characteristics**
>
> **DEFINITION**
>
> Sexual dysfunction is defined as a state in which a person experiences a change in sexual function that is viewed by the person as unsatisfying, unrewarding, or inadequate. The definition includes physiologic, psychological, and social components.
>
> **RELATED FACTORS**
>
> Attitudes
> Anxieties and fears
> Sexual knowledge and skills
> Social skills
> Sexual life-style
> Ethnic status
> Religion
> Sexual orientation
> Socioeconomic status
> Social roles
> Sexual abuse
> Aging
> Changes in body and body image
> Prescription and nonprescription medication
> Substance use and abuse
>
> **DEFINING CHARACTERISTICS**
>
> Lack of desire
> Primary orgasmic dysfunction
> Secondary orgasmic dysfunction
> Vaginismus
> Dyspareunia
> Primary erectile dysfunction
> Secondary erectile dysfunction
> Premature ejaculation
> Inhibited ejaculation
> Difficulty communicating about sexuality
> Sex role conflicts
> Interpersonal conflict
> Seeking attention or confirmation
> Isolating behavior

manner in which the nurse listens and the language and labels the nurse uses will either invite or close the door on the client's disclosures.

Nurses have experienced the same socializing process around sexuality that clients have experienced. Nurses, too, have personal values, beliefs, and experiences that may make listening to another's sexual history uncomfortable. This discomfort may show in the nurses' facial or body language. Clients may use language that is uncomfortable for the nurse to hear or so far out of the nurse's realm of experience that the nurse does not understand the meaning. The nurse, in turn, may use words for the client's sexual behavior that frighten the patient. Words such as *perversion, deviant,* and *abnormal* have a judgmental tone. They label, rather than describe. Labels such as *frigid* or *impotent* have powerful negative connotations in the vernacular. The most helpful posture for the nurse is to assess the patient's feelings and to use language that accurately describes sexual behavior, rather than labels that judge.

There are five appropriate and helpful assessment questions a nurse can ask a client.[1]

1. What is the sexual problem from your point of view?
2. How long has this been a problem?
3. What do you think is the cause of the problem?
4. What have you done about it up to now?
5. What do you want to be different?

It is also essential to carefully assess the client's health history and determine the use of prescription and non-prescription drugs. This includes clarifying dosage levels, frequency, and length of use.

Nursing Diagnosis

After a complete analysis of the assessment data, the nurse is then ready to establish a nursing diagnosis of sexual dysfunction. The accuracy of the nursing diagnosis is partially a reflection of the ease with which the client and the nurse have been able to confront their anxieties around discussing the client's sexual dysfunction. An example of a nursing diagnosis for a particular client is sexual dysfunction (rarely has orgasms) related to anxiety and misinformation.

Client Goals and Nursing Interventions

Clients bring a sexual history, sexual worries and concerns, and some degree of accurate or inaccurate sexual knowledge into the health-care setting. Communication skills around sexual concerns range from nonexistent to excellent. Clients may present with sexual dysfunctions in any inpatient or outpatient setting. Because personal sexual thoughts and behaviors are generally private, the client "goes public" by revealing a sexual dysfunction to a health care provider. The nurse may well be the first person ever to hear a client's sexual concerns. The sexual concerns may become a primary focus of the health care or become a less central issue.

There are factors in nurses' own personal histories and beliefs about sexuality that may interfere with this interaction. Nurses may avoid responding to clients' sexual concerns because of their own discomfort in talking about sex. They may have strong reactions to a client's sexual attitudes and practices. They may have no experience dealing with the sexual issues of persons with sexual life-styles different from their own. Nurses may believe that they have to be experts in the field of human sexuality before they can invite clients to pre-

sent their sexual concerns. However, assessing for sexual concerns does not mean the nurse has to treat the concern. In addition, nurses can prepare themselves for this role by examining their own sexual values and beliefs, understanding their own sexual histories, learning about human sexuality, and assessing the limits of their competency to deal with sexual concerns. They can familiarize themselves with the specific sexual health concerns of persons from different cultural, ethnic, and religious backgrounds. They can familiarize themselves with the sexual health needs of people of all sexual orientations or affectional preferences.

Although client goals for those with the nursing diagnosis of sexual dysfunction vary with the unique situation, there are some commonalities. It is expected that the client will feel more comfortable in discussing sexual concerns. New information about sexual functioning will be learned or previous misinformation will be corrected. The client gains an understanding of stress or other underlying etiologic factors. Finally, the client will learn new behavioral strategies and techniques.

Woods describes the different roles nurses have in assisting clients with sexual health.[16] These roles are determined by the nurse's personal comfort level, expertise, and the health care setting. The nursing roles include (1) influencing the health care setting, (2) giving permission and validating feelings, (3) teaching, (4) counseling new behavior strategies, and (5) providing resources. The nursing role thus runs from the most simple to the most complex, from one-time, intake contact to ongoing therapist.

The nurse can influence the health-care setting and, thereby, anticipate clients' sexual concerns in a number of ways. Written and verbal communications can validate sexuality as a part of total health care. Brochures and handouts dealing with sexuality as it relates to the specific health care setting can be prominently displayed. Intake forms and health assessment forms should include questions that elicit clients' sexual concerns. Such questions can include: "Your sexual health is important to us. Are there any sexual concerns you would like help with?" "How has this (presenting health concern) affected your sexuality?" Privacy to talk, assurances of confidentiality, and time to talk are important signals to clients that sexuality concerns are valued.

The nurse can encourage a client to discuss sexual concerns by validating the client's fears or anxieties in talking about the concern. Signaling this kind of permission to talk about a sexual concern empowers a client. Validating and normalizing sexual fears and anxieties is the most common form of nurse–client interaction in dealing with sexual concerns. A client may worry about sexual fantasies that involve a person other than the client's sexual partner. The nurse may reassure the client that such fantasies are common and are quite separate from reality. Clients may be looking for permission to continue a sexual behavior, to stop a sexual behavior, or to change a sexual behavior.

Clients have a responsibility not to violate their own or others' moral codes or legal codes with their behaviors.

Giving information is an educational function. The role of educator about sexual health concerns involves a different level of expertise from permission giving. Information needed may include such topics as fertility, fertility control, and the effects of medication on sexual desire and sexual functioning. Clients need information and education in adapting their sexual behaviors to changes in life stage, body changes caused by illness or surgery, or changes in sexual beliefs and attitudes.

The nurse may counsel new behavioral strategies, that is, make specific suggestions that clients are encouraged to try on their own. This implies an even higher level of sexual knowledge and intervention skills for the nurse. Examples of specific suggestions include suggesting ways for a woman to talk to a sexual partner about her feelings after a mastectomy. A man who is ejaculating sooner than he desires is given specific techniques for attempting to lengthen the time between his arousal and ejaculation.

A final role for all nurses is that of resource person. Nurses can develop a resource and information bank. Such a resource bank can be used for the nurse's own professional growth and development, for client education and intervention, and for the growth and education of other health care persons in the nurse's work environment. Bibliographies, addresses of book stores that carry educational books on sexuality, community resource agencies for sexual health, law enforcement numbers, therapists and their specialities, all are invaluable resources to have at hand in the health care setting.

Evaluation

Criteria for evaluation must often compete with unrealistic societal expectations for sexual behavior. For example, client expectations for the number of orgasms or duration of erection may be based on fears of being in some way abnormal or inadequate. The criteria are thus stated in behavioral terms that are free of the expectations of sexual myths and misinformation. Even when nurse and patient seem to agree on how the success of interventions will be evaluated, the client may continue to harbor secret expectations of "the way it is supposed to be."

There must be sufficient opportunity to monitor the client's progress in meeting the intervention goals. When a client's discomfort with dealing with sexual issues is high, noncompliance becomes a major issue. This is also true if the client is also dealing with a sexual partner who is uncomfortable with, or threatened by, the intervention.

In modifying an intervention plan based on evaluation feedback, the client may need permission and encouragement to try other intervention strategies. For example, it may be very difficult for a client with rigid sexual beliefs and behaviors to tolerate changes in that system. The nurse's suggestions for modifying an intervention initially may not be acceptable to the client (Chart 2).

CHART 2
Sexual Dysfunction: Summary of the Nursing Process

NURSING INTERVENTIONS	OUTCOME CRITERIA
CLIENT GOAL: FEEL COMFORTABLE DISCUSSING SEXUAL CONCERNS	
Influence the health care setting so that sexual concerns can be acknowledged	
Include sexual health as part of nursing assessment	
Utilize interventions that give permission to discuss feelings about sexuality	Brings up sexual concerns
CLIENT GOAL: GAIN AN INCREASED UNDERSTANDING OF SEXUAL FUNCTIONING	
Assess for inaccurate information	
Discuss information relevant to client's sexual concerns (e.g., effect of medications on sexual function)	
Share educational resources	
Refer to sources of further information	Verbalizes accurate information about sexuality
CLIENT GOAL: UNDERSTAND MORE ABOUT ISSUES INVOLVED IN ETIOLOGY OF SEXUAL DYSFUNCTION	
Discuss stress, medication, and other causes of sexual dysfunction	
If appropriate, refer for medical evaluation of possible causes of sexual dysfunction	Seeks medical evaluation
CLIENT GOAL: LEARN NEW BEHAVIORAL STRATEGIES	
Counsel client concerning relationship issues that may interfere with sexual functioning	
Make specific suggestions concerning new behaviors for increasing sexual functioning	Discusses concerns with partner Tries and evaluates specific suggestions

CASE STUDY

A 47-year-old man came to an outpatient mental health clinic and requested to talk with a male nurse or male doctor. He had just moved to this community and had no regular doctor. He seemed hesitant and anxious. He described himself as being "stressed out" over the move and as not expecting such an intense reaction to this change in his life. He and his wife of 25 years had grown children, and this was the first time they had been away from family and friends and living in a community new to them. He described the marriage as good; however, he recently could not "satisfy" his wife sexually. He stated he "didn't feel like a man" and that his wife might be better off with someone else. He described his wife as frustrated and angry with their sex life.

The initial assessment revealed that he had erections upon awakening in the morning; however they did not last long enough to attempt intercourse. He occasionally tried to masturbate, but was unsuccessful. He was also uncomfortable talking with his wife about the problem. When asked about prescription drugs and alcohol use, he stated that he was drinking at least two beers a day, which was more than usual for him. He was taking no medication.

The initial diagnosis was sexual dysfunction (erectile dysfunction) related to stress from the move. Together the client and the nurse decided upon two initial goals for the client: (1) experience increased comfort level in talking about his sexual concerns, and (2) understand the diagnosis and options for treatment.

The nurse praised the client for asking for help with his sexual concerns and explained that he was not alone with this problem and that it was helpful to discuss his feelings about himself as a sexual person. The client was assured that it was not unusual to have feelings of anxiety, sadness, or depression, especially when he was not able to be sexual in his usual manner. He was told that it was sometimes easier to talk with a spouse after talking to a health care provider first. The nurse also explained that further tests needed to be done and described the procedure and rationale. The client was encouraged to ask questions as they came up about the tests and procedures. The nurse also shared information about the effects of stress and alcohol on sexual behavior. Information was given about the psychological and physiologic causes of erectile dysfunction. A specific medical assessment to rule out any related organic causes was recommended. The client and the nurse worked out a plan to review treatment options upon receipt of the medical report.

SUMMARY

Sexual functioning and, therefore, sexual dysfunction can be related to physiologic, psychological, sociologic, and spiritual aspects of life. Because of the range of societal and individual attitudes and behaviors around sexuality, a definition of sexual dysfunction must be client centered. A dysfunction must be viewed from the client's description of unsatisfying or inadequate feelings or behaviors.

Sexual attitudes, sexual anxiety and fears, sexual information and skills, and social skills, all are factors related to sexual dysfunction. The most common female sexual dysfunctions are primary and secondary orgasmic dysfunction, vaginismus, and dyspareunia. The most common male sexual dysfunctions are primary and secondary erectile dysfunction, premature ejaculation, and inhibited ejaculation. Sexual dysfunctions may also arise from aging, changes in body and self-image, changes in life-style, and conflicts in values.

Assessment of sexual dysfunction is a process by which nurse and client gather data to decide the most appropriate goals and interventions. Sexual data gathering may be influenced by denial, embarassment, or lack of knowledge and communication skills around sexuality. The assessment questions are designed to elicit information from the client about the nature of the dysfunction, its duration, the client's perception of the cause, attempts to alleviate the symptoms, and the desired outcome. Particular attention is paid to the client's health history and medications.

The nursing diagnosis and the goals for intervention are clarified in behavioral terms. Care is taken to ensure that the goals are realistic and free of overt or covert sexual myths and societal expectations. Intervention strategies reflect the many facets of the nursing

Research Highlights

Major progress has been made in recent years in the treatment of erectile dysfunction in men. Because of assessment and treatment techniques being developed in the medical field, the focus on the causes of erectile dysfunction are shifting to include medical as well as psychological causes.

Slag and his colleagues studied the erectile dysfunctions of 188 men in a medical outpatient clinic.[12] The age of the sample was 59.4 plus or minus 1.3 years. Only 14% of the evaluated men showed psychogenic causes of their dysfunction. The following medical diagnoses were identified for the remaining men: medication effect, 25%; neurologic, 7%; urologic, 6%; primary hypogonadism, 10%; secondary hypogonadism, 9%; diabetes mellitus, 9%; hypothyroidism, 5%; hyperthyroidism, 1%; hyperprolactinemia, 4%; miscellaneous, 4%; and unknown causes, 7%. Screening for alcoholism revealed 7% of the men to be alcoholic. The study points out the prevalence of related medical factors in erectile dysfunction, particularly in older men. The authors note that general medical and psychological assessments may well miss hormonal and medication factors influencing erectile dysfunction. This study points out the complexity of the etiology of erectile dysfunction. Therefore, the nurse should be sure that there is an opportunity for thorough and in-depth assessments of both medical and psychological aspects.

role: encouraging disclosure of sexual concerns, sharing information, offering specific suggestions, and acting as community health-care resource person.

Evaluation of the intervention strategies includes the opportunity to modify them if necessary. Attempts to be flexible and creative in designing modifications may meet with resistance on the part of clients who have a narrow definition of the purpose of sex and sexuality.

References

1. Annon J. The behavioral treatment of sexual problems, vol 1. Brief therapy. Honolulu: Enabling Systems; 1975.
2. Calderone M, Johnson E. The family book about sexuality. New York: Harper & Row; 1981.
3. Dickman G, Livingston C. Sex and the female ostomate. Los Angeles: United Ostomy Association; 1982.
4. Hammond DC. Screening for sexual dysfunction. Clin Obstet Gynecol. 1984;27:732–737.
5. Hogan R. Human sexuality: a nursing perspective. New York: Appleton–Century–Crofts; 1980.
6. House WC, Pendleton L. Sexual dysfunction in diabetes. Postgrad Med. 1986;79:227–235.
7. Kapland HS. Disorders of sexual desire. New York: Simon & Schuster; 1979.
8. Kinsey AC, Pomeroy WB, Martin CW. Sexual behavior in the human male. Philadelphia: WB Saunders; 1948.
9. Kinsey AC, Pomeroy WB, Martin CW. Sexual behavior in the human female. Philadelphia: WB Saunders; 1953.
10. Kim MJ, McFarland GK, McLane AM. Pocket guide to nursing diagnosis. 3rd ed. St Louis: CV Mosby; 1989.
11. LaFerla JJ. Inhibited sexual desire and orgasmic dysfunction in women. Clin Obstet Gynecol. 1984;27:738–749.
12. Slag MF, Morley JE, Elson MK. Impotence in medical clinic outpatients. JAMA. 1983;249:1736–1740.
13. Steege JF. Dyspareunia and vaginismus. Clin Obstet Gynecol. 1984;27:750–759.
14. Stockdale-Woolley R. Sexual dysfunction and COPD: problems and management. Nurse Pract. 1983;2:16–17, 20.
15. Thompson WL. Sexual problems in chronic respiratory disease. Postgrad Med. 1986;79:41–44, 47, 50–52.
16. Woods NF. Human sexuality in health and illness. 3rd ed. St Louis: CV Mosby; 1984.
17. Zilbergeld B. Male sexuality. Boston: Little, Brown & Co; 1978.

SLEEP PATTERN DISTURBANCE

Martha J. Lentz

DEFINITION AND DESCRIPTION

A child awakens during the night, a young adult cannot get to sleep, or an older adult awakens in the early morning and tries but cannot return to sleep. All of these people are experiencing disruption in the desired pattern of sleep. To understand the different alterations in sleep patterns that can occur, it is necessary to consider what are typical patterns of sleep and how typical patterns of sleep vary across the life span.

Sleep is only one portion of the sleep–wake cycle and needs to be considered in the context of the person's total daily experience. As can be seen from the examples just cited, not being able to go to sleep at a desired time or awakening too early results in alterations in the timing of sleep within the total day's sleep–wake cycle. In assessing a client's pattern of sleep, not only the amount, but the location in the daily sleep–wake cycle is significant. In addition, within-sleep pattern alterations of sleep stages can also exist. Such within-sleep alterations, which can only be evaluated by electrophysiologic measurement, may also influence the person's waking experience. *Sleep pattern disturbance* then can be defined as a deviation in the amount of sleep or timing of the sleep period from that desired by the client and needed for adequate daytime functioning.

THEORY AND RESEARCH
Electrophysiology of Sleep

Sleep stages are defined by characteristic patterns of brain waves that predominate in each 20- to 30-second epoch of electroencephalographic (EEG) recording. Five sleep stages have been defined (Fig. 13-24). Stage 1 through stage 4 are classified as non-rapid eye movement (non-REM or NREM) sleep. The fifth stage is called REM (rapid eye movement) sleep and takes its name from the rapid eye movements that occur during this sleep. REM sleep is the stage in which most dreaming occurs, particularly dreams that are more bizarre combining person, place, and events that could not exist together in everyday life.

As a person enters sleep and progresses through the first four sleep stages the brain waves become progressively slower and higher in amplitude. When awake, brain activity shows desynchronized activity with low-amplitude, high-frequency waves occurring at 18 to 30 cycles per second (cps). If the eyes are closed and the person is quiet, alpha-rhythm predominates at 8 to 14 cps and with a larger amplitude. As the person becomes drowsy the brain waves slow further, developing theta-waves that occur at 4 to 7 cps, with still higher amplitude. The eyes develop long slow-rolling movements as stage 1 sleep is entered, the percentage of alpha-waves decreases to less than 50% per 30-second epoch. When awakened from stage 1 sleep, an individual will probably deny having been asleep.[10]

As the brain waves slow further, sleep deepens and the person enters stage 2 sleep. Stage 2 sleep is characterized by two distinct wave forms—sleep spindles and K-complexes. Sleep spindles are bursts of activity of 12 to 14 cps and are named sleep spindles because, as recorded on polygraph paper, they look like a spindle. This is the only waveform that is entirely unique to sleep and is never seen during waking. The K-complexes are large waves exceeding 75 μV and lasting half a second, that occur spontaneously in stage 2 sleep. In waking, K-complexes can be evoked by external stimulation. When awakened from stage 2 sleep, individuals generally agree that they have been asleep.[10]

As sleep deepens further, the person becomes more difficult to arouse, brain waves are very slow and synchronized. Delta-waves, which characterize stages 3 and 4, are waves lasting longer than half a second and are 75 μV or greater in amplitude. Stage 3 contains 20% to 50% delta-waves per 30-second epoch, and stage 4 has more than 50% delta-waves per 30-second epoch. These stages are often considered together and may be called delta sleep or slow-wave sleep.[10]

The fifth stage of sleep is REM sleep. This sleep is often called dream sleep or paradoxical sleep. It is called dream sleep because this is when dreaming in vivid or bizarre appearance takes place. When awakened from REM sleep, individuals will often report that they have been dreaming. This sleep is also called paradoxical sleep because the brain waves are nearly as fast as in the awake stage, but the person is most resistant to arousal from external stimulation. Electromyographic (EMG) levels reach the lowest levels, as there is central atonia with occasional twitches of the extremities. All these changes accompany the characteristic bursts of rapid eye movements. Each of the sleep stages recur across the night in a cyclic manner.[10]

Sleep Stage Distribution

During sleep, the individual typically passes through each of the sleep stages in a cycle lasting approximately

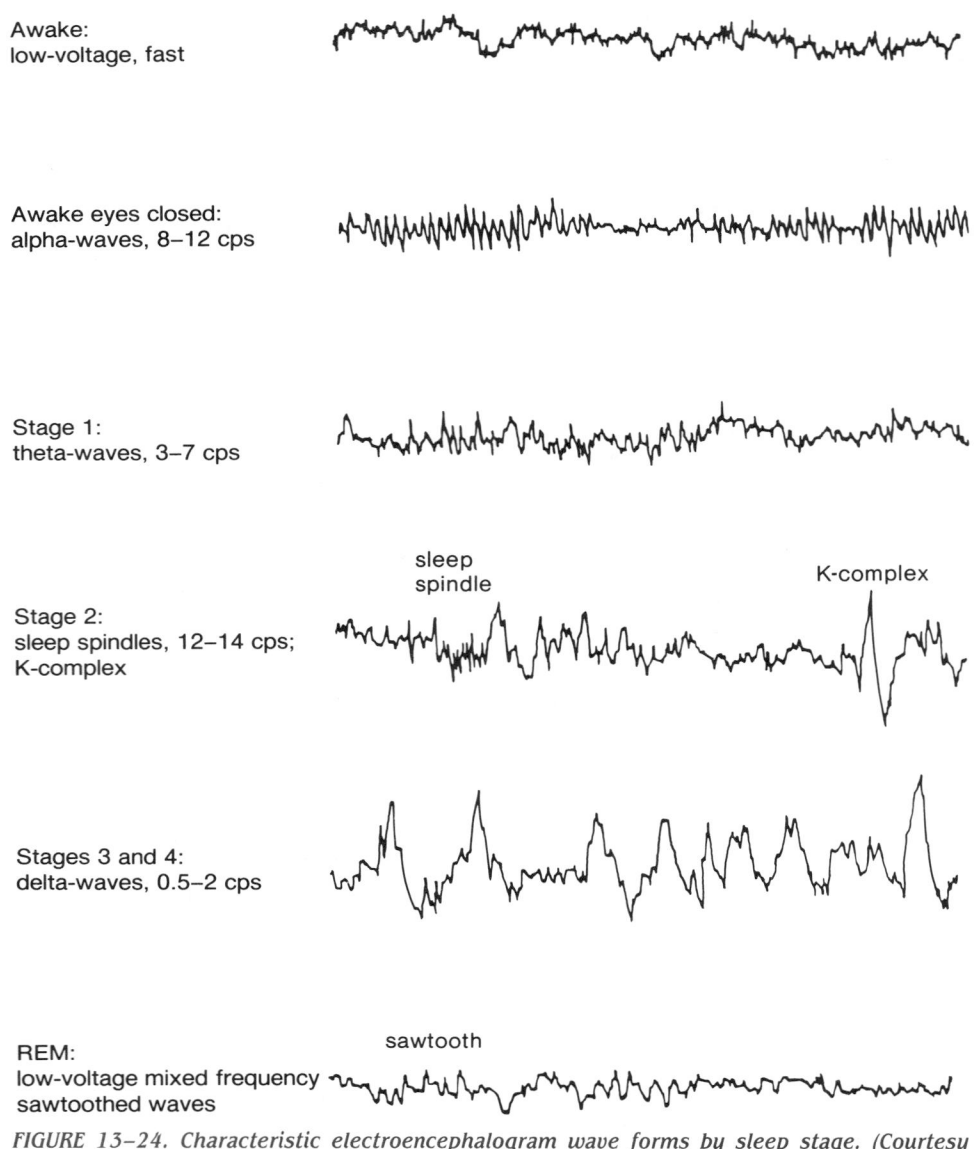

Awake:
low-voltage, fast

Awake eyes closed:
alpha-waves, 8–12 cps

Stage 1:
theta-waves, 3–7 cps

Stage 2:
sleep spindles, 12–14 cps;
K-complex

sleep
spindle

K-complex

Stages 3 and 4:
delta-waves, 0.5–2 cps

REM:
low-voltage mixed frequency
sawtoothed waves

sawtooth

FIGURE 13–24. Characteristic electroencephalogram wave forms by sleep stage. (Courtesy University of Washington School of Nursing, Sleep Laboratory)

60 to 120 minutes for the young adult. The amount of time spent in each stage varies individually and with age. The percentage of time spent in each of the sleep stages differs from the first third of the sleep period to the last third of the sleep period.

Infants typically spend a much greater proportion of the total day in sleep and have much greater proportion of REM sleep (often called active sleep) than do adults. By the time children are of school age they will have essentially adult values of sleep. The typical young adult will spend approximately 50% of sleep time in stage 2, 20% in stages 3 and 4, and 25% in REM. Most stage 3 and 4 sleep will occur in the first half of the night. The REM periods will increase in length during the last half of the sleep period. In older adults, sleep is less consolidated than in younger adults. The older adult typically changes sleep stages more often and

enters stage 1 or awakens more frequently than young adults (Fig. 13-25). Stages 3 and 4 decrease and may disappear by the time individuals are in their 60s. Sleep efficiency decreases, more time is spent in bed to obtain the same amount of sleep obtained by younger adults. Using objective EEG measures of sleep, women appear to maintain their sleep stage structures better than men, but complain more of sleep disturbances.[7,17]

Physiological Changes Within Sleep

Sleep is often thought of as just involving brain activity. As described in the foregoing, sleep stages are primarily based on alterations in electrical brain wave activity; however, physiologic changes throughout the body accompany sleep. Physiologic changes start to occur be-

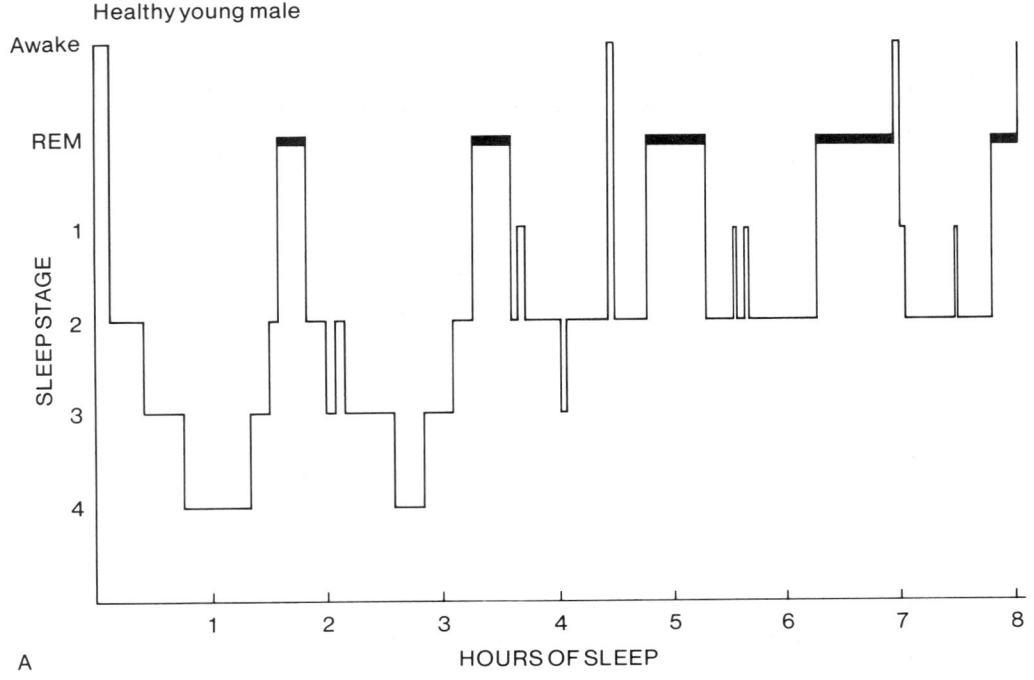

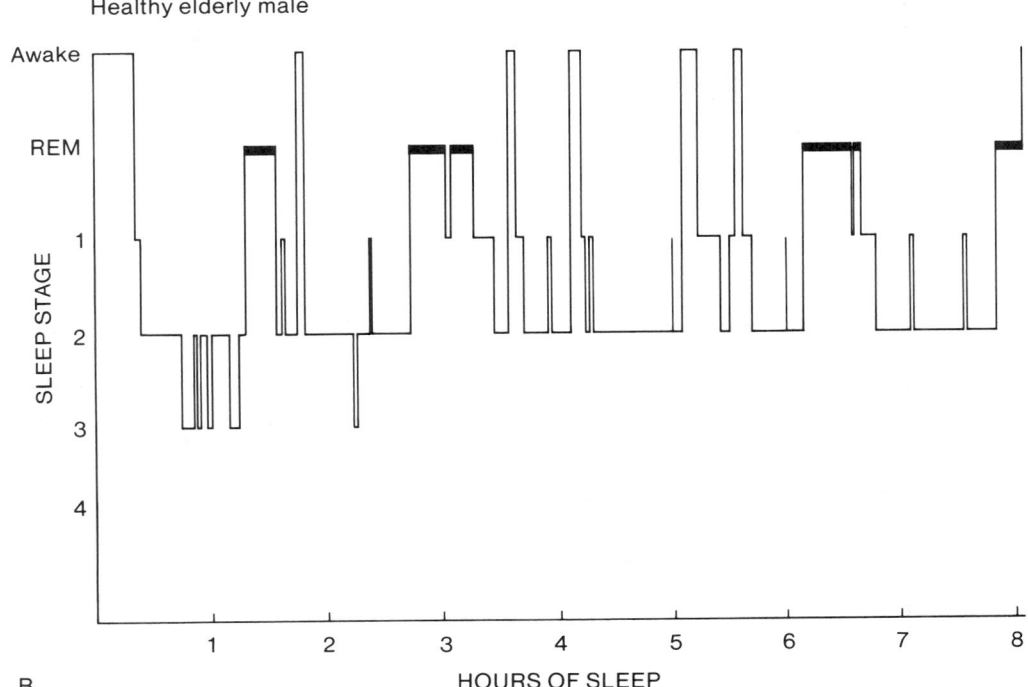

FIGURE 13–25. (A) Hypnogram of one-night's sleep of young male. Note that there are only two awakenings and distribution of stage 3, stage 4, and REM sleep. (B) Hypnogram of one night's sleep of elderly male. Note multiple awakenings, increased stage shifts, and small amount of stage 3 sleep. (Courtesy University of Washington School of Nursing, Sleep Laboratory)

fore sleep; approximately an hour before sleep the body temperature begins to fall, and the rate of temperature fall accelerates with sleep onset.[4] As the person enters stage 2, muscles relax and respiration becomes slow and regular. Blood pressure and pulse rate are low-

ered.[15] During stages 3 and 4, there is a surge in growth hormone secretion.[16] Throughout NREM sleep a stable low level of physiologic activity is maintained (Table 13-16).

The stability and level of physiologic activity change

Table 13-16

Characteristics of sleep stages and associated physiologic characteristics

SLEEP STAGE	POLYSOMOGRAPHIC INDICES	PHYSIOLOGIC CHARACTERISTICS
Stage 1	Less than 50% alpha-wave Appearance of theta-waves Long slow-rolling eye movements High electromyogram (EMG)	Lowered body temperature Decreased heart rate and blood pressure Decreased respiratory rate
Stage 2	Sleep spindle 12–14 cps Spontaneous K-complex greater than 75 μV, last a minimum 0.5 sec Lowered EMG level	Lowered body temperature Decreased heart rate and blood pressure Slow deep regular respiration
Stage 3	Delta-wave 75 μV, $\geq$0.5 sec; occupy 30%–50% of epoch	Lowered body temperature Decreased heart rate and blood pressure
Stage 4	Delta-wave 75 μV, $\geq$0.5 sec; occupy >50% of epoch	Growth hormone released Few body movements
REM	Fast mixed frequency waves Rapid eye movements Very low EMG levels	Reduced autonomic control of heart rate, blood pressure, respiration and thermoregulation Penile erection Increased brain blood flow

dramatically when a person enters REM sleep. With the onset of REM sleep, a central atonia occurs, the postural muscles of the neck and the muscles of the jaw relax. This central atonia is accompanied by occasional jerking movements of hand, wrists, feet, and ankle.[6] Autonomic control is reduced; thermoregulation is lost; blood pressure, heart rate, and respiration become more variable.[15]

RELATED FACTORS

Difficulties initiating and maintaining sleep may be transient or persistent and may be associated with age (discussed earlier); psychophysiologic arousal; psychiatric disorders; drug or alcohol use; travels across time zones; or shift work.

Transient sleep disruption from psychophysiologic arousal may last up to three or four weeks and is associated with a specific event or situation. Such situations can include loss of a loved one, beginning a new job, moving to a new school, ending of a relationship, or travel and vacations. These events or situations result in an acute emotional arousal, with the person experiencing difficulty in falling asleep, staying asleep, or awakening too early in the morning.[1]

Difficulty in initiating and maintaining sleep is often associated with psychiatric disorders. Some examples of conditions having altered sleep patterns are mood disorders, such as bipolar disorder and major depression. In bipolar disorder during a manic episode, the client may sleep only a few hours a night, but report not needing more sleep. In a major depressive episode, a client may experience inadequate sleep or hypersomnia on a daily basis. With a melancholic type of depression, early-morning awakening may be experienced. Sleep pattern disturbance also may occur in conjunction with organic mental syndromes (e.g., delirium with disturbance of the sleep–wake cycle). Treatment of the psychiatric disorder results in an improvement of the sleep pattern.

Many drugs have the potential to affect sleep, particularly those that alter the level of neurotransmitters (norepinephrine or serotonin) or alter receptor sites. For example, tricyclic antidepressants and monamine oxidase inhibitors, by their action on serotonin pathways, are associated with decreased REM sleep. Lithium also decreases REM sleep and increases slow-wave sleep. Commonly consumed drugs, such as caffeine and alcohol, also affect sleep composition and timing. Many other drugs, even those without expected central effects, do influence sleep composition and duration. When evaluating sleep pattern disruption, attention to all drugs being used is usually warranted as a possible source of sleep imbalance. Altered sleep patterns secondary to drug or alcohol use are best dealt with by treating the initiating causes.[11]

Traveling across time zones or working non-daytime shifts requires that an individual initiate and maintain sleep during times that they would normally be awake. The socially desired time of sleep is thus out of phase with the usual circadian timing of sleep. For each hour of time zone shift, approximately one day is required for adjustment to the new time. Adjustment is easier when travel is in a westward direction, because there is a delay in timing, as opposed to eastward travel, which requires an advance in the circadian timing. Adjustment to shift work is similar, but with the added difficulty that the surrounding social cues do not support the individual's need to change the timing of the sleep period.

Other medical conditions may result in sleep pattern

disruption by requiring the person to awaken to breathe, as in sleep apnea in which breathing repeatedly stops, or because of sudden body movements, as in nocturnal myoclonus in which there is rapid repeated jerking of the legs. The presence of pain or the inability to maintain a sleep conducive position may also disrupt sleep.

DEFINING CHARACTERISTICS

Because sleep is not a single unitary activity, but rather, represents a complex of neurologic and behavioral patterns, there are correspondingly a number of different elements that can be seen as alterations in sleep patterns. The timing of sleep disruptions can serve as a starting place for identifying characteristics of different patterns of sleep alterations. The sleep alteration may be one of difficulty initiating or maintaining sleep, or it could be characterized by excessive daytime sleeping. A disordered sleep–wake schedule can include timing of consolidated sleep to a non-socially acceptable time, as when a person cannot sleep before 3 A.M., but then has a normal sleep period of seven to eight hours duration. A disordered sleep–wake schedule is encountered during travel across time zones or when doing shift work.[1]

In addition to the timing of sleep, the duration of the sleep disruption and the presence of other conditions provides information. Persistent psychophysiologic disruption of sleep lasts longer than three to four weeks and probably represents a mutual reinforcement of chronic somatized tension, anxiety, and a negative conditioning to sleep. Lying down to attempt sleep can result in a worry or dread of being unable to sleep that increases arousal to the point that the person is indeed unable to initiate sleep. Persons with a long history of sleep difficulty will often identify the onset of poor sleep in relation to a specific stressful event, thus supporting the idea of the learned or conditioned development from the transient psychophysiologic arousal sleep alterations.[1] The presence of excessive daytime sleepiness, or even decreased daytime alertness, is a clear indicator of difficulty with achieving adequate sleep (Chart 1).

NURSING PROCESS AND RATIONALE

Assessment

The "gold standard" for determining sleep duration and pattern is by electrophysiologic measurements. However, nurses seldom have access to electrophysiologic sleep measurements when trying to evaluate a client's sleep status and, thus, must rely on other techniques, primarily self-report and observations.[12]

SELF-REPORT

Self-report of sleep may be obtained by a general question, such as, "Did you have a good night's sleep?"

CHART 1
Sleep Pattern Disturbance: Definition, Related Factors, and Defining Characteristics

DEFINITION

Sleep pattern disturbance is a deviation in the amount of sleep or timing of the sleep period from that desired by the client and needed for adequate daytime functioning.

RELATED FACTORS

Age
Psychophysiologic arousal
Psychiatric disorders
  Mood disorders: bipolar and depression
  Organic mental syndromes: delirium
Drug use
Alcohol use
Travel across time zones
Shift work
Other health conditions

DEFINING CHARACTERISTICS

Timing of sleep
  Difficulty initiating sleep
  Early morning awakening
  Unable to sleep at desired time
Inability to maintain sleep
Length of time sleep difficulty has been experienced
  Short-term or situational: fewer than three to four weeks
  Chronic: longer than four weeks
Daytime sleepiness or lowered level of alertness

However, general questions that ask about difficulty with going to sleep or staying asleep are especially likely to result in underreporting of sleep problems by men.[14] A specific rating scale or structured questions on the timing of sleep events may also be used. Specific questions (e.g., "How long did it take you to go to sleep?" or "How many times did you awaken?") elicit responses that are in closer agreement with electrophysiologic sleep measures. Good sleepers are usually able to accurately estimate the number of minutes it takes to fall asleep and the number of awakenings during the night. The number of nighttime awakenings reported will closely reflect awakenings of four minutes or longer.[2] Persons experiencing insomnia are often less able to estimate the length of time taken to fall asleep. This may be the result of several factors. Because they do take longer to fall asleep, they are trying to estimate a greater range of time and the transition to sleeping may be less discrete. The person experiencing insomnia often has several initial brief periods of stage 2 sleep, with episodes of being awake, before achieving consolidated stage 2 sleep.[5] Even good sleepers have difficulty accurately identifying that they have really been asleep when awakened from stage 2 and stage 4 sleep and asked if they have been asleep or awake. Furthermore, even when correct about sleep status, they lacked confidence in the accuracy of their perceptions of having been asleep. They were, however, accurate and confident in reporting having been awake when they were contacted during an awake episode and asked if they had been asleep or awake.[13] The uncertainty of having been asleep when awakening may contribute to clients, who experience intermittent nighttime awakening, reporting that they have not slept at all during the night.[8]

Information about the perceived adequacy of sleep (i.e., how well rested the person felt upon awakening) can only be elicited from the perspective of the client's experience. Questions about daytime performance and feelings of fatigue also provide further information on the quality of the sleep experience. The best test of sleep adequacy is whether or not the person feels rested, alert, and able to function in the manner desired during the day. The daytime functioning information is particularly relevant in hypersomnia (excessive sleepiness) conditions, such as in sleep apnea. In conditions such as sleep apnea, the nighttime sleep is extremely fragmented, but the individuals are so fatigued that they are unaware of the extreme sleep disruption, and daytime performance decrements will be their primary complaint.

OBSERVATION

Observational techniques are often used by nurses to assess the sleep status of clients. Observations are typically made every half hour to every hour. Specific client behaviors that are used to indicate sleep are relaxed recumbent posture, eyes closed, and slow, even respirations. In some situations when the nurse is making observation, the client is asked to speak or lift a hand if awake. If the client movement is detected, it is important to distinguish between intentional movement and the involuntary movements of finger, wrists, feet, and ankles associated with REM sleep. Major movements that may be associated with sleep stage changes and involve turning over or repositioning require a longer period of observation to see if the respirations and posture indicate continued sleep.

Nursing Diagnosis

The diagnostic category of sleep pattern disturbance is utilized in making a specific nursing diagnosis for a particular client. The nursing diagnosis will usually include both a statement of the particular pattern of sleep alteration and a secondary statement related to factors influencing or contributing to the occurrence of that pattern. For example, a diagnosis might be stated as: sleep pattern disturbance related to poor sleep hygiene.

Client Goals and Nursing Interventions

Sleep is a complex phenomenon, because many things both internally and externally can influence a person's ability to achieve a good night's sleep. Fortunately, a number of rather simple acts and avoidances can contribute to improved sleep. The collection of activities are often referred to as sleep hygiene. They include avoiding arousing activities immediately before trying to sleep; avoiding doing irritating activities (e.g., working on an unpleasant project such as filling out income tax forms); avoiding interesting activity, such as reading an exciting murder mystery that can waken such a high level of interest that sleep is difficult to initiate. In addition, chemical stimulants, such as caffeine and alcohol, should be avoided. Alcohol is often taken by people to try and improve sleep because of its initial depressant effect. The result, unfortunately, is that even though the person may fall asleep quickly, arousal rebound with awakening in the night and difficulty returning to sleep is often experienced. Many medications also contain stimulating substances and should be avoided before the sleep period.

Although many activities, such as the foregoing, interfere in easily obtaining sleep onset, there are also many activities that can assist in achieving sleep. Exercise that causes a sense of fatigue is desirable at some time during the day, but should cease approximately two hours before trying to sleep. Development of an environment that is conducive to sleep, including a comfortable sleeping surface, either hard or soft, in an area of reduced light and noise is useful. When in the sleeping area, all cues should indicate that it is a place for sleep, rather than, for example, watching television. The sleeping area should be a secure as well as a comfortable place. People who live alone or in high crime areas may report waking up to every little sound, and they are essentially remaining vigilant to protect themselves against environmental threat at the expense of good sleep. A good dead bolt on the bedroom door and a telephone at the bedside to call for help may be the best sleeping aids for them.

Of great importance to good sleep is a regular sleep schedule. Levels of sleepiness vary across the 24 hours, and it is much easier to initiate sleep in conjunction with a sleepy phase than an awake phase. A regular sleep schedule contributes to a regular timing of body rhythms and allows the timing of trying to initiate sleep to coincide with an increased sleepiness phase.

Evaluation

Nurses can evaluate the extent to which their interventions have been effective by noting how well the client initiates and maintains sleep during the desired time for sleep. The client's reported satisfaction with sleep, feeling of alertness, and capacity to function adequately during the daytime provide further information on the effectiveness of sleep measures (Chart 2).

CHART 2
Sleep Pattern Disturbance: Summary of the Nursing Process

NURSING INTERVENTIONS	OUTCOME CRITERIA
CLIENT GOAL: UNDERSTAND PROBABLE CAUSE OF SLEEP PATTERN ALTERATION	
Obtain history of client's usual sleep pattern (time, presleep routine)	Specific probable causes are identified
Check for environmental factors disrupting sleep (e.g., light, noise)	
Assist client to identify subjective experience which might interfere with sleep (e.g., worries, pain, anxiety)	
Identify medication effects that might interfere with sleep (include prescription and nonprescription)	
Identify consumption of stimulants or depressants that have rebound (e.g., caffeine, alcohol, nicotine)	
Assist client to identify daytime activities that interfere with sleep (e.g., exercise, naps)	
CLIENT GOAL: INITIATE SLEEP IN LESS THAN 20 MINUTES	
Schedule sleep period for usual sleep time	Goes to sleep in less than 20 minutes
Provide opportunity for presleep routines	
Provide quiet, secure, comfortable sleep environment	
Encourage client to limit intake of caffeine, alcohol, and nicotine to early in day	
Provide opportunity for client to deal with anxiety and worries during the day	
CLIENT GOAL: EXPERIENCE FEW NIGHTTIME AWAKENINGS	
Maintain quiet secure sleep environment	Reports few awakenings
When in hospital setting, minimize and group necessary procedures and assessments	Reports having slept soundly
	Is rested
Encourage client to continue limiting caffeine, alcohol, and nicotine to early in day	

Research Highlights

Daily or nightly, nurses endeavor to assess clients' sleep status. Although electrophysiologic measurements of brain activity is considered the standard for determining sleep status, this procedure is rarely if ever accessible to the nurses. An important research question thus becomes how comparable are different sleep assessment techniques. Kupher and colleagues[9] compared nurses' evaluation of sleep with electroencephalographic (EEG) measures of sleep. Clients hospitalized with the diagnoses of depression (N = 12), schizophrenia (N = 7), or manic-depressive disorder (N = 1) were evaluated for a total of 450 nights. Standard EEG measures were used. The nurses used the established protocol of observing the client every half hour and determining if the client was awake or asleep. Criteria used included eyes closed, relaxed and immobile posture, regular respiration, and apparent unresponsiveness to environmental stimuli. There was good agreement in nursing assessment of sleep status with the EEG measures for the seven clients who had a diagnosis of schizophrenia and for four of the twelve clients who had a diagnosis of depression. There was poor agreement on the observed versus EEG measures for the remainder of the clients. The nurses generally erred in reporting the clients were asleep, when the EEG indicated they were awake. However, on several occasions the nurses evaluated the clients as being awake, but the

EEG measures indicated that the clients were sleeping. The authors concluded that the immobility of the clients with depression resulted in the nurses erroneously perceiving them as being asleep. This study has several strengths in its design, including the use of a standard protocol with which the nurses were familiar and the measurements being made across many nights.

Another group of investigators, Dotson and colleagues,[3] studied nurses' assessment of sleep and self-reported sleep in a group of clients post-burn injury. Self-report questions were phrased in a general form, except for one question that asked the number of times awakened. This general approach could bias the responses as discussed earlier.[14] The nurses' sleep score was calculated by assigning numerical values to nurse reports of patient awake or sleeping, eyes open or shut, spontaneous talking, motor movement, respiration pattern, and number of times the nurse awakened the client for care. However, no information was provided on how these numerical values were derived. Low correlations were reported between these numerical values and client self-report. The reliability of the self-report measure is not clear because results of correlation across the nights of self-report are not presented. This is an interesting study, but flaws in reporting it make it difficult to know how to interpret the results. This issue certainly warrants further research.[3]

CASE STUDY

Elaine, a 36-year-old woman, complained of difficulty getting to sleep and maintaining sleep. She also reported morning fatigue. Her problem of getting to sleep had initially begun five years earlier, following the death of her father. She reported dreading going to bed and being unable to sleep. She often read and watched television in her bed as a means of going to sleep. She typically took 2 oz of alcohol to help her sleep. Upon questioning, Elaine reported that it took her up to one hour to go to sleep, and that she awakened at about 3:00 A.M. and was unable to return to sleep for at least an hour. Her usual bedtime was 11:00 P.M., and she used an alarm to awaken at 7:00 A.M. weekdays and awakened spontaneously by 8:00 A.M. on weekends. Her nursing diagnosis was sleep pattern disturbance with (1) delayed sleep onset related to learned chronic psychophysiologic arousal and (2) nocturnal awakenings related to arousal rebound secondary to alcohol use. A plan of care was developed that included mild exercise in the early evening to promote physical fatigue and decrease tension. Elaine removed her television from her bedroom and rearranged her bedroom to conform more closely to what she thought was a comfortable quiet place for sleep. If she was unable to get to sleep within 20 minutes she got up and did a boring task for 15 to 20 minutes before returning to bed. She discontinued using alcohol before sleep. After several months she reported rarely awakening for long periods in the middle of sleep time. She has continued to have some difficulty in getting to sleep initially, but has been better able to tolerate it because of the greater amount of sleep obtained in the absence of midsleep awakenings.

SUMMARY

Sleep is a complex of neurologic and behavioral patterns, any of which may be involved in sleep pattern disturbance. The understanding of usual sleep patterns across the life span and conditions commonly related to sleep pattern disturbance can help to suggest what may be happening within, or contributing to, the sleep pattern disturbance. Careful evaluation of the related conditions, the client's self-reported sleep experience, and daytime alertness, coupled with careful observation will assist in the identification of an appropriate nursing diagnosis.

References

1. Association of Sleep Disorders Centers. Diagnostic classification of sleep and arousal disorders. 1st ed. Prepared by the Sleep Disorders Classification Committee, HP Roftworg, Chairman. Sleep. 1979;2:1–137.
2. Baekeland F, Hoy P. Reported versus recorded sleep characteristics. Arch Gen Psychiatry. 1971;24:548–551.
3. Dotson CA, Kibbee E, Eland JM. Perception of sleep following burn injury. J Burn Care Rehabil. 1986;7:105–108.
4. Gilberg M, Akerstedt T. Body temperature and sleep at different times of day. Sleep. 1982;5:378–388.
5. Hauri P, Almstead E. What moment of sleep onset for insomnia? Sleep. 1983;6:10–15.
6. Jacobsen A, Kales A, Lehmann D, Hoedemaker F. Muscle tones in human subjects during sleep and dreaming. Exp Neurol. 1964;10:418–424.
7. Karacan I, Thornby S, Anch M. Prevalence of sleep disturbance in a primarily urban Florida county. Soc Sci Med. 1976;10:239–244.
8. Knab B, Engle R. Perception of waking and sleeping: possible implications for evaluation of insomnia. Sleep. 1988;11:265–272.
9. Kupfer DJ, Wyatt RJ, Snyder F. Comparison between electroencephalographic and systematic nursing observations of sleep in psychiatric patients. J Nerv Ment Dis. 1970;151:361–368.
10. Rechtshaflen A, Kales A. Manual of standardized terminology, technique and scoring system for sleep stage of human subjects. Berkeley: Brain Information Service/Brain Research Institute, University of California Press; 1968.
11. Reynolds C III, Kupfer D. State-of-the-art review. Sleep research in affective illness. State of the art circa 1987. Sleep. 1987;10:199–215.
12. Richards K. Techniques for measures of sleep in critical care. Focus Crit Care. 1987;14(4):34–40.
13. Rosekind MR, Schwartz GE. The perception of sleep and wakefulness I: accuracy and certainty of subjective judgments. Sleep Res. 1988;17:89.
14. Ruler A, Lack L. Gender differences in sleep. Sleep Res. 1988;17:244.
15. Snyder F. Changes in respiration, heart rate, and systolic blood pressure in human sleep. J Appl Physiol. 1964;19:417–422.
16. Takahashi Y, Kipnis D, Daughaday W. Growth hormone secretion during sleep. J Clin Invest. 1968;47:2079–2909.
17. Williams R, Karacan I, Hursch C. Electroencephalography (EEG) of human sleep: clinical application. New York: John Wiley & Sons; 1974.

SOCIAL INTERACTION, IMPAIRED

Jan Westwell and Mary-Lou Martin

DEFINITION AND DESCRIPTION

Social interaction does not refer to a single social exchange but rather to a series or pattern of interaction. Each interaction that occurs is unique and takes place within a context. Interaction consists of both verbal and nonverbal communication and is a multidimensional dynamic process that involves at least two individuals. All individuals in the interaction contribute to the process and outcome of the interaction. Although one individual may have overt difficulty in interacting, never is the interaction a reflection of just one person. There is always more than one version about what occurred in an interaction. Each participant's perception of the interaction is unique and understood in terms of his or her view of reality. Sociocultural beliefs, values, and norms influence what is accepted as appropriate social interaction. In addition, individuals bring personal values, beliefs, expectations, conflicts, and styles to the interaction.

The establishment and maintenance of positive social interaction with others is implicit in mental health. *Impaired social interaction* is the state in which an individual participates in an insufficient or excessive quantity or ineffective quality of social exchange. Impaired social interaction occurs when the individual, or those involved in the interaction, identify dissatisfaction with their social exchange. One area of dissatisfaction may be with the quantity of social exchange. The individual may experience an unsatisfying or inadequate frequency or duration of interaction or, conversely, experience an excess in frequency or duration of social exchange. Another area of dissatisfaction may be in the quality of the interaction, for example when some need or expectation has not been met.

The following examples may indicate a pattern of impaired social interaction: a 12-month-old infant who does not respond to the voice or touch of the parents; a six-year-old child who is unaware of social norms, frequently appears awkward, and is regularly shunned by peers; an adolescent who is aggressive towards others and has no friends; a 20-year-old woman who is embarrassed and awkward with men; a gregarious man in his mid-30s who has numerous acquaintances, but no intimate and interdependent relationships; a woman who does not initiate or respond to social contact; a senior citizen who gradually withdraws, and others no longer seek her company; a person who constantly interrupts others, making derogatory remarks; and a middle-aged man who is unable to control abnormal involuntary muscle movements and finds others avoid him. These examples reflect some of the many characteristics that people with impaired social interaction may exhibit (Fig. 13-26).

THEORY AND RESEARCH

As evident from the definition and description, social interaction is a complex phenomenon. The approaches that follow will assist the nurse in conceptualizing social interaction and will provide direction for nursing care.

Various theorists have described different components and aspects of interaction. One approach to viewing interaction was proposed by Sullivan,[20] who regarded interpersonal behavior as the expression of personality. In this theory, personality is regarded as evolving from the individual's social relationships with others. "Personality is the relatively enduring pattern of recurrent interpersonal situations which characterize a human life" (reference 20, pp 110, 111). The process of socialization begins at birth when the infant becomes part of an interpersonal situation. The uniqueness of each individual is defined by the accumulation of social interaction experiences. Although a person may avoid contact with others, memories of past interpersonal exchanges will continue to influence that person's experience of the world.

Another approach to understanding interaction asserts that a minimum of eight levels of awareness operate in an ordinary interaction.[5] These levels are operating constantly, and the degree of awareness about each level fluctuates. The first level is called bodily awareness. Usually, the individual is not focusing awareness on body systems; it is only when something (e.g., heart rate) reaches a certain threshold (e.g., tachycardia) that awareness is focused on a body system. The second level of awareness, self-consciousness, refers to the individual's awareness of external appearance. The individual asks questions such as: Am I being perceived the way I want? Do I make sense? At the third level, called ego intersubjective awareness, the individual is socially conscious and judges the self against his or her interpretations of other people's responses. The fourth level is called consciousness of kind or "my people versus aliens." Here, the individual evaluates the person with whom he or she is interacting based on their relationship. The individual recognizes and expe-

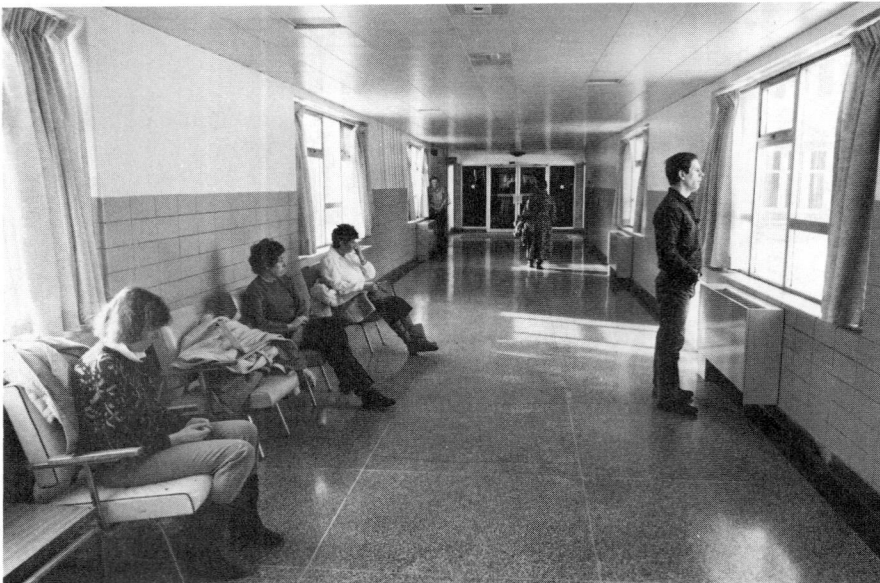

FIGURE 13–26. Many psychiatric clients have difficulty initiating and maintaining social exchange.

riences a sense of belonging to "my people." "Aliens" are everybody else. As would be expected, the individual's interactions are different with people in the two categories. At the fifth level the individual has awareness of participating in "something." The "something" is dependent upon the individual's role and the roles of the others within the context. Factors that compose the meaning of the "something" are: (1) What is the occasion? (2) Who are the participants? (3) When is it taking place? (4) Where are the participants in relation to their environment? and (5) What is the meaning of the participants' behavior? At the sixth level the individual has awareness of a larger relational context (i.e., people other than those currently participating may become involved later). People are stereotyped and responded to, based on the assumptions made about that particular stereotype. At the seventh level the individual has awareness of being a powerless part of a much larger whole (i.e., one individual is unable to change the course and direction of the world). At the eighth level, called cosmic species awareness, the individual is aware that, despite the complexities of the world, each individual has the power to preserve or destroy life. At this level, the individual's concerns are the unity and interdependence of people as a species. These eight levels of awareness, although abstract, reflect the multidimensional nature of interaction.

It has been noted that an individual cannot not communicate (i.e., not speaking when spoken to conveys a message).[24] The communication of one individual serves as a stimulus for the other and vice versa. Communication is meaningless if it is bereft of context. The individual's processing of verbal and nonverbal information is critical for understanding the context, in interpreting, and in engaging in social exchange. A major feature of schizophrenia is the person's inability to process the verbal and nonverbal information.[8] Because of this inability, the person with schizophrenia often mis-

interprets the roles and expectations of others. An example would be if a nurse were taking a group of clients outside and asked one client: "Would you like to go out?" This question could be misinterpreted and result in confusion if the social context was not understood.

The individual's pattern of relating is also associated with cognitive capabilities and maturational stage. Assessment of cognitive functioning and maturational stage may be crucial to understanding the client's experience and learning abilities. For example, an individual with neurologic impairment may be less able to process sensory input and less able to respond to social cues appropriately than can one without such impairment. The pattern of relating will depend upon the participant's perceptions, the phase of the relationship, and the context of the social exchange.

RELATED FACTORS

All individuals experience difficulty in their social interaction at one time or another. A nursing diagnosis of impaired social interaction is identified when a severe disruption in the individual's social interaction pattern is present. Impaired social interaction is likely to be observed in clients with psychiatric diagnoses[1] of personality disorders, schizophrenia, mood disorders, organic mental disorders, psychoactive substance use disorders, delusional (paranoid) disorders, somatoform disorders, mental retardation, and anxiety disorders. Many individuals with psychiatric diagnoses may have difficulties with reality testing, judgment, regulating and controlling impulses, thought processes, and use of defense mechanisms. These difficulties can have an impact on social interaction. Impaired social interaction may also be observed in persons who have physical disabilities, neurologic impairments, and sensory impairments. Persons who have disabilities or chronic illness, or who have experienced the loss of a significant other may be vulnerable to decreased opportunities for social interactions.

Learning about how to interact with others is an ongoing process throughout life. Social skills are learned and involve developmental tasks appropriate to the individual's stage of maturation. Failure to develop intimacy and interdependency with others may be associated with impaired social interaction. If an individual's needs (e.g., related to mastery, self-concept, and trust) have not been met in the childhood years, the adult may have difficulty interacting successfully. Persons who do not behave as expected for their age (such as those with developmental delays) may also experience social interaction difficulties.

Persons with psychiatric illnesses may have difficulty—depending upon the onset and the severity of their illness—acquiring the knowledge and skills related to social interaction. Even if the person has acquired some of the knowledge and skills for social interaction, his or her intrapsychic and interpersonal problems may influence the interaction. An example is the insecure person who interprets all social exchanges as threatening and devaluing.

Sociocultural values and beliefs influence social interaction. Impaired social interaction is most likely to occur when there is dissonance or inconsistency between an individual's pattern of relating and that of others.

DEFINING CHARACTERISTICS

Manifestations of impaired social interaction can vary depending upon the type and degree of impairment. It is artificial to separate the quality and the quantity of social interaction, because they are interrelated. An excess of quantity (e.g., monopolizing the conversation) may affect the quality of the interaction. It may be difficult to determine if the particular features of impaired social interaction are behavioral manifestations of the impairment or whether they are contributing causes of impaired social interaction. For example, poor conversational skills could be assessed as a defining characteristic or as a cause, depending upon the nurse's conceptualization and the client's situation.

Impaired social interaction does not refer to a single social exchange. Ineffective social behaviors, such as minimal social involvement, poor conversational skills, or inappropriate interpersonal skills, will be evident in a pattern of social exchange. Minimal social involvement could include difficulty initiating or maintaining social exchange. Poor conversational skills could include ineffective listening, interrupting others, ignoring others, monopolizing conversations, and making irrelevant or derogatory remarks. Inappropriate interpersonal skills could include too intense or too little eye contact, not observing usual social distances, unusual behaviors, or an inability to interpret and respond appropriately to social cues within the context. A pattern of ineffective social behaviors may result in an insufficient quantity of social exchange. This may also indicate a diminished social network. An excessive quantity of social exchange may be demonstrated by an unmanageable social network, lengthy interactions, or verbosity. Some individuals may continually seek social contact regardless of others' responses. Such individuals may or may not have a subjective awareness that something is affecting the interaction (Fig. 13-27).

The individual who subjectively feels dissatisfied or whose participation in social exchanges consistently leaves others dissatisfied may be described as experiencing an ineffective quality of social exchange. Such individuals may report that they are misunderstood by

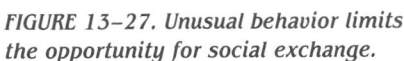

FIGURE 13–27. *Unusual behavior limits the opportunity for social exchange.*

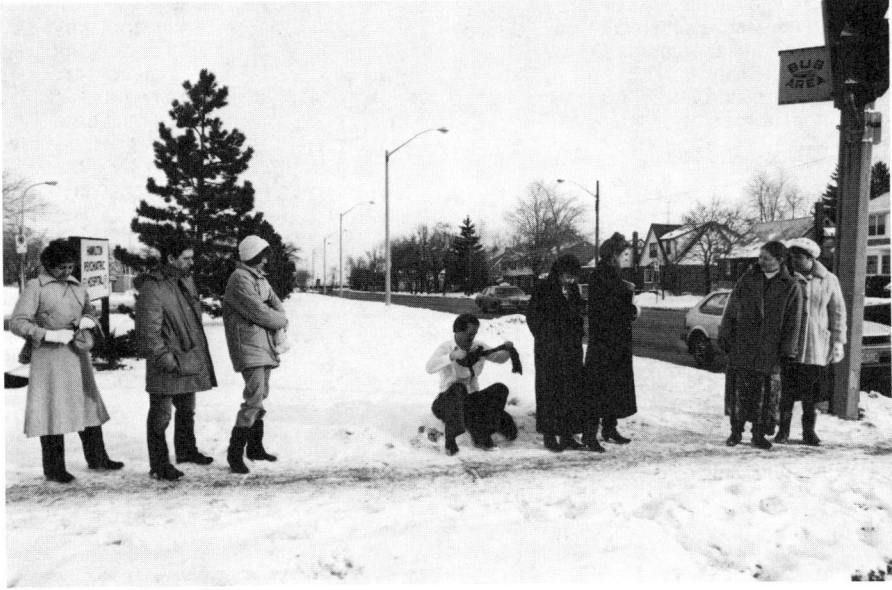

others or that people do not respond in an expected manner (Chart 1).

NURSING PROCESS AND RATIONALE
Assessment

The nurse seeks to understand the subjective meaning of social interaction for the client. A trusting relationship is essential for the client to disclose the meaning of his or her experience. Examination of the nurse's personal experience and participation in interactions with the client can facilitate the nurse's understanding of the interaction process and the client's experience. An example may be the client who frequently criticizes the nurse, demanding that the nurse comply with requests immediately. The nurse may feel defensive and enraged in response to the client's criticism and demands, and behave by withdrawing, avoiding, dominating, or demeaning the client. If this interaction process is recognized, the nurse may be able to stop acting-out his or her feelings and remain therapeutic. Clinical supervision and other means of increasing self-awareness will assist the nurse to understand his or her experience with the client.

The nurse's assessment of numerous client contacts and situations provides an understanding of the client's social interaction pattern. Factors to consider may include: Is the client socially active? Does the client have friends? Do others seek his or her company? The client may or may not be able to identify problems in his or her style of interaction. Much of the assessment, therefore, may be dependent upon the nurse's knowledge about interaction, his or her observation of the client, and experience of interacting with the client. The nurse can assess the degree of comfort experienced when interacting with the client, the clarity and the appropriateness of the communication, and the sense of mutuality of the interaction. It is likely that if the nurse wishes to avoid contact or frequently becomes angry and defensive with the client, that others may also have similar experiences. The nurse's personal experience can be compared with members of the

---

CHART 1
Impaired Social Interaction: Definition, Related Factors, and Defining Characteristics

DEFINITION

Impaired social interaction is the state in which an individual participates in an insufficient or excessive quantity or ineffective quality of social exchange.

RELATED FACTORS
Psychiatric disorders

Personality disorders
Schizophrenia
Mood disorders
Organic mental disorders
Psychoactive substance abuse disorders
Delusional (paranoid) disorder
Anxiety disorders
Mental retardation
Somatoform disorders

Other factors

Physical disabilities
Neurologic impairments
Sensory impairments
Chronic physical illness
Sociocultural disparity
Absence of significant others
Lack of opportunity to interact with others
Lack of communication and conversational skills
Lack of interpersonal skills
Language barrier
Aggressiveness
Grief
Impaired self-concept
Anxiety
Anger

Dysfunctional family in childhood
Inadequate learning experiences
Sensory or perception alteration

DEFINING CHARACTERISTICS

Avoidance of social situations
Does not initiate social contact
Does not maintain involvement in social exchange
Low self esteem
Discomfort in social situations
Minimal social involvement
Anxiety
Inability to trust others
Age-inappropriate behavior
Lack of close interdependent relationships
Verbal report of an unmanageable social network
Report of dissatisfaction with social exchange or social relationships
Report of frequently feeling misunderstood
Report by others of dissatisfaction with the social exchange involving the individual

Poor conversational skills

Ineffective listening
Interrupting others
Ignoring others
Inappropriate speech content (e.g., irrelevant or derogatory comments)
Monopolizing conversations

Inappropriate interpersonal skills

Too intense or too little eye contact
Disrespect for social distance
Unusual postures and gestures
Not responding to social cues
Overbearing, aggressive behavior

> ## CHART 2
> ## Impaired Social Interaction: Summary of the Nursing Process
>
> | NURSING INTERVENTIONS | OUTCOME CRITERIA |
> |---|---|
> | **CLIENT GOAL: EXPERIENCE INCREASED AWARENESS OF SUBJECTIVE EXPERIENCE AND MANNER OF PRESENTATION** | |
> | Establish therapeutic nurse–client relationship | Discusses experience |
> | Discuss thoughts, feelings, and sensations related to unsatisfying social exchanges | Reports more satisfying social exchanges |
> | Discuss potential responses by others to client's manner of presentation | Evidences body language congruent with verbal communication |
> | Assess knowledge about communication skills and ability to use in social exchange | Verbalizes understanding of communication techniques |
> | **CLIENT GOAL: EXPERIENCE INCREASED COMFORT IN SOCIAL INTERACTION** | |
> | Assess level of anxiety | Greets acquaintances appropriately |
> | Identify problematic issues in social exchange | Engages in social exchange |
> | Explore and acknowledge client's experience | Speaks clearly with culturally appropriate affect |
> | Practice role-playing | Exchanges comments in culturally appropriate manner |
> | Videotape role-playing | Gives and obtains information |
> | | Verbalizes usefulness of social skills group |
> | | Reports decrease in anxiety |
> | | Demonstrates increased comfort in social interaction |
> | **CLIENT GOAL: DEVELOP SATISFYING INTERPERSONAL RELATIONSHIPS** | |
> | Establish therapeutic nurse–client relationship | Participates in planned nurse–client interactions |
> | Explore client's subjective experience with a specific social exchange | Identifies factors related to problematic situations |
> | Teach social skills | Establishes satisfying relationships with others |

health-care team, the client's significant others, and the client. Questions that may facilitate the client examining his or her style of interaction may be: Do people respond to you the way you would like them to? Are your interactions with others often puzzling? Are your relationships with others generally satisfying? Behaviors such as those listed in the section on defining characteristics (see Chart 1) may help the nurse to identify problematic behavioral manifestations. Assessment of family interaction can also be useful; similar interaction patterns may be experienced within the therapeutic nurse–client relationship. It is critical for the nurse to remember that, although many psychiatric clients have overt difficulty with their social exchange, the interactional process is a shared responsibility. The nurse must examine his or her participation in the interactional process and determine the impact of this participation.

Nursing Diagnosis

A nursing diagnosis of impaired social interaction is formulated when the client has identified, or the nurse has observed or experienced, a pattern of unsatisfactory social exchange with the client. Some examples of diagnostic statements are: impaired social interaction related to lack of interpersonal skills; impaired social interaction related to sociocultural value disparity; impaired social interaction related to negative self-concept and anxiety; and, impaired social interaction related to feelings of anxiety.

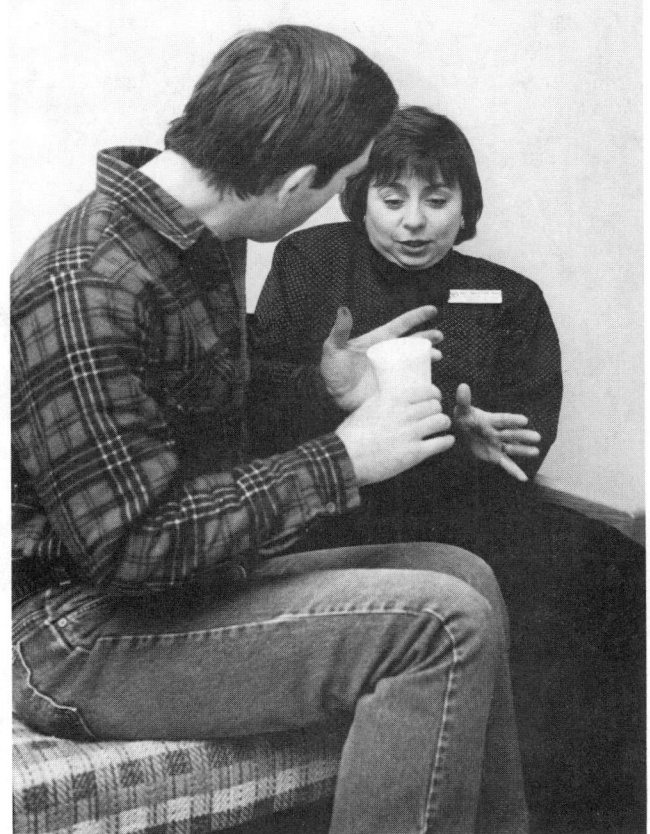

FIGURE 13–28. Interpersonal competencies necessary for social living and problem solving may need to be learned.

Client Goals and Nursing Interventions

The client with impaired social interaction may benefit from a variety of therapeutic modalities. Essential to effective intervention and goal attainment is the establishment of a nurse–client relationship. This involves the assignment of a nurse to the client on a consistent basis. The nurse who possesses therapeutic qualities and meets regularly with the client can begin to develop a trusting nurse–client relationship. It is important that the nurse recognize and demonstrate respect for cultural, religious, and social differences.

Individual counseling or therapy can assist the client to identify his or her subjective experience, relate it to events, make sense of what happened, and explore alternate ways of interacting. One model to facilitate this process is investigative counseling.[16] Clients with impaired social interaction may lack the interpersonal competencies necessary for social living and problem solving (Fig. 13-28). Nursing as a therapeutic interpersonal process can help facilitate the development of interpersonal competencies.

A variety of group strategies have been developed that facilitate the acquisition of knowledge and skills required for social exchange by individuals. Group therapy may facilitate the individual's understanding of self and others, which may lead to increased interpersonal skills. Social skills training includes clinical strategies such as communication skills training, modeling, behavioral rehearsal, social reinforcement, and homework assignments. Social skills training provides the client with information about interaction, opportunities to practice strategies, and to receive feedback. The goal of these interventions is to increase the individual's social competence.

Evaluation

Evaluation of outcome criteria may include (1) the client's subjective report of increased satisfaction with social exchange and (2) others' observation and report of increased satisfaction with their interactions with the client. These evaluation criteria imply that the client has developed some awareness of his or her participation in an interaction and the impact this participation may have had in the interaction. It is not uncommon for change in the client's social interaction pattern to be gradual and variable, influenced in part by how others respond to these changes (Chart 2).

Research Highlights

Two classic studies[13,14] examined interaction between the nurse and client. Both studies found that nurses were less therapeutic in their client interactions than expected.

More recent studies have focused on various aspects of social interaction. Rook[18] identified the negative side of interaction and its impact on psychological well-being. Although the study sample was limited to 68 to 89-year-old widowed women, results indicated that negative social interaction had greater impact on psychological state than positive social interaction. Well-being was found to be unrelated to the frequency of interaction. Brier and Strauss[7] examined the role of social relationships in clients recovering from psychotic episodes and found that clients' needs and social interaction abilities changed during the recovery period. A two-year participant observation study[19] examined criteria necessary for mentally retarded individuals to "appear normal" in their social interactions. The study found that social interaction skills could not be taught as a set of rules or responses. The researchers concluded that interaction was a complex task involving the assessment of social context and the relationship.

Numerous studies have investigated the impact of social skills training with psychiatric clients. Some studies[2-4] indicate that interaction by nurses with clients can improve social competence and prevent regression. Other researchers[23] have demonstrated that social skills training improves clients' social skills and decreases the number of relapses or rehospitalizations. Many types of content and various formats to teach social skills have been described in the literature.[6,9-12,15,17,21,22]

Beard and coworkers[3] conducted an experimental investigation that studied the social competency of chronic psychiatric inpatients in a Veterans Administration Hospital. Social competence was defined as the ability to know, remember, and do what was expected, complete tasks, and to adhere to hospital routine. The control group received routine hospital care, and the experimental group participated in daily activity groups. The activity group involved (1) the manipulation of concrete objects in the environment, such as finger painting, modeling clay activities, building activities, perception activities, and touch and texture puzzles; and (2) activities geared toward preparation for more independent living, such as pictures for projective techniques (i.e., pictures depicting a family or community scene were used to tell a story), activities in a homelike setting, and socialization activities in the community. The findings disclosed a statistically significant difference between the experimental and control groups on social competence. The experimental group increased their social competence, and most moved from a closed ward to either an open ward or community home. The results support that nursing intervention with use of activity groups can assist clients to increase their social competence and enhance their independent-living skills. The researchers suggest that nurses are in a unique position to assist clients in increasing their cognitive and social functioning through nurse–client interaction in planned activity groups. Additional research is needed to understand social interaction and further clarify the variables that influence social interaction.

CASE STUDY

Frank, a 30-year-old, single unemployed male, was admitted to a tertiary care psychiatric hospital. His psychiatric diagnosis was chronic schizophrenia, undifferentiated type. As had occurred in the past, the police brought him to hospital because people in the community had complained that he was verbally aggressive, requesting cigarettes and money. Boarding home arrangements between hospitalizations have failed, as Frank has been unable to get along with the boarding home operator or residents. His parents live nearby but have been only minimally involved. He has no close relationships with others.

Nursing staff described Frank as a difficult client because of his poor interpersonal skills, angry outbursts, and attempts to elope. Other clients avoided him. He had an unusual gait, unusual gestures, and frequently placed himself too close to others. The only time he approached others was when he wanted cigarettes or money. The major nursing diagnosis was impaired social interaction related to knowledge deficit about social norms manifested by lack of interpersonal skills.

The primary nurse assigned to Frank established a therapeutic relationship through nurse–client interactions. The nurse's approach was caring, accepting, and nonjudgmental. Initially the nurse met with Frank while he paced in the hallways. The initial client goals were (1) to be able to identify his primary nurse and (2) to approach the primary nurse without always requesting cigarettes or money. The nurse and Frank mutually established the long-term goal of communicating with others in a less aggressive manner. Through modeling the nurse demonstrated appropriate social skills. The nurse and Frank problem-solved about how he could best manage his cigarettes and money. The nurse encouraged Frank to verbalize his feelings and thoughts, rather than acting them out. Eventually, the nurse was able to meet with him in an interviewing room for five minutes twice daily. Through role-playing and feedback the nurse assisted Frank to practice initiating conversation in different situations, without asking for cigarettes or money. Incidents of verbal abuse decreased. Frank frequently approached his primary nurse without asking for a cigarette, although he continued to request cigarettes from others. Before discharge, the nurse was able to begin to explore with Frank the impact his behavior may have on other people and possible ways of interacting. He was discharged with follow-up care in a day-treatment facility.

SUMMARY

Learning how to interact successfully with others is an ongoing process. Impaired social interaction refers to a pattern of unsatisfying social exchange. Many individuals, particularly clients with psychiatric disorders, experience difficulty in their social interactions.

The nursing care of individuals with impaired social interaction involves the development of a therapeutic nurse–client relationship. Individual and group therapies will facilitate the client's self-awareness, knowledge, and skill in effective communication; comfort in social exchanges; and ultimately, the ability to establish and maintain a satisfying interpersonal relationship.

References

1. American Psychiatric Association. Diagnostic and statistical manual of mental disorders, 3rd ed. Washington, DC: American Psychiatric Association; 1987.
2. Beard M, Bidus D. A study of the effects of remotivation on social competence, social interest and personal neatness. J Psychiatr Nurs Ment Health Serv. 1968;6:197–201.
3. Beard M, Enelow C, Owens J. Activity therapy as a reconstructive plan on the social competence of chronic hospitalized patients. J Psychiatr Nurs Ment Health Serv. 1978;16:33–41.
4. Beard M, Metts F, Byrd D. Effects of sensory stimulation and remotivation on schizophrenic persons. J Psychiatr Nurs Ment Health Serv. 1972;10:5–8.
5. Boughey H. Ashtaavadhaana: mapping eight levels of social awareness toward a geography of salient environments. Envir Behav. 1985;17:411–444.
6. Brady JP. Social skills training for psychiatric patients, II: Clinical outcome studies. Occup Ther Ment Health. 1985;5:59–74.
7. Brier A, Strauss JS. The role of social relationships in the recovery from psychotic disorders. Am J Psychiatry. 1984;141:949–955.
8. Dawson D, Bartolucci S, Blum H. Language and schizophrenia: towards a synthesis. Comp Psychiatry. 1980;21:81–90.
9. Denton PL. Teaching interpersonal skills with videotape. Occup Ther Ment Health. 1982;2:17–34.
10. Fecteau GW, Duffy M. Social and conversational skills training with long-term psychiatric inpatients. Psychol Rep. 1986;59:1327–1331.
11. Foxx RM, McMorrow MJ, Bittle RG, Fenlon SJ. Teaching social skills to psychiatric inpatients. Behav Res Ther. 1985;23:531–537.
12. Knibbs J, Hardiman F. Ment Health Forum: A sense of security . . . schizophrenic patients . . . social skills training. Nurs Mirror. 1983;9:157.
13. Mathews BP. Measurement of psychological aspects of the nurse–patient relationship. Nurs Res 1962;11:154–162.
14. Methven D, Schlotfeldt R. The social interaction inventory. Nurs Res. 1962;11:83–88.
15. Miller TW, Wilson GL, Dumas MA. Developments and evaluation of social skills training for schizophrenic patients in remission. J Psychiatr Nurs Ment Health Serv. 1979;17:42–46.
16. Peplau HE. Interpersonal relations in nursing. New York: GP Putnam's Sons; 1952.
17. Rawat R. Ment Health Forum: Social skills training. Nurs Mirror. 1983;9:157(12).
18. Rook KS. The negative side of social interaction: impact on psychological well-being. J Pers Soc Psychol. 1984;46:1097–1108.
19. Rumelhart MA. The normalization of social interaction: when shared assumptions cannot be assumed. Qual Sociol. 1983;6:149–162.
20. Sullivan HS. The interpersonal theory of psychiatry. New York: WW Norton & Co; 1953.
21. Topf M, Dambacher B. Teaching interpersonal skills: a model for facilitating optimal interpersonal relations. J Psychiatr Nurs Ment Health Serv. 1981;19:29–33.
22. Vousden M, Fisher P. Ment Health Forum: Actions speak louder than words. Nurs Mirror. 1983;9:157(12).
23. Wallace CJ, Liberman RP. Social skills training for patients with schizophrenia: a controlled clinical trial. Psychiatr Res. 1985;15:239–247.
24. Watzlawick P, Beavin JH, Jackson DD. Pragmatics of human communication: a study of international patterns, pathologies and paradoxes. New York: WW Norton & Co; 1976.

SOMATIZATION

Joanne Davis Whitney

DEFINITION AND DESCRIPTION

Somatization is the expression of psychological conflicts through physical concerns. A person who somatizes is focused on somatic symptoms such as pain or body functions (e.g., digestion, elimination). Somatization has been associated with various clinical problems and psychological disorders;[18] it is recognized as having a high prevalence in many countries. Clinically, the term somatization has multiple meanings and uses.[3] However, it is frequently used in a general way to describe clients who use somatic complaints and concerns as a method of coping.[18] A focus on somatic symptoms may permit the client to achieve personal gain. A person may escape from daily home obligations because the condition or symptom is exacerbated. In a similar way a client may avoid interpersonal contacts because the physical problem is so troublesome that they "must stay at home" and, therefore, be isolated. Somatization can serve various purposes for a person, but it is generally perceived as an ineffective means of coping with psychological distress.

THEORY AND RESEARCH

There are several theories that help to explain why somatic behavior develops and is a sustained pattern for some persons. Explanations are based on developmental theory, psychodynamic theory, stress theory, and the way physiologic sensations are perceived.

In the context of *developmental theory* it is proposed that the person never learned or developed adequate verbal or cognitive skills to express unpleasant emotions or psychological distress.[14] This leads to the expression of feelings in somatic ways, rather than through cognitive strategies. The way in which children are socialized by their families and social environment to deal with physical and emotional pain appears to influence later ability or style of coping with emotions.[14] It is also likely that a link exists between parents who model somatic behavior and its presence in offspring, during both their childhood and adult years.[16] Psychosomatic families have been described who demonstrate a lack of language for emotions, an inability to work out conflict verbally, and denial that psychological problems exist.[5,14,24]

Psychodynamic theory identifies somatization as the result of the unconscious gratification and meaning that body symptoms or physical suffering provide.[3] This theory explains somatization as being influenced by early life experiences, and it examines the relationship between somatization and inhibition of anger, use of somatic complaints as a defense mechanism, or for achievement of primary or secondary gain. In each case, somatization serves to decrease intrapsychic conflict. Used as a defense, against low self-esteem for example, somatization allows the person to believe something is wrong with the body or body part, rather than with the "self." When somatization achieves primary gain, there is a decrease in intrapsychic conflict, while secondary gain legitimizes interpersonal advantages (e.g., attention, support) because of the physical illness.[3]

Stress theory suggests that psychosocial stressors are important antecedents to somatization.[9] Although other factors may also contribute to the appearance of somatic behavior, when individuals who somatize experience increased stress, there is likely to be an increase in medical contacts without the presence of physical disease.[22,29] Here, somatization may represent a chronic response to stress, but intensifies as an acute phenomenon, which diminishes as the stress decreases. Higher life stress has been measured in adolescents who report recurrent pain without an identifiable organic cause.[10] This indicates a need to evaluate psychological stressors and not dismiss their importance in comparison with organic causes.

Somatization is also thought to be related to *perception* of physiologic sensations.[19] Hence, the person may have a heightened awareness of normal sensations and may amplify and misinterpret the physical symptoms of emotion.[3] The lack of recognition and understanding of emotional distress and related physical symptoms, such as nausea or fatigue, lead the person to believe that the primary problem is physical, rather than emotional. It should be noted that cultures differ in their emphasis on the physical, rather than emotional, symptoms of distress. In some societies emphasis on physical symptoms is the norm and not considered to be abnormal.

RELATED FACTORS

Somatization is associated with several psychological disorders. These include somatization disorder, conversion disorder, somatoform pain disorder, hypochondriasis, and undifferentiated somatoform disorder.[1,21] Several authors have described the occurrence of somatic complaints in clients with depression.[14,15,28,31] In a study of nursing diagnoses of depressed psychiatric in-patients, somatization was the diagnosis most frequently identified.[30] In depressed clients, the somatic focus can mask the underlying depression, which both client and health-care provider fail to recognize.[2] There is a risk that the physical complaint will be treated symptomatically, while the underlying depression is left untreated.[15]

Somatization has been observed to coexist with depression in clients with chronic medical illness.[6,13,31] In a study of medical inpatients referred to a psychiatric liaison service, 38% focused on somatic symptoms.[13] Nearly one-half of the clients with somatic complaints had major depression, a rate that exceeded nonsomatizing clients 2.5 times. Depression and chronic medical illness, both alone and combined, were found to be significant contributors to somatic complaining in elderly persons who attended lunch programs in senior centers.[31] Somatic complaints tended to be related to a number of body systems; there was a strong positive association between the number of chronic illnesses a person had and somatic complaining.[31] Mild somatic signs should not automatically be attributed to depression, but persistent, severe symptoms that are exaggerated in proportion to the physical illness should raise concerns that depression may be present.[6]

The attitudes about and implications of illness vary among ethnic groups.[9] Whether or not a person engages in somatic behavior appears to have a basis in cultural norms. Somatization may occur because it is the norm, and it is generally more acceptable to have a physical, rather than emotional, problem.[18] Studies of certain developing Middle Eastern countries and also Hispanic groups in the United States and South America have demonstrated clients who report a prevalence of physical complaints such as weakness, dizziness, and gastrointestinal symptoms.[7,8,11] In many non-Western countries the presenting manifestations of psychological problems are in the form of vague physical symptoms.[14,25] A somatic focus may be made more likely because some languages lack words to describe emotional states, or there is a culturally based physical interpretation and understanding of emotional states.[14] Several other factors have been related to somatization. Age is believed to be associated with a willingness to take on the sick role. It has been suggested that the older a person is, the greater entitlement that is felt for being ill. Older people, therefore, are more likely to adopt a pattern of somatization. A rural background,[3] history of childhood physical abuse or emotional neglect,[4] gaining attention through illness while growing up, or having somatization modeled by family members are also related factors.[18,23]

DEFINING CHARACTERISTICS

The presentation of somatization will vary with the individual client, but certain behavior patterns are indicative of the problem. The repeated focus on a partic-ular symptom or on multiple physical symptoms is the hallmark of somatization. Physical symptoms involved in somatization include, but are not limited to, pain, dizziness, loss of balance, fatigue, gastrointestinal distress, and localized weakness.[19] The symptom is often presented in an exaggerated way, and the client's concern may be excessive in light of the actual severity of physical illness. There, in fact, may be no objective findings to explain the client's subjective complaints. The client may demonstrate dramatic physical manifestations such as falling or collapsing. On the other hand, complaints may be presented in a vague way as, for example, in complaints of general weakness or tiredness.

The client's history will often provide insight into the use of somatization as a behavioral response. The client may have an extensive history of medical contacts or surgical interventions.[26] The client's history may also reveal an increase in physical symptoms as a response to identifiable precipitants. Somatization may occur only episodically in relation to the occurrence of stressful situations.

Additional characteristics can be related to interpersonal gain achieved by the symptom. This includes observations that the client's support from others is dependent on the symptom, and complaints may increase in the presence of selected individuals. The symptom may enable the client to avoid an offensive activity or interaction. Finally, when the client is given psychological support, physical symptoms frequently abate.

A recent nursing study of clients identified as having somatic behavior showed a cluster of defining characteristics.[32] It was found that somatizing clients reported multiple physical problems as well as repeated symptoms with a focus on body functions; concern with physical symptoms did not match observed severity of illness; symptoms often were linked to an identifiable precipitant; activities were avoided because of the symptom, and the physical problem brought the client a considerable amount of support.[32] This cluster of defining characteristics suggests the use of somatization as a mode of coping. It emphasizes the role secondary gain may play in sustaining somatic behavior (Chart 1).

NURSING PROCESS AND RATIONALE

Assessment

In considering therapeutic approaches for the somatizing client, the importance of somatization as a long-term communication style needs to be recognized. It is also critical to appreciate that the somatic behavior is likely to be motivated by emotions, such as sadness or anger, that the client is unable to express verbally.[17] Somatic behavior is often easily recognized because it is an overt expression, but identifying underlying emotions presents a greater challenge. In assessing the somatizing client, it is therefore useful to explore the client's feelings and the meaning the behavior has for the individual. Because clients who somatize may be

CHART 1
Somatization: Definition, Related Factors, and Defining Characteristics

DEFINITION

Somatization is the expression of psychological conflicts through physical concerns.

RELATED FACTORS

Somatization disorder
Conversion disorder
Somatoform pain disorder
Hypochondriasis
Undifferentiated somatoform disorder
Depression
Cultural factors
Physical illnesses
Advanced age
Rural background
Childhood abuse or neglect
Somatization modeled in family of origin
Somatization reinforced in family interactions
Family lacks language of emotions
Family difficulties in working out conflicts verbally
Overwhelming situational stressors
Difficulty coping

DEFINING CHARACTERISTICS

Reports particular physical symptom repeatedly
Reports multiple physical symptoms
Obtains environmental support by way of symptoms
Concern with physical problems not commensurate with severity of physical illness
Responds with physical symptoms following identifiable precipitant
Focuses on bodily functions
Subjective complaints inconsistent with objective findings
Activities or interactions avoided because of symptom
Physical complaints expressed in an exaggerated way
Physical symptoms decrease with psychological support
Extensive history of medical contacts and surgical interventions
Pain or other difficulties indicated nonverbally
Increase in complaints of physical symptoms in the presence of certain individuals
Physical complaints presented in a vague way
Physical complaints presented in a dramatic way

depressed, feelings of worthlessness, loss of interest in usual activities, suicidal ideation, psychomotor agitation or retardation, anorexia, and insomnia are important areas for assessment.[6]

In assessment, the nurse should be aware of the tendency to create a dichotomy between physical and psychological etiologies of somatization. Knowledge that somatization often occurs with physical illness helps to decrease the likelihood that clients will be diagnosed as either physically ill *or* somatizing, without considering the possibility that both may exist.

Establishing a relationship with the client is a fundamental component of care that provides a basis for assessment and intervention.[9,20,27] Trust is built within the context of the relationship. Establishing relationships with these clients may be difficult because they often have problems with interpersonal relationships and with articulation of their feelings. However, even limited contact will allow the nurse to gradually assess the use of physical symptoms and gain understanding of the feelings they represent.[9]

Nursing Diagnosis

The initial diagnosis may be broad (e.g., somatization) until there is sufficient information to allow individualizing the diagnosis. As related factors are clarified the diagnosis becomes more specific and useful for guiding care. For example, somatization related to an inability to work out family conflicts verbally, or somatization related to a learned pattern of coping through the use of physical complaints, are diagnoses that can begin to direct care. In addition, the diagnosis can further identify the impact on daily living. An example of a diagnosis that includes information about the influence on the client's life is somatization related to cultural background and home stressors preventing adequate management of work and home responsibilities.

Client Goals and Nursing Interventions

Specific interventions will depend on the individual client. In general, clinical approaches may be most effective if the focus is not on the somatizing behavior, but on helping the client to gain insight into feelings and to develop new or different ways to cope with psychological distress. Because somatizing is likely to represent a firmly established behavior pattern, limiting or restricting somatic complaints may be interpreted by clients as not listening or not having concern for their problems. In addition, complete removal of the symptoms may not be possible or even desirable.[17] For some clients, removal of the symptom might have serious implications, for example, the client who uses somatization to control aggression or violence. Stripping a person of self-protective devices, no matter how maladaptive they appear, is not helpful, unless some more adequate coping tools are substituted.[20] Acknowledging and briefly assessing physical complaints without dwelling on them can help to reduce the client's focus on the symptom.[26] With this approach, the nurse listens sensitively to the client, but takes care to avoid overly active interventions. Encouraging the client to verbalize concerns in a nonsomatic way can be a gradual modification of this approach.[12]

If the somatic behavior achieves secondary gain, enlisting the client's active participation in care is important. The nurse–client relationship needs to be one of mutual participation. This not only helps to support the client to make decisions, but will also tend to undermine the use of somatization to obtain gratification and sustain dependency needs. Secondary gain can also be discouraged by not allowing the client to meet social needs through somatization. The nurse manifests concern about the problem, but strongly encourages the client to be "in bed" if the physical symptom is so serious.

Behavior modification may be a useful approach, particularly in clients who respond to support. It is most effective if positive reinforcers for somatization can be eliminated (e.g., secondary gain). Appropriate behaviors, for example, increasing activity and managing daily activities, can then be rewarded and supported.[20]

If at all possible, it is valuable to explore symptom meaning with the client. One technique when somatic complaints occur is to ask the client, "If that (symptom or complaint) were an emotion, what would it be?" Exploring emotions can help the client gain insight into the meaning of behavior. At the same time an educational approach may be beneficial in helping the client to better understand the basis for behavior.[9,27] The nurse can describe how sickness is viewed in society and why people may be more comfortable with physical rather than emotional distress. Data on the way feelings and illness were expressed in the client's family can provide information that enhances insight. The client who understands the beginnings of, and reasons for, somatic behavior may then be more receptive to learning other ways to express and manage emotions (e.g., increasing assertiveness and engaging in alternative patterns of communication).

Nursing interventions for clients who somatize are directed toward decreasing physical symptoms, increasing the client's ability to recognize and express feelings, and developing alternative means of meeting needs. Interventions also concentrate on comprehending the source(s) of somatic behavior. Somatization is a complex phenomenon and requires careful consideration and choice of therapeutic alternatives based on individual assessment.

Evaluation

Evaluation of the client's progress is based on outcome criteria that relate to client goals and nursing interventions. Although these are individualized, depending on the specific situation, there are some general behaviors that mark improvement. A gradual increase in ability to manage and engage in daily activities and a decrease in somatic complaints are indicative of progress. Improvement in these areas can be seen as the client develops alternative coping strategies and learns to meet needs in new ways. Demonstration of the use of different coping methods, the ability to recognize and articulate feelings, and a willingness to explore past events that may have influenced the manner in which psychological concerns are expressed, are also signs of progress (Chart 2).

CASE STUDY*

A 72-year-old married woman, Ruth R, was admitted to an inpatient psychiatric unit of a large community hospital with a diagnosis of possible dementia or depression. She had had one previous psychiatric hospitalization. Recent life events included the sale of the couple's home, which had happened so quickly they had insufficient time to make new housing arrangements. The client also reported a change in the husband's behavior, which she described as bizarre and

* The author expresses appreciation for the helpful assistance of Jackie Gerike, RN, BSN, and Donna Poole, RN, MSN, who provided information for this case study and on the clinical care of the client who experiences somatization.

CHART 2
Somatization: Summary of the Nursing Process

NURSING INTERVENTIONS	OUTCOME CRITERIA
CLIENT GOAL: EXPRESS DIMINISHED SOMATIC BEHAVIORS	
Acknowledge symptom(s) without undue emphasis	Has fewer somatic complaints
Involve client as active participant in care	
Reduce rewards for focus on somatic behaviors	
CLIENT GOAL: INCREASE USE OF ALTERNATE STRATEGIES FOR COPING WITH PSYCHOLOGICAL CONCERNS	
Support client in trying new ways of handling concerns	Responds to stressful situations with fewer somatic complaints
Introduce client to new coping alternatives as appropriate (e.g., assertiveness, relaxation)	Demonstrates ability to use varied coping skills
CLIENT GOAL: GAIN UNDERSTANDING OF FEELINGS	
Assist client to explore emotions	Begins to articulate feelings
Encourage expression of feelings in ways other than through physical symptoms, especially verbally	Recognizes relationship of physical symptoms and psychological concerns

Research Highlights

The multicultural nature of society in the United States presents unique challenges to health-care providers. Familiarity with cultural variations in beliefs about illness and illness behaviors has important implications for assessment and treatment in clinical practice. A study by Escobar and associates compared symptom profiles of clients with major depression in the United States and in Colombia, South America.[8] The researchers were particularly interested in gaining information about the phenomenology of affective disorders for Hispanics in their native setting. The sample comprised 41 clients in Bogota, Colombia and 32 clients in the United States. The clients were participants in a larger study evaluating antidepressant agents. All subjects were newly admitted to the treatment facilities and met the diagnostic criteria for major depression. Data were collected using a structured clinical interview, the Hamilton Psychiatric Rating Scale for Depression, and a symptom profile for depressive disorders developed by the researchers. The symptoms of depression were very similar between groups, but depressed Colombian clients had significantly higher somatization scores than subjects in the United States. The researchers could not explain the difference in somatization by socioeconomic status. They suggested that other factors were important to consider, (e.g., stigmatization of mental illness by Hispanic societies, a lack of psychological sophistication, and the use of somatization to legitimize health-seeking behaviors). The researchers noted that because Hispanic Americans tend to preserve many of their cultural values over several generations, it is important to recognize these factors and their potential relationship to somatization and meaning for the client.[8]

erratic during the previous two weeks. She was anxious and tearful. Her physical examination was normal with the exception of a mild systolic murmur. Psychological testing revealed acute distress, disorganization, confusion, marked dependence on her husband, and self-criticism. Early in her hospitalization, Ruth focused on multiple physical problems but was particularly obsessed with her bowels. She ruminated over her clothing and appearance and frequently felt she was "going to collapse." At times she described her body as "totally shut down." Her complaints were exaggerated and were not validated by physical findings. Worry about her husband and his ability to manage while she was in the hospital was causing her a great amount of distress.

Somatization related to situational stressors and inability to cope was one of the priority nursing diagnoses for Ruth. In the mornings she would often lie immobile on her bed, expressing concern about her physical problems. Because she felt she was not being listened to, an approach was used in which staff first listened to her concerns before any demands on her were made. Her somatic complaints were acknowledged, and she was assured related needs would be taken care of (e.g., prescribed stool softeners given). The expectation that she be involved in her care and that her help was necessary was emphasized. Activities of daily living were broken down into small, less overwhelming tasks that she could accomplish (e.g., brush teeth). She was encouraged to make her own decisions, but also was given support and reassurance. When she felt she could not enter a group meeting, she was accompanied by a nurse. Arrangements were made for her to telephone her husband each day. During her hospitalization he began outpatient therapy for depression, which helped reduce some of her worries. Her somatic complaints decreased as she received psychological support through individual sessions with nurses and through groups. Her self-confidence increased. Her anxieties were addressed individually, and outside support was obtained if necessary. For instance, Ruth had concerns of a legal nature, thus a meeting with an attorney was arranged. By discharge, her somatic complaints had decreased, and she was functioning independently. Discharge plans included outpatient couple therapy, individual follow-up with a psychiatrist, and medication [nortriptyline (Aventyl), levothyroxine (Synthroid)]. This client demonstrated somatic behavior as part of a response to recent stressors. The use of somatization was decreased by helping her to manage anxiety through more appropriate and effective strategies.

SUMMARY

Somatization occurs when psychological concerns are expressed in a somatic idiom. This behavior usually represents a chronic style of coping through which the client is enabled to meet emotional needs and gain attention and support. It is also likely to have a firm foundation in the client's family history or cultural background. Nursing interventions for clients who somatize center around increasing the client's awareness and understanding of emotions and assisting them to develop new methods to meet needs and manage stress.

References

1. American Psychiatric Association. Diagnostic and statistical manual of mental disorders. 3rd ed. Washington, DC: American Psychiatric Association; 1987.
2. Anstett RE, Poole SR. Depressive equivalents in adults. Am Fam Pract. 1982;25:151–156.
3. Barsky AJ, Klerman GL. Overview: hypochondriasis, bodily complaints and somatic styles. Am J Psychiatry. 1983; 140:273–283.
4. Blumer D, Heilbronn N, Pedraza E, Pope G. Systematic treatment of chronic pain with antidepressants. Henry Ford Hosp Med J. 1980;28:15–21.
5. Brodsky CM. Sociocultural and interactional influences on somatization. Psychosomatics. 1984;25:673–680.
6. Cavanaugh SVA. Diagnosing depression in the hospitalized client with chronic medical illness. J Clin Psychiatry. 1984;45:12–16.
7. Escobar JI. Cross-cultural aspects of the somatization trait. Hosp Commun Psychiatry. 1987;38:174–180.

8. Escobar JI, Gomez J, Tuason VB. Depressive phenomenology in North and South American patients. Am J Psychiatry. 1983;140:47–51.

9. Ford CV. The somatizing disorders, illness as a way of life. New York: Elsevier Biomedical; 1983.

10. Greene JW, Walker LS, Hickson G, Thompson J. Stressful life events and somatic complaints in adolescents. Pediatrics. 1985;75:19–22.

11. Harding TW, De Arango MV, Baltasar J. Mental disorders in primary health care: a study of their frequency and diagnoses in four developing countries. Psychol Med. 1980;10:231–241.

12. Holt RE, LeCann AF. Use of an integrative interview to manage somatization. Psychosomatics. 1984;25:663–669.

13. Katon W. Depression: relationship to somatization and chronic medical illness. J Clin Psychiatry. 1984;45:4–11.

14. Katon W, Kleinman A, Rosen G. Depression and somatization: a review. Part I. Am J Med. 1982;72:127–135.

15. Katon W, Kleinman A, Rosen G. Depression and somatization: a review. Part II. Am J Med. 1982;72:241–247.

16. Krietman N, Swinsbury P, Pearce K, Costain WR. Hypochondriasis and depression in outpatients at a general hospital. Br J Psychiatry. 1965;111:607–615.

17. Lichstein PR. Caring for the patient with multiple somatic complaints. South Med J. 1986;79:310–314.

18. Lipscomb PA, Katon W. In: Cameron OG, ed. Presentation of depression: depression in medical and other psychiatric disorders. New York: John Wiley & Sons; 1987.

19. Lloyd GG. Psychiatric syndromes with a somatic presentation. J Psychosom Res. 1986;30:113–120.

20. Lowy FH. Management of the persistent somatizer. Int J Psychol Med. 1975;6:227–239.

21. Maue FR. Functional somatic disorders. Postgrad Med. 1986;79:201–210.

22. Mechanic D, Volkart EH. Stress, illness behavior and the sick role. Am Sociol Rev. 1961;26:51–58.

23. Mechanic D. Development of psychological distress among young adults. Arch Gen Psychiatry. 1979;36:1233–1239.

24. Minuchin S, Rosman BL, Baker L. Psychosomatic families: anorexia nervosa in context. Cambridge: Harvard University Press; 1978.

25. Racy J. Somatization in Saudi women: a therapeutic challenge. Br J Psychiatry. 1980;137:212–216.

26. Smith GR, Monson RA, Ray DC. Patients with multiple unexplained symptoms. Arch Intern Med. 1986;146:69–72.

27. Smith RC. A clinical approach to the somatizing patient. J Fam Pract. 1985;21:294–301.

28. Stoudemire A, Kahn M, Brown JT, Linfors E, Houpt JL. Masked depression in a combined medical–psychiatric unit. Psychosomatics. 1985;26:221–228.

29. Tessler R, Mechanic D, Dimond M. The effect of psychological distress on physician utilization: a prospective study. J Health Soc Behav. 1976;17:353–364.

30. Thomas MD, Sanger E, Whitney JD. Nursing diagnosis of depression: clinical identification on an inpatient unit. J Psychosoc Nurs Ment Health Serv. 1986;24:6–12.

31. Waxman HM, McCreary G, Weinrit RM, Carner EA. A comparison of somatic complaints among depressed and non-depressed older persons. Gerontologist. 1985;25:501–507.

32. Whitney JD, Sanger E, Thomas MD, Wolf-Wilets V. A validation study of the nursing diagnosis "somatization". Arch Psychiatr Nurs. 1988;2(6):345–349.

SPIRITUAL DISTRESS

Billie M. Severtsen

DEFINITION AND DESCRIPTION

Spiritual distress is defined as a disruption in the life principle that pervades a person's entire being and that integrates and transcends one's biologic and psychological nature. This life principle is the force that enables an individual to make meaning out of the various events that occur in the course of a lifetime. According to Berger and Luckmann,[1]

> Human knowledge is given in society as an a priori to individual experience, providing the latter with its order of meaning. This order, although it is relative to a particular socio-historical situation, appears to the individual as the natural way of looking at the world (reference 1, p 8).

Thus, a person looks at the world through a kind of prism of meaning that he or she has developed and that provides a certain view or apprehension of what is perceived as universal or ultimate truth.

THEORY AND RESEARCH

Spiritual refers to whatever gives life its ultimate meaning. It does not necessarily concern what is thought of as religious sects or even a world religion, although spiritual concerns may certainly include religion. Ultimate concerns, according to Tillich, may center around one's work, one's family, one's career, one's country, or one's church.[7] These issues are much more powerful than a stated belief in a creed or a set of religious doctrines. James Fowler integrates Tillich's concept of spirituality in his work.[3]

> Faith, it appears, is generic, a universal feature of human living, recognizably similar everywhere despite the remarkable variety of forms and contents of religious practice and belief. Faith, classically understood, is not a separate dimension of life, a compartmentalized speciality. Faith is an orientation of the total person, giving purpose and goal to one's hopes and strivings, thoughts and actions (reference 3, p 14).

Spiritual growth and mental or emotional growth are similar phenomena. Peck[5] makes "no distinction between the mind and the spirit, and therefore, no distinction between the process of achieving spiritual growth and achieving mental growth. They are one and the same" (reference 5, p 11). Other authorities such as

Viktor Frankl[4] maintain that the central core of a person is spiritual and that this core is surrounded by a "psyche" (emotions) and "soma."

Faith or the spiritual life principle is not only religious and philosophical but also social and relational (Fig. 13-29). This means that faith or spirituality is seen as people interact with one another in communities. It is an integral part of everyday life; therefore, lifetime events that challenge an individual's faith or disrupt the meaning matrix that he or she has created cause spiritual distress.

Fowler has identified six stages of faith through which individuals pass as they mature.[3] *Intuitive–projective* faith corresponds with the developmental task of the child learning to trust, *mythic–literal* faith parallels the child's attempt to seek autonomy, and *synthetic–conventional* faith corresponds with the attempt of the adolescent to develop an identity out of role confusion. Young adults typically reflect upon spiritual values and fine-tune their faith to the values they have chosen. Fowler calls this *individuative–reflective* faith. As people enter midlife, their ultimate concerns tend to become fixed or settled, either in *conjunctive* or *universalizing* faith. Ultimate concerns, therefore, are perceived differently in different developmental levels, and the faith that supports and gives meaning to the life of the individual is viewed, at least partially, from a developmental framework. In other words, the developmental crisis that precipitates the individual to move toward a newer, more mature way of coping also precipitates the individual to perceive both ultimate concerns and meaning in a new way. Early spiritual development, for example, is closely related to trust. By contrast, an adolescent concerned with self-consciousness in a developmental sense also sees faith as something to be questioned and clarified until it becomes personalized.

Fowler[3] based his study on earlier classic scholarly works by theologians such as Paul Tillich, Richard Niebuhr, and Wilfred Cantwell Smith. These writers have tried to expand the idea of spiritual beyond the concept of religious sect or even organized religion into the area of centering or ultimate concerns. Whatever gives life meaning and serves as a source of strength and hope can be classified as a centering concern. In addition to a Higher Being or God, a person, a community, an activity, an attitude, or an experience can be a source of the spiritual in an individual's life, according to this view. Steeves and Kahn[6] have explored the area of meaning, treating it as a phenomenon that often

450

FIGURE 13–29. *Spirituality is not only religious and philosophical, but also social and relational. Individuals demonstrate spirituality as they interact with others in communities.*

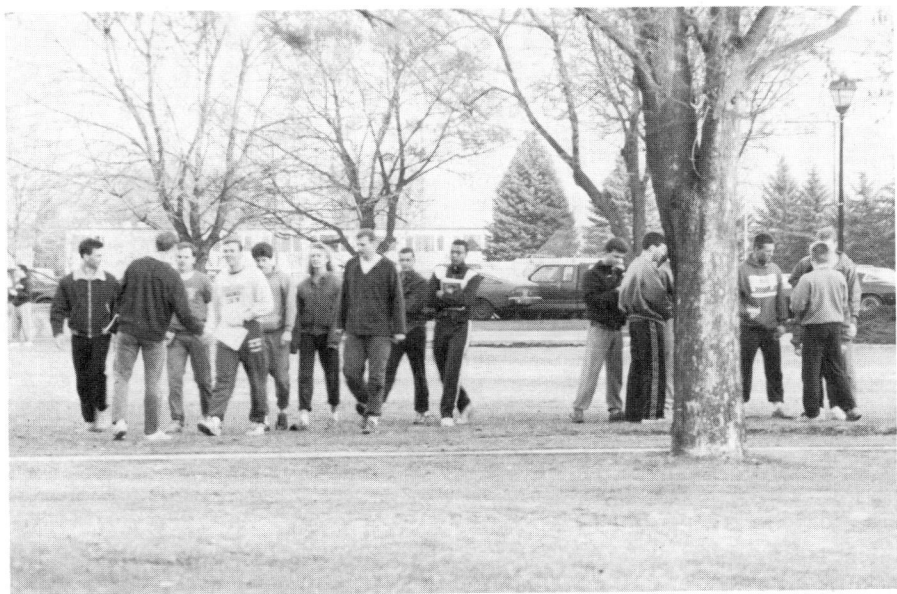

occurs as a result of suffering. They report it as a relatively common event that often occurs in hospice settings. Frankl,[4] by contrast, explores the area of meaning as a process. In this model the free choosing of one attitude response over another as a response to suffering or crisis becomes the meaning component of the event.

RELATED FACTORS

The most characteristic factor related to the development of spiritual distress is *loss*. Although loss may be perceived by people as major or minor, temporary or permanent, and of ultimate or superficial concern, it is a phenomenon that almost automatically forces individuals to readjust the matrix of meaning which they have created in their lives (Fig. 13-30). When a loss occurs in the life of an individual, ultimate concerns are often addressed causing a person to rethink or redefine values, meanings, or whatever it is that has centering power in his or her life. As a result of events surrounding illness, the nature of therapy, or of suffering, a normal individual may seriously question his or her value system. For example, if an adolescent experiences a schizophrenic break and is hospitalized, the parents of the adolescent may suffer spiritual distress. The values of this couple about having children, about parenting, or about even existing as a family unit have been seriously challenged because of their child's illness.

Environmental change may lead to spiritual distress, as when an individual is separated from a religious or cultural community. People are strongly influenced in their choice of values or ultimate concerns by the kinds of value choices that are made in their communities. If they are separated from those groups, the values that fit well within the context of a particular community may

be questioned or even discarded, leaving the person disrupted or disconnected from what had previously given life much of its meaning. For instance, immigrants who leave a familiar place may suffer the symptoms of spiritual distress in their new home, even though they may be much better off in an economic sense than they were in their old environment.

Finally, if a person is depressed, anxious, or unhappy over the *inability to successfully manage a stressful situation*, he or she may experience spiritual distress. Until the stressful situation is adequately resolved, the person will feel uncomfortable. Grief work, that is, the process of giving up the intense emotional attachments that bind people to the things that they have lost, and the reinvesting of those same intense ties into something new or different, is often a long and tedious process that can cause individuals to question the ultimate

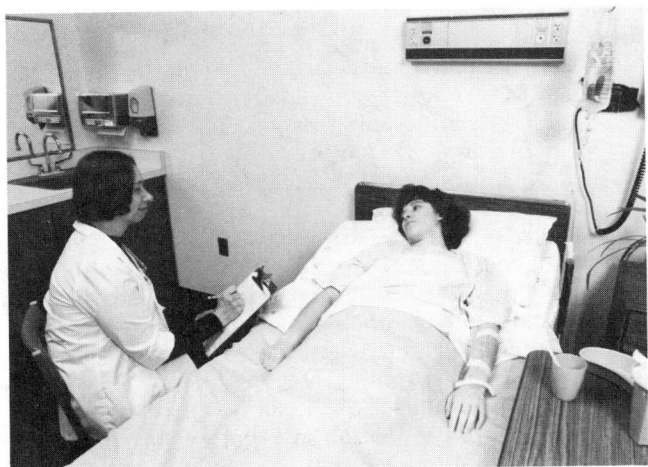

FIGURE 13–30. *Loss is a common related factor of spiritual distress, and illness and the nature of therapy often signifies a loss to the client.*

meaning of their lives. As the loss is resolved and the grief work completed, meaning returns to the particular universe of the individual, although probably in a somewhat different framework than before the original loss occurred. The spiritual distress experienced by the person during grief work will most likely also abate as meaning is again found.

DEFINING CHARACTERISTICS

Certain behaviors may indicate the presence of spiritual distress. Clients may express dissatisfaction or disillusionment with their system of faith. This may take the form of questioning previously held commitments to certain values. A person might say, for example, how stupid it is to believe in a loving or caring God after the individual has lost a close friend or family member to suicide. A hospitalized patient may question the psychiatric treatment. A client might also question existence itself, saying that life is no longer worth living or that he did not ask to be born.

The questioning of one's relationship with a deity is another way of demonstrating spiritual distress. Blaming or exhibiting little trust in the religious values that previously had seemed satisfactory is often the manner in which people will indicate that their relationship with whatever they perceive of as God is unsatisfactory. A client may say something like, "What good are prayers anyway?" This may indicate a disrupted relationship if prayers were previously perceived as useful by the client. Hostile verbalizations toward religious authority figures, such as a priest or rabbi, may indicate decreased trust in the framework of faith represented by that particular religious sect. If the religion represented an important ultimate concern to the client earlier, the hostile behavior is indicative of distress.

Conversely, the patient might seek out an alternate belief system. The original hopelessness of the situation that initially promoted the spiritual distress may be replaced by the search for a new system or framework of meaning. The individual may seek advice from a variety of people to satisfactorily explain what has happened. Here, the person seeks to restructure his or her framework of meaning by asking other people to interpret his or her situation. Support groups often function in this way, that is, they assist an individual who is making an attempt to form a new set of centering concerns. Likewise, a traumatic event, such as the loss of a loved one, might cause a Christian who had always assumed that each single life had innate dignity and worth, to embark upon a study of eastern religions such as Buddhism or Taoism with their traditions of collective humanity and karma.

Finally, individuals experiencing spiritual distress usually appear to be unhappy, lonely, or hopeless. They may complain of somatic symptoms such as fatigue, headache, insomnia, or loss of appetite. They may blame themselves for the problem, saying, for example, "It's all my fault," or "I have only myself to blame," or they may deny responsibility for what is happening or has happened, as indicated by comments like, "It's not really fair at all," or "I did nothing to deserve this" (Chart 1).

CHART 1
Spiritual Distress: Definition, Related Factors, and Defining Characteristics

DEFINITION

Spiritual distress is a disruption in the life principle that pervades a person's entire being and that integrates and transcends one's biologic and psychological nature.

RELATED FACTORS

Losses, such as those involved in
Illness
Treatment/therapy
Suffering/pain

Environmental change, especially separation from religious or cultural community

Inability to manage a stressful situation

DEFINING CHARACTERISTICS

Dissatisfaction with meaning of life and belief system
Questions previously held values
Questions meaning of existence
Questions treatment protocol
Questions meaning of suffering
Expresses conflict about own beliefs

Questions relationship with deity
Blames deity for loss
Shows hostility toward religious authority figures
Questions previous trust placed in deity

Searches for alternative ultimate concerns
Seeks different belief system
Changes usual spiritual practices
Seeks advice from counselor or support group
Seeks spiritual assistance

Demonstrates emotional distress
Appears unhappy
Appears lonely or isolated
Appears depressed
Demonstrates anxiety
Blames self
Avoids responsibility for situation

Demonstrates somatic symptoms
Headache
Fatigue
Sleep disturbance
Gastrointestinal distress
Tightness in chest

NURSING PROCESS AND RATIONALE
Assessment

Routine historical questions often provide the psychiatric nurse with clues to whatever it is in the client's life that has assumed the importance of ultimate concern. As stated earlier, an ultimate concern may be specifically religious, as in a client who shares that certain religious practices are of great importance or help in this situation. However, a centering concern may include areas that are not specifically religious. For example, a client might state or imply that his family is of paramount importance to him and that being separated from them is very distressing to him. Here, the nurse can validate his view by clarifying his statement. "I understand you to say that your wife and children are vitally important to you and that the thought of separation from them for a long time is very painful for you to think about," is an example of clarifying what the client means.

Spiritual distress almost always occurs within the larger context of loss, and the loss is often abrupt or unexpected. It is, therefore, helpful for the nurse to consider the loss that has occurred in the client's life. An important loss, that is, a loss that disrupts the meaning framework that the client has formulated for his life, is the most likely kind of loss to cause spiritual problems, even though the client may not view the loss as a spiritual one. For example, an individual who is proud of her healthy life-style is, because of a bipolar disorder, placed on a long-term regimen of lithium. She may not see the medication dependency as a spiritual loss and may indeed state that her spiritual beliefs are distinctly different from the issues of a psychiatric diagnosis and the need for lifelong medication. But her ultimate or centering concern may have been severely disrupted if staying healthy (which she defines as being medication free) is a major source of strength and hope in her life. An important goal, then, for clients experiencing spiritual distress, is to develop an attitude toward the loss that restores meaning to the person's life. Just as loss is the predominant theme in the development of spiritual distress, so the process of choosing an attitudinal response to the loss that will restore meaning is the way to reach adequate resolution of the problem.

Nursing Diagnosis

This nursing diagnosis can be made more specific for a client as, for example, spiritual distress related to being apart from friends and family after a job-related move.

Client Goals and Nursing Interventions

When the diagnosis of spiritual distress is made, the chief role of the nurse is that of therapeutic communi-cator. The nurse remains available and supportive as the client explores what the loss means, both in a cognitive and an emotional sense (Fig. 13-31). During this time, the client usually is also progressing through the classic stages of adaptation, i.e., denial, hostility, and reorganization, described by Engle.[2] The supportive nurse will not only remain available to talk with the client, but will also encourage interaction with those people, or those things (activities) that provide meaning. Talking with religious advisors, praying, or reading devotional literature may be extremely meaningful for one client, as talking with good friends, listening to music, reading, meditating, or being in a favorite environment may provide meaning to another person (Fig. 13-32).

As clients begin to understand the full import of the loss on the meaning that life previously had, they will generally begin to "try out" various attitudinal responses to the problem. The young woman, mentioned earlier, who must remain on lithium indefinitely, may respond to her condition by criticizing her psychiatrist, by refusing to follow the medication protocol, by researching other treatment options, or by emphasizing other aspects of her healthy life-style such as relaxation exercises. As clients consider various attitudinal or value responses that can be made to the situation,

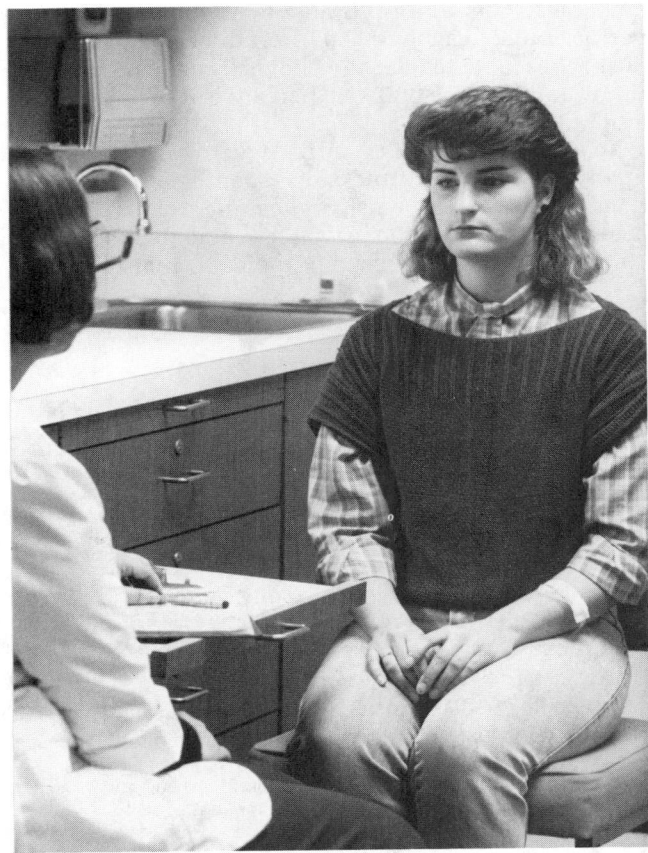

FIGURE 13–31. After assessment of spiritual distress, the nurse's chief role is that of therapeutic communicator, helping the client to explore the meaning of loss.

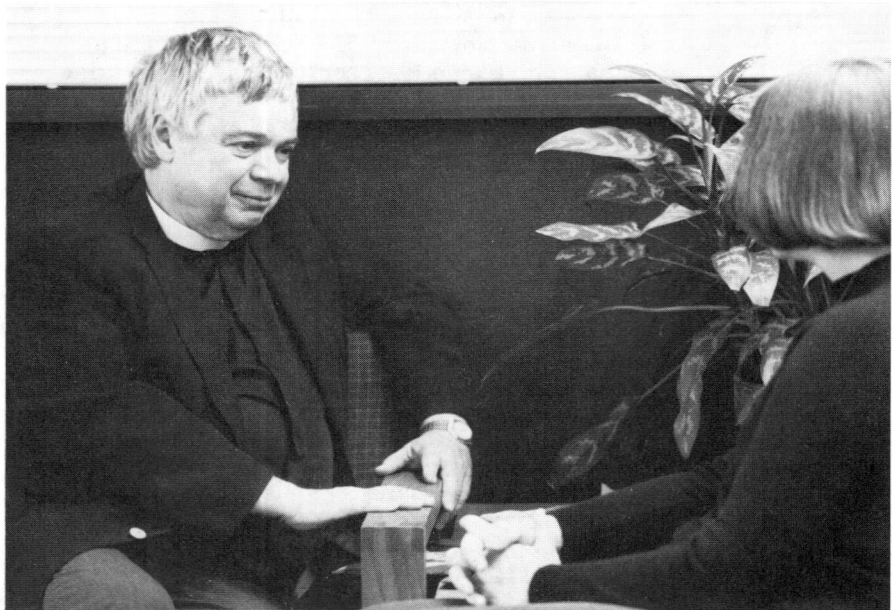

FIGURE 13–32. The best spiritual advisor is the individual who is best able to offer the client strength and hope in the situation at that time.

they will benefit from nonjudgmental and understanding communication. It should be emphasized again that, although supportive communication may come from a specifically religious source, it may also come in an equally helpful form from a family member, a support group colleague, a good friend, or a nurse. Whoever is best able to offer the client strength and hope in the situation is the best spiritual advisor for him or her at that time.

To adequately resolve spiritual distress, clients must finally choose an attitudinal response to their situations that restores a sense of meaning. When meaning is restored, so is the life principle that defines spiritual. An attitudinal choice usually indicates that the client

has reinvested the emotional ties previously invested in the loss object into a new area of centering concern. For example, the medication-dependent client might choose to make the regular practice of meditation as meaningful in her life as her earlier independence from medication had been. She might also say how important her family, her counselor, or her nurse had been in the process of reaching this conclusion.

Evaluation

Clients' communications illustrate that the relationships with those who assisted them to reform their ul-

---

CHART 2
Spiritual Distress: Summary of the Nursing Process

NURSING INTERVENTIONS	OUTCOME CRITERIA
CLIENT GOAL: DEFINE ULTIMATE CONCERNS	
Be available to communicate with client in a supportive, nonjudgmental, and understanding way	Expresses that sense of meaning in life occurs in relation to identified ultimate concerns
CLIENT GOAL: EXPLORE THE COGNITIVE AND EMOTIONAL MEANING OF ANY LOSS OR ENVIRONMENTAL CHANGE IN LIGHT OF ULTIMATE CONCERNS	
Assist client to discuss meaning of these events	Discusses the meaning of these events in relationship to identified ultimate concerns
Provide opportunity for client to explore ultimate concerns	
CLIENT GOAL: CHOOSE A WAY OF RESPONDING TO EVENTS	
Explore with client various possible attitudinal responses toward loss or environmentally changed events	Explores various attitudinal responses and ways of handling the problem or situation
Encourage dialogue between client and supportive others about sources of meaning in client's life	Demonstrates a reinvestment of emotional ties and of meaning in new concerns
Affirm client's ability to respond to loss and recreate meaning in life	

timate concerns (their "spiritual communities") have been established or reestablished. At this time, clients will also probably experience a dramatic reduction of the symptoms of spiritual distress such as unhappiness, loneliness, fatigue, or depression. A decrease in somatic symptoms (e.g., insomnia, headache, inability to eat) will usually be seen. Disruption in the life of a person, according to Frankl,[4] may produce somatic or emotional symptoms. If the spiritual core is healed (through the development of meaningful attitudes toward the disruption), a reduction of other symptoms can be anticipated.

Clients may delay, temporarily or permanently, the acceptance of responsibility for the loss causing the spiritual distress. Similarly, the individual may be trapped in a state of chronic denial or hostility as a reaction to the loss. Just as meaning as an attitudinal response must be identified by the *client* as opposed to the psychiatrist, the family, or the psychiatric mental health nurse, so the nurse must remain available to the client. No satisfactory resolution to spiritual distress can be obtained unless the client discovers the meaning of the situation for himself or herself. Thus, although support and availability are important tools, the nurse should not push the client to a premature meaning choice—even when the individual is uncomfortable (Chart 2).

CASE STUDY

Hazel, a 58-year-old divorced woman, was hospitalized with a psychiatric diagnosis of cyclothymic disorder. Eight years earlier she had experienced a depression that had been successfully treated with psychotherapy. Her family reported that over the past two to three years she has had some periods of being very expansive, distractible, and talkative, as well as other periods of being depressed, sleeping a lot, and having little interest in things. She had not sought treatment during this time; but then, one of her expansive periods coincided with a daughter's traumatic divorce. Hazel invited this daughter and her three children to come live with her. Hazel began taking the children every-

where and, although she initially seemed to enjoy having them around, she became easily overwhelmed by the noise and activity. This was compounded by disagreements with her daughter about how to raise the children and what the routines in the house should be.

On admission to the hospital, Hazel was talking rapidly and wringing her hands, was unkempt, and paced the floor. She expressed feelings of sadness, could not eat or sleep, and her family reported a considerable weight loss in the past several weeks. Her initial nursing diagnosis was agitation related to recent stressors. An effort was made to decrease stimuli in her environment and to monitor her activities of daily living to ensure good hygiene, adequate nutrition, and sufficient rest. As the client became less agitated, she expressed to the psychiatric clinical nurse specialist her distress about her inability to do more to help her daughter. Hazel anguished about not being "responsible and helpful." It was important to her to be in control of a situation and to be able to help others, and she felt a religious obligation to do so. As she herself had been divorced, she remembered how difficult it was and felt that everyone, including people from her church, had turned their backs on her. She felt she was doing the same thing to her daughter by not being better able to handle the situation. The clinical nurse specialist made a nursing diagnosis of spiritual distress related to difficulty in living up to her self-ideal of being helpful to her divorced daughter. Hazel was encouraged to talk about what "responsibility" and "being helpful" meant to her and came to realize that there were other ways of maintaining these values than having her daughter live with her. A series of three sessions was held with the divorced daughter and the three other adult children to work out arrangements that would extend help within the family without burdening Hazel. In addition, Hazel sought out the chaplain for religious guidance.

SUMMARY

Spiritual distress occurs when loss is experienced, causing the meaning matrix that individuals develop for their lives to become disrupted. Ultimate concerns are, therefore, challenged and sources of strength and hope diminished. Following assessment, nursing intervention is designed to support the client in exploring

Research Highlights

Steeves and Kahn observed a recurrent phenomenon in their work with individuals who were terminally ill.[6] Those who were grieving the anticipated loss of their own life or the life of someone close to them often reported on everyday incidents that seemed to change their perception of their situation. For example, one woman whose husband was dying reported that as she worked in her garden, she became peaceful and content and felt in contact with forces greater than herself. Such incidents seemed to be reported in individuals who were adjusting well but not in those who were having a difficult time dealing with their suffering.

Because of the significance of this phenomenon,

Steeves and Kahn believed it warranted exploration. Drawing on a review of diverse literature and the incidents they had observed, they developed a concept called "experiences of meaning" and stated it as a series of assumptions. One assumption, for example, was: "Experiencing meaning is a positive thing, in that individuals are not totally fulfilled without having experiences of meaning. Also, individuals are better able to cope with suffering when they have experiences of meaning in their lives" (reference 6, p 116). They saw their work in developing this and other assumptions as the first stage of a process that could lead to discussion and the development of research questions.

the loss and finally choosing an attitude, or a value response to the crisis, thereby creating another meaning matrix.

References

1. Berger PL, Luckmann T. The social construction of reality; a treatise in the sociology of knowledge. Garden City, NY: Doubleday & Co; 1966.
2. Engle G. Grief and grieving. Am J Nurs. 1964;64:(9):93–98.
3. Fowler JW. Stages of faith; the psychology of human development and the quest for meaning. San Francisco: Harper & Row; 1981.
4. Frankl V. The unconscious God. New York: Washington Square Press; 1975.
5. Peck MS. The road less traveled; a new psychology of love, traditional values and spiritual growth. New York: Simon & Schuster; 1978.
6. Steeves RH, Kahn DL. Experience of meaning in suffering. Image. 1987;19:113–116.
7. Tillich P. Dynamics of faith. New York: Harper & Row; 1957.

SUBSTANCE ABUSE
(ALCOHOL)

Britt Finley

DEFINITION AND DESCRIPTION

Substance abuse (alcohol) as a nursing diagnosis refers to a pattern of behavior characterized by excessive drinking of alcohol, which occurs at regular daily intervals, regular weekend intervals, or during binges (intoxicated for at least two successive days) interspersed with periods of nonexcessive drinking; difficulty in stopping or reducing the amount of alcohol use; pattern of pathologic alcohol use extending for at least one month; impaired social or occupational role functioning associated with substance abuse (alcohol), or any combination thereof. Substance abuse (alcohol) can be manifested in the spiritual–belief, cognitive–perceptual, biologic, and psychosocial aspects of individuals, families, and groups.

THEORY AND RESEARCH

A number of theories are in use to explain substance abuse (alcohol). These are the biologic–genetic model, learning and social model, the psychodynamic model, and the multidimensional model.

Biologic–Genetic Model

According to the biologic–genetic model there is a specific genetic vulnerability for alcoholism.[1] This is suggested by familial patterns in blood acetaldehyde levels after alcohol ingestion, as well as by the presence of characteristically low monoamine oxidase in clients with alcoholism and in their family members.[20] Research on a genetic marker for alcoholism has investigated (1) blood groups and serum proteins, (2) color vision defects, (3) phenylthiourea taste sensitivity, and (4) secretion of ABO blood group substance. These studies have shown no hard evidence for an association between alcoholism and inherited factors.[39] Twin and adoption studies suggest a modest genetic influence for men in both normal drinking and alcoholism, although evidence is lacking in studies for women.[32]

Learning and Social Model

The learning and social model proposes that alcoholism is a process developed within a social context. Supporting research has used both animal and human sub-jects. A conditioning model of alcohol tolerance has demonstrated that cues from the environment (odor, sight, taste) produce a stimulus that results in alcohol consumption, and when ethanol is not available for consumption, a psychological compensatory response called craving is produced.[29] Colonies of rats have been studied for alcohol use, and it was demonstrated that those rats who had low dominance standing and chronic inactivity were the ones who overconsumed alcohol.[10]

Psychodynamic Model

The psychodynamic model of alcoholism proposes that problematic infant and child rearing practices produce psychosexual maldevelopment and dependence–independence conflicts. The individual may be dependency-conflicted or overly dependent.[23] It is believed that while habitual alcohol use is in process, the client uses behavior such as exaggeration, denial, rationalization, impulsivity, hedonism, resentment of authority, and affiliation with socially deviant groups. The complications of these behaviors are decreased work efficiency, job loss, alienation of friends and family, legal difficulties, and hospitalization.[27]

Multidimensional Model

The conception of alcoholism that receives most support is a blending of these models into a multidimensional model that allows the interaction of biologic, behavioral, and sociocultural factors. The biologic–genetic model is implemented in teaching about any possible genetic risk of alcoholism and the identification of the relatives with alcoholism in a genogram. Such health education reduces the sense of shame about the disease. The biologic model relates the medical disease of alcoholism in the progression from occasional initial relief drinking to an increase in alcohol tolerance, and from loss of memory during heavy drinking periods (blackouts) to an urgency of drinking. This illustration of the sequelae of the disease shows the client that a pattern has been delineated by the predictable nature of the disease. This identification increases the sense of hope that the disease process can be arrested. The behavioral model is helpful in identification of high-risk situations for drinking, for example, when the individual is most likely to be ritualistically drinking. The psychodynamic model provides understanding in addressing low self-esteem and the resultant intrapersonal dilemmas, as well as independence–dependence ambivalence. Heterogeneity among persons with alcohol-related problems can best be served by this multidisciplinary perspective.[23]

RELATED FACTORS

The development of substance abuse (alcohol) is related to sociocultural, psychobehavioral, physical, and spiritual factors.

Sociocultural factors are present in peer interaction around drinking as a primary activity for entertainment. This leads to the preference of drinking for social interaction. The early attitudes toward alcohol is shaped by media commercials, television portrayal of alcohol use as a coping skill, and the belief that the use of alcohol to reduce life's stress is socially acceptable.[30]

Psychological factors include the cognitive and behavioral aspects. Logical thinking is replaced by denial and negativity which can lead to further misuse of alcohol. The misuse of alcohol can become a major pattern for coping with life's problems. Family modeling of alcohol use is thought to encourage alcohol use by the offspring. As children begin to drink, their developmental task fulfillment is compromised and the potential for self-actualization is hampered.[30] The aging person who has never used alcohol before may begin to drink in an effort to assist with the crisis of relocation, retirement, death of a spouse, or loss of health. This group of clients is identified as having late-onset alcoholism, as opposed to early-onset alcoholism, a condition that persists throughout adulthood.[19]

The physical dimension includes related factors such as genetic predisposition, a routine of poor health habits, and a significant change in tolerance that results in increasing amounts of alcohol consumption before intoxication occurs.[30] As the client continues to drink, there may be less food intake because the calories in alcohol will dull the appetite. Loss of health can lead to an increased use of alcohol in an attempt to reduce the stress of an illness, particularly one involving physical pain.

Alcohol abuse can be related to spiritual depletion with a loss of life's meaning.[34] Rather than engaging in life, the client spends time and energy resources ingesting alcohol. This focus is cyclic, leading to a further loss of values and objectivity. Other people, other interests, and other activities become less important as the use of alcohol as a central focus gains prominence. Families who are in chaos and crisis, with each member feeling powerless, often use alcohol to create a sense of relief from despair.[14] Unfortunately, alcohol abuse in these families increases the potential for domestic violence, and the crisis is escalated, rather than diminished.[12]

DEFINING CHARACTERISTICS

Defining characteristics of substance abuse (alcohol) can vary. Alcoholism can be divided into several subtypes. Gamma alcoholism applies to binge drinkers who alternate periods of sobriety and drunkenness, in contrast with beta alcoholism, that is manifested by physical complications of *chronic* alcohol use, such as cirrhosis, gastritis, and polyneuropathy without physical dependence on alcohol.[7] For example, the client with gamma alcoholism could be a college student who engages in acute heavy episodic drinking. There are few physiologic manifestations and no withdrawal symptoms. However, these persons are prone to accidents. The client with beta alcoholism, on the other hand, for example, could be a housewife who is a maintenance drinker. These clients experience withdrawal symptoms, and their physiologic state becomes compromised.

The physical problems that may occur are trauma, alcoholic hypoglycemia, alcoholic hyperglycemia, alcoholic hepatitis, cirrhosis, gastritis, and hypothermia.[13] Alcohol breath odor, alcoholic blackouts (loss of memory without passing out), or rambling speech with hostile or grandiose content alerts the nurse to substance abuse (alcohol).[16] The pathophysiology of chronic or acute heavy drinking affects every physiologic system.[13] A flushed face caused by the vasodilation effects of alcohol, numerous bruises from falling or from fights, and any illness that is not responding as it should because of a deficit in self-care may also be clues in the appraisal of alcohol abuse.[11]

Impaired occupational functioning is dependent upon problems with the work role. For purposes of illustration, the characteristics that should alert nurses or health-care administrators to alcohol misuse or dependence by nurses will be used. Background indicators include family history of drug or alcohol abuse, frequent changes in work site, and prior reputation as a good employee. Behavioral manifestations include sloppy charting, excuses for days off or sick days following days off, social isolation, frequent bathroom visits to drink, irritability and mood swings, alcoholic blackouts, frequent emergencies, marital or family problems, and loss of interest in personal grooming. Physical signs include weight loss, unsteady gait, slurred speech, and hand tremor.[38]

Impaired social functioning can include poor judgment, divorce, arrests for violent crimes, arrest for driving under the influence, social isolation, and making promises that are not kept.

Psychosocial difficulties manifested by the client can include depression, suicidal threats, ambivalence, grandiosity, and social withdrawal. Preoccupation with alcohol in conversation, for example, frequent references to being drunk, is also a clue.[11] Behavioral manifestations in adolescents are poor school grades, discipline problems, excessive fighting, truancy, vandalism, and hyperactivity.[6]

The pathologic pattern of alcohol abuse is seen in binges, loss of control over the amount drunk, blackouts, and an inability to stop drinking, despite its untoward effects and innumerable resolutions made by the person to quit sometime in the future[1] (Chart 1).

NURSING PROCESS AND RATIONALE

Assessment

Assessment may be quick or in-depth. A quick assessment is for emergency conditions and withdrawal. An in-depth assessment of alcohol use should be conducted for clients in any of the high-risk groups. The high-risk groups for the development of alcoholism are those who (1) have a positive family history for alcoholism, (2) had a family of origin with a moral prohibition against alcohol but are now in a drinking cultural context, (3) have a spouse with either an abstinence or alcoholism history in the family of origin, (4) are Irish or Scandinavian, since they report a high rate of alcoholism, (5) certain tribes of Native Americans, (6) have female relatives with recurrent depression in more than one generation, or (7) are heavy smokers because heavy drinking is often associated with heavy smoking.[11,17]

The assessment should include the existence of potential overlapping problems, such as drug abuse. In addition, pathologic gambling,[25] spouse abuse,[2] child neglect or abuse,[41] eating disorders,[5] and depression[4] have all been identified as frequently being associated with alcoholism. The assessment should also include the potential existence of personality disorders because the presence of overlapping symptoms of personality characteristics and the use of alcohol has been established.[40] Rawlings[40] has identified seven subtypes: (1) the chronic severe distress group resembles borderline personalities and uses alcohol to reduce tension; (2) the passive–aggressive sociopaths are resentful and self-centered; (3) the antisocial sociopaths alternate between hostility and superficial friendliness; (4) the reactive depressive group are passive–aggressive and depressed after antisocial activities; (5) the severely neurotic psychophysiologic type are dependent people who focus on physical illness, in contrast to (6) the paranoid alienated type who are violent when drunk and are hostile, suspicious persons; and (7) the final group of mixed character dysphoria-type who worry about inadequacies and are nondisclosing.[40]

An in-depth history is useful and the nurse should seek information that will form a baseline of data. Intellectual functioning, physical functioning, social functioning, spiritual functioning, and alcohol use itself must be assessed. (1) Questions that may assess intellectual functioning are: How do you view your drinking? Has drinking presented any problems for you? How do you spend your leisure time? (2) Physical functioning may be assessed by asking these questions: What is your general health? changes in appetite? bowel habits? weight changes? vomited blood? Have you had any heart problems? chest pains? coughed up blood? Do you have tingling pain or numbness in your legs or arms? tremors? seizures? hearing or seeing things? blackouts? Are you taking any drugs or prescribed medication? (3) Social functioning may be assessed by asking these questions: Have you had any arrests? fights? accidents? What is your living arrange-

---

CHART 1
Substance Abuse (Alcohol): Definition, Related Factors, and Defining Characteristics[11,27]

DEFINITION

Substance abuse (alcohol) is a pattern of behavior characterized by excessive drinking of alcohol, which occurs at regular daily intervals, on regular weekend intervals, or during binges (intoxicated for at least two successive days), interspersed with periods of nonexcessive drinking; difficulty in stopping or reducing amount of alcohol use; pattern of pathologic alcohol use extending for at least one month; and/or impaired social or occupational role functioning.

RELATED FACTORS

Sociocultural factors (e.g., peer pressure, media promotion of drinking)
Psychological factors (e.g., use of alcohol to cope with stress, denial of use and consequences)
Physical factors (e.g., genetic predisposition, poor health)
Spiritual factors (e.g., loss of purpose and objectivity)

DEFINING CHARACTERISTICS

Impaired social functioning (e.g., arrests, social isolation)
Impaired occupational functioning (e.g., poor job performance)
Psychological difficulties (e.g., suicidal threats, grandiosity)
Pattern of pathologic alcohol use (e.g., binges, blackouts)
Physical problems (e.g., trauma, hypoglycemia, gastritis)

ment? Do you have an occupation? Whom do you feel close to? (4) Spiritual functioning can be assessed by these questions: Are you affiliated with a religious group? How often have you felt extreme alienation? (5) Questions that will form the data base about drinking are: When did you have your first full drink of alcohol? How was that experience? When did you first experience problems related to alcohol use? When was your last drink? Describe your drinking pattern last year?[11]

The appraisal for an emergency room trauma client who has alcohol on his breath or who is admitted for treatment should be quickly done to ascertain the health status. These questions have two categories: impending withdrawal assessment and potential emergency conditions. To find out past withdrawal history ask: What reactions have you had when you stopped drinking in the past? hear or see things? convulsions? To make a judgment about immediate intervention ask: When did you have your last drink? How much have you been drinking? When did this drinking episode start? Are you taking any medication?[11] Potential emergency conditions can be asked about with these questions: Have you recently been hurt? Do you have any chronic health problems?[11]

Nursing Diagnosis

The formulation of the specific nursing diagnosis is based on the assessment information. The nursing diagnosis of substance abuse (alcohol) related to low self-worth would be appropriate if the client discussed use of alcohol to cope with shame, confusion, and sense of inadequacy in his life. The nursing diagnosis of substance abuse (alcohol) related to unresolved grief would be appropriate if the nursing history revealed the use of alcohol as a coping strategy following the loss of a significant other, job, or health change. The client who discloses an inability to sleep which has resulted in alcohol abuse could have a diagnosis of substance abuse related to difficulty in sleeping.

A major difficulty in formulating a nursing diagnosis may be the client's denial of the problems related to alcohol abuse. Clients with middle-stage and late-stage alcoholism have elaborate shields from acknowledging the problems caused by alcohol use. For example, depression or low self-worth, loss of significant others, vocational stress, health problems, and sleep disturbances can be consequences of substance abuse (alcohol) as well as contributing factors to the abuse. As the client abstains from alcohol, the primary related factors will be more easily understood.

Client Goals and Nursing Interventions

The client goals are to recognize and accept the drinking problem, develop adaptive coping strategies, eliminate the need to use alcohol as a means of escape, im-

prove self-concept, and gain personal hope. As the nurse uses interventions aimed at these goals, success will be facilitated by functional attitudes. Functional attitudes that assist the nurse in being therapeutic with these clients are firmness, optimism, warmth, hopefulness, patience, and persistence, as opposed to such dysfunctional attitudes as rigidity, helplessness, coldness, suspiciousness, hopelessness, impatience, and giving up.[9]

The goal of having the client recognize and accept the drinking problem requires intervention addressing the client's denial. By teaching the risk factors, sequences, and defining characteristics of alcoholism, and the heterogeneity of responses to drinking, the client will be able to identify his or her own risk factors, defining characteristics, and pattern of adaptation to abusive drinking. Clients can be requested to document their drinking and problems related to drinking; and list the costs and benefits of their drinking along social, financial, physical, spiritual, and mental dimensions. Significant others can be encouraged to explain to the client the problematic impact of the alcohol abuse. The client is assisted to describe the ways that behavior changes when drinking and what is disliked about the drinking.

To be successful in meeting the goal of acceptance of the drinking problem, the nurse will need to confront the client's fears. Fear of being rejected because of being an alcoholic is common.[11] The stereotype of the person with alcoholism as that person's not being worthwhile is very stigmatizing. This stereotype can be challenged by the client seeing successful recovering alcoholics in Alcoholics Anonymous. The client can say, "I'm an alcoholic. Alcoholics are worthwhile people. I'm a worthwhile person." Another method to reduce stigma is for the alcoholic to split the concept into reference to a recovering, sober, or "wet," intoxicated alcoholic; once the person can accept the fact of not being a drinking alcoholic the diagnosis may be accepted.[16] Teaching–learning theory is employed in nursing interventions throughout the client's treatment.

Another aspect that influences the client's compliance with alcoholism treatment is the health beliefs about himself or herself and health attitudes held. Attitudes about the clients' perceived severity of their drinking, their satisfaction with the professional relationships, and expectations of improvement all increase compliance.[35] The nurse can do much to influence these beliefs by teaching about alcoholism as a treatable disease, facilitating the client's identification of his own disease and its behavioral, physical, spiritual, and cognitive consequences. Reality orientation about the severity of drinking can also be effected by hearing from family members, employers, physicians, and clergy. This structured information sharing is a technique called "intervention" and is used to encourage the alcoholic to seek treatment. Sharing information about the client's condition in a realistic, straightforward manner is beneficial.

The client goal of developing adaptive coping strategies and eliminating the need to use alcohol as a means of escape may involve family treatment. Family treatment for alcoholism is integral to recovery. There are several treatment modes: spouse involvement, children of alcoholics, parents of alcoholics, or the family as a system itself. The life-style changes that recovery from alcoholism involve will be enhanced by family treatment.[22] The nurse may be involved in conducting family therapy or in making the appropriate referral. It is thought that alcohol abuse creates stress leading to family dysfunction.

Spiritual development is an additional aspect to developing adaptive coping strategies for recovery. The basic premise of Alcoholics Anonymous is a spiritual awakening. Health professionals, including nurses, are seeing the value of assisting clients in finding spiritual meaning in their daily lives.[34] Light believes that spiritual isolation and impoverishment of alcoholics are the two most important single factors in the development of alcoholism. Relying on a higher power means that the grandiosity of the person as being independent and superior must be set aside.[26] Previously blocked spiritual expression is important to recovery and should be encouraged by the nurse. If the client has these interests and capabilities, aesthetic activities that involve creativity also can be used (e.g., poetry, drawing).

Social integration, rather than the previous social isolation, is accomplished by networking with groups and individuals who support alcohol recovery.[15] These interventions will meet the goal of facilitating the client's improvement of self-worth and gaining personal hope. Examples of this would be referral to self-help groups (Alcoholics Anonymous, Al-Anon, Alateen, Women for Sobriety), hobby groups, business groups, and civic groups.

Clients cease growth when the use of alcohol becomes a primary coping skill. These persons have low self-esteem and fear of rejection. The defense mechanisms of denial, projection, and reaction formation are used. A foundation of faulty attitudes and beliefs keep them in isolation, and they fail to do adequate reality testing.[26] Rational–emotive therapy can be useful in dispelling faulty cognition and self-talk[36] (see Chapter 42).

Adaptive coping strategies to achieve an alcohol-free environment are important. The client will need to identify affective triggers for alcohol use and design other options to process the feeling. An example might be the previous reliance on alcohol when anger or boredom was present. Alternatives such as assertiveness training, meditation, and conflict management will be helpful.

The client will also need to identify high-risk situations for alcohol use and the frequent rituals that culminate in its use. If the person always stopped at a bar after work, a new route home that does not pass the bar could be useful. The first holidays, birthdays, and other traditional celebrations (sometimes that includes every Friday night) will need very specific planning to prevent relapse. The client should role-play how to turn down a drink by saying, "No, I don't want a drink" or "I don't drink anymore." The client should practice asking for nonalcoholic beverages. The previous drinking friendship network may also be too high-risk, and the need for new relationships can be met through Alcoholics Anonymous or other appropriate groups. The client needs to understand that the alcoholism cannot be cured, although it can be arrested without further progression if an alcohol-free and drug-free life-style is adopted.

Grief work is important. Previous grief may have been unresolved because of the presence of alcohol, and in recovery, these issues may be integrated. The first grief issue may be the loss of alcohol, which has been a central life focus.[37] Mourning for the childhood loss of parental love and the resultant shame are examples of important and necessary core psychodynamic issues to be resolved.[24] A goal is to assist the client in increasing self-care competence.

A regular exercise program,[31] assertiveness training,[18] nutritional supplementation,[8] problem-solving techniques,[8] and journal writing[36] are used to enhance recovery. These skills can produce a sense of mastery and allow for the internalization of locus of control.[21]

FAMILY ISSUES

As the client begins to achieve control over the drinking, to implement new coping strategies, and to increase a sense of competence and hope, a new phase of life is entered. The sobriety initially brings a new sense of relief to the family and, yet, the adaptation to alcohol-free interactions in the family requires adjustment.

Five major family problem areas of sobriety have been identified by Estes.[12] The first is the reinstatement of the husband or wife into family roles through the development of trust, rather than the suspicion typical of the drinking phase. Sexual readjustment is often difficult for the spouse as bitterness over possible infidelity remains. The second problem area is communication difficulty and learning new styles of relating that are not based on the blaming pattern that was previously employed. The affective responses of the spouse are the third problem area because of lingering resentments, and the unresolved anger related to the drinking days of the marriage. The client's disruptive traits and behavior constitute the fourth problem area. Irrational behavior in reaction to stress has been called a "dry drunk." This response pattern can be as disruptive to the spouse as the drinking was, particularly if mutual blaming is precipitated. The final problem area has to do with situations involving alcohol or alcohol-related problems. Confronting the consequences of alcohol-related problems, worrying about relapse, and learning to be in a social drinking context are typical in this phase.[12]

Evaluation

The complex individual and family responses to alcohol and the physical, emotional, spiritual, and behavioral interventions put in place will require continual evaluation for effectiveness. The client needs to progress from denial of the alcohol abuse to an awareness of the specific damage that it is causing. An alcohol-free and drug-free life-style is necessary.[33] Following this perception, identification of the necessary life-style changes and options to modify life's stress need to be identified specifically. The client should report using abstinence skills successfully at work and in daily life activities. Problem-solving, reduction in impulsivity, adequate occupational role performance, and interpersonal intimacy will be evaluated in this phase of recovery. The improvement of self-concept and attainment of personal hope will be evaluated through the report of a belief that personal change is possible. This belief will be documented by the successful completion of short-term goals and the discussion of personal insight gleaned from creative activity. The contrast of the self-image before treatment, which was narrowly focused on destruction through alcohol abuse, with the recovery self-image, alive with satisfaction gained from personal integration, is striking. This is for many addiction nurses the most exciting evaluation data available (Chart 2).

CASE STUDY

A 38-year-old male mechanic was referred to outpatient therapy with an addictions nurse after a visit to an emergency room for hypothermia and dehydration. He had been married for 14 years, and the marriage has been chronically strained. Mr. and Mrs. S had a 6-year-old daughter and 2 sons, ages 9 and 13. Mr. S stated his wife was physically and verbally abusive to both him and the children. His reason for remaining in the marriage was to "protect" his children from

Mrs. S. He portrayed himself as a "people pleaser" who did not know how to handle conflict. Because his wife worked a different work shift than he did, most of Mr. S's time was spent with his children. The S's lived in a remote rural area.

On the winter night of the emergency room visit, Mr. S had gone out with his male friends. They had gone to three bars and Mr. S drank in each of them. His last memory was of being a passenger in the back of a pickup truck at 1:30 A.M. When he was taken home by his friends, they found him unresponsive and thought he was hypothermic. Mr. S had no memory of being in a coma and of the police taking him to the emergency room. His blood alcohol level was found to be 0.240. His next memory was of being delivered back to his house where his wife kicked him and verbally abused him about his drinking. As Mr. S described this last incident, he cried and stated his concern that the children had seen the abuse.

Mr. S's drinking history revealed an alcoholic paternal grandfather, and being unable to stop drinking without a struggle, morning drinking, and numerous marital problems created because of drinking. He had never had physical withdrawal symptoms. His drinking pattern was periodic binge drinking. The primary nursing diagnosis was substance abuse (alcohol) related to lack of assertiveness and ambivalence about marriage. The nursing goal of helping the client recognize and accept the drinking problem was met in this phase by teaching and crisis intervention. Didactic teaching about alcoholism was accomplished by videotapes, audiotapes, written assignments, and reading. Crisis intervention was used to help identify the perception of the hypothermia as being related to alcohol abuse. Psychotherapy was employed to identify the marital ambivalence, which was related to alcohol abuse. Mr. S described his drinking as "alcoholic" and began to read a great deal about the disease. He described the function of alcohol in his life as being related to the ambivalence toward his marriage. The part of him that was angry at his wife could attain revenge by drinking, and the part of him that was afraid to

CHART 2
Substance Abuse (Alcohol): Summary of the Nursing Process[28]

NURSING INTERVENTIONS	OUTCOME CRITERIA
CLIENT GOAL: RECOGNIZE AND ACCEPT THE DRINKING PROBLEM	
Teach about the disease of alcoholism	Reports comparison of his drinking with the disease pattern
Ask client/family members to list the social, financial, physical, spiritual, and mental consequences of the drinking problem	Identifies dysfunction and self-limitation caused by drinking
Refer to Alcoholics Anonymous	Attends AA meeting and reports optimism about recovery
CLIENT GOAL: DEVELOP ADAPTIVE COPING STRATEGIES AND ELIMINATE THE NEED TO USE ALCOHOL AS A MEANS OF ESCAPE	
Offer family therapy as a treatment modality	Discusses family dysfunction as an adaptation to alcohol abuse
Encourage appropriate referrals for social network	Identifies social activity at which drinking will occur
CLIENT GOAL: IMPROVE SELF-CONCEPT AND GAIN PERSONAL HOPE	
Assist client to increase self-care competence gradually	Participates in exercise program, relaxation, and good nutrition
Ask client to identify and acknowledge success, skills achieved and small gains made	Demonstrates improved self-esteem
Assess for medical problems if recovery is not proceeding successfully and make appropriate referrals	Receives appropriate treatment for health problems

Research Highlights

In an effort to identify the alcoholic clients' problems seen by medical–surgical nurses, Bartek et al. designed an exploratory study that involved an open-ended questionnaire.[3] By using a random method, 50 hospitals were chosen for the study and directors of nursing were asked to submit the names of medical–surgical nurses. A total of 20 directors responded and 236 subjects from the list agreed to participate. The questionnaire asked for three difficult physiologic problems of hospitalized alcoholic clients, factors that made the problem difficult, nursing intervention for the problem, and effectiveness of the intervention. This same information was asked for psychosocial client problems.

The data were analyzed by using a 12 nursing diagnoses scheme. The technique for placing the data into nursing diagnostic categories was a group process. To test the inter-rater reliability of this process, one member independently coded the data, with a resultant 92% concordant responses for the group process identification of nursing diagnosis.

The three most difficult physiologic nursing diagnoses were potential for injury, alteration in nutrition and elimination, and fluid volume deficit. The most common factor that made care difficult for the diagnosis of potential for injury was the client's coping behavior. The nurses saw the client as "temperamental," "immature," "demanding," and "aggressive." The most common nursing intervention for potential of injury was to intervene for safety. The factors that made care difficult for the nursing diagnosis of alterations in nutrition and elimination were the client's physical problems and coping behaviors. Examples of the physical problems cited were

pain, vomiting, and frequent stools, and the coping behavior examples were lack of trust, low self-esteem, and feelings of abandonment. The nursing interventions chosen most often for this diagnosis were (1) provide nutrition, (2) administer medication, and (3) use communication techniques with client. Interventions into the nursing diagnosis of fluid volume deficit were difficult because of nurse's feelings or perceptions. The nurses reported they had difficulty viewing alcoholism as a disease and were unable to remain caring or nonfrustrated. This resulted in the feeling of being inadequate to cope with the client's problem.

The three most difficult psychosocial nursing diagnoses were ineffective individual coping, ineffective family coping, and noncompliance. The factor that made care difficult for the diagnosis of ineffective individual coping was the client's coping behavior. An example of ineffective coping behavior cited by the nurses was noncompliance with the medical treatment and continued alcohol abuse. The most frequently cited intervention technique for the diagnosis of ineffective individual coping was the use of a diplomatic, nonjudgmental approach. Ineffective family coping was made difficult because of the deterioration of significant relationships. The intervention most commonly used for this nursing diagnosis was use of communication techniques with the family. This refers to the nurse emotionally supporting the family and bringing family members together for the client. Noncompliance was difficult because of the nurse's feelings and perceptions and the patient's coping behavior. The nursing interventions used were social support for the patient and providing education.

leave her could ensure his continued dependency because of drinking. The crisis of the winter night hypothermia was successful in helping him acknowledge this pain.

Mr. S was highly motivated to gain control of his drinking and maintain consistent sobriety throughout the year. He attended Alcoholics Anonymous. He began to write songs and made nondrinking friendships. He and his wife were referred for marital therapy, but Mr. S's passive–aggressive style sabotaged these efforts. Mr. S took responsibility for his initial decision of marrying, saying "I only married her so I could get out of debt. She had a good job." He saw himself as now being capable of meeting his own financial needs and regretted the exploitation of his wife. He separated from his wife and became the custodial parent. He began to have a sense of empowerment and dealt with the chronic sorrow of his childhood poverty. He joined a singing group and took up stamp collection as hobbies. He began to date another woman and was hopeful that he could establish a friendship based on caring and self-reliance.

The nursing goal of developing new coping strategies and eliminating the use of alcohol as a means of escape was met through the nursing interventions of appropriate social network referral, marital therapy, and an analysis of drinking. The goal of improving self-concept and a sense of hope was met by gradual increase in competence through self-care and contrasting the behaviors found in his life during alcohol abuse and the behaviors present in recovery.

SUMMARY

Substance abuse (alcohol) can occur in numerous nursing settings. The multidimensional understanding of this nursing diagnosis underlies the nursing interventions. After assessment, the nursing strategy is to assist the client in recognition and acceptance of the drinking problem, development of adaptive coping strategies, elimination of the need to use alcohol as a means of escape, an improvement of self-concept, and gaining a sense of hope.

References

1. American Psychiatric Association. Diagnostic and statistical manual of mental disorders. 3rd ed. Washington DC: American Psychiatric Association; 1987.
2. Baker SA. Family violence and chemical dependency. Focus. 1987;10:3.
3. Bartek JK, Lindeman M, Newton M, Fitzgerald P, Hawks JH. Nurse-identified problems in the management of alcoholic patients. J Stud Alcohol. 1988;49:66.
4. Berner P, Lesca OM, Walter H. Alcohol and depression. Psychopathology. 1986;19(supp 2):177–183.
5. Bulik CM. Drug and alcohol abuse by bulimic women and their families. Am J Psychiatry. 1987;144:12.

6. Bullard JD. Maternal-child nursing. In: Bennet G, Vourak DS, eds. Substance abuse. New York: John Wiley & Sons; 1983.

7. Chafetz ME. The alcoholic patient: diagnosis and management. Oradell, NJ: Medical Economic Books; 1983.

8. Chappel J. Alcohol and drug dependencies. Consultant. 1987;27:60–64.

9. Einstein S. Intervening in the use and misuse of drugs and alcohol: critical issues, specious actions, misplaced faith and ironic outcomes. Int J Addict. 1986;21:4–5.

10. Ellison GP, Potthoff AD. Social models of drinking behavior in animals. In: Galanter J, ed. Recent developments in alcoholism. New York: Plenum Press; 1984.

11. Estes N, Smith-DiJulio K, Heinemann ME. Nursing diagnosis of the alcoholic person. St Louis: CV Mosby; 1980.

12. Estes NJ, Grisham KJ. Sobriety: problems, challenges and solutions. In: Estes NJ, ed. Alcoholism development, consequences and interventions. St Louis: CV Mosby; 1986.

13. Field KL. Medical-surgical nursing. In: Bennet G, Vourakis C, Woolf DS, eds. Substance abuse. New York: John Wiley & Sons; 1983.

14. Finley BG. The family and substance abuse. In: Bennet G, Vourakis C, Woolf DS, eds. Substance abuse. New York: John Wiley & Sons; 1983.

15. Flagan RW, Mauso AL. Social margin and reentry: an evaluation of a rehabilitation program to skid row alcoholics. J Stud Alcohol. 1986;47:413–423.

16. Forchuk C. Cognitive dissonance: denial, self-concepts and the alcoholic stereotype. Nurs Papers. 1984;16:3.

17. Forten ML. Community health nursing. In: Bennett G, Vourakis C, Woolf DS, eds. Substance abuse. New York: John Wiley & Sons; 1983.

18. Gorski TT. Relapse prevention planning: a new recovery tool. Alcohol Res World. 1986;11:2–11.

19. Hall EP. Substance abuse in the aging. In: Bennet G, Vourakis C, Woolf DS, eds. Substance abuse. New York: John Wiley & Sons; 1983.

20. Hesselbrock VM, Shaskan EG, Meyer RE. Biologic and genetic factors in alcoholism. Rockville, MD: National Institute on Alcohol Abuse and Alcoholism, 1983.

21. Huckstadt A. Locus of control among alcoholics, recovering alcoholics and nonalcoholics. Res Nurs Health. 1987;10:23–38.

22. Jauzen C. Use of family treatment methods by alcoholism treatment services. Alcohol Health Res World. 1985/1986;10:2.

23. Keller M. Multidisciplinary perspectives on alcoholism and the need for integration. In: Freed E, ed. Interfaces between alcoholism and mental health. New Brunswick, NJ: Rutgers Center for Alcohol Studies; 1982.

24. Lerner R. Shame. Changes. 1987;2:3.

25. Lesieur HR, Blume SB, Zoopa RM. Alcoholism, drug abuse, and gambling. Alcohol Clin Exp Res. 1986;10:3.

26. Light WJG. Psychodynamics of alcoholism. Springfield, IL: Charles C Thomas; 1986.

27. Ludwig AM. Principles of clinical psychiatry. 2nd ed. New York: Free Press; 1986.

28. McFarland G, Wasli E. Nursing diagnosis and process in psychiatric mental health nursing. Philadelphia: JB Lippincott; 1986.

29. Melchior CL, Takakoff B. A conditioning model of alcohol tolerance. In: Galanter M, ed. Recent developments in alcoholism. New York: Plenum Press; 1984.

30. Metzger L. From denial to recovery. San Francisco: Jossey-Bass; 1988.

31. Murray PA. Fitness and recovery. Alcohol Health Res World. 1986;11:32.

32. Murray RM, Clifford CA, Gurling HMP. Twin and adoption studies. In: Galanter M, ed. Recent developments in alcoholism. New York: Plenum Press; 1983.

33. Pomerleau O, Pertschuk M, Stinnet J. A critical examination of some current assumptions in the treatment of alcoholism. In: Freed EX, ed. Interfaces between alcoholism and mental health. New Brunswick, NJ: Rutgers Center on Alcohol Studies; 1982.

34. Prugh T. Alcohol, spirituality, and recovery. Alcohol Health Res World. 1985/1986;10:2.

35. Rees DW. Health beliefs and compliance with alcoholism treatment. J Stud Alcohol. 1985;46:6.

36. Reruche MA. Alcohol dependence syndrome in women's perspective on disability and rehabilitation. J Rehabil. 1986;52:67–70.

37. Secretary of Health and Human Services. Sixth special report to the US Congress on alcohol and health. Rockville, MD: National Institute on Alcohol Abuse and Alcoholism; 1987.

38. Sullivan E, Bissel L, Williams E. Chemical dependency in nursing. Menlo Park: Addison–Wesley; 1988.

39. Swinson RP. The genetic markers and alcoholism. In: Galanter M, ed. Recent developments in alcoholism. New York: Plenum Press; 1983.

40. Wallace J. The other problem of alcoholics. J Subst Abuse Treat. 1986;3:167.

41. Williams CN. Child care practices in alcohol families. Alcohol Health Res World. 1987;12(summer):77.

SUBSTANCE ABUSE

(DRUGS)

Britt Finley

DEFINITION AND DESCRIPTION

Substance abuse (drugs) as a nursing diagnosis refers to a pattern of behavior characterized by frequent need and use of drugs for personal functioning; difficulty in reducing or stopping the amount of drug used; periodic unsuccessful efforts to stop the use of the drug; episodes of complications from drug misuse; or frequent use of drugs causing impairment of functioning for at least one month. Substance abuse (drugs) can be manifested in the psychosocial, biologic, cognitive–perceptual, and spiritual–belief aspects of individuals, families, and groups.

THEORY AND RESEARCH

Psychoanalytic

In general, the psychoanalytic view is that chemical dependence results from efforts to cope with the oral stage of psychosexual developmental difficulties.[1] This view holds that the client is acting out of the unconscious independence–dependence conflict. The impaired reality testing, poor impulse control, egocentrism, inability to negotiate the tension of reality and pleasure drives, and fear of interpersonal intimacy seen in some substance-abusing clients is explained as fixated oral development.

Biologic

The biologic understanding of drug use is increasing. The view attributes the abuse of substances to the biophysiologic interrelationships of the abuser and the substance. The research on endogenous opioids, endorphins, is an example of the biologic view of substance abuse. It is hoped that this research will assist in understanding biologic causes of increased susceptibility to opiate abuse, as well as the mechanisms of opiate addiction. Opiate receptors have been discovered for endogenous opioids, and the functional actions and cellular sources of endogenous opioids have been defined.[28] The search for biological and genetic markers is another example of the biologic model, which may eventually identify persons at risk so that appropriate counsel may be given.[41] Examples of markers under current review are pharmacogenetic differences in enzyme metabolism, in antigens, and in blood groupings, and DNA polymorphisms. Genetic linkage research refers to the precise location of genes within the same chromosome and can determine which members of an at-risk family possess the gene that produces susceptibility. Studies have been conducted on the association of disease and genetic status such as changes in addicts' lymphocytes and the level of chromosome aberrations.[41]

Biological differences in drug responses based on gender are being investigated to better understand misuse and dependency.[14] The menstrual cycle as a significant correlational variable has been included in the design of psychopharmacologic research. Currently there are mixed reports on the cycle-related changes in drug use and its effects.[24]

The biologic model is used to explain the positive reinforcement that leads to abuse and addiction. The strong abuse potential of cocaine is related to the direct stimulation of the brain's reward system in the hypothalamus. Cocaine prolongs the dopamine activity in the synapse by blocking the dopamine re-uptake mechanism, just as does the dopamine involvement in food and water reinforcement mechanisms.[45]

Stress–Adaptation

Stress theory suggests that substance use is a coping mechanism to decrease negative affect or increase positive affect. The adaptive orientation to addiction emphasizes homeostasis as a motivator for drug use. The individual copes with the environmental demands by augmenting the inadequate available resources with drugs. This view of addiction emphasizes the stages of change and looks at the different learning within each stage, from drug initiation to maintenance. High-risk situations both for initiating use (peer pressure) and relapse (drug hunger produced from drug-related cues) receive consideration within this theory.[22]

Gender difference and its interrelatedness to heroin use as an adaptive mechanism has been researched by Tucker.[43] She found gender differences in use patterns of heroin addicts and attributed this to social support and environmental demand differences between the sexes. Whereas males were often polydrug users before initiating heroin use, females were more likely to begin

465

their drug use with heroin. Tucker postulated that female heroin initiation began as an adaptation to the social situation of being with a man who used heroin. The female's adaptation to a support system that encouraged heroin use was to begin her own use. The sustained drug-use pattern was also different: females used heroin within an environmental demand context and were less likely than men to use heroin daily as well as less likely to overdose on heroin.

Family Dysfunction

Some theorists understand drug abuse as originating from family dysfunction. For a full discussion of a family system view of an adult substance abuser, see Chapter 16. Adolescent drug abuse may be an outcome of family process when the marital coalition is weak, intergenerational boundaries are confused, and there is a low level of individuation of the members.[42] The diffuse psychological boundaries and low self-esteem in such families mean that strong feelings are frightening, and family members allow expression of feelings only while under the influence of a drug. Such families are best described as systems whose members have a sense of loneliness, worthlessness, and deprivation. Chemical dependence can have a multigenerational history. The parents in their families of origin have had limited experience with problem-solving skills, interdependency, and conflict management. As marriage partners, they do not know how to make joint decisions and have generally unsatisfactory marriages. There may be a high incidence of incest as the opposite-sex parent attempts to establish intimate relationships with the child. The same-sex parent is described as rejecting, whereas the opposite-sex parent rarely attempts to change the drug dependence that limits the independence potential of the child. Conflicts relating to jealousy of the same-sex parent toward the addicted child evolve.[42]

When the parents cannot cooperate in dysfunctional families, mutual limit setting is impossible, and the adolescent addict is unsupervised. Attention is gained through negative behavior, which serves to maintain the family homeostasis, and individuation and separation are difficult to establish for the child. The crisis created by the addict may be the only way the family members interact. The separation from the family of the addict through marriage or other means is often sabotaged, and as an adult, the addict may return home.[42]

RELATED FACTORS

The development of substance abuse/dependence has five major related factors: spiritual, physical, sociocultural, family, and psychobehavioral. Spiritual factors related to substance abuse (drugs) may be the loss of control over life's experience and the resultant meaninglessness. This may result in substance use that, in turn, creates more uncontrolled, stressful events.[29]

Physical related factors, including genetic susceptibility, poor health habits, and pain, may result in drug abuse. Drug use may begin with the loss of health, especially when it involves pain. Poor health habits also contribute to substance abuse, and an important predictor of current substance use is past drug use.

More than one third of all men and one fifth of all women have had experience with cocaine by the time they have reached their mid-20s. However, this use is generally limited to fewer than ten trials. The frequency of adolescent marijuana use is the most significant predictor for frequent cocaine use in young adulthood.[17]

The sociocultural-related factors include cultural norms that support drug use as a valued activity. The role-modeling of drug use by culturally powerful significant others creates acceptance and prestige of drug-taking behavior. For a fuller discussion of the cultural theory of substance abuse, see Chapter 16.

Families in chaos and turmoil may begin the use of drugs to reduce the possibility of structural change in the family system, thereby maintaining the status quo. While family members are focused on drug use as a problem of an individual member, they are free to ignore the underlying issues of personal unhappiness with one another and the dysfunctional family system roles and rules.[42]

Attempts to identify behavioral or social-risk factors for drug use have begun to be well researched, and it is apparent that there is no single specific trigger or event that predicts drug use in a given person.[29] Socialization to nontraditional norms, disruption in normal child–parent relationships, lack of involvement in organized groups, physical pain, and mental anguish all have been shown to be predisposing factors in initial drug abuse.[12] Research on high school marijuana and cocaine users shows common variables in terms of background and life-style factors. Included among the strongest predictors of use were truancy, evenings out for recreation, and political views.[30]

DEFINING CHARACTERISTICS

The client with a nursing diagnosis of substance abuse (drugs) may present a variety of problems—family, employment, health, and financial. Impaired social functioning will be manifested by interpersonal difficulties with family and friends. Personal values may conflict with societal values, as demonstrated by criminal delinquent behavior and traffic accidents.

Impaired occupational functioning may be manifested. Frequent job loss, absenteeism, and an inability to perform in the job can be present. The client may be underemployed, using only a portion of his or her potential in the work place. Difficulty with coworkers and supervisors may be reported. Injury at work because of impaired psychomotor coordination is also a clue to substance use.

The physical problems that are manifested will vary depending on the specific properties of the substance used, as well as the amount and method of use. For example, the consequences of cocaine use relate both to the level of cocaine use and the route of injection (intranasal, intravenous, smoked, or oral). The most common route is "snorting" or inhaling. Chronic rhinitis and ulcerated or perforated nasal septum can develop after this recurrent means of administration. The smoking of cocaine free base is the most effective method of rapidly delivering high concentrations of cocaine and is gaining in popularity.[9] Crack, a purified freebase form of cocaine, is always smoked. Although cocaine is 15% to 25% pure, crack is as much as 90% pure. The "snorting" of cocaine produces euphoria in one to three minutes for a period of 30 minutes; crack's high begins in four to six seconds and lasts five to six minutes.[1] Physical signs of cocaine use are an increase in heart rate and blood pressure; heart attacks related to coronary spasm and brain hemorrhage have also been reported. Bowel injury because of impaired bowel circulation may result in severe colitis and ulcerated bowel. Paranoid thinking related to cocaine may trigger violence, even homicide. In addition, sexual dysfunction is common in heavy cocaine abusers.[28] The withdrawal syndrome of cocaine is manifested by sleep disturbance, eating disturbance, strong craving, tremor, muscle pain, and electroencephalogram (EEG) changes.[28]

Maladaptive behavior and feelings are typical in the substance abuser. Use of drugs can mask, imitate, or mimic psychopathology.[34,39] The stigma of addiction as well as concerns about the loss of control over drug use may tax the addict's vulnerable self-esteem. Drug abusers have been defined as having external locus of control, low self-concept, feelings of disillusionment, and personal stress[4] (Chart 1).

CHART 1
Substance Abuse (Drugs): Definition, Related Factors, and Defining Characteristics

DEFINITION

Substance abuse (drugs) is a pattern of behavior characterized by a frequent need and use of drugs for personal functioning; difficulty in reducing or stopping the amount of drug used; periodic, unsuccessful efforts to stop use of drug; episodes of complications from drug misuse; or frequent use of drugs causing impairment of functioning for at least one month.

RELATED FACTORS

Physical (e.g., increased genetic susceptibility to opiate use)
Psychobehavioral (e.g., poor impulse control, sense of powerlessness)
Family (e.g., intergenerational use of substances)
Spiritual (e.g., loss of sense of purpose)
Cultural (e.g., acceptance of drug use as a normative behavior)

DEFINING CHARACTERISTICS

Impaired social functioning (e.g., disrupted friendships)
Impaired occupational functioning (e.g., job loss)
Physical problems* (e.g., nasal septum erosion)
Maladaptive behavior patterns or feelings (e.g., high dependency needs/low tolerance for frustration)

* Problems depend on type of drug and length of its use.

NURSING PROCESS AND RATIONALE

Assessment

The assessment for substance abuse (drugs) needs to review seven factors: use of drug(s), loss of control, life impact, previous treatment, client's perception of problems, client's needs and requests, and perception by significant others. The areas of information to be gathered in terms of use are the frequency, patterns of abuse, social context, and specific drugs used. Questions need to be specific, for example: Have you been drinking? Smoking? Inhaling? Taking drugs intravenously? Using marijuana? When did you last use a drug(s)? How much? How much did you use yesterday? Were you alone? What happens when you use the drug? Polydrug abuse as well as a need for detoxification should be assessed. Loss of control will be indicated by the data on sequelae of cessation and attempts to stop. Questions include: Can you handle more drugs than before? Do you ever use more than you intend? What happens when you stop? The life impact factors of health, legal, financial, and occupational problems, as well as those involving family and friends require these types of questions: What do your friends say about your drug use? Have there been problems at home lately? Have you been having financial difficulties? How's work for you? Previous treatment course, compliance, and complication information may be addressed by asking: Have you ever gone to anyone for help about your problems? What happened? When? Are you going to AA? To determine judgment, insight, and client's perception of the problem, ask: What brings you here? Has your drug or alcohol use caused problems? To determine the client's needs and requests, ask: What do you want to see happen? To assess the significant other's perceptions of abuse duration, severity, and past treatment, ask: Could you describe the problem? What do you want to see happen?

Nursing Diagnosis

The information from the client concerning life impact, client's perception of the problems, client's needs and requests for help, as well as perception by significant others, guides the nurse in making a specific client-related nursing diagnosis. Substance abuse (drugs) related to emotional immaturity could be a specific diagnosis for an adolescent or young adult who began early addictive drug use in a social–recreational use pattern that has expanded to compulsive use. The use of drugs will delay the client's ability to complete normal developmental tasks, and it is thought that personality is arrested at the age at which drug abuse began.[25] Substance abuse (drugs) related to need to escape could be an appropriate nursing diagnosis for the client who describes being burdened by life stress, and, therefore, unable to cope with the pressure and demands, uses drugs as an attempt to cope. Such a client may have a maladaptive response to a crisis, such as loss of a parent or mate. The unresolved grief creates too much distress for such a client, and the substance abuse reduces the awareness of the burden. Unfortunately, as long as the client is self-medicating, the resolution of the grief will also be hampered.

Client Goals and Nursing Interventions

The nursing goals are to meet physiologic and safety needs and develop alternative coping skills and lifestyle to reduce or eliminate drug misuse.[20]

The nursing interventions useful for meeting physiologic and safety needs vary with the biologic responses to the substance used and, therefore, will be drug-specific. An example of such a difference is the usefulness of being highly focused with short reality-oriented sentences when dealing with a client who is disoriented following lysergic acid diethylamide (LSD) ingestion. This is in contrast to providing a quiet environment free from stimuli, for the phencyclidine (PCP)-abusing client where the client can be unobtrusively monitored.[20]

The first determination made in meeting the physiologic and safety needs is assessment of the level and type of drug present in the substance abuser's system. Comprehensive examination of all body systems assists in the identification of physiologic responses to both episodic and continuous substance use.[2] Drug usage may be detected by body fluid examination, behavioral observation (mood changes, poor psychomotor coordination), or physiologic signs of use (needle marks, pupil size). Pupil diameter varies according to the substance used. Dilated pupils may result from use of phencyclidine, marijuana, or stimulants, and from sedative–hypnotic, alcohol, and opiate withdrawal. Opiate intoxication causes the pupils to become extremely small. Nystagmus is present in alcohol, sedative, or PCP intoxication. The test for nystagmus is to ask the subject to hold the head in a fixed position while tracking the examiner's finger or small flashlight across the visual field 12 to 20 cm from the face.[39]

Assessment for intoxication requires knowledge of how the drugs within a specific classification influence the biologic system. Opiate intoxication manifests in euphoria, drowsiness, and respiratory depression. Barbiturate intoxication causes respiratory depression, relaxation, and slowed physical and cognitive activity. Cocaine intoxication signs are elevated blood pressure, increased heart rate, insomnia, diaphoresis, and pressured speech.[1]

Withdrawal occurs when physiologic dependence on the substance has been developed. Withdrawal signs for barbiturates are malaise, nausea, vomiting, insomnia, and tremulousness, which may progress to seizures, hallucinations, and delirium. Heroin withdrawal produces sniffling, gooseflesh, lacrimation, and sneezing in the mild forms. In severe heroin withdrawal, there are body aches and severe agitation. Cocaine withdrawal manifests by irritability, restlessness, and lack of energy.[1]

While the client is experiencing physiological disequilibrium, the nurse collaborates with the physician to treat altered sensory–perception, fluid–electrolyte imbalance, pain, and sleep disturbances (Fig. 13-33). The nursing interventions also aim at protecting the client from additional injury. An example of this would be turning the intoxicated, vomiting client on his side with the face down to avoid aspiration of vomitus. For the comatose substance abuser, maintaining the respiratory–circulatory integrity is vital.

Idiosyncratic drug reactions can produce violent behavior. The nursing guidelines for intervention into this situation are similar to dealing with other violent clients. The nurse must be cautious with motor move-

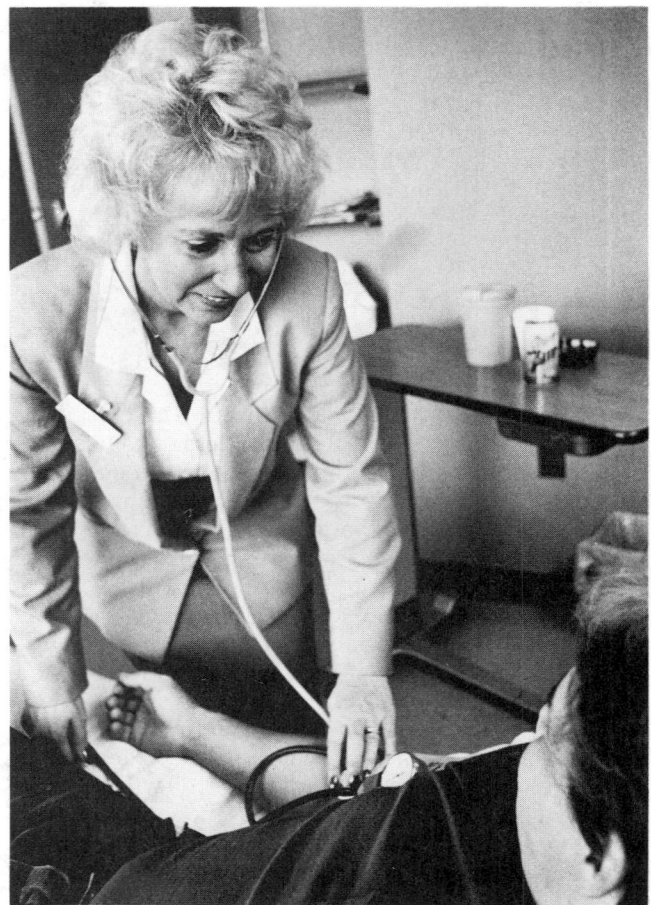

FIGURE 13–33. The psychiatric mental health nurse must assess the client's physiologic status. (Photograph © 1988 by Jeffrey J. Smith)

ments and not make sudden motions or argue with the client. The voice used should be calm. Attempt to show the client that the nurse is an advocate, and have the client verbalize about positive affective relationships.[10]

While the client is on an inpatient unit, the establishment of a drug-free milieu is critical. Each treatment center will employ admission procedures to search the client for drugs, and the search may include body orifices as well as a clothing search. The monitoring of visitors to be certain there are no drugs will also vary by treatment setting. Some units prohibit visitors or gifts sent to the client to ensure drug security, whereas others will request only that visitors not bring drugs to clients. Institute security procedures so that clients are not getting drugs from the medical supplies of the unit or from other clients. The nurse must actively plan the physical environment of the substance abuse unit to ensure structural integrity that promotes safety (Fig. 13-34).

The nursing interventions aimed at developing alternate coping skills and lifestyles to reduce or eliminate drug abuse will start with a client's commitment to abstinence. Before the client is willing to make a commitment to abstinence, denial must be addressed. Denial includes the unwillingness of the client to accept responsibility for the substance use and its consequences. The commitment to the abused substance is quite high, hence the cycle of addiction. That is, the object relationship with the substance is strong, and the substance may be the only "friend" for the client.[47] Confrontational techniques can be used together with a caring attitude. Metzger has identified two levels of confrontation.[26] Soft confrontational techniques hook the client's inherent values in addressing the abuse. An example of this would be: "You were doing well in your job until your marijuana use increased." Soft confrontation also emphasizes the negative consequences of the drug use. An example is: "Every time you use cocaine you get violent." Hard confrontation requires a tough stance and incorporates information

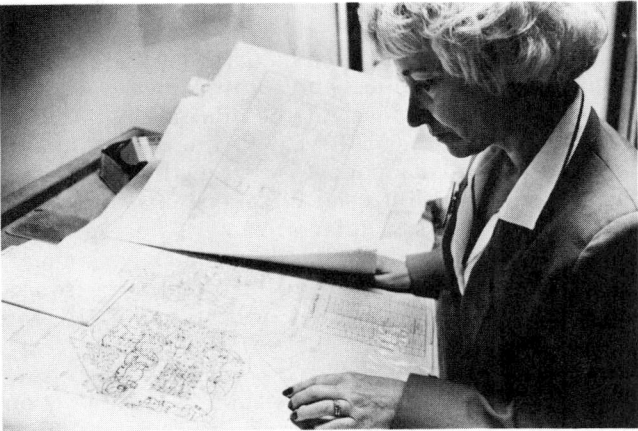

FIGURE 13-34. *The nurse has a role in actively planning the physical environment of the substance abuse unit to ensure the structural integrity that promotes safety. (Photograph © 1988 by Jeffrey J. Smith)*

the professional has gained through assessment. An example would be: "Many drug users lose weight because of the decreased appetite. You look about 40 pounds underweight."

The element of hope is an important aspect of facilitating an alternate life-style. Each informational sharing with the client should emphasize the benefits and possibilities of recovery.[26] Some treatment settings employ personnel who are themselves recovering substance abusers and, in this way, the client can see functioning role models who offer hope by their example.

Education about addiction and the drug or drugs that have been abused will increase the awareness of abuse (Fig. 13-35). As information about the substance is gained, the client can understand the responses more clearly. This will also diminish denial.

Social skills training for both the abuser and spouse, and assertiveness training, relaxation, and desensitization, has been helpful in changing substance abuse responses.[6,21] The National Institute on Drug Abuse has published a structured curriculum for recovery training, *Addict Aftercare: Recovery Training and Self-Help.*[46] Various other techniques that can be helpful in recovery are: meditation,[11] yoga,[36] exercise,[37] biofeedback,[36] problem-solving,[35] acupuncture,[38,40] massage,[36] and creative writing.[19]

Focus must be placed on the "here and now."[25] Short-term behavioral contracts for new interactions, other than drug use, can be very useful.[23] An example of this is establishing the goal to complete the daily job activities without the use of any substances. In making the goal realistic, the nurse would establish with the client when during the day the substance use routinely occurred and what the ritual surrounding the use was. The reinforcement for abstinence would also be mutually planned (e.g., going for a relaxing walk). The contract would include maintaining abstinence, a concrete plan to avoid the ritualistic drug use, and a reinforcement for abstinence. Another example of a short-term behavioral contract is the contingency contract that states that if a certain behavior is manifested, then a predictable consequence will be put in place. An example of contingency contracting is for the client and the outpatient nurse therapist to contract for the consequences of urine testing positive for drug use. Frequently, the consequence contracted will be based on the vocational or legal situation of the client. A client who is on probation for criminal charges may have his or her probation officer notified so legal repercussions can be put in place. A chemically dependent nurse, for example, whose professional license is being monitored, may contract to have the Board of Nursing notified. This mechanism operates as a constraining influence in impulsive substance use because the direct outcomes are significant to the client. This contract augments the desire of the substance abuser to remain free from drug use of any kind.

The role of nutrition in the treatment of substance abuse is well researched. The sequelae of chronic drug use are manifested in the central nervous system even

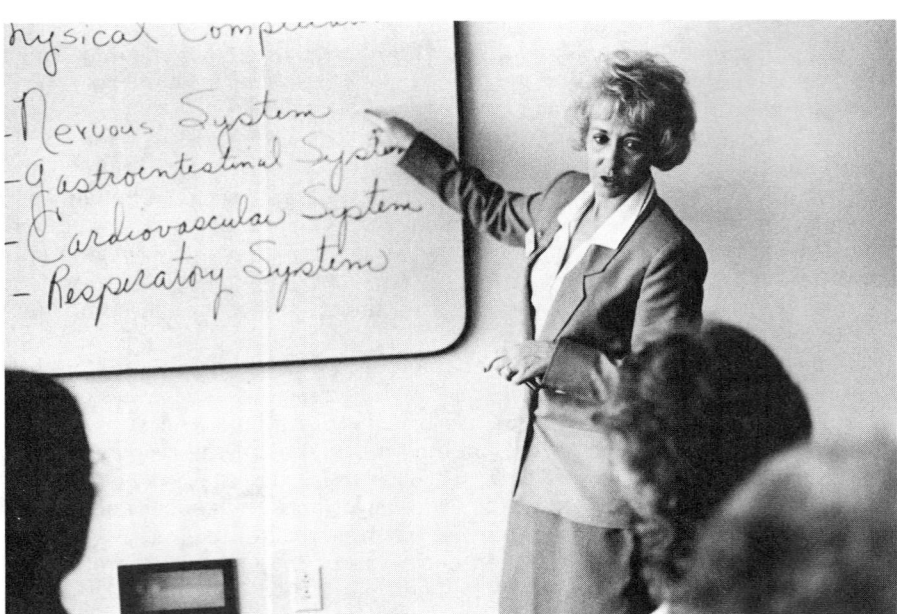

FIGURE 13–35. Education about addiction and drugs increases the client's awareness of abuse and aids the client in understanding his or her responses. (Photograph © 1988 by Jeffrey J. Smith)

after the drug use has been stopped.[7] There is a relationship between the action of substance use and the level of opioids in the brain. Substance abuse creates a decrease in opioid levels, and this deficiency is thought to be related to craving. Nutritional supplemental formulas improve the brain nutrition through increasing amino acid levels, and vitamins have been found to reduce craving and increase the substance abuser's response to supportive treatment.[5] Chronic use of psychoactive drugs affects the brain and creates an imbalance of neurotransmitters. Amino acid nutritional supplements with vitamins are beneficial.[45] These supplements may need to be continued for one to three years.

Hypoglycemia is a trigger to relapse and must be avoided. Nutritional classes that cover the important reasons to be aware of good nutrition, how to read food labels, and how to maintain good nutrition are an important element in recovery treatment.[13] The client should also be taught to avoid caffeinated beverages, as these increase anxiety, create sleep disturbance, and are potentials for abuse. Transitory hypertension in early withdrawal can be helped by low-sodium diets.[4] The nursing target is to increase the client's nutritional self-care so that the client can recover from the depletion resulting from the substance abuse, as well as avoid relapse. Hoffman and Estes investigated recovering substance abusers and found that the most frequent somatic experience related to recovery concerned eating patterns.[15] Food binges during recovery may be related to alcohol- or drug-induced nutritional deficits, and excessive carbohydrate intake may be related to previous high-caloric intakes through alcohol. Nutritional nursing measures are thus of utmost significance in substance abuse treatment, and they increase the client's sense of hopefulness about the recovery process.

The substance abuser has a history of poor interpersonal relationships. Psychotherapy, group therapy, family therapy, and attendance at Alcoholics Anonymous (AA) or Narcotics Anonymous (NA) is useful. Psychotherapy needs to include discussion of the insights the client is having as the "new" responses are practiced.[25] Group therapy is encouraged to allow the individual exploration and interpretation of feeling states in a safe environment.[8] Psychodrama, in which enactment of experiences occurs, has proved very helpful and insight-producing for these clients and may promote more improvement in the area of activity than does group therapy.[46] Family therapy using structural theory and strategic therapy has produced promising results.[18,23] These therapies address the family process that is created by the homeostatic balance influenced by drug use. Active participation in a 12-step self-help group also enhances relationship potential while at the same time it gives concrete examples of coping with substance abuse.

The client who is addicted has been characterized as having an "unlived life," and spiritual awakening can enable the process of insight and integration.[32] The integration of spiritual beliefs with the determination that the spiritual component is a strength is a valuable nursing intervention used for all clients, including substance abusers.[31] Referral to a 12-step self-help group such as NA will facilitate spiritual development, as the first step involves gaining assistance from a "higher power." For a fuller description of NA, see Chapter 16.

Relapse prevention research is offering insight into the long-term commitment required in the reduction and elimination of drug misuse.[33] Drug substitution is an example of ineffective coping that leads to relapse. Clients should be taught that both the nonmedical and medical use of some drugs can result in relapse. Specific drugs to be avoided are all intoxicating substances, including alcohol, as well as over-the-counter agents to produce sleep, excitement, or weight loss.[27] Teaching the client to call the clinic after treatment discharge if relapse occurs may limit its duration.[33]

After early recovery, clients frequently report disturbing dreams that portray relapse. Intervention into this concern has been teaching the technique for lucid dreaming, which is learning to remember that the experience is a dream. The client may respond, "No, I don't do that anymore" to the offer of alcohol or drugs.[36] A frank discussion of ambivalence toward renewing chemical use and support of continued abstinence is also helpful. Reinforcement of measures to confront trigger cues for substance abuse is also necessary. This can be accomplished by having the client review the occurrences of the day preceding the dream to see if there was adequate self-care. An example of this would be becoming frustrated with a spouse and not acknowledging the tension, being overly compliant at work, or having unrealistic expectations of oneself. The nurse can reframe the dream to see that the client is no longer in denial about the substance use and is saying, "Wake up to the fact that there are still parts of me that want to use alcohol or drugs!" This warning can be useful when its purpose is to alert the client to renewing abstinence efforts.

The nurse collaborates and consults with other health providers in care for the substance abuser,[3] since the multivariant nature of substance abuse requires an interdisciplinary team. The nurse must create trust and facilitate communication structures so both interdisciplinary staff and clients can speak directly with one another to enhance client recovery. The staff needs to be straightforward with one another and supportive of one another as well as the client.[2]

Figure 13-36 shows the psychiatric mental health nurse in an interdisciplinary team meeting.

Evaluation

The effectiveness of nursing interventions aimed at meeting physiologic and safety needs are measured by the following outcome criteria: physiologic integrity is preserved and promoted; safety needs are protected; and abstinence from drug use other than those prescribed is achieved. The outcome criteria for nursing interventions aimed at developing alternative coping skills and life-style that reduces or eliminates drug use are the following: the reporting of substance use as a problem that the client desires to change, the identification of hopefulness about recovery, the successful completion of short-term contracts for abstinence, the use of good nutritional habits, and an increase in self-expression individually and in groups (Chart 2).

CASE STUDY

Mrs. Lorraine F is a 48-year-old director of a nonprofit service organization. She weighs 216 lb and is 5'7" tall. She has been married for 28 years to a self-employed businessman and has four daughters. She presented for outpatient counseling for emotional problems related to marriage difficulties. Mrs. F is an active Mormon and believes that their temple marriage united them as man and wife throughout eternity as well as in the here and now. She complained of many financial, job, and family problems. The psychiatric nurse therapist began to assess the client's perceptions. She not only had a rigid, domineering husband, but had experienced the death of a child—from congenital heart abnormalities—that she had never resolved. As the client gained

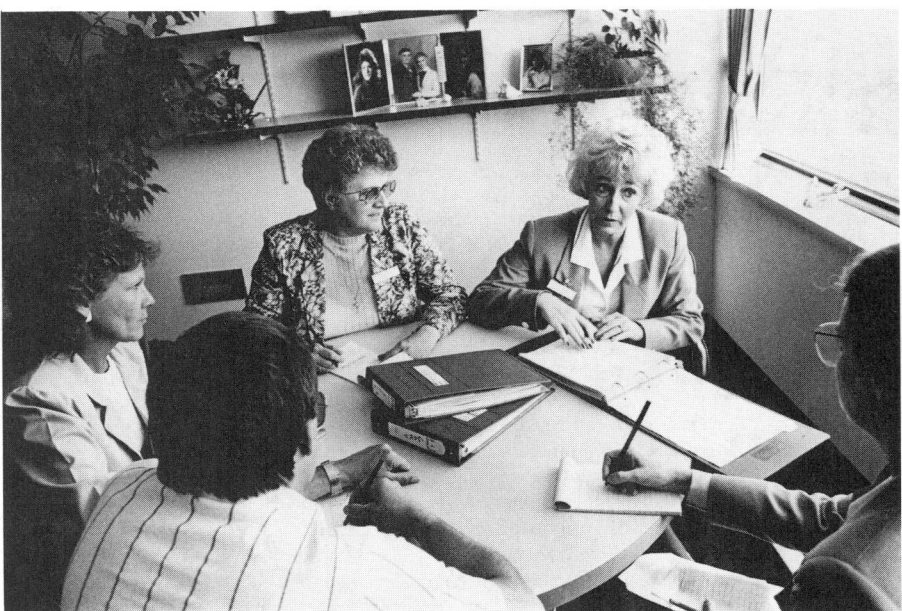

FIGURE 13–36. Nurses collaborate with other health care providers in caring for the substance abuser. (Photograph © 1988 by Jeffrey J. Smith)

CHART 2
Substance Abuse (Drugs): Summary of the Nursing Process[4,10,20,23,33]

NURSING INTERVENTIONS	OUTCOME CRITERIA
CLIENT GOAL: MEET PHYSIOLOGIC AND SAFETY NEEDS	
Observe for decreased respiratory function and drowsiness, pressured speech, and seizures, and provide appropriate measures based on intoxication or withdrawal phase	Physiologic integrity is preserved and promoted
Utilize interventions appropriate to client who is violent or disoriented	Safety needs are protected
Prevent uncontrolled access to drugs	No use of drugs other than those given by prescription is reported
CLIENT GOAL: DEVELOP ALTERNATIVE COPING SKILLS AND LIFE-STYLE TO REDUCE OR ELIMINATE DRUG ABUSE	
Use confrontation techniques to reduce denial	Reports substance abuse is a problem
Emphasize the possibility of recovery	Identifies hope for recovery
Utilize social skills training (e.g., assertiveness)	Reports increased confidence in social situations
Develop short-term behavioral contracts for abstinence	Successfully completes contract
Provide dietary counseling to avoid relapse	Reports good nutritional habits
Refer for therapy to improve interpersonal and intrapersonal relationships	Expresses positive self-concept
Educate about relapse prevention	Reports a plan to deal with urge to use drugs

trust in the nurse, childhood sexual molestation came to light. Initially, there was denial of drug use; however, Mrs. F later acknowledged that she had been taking 0.5 mg of alprazolam (Xanax) three times a day for 1½ years, as prescribed by her physician. Mrs. F did not drink alcohol or use any other drugs. A primary psychiatric diagnosis formulated by the psychiatrist was hypnotic dependence (benzodiazepine).

The medical–psychiatric treatment for benzodiazepine dependency requires inpatient treatment because the withdrawal symptoms can include anxiety, tremors, nightmares, seizures, and delirium.[44] After admission to the inpatient unit, Mrs. F was given decreasing amounts of phenobarbital to gradually withdraw her over a two-week period. No adverse effects of alprazolam withdrawal occurred. Once in the hospital, Mrs. F related that she had used a variety of prescription drugs for anxiety, such as diazepam (Valium)

and prazepam (Centrax). The nursing diagnoses formulated were substance abuse (benzodiazepine) related to financial, marital, and job stressors, and altered nutrition, more than body requirements, related to need for escape.

Interventions related to the substance abuse were to provide protection of physiologic integrity during benzodiazepine withdrawal by observation of central nervous system functioning and to limit the use of drugs other than those prescribed. Nursing interventions to develop alternative coping skills to deal with the financial, marital, and job stress were multifaceted. Mrs. F joined a women's support group and began to receive encouragement for viewing herself as important and worthy of respect. She decided that her stressful job was not in her best interest and after saying "I know I will die unless I stop working so hard," made plans to resign. The time gained from leaving her job was used for her own personal work and pleasure; she

Research Highlights

Hutchinson used qualitative field research in an effort to understand the recovery process of chemically dependent nurses.[16] Observation of nurses for a year in their self-help group was combined with in-depth interviews with 20 chemically dependent nurses. The three stages of recovery were found to be: surrendering, accepting, and committing. Surrendering involved three phases. The first stage was the acknowledgment that the nurse was powerless over her abuse. There was a willingness to say, "I'm an addict" and reduce denial. Confession followed the acknowledgment; this is the review of the chemical experience and feelings about the experience. The final phase of surrendering was prayer, a communication between the self and higher power, which extended throughout the recovery process. The second stage, accepting, was found to have three phases: disease, self, and reality. The acceptance of drug dependence as a chronic,

life-threatening illness was followed by self-acceptance. Accepting reality was the understanding that reality could, and should, be faced in a drug-free state. The final stage of commitment had two parts: accepting new attitudes and new behaviors. The new attitudes were concerned with self-care and self-responsibility. The new behaviors were congruent with the new attitudes. The self-integration of recovery from chemical dependency in nurses was found to be a cyclic process, and relapse diminished as that self-integration was strengthened.

This study supports the hopefulness that professionals can have about the potential for altering life-style such that drug use is no longer necessary. The delineation of each phase of recovery is a pragmatic concept in the establishment of sequential realistic behavioral targets for nursing interventions.

began daily walking and resumed her piano and church organ playing. Mrs. F signed a behavioral contract to attend a nonsmoking AA group, remain active in her church, and participate in weekly counseling sessions.

The weekly counseling sessions continued to clarify the marital ambivalence and sexual self-esteem ramifications of the childhood molestation. Realistic expectations of herself in her role as a wife, creative activity to promote self-esteem, and increased spiritual counseling from her Bishop were useful in promoting a drug-free lifestyle. The client terminated weekly counseling with more mature responses to her interpersonal and intrapersonal conflicts. These adaptations were possible because Mrs. F was no longer using benzodiazepines as her primary coping mechanism.

Five years after her initial visit to the nurse, Mrs. F remains conflicted and ambivalent about her marriage. She is active in her church and is receiving a great deal of social support. No relapse has occurred and Mrs. F has lost weight. Although she no longer regularly attends psychotherapy, she does go periodically to the inpatient treatment aftercare programs. She feels they are her "family" and the bonding to both staff and previous clients remains high. She also periodically attends AA meetings. Recently, she called the nurse for relapse prevention counseling created by the stress of personal intimacy issues within the marriage.

SUMMARY

Biologic, psychological, and stress–adaptation theory provide a framework for understanding substance abuse (drugs). The related factors of this nursing diagnosis include cultural norms that encourage use, spiritual distress about life's meaning, physical genetic predisposition, and disruption in normal child–parent relationships. The defining characteristics are manifested in multiple domains: financial, health, employment, and family life. The physical manifestations will depend on the drug used. The nursing interventions are aimed at providing safety during intoxication and withdrawal, and promoting a drug-free lifestyle. Collaboration of the other team members is critical to the client's care.

References

1. Ace AM, Smith D. Crack. Nursing '87. 1987;5:614–616.
2. American Nurses Association, Drug and Alcohol Nursing Association, National Nurses Society on Addictions. The care of clients with addictions. Kansas City: American Nurses Association; 1987.
3. American Nurses Association and National Nurses Society on Addictions. Standards of addictions nursing practice with selected diagnoses and criteria. Kansas City: American Nurses Association; 1988.
4. Bennett G, Graves SE, Kavanaugh MT, Vourakis C. An overview of substance abuse treatment. In: Bennett G, Vourakis C, Woolf DS, eds. Substance abuse. New York: John Wiley & Sons; 1983.
5. Blum K, Topel H. Opioid peptides and alcoholism: genetic deficiency and chemical management. Funct Neurol. 1987;1:71–83.
6. Caddy GR, Block T. Behavioral treatment methods for alcoholism. In: Galunter M, ed. Recent developments in alcoholism, vol 1. New York: Plenum Press; 1983.
7. Carlen PL, Wilkinson DA, Wortzman G, Holgate R. Partially reversible cerebral atrophy and functional improvement in recently abstinent alcoholics. Can J Neurol Sci. 1984; 11:441–446.
8. Cooper DE. The role of group psychotherapy in the treatment of substance abuse. Am J Psychother. 1987;41:66.
9. Fischman MW. The behavioral pharmacology of cocaine in humans. In: Grabowski J, ed. Cocaine: the pharmacology, effects and treatment of abuse. Rockville: National Institute on Drug Abuse; 1984.
10. Gallant DS. Alcohol and drug abuse curriculum guide for psychiatric faculty. Rockville, MD: National Institute on Alcohol Abuse and Alcoholism; 1982.
11. Ganguli HGL. Meditation subculture and drug use. Hum Relat. 1985;38:953.
12. Gorsuch RL, Butler MC. Initial drug abuse: a review of predisposing social psychological factors. Psychol Bull. 1986;83:120–137.
13. Graves JR. The role of nutrition in the treatment of alcoholism. In: Parvez S, Burov Y, Parvez H, Burns E, eds. Progress in alcohol research, vol 1. Utrecht: VNU Science Press; 1985.
14. Hamilton JA. An overview of the critical rationale for advancing gender-related psychopharmacology and drug abuse research. In: Ray BA, Braude MC, eds. Women and drugs: new era for research. Rockville, MD: National Institute on Drug Abuse; 1986.
15. Hoffman AL, Estes NJ. A tool for measuring body and behavioral experiences. Alcohol Health Res World. 1986;10:3.
16. Hutchinson S. Towards self-integration: the recovery process of chemically dependent nurses. Nurs Res. 1987; 36:339–343.
17. Kandel DB, Murphy D, Karus D. Cocaine use in young adulthood: patterns of use and psychological correlates. In: Kozel NS, Adams EH, eds. Cocaine use in America: epidemiologic and clinical perspectives. Rockville, MD: National Institute on Drug Abuse; 1985.
18. Levin SB, Raser JB, Niles C, Reese A. Beyond family systems—towards problem systems: some clinical implications. J Strat System Ther. 1986;5:62–69.
19. McDonald E. Creative writing therapy used to assist chemically dependent adolescents express feelings. In: International perspective—past, present, future. Calgary, Alberta: Alberta Alcohol and Drug Abuse Commission; 1986.
20. McFarland GK, Wasli E. Nursing diagnoses and process in psychiatric mental health nursing. Philadelphia: JB Lippincott; 1986.
21. McGarty R. Use of strategic and brief techniques in the treatment of chemical dependency. J Strat System Ther. 1986;5:20–29.
22. Malley DM, Johnson LD, Bachman JG. Cocaine use among American adolescents and young adults. In: Kogel NJ, Adams EH, eds. Cocaine use in America: epidemiological and clinical perspectives. Rockville, MD: National Institute on Drug Abuse; 1985.
23. Marlott GA. Coping with substance abuse: implications for research, prevention and treatment. In: Shiffman S, Willis TA, eds. Coping and substance use. New York: Academic Press; 1985.
24. Mello NK. Drug use patterns and premenstrual dysphoria. In: Ray BA, Braude MC, eds. Women and drugs: new era for research. The second triennial report to Congress from the Secretary, Department of Health and Human Services. Rockville, MD: National Institute of Drug Abuse; 1987.
25. Mendelson SH, Mello N. The diagnosis and treatment of alcoholism. New York: McGraw-Hill; 1986.
26. Metzger L. From denial to recovery. San Francisco: Jossey-Bass; 1988.

27. Mulry JT. Drug use in the chemically dependent. Postgrad Med. 1988;83:279–283.

28. National Institute on Drug Abuse. Drug abuse and drug research: the second triennial report to Congress from the Secretary, Department of Health and Human Services; 1987.

29. Newcomb MD, Maddolician E, Bealter PM. Risk factors for drug use among adolescents: concurrent and longitudinal analysis. Am J Public Health. 1986;76:525–531.

30. O'Malley DM, Johnston LD, Bachman JG. Cocaine use among American adolescents and young adults. In: Kogel NJ, Adams EH, eds. Cocaine use in America: epidemiological and clinical perspectives. Rockville, MD: National Institute on Drug Abuse; 1985.

31. Peterson EA. How to meet your clients' spiritual needs. J Psychosoc Nurs. 1987;25:34–37.

32. Prugh T. Alcohol, spirituality and recovery. Alcohol Health Res World. 1985/86;10:29.

33. Rounsaville B. Clinical implications of relapse research. In: Tims FM, Leukefeld CG, eds. Relapse and recovery in drug abuse. Rockville, MD: National Institute on Drug Abuse; 1986.

34. Rounsaville BJ, Kosten TR, Weissman MW, Keeber HD. Evaluating and treating depression in opiate addicts. Rockville, MD: National Institute on Drug Abuse; 1985.

35. Sanchez-Craig M. A therapist manual for secondary prevention of alcohol problems. Toronto: Addiction Research Foundation; 1985.

36. Seymour RB, Smith DE. Drug free. New York: Sarah Lazin Books; 1987.

37. Siegler M, Osmond H, Newell S. Models of alcoholism. In: Freed EX, ed. Interfaces between alcoholism and mental health. New Brunswick: Rutgers Center of Alcohol Studies; 1982.

38. Smith DE. Decreasing drug hunger. Prof Counsel. 1986; 12:15.

39. Smith DE, Wesson DR. Substance abuse in industry: identification, intervention, treatment and prevention In: Smith DE, Wesson DR, Zerkin EL, Novey JH, eds. Substance abuse in the workplace. San Francisco: Haight-Ashbury Publications; 1984.

40. Smith MD. Acupuncture treatment for cigarette smoking. In: Alcohol, drugs, and tobacco: an international perspective—past, present, future. Calgary, Alberta: Alberta Alcohol and Drug Abuse Commission; 1986.

41. Sparkes RS. Polymorphic gene marker studies. In: Braude MC, Chao HM, eds. Genetic and biological markers in drug abuse and alcoholism. Rockville, MD: National Institute on Drug Abuse; 1986.

42. Textor MR. Family therapy with drug addicts: an integrated approach. Am J Orthopsychiatry. 1987;57:495–507.

43. Tucker MB. Coping and drug use among heroin-addicted women and men. In: Shiffman S, Willis TA, eds. Coping and substance use. New York: Academic Press; 1985.

44. Wesson DR, Smith ED. Abuse of sedative hypnotics. In: Lowinson JH, Ruiz P, eds. Substance abuse clinical problems and perspectives. Baltimore: Williams & Wilkins; 1981.

45. Wise RA. Neural mechanisms of the reinforcing action of cocaine. In: Grabowski J, ed. Cocaine: pharmacology, effects, and treatment of abuse. Rockville, MD: National Institute on Drug Abuse; 1984.

46. Zackon F, McAuliffe WE, Ch'ien SMN. Addict aftercare recovery and self help. Rockville, MD: National Institute on Drug Abuse; 1985.

47. Zimburg S. The clinical management of alcoholism. New York: Brunner/Mazel; 1982.

SUICIDE POTENTIAL

Geraldine M. Spillers

DEFINITION AND DESCRIPTION

Suicide potential is the possibility that the client will kill himself or herself voluntarily and intentionally.[12] Frequently associated with suicide potential are other terms such as *suicidal ideation* (having thoughts of committing suicide or thoughts of methods by which to commit suicide), *suicide attempt* (self-destructive behavior that could be lethal), *suicidal gesture* (self-destructive behavior that usually is not lethal and often is viewed by others as manipulative behavior), and *self-destructiveness* (behavior by which one damages self immediately, impulsively, or chronically).[21]

Suicide is one of five leading causes of death in the United States and the second most frequent cause of death for individuals 15 to 25 years old. About 12% of those who threaten or attempt suicide actually kill themselves. Many authorities in the field of suicidology agree that current statistics may greatly understate the actual occurrence of suicide. For example, many auto and other accidents may have suicidal intention. Also, because of social stigma, insurance coverage issues, and differing legal criteria for classifying cause of death, suicide may not be recorded as the cause in many cases.

THEORY AND RESEARCH

One in every eight suicide attempts is fatal. The number of attempts and completions has increased dramatically over the past decade. Although certain groups still appear to be high risk, the statistical gap is rapidly narrowing between ages, sexes, races, and economic, social, and religious groups.

A number of theories have been developed to explain suicide, to predict suicide potential, and to improve prevention programs. Theorists from different perspectives agree on one issue: there is no one single causative factor for or predictive of suicide.[11,22] Current theories fall into one of three categories: psychophysiological, psychodynamic, and psychosocial.

In the *psychophysiological* category, biochemical data have emerged independently from different studies of depression and other affective disorders and their

correlation with suicide. (Of all the psychiatric disorders, the affective disorders are most consistently associated with suicide.[2,3]) Urine levels of cortisol have been found to be significantly elevated in depressed patients just prior to death by suicide. It is thought that the increased cortisol levels may result from increased psychological stress and the failure of psychological defenses to manage the stress.[2,6] Several studies have focused on neurotransmitters in the brain, especially norepinephrine and serotonin, and their relation to depression with suicidal behavior.[6,7,24] By different mechanisms, psychotropic drugs such as monoamine oxidase inhibitors (e.g., phenelzine) and tricyclic, tetracyclic, and other antidepressants (e.g., imipramine, maprotaline) increase effective levels or function of neurotransmitters. As a result, the patient experiences mood elevation and is better able to deal with psychosocial stressors.[8] Other studies have investigated a relation between electrolyte level and manic–depressive illness with suicidal behavior. Sodium promotes neurotransmission in the brain; imbalances in sodium may thus result in extreme mood disorders. Lithium carbonate affects sodium balance and is highly successful in controlling and preventing recurrent episodes of manic–depressive illness.[6,7]

The *psychodynamic* view of suicide focuses on the individual personality. Sigmund Freud considered suicide to be an outcome of intrapsychic phenomena to which all persons are vulnerable. He viewed self-destructive behavior as the result of interaction between two basic instincts: Eros (will to live) and Thanatos (will to die). Through the defense mechanisms of identification, introjection, and regression, the suicidal person kills someone within, a significant other who is loved and lost. Failure to achieve separation–individuation of the ego would render a person more vulnerable to suicide or self-destructive behaviors. Alfred Adler characterized suicidal persons as narcissistic, attempting to hurt others by hurting self. Karl Menninger maintained that under sufficient stress and conflict, the wish to die wins over the wish to live. He identified three major categories of suicide potential: (1) chronic—the addiction to martyrdom and psychosis; (2) focal—self-mutilation; and (3) organic—the development of a chronic or terminal illness.[11]

From the *psychosocial* framework, self-destructive behavior is viewed with the belief that something is wrong with the relation between the individual and his or her sociocultural system. Throughout life, it is the family system (origin, nuclear, extended) that is the

---

The opinions in this section are those of the contributor and do not necessarily reflect those of the National Institutes of Health, USPHS.

primary context for all relationships.[5] The individual physiological and psychodynamic traits are formed by interacting with the family, significant other, and sociocultural systems. Commonly referred to as the "father of sociology," Emile Durkheim (1858–1917) established a model for the psychosocial study of suicide. In his schema, all suicides fall into one of three basic groups. In *altruistic* suicide, the victim is highly enmeshed with a social group and gives his or her life as a martyr to advance the cause of that group. This form of suicide is viewed as honorable in certain cultures and religious and sociopolitical contexts. In *egoistic* suicide, the individual has suffered from a lack of meaningful interactions with others and has become isolated and without resources. *Anomic* suicides result when society experiences a period of disintegration, such as economic depression, or when a familiar relation between an individual and society changes suddenly. A stable role for an individual that is changed abruptly by death, loss, or unemployment may result in crisis and self-destructive behavior.[24]

The psychosocial perspective attempts to find meaning behind the statistics of suicide. During the last 20 years in the US, suicide rates have risen sharply for all demographic groups, but especially for the adolescent and elderly populations.[20] The field of family therapy considers suicidal behavior as a symptom of family dysfunction[5] or as a problem for the family, and therapy is aimed at promoting healthy function of the family system.

The psychophysiological, psychodynamic, and psychosocial factors can interact in complex ways. Multiple etiologies may be involved in producing suicide potential.

RISK FACTORS

Suicide and suicide potential occur in a number of psychiatric conditions: major depression, bipolar disorder (manic or depressive episode), schizophrenia, dementia, delirium, psychoactive substance-abuse disorders, and personality disorders.[1] The highest incidence of suicide potential and fatal acts occurs in persons with major depression: three times the rate for those with any other psychosis (including schizophrenia) and six times that for persons with personality disorders.[24] Clients can be at particular risk as they are recovering from depression and have increased energy levels.

It is important to remember that the majority of people who commit suicide have not sought psychiatric treatment and therefore first come to the attention of nonpsychiatric professionals. Individuals experiencing confusion, disorientation, altered sensory perceptions, severe anxiety, or panic are high risk for self-harm because of their impaired judgment and reality testing skills. The need for assessment of risk and concern for immediate safety also encompasses individuals experiencing delusions or auditory hallucinations commanding self-harm.

Individuals with borderline personality disorder frequently experience suicidal ideation and make suicidal gestures, often nonlethal self-mutilation (i.e., wrist cut-

ting). Suicide gestures are made repeatedly and often are labeled by others as manipulative behavior. Stress tolerance is low, and impulse control is poor in this group. However, the presence of other risk factors certainly can lead to more lethal attempts and accidental completion.[1,15] There is some evidence that individuals whose parents or siblings committed suicide are at higher risk, especially if grieving, guilt, or anger is unresolved.[24]

A significant number of people, particularly men, who commit suicide have suffered from one or more chronic physical illnesses. In those with a chronic disease, the older the individual, the greater the risk of suicide. Studies have identified four high-risk groups of clients with chronic illness. Those suffering from diseases of the central nervous system (epilepsy, multiple sclerosis, stroke, head injuries, Huntington's chorea) and cancer have the highest suicide rate. Two other groups at risk are elderly men with genitourinary diseases and individuals having peptic or duodenal ulcers necessitating gastrectomy. The incidence of suicide related to Cushing's disease with concurrent depression has been decreasing in recent years because of timely treatment of the depression. However, several other metabolic and endocrine disorders can cause depression and therefore increase the risk of suicide potential.[25] Researchers speculate that the correlation between suicide and certain chronic diseases may reflect concurrent depression and inadequate resources to manage the stress. One study of 175 suicide victims found that 42% had contact with the medical profession for chronic illness management during the 6 months prior to death. Assessment for depression and for support system adequacy should not be overlooked in those with chronic physical illness.[10,25]

Many studies have identified alcoholism as a significant factor related to suicides, second only to depression. Alcoholism and depression coexist in many with suicide potential. Eighty per cent of alcohol-related suicides are men over the age of 40. In one important study, the mean duration of alcohol abuse prior to suicide was 20 years.[14] Another study of 100 alcohol-related suicides reported that 92% had verbalized their suicidal ideation more than once. The single factor most frequently associated with alcohol-related suicides was the loss of a significant relationship: 26% of victims had such a loss within 6 weeks of their suicide.[14]

Additional factors frequently associated with suicide potential are loss of a significant other, loss of economic status, lack or loss of self-esteem, internal conflicts or guilt, unstable lifestyle with poor impulse control, and lack of social support system and resources to manage stress.[11] The highest-risk populations by age are those individuals 15 to 25 years old and those over age 60. The elderly have factors such as loss of a spouse, chronic illness or disability, and economic losses that contribute to risk for suicide potential.[23] In recent years, the incidence of adolescent suicides has risen sharply, with more teens committing suicide in pairs or groups. The adolescent is especially vulnerable to develop suicide potential after the loss by suicide of a friend.[20] Considering gender as a risk factor, men have a higher suicide rate than women, but in the US, women have a much higher rate of suicide attempts. In addition, men tend to use far more lethal methods such as hanging and firearms.[11] In past decades, racial minorities were thought to have a higher suicide rate, but recent studies indicate that related factors such as losses of economic status, support systems, and family members may be more significant than race in predicting risk for suicide.[20]

The following personality characteristics have been noted consistently in psychological testing of those recovering from suicide attempts: rigid in cognitive function, perceiving the world in terms of highly polarized concepts, inflexible attitudes, perceiving the environment and others as powerful over self, and the belief that in suicide, the self will achieve power over the environment and others.[17,24]

Cultural factors can influence the nature and frequency of suicide potential. Suicide in the US elderly population has increased more than 60% in the last 20 years.[20] In China, elderly suicide is extremely rare. In Asian societies, the elderly remain an active, integrated, even revered part of the extended family, whereas in recent times, there has been a trend in America for the elderly to become more isolated and to be viewed as having diminished productive value. The suicide rate for adolescents world-wide has been correlated with the permissiveness of society, divorce rates, and family dysfunction.[5]

Only one country, Great Britain, has substantially reduced its suicide rate over the last three decades. This success has been attributed to a popular movement called the Samaritans. The program centers throughout the British Isles offer counseling and volunteers who befriend suicidal clients. The program is thought to be so successful because of the large number of community volunteers involved.[24]

Altruistic suicide continues in some societies, where suicide is viewed as advancing a cause or atoning for the sins of the society. This also is the explanation for the behavior observed with mass suicides of certain cult organizations.[20] Fatalistic suicide occurs in societies that have a high level of racism, genocide, and intolerance of religious freedom.[20] The epidemiology of suicide throughout the world reveals that the lowest rates occur in agricultural societies with low divorce rates. The highest rates occur in cultures with restrictive, highly regulated governments; with alcoholism as a major health problem; with high divorce rates; in large urban–industrial communities; and with a high degree of enmeshment between individual identity and social role.[20]

DEFINING CHARACTERISTICS

A client experiencing suicide potential may exhibit a wide range of behaviors, depending on the nature and etiology of the disturbance, age, sociocultural environment, and the context of the immediate situation. If the client is able and willing to verbalize, clues may be clear and direct, such as, "I'm just going to kill myself" or "If I had a gun, I would shoot myself." Verbal clues can also be less direct, such as, "I'm not really worth your time" or "My parents would be much better off without me." There are often behavioral clues, such as writing farewell letters, giving away treasured possessions, self-destructive or reckless activities, making a will and closing bank accounts, increased or unusual preoccupation with religious activity, or appearing cheerful or peaceful after a period of agitated depression. When questioned directly, a client may refuse to confirm or deny the presence of suicidal ideation. It is not uncommon for statements and nonverbal behavior to be incongruent when the patient is ambivalent, manipulative, or in denial of crisis or wishes to avoid confronting and labeling of suicide potential.

There are some characteristics shared by most suicidal clients. Ambivalence about living vs dying is frequently strong. Feelings of hopelessness and helplessness are usually overwhelming. "Tunnel vision,"[22] with inability to see any alternative solutions to the current problems or stressors, is usually observed. If the client is sharing information, certain factors frequently will be described, such as increased social isolation, decreased resources, significant stressors, recent losses or anniversary of a significant loss, low self-esteem, and chronic unmet needs.

Behaviors related to meeting physiological needs, maintenance of safety, or activities of daily living may be disturbed. For example, a client who is an insulin-dependent diabetic may refuse to take insulin injections. Refusal to eat or drink may be further evidence of self-destructive wishes. Lack of appetite, sleep disturbances, neglect of hygiene and grooming, and anhedonia are common. Concentration and cognitive abilities may be impaired, making the completion of a simple task or attentiveness to safety impossible. Obsessive rumination about trivial events or feelings of unfounded guilt and remorse often accompany severe depression with feelings of worthlessness.

Suicidal clients can be withdrawn and isolative with sad mood, depressed or flat affect, poor eye contact, latency of speech, and profound psychomotor retardation. On the other hand, a suicidal client can present with psychomotor agitation, hypomania or rapid mood swings, loud and pressured speech, and irritable and demanding behavior. Hostility, threats, or aggressive acts to harm others or the environment also can be exhibited. Clients experiencing a psychotic process may describe, or respond with bizarre nonverbal behavior to, delusions or auditory hallucinations commanding self-harm. Behaviors such as burning self with cigarettes, head pounding, and other serious self-mutilation are not uncommon in individuals with a psychotic process. Males who are experiencing acute psychosis, suicidal ideation with command hallucinations, and severe sexual identity disturbance have been known to mutilate their testicles.

Those clients who are experiencing disturbed interpersonal relationships frequently threaten suicide in an attempt to effect change in another's behavior. Self-mutilating gestures or life-threatening acts may be dramatic and impulsive (Chart 1).

NURSING PROCESS AND RATIONALE
Assessment

The first priority in assessing for suicide potential is being attentive to clues. References to suicidal thoughts and feelings may be direct, indirect verbal, or nonverbal, as previously mentioned. The nurse's

---

CHART 1
Suicide Potential: Definition, Risk Factors, and Defining Characteristics

DEFINITION

Suicide potential is the possibility that the patient will kill himself or herself voluntarily and intentionally.

RISK FACTORS

Depression
Other mood disorders
Schizophrenia
Other psychoses
Neurologic disorders
Delirium
Dementia
Use or withdrawal of alcohol or other substances
Organic brain disorders
Hallucinations, delusions
Stress, acute or chronic
Isolation
Loss of significant other
Loss of self-esteem
Loss of physical health, function
Cultural factors
Spiritual distress
Anxiety
Personality disorders
Impulse control disorders
Internal conflicts, guilt
Family dysfunction, crisis
Loss of resources, social and economic
Unmet needs

DEFINING CHARACTERISTICS

Ambivalence
Withdrawn, isolative behavior
Impaired concentration
Cognitive constriction, tunnel vision
Psychomotor agitation
Psychomotor retardation
Anxious
Attentive to internal stimuli
Verbalizes suicidal thoughts, feelings, plan
Verbalizes references to death, dying
Gives away possessions
Anger, hostility
Impulsive behaviors
Depressed affect
Appetite disturbances
Hopeless–helpless
Disturbed sleep patterns

---

avoidance of direct questioning when suicidal ideation is revealed can communicate anxiety or indifference to the client and lead to incomplete assessment of suicidal risk. Statements of concern followed by direct questions often are helpful, such as "I'm concerned about your safety. Are you having thoughts of killing yourself?" or "You sound pretty hopeless right now. Have you had thoughts of suicide?" The client in crisis who is having difficulty verbalizing generally finds it easier to respond with thoughts rather than feelings. Specific directions to describe detail are helpful to the anxious, overwhelmed client. Some clients are reluctant to share their suicidal thoughts, feeling ashamed or frightened about loss of control. Framing questions can be useful, such as, "Sometimes, people in similar situations feel like harming themselves. Is that true for you?" or "A crisis can cause some people to lose control. Are you in danger of doing something to harm yourself now?" If the client is withdrawn, several statements of observation and concern followed by periods of silence usually are effective.

Accurate assessment of suicidal risk involves learning more about:

1. The suicidal plan, especially the method, availability, specificity, and lethality. The highest-risk client has thought through every detail, has the method readily available, is determined that no opportunity for rescue is possible, has put final affairs "in order," and has selected a highly lethal method such as a gun, hanging, gas or carbon monoxide poisoning, or overdose of a lethal, rapid-acting drug. Have there been previous attempts? What were the circumstances, severity, and recovery course?
2. The recent events, especially in the last 24 hours and past months. Are there losses or potential losses of significant others, employment, resources?
3. The significant others and living arrangements. Ask about marriages, divorces, children, and support system of friends. How does the client describe these relationships? How does the client think significant other(s) would react to a suicide attempt? What is the relationship with parents, brothers, and sisters? Is this the anniversary of the death of a significant other? Is the client living alone and, if so, for how long?
4. The nature of this crisis experience. Is the client able to manage the activities and demands of daily living and still able to work, or is he or she completely overwhelmed and immobilized? Is this a single crisis or one of many?
5. The coping strategies and patterns of managing stress. How does the client respond to stress and reduce anxiety on a daily basis? Is anxiety chronic because of a long pattern of unmet needs, or is it related to a single traumatic event? Does the client use alcohol or other substances, including prescription medications? Has the lifestyle been relatively stable, or is it unstable, with impulsive, self-destructive behaviors as the norm?
6. The resources available, both internal and external. Is client able to provide for basic needs such as

food, clothing, housing, and health care? Does a significant other provide major support? What is the current financial and employment status? Does the client have physical limitations? What are client's strengths? Are there beliefs or values, including spiritual–religious beliefs, that influence him or her? How does the client describe self-concept, self-esteem?

7. The psychiatric history and current symptoms of illness. Is the client in therapy? What is the nature of the relationship with the therapist? How does the client describe his or her experience with treatment, including hospitalizations: negative or valuable? Are symptoms of a mental illness related or observed? What past and current medications have or have not been helpful? How do symptoms affect the relationships and activities of daily living?

8. The medical–physical history and current symptoms of illness. Is a chronic or terminal illness present? Has there been a recent serious illness or series of such illnesses? Are there current symptoms that may be related to a metabolic disorder? Has the client consulted a physician or health care agency in the last 6 months? How do symptoms affect relationships and activities of daily living? Are there significant issues related to reproductive or sexual activity? Are there disturbances in appetite, sleep, or elimination?

All of the above subjects must be explored, will usually overlap, and need not be addressed in any specific order. Demographic data (sex, age, race, religion, education, socioeconomic and marital status) are important parts of assessment but should not be viewed as isolated predictors of suicidal risk.[11,19,24]

Nursing Diagnosis

To be useful, the nursing diagnosis of suicide potential must be made more specific by relating the findings in the assessment.[12] For example, the client may be experiencing a mood disorder such as depression and difficulty with a chronic physical illness. The complete nursing diagnosis then would be suicide potential related to depression and loss of physical health or function. For the client with schizophrenia experiencing delusions and command auditory hallucinations to harm self, the nursing diagnosis would be suicide potential related to delusions and auditory hallucinations. A client in the acute stage of alcohol withdrawal may be delirious with suicidal references or impulsive gestures. The nursing diagnosis then would be suicide potential related to alcohol withdrawal and delirium. Once this withdrawal is complete, further assessment may indicate that suicide potential is still present but the related factors would be different, e.g., suicide potential related to loss of a significant other.

Other examples of related factors found in assessment and included to make the nursing diagnosis more specific are multiple losses, chronic low self-esteem, borderline personality disorder with poor impulse con-

trol, and panic disorder. Family crisis or dysfunction often precipitates suicide potential in adolescents and can be included in the nursing diagnosis to increase specificity.

Client Goals and Nursing Interventions

To achieve successful intervention, the nurse must develop self-awareness of attitudes about suicide and avoid making and communicating judgments. For example, telling the client, "Life is really worth living" is not necessarily helpful. What is viewed by the nurse as a minor stressor may be an overwhelming stressor for the client.

With the initial assessment complete, a decision on the appropriate *level of observation* is made. The level of observation, precautions to be taken, and limits on activity or freedom of movement must be reviewed with the client, emphasizing the rationale for maintaining a safe environment. The desired outcome is for the client to feel safe, in control of, and responsible for his or her behavior related to safety. Clients in an emergency room or medical unit after a suicide attempt require maximum observation pending thorough assessment by a mental health professional. This means a nurse has the client in view at all times, including in the bathroom. This is sometimes termed *one-to-one* (1:1) care. Clients treated on a medical–surgical unit for serious complications of the attempt are high risk, especially when expressing, "I wish you hadn't saved me" or when they are confused, delirious, nonverbal, or psychotic. The psychotic client with lethal self-mutilation and active hallucinations is extremely high risk, and one-to-one nursing care is required. If the client is impulsive or nonresponsive to verbal directions in any setting, restraints may be required. One-to-one nursing care is maintained when restraints are used, and the rationale for safety is always communicated. Some clients require involuntary civil commitment to a secure unit if a danger to self and refusing treatment. Maximum observation is required until the client can agree to participate in treatment and sign a contract (discussed below). Other measures may be helpful or necessary for safety, such as closing or locking the doors to the unit, posting suicide precaution notices in appropriate locations for staff, and ensuring that the suicide observation status is reviewed in each shift report.

When a client agrees to voluntary treatment on a psychiatric unit, one-to-one suicide precautions may still be necessary for a short duration. Seclusion or restraints are measures of last resort when all other behavioral interventions have failed to maintain safety, and such measures must always include continued one-to-one nursing care. A period of maximum observation is not merely standing guard but is an opportunity to begin returning control to the client, to establish rapport, to communicate expectations for safety, and to begin to develop a care plan with the client.[4] Less restrictive interventions may be sufficient to ensure safety and more appropriate to promote an outcome of increased responsibility. For example, expecting the client to remain in visual contact in selected areas may be effective. Expecting the client to sign an observation record and make verbal contact at 15-minute intervals is another intervention. Such close observation provides structure and helps the client gradually assume responsibility for his or her own safety. The level of observation should be discussed with the health care team and with the client every 24 hours. Precautions to ensure safety may need to be reinstituted at some point, as when there are sudden changes in behavior, denial of crisis or lethality of the attempt, or statements incongruent with nonverbal behavior. For example, the client recovering from depression faces a period of much higher risk as the depression "lifts" and he or she has more energy.[8]

Another highly effective intervention is use of the written *contract*. The client participates in the development of and signs a contract to refrain from harming self and to verbalize feelings of self-harm rather than impulsively acting them out. An even more detailed contract is especially effective with borderline patients or patients who are impulsive and manipulative and attempt to sabotage treatment efforts. A contract may cover a wide variety of specific behaviors and alternatives and goals to be met and is revised at intervals. A contract outlines in a clear, concrete manner the defined problem(s) for the client, the goal(s) to be achieved with target date, and the specific responsibilities of both client and nurse. The contract is signed by both and shared with and followed by other staff. Written contracts are a therapeutic process that can promote several desirable outcomes such as achieving success with alternative behaviors, learning the benefit of adult role relationships, learning problem-solving skills, and accepting responsibility for and the consequences of behavior. The use of written contracts also is successful in reducing the length of hospital stay when initiated within 48 hours of admission.[9,18] Written contracts are useful in the outpatient setting to promote outcomes noted above and to increase the commitment to continuing treatment.

Health teaching occurs throughout the treatment process, and its focus is determined by the factors identified as the etiology of suicide potential. For example, a client may need to learn facts about depression, loss and grieving, hallucinations, or alcoholism or other substance abuse. Frequently, a client needs to learn different coping methods to manage stress, anxiety, anger, disappointment, or conflict resolution. Learning new communication skills and how to increase self-esteem often is essential. Cognitive therapy may be appropriate to begin changes in the client's feeling–thought–behavior patterns. Assertiveness and affirmation teaching with skill practice sessions are helpful. Teaching in group sessions promotes learning from shared experience, decreasing feelings of isolation. Promoting the concept that the client can make choices may help decrease the client's perception of self as a victim who is helpless. The need for prescribed medications should be discussed along with review of ways to minimize common side effects and the impor-

tance of seeking consultation before deciding to discontinue medications.

Family therapy is strongly recommended, especially for adolescents. Changes in family communication patterns can provide substantial support needed to decrease suicide potential.

Throughout treatment, discharge planning is in process, with the goal of gaining the client's commitment to outpatient therapy and appropriate use of recommended resources. Reviewing the care plan with the client prior to discharge can be valuable to evaluate outcomes and revise goals for follow-up therapy. If the client experiences shame or embarrassment about psychiatric treatment for a suicide attempt, it is helpful to role play situations that might arise and frame the hospital experience in a context of productive outcomes.

Evaluation

As an initial outcome of feeling safe with the nurse's presence, the client will more fully express thoughts and feelings about suicide and refrain from impulsive acts to harm self and may initiate contact to verbalize. In the early stages of recovery, clients who have been severely withdrawn or immobilized will begin to assume more physical self-care activities. As care continues, the client will explore issues related to the suicide potential or attempt and begin to interact more with others in the environment. When forming a written contract with the client, the nurse should observe for outcomes such as sustained eye contact; absence of hesitation with responses; affirmative statements of commitment to safety; statements reflecting ownership of thoughts, feelings, and behaviors; and hopeful expressions about living. The nurse should validate the contract by asking simple, direct questions about the patient's ability to maintain safety. The client will follow the contract by seeking out the nurse and verbalizing thoughts rather than impulsively acting out.

Active work toward goals will include the client being able to identify stressful experiences and use alternative behaviors to manage anxiety. The client will report feelings of increased competence with new knowledge and skills, including knowledge about medications. Toward the end of the acute phase of treatment, the client will report an absence of suicidal feelings, review goals for outpatient therapy, and relate knowledge of community resources to be utilized (Chart 2).

CASE STUDY

A 48-year-old woman was hospitalized after a suicide attempt with a potentially lethal drug overdose. She was found by her husband and two adolescent sons when they returned 2 days early from a camping trip. It was her first suicide attempt, but she had been hospitalized for an episode of severe depression 5 years previously. This attempt coincided with the anniversary of the suicide death of her mother. Over the last 6 months, she had withdrawn from social activities, experienced the loss of her job as a

---

CHART 2
Suicide Potential: Summary of the Nursing Process

NURSING INTERVENTIONS

OUTCOME CRITERIA

CLIENT GOAL: FEEL SAFE AND SECURE AND NOT ACT TO HARM SELF

Assess current suicide risk
Implement appropriate level of observation–precautions; 1:1,
  if needed
Acknowledge feelings and experience and explain precautions
Communicate simple expectations, clear limits of no self-harm
Provide structure; prevent isolation with frequent interaction
Make immediate environment safe
Prevent impulsive acts; offer alternatives to decrease anxiety

Verbalizes thoughts, feelings of suicide
Refrains from impulsive acts to harm self
Remains in visual contact, if so directed
Initiates verbal contact; signs in at intervals
Makes written no-harm contract

CLIENT GOAL: ATTEND TO ACTIVITIES AND TO OTHERS IN THE ENVIRONMENT

Assess suicide potential every 24 hours
Revise level of observation and written contracts when
  appropriate
Assist with activities of daily living as needed, promoting self
  care
Begin involvement in unit activities; observe interactions with
  others
Involve in goal-setting; explore issues, strengths, and
  resources
Engage in family therapy

Shows interest in self-care; attends to hygiene,
  grooming, nutrition
Verbalizes issues related to suicide potential
Maintains responsiblity of no-harm contract
Interacts with others, including family and friends

**CLIENT GOAL: INCREASE FOCUS ON PROBLEM-SOLVING, THEREBY EXPERIENCING LESS HOPELESSNESS AND
HELPLESSNESS**

Involve in active problem solving
Encourage participation in groups, activities with others
Share observations of progress, behavior, strengths
Review alternative behaviors to manage stress
Promote active decision making; offer, make aware of choices

Identifies anxiety and stress and uses alternative
  behavior to manage
Reports feeling some hope and increased competence
  with feelings, behaviors, and communication with
  others

CLIENT GOAL: INCREASE KNOWLEDGE ABOUT SUICIDE POTENTIAL AND RELATED ISSUES

Teach skills related to primary issues: cognitive, assertive,
  stress management
Teach techniques for reduction of symptoms related to illness
Teach availability and resources to use in crisis
Teach benefits of follow-up therapy to resolve issues
Teach purpose, side effects, schedule of medications

Reports absence of suicidal feelings
Communicates feelings of competence related to new
  patterns of behavior and skills
States plan to seek further therapy and use community
  resources
Verbalizes understandings of purpose, side effects,
  schedule of medications

---

teacher, stopped seeing her therapist, and discontinued medication. After being medically stabilized, she agreed to transfer to the psychiatric unit. She was lethargic and non-verbal except to repeat, "Why did they come home early? They would be better off without me." Her husband and sons were anxious, frightened, angry, and felt helpless. The major nursing diagnosis was suicide potential related to depression and multiple losses. Suicide precautions were implemented to help her feel safe and secure. Initially, she required structure and supervision to complete her hygiene and grooming, complaining that she didn't care. Gradually, she began to talk, describing feelings of helplessness, unresolved grief since her mother's suicide, and that her husband and children did not really need her and a belief that she should die like her mother. She resumed her antidepressant medications and attended medication teaching group. Gradually, she became more involved in unit activities and attended other groups to learn new skills. Cognitive, assertiveness, and affirmation groups helped her to share experiences and focus attention on her self-esteem. Several family conferences helped to identify patterns and

issues in the family relationships that were problematic for all members. As her mood improved and stabilized, she began to feel more hopeful, explored options for a return to work, and reestablished contact with a church group that had previously been of value. Discharge planning included return to her individual therapist, who could also monitor the medication regimen, and family therapy sessions twice a month.

SUMMARY

Suicide potential can occur as the result of many factors in both the psychiatric and the general populations. It has been explained through psychophysiological, psychodynamic, and psychosocial theories. Thorough assessment is followed by nursing diagnosis and interventions that protect the client from self-harm and enable the client gradually to assume increased

Research Highlights

Although the subjective meaning of suicide attempts has received much attention in the literature, there have been few attempts to understand suicide attempts using a phenomenologic approach. Pallikkathayil and McBride conducted a phenomenologic study focused on the subjective meaning of suicide.[16] The principal purposes were: (1) to describe the common themes expressed in reasons given for the drug overdose and to see if there is a relation between the themes and scores on the Suicide Intent Scale; (2) to describe the extent to which subjects communicated their suicidal intent or action; and (3) to describe common feelings reported by the subjects both before and after the suicide attempt. A convenience sample of six male and nineteen female subjects was obtained from three hospitals in a large metropolitan area. All subjects were over 18 and had attempted suicide by drug overdose. Eighty percent were under 30 years of age. Two instruments were utilized. The Suicide Intent Scale (SIS), designed to measure the intensity of the person's wish to die at the time of the suicide attempt, had estab-

lished validity and reliability. The other instrument was an open-ended interview protocol, critiqued for content validity. Content analysis was performed to determine themes for suicidal purpose. Significant clinical findings were: (1) patients were eager to talk to the researcher about their suicidal crisis; (2) 21 of the 25 subjects took their own prescription drugs for overdose; 15 of the 25 subjects thought about their suicide attempt for less than 1 day and the rest for less than 1 hour; and (3) a strong correlation existed between stated suicidal purpose and the SIS score. Those who scored high on the SIS and who verbalized a desire to die during the interview were considered priority candidates for intensive follow-up.[16]

A demographic finding that 88% of the subjects in this study were single or separated was thought to lend strong support to the suggestion that social isolation may be closely related to suicide potential. However, another study found that amount of religious activity may be more significant than amount of social support as a factor influencing suicide potential.[13]

responsibility for remaining safe. Further interventions are directed at developing alternatives to suicidal behavior, learning to manage stress-producing symptoms, and increasing knowledge and skill to alleviate anxiety, gain insight, and utilize supportive resources.

References

1. American Psychiatric Association. Diagnostic and Statistical Manual of Mental Disorders. 3rd ed, revised. Washington, DC: American Psychiatric Association; 1987.
2. Asberg M, Nordstrom P, Traskman–Benz L. Biological factors in suicide. In: Roy A, ed. Suicide. Baltimore: Williams & Wilkins; 1986.
3. Beck AT. Depression: cause and treatment. Philadelphia: University of Pennsylvania Press; 1967.
4. Blythe MM, Pearlmutter DR. The suicide watch: a re-examination of maximum observation. Perspect Psychiatr Care. 1983;21:3.
5. Bowen M. Family therapy in clinical practice. New York: Jason Aronson; 1978.
6. Bunney WE, Fawcett JA. Biochemical research in depression and suicide. In: Resnik HLP, ed. Suicidal behaviors. Boston: Little, Brown; 1968.
7. Bunney WE, Fawcett JA. Possibility of a biochemical test for suicide potential. Arch Gen Psychiatry. 1965;13:212.
8. Campbell L. Depression: acute care in the hospital. Am J Nurs. 1983;86(3).
9. Cook D, Skeldon I. The use of a contract admission procedure on an acute psychiatric admission ward. Br J Psychiatry. 1980;136:463.
10. Field WE. Physical causes of depression. J Psychosoc Nurs Ment Health Serv. 1985;23(10):7.
11. Hatton CL, Valente SM, Rink A. Suicide: assessment and intervention. New York: Appleton-Century-Crofts; 1977.
12. McFarland G, Wasli E. Nursing diagnosis and process in psychiatric mental health nursing. Philadelphia: JB Lippincott; 1986.
13. Mullis MR, Byers PH. Social support in suicidal patients. J Psychosoc Nurs Ment Health Serv. 1987;25(4):16.
14. Murphy GE: Suicide in alcoholism. In: Roy A, ed. Suicide. Baltimore: Williams & Wilkins; 1986.
15. O'Brien P, Caldwell C, Transeau G. Destroyers: written treatment contracts can help cure self destructive behaviors of the borderline patient. J Psychosoc Nurs Ment Health Serv. 1985;23(4):19.
16. Pallikkathayil L, McBride AB. Suicide attempts: the search for meaning. J Psychosoc Nurs Ment Health Serv. 1986;24(8):13.
17. Piotrowski ZA. Psychological test prediction of suicide. In: Resnik H, ed. Suicidal behaviors. Boston: Little, Brown; 1968.
18. Rosen B. Written treatment contracts: their use in planning treatment programs for inpatients. Br J Psychiatry. 1978;133:410.
19. Roy A. Suicide in schizophrenia. In: Roy A, ed. Suicide. Baltimore: Williams & Wilkins; 1986.
20. Sainsbury P. The epidemiology of suicide. In: Roy A, ed. Suicide. Baltimore: Williams & Wilkins; 1986.
21. Schultz JM, Dark SL. Manual of psychiatric nursing care plans. 2nd ed. Boston: Little, Brown; 1986.
22. Shneidman ES. Some essentials of suicide and some implications for response. In: Roy A, ed. Suicide. Baltimore: Williams & Wilkins; 1986.
23. Smoyak SA. Old age. In: Critchley DL, Maurin JT, eds. The clinical specialist in psychiatric mental health nursing. New York: John Wiley & Sons; 1985.
24. Snyder SH. Biological aspects of mental disorder. New York: Oxford University Press; 1980.
25. Whitlock FA. Suicide and physical illness. In: Roy A, ed. Suicide. Baltimore: Williams & Wilkins; 1986.

SUSPICIOUSNESS

Jean Scheideman

DEFINITION AND DESCRIPTION

Suspiciousness incorporates such qualities as cynicism, hostility, and negativism. It is a mode of interacting manifested by mistrust of others, a belief that people are basically evil and out to get what they can for themselves at the expense of others.

A milder form of suspiciousness can occur in everyday situations. The mother of a 15-year-old becomes suspicious when her daughter suddenly volunteers to do the dishes. A wife becomes suspicious when her husband uncharacteristically presents her with flowers. A homeowner becomes suspicious when a company's bid to reroof his house is half that of the competitor. Behind each of these instances is a questioning of the other's motivation. It is when the lack of trust of others becomes generalized in relationships that suspiciousness can create problems for an individual. In an even more severe form, of course, there can be delusions of persecution (see nursing diagnosis entitled Delusions). The focus here is on suspiciousness that creates problems in relationships but is less severe.

THEORY AND RESEARCH

Erikson described the development of the opposite of suspiciousness, namely trust.[4] He named the first developmental crisis "basic trust vs basic mistrust" and regarded it as fundamental to all other developmental stages. When nurturance is consistent, infants learn not only to trust themselves but to rely on the consistent presence of the nurturing figure. A child who is raised in an environment where trust is not fostered grows up to be insecure and alienated from others.

Parents in whom rigidity and sarcasm are prominent features contribute to the growth of suspiciousness in their children. Victims of criminal assault or robbery, persons living in abusive or alcoholic families, and persons living in an alien society may experience heightened mistrust.[7] Families who are highly dogmatic may either foster guilt in their children or nudge them toward seeing the world from a "we vs they" position. The opportunity to develop a healthy self-concept with a sense of optimism and openness toward others can be diminished in these situations.

To determine whether genetic factors influence the personality trait of suspiciousness, extensive questionnaires were mailed to 5967 adult twin pairs in Austra-

lia.[6] Questionnaires were returned by both members of 3810 pairs and were used to study a "suspiciousness" factor obtained from the Eysenck Personality Questionnaire.[5] Levels of suspiciousness were significantly higher in males than in females. Divorced or separated individuals were more suspicious than married individuals. Suspiciousness was negatively correlated with age and education, positively correlated with neuroticism and alcohol consumption (in males only), and uncorrelated with extroversion. The researchers concluded that additive genetic factors probably play an important role in influencing levels of suspiciousness.[6]

In a study to identify clients who are most likely to become dangerous on an acute care unit, suspiciousness was cited as one predictor of violence.[11] Suspicious clients were found to present a dilemma: they react poorly to a setting with many rules and restrictions, yet their symptoms often lead them into treatment facilities that have such rules.

In a population of clients with paranoia, those with a high level of suspiciousness had shorter hospitalizations and better recovery of social functioning but a poorer prognosis for full remission than those with lower levels of suspiciousness.[9] However, clients who are suspicious are not easy to study over time, because they tend not to stay in treatment.[9]

RELATED FACTORS

Suspiciousness can begin in the first stage of development. In addition, children who grow up in families where mistrust exists between members of that family and other households learn to be less trusting. A child takes on attitudes of significant figures, thus perpetuating values from one generation to another.

Some individuals who were previously trusting may become suspicious as a result of circumstances in their adult life. When there is impairment in vision or hearing loss, the resulting misinterpretation of stimuli can lead to suspiciousness. This is especially true in the elderly, who often suffer from social isolation in addition to the sensory impairment.

Stress is also a factor contributing to suspiciousness. Anxiety occurs in individuals as a reaction to something that is perceived or felt to be a danger. A common way of handling this uneasy feeling is to become angry and blame others in the environment. Stress therefore exacerbates suspiciousness by narrowing the individual's repertoire of coping behaviors and increasing the chance that an automatic negative response of anger, hostility, or suspiciousness will be triggered.

The development of suspicion directed at friends and family is a common early symptom of organic brain syndrome.[8] DSM-III-R conditions characterized by suspiciousness include amphetamine intoxication, cannabis intoxication, cocaine intoxication, hallucinogen hallucinosis, organic personality syndrome, paranoid personality disorder, and schizotypal personality disorder.

DEFINING CHARACTERISTICS

Clients who are suspicious are likely to withhold information, to resist recommendations for treatment, and to misinterpret actions in the environment. One client being screened for admission to a psychiatric facility replied to initial questions about his eating and sleeping patterns but balked at those about his family saying, "Now that's too personal. It goes against my constitutional rights."

Such clients tend to remain aloof, guarded, and alone. They may scan the environment with a sense of urgent hypervigilance and yet refuse to speak about what troubles them. Body language that serves to put distance between people may occur. For example, eye contact may be avoided, and the client may sit or stand farther away than might be culturally expected. There may be great sensitivity to the slightest nuances that suggest rejection. Special meaning may be imputed to coincidental events. Suspicious individuals may denounce others in the environment who are laughing or talking together for ridiculing them. They may be hesitant to eat food prepared by others. Clients who are suspicious may fear that falling asleep will be dangerous and therefore erect barricades to prevent others from entering their rooms during the night.

Those whose suspiciousness is related to cognitive impairment may misplace items and accuse nursing staff, other clients, or family members of having stolen them. Those with sensory impairment may misinterpret something they have only partially seen or heard and attribute malevolent motives to others (Chart 1).

NURSING PROCESS AND RATIONALE
Assessment

Because clients who are suspicious tend to remain aloof and to be hesitant to share information, body language such as muscle tenseness, hypervigilance, and averted gaze may be the most obvious indicators of the condition. In addition, nurses may be acutely aware of feeling highly anxious themselves when approaching clients who use distancing maneuvers as a way of screening themselves from interpersonal contact. Because stress tends to increase suspiciousness, clients newly admitted to an inpatient facility are particularly prone to suspect that hospitalization will not serve

---

CHART 1
Suspiciousness: Definition, Related Factors, and Defining Characteristics

DEFINITION

Suspiciousness is a mode of interacting manifested by a mistrust of others, a belief that people are basically evil and out to get what they can for themselves at the expense of others.

RELATED FACTORS

Socially isolated childhood
Dysfunctional family
Sensory impairment
Stress
Amphetamine, cannabis, or cocaine intoxication
Hallucinogen hallucinosis
Organic personality syndrome
Paranoid personality disorder
Schizotypal personality disorder
Social isolation

DEFINING CHARACTERISTICS

Isolation
Misinterpretation of actions in the environment
Use of distancing maneuvers, such as lack of eye contact
Sense of hypervigilance
Hypersensitivity to rejection
Fear of eating or falling asleep
Guarded, aloof manner
Negative or accusatory remarks about others
Hostility
Irritability
Defensiveness

---

their best interests. The response may range from quiet resignation to angry outbursts that can escalate from verbal to physical abuse.

Nursing Diagnosis

An example of a nursing diagnosis for a particular client would be suspiciousness related to organic personality syndrome and hearing impairment.

Client Goals and Nursing Interventions

The primary goal in working with clients who are suspicious is to prevent overt aggression. There is need to accept their guardedness, their lack of verbal communication, or their sullen glances in order to avoid more overtly aggressive behavior. At the same time, care is necessary to avoid power struggles if at all possible, for that would further increase the client's anxiety. Allowing clients to have as much control as possible over their own care is beneficial and gives them time to anticipate events. For example, clients may be given options in deciding what time of day and in what site an injection will be given.

It may be helpful to pick out one staff member who seems to have better rapport than others and use this person as the main contact. These clients are so likely to put a negative interpretation on what they hear that the contact person must be scrupulous in explaining procedures, following through on what is said, and answering questions clearly and honestly. Progress may eventually be made in teaching clients to check out their suspicions realistically. This process is facilitated by raising doubt as to what a client is saying. Gently questioning material rather than attempting to reason is the technique of choice, because it avoids placing a client in a defensive position.

To distract clients from ruminating on their problems, focus might best be placed on events in the here and now. A simple game or task can serve this purpose. One client enjoyed watering the plants. Another helped fold the menus for the next day. Usually, these clients respond best to activities on the group periphery rather than in the spotlight.

Whatever the intervention, two factors are important. First, the relationship between the client and the nurse should be fashioned to maintain neutrality and distance. These clients often are out to defeat whatever approach is attempted. They are frightened by premature or enthusiastic offers of help and need to know that the nurse is competent. They tend to respond better if something is suggested in a tentative if not skeptical manner. "Sometimes people find this useful" or "I'm not sure this will work for you" are phrases that allow clients to feel more in control of their own treatment.

Second, it takes time if trust is to grow in a person who has never known it. Short hospitalizations and frequent changes in health care workers create difficulties. Programs that provide case managers in regular contacts tend to be more effective in meeting the needs of these clients.

Evaluation

Progress may be slow and setbacks frequent. A client who is doing relatively well may develop a heightened degree of suspiciousness with developments that bring stress and new demands for adaptation. Evaluation is ongoing when the client's level of functioning is monitored by mental health workers who are involved with the person long enough for trust to be established. Such changes as fewer acts of aggression and better integration into the community may suggest a lessening of suspiciousness (Chart 2).

CASE STUDY

Joe is a 37-year-old man who showed high suspiciousness when he was ordered to attend a day treatment program as part of a 90-day less-restrictive court order. Because of his unwillingness to sign releases for information about previous psychiatric treatment, little was known about him until he reluctantly agreed to allow medical records to be sent from another hospital. These records described a man so suspicious and isolated that at one point in the past, he had

CHART 2
Suspiciousness: Summary of the Nursing Process

NURSING INTERVENTIONS	OUTCOME CRITERIA
CLIENT GOAL: EXPERIENCE A BEGINNING SENSE OF TRUST	
Limit the number of staff who interact with the client	Exhibits more relaxed body language
Respect need for space and privacy	Shows improvement in eating and sleeping
Approach the client in a neutral, low-key manner	Verbalizes concerns with staff
Explain procedures and follow through with what is said	
Allow the client as much control as possible	
CLIENT GOAL: ENGAGE IN ACTIVITIES IN THE HERE AND NOW	
Direct client to simple tasks or games when appropriate	Spends more time interacting with others
Offer positive feedback for acceptable behavior	Exhibits ability to focus on tasks or games
	Verbalizes about matters in the here and now
CLIENT GOAL: INCREASE KNOWLEDGE ABOUT OWN BEHAVIOR	
Teach client ways to recognize and handle feelings	Reports on feelings rather than acting on them
Teach ways to check out suspicions	Checks with others on suspicions
Teach medication management	Follows recommendations of medication regimen
FAMILY GOAL: EXPERIENCE FEWER PROBLEMATIC INCIDENTS OF CLIENT'S SUSPICIOUSNESS WITH FAMILY	
Teach client's family more effective and satisfying strategies for dealing with the client	Family experiences fewer problematic incidents in interactions with client
Offer support to the family and identify resources for help	Family and friends report greater understanding or less discomfort with the client

Research Highlights

Studies support the premise that high levels of suspiciousness are associated with deleterious health outcomes. Level of hostility (Ho) was assessed by a 50-item subscale of the Minnesota Multiphasic Personality Inventory of 1877 employed middle-aged men who were free of coronary heart disease.[10] After adjustment for age, blood pressure, serum cholesterol, cigarette smoking, and intake of ethanol, the relative probability of serious coronary heart disease within 10 years was 0.68 for men with Ho scores less than 10 in comparison with men with higher scores. Because the person with a high score on the Ho scale "has little confidence in his fellow man" and "sees people as dishonest, unsocial, immoral, ugly, and mean," it was also conjectured that the Ho score may be inversely related to the quantity and quality of social supports.[10]

In another study, scores on Factor L of the Sixteen Personality Factor Questionnaire, a measure of suspiciousness that is closely related to the Ho scale, predicted survival in a stratified random sample of 500 older men and women drawn from subscriber lists of a health insurance plan.[1,3] In follow-up of approximately 15 years, those individuals with scores indicating higher levels of suspiciousness had greater mortality risk.[1]

Beard tested the premise that a decrease in the level of interpersonal trust as measured by personality inventory may lead to heart disease.[2] High-trust scorers had lower cholesterol, smaller body mass index, lower diastolic blood pressure, and lower clinical variables. These findings suggest that trust may produce a general sense of well-being, thereby reducing the physiological tendency to defend against threat.[2] Conversely, the stress resulting from low levels of trust may elicit physiological arousal without opportunity for the musculoskeletal discharge of the state of arousal. Furthermore, chronic arousal is known to be damaging to the cardiovascular system.[2]

tied himself to the chair in his apartment in order to prevent himself from jumping through the window. The nursing diagnosis was suspiciousness related to isolation and chronic mental illness.

In the day treatment setting, he kept his belongings in a pack strapped to his side and sat in the same chair, refusing offers of coffee or food. He wore layers of clothing with three or four shirt collars emerging from under a sweatshirt and leather jacket. Joe was at the door each morning waiting to be let inside. He went directly to his chair and spent much of the time with his eyes either partially closed feigning rest or searching the room as if noting the whereabouts of others. For the first week or two, he occupied a chair between two empty ones, because clients were wary of him, and staff were sensitive to his need for personal space and privacy. Occasionally one staff member approached Joe and spoke briefly to him in a low key way.

After a few weeks, he took off his pack and joined others outside for a cigarette. Finally, one day, he raised his hand and volunteered to work on the maintenance crew. Cleaning the kitchen became his daily task. Although he never initiated conversation, he began to eat with other clients and to respond to attention by smiling and answering direct questions. One month after his court order was over, he was still attending the program voluntarily.

SUMMARY

Suspiciousness occurs in persons who have a basic lack of trust. They grow up believing that the world is a dangerous place, with evil lurking at every turn. Many of these people remain outside the mental health system, for they do not trust others enough to seek help. Clients who are suspicious tend to be difficult persons, for they arouse fear and anger in others. Their behavior is often associated with psychotic delusions and aggression. Interventions aimed at evoking a sense of trust are the focus of nursing care. A neutral, matter-of-fact approach that respects clients' needs for space and privacy is important. Such an approach includes an opportunity to demonstrate that the nurse is trustworthy and consistent, able to take care of personal needs without need to control the client.

References

1. Barefoot JC, Siegler IC, Nowlin JB, Peterson BL, Haney TL, Williams RB Jr. Suspiciousness, health, and mortality: a follow-up study of 500 older adults. Psychosom Med. 1987;49:450–457.
2. Beard MT. Trust, life events, and risk factors among adults. Adv Nurs Sci. 1982;4:26–43.
3. Cattell RB, Eber HW, Tatsuoka MM. Handbook for the Sixteen Personality Factor Questionnaire (16 PF). Champaign, Illinois: Institute for Personality and Ability Testing; 1970.
4. Erikson EH. Childhood and society. New York: WW Norton; 1963.
5. Eysenck HJ, Eysenck SBG. Manual of the Eysenck Personality Questionnaire. London: Hodder and Stroughton; 1975.
6. Kendler KS, Heath A, Martin NG. A genetic epidemiologic study of self-report suspiciousness. Compr Psychiatry. 1987;28:187–196.
7. Patrick M. Daily living with cognitive deficits and behavioral problems. In: Carnevali DL, Patrick M: Nursing management of the elderly. 2nd ed. Philadelphia: JB Lippincott; 1986.
8. Price BH, Mesulam M. Psychiatric manifestations of right hemisphere infarctions. J Nerv Ment Dis. 1985;173:610–614.
9. Ritzler BA. Paranoia—prognosis and treatment: a review. Schizophr Bull. 1981;7:710–728.
10. Shekelle RB, Gale M, Ostfeld AM, Paul O. Hostility, risk of coronary heart disease and mortality. Psychosom Med. 1983;45:109–114.
11. Werner PD, Rose TL, Yesavage JA, Seeman K. Psychiatrist's judgments of dangerousness in patients on an acute care unit. Am J Psychiatry. 1984;141:263–266.

WELLNESS-SEEKING BEHAVIOR

Maisie Schmidt Kashka and Mary I. Huntley

DEFINITION AND DESCRIPTION

The diagnostic category that NANDA has termed *health-seeking behavior* is here termed *wellness-seeking behavior*.[2] *Wellness-seeking behavior* is defined as a state in which an individual in stable health is actively seeking ways to alter personal health habits or the environment to move toward a higher level of health. Furthermore, *stable health status* is defined as: age-appropriate illness prevention measures *achieved*, client reports good or excellent health, and signs and symptoms of disease, if present, are controlled.[1,2] In this definition, illness prevention measures have been achieved (or are being implemented); therefore, a client with this diagnosis would not knowingly be engaging in "at-risk" behaviors. This does not preclude an individual with a chronic illness from demonstrating wellness-seeking behaviors. Clients who have learned the adaptation that comes from living with a chronic illness may be ready to attain new and advanced levels of wellness despite physical or psychosocial restrictions or disabilities. Often, it is the very individuals who have had to cope with illness and have asked the hard questions about life and relationships who may, in fact, be working toward high-level wellness, even as they struggle with physical or mental illness.

The diagnosis, wellness-seeking behavior, challenges the psychiatric mental health nurse to think about wellness-seeking behavior for psychiatric mental health clients. Wellness-promoting interventions used by the nurse during therapy facilitate mental health client's progress toward health. Once the person has reached "stable health," the diagnosis of wellness-seeking behavior can become appropriate. Nurses in psychiatric mental health settings must assess and recognize the client's potential and readiness for this diagnosis. A goal in psychiatric mental health nursing, as in all other specialties in nursing, is to facilitate the client's use of resources that can extend beyond the initial treatment milieu.

THEORY AND RESEARCH

Perspectives on health and wellness that have emerged over the past 15 years are helpful in providing a rationale for conceptualizing the diagnosis, wellness-seeking behavior.

Health and Illness

Laffrey and coworkers[13] have identified two primary views of health. One is termed the *pathogenic paradigm* and states that health is "any behavior that is disease related, whether it is to prevent or cure," whereas the second is termed the *health paradigm* and "espouses an organismic view of human beings who are seen as autonomous, responsible, and having potential for growth. . . . Health is a fluid, flexible process, a subjective phenomenon of each human being" (reference 13, pp 96–97). The nursing diagnosis of wellness-seeking behavior is very useful in this latter paradigm.

Health can be classified under four different models.[23] These four models have been called (1) the clinical model, (2) the adaptation model, (3) the role performance model, and (4) the eudaimonistic model.[23] *Eudaimonistic*, a term of Greek origin, refers to the theory or act of happiness. The eudaimonistic model describes the kind of health first described by Dunn in 1961 as "wellness."[7]

Wellness

Dunn identified health-promoting behavior by the term *high-level wellness* to describe the optimum state of health achieved by self-actualizing individuals. Dunn defined high-level wellness as "an integrated method of functioning which is oriented toward maximizing the potential of which the individual is capable. It requires that the individual maintain a continuum of balance and purposeful direction within the environment where he is functioning" (reference 7, pp 4, 5). According to Dunn, the individual striving for high-level wellness is a person with life goals and purpose ever striving to better him- or herself. This advanced state is not a goal that is obtained, but rather a *process* toward which the individual continually aspires.

Wellness and Nursing

Nurses have used the term *wellness* in discussing health and wellness-seeking behavior. Clark[3] defines *wellness* as "a process of moving toward greater awareness of oneself and the environment leading toward ever-increasing planned interactions with the dimensions of nutrition, fitness, stress, environment, interpersonal relationships, and self-care responsibility" (reference 3, p 3). As part of Huntley's[10] grounded theory study, educated well older women were asked to define wellness. Six themes emerged which collectively formed the following definition, also compatible with other works:[3,7,20,23] "wellness is a chosen, balanced state of mind, body, and spirit in which the person is able to cope with adverse stimuli, is able to experience feelings of security and contentment, and expresses a positive and hopeful attitude about life" (reference 10, p 92). Wellness in this definition was further conceptualized as "enjoyable unity."

Oelbaum[19] utilized Dunn's concept of wellness to list 26 hallmarks of adult wellness; she emphasized that wellness could exist concurrently with physical illness if the person was maximizing his or her potential. Pender[20] also utilized Dunn's concept of wellness as part of her conceptualization of health promotion. Pender perceived health behaviors stemming from either an actualizing tendency or a stabilizing tendency. The actualizing tendency is seen as the underlying motivation for movement toward high-level wellness, whereas the stabilizing tendency underlies health protection activities. Both tendencies are necessary for the individual to maintain and advance health status. Pender combined these tendencies in the following definition of *health*: ". . . the actualization of inherent and acquired human potential through goal directed behavior, competent self-care, and satisfying relationships with others while adjustments are made as needed to maintain structural integrity and harmony with the environment" (reference 20, p 27). Criteria for evaluating health based on Pender's definition are discussed in the assessment portion of this section. Pender[20] also formulated the areas in which wellness-seeking behaviors occur that can advance the individual to new levels of wellness. The areas emphasized by Pender include modification of life-style, exercise and physical fitness, nutrition and weight control, stress management, and social support.

Psychiatric mental health nurses contribute substantially to wellness-seeking behaviors, particularly in the modification of life-style, stress management, and social support. Life-style modification can be accomplished only through sustained behavior change. This means that the same principles used with psychiatric mental health clients to change unhealthy behaviors can be used to motivate behaviors in healthy individuals that will move them to still higher levels of wellness. Pender emphasized the use of self-confrontation, cognitive restructuring, social modeling, and behavior modification techniques as useful tools in assisting clients to adopt wellness life-styles. Psychiatric mental health nurses use some of these interventions in their practice on a daily basis. Many psychiatric mental health units include stress management sessions as part of the therapeutic milieu; therefore, many psychiatric mental health nurses are already familiar with these techniques. Because psychiatric mental health nurses work with both clients and families on issues of relationships, techniques for evaluating and improving social support systems become an even more important part of their practice.

The health of the family affects the health of the individual and of society itself.[6] Psychiatric mental health nursing has always emphasized the effect of family dynamics upon individual functioning. Therefore, the influence of family health practices and life-style is a legitimate reason for incorporating family health promotion into psychiatric mental health nursing practice.

The importance of wellness-seeking behaviors cannot be overemphasized because the major causes of death are related primarily to life-style behaviors, rather than events or illnesses over which persons have no control.[14,24] Five areas need to be considered: diet, smoking, lack of exercise, alcohol abuse, and control of hypertension. A landmark study[14] found that seven personal health practices were highly correlated with physical health and increased longevity (especially for men). These health practices, often used to assess life-style, were (1) sleeping seven to eight hours daily, (2) eating breakfast almost every day, (3) never or rarely eating between meals, (4) currently being at, or near, height-adjusted weight, (5) never smoking cigarettes, (6) moderate or no use of alcohol, and (7) regular physical activity.

The health belief model, first described in the early 1950s, has been widely used to explain health behavior. Mikhail[17] reviewed the health belief model and found that, although this model does provide some insight into health behavior and motivation, it does not always provide a full explanation for health-related behaviors. Mikhail asserted that more research is needed to explore the conditions under which health beliefs are formed and identify strategies to influence those beliefs.

RELATED FACTORS

First and foremost, wellness is a process that is lived. It is not a product that is achieved as a result of health promotion activities. As a result of that lived process, the client will grow to new levels of being and, often, experience a sense of well-being as a part of that growth. There are two major categories of factors that influence the experience of wellness-seeking behavior: personal factors and environmental factors. Personal factors include values, education, socioeconomic status, and life circumstances. Environmental factors include community resources and work place resources.

Personal Factors

There are numerous personal factors that can affect whether or not a person will choose to engage in wellness-seeking behaviors that can lead to high-level wellness. These factors include all those personal resources an individual brings to any situation.

VALUES

Persons learn different values. In considering wellness-seeking behavior, one might ask if the client values absence of disease (neutral health)[1] or wellness. Most people value absence of disease, and many people are willing to engage in those behaviors that will maintain a disease-free state. However, to go beyond health protection or health maintenance behaviors to health promotion behaviors requires a valuing of wellness or positive health. Some chronically ill individuals engage in wellness-seeking behaviors aimed at personal growth, rather than behaviors just aimed at staying alive; such clients value wellness and are wellness-seeking. Personal values are affected by the health values and behaviors modeled by parents and other significant persons in an individual's life, as well as the impact of the value the culture itself places on health. Because wellness-seeking behavior is a proactive process, it involves a value choice—a choosing to engage in those behaviors that promote positive change and personal growth in the physical, mental, emotional, and spiritual spheres.

EDUCATION

Our values are often significantly influenced by the educational process. An emphasis on health and wellness in the school system not only teaches the facts about health, it says to the child that health is important, just as English, history, and math are important. Furthermore, the skills learned in the educational process enable the individual to continue to learn about health throughout his or her life. Persons who cannot read have not only been deprived of the content of the health classes taught in schools, but also cannot be lifelong learners about health. Such individuals are also likely to have jobs that will provide health insurance benefits; therefore, even health protection may not be available to them. The more educated the person the more likely he or she has some basic health information and engages in some healthful behaviors.

SOCIOECONOMIC STATUS

One of the moral and ethical dilemmas facing nurses and others who believe in wellness as an ultimate goal is the question: Is health promotion only for the upper and middle classes? Those struggling for existence, who are homeless, or who are working for minimum wage, usually do not have the means to focus on wellness. The homeless person eating from a "soup kitchen" cannot choose his or her diet. Furthermore, the homeless person dependent on clothing donations cannot choose footwear appropriate for many hours of walking. Even health protection and health maintenance are often beyond the reach of the poor.

LIFE CIRCUMSTANCES

The stressors present in a person's life at any given time can affect the capacity for wellness-seeking behaviors. Demands of job or family can so fill an individual's life that there is no time to choose and focus upon health promotion goals. Often, when such life circumstances as an ill family member or increased job demands exist, the individual can only focus on remaining illness-free during the stressful time. Such persons often do not have the time and energy to engage in those wellness-seeking behaviors. In such circumstances, health protection or maintenance behaviors may be the only realistic option. Such clients can, however, be encouraged to maintain wellness as a value so that when life circumstances change, they may be able to use the past stressful experience as a departure point for growth.

Environmental Factors

COMMUNITY RESOURCES

Churches, schools, and other community institutions can, and often do, offer programs aimed at wellness. In affluent communities, there are private fitness centers (aimed at physical wellness) designed to profit from the middle- and upper-class emphasis on health promotion. However, nonprofit organizations such as the YWCA and the YMCA also provide opportunities for those with more limited financial resources to engage in physical fitness and other health promotion activities. The programs offered by nonprofit organizations may be more holistic in their approach, with classes in stress management, meditation, and leisure, as well as traditional physical fitness activities.

WORKPLACE RESOURCES

Wellness-oriented programs are now often found in business and corporate settings, with large companies sometimes investing several million dollars into onsite corporate fitness programs.[9] In such settings, it is the company that is seeking to stimulate employee wellness-seeking behaviors because improvements in lifestyle will ultimately also produce healthier and more productive employees. Greiner[8] noted that the executive officer of one large corporation stated that his company saved three dollars for every one dollar spent on health promotion and wellness. Furthermore, a state department of health found that employees who were smokers used 1.5 more sick days per month than did the employees who did not smoke; the smokers cost this department an estimated 11,931 dollars per year.[8] As a result of such expenses, employee wellness motivation becomes an important consideration.

Thus, many factors impinge on an individual's ability

or desire to engage in wellness-seeking behavior. Because wellness implies that the person is moving toward self-actualization, any factor that would hinder self-actualization would also affect wellness-seeking behavior.

DEFINING CHARACTERISTICS

The defining characteristics of wellness-seeking behavior are the following:[2]

1. Expressed or observed desire to seek a higher level of wellness
2. Expressed or observed desire for increased control of health practice(s)
3. Expression of concern about the effect of current environmental conditions on health status
4. Expressed or observed desire for familiarity with community wellness resources in an individual desiring a higher level of wellness
5. Demonstrated or observed desire for knowledge of health promotion behaviors in an individual desiring a higher level of wellness

The primary defining characteristic of wellness-seeking behavior is the client's own expression of a desire to achieve a higher level of wellness. Unless the nurse knows that the client desires to move toward this goal, the defining characteristics might also be present in a client only wishing to remain illness-free. Wellness by definition is a holistic concept. In other words, a wellness-oriented individual would generally not embark on an exercise program while continuing to abuse nicotine, since the abuse of nicotine itself indicates that the individual has not achieved a stable health status and remains at risk for all those disorders caused, or complicated, by nicotine use. Because wellness is a process, not a product, persons aiming to seek higher levels of wellness may change behaviors in all the areas for health promotion advocated by Pender.[20] Likewise, individuals with health problems that have been controlled to the maximum that they can be controlled (clients with cancer, spinal cord injury, and such), can exhibit the desire to achieve the maximum of which they are capable. Such clients are wellness-oriented and are exhibiting wellness-seeking behavior. The paraplegic person who takes up wheelchair basketball to get more physical activity and engages in an activity that also provides interpersonal contact with others is exhibiting wellness-seeking behavior.

The other characteristics imply a perceived need by the client to change a health practice or environmental condition, or to gain knowledge about health promotion or community resources. Once again, note that even though a client perceives a need to move to a higher level of wellness, this is done from a *stable health status*[1,3] (Chart 1).

CHART 1
Wellness-Seeking Behavior: Definition, Related Factors, and Defining Characteristics

DEFINITION

A state in which an individual in stable health is actively seeking ways to alter personal health habits or the environment to move toward a higher level of health.

RELATED FACTORS

Personal factors
    Values
    Education
    Socioeconomic status
    Life circumstances
Environmental factors
    Community resources
    Workplace resources

DEFINING CHARACTERISTICS

Desire to seek new level of wellness
Desire for increased control of health practices
Concern about effect of current environment on health
Desire for information about community resources
Desire for knowledge about health promotion behaviors

NURSING PROCESS AND RATIONALE
Assessment

Although any movement toward wellness made by a client could be termed "wellness-seeking," assessment begins with a determination of the client's present health status (i.e., is he or she in present stable health or expressing motivation to move toward a more healthful state?). Brubaker[1] emphasizes the necessity of starting from a point of stable health in her statement: "Accepting any movement upward on the health continuum as health promotion, no matter what the starting point, produces an undifferentiated, and, therefore, useless term and is thus rejected" (reference 1, p 12). If the client is in stable health, the next consideration is the client's own conception of health. The level of wellness-seeking behavior desired by the client will vary depending on his or her conception of health. The term *conception* is used to note a broader, more general definition of health as opposed to a narrower perception of one's own health status. The following questions assist the psychiatric mental health nurse in assessing the client's conception of health:

1. Does the client believe that health is merely absence of disease?

2. Does he or she believe that health is the ability to fulfill the expectations of all his or her life roles?

3. Does he or she believe that health is the ability to adapt to life stressors experienced by persons in social and physical environments?

4. Does the client believe that health is something more than all of these other beliefs—believing that health is a process leading to a maximization of potential, characterized by self-actualization, well-being, and a "zest for life"?

Clients whose conception of health is the clinical model might well focus on behaviors specifically related to health risks. For example, a well client in the midlife years whose family has a history of adult-onset diabetes and whose weight is in the upper limits of normal, might exhibit wellness-seeking behavior by inquiring about his or her risk of developing diabetes and the appropriate risk reduction measures. Clients concerned with role performance might seek those health behaviors that would most prepare them to meet the multiple-role demands experienced in the present complex society. Likewise, a client conceiving of health as adaptation might focus on the potential for growth resulting from life and environmental adaptations. Finally, clients with a eudaimonistic conception of health will be concerned with issues of personal growth and actualization. Such clients might be concerned with developing new direction and life purpose.

The following questions were developed from Pender's criteria (reference 20, p 27) and may be used by the nurse to assess an individual's level of wellness.

1. Does the client history document personal growth and positive change over time?

2. Can the client identify both short-term and long-term goals that continue to guide his or her behavior?

3. Has the client been able to prioritize his or her identified goals?

4. Is the client aware of alternative behavioral options that can be utilized to accomplish goals?

5. Does the client perceive optimum health as one of life's primary purposes?

6. Is the client actively engaged in satisfying and fulfilling interpersonal relationships?

7. Does the client actively seek new experiences that expand knowledge or increase competencies for personal care?

8. Does the client history document high tolerance for new and unusual situations or experiences?

9. Does the client derive satisfaction from the experience of daily living, exhibiting a zest for living?

10. Does the client expend more energy in acting on the environment than in reacting to it?

11. Does the client identify barriers to growth and have a constructive plan for removing or ameliorating them?

12. Does the client monitor him or herself and accept feedback from others to determine personal and social effectiveness?

13. Is the client maintaining conditions of internal stability compatible with continuing existence?

14. Does the client anticipate internal and external threats to stability and take appropriate preventive actions?

Nursing Diagnosis

The nursing diagnosis of wellness-seeking behavior can be arrived at after completion of the assessment. As can be noted from the previous discussions concerning the defining characteristics and the assessment, when a client in a stable health state expresses a desire to move toward high-level wellness, the diagnosis of wellness-seeking behavior is appropriate. Sometimes this desire can be expressed by the client in terms of questions about fitness programs, diet, or a desire to discuss future goals, for example, wellness-seeking behavior (fitness program) related to worksite resources. Perhaps a chronically ill client may express the desire to achieve a level of psychological health that is not possible for him or her in the physical area, for example, wellness-seeking behavior (psychological health) related to increased opportunities for exploring emotions. It is often those clients who have had to face the difficulties and challenges of chronic illness who begin to ask the kind of questions about life that lead them to begin to seek health beyond mere absence of disease. Indeed, sometimes the absence of disease is not possible, in which case, the client may "rise above" the illness and begin to actualize in other areas; for example, wellness-seeking behavior (stress management program) related to chronic pain.

Client Goals and Nursing Interventions

In assisting clients to make the necessary changes to attain new levels of health, it is important to remember that people tend to choose those patterns of behavior that will cost them the least and gain them the most. Therefore, in counseling clients on new patterns of health behavior, it is very important to assist the client to assess the costs and benefits of any health behavior.

Hobson and associates[9] suggest that the motivational process for wellness-seeking behavior has three components: (1) the energizing of the wellness-seeking behavior, (2) the direction of the behavior, and, (3) the sustaining of the behavior. They suggest that *energizing of wellness-seeking behavior* may occur as a result of an aggressive communication addressing the advantages of fitness including the psychological and physiologic improvements that can occur. Participants in fitness programs were better able to handle stress, slept better, experienced a higher energy level, had more physical strength, and felt better about themselves.[9] "Interestingly, improvement of self-concept began to occur immediately once the fitness program was started. It seems that people feel better about themselves when they are doing something positive for their health" (reference 9, p 82). This finding lends support to psychiatric mental health nurses emphasizing the need for fitness activities for psychiatric mental health clients. The second component, *direction of behavior*, is important because the individual needs to find a program that offers the most in terms of financial cost and time. Companies that offer corporate health programs understandably want their employees to use those programs. Finally, the third motivational component of wellness-seeking behavior is the most critical because it is concerned with the individual's *ability to sustain over time the behaviors* that are to become a part of the life-style. Keeping the fitness participant apprised of his or her physical improvements can act as a behavioral reinforcement for the behavior. Another reinforcer of sustained wellness-seeking behavior occurs when the behavior is socially reinforced by small-group activities that also offer opportunities for social interaction. Engaging in fitness activities with another person or a small group can be a powerful motivator.[9]

A concern of a physical fitness program, for any age group, is the potential for injury, because injuries can interrupt the newly established routine and the beginning social support. Injuries occur when the skills demanded of an activity exceed the capabilities of the person performing the activity, if only for a moment.[22] One way to minimize the potential for such injuries is to ensure that fitness programs are supervised by professionals qualified to understand the requirements of human performance. Therefore, nurses encouraging clients to investigate fitness programs need also to recommend those programs that employ professionals as supervisors of these activities.

Because health practices are interrelated and do not exist in isolation from each other, it becomes very important to look at wellness-seeking behavior in the context of multiple health practices. There is a greater likelihood that a targeted health practice will be maintained if the new behavior fits into the person's overall wellness life-style.[21]

For the nursing diagnosis, wellness-seeking behavior, the following goals and interventions are applicable:[12,23]

Clinical Wellness-Seeking Behavior
Goal: The client will perform primary prevention activities (disease prevention, health risk reduction) that will move him or her to a higher level of wellness.
NURSING INTERVENTIONS
1. Assess those conditions for which the client may be at risk, perhaps by using a Health Risk Assessment instrument.
2. Assess the client's present state of health knowledge.

3. Engage in teaching activities that will facilitate the client's acquisition of knowledge of primary prevention activities.
4. Assist the client in joining those activities most appropriate to his or her age, resources, and interests.
5. If possible, assist the client in joining activities that will involve others engaging in primary prevention activities.

Role Performance Wellness-Seeking Behavior
Goal: The client will demonstrate the ability to expand his or her role performance to new and higher levels.
NURSING INTERVENTIONS
1. Explore with the client his or her present roles and the ways in which they might be expanded to new levels.
2. Explore with the client resources available that are helpful in role expansion.
3. Assist client in determining what group or therapeutic strategies might be helpful in assisting the movement toward role expansion.

Adaptive Wellness-Seeking Behavior
Goal: The client will demonstrate the ability for creative adaptation resulting from effective interaction with physical and social environments.
NURSING INTERVENTIONS
1. Explore with the client ways in which his or her physical and/or social environment could become more growth-producing.
2. Assist client in finding the resources that might assist in new adaptations.
3. Support the client as he or she explores new social settings and environments.

Eudaimonistic Wellness-Seeking Behavior
Goal: The client will engage in activities aimed at enhancement of well-being, self-fulfillment, and development of his or her maximum potential.
NURSING INTERVENTIONS
1. Explore with the client his or her conception of life purpose and direction.
2. Assist the client in finding resources that can assist in his or her growth and development.
3. Assist the client in finding social resources that will support his or her personal growth.

Evaluation

Evaluation of wellness-seeking behavior will refer back to the client goals that were established as part of the nursing care plan. To evaluate, the following questions might be asked: Did the client move to a new or higher level of wellness? Were the activities associated with wellness-seeking behavior successful? Has the client moved to another dimension of health–wellness, that is, has he or she moved from one dimension of health, such as clinical, to another? Is the client now open to an even greater possibility for wellness, such as eudai-monistic? (Chart 2).

CASE STUDY

Marie is a volunteer at the Women's Shelter. The Shelter provided her with crisis intervention two years ago when she decided that being in an abusive spouse relationship was no longer acceptable to her. Psychotherapy helped her gain insight related to her relationships with men and women and her situational low self-esteem. She is now divorced and lives with her two children, ages 10 and 8. Her job provides an adequate salary for the family's needs.

During one of her volunteer days at the Shelter, she asked the psychiatric nurse consultant for assistance in exploring some future life directions. The nurse asked her several questions about her health status; roles in her life; and her home, work, and community environments. The nurse was interested in *assessing* the whole situation, rather than responding only to Marie's immediate concern. From Marie's responses, the nurse learned that Marie is at risk for adult-onset diabetes; otherwise, the data provided indicated she is in stable health. The nurse also learned that Marie is functioning well in her family, work, and volunteer roles; however, she is aware of being present-, not future-oriented. Her environmental situation is influenced by her concern about future roles. She wonders if she should work toward another degree to improve her job situation and how this would affect her family.

This situation illustrates a client in stable health who is exhibiting wellness-seeking behavior according to two conceptions of health: the clinical model and the role performance model. Marie was aware that her family history of diabetes suggested that one day she may be diabetic; however, she was unaware that a diet and exercise program could reduce the risk of developing it. Therefore, Marie's initiation of health risk reduction activities is an example of behaviors associated with the clinical model. Marie's behaviors associated with examining her future roles are related to the role performance model. The nursing diagnoses identified were wellness-seeking behavior related to a desire to reduce a health risk and wellness-seeking behavior related to anticipatory role transitions.

Marie had been focused on the past for several years. She now perceives herself as a well person (stable health). However, she had not been future goal-oriented in her thinking. She had not thought about being able to prevent the onset of diabetes or about role changes that would be occurring. For example, in ten years her mother role will change, because it is likely that both of her children will have graduated from high school. Forming life goals—short-term as well as long-term—is a strategy advocated by mental health experts; preparation for anticipated changes provides opportunities for the person to meet new roles more successfully. Marie is initiating discussion with an appropriate health care professional.

General goals focused on Marie's desire to take the steps necessary to reduce the diabetes health risk and to begin planning for future role transitions. Specific behavioral outcome criteria were identified for each client goal. Because one of the goals focused on reduction of the diabetes health risk, the outcome criteria included Marie's verbalizing her thoughts and feelings about diabetes, attending a diabetes education program, and making a follow-up appointment with the nurse to report on her progress. Outcome criteria related to her goal for planning for future role transitions included Marie's being able to state past and present goals, discussing her current aspirations, stating her plans for the future, and finally, utilizing the resources available to her for goal fulfillment. All of the outcome criteria were measurable, thus facilitating the nurse's evaluation.

The nurse assisted Marie to talk about her thoughts and feelings concerning diabetes and referred her to a diabetic education resource. She also encouraged Marie to make a follow-up appointment to report back to the nurse the progress she had made. As part of nursing interventions, the nurse also discussed past, present, and future goal planning with Marie to facilitate further present and future role performance. Marie's dreams and aspirations were also discussed, and the nurse reinforced Marie's desire to begin to plan for her future roles. Community resources that might assist Marie in formulating role transition behaviors were suggested by the nurse. The nurse was careful not to give Marie advice on her future plans, but rather gave her the opportunity to explore the options available.

Marie attended a diabetes education program series and made needed changes in her nutritional and exercise activities. She also was able to utilize this information for her

---

CHART 2
Wellness-Seeking Behavior: Summary of the Nursing Process

NURSING INTERVENTIONS	EXPECTED OUTCOMES
CLIENT GOAL: ENGAGE IN ACTIVITIES THAT ACHIEVE AND ENHANCE WELLNESS	
Determine client's present health status	Performs primary prevention behaviors
Assess client's conception of health	
Assess areas of potential growth for client	
Assess client's present level of health promotion behaviors	
Assist client in a health risk reduction evaluation	
Teach client about health promotion activities	
Encourage client to join with others in health promotion activities	Demonstrates ability to expand role performance
Assist client in finding available community resources for health promotion	Adapts creatively to environment

children, teaching them about ways to reduce the diabetes risk in their family.

Marie had several discussions with the nurse concerning her desire to establish new goals and life direction that would facilitate her future adjustment after her children leave home. She consulted with the Women's Center at the local university to explore her options about returning to college to further her education. Her current employer was also a resource for the influence that education might have on her future work role. At present, Marie stated she has applied for a scholarship and plans to take her first course the following year.

The nurse in this situation not only assisted Marie with the presenting problem and concern, but she also used her knowledge to assess in two areas. She assessed whether or not Marie was in stable health. Then she asked Marie ques-

Research Highlights

Health can be investigated as either a dependent or an independent variable. Health can be examined as it relates to fullness of life, in which case, "the operational definitions could include such behaviors as a sense of humor, joy, curiosity, a willingness to explore alternatives, the enjoyment of sex, or creativity" (reference 26, p 6).

Nemcek[18] analyzed health promotion research on well adults completed by nurses between 1970 and 1985. She found a rising interest in health promotion and resulting research since 1970. Health promotion in well adults "has been more extensively researched between 1983 and 1985 than any time prior. It is a contemporary concern to nurse researchers" (reference 18, p 474). All of the research surveyed by Nemcek included women as subjects and focused on assessment, particularly assessment of health promotion parameters. She concluded that "further work is needed in all the functional health patterns to provide nurses with a whole person knowledge base in the field of health promotion practice" (reference 18, p 475).

Walker and coworkers[25] have developed an instrument measuring a life-style reflective of health promotion. Building upon the assessment tool included in Pender's book, the Health-Promoting Lifestyle Profile (HPLP) measures health promotion activities in six areas: self-actualization, health responsibility, stress management, interpersonal relations, exercise, and nutrition. Although a new instrument, the HPLP has great potential for nurses interested in exploring the correlates of a wellness life-style. Kashka[11] used this instrument in her exploration of the relationship of purpose and meaning in life and a wellness life-style and found that there was a relationship between these constructs in adult employed women.

Mikhail[17] provides a review of research using the health belief model. Her review summarizes research design, sample size, specific health behavior, statistical procedure, and results related to specific health belief model components.

Cox and associates[4] have developed an instrument to measure motivation in health behavior. The Health Self-Determinism Index (HSDI) is composed of four subscales (self-determined health judgments, self-determined health behavior, perceived competency in health matters, and internal–external cue responsiveness) and measures intrinsic motivation. They found, in a study of 379 older adults, that "general well-being, education, perceived health status, race (only blacks and whites), and sex were the significant predictors of the elders' total HSDI score" (reference 4, p 10). They also found that the more an individual was intrinsically motivated, the less

likely that nicotine was used. Furthermore, the more intrinsic the orientation of an individual and the more intrinsic in judgment and cue responsiveness, the less likely tranquilizers were used. Responsiveness to internal cues was related to self-determination of health judgment. Well-being was an important predictor of three of the four subscales. "Clearly, elders are better able to be more self-determined in their choice of health behaviors, feel more competent about their decisions or actions, and respond more to inner-directed forces if they have a greater sense of well-being" (reference 4, p 13). Furthermore, "better health is more apt to allow for independent decision making and self-reliance in the elderly" (reference 4, p 13).

Rakowski[21] in his analysis of the 1979 health practices survey, found no single predictor of personal health practices across age–sex groups, and also found that even within groups, no clear predictor could be found, although education seemed to be a strong influence across age–sex lines. He suggests that "any given predictor variable will be important for someone, but no one predictor will be important for everyone—or even a large majority . . . it may then become more appropriate to study health practices individually and within each subgroup, rather than collectively" (reference 21, p 386).

McBride[15] is specifically concerned with the direction of research about health behavior in women, especially as it relates to the mental health of women. Special attention needs to be paid to the multiple roles engaged in by women and the effect these multiple-role demands have upon their health. In examining wellness-seeking behavior, the question might be asked: What are the wellness-seeking behaviors of women experiencing multiple role demands?

Dana and Hoffman[5] in their assessment of instruments purporting to measure health, found that instruments tended to measure those attributes of health that are most easily quantifiable, such as nutrition, exercise, stress, safety, smoking, and drug use. They point out that reliability and validity are often not well-established for instruments measuring various aspects of health, and moreover, that there is not a consensus of opinion on the definition of health. Dana and Hoffman do, however, advance eight major concepts of holistic health: seeking of wholeness in life, an individual is more than the sum of parts, good health is more than physical well-being, health is not the mere absence of disease, disease is multicausal, illness can be a positive learning experience, health maintenance and prevention are more important than treatment of disease, and self-responsibility is an important aspect of health.

tions to assess her conception of health. The nurse learned that Marie was exhibiting behaviors associated with two of the models of health—clinical and role performance. Marie's situation illustrates that the models of health are fluid. There is movement back and forth because wellness is a process. Marie's working at the shelter as a volunteer is an example of her behavior in the eudaimonistic health model. She is sharing her growth with others so that they too may grow from an unhealthy situation. Before Marie's discussion with the nurse, one might have assessed that she was exhibiting behaviors primarily in the eudaimonistic model. Therefore, as new situations arise and when people are confronted with new stimuli, their conception of health may change. Marie's situation exemplifies the back-and-forth, up-and-down, or spiraling movement that occurs in the process of wellness-seeking behavior in each model.

SUMMARY

Wellness-seeking behavior as a nursing diagnosis in psychiatric mental health nursing practice, as well as in other areas of practice, is gaining recognition and action by nurses. Nurses have knowledge to assist persons in viewing health as more than the absence of illness. A wellness orientation from the nurse's perspective will facilitate the process of wellness in others. Wellness-seeking interventions have the potential of creating a healthier society. A healthier society will have less need for costly, highly technical illness care. Additionally, citizens in a healthy society can enjoy a higher quality of life. Nurses have an important and significant role in facilitating persons to take charge of their health, to view wellness as a process, and to use the health care system in a health-oriented rather than a pathogenic-oriented manner.

References

1. Brubaker B. Health promotion: a linguistic analysis. ANS. 1982;5:1–14.
2. Carroll-Johnson R, ed. Classification of nursing diagnosis: proceedings of the eighth conference. Philadelphia: JB Lippincott; 1988.
3. Clark CC. Wellness nursing: concepts, theory, research, and practice. New York: Springer; 1986.
4. Cox CL, Miller EH, Mull CS. Motivation in health behavior: measurement, antecedents, and correlates. ANS. 1987;9:1–15.
5. Dana RH, Hoffman TA. Health assessment domains: credibility and legitimization. Clin Psychol Rev. 1987;5:539–555.
6. Duffy ME. Health promotion in the family: current findings and directives for nursing research. J Adv Nurs. 1988; 13:109–117.
7. Dunn HL. High-level wellness. Arlington, VA: Beatty; 1961, 1973.
8. Greiner PA. Nursing and worksite wellness: missing the boat. Holis Nurs Prac. 1987;2:53–60.
9. Hobson CJ, Hoffman JJ, Leonard LM, Freismuth PK. Corporate fitness: understanding and motivating employee participation. Fitness in Business. 1987;80–85.
10. Huntley MI. Laughter and wellness as perceived by older women: grounded theory [Dissertation]. Denton, Texas: Texas Woman's University; 1988.
11. Kashka MS. The relationship between purpose and meaning in life and health promotion activities in adult employed women [Dissertation]. Denton, Texas; Texas Woman's University; 1987.
12. Laffrey SC. Health promotion: relevance for nursing. TCN. 1985;7:29–38.
13. Laffrey SC, Loveland-Cherry CJ, Winkler SJ. Health behavior: evolution of two paradigms. Public Health Nurs. 1986;3:92–100.
14. Matarazzo JD, et al. Behavioral health: a 1990 challenge for the health sciences. In: Matarazzo JD, et al, eds. Behavioral health: a handbook of health enhancement and disease prevention. New York: John Wiley & Sons; 1984.
15. McBride AB. Mental health effects of women's multiple roles. Image. 1988;20:41–47.
16. McFarland G, Wasli E. Nursing diagnoses and process in psychiatric nursing. Philadelphia: JB Lippincott; 1986.
17. Mikhail B. The health belief model: a review and critical evaluation of the model, research, and practice. ANS. 1981;4:65–82.
18. Nemcek MA. Research trends in the health promotion of well adults. AAOHN J. 1986;34:470–475.
19. Oelbaum CH. Hallmarks of adult wellness. Am J Nurs. 1974;74:1623–1625.
20. Pender NJ. Health promotion in nursing practice, 2nd ed. Norwalk, CT: Appleton & Lange; 1987.
21. Rakowski W. Predictors of health practices within age–sex groups: national survey of personal health practices and consequences, 1979. Public Health Rep. 1988;103:376–386.
22. Rivara FP. Epidemiology of childhood injuries. In: Matarazzo JD, et al, eds. Behavioral health: a handbook of health enhancement and disease prevention. New York: John Wiley & Sons; 1984.
23. Smith JA. The idea of health. New York: Teachers College Press; 1983.
24. United States Public Health Service. The 1990 health objectives for the nation: a midcourse review. Washington, DC: USPHS; 1986.
25. Walker SN, Sechrist KR, Pender NJ. The health-promoting lifestyle profile: development and psychometric characteristics. Nurs Res. 1987;36:76–81.
26. Winstead-Fry P. The scientific method and its impact on holistic health. ANS. 1980;2:1–7.

Clients With Major Psychiatric Disorders and the Nursing Process

14

Mary Kunes-Connell

Clients With Disorders Usually First Evident in Infancy, Childhood, and Adolescence

OBJECTIVES

After reading this chapter, the reader will be able to:

1. *List common disorders evident during infancy, childhood, and adolescence*
2. *Describe the dynamics and behaviors associated with conduct disorders in children and adolescents*
3. *Identify possible nursing diagnoses and related factors associated with conduct disorders*
4. *Examine general treatment strategies and nursing interventions for children displaying behaviors associated with conduct disorders*
5. *Utilize the nursing process to identify, describe, and plan care for a child experiencing a behavioral disorder*
6. *Examine the etiologies and characteristics of the child or adolescent with mental retardation*
7. *List possible nursing diagnoses and related etiologies associated with mental retardation*
8. *Discuss treatment approaches to the child or adolescent with mental retardation.*

INTRODUCTION

Most adults acknowledge the difficulty and hardships faced by even the most healthy of children and adolescents growing up in today's society, who are confronted with situations requiring a formulation of a coherent self-identity, healthy interpersonal behavior patterns, a clear sense of values, and adaptive role behaviors in the family and societal system. Environmental situations and demands challenge these youths' physical, cognitive, social, and emotional abilities. Most accept these challenges by developing the skills and abilities necessary for good personal adjustment. Of the 66.8 million individuals younger than age 18, it is estimated that 82% will adequately adjust to the demands.[8,9,22,31] However, it must be remembered that even these children develop certain problem behaviors throughout the course of their growth and development, for example, negativism and other oppositional behaviors, fears, and nightmares.[8,9] The difference between these youths and those 18% requiring professional services is that most of these childrens' problem behaviors are episodic and do not seriously interfere with their personal, family, or social adjustment. The 18% (approximately 8 million), however, display behaviors reflecting a much poorer adjustment to life's demands[9,22,30] and are in need of professional mental health services. This figure may be on the increase by the year 2000 because today's youth seem to be experiencing serious, more complex disorders, including psychosis, autism, mental retardation, eating disorders, and conduct disorders.[9] Without professional treatment, these disorders do not necessarily remit and may serve only to increase the child's or adolescent's risk of future emotional, cognitive, or psychosocial disorders.[8]

DIFFERENTIATION BETWEEN NORMAL CHILD OR ADOLESCENT BEHAVIOR AND BEHAVIOR INDICATIVE OF EMOTIONAL DISORDERS

When discussing child and adolescent behavior, questions often arise concerning the differentiation between behaviors considered to be a part of the child's or adolescent's "normal" development and behaviors considered to be symptoms of emotional disorders. In fact, Offer and associates[24] in their research concluded that most mental health professionals are unable to distinguish "normal" from "abnormal" adolescent behaviors. This study is an example of the growing body of evidence indicating the need for a definitive set of criteria that will enable the professional to screen those children and adolescents displaying serious emotional and behavioral disorders from those displaying normal behaviors in response to the negotiation of developmental tasks.

There is little agreement on what criteria should be established; however, the literature does point to a number of characteristics that could serve to define serious emotional disorders in children and adolescents. The criteria most often discussed center on the following characteristics of the displayed behaviors.[1,8,13,19,25]

The Disordered Behaviors are Repetitive and Serve as Persistent Patterns of Coping with Societal Demands. Most children will, at some point, display negativity, rebelliousness, preoccupation with appearance and food, irritability, nightmares, sleepwalking, temper tantrums, or other behaviors that, on the surface, would appear to be dysfunctional. A closer look discloses that these behaviors are usually episodic and serve as a temporary response to an identifiable stressor (e.g., relocation, death of parent, divorce). Once the child has worked through the stressor, these behaviors abate, and more appropriate behaviors are substituted.[8,12,13] Furthermore, Schwartz and Johnson[25] point out that many acting-out behaviors (e.g., thumbsucking, nightmares) tend to diminish as the child's age increases. This, in part, may be because as the child grows and develops, his cognitive, social, and problem-solving skills become more refined, allowing the child to forego the more physical modes of expression.

The Disordered Behaviors Extend Beyond Age-Appropriateness Either for the Type or Frequency of the Displayed Behavior. Many "abnormal" behaviors are, in reality, normal behaviors for certain periods of development. It is not abnormal for a 3-year-old or a 12-year-old to be negativistic and oppositional. On the other hand, it is not necessarily appropriate for a 10-year-old to wet the bed. It is imperative that the nurse have a firm grasp on normal growth and developmental patterns to make accurate comparisons of the displayed behaviors.

The Disordered Behaviors Are of Such Intensity That They Become Detrimental to the Child's Daily, Interpersonal, or School Functioning, Significant Others, or Society in General. Most acting-out behaviors do not violate society's norms or seriously impair the child's functioning, even though the child may experience consequences of his behavior. On the other hand, behaviors that are self- or other-destructive create a situation whereby the child's or other's safety becomes a priority reason for seeking treatment.

The Disordered Behaviors often Deviate from Social or Cultural Norms. Hearing voices, vandalism, truancy, promiscuity, and similar behaviors are deviant in that they defy those norms that are considered socially or culturally acceptable. These behaviors do not always imply emotional disorders. However, many children and adolescents have limited abilities to verbalize their feelings and rely on acting-out behaviors to express their inner needs and feelings. Usually, these acting-out behaviors do not defy norms; however, when they do, the child or adolescent "stands out" and comes to the attention of the professional or legal system for evaluation.

These four criteria are not exhaustive; however, they provide an initial guideline to distinguish behaviors indicative of normal development from those reflecting more serious disorders.

DISORDERS EVIDENT IN CHILDREN AND ADOLESCENTS

A review of the literature[1,8] reveals two important characteristics for disorders experienced by children and adolescents: (1) Many disorders have an age-specific onset; that is, it would be rare to see certain disorders occurring before a specific age (e.g., pica rarely occurs before 12 months of age). (2) A number of disorders clearly cross all age groups; that is, the onset of behaviors may occur at a number of different points along the age continuum (e.g., the onset of mental retardation can occur at any age, whereas conduct disorders commonly have their age of onset in either childhood or adolescence). Table 14-1 differentiates those disorders common to children and adolescents that may have an onset at a number of different points along the age continuum, from those that have a more age-specific onset. Because a discussion of each disorder possibly affecting the child or adolescent is beyond the scope of this chapter, emphasis will be placed on two disorders that tend to have potential

long-term implications for the child or adolescent: mental retardation and conduct disorders.[8,12,13] This chapter will focus on an overall discussion of the etiologies, assessment, nursing diagnoses, and treatment approaches for the child or adolescent with a diagnosis of mental retardation or conduct disorders.

Mental Retardation

Mental retardation is neither a psychopathologic nor an emotional disorder. Rather, it is a label for intellectual–cognitive deficits impairing an individual's ability to adapt to the daily-living, social, and work demands of the environment. The essential diagnostic criteria for mental retardation include intellectual deficits, as determined by intelligence quotient (IQ) testing, and adaptive difficulties, as determined by adaptation scales, developmental testing, and clinical observations.[2,10,11] It is estimated that approximately 3% of all individuals in the United States are affected by mental retardation.[19] A number of these individuals are concurrently diagnosed with an Axis I diagnosis (e.g., schizophrenia) and an Axis II diagnosis of mental retardation. When clients enter the mental health system with co-morbidity, the nurse must bear in mind that the psychopathology cannot be treated in isolation from the retardation. The cognitive deficits affect clients' capabilities to express themselves verbally and utilize the problem-solving process to negotiate developmental demands. Mental retardation has often been given only cursory coverage in nursing education; as a result, some psychiatric nurses are frustrated with the challenge presented by mentally retarded youth. It is

TABLE 14–1
Relationship between age of onset and type of disorder evident in children and adolescents[2]

AGE GROUP	DISORDERS WITH VARIABLE ONSET	DISORDERS WITH AGE-SPECIFIC ONSET
Infancy (0–1 yr) Toddlerhood (13–36 mo) Preschool (3–5 yr) School-age (5–12 yr) Adolescence (12–18 yr)	Depression / Autistic disorder / Mental retardation / Elective autism / Avoidant disorder / Separation anxiety disorder / Substance abuse / Obsessive compulsive disorder / Conduct disorders	Rumination disorder of infancy / Reactive attachment disorder / Pica / Reactive attachment disorder / Developmental coordination disorder / Developmental expressive language disorder / Functional enuresis / Receptive language disorder / Functional encopresis / Gender identity disorder / Attention deficit disorder / Developmental articulation disorder / Gender identity disorder of childhood / Oppositional disorder / Developmental reading disorder / Expressive writing disorder / Tourette's syndrome / Anorexia nervosa / Bulimia nervosa / Gender identity disorder of adolescence / Identity disorder

essential that nurses have a basic knowledge of mental retardation, of its impact on the child and family, and of nursing strategies when working with the retarded child or adolescent.

ETIOLOGIES

If two children both have a diagnosis of mental retardation, they are unlikely to have the same degree of handicaps. The American Association of Mental Deficiency[11] and DSM-III-R[2] delineate four levels of retardation, ranging from mild to profound. Each level carries with it certain manifestations differentiating the degree of handicap for the youth. Table 14-2 identifies the four categories of retardation along with the behavioral manifestations for each level.

There is no one cause that explains all forms of retardation. Five general factors that could lead to the development of retardation include: (1) Many forms of retardation are associated with *genetic abnormalities.*[19,25] Some genetic abnormalities result in metabolic disturbances leading to neural degeneration or the in-

ability of the body to rid itself of toxins, leading to various forms of brain damage. Disorders such as Tay-Sachs disease or phenylketonuria are primary examples.[19,25] Other genetic disorders involve chromosomal abnormalities that ultimately influence intellectual growth and development. It is believed that intelligence has a genetic component to its development;[19,25] therefore, any chromosomal disruption may alter brain size, brain structure, or brain metabolism, or all three. Chromosomal disorders include Down syndrome and Klinefelter syndrome. (2) *Prenatal variables,* such as alcohol or drug use (prescription and nonprescription), malnutrition, radiation, and infection or illness, all may negatively influence intellectual development. These factors may affect overall birth weight, brain size and weight, and central nervous system (CNS) development.[19,25] (3) *Perinatal factors,* such as head injury during the birth process or anoxia, can decrease oxygen to the brain, causing focal or general brain damage.[19,25] (4) *Physical* or *physiologic trauma,* such as head injury, ingestion of poisons, and excessive drug or alcohol use, may increase the risk of brain damage throughout a

TABLE 14–2
Behavioral manifestations of mild, moderate, severe, and profound levels of mental retardation[2,17,19,25]

ACTIVITY OF DAILY LIVING SKILLS	SOCIAL/INTERPERSONAL SKILLS	EDUCATIONAL SKILLS/ PROBLEM-SOLVING SKILLS	MOTOR/ COORDINATION SKILLS
MILD RETARDATION			
Can be taught independent activities of daily living Can be taught to live independently	Can develop social skills Can develop ability to verbalize rather than act out feelings and needs	Can succeed in reading, math, and spelling skills Can succeed in vocational education Limited abilities for abstract thinking	Has gross and fine motor abilities —can often do semiskilled manual labor —can do unskilled manual labor
MODERATE RETARDATION			
Requires some assistance with activities of daily living Requires some structure in living arrangements (e.g., halfway house)	Simple work mastery Some ability to act out versus verbalization of feelings and needs	Can learn words, numbers, and signs that facilitate basic survival Poor abilities for abstract thinking	Follows simple two- to three-word instructions Poor fine motor skills, good gross motor skills Can participate in unskilled labor requiring repetitive tasks
SEVERE RETARDATION			
Possibility of teaching some ADL skills with long-term consistent behavior modification Requires great deal of assistance Requires structured living arrangements	Some expressive skills: says a few words Strong nonverbal acting out of needs/feelings	Rarely can learn to read, write, spell, or use math No ability to abstract	Poor gross and fine motor skills; uncoordinated
PROFOUND RETARDATION			
Unable to complete ADLs independently Typically requires institutional placement and full-time care	Unable to relate verbally to others	No success in academic skills No ability to abstract	No fine or gross skills

person's life.[19,25] (5) Finally, *social deprivation* has been postulated to produce a level of retardation. Schwartz and Johnson[25] summarize a number of research studies implicating the social environment (e.g., poverty, institutional environments, and isolation) in cognitive development. The interplay of the environment with other factors (i.e., nutrition, illness) in producing retardation should be considered.[19,25]

ASSESSMENT

To accurately evaluate the status of the mentally retarded, the health care professional performs a thorough and comprehensive assessment, including complete history and physical examination, psychological and educational testing, social and problem-solving assessment, an evaluation of self-care skills, and an evaluation of the family's coping responses.

History and Physical Examination.
The history and physical examination are important elements to determine or rule out possible causes of the retardation. It is important to interview family members or significant others to determine a history of retardation. Affirmative responses to this line of inquiry might suggest to the nurse the possibility of genetic abnormalities. Furthermore, it is vital to gather information on any prenatal, perinatal, or postnatal difficulties. Prenatal questions should be directed toward prenatal care received, nutritional problems, illnesses and infections during pregnancy, and use of medications or drugs during pregnancy. The nurse should inquire about any difficulties or complications during labor or the postpartum period. It is also important for the nurse to have an understanding of the child's ability to meet developmental milestones (e.g., walking, talking, feeding self). In addition to clues for the etiology, this line of questioning may provide evidence for the level of retardation being experienced by the child.

A complete physical examination should entail a neurologic examination and blood workup. Because brain damage can have a negative effect on all systems, it is necessary to determine all levels of deficits before planning care.

Psychological and Educational Testing.
It is imperative that a suspected case of mental retardation be validated through IQ testing by specialists. Because IQ is one of the diagnostic criteria for retardation, a case cannot be confirmed merely by one's clinical observations. Accurate IQ testing requires the use of standardized intelligence tests. The most popular IQ test is the Stanford–Binet Intelligence Scale.[2,17,19,25] In addition, educational testing of the school-aged (and often, the preschool-aged) child is essential. Because the mildly retarded child often reaches the fifth or sixth grade level of functioning and the moderately retarded child can, at times, accomplish skills equivalent to the third grader, standardized educational tests can help to differentiate levels of retardation.[19,25] Tests such as the

Wechsler Intelligence Scale for Children, Revised (WISC-R) are accepted methodologies for evaluating the educational potential of the child.[19,25]

Social and Problem-Solving Assessment.
Cognitive abilities directly affect the ability to socialize and express self. The effect of cognitive defects on the ability to verbalize and relate to others must be evaluated to be able to determine the level of the child's ability to engage in a therapeutic relationship and work through problem behaviors. An assessment of verbal skills is essential, since verbal skills address the child or adolescent's ability to do the following:

1. *Express basic physiologic and psychosocial needs.* When children are unable to verbalize their needs effectively, frustration begins to build. Unable to express either their needs or their frustration, they often act them out in some aggressive or otherwise unacceptable manner. There may be no satisfaction for the children because, in addition to their needs not being met, they often receive negative consequences for the acting-out behavior.[17,19]
2. *Express emotions.* Emotions are abstract concepts, the verbal expressions of which require higher levels of cognitive functioning. If these cognitive levels are impaired, the child does not have the necessary skills to process the feelings being experienced internally and to externalize it through verbal expression.
3. *Problem-solving complex situations.* Problem-solving requires skills to perform certain steps, including the ability to identify the problematic situation; identify the feelings experienced with the situation; connect behaviors with the feelings; identify what makes behaviors inappropriate; generate alternative behaviors; test behaviors; and evaluate the effectiveness of the newly tried behaviors. These are complex steps requiring the ability to abstract and connect past situations with the present. However, as Lubetsky[17] points out, retarded individuals often lack that ability to abstract the situations or generate alternatives without having previously experienced the situation. The retarded child, rather than verbalizing his feelings and solutions, acts out his responses behaviorally.

Self-Care Abilities.
Steele's[28] study of self-care skills in 46 retarded adolescents indicated that even the mildly retarded often lacked skills necessary to function at a basic wellness level. Skills such as the ability to weigh self, to take care of minor cuts or colds, and to exercise, were either not known to the adolescent or, if known, not practiced.

It is necessary for the psychiatric mental health nurse to have baseline data on the level of independence in performing self-care skills. The youth should be observed for the level of ability to meet nutritional, elimination, hygiene, and grooming needs. Furthermore, it is necessary to assess the present living arrangements for the youth (that is, family versus boarding house versus institutionalization), and to evaluate the success or failure of these arrangements.

To assist the nurse in assessment of self-care or other general adaptive abilities, a number of rating scales have been recognized as useful in supplementing the interview and clinical observation of the nurse. Scales such as the Adaptive Behavior Scale and the Vineland Social Maturity Scale are useful in comparing the child's actual behavior with the developmental norms in a number of areas, including physical development, self-care behaviors, ability to follow rules, and ability to socialize.[2,19,25]

NURSING DIAGNOSES

Nursing diagnoses for the child or adolescent with mental retardation include impaired verbal communication, aggression, impaired social interaction, altered growth and development, self-care deficit(s), and self concept disturbance; nursing diagnoses for the family system affected by the situation include dysfunctional family processes. The mentally retarded child or adolescent often enters the mental health system with a multitude of problems. When formulating a plan of care, it is necessary for the psychiatric mental health nurse to identify those diagnoses that provide the opportunity for comprehensive treatment planning. For the individual whose diagnosis is mental retardation, nursing diagnoses such as altered growth and development and self-care deficits must always be considered, as these diagnoses are usually identified. When the child or adolescent enters the mental health care system, a frequent presenting problem relates to the child's or adolescent's inability to cope effectively with his or her new environment.[14,21] This inability to cope with environmental demands relates to the child's or adolescent's inability to effectively communicate needs and feelings.

To express themselves, mentally retarded children or adolescents may cope through physical acting-out behaviors. The retarded child's or adolescent's acting-out behaviors tend to be stereotyped, repetitive, persistent, and injurious to self or others, leading to nursing diagnoses of bizarre behavior, aggression, altered impulse control, and potential for injury. These behaviors, to some extent, are an attempt to relieve the anxiety and protect the ego from the overwhelming sense of powerlessness experienced by the child.[14,19,21,23] These behaviors, by their intimidation, aid children's attempts to control their situation. In addition to their destructive tendencies, these actions become learned patterns of behavior, creating long-term problems for the family situation or school setting in terms of their ability to manage the behavior and maintain the safety of the child.

The child rarely enters the mental health system alone. The cognitive deficits and ensuing behaviors create a great deal of emotional distress for the family. Although many families adjust quite well, others manifest behaviors indicative of the nursing diagnosis dysfunctional family processes. Beavers and coworkers,[4] in their study of functional versus dysfunctional family coping, point out the strong desire of dysfunctional families to compensate for their own perceptions of failure and powerlessness by rigidly controlling the child's life. Furthermore, these parents often view the child as "retarded" and helpless, thereby creating a need to overprotect. This familial pattern of behavior, in turn, creates a sense of submissiveness and dependency in the child. Ultimately, children cannot progress in this type of family situation because they are not allowed to capitalize on strengths. The child's frustration builds, thus increasing acting-out behaviors, which, in turn, results in an increased sense of powerlessness, inadequacy, and failure. The cycle of dysfunctional parent–child interactions continues.[4,19]

INTERVENTIONS AND EVALUATION

The acting-out behaviors of the mentally retarded child tend to be negative, socially unacceptable, and aggressive. These behaviors range from self-stimulating behaviors to alleviate anxiety (repetitive rocking, rubbing, stroking) to aggressive behaviors designed to gain attention (hitting, kicking, spitting, encopresis). The goal of any program should center on decreasing socially unacceptable or destructive behaviors and increasing behaviors that enable a successful adaptation to society. Because the child or adolescent often does not possess the skills necessary to "work through" these behaviors or verbalize feelings and needs, behavior modification is the therapy of choice.[12,19,21] Behavior modification operates on two premises: that a behavior can be learned and unlearned when paired with the appropriate positive or negative reinforcement for the behavior (operant conditioning); and that appropriate behaviors can be learned through a modeling–feedback or reinforcement process (social learning).[12,26]

The first step in either approach is a thorough assessment of the child's target behaviors for intervention. As the psychiatric mental health nurse performs this assessment, a number of questions must be answered:

- Is the goal the reinforcement or the alleviation of certain behaviors or both?
- What specific behaviors need to be reinforced?
- What behaviors need to be eliminated?
- What would the child consider rewards for good behavior (e.g., food, time with peers or staff, television, music)?
- What would the child not like to have taken away from him?
- What is the child's attention span?

The answers to these questions facilitate identifying and prioritizing target behaviors. When developing a behavior modification program, it is necessary to pinpoint specific, concrete behaviors. It is also necessary to deal with only a few behaviors at any one time. Attempts to focus on several behaviors do not allow the mentally retarded child to discriminate which behaviors are truly being reinforced or extinguished. A guideline to prioritizing target behaviors would be to focus on the elimination of those that are destructive to the individual or others or the reinforcement of the most socially acceptable behaviors. For example, although a 9-year-old mildly retarded boy demonstrated a number of socially unacceptable behaviors including grunting, playing with food, inappropriate sexual talk, and inappropriately hitting/touching female clients, it was the sexual talk and touching/hitting behaviors that tended to be the most disturbing.

Second, accurate answers to the reward questions enhance compliance with the program because the child is more likely to follow through with appropriate behaviors if the rewards or punishments have meaning to him or her. For example, this same 9-year-old enjoyed television time. Therefore, the 7:00 PM television time became an earned reward when the child was able to spend the 6:30 to 7:00 PM activity time with peers without sexual talk or inappropriate touch. Because this child disliked "rest time in his room" this consequence was used as a negative reinforcement for

15 minutes when the client displayed the foregoing behaviors during the activity time.

Rewards are positive reinforcers and serve to enhance behaviors; therefore, the psychiatric mental health nurse must be careful to avoid rewarding any negative behaviors. For instance, if a nurse, believing that the client's negative behavior was a plea for attention, continued to give attention by spending time with the client during his "time-out" period, this would serve to gratify the child's need for attention, leading to continuation of the behavior. On the other hand, punishment should alleviate unwanted behaviors. It should not be corporal; rather, it should emphasize the loss of a privilege (e.g., game time), the use of seclusion, or time-out period.[12,19] When using seclusion or time-out the nurse must keep in mind the principle of least-restrictive environment for treatment. Therefore, time-out periods should be spent in the child's room or by spending a brief (five- to ten-minute) period in a chair in a nonstimulating area. Box 14-1 presents one sample protocol for interventions used when the

---

BOX 14–1
Plan of Care for Interrupting Escalating Behavior

BEHAVIOR	STAFF INTERVENTION
ANXIOUS BEHAVIOR Characterized by increased motor activity, pressured speech, increased volume of voice tone, inability to remain on task	1. Sustain a supportive approach 2. Recognize that something unusual is happening and verbally identify what you observe 3. Sustain a nonjudgmental attitude and attempt to diffuse anxiety by distracting child, but do not push child into another activity 4. Staff should remain calm and communicate concern to child; voice tone should be calm and matter-of-fact
DEFENSIVE/DISRUPTIVE BEHAVIOR Characterized by refusal to follow directives, verbally abusive behavior, escalating physical movement (e.g., running up and down halls), threatening to harm self or others, disorganized behavior	1. Verbally identify behavior in a calm matter-of-fact voice 2. If behavior persists, ask the child to take a form of "time-out" Chairtime: child is asked to sit quietly in a chair in hall or corridor or in an area away from the group, typically 3 min in length, but not more than 5 min Time-out: child is asked to stand in an area of room facing away from group up to 3 min Room-time: child is asked to go to room typically 3 min but not more than 5
OUT-OF-CONTROL BEHAVIOR WITHOUT ACTUAL PHYSICAL AGGRESSION TOWARD SELF OR OTHERS Characterized by refusal to take a time-out along with verbal threats to harm others	1. Tell child to go directly to time-out for a specified period of time, typically 5 min, but not more than 15 2. If child refuses, staff should assist child to the quiet room where the door remains open 3. Under rare circumstances where extremely disruptive disorganized behavior persists or if child becomes actively violent toward self or others, the door will be closed and the usual locked seclusion will be followed and/or therapeutic holding will be implemented
VIOLENT ACTING-OUT BEHAVIOR Active endangerment of self and others characterized by assaultive, aggressive, self-injurious behaviors, destruction of property, inciting others to act out, blatant out-of-control and riotous behavior	1. Staff will implement measures to place patient in seclusion or 2. Staff will implement therapeutic holding of client

(Used with permission from Young Adolescent and Children's Program, AMI Saint Joseph Center for Mental Health, Omaha, NE.)

child's behavior begins to escalate. This sample protocol attempts to decrease escalating behavior while keeping in mind the principle of least-restrictive environment. However, the manifestation of severely destructive behaviors might result in a period of seclusion (20 to 30 minutes). For example, as stated earlier this 9-year-old received brief 15-minute periods in his room when displaying touching or sexual talk behaviors. However, this client periodically displayed hitting, kicking, and encopretic behaviors. These behaviors, considered more destructive, required a 30-minute seclusion in a time-out room.

Operant-conditioning techniques have proved quite effective when working to alter behaviors. Even more effective, however, is the combined use of operant conditioning and social learning theory.[12,19,26] Modeling appropriate interpersonal behaviors (e.g., eye contact, table manners, facial expressions, tone of voice) for the child, followed by rehearsal and feedback, has been shown to be effective in teaching social skills and improving interpersonal relationship building.[12,26] (Refer to Chapter 23 for a detailed discussion of the use of modeling with children and adolescents.) When modeling certain behaviors, the psychiatric mental health nurse must remember to positively reinforce demonstrations of them. Positive reinforcement increases the behaviors' frequency of occurrence, eventually habituating the behaviors for the child. Certain guidelines need to be considered:

- Consistency is the essential ingredient in the success of the program. Behaviors cannot be unlearned rapidly; they require time, patience, and repetition of rewards.
- The program must be evaluated at least weekly to revise those rewards or punishments and time frames that are not producing the desired behaviors. The evaluation should determine if the target behaviors are increasing or decreasing and if the child is displaying social skills appropriate to gaining acceptance by others.

Family therapy is also a key to the successful care of the retarded child. Family therapy should take the form of psychoeducation, support, and referral. Beavers and associates[4] point out that successful coping is correlated with a knowledge of the disorder and its treatment. Education should emphasize information on (1) mental retardation, including its causes and symptomatology; (2) various treatments for retardation; (3) behavior modification and its implementation in the home setting; and (4) resources available in the community. Education of families can occur in the one-to-one or group setting.

When educating families, it is important to provide them with materials and sources to which they can refer when the child returns home. Handouts, brochures, books, or tapes on this subject serve as reminders and reinforcers for families as they work with the child on a day-to-day basis.

Supporting the family by means of crisis intervention, stress management, and parenting groups becomes important to the success of the child's care. Dauz-Williams and colleagues[6] report the success of family crisis intervention and stress management in a study of two families with retarded children. The results of programs designed to educate and provide support simultaneously to family members indicates that the families verbalized decreased anxiety about their child's behaviors and how to deal with them. Each family also demonstrated a high compliance with a successful behavior modification program.

Parenting support groups are vehicles for validation and support from others going through similar experiences. Parents often feel as if they are the only ones going through these situations. To hear others facing similar situations decreases their sense of aloneness. A supportive parent group should:

- Allow parents to ventilate their feelings in an open, trusting climate
- Avoid belittling judgments about parental feelings or behaviors
- Avoid blaming parents for the child's behavior
- Redirect parents' tendency to blame themselves
- Focus on parental strengths versus parental inadequacies.

Conduct Disorders

Many youths involved in the mental health system demonstrate some form of maladaptive behavior (e.g., runaway behavior, truancy, and sexual acting out). These behaviors can be underlying symptoms for severe psychopathologic disorders (e.g., depression, schizophrenia) or can represent a child or adolescent disorder considered to be quite prevalent in our society, that is, conduct disorders. It is believed that 4% to 10% of the child and adolescent population (2.6 to 6.6 million) has some degree of conduct disorder.[7,13,33] However, many of these individuals will remain untreated because treatment often occurs only when the child comes into contact with the law. Parental referral is not as frequent because the family system also tends to be dysfunctional.

The DSM-III-R differentiates three types of conduct disorders including group type, solitary aggressive type, and undifferentiated type.[2] Conduct disorders, according to Kazdin,[13] may be evaluated on the following dimensions:

- Inability versus ability to engage in relationship or attachment behaviors
- Clusters of aggressive or nonaggressive modes of conduct that are in opposition to social norms or legal sanctions
- Behaviors that are persistent and markedly interfere with personal and social functioning. The DSM-III-R[2] defines *persistent* as behaviors having at least a six-month duration

- Negative, disruptive behaviors occurring as a part of group behavior or as individual behavior
- Behaviors that tend to be longer-term or extend beyond the age at which the behavior is expected to dissipate.

The prevalence and long-term severity of this disorder mandates that nurses be aware of the essential characteristics and treatment strategies in an attempt to decrease the potential for long-term disability arising from the disorder.

FAMILY DYNAMICS AS CAUSATIVE FACTORS IN CONDUCT DISORDERS

Genetic predisposition has been hypothesized for conduct disorders, based on the presence of behavioral problems in relatives of children with this problem.[13,25] However, a counterargument to this hypothesis is that children raised in an environment in which others exhibit disordered behaviors see these behaviors as models for their own actions, thereby increasing the risk for development of behavioral disorders.[13,25,27,29] Much research has concentrated on the role of the family, that is, both structural and functional variables in the family as critical predictors of conduct disorders in children.[7,13,25,27,29]

Structural Variables. The absence of a parent correlates with the onset of conduct disorders, not so much because of the absence, but because of the conflict that often precedes and accompanies it. Negative, hostile, or aggressive behavior, or all, may be common in the household. The child becomes accustomed to this behavior as a way of interacting with others and resolving conflict—it becomes the child's mode of conduct.

Family Role Variables. Family systems can demonstrate pathological communications leading to the formation of conduct disorders. Several family variables correlate with this disorder. Inconsistent limit setting and disciplinary practices can create confusion for the child. It has been hypothesized that families of children with conduct disorders tend toward the extremes of limit setting, varying from rigid rules to laissez-faire parenting.

Singer[27] hypothesizes that in a behavior-disordered family one parent takes on the role of rule maker, while placing the burden for reinforcement on the other parent. There would be no issue if both parents were in agreement; however, the parent who enforces the rule often does not agree with it and fails to follow through or subtly undermines its reinforcement. The situation is even more complicated when parents initially reinforce a rule, but when confronted by the child's continued negative behavior, back down and allow the behavior. The child becomes confused about boundaries for behaviors and is unable to develop and validate a consistent set of socially acceptable behaviors. Similarly, families who are too permissive do not allow children to develop superego functioning. Without this

ability they are not given the opportunity to develop a set of internal controls over behaviors.[27,29]

Tolan,[30] Kazdin,[13] and Faulstich[7] cite specific observation of parent–child interactions that correlate with conduct disorders: (1) Conflict resolution is not a collaborative effort. Rather, it takes on a defensive, autocratic flavor, whereby one member dictates what will occur in the family. (2) Families tend to demonstrate an emotional distance and, in fact, tend to negatively reinforce any display of affection or feelings.[27,30] (3) Coercion and punishment are the modes of parental behavior when dealing with the behavior exhibited by the children. The parental focus is on the negatives of the child with little acknowledgment given to positive behaviors.[27] (4) Unintentionally, parents may serve to reinforce negative, disruptive behaviors by giving constant attention to children when they display these behaviors. If children believe that the only way to receive attention is through the manifestation of negative behaviors, then, parents positively reinforce these behaviors through their constant acknowledgment of behavior. The pathologic communication styles of families result in a pattern of childhood behavior that tends to mirror that of the family system. The child's behaviors become manipulative, negative, and aggressive.

ASSESSMENT

An understanding of the etiological factors can serve as a framework for the assessment of individual and family behavior when the psychiatric mental health nurse suspects conduct-disordered behavior. Assessments should explore, in some depth, a family history and background of the disordered pattern and its duration, frequency, and intensity, as well as the communication structure in the family system. These general assessment categories will allow a comprehensive evaluation of the child and family system behavior and determine family or environmental factors that might influence or strongly suggest conduct-disordered behavior. Chapter 23 provides a series of general questions that can be used to elicit an overview of the child's and family's perception of the displayed behaviors in a number of environments (family, school, peer environment). If nurses suspect conduct disorders, they should focus on issues related to the duration and intensity of behaviors, the consequences of behaviors, rules, and general parent–child interactions. Box 14-2 identifies potential interview questions and behavioral observations for evaluating the child and family.

NURSING DIAGNOSES AND INTERVENTIONS

Data collection with children manifesting conduct-disordered behaviors can reveal a number of common themes. Diagnoses related to behavioral issues tend to dominate the nursing diagnosis list. Because the child or adolescent enters the mental health system with multiple behavioral problems, it is essential that the nurse identify those diagnoses that will allow the formulation of a comprehensive treatment plan. It should

---

BOX 14–2
Conduct Disorders: Assessment Guidelines and Observations
for Interviewing the Child and Family[7,13,15,16,33]

ASSESSMENT GUIDELINES	OBSERVATIONS

ASSESSMENT GUIDELINES

FAMILY HISTORY

1. Are there any family members who have displayed behaviors including school problems, aggressiveness, or other acting out behaviors?
2. Have any family members been in trouble with the law? If so, describe.
3. Is there any history of chemical use/abuse in the family? If yes, describe.

CHILD/ADOLESCENT BEHAVIOR PATTERNS

1. Describe the child's present behaviors. How have the behaviors caused problems for the child/family?
2. Is the child, or has the child been, in trouble with the law? If yes, describe.
3. How long has the child displayed these behaviors?
4. Has any event recently increased the frequency or intensity of the child's behaviors?
5. Has the child ever physically hurt someone or acted out in an aggressive way? If yes, describe.
6. Are you aware (or do you suspect) your child of using/abusing drugs/alcohol?
7. What limits do you set in the home?
8. Are these limits effective? Describe.

PARENT–CHILD COMMUNICATION PATTERNS

1. Who are the members of the family?
2. Who sets the rules in the family?
3. Who does the disciplining?
4. What forms of discipline are used?
5. How effective is the discipline?
6. When there is an argument/conflict in the family, how is it settled?
7. During a day how much time would you say that you spend with your child?

OBSERVATIONS

1. Supplement interview with standardized behavior checklist such as:
   MMPI[12]
   Adolescent Antisocial
   Self Report Behavioral
   Checklist[12,13]
2. Observe response to rules and limits on unit
3. Observe interaction with peers, staff, family

Observe Parent–Child Interaction For

1. Verbal/nonverbal display of affection versus detachment
2. Degree of openness versus degree of suspicion
3. "Rules" of family communication (i.e., who speaks for family)

---

be noted that when working with a diagnosis, such as manipulation, the nurse is simultaneously intervening in other related behavioral issues. Furthermore, it is not appropriate for the nurse to intervene only with the child; family intervention is essential for positive long-term response to treatment. Among the most common nursing diagnoses associated with the child or adolescent with conduct disorders are manipulation and dysfunctional family processes, which represent the major behavioral manifestations of these children. However, these nursing diagnoses would need to be made more specific by using data from the child's and family's situations to serve as guidelines for individualized interventions.

Manipulation is defined as "a mode of interacting involving attempts to control others to meet one's own immediate desires and feelings."[21] The child or adolescent, with long-term parent–child interactional patterns that are inconsistent, ineffective, manipulative, defensive, evasive, and void of emotions, may demonstrate an inadequate superego development. The superego plays a strong role in the ability to control impulses and determine the appropriateness of behavior. In addition, such interactions cause the child to be

confused and to mistrust others' ability to follow through with their promises.[27] The combination of poor superego development and mistrust in others is manifested in behaviors that attempt to give the child a sense of control over the self and success in getting needs met, without having to rely on others who have already proved unreliable, resulting in manipulation. Manipulation can be displayed in a wide range of behaviors. Overt aggressive behaviors manipulate the environment through intimidation. Youths displaying conduct disorders might use verbal aggression (vulgarities, angry tone of voice, threats) or nonverbal aggression (assaults, fights, property destruction, vandalism, firesetting) to control another's response and avoid problem solving.[2,5,7,32,33] A more covert form of manipulation is manifested in behaviors that are antagonistic.[13] The child may be demanding or argumentative, may play parents and staff against each other, or may engage in tattling and teasing.[2,13] Other children display more passive behaviors (silent treatment, poor follow-through with rules and requests, gossip, lying, and setting up peers to get into trouble, then sitting back to observe the results).[2,13] Seductive behaviors use enticement to persuade others to meet needs. Excessive compliments and flattery are dominant manipulative behaviors. The youth may be sensitive to another's vulnerabilities and may use these vulnerabilities to his or her advantage. The youth makes the other individual believe that he or she is the only one that the child can trust and count on and that "good" people do not let you down.[5]

The management of manipulation requires a consistent, predictable milieu. Clear messages about expectations of behavior and the consequences for inappropriate behavior must be given. Staff reliability in following through with realistic expectations and limits becomes the key to successful treatment. Chapter 23 emphasizes the key ingredients to successful limit setting and discipline. When working with the conduct-disordered child, a number of methods can be used to accomplish successful behavior modification. One step in behavior modification is *behavior contracting*. The contract should reinforce prosocial behaviors, while providing a mechanism for adaptive problem solving. The contract is most successful because it provides a consistency of approach through clear, unambivalent messages about acceptable and nonacceptable behavior, a mechanism for controlling and modifying maladaptive behavior, and a sense of control for the client, for the choice of consequences is contingent on the client's choice of follow-through with the contract.[5,7,16,18,19] A successful contract has the following:

- Mutual collaboration on identification of acceptable, prosocial behavior and prioritizing of behaviors for contracting (too many behaviors become unwieldy and make it difficult to formulate a clear contract)
- Identification of expected client behaviors
- Identification of situations for which the behaviors are expected
- Identification of a reward "for follow-through" and a "pay-back" system for no follow-through[7,18,20,31]

It is important that the contract includes a mechanism by which the child or adolescent learns the steps of problem solving. This might be attendance at individual and group therapy during which the problem-solving process can be facilitated by implementing certain techniques.

1. Confrontation and feedback when observing manipulative behaviors
2. Facilitation of the client's ability to verbalize reasons for behavior
3. Facilitation of reality-testing by the client concerning potential or actual consequences of behavior
4. Exploration and rehearsal of alternative behaviors and responses[3,5,7,12,13,16,32]

Approach these steps in a supportive, nonargumentative, and nondefensive manner such that the child experiences open channels of communication.

Pathologic parent–child communication patterns perpetuate the family's continued behavior. Therefore, when there is a nursing diagnosis of dysfunctional family processes, the nurse must educate parents on methods to manage behavior (e.g., behavioral contracts, limit setting) while addressing the issue of parent–child communication. The nurse can do this by (1) pointing out inconsistencies in parent–child interactions, (2) discussing the effects of these patterns on the child's behavior, (3) offering suggestions for alternative parenting techniques, (4) educating the family on limit setting and disciplining techniques, and (5) providing role model consistency when working with the child and family.[7,27,29,30,32] Consistency and firmness of approach, coupled with support, are essential ingredients in successful implementation of contracting and family therapy.

EVALUATION

Effectiveness of interventions can be observed when the child or adolescent decreases the need to act out impulses and increases the use of effective problem-solving skills in stressful situations. The psychiatric mental health nurse observes for an increase in prosocial behaviors with family, staff, teachers, and peers.

Effectiveness of family interventions can be demonstrated in the parents' utilization of more effective, consistent limit setting. Also, the ability to use active listening and conflict resolution skills in confrontations with the child or adolescent demonstrates the effectiveness of parent training sessions.

CASE STUDY

Jim L is an 11-year-old boy admitted to a mental health facility with a diagnosis of conduct disorder. He was admitted as part of a court evaluation for stealing, his second offense this past year. Jim now lives at home with his biologic mother and 9-year-old sister. Jim's parents have been divorced for six years; Jim has frequent contact with his father. Mrs. L states that Jim has shown a number of disruptive behaviors over the past year. At home he rarely completes chores, frequently fights with his sister, and has threatened his mother. His mother states that he lies about the smallest things and that she has had several calls from school about his fighting with other children and behaving disruptively in class. Mrs. L adds that Jim has been caught stealing tapes from a local record store twice.

Mrs. L states that Jim does not always follow through with her limits. She acknowledges frustration in disciplining because she works full-time and is tired when she comes home. Discipline consists of grounding and loss of privileges. Mrs. L notes that her ex-husband is more lenient in his disciplining techniques.

Initial observations of Jim's behavior on the unit include defiance of rules, sarcasm, and poor follow-through in activities. Jim's roommate has reported that several of his personal belongings are missing.

On the basis of the initial interview and behavioral observations, the nursing staff identified manipulation of his environment as a way of coping with the anger over the family situation. A second nursing diagnosis identified was dysfunctional family processes, with particular emphasis on a dysfunctional mother–child interaction.

NURSING CARE PLAN 14-1

JIM

NURSING INTERVENTIONS	OUTCOME CRITERIA

NURSING DIAGNOSIS: Manipulation related to inability to deal with feelings of anger toward present family situation

CLIENT GOAL: Identify behaviors that are manipulative in nature

- When observing manipulative behaviors confront Jim with these behaviors
- Explore with Jim what he accomplishes when using these behaviors
- Explore the self-defeating nature of these types of behaviors in relation to family and peer relationships, as well as legal consequences
- Use 1:1 and group therapy to correlate feelings (i.e., anger) with manipulative behaviors
- Correlate manipulation with need to control his environment
- Help Jim to identify situations where he feels out of control
- Explore ways to promote a more positive sense of control at home, at school, and with peers
- Explore alternatives to acting out feelings, e.g., journal, sports

Outcome Criteria:
Verbalizes those behaviors that are self-defeating
Connects his manipulative behaviors to particular family situations or feelings
Practices more positive responses to anger

CLIENT GOAL: Display decreased manipulation when interacting with peers or authority figures, i.e. staff or parents

- Channel Jim to one staff member for all manipulative requests
- When identifying inappropriate behaviors, set the following limits:
  - Identify the behaviors and explain the reason for their inappropriateness in the situation
  - Set consequences for the behaviors related to the inappropriate behavior, i.e., fighting with peer would necessitate 15 min in room as a time-out
  - After Jim follows through with consequences, use 1:1 time to explore reasons for limit and alternatives to present behavior
- Provide positive feedback when noting appropriate behaviors with peers, staff, and family

Outcome Criteria:
Decreases manipulative behaviors on the unit

NURSING DIAGNOSIS: Dysfunctional family processes related to divorce situation, inconsistencies in limit setting, and communication between mother and Jim

FAMILY GOAL: Increase ability to resolve conflicts

- In parenting groups and individual sessions with mother:
  - Identify present ways that the mother responds to Jim when she is experiencing conflict with him
  - Explore the self-defeating responses that mother may be using in dealing with Jim
  - Educate the mother on verbal and active listening techniques:
    - Responses that further communication with Jim
    - Responses that enhance a discussion of feelings
    - Avoidance of lectures, threats, derogatory remarks
- Explore situations that evoke conflicts in the home and identify and rehearse communication techniques that foster a positive conflict resolution
  - Avoid advice-giving
  - Use I-messages to express feelings to Jim

Outcome Criteria:
Mother uses active-listening techniques when communicating with Jim
Mother practices conflict resolution techniques when experiencing actual conflicts with Jim

Continued

NURSING CARE PLAN 14–1

JIM *Continued*

NURSING INTERVENTIONS	OUTCOME CRITERIA

- Use active listening to understand Jim's position in the conflict
- Identify alternatives mutually with Jim
- Choose one alternative to the conflict situation and act on this alternative
- Mutually evaluate the effectiveness of the alternatives
- Rehearse the conflict-resolution techniques in actual situations with Jim

A combination of individual, group, and family therapy was utilized throughout Jim's hospitalization. In working with Jim, the focus of the plan of care was on decreasing the manipulative behaviors, while facilitating a more positive response to his anger with his family situation. To promote a positive family interaction, the care plan emphasized educating the mother and Jim on communication. Secondly, the staff worked intensively with the mother to improve her parenting skills, especially in the areas of limit setting and conflict resolution (see Nursing Care Plan 14-1 for a sample care plan for Jim).

Research Highlights

A child with a diagnosis of mental retardation or other developmental delays affects the entire family system. For the nurse to facilitate optimal functioning in this system, an effort must be made toward understanding how the family copes when confronted with a retarded child. Because the child's primary perception of and interaction is with the family, the family's level of adjustment and coping will play a major role in the child's ability to adjust. The purpose of a study conducted by Beavers and associates[4] was to determine characteristics of families that would correlate with positive or negative levels of adjustment. By using both clinical observations and family-rating scales, 40 families were ranked for their level of adjustment while rearing a retarded child. These families were further subdivided into four groups of ten families based on the age similarities of the retarded children. An analysis of the data revealed that the families could be ranked along a continuum of adjustment, ranging from optimal functioning to borderline dysfunctional. The authors attempted to correlate salient characteristics of the families at each level of adjustment.

Characteristics that separated families with a more healthy adjustment from those experiencing a dysfunctional level of coping included

1. *Family Structure.* Those demonstrating a healthy adjustment to the situation tended to have a spouse or partner with whom they could share care taking responsibilities. Parents demonstrating a poorer adjustment often were single parents. It would appear that the need to distribute responsibilities and have support systems is important for effective functioning.
2. *Realistic Expectations and Rules.* Families with a positive adjustment developed their expectations based on the strengths and limitations of the child. This family type was also flexible and able to alter expectations and rules when needed. The essential ingredient in a healthy family would appear to be flexibility versus rigid control of the child.
3. *Lack of Labeling.* The family's perception of the child is that of an individual with unique needs. These families do not focus on only the child's retardation but see the child as a person with unique needs. The siblings are also taught to view each other in this way.
4. *Knowledge of the Child's Disorder.* When the family has a clear understanding of the etiology, behaviors, and problems or potential problems associated with the disorder, the family is better able to plan successful home management strategies.
5. *Support Systems.* Healthy family adjustment seems predicated on the ability of the family to utilize interpersonal and community resources.

These would appear to be important factors in successful adjustment. An understanding of these characteristics may serve as a framework for assessment and intervention when working with these children and their families. It is necessary for the psychiatric mental health nurse to sort out the family's perception of the child, and the child's strengths, limitations, and needs, as well as the family's perception of the child and their ability to function as a cohesive unit. The nurse's roles are important in increasing the family's understanding of the child's disorder to dispel myths about retardation. Finally, the nurse must evaluate the family's support system to maximize the family's use of appropriate support systems.

SUMMARY

Children and adolescents in today's society are faced with numerous intrapersonal, interpersonal, and environmental stressors, and most of them successfully adjust. However, 18% of the population is not so fortunate. Instead, they experience overwhelming feelings of anxiety and powerlessness. These feelings are manifested in a number of emotional, behavioral, and thought disorders. The nurse's energy should be directed toward providing the youth with skills necessary to successfully adapt in society. The child often serves in the role of "communicator" for the family's chaos; therefore, family support and intervention are clearly indicated if the child is expected to reach a healthy level of adjustment.

References

1. Achenbach T. Assessment and taxonomy of child and adolescent psychopathology, vol. 3. Beverly Hills: Sage Publications; 1985.
2. American Psychiatric Association. Diagnostic and statistical manual of mental disorders, 3rd ed, revised. Washington, DC: American Psychiatric Association; 1987.
3. Barile L. A model for teaching management of disturbed behavior. Psychosoc Nurs Ment Health Serv. 1982;20:9–11.
4. Beavers J, Hampson RB, Hulgus YF, Beavers WR. Coping in families with a retarded child. Fam Process. 1986;25:365–377.
5. Chitty KK, Maynard CK. Managing manipulation. J Psychosoc Nurs Ment Health Serv. 1986;24:9–13.
6. Dauz-Williams P, Harrison-Elde J, Hill S. Media approach to family training in behavior management: two families. Issues Compr Pediat Nurs. 1986;9:59–77.
7. Faulstich ME, Moore JR, Roberts RW, Collier JB. A behavioral perspective on conduct disorders. Psychiatry. 1988;51:398–413.
8. Gelfand DM, Peterson L. Child development and psychopathology. Beverly Hills: Sage Publications; 1985.
9. Gould MS, Wunsch-Hitzig R, Dohrenwend B. Estimating the prevalence of psychopathology: a critical review. Am Acad Child Psychiatry. 1981;20:462–476.
10. Grossman H. Manual of terminology and classification in mental retardation. Washington, DC: American Association of Mental Deficiency; 1973.
11. Grossman H. Manual of terminology and classification in mental retardation. Washington, DC: American Association of Mental Deficiency; 1977.
12. Johnson J, Rasbury MC, Siegel LJ. Approaches to child treatment: introduction to theory, research, and practice. New York: Pergamon Press; 1986.
13. Kazdin A. Conduct disorders in childhood and adolescence, vol. 9. Newbury Park: Sage Publications; 1987.
14. Kim MJ, McFarland G, McLane AM. Pocket guide to nursing diagnosis, 3rd ed. St Louis: CV Mosby; 1989.
15. Kulik J, Stein KB, Surbin TR. Dimensions and patterns of adolescent behavior. Counsel Clin Psychol. 1986;32:375–382.
16. Kunes-Connell M. Adolescent disorders. In: Norris J, Kunes-Connell M, Stockard S, Ehrhart P, Newton G, eds. Mental health nursing: a continuum of care. New York: John Wiley & Sons; 1987.
17. Lubetsky M. The psychiatrist's role in the assessment and treatment of the retarded child. Child Psychiatry Hum Dev. 1987;16:261–271.
18. Lyon GG. Limit setting as a therapeutic tool. In: Backer B, et al., eds. Psychiatric mental health nursing: contemporary readings. Monterey, CA: Wadsworth Health Science, 181–193; 1985.
19. Matson J, Frame C. Psychopathology among mentally retarded children and adolescents. Beverly Hills: Sage Publications; 1986.
20. McEnany GW, Tescher BE. Contracting for care: one nursing approach to the hospitalized borderline patient. J Psychosoc Nurs Ment Health Serv. 1985;23:11–15.
21. McFarland G, Wasli E. Nursing diagnosis and process in psychiatric nursing. Philadelphia: JB Lippincott; 1986.
22. National Association of Private Psychiatric Hospitals. In perspective: child and adolescent psychiatric hospitalization. Washington, DC: NAPPH; 1988.
23. Norris J, Kunes-Connell M. Self-esteem disturbance. Nurs Clin North Am. 1985;20:745–762.
24. Offer D, Ostrov E, Howard K. The mental health professional's concept of the normal adolescent. Arch Gen Psychiatry. 1981;38:149–152.
25. Shwartz S, Johnson J. Psychopathology of childhood: a clinical–experimental approach, 2nd ed. New York: Pergamon Press; 1985.
26. Ross SD, Edleson JL. Working with children and adolescents in groups. San Francisco: Jossey–Bass; 1987.
27. Singer M. Delinquency and family disciplinary configuration: an elaboration of the superego lacunae concept. Arch Gen Psychiatry. 1984;21:795–798.
28. Steele S. Assessment of functional wellness behavior in adolescents who are mentally retarded. Issues Compr Pediatr Nurs. 1986;9:331–340.
29. Stierlin HW. A family perspective on adolescent runaways. Arch Gen Psychiatry. 1973;29:56–62.
30. Tolan P, Cromwell R, Brasswell M. Family therapy with delinquents: a critical review of the literature. Fam Process. 1986;25:619–650.
31. US Office of Technology Assessment. Children's mental health: problems and services. Durham, NC: Duke University Press; 1986.
32. Webster-Stratton C. Intervention approaches to conduct disorders in young children. Nurse Pract. 1982;234:23–34.
33. Webster-Stratton C. Recognizing and assessing conduct disorders in children. Maternal Child Nurs. 1983;8:330–335.

15

Joan Norris

Clients With Organic Mental Syndromes and Disorders

OBJECTIVES

After reading this chapter, the reader will be able to:
1. Differentiate delirium and dementia
2. Describe various intoxication and withdrawal syndromes related to psychoactive substance dependence and abuse
3. Identify etiologic and influencing factors in organic mental disorders
4. Discuss the significance of the problem of organic mental disorders
5. Identify the components of a comprehensive assessment for making a nursing diagnosis and formulating a plan of care for clients with delirium, dementia, psychoactive substance intoxication, and withdrawal
6. Identify common nursing diagnoses, related client goals, and expected outcomes for clients with organic mental disorders
7. Implement appropriate nursing roles and functions in the supportive care of clients with organic mental disorders
8. Formulate a plan for family education and support
9. Apply knowledge of nursing in organic mental disorders to a case situation involving alcohol withdrawal delirium
10. Describe research findings applicable to the caregivers of clients with organic mental disorders.

DEFINITIONS AND DESCRIPTIONS

Organic mental syndromes and disorders can best be described as psychological or behavioral conditions that have an organic basis and result in either temporary or permanent brain dysfunction. These disorders may result from trauma, infection, or circulatory disturbances of the brain itself or from a systemic toxin, biochemical deficiency, or psychoactive substance abuse. The DSM-III-R differentiates syndromes and disorders on the basis of whether a specific etiology can be known or presumed. Thus, delirium is referred to as a general syndrome but alcohol withdrawal delirium or delirium tremens is referred to as a specific disorder caused by cessation of drinking by an alcohol-dependent person.[1] Organic mental syndromes include delirium, dementia, amnestic syndrome, intoxication, withdrawal, and other organic syndromes characterized by delusions, hallucinations, anxiety, or mood or personality changes. Organic mental disorders are listed under three classifications: dementias arising in the senium and presenium (primary dementia of the Alzheimer's type and multi-infarct dementia), psychoactive substance-induced disorders (see Box 15-1) and organic mental disorders related to physical conditions

(Axis III). These Axis III disorders include all of the organic mental syndromes listed but are referred to as disorders because of the associated physical conditions or other etiologies. These would be specified, for example, as dementia associated with aquired immune deficiency syndrome. The primary focus of this chapter will be on the general syndromes of delirium and dementia and the psychoactive substance-induced disorders. Clients with Alzheimer's disease are covered in Chapter 26.

Delirium

Delirium has a relatively abrupt onset in response to an injury, toxic state, or illness, which may be life threatening. Disturbances of thought and perception are manifested by confusion and disorganization with related emotional responses. The client's thinking may be unclear, interrupted, distractable, slowed, and unfocused. Speech is likely to be illogical or incoherent. Sensory input can be misperceived as illusions. Visual or auditory hallucinations are common in delirium, and other senses may be affected. Generally, clients are very frightened by hallucinations and may respond impulsively in their attempts to flee from or ward off the threat. Delusional thinking may occur. For instance, the delirious person may interpret the presence of restraints as being tied up by kidnappers and held for ransom. The level of consciousness is variable, and the client may fluctuate from stuporous to relatively alert or agitated throughout the day. Various abnormal movements such as tremors or picking at the sheets may occur.[1,9]

Dementia

In dementia, cognitive deficits are the primary symptoms, and the client generally remains alert while experiencing declining memory, orientation, judgment, and ability to think abstractly. This decline results in concreteness: inability to interpret proverbs and to identify and discriminate the distinct meanings of words. Later, the ability to find and use words accurately may be impaired. Behavior changes are a result of poor judgment and impulse control, leading to inappropriate language, dress, and actions. If cognitive deficits are mild, the person may develop elaborate strategies to conceal or overcome the problems and will experience anxiety and depression based on awareness of the losses. Primary degenerative dementia (Alzheimer's disease is the most common type) is characterized by gradually declining cognitive functioning, whereas a dementia caused by an abrupt trauma to the brain will be directly associated with the onset of the causative factor.

Delirium and dementia can occur at any age but are more commonly seen in the elderly. They may occur together, so a medical diagnosis of dementia will not be made until after any delirium has cleared. For further

TABLE 15–1
Similarities and Differences between Delirium and Dementia Based on DSM-III-R Description

DELIRIUM	DEMENTIA
ONSET	
Abrupt (hours to days)	Abrupt only if cause is trauma, toxin, or other direct injury or deficit. Gradual onset is characteristic of primary degenerative dementias (months to years of deterioration)
DURATION	
Brief (usually 1 week–1 month)	Long-term
SIGNS AND SYMPTOMS	
Lowered level of consciousness	May be fully alert
Impaired memory	Impaired memory
Disorientation	Personality changes
Intensity fluctuates throughout the day	Impaired social or work function based on intellectual decline
Disturbance in two or more of the following:	Disturbance in one or more of the following:
Perception	Ability to abstract
Speech	Judgment
Sleep–wakefulness	Motor skills
Psychomotor activity	Identification of objects
ETIOLOGY	
Evidence of specific organic influencing factors such as toxicity or anoxia	Evidence or presumption of organic influencing factors most commonly involving the central nervous system

information clarifying similarities and differences in symptoms of delirium and dementia, see Table 15-1.

Psychoactive Substance-Induced Intoxication and Withdrawal

Psychoactive substance-induced organic mental disorders are divided into intoxication—pertaining to excessive intake of alcohol or drugs—and withdrawal— occurring in response to reduction or interruption of alcohol or drug intake in a person dependent on the substance. Each diagnosis includes the name of the specific substance involved if known. There are additional disorders, complications of chronic alcohol abuse, that are based on vitamin B_1 (thiamine) deficiencies. Wernicke's encephalopathy is a state of delirium induced by this vitamin deficit, whereas Korsakoff's disease (alcohol amnestic disorder) is the dementia resulting when the vitamin deficiency is not treated adequately in time to prevent permanent damage (Box 15-1).

BOX 15–1
Predominant Symptoms of Psychoactive Substance-Induced Organic Mental Disorders[1,5,11]

ALCOHOL
Intoxication. Slurred speech, poor coordination, talkativeness, poor attention span, and mood changes
Withdrawal (2 days to 1 week or more after reducing/stopping intake in a dependent person). Gross tremor; nausea and vomiting; elevated temperature, pulse rate, and blood pressure; anxiety; and diaphoresis
  Delirium (delirium tremens) includes withdrawal with agitation, hallucinations, and possibly delusions
  Hallucinosis refers to auditory hallucinations without delirium in withdrawal
Delirium (thiamine deficiency/Wernicke's encephalopathy). Symptoms of delirium and memory loss
Dementia (amnestic disorder/Korsakoff's disease). Symptoms of dementia with severe memory loss

BARBITURATE, SEDATIVE-HYPNOTIC, OR ANTI-ANXIETY AGENT
Intoxication. CNS depression (similar to alcohol induced), irritability, poor memory, lowered inhibitions, diaphoresis
Withdrawal (2 to 14 days, depending on specific substance dependence). Gross tremors, orthostatic hypotension, elevation of pulse, anxiety, depression, irritability, diaphoresis
  Delirium. Similar to alcohol induced (delirium tremens)

OPIATE
Intoxication. Pinpoint pupils, euphoria, lethargy, slurred speech, poor memory and attention span, decreased motor activity and coordination
Withdrawal (6 to 8 hours after last dose or after a narcotic antagonist is administered to a narcotic-dependent person). Dilated pupils; increased temperature, blood pressure, and pulse rate; yawning; watery eyes; nasal discharge; diaphoresis; cramping and diarrhea; and insomnia

AMPHETAMINE OR COCAINE
Intoxication. Agitation, elation, talkativeness, hyperalertness, grandiosity, dilated pupils, increased blood pressure and pulse rate, diaphoresis, chills, nausea and vomiting
Withdrawal. Fatigue, depression, difficulty sleeping or increased dreaming
Organic delusional syndrome. Hostility, aggression, anxiety, suspicion, delusions of persecution

PHENCYCLIDINE (PCP)
Intoxication. Nystagmus, elevated blood pressure and pulse, obliviousness to pain, ataxia, slurred speech, anxiety, agitation and mood swings, slowed time perception, synesthesia (experience of a sensory stimuli in another mode; i.e., SEEING a symphony); may become belligerent, impulsive, and assaultive
Delirium. Symptoms of delirium

HALLUCINOGEN (E.G., LSD, MDP, MESCALINE)
Intoxication. Hallucinations, dilated pupils, elevated pulse and blood pressure, diaphoresis
Hallucinosis. Alertness with perceptual changes, feelings of depersonalization and unreality, hallucinations, and synesthesia
Organic delusional syndrome. Delusions are prominent in an alert person beyond 24 hours after hallucinogen ingestion
Mood disorder. Feelings of anxiety, guilt, depression, restlessness, talkativeness and insomnia; may fear "going crazy"

CANNABIS
Intoxication. Rapid pulse, intensified sensory perceptions, apathy, slowed sense of time, dry mouth, and increased appetite. May develop anxiety and suspiciousness

TOBACCO
Withdrawal. Craving, irritability, anxiety, difficulty in attention, headache, restlessness

CAFFEINE
Intoxication (intake of 250 mg or more). Tension, restlessness, flushing, diuresis, twitches, gastrointestinal distress, irregular pulse, and sleep disturbances

SIGNIFICANCE

Clients with organic mental disorders are likely to be a continuing focus of nursing practice. The numbers of older persons are increasing, and the proportion of elders (over 65 years of age) in the US population has increased considerably. This age group is more vulnerable to both delirium and dementia. The number of persons with alcoholism in the US is projected to be 10 million.[2] The estimated prevalence of alcoholism in general hospital clients ranges from 5% to 75%, depending on the type of hospital. Many of these clients are alcohol dependent and will experience withdrawal symptoms.[11] Overall, it is estimated that about 3 million Americans have organic mental disorders, and many others are significantly influenced by the problem in their roles as caregivers and family members. Nurses in general hospitals, psychiatric settings, and the community will all be confronted with the problems of these clients and their families.

ASSESSMENT

Assessment of clients with organic mental disorders requires a comprehensive focus including physical, safety, psychosocial, and supportive factors. Once the causative condition is stabilized, it becomes essential to assess the overall functional status and self-care capacity of the client.

Physical and Diagnostic Factors

Physical factors frequently are associated with organic mental disorders. These associations may be directly causal, may occur as complications, or may be secondary outcomes of impaired self-care capacity. Physical problems that may result in organic mental disorders include brain trauma or tumors, degenerative neurologic disorders, infections of the brain or central nervous system, cerebral anoxia resulting from cardiopulmonary or circulatory problems, nutritional or endocrine deficiencies, toxic metabolic states, and substance abuse.[1,8,9] Family members can be helpful in identifying the onset and duration of physical complaints or problems such as vertigo, headache, motor coordination difficulties, exposure to toxins in the home or work place, prior medical conditions, and patterns of alcohol and drug use. Diagnostic tests ordered by the physician may include a lumbar puncture and cerebrospinal fluid examination to measure intracranial pressure and check for the presence of abnormal substances (i.e., blood, protein, bacteria). A computed tomography (CT) scan may be used to examine brain structures and to seek signs of hemorrhage or tumor. An electroencephalogram (EEG) may be done, recording the electrical activity of the brain while the client is awake and asleep.

Physical needs and safety of the confused client are significant aspects of assessment. The nurse needs to determine the extent of the confusion and to provide for adequate observation and supervision to prevent injury to the client and wandering. Adequacy of self-feeding, intake, and output must be monitored continually and vital signs recorded regularly.

Mental Status and Psychosocial Functioning

Levels of consciousness are basic indicators of brain function. These levels may be broadly categorized as: (1) alert, awake, and responsive; (2) lethargic: drowsiness that may alternate with agitation and irritability; (3) stuporous: unresponsive to any but very strong stimuli; or (4) comatose: unresponsive to all stimuli. Orientation is assessed by checking the client's awareness of own name (person), current surroundings (place), and the day, month, and year (time). The Glasgow Coma Scale provides a more quantifiable rating system for level of consciousness using eye opening and motor and verbal responses.[12]

Mental status components are key areas for assessment and include appearance, behavior, speech, affect, and, most importantly in dementia, cognitive function and memory. From these data, an estimate of cognitive functioning can be made, or the client may be referred to a psychologist for further testing. There also are several brief tests of mental status that can be used to monitor functioning, such as the Mental Status Questionnaire (MSQ)[6] and the Mini Mental State (MMS).[3]

Behavioral and social skills should be noted, because lowered inhibitions, poor memory, and decreasing awareness of social customs may result in inappropriate language, gestures, or actions in eating, toileting, and social behaviors. Antecedent cues to inappropriate behavior should be noted, as it may be possible to anticipate and avoid some problems or to provide guidance or redirection in specific situations. It is useful to determine the person's level of distractability and those stimuli that consistently gain attention. These activities can then be used to distract the person from inappropriate behaviors. It is equally important to determine those activities the person can perform independently and the specific kinds of assistance that will be needed from others once the person's behavior is stabilized.

Family and Social Support

Prior to discharge planning, it is helpful to identify the various components of the client's social support network. This will vary widely and have a significant impact on the options for care in the community. The essential information to be obtained is: (1) what kinds of assistance are available? and (2) to what extent can these compensate for the client's self-care deficits? Some persons with severe deficits can be managed successfully in their own homes with supportive family and environmental management, whereas others, with fewer disabilities, may require institutionalization because family members are not available for assistance or because of factors such as hostile behavior, wandering, or ingestion of hazardous objects.

TREATMENT MODES AND NURSING ROLES

Treatment of organic mental disorders often is largely supportive rather than curative, particularly when etiologic factors are unknown or irreversible. In delirium, the client is in acute distress, requiring intense supervision and physiological support measures. Identification and treatment of the causative factor may be a significant aspect in the client's eventual outcome. The quality of nursing care may determine whether the client's physical and safety needs are maintained until the delirium subsides. This is also true of emergency treatment for intoxication, which may involve overdose, untoward reactions, or bizarre behavioral responses. Withdrawal reactions from alcohol, sedatives, and hypnotics can induce a state of delirium. Psychoactive substance-induced problems will require follow-up treatment of the underlying substance abuse disorder after detoxification.

In dementia, the supportive care is oriented toward maintaining physical and functional status on a long-term basis. Discharge planning and placement is vital to this approach, because most dementias are not "cured," but client health status can be maintained and, in many cases, improved.

Physical Support

Monitoring and support of physiological and safety needs takes priority in the client with an altered level of consciousness. Nutrient and fluid needs may be met through direct assistance or supplemental intravenous or nasogastric feedings. Elimination is monitored for adequacy of renal output and to avoid constipation. Intake and output records are carefully maintained. Circulation and joint mobility can be maintained through skin care, back massage, passive range of motion, and frequent turning and repositioning. While providing physical care, it is important to communicate with confused, stuporous, or comatose clients by giving brief, clear explanations of the nurse's actions. Orienting cues should be provided at all possible opportunities. For instance, "Good morning, Mr. Smith. It's Monday morning and time for your breakfast now. I'm looking out the window, and it's a snowy December day. . . ." A warm, reassuring manner is helpful in explaining environmental stimuli to delirious clients. For example, "You are in the hospital. I'm a nurse. I'll stay here with you." It may be necessary to interpret reality if distressing illusions or hallucinations are present. If information is repeated often enough and

calmly enough, many clients will become less fearful and agitated.

Pharmacologic Aspects

A wide variety of pharmacotherapeutic agents may be employed in organic mental disorders, depending on the type of disorder and the causative agent. It is essential for the nurse to observe carefully for both therapeutic effects and side effects. With elderly patients and those with other physiological complications, it is particularly important to achieve effective therapeutic drug levels with the smallest possible dosage and minimal side effects. Nursing observations can be particularly helpful in determining this therapeutic balance. Box 15-2 describes pharmacotherapeutic approaches commonly used in organic mental disorders.

Health Maintenance

Health maintenance or functional needs include those of basic self-care, community living, and cognitive skills. Basic self-care needs refers to the person's ability to toilet, feed, bathe, dress, groom, and ambulate independently. Community living requires more advanced skills, such as the ability to prepare meals, obtain groceries and assistance in emergencies (i.e., use the telephone), and maintain a clean, safe environment. Cognitive skills include orientation and the ability to make good judgments, to manage one's money, and to recall and follow directions (i.e., in taking prescribed medications).[10]

The person with adequate self-care and community living capabilities generally can live independently with some assistance. Cognitive deficits such as poor judgment in making contracts or inability to manage financial affairs often can be dealt with through court appointment of a conservator or by a member of the family obtaining power of attorney to manage these affairs. Inability to follow a medical regimen correctly or to take prescription drugs accurately requires family supervision or home nursing visits. Individuals who lack community living skills will require significant supervision and assistance from family or other caregivers and will need to live in supervised group or family settings. The client who lacks basic self-care skills will require consistent physical care and supervision by family caregivers or placement in a long-term care setting. If family members are planning to provide complete care at home, it is important to assess their knowledge of the client's condition and care needs, their skills in providing the needed care and procedures, and their awareness of community resources available in the form of respite care, support groups, and other agencies that provide related types of assistive services. Social workers may be helpful to families in finding community resources or agency placements. Nurses must assume responsibility for assessing and

---

BOX 15–2
Pharmacotherapeutic Approaches
in Organic Mental Disorders[5,15]

SUBSTANCE-INDUCED DISORDERS

ALCOHOL AND/OR SEDATIVE-HYPNOTICS
Intoxication. Withold CNS depressants because of cross-potentiation
Withdrawal. Phenytoin may be used for grand mal seizures; benzodiazepines or haloperidol decrease the severity of withdrawal symptoms

HEROIN OR OTHER OPIATES
Overdose. Use of a narcotic antagonist such as naloxone
Withdrawal. May be accomplished gradually by slowly reducing the customary dosage of the opiate itself (i.e., morphine or a synthetic such as meperidine [Demerol]) or by substituting oral methadone in orange juice so dosage decrements are not obvious
Methadone maintenance. Substitution of a longer-acting narcotic to achieve a controlled, legally sanctioned addiction, permitting resumption of work and social roles (often when other attempts to detoxify and abstain have failed)

PHENCYCLIDINE (PCP)
Toxicity. Haloperidol or diazepam may be used to reduce delusional and agitated behavior

HALLUCINOGEN
Intoxication. Chlorpromazine or diazepam are commonly used to treat "bad trips" or "flashbacks"

DELIRIUM
Specific treatment. Addressed to specific causes or influencing factors, such as intravenous fluids and electrolytes to correct imbalance, chelating agents for heavy-metal toxicity, physostigmine for anticholinergic toxicity
Supportive therapy. Antiepileptic agent such as phenytoin, phenobarbital, or benzodiazepines for control of seizures; benzodiazepine, haloperidol, or chlorpromazine for control of agitation, hallucinations, and anxiety

DEMENTIA
Specific treatment. Pentoxifylline, nimodipine, lecithin, and physostigmine have been tried to improve memory; deanol has been given to increase cholinergic activity and reduce anxiety; vasodilators such as papaverine/ergoloid may be used to improve circulation and cognition
Supportive therapy. Tricyclic antidepressants may be used to treat or to rule out depression as a diagnosis; oxazepam or haloperidol may be used to reduce anxiety and agitation

---

meeting the education and training needs of family caregivers.

Environmental Management

The environment for the organically mentally impaired person should be safe, well lighted, and clearly structured and should minimize confusing or ambiguous stimuli. This is true for the delirious client in a detoxification unit or acute hospital and also for the confused client in the home or long-term care setting. Hazards such as clutter, throw rugs, uneven floors, and rickety stairs must be removed or repaired to prevent falls. Lighting should be bright enough to eliminate shadows and distortions, which can be frightening to the confused person, as well as a source of falls. Structure to promote orientation can be provided in a number of ways such as use of large visual cues (calendars, clocks, names on rooms and common areas), a consistent routine, a clearly posted schedule of the day's activities, and frequent communication throughout the day as to the time and the place of any upcoming events. Assigning clients who know the environment well to assist in orientation to the new setting (a buddy system) may be helpful until newer arrivals learn the routines and physical layout. Extraneous noises and stimuli should be minimized to prevent overload and misinterpretation. Clients who become upset or overstimulated should be moved to a less-stimulating environment and assisted in performing a simple task such as making their beds, dusting or sweeping, or going for a walk until they regain a sense of comfort and control.

Clients with dementia need a familiar routine and surroundings. If they are taken to group gatherings or if family members get together, it is important for someone familiar to remain near to provide orienting cues, introductions, and tactful cues as to expected behaviors. Otherwise, the person's deficits in memory and judgment may be distressing and embarrassing to the client and to others. A balance of activity is an important component of environmental care. Even the most regressed clients may profit from an activities group that focuses on self-care and grooming activities.* Previously unresponsive clients may respond to individual or group activities that emphasize bodily care such as brushing and setting hair, applying cosmetics for women, or shaving and grooming for men. Massage and other activities involving touch can be a means of communicating caring when words are no longer clearly understood (Fig. 15-1). For other clients, activities such as baking, crafts, or trips "down memory lane" featuring pictures of old movie stars and the music of "times gone by" will stimulate interest and discussion. Activities and participants should be carefully selected so that clients are placed appropriately according to cognitive skill level. It also is important that activities not be presented as tests of memory but instead as an overview of a particular time that lets the music or ideas jog memories of those who wish to share them.

Family Education and Support

During the diagnostic phase of organic mental disorders, family members will be very anxious and concerned. They are easily confused and frightened by the vague and threatening possibilities being explored during diagnostic testing and evaluation. At this time,

---

* Tappen R, personal communication, March 1987.

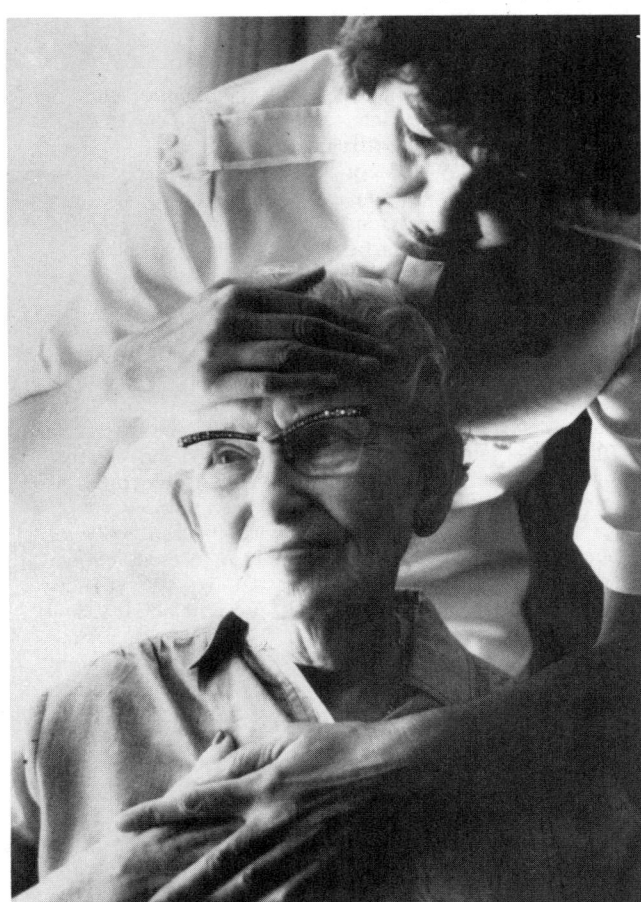

FIGURE 15–1. Consider the power of touch to communicate when words fail. ("Healing Hands" by Nancy Anne Dawe; part of the Modern Maturity Seasoned Eye II Photography Exhibition. Reprinted with permission from Modern Maturity 1988; 33(1):45.)

nurses need to be very aware of family needs for information, for clarification of misunderstandings, and for emotional support. Because the symptoms of confusion, delirium, or dementia are so obvious and so overwhelming, there is much frustration experienced while physicians attempt to identify and treat possible causes, sometimes successfully, but other times with guarded or negative outcomes.

For family members of clients with substance-induced organic mental disorders, it is particularly important to recommend a family program through a substance abuse treatment center. Alcoholism and drug abuse are called family diseases because the substance abuser's problem influences all the other members of the family in numerous ways. It is vital that the family gain sufficient information and strength to cope with its problems whether or not the substance abuser is willing to seek treatment. There are numerous community agencies and self-help groups that can provide additional support as needed, such as Al-Anon or a family services agency.

Family members of clients with dementia generally experience a long process of gradually developing awareness of the client's problems. Initially, the client may become forgetful, begin to get lost in strange places, and have difficulty at work or in tasks such as making change or paying bills. Withdrawal, depression, anxiety, or denial of problems may occur. Often, other people will recognize the problems before family members do. Many families describe a process of vague awareness of the problem but minimize or deny it until a serious incident occurs such as the person's becoming lost or profoundly agitated and confused by new surroundings. Even though two or more physicians have confirmed a diagnosis such as Alzheimer's disease, some family members may continue to deny the disorder by shopping for doctors with other opinions, by intensively trying to make the client better, or by withdrawing from the situation. When the family is ready to confront the serious decisions and client problems to be addressed, they will require education and support about the client's condition and likely progression, approaches to various problems that other caregivers have found to be effective, alternative sources of care from daycare to the various types of long-term care placements available, and ways to cope and care for themselves in a highly stressful situation. There are numerous helpful resources such as books focused on caregiving (i.e., The 36-Hour Day[13]), local self-help groups, and caregiver support groups.

COMMON NURSING DIAGNOSES

Major nursing diagnoses associated with organic mental disorders include altered perception/cognition (confusion, delusions, hallucinations, or memory loss). Because of the primary distortions of thought and perception and variations in specific areas of brain alteration, there are a number of other nursing diagnoses that can be identified. Anxiety is common as the client vaguely perceives the various threats to self and health. Altered nutrition and potential fluid volume deficit* may occur related to changes in appetite and cognitive dysfunction. Bowel incontinence,* constipation,* diarrhea,* or altered patterns of urinary elimination* may occur related to cognitive difficulties and diminished neurologic control. Role performance disturbance at work and in social situations can occur. Agitation and sleep pattern disturbance also are common. Those clients who retain awareness of their surroundings may experience disturbance in self-esteem. Clients can exhibit defensive coping or depression. Ineffective individual coping may be present secondary to the numerous cognitive deficits involved.[14] Other nursing diagnoses include emotional lability, altered impulse control, knowledge deficit, and impaired social interaction.

Ineffective family coping* may occur in response to the problems inherent in trying to deal with the client's extensive deficits while balancing the various individ-

---

* Other NANDA nursing diagnosis.

ual and developmental needs of all family members. Coping may be compromised (ineffective family coping: compromised)* on the basis of inadequate information, family disorganization, or exhaustion of the support capacity of primary caregivers. Coping may also be severely disabled (ineffective family coping: disabling)* because of chronically unexpressed guilt, disagreement among family members on coping styles, or highly ambivalent family relationships. Dysfunctional family processes may undermine family strengths such as those defined by Otto: meeting physical, spiritual, and emotional needs of members; demonstrating respect for others' views and autonomy; expressing and accepting feelings; meeting security needs; and maintaining flexible roles and functions.[14] The family may be in crisis, communication may be impaired, and they may be unable to meet members' needs for nurturance and security. The family may also have specific knowledge deficits about caregiving techniques or available resources. The burdens of caregiving may lead to diversional activity deficit on the part of family members. They may suffer caregiver burnout and lose their effectiveness in caring.

---

* Other NANDA nursing diagnosis.

CASE STUDY

John J, age 52, was admitted with a compound fracture of the femur and possible internal injuries after a car accident. His admission blood alcohol level was 0.21. On the second postoperative day, he slept poorly, was noticeably tremulous, complained of nausea, and began to ask staff members if there was someone hiding in the corner or if they saw a dog under the bed. Recognizing these symptoms as indicative of delirium tremens, the charge nurse contacted the physician, who ordered diazepam immediately and every 6 hours and intravenous fluids with B complex vitamins added. Mr. J became increasingly vigilant and agitated, occasionally getting up to look under the bed or peering out the door, disconnecting his intravenous needle and tubing in the process. His vital signs were: temperature 101°, pulse rate 116, respirations 24, and blood pressure 148/90. His wife was present and very frightened by his behavior. She indicated that he had been a heavy drinker for more than 20 years, but nothing like this had ever happened before. She indicated a need to be present, but her anxiety level was high and she kept saying, "I don't know what to do when he says these crazy things about seeing animals and people everywhere." The nurse called the physician for permission to use restraints for Mr. J's safety because he was disoriented and extremely confused and responded impulsively to the vivid hallucinations (see Nursing Care Plan 15-1 for a sample care plan for John J).

Research Highlights

Family caregivers of the severely and chronically ill are themselves at risk for stress-related physical and socioemotional problems. Caregivers of adults with dementia experience long-term frustration as they struggle to maintain the client's health and safety in the face of deteriorating cognitive awareness, personality, and functioning. A study of family caregivers of adults with dementia by George and Gwyther[4] sought to measure aspects of the caregiving burden and to identify characteristics of clients and caregivers associated with various levels of burden. Five hundred ten caregivers volunteered to participate. They had been contacted from the mailing list of a family support program. Eighty-nine per cent of those contacted agreed to participate. Members of the sample were predominantly women (71%) and older (mean age of 57) and tended to be more highly educated and to have higher income than the general population. Nonwhites tended to be underrepresented in this sample. Fifty-four per cent of this group were spouses, 32% were adult children, and 14% were other family members. Fifty-three per cent of the caregivers lived with the client, 34% of clients were in a nursing home, and 13% of the remaining clients lived with someone other than the caregiver responding. Survey items focused on the duration of illness, the severity of the symptoms manifested by the client, and four measures of the caregiver's well-being: physical and mental health, financial resources, and social participation. Comparisons of the caregivers' mean scores with normative data from the general population permitted the researchers to estimate the influence of caregiving on well-being. Significant findings included an association between the severity of client symptoms and both lower self-ratings of health and time spent relaxing and high self-report of stress symptoms. A highly important finding was that those caregivers reporting a perceived need for more social support had significantly lower scores ($p = <0.01$) on all indicators of well-being with the exception of number of physician visits. Caregivers who resided with the demented adult reported the highest levels of stress symptoms and of psychotropic drug use with the lowest levels of affect, life satisfaction, and social participation.[4]

The study findings strongly imply a need for assessment of caregivers' perceptions as to the adequacy of the social support they receive. Recognizing the influence of perceived lack of support on numerous aspects of caregiver well-being will alert the nurse to caregivers in distress. By enhancing social support, caregiver stress and burden may be reduced, and irritability and neglect (and in some cases, abuse) of clients may be prevented.

NURSING CARE PLAN 15–1

JOHN J

NURSING INTERVENTIONS	OUTCOME CRITERIA

NURSING DIAGNOSIS: Altered perception/cognition (confusion, hallucinations) related to alcohol withdrawal

CLIENT GOAL: Experience improved cognition and perception

- Reorient calmly and frequently
- Assist in interpreting the environment (e.g., "You are in the hospital. I'm your nurse")
- Maintain adequate lighting to reduce shadows and illusions
- Reduce excess environmental stimuli and abrupt noises

Demonstrates:
  Ability to test reality
  Accurate perception of environment
  Orientation to time, person, and place

NURSING DIAGNOSIS: Potential fluid volume deficit* and altered nutrition related to cognitive dysfunction

CLIENT GOAL: Maintain adequate fluid and nutritional intake

- Maintain accurate record of food and fluid intake and output
- Weigh John on admission and weekly
- Encourage and assist with small amounts of high-caloric liquids frequently
- Follow safety precautions in feeding to avoid choking or aspiration

Demonstrates:
  Adequate hydration
  Caloric intake of 1200+
  Maintenance of body weight
  No signs and symptoms of electrolyte imbalance

NURSING DIAGNOSIS: Agitation related to perception of environmental threats and hypervigilance

CLIENT GOAL: Experience reduced restlessness and agitation

- Use calm, reassuring manner and voice
- Remain with John to interpret the environment. Use gentle touch, soothing gestures of being cared for (i.e., backrub, holding hand, cool cloth to cover forehead and eyes)
- Limit use of restraints to minimum essential for safety

Demonstrates:
  Absence of hallucinations
  Reduction in tremors
  Orientation
  Ability to relax

NURSING DIAGNOSIS: Potential for injury related to altered thought processes

CLIENT GOAL: Experience no self injury

- Monitor vital signs every 2–4 hours until stabilized for 24 hours or more
- Observe every 15 minutes for safety
- Use restraints as necessary to prevent wandering, self-injury, or accidents
- Encourage a family member to be present when possible

No evidence of self injury

NURSING DIAGNOSIS: Dysfunctional family processes related to inadequate understanding of client condition and inability to act effectively based on needs

FAMILY GOAL: Understand John's condition and provide support

- Contact physician and encourage conferring with the wife on John's diagnosis and prognosis
- Clarify and reinforce the physician's discussion of the diagnosis

Wife will demonstrate understanding of John's condition and prognosis:
  Delirium tremens are time limited

---

* Other NANDA nursing diagnosis.

Continued

NURSING CARE PLAN 15-1

JOHN J *Continued*

NURSING INTERVENTIONS	OUTCOME CRITERIA
■ Role model and teach basic skills of reorienting, reassuring, and reality testing ■ Involve wife/family in care according to desires and capability ■ Reinforce and give feedback on participation and the value to John of a familiar, reassuring person ■ Assist and encourage wife in maintaining health and meeting own needs for food, rest, and sleep ■ Stress importance of follow-up treatment for alcoholism and available resources (AA, local treatment programs, and family counseling) ■ Discuss importance of family education and support whether John seeks treatment or not	Life-threatening but good prognosis Wife will demonstrate ability to participate in care effectively: Remain calm Offer reassurance and reality testing Assist safely with feeding and observation Understand the importance of follow-up treatment and available resources for: Alcohol treatment Family treatment

SUMMARY

The following are key concepts and principles related to the care of clients with organic mental disorders: (1) the extent and nature of the specific organic causes will determine the degree and duration of cognitive and behavioral deficits; (2) maintaining physical needs and safety of the client is a priority; (3) nursing care is significant in maintaining or improving the functional abilities of clients regardless of the extent of the organic mental damage; (4) the extensive cognitive and self-care deficits occurring in organic mental disorders make comprehensive nursing care essential in order to maintain the physical, emotional, and safety needs of the client; and (5) family members require education, support, and resource information in order to assist effectively in meeting client needs.

References

1. American Psychiatric Association: Diagnostic and statistical manual of mental disorders. Ed 3, revised. Washington, DC: American Psychiatric Association; 1987.
2. Estes NJ, Heineman ME. Alcoholism—development, consequences and interventions. Ed 2. St Louis: CV Mosby; 1982.
3. Folstein MF, Folstein S, McHugh P. Mini-Mental State: a practical method for grading the cognitive states of clients for the clinician. J Psychol Res. 1975;12:189–198.
4. George LK, Gwyther LP. Caregiver well-being: a multi-dimensional examination of family caregivers of demented adults. Gerontologist. 1986;26:253–259.
5. Hall SM. Drug abuse and addiction. In: Pagliaro AM, Pagliaro LP, eds. Pharmacologic aspects of nursing. St Louis: CV Mosby; 1986.
6. Kahn RL, Goldfarb AI, Pollack M, Peck A. Brief objective measures for the determination of mental status in the aged. Am J Psychiatry. 1960;117:326–328.
7. Kim MJ, McFarland GK, McLane AM. Pocket guide to nursing diagnosis. 3rd ed. St Louis: CV Mosby; 1989.
8. Kolata GB. Clues to the cause of senile dementia. Science. 1981;211:1032–3.
9. Kolb LC, Brodie HKH. Modern clinical psychiatry. 10th ed. Philadelphia: WB Saunders; 1982.
10. Lamy PP, ed. Organic brain syndrome. Elder Care News. 3(3), 1983.
11. Lerner D, Fallon HJ. The alcohol withdrawal syndrome. N Engl J Med. 1985;313:951–952.
12. Luckman J, Sorensen KC. Medical–surgical nursing: a psychophysiologic approach. 3rd ed. Philadelphia: WB Saunders; 1987.
13. Mace NL, Robins PV. The 36-hour day. Baltimore: Johns Hopkins University Press; 1981.
14. McFarland GK, Wasli E. Nursing diagnoses and process in psychiatric–mental health nursing. Philadelphia: JB Lippincott; 1986.
15. Pajk M. Alzheimer's disease: inpatient care. Am J Nurs. 1984;84:217–228.

16

Britt Finley

Clients With Psychoactive Substance Use Disorders

OBJECTIVES

After reading this chapter, the reader will be able to:

1. *Discuss the prevalence of psychoactive substance use disorders among client populations*
2. *Define substance abuse as a pattern from experimental use to compulsive use*
3. *Explain psychological dependence, tolerance, and physical dependence properties of depressants, stimulants, and psychotomimetics*
4. *Contrast the etiologic explanations of substance use and abuse, including the genetic influence, behavioral learning theory, family systems model, psychoanalytic theory, cultural influence, and moral explanations*
5. *List behavioral, physical, and social indicators of substance use*
6. *Discuss chemical use assessment*
7. *Describe treatment settings and modalities available for substance abuse*
8. *Explain the variety of nursing activities pertinent to substance use*
9. *List relevant nursing diagnoses that accompany psychoactive substance use disorders.*

DESCRIPTION

The use of alcohol and drugs in America has become widespread. Alcohol abuse is the third leading cause of death in North America.[54] Substance use is now of such proportions that 19 of the 226 health objectives set by the U.S. Public Health Service to be achieved by 1990 focused on alcohol and drug misuse.[49] Success in achieving these objectives has been mixed. The objective to reduce annual fatalities from alcohol-related motor vehicle accidents to fewer than 9.5:100,000 has been met, and the decline in per capita consumption of alcohol has reduced the annual cirrhosis mortality to 12:100,000 of the population. On the other hand, drugs other than alcohol were responsible for 3.3 deaths per 100,000 (against the objective of 2:100,000),[55] and although high school seniors report less use of marijuana, amphetamines, heroin, and sedatives than before, the use of cocaine, cigarettes, alcohol, and binge drinking remains of concern. Clearly, health problems related to alcohol and drug use continue to exist.

The extent of substance use can be measured through economic costs. Studies show that the total annual costs of drug abuse is close to 100 billion dollars.[41] Problem drinkers are 21% less productive than other workers. Fetal alcohol syndrome (FAS) causes serious birth defects in one to three cases per 1000 births, resulting in high treatment costs.[40] Violent crime and property crime are also heavily related to alcohol and drug abuse, and the total social costs related to such crimes are very high.[42]

The direct health care cost of alcohol and drug abuse is substantial. The economic health costs of alcohol misuse and alcoholism alone approached 120 billion dollars in 1983.[42] An index for the extent and consequences of substance abuse is the presence of medical emergencies. In 1984, the National Institute on Drug Abuse reported that the most prevalent type of drug-related emergency room visit was alcohol in combination with other drugs, and the second was heroin or morphine followed by diazepam (Valium), cocaine, and nonnarcotic analgesics.[44] Drugs can also cause medical emergencies through injury in accidents, falls and deaths. It is estimated that 50% of all motor vehicle accidents are alcohol related, and 20% have other drug involvement. Twenty-five percent of all fire injury is alcohol related, 40% of all falls, and 10% to 20% of all aviation, rail, and marine accidents.[60]

Depending on the health care agency, 25% to 50% of the general client population will have alcohol- or drug-related problems.[42] Psychiatric mental health nurses will encounter a high prevalence of substance use problems in their clients. Nurses who kept statistics on their clients in one state psychiatric hospital found that nearly 80% of all clients presented with alcohol or drug use, or a combination, as a contributing factor.[33]

Substance use patterns vary according to sex, age, and ethnic background. Women generally have less reported drug abuse and dependence than men; about 25% of all those with a diagnosis of drug abuse, who are in treatment, are women. Recently, however, there has been an increase in drinking among women aged 35 to 64 years. People who are over 65 years of age have a lower prevalence of alcohol abuse. The homeless, who include women, children, mentally ill, and the elderly, have a high rate of alcohol problems. There is a higher rate of alcohol use and abuse among Hispanic males, American Indians, and Alaskan Natives than the general public. Black men drink less than white men, but black women who drink consume more than white women who drink.[40] In summary, there is variation among those who abuse substances.

Nurses, similar to other health care workers, can themselves become chemically dependent. A National Council of State Boards of Nursing review of disciplinary actions against nurses showed that 67% of the 2255 cases were related to chemical dependency.[3] The National Nurses Society on Addictions has formulated a position paper on the impaired nurse that states that there are probably 40,000 nurses who suffer from alcoholism.[58] The American Nurses Association (ANA) has created guidelines in assisting with this problem. The publication is entitled *Addictions and Psychological Dysfunctions in Nursing: The Profession's Response to the Problem.*[1]

PSYCHOACTIVE SUBSTANCE USE BEHAVIOR

Sequence of Substance Use

The sequence of substance use appears to be fairly well defined, both by choice of drug used as well as by the pattern of its use. The progression of drug use by choice of drug appears to be (1) wine or beer; (2) cigarettes or hard liquor; (3) marijuana; and (4) illicit drugs other than marijuana, such as cocaine. The younger the person is when drug involvement begins, the higher the likelihood of moving on through the sequence to illicit drug use.[41] The pattern for a particular drug (Table 16-1) tends to begin with *experimental use* which is a short-term trial and may progress to *social–recreational use*, which is defined as drug use among friends who share a social experience. The next phase of development is *circumstantial use*, aimed at use of the drug to deal with a particular problem situation. *Intensified use*, which is a long-term daily use, may be followed by *compulsive use*, a pattern of high frequency and intensity with psychological and perhaps physical dependency.[22,36] Simultaneous multiple-drug use is the most common type—for example, alcohol and marijuana.[41] The continuum of drug use and abuse goes from nonuse to compulsive use and abuse within each drug classification.

Age of Initiation

It has been shown that there are drug-specific ages for initiation of use. Early adolescence is a time of experimentation. Generally, after the age of 25, there is no initiation of alcohol or cigarette use and no initiation of the use of illicit drugs, with the exception of cocaine. Prescribed psychoactive drugs and cocaine may be initiated after age 25. The order of persistence in drug use from the middle to late 20s is alcohol (the most persis-tent or continually used), followed by cigarette use, marijuana, and cocaine. The degree of earlier drug involvement is the most powerful predictor of persistence of use.[51] There is recent evidence however, that some elderly people develop alcohol problems only late in life. For example, individuals in this group may begin drinking at age 31, maintain alcohol use until 74, and then experience heavy alcohol use.[31]

TERMINOLOGY

The term *abuse* has been defined by the ANA as "an instance or pattern of conduct that exceeds a given norm determined by variables such as age, personality, culture, and health conditions."[2] The term *addiction* has been defined by the ANA to be "an illness characterized by compulsion, loss of control, and continued patterns of abuse despite perceived negative consequences; obsession with a dysfunctional habit."[32]

Psychological dependence (craving, habituation) is a term that means that the drug user's drug of choice provides reinforcement for continued use. For example, the psychotomimetics, such as marijuana and lysergic acid diethylamide (LSD), allow escape from reality and the production of an interior fantasy by which the hesitant, shy individual feels more confident.[32] This psychological dependence leads the addict to use the substance regardless of the negative consequences. The early peak experiences with the substance may be very positive, and the addict believes that it will always

TABLE 16–1
Patterns of substance use and application: cocaine free-base use

| USE PATTERNS | APPLICATION: COCAINE FREE-BASE SMOKING | | |
	Dose/Duration of Use	Set of User	Setting of Use
Experimental (use is short-term, nonpatterned)	Total intake less than 1 g: maximum frequency of 10 episodes of smoking with varying intensity	Satisfy curiosity; seeking drug effects (e.g., euphoria, stimulation)	Social event with close friends
Social–Recreational (use occurs in social gatherings)	Variable—dependent upon supply of drug	Engage in socialization; share pleasant experience with friends and acquaintances	"Free-base party"; host supplies drug for guests
Circumstantial–Situational (use is task-specific, self-limited)	Variable—differing* doses and duration of use; self-limited use	Increase work performance;* elevate mood to relieve depression	
Intensified (use is long-term, patterned)	At least one smoking episode per day—"runs" or "binges" of continuous smoking; average daily use: 5–6 hr; duration: 1–2 mo	Obtain relief from persistent problems or stressful situation; maintain a self-prescribed level of performance	Alone or with one other user
Compulsive (use is highly frequent with intense levels of long duration; substance-specific dependence)	Variable—sufficient to forestall abstinence-like syndrome; 3 mo–4 yr	Elicit euphoria and stimulation; avoid discomfort or depression of withdrawal	

* Dose and set of situational use not observed for free-base smokers. More typical pattern for intranasal use; free-base smokers manifested a preoccupation with drug-seeking and drug-taking behavior during smoking episodes; they did not exhibit self-limited use.
From Hoffman AL. Substance use/abuse disorder: educational issues. In: Proceedings: third annual national conference for nurse educators on alcohol and drug abuse. New York: National Council on Alcoholism; 1984:56.
Reproduced with permission of the National Council on Alcoholism Inc.

be experienced, despite the transition to shame, guilt, and despair that follow its use.[31]

Drug tolerance is an important concept in psychoactive substance use disorders. Over time, the brain and body adapt to higher levels of the substance and more of the substance is required to produce the initial effect of the drug. Other factors that impinge on tolerance are the behavioral state and the environmental context of the drug administration.[29] Cross-tolerance often develops for drugs within the same classification.[31]

Physical dependency is the result of continued use of a substance in which the termination of that substance may result in a syndrome of physiologic responses specific to that substance. Administration of the drug or a chemically related drug will stop the withdrawal symptoms. This is an important reason for continued drug use.[31]

The DSM-III-R classification for psychoactive substance use disorders places pathologic use in either psychoactive substance dependence or psychoactive substance abuse categories. The DSM-III-R category of drug dependence is used when there is a pattern of pathological abuse, impairment of function, and tolerance or withdrawal phenomena. The dependence is on a continuum from mild to severe, as well as from partial remission to full remission.[4] The drug abuse criteria are used when the individual has never met the criteria for drug dependence and has either (1) continued drug use despite knowledge of social, occupational, or physical problems caused by drug use or (2) used them recurrently in situations involving physical hazards, for example, driving a car under the influence.[4]

An illustration of the history of drug abuse patterns in chemically dependent nurses and the DSM-III-R criteria for substance abuse disorder is found in Box 16-1.

TYPES OF SUBSTANCES USED

The substances used may be psychodepressants, psychostimulants, or psychotomimetics. They may be used in combination with one another or separately (Table 16-2). Because of the possibility of polydrug use, complete histories of the substance abuser must be taken to determine withdrawal syndromes and overdose dangers. Because alcohol is most frequently used with other drugs, especially tranquilizers, the alcohol–drug interaction is important. The combined central nervous system depressant effect of alcohol and tranquilizers increases the adverse effects of delayed reaction times of perception, cognition, and information processing. Marijuana and alcohol are often used together, and research has demonstrated that ability to perform complex movements, such as those used in driving a car or piloting a plane, are more impaired as a result. Alcohol used in combination with antipsychotics results in decreased respirations, motor activity, and increased response time for avoidance and escape responses. Combined use of morphine and alcohol also acts in a synergistic fashion, and it is thought that death is more likely from repeated use of this combination because of the sensitized response to alcohol from the morphine.[37]

THEORIES OF SUBSTANCE USE

Explanations of substance use, abuse, or dependency include: genetic explanations, behavioral theory, family systems theory, psychoanalytic theory, and cultural influences.

Genetic Explanations

Research on the genetic influence on alcohol abuse and alcoholism is more developed than research on the genetic influence on drug abuse. Genetic research is demonstrating a link between alcoholism in parents and the incidence in offspring. Research designs focused on nonalcoholic foster parents raising children whose biologic parent was alcoholic. In these studies, the prevalence of alcohol use in the children was higher than when the biologic parents were not alcoholic. There are also indicators of genetic differences in the electrophysiology measured by electroencephalographic (EEG) patterns: in comparison with the control group, sons of alcoholics showed a significant excess of fast EEG activity.[40] In another study, subjects with a low risk and those with a high risk for alcoholism were given alcohol; EEG alpha activity was then recorded. High-risk subjects showed greater decrease in alpha frequency in response to alcohol, thereby supporting the idea that high-risk individuals are more physiologically sensitive to alcohol than control subjects. The evoked potential (EP) and event-related potential (ERP) techniques of measuring EEG responses also revealed that even nonalcoholic sons of alcoholic fathers have different brain electrical patterns. Experts have concluded that this demonstrates a genetically influenced susceptibility to alcoholism.[40]

There has not yet been sufficient neuropsychological testing completed to say if significant genetic differences exist between nonalcoholic young adults at risk for alcoholism and offspring of nonalcoholics. The genetic susceptibility to alcoholism has been hypothesized to be related to levels of monoamine oxidase (MAO), an enzyme that degrades monoamines, as well as acetaldehyde, the product of enzymatic metabolism of alcohol. Platelet MAO levels have been reported to be lower in alcoholics than in controls, and one study, which has yet to be replicated, showed that those with the severe form of alcoholism had significantly lower MAO levels.[40] Three studies have reviewed levels of acetaldehyde to investigate its etiologic role in alcoholism. Although it appears that acetaldehyde levels are higher in alcoholics than in controls, after alcohol consumption, there is no clear evidence that this is either the cause or the consequence of alcoholism.[40]

BOX 16–1
Diagnostic Criteria for Substance Abuse Disorder, Dependence with Illustration from a Study of Chemically Dependent Nurses

SUBSTANCE DEPENDENCE*

A. At least three of the following
   1. Tolerance: Need to markedly increase amounts of the substance to achieve intoxication or desired effect, or markedly diminished effect with continued use of the same amount
   2. Substance often taken in larger amounts or over a longer period than the person intended

   3. Persistent desire or one or more unsuccessful attempts to cut down or control substance use

   4. Much time spent in activities necessary to get the substance, taking the substance, or recovering from its effects

   5. Frequent intoxication or withdrawal symptoms when expected to fulfill major obligations at work, school, or home
   6. Important social, occupational, recreational activities given up or reduced because of substance abuse

   7. Continued substance abuse despite knowledge of having a recurrent social, psychological, or physical problem that is caused or exacerbated by the use of the substance
B. Some symptoms of the disturbance have persisted for at least one month, or have occurred repeatedly over a longer period

ILLUSTRATION†

The nurses interviewed varied in the amount of time from the initial recreational use of the drug to the drug commitment phase. The nurses went through a quick process of addiction from the stage of drug use commitment phase to the stage of compulsive use.

These nurses felt that daily life was painful either because of work, general low esteem or physical pain. The nurses who were obsessed with getting alcohol or drugs quickly owing to a crisis situation developed addiction faster than those who used them only to offset stress and "feel better." The critical agenda of taking a drug to address a life problem evolved into a pattern which was life-inhibiting. Revoking of license, overdose, suicide, or death were consequences of the alcohol or drug user.

The dialogue with the self to justify the alcohol or drug as necessary to exist was well documented. Initially the nurse would say, "I can take these pills from the doctor, but if I ever steal drugs from the unit, I'll quit." Later the nurse would say, "I need these drugs to get through the shift, but I'll never take drugs from a patient in pain." Later nurses replaced narcotics in vials with sterile saline.

The commitment of making a decision to use drugs as part of a life-style for the nurses involved finding physicians who would prescribe drugs or stealing hospital drugs to make money to support their habit. Nurses rarely used street drugs. Forging, stealing, and lying to get drugs was routine. Elaborate strategies were created to forge prescriptions and steal drugs from the workplace.

Physical dependence was a complicating variable. This was difficult to document because of the denial, "conning" behavior, and disengagement of the nurses.

Drinking at home before or after work evolved to the nurses drinking at the work place and hiding alcohol in secret areas. Nurses reported disengaging from their friends, coworkers, the nursing profession's values, and themselves. The secret behaviors are due to the need to avoid discovery. One woman said, "I withdrew more and more from my family and friends. I would not let anyone help me or get to me. In a way I became a totally different person. I was totally into myself."

The nurses began to have severe relationship disturbances, compromised work performance, and trouble with the legal system or board of nursing. Despite these consequences, the nurses surrendered themselves to the use of alcohol or drugs. Nurses said, "You drink to live. Using drugs is like survival. I would give my life to use."

---

* Adapted from American Psychiatric Association, diagnostic and statistical manual of mental disorders, 3rd ed, revised, Washington, DC: American Psychiatric Association; 1987.
† Adapted from Hutchinson S. Chemical dependent nurses: the trajectory towards self-annihilation. Nurs Res.; 1986;35:196–200.

Behavioral Theory

The behavioral model of addiction describes drug-taking behaviors as learned behaviors. Individual expectations surrounding the continued use of alcohol and other drugs, in addition to the environmental reinforcers coming from friends and the drinking situation, serve to enhance the drug pattern use. Drug abusers use drugs to cope with low self-esteem, personal stress, external locus of control, and feelings of disillusion.[28] Complex learning mechanisms involve biological, psychological, and social reinforcement for drug use by the drug user and eventual abuser.[15,16] Social learning theory is also used to explain that offspring of drug-abusing parents see specific role models of addiction in their parents and, thus, develop their own adult addiction.

TABLE 16-2
Classification of drugs according to potential drug-dependence

	DEPRESSANTS		STIMULANTS	
	Sedatives	Opiates	Amphetamines	Cocaine
Psychological dependence	++	++	++	++
Tolerance	++	++	++	0/+
Physical dependence	++	++	+	+?

Key: ++ = marked presence; + = presence; 0 = absence; ? = questionable; − = sensitization or reverse tolerance; / = evidence of either.
Reprinted with permission of The Free Press, a Division of MacMillan, Inc. from Ludwig AM. Principles of clinical psychiatry, 2nd ed. Copyright 1986 by The Free Press.

Family Systems Theory

The family systems model explains addiction as having its roots in family dysfunction, with the family adapting to the chemical dependency of its member through maladaptive responses. The difficulties in the marital relationship results in pain, and the genetically vulnerable mate begins to use chemicals to offset the frustration; this, in turn, creates new disharmony. Soon the family is in a rigid disorganization that makes problem solving impossible, and one family crisis follows another. The conceptualization of addiction as a cyclic process of the failure of the family to form an interpersonal intimate system is well recognized.[7,56] At times, when the system's equilibrium is in danger, the addict creates a situation that focuses attention on him or her, and the system, although dysfunctional, is maintained.

The structural role for children in addicted families may be that of the parental child (the caretaker), the good child, or the symptomatic child (the addict).[10] The children raised in the substance-abusing family may have loss of self-esteem, interpersonal fear, distorted perceptions, guilt, denial, suppression and repression, identity confusion, all-or-nothing thinking, substance abuse, and enmeshment with the family.[36,40,56]

The wife or husband of the substance abuser is called the "codependent" or "enabler." It is thought that adaption to the stress of the addiction process leads the chief enabler (the person assisting the addicted family member) to behave in a manipulative and powerless manner.[40]

Psychoanalytic Theory

According to psychoanalytic theory, the meaning of drug use, abuse, and dependence lies in certain mental processes. The compulsivity of drug use functions as an "artificial affect defense" to numb overwhelming feelings.[67] Drugs to self-medicate the feelings of jealousy,

panic attacks, shame, or rage are the hypnotics and narcotics. Helplessness, depression, and emptiness may be defended with stimulants (cocaine). The psychedelics are employed against meaninglessness and isolation. Alcohol temporarily helps guilt and longing to be diminished.

The trigger for drug use may be the disappointment of unrealistic expectations. The addictive person is unable to resolve a crisis because of an infantile neurosis, having oedipal and pre-oedipal roots. It is thought that the trauma in the middle or late second year of life creates narcissistic expectations and aggressions toward the self.[67] The basic feelings of inadequacy and unworthiness are denied, and the protection of control, compliance, and self-reliance is put in place. The basic unmet needs create ambivalence about everything.[31] The use of substances facilitates the denial of inadequacy and attempts to mask the feelings of grief, rage, and sense of loss. The reaction formation of grandiosity is manifested.[69] Light summarizes the psychodynamics of addiction by saying:

> Addictive behavior in general derives from a combination of oral-dependency, loss of power and control, obsessive–compulsive, passive–aggressive and sadomasochistic traits, which lead to self-destructive and immature acting-out of conscious and preconscious impulses (reference 31, p 168).

Cultural Influences

Cultural influences may play a role in substance use. Attitudes in a society, for example, toward the mood altering experience, as well as the substance itself, are important.[20] For example, some connect the Jewish ideal of self-control and rationality to their high rates of sobriety, in contrast with the higher rate of alcoholism among the Irish who value the mystical and tragic.[45,46] Drinking in some societies occurs within ceremonial and social contexts. In Latin America and South Amer-

properties

PSYCHOTOMIMETICS			
Psychedelics	Anticholinergics	Inhalants and Solvents	Unclassified
+ ++/−	+/0 +	+/0 ++	++ ?
0	0/+?	0	0

ica the community party or fiestas are the scene of most drinking. These festivals affirm group identity, and the drinking is rarely disruptive.[20]

Moral Explanations

The moral explanation of addiction holds that bad habits and values determine if a person becomes an addict. Psychiatrist Szasz in agreement with this view observes that "excessive drinking is a habit."[59] Peele[46] also supports the view that addiction is a value-driven activity and results from an accumulation of choices. He believes addicts can be characterized as having disregard for social consequences, having uninhibited aggression, and being sensation seeking. He supports the development of prosocial values inherent in the "Just Say No" campaign against drugs, which Nancy Reagan inaugurated.[56] In Singapore, a major international seaport with a multiethnic population and relative ease of access to illicit drugs and alcohol, the prevalence of substance use disorders is reported to be very low. This, according to residents, is explained by strict laws, social values, and morals. For example, penalties for the possession of specified quantities of illicit drugs include the death penalty, and persons engaging in excess alcohol consumption may be shunned by others.

NURSES' BELIEFS

Research to determine registered nurses' beliefs about the alcohol abuser has recently been completed. A national randomly selected sample of 1026 ANA members participated in a mail survey, which revealed the predominant belief that alcoholism has a psychological basis, as well as one that is genetic or physical. There was, however, little belief in moral weakness as a cause. Master's prepared nurses and diploma graduates identified alcoholism as having a psychological or

physical basis more often than nurses with doctoral degrees or baccalaureate degrees. Associate degree nurses chose medical treatment more frequently than diploma, bachelor's degree, or master's degree nurses. There were no subject differences in perception based on clinical specialty, institution, position held, or residential state. When compared with a more positive view about alcohol abuse than reported in other studies, there was a greater tendency to see alcoholism as an illness with the moral weakness view less predominant.[57]

ASSESSMENT

The target of assessment includes these determinations: (1) the presence of drug intoxication and overdose, (2) the presence of drug withdrawal, or (3) the presence of substance abuse or substance dependence.

Psychoactive Drug Intoxication and Overdose

Intoxication or an overdose is often a medical emergency, especially if stupor is present. Likewise, drug withdrawal may also constitute a medical emergency, and quick assessment is required for client safety. Drug overdose and drug intoxication signs and symptoms are drug specific and require knowledge of specific drug actions for assessment.

Psychoactive substance abuse and dependence disorders are distinguished, in the DSM-III-R classification, from psychoactive substance-induced organic mental disorders. The term psychoactive substance-induced organic mental disorders describes the effect of substances on the central nervous system. The term psychoactive substance use disorders is used to define the maladaptive behavior associated with more-or-less regular use of substances. Persons who have psychoac-

BOX 16-2
Stimulant Intoxication and Overdose: Signs, Symptoms, and Diagnostic Aids

SIGNS	SYMPTOMS	DIAGNOSTIC AIDS
MOST COMMON	**MOST COMMON**	
Tachycardia	Anorexia	Blood or urine levels of amphetamine
Hyperpyrexia	Euphoria	or cocaine
Diaphoresis	Irritability	
Dilated pupils	Manic affect	
Hypertension	Paresthesia	
Dry mouth	Restlessness	
Tremor	Insomnia	
Hyperactivity	Labile affect	
IN HIGHER DOSES	**IN HIGHER DOSES OR AFTER PROLONGED USE**	
Delirium	Auditory, visual, and sometimes tactile hallucinations	
Seizures followed by	Paranoid ideation or psychosis	
coma		
Hyperactivity	Stereotyped activity	

From Gallant DS. Alcohol and drug abuse curriculum guide for psychiatric faculty. Rockville, MD: National Institute on Alcohol Abuse and Alcoholism, DHHS Publication No. (ADM) 82-1159; 1982:59.

tive substance use disorders will frequently also have a psychoactive substance-induced organic disorder such as intoxication.[4] Physical assessment and diagnostic tools will depend on classification of the drug suspected and the possible presence of dependence/abuse/organic disorders (Boxes 16-2 through 16-6).

Psychoactive Drug Withdrawal

The essential feature of these disorders is the characteristic withdrawal symptom, which is drug-specific and occurs because of the recent cessation or reduction in the use of the drug.[4] The severity of the withdrawal depends on the amount and pattern of use as well as the individual physiologic differences of the user. The duration of time between the last drug intake and the presence of withdrawal symptoms depends on the half-life of the drug. Benzodiazepine withdrawal occurs five to seven days after medication is discontinued or reduced, and alcohol withdrawal starts within the first two days after the last drink. Opiate withdrawal usually begins 6 to 12 hours after the last use.[26]

BOX 16-3
Hallucinogen Intoxication: Signs, Symptoms, and Diagnostic Aids

SIGNS	SYMPTOMS	DIAGNOSTIC AIDS
Dilated pupils	**LOW TO MODERATE DOSES**	None is widely available
Hypertension		Some laboratories can do urine or blood levels.
Hyperreflexia	Anxiety	GC with a nitrogen detector or GC–MS
Tremor	Visual distortions	instruments are required for those drugs
Hyperpyrexia	Hallucinations	that can produce behavior changes at
Tachycardia	Changes in body image	specified blood levels
Facial flush	Labile affect	
Conjunctival injection (marijuana)	Paresthesia	
	Synthesias*	
IN HIGHER DOSES	Time–space distortions	
	Rambling speech	
Toxic psychosis	Easy suggestibility	
Seizures (rare)		
Depersonalization	**IN HIGHER DOSES**	
Paranoid ideation	Acute panic reactions (not always	
	dose related, however)	

* The patient may complain of "feeling sounds" or "hearing colors."
From Gallant DS. Alcohol and drug abuse curriculum guide for psychiatric faculty. Rockville, MD: National Institute on Alcohol Abuse and Alcoholism, DHHS Publication No. (ADM) 82-1159; 1982:61.

BOX 16–4
Phencyclidine (PCP, Angel dust) Intoxication and Overdose: Signs, Symptoms, and Diagnostic Aids

SIGNS	SYMPTOMS	DIAGNOSTIC AIDS
LOW DOSES	**LOW TO MODERATE DOSES**	Blood and urine levels of phencyclidine. Either GC apparatus with a nitrogen detector or GC–MS is required for detection of blood or urine levels in the low nanogram range. Otherwise, laboratory false-negatives can confuse the diagnosis. Test may be positive for a week after the last dose.
Dysarthria	Abnormal acuteness of sense of hearing	
Horizontal and vertical nystagmus	A floating feeling	
Gait ataxia	Aggressiveness	
Tachycardia	Euphoria	
Increased deep tendon reflexes	Analgesia	
	Body distortions	
HIGHER DOSES AND OVERDOSE	Nausea	
	Feelings of great strength	
Blank stare	Amnesia	
Facial grimaces		
Hypertension	**HIGHER DOSES**	
Muscle rigidity, spasms	Inability to speak	
Seizures	Labile affect	
"Eyes open" coma, levels of consciousness may fluctuate	Vomiting	
Drooling	Psychotic reactions, delirium, schizophreniform psychosis	
	Paranoid delusions	
	Hallucinations	

From Gallant DS. Alcohol and drug abuse curriculum guide for psychiatric faculty. Rockville, MD: National Institute on Alcohol Abuse and Alcoholism, DHHS Publication No. (ADM) 82–1159, 1982:62.

Cues for Presence of Dependence and Abuse in Clients

Because of the prevalence of alcohol and drug abuse and addiction, it is advisable to assess all clients for the existence of alcohol or drug-related problems such as physical evidence of alcohol, poor health, multiple arrests, job loss, or marital problems. Additional clues that indicate a need for a more directed chemical dependency assessment are drinking in relation to stress, history of car accidents, family history of alcoholism, intermittently elevated blood pressure, gastritis, blood alcohol levels of 9 mmol/L, serum glutamic-oxaloace-

BOX 16–5
Hypnosedative Intoxication and Overdose: Signs, Symptoms, and Diagnostic Aids

SIGNS	SYMPTOMS	DIAGNOSTIC AIDS
LOW DOSES	**LOW TO MODERATE DOSES**	Blood and urine levels of depressant drugs
Horizontal and, less frequently, vertical nystagmus	Dizziness	EEG-nonspecific depressant effect
Dysarthria	Paradoxical excitement or violence	
Ataxia	Confusion	
Depressed respiratory rate	Lethargy, drowsiness	
Hypotension	Clumsiness	
Depressed deep tendon reflexes		
Stupor	**HIGHER DOSES**	
Hypotonia	Irritability	
Dysmetria	General sluggishness	
	Inability to concentrate	
HIGHER DOSES AND OVERDOSE		
Coma		
Shock		
Respiratory arrest		
Pupils may be slightly constricted* or unchanged		

* Except for glutethimide (Doriden), which may present with dilated pupils or anisocoria.
From Gallant DS. Alcohol and drug abuse curriculum guide for psychiatric faculty. Rockville, MD: National Institute on Alcohol Abuse and Alcoholism, DHHS Publication No. (ADM) 82–1159; 1982:63.

BOX 16–6
Opiate Intoxication and Overdose:
Signs, Symptoms, and Diagnostic Aids

SIGNS	SYMPTOMS	DIAGNOSTIC AIDS
MOST COMMON	**LOW DOSES**	Naloxone (Narcan) reverses signs and symptoms of overdose and intoxication
Miosis*	Euphoria	
HIGHER DOSES	Floating feeling	
Nodding†	Sleepiness	
Hypotension	Anxiety	
Hypothermia		
Depressed respirations		
Shock		
Needle marks, tracks		
Cyanosis		
Tachycardia		
OVERDOSES		
Pulmonary edema		
Coma		
Apnea		

---

* With meperidine (Demerol) the pupils may sometimes be dilated.

† The head falls to chest and jerks back several times each minute.

From Gallant DS. Alcohol and drug abuse curriculum guide for psychiatric faculty. Rockville, MD: National Institute on Alcohol Abuse and Alcoholism, DHHS Publication No. (ADM) 82–1159; 1982:59.

---

tic transaminase (SGOT) of 0.09 μmol · 5^{-1}/L, high normal corpuscular volume, or γ-glutamyltransferase of 5.07 μmol · s^{-1}/L.[8] Other physical signs could be thick red skin on the nose created from chronic vasodilation, bruises from repeated falls, infections that are slow to heal, slurred speech, poor sleep, changes in personal grooming, and financial distress.[63] The specific medical complications of alcohol and drug abuse that should alert the health provider to do an assessment for chemical use are endocarditis caused by pneumococci, staphylococci, or gram-negative bacteria from IV drug use; multiple microinfarcts in the lungs from insoluble material in the IV drugs that adheres to the lung; hepatitis (the most common medical complication of drug abuse); cirrhosis (from chronic alcohol abuse); gonorrhea or syphilis (drug abusers have a higher incidence); bacteremia; crash injuries and fractures; and chronic constipation (result of opiate drugs).[12]

A recent study demonstrated a 70% recognition rate for alcohol abuse and alcoholism by emergency room nurses admitting patients to a medical floor of a large county-operated hospital. The nurses who provided inpatient care at the hospital, however, had only a 58% recognition rate for patients with alcoholic problems.[11]

Client Interview Regarding Substance Use

The interview of clients suspected of substance use disorders should include an alcohol and drug history of substance use, when use began, which types or combinations of substances are used, how often use occurs, and amounts used. Questions should begin with the less threatening subject; for example, ask about the amount of coffee and cigarettes before asking about wine and beer use and about legal drug use before that of illegal drugs. It is also important to ask about how significant others respond to the use, as well as about the client's own response to use.[26] Initially, the clinician should not attack the denial mechanisms. For more specifics about the nursing assessment of the substance abuser see the nursing diagnoses entitled Substance Abuse (Alcohol) and Substance Abuse (Drugs).

The most widely used detection instrument to assess alcoholism is the Michigan Alcoholism Screening Test (MAST). This 25-item questionnaire reviews lifetime consequences of alcohol use.[26] It is used to provide a clearer picture of alcohol use when the initial history of alcohol use appears problematic (Box 16-7). Other clinicians prefer to use the CAGE clinical interview to make a diagnosis of alcoholism. The acronym "CAGE" comes from the focus on cutting down, annoyance by criticism, guilty feeling, and eye-openers. The questions are: Have you ever felt you ought to *cut* down on your drinking? Have other people *annoyed* you by criticizing your drinking? Have you ever felt bad or *guilty* about your drinking? Have you ever had a drink first thing in the morning to steady your nerves or to get rid of a hangover (*eye-opener*)?[14]

Additional assessment information can be gleaned from laboratory testing of body fluids. Gold and Dalkis recommend drug testing with radioimmunoassay (RIA), enzyme assays, or computer-assisted gas chromatography–mass spectrometry (GC–MS) for differential diagnosis of almost every psychiatric patient.[19]

Psychiatric Manifestations Associated With Drug Use

Psychiatric symptoms of illicit drug use have been identified, and laboratory testing can be a significant factor in diagnosis. Marijuana use may result in panic attacks and anxiety reactions, impaired recent memory, depression, and acute toxic psychosis. High rates of major and minor depressions can be associated with chronic opiate use. The use of stimulant drugs can create a state very much like the manic episode of bipolar disorder. Cocaine abuse results in behavior similar to that of major depression. Phencyclidine (PCP) can cause an acute psychosis. Conduct-disordered behavior, hallucinations in 50% of cases, and euphoria are the immediate effect of volatile fume use. Abuse of

---

BOX 16–7
Michigan Alcohol Screening Test (MAST)

POINTS		QUESTIONS
(0)	1.	Do you enjoy a drink now and then?
(2)	2.	Do you feel you are a normal drinker?*
(2)	3.	Have you ever awakened the morning after some drinking the night before and found that you could not remember a part of the evening before?
(1)	4.	Does your spouse (or parents) ever worry or complain about your drinking?
(2)	5.	Can you stop drinking without a struggle after one or two drinks?*
(1)	6.	Do you ever feel bad about your drinking?
(2)	7.	Do friends and relatives think you are a normal drinker?*
(0)	8.	Do you ever try to limit your drinking to certain times of the day or to certain places?
(2)	9.	Are you always able to stop drinking when you want to?*
(4)†	10.	Have you ever attended a meeting of Alcoholics Anonymous (AA)?
(1)	11.	Have you gotten into fights when drinking?
(2)	12.	Has drinking ever created problems with you and your spouse?
(2)	13.	Has your spouse (or other family member) ever gone to anyone for help about your drinking?
(2)	14.	Have you ever lost friends or girl or boyfriends because of drinking?
(2)	15.	Have you ever gotten into trouble at work because of drinking?
(2)	16.	Have you ever lost a job because of drinking?
(2)	17.	Have you ever neglected your obligations, your family, or your work for 2 or more days because you were drinking?
(1)	18.	Do you ever drink before noon?
(2)	19.	Have you ever been told you have liver trouble? Cirrhosis?
(2)	20.	Have you ever had delirium tremens (DTs), severe shaking, heard voices, or seen things that were not there after heavy drinking?
(4)	21.	Have you ever gone to anyone for help about your drinking?
(4)	22.	Have you ever been in a hospital because of drinking?
(0)	23. a.	Have you ever been a patient in a psychiatric hospital or on a psychiatric ward of a general hospital?
(2)†	b.	Was drinking part of the problem that resulted in hospitalization?
(0)	24. a.	Have you ever been seen at a psychiatric or mental health clinic, or gone to any doctor, social worker, or clergyman for help with an emotional problem?
(2)†	b.	Was drinking part of the problem?
(2)	25.	Have you ever been arrested, even for a few hours, because of drunk behavior?
(2)	26.	Have you ever been arrested for drunk driving after drinking?

* Negative responses are indicative of alcoholism.
† Positive response would be diagnostic of alcoholism.

A total of 4 or more points is presumptive evidence of alcoholism, while a 5-point total would make it extremely unlikely that the individual was not alcoholic. However, a positive response to 10, 23, or 24 would be diagnostic; a positive response indicates alcoholism.

From Gallant DS. Alcohol and drug abuse curriculum guide for psychiatric faculty. Rockville, MD: National Institute on Alcohol Abuse and Alcoholism; 1982:53–54.

LSD has been associated with schizoaffective disorders, major depressions, and severe panic and anxiety reactions. Alcohol and sedative–hypnotic use may result in attacks of anger and depression.[19] Thus, it is critical to completely assess for substance use and abuse in psychiatric clients.

The addicted client may have a coexisting psychiatric illness and, therefore, those DSM-III-R diagnoses that have an associated risk for addiction require special attention. Psychiatric conditions, such as major depression, bipolar disorder, and antisocial personality disorder, have been found in conjunction with alcoholism.[28,50] Clients with anxiety disorders (agoraphobia with panic attacks, panic disorder, simple or social phobia, or generalized anxiety disorder) have also been found to abuse alcohol.[61] Mood disorders occur more commonly among abusers of central nervous system stimulants.[38] Clients with schizophrenia may also de-

velop alcoholism. Freed did an extensive review of the literature available on the drinking patterns of schizophrenics and showed that "not an insignificant proportion of schizophrenics are intemperate" and the use of alcohol may hide psychotic manifestations of chronic schizophrenia.[16]

The substance abuser may use more than one substance or may have a secondary psychiatric diagnosis. Ten percent to twenty percent of alcoholic clients may also have coexisting drug abuse.[41] A study of clients entering Phoenix House Foundation, a therapeutic community treatment for substance abusers, showed 17% had a substance diagnosis only, 9% had a psychiatric diagnosis only, and 67% had both a substance diagnosis and another psychiatric diagnosis.[27] In one study of hospitalized alcoholics, male alcoholics were more likely to have a diagnosis of antisocial personality and substance abuse disorder, whereas female alcoholics were more likely to have the diagnosis of major depression or phobia.[21]

TREATMENT MODALITIES AND NURSING ROLES
Treatment Settings

Treatment settings include community and hospital systems. The types of hospital programs are alcoholism and drug rehabilitation programs in general hospitals, free-standing inpatient hospital programs, and aversion-conditioning hospitals. Other potential treatment settings include therapeutic communities, halfway houses, vocational rehabilitation clinics, outpatient clinics, community human service agencies, the police–court system, the business and industrial system, and Alcoholics Anonymous.[44]

The inclusion of both alcohol and drug abusers in the same setting is typical. The reasons for this are the polydrug use pattern of clients, the professional view that alcoholism is a type of drug abuse, and economic pressures not to offer treatment for only one type of drug abuse. Tobacco dependence and heroin addiction are exceptions to this rule and may be exclusively treated.[10]

In 1982, all known alcoholism, drug, and combined alcoholism–drug treatment units in America, both private and public, were surveyed by the National Institute of Drug Abuse.[41] The general profile of the treatment units showed that 12% were in general hospitals, 21% were in community mental health centers, and 45% were free-standing. The facility utilization rate was 84.3% for all units, and about 78% of all patients at the survey time were receiving outpatient care. Twenty-three percent of the units were owned by local or state governments, and 65% of the units were nonprofit. The demographic characteristics of the patients showed that 78% were male. There were 70.9% white clients, 15.6% black, and 9.3% Hispanic. Clients aged 65 or over comprised 2.2% of all the groups, and 4.9% were aged 18 or below.

Approximately 15% to 20% of substance abusers have no present or past psychiatric problems. This group is identified as being low-severity clients. Sixty-five percent of substance abusers have moderate symptoms of depression/anxiety at admission, with little prior history of problems, and are labeled the mild severity client group. High severity clients make up 15% to 20% of the substance abusers and are those with serious cognitive impairment and depression/anxiety symptoms. Each grouping of clients responds to different treatment approaches. High severity clients have very minor rates of improvement. An example of treatment difficulty for this group is their need for psychotropic medication for psychopathology, whereas drug abuse treatment settings generally prohibit medication use. This population may actually increase their dysfunction in extended treatment modalities (e.g., encounter groups which may be harmful). Low severity clients do quite well in all programs and, because of cost, may choose outpatient treatment. Mild severity clients do well in outpatient programs if they are without serious employment or family problems; however, those who also have serious legal problems may require inpatient treatment.[41]

Because the treatment of addiction is a long-term process, a client or family may be seen in several treatment settings as the presenting needs change.[36] The most effective treatment programs have these seven traits: a treatment philosophy that is implemented consistently and logically, inpatient medical care resources, aggressive postdischarge follow-up, involvement of significant others of the addicted in counseling, adjunctive use of disulfiram (Antabuse) for those with alcohol problems, behaviorally oriented therapy in addition to verbal therapies, and community networking.[41] Other important characteristics that nurses should look for in treatment referral sources are those which are directed at specific client needs, help clients overcome dependence, and facilitate change.[65]

To decide which treatment setting is best suited for client needs, the nurse assesses the severity of dysfunction in the areas of medical condition, employment, alcohol and drug use, legal status, psychiatric conditions, and family relations.

Explanation of the effectiveness of different treatment designs for special populations (adolescents, geriatrics, women, dual diagnosis) has begun. Treatment of adolescent drug abuse significantly decreases this abuse when the following characteristics are present: treatment of a large adolescent population; relative large budget; therapist–counselors have at least two years experience with adolescents; use of therapy methods such as music and art therapy; confrontational group and crisis intervention; provide vocational counseling, birth control services, and recreational services; and are perceived by clients as encouraging free expression.[17] The social learning inpatient model of treatment for the geriatric alcohol abuser which entails alcohol education and training in self-management and problem-solving skills with marital therapy has been found to produce successful abstinence between two and three years after the program for 50% of the group, with an additional 12% reporting reduced alcohol intake.[9] One evaluation reviewed an inpatient women's addiction treatment program in which women had their own special three-week program consisting of relaxation therapy, individual counseling with female counselors, group therapy, and educational classes. No differences were noted in the patient outcomes from the all-women's group, in comparison with mixed women's group, men's group, or mixed men's group.[13] In one treatment center, the male alcoholics' response to three outpatient treatment interventions was addressed by random assignment to (1) medication only, (2) untreated medical monitoring, or (3) active support. After 12 months, all groups had improved social function and reduced alcohol misuse, regardless of treatment intervention.[48]

A unique outpatient treatment program for psychiatrically impaired substance abusers employed techniques from substance abuse treatment (AA or NA referral, skills training) and psychiatric treatment (individual psychotherapy, family counseling, day treatment). Patients with personality disorders and those who were abusing both alcohol and drugs dropped out of the program. Those clients with past outpatient treatment were likely to remain in the program, which supports the view that psychotherapy may be helpful, even when immediate abstinence is not in place.[30] The use of psychotherapy for opiate addicts receiving methadone maintenance has shown mixed results.[52]

The Generalist and Specialist Nursing Role

The nursing role within addiction treatment settings may be at the generalist or specialist level, and it may involve roles of clinician, educator, supervisor, consultant, and researcher. Within the treatment domain, the nurse identifies the addicted client or family member and encourages the client to seek treatment. Within the initial referral, the nurse provides data about the treatment options and their congruency with the presenting clinical picture. Advocacy for the client within the setting is also a nursing function. The nurse may participate in treatment by giving educational classes about alcohol and drugs and addiction itself, as well as providing family, group, or individual therapy, counseling, and behavior modification. The nurse may also be responsible for assisting with medical detoxification from physical consequences of substance use. During recovery, nursing interventions require collaboration with a variety of community resources.

In 1988, the American Nurses Association and National Nurses Society on Addictions published the document *Standards of Addictions Nursing Practice with Selected Diagnosis and Criteria*. This document is for generalist nurses and lists 26 nursing diagnoses common to addicted client populations. They are grouped in the biologic, cognitive, psychosocial, and spiritual responses.[3] Within each response, defining characteristics and criteria are given for the nursing diagnoses (Box 16-8).

The use of the nursing diagnoses substance abuse (drugs) and substance abuse (alcohol) is very useful at a higher level of abstraction that allows the inclusion of related factors and the integration of the biologic, cognitive, psychological, and spiritual patterns of functioning. Refer to those nursing diagnoses for more specific nursing measures.

Biological Treatment Modalities

COMATOSE CLIENT

The client with substance abuse who experiences a medical emergency may be exhibiting decreased levels of consciousness. Supportive care should begin as soon as possible and the client may be aroused and returned to consciousness. Clients who do not respond to verbal or noxious stimuli or who return to sleep when the stimuli is removed should immediately have vital signs taken again. Emergency cardiopulmonary resuscitation must be started immediately if the comatose client is apneic, with absent heart sounds, or has severe hypotension. Establishment of an intravenous line and drawing blood for evaluation of glucose, alcohol, sodium, potassium, creatinine, blood urea nitrogen, and hematocrit levels, and for a complete blood count and drug screen is the next priority. Medication with a narcotic antagonist such as naloxone (Narcan) may produce improvement in respiratory rate if there is a narcotic overdose. Thiamine may also be administered if acute alcoholic encephalopathy is suspected.[19]

Once the client is stabilized, a complete physical examination for trauma, pneumonia, and physical signs of alcoholism or addiction is begun. Because an intoxicated client often refuses medical therapy, restraint

---

BOX 16-8
Nursing Diagnoses Common to Addicted Client Populations[3]

BIOLOGIC RESPONSES	COGNITIVE RESPONSES	PSYCHOSOCIAL RESPONSES	SPIRITUAL RESPONSES
Sensory–perception alteration	Knowledge deficit	Impaired communication	Spiritual desires
Potential for injury	Alteration in thought processes	Ineffective individual coping	Powerlessness
Self-care deficit	Noncompliance	Alteration in self-concept	Hopelessness
Sexual dysfunction		Anxiety	Grief
Sleep pattern disturbance		Fear	
Alteration in nutrition: less than body requirements		Social isolation	
Alteration in comfort: pain		Dysfunctional family process	
Altered growth and development: biologic		Altered parenting	
		Altered growth and development: psychosocial	
		Potential for violence	

may be necessary. The use of a quiet room for frequent neurologic vital sign monitoring may reduce aggression. The restraint of a lethargic patient should be in prone or lateral decubitus position to avoid aspiration. X-ray films may also be obtained when fractures are suspected.[34]

Seizures caused by the drug itself can result from methaqualone (Quaalude), heroin, phenothiazines, stimulants, phencyclidine, or meperidine. Hypoxia from drug overdose may also result in seizures. The client should be protected from aspiration and from doing harm to self or others. No restraint of movement during a seizure should be attempted.

CLIENT IN WITHDRAWAL

The opiate withdrawal syndrome is controlled by providing the client with enough drug (methadone) to eliminate withdrawal without causing a "high" or mental clouding. Once stabilized, the drug is withdrawn gradually until a drug-free state exists. Because those who are heroin-dependent are often also dependent on sedatives or alcohol, assessment for those withdrawal syndromes is indicated.[19]

Withdrawal from sedative hypnotics and minor tranquilizers can be life-threatening. The individual is slowly withdrawn from the addictive agent or a long-acting barbiturate (phenobarbital) with subsequent withdrawal is substituted. In cases of multiple dependence, the safest technique appears to be withdrawal of one drug at a time. For example, if the client is addicted to methadone and barbiturates, the methadone dose will remain constant, while the barbiturate dose is gradually decreased. Once the barbiturates have safely been completely withdrawn, the methadone dose is reduced.[34]

DISULFIRAM (ANTABUSE)

Alcoholism treatment may include treatment with disulfiram (Antabuse) which interferes with the metabolism of alcohol. The resultant levels of acetaldehyde can produce syncope, hypertension, dyspnea, flushing, and nausea and, in rare instances, heart failure and death has also occurred. Therefore, it is necessary to be free of alcohol for 12 hours before initiating disulfiram therapy. The dose and frequency of administration may vary. The usual maintenance dose is 250 mg daily or three times a week. The client must be warned that should any alcohol be ingested, a reaction is likely and teaching about avoiding alcohol in foods, elixir medication, and alcohol products, such as after-shave lotion, is imperative. Should the client drink alcohol, the reaction is dependent on the dose of disulfiram and alcohol, and can be a serious medical emergency. For that reason, disulfiram is usually not given to the person who is in the last phase of chronic alcoholism and unable to stop the use of alcohol. The value of disulfiram is that it helps produce the sobriety on which treatment participation is built. Return of clear thinking and sensory perception may take weeks or months of sobriety. It is estimated that up to 200,000 persons with alcoholism in the United States take disulfiram regularly.[34]

NUTRITION

Substance abusers often have nutritional difficulty because of the impaired self-care, which affects food intake, as well as the nutritional implications of the substance itself. Alcohol contains calories and, therefore, an alcoholic may derive "empty" energy from alcohol without the nutritional vitamin, mineral, and protein balance. Maldigestion and malabsorption also are the result of alcohol intake. Protein and amino acid metabolism is significantly altered by heavy use of alcohol. Magnesium, calcium, thiamine, and vitamin A levels become deficient in alcoholism. The nutritional rehabilitation of the substance abuser will include emergency vitamin, fluid, and electrolyte replacement, as well as diet therapy in long-term management[66] (see nursing diagnoses entitled Substance Abuse (Alcohol) and Substance Abuse (Drugs)).

Sociotherapy

THERAPEUTIC COMMUNITIES

Cohen[12] uses the term *sociotherapy* to refer to the treatment of substance abuse that emphasizes social interaction. Therapeutic communities, drop-in centers and hotlines, and Alcoholics Anonymous, Al-Anon, and Alateen are examples of this type of therapy.

The therapeutic community form of substance abuse treatment was started in the late 1950s by Charles Diedrich when he formed Synanon.[41] He believed that the emotional immaturity of the drug abuser required living within a structured community for one to two years before autonomous function was possible. The functioning therapeutic community is marked by pacing the resident from a no-privilege status for a neophyte to the personal freedom of those who have graduated from the community. Cohen believes that this form of treatment produces drug-free clients, with low recidivism rates, who are also gifted workers with the drug-dependent. Traditionally, nurses have not played a part in these types of therapeutic communities because they were run by the residents. Recently, there has been more professional input in these communities.[41]

DROP-IN CENTERS AND HOTLINES

Drop-in centers and hotlines may provide crisis intervention for those who do not seek assistance from the traditional health care systems because they do not see themselves as "sick."[12] Nurses may staff these centers as volunteers since there is usually no charge for service.

ALCOHOLICS ANONYMOUS, AL-ANON, AND ALATEEN

In 1935, a surgeon and a businessman formed Alcoholics Anonymous (AA). Its basic beliefs are contained in its "12 steps" (Box 16-9).

Alcoholics Anonymous provides social support for the addicted person, whereas Al-Anon was created to help family members of the alcoholic. Alateen is the organization for the teenage children of a parent with alcoholism. Another 12-step self-help group is Adult Children of Alcoholics. Other addictions may have their own 12-step program [e.g., Narcotics Anonymous (NA)] depending on the community. The social network provided by these groups is extremely helpful.[67] A survey of its members conducted by the General Service Office of Alcoholics Anonymous found that those who attend meetings increased their chances of remaining sober, chances that increased with length of sobriety. Forty percent of those with less than a year's sobriety had a chance of remaining sober another year. On the other hand, those with five years sobriety had an approximately 90% chance of remaining sober for another year.[43]

The nurse's role in relation to AA treatment is to be familiar with the organization, to make appropriate referrals, and to share with clients positive expectations about the help it offers.

Psychotherapy

SUBSTANCE ABUSE COUNSELING

Traditional dynamic psychotherapy, which is insight-oriented, has not been considered the most useful therapy for the substance abuser. Alcoholism counseling is focused on the present and oriented toward realistic short-term behavioral changes that can produce positive results.[40] Weinberg[65] delineated stages for counsel-

---

BOX 16–9
Twelve Steps of Alcoholics Anonymous

1. We admitted we were powerless over alcohol—that our lives had become unmanageable.
2. Came to believe that a Power greater than ourselves could restore us to sanity.
3. Made a decision to turn our will and our lives over to the care of God *as we understood Him.*
4. Made a searching and fearless moral inventory of ourselves.
5. Admitted to God, to ourselves, and to another human being the exact nature of our wrongs.
6. Were entirely ready to have God remove all these defects of character.
7. Humbly asked Him to remove our shortcomings.
8. Made a list of all persons we had harmed, and became willing to make amends to them all.
9. Made direct amends to such people wherever possible, except when to do so would injure them or others.
10. Continued to take personal inventory and when we were wrong promptly admitted it.
11. Sought through prayer and meditation to improve our conscious contact with God *as we understood Him,* praying only for knowledge of His will for us and the power to carry that out.
12. Having had a spiritual awakening as the result of these steps, we tried to carry this message to others, and to practice these principles in all our affairs.

---

ing the substance abuser: assessment, recognition and acceptance, sobriety and beyond. In the assessment phase, primary data is collected about the family relationships, because intoxicated behavior leads to poor interpersonal relationships with a spouse and children. After assessment, the goal is for the client to accept the need for change, based on what he or she says is disliked about substance abuse behavior, and to assist the client in stopping the abuse. The third stage, sobriety, is the substitution of an activity to replace substance use, for example, coaching how to decline alcohol or drugs in social settings.

GROUP THERAPY

Group therapy is usually particularly useful with the substance abuser. Vannicelli[62] describes explicit treatment contracts that spell out what group members can expect as the cornerstone to effective group process. This clarity about ground rules allows clients to succeed. She suggests the following rules: (1) a commitment of at least three months, (2) timely attendance, (3) advance notice for terminating group, (4) abstinence commitment, (5) commitment to talk about personal difficulties, (6) commitment to talk about group interpersonal process, (7) outside-of-group limitations on behavior, and (8) the nature of group leader communication with outsiders.

FAMILY THERAPY

Recently, clinicians have recognized that family members are in need of therapy themselves as individuals and as a family unit.[7,40] Patterns of family interaction that require intervention include denying the substance abuse, avoiding conflicts that may precipitate abuse, excusing the substance abuse, protecting the abuser from the consequence of misuse, and controlling situations so substance use will not occur.[68]

Often, those who were children in the substance-abusing family will seek counseling as adults. Mansmann and Newhausel[35] have divided the stages of recovery for adult children of alcoholics into survival, emergent awareness, care issues, transformation, integration, and genesis. (1) *Survival* as an adult from a substance-abusing family may be manifested by psychosomatic illness, depression, eating disorders, as well as other dysfunctions. (2) *Emergent awareness* occurs when denial about the childhood experience begins to lessen. The use of reading materials and support groups is indicated in this phase. (3) *Care issues* occur when the client connects the influence of the past with the present. Talking with family members, support groups, and group therapy can be useful interventions. (4) *Transformation* is the stage at which the behavioral changes produced by early child responses to stress changes to more functional adult responses. (5) *Integration* allows the potential of new behavior to be implemented. Examples of integration would be reduction in a need to control, or an increase in the ability to be playful or assertive. (6) *Genesis,* the final phase, occurs when the resolution of past injury allows self-congruence and positive self-esteem.

Nursing roles within the psychotherapy treatment modalities may include being the counselor, group leader, or family therapist, depending on specialist training and treatment setting.

Chemical Aversion Therapy

Aversion conditioning is a technique of behavior modification used to treat substance abuse and maladaptive behavior. The purpose of such therapy is to assist in abstinence by learned association between an unpleasant experience and the abused substance. Aversion therapy is most frequently used in alcoholism treatment, although it can be used to treat drug abuse. Chemical aversion conditioning (CAC) therapy is used in treating alcoholism, and the drug used as the conditioning agent most often is emetine hydrochloride. The treatment is repeated presentation of the stimulus (alcohol) with resultant response (nausea and vomiting induced by emetine). The client with alcoholism is typically given five treatments every other day over a ten-day period in the hospital. In the session, the client is in a barlike room and given his preferred alcoholic beverage and instructed to drink rapidly. The emetine produces vomiting and, therefore, the client is negatively conditioned to the sight, smell, and taste of alcohol. The usefulness of CAC treatment has not yet been established.[39] It is typically administered in conjunction with other treatment modalities, and this makes the specific effects of CAC more difficult to measure. Potential risks with the use of emetine include gastrointestinal, neuromuscular, and cardiovascular effects: CAC is recommended for use only when less intrusive therapies have failed.[39] The nursing role with CAC is to administer the drug, watch for untoward effects, and assist in the sessions.

RELAPSE AND RECOVERY

Terms

There are a variety of ways to view relapse and its antithesis, recovery. *Relapse* may be seen as the moment in time when drug use again begins or as a process in which drug use occurs over time. As a process, it would refer to the same intensity of addiction and use and, subsequently, the same or worse consequences associated with its use as before the drug-free period. For example, relapse in a methadone maintenance client would be the daily resumption of frequent opiate use. *Recovery*, on the other hand, is the moment drug use is stopped or as the process over time in which drug use ceases.

Metabolic and Genetic Explanations and Relapse

Just as drug dependence is genetically influenced, so is relapse. Opiate dependence may be genetically related to endorphin deficiency and, therefore, only narcotic

use would create a sense of normality.[41,53] Abstinence in these cases would be quite difficult. The metabolic result of opiate use appears to be decreased endorphin levels, and this deficiency, when coupled with the genetic low level, may make lifetime use of methadone necessary.[41] Alcoholism may relate to metabolic alterations that create heavy alcohol use if abstinence is broken, and the ingestion of one drink may lead to heavy, serious alcohol use.[67] Practitioners may use the genetic basis of relapse in order to be nonjudgmental in explaining that "controlled" use of substance is not possible.

Social Support, Stress, and Relapse

The role of stress, coping responses to stress, and the buffering effects of social support is being researched as it relates to relapse. Drug abusers' networks may not be supportive of abstinence because of the drug use of its members; this would lead to shorter periods of abstinence.[64] The nursing implications of this research will be to assist clients to increase networks supportive of abstinence and to teach specific coping strategies for specific stressors.

Conditional Craving and Relapse

In the regular substance abuser, stimuli pertinent to drug use have been repeatedly paired with the use of the drug and subsequent drug effects. The process of gulping the first drink, or "cooking up heroin" produces strong conditional stimuli that reinforce the use.[5] Nursing implications are to teach about the occasions of drug-craving, to identify common craving situations, and to suggest alternatives to respond to and limit drug craving. Complete abstinence is the goal to be reinforced, as it will reduce craving. However, if the substance-abusing client begins to believe he or she is no longer addicted, that too may result in drug use.[68]

CASE STUDY

Mr. Robert A is a 37-year-old man with a diagnosis of alcohol dependence, cannabis dependence, nicotine dependence, and cocaine dependence. His DSM-III-R psychiatric diagnosis is polysubstance dependence. His history reveals continuous use of alcohol, tobacco, and marijuana since the age of 18, and periodic abuse of cocaine. Psychological dependence is manifested in a compelling desire to use alcohol, marijuana, and nicotine, and an inability to stop; he smokes two packs of cigarettes a day and also uses marijuana daily. He has had no other major illnesses and no symptoms of physiologic addiction to alcohol.

Mr. A owns a small business, has been married for 15 years, and has 10- and 4-year-old sons. He presented for outpatient treatment following the crisis of an extramarital affair with a younger woman who, like his wife, was concerned about his drinking pattern. He saw a psychologist for five sessions and decided that he did wish to reunite with his wife and children, and would comply with his wife's request that he explore his alcohol use.

NURSING CARE PLAN 16-1

MR. ROBERT A

NURSING INTERVENTIONS	OUTCOME CRITERIA

NURSING DIAGNOSIS: Substance abuse (alcohol, cannabis, nicotine, cocaine) related to genetic predisposition, inadequate coping skills, and poor self-image

CLIENT GOAL: Recognize and accept his substance abuse problem

■ Teach about the disease of drug dependence ■ Ask for daily recording of substance use ■ Establish targets for substance use (only 7 drinks a week and never more than 5 per occasion) ■ Invite Robert to list subsequent negative consequences owing to substance abuse	Contrasts own drug use pattern with the disease of chemical dependence and identifies his own substance dependence

CLIENT GOAL: Improve self-concept and gain personal hope

■ Identify stressful areas when drug use likely and develop alternatives	Lists high-risk situations and his specific plans to maintain abstinence
■ Offer referral for spiritual growth	Values power outside of self as assistive
■ Clarify boundaries between self and others and reduce shame	Respects boundaries of self and others

CLIENT GOAL: Develop alternative coping strategies and eliminate need to use drugs as a means of escape

■ Engage in grief work to resolve previous losses	Clarifies denial about childhood issues
■ Offer parent effectiveness training to broaden resources as a father	Reports increased effectiveness in parental role
■ Refer for rational emotive therapy to address illogical, irrational thoughts and resultant feelings	Reports new possibilities being explored in his life
■ Support ability to see full choices available	Integrates new behaviors

---

Mr. and Mrs. A attended the first visit with the nurse therapist together. A genogram identified alcoholic fathers for both partners. The nurse began addressing the disease concept of drug dependence and asked both partners to record their daily use of alcohol and marijuana. Mr. A, certain that alcohol and marijuana use was a behavior over which he had control, contracted to have only seven drinks in a week, never more than five drinks on any one occasion, and no marijuana use. During the first week, no drinking was reported; however, the abusive pattern subsequently returned, with no more than two abstinent days during the next six weeks. After reviewing the documentation, Mr. A also stated that his early denial and need to minimize his alcohol use had further compromised his reports, nor did he stop marijuana or tobacco use.

The following nursing diagnoses were formulated: substance abuse (alcohol) and substance abuse (drugs) related to genetic predisposition, inadequate coping skills, and poor self-image.

Attempts to strengthen the marital coalition during conjoint therapy sessions were partially successful. Both partners were creative, insightful, and articulate, able to express their feelings of anger, sadness, and guilt, mixed with love and hopefulness. Each felt bonded to the other, and they were able to be playful together, although this often involved alcohol and marijuana use. They frequently displayed the classic substance abuse–codependent roles. Sufficient improvement was made in the marriage that the couple chose to terminate conjoint therapy. However, the nurse was candid about the compromised level of functioning possible because the drug dependence was still in process, and encouraged them to return for assistance should they find it necessary in the future.

Mrs. A returned for individual counseling four months later and, after a year, had made the decision that a husband under the influence of drugs was counterproductive to her own growth. Mr. A consented to admission for inpatient alcohol and drug treatment, and was admitted on a weekend after a drunken episode at Christmas, which also involved cocaine. However, he was hostile to his wife and the staff and stayed less than eight hours before demanding release. Mrs. A told him that he could not come home and that she would not discuss possible reconciliation until he began counseling. Mr. A subsequently came for weekly individual sessions on an outpatient basis for more than a year.

The nursing diagnoses were substance abuse (alcohol) and substance abuse (marijuana, cocaine). The treatment goals for Mr. A were that he would (1) recognize and accept the substance abuse problem; (2) improve his self-concept and gain personal hope; and (3) develop adaptive-coping strategies and eliminate the need to use drugs as a means to escape.

The first goal was accomplished by having Mr. A read about alcoholism. He also had to confront reality about the problems his drinking was causing and was asked to monitor the loss of control over his intake that he experienced and the resulting negative consequences. He described his alcohol use as "a tomb created by a shaft opening into the bowels of the earth with only death the end, dark, ugly." He reported that the Christmas-time episode that had resulted in his wife's intervention was his "crying out to be freed by the illusion created by alcohol" and was "the biggest favor she's ever done me—I realized I was loved, and that I could

sacrifice my old life of being imprisoned and penned in and begin to believe in myself." He was thus successful in identifying his addiction.

The second goal was achieved by reinforcing his success in abstaining from alcohol and drugs, teaching him new behaviors to cope with stressors, and referrals for spiritual growth. Mr. A was able to grieve by recalling the initial powerlessness of a chaotic childhood and how he learned to survive by "rolling with the punches." He became aware of how "really sad I am that it had to be that way," and "I don't want that to be the life I give to my kids. I can use these lessons and let go." He replaced his early avoidance of conflict patterns that resulted in placation, devious oppositional behavior, and subsequent substance abuse.

Mr. A has maintained sobriety with occasional drinks on several occasions. He continues to smoke cigarettes and uses marijuana about twice a month. He has come to see himself as an optimistic, self-confident, and nurturing husband and father. Mrs. A has taken graduate courses in her area of expertise and is productive at work; she no longer uses marijuana and is pleased with her life (see Nursing Care Plan 16-1 for a sample care plan for Mr. Robert A).

SUMMARY

The prevalence of substance use disorders is widespread in America and produces substantial damage to society in terms of crime, health, and social consequences. The nurse frequently has clients with these disorders, especially in psychiatric mental health settings. The sequences of progressive drug use is (1) beer

Research Highlights

Potamianos and associates[47] investigated staff and patient perceptions of problem drinkers in an English general hospital setting. A sample of 275 subjects was included: hospital staff physicians, nurses, patients referred to the hospital for alcohol-related problems, and local physicians. Each subject was asked to rate the "typical problem drinker" according to a seven-point Likert-type scale. The number 1 referred to the first attribute, and the number 7 referred to the opposite attribute. There were 12 pairs of terms including happy childhood—unhappy childhood; responsible—irresponsible; unlikely to become dependent on other drugs—likely to become dependent on other drugs. The instructions then called for the subject to rate the "self" and the "ideal self" according to the same scale.

There was a significant difference in the views of nurses, hospital staff physicians, general practitioners, and patients regarding problem drinkers. The patients had the most positive view of the problem drinker, and nurses had the most negative view. For each professional group, the mean difference between scores given the "problem-drinker" and the "self" were larger than the differences between the scores given the "self" and the "idealized self." That is, there was greater disparity be-

tween how professionals perceived the problem drinker and their own self than the difference in their idealized self and their self. The patient group had the opposite finding in that the difference was greater between the idealized self and the self than it was between the self and the problem drinker.

The psychological distance between professional and patient indicated by this British study could potentially affect the empathic capability of health professionals. It would be interesting to replicate this study in America. Is a problem drinker less or more stigmatized in England than in America? In addition, the replication of the study in a substance abuse treatment center would give an opportunity to see if addiction professionals have different views about the problem drinker than those who work in a general hospital setting.

The attitude of the health professional is an essential component in provision of health promotion and disease prevention. When the target of intervention is a stigmatized group, such as the substance abuser, a negative attitude is counterproductive. In these cases, both the health provider and the client may hold views that sabotage the interactional potential for recovery.

or wine, (2) cigarettes or hard liquor, (3) marijuana, and (4) illicit drugs. The pattern of use may move from social–recreational use to circumstantial use. This is followed by intensified use to compulsive use. Genetic influence, behavioral learning, family system patterns, and interpersonal factors are important influences in substance use and abuse. Assessment for substance use disorders includes the determination of drug abuse, dependence, overdose, and withdrawal. The appropriateness of treatment in community or institutional settings is dependent on the pattern of substance use. The family and drug-dependent individual are included in treatment. The nurse working with individuals with substance use disorders may be prepared at either the generalist or specialist level. Biologic treatment modalities, sociotherapy, psychotherapy, family therapy, and chemical aversion conditioning are possible treatment interventions. Relapse and recovery can be influenced by genetic, social support, and behavioral-conditioning factors.

References

1. American Nurses' Association. addictions and psychological dysfunction in nursing: the profession's response to the problem. Kansas City, MO: American Nurses' Association; 1984.
2. American Nurses' Association, Drug and Alcohol Nursing Association, National Nurses' Society on Addictions. The care of clients with addictions, dimensions of nursing practice. Kansas City, MO: American Nurses' Association; 1987.
3. American Nurses' Association, National Nurses' Society on Addictions. Standards of addiction nursing practice with selected diagnosis and criteria. Kansas City, MO: American Nurses' Association; 1988.
4. American Psychiatric Association. Diagnostic and statistical manual of mental disorders, 3rd ed, revised. Washington, DC: American Psychiatric Association; 1987.
5. Babor TF, Cooney NL, Laveruian RJ. The drug dependence syndrome as an organizing principle in the explanation and prediction of relapse. In: Tims FM, Leukefeld CG, eds. Relapse and recovery in drug abuse. Rockville, MD: National Institute on Drug Abuse; 1986.
6. Bennet G, Graves SE, Kavanaugh MT, Vourakis C. An overview of substance abuse treatment. In: Bennet G, Vourakis C, Woolf D, eds. Substance abuse. New York: John Wiley & Sons; 1983.
7. Brolsma JK. Family therapy in the treatment of alcoholism. In: Estes NK, Heinman ME, eds. Alcoholism: development, consequences and interventions. St Louis: CV Mosby; 1986.
8. Brown RL, Carter WB, Gordon MJ. Diagnosis of alcoholism in a simulated patient encounter by primary care physicians. J Fam Pract. 1987;25:260.
9. Carstensen LL, Rychtarik RG, Prue D. Behavioral treatment of the geriatric alcohol abuser: a long term follow-up study. Addict Behav. 1985;10:307–310.
10. Cleveland M. Families and adolescent drug abuse: structural analysis of children's roles. Fam Process. 1981;20:295–304.
11. Cohen M, Kern JC, Hassett C. Identifying alcoholism in medical patients. Hosp Commun Psychiatry. 1986;37:399.
12. Cohen S, Callahan JF. The diagnosis and treatment of drug and alcohol abuse. New York: Haworth Press; 1986.
13. Douglas SS, Pesheau G. Evaluation of an inpatient women's addiction group. In: Alcohol, drugs and tobacco: an international perspective—past, present, future. Calgary, Alberta: Alberta Alcohol and Drug Commission; 1985.
14. Ewing JA. Detecting alcoholism: the CAGE questionnaire. JAMA. 1984;14:1905–1907.
15. Florenzo RU, Pemjean A. Recent advances in knowledge about alcohol problems: social and behavioral sciences. In: Proceedings of the 34th International Congress on Alcoholism and Drug Dependence, Alberta Alcohol and Drug Abuse Conference; 1988.
16. Freed EX. Alcoholism and schizophrenia: the search for perspectives. In: Freed EX, ed. Interfaces between alcoholism and mental health NIAAA–RMCAS alcoholism treatment series, No 4. New Brunswick, NJ: Publication Division, Rutgers University Center of Alcohol Studies; 1982.
17. Friedman HS, Glickman NW. Program characteristics for successful treatment of adolescent drug abuse. J Nerv Ment Dis. 1986;174:664–672.
18. Gallant DS. Alcohol and drug abuse curriculum guide for psychiatric faculty. Rockville, MD: National Institute on Alcohol Abuse and Alcoholism; 1982.
19. Gold MS, Daekis CA. Role of the laboratory in the evaluation of suspected drug abuse. J Clin Psychiatry. 1986;47:17–23.
20. Gordon AJ. Alcohol use in the perspective of cultural ecology. In: Galanter M. ed. Recent developments in alcoholism, vol 2. New York: Plenum Press; 1984.
21. Hesselbrock MM, Neyer RE, Keener JJ. Psychopathology in hospitalized alcoholics. Arch Gen Psychiatry. 1985;42:1050–1055.
22. Hoffman A. Substance use/abuse/disorder. In: Current issues in alcohol and drug abuse nursing: research, education, and clinical practice. New York: National Council on Alcoholism; 1984.
23. Hoffman AL, Heinemann ME. Alcohol problems in elderly persons. In: Estes NJ, Heinemann ME, eds. Alcoholism development, consequences and intervention, 3rd ed. St Louis: CV Mosby; 1986.
24. Hutchinson S. Chemically dependent nurses: the trajectory toward self-annihilation. Nurs Res. 1986;35:196–200.
25. Jackimczyk KC, Roberts MR. Approach to the intoxicated patient. Top Emerg Med. 1984;6:9–13.
26. Jacobson GR. Detection, assessment and diagnosis of alcoholism—current techniques. In: Galanter M, ed. Recent developments in alcoholism. New York: Plenum Press; 1983.
27. Jainchill N, DeLeon G, Pinkham C. Psychiatric diagnoses among substance abusers in therapeutic community treatment. J Psychoactive Drugs. 1986;18:209–213.
28. Jurich AP, Polson CE. Reasons for drug use: comparison of drug users and abusers. Psychol Rep. 1984;55:371–378.
29. Kalant H. Tolerance and its significance for drug and alcohol dependence. In: Harris LS, ed. Problems of drug dependence, 1986. Rockville, MD: National Institute on Drug Abuse; 1987.
30. Kofoed L, Kania J, Walsh T, Atkinson RM. Outpatient treatment of patients with substance abuse and coexisting psychiatric disorders. Am J Psychiatry. 1986;14:867–869.
31. Light WJH. Psychodynamics of alcoholism. Springfield, IL: Charles C Thomas; 1986.
32. Ludwig AM. Principles of general psychiatry. New York: Free Press; 1986.
33. McKelvy MJ, Kane JS, Kellison K. Substance abuse and mental illness. J Psychosoc Nurs. 1987;25:23.
34. McNichol RW, Logsdon SA. Disulfiram: an evaluation research model. Alcohol Health Res World. 1988;12:203–209.
35. Mansmann PA, Newhausel PA. Life after survival. Malvern, PA: Genesis Publishing; 1986.
36. Metzger L. From denial to recovery. San Francisco: Jossey-Bass; 1988.
37. Moskowitz H. Adverse effects of alcohol and other drugs on

human performance. Alcohol Health Res World. 1985; 9(4):11–15.

38. Mirin SM, Weiss RD. Affective illness in substance abusers. Psychiatr Clin North Am. 1986;9:503–514.

39. National Center Health Services Research and Health Care Technology Assessment. Chemical aversion therapy for the treatment of alcoholism. Rockville, MD: US Department of Health and Human Services; 1988.

40. National Institute on Alcohol Abuse and Alcoholism. Sixth special report to the U.S. Congress on alcohol and health. Washington DC: US Department of Health and Human Services, Alcohol, Drug Abuse, and Mental Health Administration, DHEW Pub. No (ADM) 87-1519; 1987.

41. National Institute on Drug Abuse. Drug abuse and drug abuse research: The first in a series of triennial reports to Congress. Washington DC: US Government Printing Office; 1984.

42. Niven R. Alcoholism: the costs of the problem and its treatment. In: Alcohol, drugs and tobacco: an international perspective. Proceedings of the 34th International Congress on Alcoholism and Drug Dependence. Calgary, Alberta: Alcohol and Drug Abuse Commission; 1985.

43. Patrick GM, Jackson JK. Characteristics of alcoholics in Alcoholics Anonymous. In: Alcohol, drugs, and tobacco: an international perspective—past, present, and future. Calgary, Alberta, Alberta Alcohol and Drug Abuse Commission; 1985.

44. Pattison EM. The selection of treatment modalities for the alcoholic patient. In: Mendelson JH, Mello NK, eds. The diagnosis and treatment of alcoholism, 2nd ed. New York: McGraw-Hill; 1985.

45. Peele S. The moral vision of addiction: how people's values determine whether they become and remain addicts. J Drug Iss. 1987;17:187–215.

46. Peele S. The meaning of addiction. Lexington, MA: Lexington Books; 1985.

47. Potamianos G, Winter D, Duffy SW, Gorman DM, Peters TJ. The perception of problem drinkers by general hospital staff, general practitioners, and alcoholic patients. Alcohol. 1985;2:563–566.

48. Powell BJ, Penich EC, Read MR, Ludwig AM. Comparison of three outpatient treatment interventions: a twelve-month followup of male alcoholics. J Stud Alcohol. 1985;46:309–312.

49. Public Health Service. Promoting health/preventing disease: objectives for the nation. Washington, DC: US Department of Health and Human Services, Public Health Service; 1980.

50. Radonco-Thomas S, Boixin D, Chabot F, et al. Nosology and diagnosis of alcoholism, issues and perspectives in subtyping (DSM III) simple alcoholism and alcoholism associated with other psychopathologies. Prog Neuropsychopharmacol Biol Psychiatry. 1986;10:129–134.

51. Raveis KH, Kandel DB. Changes in drug behavior from the middle to the late twenties: initiation, persistence, and cessation of use. Am J Public Health. 1987;77:607–611.

52. Rounsville B. Clinical implications of relapse research. In: Tims FM, Leukefield CH, eds. Relapse and recovery in drug abuse. Rockville, MD: National Institute on Drug Abuse; 1986.

53. Rounsville BJ, Kosten TR, Weissman MW, Keeber HP. Evaluating and treating depression in opiate addicts. Rockville, MD: National Institute on Drug Abuse; 1985.

54. Seymour RB, Smith DE. Drug free. New York: Sara Lazin Books; 1987.

55. Silverman MM. Status of the 1990 objectives on misuse of alcohol and drugs. MMWR. 1987;36:720–723.

56. Stanton MD, Todd TC, et al, eds. The family therapy of drug abuse and addiction. New York: Guilford Press; 1982.

57. Sullivan EJ, Hale RE. Nurses' belief about the etiology and treatment of alcohol abuse: a national study. J Stud Alcohol 1987;48:456–460.

58. Sullivan E, Bissell LC, Williams EW. Chemical dependency in nursing. Menlo Park, CA: Addison-Wesley; 1988.

59. Szasz TS. Bad habits are not diseases. In: Freed EX, ed. Interfaces between alcoholism and mental health, NIAAA-RUCAS alcoholism treatment series. New Brunswick, NJ: Publications Division, no. 4. Rutgers Center of Alcohol Studies; 1982.

60. Tremble JG, Walsh JM. A new initiative for solving age-old problems. Alcohol Health Res World. 1985;9(4):2–5.

61. Thayer BA, Parrish RT, Himle Z, Cameron OG, Curtis GC, Neese RM. Alcohol abuse among clinically anxious patients. Behav Res Theory. 1986;24:357–359.

62. Vannicelli M. Group psychotherapy with alcoholics: special techniques. In: Estes NJ, Heinmann ME, eds. Alcoholism: development, consequences and interventions, 3rd ed. St. Louis: CV Mosby; 1986.

63. Wade M. Meeting the challenge of alcohol and drug abuse in the older adult. Home Health Care Nurse. 1987;7:19–20.

64. Wesson DR, Havassay BE, Smith DE. Theories of relapse and recovery and their implications for drug abuse treatment. In: Tims FM, Leukefeld CG, eds. Relapse and recovery in drug abuse. Rockville, MD: National Institute on Drug Abuse; 1986.

65. Weinberg JR. Counseling the person with alcohol problems. In: Estes NJ, Heinemann ME, eds. Alcoholism development, consequences and interventions, 3rd ed. St Louis: CV Mosby; 1986.

66. Worthington-Roberts B. Alcoholism and malnutrition. In: Estes NJ, Heinemann ME, eds. Alcoholism development, consequences and interventions, 3rd ed. St Louis: CV Mosby; 1986.

67. Wurmser L. Psychodynamics of substance abuse. In: Lowinson JH, Ruiz P, eds. Substance abuse: clinical problems and perspectives. Baltimore: Williams & Wilkins; 1981.

68. Zackon F, McAuliffe WE, Ch'ien JM. Addict after-care: recovery training and self-care. Rockville, MD: National Institute on Drug Abuse; 1985.

69. Zimburg S. The clinical management of alcoholism. New York: Brunner/Mazel; 1982.

17

Melodie A. Lohr

Clients With Schizophrenia

OBJECTIVES
After reading this chapter, the reader will be able to:
1. Describe schizophrenia and related disorders
2. Discuss theories of the etiology of schizophrenia
3. Describe pharmacotherapeutic and psychotherapeutic interventions in the disorder
4. Discuss problems in the nursing management of clients with schizophrenia.

DESCRIPTION

Schizophrenia is a condition marked by a severe and often irreversible deterioration in personality, affect, and intellectual functions. The modern conception of schizophrenia begins with Emil Kraepelin who, in the late 1800s, combined "hebephrenia" and "catatonia" with certain paranoid states and, borrowing the term from Morel, called the condition *dementia praecox*.[14] Kraepelin conceptualized the condition to consist of largely irreversible intellectual deterioration beginning around or shortly after adolescence. Bleuler, in the early 1900s, modified Kraepelin's concept by including cases with a much better prognosis and, in 1911, renamed the condition *schizophrenia* (meaning "splitting of the mind"). Actually, Bleuler believed that there was more than one form of schizophrenia, and referred to the "group of schizophrenias." Many investigators today also believe that schizophrenia is not a single disease, but rather, a group of related conditions. Bleuler considered that there were basically four mental processes involved in the disordered cognition of schizophrenic clients, sometimes called the four "As" of schizophrenia, consisting of disturbance of *association* (loosening of associations), disturbance of *affect* (flattened or inappropriate affect), *ambivalence* (in which conflicting ideas are embraced without conscious conflict), and *autism*. In the mid-1900s, Kurt Schneider proposed that schizophrenia could be diagnosed according to primary and secondary criteria,[6] listed in Box 17-1. The primary criteria were called *first-rank symptoms*. Although Schneider did not consider the presence of first-rank symptoms essential for the diagnosis of schizophrenia, they were strong indicators, whereas the secondary criteria, or *second-rank symptoms*, of schizophrenia, although frequently a component of the syndrome, were considered much weaker indicators. Schneiderian criteria form a large component of many popular diagnostic schemes for schizophrenia, including the DSM-III-R.[1] Diagnostic criteria for the active phase of schizophrenia in the DSM-III-R[1] include: either (1) delusions, prominent hallucinations, incoherence/loosening of associations, catatonic behavior, inappropriate/flat affect (at least two); or (2) bizarre delusions; or (3) prominent hallucinations, for at least one week.

Subtypes

Schizophrenia has been subdivided in many different ways. The simplest subclassification schemes have divided schizophrenia into two forms. One diagnostic scheme of this sort subdivides schizophrenia into *paranoid* and *nonparanoid* forms, depending upon whether symptoms of paranoia dominate the clinical picture. Another such scheme has been described as type I versus type II, or *positive* versus *negative* schizophrenia.[2,3,7,10] Type I, or positive, schizophrenia consists of so-called positive or productive symptoms, such as delusions, auditory hallucinations, and incoherent thought and speech. The second, called type II, or negative schizophrenia, consists of so-called negative, core, or defect symptoms, such as social withdrawal, alogia (poverty of thought and speech), anhedonia (inability to experience pleasure), flattening of affect, attentional impairment, and lack of motivation. Type I schizophrenia has been considered to have a better prognosis, a better response to neuroleptic medications, and little evidence of structural brain abnormalities, whereas type II schizophrenia is thought to have a poor response to neuroleptics, poor prognosis, and evidence of ventricular enlargement on the computed tomography (CT) scan. Many, if not most, schizophrenic clients do not fit neatly into one or the other of these two groups, having instead a combination of positive and negative symptoms.

A more commonly used subtyping scheme is that employed in the DSM-III-R,[1] in which schizophrenia is considered to occur in five main forms:[22] (1) a *catatonic* form, marked by disturbances such as excitement, negativism, rigidity, or stupor; (2) a *disorganized* form, marked by incoherence, flat, silly, or inappropriate affect, and a lack of systematized delusions (this form corresponds to what has formerly been called hebephrenic schizophrenia); (3) a *paranoid* form, marked by preoccupation with systematized delusions or with frequent auditory hallucinations related to a single theme, but without marked disorganization; (4) an *undifferentiated* form, in which the client does not fit into any of the foregoing groups, but still meets criteria for schizophrenia; and, finally, (5) a *residual* form, in which the client has had an episode of schizophrenia in the past, but not currently, although there are still

---

BOX 17-1
Schizophrenic Symptoms According to Kurt Schneider

FIRST-RANK SYMPTOMS

Audible thoughts
Voices arguing or discussing
Voices commenting
Somatic passivity experiences
Thought withdrawal and other experiences of influenced thought
Delusional perceptions
All other experiences involving "made" volition, affect, or impulses

SECOND-RANK SYMPTOMS

Other disorders of perception
Sudden delusional ideas
Perplexity
Depressive and euphoric mood changes
Feeling of emotion impoverishment

(Adapted from Berner P, Gabriel E, Hatschnig H, et al. World Psychiatric Association diagnostic criteria for schizophrenia and affective psychoses. Washington, DC: American Psychiatric Press; 1983.)

symptoms of social withdrawal or eccentric behavior (this corresponds to what was formerly called "simple" schizophrenia). One of the problems with this diagnostic scheme, apart from the fact that it has not been fully validated, is that some clients will appear to have one subtype of schizophrenia at one time during the course of their illness, and a different form at another time.

Symptoms

Many different symptoms have been described in schizophrenia (Box 17-2). Schizophrenia is sometimes called a *cognitive* disorder, meaning that there is an impairment in cognition or thought. This impairment has been divided into two forms: disorder of the *form* of thought (or *formal thought disorder*), and disorder of the *content* of thought. Formal thought disorder includes such symptoms as incoherence, tangentiality, loosening of associations, word salad, derailment, and illogicality; in other words, disorders marked by disorganization of language.[2] In contrast, *disordered thought content* usually means hallucinations, delusions, illusions, and other conditions in which cognitive dysfunction occurs without abnormalities in syntax. Disorders of the form and the content of thought can occur either separately or together in any given client with schizophrenia. Apart from disordered cognition, schizophrenic clients also have *disordered affect*, often in the form of flattened or inappropriate affect. Clients often demonstrate *disordered behavior*, especially in catatonic schizophrenia. Finally, schizophrenic clients frequently suffer from a number of negative symptoms, such as social withdrawal. It is worth remembering that no single symptom is pathognomonic of schizophrenia, with every symptom seen in many conditions apart from schizophrenia. It is the combination of symptoms, in the absence of organic factors, that allows the diagnosis of schizophrenia to be made.

Although there is some evidence that schizophrenia and mood disorders are separable conditions (and, indeed, the presence of significant affective symptomatology is an exclusion criterion for the diagnosis of schizophrenia in the DSM-III-R), many individuals appear to manifest both schizophrenic and affective symptoms.[23,40] These clients are often said to have *schizoaffective disorder*. In some cases, manic symptoms predominate (*schizoaffective disorder, bipolar type*), and in others depressive symptoms are more apparent (*schizoaffective disorder, depressive type*). Although these conditions have been considered to be related to schizophrenia, it is not clear exactly what they represent, and some investigators believe they are more closely allied with mood disorders. In general, the prognosis of these conditions, although worse than mood disorders, is better than for schizophrenia. According to the DSM-III-R,[1] four things are needed for the diagnosis of schizoaffective disorder:

1. During an episode, mania or major depression *and* schizophrenia were present *at the same time.*
2. During another episode (or another part of the same episode), delusions or hallucinations were present *without mood symptoms* for at least two weeks.
3. The episodes involving mood disorder make up a substantial part of the active illness, and do not simply occur transiently during the psychosis, or only during residual illness.
4. An organic cause has been ruled out.

A typical case is diagrammed in Figure 17-1. (See also Chapter 19.)

Epidemiology

Schizophrenia has been diagnosed in individuals all over the world. For a number of years it was thought that the lifetime prevalence (that is, the percentage of persons who are likely to develop the disorder some time during their lives) of schizophrenia is about 1% in most areas of North America, Europe, and Asia.[7] It now appears that there are certain areas in the world, such as western Ireland and a certain region in northern Sweden, that have a much higher prevalence, perhaps as high as 3%, and there are also areas that probably have a lower prevalence than 1%. The lifetime risk of developing schizophrenia is about the same for men as for women, although there is evidence that men have, in general, an earlier age of onset than women, namely, 18 to 25 years compared with 26 to 45 years for women.[24] The point prevalence of schizophrenia appears to be approximately 2% worldwide, and the incidence is somewhere in the range of 30 cases per 100,000 per year.[17]

Course

Schizophrenia usually first appears in late adolescence or early adulthood, with approximately 50% of cases having an onset before the age of 25, although there are a number of cases in which the disease appears to develop after the age of 45.[34] Sometimes there are prodromal symptoms, such as social withdrawal or eccentric behavior for years before the onset of clear-cut psychosis. In other clients, the premorbid functioning is excellent without a hint of the oncoming illness. The initial episodes of schizophrenic illness are often precipitated by stress and, to a lesser extent, so are many later episodes. There is some evidence that decreasing stress can decrease the number and severity of subsequent exacerbations of the illness.[19] Many clients also have a history of drug and alcohol abuse before or during the illness, which may be an attempt to self-medicate, but frequently complicates the diagnosis and clinical course.

The course of the illness is highly variable.[16,38] It has been estimated that in approximately one third of cases, the clients may return to the previous level of functioning after a short period of illness. Another third have a history of remissions and exacerbations throughout their lives, and the final third appear to

BOX 17-2
Signs and Symptoms Described in Schizophrenia*

HALLUCINATIONS: A sensory perception that occurs in the absence of a corresponding stimulus

(See nursing diagnosis entitled Hallucinations for further information)

ILLUSIONS: Misperceived or misinterpreted sensory stimuli

Deja vu: the feeling that a novel situation is familiar and has been previously experienced
Jamais vu: the feeling that a familiar situation is strange or novel
Hypersensitivity to light, sound, temperature, smell
Misperceptions of sights, sounds, feelings, movements, and the passage of time

DELUSIONS: Beliefs strongly held in spite of overwhelming evidence to the contrary, and against the normal values of the individual's culture and family

(See nursing diagnosis entitled Delusions for further information)

AFFECTIVE DISTURBANCES: Disturbances of the feeling state of an individual

Flattened affect: decreased emotional range
Inappropriate affect: affect that does not correspond to that expected in a given situation; sometimes of a silly or giddy nature
Anhedonia: diminished ability to feel pleasure
Paranoia: excessive fear, inappropriate to the environment

FORMAL THOUGHT DISORDER (DISORGANIZED LANGUAGE): Language that suffers from impaired syntax

Incoherence: a general term for incomprehensible speech
Derailment: speech in which the meaning of a sentence or group of sentences does not follow that of the previous sentences
Fragmentation of speech: speech in which there is disruption of sentence structure
Word salad: a severe form of fragmentation of speech in which seemingly unrelated words are strung together
Neologism: the invention of new words
Blocking: an interruption of speech in the middle of a thought
Mutism: inhibition of speech

NEGATIVE SYMPTOMS: Symptoms in which some function is diminished or lost

Social withdrawal: asocial behavior marked by social isolation
Attentional impairment: diminished ability to maintain attentional focus
Apathy: diminished interest in events or surroundings
Alogia: poverty of speech or of speech content
Abulia: impaired ability to make decisions or act independently
Hyposexuality: loss of interest in sex

BEHAVIORAL ABNORMALITIES: Disturbances in behavior, most often observed as a part of the catatonic syndrome

Stupor: markedly diminished responsiveness to the environment
Rigidity: excessive muscular tension
Waxy flexibility: moldable posturing, in which the client's body can be placed in strange postures that are maintained for long periods
Mannerisms: bizarre ways of performing normal activities
Stereotypy: complex repetitive purposeless acts
Echopraxia: repetition of movements observed in another person
Echolalia: repetition of words or other sounds
Automatic obedience: compliance with requests or commands without conscious intervention
Negativism: the opposite of automatic obedience, in which clients perform the opposite of what is requested, or pull or turn away

OTHER FEATURES

Excessive water drinking
Deterioration in personal hygiene

---

* No single symptom or sign is pathognomonic of schizophrenia.

have a chronic unremitting or deteriorating course throughout life, although there is some evidence that the percentage of patients with a chronic deteriorating course may be lower than one third.[16] The prognosis is better if the clients had good premorbid functioning, an acute onset, and significant affective component to the illness. Many schizophrenic clients in later life appear to develop "schizophrenic burnout" in which the disease becomes less marked by positive symptoms, and more by negative symptoms.

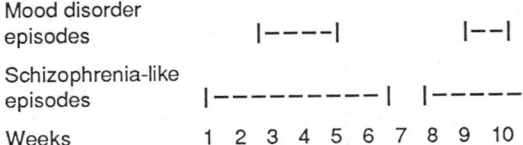

Mood disorder episodes	I----I		I--I
Schizophrenia-like episodes	I---------I	I-----I	
Weeks	1 2 3 4 5 6 7 8 9 10		

FIGURE 17–1. Schematic of a typical case of schizoaffective disorder. Note: (1) co-occurrence of mood disorder and schizophrenia; (2) at least two weeks of hallucinations or delusions without mood disorder; (3) mood disorder is a significant component of illness (about 40% of the episodes in this case).

ETIOLOGY

Genetic and Environmental Factors

Evidence that schizophrenia is, at least partially, a genetic disorder comes from the following findings:[13,27,41] (1) Family members have a higher risk for developing the condition. The risk for full siblings of a schizophrenic person to develop schizophrenia is 7% to 8%, the children of one schizophrenic parent have a 9% to 12% risk, and the children of two schizophrenic parents have a 35% to 45% risk. (2) The concordance rate for twins (i.e., the percentage of cases in which both twins have the condition) is much higher for monozygotic (identical) twins (about 50%) than for dizygotic (fraternal) twins (10%–15%). (3) The prevalence of schizophrenia is higher in biological than in adoptive relatives of schizophrenic clients, and the biological relatives of adopted schizophrenics have a higher prevalence of schizophrenia than those of control adoptees.[41] In spite of this evidence for a genetic component, the fact that only about half the time will both members of a set of identical twins have the disorder means that *environmental influences* are also important in the development or manifestation of the disorder.

For some as yet unknown reason, it is more common for schizophrenic individuals to be born in the late winter and early spring months, which some investigators have proposed may be related to viruses that are common at these times of year, although the evidence for this is poor.[17]

Psychological Theories

Many different psychological theories have been offered for schizophrenia. Some theories have conceptualized schizophrenia to result from problems with attention or information processing, because it has been noted that these persons perform poorly on tasks requiring sustained attention.[4,8,11,12,36,37] Thus, the person with schizophrenia may suffer from an impairment in selectively directing attention, perhaps resulting from a dysfunctional attention "filter," or from states of sensory overload, which leads to disorganization of mental functioning. There also appears to be impairment in information processing, such that there is too much information flow, poor retrieval, or deficits in cognitive constructs.

Psychoanalytic Theories

There have been many psychoanalytic theories of schizophrenia.[32] Some of these theories have focused on psychological conflict between unconscious defenses and unacceptable impulses, whereas other theories have focused more on ego function deficits—in which impaired ego development leads to poor ego boundaries—and the use of primitive defense mechanisms such as projection, distortion, denial, and splitting. Many recent psychoanalytic theorists maintain that primitive or disturbed ego functioning is important in the genesis of schizophrenic symptoms, in particular, impaired separation–individuation of internalized representations of the self from those of the mother.

Family Theories

There have been many different family theories of schizophrenia. Some theories, such as those of Bateson and coworkers,[5] have focused on what have been termed double-bind communications, in which a child in an intense relationship is given two conflicting messages (often one is verbal and the other nonverbal) to which a response is required. When this happens repeatedly in certain vulnerable individuals, psychosis develops as they attempt to respond to a situation in which they will always be wrong, one way or another. Jackson and Weakland[21] have proposed that a schizophrenic individual serves to maintain homeostasis or equilibrium in certain families. Although initial reports indicated that there is a high relapse rate for schizophrenic clients who have families that are high in expressed emotion (EE); (i.e., families that are highly critical or overinvolved with the client),[42] more recent studies suggest that high household EE may not be a predictor of relapse.[19,31] (See nursing diagnosis entitled Family Coping, Potential for Growth.) Although it is not always clear whether family pathology represents a cause or an effect of the schizophrenic illness, in general, many families show poor boundaries, role confusion, and ambivalence. Although family theories of schizophrenia are interesting, with the exception of studies of expressed emotion, there have been few well-controlled research studies to support or refute them. At present, many of the ideas remain speculative.

Biologic Findings

Although the biological basis of schizophrenia is unknown, over the past 30 years, a number of important discoveries concerning the neurobiology of schizophrenia have been made. A subset of clients appear to have enlarged lateral cerebral ventricles on CT scan. Many schizophrenic individuals, as well as some of their nonschizophrenic family members, show problems in eye tracking when their eyes are carefully examined while following a moving object. Some schizophrenic clients have a lower IQ, but many do not, and often schizophrenic clients are quite intelligent. Evidence is gradually accumulating that indicates that certain areas of the brain are more likely to be involved in the disease process than other areas.[39] These include the frontal lobes, especially the prefrontal cortex (dysfunction of which may relate more to the negative symptoms of schizophrenia), and the limbic system, particularly the nucleus accumbens, hippocampus, and amygdala (dysfunction of which may relate more to the positive symptoms of schizophrenia). For those schizophrenic clients who have movement disorders, there is evidence that the basal ganglia may also be involved.

Much research into schizophrenia over the past two decades has centered on what has been called the dopamine hypothesis of schizophrenia.[15,28,33] Basically, this hypothesis states that certain symptoms of schizophrenia (especially the positive symptoms described earlier) are due to excessive transmission of nerve impulses through nerve cells that use the chemical messenger dopamine as a neurotransmitter. In particular, the dopamine nerve cells thought to be involved are those that travel from the brain stem to the frontal cortex and to the limbic system. This hypothesis was based on two main discoveries: (1) different neuroleptic medications blockade dopamine receptors at concentrations that correspond to their ability to reduce psychosis,[9,35] and (2) drugs that can mimic schizophrenia, such as amphetamine, stimulate dopamine receptors.[15] Although there is much evidence supporting the role of excessive dopamine in schizophrenia, there is some evidence indicating that certain symptoms, such as the negative symptoms, are due, if anything, to a decrease, rather than an excess, in dopaminergic transmission in the brain. There is also evidence that other chemical messengers, such as norepinephrine (noradrenaline), are also important in schizophrenia.[18,20,25] The evidence showing that there is abnormal neurochemical transmission in the brains of some schizophrenic clients is what is being referred to when some people speak of a "chemical imbalance" in the brain.

Because there are many different theories of schizophrenia, involving psychological, family, environmental, genetic, and biologic factors, some investigators have proposed that there are a spectrum of vulnerabilities for the development of schizophrenia. Thus, some individuals possess high genetic vulnerability, some high family vulnerability, and so on, and the combination and interaction of these may determine whether a given individual will develop the illness.

ASSESSMENT

The assessment of clients with schizophrenia is often complex, because it involves so many different areas of functioning. Perhaps the most critical area to assess is that of cognition, since suspiciousness and disorganization can make the implementation of any treatment

plan particularly difficult. Other important areas of functioning to be assessed include the client's perceptions (including hallucinations), mood and affect, activity level, nutrition, sleep, and self-care needs.

It is important to try to understand the capabilities and level of functioning of a client, to determine what realistic goals may be. On the other hand, it is also important not to assume that simply because a client has returned to a level of previous function, no further improvement can be achieved. It is a common fallacy to believe that when the client with schizophrenia has resumed a previous level of function, then that is all that can be expected, and any further expenditure of energy on the client is not worthwhile. With adequate time and effort, clients can often do much better than would be commonly anticipated.

TREATMENT MODALITIES AND RELATED NURSING ROLES
Pharmacologic Treatment

The mainstay of treatment for schizophrenia is the use of neuroleptic medications. Although most schizophrenic clients respond, at least partially, to neuroleptic medications, in many clients, especially those with predominantly negative symptoms, the response is poor. Also, clients often do not respond immediately to neuroleptics, with some clients requiring up to six weeks to show a response (see Chapter 39). Many do well with oral neuroleptic medications, but some clients, who have problems complying with oral drugs, may fare better with intramuscular injections of long-acting depot neuroleptics such as depot fluphenazine or depot haloperidol. It has been shown that nearly 75% of clients will relapse within $1\frac{1}{2}$ years after discontinuing neuroleptics, whereas only about 25% relapse if neuroleptics are continued. Other drugs that have been used in the treatment of schizophrenia include lithium, carbamazepine (Tegretol), reserpine, and propranolol (Inderal). Antidepressants have been used for clients with depressed or flattened affect, and stimulants, such as methylphenidate, have been used for negative symptoms. Electroconvulsive treatment has also been used for rare clients with severe acute schizophrenic episodes, but this has been found to be generally ineffective in chronic schizophrenia. Benzodiazepines, such as lorazepam, have been used in the treatment of catatonia. (For a more comprehensive discussion of psychopharmacologic interventions in schizophrenia, see Chapter 39.)

Many clients suffer from extrapyramidal side effects (EPS) of neuroleptic medications, including acute dystonic reactions (such as oculogyric crises of the eyes, trismus of the jaw, and torticollis of the neck), neuroleptic-induced parkinsonism (including tremor, rigidity, and slowing of movements), and akathisia (motor restlessness). These side effects are usually treated with an anticholinergic drug such as benztropine, trihexyphenidyl, orphenadrine, and others. Akathisia is sometimes also treated with propranolol or with a benzodiazepine. Tardive dyskinesia, a movement disorder marked by choreoathetoid movements, predominantly of the hands and face, occurs in approximately one of four clients treated with neuroleptics long-term, and there is no known generally effective treatment at this time. (See Chapter 39 for a further discussion of neuroleptic side effects.)

The role of nurses in pharmacotherapy of schizophrenia is often quite complex, requiring careful individualized assessments of clients. For example, nurses must be familiar not only with neuroleptic drugs, but with drug interactions and the use of medications for treating side effects. Many schizophrenic clients require as-needed (prn) medication. It often requires careful consideration to determine whether the prn should be a neuroleptic or an anticholinergic medication because that decision involves differentiating between akathisia and a worsening of the psychosis. Another problem concerns clients who may benefit more from a behavioral intervention, such as a time-out, than from a pharmacologic intervention.

Milieu Therapy

A *therapeutic milieu* is a structured environment actively maintained by the nursing staff and designed to meet the needs of a specific population of clients. For schizophrenic clients, the milieu should be designed to promote repair of the clients' deficits in ego functioning, such as controlling aggression and destructiveness, promoting reality testing, and identifying appropriate amounts of stimulation. The milieu atmosphere should promote direct communications and community feeling, while enhancing the individual's ability to make decisions and function autonomously. Milieu therapy may also be associated with several problems that should be watched for and guarded against, including regression and under- or overstimulation. It must be noted, however, that the therapeutic milieu, being an artificial environment, may not by itself be enough to prepare the client for community living.

In general, the milieu of a ward is strongly influenced by the nursing staff, and it is important for all nurses to be aware of the powerful effects the milieu can have on clients. Schizophrenic clients are particularly sensitive to changes in the milieu, much more sensitive than might at first be assumed from their degree of psychosis.

Group Therapy

Group therapy, in both inpatient and outpatient settings, may be helpful for schizophrenic clients. Again, an attempt should be made to avoid overstimulation of the client, hence, directly threatening topics should be avoided. Groups are often constructed according to the functional level of the client, with some groups geared toward promoting skills required in daily living, other groups that focus upon medications and side effects, and still others in which issues such as understanding and coping with schizophrenia are addressed. Nurses often run groups in both inpatient and outpatient settings, and such groups should be tailored to the needs of the specific schizophrenic population involved. For example, in severely disturbed clients, the issues addressed should be as nonthreatening as possible. In less disturbed clients, groups can center on activities of daily living, and in still higher functioning clients, the focus can be on what schizophrenia is and how to live with it.

Individual Therapy

Although therapeutic approaches differ in detail, dependent upon the psychotherapeutic framework of the therapist, as a general rule, individual therapy with schizophrenic clients tends to be supportive. Developing a therapeutic relationship can be difficult with schizophrenic clients, especially with those who are paranoid. Also, the psychiatric nurse therapist must be careful, in supporting the client, to avoid supporting maladaptive or primitive thoughts or behavior. As with group therapy, it is often helpful to focus on performance of daily-living activities, such as shopping and paying bills. The psychiatric nurse therapist can also serve as a role model for appropriate behavior in a variety of different situations. Although intensive, insight-oriented psychotherapy has been used with some success in some schizophrenic clients, as a general rule such an approach should be used only with extreme caution, and then, only in the higher-functioning clients, as it may cause regression, acting out, and withdrawal.[27,32]

Family Therapy

Family therapy may be helpful, especially in reducing the rate of relapse of schizophrenic clients. Often, the schizophrenic client becomes the focus for problems that involve the family as a whole, and the identification of such family problems through a process of clarification of family boundaries and roles may be beneficial to the entire system, including the schizophrenic family member. Sometimes it is helpful to have groups composed of several schizophrenic clients and their families, called "multiple-family groups." Families of schizophrenic clients are often desperate for help and support, and one of the nurse's roles is often to provide support to the family, in terms of helping them understand schizophrenia as a disease process, allowing them to see that there are others who have similar problems, and giving them a sense of hope about the future.

Other Therapies

There are a variety of other therapies that have also been reported as helpful in schizophrenia, including occupational therapy, recreational therapy, rehabilitation therapy, dance therapy, art therapy, and psychodrama.

COMMON NURSING DIAGNOSES

Schizophrenia causes such pervasive dysfunction in so many areas of mental experience and behavior, that there are many different nursing diagnoses that are commonly associated with it. The most common are bizarre behavior, defensive coping (especially projection, distortion, and denial), emotional lability, fear, altered impulse control, noncompliance, altered perception and cognition (especially hallucinations, confusion, and delusions), regressed behavior, impaired resource management (including difficulty managing time and finances), disturbance in self-concept, self-care deficits (especially in daily-living skills such as personal hygiene, dressing, grooming), and suspiciousness. Other common nursing diagnoses include aggression, anxiety, impaired communication, depression, potential for elopement, guilt, altered health maintenance, potential for injury, loneliness, manipulation, altered nutrition, sexual dysfunction (especially reduced sexual drive, often secondary to neuroleptic medications), impaired social interaction, substance abuse (drugs, alcohol), and suicide potential.

CASE STUDY

Ed C is a 32-year-old man with a 10-year history of chronic paranoid schizophrenia. During childhood he was very social and did quite well in school, but after adolescence he started to become more isolative, preoccupied with magic and the occult, although such subjects were far from his family's beliefs. He would stay in his room in bed for days at a time, and while at the dinner table would suddenly blurt out statements such as "Stop looking that way!" or "Did you poison this chicken?" He entered college and did moderately well the first year, but failed most of his courses the second year. It was during his second year of college that he disappeared for several days and was discovered by the police walking along the expressway in the cold with no shoes on, muttering to himself. He claimed that the dean of his college was working with the CIA to extract information from his head about the workings of plants which, if ground up, could stop all disease. He was disheveled, with blisters on his feet, and would glance around behind himself and smile for no apparent reason. He claimed he knew about the CIA plot because something called "the group" had told him about it. This group he claimed was talking to him, even during the interview, but he would not disclose what these voices said. He was clutching a comb that he would occasionally place up to his ear, stating that the teeth of the comb were real teeth talking to him.

During his initial admission he was placed on a therapeutic regimen of haloperidol (Haldol), 10 mg twice a day, and, over several weeks, the voices diminished in intensity and he no longer spoke of the CIA plot. The dosage of haloperidol was increased to 10 mg three times a day, following which he had a dystonic reaction consisting of his tongue protruding from his mouth and his eyes rolling up into his head (oculogyric crisis), relieved by an intramuscular injection of 2 mg of benztropine mesylate (an anticholinergic drug). He was maintained on benztropine 2 mg bid for the next several days. The haloperidol dosage was not changed during this time. He continued to be withdrawn and isolated. His care for the nursing diagnosis of delusions is outlined in Nursing Care Plan 17-1.

SUMMARY

Schizophrenia is a mental disorder marked by a severe and often irreversible deterioration in personality, affect, and intellectual function that may affect as much as 1% of the population. The basis for the disorder is unknown, although impaired ego functions, deficits in attention and information processing, family difficulties, and dysfunction in dopamine transmission, especially in the frontal lobes and limbic system, all have been considered to play a role in the development of

Research Highlights

A recent epidemiologic study by Mednick and coworkers of persons at high risk for developing schizophrenia suggests that the second trimester may be a particularly critical period in brain development.[29] These researchers investigated psychiatric hospital diagnoses for all persons in greater Helsinki, who had been exposed to the type A2 influenza epidemic that occurred in Finland in 1957. They determined that those persons exposed to the epidemic during the second trimester of fetal development were at increased risk of later being admitted to a psychiatric facility with the diagnosis of schizophrenia. These investigators further went on to suggest that the timing of an insult to fetal development may be more important than the nature of the insult itself. Thus, it is possible that some cases of schizophrenia may be related to trauma, infection, or exposure to toxins during fetal development, especially during the second trimester. If it does turn out that developmental insults are an important risk factor for the development of schizophrenia, then it would be possible to begin primary preventive programs, especially in families of persons with schizophrenia who are already at higher risk for having children with schizophrenia. Although such considerations are in the future, nurses would play a very important role in any such primary preventive measures for schizophrenia, in terms of client guidance and education.

NURSING CARE PLAN 17–1

ED C

NURSING INTERVENTIONS*	OUTCOME CRITERIA

NURSING DIAGNOSIS: Delusions related to chronic paranoid schizophrenia

CLIENT GOAL: Begin to demonstrate some trusting behavior by initiating interactions with staff and other clients

■ Build trusting relationship with Ed by initiating brief supportive contacts	Increases time spent in contact with nurses
■ Encourage contact with other clients	Feels more comfortable with other clients and increases contact with them
■ Maintain adequate distance from Ed	Feels safe with staff, and not threatened

CLIENT GOAL: Increase sense of self worth

■ Accept client's limitations when delusions remain	
■ Maintain a stable environment for Ed by explaining client schedule and letting Ed know when you are leaving and when you will be back	Increased feeling of stability and comfort with staff
■ Generally talk about neutral subjects with Ed	
■ Reflect back the feeling expressed by the delusion	
■ Offer positive feedback for involvement in constructive activities	

* See also nursing interventions for nursing diagnosis: altered perception/cognition (delusions).

---

the disorder. The mainstay of treatment is the use of neuroleptic medications, although other drugs such as lithium are also occasionally of benefit. Group, individual, and family therapy may also be beneficial, especially when used in conjunction with neuroleptic medications.

References

1. American Psychiatric Association. Diagnostic and statistical manual of mental disorders, 3rd ed, revised. Washington, DC: American Psychiatric Association; 1987.
2. Andreasen NC. Thought, language, and communication disorders. I. Clinical assessment, definition of terms, and evaluation of their reliability. Arch Gen Psychiatry. 1979;36:1315.
3. Andreasen NC, Olsen S. Negative v positive schizophrenia: definition and validation. Arch Gen Psychiatry. 1982;39:789.
4. Baribeau-Braun J, Picton TW, Gosselin J-Y. Schizophrenia: a neurophysiological evaluation of abnormal information processing. Science. 1983;219:874–876.
5. Bateson G. Minimal requirements for a theory of schizophrenia. Arch Gen Psychiatry. 1960;2:477–491.
6. Berner P, Gabriel E, Hatschnig H, et al. World Psychiatric Association diagnostic criteria for schizophrenic and affective psychoses. Washington, DC: American Psychiatric Press; 1983.
7. Berrios GE. Positive and negative symptoms: a conceptual history. Arch Gen Psychiatry. 1985;42:95.
8. Callaway E, Naghdi S. An information processing model for schizophrenia. Arch Gen Psychiatry. 1982;39:339–347.
9. Creese I, Burt DR, Snyder SH. Dopamine receptor binding predicts clinical and pharmacological potencies of antischizophrenic drugs. Science. 1976;192:481–483.
10. Crow TJ. The two-syndrome concept: origins and current status. Schizophr Bull. 1985;11:471.
11. Freedman R, Adler LW, Gerhardt GA, et al. Neurobiological studies of sensory gating in schizophrenia. Schizophr Bull. 1987;13:669–678.
12. Geyer MA, Braff DL. Startle habituation and sensorimotor gating in schizophrenia and related animal models. Schizophr Bull. 1987;13:643–668.
13. Gottesman II, Shields J. Schizophrenia: the epigenetic puzzle. Cambridge: Cambridge University Press; 1982.
14. Hamilton M. Fish's schizophrenia. Bristol: Wright PSG, 1984.
15. Haracz JL. The dopamine hypothesis: an overview of studies with schizophrenic patients. Schizophr Bull. 1982;8:438–469.
16. Harding CM, Zubin J, Strauss JS. Chronicity in schizophrenia: fact, partial fact, or artifact? Hosp Commun Psychiatry. 1987;38:477–486.
17. Hare EH. Epidemiology of schizophrenia and affective psychoses. Br Med Bull. 1987;43:514.
18. Hartmann E. Schizophrenia: a theory. Psychopharmacology. 1976;49:1–15.
19. Hogarty GE, McEvoy JP, Munetz M, et al. Dose of fluphenazine, familial expressed emotion, and outcome in schizophrenia. Arch Gen Psychiatry. 1988;45:797.

20. Hornykiewicz O. Brain catecholamines in schizophrenia: a good case for noradrenaline. Nature. 1982;299:484–486.
21. Jackson DD, Weakland J. Schizophrenic symptoms and family interaction. Arch Gen Psychiatry. 1959;1:618–621.
22. Kendler KS, Gruenberg AM, Tsuang MT. Outcome of schizophrenic subtypes defined by four diagnostic systems. Arch Gen Psychiatry. 1984;41:149.
23. Levitt JJ, Tsuang MT. The heterogeneity of schizoaffective disorder: implications for treatment. Am J Psychiatry. 1988;145:926–936.
24. Loranger AW. Sex difference in age at onset of schizophrenia. Arch Gen Psychiatry. 1984;41:157.
25. Mason ST. Designing a non-neuroleptic antischizophrenic drug: the noradrenergic strategy. Trends Pharmacol Sci. 1983;4:353–355.
26. May PRA, Tuma AH, Dixon WJ. Schizophrenia: a follow-up study of the results of five forms of treatment. Arch Gen Psychiatry. 1981;38:776–784.
27. McGuffin P, Murray RM, Reveley AM. Genetic influence on the psychoses. Br Med Bull. 1987;43:531–556.
28. McKenna PJ. Pathology, phenomenology and the dopamine hypothesis of schizophrenia. Br J Psychiatry. 1987;151:288–301.
29. Mednick SA, Machon RA, Huttunen MO, Bonett D. Adult schizophrenia following prenatal exposure to an influenza epidemic. Arch Gen Psychiatry. 1988;45:189–192.
30. Meltzer HY, Sommers AA, Luchins DJ. The effect of neuroleptics and other psychotropic drugs on negative symptoms in schizophrenia. J Clin Psychopharmacol. 1986;6:329.
31. Parker G, Johnston P, Hayward L. Parental "expressed emotion" as a predictor of schizophrenic relapse. Arch Gen Psychiatry. 1988;45:806.
32. Pao P-N. Schizophrenic disorders. New York: International Universities Press; 1979.
33. Pearlson G, Coyle JT. The dopamine hypothesis and schizophrenia. In: Coyle JT, Enna SJ, eds. Neuroleptics: neurochemical, behavioral and clinical perspectives. New York: Raven Press, 1983:297–324.
34. Rabins P, Pauker S, Thomas J. Can schizophrenia begin after age 44? Compr Psychiatry. 1984;25:290.
35. Seeman P, Lee T, Chau-Wong M, Wong K. Antipsychotic drug doses and neuroleptic/dopamine receptors. Nature. 1976;261:717–718.
36. Sengel RA, Lovallo WR. A random process model of cognitive deficit in schizophrenia. Schizophr Bull. 1980;6:576–585.
37. Siegel C, Waldo M, Mizner G, Adler LE, Freedman R. Deficits in sensory gating in schizophrenic patients and their relatives. Arch Gen Psychiatry. 1984;41:607–612.
38. Stephens JH. Long-term prognosis and followup in schizophrenia. Schizophr Bull. 1978;4:25.
39. Stevens JR. An anatomy of schizophrenia. Arch Gen Psychiatry. 1973;29:177.
40. Tsuang MT, Simpson JC. Schizoaffective disorder: concept and reality. Schizophr Bull. 1984;10:14.
41. Tsuang MT, Winokur G, Crowe RR. Morbidity risks of schizophrenia and affective disorders among first degree relatives of patients with schizophrenia, mania, depression and surgical conditions. Br J Psychiatry. 1980;137:497.
42. Vaughn CE, Leff JP. The influence of family and social factors on the course of psychiatric illness. Br J Psychiatry. 1976;129:125–137.

18

Georgia Whitley

Clients With Delusional (Paranoid) Disorder

OBJECTIVES

After reading this chapter, the reader will be able to:
1. *Describe delusional (paranoid) disorder*
2. *Discuss the assessment of clients who may have a delusional (paranoid) disorder*
3. *Identify treatment modalities and related nursing roles in the care of clients with delusional (paranoid) disorder*
4. *List nursing diagnoses most commonly identified in clients with delusional (paranoid) disorder*
5. *Develop client goals that are appropriate for clients with delusional (paranoid) disorder*
6. *Select nursing interventions that are appropriate for clients with delusional (paranoid) disorder*
7. *Evaluate the effectiveness of nursing interventions for clients with delusional (paranoid) disorder.*

DESCRIPTION

Delusional (paranoid) disorder is distinguished by the presence of persistent, nonbizarre delusions that are not due to any other mental disorder, such as a schizophrenic, schizophreniform, mood, or organic mental disorder.[1] The delusional behavior is the most typical feature of these clients' behavior; auditory or visual hallucinations are not prominent.[1] Types of delusional disorder are distinguished by the delusional themes commonly seen and include erotomanic, grandiose, jealous, persecutory, and somatic (Box 18-1).[1] The occurrence of more than one delusional theme in the same individual is frequent. The most common type is persecutory with delusions ranging from simple to complex and usually following a theme. Individuals may believe that there is a conspiracy against them or that they are being cheated, spied upon, followed, poisoned, drugged, maligned, or harassed. Small incidents may be exaggerated and integrated into the delusional system. The delusions may become focused upon jealousy in which the individual becomes convinced, without cause, that the significant other is unfaithful. Ordinary events can become distorted into evidence of the partner's unfaithfulness.

The personality of the client with a delusional (paranoid) disorder may be characterized by resentment and anger, which can lead to violent behavior. Delusions that involve power, wealth, or prestige are common, as are ideas of reference in which the individual incorrectly interprets events or conversations as related to self. These individuals frequently contact public officials to seek correction of perceived injustices or to initiate legal actions. They are often described as seclusive, eccentric, and suspicious, and frequently live in social isolation.

Delusional disorders usually occur in middle or late adult life, with onset between 40 and 55 years of age, but they can also occur at a younger age. The course of the disorders is variable, with chronicity seen with some clients; however, waxing and waning of symptoms is common. Some clients have remission with no relapse, whereas others have remissions with subsequent relapses. The delusional individual usually has some degree of difficulty with interpersonal relationships; thus, marital and social relationships are frequently impaired. Intellectual functioning may be adequate, as may occupational functioning, depending upon the degree of interpersonal demands within the work situation. Severe stress involving drastic environmental changes or sensory deprivation may predispose individuals to the development of a delusional disorder.

A psychodynamic view of paranoid delusions holds that the delusions result from anxiety and give structure or logic to anxieties and doubts about the self.[3] Freud's original theory of paranoia related the delusional thinking in both sexes to projection and reaction formation in relation to unacceptable homosexual wishes.[2,3] Freud's premise was that the homosexual wish is unacceptable to the ego and undergoes projec-

---

BOX 18-1
Types of Delusional (Paranoid) Disorder[1]

TYPE	DESCRIPTION
EROTOMANIC	An erotic delusion in which one is loved by another Usually delusion of romantic, spiritual love rather than sexual love Usually about a person of higher status (famous person, boss, or even a stranger) Client may try to contact the person (calls, letters, gifts, visits, surveillance, stalking) Client may come into contact with the law because of efforts to pursue the person who is object of delusion
GRANDIOSE	Belief that one possesses great, unrecognized talent or insight or has made an important discovery Frequently seeks out governmental agencies Less common delusion of a special relationship with a prominent person (movie star, the President) May have religious content, and individuals with such delusions sometimes become leaders of religious cults
JEALOUS	Convinced without evidence that partner is unfaithful Collects physical "evidence" Confronts partner Tries to restrict or watch activities of partner May physically attack partner or suspected other "lover"
PERSECUTORY	Convinced, without cause, that other person is engaged in harmful acts toward the client Convinced that others are poisoning the client Convinced without cause that others are talking about the client
SOMATIC	Convictions that one emits a foul odor from body (skin, mouth, rectum) Conviction that one is infested with insects in or on the skin or has an internal parasite Convinced that certain parts of the body are misshapen and ugly or that certain parts are not functioning Usually consult nonpsychiatric physician for treatment

tion, becoming "he (she) hates me, therefore I must fear him (her)."

The paranoid person possesses an intolerance of hostile, aggressive, and omnipotent impulses that are unacceptable to the ego. To deal with these impulses, the individual projects them onto other persons or situations outside the self. The feelings of omnipotence expressed in delusional disorder relate to a fixation at, or a regression to, the narcissism more typical of 12 to 18 months of age.

Interpersonal theory, developed by Sullivan, describes a process by which the individual learns in childhood that it is best not to express anger and resentment, which leads to negative attitudes toward other people and life in general.[6] These attitudes inhibit the development of interpersonal relationships in which feelings and thoughts can be expressed, validated, or corrected. The individual projects weaknesses onto others and protects self-esteem by proclaiming how unworthy others are. The paranoid behaviors develop as blame is transferred from the self to others.

ASSESSMENT

When interviewing the individual to determine whether delusions are present, the health professional evaluates the client's statements for patterns of denial, rationalization, and projection. The client may say, for example, "I do not need treatment," and may blame others for events and circumstances. The client's need to maintain control and distance during the interview, as well as an aura of superiority and aloofness, may be evident. The individual may show anger, hostility, and aggression as a response to the fear and anxiety that is felt. Suspicion and lack of trust are manifested by the client through furtive glances at the surroundings and a wary approach toward others. Individuals with delusional disorder tend to be secretive about possessions and actions and frequently fear that others are trying to cause harm or take property. They may share only minimal information and often scrutinize all words and actions of others for possible negative intentions. They may use sophisticated language, discuss achievements, or tell about important people that are known, in an attempt to elevate self-esteem and control frightening situations.

As clients tell about life situations, unnecessary detail may be included with the exclusion of important data. Delusional material is often presented in a fashion in which logical connections are absent and logical conclusions cannot be drawn. The nurse may become aware of an emotional distancing when interacting with individuals with delusional disorder. In addition, clients may project angry feelings onto the nurse or other staff members. The nurse must evaluate the situation with the understanding that this behavior is not a personal response, but is generated by the client's fears.

TREATMENT MODALITIES AND RELATED NURSING ROLES

Many persons who have delusional disorder never come to the attention of mental health care professionals. They live a seclusive or eccentric life-style that they have adopted to deal with their delusions. Changes in the life situation that cause additional demands and stress may cause the behaviors to become more pronounced and may cause the individual to be brought to mental health professionals for assistance. These clients become psychiatric inpatients usually only in these crisis situations and are more commonly seen by health care professionals in outpatient settings.

Because the client may be fearful, the behavior of the nurse must promote trust and provide the opportunity for the client to trust. Focusing on the client's feelings, rather than on concrete details, is most helpful. Conversational themes that indicate anxiety and low self-esteem may be reflected back to the client, with an opportunity to explore these feelings. The nurse consciously steers away from any arguments about the content of delusions. Appropriate responses include a realistic report of how the nurse perceives reality, without a disagreement about the client's perceptions of reality. Being open, honest, and reliable with this client assists in establishing whatever trust is possible and is especially important because the client is on guard against any secretive or unknown activities. Letting the client know what is planned, as well as following through as anticipated, helps the client know that one can rely upon the nurse and what is promised.

An individual with a delusional (paranoid) disorder has a need to maintain control and interpersonal distance. The nurse must respect the client's need for privacy and emotional distance by allowing the client to set the pace for interpersonal interactions, being careful not to be overly emotional or assertive. The client is usually able to interact socially only gradually and, initially, with a limited number of persons. Because of low self-esteem, recognition and praise in appropriate situations will increase feelings of self-worth. If the client behaves in a suspicious and questioning manner, matter-of-fact answers and continuation of normal activities in a calm manner are indicated. Responding with kindness and in a helpful manner will eventually help decrease client fears and suspicions.

After communication has been established, the client is encouraged to discuss mistrust of others. Doubt may be interjected by the nurse about the reality of any delusional materials presented. The client needs to learn to handle stresses in positive ways, rather than using defensive maneuvers such as denial and projection. Counseling with family members and employers to help them understand the client's behavior and to give direction for how to be supportive will help reduce stress for the client and others. Health teaching with the client will include positive ways of handling stress, such as talking over concerns with appropriate persons, participation in physical activities (sports, walking, jogging, swimming), use of music for relaxation, and progressive muscular relaxation. If the client has a sensory impairment that adds to isolation and stress, corrective measures such as hearing aids, contact lenses, or glasses are indicated. Other environmental hazards or necessities should be investigated and handled through use of community resources.

Some delusional systems are long-term and will not be eliminated by therapy. The goal with a client who has a fixed delusion is to help the client minimize the delusional system and its impact and maximize the focus of life on reality. Therefore, after initial assessment, discussions of the delusions are not encouraged. If medication therapy is deemed helpful, the physician may order neuroleptics to decrease anxiety and thereby reduce the delusions. Commonly used drugs include haloperidol (Haldol), chlorpromazine (Thorazine), and thioridazine (Mellaril). Because acutely ill clients with a delusional disorder frequently are unwilling to take pills, liquid medication may be the form of choice. The client and family members need to be taught about expected therapeutic effects of the medication, as well as possible side effects.

COMMON NURSING DIAGNOSES

Nursing diagnoses commonly found in clients with delusional disorder include:

- Ineffective individual coping
- Impaired social interaction
- Altered perception/cognition (delusions) (suspiciousness)
- Aggression (specify).

CASE STUDY

Bill, a 46-year-old tax accountant, came to the mental health clinic accompanied by his elderly parents. The family attorney and his parents had insisted that he seek help for his difficulties. Bill, who lives alone in his condominium, had been complaining that the four young, male graduate students who live next door to him have been brainwashing him for the past three years. Bill had built walls around his patio and otherwise fortified his condominium against his

neighbors' "brainwashing techniques." The neighborhood condominium association informed Bill that he could not make these changes in his property because of the restrictions of the association. Bill feels that the officers in the association are colluding with the four young men in their attempts to brainwash him. He sought the counsel of the family attorney to start legal proceedings against the association and his neighbors. The attorney was unable to persuade Bill that his thoughts and desire to sue were unreasonable and contacted Bill's parents. They were somewhat aware of Bill's problems and appreciated the assistance offered by their attorney relative to what to do about getting help for Bill. Together they persuaded him to come to the clinic.

Bill's psychiatric diagnosis is delusional (paranoid) disorder, persecutory type. Nursing diagnoses for Bill include ineffective individual coping related to inadequate coping methods and delusions; and impaired social interaction related to inability to engage in satisfying personal relationships, delusions, and unacceptable social behavior (see Nursing Care Plan 18-1).

SUMMARY

Delusional (paranoid) disorder is distinguished by the presence of nonbizarre delusions that are not due to any other mental disorder. Types of delusional disorder include erotomanic, grandiose, jealous, persecutory, and somatic. Delusional disorder generally occurs in middle or late adult life and may be chronic. Psychoanalytic theory describes the paranoid person's intolerance of hostile, aggressive, and omnipotent impulses that are unacceptable to the ego. To deal with these impulses, the individual projects them to persons or situations outside the self. Interpersonal theory describes the projections of weaknesses onto others as a protection of one's own self-esteem resulting in proclamations of the unworthiness of others. Paranoid behaviors develop as blame is transferred from self to others.

Therapy initially focuses on establishing a trusting relationship between the nurse and the client. Focusing on feelings and encouraging expression and exploration assist the client to deal with feelings in ways other than delusions. Because social isolation is common, gradual and limited social interactions are initiated as tolerated by the client. Self-esteem is increased

Research Highlights

The following are research problems derived from the study of nursing care of persons with delusional disorder:

1. Develop and validate an instrument that identifies persons at risk for developing delusions
2. Validation of nursing diagnoses specific to suspicious behavior patterns
3. Exploration of outcomes of nursing interventions with persons with delusional disorder
4. Comparison of treatment outcomes of therapy with

two groups, one that includes and one that does not include medication
5. Family studies of persons with delusional (paranoid) disorder
6. Study of the relationship of life events to the occurrence of delusional disorder
7. Study of the effects of client education upon treatment compliance by persons with delusional disorder.

BILL

NURSING INTERVENTIONS	OUTCOME CRITERIA

NURSING DIAGNOSIS: Ineffective individual coping related to delusions

CLIENT GOAL: Experience less preoccupation with delusional thought

- Focus on feelings and encourage expression of feelings
- Do not *argue* about content of delusions; interject *doubt* if appropriate
- Give honest perceptions of reality in feedback to Bill
- Be open, honest, and reliable in interactions with Bill to avoid generating any fearful or suspicious feelings
- Respect Bill's need for privacy and emotional distance as necessary
- Respond to suspicions of Bill with matter-of-fact answers and in a calm manner
- Encourage Bill to express feelings with others

Expresses and discusses feelings

CLIENT GOAL: Develop adaptive coping strategies

- Provide health teaching regarding positive ways of handling stress: talking over concerns with appropriate persons, participation in physical activities (sports, walking, jogging, swimming, biking), use of music for relaxation, and progressive muscular relaxation
- If indicated, teach Bill and family therapeutic value of medication therapy and daily routines that promote compliance
- Do not encourage discussion of delusional material after initial assessment

Uses constructive coping strategies

NURSING DIAGNOSIS: Impaired social interaction related to inability to engage in satisfying personal relationships, delusions, and unacceptable social behavior

CLIENT GOAL: Develop meaningful relationship(s)

- If possible, assist Bill to identify person(s) with whom relationship is desired and feasible
- Support Bill in initiating interactions on a regular basis

Interacts with identified person(s) on a regular basis

CLIENT GOAL: Identify new or previous leisure interests

- Complete leisure assessment; select one activity and plan ways to participate; support client in initial attempts

Engages in a leisure activity that involves some degree of social interaction

CLIENT GOAL: Experience support from significant others

- Counsel family members and employer, if appropriate, to help them understand Bill's behavior and to give direction as to how to be supportive of Bill
- Provide opportunity for Bill and significant others to talk and focus on feelings/ stresses

Explores factors relative to positive adjustments with family and employer

CLIENT GOAL: Engage in positive behaviors and eliminate negative behaviors

- Plan daily schedules with Bill that minimize environmental factors that stimulate suspicions; focus daily living patterns upon positive routines and positive factors in Bill's life

Uses positive factors in environment; negative stimuli are decreased or eliminated

---

Clients With Delusional (Paranoid) Disorder

through appropriate recognition and praise. Health
teaching includes positive ways of handling stress to
avoid reverting to delusional behaviors when stressed.

References

1. American Psychiatric Association. Diagnostic and statistical manual of mental disorders, 3rd ed, revised. Washington, DC: American Psychiatric Association; 1987.
2. Freud S. Psychoanalytic notes on an autobiographic account of a case of paranoia dementia paranoides, vol 12. London: Hogarth Press; 1959.
3. Freud S. The complete psychological works of Sigmund Freud, vol 14. London: Hogarth Press; 1959.
4. Kim M, McFarland G, McLane A. Pocket guide to nursing diagnoses, 3rd ed. St Louis: CV Mosby; 1989.
5. McFarland G, Wasli E. Nursing diagnoses and process in psychiatric mental health nursing. Philadelphia: JB Lippincott; 1986.
6. Sullivan HS. Clinical studies in psychiatry. New York: WW Norton; 1956.

19

Georgia Whitley

Clients With Psychotic Disorders Not Elsewhere Classified

DESCRIPTION
ASSESSMENT
TREATMENT MODALITIES AND RELATED NURSING ROLES
COMMON NURSING DIAGNOSES
CASE STUDY

OBJECTIVES

After reading this chapter, the reader will be able to:

1. Describe psychotic disorders not elsewhere classified
2. Discuss the assessment of clients who may have a psychotic disorder not elsewhere classified
3. Identify treatment modalities and related nursing roles in the care of clients with psychotic disorders not elsewhere classified
4. List nursing diagnoses most commonly identified in clients with psychotic disorders not elsewhere classified
5. Develop client goals that are appropriate for persons with psychotic disorders not elsewhere classified
6. Select nursing interventions that are appropriate for clients with psychotic disorders not elsewhere classified
7. Evaluate the effectiveness of nursing interventions for persons with psychotic disorders not elsewhere classified.

DESCRIPTION

The diagnostic class, *psychotic disorders not elsewhere classified*, encompasses disorders that do not fit into the categories of organic mental disorders, schizophrenia, delusional disorder, or mood disorder with psychotic features.[1] Four specific categories exist in this class: brief reactive psychosis, schizoaffective disorder, induced psychotic disorder, and schizophreniform disorder.[1] A fifth category, psychotic disorder not otherwise specified, describes psychotic disorders that do not meet the criteria for any specific psychotic disorder or when there is not adequate information on which to base a specific diagnosis.[1] These psychotic disorders are distinguished by one or more of the following characteristics: mood changes, regressive behavior, personality disintegration, reduced levels of awareness, difficulties in functioning, and impairment in reality testing (Box 19-1 gives additional information). These characteristics of psychotic disorders provide an extensive range of needs of nursing care for these clients. Boundaries between diagnostic categories are not always clear. The focus of nursing assessment, diagnosis, and intervention are guided by the individual needs and behaviors of the client.

Because this classification includes four specific categories and a residual one, causative and epidemiologic factors, as well as course of illness are considered separately for each category. *Brief reactive psychosis* usually occurs in late adolescence or early adulthood with acute psychotic symptoms usually present for one to two days but not more than one month. Secondary symptoms such as lowered self-esteem or mild depression may persist for a few weeks with an eventual return to pre-illness level of functioning. Preexisting personality disorders (paranoid, histrionic, narcissistic, schizotypal, borderline) and major stress are predisposing factors in this disorder.[1]

In *schizoaffective disorder*, at one time, the client presents with both a schizophrenic and a mood disturbance and, at another time, with psychotic symptoms without a mood disturbance. The typical age of onset is thought to be early adulthood, with a tendency toward a chronic course. This disorder is diagnosed less frequently than schizophrenia.[1]

In *induced psychotic disorder*, a delusional system develops in the client as a result of a relationship with a person with an established delusion. If the relationship is discontinued, the delusional beliefs of the client will decrease or disappear. This disorder was formerly termed "folie à deux." The age of onset is variable, with a chronic course if the relationship cannot be altered. This is a rare disorder that occurs most frequently in females.

Schizophreniform disorder is characterized by the same features as schizophrenia, but with a total dura-

---

BOX 19–1
Psychotic Disorders Not Elsewhere Classified[1]

TYPES	CLINICAL MANIFESTATIONS
BRIEF REACTIVE PSYCHOSIS	Sudden onset of a psychotic disorder of *at least a few hours but no more than one month duration* with eventual *full return to previous level of functioning;* symptoms occur immediately *after a recognizable psychosocial stressor* Characterized by emotional turmoil and one of the following: (1) incoherence or loose associations, (2) delusions, (3) hallucinations (4) catatonic or disorganized behavior Behavior may be bizarre, suicidal, or aggressive and affect is often inappropriate Usually occurs in *adolescence or early adulthood*
SCHIZOAFFECTIVE DISORDER	Client presents symptoms of schizophrenia and of a mood disorder concurrently, but at another time presents hallucinations and delusions without mood symptoms Typical age of onset is thought to be *early adulthood* Appears to be a *chronic* course of illness
INDUCED PSYCHOTIC DISORDER	Client develops a delusional system as a *result of a close relationship with another person who has an already established delusion* If the relationship with the person with the delusion is interrupted, the client's delusions will diminish or disappear The course of the illness is usually *chronic* because it usually involves a long-term relationship that is not easily altered
SCHIZOPHRENIFORM DISORDER	Identical with manifestations of schizophrenia, with the exception that the *duration* (onset, acute phase and residual phases) *is less than six months* Characterized by emotional turmoil and confusion, acute onset, and resolution, with *a likelihood of returning to previous levels of functioning*
PSYCHOTIC DISORDER NOT OTHERWISE SPECIFIED (ATYPICAL PSYCHOSIS)	Age of *onset is variable* Psychotic symptoms are present but do not meet the criteria for any other nonorganic psychotic disorder Used when there is inadequate information to make a specific diagnosis

tion of fewer than six months. The client with schizophreniform disorder may experience vivid hallucinations, fear, confusion, and emotional distress. The relationship between schizophrenia and schizophreniform disorder is not clear, with some family and genetic studies suggesting that this disorder is distinct from schizophrenia, and some studies suggesting a relationship between the two disorders.[1]

The category *psychotic disorder not otherwise specified (atypical psychosis)* is appropriate when the client demonstrates psychotic symptoms, but does not demonstrate symptoms related to any of the other nonorganic psychotic disorders. This category is used when there is inadequate information available to the health team to enable the establishment of a specific diagnosis. If further data becomes available the diagnosis can be changed.

Psychoanalytic theorists state that psychotic behavior occurs when the ego can no longer withstand internal and external pressure arising from both the id and external reality. The psychotic individual may have a fragile ego related to inhibited ego development.[2] Life situations that threaten self-esteem, produce guilt, or stimulate angry or erotic impulses increase anxiety. Dysfunctional use of defenses to cope include escapes from reality through delusions, hallucinations, and other psychotic behaviors. The individual will try to repress the unacceptable impulses and thoughts and may begin to neglect activities of daily living. If anxiety escalates to the panic level, repression may begin to fail, and the individual may have difficulty distinguishing self from environment, communication becomes very disturbed, and capacity to relate to others is minimal.

According to interpersonal theorists, inadequacies and impairments in the parent–child relationship predispose the individual to behavioral problems in later years. Development of the child's self-concept depends upon the appraisals of significant others.[5] Intense anxiety in the parent–child relationship may lead to a negative self-concept and a lack of a sense of trust in the self and others. Anxiety may become an ever-present force in the life of this individual. A psychotic episode may be precipitated when dissociated (unconscious) portions of the self come into awareness and generate additional anxiety. An escape into psychosis is more comfortable than trying to cope with the negative, unacceptable parts of the self.

ASSESSMENT

The client who is experiencing a psychotic disorder not elsewhere classified requires a comprehensive assessment of individual functioning as well as an environmental evaluation of the family and social system by the mental health team. Safety needs and general physical needs may emerge as priorities because of the perceptual and problem-solving difficulties of the client. Abilities to meet basic needs and carry out activities of daily living may be impaired and require careful as-

sessment. Thought disorders and alterations in perceptions should be assessed for implications for client safety. Distortions of reality may lead to impulsive acts that are harmful to self or others. If the client receives psychotropic medications, the nurse will observe for therapeutic effects. Assessment of the home environment and the client's significant others will aid the health team in identifying the client's external support system, as well as needs for interventions within the system.

TREATMENT MODALITIES AND RELATED NURSING ROLES

Initially, the client may need to be hospitalized because of the severity of symptoms. The first treatment considerations concern the provision of safety for the client and others. If the client is agitated, a low-stimulus environment devoid of objects with which to harm self or others is provided. Observation and monitoring of behavior is necessary during this time.

The client may require special attention in relation to physical needs. Food and fluid intake need to be monitored. If the client is agitated, food can be provided in a quiet setting away from others. Portable food and fluids may be necessary if the client is unable to sit and eat in the customary manner. Food should be ready to eat and at a safe temperature for consumption, because the client may not attend to these details and could be harmed. Urinary and bowel elimination must be monitored, as it may be necessary to provide the client the opportunity to use the bathroom for elimination. Adequate roughage, fluids, and exercise must be provided to prevent constipation, especially if the client is receiving antipsychotic medication therapy.

Activity levels of the clients may range from stupor to hyperactivity. The hyperactive client needs a quiet environment, with provision for rest periods during the day and adequate sleep during the night. Bedtime rituals and other sleep-promoting activities as well as medication therapy, when indicated, are appropriate for the hyperactive psychotic client. The client who is withdrawn or slowed will need assistance with adequate activity. For the stuporous client this may mean passive range-of-motion exercise. Other clients may simply need assistance or encouragement for moving about or walking. If the client is receiving antipsychotic medication, the pulse and blood pressure should be monitored for postural hypotension, tachycardia, and arrhythmias.

If the client is unable or unmotivated to care for personal hygiene needs, staff members must tactfully assist the individual with oral hygiene, bathing, hair care, and dressing to maintain an acceptable appearance. Because a lowered self-esteem may be a predisposition to a psychotic disorder, the staff needs to help the client perceive the self realistically and to assist in identifying and building upon strengths. If the client is withdrawn, interaction needs to be patterned into daily routines, beginning with one-to-one relationships, with gradual extension to small then larger group activities and settings. If a client is overstimulated, one-to-one interactions of low intensity are appropriate until the individual is able to tolerate interactions with others without additional overstimulation.

When the client has hallucinations or delusions, the staff needs to provide reality orientation and assist the individual to feel safe and secure. Many psychotic experiences are very frightening and cannot be decreased until the accompanying fear and anxiety are diminished.

The home environment and interactions with significant others are explored, both as potential stressors that relate to the psychotic episode of the client and as a support system in the recovery process. Drug therapy needs to be explained to the client and the family, with both therapeutic effects and possible side effects included. A plan for continuing care, as necessary, should be established, with consensus from the client, family, and health team members. Drug therapy with antipsychotics is continued until the acute psychotic episode is over and the client begins to stabilize in functional abilities. Individual psychotherapy, group therapy, or family therapy may be initiated as the client becomes oriented to reality. These therapies are frequently helpful after the acute phases of the illness.

After short-term hospitalization, the client may be referred to day treatment or outpatient treatment. Depending upon the length of the illness, and the client's prior level of functioning and support system, the client may find rehabilitative services such as vocational rehabilitation, half-way houses, or foster home care helpful.

COMMON NURSING DIAGNOSES

The following nursing diagnoses are commonly found in clients with psychotic disorders not elsewhere classified:

- Aggression (extreme/violence)
- Self-care deficit: bathing/hygiene, dressing/grooming, feeding, toileting
- Altered perception/cognition (delusions/hallucinations)
- Anxiety
- Self-concept disturbance
- Altered impulse control
- Noncompliance
- Impaired communication
- Ineffective individual coping
- Suspiciousness
- Manipulation.

CASE STUDY

Shelia, a 38-year-old office manager for a large computer company, was hospitalized for psychiatric treatment. Her psychiatric history included a major depressive episode about six months previously in which she lost energy and motivation to do anything, had difficulty sleeping, lost her appetite, and could not concentrate enough to read or watch television. At that time, she had recently broken up with her live-in boyfriend. After he moved out, she became delusional, being extremely frightened that someone would break into her home and harm her or steal her possessions. She bought a burglar alarm system, installed new locks, got an unlisted phone number, and purchased a gun for protection. She was too frightened to leave the house to go to work and stayed home with the doors locked and the shades drawn. Shelia felt that she heard voices of neighbors and strangers alike threatening to harm her or steal from her. Her sleep was disturbed, and she was up each morning by 4:00 or 5:00 AM. During the initial illness, Shelia dropped from her normal weight of 118 lb to 97 lb. At that time, Shelia was hospitalized for three weeks and was treated with antipsychotic and antidepressant medication. She continued the medication therapy upon discharge and was seen as an outpatient. She regained most of the weight she had lost and returned to her job. During a recent outpatient session, Shelia told her therapist that she thought that people were plotting to harm her or steal from her and that she

Research Highlights

Following are some suggestions for nursing research in areas related to the care of clients with psychotic disorders:

1. Investigate the relationship between stressful life situations and the occurrence of psychotic disorders not elsewhere classified
2. Conduct a retrospective client survey of persons who experienced a psychotic disorder not elsewhere classified to determine which nursing interventions clients perceived as assisting in their recovery
3. Conduct a descriptive study of nursing interventions that are effective in diminishing delusions, hallucinations, and other psychotic behaviors

4. Study the therapeutic milieu to determine which characteristics are helpful in the management of clients with psychotic behavior not elsewhere classified
5. Evaluate client compliance in taking antipsychotic medication after discharge when the inpatient diagnosis was a psychotic disorder not elsewhere classified
6. Compare posthospitalization adjustments of clients with psychotic disorders not elsewhere classified who are compliant with their medication regimen with similar clients who are noncompliant with their medication regimen.

NURSING CARE PLAN 19–1[3,4]

SHELIA

NURSING INTERVENTIONS	OUTCOME CRITERIA

NURSING DIAGNOSIS: Aggression related to fear and tension

CLIENT GOAL: Express no violence toward self or others

■ Encourage Shelia to express and discuss fears ■ Mutually develop strategies for appropriate nonverbal ways of dealing with tension ■ Administer psychotropic medications as indicated	Expresses fears No evidence of violence toward self or others

NURSING DIAGNOSIS: Altered cognition/perception related to psychological conflicts and stress

CLIENT GOAL: Have decreased frequency and duration of irrational thinking and replace with reality-based thoughts

■ During assessment, allow Shelia to express irrational thoughts ■ Focus on feelings engendered by irrational thinking ■ Refocus Shelia on here-and-now realities after discussing delusions and feelings related to irrational thinking ■ Teach Shelia thought-stopping and thought-switching as techniques for dealing with irrational thoughts	Corrects irrational thinking and focuses on reality-based thinking
■ Provide safe, secure environment ■ Initially assist Shelia to describe auditory hallucinations and to specifically identify what, who, when, where, and how of hallucinations ■ Share your own perceptions of reality with Shelia matter-of-factly; do not argue with Shelia about her perceptions ■ Teach Shelia to use work or diversional activities to maintain a focus on reality	Experiences decreased auditory hallucinations through participation in work or diversional activities

NURSING DIAGNOSIS: Self-esteem disturbance related to lack of positive feedback

CLIENT GOAL: Experience increased self-esteem

■ Spend time with Shelia; communicate acceptance and unconditional positive regard
■ Assist Shelia to focus on strengths and potentials
  Help Shelia to identify and to list strengths
  Encourage participation in activities with potential for success
  Give positive feedback as well as encouraging Shelia to develop own opinions of self-worth
■ Assist Shelia to practice assertive communication skills
■ Help Shelia set up schedule of positive reinforcement for self: leisure time, buys something new, takes self out to eat
	Experiences increased self-esteem demonstrated by: participates successfully in activities; accepts appropriate positive feedback; uses assertive communication skills; self-provision of positive reinforcement

NURSING DIAGNOSIS: Ineffective individual coping related to crisis and inadequate coping methods

CLIENT GOAL: Objectively assess life situation

■ Encourage Shelia to describe life situation	Analyzes life situation realistically Continued

NURSING CARE PLAN 19-1[3,4]

SHELIA *Continued*

NURSING INTERVENTIONS	OUTCOME CRITERIA
CLIENT GOAL: Develop an awareness of emotional responses to stressful situations	
■ Assist Shelia in describing emotional responses to stressful situation	Achieves realistic perception of own responses to stress
CLIENT GOAL: Construct a plan for dealing with stressful situations	
■ Teach Shelia problem solving skills in relation to stressful situations 　Identify strategies 　Role-play responses 　Identify and implement anxiety-reducing activities	Uses coping resources to resolve stress-producing situation

had not gone to work for the past two weeks. She did not appear depressed. Shelia's parents stated that Shelia's behavior had been very bizarre for the previous two weeks and agreed that hospitalization was necessary. The DSM-III-R diagnosis for Shelia was schizoaffective disorder. Nursing diagnoses for Shelia included aggression related to fear and tension; altered cognition/perception related to psychological conflicts; self-esteem disturbance related to lack of positive feedback; and ineffective individual coping related to crisis and inadequate coping strategies (see Nursing Care Plan 19-1 for a sample care plan for Shelia).

SUMMARY

Five categories exist in the diagnostic class, psychotic disorders not elsewhere classified: (1) brief reactive psychosis, (2) schizoaffective disorder, (3) induced psychotic disorder, (4) schizophreniform disorder, and (5) psychotic disorder not otherwise specified (atypical psychosis). Life situations in which the individual is unable to cope and the anxiety level increases to an intolerable level may cause the person to escape from reality through psychotic behaviors. Safety needs and

general physical needs are initial priorities in the care of these individuals. Reality orientation and a safe, secure environment will help the client deal with hallucinations or delusions. Acutely psychotic individuals are initially hospitalized then referred to day treatment, outpatient treatment, or other rehabilitative services.

References

1. American Psychiatric Association. Diagnostic and statistical manual of mental disorders, 3rd ed, revised. Washington, DC: American Psychiatric Association; 1987.
2. Friedman AM, Kaplan HI, Sadock BJ, eds. Comprehensive textbook of psychiatry, 3rd ed. Baltimore: Williams & Wilkins; 1980.
3. Kim M, McFarland G, McLane A. Pocket guide to nursing diagnoses, 3rd ed. St Louis: CV Mosby; 1989.
4. McFarland G, Wasli E. Nursing diagnoses and process in psychiatric mental health nursing. Philadelphia: JB Lippincott; 1986.
5. Sullivan HS. The interpersonal theory of psychiatry. New York: WW Norton; 1953.

20

Jennifer A. Turner
Sharon A. Link

Clients With Mood Disorders

OBJECTIVES

After reading this chapter, the reader will be able to:

1. *Define types of mood disorders*
2. *Identify the epidemiologic characteristics of major depression and bipolar disorder*
3. *Describe the psychodynamics of mood disorders*
4. *Differentiate the characteristics of major depression and bipolar disorder over the life span*
5. *Select nursing diagnoses most commonly found in clients with major depression and bipolar disorder*
6. *Discuss current treatment modalities and related nursing roles*
7. *Develop a nursing care plan for a client with a mood disorder.*

TYPES OF MOOD DISORDERS

Affect can be defined as an immediately expressed and observed emotion, in contrast to *mood*, which is a pervasive and sustained emotion that markedly colors the person's perception of the world.[5] A disturbance of mood is the central feature of a *mood disorder*. A *mood syndrome* pertains to mood and related symptoms that occur together over a time period. A *mood episode* refers to a mood syndrome that is not due to a known organic factor and is not a part of a nonmood psychotic disorder.[5] Mood disorders are determined by the patterns of mood episodes. Mood disorders can be classified as depressive disorders or bipolar disorders.[5]

Depressive Disorders

The depressive disorders include major depression and dysthymia. *Major depression* is a mood disturbance in which there is one or more major depressive episodes that have the essential feature of depressed mood or loss of interest or pleasure in almost all activities. Associated symptomatology includes sleep and appetite disturbances; change in weight; loss of energy; psychomotor agitation or retardation; feelings of helplessness, hopelessness, and worthlessness; excessive or inappropriate guilt; decreased ability to concentrate; and suicidal ideation or attempts. These symptoms represent a change from previous functioning and occur most of the day, nearly every day, during a two-week period.[5] Major depression is subclassified as single episode or recurrent. The severity of a major depression is identified as mild, moderate, severe without psychotic features, or severe with psychotic features. *Dysthymia* is a chronic disturbance in mood characterized by depressed mood for most of the day, more days than not, for at least two years. A major depression that may be superimposed on a more chronic dysthymia is called a "double depression."

Bipolar Disorders

Bipolar disorders refer to mood disturbances that are characterized by mood swings from elated, expansive, or irritable mood with erratic hyperactivity (bipolar disorder, manic), to severely depressed (bipolar disorder, depressed). Bipolar disorders may also be classified as bipolar disorder, mixed; cyclothymia; or bipolar disorder not otherwise specified. The central feature of bipolar disorder is one or more manic episodes, which are usually, but not always, accompanied by one or more major depressive episodes. In cyclothymia there is a more chronic mood disturbance of at least two years duration (one year for children and adolescents). There may be numerous periods of depressed moods or loss of interest or pleasure, as well as numerous hypomanic episodes (which are less intense than manic episodes). Bipolar disorders may also be subclassified as

bipolar I or bipolar II. Bipolar I is characterized by periods of mania, often accompanied by periods of depression. Bipolar II involves milder hypomanic periods and severe depressive periods, which often require hospitalization.[1,2] The danger of suicide and suicidal attempts is highest in those with bipolar II disorder.

EPIDEMIOLOGY

Mood disorders—specifically major depression, bipolar disorder, and dysthymia—affect 10 to 15 million Americans (5%–7%) at any given time. Some studies have estimated that one in four persons will experience some type of mood disturbance during his or her lifetime.[4] Many of those disturbances are mild and self-limiting, and the person does not seek help. In certain individuals, however, these minor episodes constitute a risk factor for subsequent major episodes.[4] Recent studies have yielded significant sociodemographic characteristics and other factors that may be associated with major depression and bipolar disorder (Table 20-1).

The National Institute of Mental Health (NIMH) Epidemiologic Catchment Area Study (ECA) surveyed over 18,000 nonhospitalized adult subjects from five locations. Results of that study indicated that a six-month prevalence of all mood disorders was 5.8%, and a lifetime prevalence of all mood disorders was about 8.3% of the population.[38] By extrapolation, the total expected number of people affected in the United States is between 9.6 million with six-month prevalence and 13.7 million with a lifetime history of a depressive disorder.[38]

The ECA program study assessed the lifetime prevalence of suicide attempts. Results showed that in individuals with no lifetime history of any mental disorder, the rate of suicide attempts was 1%. Among those with a lifetime history of a depressive disorder, the rate of suicide attempts was 18% for those with major depression, 24% for those with bipolar disorder, and 17% for those with dysthymia.[38] It is estimated that 16,000 suicides in the United States annually are associated with depressive disorder. Murphy found that mood disorders were associated with increased general mortality and, to a small degree, also with natural death. The relationship between depression and death was significantly more pronounced for men.[34]

Major Depression

Major depression affects approximately 7% of the adult population. Epidemiologic studies identified 13% to 20% of the population with depressive symptoms.[8] There is a progressive increase in prevalence of depression for each cohort of individuals born during successive decades this century.[21,27,40] Studies of depression also show an earlier age at onset of depression among younger cohorts, suggesting the rate of depressive disorders may be rising in successively younger

TABLE 20–1
Epidemiology of mood disorders[39,56,57]

EPIDEMIOLOGICAL CATEGORY	MAJOR DEPRESSION	BIPOLAR DISORDER
Lifetime risk	8–12% men 20–26% women	0.6–0.9% in industrialized nations 1.2% in American adults
Incidence	247:100,000–598:100,000/yr (women) 82:100,000–201:100,000/yr (men)	7.4:100,000–32:100,000/yr (women) 9:100,000–15.2:100,000/yr (men)
Sex	2:1 women/men	Almost all studies show almost equal distribution
Age of onset	Range 25–44 yr Age of highest risk is 18–44 yr, particularly 18–24 yr	Increasing incidence until aged 35; range 24–31 yr; 20% in adolescence; 20%–50% after aged 50
Race	Equally affects white/black	Most studies show no strong association
Marital status	2.5:1 separated or divorced; discord among married couples increases risk	More common among single or divorced individuals; hypothesized that marital status may change as result of this disorder
Social class	No particular pattern; depressive symptoms more common in lower social class	Most studies show may occur more frequently in upper socioeconomic class
Family studies	1.5 to 3 greater risk of depression among relatives of depressed probands compared with those in control	Have both bipolar and unipolar first-degree relatives in roughly equal frequencies

aged groups.[38,56] Also, for each birth cohort, the rates of depression for female subjects are greater than those for male subjects.[27]

Studies investigating children at high and low risk for depression show 6 to 17-year-old individuals of depressed parents at high risk.[56] A two- to threefold increase in major depression is evident in these children. The rate of concordance of depression in monozygotic twins is 50% compared with 23% in dizygotic twins.[21]

Bipolar Disorder

There has long been an acknowledged, but unexplained, connection between bipolar disorder and creativity and accomplishment. Many great artists, writers, musicians, religious and political leaders are either known or suspected to have been bipolar.[14] It has been estimated that approximately 1.2% of American adults, or between 1 and 2 million Americans, have bipolar disorder.[4] There is an increased incidence of bipolar disorder in first-degree relatives of persons with this disorder. Twin studies have shown that in monozygotic twins, if one twin develops bipolar disorder, the other twin has an approximate 80% chance of developing the illness. If one member of a pair of fraternal twins develops the illness, the other twin has an approximate 20% chance of developing the illness.[28] These results have tended to lend evidence to a genetic theory of transmission. A study by Akiskal concluded that early, abrupt onset of a psychotic depression in an individual with a family history of bipolar disorder was so predictive that those individuals were started and maintained on lithium regimen after the episode had

been controlled.[3] DSM-III-R criteria for a major depressive episode and for a manic episode and the nursing diagnoses associated with each are shown in Tables 20-2 and 20-3, respectively.

ETIOLOGIC EXPLANATIONS
Psychoanalytic Theory

Abraham identified the role of ambivalence and the role of significant others in the predisposition to depression, viewed as a recurrence of childhood behavior that is inappropriate to adult behavior. He elaborated the role of early love relations in the development of later psychopathology.[17]

Freud believed depression was anger turned inward. The therapeutic aim was to redirect the anger outward. Later Freud amended his theory and added that depression resulted from an overly severe superego. Two additional attributes have since been added. These are pathologic dependency and self-inhibition.[17] Freud believed that inhibition of functions, including interest in the external world, was a result of the narcissistic wound that absorbed nearly all the ego energy. Mania, in psychoanalytic terms, is best understood as a defense against depression. This defense involves both a denial and a reversal of affect. As depression is seen as a reaction to narcissistic injury and loss, mania appears to be the ego's insistence that the injury has been repaired, the superego conquered, and narcissistic supplies replenished. This is only transient, however, and depressive feelings usually return.[31]

TABLE 20-2
DSM-III-R criteria for major depressive episode and associated nursing diagnoses

DSM-III-R CRITERIA[5]	NURSING DIAGNOSES
Depressed mood	Disturbance in self-esteem (chronic, low self-esteem); depression; loneliness; anger
Diminished interest or pleasure in all activities most of the day	Activity intolerance (psychological)*; depression
Significant weight loss or weight gain	Nutrition altered, either more or less than body requirements
Insomnia or hypersomnia	Sleep pattern disturbance
Psychomotor agitation or retardation	Agitation; activity intolerance (physiologic)
Fatigue or loss of energy	Fatigue*
Feelings of worthlessness or excessive or inappropriate guilt	Hopelessness; powerlessness; guilt
Diminished ability to think or concentrate	Altered perception/cognition; confusion; memory loss
Recurrent thoughts of death	Aggression (extreme/violence); suicide potential
Depressed mood with psychotic features	Altered perception/cognition; delusions; hallucinations
	Other: anxiety; communication, impaired; ineffective individual coping; fear; dysfunctional grieving; altered health maintenance; loneliness; postoverdose syndrome; sexual dysfunction; impaired social interaction; self-care deficit; somatization

* Other NANDA nursing diagnosis.

Interpersonal Theory

The interpersonal theory of depression emphasizes the role of environmental and familial factors in its development.[23] Meyer believed the client's response to environmental change and stress was a result of early developmental experiences within the family system and in social groups. Sullivan emphasized the significance of interpersonal processes that occur between people at any time.

Interpersonal difficulties are identified as both an antecedent (e.g., parental neglect, abuse) and a consequence of depression. Examples of interpersonal antecedents occurring during childhood include family disharmony, parental neglect, abuse and rejection, and loss of a parent. Children with one or more depressed parents have an increased chance of developing depression.[23]

Significant interpersonal antecedents occurring in adulthood include separation, divorce, other marital problems, losses (especially of loved ones or those associated with a strong interpersonal relationship), and the absence of supportive social relationships.[20,43]

An interpersonal consequence of depression is the effect it has on interpersonal difficulties. Briscoe and

TABLE 20-3
DSM-III-R criteria for a manic episode and associated nursing diagnoses

DSM-III-R CRITERIA[5]	NURSING DIAGNOSES
A distinct period of abnormally and persistently elevated, expansive, or irritable mood	Emotional lability
Inflated self-esteem or grandiosity	Self-esteem disturbance; chronic low self-esteem
Decreased need for sleep	Sleep pattern disturbance
More talkative than usual or pressure to keep talking	Impaired communication
Flight of ideas or subjective experience that thoughts are racing	Impaired communication; altered perception/cognition
Distractibility	Altered perception/cognition
Increase in goal-directed activity (either socially, at work or school, or sexually) or psychomotor agitation	Impaired social interaction; bizarre behavior; agitation
Excessive involvement in pleasurable activities that have a high potential for painful consequences	Altered impulse control
May have psychotic features along with disturbance of mood (delusions, hallucinations, or catatonic symptoms)	Altered perception/cognition; delusions
	Altered perceptions/cognition; hallucinations
	Self-care deficit
	Other: aggression; anger; ineffective individual coping; emotional lability; dysfunctional family processes; altered health maintenance; knowledge deficit; manipulation; noncompliance; nutrition, altered, less than body requirements; substance abuse (alcohol); substance abuse (drugs)

Smith studied the hypothesis that divorce was a consequence, rather than an antecedent of depression. Their interviews concluded that depression contributed to the marital disruption of 17 of the 45 subjects.[23]

Cognitive Theory

The cognitive theory of depression, originated by Aaron Beck, identifies depression as stemming from a world view based on false beliefs about one's self, the future, and the world. A central feature of this theory is that the depressed individual's negative view is usually a distortion of reality.[46] Therefore, other symptoms typical of depression (motivational deficits, suicidal impulses, sadness) are generated by distorted thinking patterns.[23]

Beck identifies cognitive triad, silent assumptions, and logical errors as necessary elements to the psychopathology of depression. The *cognitive triad* includes the negative view by depressed clients of themselves, their future, and their world, along with the belief that they are doomed for unhappiness. *Silent assumptions* are irrational beliefs or rules that significantly affect the depressed person's emotional, behavioral, and thinking patterns. *Depressive assumptions* are inferred by examining the situation, emotions, and themes associated with the various negative automatic thoughts.[23]

According to cognitive theory, a depressed person will utilize these dysfunctional assumptions more than adaptive assumptions. As the degree of depression becomes more severe, the individual's ability to think logically decreases immensely. Examples of *logical errors* include arbitrary inference (drawing conclusions without adequate evidence); selective abstraction (focusing on a specific negative detail while ignoring others); overgeneralization (drawing a general conclusion on a single incident); magnification or minimalization (overestimating or underestimating the importance of an event); personalization (relating events with oneself without evidence); and all-or-none thinking (thinking in absolute terms).[46]

Behavioral Theory

The dominant behavioral theory of depression is the social learning theory which postulates that psychological functioning can best be understood in terms of continuous reciprocal interactions among personal factors, such as cognitive processes, behavioral factors, and environmental factors.[19] Individuals are recognized as being in control of their behavior. The central key of behavioral theories of depression is that being depressed is a consequence of a decrease in person–environment interactions that have positive outcomes for a person, or an increase in the rate of punishing experiences, or a combination of such.[19]

Learned Helplessness Theory

Seligman's theory of learned helplessness as a cause of depression originated from laboratory studies involving animals. Human studies led to the assumption that learned helplessness was a model of depression. The main concept of this theory is that when individuals believe they have no control over their situation, are unable to reduce suffering or to gain praise or reinforcers in their environment, they experience feelings of helplessness and powerlessness.[30] If individuals have little success in mastering their environment, they develop hopelessness, passivity, and lack of assertiveness, and the susceptibility to depression increases.[30]

Abramson and coworkers designed a more complex version called attributional reformulation of learned helplessness. Individuals react to uncontrollable events by displaying distinct explanatory or causal styles. The result of this process is the individual experiencing passivity, cognition deficits, sadness, anxiety, hostility, decreased aggression, decreased neurochemical balance, and increased susceptibility to disease.[36]

Biologic Theories

The most common biologic theories concern monoamine and other neurotransmitter systems, neuroendocrine factors, limbic system defects, circadian rhythm, and genetic transmission. Neurotransmitters originate from the brain to provide the means by which the brain changes and regulates mood, behavior, and virtually all bodily functions.[52] Neurotransmitters may be implicated in mood disorders caused by faulty synthesis of transmitters, dispatching wrong amounts, excesses not broken down or withdrawn, or by receptor neurons malfunctioning.[14]

James and Cohen-Cole, in a review of the literature,[21] found the monoamine hypotheses to be the most widely accepted biologic explanation of depression. This hypothesis is founded on the discovery that drugs (such as reserpine) that are capable of causing or alleviating depression, affect monoamine neurotransmission.[21] Neurotransmitters that have been implicated in mood disorders include (1) norepinephrine, (2) serotonin, (3) dopamine, and (4) acetylcholine. Both unipolar and bipolar research subjects have been found to react with a similar exaggerated release of norepinephrine when clinically stressed, although at rest, their levels are dissimilar.[14] Low levels of serotonin have been noted in individuals exhibiting impulsive violence and suicidal behavior. This appears to be an inherited biochemical trait.[14]

Most neuroendocrine research points to an overactive hypothalmus–pituitary–adrenal axis. Simmons-Alling found that theories involving the limbic system are based upon a hypothesis of "kindling" of electrical activity (or seizure) in the limbic system that interferes with neurotransmission, forming the rationale for the use of anticonvulsants in mood disorders.[49]

Ryan and associates found that in the human body there seems to be a characteristic daily rhythm to most every function. Though disruptions in the body's daily cycles have not been found to cause mood disorders, there are reasons to investigate them. They cite the cyclic nature of rapid cycling bipolar and seasonal affective disorders, as well as the recurrent nature of mood disorders in general. In addition, symptoms of depression may include diurnal variation and variations in the sleep–wake cycle.[45]

Genetic Theory

Family, twin, and adoptive studies had suggested a genetic basis in bipolar disorder. In 1987, the National Institute of Mental Health announced a major breakthrough in the field of genetic research. Bipolar disorder was found to be linked to DNA markers on chromosome 11 in the Old Order Amish (OOA).[48]

ASSESSMENT
Data Collection

Data collection includes a chronology of events that lead the client to seek treatment at this time and the client's perception of the problem. Typically (but not always) a client with a mood disorder will present with a subjective complaint of an alternation of mood (Box 20-1). There are also biologic, psychological, and sociological manifestations of mood disorders. Biologically, there may be alterations in eating patterns, elimination habits, sleeping patterns, psychomotor activity, level of energy, menstrual cycle, and libido. There may also be a seasonal component associated with the presenting problem. Psychologically, there may be affective and cognitive changes. Psychotic symptoms that are mood congruent may also be present. Socially, there may be changes in behavior that affect social interaction and communication. Suicidal or homicidal ideation may be present, and assessment for potential is critical. Any recent losses or life changes should be noted.

Past psychiatric history is a key part of the assessment process as it helps to provide a longitudinal picture of the client. Previous psychiatric treatment (both outpatient and hospitalizations), treatment modalities utilized, and responses to treatment are extremely important. Any family history of psychiatric illness is noted.

Psychosocial history is also obtained from the client. Relevant factors assessed include (1) personal data, (2) educational and vocational data, (3) family history, (4) ethnic and cultural factors, and (5) coping mechanisms used by the client.

The medical history comprises the past medical history, current physical findings, current laboratory findings, and medication usage. A dexamethasone suppression test, the corticotropin-releasing hormone infusion, or a thyroid-releasing hormone infusion may be performed.[52] The use of prescribed medication,

over-the-counter drugs, and illegal substances is identified because mood disorders may be drug-induced or related to physiologic dysfunction.[9] Disruption in affect or mood may be found in many psychiatric disorders (Table 20-4).

Assessment Scales

Inventories or scales can be utilized to assist in assessing the presence or severity of a manic or major depressive episode. These include the Minnesota Multiphasic Personality Inventory–Mania Scale, the Hamilton Rating Scale for Depression, the Zung Self-Rating Depression Scale, the depressive subsection of the Schedule for Affective Disorders and Schizophrenia, and the Geriatric Depression Scale.[30,43,52]

Mental Status

Clients with major depression often have an overall unkempt appearance because of disinterest in how they look, a dull facial expression with furrows between the eyes, the corners of the mouth turned downward, and Veraguth's fold (a peculiar triangle-shaped fold in the nasal corner of upper eyelid).[29,33] They may have poor eye contact, usually looking downward or staring into the distance. Retardation (paucity of movement with slumped shoulders) is more frequently observed in younger clients, whereas agitation (restlessness, pacing, and handwringing) is more common in the elderly.[29] The clients often speak in a very low, toneless voice in a slow manner or even in inaudible monotones. Clients may have crying episodes and may be irritable. The mood exhibited by clients with major depression encompasses an aura of sadness, gloom, despair, pessimism, and hopelessness. The relationship of the mood to the content of the conversation should be noted. The severity of the depression and the immediate risk of suicide are assessed by inquiry into the client's thoughts about death, any possible plans or written notes, availability of means to attempt suicide (firearms, drugs), and any previous attempts. The client may exhibit delusions of deserved punishment, of being controlled, or of persecution.[5] Occurrence of dreams (especially of the past) is not uncommon.[33] Assessment of hallucinatory material involves themes of guilt, punishment, personal inadequacy, death, nihilism, and disease.[3,5,24] Indecisiveness and decreased ability to concentrate may be evident. Orientation and memory are more impaired in the elderly.

The client with a bipolar disorder may present with either a major depressive episode or a manic episode. A client presenting with a depressive episode would appear as previously described under assessment for major depression. A client presenting with a manic episode may be dressed rather flamboyantly and with garish makeup. There may be hyperactivity (at times to the point of being aggressive), and hyperverbal with pressured speech. The mood may be elated or irritable.

BOX 20-1
Characteristics of Mood Disorders Across the Lifespan

MAJOR DEPRESSION	BIPOLAR DISORDER

CHILDREN

MAJOR DEPRESSION

Intense anxiety symptoms: inability to sit still, frequent picking/rubbing on skin
High degree of somatization
High degree of appetite changes and sleep disturbances
Depression expressed by reported sadness, appearing sad, frequent crying, poor self-concept as expressed by negative comments about body
High degree of social withdrawal
High percentage of severe neglect and/or abuse[12]

BIPOLAR DISORDER

Syndrome called manic-depressive variant syndrome of childhood: family history of affective dysfunction, hyperactivity, affective storms (disruptive temper outbursts), impairment in interpersonal relationships; secondary symptoms: sleep disturbance, short attention span, enuresis, some evidence of neuropathology[25]

Family history positive for bipolar manic illness with other family members exhibiting seemingly related symptoms of dysphoria, alcoholism, and learning disabilities; clinical symptoms: disturbance of affect/dysphoria, hyperexcitability, lability, disturbance of academic achievement, distractibility, poor concentration, impulsivity, transient rage outbursts; psychological test pattern with high verbal abilities and significantly lower performance scores[25]

ADOLESCENCE

MAJOR DEPRESSION

Increased antisocial behaviors: aggression, leaving home, reluctance to cooperate with family, substance abuse
Decrease in social activities
Difficulty with school, difficulty concentrating
Depression manifested by sulkiness, increased emotionality, inattention to personal appearance
Psychomotor agitation: pacing, hand-wringing
Psychomotor retardation: decreased speech, slow to respond
Sleep disturbances: hypersomnia
Anorexia is frequent

BIPOLAR DISORDER

Often presents differently than adult-onset mania with more symptoms especially delusions and ideas of reference
May appear explosive and/or disorganized
Behavioral dyscontrol with physical aggressiveness and conflict with law (more frequently than in adults); (follow-up an average of 15 years later showed equivalent or superior outcome compared with adult onset mania); 20% of adolescents hospitalized with a depressive episode developed mania within a three-year follow-up[25]

ADULT

MAJOR DEPRESSION

Anhedonia
Diurnal variation
Psychomotor retardation
Poor appetite
Fatigue
Hopelessness

BIPOLAR DISORDER

Distinct period of abnormally and persistently elevated, expansive, and irritable mood
Inflated self-esteem or grandiosity
Decreased need for sleep
Delusions, hallucinations
More talkative than usual or pressure to keep talking
Flight of ideas or subjective feelings that thoughts are racing
Distractibility
Decreased goal-directed activity
May have psychotic features
Excessive involvement in pleasurable activities which have high consequence for painful consequences

ELDERLY

MAJOR DEPRESSION

Increased somatization and increased concern over physical problems
Increased vegetative signs: poor appetite, easy fatigability, sleep disturbances (especially early in morning), weight loss, decreased interest in everyday tasks
Increased agitation
Increased complaints of pain
Increased memory impairment, decreased concentration, slowed thinking
May be mistaken for dementia

BIPOLAR DISORDER

Manic episodes tend to be atypical
Overactivity not as pronounced and may be mistaken for agitated depression
Manic and depressive symptoms may be mixed at any time
Speech may be more circumstantial or with obsessional quality as contrasted with pressured flight of ideas in younger clients
Paranoid delusions more common
Manic episode may be mistaken for delirium, especially if dementia coexists
More susceptible to neurotoxic effects of lithium: confusion, lethargy, ataxia, tremor and GI effects (nausea and vomiting, abdominal pain, diarrhea)
Depression more frequent than mania

FIXED, CORE SYMPTOMS FOR ALL AGES

Diminished ability to concentrate, sleep disturbance, suicidal ideation[12]

TABLE 20–4
Phenomena commonly associated with depression, mania, or addiction*

	DEPRESSION	MANIA	DEPRESSANTS	STIMULANTS	OPIOIDS
Agitation	x	x	i/w	i	w
Anhedonia	x		w	w	i/w
Anorexia	x		w	i	i/w
Anxiety	x	x	w	i	w
Apathy	x		i	w	i
Crying spells	x		i	w	w
Confidence		x	i	i	
Depressed libido	x		w	w	i/w
Distraction	x	x	w	i	i/w
Grandiosity		x	i	i	
Guilt	x		w	w	w
Hostility		x	i/w	i	i/w
Hyperactivity		x	w	i	
Hypersexuality		x	i	i	
Irresponsibility	x	x	i/w	i/w	i/w
Insomnia	x	x	w	i	
Lethargy	x		i	w	i
Memory problems	x		i		
Paranoia		x	w	i	
Sluggishness	x		i	w	i
Weight loss	x	x	i/w	i	i/w

(From Cameron D. Presentations of depression: depressive symptoms in medical and other psychiatric disorders. © New York: John Wiley & Sons; 1987. Reprinted with permission of John Wiley & Sons.)
* i, intoxication; w, withdrawal; x, often present.

Flight of ideas, in which a client appears to skip from one topic to another, and loosening of associations may be present. There may be mood-congruent delusions and hallucinations. Insight and judgment during mania are typically quite poor, resulting in great risk of inappropriate behavior and social crises.

Rapid Cycling in Bipolar Disorder

Rapid cycling is relatively uncommon and may be defined as four or more episodes or cycles per year. These cycles may be hours, days, weeks, or months in length. It is more common in women (92% of rapid cyclers in one study), especially those with low thyroid indices.[2,54] The largest group of rapid cyclers are clients in whom rapid cycling is associated with tricyclic antidepressant treatment. The mere initiation of antidepressant treatment in some appears to alter the body's circadian rhythm. Rapid cycling may also begin on its own and continue relentlessly over the years. Rapid cyclers have been noted to respond poorly to lithium, but Tegretol may be of some use.

TREATMENT MODALITIES AND RELATED NURSING ROLES

Psychoanalytic Therapy

Psychodynamic (expressive) psychotherapy is based on psychoanalytic theory. The aim is to examine the repetitive dysfunctional patterns of behavior and cognition that led the individual to a major depression or that occur during mania. Expected outcome of the therapy would be to increase insight into those behaviors and cognitions and to alter dysfunctional patterns. Psychoanalysis is the most intensive open-ended form of therapy. It utilizes free association, the aim of which is to ultimately alter the character structure of the individual. Psychoanalysis would not be attempted with a client in a manic episode or with a client experiencing a major depression with psychotic features. Early in treatment a combination of therapies might be utilized.

Interpersonal Therapy

Interpersonal psychotherapy is a short-term therapy focused at reducing symptoms and improving interpersonal functioning. The following problems experienced by a depressed person, for example, are addressed: (1) interpersonal problems associated with the depression, (2) depressive symptoms, and (3) demoralization that occurs in relation to (1) and (2). The client and therapist explore circumstances associated with the development of the depressive symptoms and ways of dealing more effectively with these circumstances in the future. This structured therapy usually focuses on one or two current interpersonal problems. Four problem areas that are common in depressed clients are grief, interpersonal role disputes, role transitions, and interpersonal deficits.[11,43] Other interpersonal problems may exist. The therapist has a lead role and pursues change in the client by utilizing education, problem solving, social manipulation, and management of the demoralization experienced by the client.

Cognitive Therapy

Cognitive therapy focuses on changing faulty thinking related to negative expectations of self, environment, and the future to more realistic and logical conditions[18,47] (see Chapter 42). The cognitive therapist works with the client to examine the validity of thoughts by providing tools to enable the client to overcome present problems and prevent reoccurrence. A cognitive framework can be used by nurses to mobilize depressed clients into activity. For example, step (1) nurse invites client to participate in special activity; step (2) if client refuses, nurse emphasizes the importance of client stating reasons for not wanting to participate; step (3) nurse and client work together to evaluate validity of these reasons; step (4) nurse invites client to test validity of his or her ideas by participating in activity; and step (5) nurse helps client recognize how favorable outcome contradicts his or her negative predictions.[32]

Behavioral Therapy

Behavioral therapy uses learning theory, behavioral analysis, reinforcement, and behavior modification as its primary concepts (see Chapter 41). For example, the therapist does a thorough assessment including the intensity of the client's depression, identifying specific behavioral deficits and excesses, identifying the personal and environmental factors that precipitate and maintain the depression, and developing the treatment plan.[11] Common therapeutic techniques used to help the depressed client overcome behavioral deficits are assertiveness training, role-playing, social skills training, stress management, and cognitive skills.[23] Therapeutic techniques used to reduce behavioral excesses are thought-stopping techniques, desensitization, and deconditioning.

Early in therapy the client is taught relaxation techniques to help cope with the unpleasantness of situations or to counter aversive situations that precipitate a depressed feeling. Another effective tool is the use of a pleasant event schedule (PES) by the client. The client identifies social, entertaining, and educational activities, the frequency with which they occur, and the degree of enjoyment experienced. In each session, the therapist and client choose several activities. Before the next session, the client participates in an activity and monitors the mood with the activity. This helps the client to focus on the relationship between mood and event. The therapist provides feedback to the client on the positive feelings related to activity.[11]

In the past decade, there has been a movement by mental health professionals toward integration of various psychotherapeutic approaches. This emergence of integrative psychotherapy addresses the complementary nature of different therapeutic approaches; the advantages of identifying interactions among cognition, affect, and behavior in clients; the importance of an empirically based therapy; the need for a common language of the therapeutic process; the need for common therapeutic principles; and the view that there are stages of psychotherapy.[7] The impact of this movement on the treatment of mood disorders is too early to identify. As this concept develops, the quality and quantity of psychotherapy research will increase.

Chemotherapy

Chemotherapeutic agents used in the treatment of major depression and bipolar disorder tend to fall under three broad categories: antidepressant agents, antimanic agents, and neuroleptics (see Chapter 39). Antidepressant medications include tricyclics, the monoamine oxidase (MAO) inhibitors, and the newer atypical agents. Tricyclic antidepressants (TCAs) are an effective pharmacologic treatment of severe depressions involving more biologic symptoms such as insomnia, anorexia, increased rapid eye movement (REM) sleep, loss of drive or sexual pleasure, circadian rhythm changes, mood alteration, and increased secretion of steroids and hormones.[6]

Antimanic agents include lithium carbonate and newer anticonvulsant medications. Lithium carbonate is the most frequently used medication for the treatment of mania. It is also used prophylactically to prevent recurrence of mania and depression.

Alternatives to lithium are currently being explored. The most commonly used alternative drugs are the anticonvulsant drugs, such as carbamazepine, valproic acid, and clonazepam. Carbamazepine has been found to be especially useful in the treatment of rapid cycling.[37]

Antidepressants and lithium may be used both in the acute phase of illness and to prevent recurrence. Studies have shown that both major depression and mania tend to recur. As a result, lithium and antidepressants are often used over extended periods to reduce the frequency and intensity of subsequent episodes.[44] However, noncompliance with medication tends to be a serious problem with bipolar clients.[2,10]

Antipsychotic medications may be used during the psychotic phase of a major depression or manic episode. These medications are used in conjunction with antidepressants in a psychotic depression, or lithium during a manic episode with psychotic features or extreme agitation.

Electroconvulsive Therapy

Electroconvulsive therapy (ECT) is a specialized therapy used in the treatment of both major depression and mania.[35] It is most commonly used in the treatment of severely depressed clients when delusions or extreme suicidal ideation is present. Several side effects and medical complications can occur and some clients may be at increased risk (see Chapter 40). Despite these risks ECT is generally accepted as a relatively safe procedure when performed by a well-trained physician.[35]

Phototherapy

The use of bright light or full-spectrum light has been used in the treatment of seasonal affective disorder (SAD). This disorder is characterized by recurrent depressions that occur typically in winter and are associated with increased somnolence, fatigue, weight gain, and carbohydrate craving. A reversal of the symptoms with possible hypomanic or manic symptoms occurs during the spring or summer.[41,42,51] The DSM-III-R addresses this phenomenon as a subgroup under the categories of major depression and bipolar disorder. It can affect children as well as adults.[42] The client is exposed to bright artificial light for five to six hours each day. Antidepressant effects disappear within two to four days after light therapy is discontinued.[42,43] Antidepressant effects of phototherapy have been found to be greater when light is applied to the eyes than to the skin.[53] (A pattern opposite SAD has also been identified in which clients may become depressed in the summer and euthymic, hypomanic, or manic at other times. Temperature may influence these depressions and may be used in their treatment.[55])

Manipulation of Sleep

Alterations in sleep have long been known to accompany mood disorders. Rapid eye movement (REM) sleep occurs earlier in clients with a major depression. The REM period lasts longer and produces a greater number of rapid eye movements. There is also an alteration of the timing of electroencephalogram (EEG) delta-wave activity, which shifts from the first to the second non-REM period.[15] Manipulation of sleep has been used to lift even the most severe depressions. Interventions include (1) deprivation of REM sleep, (2) total sleep deprivation, (3) partial sleep deprivation, and (4) advancing the sleep cycle. Individuals are so sensitive to the effects of increased sleep that even a nap the following day can undo beneficial effects of partial sleep deprivation. Deprivation of REM sleep for a few weeks, however, may confer lasting antidepressant effects. Sleep deprivation may also be combined with drugs to treat depression. Lithium combined with partial sleep deprivation and clomipramine combined with total sleep have shown promising results.

Research involving the sleep of bipolar clients is not as extensive. It has been noted that bipolar depressives tend to sleep longer than unipolar depressives, but they tend to be alike in having shortened REM latency and increased rapid eye movements. The hyposomnia of mania has been commonly regarded as a consequence of the activating effects of the manic state. It has been noted that sleep deprivation may precipitate mania. This suggests that stressful emotional experiences, as well as pharmacologic agents, may result in sleep loss and thereby precipitate mania.[15]

Interpersonal Interactions

Clients with bipolar disorder, manic, are well known on inpatient units for their ability to create havoc and induce great discomfort in those around them. Five types of interpersonal maneuvers have clear implications for the nurse who must deal with these clients: (1) manipulation of the self-esteem of others, (2) perceptiveness to vulnerability and conflict, (3) projection of responsibility, (4) progressive limit testing, and (5)

alienating family members.[22] These clients tend to rapidly establish superficial relationships with others; may appear to be bright, cheerful, and entertaining; may flatter those around them; and may possess an uncanny ability to sense issues of self-esteem in others and to use that knowledge as a way of exerting interpersonal leverage. A characteristic related to the ability to appeal to the self-esteem issues of others is their uncanny ability to perceive vulnerability and conflict. This ability is related to both individuals and groups. They are then able to bring covert conflict into the open, manipulating the situation to cause acute discomfort in all concerned. They tend to see staff in terms of good and bad, readily setting up splitting situations.

These clients are also adept at projecting responsibility for their own actions onto others. This is especially likely to occur when the staff member's feelings of self-worth is based upon how well the client is doing. The staff member becomes progressively more invested in a favorable outcome for the client and deflection of responsibility is facilitated.

Testing and challenging of limits is another characteristic of interaction with others. When demands are not met, the other person is regarded as unreasonable or unfair. Finally, these clients tend to distance and alienate themselves from other family members. Anger is the characteristic response of spouses. Marriages are much more likely to end in divorce as a result of a manic phase of bipolar disorder. Spouses tend to view manic behavior as willful and spiteful. Conversely, behavior during the depressive phase is more likely to be viewed by the spouse as part of an illness over which the client has little control.

A knowledge of characteristic interactions initiated by clients experiencing a manic episode is crucial to the nurse's psychotherapeutic work with them. Frequent staff meetings may constructively deal with attempts to divide staff. Acknowledging conflict can decrease efforts to manipulate. Considering one's own role in interacting with these clients decreases their ability to target the psychiatric nurse's own self-esteem. Finally, establishing firm, unambiguous limits and strictly adhering to them decreases further challenging of limits (see Chapter 33).

CASE STUDY

Susan, a 24-year-old young woman, was admitted to the psychiatric inpatient unit. She was accompanied by her second husband to whom she had been married for two years. He reported that for the past two to three months, Susan had begun to act "hyper" and to do uncharacteristically "crazy" things. He said that Susan had admitted to stealing from her customers while working as a door-to-door cosmetics saleslady, and to being sexually promiscuous with near strangers. The night before admission, he stated Susan had sprayed him in the face with mace during an argument, then drove off recklessly with her frightened 4-year-old daughter. Her husband was alarmed by her behavior, as Susan had always been a caring wife, mother, and homemaker. He voiced uncertainty about the future of their marriage. On admission to the unit, Susan was noted to have

SUSAN

NURSING INTERVENTIONS	OUTCOME CRITERIA

NURSING DIAGNOSIS: Sleep pattern disturbance related to extreme hyperactivity

CLIENT GOAL: Reestablish adequate sleeping patterns

- Provide quiet, comfortable environment with minimal stimulation
- Observe for signs of fatigue
- Allow for periodic rest periods until regular nighttime sleeping schedule is reestablished
- Avoid caffeine intake

Reports return of "normal" sleep schedule
Reports feeling rested following sleep

NURSING DIAGNOSIS: Altered nutrition (less than body requirements) related to an increase in nutritional needs because of hyperactivity and decrease in dietary intake

CLIENT GOAL: Consume well balanced, high-caloric diet

- Identify food preferences including foods high in complex carbohydrates and protein[26]
- Offer frequent high-calorie meals and fluids, including finger foods that can be eaten while Susan is active
- Monitor intake and weigh daily

Establishes an eating pattern of 4–6 small meals a day
Increases intakes of high-caloric food and drinks
Weight stabilizes

NURSING DIAGNOSIS: Noncompliance (failure to take lithium carbonate as prescribed)

CLIENT GOAL: Reestablish compliance with taking lithium carbonate as prescribed

- Administer psychotropic medication as prescribed
- Observe Susan's response to the medication including possible side effects
- Monitor associated laboratory tests
- Educate Susan about medication and diagnosis when condition has stabilized
- Determine factors involved with Susan's noncompliance

Establishes therapeutic lithium level
Reports possible side effects
Verbalizes purpose and desired effects of medication
Demonstrates acceptance

NURSING DIAGNOSIS: Emotional lability related to bipolar disorder, manic

CLIENT GOAL: Reestablish emotional stability

- Give simple, truthful responses
- Use firm, calm approach in communicating with client
- Do not argue with Susan
- Provide consistent, structured environment under close staff supervision
- Avoid group activities for Susan until she is stabilized

Demonstrates more appropriate affect
Verbalizes feelings of increased self-control

NURSING DIAGNOSIS: Altered perception/cognition related to distractibility

CLIENT GOAL: Increase attention span

- Decrease environmental stimuli
- Provide five-minute interactions with Susan using short words and sentences

Responds to simple communication

Continued

SUSAN *Continued*

NURSING INTERVENTIONS	OUTCOME CRITERIA
■ Increase exposure to milieu slowly as distractibility decreases	Participates in milieu activities

NURSING DIAGNOSIS: Altered impulse control related to hypersexuality

CLIENT GOAL: Return to premorbid sexual functioning

■ Observe Susan's behavior closely while interacting with others in the milieu	Displays appropriate behavior on the unit
■ Protect Susan using firm structure when sexually provocative behavior is noted	
■ Encourage Susan to ventilate feelings regarding previous sexual activity once control has returned	Verbalizes feelings related to and understanding previous sexual activity

NURSING DIAGNOSIS: Agitation related to bipolar disorder, mania

CLIENT GOAL: Return to normal activity level

■ Monitor for signs of increasing activity or agitation	Reports feeling less agitated
■ Decrease stimuli in Susan's environment	Demonstrates appropriate activity level
■ Seclude or restrain if less restrictive measures unsuccessful	

NURSING DIAGNOSIS: Dysfunctional family processes related to Susan's behavior

CLIENT GOAL: Improve communication within family

■ Allow Susan to ventilate feelings regarding her behavior once mania has ceased	Demonstrates improved communication within family system
■ Encourage family to ventilate feelings regarding Susan's manic behavior	Demonstrates constructive interaction
■ Provide information for husband regarding Susan's diagnosis, prognosis, treatment, and appropriate support groups	
■ Help husband make contact with acceptable support group	
■ Refer for family therapy, if needed	

NURSING DIAGNOSIS: Knowledge deficit (pertaining to the illness)

CLIENT GOAL: Increase comprehension of nature of bipolar disorder and course of illness

■ Provide patient education focusing on early signs, environmental factors that can lead to full-blown mania, alternative coping methods, and available self-help groups	Recognizes early signs
	Reports increased internal locus of control
	Names appropriate self-help groups in community
■ Provide positive reinforcement for increased initiative in acquiring additional information about her illness	Demonstrates acceptance of and responsibility for own illness

Research Highlights

Egeland and associates[16] began a study of bipolar disorder in the Old Order Amish (OOA) in 1976. The OOA was an appropriate population to study because of their homogeneity, stability, large family pedigrees, and excellent genealogy records. With strong religious and moral traditions, there is virtually no criminal behavior, violence, marital separation or divorce, alcoholism, or difference in socioeconomic or educational status to cloud the picture.

The OOA hospital and genealogy records were reviewed. Families were interviewed. Five researchers independently reviewed records and made diagnoses using specific research diagnostic criteria. Although the prevalence of bipolar disorder was found to be the same in the OOAs as in the general American population,[16] the results seemed to indicate that the disorder was carried by a dominant gene with incomplete penetrance. The next step was to look for a genetic marker. Thirty-two bipolar disorder families had been found. The DNA study was based on one large composite that encompassed three of the original 50 families who had settled in Lancaster County, Pennsylvania between 1720 and 1750. These families had 81 members, 19 of whom were diagnosed as having mood disorders. Fourteen of the 19 had some form of bipolar disorder. The scientists were able to locate and correlate a gene at the tip of the short arm of the chromosome 11 with the occurrence of bipolar disorder. The results seemed to indicate that bipolar disorder was carried by a dominant gene with only partial penetrance. Although there would be a 50% chance of passing along a strong predisposition to offspring, 63% of those with the gene had developed the disorder.[16]

This discovery was the first demonstration of a possible genetic basis for one of the major mental disorders, an essential step in identifying neurobiologic abnormalities that lead to the expression of this illness. The researchers caution that these results have been found in one pedigree only, that similar studies are ongoing, and that different family genes can be responsible for a genetic predisposition to a disease.[16,48]

rapid, pressured speech. She was grandiose with a labile affect, agitated, intrusive, and easily distractible. She slept intermittently, averaging three to four hours a night. She ate very little and reported a ten-lb weight loss in the past month. Susan's past psychiatric history revealed she was hospitalized for mania at ages 16, 19, and 21. Lithium carbonate had been prescribed, but she had been noncompliant for the past six months. She also admitted to infrequent cannabis abuse. Susan's past medical history was significant for two full-term pregnancies. The first, at age 16, resulted in the birth of a son who was given up for adoption. The second resulted in the birth of her daughter. Susan also reported that ten months before admission she had undergone a laparoscopy as part of an infertility workup. That resulted in a diagnosis of blocked fallopian tubes, making subsequent pregnancies improbable. The nursing diagnoses for Susan were sleep pattern disturbance, altered nutrition, noncompliance, emotional lability, altered perception/cognition, altered impulse control, agitation, dysfunctional family processes, and knowledge deficit (see Nursing Care Plan 20-1 for a sample care plan for Susan).

SUMMARY

The DSM-III-R subclassifies mood disturbances as depressive disorders and mood disorders with the major illnesses being major depression and bipolar disorder. These conditions affect a substantial portion of the American population. There are multiple theories of causation addressing major depression and bipolar disorder. These disorders can be acute or chronic, and both are manifested by changes in the biologic, psychological, and sociologic functioning of the client. Mood disorders are treated with a variety of psychosocial therapies and biologic therapies. Nursing care involves a thorough assessment, nursing diagnosis, and nursing intervention.

References

1. Akiskal HS. Characterlogic manifestations of affective disorders: toward a new conceptualization. Integrative Psychiatry. 1984; May/June:83.
2. Akiskal HS. The clinical management of affective disorders. In: Cavernar JO, ed. Psychiatry, vol 1. Philadelphia: JB Lippincott; 1988.
3. Akiskal HS. The clinical significance of the "soft" bipolar spectrum. Psychiatr Ann. 1986;16:667–671.
4. Akiskal HS, Webb WL. Affective disorders: recent advances in clinical conceptualization. Hosp Commun Psychiatry. 1983;34:695–702.
5. American Psychiatric Association. Diagnostic and statistical manual of mental disorders, 3rd ed, revised. Washington, DC: American Psychiatric Association; 1987.
6. Baldessarini R, Cole J. Chemotherapy. In: Nicholi A, ed. The new Harvard guide to psychiatry. Cambridge, MA: Belknap Press; 1988.
7. Beitman BD, Goldfried MR, Norcross JC. The movement toward integrating the psychotherapies: an overview. Am J Psychiatry. 1989; 146:138–147.
8. Blazer D, Swartz M, Woodbury M, et al. Depressive symptoms and depressive diagnoses in a community population. Arch Gen Psychiatry. 1988;45:1078–1084.
9. Bloodworth RC. Hazards of marijuana: a psychiatrist's viewpoint. Brawner Byline. Winter, 1981–82.
10. Cameron D. Presentations of depression: depressive symptoms in medical and other psychiatric disorders. New York: John Wiley & Sons; 1987.
11. Canter A. Contemporary short-term psychotherapies. In: Munoz RA, ed. Therapeutic potential of mood disorders. San Francisco, Jossey-Bass; 1984.
12. Carlson GA, Kashani JH. Phenomenology of major depression from childhood through adulthood: analysis of three studies. Am J Psychiatry. 1988;145:1222–1225.
13. Cassem NH. Depression. In: Hacket TP, Cassem NH, eds. Massachusetts General Hospital handbook of general psychiatry. Littleton, MA: Year Book Medical; 1987.

14. When symptoms become the focus of your life. Discover. 1986;10.

15. Doghramji K. Sleep disorders: a selective update. Hosp Commun Psychiatry. 1989;40:29–40.

16. Egeland JA, Gerhard DS, Pauls DL, et al. Bipolar affective disorders linked to DNA markers on chromosome 11. Nature. 1987;325:783–787.

17. Freud S. Mourning and melancholia. In: Strachey J, ed. The standard edition of the complete psychological works of Sigmund Freud. London: Hogarth Press; 1915.

18. Gordon VC, Gordon EM. Short-term group treatment of depressed women: a replication study in Great Britain. Arch Psychiatr Nurs. 1987;1(2):111–124.

19. Hoberman HM, Lewinson PM. The behavioral treatment of depression. In: Beckham EE, Leber WR, eds. Handbook of depression: treatment, assessment, and research. Homewood, IL: Dorsey; 1985.

20. Ilfeld FW Jr. Current social stressors and symptoms of depression. Am J Psychiatry. 1977;134:161–166.

21. James ME, Cohen-Cole SA. Major depression: current perspectives. Emory Univ J Med. 1989;3:110.

22. Janowsky D, et al. Playing the manic game. *Arch Gen Psychiatry*. 1970;22:252–261.

23. Jarrett RB, Rush JA. Psychotherapeutic approaches for depression. In: Cavenar JO, ed. Psychiatry, vol 1. Philadelphia: JB Lippincott; 1988.

24. Kerr NJ. Sign and symptoms of depression and principles of nursing intervention. Pers Psychiatr Care. 1987/88;24:(2)48–63.

25. Kestenbaum CJ. Children at risk for manic–depressive illness: possible predictors. Am J Psychiatry. 1979;136:1206–1208.

26. Kim MJ, McFarland GR, McLane AM. Pocket guide to nursing diagnosis, 3rd ed. St Louis: CV Mosby; 1989.

27. Klerman G, Lavor PW, Rice J, et al. Birth–cohort trends in rates of major depressive disorder among relatives of patients with affective disorder. Arch Gen Psychiatry. 1985;42:689–693.

28. Kolata G. Manic–depression: is it inherited? Science. 1986;232:575–576.

29. Lehmann HE. Affective disorders: clinical features. In: Kaplan HL, Sadock BJ, eds. Comprehensive textbook of psychiatry/IV. Baltimore: Williams & Wilkins; 1985.

30. Lum TL. An integrated approach to aging and depression. Arch Psychiatr Nurs. 1987;2:211.

31. MacKinnon R, Michels R. The psychiatric interview in clinical practice. Philadelphia: WB Saunders; 1971.

32. Manderino MA, Bzdek VM. Mobilizing depressed clients. J Psychosoc Nurs. 1986;24:23–28.

33. Margolin CB. Assessment of psychiatric patients. J Emerg Nurs. 1980;6(4):30–33.

34. Murphy J, Monson R, Olivier D, Sobol A, Leighton A. Affective disorders and mortality. Arch Gen Psychiatry. 1987;44:473–480.

35. National Institute of Mental Health. Electroconvulsive therapy. Consensus development conference statement 1985;5(11):8.

36. Petersen C, Seligman, ME. The learned helplessness model of depression: current status of theory and research. In: Beckham EE, Lebor WR, eds. Handbook of depression: treatment, assessment, and research. Homewood, IL: Dorsey; 1985.

37. Post M, Ballenger J. Carbamazepine (Tegratol) and affective illness. Curr Affect Illness. 1983;2:7.

38. Regier DA, Hirschfield RM, Goodwin FK, et al. The NIMH depression awareness, recognition, and treatment program: structure, aims and scientific basis. Am J Psychiatry. 1988;145(11):1351–1357.

39. Regier D, Myers J, Kramer M, et al. The NIMH epidemiologic catchment area program. Arch Gen Psychiatry. 1984;41:934–941.

40. Rice J, Reich T, Andreasen NC, et al. The familial transmission of bipolar illness. Arch Gen Psychiatry. 1987;44:441–447.

41. Rosenthal N, Sack DA, Carpenter CJ, et al. Antidepressant effects of light in seasonal affective disorder. Am J Psychiatry. 1985;142:163–170.

42. Rosenthal N, Carpenter CJ, James SP, et al. Seasonal affective disorders in children and adolescents. Am J Psychiatry. 1986;143:356–358.

43. Rounsaville BJ, Klerman GL, Weissman MM, Chevron ES. Short-term interpersonal psychotherapy (IPT) for depression. In: Beckham EE, Lebor WR, eds. Handbook of depression: treatment, assessment, and research. Homewood, IL: Dorsey; 1985.

44. Runck B. NIMH report—conference recommends pharmacologic prevention of recurring mood disorders. Hosp Commun Psychiatry. 1984;35:871–873.

45. Ryan L, Montgomery A, Meyers S. Impact of circadian rhythm research on approaches to affective illness. Arch Psychiatr Nurs. 1987;1:236–240.

46. Sacco WP, Beck AT. Cognitive therapy of depression. In: Beckham EE, Leber WR, eds. Handbook of depression: treatment, assessment, and research. Homewood, IL: Dorsey; 1985.

47. Schrodt GR Jr, Fitzgerald BA. Cognitive therapy with adolescents. Am J Psychother. 1987;41:402–408.

48. Science Press Seminar. Feb 25 1987. NIMH Public Affairs Branch, Office of Science Information.

49. Simmons-Alling S. New approaches to managing affective disorders. Arch Psychiatr Nurs. 1987;1:219–224.

50. Slaby A. Handbook of psychiatric emergencies, 3rd ed. New York: Elsevier Science Publishing; 1986.

51. Thompson C, Issacs G. Seasonal affective disorder—a British sample symptomatology in relation to mode of referral and diagnostic subtype. J Affective Disorders. 1988;14:1–11.

52. Tirrell C, DeForest D. Neuroendocrine factors in affective disorders. Arch Psychiatr Nurs. 1987;1:225–229.

53. Wehr T, Skwerer RG, Jacobsen FM, et al. Eye versus skin phototherapy of seasonal affective disorder. Am J Psychiatry. 1987;144:753–757.

54. Wehr T, Sack DA, Rosenthal NE, et al. Rapid cycling affective disorders: contributing factors and treatment responses in 51 patients. Am J Psychiatry. 1988;145:179–184.

55. Wehr T, Sack DA, Rosenthal NE. Seasonal affective disorder with summer depression and winter hypomania. Am J Psychiatry. 1987;144:1602–1603.

56. Weissman MM. Advances in psychiatric epidemiology: rates and risks for major depression. Am J Public Health. 1987;77:445–451.

57. Weissman MM, Merikangas KR, Boyd JH. Epidemiology of affective disorders. In: Cavenar JO, ed. Psychiatry, vol 1. Philadelphia: JB Lippincott; 1988.

21

Joan M. Baker

Clients With Anxiety Disorders

OBJECTIVES

After reading this chapter, the reader will be able to:

1. Describe and differentiate the anxiety disorders on the basis of symptoms, prevalance, and course
2. Discuss four major theoretical explanations of anxiety disorders
3. Discuss problems related to the assessment of the anxiety disorders
4. Identify and evaluate current treatment methods and describe the most efficacious treatments for each disorder
5. Explain the nurse's role in treatment implementation
6. Discuss nursing diagnoses that could be formulated with clients having an anxiety disorder
7. Identify some areas of research needed in the work with clients with anxiety disorders.

INTRODUCTION

More Americans experience anxiety disorders than any other group of disorders, according to one source.[18] Community prevalence studies find that the occurrence of all anxiety disorders in the general population ranges from 2.9% to 8.4%, and if all these people were to seek help, health care providers would be unable to meet the demand.[14]

Anxiety disorders, as described in Diagnostic and Statistical Manual of Mental Disorders, Third Edition, Revised (DSM-III-R), include a group of nonpsychotic disorders classified as follows: panic disorder with and without agoraphobia, agoraphobia without history of panic disorder, social phobia, simple phobia, obsessive compulsive disorder, post-traumatic stress disorder, and generalized anxiety disorder.[2] Although all these disorders will be discussed, the phobias will be addressed in more detail in this chapter.

ANXIETY

Anxiety is an everyday experience for everyone.[4] Anxiety can be a motivating force that enhances the ability to cope with stressors. On the other hand, too much or too little anxiety can be maladaptive.[4,15]

ANXIETY DISORDERS

The characteristic features of anxiety disorders are symptoms of anxiety and anxiety avoidance behaviors.[2] Anxiety is usually predominant in panic disorder and generalized anxiety disorder. Avoidance behaviors are actions taken by an individual to avoid the experience of anxiety. All phobic behaviors and most obsessive compulsive disorder behaviors are characterized by avoidance. In post-traumatic stress disorder, both anxiety symptoms and avoidance behaviors are common.[2]

The DSM-III-R categories of anxiety disorders and pertinent information related to each disorder are listed in Table 21-1. In general, anxiety disorders are often related to depression, occur in younger people, have a chronic course with variable impairment in social and occupational functioning, and are thought to occur more often in females. Anxiety disorders may be difficult to differentiate from a wide variety of other physical and mental disorders that also present with anxiety.[5,11]

Panic Disorders (With and Without Agoraphobia)

Panic disorders are syndromes of unpredictable, irrational episodes characterized by extreme apprehension or terror.[4] The disorder usually begins with an unexpected panic attack with an unclear cause. Recurrent anxiety reactions may become associated with specific situations.[5] The person experiences intense fear throughout the attack, which may last from minutes to hours. Panic disorder can occur with or without agoraphobia (fear of public places). Although a panic attack can be a one-time occurrence, more often, panic attacks occur periodically for weeks or months and have been known to wax and wane for years.[2]

A person may be said to have panic disorder if he or she meets the following criteria:[2] (1) one or more unexpected panic attacks not triggered by being the focus of others' attention; (2) four attacks within a 4-week period or one or more attacks followed by at least a month of persevering fear of having another attack; (3) at least four of the following symptoms during one or more of the attacks: shortness of breath/smothering sensation; dizziness, unsteadiness, faintness; choking; palpitations/increased heart rate; trembling/shaking; sweating; nausea/abdominal distress; depersonalization/derealization; numbness/tingling; hot flashes/chills; chest pain/discomfort; fear of dying, fear of going crazy/losing control (fewer than four symptoms is considered to be a limited symptom attack and is not diagnostic of panic disorder); (4) in at least some of the attacks, at least four of the symptoms developed suddenly and increased in intensity within 10 minutes of when the first symptom was noted; and (5) no organic or chemical cause can be found.

In panic disorder with agoraphobia, the person meets the criteria for panic disorder and additionally has a fear of public places from which escape might be difficult or embarrassing or where help (in case of a panic attack) might not be available. The person either restricts travel (becomes homebound), needs a travel companion when away from home, or endures the situation despite high anxiety.[2] Panic disorder with agoraphobia is the most troubling phobic disorder seen in adult psychiatric clinics.[4]

Although there is controversy around predisposing factors, the current thinking is that separation anxiety in childhood, sudden loss of social supports, disruption of significant interpersonal relationships, increased incidence of depression, alcohol abuse, and cardiovascular problems may contribute to the emergence of panic disorder.[2,5] There is evidence of an association between mitral valve prolapse and panic disorder. In seven studies conducted between 1978 and 1983, the pooled rate for mitral valve prolapse was 23% in clients with panic disorder of agoraphobia, whereas the rate in the general population was 5.3%.[6] Studies on the cause of this association have produced inconclusive results.[6]

Agoraphobia Without History of Panic Disorder

A phobic disorder is characterized by a persistent and irrational fear of a specific object, situation, or activity.[11] Usually, the phobic person is aware that the fear is unrealistic but still avoids its target. Encountering what is feared leads to severe anxiety.[4]

Agoraphobia is the fear of being in public places

TABLE 21-1
DSM-III-R categories of anxiety disorders with pertinent features[2,5,14]

ANXIETY DISORDER	AGE AT ONSET	COURSE	IMPAIRMENT	PREDISPOSING FACTORS	PREVALENCE (SEX RATIO)
Panic disorder (with and without agoraphobia)	Late 20s	Panic attacks several times per week up to daily May last for weeks to years May remit and recur	With agoraphobia, there is constriction in lifestyle; may become housebound May be unable to leave house without a companion	Separation anxiety disorder in childhood Sudden loss of social supports Disruption of significant interpersonal relationships Often associated with depression	Without agoraphobia, found in 1% of population, equal in males and females With agoraphobia, found in 2%-5% of the population and twice as often in females
Agoraphobia without history of panic disorder	20s-30s	Persists for years	Severe in clinical samples	Separation anxiety disorder in childhood Stress Needs additional study	Rare in clinical samples 0.6% in general population More common in females
Social phobia	Childhood through early adolescence	Chronic	Inconvenient; some mild interference with social/occupational areas	Has not been well studied	1.7% in community prevalence studies More males than females in clinical samples
Simple phobia	Childhood through fourth decade; mean age of onset is in the midteens	Childhood phobias often disappear without treatment Those that persist into adulthood rarely remit without treatment	Usually mild, depending on convenience of avoidance	Has not been well studied	7% in the general population Diagnosed more often in females
Obsessive compulsive disorder	Childhood through early adulthood 65% of disorders appear before age 25	Chronic waxing and waning of symptoms	Moderate to severe Compulsive acts may become major life activity	May be associated with depression or stressors Needs further study	1%-2% of psychiatric patients Equal distribution in males and females
Post-traumatic stress disorder	Any age	Symptoms start immediately or soon after trauma Re-experiencing of symptoms may develop months or years later	Mild to severe Phobic avoidance may affect marriage and family relationships Self-defeating actions, suicide, substance abuse	Pre-existing psychopathology Extreme stressor Often associated with depression	Data unavailable
Generalized anxiety disorder	20s-30s	Usually present for many years Needs further study	Usually only mild	In clinical populations, sometimes follows a major depressive episode	Not common Equal in males and females

where escape may be blocked or help unavailable (in the event of development of symptoms that could be embarrassing or incapacitating).[2,11] Examples of agoraphobic situations include being in a crowd, on a bridge, or in an elevator; traveling in a train, bus, or car; and flying on airplanes.[2,5] The person is usually fearful of developing a symptom attack that could incapacitate him or her (e.g., heart attack) or cause embarrassment (e.g., loss of bowel or bladder control or vomiting).

Sometimes, this condition occurs when a person is fearful that a symptom *could* develop, even though it never has.[2]

Whether this disorder is a variant of panic disorder with agoraphobia is not clear.[2] Most clinical impressions support the idea that agoraphobia develops subsequent to panic attacks and that the avoidance behavior is related to having a panic attack where aid would not be available.

Social Phobia

People who develop social phobias have a persistent fear of one or more situations where they feel others are scrutinizing or criticizing them or where they fear they may behave in an embarrassing manner. Gaze aversion is common. Many fear they will shake, blush, vomit, or see others vomit.[2,14] Examples of social phobia include fear of eating in public, fear of public speaking, and fear of using public lavatories.[2,5,14] The fears are specific to social situations and are not related to any other medical or psychiatric disorder (e.g., not to fear of having a panic attack), and the person realizes that the fear is excessive or unreasonable. At some point in the disturbance, exposure leads to an immediate anxiety response. Avoidance is the way most people deal with this disorder, although if avoidance is not convenient or possible, the person may try to endure the situation despite intense anxiety. The avoidant behavior can interfere with the individual's social and work life.

Simple (Specific) Phobia

Simple phobia is characterized by a fear of a specific object or situation other than those associated with other anxiety disorders. Typical examples of simple phobias include those involving animals (e.g., dogs, snakes, insects, mice), blood injury (e.g., witnessing blood or tissue injury); closed spaces (claustrophobia), heights (acrophobia), and air travel.[2] Exposure to the stimulus will immediately provoke an anxiety response. The person uses avoidance to deal with the object or situation or endures the situation with intense anxiety. The diagnosis of simple phobia is made when the avoidant behavior interferes with the person's routine or relationships or if the phobic individual has a marked distress about the fear.[2]

Obsessive Compulsive Disorder

The essential features of obsessive compulsive disorder are obsessions (repetitive, intrusive, senseless ideas, thoughts, impulses, or images) or compulsions (repetitive purposeful and intentional actions performed in response to an obsession according to certain rules or in a ritualistic way).[2] The obsession(s)/compulsions(s) cause marked distress and take more than an hour per day or interfere with daily functioning or social relationships.[2] Any attempt to resist a compulsion increases anxiety.[5] A majority of the people with obsessive compulsive disorder who are seen clinically have both obsessions and compulsions.[14]

Ritualistic behaviors involve washing and cleaning, checking, and primary obsessional slowness.[14] Individuals whose rituals involve washing and cleaning usually have concerns related to contamination from bodily secretion, germs, dirt, or chemicals. It is common for them to seek reassurance from others about performing their ritualistic behavior in a proper way or about not having taken some harmful action. The effect of this reassurance is transitory, and the person will seek it continually unless the reassurance is withheld.[14] Individuals whose ritualistic behaviors involve checking usually have concerns about death, disease, or disaster. They must check the possibility of danger repeatedly or in a certain way to avert anxiety.[14] For example, Joe J was a 26-year-old truck driver whose compulsion caused him to be fired from his job when he could no longer control his urge to stop the truck every 500 feet and get out to check if he had hit anything on the highway. He said, "It was stupid and irrational, but I couldn't help it." Primary obsessional slowness is rare and very disabling. The individual may take hours to complete a task others finish in minutes. An example would be taking 2 hours to wash one's face.[10]

The main difference between phobias and obsessive compulsive disorder is that in a phobia, the person must avoid something to ward off the anxiety, whereas in obsessive compulsive disorder, one must do or think something to deal with the anxiety.[4]

Post Traumatic Stress Disorder

Post traumatic stress disorder involves the development of symptoms after a traumatic event that is not within the range of usual human experience (e.g., a threat to one's life; sudden destruction of one's home or community; seeing someone seriously threatened, injured, or killed; or learning of serious harm to a significant other). Examples of such trauma include rape, war, and floods.[2]

Symptoms of post traumatic stress disorder involve re-experiencing the trauma (e.g., dreams), reliving the event while in a dissociative state, avoidance of stimuli associated with the trauma, and a generalized emotional "anesthesia." The person also suffers from increased arousal, including difficulty falling or staying asleep, nightmares, hypervigilance, and an exaggerated startle response. There may be difficulty in concentrating or in task completion. There may be changes in aggression, which can range from inability to express anger to explosive outbursts.[2]

Generalized Anxiety Disorder

Generalized anxiety disorder is characterized by an unrealistic or excessive feeling of anxiety about two or more areas of life that persists for 6 months or longer. The person reports feeling worried more days than not. When anxious, the person shows signs of motor tension, autonomic hyperactivity, vigilance, and scanning.[2] The main difference between panic disorder and generalized anxiety disorder is the absence of discrete panic attacks in the latter.[5]

ETIOLOGY
Psychodynamic Theory

According to psychodynamic theory, children learn to repress "unacceptable" wishes when such wishes arouse intense anxiety because of disapproval from significant others. The anxiety may be related to intrapsychic or interpersonal events. When an adult encounters a situation that threatens to arouse a repressed wish or behavior that was intensely forbidden in childhood, anxiety occurs, and the person will use defense mechanisms to ward off the arousal of the wish or behavior and the related anxiety.[4] Thus, reality is distorted, and anxiety is relieved. The symptoms are symbolic of the client's attempt to manage the anxiety.[4] In phobias, for example, one view is that the defense mechanisms of displacement and avoidance are thought to be used to deal with Oedipal conflict and castration fears.[15] The anxiety is displaced onto an external object or situation, which the person is then able to avoid.[4] This theory has lost much of its former popularity.

Behavioral Theory

In the behavioral framework, anxiety disorders are viewed as learned responses to anxiety-provoking experiences.[15] A painful experience conditions the person to avoid similar experiences that evoke anxiety.[4] This preventive action is called a conditioned avoidance response.[7] It becomes maladaptive when, through generalization, harmless objects or situations arouse anxiety, and avoidance of the harmless object relieves the anxiety. Therefore, the person never gets close enough to the object or situation to learn that it is harmless and to unlearn the maladaptive response.[4] Extinction of the conditioned avoidance response involves making it impossible to use that response so that the person experiences progressively less anxiety and eventually overcomes the fear.[7] Behavioral formulations of phobias, compulsive rituals, and similar behavior utilize some version of conditioned avoidance response. Treatment based on behavioral therapy has been very successful.

Social Learning and Cognitive Theories

The theoretical frameworks of social learning and cognition propose that the thought processes intervening between a stimulus and a response are as important as the stimulus. For example, a phobia may reflect a person's self-image of helplessness and powerlessness. The treatment based on these models focuses on restoring the individual's self-esteem and removing blocks to personal or professional growth.[4,20]

Psychobiologic Theory

Anxiety states have been produced in laboratory settings by exposure to a phobic stimulus, infusions of sodium lactate; oral administration of caffeine, carbon dioxide (CO_2) inhalation, and hyperventilation.[17] So far, there is no unifying theory to explain all induced states. One recent study of repeated CO_2 exposure involving client's with panic disorder presented evidence that these client's have more anxiety after CO_2 inhalation than do controls and, interestingly, that the anxiety response diminished as the CO_2 exposure increased.[19] The investigators encourage further study of the possibility that anxiogenic (anxiety-causing) agents may be anxiolytic (anxiety-reducing).[19] Current and future research in the psychobiology of anxiety and the neural and molecular mechanisms in anxiety should lead to a better understanding of the causes of anxiety and to more effective diagnosis and treatment based on those theories.

ASSESSMENT

Because anxiety is a universal experience, it is not easy to separate the symptoms accurately under a specific diagnostic category. Even if the symptoms are clear-cut, their cause may not be.

One of the first tasks in assessment is to make sure associated conditions have been considered and ruled out. Medical conditions associated with anxiety and which may erroneously be diagnosed as a primary anxiety disorder include disorders of the central nervous, endocrine, or cardiovascular systems and drug-related disorders.[4] For example, a person who drinks two to five cups of caffeinated coffee per day may present a clinical picture similar to panic disorder or generalized anxiety disorder.[21] Other psychiatric syndromes must also be considered. For example, it often is difficult to determine whether a person is depressed with anxiety or vice versa.[11] When other conditions have been eliminated, one must determine whether the anxiety is maladaptive rather than simply a temporary response to a particular stress. The final decision is to determine into which category of anxiety disorder the symptoms and behavior best fit according to the DSM-III-R.

Assessment involves taking a thorough history of the client's life including childhood background, family issues, marital issues, sleep problems, somatic complaints, drug and alcohol use, current medications, prior psychiatric illnesses, social and occupational functioning, and onset and extent of anxiety symptoms. A physical examination is performed to rule out physical causes (including blood studies, an electrocardiogram, and an electroencephalogram when indicated). Finally, a battery of psychological tests is administered to help rule out other psychiatric disorders and to determine the client's intellectual functioning. A comprehensive assessment tool specific to anxiety disorders is the Anxiety Disorders Interview Schedule–Revised (ADIS-R). This interview guide is designed to assist in the differential diagnosis of the anxiety disorders and to provide detailed information regarding the patient's level of functioning.[9]

A person with a phobia will often report some restriction in activities. The phobia may disappear or diminish a great deal when the individual is with someone he or she can trust. The absence of this trusted other often leads to feelings of helplessness and dependence.[4] It is not uncommon for the person to report that the irrational fear began suddenly and then became more generalized.

TREATMENT

The DSM-III-R categories of anxiety disorders attempt to distinguish the various disorders clearly. However, current studies indicate that panic, as well as generalized anxiety, occur in most of the anxiety disorders.[18] There also is a fair amount of agreement in the literature that agoraphobia in various degrees accompanies panic attacks in most patients. These three categories often seem to merge with one another and with depression.[18] Broad treatment approaches therefore have been most successful and include pharmacologic therapies and behavioral and psychological therapies.[11]

Pharmacologic Therapies

Antidepressants, anxiolytics, and beta-adrenergic receptor blockers are often used to treat anxiety disorders. The efficacy of other drugs is also being studied.

Antidepressants such as imiprimine (Tofranil), a tricyclic antidepressant, and phenelzine (Nardil), a monoamine oxidase (MAO) inhibitor, are the medications chosen most often for panic disorder and are also viewed as effective in the treatment of post-traumatic stress disorder.[11,18] Imiprimine enhances the treatment effect of exposure (discussed below) in agoraphobia.[18] Reports have indicated that clomiprimine (Anafranil) is effective in the treatment of obsessive compulsive disorder. Clomiprimine alone is probably not as effective as behavioral treatments alone.[18] Other tricyclic antidepressants and MAO inhibitors need to be studied to determine their efficacy in the treatment of anxiety disorders.

Anxiolytic agents include the benzodiazepines such as alprazolam (Xanax) and clonazepam (Clonopin) which, in moderate doses, produce tranquilization and muscle relaxation. Psychological dependence on these drugs is problematic.[11] Benzodiazepines are considered effective in the treatment of panic attacks, agoraphobia, and generalized anxiety disorder.[18] Buspirone (Buspar), a fairly new nonbenzodiazepine anxiolytic, has no sedating effects or withdrawal symptoms and may provide a useful alternative to benzodiazepines in treating generalized anxiety disorder.[18]

Beta-adrenergic receptor blockers such as propranolol (Inderol) relieve various somatic symptoms of anxiety.[11] Beta blockers have been considered effective in the treatment of generalized anxiety disorder but not

as effective as benzodiazepines. Interest in these drugs therefore has declined somewhat.[16] Generalizations from studies of these drugs are limited by the small doses and short periods of administration.[16] There are also vague and conflicting reports of clinical impressions about beta blockers. Some patients respond well; others do not seem to. More carefully delineated and controlled studies need to be done with specific disorders, such as social phobias, where results with these drugs have so far been inconclusive.[16] Who can be helped by these drugs and under what conditions are questions that need to be addressed specifically.

Other drugs have shown various degrees of promise in treating anxiety disorders. Carbamazapine (Tegretol), an anticonvulsant, which may reduce help-seeking behaviors and dysphoria in panic attacks, was also effective in addressing anxiety in seven of ten war veterans suffering from post-traumatic stress disorder.[18] Clonidine (Catapres), an alpha-2 receptor agonist, has been effective in reducing the hyperactivity seen in this disorder. Verapamil (Isoptin), a calcium channel-blocking agent, has been modestly effective in reducing panic attacks.[18] Studies of patients with social and simple phobias have not proved drugs to be effective.[18] More studies are needed in this area as well as further comparison studies between drug and behavioral therapies.[16]

Behavioral and Psychological Therapies

Exposure is a treatment of choice in anxiety disorders where avoidance behavior is creating a problem. It is extremely useful in obsessive compulsive disorder and phobias. This treatment involves exposing the willing person to the stimulus that has evoked anxiety until the anxiety subsides while preventing the usual avoidance response.[14] The best chance of success comes with identification of all of the ways the client avoids the stimulus and then prevention of avoidance until the anxiety lessens.[13,14]

There are two types of exposure: live and fantasy.[14] Live exposure involves confronting the real object or situation and is thought to be the most valuable, although studies in this area conflict.[14] Fantasy exposure, which involves having the person visualize the object or situation, is especially useful when real stimuli may not be available, such as in the case of a person who is afraid of thunderstorms.[14]

Desensitization and flooding are two methods of exposure. Desensitization involves gradually introducing the avoided object or situation and may or may not be preceded by relaxation exercises. Flooding involves rapidly confronting the worst possible situation in order to enable the client to accept the feared event.[3] If flooding is too frightening, the client may become noncompliant with the treatment. It is important to involve the client in the treatment program and to proceed at a pace the person feels able to tolerate. The overall goal is prolonged exposure with eventual reduction of the anxiety in the presence of the feared object or situation. Avoidance prevention is used along with exposure so that the treatment is not interrupted.[14]

Self-directed exposure can be as effective as a therapist-directed program and represents a tremendous cost savings.[18] Self-management can be considered for clients who are not suicidal or on drugs or alcohol; are in good physical condition; are clear and specific about the help they want in order to improve their quality of life; and are committed to cooperate with the treatment program, including performing the assigned homework. The therapist helps to develop and explain the program and then turns it over to the client to manage.[12] As with any exposure plan, the anxiety will diminish but will not disappear entirely. If a relapse occurs, a booster session with the therapist or a revised plan may be in order.[12]

In planning a self-managed exposure program, it is important to help the client identify exactly what is feared (avoidance profile), to specify the goals to be achieved, to allow enough time to complete the exposure (long exposure periods reduce fear more than shorter ones), to know what sensations the client experiences when frightened, and to have the client choose some new tactic to cope with the anxiety instead of avoid it. For example, a person might choose to tense and relax muscles instead of giving in to the feeling of wanting to run away.[12,14] Clients on a self-managed program can benefit from a self-help book on self-directed exposure.[12]

Problem solving and assertiveness training involve assisting the client with coping skills. Problem solving involves discussing stressful life situations and ways to cope with those situations, setting goals, and trying out new coping behaviors. Studies in this area indicate that clients rate problem solving as valuable. However, if problem solving was done without exposure, the program was unreliable in reducing avoidance behaviors.[14]

Assertiveness training involves teaching clients to state their opinions, ideas, and feelings without resorting to passive or aggressive behavior. In studies of such training, assertiveness was increased. However, phobias and anxiety improved only when assertiveness training was accompanied by exposure.[14]

Cognitive approaches involve altering thoughts to prepare the client for changes in behavior. Two techniques may be used: identifying and challenging irrational ideas or changing the client's internal dialogue (self-talk).[14] Studies done with phobics and people with obsessive compulsive disorder indicate this method has limited effect when used alone.[14] Recent reports indicate positive results with cognitive techniques combined with other techniques, such as relaxation, in clients with panic disorder or generalized anxiety disorder.[18]

Other approaches in the treatment of anxiety disorders, such as relaxation, education, social skills training, group therapy, marital counseling, and individual psychotherapy, have produced various results. Their use would seem indicated whenever the circumstances seem appropriate; e.g., family therapy sessions with significant others who may inadvertently be supporting phobic avoidance behaviors and thus helping the client maintain the illness. A combination of treatment strategies should be used whenever indicated. Further research will be directed toward identifying the most effective combinations of treatment. Nurses have the opportunity to be proactive in investigating such areas of clinical concern.

Nursing Role

The psychiatric mental health nurse generalist will focus primarily on teaching about the effects and side effects of medications, helping the client learn new coping skills to manage anxiety (e.g., relaxation, assertiveness), and counseling the client about compliance with the behavioral program and difficulties in implementing the program.[1] Because many clients with anxiety disorders have a related depression, it is crucial to assess the individual's suicidal thoughts and feelings and to take steps to assure that the client does no self-harm.

The psychiatric mental health nurse specialist will additionally be concerned with counseling specific clients in modifying or eliminating dysfunctional behaviors. In counseling a client with a disabling phobia, the first step involves fully assessing the avoidance operations. Next, the nurse teaches the client about the methods and rationale of exposure, emphasizing the necessity for the client to remain in the anxiety-provoking situation until the anxiety subsides. The nurse can specifically prescribe the first few exposure tasks and then turn the program over to the client, if indicated. A client diary of the exposure tasks performed and the outcomes of those tasks can help the client keep track of progress.[13] It is important to warn the client that setbacks may occur but can be managed by returning to a less threatening level of exposure and repeating the task.[14]

Too sudden an exposure can lead to fear and noncompliance in the client with a disabling phobia.[14] A client can often be encouraged to "keep at it" by learning to carry out exposure in a manageable way. For example, flooding may be too threatening, in which case, the nurse can help the client develop a plan where exposure increases gradually and encourage the client to engage in the task by attending to it and feeling it in all its aspects. It also is important that the client endure rather than avoid the exposure and vary the exposure so that none of the relevant cues creates a fear response; e.g., look at object, feel object.[14] The nurse specialist may model behavior for the client who is unclear or needs encouragement.[14] An example of modeling by the nurse in the case of overcoming a fear of dogs would include looking at the dog while touching the dog (with gloves if necessary and then with bare hands), petting the dog, picking up the dog, and finally holding the dog for an extended period of time. Once the client has developed confidence, the client is encouraged to confront the feared object or situation on his or her own, without aid.[14] It is important that no benzodiazepines or alcohol be used during exposure, because this tends to make the exposure less effective. Encouraging and praising the client for his or her efforts may help maintain motivation. The counseling sessions may be expanded to include the client's family and significant friends. Such counseling sessions can help the client to understand and benefit more fully from the treatment program and may help educate family and friends on how to stop supporting the client's avoidance behaviors.

COMMON NURSING DIAGNOSES

The following nursing diagnoses may be useful in working with clients experiencing anxiety disorders: anxiety, bizarre behavior, ineffective individual coping, dysfunctional family processes, defensive coping, depression, diversional activity deficit, fear, guilt, hopelessness, altered impulse control, knowledge deficit, loneliness, altered parenting, post-trauma response, powerlessness, rape trauma syndrome, ritualistic behavior, self-concept disturbance, sleep pattern disturbance, impaired social interaction, somatization, substance abuse (alcohol), substance abuse (drugs), suicide potential, suspiciousness, and aggression (violence).

CASE STUDY

Sloane P, a 28-year-old woman, was brought to the outpatient anxiety clinic by her husband, Frank. For the past 3 years, she had refused to leave their apartment except for short periods, and on those occasions, she would go out only if Frank accompanied her. Even then, she did not like to go very far away from their apartment or to be gone very long. Frank had been hoping Sloane would "snap out of it" and had inadvertently fallen into a pattern of supporting Sloane's behavior. Sloane expressed fear that "something terrible" would happen to her if she went out, although she could not say what that terrible thing was. Sloane's brother, Steve, who lived in another state, visited Sloane and Frank last week. He had not seen them for 5 years and was astonished at the behavior of his sister. He persuaded Frank that Sloane needed professional help.

Both Sloane and Frank felt they had a good marriage. Frank did admit that Sloane's reluctance to leave their apartment had been more than inconvenient at times. For example, Sloane worked at home in her own accounting business, but because she would not leave their apartment, Frank picked up and delivered the accounting books for each firm every month. Frank also did most of the shopping and attended business social functions alone, and they had not gone on a vacation for 3 years. Both agreed that Sloane had grown too dependent on Frank.

After a thorough medical work-up, history, and psychological evaluation, the DSM-III-R diagnosis was panic disorder with agoraphobia. Mary J, R.N., M.N., was assigned as Sloane's nurse therapist. The recommendation from the treatment team was a desensitization program and a family conference to help Frank and Sloane discuss some changes in their relationship and assess need for further family therapy.

Mary met with Sloane to determine a picture of Sloane's avoidance behavior and developed the accompanying nursing care plan (see Nursing Care Plan 21-1 for a sample care plan for Sloane P).[15]

SUMMARY

More people experience anxiety disorders than any other group of disorders. Everyone experiences symptoms of anxiety; when the psychological and physiological responses to anxiety become maladaptive, then a diagnosis of anxiety disorder is made. Anxiety disorders are frequently associated with depression and are characterized by overt symptoms of anxiety or by anxiety avoidance behaviors. Because anxiety is universal, anxiety disorders may be difficult to differentiate from other physical and mental disorders that also present with anxiety. There is controversy about the causes and treatment of anxiety disorders, as well as the definitions of the disorders themselves. Exposure is the treatment of choice for disorders with avoidance behaviors. Self-directed avoidance exposure programs can be as effective as therapist-directed programs and

Text continued on page 588

Research Highlights

The field of anxiety disorders is one where clear, well-delineated studies need to be done. Nursing research can be very effective in helping to sort out prevention and treatment strategies that will improve the way anxiety is dealt with on all levels. Answers to the following questions could be identified through systematic study. It is hoped that this list of questions will stimulate further ideas in the reader's mind.

1. What coping skills need to be taught to clients with anxiety disorders?
2. What is the best method for teaching coping skills?
3. Are there family interactions that facilitate the development or maintenance of an anxiety disorder? What do family members need to do differently?

4. What impact does life with a parent with an anxiety disorder have on children?
5. What nursing diagnoses and client outcomes are most critical in working with clients with anxiety disorders?
6. What concepts need to be taught in grades K–12 about anxiety and its management? (An anxiety education program could be similar in format to alcohol, drug, and sex education.)
7. What do parents need to know about predisposing factors; e.g., symptoms of childhood separation anxiety and how to respond to the child showing such symptoms?
8. What are the factors that lead to relapse, and what is the best way to address these factors?

NURSING CARE PLAN 21–1

SLOANE P

NURSING INTERVENTIONS	OUTCOME CRITERIA

NURSING DIAGNOSIS: Ineffective individual coping related to anticipatory anxiety about public places and social interaction

CLIENT GOAL: Identify one specific avoidance behavior that can be targeted by exposure treatment

- Teach Sloane principles of desensitization and exposure
- Emphasize avoidance prevention, engagement, and endurance and prepare Sloane for setbacks and how to deal with them
- Teach about relaxation as a tool to prepare for desensitization and exposure

Prioritizes avoidance behaviors
Selects one behavior to change by exposure program

CLIENT GOAL: Implement a self-managed exposure program with the assistance of spouse

- Teach relaxation techniques to be used prior to exposure at client's option
- Meet with Sloane and Frank to specify a desensitization program related to one specific avoidance behavior identified by client (grocery shopping in supermarket)
- Encourage Sloane to shop at corner supermarket every day until 1 hour exposure is tolerated. (Does not have to buy; goal is to "shop.") Start with 15-minute exposure and increase by 15 minutes each day until able to tolerate for 1 hour
- Encourage Frank to accompany Sloane on first shopping trip and then gradually distance himself from her each day; e.g., wait at end of aisle, then at the cashier, then outside the store, and finally stay home while wife walks to the store to go shopping
- Teach Frank that if Sloane requests that he do the shopping, he is to respond by saying, "The staff at the hospital said I was to remind you to do the shopping."
- Encourage Sloane to use diary to record exposure time and evaluate her progress on a scale of 1 to 3: 1 = minimal anxiety and minimal or no urge to avoid; 2 = mild to moderate urge to avoid; 3 = intense anxiety with strong urge to avoid
- Encourage Sloane to use diary to plan next day's exposure. If anxiety is intense, slow down the exposure, increase or repeat the previous day's exposure until anxiety is reduced
- Teach Sloane to plan alternative ways to handle anxiety during exposure, e.g., deep breathing, contracting and relaxing muscles, etc.

Reports a reduction in anxiety during exposure
Carries out targeted behavior independently for one hour without presence of husband
Uses alternative ways to handle anxiety in exposure setting
Reports success in using self-exposure in targeting other behaviors
Verbalizes understanding of application of exposure program to other avoidance behaviors

NURSING DIAGNOSIS: Dysfunctional family processes related to inadequate socializing, overdependence on husband, and inability to meet mutual social needs of marital partners

FAMILY GOAL: Discuss new ways of interacting with each other

- Conduct a family conference with the goal of identifying mutual and separate activities for Sloane and Frank

Couple identifies mutual activities they are willing to share

FAMILY GOAL: Express willingness to individuate by engaging in activities independent of each other

- Encourage Sloane and Frank to decide on the mutual and independent activities each is willing to pursue

Agrees to a minimum number of shared activities per week
Continued

NURSING CARE PLAN 21-1

SLOANE P *Continued*

NURSING INTERVENTIONS	OUTCOME CRITERIA
■ Request Sloane and Frank negotiate for a specific number and type of mutual activities such as eating dinner in a restaurant, going to a movie, or attending church	Identifies separate activities each person agrees to pursue independently or with other people Agrees to a minimum number of independent activities per week Demonstrates ability to negotiate about mutual activities

FAMILY GOAL: Make a decision in regard to continuing family counseling

■ Encourage couple to summarize work done in first family session ■ Recommend two additional family counseling sessions to evaluate exposure program and individuation of Sloane and Frank	Agrees to continue family sessions according to therapist recommendation

result in tremendous cost savings for the patient. The roles of treatments (such as relaxation, education, assertiveness training, cognitive therapy, behavioral therapy, family therapy, medication therapy, group therapy, and one-to-one therapy) in anxiety disorders are not thoroughly understood. Future research should identify those therapies or combination of therapies that best address these disorders.

References

1. American Nurses' Association. Standards of psychiatric and mental health nursing practice. Kansas City: American Nurses' Association; 1982.
2. American Psychiatric Association. Diagnostic and Statistical Manual of Mental Disorders. 3rd ed, revised. Washington, DC: American Psychiatric Association; 1987.
3. Bech AT, Emery G, Greenberg RL. Anxiety disorders and phobias. New York: Basic Books; 1985.
4. Berger DM. Anxiety and related disorders. In: Greben SE, Rakoff VM, Voineskos G, eds. A method of psychiatry. Philadelphia: Lea & Febiger; 1985.
5. Cameron OD. The differential diagnosis of anxiety. Psychiatr Clin North Am. 1985;8:3–23.
6. Crowe RR. Mitral valve prolapse and panic disorder. Psychiatr Clin North Am. 1985;8:63–71.
7. Curtis GC. Anxiety and anxiety disorders. Psychiatr Clin North Am. 1985;8:159–168.
8. Curtis GC. New findings in anxiety. Psychiatr Clin North Am. 1985;8:169–175.
9. DiNardo PA, Barlow DH. Anxiety Disorders Interview Schedule–Revised (ADIS-R). Albany: Phobia and Anxiety Disorders Clinic, University of Albany, State University of New York; 1988.
10. Insel TR. Obsessive–compulsive disorders. Psychiatr Clin North Am. 1985;8:105–117.
11. Jack RA, Matthew RJ. Anxiety disorders: diagnosis and treatment. Compr Ther. 1985;7:31–37.
12. Marks IM. Living with fear. New York: McGraw-Hill; 1978.
13. Marks IM. Behavioral aspects of panic disorder. Am J Psychiatry. 1987;144:1160–1165.
14. Marks IM. Fears, phobias, and rituals. New York: Oxford University Press; 1987.
15. McFarland GK, Wasli EL. Nursing diagnosis and process in psychiatric mental health nursing. Philadelphia: JB Lippincott; 1986.
16. Noyes R Jr. Beta-adrenergic blocking drugs in anxiety and stress. Psychiatr Clin North Am. 1985;8:119–132.
17. Rainey JM, Nesse RM. Psychobiology of anxiety and anxiety disorders. Psychiatr Clin North Am. 1985;8:133–144.
18. Roy–Byrne PP, Katon W. An update on treatment of anxiety disorders. Hosp Community Psychiatry. 1987;38:835–843.
19. Van den Hout MA, van der Molen M, Griez E, Lousberg H, Nansen A. Reduction of CO_2 anxiety in patients with panic attacks after repeated CO_2 exposure. Am J Psychiatry. 1987;144:788–791.
20. Wolfe JL. Women. In: Ellis A, Bernard ME, eds. Clinical applications of rational-emotive therapy. New York: Plenum Press; 1985.
21. Wolkowitz OM, Paul SM. Neural and molecular mechanisms in anxiety. Psychiatr Clin North Am. 1985;8:145–158.

22

Maryanne Godfrey

Clients With Personality Disorders

OBJECTIVES

After reading this chapter, the reader will be able to:

1. *Define* personality disorders
2. *Describe characteristics of various personality disorders*
3. *Describe two approaches to assessment for personality disorders*
4. *Discuss psychiatric treatment modalities for clients with personality disorders*
5. *Identify common nursing diagnoses for clients with personality disorders*
6. *Discuss strategies for nursing interventions for clients with personality disorders.*

DESCRIPTION

"*Personality* can be defined as those enduring and consistent attitudes, beliefs, values, and patterns of adaptation that distinguish one person from another" (reference 2, p 133). It is when this constellation, or some part of it, becomes fixed, rigid, unyielding, and maladaptive that a personality disorder exists. Therefore, individuals with personality disorders have a characteristic style of interacting that is maladaptive and persistent over time.

Types

The DSM-III-R[1] recognizes eleven distinct types of personality disorders categorized into three main clusters. The first cluster, *odd and eccentric,* includes paranoid, schizoid, and schizotypal. Individuals with these personality disorders infrequently come into contact with health professionals. They tend to be alienated from society and experience difficulties in their social interactions. Their behavior is withdrawn and isolative. They are emotionally distant, and it is difficult to get to know them. Socially, they are aloof, avoiding social situations or intimate relationships. The second cluster, *dramatic and emotional,* includes antisocial, borderline, histrionic, and narcissistic personality disorders. Individuals with these disorders may be marginally functional in society. They tend to have a high profile in the health care setting because they are emotionally explosive, with interpersonal relations that tend to be intense and unstable. Socially, they avoid being alone, but have difficulty tolerating emotional closeness. Their behavior is often dramatic and demanding. Mental health contacts may be secondary to involvement with the legal system. The third cluster, *anxiety and fear-based,* includes avoidant, dependent, obsessive–compulsive, and passive–aggressive personality disorders. Individuals with these personality disorders appear socially inept. They have difficulty expressing emotions and are sensitive to rejection. Interpersonal relations range from icy cold to extreme neediness. These individuals frequently come into contact with health professionals as a result of another problem, such as depression or physical illness.

Clients with personality disorders come to medical or psychiatric settings bringing with them a unique set of problems. However, they rarely come for treatment of their personality disorders. Rather, the disorder is disguised among a constellation of physical and emotional complaints. Frequent presentations include depression, situational crisis, vague physical complaints, and chronic pain. Early indicators that a personality disorder may be present include difficulty establishing a nurse–client relationship, disagreements among team members, a reluctance by the nurse to provide client care, or difficulty accomplishing treatment objectives. Misdiagnosis of individuals with personality disorders is common, as is difficulty in implementing an appropriate treatment regimen.

The prevalence of personality disorders has been estimated to be between 5% and 15% in the general population and between 33% and 50% in psychiatric clients.[5] Specific personality disorders, characteristic behaviors, and primary affects are summarized in Table 22-1.[1,10]

ASSESSMENT

There are two systems for identifying personality disorders: the dimensional and the categorical.[5,10] The dimensional system relies on a group of traits along a continuum based on psychological testing and the norms of numerous individuals. The primary aim is to identify those traits that most clearly define personality types and associated behavior. Pathologic traits are seen on a continuum with nonpathologic traits. An example of the dimensional type is the Minnesota Multiphasic Personality Inventory (MMPI), a test of over 500 items. The answers are used to define personality traits and habits of the individual. The dimensional method of personality testing is cross-sectional rather than longitudinal and does not take into account an individual's history or clinical data. Rather, it reflects what is happening at the time of the test. Dimensional methods are useful as adjuncts to clinical assessment, but they are not used exclusively, nor are they thought to be predictive of behavior.

The second system is categorical. This is a descriptive approach relying on a disease model of grouping symptoms to describe specific personality disorders. The DSM-III-R is the most recent effort to provide standardized criteria for the establishment of a psychiatric diagnosis of personality disorders.[1] The DSM-III-R establishes a prototype for each disorder that gives a profile of symptoms that must be present to make a diagnosis. The criteria, however, are not always specific enough to differentiate one personality disorder from another.[12]

TREATMENT MODALITIES

Since clients usually come into contact with health professionals because of another problem, the personality disorder may not be the primary focus of care. Even when the personality disorder is the focus of treatment, there is insufficient research to indicate clear-cut guidelines for choice of treatment of all disorders.[12] However, a number of different treatments have been shown to have some benefit for certain disorders:[12] (1) psychodynamic therapies that focus on change of personality structure or on increasing the individual's flexibility and adaptability; (2) supportive therapy during periods of stress; (3) group or marital therapies directed toward the individual's interpersonal style; (4) behavioral and cognitive therapies focused on particular characteristics of a disorder; (5) pharmacotherapy focused on particular symptoms such as anxiety or cognitive–perceptual manifestations.[12]

TABLE 22-1
Characteristics of specific personality disorders

PERSONALITY DISORDER	CHARACTERISTIC BEHAVIOR	PRIMARY AFFECT
ODD AND ECCENTRIC		
Paranoid	Interprets reality as threatening; negativistic; high levels of suspiciousness; may be jealous, hypervigilant; angry outbursts	Angry
Schizoid	Indifferent to social relationships; restricted range of emotional experience and expression; solitary; appears cold and aloof	Constricted
Schizotypal	Peculiarities and eccentricities in thought content, appearance, and behavior; may include suspiciousness, ideas of reference; magical thinking; interpersonal relationships limited to family; few if any close friends	Constricted
Antisocial	Irresponsible, with potentially destructive behavior, physically and emotionally; little to no regard for sociocultural norms and the feelings of others	Angry, hostile
DRAMATIC AND EMOTIONAL		
Borderline	Disturbed sense of self; difficulty with interpersonal relationships; marked by anger and intense shifts in mood; threats of self-harm	Angry, depressed
Histrionic	Exaggerated and dramatic in presentation; demanding with an inability to delay gratification; seductive style	Labile
Narcissistic	Grandiose with inflated sense of self, very sensitive to approval; easily hurt; preoccupied with self, lacks empathy	Full range of affect with underlying depression
ANXIETY AND FEAR-BASED		
Avoidant	Social discomfort, fears disapproval of others, shy with fear of social blunders	Blunted, depression
Dependent	Dependent and submissive style; heavy reliance on the opinions of others; seeks approval; tense and anxious when alone; nonassertive and subordinate to others	Depressed
Obsessive–compulsive	Rigid perfectionism; preoccupation with rules; inflexible in most areas of life	Blunted, angry
Passive–aggressive	Passive resistance to social and occupational roles; procrastinates, indirect expression of ideas and feelings especially negative ones	Angry, irritable

Cowdry suggests that if medicines are to be used, they should be used in conjunction with psychotherapy.[4] He identifies target symptoms for the use of medication as affective dyscontrol, behavioral dyscontrol, or intrapsychic and interpersonal problems. He notes that medications may be useful in accessing intrapsychic difficulties, but certainly should not be considered the only treatment, nor the treatment of choice. If medications are to be used, he suggests that the initiation dosage of the medications be lower than usual protocols.[4]

Clients with personality disorders may require hospitalization, especially during periods of crisis. Hospital-based care offers a client a place to reorganize the self and mobilize defenses to return to baseline functioning. The role of the hospital staff is to help the client identify precipitants leading to hospitalization and what is necessary for the client to return to his or her daily activities of living. Hospital-based care is generally short-term with clear definition of goals and specific strategies to meet those goals. In recent times it has been thought inappropriate to spend time dealing with long-term characterological issues while the client is on a short-term stay unit.[6,8] This can be contrasted to an inpatient model of much longer duration, generally employing principles of psychoanalytic theory. Here, the inpatient setting is highly structured and the individual is known to be hospitalized for many months with the intention of actually pursuing characterological change.

NURSING DIAGNOSES AND NURSING ROLES

Common nursing diagnoses associated with clusters of personality disorders are summarized in Table 22-2. In caring for clients with personality disorders, the nurse attempts to reduce the disruptive impact of pathologic behaviors on the client and those in the client's environment. Certain guidelines are useful, particularly in the hospital setting.

1. Focusing on the task at hand gives the client a structure for what is to be accomplished during hospitalization. The presence of a personality disorder is a long-term problem and will not change during a short-term hospitalization.[6,8] Clients often avoid the objectives of treatment because of the anxiety associated with change. Focusing on the task at hand helps to diffuse anxiety and to structure realistic goals for hospitalization.
2. Providing structure assists the client to maximize functioning and prevents overreliance on the hospital.
3. Setting consistent limits is done by clearly describing how the hospital works, what can be accomplished, and what the expectations are. Because the client may expect more of a nurse than is appropriate, consistent limits help the client to avoid

TABLE 22-2
Common nursing diagnoses by clusters of personality disorders

NURSING DIAGNOSES	ODD AND ECCENTRIC	DRAMATIC AND EMOTIONAL	FEAR AND ANXIETY
Aggression		X	
Anger		X	X
Bizarre behavior	X		
Boredom		X	X
Communication, impaired	X		
Coping, ineffective individual		X	X
Defensive coping	X	X	X
Depression		X	X
Diversional activity deficit	X		
Elopement, potential for		X	
Emotional lability		X	
Impulse control, altered		X	
Injury, potential for		X	
Manipulation		X	
Powerlessness	X	X	X
Self-concept disturbance	X	X	
Sleep pattern disturbance	X		X
Social interaction, impaired	X	X	X
Somatization		X	X
Substance abuse (alcohol)		X	
Substance abuse (drugs)		X	
Suicide potential		X	
Suspiciousness	X		

disappointments from unfulfilled expectations. Discussion among staff members also helps reduce staff splitting and provides support for staff members.

4. Adopting a neutral therapeutic stance is especially useful with the client who desperately seeks the omnipotent care provider, only to radically switch to devaluing the individual in defense against the internal sense of loss and rejection. The care provider must be aware of these projections and not react in anger, but with a consistent, therapeutic response. Brief, frequent contacts are preferable to lengthy intense contacts because they help contain the emotional flooding often experienced by individuals.

5. Confrontation is to be avoided. The client lacks the internal ego structure necessary to modulate emotional responses. Frequently clients communicate that enormous amounts of care are necessary. But this is a coping mechanism that defends against underlying feelings of inadequacy and need. The client often does not understand his or her part in a situation and may deny any part at all. In an effort to maintain a working therapeutic relationship, the client needs redirection to the task at hand and the overall goals of hospitalization.

6. Preventing destructive behavior is critical to a successful hospital stay. Nurses alert to early warning signs of mood lability, and increased demands, can intervene to prevent a client's self-harm. This may include a no-harm contract, close observation, one-to-one monitoring, or physical restraints. It may also include discharge if that was part of the original treatment contract. The overall message to be communicated to the client is that the staff and clients will work together to maintain a safe environment. Therapeutic and problematic nursing actions with clients with personality disorders are summarized in Box 22-1.

CASE STUDY

Phyllis, a 28-year-old single woman, was referred for hospitalization for suicidal ideation by her outpatient therapist. Her Axis I psychiatric diagnoses were polysubstance dependence and dysthymia, and Axis II diagnosis was borderline personality disorder. Phyllis has been hospitalized 39 times during the last year with one drug overdose and multiple instances of self-mutilation. She was the eldest of eight children and was physically abused as a child. At the time of hospitalization she had little contact with her family of origin and no close relationships. Her work record had been erratic. Recent psychosocial stressors included termination with her outpatient therapist and estrangement from her female lover of three years. She reported that she has been drinking up to nine beers a day and using a variety of street drugs. Upon admission she experienced symptoms of alcohol withdrawal, necessitating the administration of chlordiazepoxide (Librium). In addition, she said that she had been depressed for a long time and has had 600 pills at home "just in case." Phyllis was confrontational and angry in interactions with staff, accusing them of incompetence. She checked information she received from one nurse with another nurse, looking for even minor discrepancies. Her nursing diagnoses included ineffective individual coping, anger, suspiciousness, manipulation, and suicide potential.

NURSING CARE PLAN 22–1

PHYLLIS

NURSING INTERVENTIONS	OUTCOME CRITERIA

NURSING DIAGNOSIS: Suicide potential related to loss

CLIENT GOAL: Refrain from self-destructive acts

■ Assist Phyllis to verbalize thoughts and feelings ■ Maintain a no-harm contract ■ Assess for suicidal ideation	Does not harm self

NURSING DIAGNOSIS: Ineffective individual coping related to borderline personality disorder

CLIENT GOAL: Attain higher level of functioning

■ Set specific time frame for hospitalization ■ Identify clear objectives for hospitalization ■ Focus on task at hand ■ Identify clear expectations for behavior	Resumes level of functioning sufficient to engage in community-based care

NURSING DIAGNOSIS: Anger related to concerns about depending on others

CLIENT GOAL: Reduce angry outbursts

■ Adopt a neutral stance ■ Acknowledge losses in Phyllis's life ■ Avoid lengthy exploration of anger ■ Clarify behavioral expectations	Talks about ideas and feelings without intense rage

NURSING DIAGNOSIS: Substance abuse (alcohol and drugs) related to borderline personality disorder

CLIENT GOAL: Gain an increased awareness of polysubstance abuse and necessary treatment

■ Assist in gaining awareness of difficulty in addressing long-term emotional issues while using alcohol and drugs ■ Refer to community drug and alcohol program	Verbalizes increased understanding of the effects of drug and alcohol on functioning Participates in community follow-up

NURSING DIAGNOSIS: Manipulation related to concerns about having needs met

CLIENT GOAL: Learn other ways to meet needs

■ Maintain clear, consistent limits ■ Identify primary nurse ■ Arrange for 15-min staff contacts every 4 hr during waking hours ■ Assist in asking for what is needed more directly	Meets needs without resorting to manipulative behavior

The hospital course focused on identifying the impact of substance abuse on everyday functioning and the identification of short-term goals to assist the patient to regain baseline functioning. The discharge plan included follow-up with a community drug and alcohol counselor and recommendation for long-term outpatient counseling. Nursing Care Plan 22-1 outlines the goals and interventions for Phyllis.

BOX 22–1
Therapeutic and Problematic Nursing Actions With Clients With Personality Disorders

THERAPEUTIC NURSING ACTIONS	PROBLEMATIC NURSING ACTIONS
Identifies client behavior and verbalizations as symptoms of an underlying problem and maintains awareness; seeks consultation and supervision as needed to sharpen diagnosis and treatment plan	Is unable to separate self from client's symptoms; personalizes interaction; is unable to accept feedback
Provides therapeutic responses, respecting the boundaries of a professional nurse–client relationship	Takes on and experiences the feelings experienced by the client: anger, devaluation; feelings can be manifested in nurse–client relationships or in relationships with other health care providers
Understands the limits of nursing treatment, expects clients to take responsibility for self	Feels overwhelmed by client expectations, takes more responsibility than necessary for client
Is comfortable with the therapeutic aspects of limit setting; is flexible and creative in setting limits; nurses share nursing diagnoses and supporting assessment data during interdisciplinary team meetings; participate in planning of client's care; interdisciplinary team meets regularly to review client management and to maintain open dialogue among members	Limit setting is inconsistent and is carried out in anger
	Nurses participate in destructive interaction with team members; unresolved disagreements about treatment objectives; lack of adequate communication

Research Highlights

As suggested earlier, the criteria for defining personality disorders is often diffuse and not well researched. There is disagreement about the extent to which psychotic phenomena can be attributed to borderline personality disorder.[7,9,11] Chopra and Beatson reported on a pilot study of 13 clients with borderline personality disorder, analyzing brief psychotic symptoms.[3] All clients met the DSM-III-R criteria for borderline personality disorder. The Diagnostic Interview for Borderline Patients[6] was administered to all the clients. The results of the interview demonstrated that psychotic symptoms were probable in all clients. The most common psychotic symptoms were of the dissociative type; derealization was present in 12, and depersonalization was present in 11. The symptoms were of varying intensity and of brief duration and were experienced during periods of stress. Seven of the 13 clients experienced non–drug-induced hallucinations, generally lasting up to several hours, not requiring medications. The authors suggest that a study of a larger group of clients followed over time could better define the extent to which psychotic phenomena are a part of the constellation of symptoms composing borderline personality disorder.

SUMMARY

The treatment of personality disorders is varied and complex. There is still much required in the study of the specific disorders. The nurse has been alerted to specific nursing interventions emphasizing optimal elements of care and general principles of intervention that can be applied to the care of individuals with personality disorders.

References

1. American Psychiatric Association. Diagnostic and statistical manual of mental disorders, 3rd ed, revised. Washington, DC: American Psychiatric Association; 1987.
2. Arana G, Nadelson C, Guggenheim F. Personality disorders. In: Guggenheim F, Nadelson C, eds. Major psychiatric disorders, overviews and selected readings. New York: Elsevier Science Publishers; 1982.
3. Chopra HD, Beatson JA. Psychotic symptoms in borderline personality disorder. Am J Psychiatry. 1986;143:(12):1605–1607.
4. Cowdry RW. Current overview of the borderline diagnosis. J Clin Psychiatry. 1987;48(suppl 8):15–22.
5. Grinspoon L, ed. Harvard Med School Ment Health Lett. 1987;4(Sept).
6. Gunderson JG, Kolb JE, Austin V. The diagnostic interview for borderline patients. Am J Psychiatry. 1981;138:896–903.
7. Jonas JM, Pope HG. Psychosis in borderline personality disorder. Psychiatr Dev. 1984;4:295–308.
8. Kellner R. Personality disorders. Psychother Psychosom. 1987;46:58–66.
9. Kolb JE, Gunderson JG. Diagnosing borderline patients with a semistructured interview. Arch Gen Psychiatry. 1980; 37:37–41.
10. Millon T. Disorders of personality: DSM III: Axis II. New York: John Wiley & Sons; 1981.
11. Tarnopolsky A, Berelowitz M. "Borderline personality": diagnostic attitudes at the Maudsley Hospital. Br J Psychiatry. 1984;144:364–369.
12. Widiger TA, Francis A. The DSM-III personality disorders: perspectives from psychology. Arch Gen Psychiatry. 1985;42:615–623.

Mental Health and Illness in Special Population Groups

23

Mary Kunes-Connell

Children and Adolescents: Developmental Issues and Concerns

OBJECTIVES

After reading this chapter, the reader will be able to:

1. Discuss intrapersonal, interpersonal, and extrapersonal variables influencing the child's or adolescent's response to stress
2. Describe techniques used to gather information related to the physical, developmental, cognitive, educational, social, and family assessment of the child or adolescent
3. Identify questions that could be used when interviewing the child or adolescent
4. Describe the possible related factors and defining characteristics associated with the nursing diagnoses of self-esteem disturbance and ineffective individual coping for children and adolescents
5. Discuss general treatment modalities and nursing interventions for children and adolescents experiencing stress, including milieu therapy, one-to-one therapy, and group therapy
6. Summarize a research study related to an aspect of mental health in children or adolescents.

INTRODUCTION

Despite the child's or adolescent's resiliency, it is increasingly difficult to grow up in a healthy way. This is evidenced by the staggering statistics on the mental health problems of children and adolescents (see Chapter 14).

As children and adolescents reach certain developmental levels, they are confronted with new ideas about themselves and their environment. Each new development task or environmental demand forces the child or adolescent to further clarify his or her sense of self as well as role performances and responsibilities. De Maio,[7] Gelfand,[11] Johnson,[18] Morrow,[23] Rickel,[30] and Rutter[32] cite a number of societal factors making developmental tasks exceedingly difficult to negotiate, thus increasing the child's or adolescent's vulnerability to the negative consequences of stress. These factors include:

■ *Changing family patterns:* The family forms the base for values from which individual beliefs, values, and philosophies are established. Furthermore, the ability to see family members deal directly with problems gives children a base for problem solving. However, the absence of a firm definition of family deprives the child of the experiences, knowledge, and validation needed to develop a repertoire of problem-solving and coping behaviors. The trend toward single-parent families, two-working-parent families, foster care, and institutional care can, in some instances, deprive the juvenile of the role-modeling necessary to respond positively to stress and change.[7,32]
■ *Media influence:* The media exerts a powerful influence on children and adolescents. Because they spend a great deal of time in front of the television, at the movies, or listening to the radio, they are bombarded with often contradictory messages, and it is hard for them to distinguish the appropriate from the inappropriate. The messages communicated by the media often mirror society's struggle with its own standards and values.[7]
■ *Shifting social mores:* Social values have shifted markedly over the past several decades and often conflict. On the one hand, children are taught to work hard to achieve the more pleasurable things in life, yet the media portrays drug buys, theft, and other crimes as means to achieve wealth. Children are told to "say no" to drugs, yet the media often portrays the "highs" associated with drug use.[7,11,18]

These, and other factors, can influence the ability of the child or adolescent to cope with a variety of developmental and environmental stressors. How they cope with stress depends on a number of intrapersonal and interpersonal variables. It is important for the mental health nurse to have an understanding of these variables and their role in the individual developmental progression and coping response of both children and adolescents.

VARIABLES INFLUENCING THE CHILD'S OR ADOLESCENT'S RESPONSE TO STRESS

Intrapersonal Characteristics

Wertlieb and co-workers,[41] in a study measuring the child's ability to cope, identify the ability to problem solve as an essential prerequisite to effective coping. This study also discusses the child's ability to effectively manage feelings as a secondary prerequisite to coping with life events and other stressors. Box 23-1 summarizes the developmental life tasks from infancy to adolescence. Any physical, emotional, or cognitive disability could compromise the child's or adolescent's ability to problem solve and manage the anxiety associated with anticipated and unanticipated life events.[18] Intrapersonal characteristics impairing the child's or adolescent's coping abilities can be divided into general categories: central nervous system (CNS) impairment and self-esteem disturbance.[32,34]

CENTRAL NERVOUS SYSTEM IMPAIRMENT

Any CNS disruption may cause an inherent impairment in the child's ability to respond adequately to the environment; several factors may increase a child's risk for CNS dysfunction. Prenatally, the mother's eating, drinking, smoking, or drug habits may affect the infant's cognitive abilities. Poor prenatal habits result in infants with lower birth weight and smaller brain mass.[34] These factors result in a retarded cognitive development, that impinges on the ability of the child or adolescent to problem solve daily life events. In addition to prenatal conditions, genetic disorders, such as phenylketonuria, homocystinuria, and Down syndrome, can have deleterious effects on the mental development of the child.[30,34,36] Neurologic deficits may also be the result of physical trauma occurring during the course of development. Accidents, head injuries, brain tumors, or spinal injuries, at any age, could result in brain damage or other CNS dysfunction affecting the child's ability to successfully respond to developmental challenges.

SELF-ESTEEM DISTURBANCE

Self-esteem has long been recognized as crucial to the mental and physical health of the child or adolescent. It does not necessarily serve as the direct link to behavior, but rather, provides a frame of reference for interpreting and acting on one's physical and interpersonal environment. When a child or adolescent has positive self-esteem, he or she is more likely to interpret and respond to the environment in positive ways.[31] Conversely, negative perception of self fosters behaviors that are most likely going to validate this negativity.

The development of self-esteem is ongoing. At each phase of a child's or an adolescent's development, it is

---

BOX 23-1
Developmental Tasks of Infancy, Early Childhood, Childhood, and Adolescence[10,11,29,37]

INFANCY (0–18 mo)

- Attempts to develop secure attachments to primary caretaker
- Begins to determine own effectiveness in getting others to meet infant's needs
- Begins to determine level of trust in relationship to environment

EARLY CHILDHOOD (10 mo–6 yr)

- Begins to develop a "sense of self"—growing perception of separateness from caretakers
- Develops sense of self-discipline (e.g., delayed gratification)
- Developing sense of individualism in decision making (e.g., ability to say "no")
- Developing cooperative abilities (e.g., play)
- Increasing use of language to meet needs
- Increasing exploration of own body
- Develops increased socializing behaviors with peers

CHILDHOOD (6–12 yr)

- Developing a sense of competency and achievement
- Developing increased responsibility for own behavior
- Understanding importance of peer relationships—seeks acceptance from peers, especially same-sexed peers; participates in mutual sharing with peers
- Increased initiative and risk taking
- Demonstrates concrete problem-solving skills

ADOLESCENCE (12–18 yr)

- Testing out family's values and developing own set of standards and values
- Increased independent decision making (symbolically moving away from family)
- Coming to grips with own sexuality and sexual roles
- Increased intimacy in peer relations
- Increased ability to utilize abstract problem-solving skills and judgment in life situations

---

important for parents, teachers, and other significant persons in the environment to ask themselves "How can I make this child feel good about himself?" or "How can I promote a positive sense of self in this child?" The answer to this question lies in the communicated messages from significant others. Constructive messages are those that convey (1) a belief in the significance and importance of the child, (2) an acceptance of the child, (3) a general trust in the child's and adolescent's judgments and decisions, (4) a sense of safety, and (5) a sense of values and standards.[14,29,33]

Interpersonal Characteristics

An environment that responds to a child's physical, emotional, and social needs in an effective, supportive, and timely fashion communicates to that child that he or she is a worthwhile person. The child develops a sense of importance and certainty about the self.

Communicating acceptance is key to self-esteem. The child or adolescent must feel accepted for who he or she is and not for what he or she can be; that is, acceptance should not be contingent on achievement, status, or other factors. Messages, such as "I love you because you get good grades, or don't make trouble," can be problematic. However, acceptance of the child does not automatically imply acceptance of all behaviors. Messages should convey that a child is still loved and accepted, even though certain behaviors are not tolerated. The child or adolescent must perceive the self as accepted and "good" despite some "not-so-good" behaviors.[14,29,33]

The focus should be placed on the strengths of an individual, since positive reinforcement of one's strengths foster positive feeling about the self. A focus

that is on only drawbacks serves to reinforce a negative self-esteem.[14,29,33]

Trust in the child's or adolescent's judgments must also be communicated. The child or adolescent must sense that he or she will not be belittled for decisions. This does not mean that others have to agree with the decisions, but rather, that the parent or significant other conveys a "listening" versus "advice" posture when the child wants to talk about decisions. If decisions do not turn out, the adult should not take on the "I told you so" posture. This reinforces feelings of ineffectiveness. Rather, a "we all make mistakes, let's learn from it" attitude facilitates a more positive sense of self.

Communicating a sense of safety by setting limits on the child's or adolescent's behavior is necessary for promoting self-esteem. Limits and expectations serve as guides for behavior. Without these, the child may not recognize personal limitations and may overstep boundaries. Inevitably, this can bring about failure. If this continues, the child could see himself as ineffective and incompetent.

Ineffective communication on the part of parents or significant others may be related to their own inability to deal with stress or with their perceptions of the child.[33,38] These situations include:

- The confrontation of parents or significant others by extreme stressors can result in a temporary impairment in coping on the part of the parent (e.g., divorce, family illness). Stress can cause the parent or significant other to invest all energies into dealing with the stressors, thereby leaving little time for attending to the needs of the children.[8,32]
- The parent's or significant other's lack of intrapersonal or extrapersonal resources to cope with even

the most minor stressors, (e.g., a parent who suffers from schizophrenia).[8]

■ The physical or cognitive "differentness" of the child (e.g., congenital defects of child, mentally retarded child).[30,34]

These situations could impinge on the quality of interactions between the child and the parent or significant other.

When families are confronted with stressful situations that overwhelm their capacities, little energy is left to invest in the child's emotional and psychological growth and development. Another variable affecting a parent's or significant other's response to a child is the emotional status of the parent or significant other. Rickel[30] and Doyle et al.[8] summarize a number of studies concerning the emotional response of the child in a dysfunctional family system. In families in which one or both parents are experiencing emotional or mental psychopathology, the atmosphere is such that the child often experiences a lack of acceptance, warmth, and adequate supervision. Thus, the child becomes more vulnerable to emotional, mental, and social maladjustment.

Finally, the atypical or "different" child often creates a distressing situation for the parents and other significant others. Parents experience a number of feelings when the child is "not okay" either physically, emotionally, or mentally. These feelings may include feelings of guilt and failure over having produced a "not-so-perfect" child, depression, anger, and embarrassment. These feelings are often projected onto the parent–child relationship in the form of emotional or physical negativity and rejections or anxious attachment. In addition to poor parent–child relationships, the atypical child often becomes the subject of peer abuse or rejection. Ridicule or rejection often leads to feelings of low self-worth and isolation.[12,29]

In essence, a dysfunctional family system or other negative parent–child interactions lead to a negative, rejecting form of communication. A child or adolescent exposed to this type of communication may adopt behaviors indicative of psychological, emotional, or social maladjustment. It is often at this point that parents, relatives, teachers, or other caretakers refer the child for evaluation or treatment.[7,17,18,30,32]

NURSING PROCESS WITH CHILDREN AND ADOLESCENTS

Assessment

Any child or adolescent referred for psychiatric treatment must have a thorough assessment to initiate an appropriate treatment plan. The evaluation of the child or adolescent is comprehensive both in the criteria used for assessment and the methods used to collect data. A variety of assessment criteria are necessary because the child or adolescent may have disorders different from the psychiatric syndromes common in adults. The common psychiatric problems affecting a child or adolescent can be behavioral, emotional, cognitive, or developmental. An assessment process must be designed to ensure the most comprehensive data collection possible.[1,2,13,34,39] Common assessment determinants serving as a general framework for the evaluation process include: physical health status, developmental status, cognitive status, educational status, emotional–behavioral–social status, and family relationship patterns.[34] Box 23-2 highlights categories forming the assessment framework.

Data collection methods should vary, because no one method has been proved to be the most effective in eliciting accurate data;[13,34,39] however, the interview is still considered one of the most important. When using the interview technique with children and adolescents, the following points should be considered:

■ The child must be interviewed, in addition to the parent or guardian.

■ It often is more productive to interview the child apart from the parent or guardian because the child or adolescent may be angry with the parent for being referred to treatment, thus increasing resistance to answering questions. The child or adolescent needs to be given some choice about the manner in which the interview is being conducted. The interview portion of the assessment combines an open-ended with a structured approach. The open-ended interview allows more of a free-flow conversation between the interviewer and interviewee. Box 23-3 depicts possible questions that could be used in an open-ended interview, and such questions can be used to obtain information related to a child's or an adolescent's present problem, educational status, recreational status, and self-concept. A drawback to this approach is that a parent or guardian or a child's perception may be influenced by a number of variables, thus hampering the clinician's ability to accurately diagnose the situation. Therefore, a structured portion of the interview might be necessary for a more objective view of the situation. The structured part of the interview might necessitate the use of standardized behavioral lists and life stress scales.[13,34]

■ The nurse requires a working knowledge of normal growth and development and of common disorders associated with childhood and adolescence to interview the child or adolescent effectively. This knowledge base facilitates the content of questions and observations that form the basis of the interview.[26]

■ The nurse must have an excellent knowledge of the normative cognitive levels of children and adolescents, which is useful when determining how to ask questions or elicit the necessary information.[26]

■ The nurse must establish rapport with the child or adolescent before asking emotionally laden questions or seeking personal information from either the parents or child. The child's or adolescent's fear

---

BOX 23–2
Child and Adolescent Assessment Criteria and Methodologies

ASSESSMENT PARAMETERS

A. Physical Assessment
   1. Medical history: history of illness, accidents
   2. Medication history: psychiatric/nonpsychiatric medications
   3. Immunologic status
   4. Recent physical/dental examination and results
   5. General nutritional and elimination status
   6. Sleep–rest patterns
   7. Exercise–activity patterns
   8. Sexual activity patterns
B. Developmental Assessment
   1. Psychomotor
   2. Language
   3. Personality–social
C. Cognitive and Psychological Assessment
   1. Intelligence assessment
   2. Thought content
   3. Perceptual abilities
D. Educational Assessment
   1. Achievement assessment (especially correlated to IQ)
   2. Assessment of motivation level and interests
   3. Attitudes toward school
   4. Quality of teacher–peer relationships
E. Social, Emotional, and Behavioral Assessment
   1. Social
      a. Quality of interpersonal relationships
      b. Degree of extroversion or introversion
      c. Social skills level
   2. Emotional
      a. Overall mood level
      b. Stability or lability of mood
      c. Expression of emotions
   3. Behavioral
      a. Life events as sources of stress
      b. Nonanticipated life events as sources of stress
      c. Response to stress
      d. Behavioral problems: duration, intensity, causes
   4. Family relationships
      a. Quality of relationships

ASSESSMENT METHODOLOGY

- Interview: parent/guardian and child (where applicable)
- Physical examination
- Neurological assessment
- Laboratory values: CBC, UA, T_3/T_4
- Radiological tests: chest x-ray, EKG, EEG

- Observation of child
- Interview of parent/guardian (e.g., Minnesota Child Development Inventory[34])
- Denver Developmental Screening[34]
- Mental status examination
- Standardized intelligence test (e.g., Wechsler Intelligence Scales—Children; Peabody Picture Vocabulary Tests[34])

- Teacher interviews
- Achievement testing (e.g., Woodcock Johnson Psychoeducational Battery)
- Observation of the child in the classroom
- Interview of the child

- Parent/guardian interview
- Behavioral evaluation checklist (e.g., Achenbach's Child Behavioral Checklist)[1,2]
- Standardized personality assessment tools (e.g., Minnesota Multiphasic Personality Inventory)[1]
- Life events scales (e.g., Coddington Life Stress Scale)[18]

---

of intrusion into his personal world or the parent's fear of being labeled a "poor parent" may produce resistance if the nurse proceeds too quickly in the interview.

The interview should be supplemented with other methods of assessment, whether they be the direct observation of the child, child–family, or child–peer relationships, self-reports, behavioral checklists, developmental scales, or psychological testing. Only through a multifaceted method can the nurse be assured of attaining a comprehensive data base for care planning. Box 23-3 illustrates possible questions that can be used by the nurse to collect data in each of the categories of the child or adolescent assessment. In addition to focusing on both the child's and family's perception of the present crisis, the tool is useful in identifying background information on the child's or adolescent's educational background, present living situations, social

and recreational status, psychological strengths and needs, developmental milestones, and physical health status. This tool also provides the nurse with the opportunity to assess interactional patterns between the child or adolescent and the family, as well as the interviewer.

Common Nursing Diagnoses

Although assessment is a ongoing process, after initial assessment, it is important for the nurse to synthesize the data collected to determine the appropriate nursing diagnoses. Because the child or adolescent often enters treatment with multiple problems, it is vital that the nurse identify nursing diagnoses that enable the implementation of the most comprehensive treatment plan. Box 23-4 lists some of the most common nursing diagnoses associated with the child or adolescent expe-

---

BOX 23-3
Psychiatric Nursing History for Children and Adolescents

FAMILY'S UNDERSTANDING OF THE PRESENT PROBLEM
1. "What caused you to bring your child here?"
2. "Has there been a recent crisis—family death, job loss, move, illness, children leaving, divorce?"
3. "Has anything like this happened before?"

Family History
4. "Tell me about the family structure (parents and siblings). Tell me about the relationship—are there any problems with any other family members (physical or emotional)? Is there or has there been any drug or alcohol abuse?"
5. "Who lives in the family?"
6. "Describe your child's adjustment to school. What school, what grade?"
7. "Describe your child's strengths."
8. "How do you feel about your child's friends?"

CLIENT'S UNDERSTANDING OF THE PRESENT PROBLEM
1. "What brought you here?"
2. "Was anything causing you difficulty at home . . . at school?"
3. "Have you felt like this at other times?"
4. "How do you feel about being here?"

PLANS FOR THE FUTURE (GOALS FOR HOSPITAL EXPERIENCE, DISCHARGE PLANS AND REFERRALS—OBTAIN INFORMATION FROM FAMILY AND CHILD IF POSSIBLE)
1. "What changes seem necessary before returning home?" "What do you expect from the hospitalization?"
2. "Has consideration been given to placement other than home?"
3. "What follow-up care is planned—day care, outpatient, home visits, etc?"

(Used with permission of AMI Saint Joseph Center for Mental Health, Omaha, Nebraska.)

CLIENT'S EDUCATIONAL STRENGTHS AND NEEDS
1. "Is there anything about school that bothers you?"
2. "Can you talk to anyone at school about your feelings or problems? Who?"
3. "If you could change school . . . how would you change it?"
4. "Tell me about your friends at school."

CLIENT'S ENVIRONMENTAL AND FAMILY STRENGTHS AND NEEDS
1. "Who worries about you in your family?"
2. "Whom do you worry about?"
3. "How does it feel living in your family right now?"
4. "Who do you talk to most in your family?"
5. "What are some of your family rules?"

CLIENT'S SOCIAL AND RECREATIONAL STRENGTHS AND NEEDS
1. "Tell me what your days are like."
2. "Do you have any hobbies or special interests?"
3. "Do you have a job?"
4. "Tell me three things you like most about your best friend."

CLIENT'S PSYCHOLOGICAL STRENGTHS AND NEEDS
1. "What type of person are you?"
2. "What type of person do others think you are?"
3. "What do you do well?"
4. "What things make you uptight?"
5. "What happens when you get uptight?"
6. "Describe overall mood (e.g., joyful, friendly, unhappy, unfriendly)."
7. "What would you like to do or be when you get older?"
8. "If you could change anything about your life or yourself, what would you change?"
9. "Have you tried drugs? Which ones? How did they make you feel?"
10. "Do you drink? What?"
11. "Do you smoke? How much?"
12. "What things make you afraid?"

(continued)

---

riencing problems. Two diagnoses—self-esteem disturbance and ineffective individual coping—are common when dealing with issues and problems facing the child and teenager and are discussed below.

SELF-ESTEEM DISTURBANCE

Self-esteem disturbance is defined as a "disturbance in the estimate one places on oneself, including one's self-worth, self-approval, self-confidence, and self-respect."[22] When a child or adolescent is confronted with consistent negative or rejecting communication by parents, teachers, or peers, the child's perception of self-worth is inevitably affected. Examples of this communication pattern might include physical or verbal abuse toward the child, inconsistent or lack of limit setting, or unrealistically high expectations placed on the child. A child or adolescent exposed to this type of communica-

tion can eventually adopt behaviors indicative of self-esteem disturbance. These include poor eye contact, self-derogatory verbalizations, evaluations of self as being ineffective in daily as well as problem situations, decreased assertiveness, lack of initiative, a decrease in appropriate risk-taking behaviors, and verbalizations of being powerless.[12,17,21,25,33]

Furthermore, these children often develop a series of self-defeating behaviors including learned helplessness, alcoholism, chemical abuse, eating disorders, depression, self-mutilation behaviors, and suicide.[21,25,33] The nurse must remember that these behaviors can result, in part, from the effect of the child's own perception of self-worth and interpretation of the environment. The child or adolescent has a need to be competent in personal decision-making skills, social skills, daily-living skills, and academic skills.

The child or adolescent who has developed low-self esteem, for whatever reason, begins to see himself as

BOX 23–3
Psychiatric Nursing History for Children and Adolescents (*continued*)

CLIENT'S DEVELOPMENTAL AND CHRONOLOGIC AGE STRENGTHS AND NEEDS
1. "Were there any problems during pregnancy, labor, and delivery?"
2. "Was there anything significant during growth and development?"
3. "Describe the child's attention span. Easily distracted?"
4. "Describe your child's activity level: constantly moving, able to sit for long periods."
5. "Does the child put a lot of energy into his reactions to new situations (e.g., new people, places)?"

NURSING ASSESSMENT: BEHAVIOR DESCRIPTION AND COMMUNICATION ABILITY OF CLIENT AND SIGNIFICANT OTHER

Interaction Pattern Observations: Client to Other Clients and Staff
1. Attitude
   Resistive or cooperative?
   Self-depreciative or complacent?
   Suspicious or trusting?
   Depressed or euphoric?
   Retiring or assaultive?
   Fearful or confiding?
   Warm/cold?
2. Mood
   Apathetic or active?
   Appropriate?
   Changeable?
   Irritable?
3. Communication
   Talkative or reticent?
   Free-flowing/guarded?
   Coherent?
   Relevant?
4. Contact with environment
   Orientation: time, place, person?
   Highly distractable/preoccupied?

5. Nonverbal communication
   Posture?
   Facial expressions?
   Motor activity?
   Mannerisms?
   Physical cues of anxiety?
6. Mental capacity
   Recent and remote memory?
   Attention and concentration?
7. Strengths

Interaction Pattern Observations: Significant Other to Child and Staff
1. Concerned/indifferent?
2. Warm/cold?
3. Physically demonstrative?
4. Talks openly with staff/guarded with staff?
5. Aggressive with staff?
6. One parent dominant?
7. Willingness to be involved in patient's care?
8. Response to separation.
9. Parental strengths.

Nursing Assessment Summary and Expected Patient/Family Outcomes
1. Reason for hospitalization
2. Family dynamics
3. Identify patient and family's perceptions and expectations
4. Identify patient's and family's potential ability to meet patient needs and cope with problems (strengths/weaknesses)
5. Identify short- and long-range goals for the patient
6. Identify short- and long-range goals for the family
7. Identify your own perceptions and expectations of patient's hospitalization based on your observation and nursing diagnosis (parenting skills needed)

ineffective. This sense of ineffectiveness becomes global. That is, the child who believes he or she is ineffective in one area begins to believe that this is true in all other areas of life. This interpretation of the self predisposes the child to behaviors associated with learned helplessness. The child begins to believe that "failures" are personal faults, but "successes" are related to factors outside of personal control. That is, the child does not associate success with self and own behaviors. Depressive behaviors are often the outcome of these feelings and beliefs.[25,33] The nurse must be acutely aware that depressed children often appear as aggressive and antisocial.

Of special interest to the mental health nurse is the child or adolescent who seems to have an extremely high self-esteem, although circumstances indicate that exactly the opposite is true. This phenomena has come to be known as *defensive self-esteem*.[12,38] Adolescent chemical abusers are often noted to display this type of self-esteem.[12] These adolescents typically project a positive image by denying or ignoring information that would reflect negatively on the self. The child or adolescent who takes on these behaviors does so in an attempt to protect the self. The child or adolescent who manifests defensive self-esteem may deny any existing problems or may blame others for the problems.[12]

INEFFECTIVE INDIVIDUAL COPING

Ineffective individual coping often goes hand-in-hand with self-esteem disturbance. As explained earlier, the self-esteem of the child and adolescent often correlates with the coping abilities of the child. Effective coping involves the ability to utilize an adaptive problem-solving process when confronted by anticipated and unanticipated life events. The steps of an adaptive coping process include:

BOX 23–4
Common Nursing Diagnoses for Children and Adolescents and Their Families

CLIENT
Aggression
Altered growth and development
Altered impulse control
Anger
Anxiety
Bizarre behavior
Body image disturbance
Boredom
Defensive coping
Depression
Diversional activity deficit
Impaired social interaction
Ineffective individual coping
Loneliness
Manipulation
Maturational crisis
Powerlessness
Regressed behavior
Role performance disturbance
Self-esteem disturbance
Situational crisis
Substance abuse (alcohol or drugs)
Suicide potential

FAMILY
Altered parenting
Anger
Anxiety
Depression
Dysfunctional family processes
Emotional lability
Family coping: potential for growth
Impaired communication
Impaired resource management
Manipulation
Powerlessness

ever, even in a rudimentary form, the skills should manifest themselves from early childhood. When the child or adolescent has not learned effective coping skills, a number of maladaptive responses begin to develop. These responses could be categorized as internal versus external problems and behaviors. Many children or adolescents internalize their emotional pain and demonstrate depressive behaviors similar to those exhibited by adults, including bland or sad affect, anhedonia, withdrawal, poor eye contact, crying, decreased energy, psychomotor retardation, poor sleep patterns, and decreased appetite.[2,3,34] Many children and adolescents who cope by internalizing their feelings often exhibit a high degree of vague somatic complaints (e.g., headaches, stomachaches).[2,34] A deadly outcome when youths internalize their feelings is suicide. Suicide is the second leading cause of death in adolescents between the ages of 15 and 19. This statistic is based on known suicides; therefore, rates may be higher when one evaluates certain accidental deaths of teenagers. The statistics on youths younger than 15 are much harder to collect, although the general consensus is that the suicide rate is considerably lower than the rates for 15 to 19 year olds. Many factors contributing to the increasing stress of children and adolescents, discussed earlier in this chapter, also seem to be predictors of suicidal vulnerability in youth. Hawton[15] and Pfeffer and coworkers[27] summarize a number of these predictors leading to an increased risk as:

- *A history of suicide in the family:* Children see family members as role models of coping behaviors, therefore, if suicide is perceived as a possible coping behavior successfully used by others, it increases the acceptability of suicide as a coping behavior.
- *Sense of alienation:* Loneliness and lack of support systems often increase the child's use of suicide as a coping behavior.
- *View of life as hopeless and negative:* Death becomes an escape from these feelings.
- *Impaired communication:* Children and adolescents use suicide as a message to say "I need help" when they are unable to communicate this need verbally.
- *Impulsivity:* Suicide may be the first impulse as a way to receive attention or relieve pain; however, the youth does not contemplate the long-term consequences of suicide—death.
- *Concept of death:* Many children and younger adolescents do not perceive suicide as permanent and terminal. Many adolescents, in general, think of themselves as invulnerable to death; therefore, suicide is just an "escape"—many do not believe that death will result.[15,27,35]

- Ability to evaluate the stressor in terms of possible positive or negative outcomes for the child's functioning
- Ability to identify emotions and the impact of these emotions on dealing with the stressful situation
- Ability to effectively manage emotions during the problem-solving process
- Brainstorm strategies to cope with stressors
- Identifying possible personal outcomes of implementing each strategy
- Identifying own intrapersonal, interpersonal, and extrapersonal resources to implement strategies
- Testing out strategies
- Evaluating the effectiveness of strategies.[1,20,41]

Granted, these steps evolve in their sophistication as the child grows both emotionally and cognitively; how-

The other end of the continuum involves the child or adolescent who externalizes his ineffective coping skills. As stated earlier, this is often exhibited as conduct disorders. These disorders are fully detailed in Chapter 14.

Interventions

Even though the general categories of interventions for children and adolescents are similar to those used when treating adults, the principles and actual techniques of treatments differ. Treatment modalities include milieu therapy, play therapy, music therapy, art therapy, one-to-one therapy, and group therapy.

MILIEU THERAPY

A key concept emerges when discussing the therapeutic milieu for children and adolescents; that is, the concept of structure.[28,35] Structure, an essential aspect of milieu therapy is founded on three concepts:

Rules
- Rules should be clearcut and simple.
- Rules are specific, yet allow for some degree of negotiation when circumstances warrant.
- Rules should be stated as positive, healthy expectations; for example, Rule: Other people's property will be respected, versus—Do not destroy other's property.
- The rules should be appropriate for the child's or adolescent's age and stage of development.
- As the child grows older, some rules should be mutually set between the caretaker and the child.[28,35]

Supportive Disciplinary Techniques
- Discipline should be carried through in a matter-of-fact, nonpunitive manner.
- Consequences for inappropriate behavior should correlate to the age and cognitive maturity of the child or adolescent. Consequences can take the form of (1) limitation of privileges, (2) decrease in personal interaction until behavior ceases, and (3) verbal interaction with the child or adolescent to discuss the behavior.
- Appropriate limit setting emphasizes behavior, rather than the child as "person."
- Limit setting should never give the message that the child is bad, but rather, the message that the behavior is not acceptable, for example, "It's OK to be angry, but I won't let you destroy your bedroom."
- Punishment is never the goal of limit setting.
- Limit setting should increase the child's awareness that certain behaviors may carry positive or negative consequences.[9,19,28,29,30,35]

Predictable Environment
- Structured daily activities and expectations as a part of the child's or adolescent's daily routine (e.g., study time, television time, bedtime, mealtime).
- Activities must provide a balance of cognitive, emotional, and social stimulation (e.g., school, recess, organized sports).
- Problem-solving techniques should take into account the level of the child's verbal skills.[16,28,35]

A natural part of being a child or adolescent is the development of a sense of identity and a sense of self-control and self-discipline. The child or adolescent, in developing a firm sense of identity, must negotiate a wide variety of psychological, social, and emotional tasks (see Box 23-1 for a summary of these tasks). Without some sense of structure and consistency, the child or adolescent can flounder in attempts at successful negotiation. There is little sense of security or validation for this trial-and-error behavior. Without directions and validations, the child or adolescent can never be sure that behaviors are appropriate and accepted by society. Usually, the home, school, or job situation provides a healthy structured environment whereby the youth can test out new behaviors and receive consistent messages that reinforce those behaviors that are healthy and self-enhancing, while altering those behaviors that are self-defeating. On the other hand, the emotionally disturbed child or adolescent has often lived in an environment that is inconsistent in its rules, limits, and routines of daily living. When this individual enters the mental health system, he or she must become a part of an environment that promotes what Yalom[42] refers to as a "corrective emotional experience."

To promote this type of experience, a unit must have a structured program providing ample opportunities for increasing an awareness of personal feelings and responses, as well as relearning behaviors and attitudes. Strategies to meet these goals must be implemented in ways that are congruent with the child's or adolescent's chronologic age, emotional, cognitive, and social development; that is, play therapy for the 5- to 6-year-old may use dolls, stuffed animals, balls, or other toys to promote an expression of feelings, whereas play therapy for adolescents would most likely consist of table games such as The Ungame that promotes an awareness of self in an atmosphere of fun. Figures 23-1 and 23-2 illustrate a possible program structure for a child or adolescent unit.

In a structured program, rules and limits are established to give the child or adolescent a sense of safety. It is important that rules and limits be reasonable (e.g., a 16-year-old writing "I will not write on the bedroom walls," 100 times as a limit for destruction of property does not allow the teen the opportunity to internalize the reasons behind the existence of such rules. A more appropriate alternative might be to have the child or adolescent take responsibility for cleaning the wall. This alternative allows the young person to understand that negative behavior carries certain consequences.

As stated previously, the methods used to achieve expression of feelings and adaptive problem-solving strategies must be tailored to the cognitive, emotional, and social needs of the child. Therefore, "talking therapy" may not always be the most appropriate medium for psychological growth. As noted in Figures 23-1 and 23-2, a portion of the child's and the adolescent's program should be devoted to strategies, such as play therapy, music therapy, and art therapy. All three therapies

TIME	Monday	Tuesday	Wednesday	Thursday	Friday	Saturday/Sunday
7–8 am	Arise/Daily Hygiene	→————————————————→				
8–8:30	Breakfast	→————————————————→				
8:30–9	Weekly/Daily Goal Setting (BG)	Daily Goal Setting (BG)	————————————————→			Arise/Daily Hygiene
9–11	Young Group-ET	————————————————→				9–9:30 Breakfast 9:30–10:30 TV Time 10:30 Playtime
	Older Group-OT/RT Activity	Music Therapy	OT/RT Activity	Music Therapy	OT/RT Activity	
11–11:30	Playtime/1:1	————————————————→			Review of Week's Goals (BG)	
11:30–noon	Lunch	————————————————→				
Noon–12:30	Quiet Time/1:1	————————————————→				
12:30–2:30	Young Group-OT/RT Activity	Music Therapy	OT/RT Activity	Music Therapy	OT/RT Activity	OT/RT Activity
	Older Group-ET	————————————————→				
2:30–3	Review of Day (BG)	————————————————→				
3–3:30	Quiet Time/1:1	————————————————→				
3:30–4	Exercise	Exercise	Stress Management	Exercise	Exercise	Exercise
4–5	Group Therapy	Art Therapy	Group Therapy	Art Therapy	Group Therapy	Art Therapy
5–5:30	Dinner	————————————————→				
5:30–6	Stress Management	Quiet Time/1:1	————————————————→			
6–7	Young Group-Story time Older Group-Study time	————————————————→			Therapeutic Game Activity (BG)	Family Time/Game Activity or Movie time
7–8	TV time/Family time	TV time Parent group	TV time/Family time	TV time Parenting Skills Group	Movie Night	
8–8:45	Self-esteem/Positive Reflection Group	————————————————→				
8:45–9:15	Prepare for bed	————————————————→				
9:15–9:30	Lights out	————————————————→				

KEY:

ET = Educational therapy   BG = Both groups
OT = Occupational therapy   YG = Young group
RT = Recreational therapy   OG = Older group

FIGURE 23–1. Sample milieu program for children's unit.

TIME	Monday	Tuesday	Wednesday	Thursday	Friday	Saturday/ Sunday
7–8 am	Arise/Daily Hygiene	———————————————————————→					
8–8:30	Breakfast	———————————————————————→					
8:30–9	Weekly/Daily Goal Setting (BG)	———————————————————————→					Arise/Daily Hygiene
9–11	Group I- Group Therapy	RT Activity	Group Therapy	RT Activity	Group Therapy	9–9:30 Breakfast 9:30–11:00 OT/RT Activity
	Group II- OT Activity	Assertiveness Training	Music Therapy	Assertiveness Training	OT Activity	
11–11:30	Stress Management	Art Therapy	Stress Management	Art Therapy	Music Therapy	Exercise
11:30–noon	Lunch	———————————————————————————→					
Noon–12:30	Quiet Time/1:1	———————————————————————————→					
12:30–2:30	Group I- OT Activity	Assertiveness Training	Music Therapy	Assertiveness Training	OT Activity	Field Trip/ Outing
	Group II- Group Therapy	RT Activity	Group Therapy	RT Activity	Group Therapy	
2:30–3	Quiet Time/1:1	———————————————————————————→					
3–5	Exercise	Study Time	Health Awareness Group-Girls/Boys	Game Therapy	Exercise	Game Therapy
5–5:30	Dinner	Cooking Activity	Dinner	———————————————————→			
5:30–6	News/Current Events	↓	News/Current Events	———————————————————→			Free Time
6–7	Study Time	Dinner with Family	Study Time	Study Time	Table Games	Stress Management
7–8	TV Time/ Family/ 1:1 Time	7–8 Parenting Group 7–9 TV Time	TV Time/ Family/ 1:1 Time	7–8 Parenting Skills 7–9 TV Time	Movie Night	Movie/Game Time
8–8:30	Self-esteem/ group	———————————————————————————→					
8:30–9	Preparation for bed	———————————————————————→					TV Time
9:00	Bedtime	———————————————————————→					Prepare for bed
9:30							Bedtime

KEY: OT = Occupational therapy   BG = Both groups
      RT = Recreational therapy

FIGURE 23–2. Sample milieu program for adolescent's unit.

carry with them a number of rules for both the children and the nursing staff. The rules are designed to give the children a feeling of freedom of expression, while giving the nurse some very specific guidelines for "stepping in." These rules impress upon the staff the need to avoid limiting behavior that is normally given consequences on the unit.

Children's Rules
1. Be active
2. Respect property and people

Nursing Rules
1. Allow the child to be free in play. The only time that play should be interrupted is when the child is physically or verbally aggressive to the point of hurting a peer, staff member, or self.
2. Accept the child's expression of feelings. Do not stifle this expression.
3. Avoid telling the child "how to play," rather, allow her or him to guide her or his own activity.
4. Be actively aware of the individual and group dynamics and use these observations as a starting point for further discussion with the child.[16,19,35]

PLAY THERAPY

Play therapy is probably one of the most useful therapeutic techniques for facilitating the child's or adolescent's ability to express feelings and impulses. Because children or adolescents often cannot, or will not, freely express their feelings or thoughts, play becomes their medium. Play therapy can be structured or unstructured.[5,34] In unstructured play therapy, the nurse provides play supplies and gives the child freedom to "do what he wants" with the supplies. Unstructured play provides a wealth of material for nursing observation and intervention. Assessments might include:

- How the child structures playtime
- How the child treats the play objects
- Content of play
- Feelings expressed during play
- Cooperative, versus competitive, versus solitary, versus parallel play activities of the child.

These assessments become the impetus for future discussions on a one-to-one or group basis.

Structured play therapy usually involves all children involved in the same activity. Games are especially useful with adolescents because the games provide a fun activity, while relaxing the individual and allowing him or her to open up more easily. Games allow an opportunity for values clarification, self-awareness, social skills training, conflict resolution, and improved problem-solving skills (e.g., Ungame, Scruples). These games confront the players with situations that force them to analyze their own feelings, experiences, and decisions. During games, the nurse may want to make the following assessments:

- Ability to cooperate in play
- Ability to follow rules
- Ability to tolerate delay
- Degree of social interactions
- Ability to problem-solve hypothetical situations
- Reactions to losing or winning
- Competitive behaviors.[5,34]

Games may be used as an adjunct to therapy, in that the game can initiate the group or individual therapy, but be interrupted when the child or adolescent responds to the activity with meaningful material for discussion.

MUSIC THERAPY

Music therapy allows those with impaired verbal and social skills an opportunity to express their various moods, as well as an opportunity to interact with others through a group activity. From the standpoint of mood expression, music may be used in a number of positive ways:

1. The child or adolescent can listen to a musical piece and "label" the feelings that are experienced when listening to the music, for example, words such as "peaceful" or "angry," then further explore these feelings.
2. In an exercise similar to the "labeling" exercise, the group can put their own words to music, which also gives the nurse the opportunity to observe the level of cooperation, interaction, and social skills of the group members.[35]
3. In a study conducted by Hinds[16] it was noted that background music during play therapy substantially decreased the children's anxiety level and increased their prosocial behaviors, including improved cooperative play, decreased aggression, improved peer interactions.
4. Music therapy can provide an opportunity for creativity and cooperation. The children or adolescents may use the music therapy time to form a "band." This activity would also allow the nurse to observe for cooperativeness, organization skills, creative potential, overall peer interaction patterns, and perceptions of self-worth.[16,35]

ART THERAPY

Art therapy is often analagous to music therapy in its goals; that is, the promotion of a healthy communication of feelings as well as a way to channel impulses. Art uses the medium of paper, clay, colors, paints, and other supplies as strategies to enhance the child's verbal and problem-solving skills.

1. Children can view artwork and "tell the story they see in the picture" or can "label" the feelings experienced when looking at the art work.
2. Children can be given art materials and, in an open-ended activity, be allowed to freely express

themselves and, following this expression, be asked to explain their own art.

3. Structured activities can be designed as, for example, having the children draw themselves or their families or drawing what they want to be when they grow up. These drawings can then be discussed individually or in a group setting.[35]

ONE-TO-ONE RELATIONSHIP WITH CHILDREN OR ADOLESCENTS

The differences in the one-to-one therapy with children or adolescents as contrasted with adults lie in the relationship-building process. Many adult clients enter the helping relationship freely and willingly because they recognize that they have problems that require help. Adults often see nurses as helpers who want to facilitate, rather than control, the direction of the relationship. Also, adults usually enter the relationship with a number of life experiences that allow building on problem-solving skills; that is, there is knowledge about the problem-solving process, even if the process cannot be applied in the here-and-now. Adults are likely to have reached the abstract level of reasoning which allows them to problem solve hypothetical situations and transfer these problem-solving abilities to real situations without ever having experienced these situations.[4,9]

Children and adolescents enter therapy with a different perspective. The characteristics that children and adolescents bring to therapy have a tremendous impact on the development of the nurse-patient relationship.

Characteristic: Children or adolescents tend not to perceive themselves as having a problem.

Impact: When children or adolescents do not perceive a problem, the need to be in therapy may not be recognized, which can lead to the belief that he or she has been "forced against his or her will." The nurse may be seen as having allied herself with the parents, whom the child now may mistrust. To set up a trusting relationship it becomes important for the nurse to:

1. Avoid taking sides, but rather, to convey to both the child or adolescent and parents that working together with both parties to facilitate problem solving is desired
2. Communicate a sense of acceptance of the child's or adolescent's feelings despite the negativity of the behaviors
3. Avoid messages that blame either the child or other family members for the problems
4. Meet the child at the child's own level; do not talk down to or patronize the child, but communicate respect for the child's potential and ability to do his or her own problem solving. The nurse must also use language appropriate to the child's or adolescent's cognitive and language skills.

Characteristic: Children often perceive the nurse as an all-powerful, all-knowing adult to whom they look for direction.

Impact: The nurse becomes a powerful role model for the child, thus, her verbal and nonverbal behavior around children must be well thought-out and consistent to gain the childrens' respect. Children perceive and pick up on discrepancies in behavior; for example, the nurse tells a child not to yell at peers, yet the child notes that the nurse is speaking in a loud, angry voice. Second, the nurse must remember that children often come from environments in which the reinforcement for behavior has been primarily negative—verbal and physical abuse, withdrawal of affection, neglect. If nurses respond in a similar manner, they do not allow children the opportunity to experience a positive growth experience. Furthermore, because the children look to nurses for directions, it may be appropriate for the nurse to take a more active, directive role than they might with the adults. That is, the nurse may have to give directions to the child by offering suggestions for the child to test out in situations.

Characteristic: Adolescents may see nurses as all-controlling individuals.

Impact: It is important that nurses facilitate, rather than dictate, the relationship. This necessitates a collaborative approach to problem identification and goal setting. It also necessitates the avoidance of an "I've been through this before—so I know what is good for you" attitude.

Characteristic: The child and adolescent's cognitive level and language abilities necessitate the need to act out feelings and situations.

Impact: Nurses must use a creative approach when facilitating problem solving, balancing verbal and nonverbal techniques if the child or adolescent is expected to benefit from therapy. Role playing, games, books, homework assignments, and journals can be used as adjuncts to a discussion of feelings and issues confronting the child. These methods provide the vehicle for the safe "acting out" of feelings and impulses that remain difficult to express on a verbal level.[4,9,10]

GROUP THERAPY WITH CHILDREN OR ADOLESCENTS

Group therapy goals center on problem identification and the development of alternative coping behaviors. Successful coping behaviors depend on the existence of (1) the ability to effectively manage feelings; (2) the ability to use the appropriate communication and social skills at the appropriate times; and (3) the ability to apply the problem-solving process in conflict situations. For the child and adolescent these skills can be effectively learned in a group setting. A method used to accomplish these goals in a group setting is the use of peer confrontation and feedback. Peers play a major role in the validation of attitudes, values, and behaviors as the child or adolescent is attempting to master the environment. As children move away from their families, they simultaneously gravitate to peers, who become the primary source of validation, support, and acceptance. Understanding the importance of peers becomes the foundation for success in a child or adolescent group setting. The group process is based on the fact that peers can provide a climate for emotional growth and behavioral change.[14]

In a group setting peers can provide the following:

- *A sense of universality:* Peers allow children or adolescents to "not feel alone" in their fears, emotions, and problems experienced because the other members of the group may have similar experiences. In essence, peers validate each other's reality.[6]
- *A sense of self worth:* The child or adolescent may get a sense of being useful to others in the group, and thereby, improve his or her feelings of self-worth, because "If I have something worthwhile to give you, then I must be an okay person."
- *Honest confrontation in a supportive atmosphere:* Adolescents can say to a peer "I've been there before, too, but it doesn't cut it to act like you're acting. I'm behind you if you want to try something new."
- *Sense of belonging:* There is a strong sense of acceptance and togetherness among children or adolescents. The child or adolescent feels accepted and respected by the group, despite some less-than-acceptable behaviors. The same feeling may not be experienced by the adolescent in relation to adults.

These factors can create a climate of safety and openness in which children or adolescents are more likely to feel free to express themselves and to experiment with new behaviors, without feeling put-down. The foregoing factors are universal and should exist, regardless of the type of group being conducted.[6,31,42]

Rose and Edelson[31] discuss "modeling" as another possible method used to achieve group goals. The modeling method can be successful in groups involving either children or adolescents. Its rationale is based on social learning theory—that is, behavior is learned by the role-modeling and feedback of others, as well as the imitation of others' behavior. The method involves the identification of target behaviors for change by an individual or individuals in the group (e.g., lack of assertiveness in social situations). Once the target behavior has been identified, the next step is to set up a role-play situation, whereby new behaviors can be addressed and practiced. In the first role-play the participants respond as they normally would in the situation; the other group members act as observers of behaviors associated with the target behavior; for example, in the assertiveness situation, the observers would evaluate the role players eye contact, body posture, voice pitch, and verbalizations. Following the role-play, the observers give the role players feedback about their behaviors, along with suggestions for change. A second role-play is then initiated in which the role players reenact the original situation with coaching done by various members of the group. Coaching involves on-the-spot feedback and suggestions to the players on aspects of the target behavior. A general group discussion then ensues about both role-plays, to provide positive feedback on the role player's efforts. Assignments may be given at the end of the session to practice the behaviors discussed in the group session. The child or teen is expected to report on his progress at the next group.[31] This type of group should be supplemented with an exploration of feelings and thoughts that lead to behaviors.

CASE STUDY

Bill is a 12-year-old boy admitted to a local mental health facility on the advice of a school psychologist. Bill now lives with his natural mother and a younger sister (6 years old). Bill's parents divorced approximately four months ago following a five-month separation. His father is a salesman and travels a great deal throughout the year; his mother recently resumed dating and has been seeing a man steadily for the past two months.

On interview, Bill's mother states that she has noted changes in Bill's behavior over the past six months with an increase in negative behaviors over the past two months. Mrs. J states that Bill has become increasingly oppositional over the past two months, frequently fighting with both her and his sister over trivial events. He has thrown items across the room when angry, often stays out past curfew, and refuses to complete his chores. Mrs. J states that some of the neighbors have been complaining that Bill has been rude to them and damages their property. Mrs. J says that Bill refuses to talk with her and is spending increasing amounts of time alone in his room.

Bill came to the attention of the school psychologist when he was caught stealing from the other children's lockers. When interviewing Bill, the school psychologist discovered that Bill has been feeling both sad and angry, but is unable to identify the reasons for these feelings. He states that he does not have fun at home or school or with friends and would prefer if everyone would just leave him alone. He states that he has made very few friends during this school year, but says that he does not care. He admits to using marijuana two to three times over the past month. He denies any suicidal ideations when asked. When reviewing his academic record, the psychologist noted that Bill's grades have declined over this term from B's to low C's and D's.

During the nursing assessment interview on admission, a number of issues surfaced concerning Bill's feelings about the recent divorce and his mother's dating. A review of the data indicated a number of problems related to anger, depression, and his inability to verbalize his own feelings. However, the nurse felt that Bill's priority problem involved his inability to effectively cope with his parents' separation and divorce. Based on a nursing diagnosis of ineffective individual coping related to feelings about parent's recent divorce, father's frequent traveling, and mother's recent dating, a sample care plan for Bill was developed (Nursing Care Plan 23-1).

During the course of hospitalization the one-to-one relationship and group therapy sessions were used to aid Bill in more appropriately managing his feelings of anger, frustration, and depression. He was helped to identify the self-

NURSING CARE PLAN 23-1

BILL

NURSING INTERVENTIONS	OUTCOME CRITERIA

NURSING DIAGNOSIS: Ineffective individual coping related to feelings about parents' recent divorce, father's frequent traveling, and mother's recent resumption of dating

CLIENT GOAL: Recognize own behavioral response to feelings such as anger (i.e., both positive and negative responses)

■ Assign nursing staff to meet Bill on a 1:1 basis daily to allow for ventilation of feelings and explore how Bill has handled anger prior to hospitalization	Verbalizes anger to nurse over present home life situation
■ In 1:1 use a variety of tools to facilitate a discussion of feelings related to Bill's parents' divorce and Bill's responses to anger, including bibliotherapy (childhood books specifically related to the topics of divorce and anger), music, or art therapy techniques)	Identifies behaviors displayed when angry and discusses the self-defeating nature of these behaviors
■ Teach Bill to keep a feelings journal to identify his anger and ways he copes with anger	
■ Use a nonjudgmental approach to facilitate trust and to encourage Bill to discuss his feelings	

CLIENT GOAL: Explore and utilize more positive ways of expressing anger and other feelings

■ Use firm, consistent limits to assist Bill in developing more positive ways to express anger; when noting that Bill's behavior indicates anger, point out behaviors that demonstrate inappropriate display of feelings and consequences for an inappropriate display of anger	Verbalizes two positive ways to express anger toward mother
■ When the consequence is set, teach Bill to expect to think about the reasons for the need to set the limit and think through alternative ways to deal with anger	Displays a decrease in acting-out behaviors
■ After the limit setting spend time on a 1:1 basis to discuss Bill's present behavior when angry as well as discussing more positive responses to the anger	
■ Offer immediate feedback when Bill expresses anger or other feelings appropriately by spending time with Bill or giving positive strokes for an appropriate expression of feelings	
■ Help Bill channel impulses into more acceptable behaviors that are age-appropriate for Bill (e.g., sports)	
■ Refer to recreational therapist for leisure assessment and discussion of other enjoyable ways to discharge feelings	
■ Teach general relaxation techniques using a behavioral therapy approach; discuss the need to recognize cues that indicate impending anger and then teach the need to respond by certain relaxation techniques	

defeating nature of his present behaviors and discuss more positive alternatives to working through home life situations.

SUMMARY

Although most children and adolescents will successfully negotiate their developmental tasks, approximately 18% of this population will experience such an overwhelming degree of anxiety to warrant formal mental health services.[13,24,40] In working with this age group the nurse must have a knowledge of factors affecting the child's or adolescent's ability to cope. Intrapersonal factors, including physical and psychological impairment, markedly influence the resources that the young person needs to meet the tasks of development.

Research Highlights

A study conducted by Offer and associates[26] focused on mental health professionals' view of normal adolescents. In this study, 62 mental health professionals including nurses, social workers, clinical psychologists, medical residents, and psychology graduate students were asked to complete the Offer Self-Inventory Questionnaire (OSIQ) as they believed a normal, healthy adolescent would respond. This questionnaire emphasized ten categories: impulse control, morals, psychopathology, body image, environmental mastery, coping abilities, mood, social relations, family relations, and vocational to educational goals. Four hundred five (405) adolescents perceived as healthy and normal and 512 adolescents exhibiting an identified disturbance were also asked to complete the questionnaire. The results of the study can be summarized as follows:

- The mental health professionals' views of "normal" adolescents differed from the healthy adolescents' views of themselves. In seven of ten categories the professional viewed the normal adolescent as demonstrating more anxiety, confusion, and a lower self-esteem than the normal adolescents' views of themselves. In only three areas—impulse control, morals,

and psychopathology—did the professionals' views and the adolescents' view closely correlate.

- In each of the ten categories, the mental health professionals' views correlated more closely with the views of the emotionally disturbed adolescent.
- The view held by the psychology graduate students about normalcy were more closely correlated with the views held by the healthy adolescents. This was postulated as possibly due to the fact that these students have had very little contact with the emotionally disturbed adolescent.

The results of this study might indicate a need for greater balance in educating mental health professionals about children and adolescents. There must, in addition to time spent in the discussion of pathology, be time devoted to the discussion of normal characteristics of adolescent behavior. Too great a focus on pathology can skew the mental health professionals' views of what is abnormal and normal. The mind set could be developed that most adolescent behaviors, including the normal behaviors, are really maladaptive responses to the adolescent developmental period.

Family relationships may also influence the ability of the child or adolescent to cope with the environment. If parents' communication and limit-setting skills are inconsistent or lacking, children receive mixed messages about their self-esteem and abilities to cope.

Second, it is important for the nurse to have a working knowledge of the profiles of behavior for the various stages of growth and development in the child or adolescent. An understanding of normal profiles serves to provide the nurse with a comprehensive frame of reference for assessment and problem identification.

Finally, a thorough understanding of each child's and adolescent's cognitive, emotional, physical, and social development serves to guide the nurse's selection of treatment strategies for the particular aged group. Milieu therapy, the one-to-one relationship, and group therapy provide a framework for structuring treatment. However, the immature cognitive and verbal skills of the child and adolescent necessitate the implementation of treatment methodologies utilizing action-oriented responses. Therefore, music therapy, art therapy, and play therapy may be required to supplement the other forms of treatment for children and adolescents.

References

1. Achenbach T. Assessment and taxonomy of child and adolescent psychopathology and psychiatry, vol 3. Beverly Hills: Sage Publications; 1985.
2. Achenbach T, McConaughy S. Empirically based assessment of child and adolescent psychopathology: practical applications. Beverly Hills: Sage Publications; 1987.
3. American Psychiatric Association. Diagnostic and statistical manual of mental disorders, 3rd ed, revised. Washington, DC: American Psychiatric Association; 1987.
4. Berlin I. Developmental issues in the psychiatric hospitalization of children. Am J Psychiatry. 1987;135:1044–1048.
5. Bernet W. The technique of verbal games in group therapy with early adolescents. J Am Acad Child Psychiatry. 1982;21:496–501.
6. Corder BF, Whiteside L, Haizlip T. A study of curative factors in group psychotherapy with adolescents. Int J Group Psychother. 1981;31:345–354.
7. DeMaio D. Technological society: its impact on youth. Top Clin Nurs. 1983;3:55–65.
8. Doyle AB, Gold D, Moskowitz D. Children in families under stress. San Francisco: Jossey-Bass; 1984.
9. Doona ME. Travelbee's interventions in psychiatric nursing, 2nd ed. Philadelphia: FA Davis; 1979.
10. Erikson E. Identity: youth and crisis. New York: WW Norton; 1986.
11. Gelfand DM, Peterson L. Child development and psychopathology. Beverly Hills: Sage Publications; 1985.
12. Gordon M. Manual of nursing diagnosis: 1986–87. New York: McGraw Hill; 1987.
13. Gould MS, Wunsch-Hitzig R, Dohrenwend B. Estimating the prevalence of childhood psychopathology: a critical review. Am Acad Child Psychiatry. 1981;20:462–476.
14. Grunebaum H, Solomon L. Peer relationships, self-esteem and the self. Intl J Group Psychother. 1987;37:475–513.
15. Hawton K. Suicide and attempted suicide among children and adolescents. Beverly Hills: Sage Publications; 1986.
16. Hinds P. Music: a milieu factor with implications for the nurse-therapist. J Psychosoc Nurs Ment Health Serv. 1980;18:28–32.
17. Hoeksema S, Seligman M, Girgus J. Learned helplessness in children: a longitudinal study of depression, achievement and explanatory style. J Person Soc Psychol. 1986;51:435.

18. Johnson J. Life events as stressors in childhood, vol 8. Beverly Hills: Sage Publications; 1986.

19. Johnson J, Rasbury W, Siegel L. Approaches to child treatment: introduction to theory, research, and practice. New York: Pergamon Press; 1986.

20. Kalfus GR, Hawkins RP, Reitz AL. A program for teaching problem-solving in a school for disturbed-delinquent youth. J Child Adolesc Psychother. 1984;1:26–29.

21. Kim MJ, McFarland G, McLane AM. Pocket guide to nursing diagnosis, 3rd ed. St Louis: CV Mosby; 1989.

22. McFarland G, Wasli E. Nursing diagnosis and process in psychiatric mental health nursing. Philadelphia: JB Lippincott; 1986.

23. Morrow L. Through the eyes of children. Time. 1988; 132(6):32–59.

24. Natural Association of Private Psychiatric Hospitals. In perspective: child and adolescent psychiatric hospitalization. Washington, DC: NAPPH; 1988.

25. Norris J, Kunes-Connell M. Self-esteem disturbance. Nurs Clin North Am. 1985;20:745–762.

26. Offer D, Ostrov E, Howard K. The mental health professional's concept of the normal adolescent. Arch Gen Psychiatry. 1981;38:149–152.

27. Pfeffer CR, Conte HR, Plutchek R, Jerrett I. Suicidal behavior in latency age children. J Am Acad Child Psychiatry. 1979;18:679–691.

28. Puskar K. Structure for the hospitalized adolescent. J Psychosoc Nurs Ment Health Serv. 1981;19:13–16.

29. Reasoner RW. Enhancement of self-esteem in children and adolescents. Fam Commun Health. 1983;6:51–64.

30. Rickel A, LaRue A. Preventing maladjustment from children through adolescence. Beverly Hills: Sage Publications; 1987.

31. Rose S, Edelson J. Working with children and adolescents in groups. San Francisco: Jossey-Bass; 1987.

32. Rutter M. Psychosocial resilience and protective mechanisms. Am J Orthopsychiatry. 1987;57:316–339.

33. Sanford L, Donovan ME. Women and self-esteem. New York: Penguin Books; 1984.

34. Schwarts S, Johnson J. Psychopathology of childhood: a clinical experimental approach, 2nd ed. New York: Pergamon Press; 1985.

35. Steinberg D. The adolescent unit: work and team work in adolescent psychiatry. New York: John Wiley & Sons; 1986.

36. Thorn G, Adams R, Brunwald E, Isselbacher K, Petersdorf R. Principles of internal medicine, 8th ed. New York: McGraw Hill; 1977.

37. Trad P. Infant and childhood depression. New York: John Wiley & Sons; 1987.

38. Turkat D. Defensiveness in self-esteem research. Psychol Rec. 1978;28:129–135.

39. US Department of Health and Human Services: National Institute of Mental Health. Psychiatric-mental health nursing: proceedings of two conferences on future directions. Washington, DC: PHS; 1986.

40. US Office of Technology Assessment. Children's mental health: problems and services. Durham, NC: Duke University Press; 1988.

41. Wertlieb D, Wegel C, Feldstein M. Measuring children's coping. Am J Orthopsychiatry. 1987;57:548–559.

42. Yalom I. The theory and practice of group psychotherapy, 2nd ed. New York: Basic Books; 1975.

24

Charlotte Naschinski

Life Events of Adulthood and Related Mental Health Needs and Treatment

OBJECTIVES

After reading this chapter, the reader will be able to:

1. Describe the adult stage of human development and related developmental tasks
2. Describe the principal features of an adult assessment
3. Identify major treatment modalities used with adult psychiatric clients and the related nursing roles
4. List nursing diagnoses commonly identified in the adult psychiatric client.

DESCRIPTION OF ADULTHOOD

A person continues to change and develop during that stage of human development referred to as *adulthood.* As described in this chapter, the period of adulthood begins with the end of adolescence and ends with the onset of old age and thus encompasses approximately 46 years (ages 18 to 64), approximately half the life span. At the end of 1986, there were 147,741,000 persons in the United States who were 18 to 64 years old, constituting approximately 61.2% of the total population.[20]

Adulthood is a period of increasing responsibilities and challenges for growth. What are the events and dynamics of this stage? Although the various stages of human development have been studied scientifically and described throughout the 20th century, it has only been in the last 30 years that adult development has been the focus of scientific inquiry. This increase in attention may in part be related to the lengthening life span as well as to a more optimistic attitude toward human psychological growth. Previously, theories of personality development asserted that events occurring during the early, formative years determined adult behavior to a large extent, leaving little room for development to continue into and throughout adulthood.

Adult Development Studies

Erik Erikson first described the stages of adulthood. Personality develops according to predictable steps within a widening social radius.[9] Each stage of the life cycle is described as coming into its ascendance, meeting a crisis, and finding a solution, although later resolution at a higher level is possible. The eight stages are named according to the task to be achieved and the consequence if the task is not achieved (see Chapter 5). The three stages that occur during adulthood are intimacy vs isolation, generativity vs stagnation, and integrity vs despair and disgust.[9]

A person enters the *intimacy vs isolation* stage when childhood and youth ends, when he or she is faced with selection of a career, forming intimate relationships with peers, and possibly marriage and establishing a family. A sufficient sense of identity is necessary to develop interpersonal intimacy as well as the ability and readiness to repudiate, isolate, and, if necessary, destroy forces and persons whose essence is personally dangerous.[10] If these tasks are not accomplished, isolation from others; stereotyped, formal interpersonal relationships; or a pattern of repeated attempts at and failures in interpersonal functioning may occur.

In Erikson's next stage of adult development, *generativity vs stagnation,* the principal task is establishment and guidance of the next generation, creativity in the arts, or achievement of life and career goals. This drive may be expressed by producing and caring for children or through other nurturing, altruistic, or creative channels. When generativity is not achieved, regression occurs, which results in feelings of stagnation and interpersonal impoverishment. Generativity is more than the production of or wish for children, artistic achievement, or accomplishment of goals: it involves moving beyond a sense of identity and an ability for intimate interpersonal relationships.

Integrity vs despair and disgust is the last of Erikson's stages of adulthood. Integrity is characterized by acceptance of one's own life and the life cycles of significant others as they are for what they are. Those who achieve integrity experience a different love of their parents, accepting them the way they are, and they accept responsibility for their own lives. Failure to achieve integrity is accompanied by the feeling that time is too short to attempt a new life and results in a sense of despair that often is hidden behind an outward display of disgust.

Other pioneers in the study of adult development are Daniel Levinson, Carl Rogers, Roger Gould, and Bernice Neugarten. The results of a study by Levinson[15] further illuminated the complexities of adult development. Midlife crises commonly occur in the fourth decade of life and are related to a perceived disparity between the real self-image and the ideal self-image.[15] If this crisis is resolved, a restabilization period follows.

According to Rogers, great disparity between the real and the ideal self-images is indicative of maladjustment. Normal development is enhanced by reducing this disparity by lessening the excessive demands of the ideal self-image and increasing the positive aspects of the real self-image.[19] The following example illustrates the effects of disparity between the real and the ideal self-image. Tom and Ellen, both in their 30s, have been married for 2 months. Ellen burst into tears when she arrived home from work one evening and found Tom vacuuming the living room and smelled dinner cooking. "You must think I'm a horrible wife and housekeeper," she cried. Patterning herself after her own mother, Ellen believed that she was solely responsible for maintaining an immaculate apartment, preparing the meals, sewing her clothes, and assuring marital intimacy. She failed to consider the facts that she was employed (unlike her mother), that she and Tom were childless, and that changes have occurred in societal expectations.

Gould emphasized the importance of time-related interpersonal changes in adulthood.[11] Although interpersonal and biologic changes are continuous throughout life, interpersonal changes are more dramatic after the age of 21. The heightened awareness of time that comes approximately at age 40 often results in a person turning toward the family and in a growing sense of satisfaction with marriage and friends.

Neugarten[18] noted the importance of the role of society and timing in adult development. Society regulates the entire life cycle, prescribing the timetable for ordering significant life events such as marriage, child rearing, and retirement. Time is at least three-dimensional in regard to the life cycle: historical time, life time (chronologic age), and social time, all intricately intertwined.[18] All of the major turning points or events in life, such as completion of formal education, marriage, and parenthood, call forth changes in self-concept, require integration of new roles, and precipitate adaptation. Life cycle events are more likely to be traumatic if they occur at a time other than what is expected, such as with the death of a child.

Concurrent with the above studies of the stages of adult development were experiments in psychiatric treatment of the family as a unit. Out of the efforts to treat dysfunctional families came descriptions of normal or functional family development that contributed greatly to understanding of the process of adulthood. For further elaboration on family systems theory and the treatment of families, refer to nursing diagnosis entitled family coping: potential for growth in Chapter 13 and to Chapter 37.

Stressful Life Event Theory

Stressful life events and their effects on adjustment and health have been studied, and a theory emerged based on the belief that excessive stress threatens an organism's existence and well being.[1] That is, excessive stress may create a detrimental discrepancy between the demand placed on the organism and the organism's ability to respond. This paradigm is derived from the association of stress with increased risk of illness and shifts attention from predisposing factors in psychopathology to precipitating factors, viewing predisposing factors as sources of vulnerability.[1] For example, loss of employment often results in depression, and certain experiences such as the early death of a parent seem to increase the probability for or potentiate the occurrence of depression.[1]

Holmes and Rahe, who developed the Social Readjustment Rating Scale, studied life stressors reported by more than 5000 clients as occurring shortly before the onset of their illnesses[12] and created a list of 43 life events scaled in terms of degree of stressfulness. Stressfulness was defined relative to the need for adaptive or coping behavior rather than to whether the event was desirable. Several studies utilizing the Social Readjustment Rating Scale found that illness, physiological and psychological, was preceded by an excess number and intensity of stressful life events.[7,8,23,25] Research conducted to determine how stressful experiences become internalized suggests that certain forms of stress suppress cellular immune functions and that different biologic effects occur in short-term stresses than in long-term stresses.[3,16] Furthermore, there appears to be an interactive effect of the magnitude of the stressor and the person's adaptive capacity on the immune response; i.e., it is the stress combined with poor coping that is immunosupressive.[16]

Understanding the relation between stressful life experiences and illness requires consideration of certain personal and social variables that can either prevent or hasten the development of illness (Box 24-1). Help-

---

BOX 24-1
Variables that Affect the Relation of Stressful Life Experiences and Illness[1]

PERSONAL VARIABLES

Experience managing stressful events
Perceived degree of control over environment
Physiological status
Psychological status
Coping skills
Help-seeking behaviors

SOCIAL VARIABLES

Current life situation
Nature of available social supports
Attitudes of peers and medical care gatekeepers

---

seeking patterns of the individual, as well as the nature of the available care system, affect the sequelae of stressful life events.

Events in Adult Development

A variety of events can present challenges for the mature adult. Although much variability exists in the course of life from one person to another, common trends and events occur as adults mature physically, economically, and interpersonally.

PHYSICAL

Physical maturity in terms of growth and ability to reproduce is essential to any definition of adulthood. Physical changes are fewer and occur more gradually in adulthood than in other stages in human development. A physical condition specific to women that may occur in adulthood is pregnancy. For a variety of reasons, such as pursuit of education or a career, many women are delaying pregnancy: the proportion of women giving birth to a first child after age 30 has increased from 3.9% of all first births in 1970 to 9.5% in 1981.[21] Although pregnancy after the age of 30 may be a desired option for a couple, it is medically considered high risk. Therefore, medical monitoring and health teaching is recommended to facilitate an uncomplicated course. Another physical change for the adult female is menopause, the cessation of ovulation and the menses. Because the maturing ovarian follicle is the source of estrogen and progesterone, postmenopausal women undergo withdrawal of these hormones. Although most women experience the menopause symptoms of hot flashes, headache, dizziness, palpitations, changes in pattern of sleep, and joint pain, only about 10% are disturbed by these symptoms. Mood changes also can occur at this time, the most common one being depression.[21] Although levels of female hormones decrease with menopause, sexual responsiveness does not necessarily decrease; indeed, it may increase secondary to the greater influence of androgens and the freedom from concern about pregnancy.[24] In the adult male, on the other hand, gonadal function usually does not cease abruptly. Rather, the decline in testicular function with accompanying loss of fertility and potency tends to be gradual.[13]

Another common physical change for the adult woman is osteoporosis, which is characterized by a loss of cortical and trabecular bone. Approximately 20 million Americans experience osteoporosis, and there are an estimated 1.3 million fractures attributable to osteoporosis annually in people 45 years of age or older.[21] The principal causes of osteoporosis are deficiencies of estrogen and calcium. Predisposing factors include increased age, female gender, small skeletal frame (in women), decreased estrogen level, and race (Asians have highest prevalence, then whites, then blacks). Factors suspected to be predisposing are alterations in the activity or level of calcium-regulating hormones, smoking, alcohol consumption, high-protein diets, lean body mass, and endocrine imbalance.[22] Treatment recommendations include estrogen replacement when necessary, calcium and vitamin supplements, and weight-bearing exercise.[21] Various drugs are being tested for possible utility.

Changes can occur over time in any body system and necessitate some adjustment for the mature adult. The needed adjustment may be minor, such as the wearing of eyeglasses, or major, such as adapting to a chronic illness. Furthermore, the person's perception of and reaction to the physical change(s) can range from acceptance with appropriate adaptation to lack of acceptance with an inappropriate or exaggerated emotional reaction.

ECONOMIC

Economic aspects of adult development center on employment. As a person enters adulthood, establishment of self in work is an important task. First, a person must select and prepare for an occupation. This task comes at a time when most people are establishing independence from the family of origin. Next, a person must make a series of decisions relative to career development; e.g., need for further education, selection of experiences within the occupation, geographic location, and development of interpersonal relationships conducive to career progression. Financial independence and growth is the desired goal in order to provide for self and possibly a family. Often, it is when this goal is being reached that the person first realizes the need to plan for retirement. This planning may involve putting together resources to augment expected social security and pension earnings. Additional financial demands may appear in later adulthood when a person's parents become disabled or have financial needs.

There has been a rapid rise recently in the participation of women in the labor force, and approximately 52% of all women are now in the labor force.[21] The most rapid shift in participation has occurred among women with children in the home; 66% of mothers with school-age children and 50% of mothers with preschool children are employed.[21] The number of women seeking employment later in life also is rising. Possible reasons for this change include the rapid rise in the divorce rate, particularly for those who have been married more than 20 years, and the greater longevity of women.

Even though their numbers are increasing in the labor force, the economic circumstances of women continue to be inferior to that of men. Women and children comprise 78% of the poor in the US. Employed women earn approximately 59% of what men earn. In fact, the average college-educated woman earns less than the average male high school dropout. Furthermore, as women approach retirement, many can expect to experience disadvantage with respect to pension plans and social security benefits related to their lower rates of employment, more intermittent employment, and lower earning power.[21]

INTERPERSONAL

Interpersonal changes are more dramatic after the age of 21 than before. As a person moves through adulthood, a number of psychosocial events with related tasks are experienced. The young adult faces acceptance of emotional and functional separation from the family of origin. The task of developing intimate peer relationships is a challenging one that entails working through issues such as sexuality, closeness vs individuality, and continuing development of a value system. Development of a marital or other mutually exclusive relationship demands realignment of relationships with family and peers. The addition of children to an adult dyad, whether by natural means, adoption, or surrogate parenting, requires learning of parental roles and increasing the family boundaries. This change may be particularly difficult if a couple has remained childless for several years; many couples present for family counseling with the complaint that one or the other is feeling neglected after the birth of a child. Additional challenges are faced by a couple with adolescent children. Again, family relationships and boundaries must change to accommodate the adolescent's growing independence. When young adult children leave home, the couple must renegotiate their relationship as a dyad, develop adult-to-adult relationships with the children, refocus on career issues, and increase involvement with the community. Even further role change is needed when couples assume the positions of in-laws and grandparents.[5]

Another common event in adulthood is loss of a spouse by death or divorce. A number of problems encountered by persons losing a spouse call for changes in self-concept and social and emotional roles: a weakened social support system, a need to work through the psychological reactions, child-rearing problems, resocialization as a single person, financial concerns, employment, and housing. The stress associated with the loss of a spouse through death or divorce often takes the form of anger, depression, loneliness, disequilibrium, regression, and ambivalent but persistent emotional attachment to the spouse.[1] The surviving spouse goes through the grieving process which, if uncomplicated, can last as long as a year or more. Successful resolution of grieving involves emotional emancipation from the lost spouse, readjustment to the environment, development of new relationships, and personal reorganization.[17]

When the loss of a spouse is through divorce, additional emotional issues may arise. The person must accept not only personal inability to resolve tensions in the marriage but also his or her own part in its failure. Relationships in the nuclear and extended family, as well as peer relationships, must be renegotiated. Feelings of hurt, anger, and guilt must be overcome sufficiently to permit the making of arrangements for finances, possessions, and the children.[5] Grieving occurs in response to the loss of a spouse and the loss of an intact family as well as to other associated losses; e.g., residence, job, finances, children.

OTHER

A number of other life events that require reevaluation of self-concept and interpersonal roles elicit other emotional responses. Individuals differ greatly in their ability to adapt to or cope with life events or stresses: some individuals experience little or no emotional difficulties during adulthood, whereas others suffer severe emotional reactions.

Anxiety is a common emotional state for mature adults and involves a perceived threat to personal, physical, or social integrity. All of the predictable turning points in adulthood can pose such threats and may thereby become related factors of the nursing diagnosis of anxiety such as threat to self-concept and threat to value system. Responses to anxiety may be constructive (such as problem solving, reframing, or seeking additional resources) or destructive (such as panic disorders, phobias, or hypochondriasis).

Depression is another emotional state common in adulthood and is often associated with loss. A number of actual or perceived losses can occur in adulthood; e.g., loss of health and life, jobs, children, spouse, role functioning. Accompanying this loss is the grieving or bereavement process, through which the individual may proceed in a functional or dysfunctional manner. Depression can be coupled with suicidal ideation and attempts.

Sexuality is another significant emotional issue for the mature adult. Several emotional reactions can occur as the developing adult establishes sexuality relative to personal and societal values. Unresolved sexuality issues may be evidenced through such behaviors as increased or decreased libido (sexual desire), promiscuity, or impotence.

Insomnia is often a problem in the middle years of adulthood.[4] Anxiety, guilt, anger, and worry related to tasks, events, or issues of adulthood may affect an individual's ability to sleep. Also, hormonal changes in women and physical changes in both sexes (nocturia, joint pain, sleep apnea) may interrupt sleep.

Psychiatric Disorders of Adulthood

When emotional reactions such as those described above become severe enough to disrupt an individual's life and functioning, psychiatric problems occur[4] that are identified by a DSM-III-R Axis I diagnosis (Table 24-1). The etiology of some of these disorders such as schizophrenia generally is related to a life-long pattern of maladjustment rather than to a single event immediately prior to the onset of the disorder. In addition, the classification of psychiatric disorders has V Codes that identify conditions not attributable to a mental disorder but which may become the focus of attention or treatment. They include:

V61.10	Marital problem
V61.20	Parent–child problem
V62.20	Occupational problem
V62.82	Uncomplicated bereavement
V62.89	Phase of life problem or other life circumstance problem.[24]

ASSESSMENT

In order to assess the relative maturity and health of a person at any point within the adult stage of human development, data are gathered about the person's cur-

TABLE 24–1
DSM-III-R Psychiatric Diagnoses Related to Emotional Problems/Issues of Adulthood[24]

PROBLEM/ISSUE	DIAGNOSIS	CODE NO.
Anxiety	Generalized anxiety disorder	300.02
	Panic disorder with agoraphobia	300.21
	Panic disorder without agoraphobia	300.01
	Social phobia	300.23
	Simple phobia	300.29
	Hypochondriasis	300.70
Depression	Bipolar disorder, mixed	296.6x
	Bipolar disorder, depressed	296.5x
	Cyclothymia	301.13
	Major depression, single episode	296.20
	Dysthymia	300.40
	Depressive disorder NOS*	311.00
Sexuality	Hypoactive sexual desire disorder	302.71
	Sexual aversion disorder	302.79
	Female sexual arousal disorder	302.72
	Male erectile disorder	302.72
	Inhibited female orgasm	302.73
	Inhibited male orgasm	302.74
	Premature ejaculation	302.75
	Sexual dysfunction NOS	302.70
Insomnia	Primary insomnia	307.42
	Dyssomnia NOS	307.40

* NOS = not otherwise specified.

rent and past physical, psychosocial, and economic status. Conclusions can then be reached about the number and intensity of life stressors as well as the person's ability to respond adequately. The variables affecting the relations of life stressors and illness presented in Box 24-1 provide the bases for the following discussion of assessment.

Physical

Physical examination provides data about the physiological status of an individual. These data are compared with developmental norms to determine the presence of or potential for health problems. While performing physical assessment, it is important to ascertain the client's perception of and reaction to physical status. Although certain findings of the physical examination may be considered normal for a middle-aged adult, such as graying of the hair, presbyopia, and decreasing cardiac output, the meaning of these changes to the person may indirectly affect health status by increasing anxiety and stress. It also is important to be alert to those symptoms that can be psychogenic or psychophysiological in origin; e.g., hypertension, nonallergic urticaria, migraine headache, duodenal or peptic ulcers, and colitis. The presence of such symptoms may be indicative of a high level of stress.

Psychological

Psychological status can be assessed in part through the mental status examination. The mental functioning and present emotional state of the person are assessed through observations of general appearance, motor behavior, speech, intellectual functioning, perception, affective state, thought processes and content, judgment, and alertness. The mental status examination is most often performed by the psychiatrist or psychiatric clinical nurse specialist. Psychological status is also assessed most often by psychiatrists, psychologists, psychiatric clinical nurse specialists, or social workers using the multiaxial evaluation system for determining the presence or absence of psychiatric diagnoses contained in the DSM-III-R. Psychological status also can be evaluated by psychologists through a variety of psychological tests such as the Thematic Apperception Test (TAT), the Rorschach Test, and the Minnesota Multiphasic Personality Inventory (MMPI).

Other psychological or personal areas to assess are coping skills and perceived degree of control over the environment. Coping skills include behaviors, cognitions, and perceptions of individuals contending with life problems. When successful, coping skills enable a person to manage external or internal demands through conquering, tolerating, or reducing the demand. Coping behaviors can include information seeking, taking direct action, inhibition of action, intrapsy-

chic defenses, and seeking help from others, including health care workers.[1] Persons whose primary locus of control is internal are more likely to perceive themselves as having control over their environment. Persons' abilities to manage stress may be enhanced by the belief that they can control and transform events in their lives. Behaviors such as extreme passivity, decreased verbalization, and verbal expressions indicating a sense of having little or no control over life suggest an external locus of control and concomitant feelings of hopelessness and powerlessness.

Socioeconomic

Social variables to assess include the person's current life situation, the nature of available social supports, and the accessibility and nature of health care. Assessment of the current life situation includes determining the person's financial resources, career status, housing situation, interpersonal relationships, family constellation, and religious and spiritual values. The review also includes assessment of the daily living environment for presence of biologic, pollutant, safety, and psychological factors that may affect coping ability and health status. Comparison of the socioeconomic assessment data with expected norms and the person's life goals can reveal discrepencies and current or potential stressors. The Holmes and Rahe Social Readjustment Rating Scale[12] is a useful tool to assess perceptions of current life situation.

Social support networks can moderate stressful life events. The presence of adequate social support has been found to contribute to fewer complications of pregnancy, faster recovery from a variety of illnesses, greater success in alcoholism treatment programs, successful coping with bereavement, and better management of life in general.[6] Social support is more than the mere presence or availability of other people. Persons can be considered as having social support when they believe that they are cared for, loved, and esteemed and belong to a network of communication and mutual obligation.[6]

A health care system that is both accessible and responsive can also moderate stressful life experiences in adulthood. It is not enough to have a health care system in place: a person must be able to use the system without undue obstacles. Attitudes of openness and acceptance in medical care gatekeepers and personnel facilitate reduction of stress and promotion of health. Furthermore, health care workers must be cognizant of and responsive to the stresses and medical care needs of the populations they serve.

In summary, assessment of the functioning and health of adults requires collection and analysis of data that will indicate whether clients are able to respond adequately to stressors. The presence of certain personal and social variables can moderate stress and so contribute to adequate functioning and health. When those same variables are absent or inadequate, the adult is more vulnerable to the effects of stress, and maladjustment or illness may result.

TREATMENT MODALITIES AND RELATED NURSING ROLES

Traditional psychotherapeutic treatment modalities, such as individual and group therapy, family therapy, and psychoanalysis, maintain certain identifiable consistencies regardless of the age of the clients (see Unit V). However, therapy should be conducted keeping in mind the psychosocial elements and nature of adulthood as described previously. Emphasis is placed on the continuing potential for growth and fulfillment. In a broad sense, psychotherapy during this stage of development involves evaluation or re-evaluation of life: taking an inventory, examination of commitments, and development of an accurate self-view as a basis for a decision to make changes or to remain on the same course of life.[4] Individual psychotherapy and psychoanalysis focus on an individual's personality and therefore, are appropriate treatment modalities to facilitate a person's ability to assess self accurately. Family therapy has as its goal improved family functioning, and group therapy facilitates improved social functioning.[10] The latter two also can facilitate a person's ability to make desired changes. Self-help and educational groups such as Overeaters Anonymous and Al-Anon are also useful in dealing with common issues or problems in adulthood.

In order to be qualified to conduct individual, group, and family psychotherapy, a nurse must have advanced specialized education. However, all nurses can provide support and encouragement to patients receiving such therapies. A nurse can play a role in self-help and educational groups; indeed, these groups often are led by nurses.

Preventive intervention programs are another type of treatment appropriate to the adult. These programs are based on beliefs that stressful life events place adaptive demands on a person and that stress is associated with an increased risk of illness. The purposes of preventive intervention programs, then, are: (1) to reduce the incidence of a particular stressful life event; or (2) to facilitate its mastery. An example of the first purpose is a program to reduce unemployment. An example of the second purpose is counseling persons grieving the loss of a job. A program designed to reduce the stress of marital disruption is described in the Research Highlights section of this chapter. Virtually all of the preventive intervention programs reported are based on mastery of stressful life events. Nurses are often involved in these programs, most frequently as interviewer, counselor, and teacher. In these roles, the nurse provides information, support, and direction to clients attempting to increase their coping skills, decision-making abilities, and perceived degree of control over the environment and social network.

NURSING DIAGNOSES

Discussion of nursing diagnoses is predicated on the view that adulthood is a continuous period of development that includes predictable events or turning points that necessitate reevaluation and change of self-concept, role performance, and interpersonal relationships. Nursing intervention is indicated when an individual needs assistance in meeting the challenges of adulthood; i.e., when there is an actual or potential alteration in human response patterns (Table 24-2).

Many challenging demands are placed on an adult that can lead to self-concept disturbance. As stated earlier, high disparity between an individual's real and ideal self-concepts can result in maladjustment. Nursing can reduce this disparity by enabling the patient to lessen the excessive demands of the ideal self-concept and increase the positive aspects of the real self-concept.

Demands also are placed on the developing adult for the integration of new roles: the young, single adult must learn intimacy with peers; the newly married must integrate roles of spouse and daughter-in-law or son-in-law; having children necessitates assuming the role of parent and later possibly of grandparent; death of a spouse brings with it roles of widow or widower and a return to being a single adult. The potential for

TABLE 24-2
Nursing Diagnoses Common in Adults According to Human Response Patterns[14]

HUMAN RESPONSE PATTERN	NURSING DIAGNOSIS
Communicating	Impaired communication
Relating	Impaired social interaction
	Role performance disturbance
	Altered parenting, actual
	Altered parenting, potential
	Sexual dysfunction
	Dysfunctional family processes
	Sexual dysfunction
Choosing	Ineffective individual coping
	Impaired adjustment*
	Ineffective family coping: disabling*
	Ineffective family coping: compromised*
	Family coping: potential for growth
Moving	Sleep pattern disturbance
Perceiving	Self-concept disturbance: body image disturbance
	Self-concept disturbance: self-esteem disturbance
	Self-concept disturbance: personal identity disturbance
	Hopelessness
	Powerlessness
Feeling	Anxiety
	Dysfunctional grieving
	Anticipatory grieving

* Other NANDA nursing diagnosis.

role performance disturbance exists. Nursing can assist an individual with role assumption and clarification when needed.

Interpersonal changes occur during the adult stage of human development. Demands are placed on an individual to communicate and relate to an ever increasing number and variety of people. In order to cope with and adjust to interpersonal demands, an individual needs decision-making, coping, communicating, and interpersonal skills. When an actual or potential alteration in the human response patterns of communicating, relating, and choosing exist, nursing intervention is indicated.

Feelings or feeling states commonly experienced in adulthood can be identified in such nursing diagnoses as anxiety, depression, and grieving. Depression often brings with it sleep pattern disturbance, hopelessness, and powerlessness. Nursing interventions can address these nursing diagnoses.

CASE STUDY

Susan K is a 38-year-old woman whose husband is at home in the terminal stages of leukemia. Mr. and Mrs. K have two sons, ages 5 and 8. Mrs. K is employed part-time as a secretary and enjoys her work. She had been accompanying her husband for his treatments, but Mr. K's condition has deteriorated, and chemotherapy has been stopped. He is expected to live for approximately 2 months, and funeral and financial arrangements have been made. Recently, Mrs. K has been seeking out the nurses in the hospice outreach program and has been complaining of a decrease in appe-

tite and of having less energy to devote to work or socialization. "I just wish there was something I could do to prevent his death. I will miss him terribly," stated Mrs. K. The nursing diagnoses formulated are: (1) anticipatory grieving related to the impending death of husband; and (2) potential for role performance disturbance related to impending death of husband. Recognizing that intervening to promote normal grief can lower morbidity and prevent dysfunction, the nurse offers to meet weekly with Mrs. K, and Mrs. K readily accepts (see Nursing Care Plan 24-1 for a sample care plan for Susan K).

SUMMARY

Adulthood spans the longest period of any of the stages of human development and includes a myriad of challenges for continuing growth. However, it has only been during the last 30 years that adulthood has been the focus of scientific inquiry. From these studies, predictable tasks, issues, crises, or turning points of adulthood have been identified, each of which places a demand on the adult to adapt.

Adults differ greatly in their ability to adapt or cope with life events. A person's ability to adapt is related to experiences with stress, current coping skills, and health status and available support system. The more able an adult is to meet the demands of adulthood, the less likely is maladjustment or illness to occur.

Nursing can provide assistance when needed in meeting the demands of adulthood. Actual or potential alterations in human response patterns are identified

Text continued on page 624

Research Highlights

One common stressful life event to which adults are vulnerable is marital disruptions. In one study designed to reduce the incidence of clinical psychopathology in the high-risk group of the newly separated, subjects were obtained via public media (newspapers, radio, posters) and through direct mailing to human service organizations and practitioners.[2] A total of 152 subjects were assigned to experimental and control groups at a ratio of two to one, respectively. All subjects received an initial interview, including completion of a symptom checklist, and subsequent interviews at 6, 18, 30, and 48 months.

Subjects in the control group were referred to community agencies as deemed necessary. Subjects in the experimental group participated in a 6-month-long treatment program that provided emotional support, crisis intervention, social interaction, referral to community agencies, and study groups that focused on career planning, legal and financial, homemaking, socialization, and self-esteem issues. Evaluative data were obtained from the pretest and post-test scores, scheduled interviews, and monthly program evaluations completed by subjects in the experimental group.

The experimental group subjects evaluated the entire program very favorably and judged the program repre-

sentatives as skillful and the study group experiences as good. The majority of the 6-month analyses demonstrated either significant differences by group for the entire study population or for only one gender. In each case of significance, subjects in the experimental group reported fewer problems and better psychological adjustment than control group subjects. The significant decrease in general psychological problem scores of the experimental group subjects persisted. The experimental group significantly reduced its psychological distress and maladjustment scores from pretest to post-test. Significant improvements were also found from pretest to post-test on the anxiety and neurasthenia subscales of the symptom checklist. No equivalent improvement was found in the control group. Analysis of 18- and 30-month data indicated that the differences in the control and experimental group members continued to exist and in some cases increased.

This intervention program was successful in reducing anxiety and fatigue and improving coping ability and physical health. Enabling the high-risk, newly separated population to cope better with stress and to maintain health reduces the chance of clinical psychopathology.

NURSING CARE PLAN 24-1

MRS. K

NURSING INTERVENTIONS	OUTCOME CRITERIA

NURSING DIAGNOSIS: Anticipatory grieving related to impending death of husband*

CLIENT GOAL: Take part in constructive and anticipatory grief work

■ Encourage Mrs. K to describe her perception of impending loss of husband	Describes her perception of impending loss of husband
■ Help her identify and express feelings	Expresses thoughts and feelings related to impending death of husband
■ Assist her to identify potential changes and problems following the death of Mr. K	Identifies potential problems and changes related to impending loss
■ Explore possible approaches to address anticipated changes and problems. Include exploration of consequences of each; e.g., what is the best that can happen if you . . . ? What is the worst . . . ?	Chooses approaches to identified potential problems and changes
■ Assist Mrs. K in identifying enjoyable activities that fit in with current demands and which provide realistic respite	Participates in enjoyable activities that provide respite
■ Assist Mrs. K in exploring any guilt she may experience while engaging in enjoyable activities	Verbalizes feelings experienced while engaging in enjoyable activities
■ Emphasize Mrs. K's legitimate need to build up resources in order to be able to support her husband and children	
■ Identify and encourage maintenance of Mrs. K's support network, including resources she may not have considered	Maintains or is receptive to supportive social network
■ If she does not have enough energy, encourage visits and concrete assistance from family members or friends	
■ Teach and encourage use of stress reduction techniques such as meditation or exercise	Practices stress reduction techniques
■ Teach Mrs. K strategies to meet the emotional needs of her children; e.g., help the boys prepare for visits with their dad	Meets emotional needs of boys, as evidenced by the boys' not feeling neglected but loved
■ Assist Mrs. K in helping her sons particpate in grieving at an age-appropriate level	Boys talk about death and dying in an open way appropriate to their age
■ Assist her in developing a weekly schedule that allows for work, time with the children, and time for self and friends	Develops weekly schedule that includes time for work, children, friends, and self
■ Assist Mrs. K to structure the interactions between the boys and their dad and between Mr. and Mrs. K according to Mr. K's status; provide analgesics prior to interactions as needed	Experiences comfortable uninterrupted interactions

* Care Plan addresses only first nursing diagnosis for Mrs. K.

from analysis of assessment data. Based on the identified nursing diagnoses, a plan of nursing care is developed to prevent or resolve the identified problem(s).

References

1. Bloom BL. Stressful life event theory and research: implications for primary prevention. Rockville: Department of Health and Human Services, ADAMHA; 1985.
2. Bloom BL, Hodges WF, Caldwell RA. A preventive intervention program for the newly separated: initial evaluation. Am J Community Psychol. 1982;11:213–218.
3. Borysenko M, Borysenko J. Stress, behavior, and immunity: animal models and mediating mechanisms. Gen Hosp Psychiatry. 1982;4:59–67.
4. Butler RN. Psychiatry and psychology of the middle-aged. In: Kaplan H, Sadock B, eds. Comprehensive textbook of psychiatry. 4th ed. Baltimore: Williams & Wilkins; 1985.
5. Carter EA, McGoldrick M. The family life cycle. New York: Garner Press; 1980.
6. Cobb S. A model for life events and their consequences. In: Dohrenwend BS, Dohrenwend BP, eds. Stressful life events: their nature and effects. New York: John Wiley & Sons; 1974.
7. Crook T, Eliot J. Parental death during childhood and adult depression. Psychol Bull. 1980;87:252–259.
8. Dooley D, Catalano R. Economic changes as a cause of behavioral disorder. Psychol Bull. 1980;87:450–468.
9. Erikson EH. Identity and the life cycle. New York: WW Norton; 1980.
10. Glick ID, Kessler DR. Marital and family therapy. Ed 2. New York: Grune & Stratton; 1980.
11. Gould R. The phases of adult life: a study in developmental psychology. Am J Psychiatry. 1972;129:521–531.
12. Holmes TH, Rahe RH. The social readjustment scale. J Psychosom Res. 1967;11:213–218.
13. Katchadourian HA. Medical perspectives on aging. In: Erikson EH, ed. Adulthood. New York: WW Norton; 1987.
14. Kim MJ, McFarland GK, McLane AM. Pocket guide to nursing diagnoses. 3rd ed. St Louis: CV Mosby; 1989.
15. Levinson D. The seasons of man's life. New York: Alfred A Knopf; 1978.
16. Locke SE. Stress, adaptation and immunity: studies in humans. Gen Hosp Psychiatry. 1982;4:49–58.
17. McFarland GK, Wasli EL. Nursing diagnoses and process in psychiatric mental health nursing. Philadelphia: JB Lippincott; 1986.
18. Neugarten B. Adaptation and the life cycle. Counsel Psychologist. 1976;6:16–20.
19. Rogers C, Dymond R. Psychotherapy and personality change. Chicago: University of Chicago Press; 1954.
20. US Bureau of the Census: Statistical Abstract of the United States: 1986. Ed 107. Washington, DC, US Government Printing Office; 1987.
21. US Department of Health and Human Services: Women's health: report of the Public Health Service Task Force on Women's Health Issues. Vol. 1. Rockville: US Public Health Service; 1985.
22. Weissinger J. The National Conference on Women's Health: executive summary. Bethesda: US Food and Drug Administration; 1987.
23. Wildman RC, Johnson DR. Life change and Lagner's 22-item Mental Health Index. J Health Soc Behav. 1977;18:179–188.
24. Williams JBW. Quick reference to the diagnostic criteria from DSM-III-R. Washington, DC: American Psychiatric Association; 1987.
25. Zautra A, Beier E. The effects of life crisis on psychological adjustment. Am J Community Psychol. 1978;6:125–135.

25

Kathleen C. Buckwalter

Psychosocial Needs and Care of the Elderly

OBJECTIVES

After reading this chapter, the reader will be able to:

1. Describe current sociodemographic trends that affect mental health care of the elderly
2. List factors contributing to underutilization of mental health services by the elderly
3. Identify elements of a comprehensive assessment for the elderly
4. Discuss how the normal aging process can interact with psychopathology and affect response to treatment
5. Identify psychosocial assessment instruments useful for assessment of the elderly
6. Discuss therapeutic objectives for working with the elderly
7. Describe the psychosocial needs of the elderly
8. Elaborate on special counseling considerations in long-term care settings
9. Discuss the advantages of group and family therapy for the elderly
10. Identify psychosocial rehabilitative strategies useful for working with the elderly
11. Discuss nursing diagnoses commonly found in the elderly with mental health problems
12. Demonstrate understanding of the assessment and intervention principles highlighted in this chapter by developing a care plan
13. Discuss needed research in psychiatric mental health nursing for the elderly.

DEMOGRAPHIC TRENDS

Epidemiologic studies clearly project a rise in the number of elderly Americans (persons over 65).[1] The current estimate is that there are more than 28.1 million persons over the age of 65.[1] By the year 2030, this number will more than double again, so that the elderly will represent more than 20% of the US population.[64] Not only is this segment of the population living longer, but with the increase in the numbers of those over 85, the elderly are becoming more frail, dependent, and vulnerable to both chronic physical diseases and mental health problems.[41] Additionally, the proportion of "old-old," those persons over the age of 85, will increase three to four times faster than the general population.[64] By the year 2050, 50% of the population is projected to live past age 85.[10] Of significance to nurses, policy makers, and health care planners is the high correlation between increased age and chronic mental and physical impairments necessitating long-term care.

Along with the rapid growth in the percentage of elderly, there has been a dramatic increase in the number of long-term care facilities. Between 1960 and 1976, the number of nursing homes increased by 140% and nursing home beds increased 302%,[46] in part because of Medicare and Medicaid legislation and the deinstitutionalization of the mentally ill. If current trends continue, the older population in nursing homes will double in 35 years from 1.3 million in 1985 to 2.8 million in 2020.[1] In the US, approximately 5% of the population over 65 resides in long-term care facilities, as do 20% of all persons over the age of 85. These trends suggest that nurses must be aware of and able to meet a complex and interdependent array of psychosocial, environmental, and physical needs of the aged.

Over the past two decades, the deinstitutionalization movement has discharged many elderly persons from mental institutions and relocated them in nursing homes.[41] Among the most challenging problems faced by nurses is the management of emotional and behavioral problems and cognitive impairment in this population.[41] Although dementia strikes only about 5% of all persons over 65 years of age, individuals with dementia account for somewhere between 50% to 75% of all persons in nursing home beds. It has been estimated that between 70% and 80% of nursing home residents have some psychiatric problem,[17] yet most long-term care facilities do not provide adequate psychosocial care for their residents.[54] Furthermore, mental problems often are the critical difference between an elderly person's ability to manage independently in the community and the need for institutionalization. This suggests a need for more and better educated geropsychiatric nurses.

The elderly traditionally have been underserved in terms of psychiatric services.[11] This neglect, which occurs in both institutional and outpatient settings, can be traced historically to Freud,[25] who emphasized the importance of early childhood experiences and who believed that personality was less amenable to change with advancing age. For example, he felt that the elderly were not suitable candidates for psychoanalysis, a therapy that favors verbal facility.[61] Furthermore, elderly individuals have been regarded as too rigid to make behavioral changes, a finding that has *not* been substantiated by research. In fact, Butler, one of the foremost advocates of mental health services for the elderly, has stated that, "the possibilities for intrapsychic changes may be greater in old age than at any other period in life" (reference 15, p 237). Several other factors also have negatively influenced the provision of psychiatric services to the elderly, including: (1) their frequent lack of ability to pay for services; (2) inaccessibility of services because of transportation or mobility problems; (3) devaluation of the potential benefits of psychotherapy by many elderly; (4) perceived stigma associated with psychiatric help in the minds of older persons; (5) a paucity of geropsychiatric nurses, physicians, and other health care professionals educated in the special mental health needs of the elderly; and (6) "ageist" biases on the part of some mental health professionals, who view the elderly as unappealing clients.[11,66]

Finally, because many health care professionals perceive mental illness as a necessary fact of life in old age, elderly persons often are not accorded comprehensive assessment and aggressive treatment.[31] Psychological disturbances in the elderly that may be secondary to physical problems frequently are mislabeled "senility" by the untrained and inexperienced clinician, who may regard most older people as normally confused, unhappy, isolated, and lonely.[68] Often, the elderly are not expected to behave responsibly and are allowed to exhibit symptoms of mental disorders such as memory problems, poor interpersonal relationships, irritability, and social withdrawal.[31]

Despite these barriers, there is evidence that the elderly *do* benefit from counseling and therapy.[12,62]

ASSESSMENT

Need for Comprehensive Assessment

Nursing assessment of the geriatric mental health client is multifaceted and challenging, in part because of the complex interplay among physical, mental, social, economic, spiritual, environmental, and treatment-related factors in this population. Thus, in addition to standard psychiatric approaches, assessment of the geriatric client should at a minimum include: (1) physical history, including risk identification regarding drugs, alcohol, and falls; (2) mental status; (3) knowledge of illness and treatment; (4) interpersonal relationships, role functioning, socialization, and support systems; (5) activities of daily living; and (6) coping mechanisms and resources.[48]

Nurses caring for geriatric clients with mental health problems must be knowledgeable about the normal aging process in order to identify pathology accurately.

For example, the elderly suffer some degree of decreased sensory acuity in all spheres. Knowledge of these sensory alterations can help nurses to modify the environment appropriately (e.g., increased nonglaring light). Sensory loss also can be linked to psychiatric disorders. For example, 40% of all persons with delusional (paranoid) disorder are believed to have a hearing disorder. The database of the geriatric mental health nurse must be comprehensive and incorporate an understanding of: (1) altered medication response and tolerance; (2) cognitive functioning alterations; (3) altered, and often diverse, manifestations of physical and psychiatric illnesses; (4) decreased rebound potential following losses and stressors (physical or psychological); (5) increased risk potential; (6) decreased stamina; (7) sociocultural stressors; and (8) altered dietary needs and capabilities.[48]

Assessment Instruments

Assessment instruments that are developed and normed on younger persons may not be reliable and valid for the elderly. For a comprehensive discussion of assessment issues in the elderly, the reader is referred to Kane and Kane's seminal text, *Assessing the Elderly*.[37] The following discussion highlights selected tools that may be most useful for the psychiatric mental health nurse assessing the geriatric client with emotional problems.

Early identification and referral of elderly who are demented will facilitate accurate diagnosis and treatment that may slow the progression of this deteriorating illness and delay nursing home placement. Early detection also is important in providing much needed help to family members. This can include support groups, respite care, and legal and financial counseling. Finally, early detection is valuable in protecting both the person with dementia and the community from potentially hazardous situations, such as driving vehicles with impaired judgment.

MENTAL STATUS EXAMINATION

The Mental Status Examination (MSE) is one of the most important diagnostic measures available to nurses for evaluating a client's mental condition. The MSE typically assesses five areas of mental function and affective relationships: (1) patterns of speech; (2) emotional reactions and mood; (3) perception; (4) thought content; and (5) cognition.[27] Cognitive ability (or disability) is particularly relevant in the mental health assessments of elderly individuals. Cognitive impairment is the central feature of dementing illnesses that occur in later life (see Chapter 26) and is the primary cause of the self-care and behavioral problems associated with them.[65] Declines in recognition, comprehension, memory, learning ability, problem solving, and orientation often are manifested in behavioral changes that increasingly limit the individual's ability

to function independently.[33] Consequently, the MSE is frequently used as a measure of the elderly person's competence to perform self-care and other activities of daily living and often is critical in placement decisions (e.g., nursing home vs community residence) when cognitive ability is questioned.[45]

Researchers and clinicians recognized the need for a brief measure of cognitive function that could be administered easily to older clients in the clinical setting (MA Smith, unpublished manuscript). The need for a gross measure of overall organic impairment led to the development of abbreviated tests that nurses can use clinically.[24,49] The most popular of the many tests in use are the Information Memory Concentration Test,[9] the Mini-Mental State Examination,[24] the Mental Status Questionnaire,[36] and the Short Portable Mental Status Questionnaire.[49] Proponents of the short MSEs emphasize the practical aspects of the tests that make them "an attractive screening instrument for ascertaining disturbances of cognition among patients" (reference 3, p 397). The scales include 10 to 30 items and can be administered in approximately 5 to 10 minutes. This brevity makes the tests practical for regular and repeated administration as well as "portable" to a variety of treatment settings. The tests "provide an objective basis for uniformity of observation and evaluation by different observers [and have] potential clinical usefulness for rapid screening purposes" (reference 36, p 326). Mini-Mental Status Examinations should *not*, however, be used to classify cognitively impaired individuals in terms of their legal status or need for long-term care.[63]

OTHER MEASURES OF COGNITION

A number of other instruments are available for measuring and "staging" clients with cognitive decline, particularly Alzheimer's disease. These tools are useful for both clinical and research purposes and include the Global Deterioration Scale,[51] the Brief Cognitive Rating Scale,[52,53] and the Alzheimer's Disease Assessment Scale.[55]

Set Test. The Set Test[29] is an easily administered quantitative verbal strategy method used with the elderly to screen for mental status changes. It neither replaces a full MSE nor pinpoints lesions in the brain. Results can be utilized to prevent overuse of medications such as psychotropic drugs, failure to control for environmental factors and safety measures, premature closure of diagnosis, prolonging of hospitalization, and an incorrect assumption that confusion is "normal" with the elderly. The Set Test cannot be used with patients who are aphasic or unable to follow simple directions.

For the Set Test, the client is asked to name as many items as possible in each of four sets: animals, cities, colors, and fruits. One point is scored for each correct item. The maximum score in each category is 10; the maximum total score thus is 40. The test is conducted in a relaxed atmosphere, and the time limit is determined by the clinical judgment of the nurse based on the state of the patient. A score of less than 15 on the Set Test correlates with other validated diagnostic measures for dementia. Fifteen to twenty-four indicates possible dementia and greater than 25 no dementia. Persons with depression score higher on this test than do individuals with dementia, and it can therefore be administered to help determine a differential diagnosis.

Geriatric Depression Rating Scale. Depression is the most common psychiatric disorder among the elderly, and it is critical that nurses be able to detect affective problems in this population. The Geriatric Depression Rating Scale (GDRS) was developed specifically as a screening device to measure depression in the elderly.[70] The GDRS is a 30-item tool with a simple yes/no response format that takes only about 5 to 10 minutes. It has well-established reliability and validity when used with the elderly. The GDRS differs from the Hamilton Depression Inventory (Ham-D) in the absence of somatic symptoms from the former's scale. The lack of diagnostic reliability of somatic complaints as indicators of depression in the elderly has been documented.[60]

Functional Ability, Social Support, and Related Measures. Because social factors can be so influential on the mental health status of the elderly, it is important that nurses take an adequate social history and be aware of instruments that measure support systems and stressors, such as the Social Provisions Scale (D Russell, EE Cutrona, manuscript in preparation), the Hassles Scale,[20] and the Geriatric Social Readjustment Rating (Life Events) Scale.[2] Ability to remain functionally independent in the community can be evaluated using the Instrumental Activities of Daily Living Scale (IADLS).[39] Activities of daily living can also be measured by tools such as the Geriatric Rating Scale,[50] a 31-item measure of resident behaviors. Comprehensive evaluation of resources can be conducted using an instrument such as the Older Americans Resources and Services Program questionnaire (OARS).[22] The OARS covers five areas: social and economic resources, physical and mental health status, and activities of daily living.

TREATMENT MODALITIES AND RELATED NURSING ROLES

Currently, the most common treatment of the elderly with emotional problems is psychopharmacologic.[7] Psychotropic medications are usually prescribed by nonpsychiatrically trained physicians, which can increase the frequency of adverse effects, untoward interactions, and iatrogenic problems. For example, Box 25-1 lists some of the more commonly prescribed drugs

---

BOX 25–1
Drugs that Can Cause Symptoms of Depression*

ANTIHYPERTENSIVES
Reserpine
Methyldopa
Propranolol
Clonidine
Hydralazine
Guanethidine

PSYCHOTROPICS
Sedatives
  Barbiturates
  Benzodiazepines
  Meprobamate
Antipsychotics
  Chlorpromazine
  Haloperidol
  Thiothixene
Hypnotics
  Chloral hydrate
  Benzodiazepines
Antidepressants
  Amitriptyline
  Doxepin

ANTIPARKINSONIANS
Levodopa

ANALGESICS
Narcotic
  Morphine
  Codeine
  Meperidine
  Pentazocine
  Propoxyphene
Nonnarcotic
  Indomethacin

CARDIOVASCULAR PREPARATIONS
Digitalis
Diuretics
Lidocaine
Procaine

HYPOGLYCEMICS (ORAL)

ANTIMICROBIALS
Sulfonamides
Isoniazid

STEROIDS
Corticosteroids
Estrogens

OTHERS
Cimetidine
Cancer chemotherapeutic agents
Alcohol

---

* Table produced by Marianne Smith, R.N., M.S.N.

---

for the elderly that can cause symptoms of depression. Other modes of therapy that can be employed by psychiatric mental health nurses should be considered, along with appropriate drug treatment (see Chapter 39), in dealing with the emotional problems of the elderly.

Therapeutic Objectives

Regardless of the modality employed, the primary therapeutic goals are to help elderly clients to function at their highest possible level and to increase their interpersonal skills and the amount and quality of their interactions with others.[67] Specific therapeutic expectations and outcomes will differ depending on the level of regression and the severity of the emotional disorder in individual clients. Thus, the objectives of therapy with the elderly may be quite diverse and can include relieving anxiety and psychological pain, maintaining or restoring adequate psychological functioning, preventing further problems, and aiding the elderly person in viewing reality more clearly.[35,47]

Three clinically useful foci or treatment aims in providing psychotherapy to the elderly are structural change, restoration of optimal level of functioning, and partial recovery.[66] Structural change entails changes in the personality through insight, adaptive intervention, and basic support. Restoring optimal functioning uses the client's defenses and adaptive methods to aid functioning in the here and now. Partial recovery is achieved by modifying the environment in an effort to decrease stress and provide more support.[66]

Not all emotional disorders found in older clients are amenable to psychotherapy. Psychological symptoms may be secondary to physical problems such as organ system failure, neurologic disturbances, nutritional deficiencies, and adverse drug interactions.[68] It is therefore very important for nurses to work closely with the primary health care providers to ensure an optimal therapeutic outcome.

Psychosocial Needs

The self-preserving strategies used earlier in life are not always possible for the older person.[56] For example, new interpersonal or sexual relationships to replace losses of spouses, friends, and companions are not always available or gratifying, and job and related role satisfactions may be curtailed. These losses become even more intense when combined with physical illness and immobility. In general, then, the psychosocial care of elderly clients entails responding to the following six basic needs: (1) for autonomy and independence; (2) for dignity, credibility, and respect; (3) for identity and individuality; (4) for communication; (5) for belonging; and (6) for touch.

Inability to meet one's basic needs can be a devastating experience, and nurses must do everything possible to preserve the autonomy, independence, and dignity of their elderly clients by attending to them in a compassionate, respectful, and understanding manner.[38] To maximize independence and to exert control over at least some aspect of one's life is another need of the elderly that is often curtailed.[5] The dependent relationships that are often fostered in institutional environments can be psychologically damaging to elderly residents, who come to view themselves as lacking self-sufficiency and the freedom to set and achieve personal goals. Fear of dependency and functional and emotional losses are factors precipitating suicide in the elderly,[44] who account for more than one-fourth of all suicides in this country (see nursing diagnosis entitled suicide potential). A sense of identity is a prerequisite for mental health, and for elderly clients to maintain their sense of individuality and identity requires that the nurse recognize, value, and respond to their individual characteristics, traits, and idiosyncrasies.[38] When elderly persons are lumped together (i.e., as clients, or the aged) or placed in some other homogeneous category, they tend to become depersonalized and to lose their identity.

Communication is another element necessary for a sense of well-being. Elderly persons need to be able to express their feelings and beliefs and be generally listened to. Listening skills are a primary factor in the establishment of any therapeutic relationship and must be developed by nurses who assess and counsel the aged.[4] Without the opportunity for communication and interaction with others, elderly persons become alienated and withdrawn and lose their sense of belonging.[5] A sense of belonging is considered a basic human need that is very applicable to the elderly, who benefit from feeling wanted and needed just for themselves. Although the elderly are the age group least touched physically by health care providers,[6] touch is an important therapeutic element to assist older persons with reality orientation and to foster a sense of identity and acceptance.

General Counseling Considerations in Long-Term Care Settings

Administrators of long-term care facilities often withhold their support for dealing with the emotional problems of elderly residents. Clients exhibiting psychiatric symptoms often are labeled "inappropriate for the facility" and transferred elsewhere rather than treated[56] or are given the physical care required but with negligible attention to meeting their psychosocial needs. Successful treatment of emotional problems in elderly residents requires close and continuing cooperation and communication between nursing staff, psychiatric mental health nursing consultants, psychiatric consultants, and administrators to create a true multidisciplinary team approach. In addition, a positive and hopeful attitude on the part of all team members is essential to the success of any therapeutic program.

In general, the following four-step problem-solving approach to the emotional problems of elderly residents is recommended: (1) assessment of the client's emotional problem and formulation of a nursing diagnosis; (2) development of a plan of intervention; (3) implementation of the plan; and (4) evaluation of the treatment. These steps require continual clarification among team members, who must also discuss the approach with the client and, when available, family members. Follow-up staff meetings enable team members to modify the treatment approach as needed to ensure attainment of therapeutic aims.[56]

Group Counseling Strategies

Group therapy has numerous advantages for dealing with the emotional problems of the elderly, including: (1) more clients can be reached by a single therapist; (2) group members can provide both support and insight for each other; (3) interpersonal skills can be tested in a nonthreatening environment;[61] (4) self-esteem and self-worth can be enhanced; (5) information and suggestions for problem solving can be provided; (6) socialization can occur; (7) reality testing and orientation can be encouraged; (8) motivation for renewing former interests and relationships is increased; and (9) intrapsychic and interpersonal conflicts can be clarified and resolved.[40] Additionally, the group approach provides an opportunity for the therapist to clarify the elderly client's diagnosis and prognosis and to supplement the goals of individual or other forms of therapy.[40]

SUPPORTIVE GROUP THERAPY

Facing reality and verbalizing feelings are important group therapy goals for the aged.[69] In supportive therapy, group members are encouraged to explore problems common to the process of aging and to ventilate feelings of rejection, loneliness, and hostility rather than to seek insight. This emphasis on support rather than ego defense mechanisms, unconscious motivations and resistances, or personality reorganization may be more appropriate than traditional psychoanalytic approaches for elderly residing in long-term care facilities.[67] Supportive groups can be effective with depressed, anxious, agitated, and withdrawn elderly persons and even with those who have compromised cognitive abilities. The supportive group approach can be described as a psychological process in which client feelings of inferiority are met with reassurance, and guilt and anxiety are relieved by a therapist who assumes an active, protective, and permissive role.[67] Supportive group therapy attempts to reestablish an emotional balance that has been upset by the many losses and crises associated with aging. Increased socialization, independence and self-sufficiency, and potential for happiness are emphasized in a supportive group therapy approach. Elderly clients benefit from tangible interactions and counseling techniques that present clear goals and purposes, such as assertiveness or interpersonal skills.[59,69]

The goals of group therapy will vary according to client composition, setting, and theoretical orientation of the therapist.[40] Although there has been little well-controlled research on the value of group therapy for the elderly, a number of early studies reported positive outcomes, even with regressed, institutionalized clients.[59,69] The reader is referred to Burnside's book, *Working with the Elderly: Group Process and Techniques,*[14] for a thorough review of group work with the elderly from a variety of theoretical perspectives and in a variety of settings.

FAMILY COUNSELING APPROACHES

Most elderly persons adhere to the American cultural ideals of independence and self-sufficiency and try to avoid burdening their adult children.[33,43] However, when other sources of support decrease (such as in times of crisis or loss of spouse or friends through relocation or death), the family often assumes a more significant helping role.[57,58] This increased reliance on family support is true for both elderly individuals living independently in the community and those residing in long-term care settings.[21] However, increased familial support is not without problems for both the elderly and the adult children involved.[19] Some of the common issues confronted in this situation may be best resolved in family counseling sessions. These single family or group sessions may deal with topics such as emotional illness in the elderly, the changing role of the female caretakers, aging as a family dilemma, and the economic, physical, and emotional burdens of older children, who may be coping with their own aging process while faced with providing long-term care for their even older relatives.[26] Ethical dilemmas such as the rights of the "old-old" (85 plus) parents vs the needs, values, and rights of the "young-old" (ages 55–75) children also can be discussed.[18] Brief, time-limited family counseling sessions promote the sharing of information and solutions to problems, enable participants to recognize the commonalities among the problems they face, and can help family members to objectify and cope with their feelings[30] (Fig. 25-1).

Many family members experience ambivalence about institutionalizing an elderly relative.[16] Counseling can help the family to arrive at a more realistic, guilt-free placement decision[40] and can facilitate positive family involvement with the long-term care staff.[13] The five main goals for family counseling and family support groups are: (1) to provide a supportive atmosphere for families of aged persons, where feelings (such as sadness, shame, grief, anger, guilt, and relief) can be shared and where similar as well as unique problems can be recognized and dealt with; (2) to provide information about the aging process and adult development, as well as available resources and services; (3) to provide assistance in and support for decision making; (4) to serve as a vehicle to teach both the elderly clients and their family members self-care activities such as assertiveness, listening, communication skills, or interpersonal skills training; (5) to provide a "safe" setting to confront such prevalent and emotional issues as sibling rivalry, unresolved childhood conflicts, and role reversals.[18] Psychotherapeutic interventions with the elderly have been positively influenced by counselors working with family members.[18] Fami-

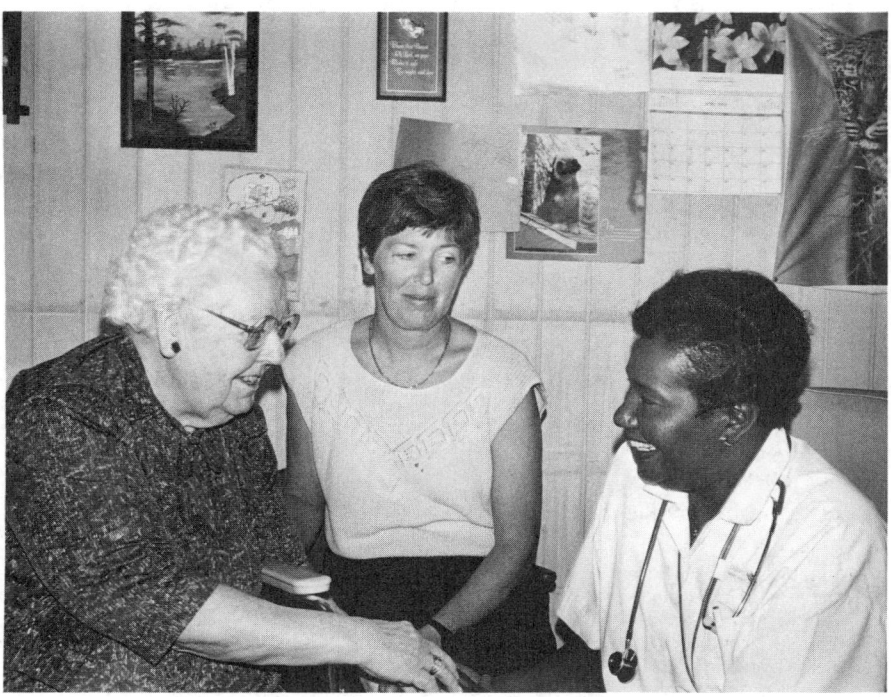

FIGURE 25–1. *Positive involvement of family members is significant in the care of the elderly client. (Courtesy of Caravilla Retirement and Skilled Care Facility, Beloit, Wisconsin, and Mary Durand Thomas)*

lies may be directly involved in these counseling efforts—as in network family therapy, multiple family group work, or family support groups—or they may be less directly involved, serving as "adjunct staff" who can be trained to approach their family member in a manner consistent with that employed by the care team. Regardless of the level of involvement, family members should always be informed about the counseling approaches and treatment techniques used with their elderly loved ones.[67]

For further reading in the area of family counseling and the elderly, the reader is referred to the book, *Counseling Elders and their Families: Practical Techniques for Applied Gerontology.*[32]

Rehabilitative Treatment Modalities

A number of psychosocial rehabilitative strategies have proved useful for the elderly (Box 25-2). And yet, too often, elderly clients with mental health problems are dismissed as hopeless by staff and family members who view the aging process as a progressive and irreversible deterioration leading inevitably to custodial care.[34] Older persons may experience what Goffman has termed a *mortification of self*[28] secondary to multiple losses involving roles, property, and self-identity. Desocialization occurs and results in many of the passive behaviors commonly displayed in long-term care settings: interpersonal detachment; apathy; decreased initiative and interest in the environment, family members, and the future; and deterioration of personal habits.[71] However, these low levels of engagement are more likely attributable to lack of opportunity than to disability.[43]

Although subjective feelings of loss of control over one's behavior and environment most often result in passivity, they may also produce inappropriate acting-out responses that label the elderly client "unmanageable" and "disruptive" and which may cause mutual withdrawal and neglect between clients, family members, and health care professionals. This abandonment is particularly unwarranted in light of recent clinical and research evidence suggesting that a combination of psychosocial rehabilitative strategies consistently incorporated into the care program can improve behavior and increase the quality of life of both community-based elderly and residents of long-term care settings. Box 25-2 presents several of the therapeutic approaches that have been found to be most efficacious in treatment of the elderly. These rehabilitative strategies are diverse but share certain characteristics that enable knowledgeable nurses to counteract the more negative effects of a long-term care environment,[67] including *psychosocial stimulation*, which encourages the revitalization of the integrity and individuality of each elderly client; *social interaction*, which can be effective in drawing individuals out of passive withdrawal or hostile rejection or channel acting out, disruptive behavior through socially acceptable and mutually rewarding interpersonal involvement (Fig. 25-2); and *positive reinforcement* related to growth and achievements, which builds each person's sense of self-control and heightens awareness of how to deal constructively with the reality of the situation (Fig. 25-3). To be successful, these approaches require consistency and caring involvement on the part of all persons coming in contact with the elderly client. Each strategy has pros and cons and should be undertaken only after individual assessment and understanding of

BOX 25–2
Summary of Treatment Modalities Useful with the Elderly

REMOTIVATION THERAPY

GOALS:
Help achieve sense of belonging
Increase feelings of self-worth, self-reliance, and personal
    value
Assist individuals to maximize their potential through
    other-directed communication and stimulating interest
    in surrounding environment and people

PROCEDURES:
Welcoming
Create a bridge to reality
Sharing the world we live in
The work of the world
Appreciation

MUSIC AND MOVEMENT

GOALS:
Improve quality of life
Increase body movement
Stimulate withdrawn persons
Stimulate reminiscence
Increase feelings of relatedness
Decrease aggressiveness, incontinence, and hallucinatory
    behavior
Improve client's appearance and self-esteem

PROCEDURES:
Listening to music
Having music in the environment
Making music

PSYCHODRAMA

GOALS:
Permit expression of emotions and ideas without feelings
    of guilt or inhibition
Explore problems in interpersonal relationships
Facilitate life review
Ease depression
Unblock and help resolve grieving
Reexperience positive roles in life's circumstances

PROCEDURES:
Resident plays a specific role
Groups of residents play interacting roles

PET THERAPY

GOALS:
Alleviate depression
Enhance self-image and identity
Help fulfill need to be loved and to love in return
Help restore emotional equilibrium

PROCEDURE:
Animals (such as dogs, cats, fish, and birds) are used as
    therapeutic catalysts

REMINISCENCE AND LIFE REVIEW

GOALS:
Increase self-esteem
Reaffirm sense of identity
Reconcile client's life and find meaning in the past to
    confront the present
Resolution of old conflicts
Personality reorganization
Restoration of meaning to a person's life
Assist elderly persons to evaluate, understand, and accept
    their lives

PROCEDURES:
Tangible reminders of the past such as pictures, mirrors,
    scrapbooks, and letters
Discussions of childhood memories, progressing to current
    memories. Possible topics include: the "Great
    Depression," military experiences, holiday
    celebrations, old-time songs or cars

SENSORY STIMULATION AND TRAINING

GOALS:
Help put the regressed person back in touch with
    surroundings
Improve sensitivity and responsiveness to the environment
Increase discrimination ability

PROCEDURES:
Structured experiences involving the five senses; e.g.,
    visual, looking in the mirror; *auditory,* listening to
    tapes; *tactile,* touching textured objects; *olfactory,*
    smelling fragrant, spicy aromas; *gustatory,* tasting
    sweet, sour, bitter foods; *kinesthetic,* moving and
    dancing

BEHAVIOR MODIFICATION AND HABIT TRAINING

GOALS:
Give maximum support to appropriate behavior and
    compensate for behavioral deficits
Increase functional levels of the elderly and also their
    sense of self-control
Reduce anxiety

PROCEDURES:
Provide an environmental cue (stimulus) that targets,
    signals, or in some way helps the resident focus on
    the appropriate, expected behavior
Provide a positive reinforcement (reward) for achievement
    of the expected behavior

---

the client are achieved. Perhaps even more important than the type of approach selected is the manner in which is delivered. Genuine concern and involvement on the part of the nurse are paramount.

COMMON NURSING DIAGNOSES

Although the elderly can experience almost any of the nursing diagnoses discussed in this text, this section highlights those that are seen most frequently and are

most amenable to psychiatric mental health nursing interventions.

Depression

The nursing diagnosis depression is applied when the elderly client suffers from a depressive disorder, a common psychiatric problem among community-dwelling elderly that can color every aspect of the person's life. Somewhere between 10% and 15% of all

FIGURE 25–2. Sharing in a music group can increase relatedness to others, elicit memories, and improve the quality of life. (Courtesy of Caravilla Retirement and Skilled Care Facility, Beloit, Wisconsin, and Mary Durand Thomas)

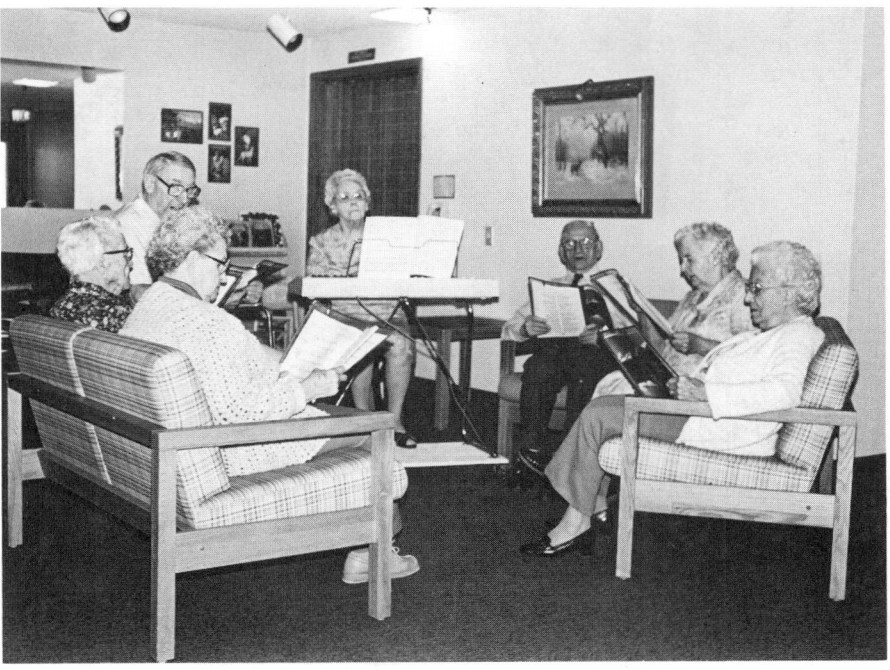

noninstitutionalized persons over age 65 are thought to be depressed and may benefit from treatment. Unfortunately, depression is frequently overlooked among the elderly because being "old and sad" are often falsely considered part of the aging process by both elderly and health professionals or because the elderly person is mistakenly believed to have an organic mental disorder (see discussion below). Also, many elderly wrongly believe that nothing can be done to improve their mood. However, careful use of antidepressant drugs and many types of cognitive and behavioral therapies have been very effective in reducing depression among the elderly.

DEPRESSION VS DEMENTIA

Although many of the symptoms of depression and dementia are similar, important differences exist. Table

FIGURE 25–3. Caring for pets helps fulfil the need to love and be loved. (Courtesy of Caravilla Retirement and Skilled Care Facility, Beloit, Wisconsin, and Mary Durand Thomas)

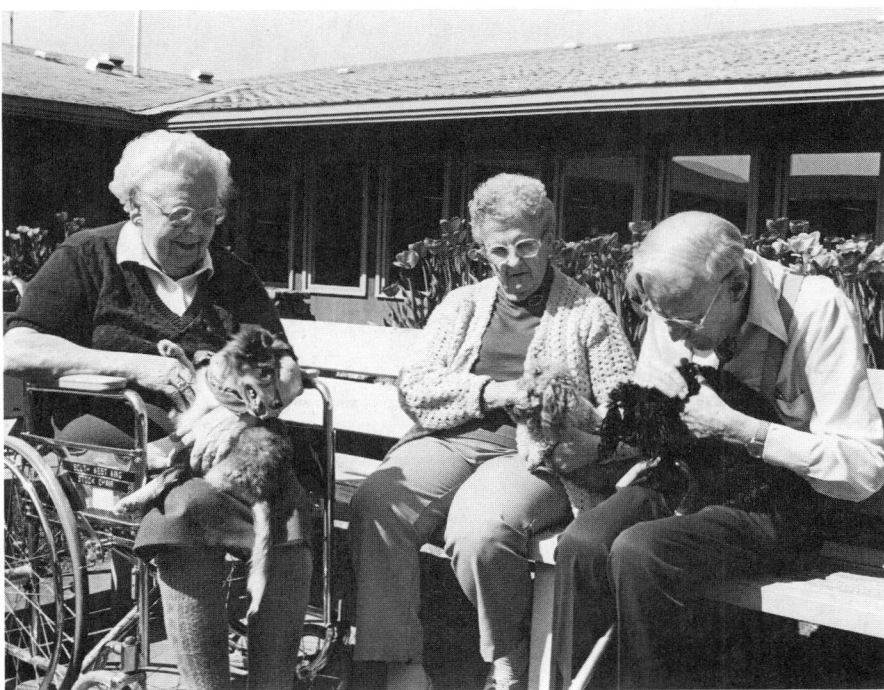

25-1 compares these two illnesses and highlights characteristics that are common to each in the elderly. It is important for nurses to be able to differentiate a highly treatable, reversible disorder such as depression from the inexorably deteriorating course of an irreversible dementia, where care, not cure, is the primary focus of nursing interventions.

Suicide Potential

Elderly people who are very critical of themselves and others are more likely to become depressed or suicidal. They are often passive, expecting others to read their minds and do what they want. Likewise, many situational changes, including many forms of loss, can put a person at risk for depression: death, financial changes, retirement, moving, or changes in health can create situational distress. In the absence of adequate support and coping, the elderly person may be more prone to becoming depressed or suicidal.

One of the most important reasons for early detection and treatment of depression in the elderly is suicide potential: the elderly have the highest suicide rate of any age group, with white men over age 80 having the greatest rate. It is difficult to predict suicide in depressed elderly because they may not give warning signals or dramatically change their behavior before a suicide attempt. Also, the elderly tend to use more lethal methods in their suicide attempts and are therefore more likely actually to kill themselves than are younger people.

Another situation for psychiatric nurses to be aware of is indirect or "passive" suicide among the elderly, who may slowly kill themselves by a variety of means such as starvation, alcohol abuse, mixing or overdosing on medications, or discontinuing needed medications. Some elderly may simply seem to give up the will to live. A number of risk factors for suicide in the elderly are similar to those of other persons throughout the life span. However, the elderly may be at increased risk because of their widowed status, social isolation, or the presence of a chronic or terminal illness.

TABLE 25–1
Comparison of Dementia and Depression

	DEMENTIA	DEPRESSION
Onset	Insidious, indeterminate	Rapid
Duration	Long	Short
Mood/behavior	Fluctuates	Consistently depressed
Response	Provides a close, but usually incorrect, answer to questions	"Do not know"
Disabilities	Concealed	Highlight
Cognition	Relatively stable	Fluctuates greatly

Altered Perception/Cognition (Memory Loss, Confusion) and Altered Impulse Control

Altered perception/cognition (memory loss, confusion) and altered impulse control frequently are related to dementia. Dementia (see Chapter 26) is not a normal part of the aging process. Persons with dementia appear confused and have problems with their thinking that are severe enough to interfere with social relationships in work, home, and community life. Dementia includes the loss of: memory, especially recent memory; judgment and impulse control; abstract thinking; and language ability. An older person with altered perception/cognition (memory loss, recent) may forget names, phone numbers, directions, conversations, or events of the day. He or she may repeat statements and have difficulty learning new information. The person writes many notes, is hesitant in responding, makes up stories, and forgets to complete a task. Persons with altered impulse control may spend large amounts of money, ignore traditional rules of conduct, and appear self-centered and lacking in concern for others. The older individual experiencing confusion may not be oriented to time, place, or person and has difficulty identifying and naming objects. Often, he or she cannot carry out activities in spite of the physical ability to do so or has difficulty understanding written information although able to read it. These problems are observed as changes in personality and behavior. The onset usually is gradual, and symptoms get worse over time, leading eventually to total dependency and, ultimately, death. The course of dementia is varied and unpredictable and may last months to many years.

The loss of mental abilities, whether because of primary degenerative dementia of the Alzheimer type or some other type of dementia, results in a number of other defining characteristics and nursing diagnoses, including: (1) impaired communication, when the person with dementia uses vague words or phrases with little meaning, has difficulty naming objects and recalling names and places; (2) personality changes, resulting in the nursing diagnoses of fear, suspiciousness, or aggression; (3) impaired social interaction, characterized by withdrawal and dependence on others; (4) behavioral changes leading to the diagnoses of altered perception/cognition (delusions, hallucinations) or bizarre behavior; (5) sleep pattern disturbance; (6) potential for injury; and (7) emotional changes that can result in diagnoses of anxiety or depression.

Suspiciousness, Bizarre Behavior, and Altered Perception/Cognition (Delusions, Hallucinations)

Suspiciousness, bizarre behavior, and altered perception/cognition (delusions, hallucinations) often occur in the elderly who suffer from chronic schizophrenia (onset in the early 20s), dementia with delusions, or delusional (paranoid) disorder. Many clients with schizophrenia now live until old age, and although most experience less intense symptoms with age, some periodically become confused and delusional. Their thinking is often of a paranoid nature, and the nursing diagnosis of suspiciousness may be identified. Likewise, elderly persons with dementias with delusions frequently exhibit paranoid behaviors and manifest suspiciousness. Forgetfulness can contribute to false beliefs that people are stealing things from them or doing things behind their backs. Often, they feel that persons who ask them about past events are attacking them at their point of greatest vulnerability.

There are a number of nursing diagnoses associated with delusional (paranoid) disorders in the elderly, including suspiciousness, bizarre behavior, delusions, or hallucinations. Sensory changes, social isolation, and other losses may precipitate delusions secondary to altered perception/cognition in the elderly. Many of the losses associated with the aging process are not under the control of the individual. The changes may be so subtle in onset that they are not recognized by the person at first. These losses create a sense of decreased control over the environment and, in turn, lead to a search for some explanation to account for them.

Anxiety, Fear, and Ritualistic Behavior

The nursing diagnoses anxiety, fear, and ritualistic behavior are often related to anxiety disorders, which occur more frequently in women than men, affecting somewhere between 10% and 15% of women over age 65. Elderly persons with anxiety disorders often complain only of physical symptoms that may mask their anxiety, but they may appear worried, nervous, fearful, or ritualistic in their behavior. Phobias are a common type of anxiety disorder among the elderly, and fear is thus a common nursing diagnosis. Panic disorders or attacks, and the related nursing diagnosis anxiety (extreme/panic), and obsessive compulsive disorders, and the related nursing diagnosis ritualistic behavior, also are seen.

Situational Crises

In situational crisis, some stressor (often a loss) sets off an emotional disturbance. This stressor can be clearly identified by the elderly person. Elderly who have had many losses may also have a physical illness that interferes with coping, or they may just have less strength to handle another loss. The stressful event can be even more upsetting than would be expected under these circumstances. The elderly person may experience difficulty in usual social or work roles. Likewise, the manifestations may be more intense and last longer than would be expected for the situation.

Sleep Pattern Disturbance

Sometimes, emotional conflicts are expressed as sleep pattern disturbances. Most elderly persons require 6 to 7 hours of sleep per night. Compared with younger persons, they sleep more lightly and awaken more, often to go to the bathroom. Gerontologic sleep pattern disturbance can be related to a variety of factors, including a move to a new environment; anxiety (worry); drug withdrawal (alcohol and sedatives); dementia; depression; physical illness, especially difficulty breathing; or pain, such as from arthritis or angina. Elderly persons who sleep too much (hypersomnia) may awaken with difficulty and often appear confused or disoriented. Older individuals who take drugs to calm their nerves, and especially those who take sleep medication over a long time, create more harmful effects than benefits with regard to their sleep cycles. Even normal changes in sleep associated with aging can be very upsetting to elderly persons. Sleep disturbances should be evaluated by the psychiatric nurse to determine the related factors.

CASE STUDY

James O, a 78-year-old widower, was brought to the community mental health center (CMHC) by his daughter, Lucille, who stated, "I think he's losing his mind." Since his wife's death 12 years ago, Mr. O has resided alone in their family home. For the past year, he has received home-delivered meals and monthly visits from a public health nurse because of visual loss. Mr. O has three adult children, but only Lucille resides in the community. His one living sister, Velma, was placed in a county care facility 5 years ago because of "senility." About a year ago, Lucille noticed the onset of memory loss in her father but attributed it to normal aging. Recently, she found her father sitting in his summer pajamas on the back porch swing in subfreezing temperatures. She has also noticed a gradual deterioration in Mr. O's hygiene and ability to prepare meals. Lucille reports that last week her father called her three times during the middle of the night, agitated and unable to sleep. She brought him to the CHMC because she fears he is "becoming senile like Aunt Velma" and is no longer able to live independently.

The psychiatric mental health nurse administered the Short Portable Mental Status Questionnaire[49] to Mr. O, whose score was 5 errors, placing him in the moderate intellectual impairment category. Mr. O was oriented to person. He communicated only in simple sentences and comprehended simple requests but became frustrated and agitated when asked to plan and carry through with more complex voluntary tasks. All vital signs were within normal limits, and Mr. O appeared physically robust with no reported medical problems other than failing vision, no known weight loss, and no medications other than an over-the-counter drug his daughter had given him to help him sleep better at night. Mr. O was referred to a local neurologist for neuropsychological testing and to rule out potential reversible causes of dementing illness such as infections or dietary insufficiencies. Following a comprehensive neurologic and psychiatric evaluation, the DSM-III-R diagnosis was primary degenerative dementia of the Alzheimer type, and the primary nursing diagnosis was altered perception/cognition (memory loss) related to pathologic changes in the cerebral cortex secondary to Alzheimer's disease. The care plan developed for Mr. O is presented in Nursing Care Plan 25-1.

NURSING CARE PLAN 25–1

JAMES O

NURSING INTERVENTIONS	OUTCOME CRITERIA

NURSING DIAGNOSIS: Altered perception/cognition (memory loss) related to changes in the cerebral cortex secondary to Alzheimer's disease

CLIENT GOAL: Maintain optimal level of cognitive/perceptual and affective functioning

■ Assess Mr. O for: Decreased short-term memory and time sense Inability to abstract and make choices and decisions Word-finding and language loss Inability to plan, initiate, and carry out goal-directed or voluntary activities or tolerate change Inability to recognize or interpret environmental stimuli Inability to tolerate multiple stimuli Increased susceptibility to fatigue Decreased knowledge of place and time Catastrophic episodes secondary to lowered stress threshold; i.e., hallucinations, threatening delusions, agitation, forgetfulness, wandering Social withdrawal or preoccupation with self Decreased ADL, legal, and financial functioning Refusal to seek appropriate medical care	
■ Create a consistent written routine, thus eliminating disturbing changes	Functions within day-to-day routine
■ Assign consistent caregivers and inform about planned routine	Develops trust in caregivers
■ Offer nonverbal reassurance and therapeutic touch	
■ Have two or three low-stimulus rest periods per day. Place Mr. O in recliner or easy chair with afghan, soft music; allow no TV or visitors at this time	Maintains optimum level of cognitive functioning
■ Minimize changes in routine, new and strange situations, large groups	
■ Do not force Mr. O to do anything	
■ Avoid potentially stressful situations for Mr. O	
■ Recognize "precatastrophic" behaviors and remove offending stimuli and/or provide rest when they occur	
■ Evaluate tasks and activities by components and simplify or eliminate when catastrophic behavior occurs	
■ Provide careful monitoring of medical conditions, medications	
■ Plan for rest prior to, during, and after unavoidable special events	
■ Minimize television, cover mirrors, eliminate pictures that could be misinterpreted	Experiences decreased number of hallucinations and threatening delusions
■ Close drapes at night	
■ Use nonverbal cues in the environment (clocks, calendars) when giving directions	Makes more accurate interpretation of environment
	Environment created supports function
■ Assist when unable to complete task and demonstration has failed	Expresses improved self-esteem
■ Do not "test" losses; i.e., asking date or time	
■ Label items with pictures	Demonstrates more accurate interpretation of environment
■ Instruct daughter Lucille and others in controlling stimuli, reminiscence, nonverbal communication skills	

Continued

NURSING CARE PLAN 25-1

JAMES O *Continued*

NURSING INTERVENTIONS	OUTCOME CRITERIA
■ Avoid caffeine	Has increased sleep at night and is less fearful late in day
■ Listen to Mr. O when he does not wish to participate in activities	Maintains optimum affective state
■ Keep planned activities short and within Mr. O's physical and mental limitations	Environment supports function
■ Keep environment and caregivers constant: do not move furniture, do not redecorate, etc.	
■ Instruct Lucille in basics of legal and financial planning for Mr. O; help her locate legal counsel	Mr. O's and Lucille's financial assets will be protected

NURSING DIAGNOSIS: Altered perception/cognition related to decreased vision and Alzheimer's disease

CLIENT GOAL: Interact functionally with environment

■ Assess Mr. O for: Intolerance to light and dark Decreased fine motor dexterity Agnosia Decreased ability to see fine objects Gait disturbance from foot placement problems Increased confusion, delusions as indication of decreased vision	
■ Provide consistent light level during day and lowered light level at night	No complaints of light intolerance; knows day from night
■ Provide for use of large-handled utensils, gross motor activities	Uses needed objects
■ Plan activities with bright colors (red, yellow) so Mr. O can see	Further visual loss is minimized; current visual level is monitored
■ Keep Mr. O's needed objects in sight in same place at all times	
■ Encourage Mr. O to wear glasses	
■ Have Mr. O wear well-fitting leather-soled shoes at same heel height as usual to maximize proprioception	No evidence of injury from bumping into objects or falls
■ Encourage use of cane for outdoor ambulation	
■ Do not move furniture. Provide for environmental consistency	

NURSING DIAGNOSIS: Sleep pattern disturbance related to Alzheimer's disease

CLIENT GOAL: Experience pre-illness sleep–wake cycle

■ Assess Mr. O for: Awakening at night and confusion regarding time, place, and person Fears or wandering at night	
■ Provide two or three rest periods during day in an armchair or recliner. (Rest periods in bed promote day/night disorientation.) Have Mr. O rest 30 minutes to 1 hour in morning and afternoon with no activities, TV, or visitors. If night wakening continues, increase number or duration of rest periods	Sleep–wake cycle approximates pre-illness state
■ Keep Mr. O up as late as possible with favorite activities, foods; plan for bedtime snacks	

Continued

JAMES O *Continued*

NURSING INTERVENTIONS   **OUTCOME CRITERIA**

- Measure blood sugar when awake at night; if low, provide a snack
- Keep consistent low-level light at night; do not turn on lamps if Mr. O awakens
- If Mr. O awakens, give snack, take to bathroom, and place back in bed
- If night wakening occurs regularly, decrease activities and stressors during day
- If Mr. O has had a high-stimulus day, anticipate night wakening and provide for safety

NURSING DIAGNOSIS: Self-care deficit related to Alzheimer's disease

CLIENT GOAL: Achieve optimum levels of self-feeding, grooming, and toileting

- Assess Mr. O for:
  Assistance and direction needed to dress, bathe, and groom
  Fear of water
  Ability to cook, clean, and shop
  Ability to toilet self
- Provide consistent scheduling of ADLs in pattern normative to pre-illness lifestyle
- Refer to OT to design program to maximize ADL function
- Allow adequate time for ADLs
- Surround bath with pleasurable stimuli and rest (i.e., music, fruit juice, rest before and after)
- If Mr. O cannot complete activity, use nonverbal demonstrations and simple sentence directions; if still unable, assist Mr. O.
- Do not stigmatize if messy
- Do not ask Mr. O to "remember" or "think about" the activity, as he will be less able to perform
- Reward Mr. O verbally or with touch when task is completed

Environment does not limit function

Well-groomed and dressed and toilets self

NURSING DIAGNOSIS: Potential for injury related to Alzheimer's disease and impaired vision

CLIENT GOAL: Be protected from harm

- Assess Mr. O for:
  Decreased judgment
  Impulsive behavior indicative of inability to inhibit
  Wandering outside and becoming lost
  Lack of concern for safety
  Changed gait and pacing
- Have ID bracelet or necklace made with name, address, and telephone and nature of disease
- Have picture of Mr. O plus information sheet ready to give to police should wandering occur
- Have nurse or family "wander" with Mr. O to record where he goes
- When taking walks, follow a consistent route
- Remove knobs from stove when not in use
- Remove can opener, blender, knives, and toaster from kitchen counter; remove guns, rifles, poisonous plants; remove housecleaning solutions
- Paint hot water tap red
- Reduce hot water heater temperature to 115° Fahrenheit
- Supervise all smoking
- Allow no liquor

No falls, burns, cuts, poisoning, or other injury
Decreased wandering
Increased feelings of security
Mr. O will be cared for in an emergency situation

Continued

NURSING CARE PLAN 25–1

JAMES O *Continued*

NURSING INTERVENTIONS	OUTCOME CRITERIA

NURSING INTERVENTIONS

- Supervise all medications
- Keep lighting level and even
- Put handrails and grabbers in bathroom
- Ensure presence of nonskid tub surface
- Remove clutter
- Remove scatter rugs
- Eliminate glaring and slippery, highly polished floors
- Have Mr. O wear well-fitting leather-soled shoes
- Provide ambulatory assistive devices as needed. Assist with walking
- Remove keys from car
- Secure doors, windows with locks that are above or below eye level
- Establish a simple, predictable routine of meals, activities, etc., if wandering occurs
- Tape red Xs to patio doors and lock
- Provide night light in the evening
- Do not leave client unattended
- Develop a workable "disaster plan" in case of emergency such as fire, flood, tornado, or illness of significant other
- Develop plans in case of death or disability of significant other

The author gratefully acknowledges the assistance of Geri Hall, R.N., M.A., in the preparation of the care plan.

SUMMARY

The elderly are the fastest growing segment of our population, yet they remain vastly underserved in terms of their mental health needs. Understanding of psychological disturbances in the elderly is complex and challenging because the disorders may be attributable to a variety of factors such as physical problems or adverse medication interactions. Therefore, assessment of the geriatric mental health client must be comprehensive and incorporate knowledge of the normal aging process as well as of the psychopathology in this population. Assessment instruments that were de-

Research Highlights

One important area in geriatric mental health about which there is inadequate information is chronic mental illness. Nurses are in an excellent position to contribute to research in this domain because of their understanding of chronic illness and because treatment for these disorders is multidimensional, multidisciplinary, and long-term. Goals for this particularly underserved client population include management of symptoms, teaching living and coping skills, and enhancing the client's quality of life, rather than curing the illness.[8] These goals are clearly compatible with professional nursing practice and research efforts.

Diseases such as schizophrenia are not fatal, and persons with schizophrena do live to become old. And yet there is a lack of literature that adequately describes such chronic mental illnesses over the life course. Nurses should be involved in longitudinal studies of the onset and life course of chronic mental illnesses that continue into old age. These studies should consider the relation of physical health and social and support factors to mental illness in the elderly. Both positive outcomes of nursing interventions (e.g., enhanced quality of life, decreased recidivism rates to institutions) and the adverse effects of therapies, such as the development of tardive dyskinesia from long-term use of neuroleptic medications, must be measured over time.

veloped and normed on younger persons may not be
valid and reliable for the elderly. Similarly, there are
some unique therapeutic objectives that should underlie treatment of elderly clients, whose psychosocial
needs may be different from those of other populations.
Group and family therapy approaches are particularly
effective with the elderly and can be conducted in a
variety of settings. A number of psychosocial rehabilitation strategies (e.g., remotivation groups, pet therapy,
reminiscence, and life review) can be employed by psychiatric mental health nurses to improve the quality of
life and adaptive capacities of the psychiatrically
impaired elderly. A number of nursing diagnoses are
applicable to the elderly, the most common being depression, suicide potential, suspiciousness, bizarre behavior, anxiety, sleep pattern disturbance, altered per-
ception/cognition (confusion, memory loss, delusions,
hallucinations), and self-care deficit. With increasing
numbers of psychiatrically impaired elderly, there is a
growing need for nursing research in all aspects of assessment and intervention strategies and health care
delivery patterns for the elderly. One vastly underre-
searched area is chronic mental illness in the elderly.

References

1. American Association of Retired Persons. A Profile of Older
    Americans. Washington, DC: American Association of Re-
    tired Persons; 1986.
2. Amster LE, Karuss HH. The relationship between life crises
    and mental deterioration in old age. Int J Aging Hum Dev.
    1974;5:51–55.
3. Anthony JC, LeResche L, Niaz U, Von Korff M, Folstein MF.
    Limits of the Mini-Mental State as a screening test for de-
    mentia and delirium among hospital patients. Psychol Med.
    1982;12:397–408.
4. Bahr RT. Touch: a means of communicating with the el-
    derly. In: Hall BA, ed. Mental health and the elderly. Or-
    lando: Grune & Stratton; 1984.
5. Bahr RT. Aging: a positive growth experience. In: Hall BA,
    ed. Mental health and the elderly. Orlando: Grune & Strat-
    ton; 1984.
6. Barnett K. A theoretical construct of the concepts of touch as
    they relate to nursing. Nurs Res. 1972;21(2):102–110.
7. Berezin MA. Psychotherapy of the elderly: introduction. J
    Geriatr Psychiatry. 1983;16(3):3–6.
8. Bellack AS, Mueser KT. A comprehensive treatment pro-
    gram for schizophrenia and chronic mental illness. Commu-
    nity Ment Health J. 1986;22(3):175–189.
9. Blessed G, Tomlinson BE, Roth M. The association between
    quantitative measures of dementia and of senile changes in
    the cerebral grey matter of elderly subjects. Br J Psychiatry.
    1968;114:797–811.
10. Brody JA. Life expectancy and the health of older people. J
    Am Geriatr Soc. 1982;30:681–683.
11. Buckwalter KC. Integration of social and mental health ser-
    vices for the elderly. Family Community Health.
    1985;8(4):76–87.
12. Buckwalter KC. Evaluation of mental health of the rural
    elderly. Cedar Rapids, Iowa: Outreach Project Final Report,
    US Administration on Aging; 1988.
13. Buckwalter KC, Hall GR. Families of institutionalized el-
    derly: a neglected resource. In: Brubaker TH, ed. Aging,
    health, and family: long term care. Beverly Hills: Sage Pub-
    lications; 1987.

14. Burnside I. Working with the elderly: group process and
    techniques. Monterey: Wadsworth Health Sciences Divi-
    sion; 1984.
15. Butler RN. Toward a psychiatry of the life cycle: implica-
    tions of sociopsychologic studies of the aging process for the
    psychotherapeutic situation. Psychiatr Res Rep. 1968;
    23:233–248.
16. Cath S. The geriatric patient and his family: the institution-
    alization of a parent—a nadir of life. J Geriatr Psychiatry.
    1972;5:25–46.
17. Cohen GD. Prospects for mental health and aging. In: Birrin
    JE, Sloane RB, eds. Handbook of mental health and aging.
    Englewood Cliffs: Prentice-Hall; 1980.
18. Cohen PM. A group approach for working with families of
    the elderly. Gerontologist. 1983;23(3):248–250.
19. Copstead LE, Patterson S. Families of the elderly. In: Carne-
    vali D, Patrick M, eds. Nursing management for the elderly.
    2nd ed. Philadelphia: JB Lippincott; 1986.
20. DeLongis A, Coyne JC, Dakof G, Folkman S, Lazarus R. Re-
    lationship of daily hassles, uplifts, and major life events to
    health status. Health Psychol. 1982;1:119–136.
21. Dobrof R, Litwak E. Maintenance of family ties to long-term
    care patients: theory and guide to practice. Rockville: Na-
    tional Institute of Mental Health; 1981.
22. Duke University Center for the Study of Aging and Human
    Development. Multi-dimensional functional assessment: the
    OARS methodology. 2nd ed. Durham, North Carolina: Duke
    University; 1978.
23. Ferris SH, Crook T. Cognitive assessment in mild to moder-
    ately severe dementia. In: Crook T, Ferris S, Bartus R, eds.
    Assessment in geriatric psychopharmacology. New Canaan,
    Connecticut: Mark Powley Associates; 1983.
24. Folstein MF, Folstein SE, McHugh PR. Mini-Mental State: a
    practical method for grading the cognitive state of patients
    for the clinician. J Psychiatr Res. 1975;12:189–198.
25. Freud S. On Psychotherapy. In: Collected Papers. Vol. 1.
    London: Hogarth Press; 1904:249–263.
26. Gelfand DE, Olson JK, Block MR. Two generations of elderly
    in the changing American family: implications for family
    services. Family Coordinator. 1978;27:395–403.
27. Ginsberg GL. Psychiatric history and mental status examina-
    tion. In: Kaplan HI, Sadock BJ, eds. Comprehensive textbook
    of psychiatry IV. Vol. 1. Baltimore: Williams & Wilkins;
    1985:487–494.
28. Goffman E. Asylums. New York: Anchor Books; 1961.
29. Goldenberg B, Chiverton P. Assessing behavior: the nurse's
    mental status exam. Geriatr Nurs. March/April 1984:94–98.
30. Goldstein R. Psychotherapy of the elderly, case #1: institu-
    tionalizing a spouse: who is the client? J Geriatr Psychiatry.
    1983;16(1):41–49.
31. Hall BA. Aging, society and mental health. In: Hall BA, ed.
    Mental health and the elderly. Orlando: Grune & Stratton;
    1984.
32. Herr JJ, Weakland JH. Counseling elders and their families:
    practical techniques for applied gerontology. New York:
    Spring Publishing; 1979.
33. Hirshfield I, Dennis H. Perspectives. In: Ragan P, ed. Aging
    parents. Los Angeles: University of California Press; 1979.
34. Hussian RA. Geriatric psychology: a behavioral perspective.
    New York: Van Nostrand Reinhold; 1981.
35. Kahana RJ. Psychotherapy of the elderly: a miserable old
    age—what can therapy do? J Geriatr Psychiatry. 1983;
    16(1):7–32.
36. Kahn RL, Goldfarb AI, Pollack M, Peck A. Brief objective
    measures for the determination of mental status in the aged.
    Am J Psychiatry. 1960;117:326–328.
37. Kane RA, Kane RL. Assessing the elderly: a practical guide to

measurement. Lexington, Massachusetts: Lexington Books; 1981.

38. Kayser–Jones JS. Psychosocial care of nursing home residents. In: Hall BA, ed. Mental health and the elderly. Orlando: Grune & Stratton; 1984.

39. Lawton MP. Assessment of behaviors required to maintain residence in the community. In: Crook T, Ferris S, Bartus R, eds. Assessment in geriatric psychopharmacology. New Canaan, Connecticut: Mark Powley Associates; 1983.

40. Lazarus LW, Weinberg J. Treatment in the ambulatory care setting. In: Busse EW, Blazer DG, eds. Handbook of geriatric psychiatry. New York: Van Nostrand Reinhold; 1980.

41. Liptzin B. Major mental disorders/problems in nursing homes: implications for research and public policy. In: Harper M, ed. Mental illness in nursing homes: agenda for research. Washington, DC: US Government Printing Office; 1986.

42. Lowenthal M, Robinson B. Social networks and isolation. In: Binstock R, Shanas E, eds. Handbook of aging and the social sciences. New York: Van Nostrand Reinhold; 1977.

43. McCormack D, Whitehead A. The effect of providing recreational activities on the engagement level of long stay geriatric patients. Age Aging. 1981;10:287–291.

44. Miller M. Suicide after sixty: the final alternative. New York: Springer Publishing; 1979.

45. Moody HR. Ethical dilemmas in nursing home placements. Generations. 1987;11:16–23.

46. Moss F, Halamandares V. Too old, too sick, too bad: nursing homes in America. Germantown, Maryland: Aspen Systems; 1977.

47. Oberleder M. Psychotherapy with the aging: an art of the possible? Psychotherapy. 1966;3:139–142.

48. Paulmeno SR. Psychogeriatric care: a specialty within a specialty. Nurs Manage. 1987;2:39–42.

49. Pfeiffer E. A short portable mental status questionnaire for the assessment of organic brain deficit in elderly patients. J Am Geriatr Soc. 1975;23:433–441.

50. Plutchik R, Conte H, Leiberman M, Baukr M, Grossman J, Lehrman N. Reliability and validity of a scale for assessing the functioning of geriatric patients. J Am Geriatr Soc. 1970;18:491–500.

51. Reisberg B. The Global Deterioration Scale for assessment of primary degenerative dementia. Am J Psychiatry. 1982;139:1136–1139.

52. Reisberg B. An ordinal functional assessment tool for Alzheimer-type dementia. Hosp Community Psychiatry. 1985;36:593–595.

53. Reisberg B, Ferris SH, Anand R, Mir P, deLeon M, Roberts E. The Brief Cognitive Rating Scale: findings in primary degenerative dementia. Psychopharmacol Bull. 1983;19:47–50.

54. Rohrer J, Buckwalter KC, Russell D. The effects of mental dysfunction on nursing home care. Social Sci Med. 28:399–403.

55. Rosen WG, Mohs RC, Davis KL. A new rating scale for Alzheimer's disease. Am J Psychiatry. 1984;141:1356–1364.

56. Sadavoy J, Dorian B. Treatment of the elderly characterologically disturbed patient in the chronic care institution. J Geriatr Psychiatry. 1983;16(2):223–249.

57. Seelback WC. Correlates of aged parents' filial responsibility, expectations and relations. Family Coordinator. 1978; 27:241–250.

58. Shanas E. The family as a social support system in old age. Gerontologist. 1979;19:169–174.

59. Silver A. Group psychotherapy with senile psychotic patients. Geriatrics. 1950;5:147–150.

60. Steur J, Bank L, Olsen EJ, Jarvik LF. Depression, physical health and somatic complaints in the elderly: a study of the Jung Self-Rating Depression Scale. J Gerontol. 1980;35:683–688.

61. Storandt M. Counseling and therapy with older adults. Boston: Little, Brown Series on Gerontology; 1983.

62. Straker M. Prognosis for psychiatric illness in the aged. Am J Psychiatry. 1973;119:1069–1075.

63. Tancredi LR. The mental status exam. Generations. 1987; 11:24–31.

64. US Bureau of the Census: Projections of the population of the United States by age, sex, and race: 1983 to 2080. Current Populations Reports, Series P-25, No. 952. Washington, DC; 1984.

65. US Congress Office of Technology Assessment. Losing a million minds: confronting the tragedy of Alzheimer's disease and other dementias. Washington, DC: US Government Printing Office; 1987: OTA-BA-323.

66. VanderZyl S. Psychotherapy with the elderly. J Psychosocial Nurs Ment Health Serv. 1983;2(10):25–29.

67. Weiner MB, Brok AJ, Snadowsky AM. Working with the aged: practical approaches in the institution and community. Englewood Cliffs: Prentice-Hall; 1978.

68. Wills R. Cognitive changes of normal aging and the dementias. In: Carnevali D, Patrick M, eds. Nursing management for the elderly. Philadelphia: JB Lippincott; 1986:241–257.

69. Wolff K. Group psychotherapy with geriatric patients in a psychiatric hospital. Psychiatr Stud Proj. 1963;3:275–277.

70. Yesavage JA, Brink TL, Rose L, Adey M. The Geriatric Depression Rating Scale: comparison with other self-report and psychiatric rating scales. In: Crook T, Ferris S, Bartus R, eds. Assessment in geriatric psychopharmacology. New Canaan, Connecticut: Mark Powley and Associates; 1983:153–167.

71. Zusman J. Some explanations of the changing appearance of psychiatric patients. Int J Psychiatry. 1967;4:216–237.

26

Sonia D. Hinds
Lillian Eleanor Wade

Clients With Alzheimer's Disease

OBJECTIVES

After reading this chapter, the reader will be able to:

1. *Define Alzheimer's disease*
2. *Describe the pathology of Alzheimer's disease*
3. *Identify the symptomatology*
4. *Identify the behavioral and physical changes according to the three stages of this disease*
5. *Describe the essential components of a nursing assessment of clients with Alzheimer's disease*
6. *Analyze the various treatment modalities*
7. *Describe the role of the nurse during the three stages*
8. *Identify common nursing diagnoses as well as nursing interventions during the three stages of the disease*
9. *Analyze a case study and nursing interventions for a client with Alzheimer's disease*
10. *Examine research findings and recommendations of a nursing research study on Alzheimer's disease.*

OVERVIEW

Alzheimer's disease was first diagnosed in a 51-year-old patient by Alois Alzheimer in 1907 and was thought to be a rare disease. In the 1960s researchers determined that it was not such a rare disease, but rather, the most common cause of dementia.[2,14] As yet, there is no cure, and numerous questions remain unanswered. With Alzheimer's disease, there is primary dementia, in which memory loss, intellectual deterioration, personality changes, and the inability to perform normal activities of daily living are evident. The dementia is characterized as insidious in onset, chronic, progressive, degenerative, and irreversible.[3,23] Caregivers of Alzheimer's sufferers describe this disease as one of the most frustrating, agonizing, dehumanizing conditions that a person can experience. It has been called Old Timer's disease, thief of minds, destroyer of personalities, wrecker of family finances, and filler of nursing homes.[18] It was referred to as "Another Name for Madness" by Marion Roach[27] in her book, which gives a moving account of her mother's battle with the disease.

Alzheimer's disease may occur as early as age 40, but it is more commonly seen among those 65 years of age and older.[15,18] It is said to be the fourth leading cause of death for people older than 65.[1] More women than men are affected, probably because women outlive men.[14] Experts describe it as a major cause of admissions to nursing homes and other long-term care facilities. Currently, this disease affects 2.5 million American adults and is the most common form of irreversible dementia.[2] It is expected that the disease will escalate as the older population increases. Nursing can play an essential role in creating and testing effective interventions that will enhance the quality of life for people with Alzheimer's disease.

ETIOLOGY

The cause of Alzheimer's disease is unknown. Several hypotheses attempt to explain the etiology of this disease, including:

1. Diminished concentration of choline acetyltransferase in the brain: This is needed for the neurotransmitter acetylcholine, the chemical necessary for normal communication between nerve cells.[7,2] Defects result in impaired memory and learning.[32]
2. Higher than normal levels of aluminum deposits in the brain: Aluminum acts as a toxin to the brain and is found in neuritic plaques and neurofibrillary tangles.[6,26]
3. Immune system dysfunction: Abnormally high levels of antibodies have been found, and it is believed that the body's immune system attacks its own cells.[17] Impaired immune function has been seen in later stages of Alzheimer's disease, causing

The authors wish to thank all the nurses, physicians, psychologists, psychiatrists, social workers, and caregivers who so graciously shared their knowledge and experiences on this subject.

the person to be susceptible to infection.[14] It is not uncommon for clients with Alzheimer's disease to die of infections, such as pneumonia, in the last stages of the disease.
4. Slow-acting virus: By identifying similar central nervous system diseases in animals, scientists are trying to determine if there is a linkage between this disease and infectious illness.[14]
5. Genetic transmission: Reports of research on Alzheimer's disease suggest that some cases are inherited.[34] It has been found that people with Down syndrome who live to the age of 40 or older develop Alzheimer's disease.[21]

PATHOLOGY

Several definite changes have been found in the brain tissue of a number of Alzheimer's sufferers upon autopsy. Three major changes seen are neurofibrillary tangles, neuritic plaques, and granulovacuolar degeneration.[29] Neurofibrillary tangles and neuritic plaques are caused by abnormal protein production in the brain.[26] The neurofibrillary tangles are pairs of thread-like nerve fibers wrapped around each other, twisting until a tangled mass of tissue is formed in the brain cells.[34] Normal cell function is impeded, resulting in cell destruction.[20] Neuritic plaques are degenerating bits of nerve cells surrounding extracellular amyloids, which are starchlike protein deposits.[34] This causes disruption in intellect and memory, depending on location and size.[31] Granulovacuolar degeneration is seen as cavities of fluid and granular material found in the pyramidal cells of the hippocampus, causing degeneration of the neurons.[30,39] Neurofibrillary tangles, neuritic plaques, and granulovacuolar degeneration are found, to some extent, in brains of people with normal aging; however, with Alzheimer's disease, these changes are in greater proportion.[29] The higher the number of plaques and tangles, the greater the disruption in intellect and memory.[33] These changes are found throughout the cerebral cortex and in large concentration in the hippocampus—the short-term memory center in the brain.[29] Another change seen in brains of persons with Alzheimer's disease is atrophy of the brain and enlarged ventricles.

SYMPTOMATOLOGY

The course of Alzheimer's disease can vary from three to as long as 20 years, with an average of six to eight years.[1] Clients with Alzheimer's disease exhibit a myriad of behavioral, psychological, and some physical changes in the later stages. The presenting symptoms for this disease coexist along with previous physical conditions and illnesses, as well as normal changes associated with aging. Generally, clients with Alzheimer's disease are in good physical health until the later stages.

The symptoms are grouped into three progressive stages. How quickly these stages progress varies among individuals. Adjustment to the different stages is dependent on the person's preexisting state of health, coping abilities, and the support of family and significant others. Box 26-1 presents a summary of major symptoms, as well as other commonly seen symptoms.

Stages of the Disease

STAGE ONE

The first stage may last two to four years. The person is usually cared for at home by family members because the initial symptoms are subtle or mild. Also, the disease may not be diagnosed until it reaches the second stage. Memory loss, which initially seems minor and is sometimes erroneously associated with the normal aging process, is identified most commonly as one of the first symptoms. Recent memory is affected, although remote memory remains intact at this point. The ability to learn and retain new information is impaired. Written notes may be utilized to compensate for what was formerly remembered easily. Difficulty with memory may involve, for example, forgetting where one's glasses or keys were placed. In addition, disorientation to time and place, inability to concentrate or engage in conversation without losing train of thought, lack of interest in surroundings, lack of spontaneity and initiative, tiredness, and an unkempt appearance may be seen. A tendency to rationalize and blame others for shortcomings may be evident. An awareness that something is wrong beyond control may lead to depression, which complicates the clinical picture. Other personality changes include becoming easily angered and irritable, particularly at the inability to communicate thoughts clearly. In the early stage, the person affected with Alzheimer's disease seeks and prefers familiar surroundings and people, and shuns the unfamiliar. As the disease progresses, the ability to perform complex tasks becomes difficult. If employed, the person may have difficulty performing on the job.

STAGE TWO

The duration of this stage is much longer than the initial stage. The first-stage symptoms become more severe, losses increase, and it becomes obvious that there is marked change in behavior. The inability to comprehend what is being said or attach meaning to spoken language increases. Paraphasia (use of words in wrong and senseless combination) and visual agnosia (inability to recognize objects) are seen. Making decisions and future plans is cause for great stress. The person with Alzheimer's disease who has difficulty coping with a stressful situation may overreact with excessive anger, frustration, or aggressive behavior. This overreaction is described as a catastrophic reaction. Supervision of daily activities may be needed. Problems with memory loss may involve not being able to find the way home while driving, forgetting to take medications, or leaving food unattended on a stove. Not only is recent memory worsened, but remote memory is affected as well. Disorientation to time and place is increased, and disorien-

BOX 26-1
Stages of Alzheimer's Disease

SYMPTOMS OF STAGE ONE
Memory loss, especially of recent events
Time disorientation
Spatial disorientation
Affect changes
Loss of sense of humor
Depression
Denial
Projection
Mistakes in judgment
Absentmindedness
Decreased concentration abilities
Lack of spontaneity
Perceptual disturbances
Carelessness in actions
Careless in appearance
Transitory delusions of persecution
Epileptiform seizures
Muscular twitchings
Hallucinations
Delusions
Irritability
Preference for familiar surroundings

SYMPTOMS OF STAGE TWO
Forgetfulness of recent and remote events
Increased inability to comprehend
Complete disorientation
Restless at night
Sundown syndrome
Increased aphasia
Agnosia (inability to recognize sensory stimuli)
Asterognosia (inability to recognize familiar objects by touch)
Apraxia (inability to carry out skilled and purposeful movement)
Perseveration phenomena (continuous repetitive motion)
Hyperorality (placing every object in mouth)
Insatiable appetite without weight gain
Alexia (inability to read)
Auditory agnosia (inability to recognize significance of sound)
Socially acceptable behaviors are forgotten
Hypertonia (excessive muscle tone)
Unsteady gait
Agraphia (inability to read and write)
Wandering
Bladder and bowel incontinence
Insensitive to needs of others
Catastrophic reaction

SYMPTOMS OF STAGE THREE
Marked irritability
Outbursts of anger
Paraphasia (use of words in wrong and senseless combination)
Seizures
Loss or diminution of emotions
Bulimia
Visual agnosia (inability to recognize objects)
Hyperetamorphosis (attempt to touch everything in sight)
Decreased appetite
Bedridden
Emaciated
Apraxia (inability to carry out purposeful movements)
Decubitus ulcers
Susceptible to infections
Unresponsive or comatose

(Adapted with permission from Williams L. Alzheimer's: the need for caring. Gerontol Nurs. 1986; 12(Feb):20–27.)

tation to person may be evident to the point that these persons do not recognize themselves in the mirror. The phrase "Take me home" or "I am ready to go home now," regardless of where the affected persons are or how long they have been in one place, is a common cry. Increased apathy, indifference, stubbornness, restlessness, irritability, suspiciousness, pacing, clinging behavior, insensitivity to the needs of others, and wandering are common. Restlessness and difficulty sleeping at night are the most common complaints about the client with Alzheimer's disease reported by caregivers. Sundown syndrome, or increased confusion in the late evening, is another problem. A person with Alzheimer's disease referred to her grandsons as "strange boys wandering around here at night." During the daytime she was able to recognize and communicate with the same grandchildren. There may be a tendency to want to repeat early behaviors. For example, a caregiver reported that her husband who was accustomed to getting up at 5 AM to go to work before becoming ill would awaken every morning at 5 AM to get dressed and try to leave his home as if going to work.

In spite of the mental confusion, clients with Alzheimer's disease are often able to retain certain skills. For example, a nursing home resident afflicted with Alzheimer's disease was able to skillfully play the piano while other residents sang hymns.

Bladder or bowel incontinence may occur for several reasons. The person may have forgotten where the bathroom is located, be unable to get to the bathroom in time, or be unable to undress to use the bathroom. If there is visual agnosia (inability to recognize objects), the person with Alzheimer's disease may not recognize the toilet. Bladder or bowel control may be maintained, however, until the third stage, when cortical control is lost.[29] Urinary tract infection may also cause bladder incontinence.

Hyperorality (placing every object in the mouth), insatiable appetite, or poor appetite, bulimia, and malnutrition may occur. Difficulty swallowing may arise because of decreased saliva and changes in esophageal motility.[4]

Toward the end of the second stage, as the body weakens, impaired gait and falls are not uncommon.

STAGE THREE

Once in the third stage, the client with Alzheimer's disease may not live more than a year. During this stage, the signs and symptoms in stages one and two continue to progress. There is intellectual and physical deterioration to the point that the affected person is unable to communicate and becomes bedridden. Consequently, institutionalization is often indicated. This stage usually terminates with an infectious disease such as pneumonia. Malnutrition, dehydration, and decubitus ulcers often lead to death.[25]

ASSESSMENT AND DIAGNOSIS

The diagnosis of Alzheimer's disease may be delayed because initial changes in the client are usually subtle.

The client may be able to compensate or cover up memory loss with jokes, witty remarks, conversation, or written notes as reminders. They may resist seeking medical attention, and family members may ignore or deny the cognitive changes in their loved one, attributing them to "old age" or being emotionally upset. Often a crisis or serious error in judgment that requires medical attention unveils the illness. If hospitalization is required, these clients find themselves in a new and unfamiliar setting in which mental confusion and disorientation may increase, causing the condition to become more obvious. The person who has been resistive to seeking medical care is now in a setting where testing can be done. An absolute diagnosis of Alzheimer's disease can be made only on the basis of an autopsy; there is no specific test that gives an absolute positive diagnosis. A complete physical examination, including a neurologic and psychiatric evaluation, should be done. Once signs of memory loss are noted, it is essential that all other causes are ruled out before the diagnosis of Alzheimer's disease is made. This is especially important because the cognitive changes of dementia may be due to a reversible or treatable condition.

The first step in the diagnostic process, then, is to look for treatable causes for failing memory and the presenting cognitive changes.[39] In the process, there needs to be differentiation between delirium and dementia. Delirium is an acute or subacute mental disturbance in which there are illusions, hallucinations, incoherence, and confusion.[8] Common disorders that cause delirium in the aged are listed in Table 26-1. Dementia, on the other hand, is a chronic condition with impairment of all cognitive functions, particularly the memory.[5] Some dementias occur spontaneously with no known cause nor effective treatment.[22] Other dementias are reversible as well as treatable.[22] Examples of dementias are multiinfarct dementia, Pick's disease, Huntington's disease, and Creutzfeldt-Jakob disease.[37] Dementias may also occur with normal-pressure hydrocephalus, Parkinson's disease, metabolic disorders, neurologic disorders, or may be drug-induced.[37]

In addition, depression in the elderly should be ruled out. The elderly commonly suffer numerous losses, especially the loss of loved ones, which may lead to depression. With depression, symptoms, such as social isolation, confusion, forgetfulness, insomnia, fatigue, and loss of appetite, are common. When depression occurs with Alzheimer's disease, however, cognitive changes occur before the depression.

The physical examination of a person with Alzheimer's disease includes a complete history from the affected person. If the person is not able to give the necessary information, a secondary source, such as family members or significant others, should be used. Information relative to the mode of onset, exact nature and progression of cognitive changes, past medical history, and family history should be obtained. Upon physical examination, the person with Alzheimer's disease may be found to be in good physical health. If other illnesses, such as diabetes, are present, the affected person may forget to take medication or maintain the prescribed diet, which will compromise

TABLE 26–1
Disorders causing delirium in the aged

DISORDER	EXAMPLES
CENTRAL NERVOUS SYSTEM DISEASE	
Neoplasm	Primary intracranial neoplasm, metastatic neoplasm (bronchogenic carcinoma, breast carcinoma)
Cerebrovascular disease	Arteriosclerosis, cerebral infarction, subarachnoid hemorrhage, transient ischemic attacks, hypertensive encephalopathy, vasculitis (lupus), cranial arteritis, disseminated intravascular coagulation
Infection	Neurosyphilis, brain abscess, tuberculosis, meningoencephalitis (bacterial, viral, fungal), septic emboli (subacute bacterial endocarditis)
Head trauma	Chronic subdural hematoma, extradural hematoma, cerebral contusion, concussion
Ictal and post-ictal states	Idiopathic seizures, space-occupying lesion, post-traumatic lesions, electroconvulsive therapy
CARDIOVASCULAR DISEASE	
Decreased cardiac output	Congestive heart failure, cardiac arrhythmias, aortic stenosis, myocardial infarction
Hypotension	Orthostatic hypotension, vasovagal syncope, hypovolemia
METABOLIC DISORDERS	
Hypoxemia	Respiratory insufficiency, anemia, carbon monoxide poisoning
Electrolyte disturbance	Kidney disease, adrenal disease, diabetes mellitus, diuretics, edematous states, inappropriate secretion of antidiuretic hormone, dehydration, starvation
Acidosis	Diabetes mellitus, kidney disease, pulmonary disease, chronic diarrhea
Alkalosis	Hyperadrenalcorticism, pulmonary disease, psychogenic hyperventilation
Hepatic disease	Acute hepatic failure, cirrhosis, chronic portahepatic encephalopathy
Uremia	Chronic glomerulonephritis, chronic pyelonephritis, acute renal failure, obstructive uropathy
Endocrinopathies	Hypothyroidism, thyrotoxicosis, "apathetic" hyperthyroidism, hypoglycemia, hyperglycemia, hypoparathyroidism, hyperparathyroidism, hypoadrenalcorticism, hyperadrenalcorticism
Deficiency states	Hypovitaminosis (thiamine, nicotinic acid, vitamin B_{12}, folate deficiency, iron deficiency)
OTHER DISORDERS	
Trauma	Burns, surgery, multiple injuries, fractures (fat embolism)
Sensory deprivation	Cataracts, glaucoma, otosclerosis, darkness (sundown syndrome)
Exogenous toxins	Medications, alcohol, withdrawal syndromes, heavy metals, solvents, insecticides, pesticides, carbon monoxide
Temperature regulation	Exposure and accidental hypothermia, heat stroke, febrile illness

(From Liston EH. Delirium in the aged. Psychiatr Clin North Am 1982;5:49–66. Used with permission)

health. Psychiatric evaluation includes screening for depression, previous history of mental illness, presence of psychiatric symptoms, and assessment of the general cognitive stage.

Diagnostic procedures, such as a lumbar puncture, computed tomography (CT) scan, or electroencephalogram (EEG), may be done. The lumbar puncture is done to rule out neurosyphilis, which, as does Alzheimer's disease, can cause aproxia (inability to carry out purposeful movements), aphasia (inability to express thoughts), and agnosia (inability to recognize items).[14] For the person with Alzheimer's disease, the CT scan typically shows cortical atrophy and ventricular dilation.[22] The EEG is usually done to obtain a baseline and is characteristically slow in the presence of Alzheimer's.[11] Box 26-2 presents a summary of recommended diagnostic testing.

Multiple drugs may be concomitantly prescribed for the elderly person, which can cause harmful side effects, such as mental confusion, disorientation, and lapses in memory. With aging, the body's ability to me-

tabolize and excrete drugs is slowed.[34] The medical history should include a thorough inventory of all prescribed and over-the-counter medications taken. If possible, the person should be instructed to bring all medications when coming for the examination. Table 26-2 lists common medications that cause delirium in the aged. Chronic alcoholism may cause memory deficit, probably from thiamine deficiency and should also be investigated.[34]

Nursing Assessment

The nursing assessment should begin the moment the client arrives for the examination. The overall presentation of self, willingness to participate in the assessment process, ability to communicate, and general appearance, all are important clues about the mental status and possible stage of the disease. A nursing physical assessment of each body system, with pertinent questions, is appropriate. The following is a summary

---

BOX 26-2
Summary of Laboratory Testing and Procedures for Alzheimer's Disease

Complete blood count with sedimentation rate
Serology study for syphilis including VDRL and FTA
Thyroid study
Metabolic screening
Vitamin B_{12} level
Folate level
Electrolyte profile
Test for human immunodeficiency virus (HIV)
Glucose level
Dexamethasone suppression test
Blood levels for specific medications client may be taking (e.g., phenytoin, digoxin level)
Chest x-ray
Electroencephalogram (EEG)
Lumbar puncture
Computed tomography (CT) scan
History and physical examination
Neurological evaluation
Psychiatric evaluation

---

of important areas to assess based on the different stages of the disease.

PSYCHOSOCIAL ASSESSMENT

Begin with assessment of the mental status. The Mini-Mental State Examination gives an overall picture of memory, concentration, abstract thinking, and judgment.[38] Impairment in recent memory with an intact remote memory may indicate early stages of the disease. For social history, information concerning work history, such as job performance (past and present), hobbies, social activities, ability to get along with others, and signs of social isolation, should be assessed. The client's self-care abilities, or the ability to carry out activities of daily living (past and present), are valuable clues. A lack of interest in personal appearance, resulting in offensive body odors and disheveled appearance, and an inability to follow written directions or remembering to take medications are evident in the second stage and should be included in the assessment. The person's sleep pattern, presence of restlessness or insomnia at night, or increased confusion should be evaluated.

NUTRITIONAL ASSESSMENT

Height and weight, as well as history of weight gain or weight loss, number of meals or foods eaten per day, and types of food should be listed. The nurse may inquire about whether the client is able to prepare meals, or to follow instructions from a cookbook, or if food is left unattended on the stove. Difficulty swallowing and the presence of agitation and restlessness that prevents the client from sitting down to eat a meal should be assessed. The presence of vitamin deficiency, dehydration, or malnutrition; loss of appetite; bulimia; hyperorality (placing every object into the mouth); and insatiable appetite should be included in the assessment.

TABLE 26-2
Common medications causing delirium in the aged

DISORDER	MEDICATION	COMMON EXAMPLES
Cardiovascular conditions	Antiarrhythmics	Procainamide, propranolol, quinidine
	Antihypertensives	Clonidine, methyldopa, reserpine
	Cardiac glycosides	Digitalis
	Coronary vasodilators	Nitrates
Gastrointestinal conditions	Antidiarrheals	Atropine, belladonna, homatropine, hyoscyamine, scopolamine
	Antinauseants	Cyclizine, homatropine–barbiturate preparations, phenothiazines
	Antispasmodics	Methanthelene, propantheline
Musculoskeletal conditions	Anti-inflammatory agents	Corticosteroids, indomethacin, phenylbutazone, salicylates
	Muscle relaxants	Carisoprodol, diazepam
Neurologic–psychiatric conditions	Anticonvulsants	Barbiturates, carbamazepine, diazepam, phenytoin
	Antiparkinsonism agents	Amantadine, benztropine, levodopa, trihexyphenidyl
	Hypnotics and sedatives	Barbiturates, belladonna alkaloids, bromides, chloral hydrate, ethchlorvynol, glutethimide, methaqualone
	Psychotropics	Benzodiazepines, hydroxyzines, lithium salts, meprobamate, monoamine oxidase (MAO) inhibitors, neuroleptics, tricyclic antidepressants
Respiratory–allergic conditions	Antihistamines	Brompheniramine, chlorpheniramine, cyproheptadine, diphenhydramine, tripelennamine
	Antitussives	Opiates, synthetic narcotics
	Decongestants and expectorants	Phenylephrine, phenylpropanolamine, potassium preparations
Miscellaneous conditions	Analgesics	Dextropropoxyphene, opiates, phenacetin, salicylates, synthetic narcotics
	Anesthetics	Lidocaine, methohexital, methoxyflurane
	Antidiabetic agents	Insulin, oral hypoglycemics
	Antineoplastics	Corticosteroids, mitomycin, procarbazine
	Antituberculosis agents	Isoniazid, rifampin

(From Liston EH. Delirium in the aged. Psychiatr Clin North Am 1982;5:49–66. Used with permission)

PHYSICAL EXAMINATION

In addition to the physical examination done by the physician, the nursing assessment may include an examination of the following body systems:

1. Musculoskeletal system: The affected person should be asked to walk across the room if able. Observe for unsteady gait, possible need for a walking aid, and a stiff, shuffling, slow gait with cupping of the hands at the side. Look for bruises or abrasions on the skin, and inquire if any falls or fractures have occurred.
2. Respiratory system: Assess for normal breath sounds. Signs of bronchopneumonia are not uncommon in the third stage of the disease.
3. Cardiovascular system: Listen for normal heart sounds. Although not affected directly by Alzheimer's disease, any preexisting changes in the cardiovascular system are useful to be aware of, for better patient care.
4. Neurologic system: If the nurse has expertise in doing this exam, a neurologic examination as part of the nursing assessment would give a more definitive picture of the client's mental status, as well as normal existent changes associated with aging.
5. Genitourinary system: Assess for continence of urine during the day and night, signs of urinary tract infection that may cause incontinence of urine, and a past history of kidney or bladder problems.
6. Gastrointestinal system: Obtain information concerning continence of feces and pattern of bowel elimination. The nurse should assess whether the person is able to find the bathroom or if feces is hidden in inappropriate places.

In assessing persons with Alzheimer's disease, the nurse should look not only for weaknesses or deficits, but should document the person's strengths and remaining abilities as well. Nursing diagnoses and appropriate interventions to maximize the person's strengths should be formulated.

ASSESSMENT OF PRIMARY CAREGIVER

Many caregivers burdened with the task of caring for a person with Alzheimer's disease receive little or no assistance from resources in the community. Many are elderly and may themselves have mental, physical, social, and financial difficulties. Assessment of the caregiving environment, which refers to the social support caregivers feel is available, community services that are used, and financial conditions that result from providing care to the person with Alzheimer's disease, is needed.[13] The nurse should inquire about physical and mental conditions the caregiver may have that interfere with care provided. The nurse should inquire about the living arrangements, such as the type of housing, number of bedrooms and living space, presence of stairs, elevators, size and composition of the

neighborhood. The daily routine of the person with Alzheimer's disease in the home should also be obtained. The foregoing information is important in obtaining a clearer understanding of the affected person's behavior and in assisting the caregiver to obtain the proper resources that are needed.

TREATMENT MODALITIES

A multidisciplinary team approach to treatment is most effective. Such a team may consist of a nurse, social worker, neurologist, neuropsychologist, and pharmacist.

Although there is no cure for Alzheimer's disease, a number of ongoing research studies are exploring ways to enhance the quality of life for affected clients. Major studies are investigating the use of acetylcholine-like drugs (acetylcholine is the neurotransmitter necessary for communication between brain cells) that block the breakdown of acetylcholine and of foods that enhance its production. In 1978 it was reported that the drug physostigmine blocks the rapid breakdown of acetylcholine, causing it to carry out its function as neurotransmitter for a longer period.[32] Improvement, however, is short-lived, and the drug has serious side effects.[32] The hormone vasopressin has been used to improve memory, with some success, but the drug causes undesirable side effects.[34] Lecithin, the dietary source of choline, has been used to increase the production of acetylcholine in the blood, but no consistent or beneficial results have been obtained.[32] To eliminate high buildup of aluminum in the brain tissue, drugs called chelating agents have been used to bond with the aluminum and eliminate it from the body.[34] These drugs are still being investigated by researchers. Experts in geriatric medicine report that short-term use of neuroleptics has been useful in controlling agitation and behavioral disturbances, such as paranoia and hallucinations, that are sometimes seen in later stages.[12] Only when conservative measures for controlling behavior have failed should neuroleptics be prescribed. Short-term, rather than long-term, use of neuroleptics is emphasized because of the possibility of tardive dyskinesia, an undesirable side effect that can have permanent effects.[12] In addition to short-term use, the lowest dosage possible to control unmanageable behavior should be prescribed, because the ability to metabolize drugs is lowered in the elderly. To control physical agitation, chlorpromazine (Thorazine) and thioridazine hydrochloride (Mellaril) are recommended.[12] Haloperidol (Haldol) may be given for psychotic and violent behavior.[35]

For restlessness and insomnia at night, chloral hydrate is recommended.[35] Experts differ in their opinion of the use of benzodiazepines for clients with Alzheimer's disease. Oxazepam (Serax) is preferred by some for restlessness and agitation because of its short half-life.[35] Others suggest that benzodiazepines with long half-lives, particularly flurazepam (Dalmane) and diazepam (Valium), increase confusion and may lead to paradoxic agitation; therefore, they should not be used for the elderly.[5,12]

If depression is present and is exacerbating the dementia, tricyclics such as doxepin hydrochloride (Adapin) and trazodone (Desyrel) are desirable because they have fewer anticholinergic effects.[35] Hydergine, a drug that contains ergoloid mesylates, is said to be useful in improving the overall functioning of the client with Alzheimer's disease.[5] However, control of emotional and behavioral factors in evaluating the effects of the drug is difficult.[5] It is most important for the nurse to be aware of common side effects of medications prescribed and to educate the client and family. For example, if the client is taking neuroleptic medications, nurses should be aware of the signs and symptoms of extrapyramidal reactions and the appropriate intervention measures, such as giving trihexyphenidyl (Artane) or diphenhydramine (Benadryl) or other antiparkinson medication prescribed by the physician.[35]

NURSING ROLES

The role of the nurse varies throughout the three stages of the disease and are described in general terms here. Specific nursing interventions based on identified problems will be addressed later.

A major nursing role includes teaching not only the client, but also the family about the disease, so that they can be empowered to be caregivers.[28] In addition to teaching, support groups for family members and caregivers of Alzheimer's patients can also be provided by the nurse. Ideally, legal issues, such as the preparation of a will and obtaining power of attorney, should be addressed when the diagnosis is made. The nurse can be instrumental in directing the family in obtaining social services if needed.

In most cases, the client is cared for at home during the early stage of the disease. A complete nursing assessment of the living arrangements, daily routine, caregiving environment, and neighborhood is necessary to formulate appropriate nursing interventions.

The role of the nurse also includes formulating nursing interventions that will allow the client to remain independent as long as possible.[4] Creativity, flexibility, and patience are needed by all involved when approaching specific nursing diagnoses. During the second and third stages, symptoms increase in severity. The nurse needs to continue ensuring physical safety, optimum health, and maintaining the dignity of the client.

The nursing diagnosis of depression related to intermittent awareness of failing memory and other implications of Alzheimer's disease may be present in the initial stage, as the client with Alzheimer's disease becomes aware of cognitive changes they are not able to control. The nurse can be supportive by informing the client and family that, although there is no cure, and the disease will become progressively worse, assistance will be given to help cope with the disease.

Death and dying and ethical issues frequently arise during the third stage. Ethical issues, such as the use of

life support and resuscitative measures need to be discussed by the family and the treatment team.

As the client with Alzheimer's disease approaches death, family members need to make preparation for the funeral, as well as work through guilt, anger, and other phases of the grieving process. The nurse needs to be aware of the dynamics at play and offer emotional support to the client and family as well.

Common Nursing Diagnoses and Interventions According to the Stages of the Disease

Nursing diagnoses commonly seen as the disease progresses in different stages are listed in the following. The nursing diagnostic categories evident in stage one are also evident in stages two and three, but in more severe form.

NURSING DIAGNOSES FOR STAGE ONE

1. Impaired communication
2. Altered perception/cognition: hallucinations, memory loss, confusion
3. Self-concept disturbance; self-esteem, role performance
4. Diversional activity deficit
5. Potential for injury
6. Fear
7. Hopelessness
8. Powerlessness
9. Emotional lability
10. Agitation
11. Impaired social interaction
12. Knowledge deficit (of family members relative to management of Alzheimer's disease)
13. Knowledge deficit (of client relative to management of Alzheimer's disease)
14. Depression
15. Family coping: potential for growth
16. Ineffective individual coping

NURSING DIAGNOSES FOR STAGE TWO

1. Sleep pattern disturbance
2. Altered nutrition, less than body requirements
3. Self-care deficit (bathing, toileting, dressing, grooming, feeding)
4. Ritualistic behavior
5. Aggression: mild, moderate
6. Suspiciousness

NURSING DIAGNOSES FOR STAGE THREE

1. Impaired physical mobility*
2. Ineffective airway clearance*
3. Impaired skin integrity*
4. Functional incontinence*

---

* Other NANDA nursing diagnosis.

Research Highlights

In 1987, Evans[9] conducted a research study to describe sundown syndrome and its determining factors. Sundown syndrome is described as increased symptoms of confusion during the evening hours. This confusion can extend into the night, causing restlessness and difficulty sleeping. Fifty-nine randomly selected, demented, and 30 undemented nursing home residents, 60 years of age and older, participated in the study. The data was collected over 2½ months with each subject observed for two-hour periods morning and late afternoon on two consecutive days, utilizing the Confusion Inventory which consists of a checklist of 48 psychomotor and psychosocial behavioral indicators of mental confusion. Manifestation of sundown syndrome, such as wandering, tapping, picking at bed clothes, and other symptoms were observed.

Psychosocial variables were measured with the Pfeiffer's Short Portable Mental Status Questionnaire (measuring the mental status of the subjects), the Face-Hand Test (used to screen for organicity), and the Philadelphia Geriatric Center Morale Scale (which is highly correlated with depression). Physiologic variables, such as medical diagnoses, medications, and night-time habits, were obtained from the medical records. Vital signs were obtained after each observation period, and observation for urine was made at that time. Additional information was obtained from the nursing staff in a questionnaire. Sensory loss was identified by gross screening for vision, hearing, and light touch. Environmental variables, such as the amount of light in the environment during the observation period, were also determined.

The mean age of the sample was 80 years. The sample was 89% black, predominantly female, single, and lived in the nursing home facility for an average of 14 months. Sundowners had a significantly shorter mean length of stay in the nursing home facility. The length of time that they were assigned to their room in the facility was shorter than nonsundowners.

Sundowners were identified by attributing a certain score on the Confusion Inventory for each behavior that was exhibited only in the evening. A mean score was obtained, and the data were analyzed. Results indicated that of the 89 subjects, 11 were sundowners, which was 12.4%, or one in eight, of the population over 60 in the nursing home facility. Eighty-two percent (82%), or more than four times as many sundowners were from the demented group. Sundowners demonstrated increased restlessness; escape behaviors; expression of feelings; talking, as well as appearing to be searching for something, and intense behavior in the evening. The Pfeiffer's Short Portable Mental Status Questionnaire revealed significantly greater mental impairment. The Face-Hand Test was significantly correlated with sundown syndrome. Results from the Philadelphia Geriatric Center Morale Scale indicated that there was no relationship between morale and sundown syndrome. Medical diagnoses and medications taken among sundowners showed no significant association with sundown syndrome.

The medical diagnoses, medications taken, vital signs, vision and hearing impairment, and touch scores showed no significant association with sundown syndrome. However, factors that were significant among sundowners were the presence of the odor of urine in the evening, and being awakened in the evening for routine nursing care (preventive measures for decubiti). Although the level of hydration was not measured, dehydration was suspected among subjects with increased body temperature and decreased diastolic blood pressure in the evening.

There was no significant difference between sundowners and nonsundowners with change in environmental light.

The results of this study support the existence of sundown syndrome, an increase in restlessness, and verbal behaviors in the late afternoon among nursing home elderly. Factors that seem to place the elderly at risk for sundown syndrome are mental impairment with dehydration, being awakened frequently in the evening, recent admissions to the facility, and being assigned to a bedroom for less than one month. This study needs to be repeated utilizing a longer and more comprehensive observation period, with other patients in home and acute settings. Nurses need to assess and document the wake–sleep cycle of persons with sleep disturbances and teach other nursing staff and family members how to cope with this problem.

CASE STUDY

Mr. B, a 68-year-old man, was admitted to a psychiatric facility during the past month for uncontrollable, violent, and disruptive behavior. At age 65, Alzheimer's disease was diagnosed. His present diagnosis is primary degenerative dementia of the Alzheimer's type—senile onset. Before hospitalization, Mr. B lived at home with his 68-year-old wife who cared for him by herself. Even though her husband became increasingly difficult to manage, Mrs. B said, "I can't bear the thought of placing my husband in a nursing home. Besides, it would cost too much money." Lately, she had not been able to assist her husband to bathe, eat, or change his clothing because he was becoming extremely aggressive and hostile. He was also unsteady on his feet and fell easily. Mrs. B said that although she loved her husband very much, she felt like a prisoner in her own home. On the night he was admitted, Mr. B attacked his wife with a knife, but did not seriously injure her. After a complete assessment and evaluation, his psychiatrist prescribed haloperidol (Haldol), 1 mg PO, q 8 hr, as needed, for severe agitation, and benzotropine mesylate (Cogentin), 1 mg IM × 1, if extrapyramidal symptoms occur. Chloral hydrate 500 mg q hs, if needed, was ordered. He was placed on close observation for unpredictable behavior. A dietary consultation was ordered because of poor appetite. During meal time he was restless. Mr. B was having difficulty adjusting to his new environment, and he isolated himself from the other residents. He was disoriented to time and place, babbled to himself as if responding to voices, paced in the hall, and rummaged through the trash cans on the ward. He was able to dress, feed, and bathe himself with some assistance. Mr. B exhibited behaviors commonly seen in the later part of the second stage of Alzheimer's disease (see Nursing Care Plan 26-1 for a sample care plan for Mr. B).

NURSING CARE PLAN 26-1

MR. B

NURSING INTERVENTIONS	OUTCOME CRITERIA

NURSING DIAGNOSIS: Impaired communication related to the disease process of Alzheimer's disease

CLIENT GOAL: Comprehend simplified means of communication

- Utilize simple sentences, speak slowly and clearly
- Utilize pictures and nonverbal cues and gestures to facilitate communication
- Utilize written messages to aid failing memory (e.g., write name in large letters and post on bedroom door)

Comprehends message sent

NURSING DIAGNOSIS: Altered perception–cognition related to cognitive deterioration

CLIENT GOAL: Demonstrate contact with reality and adjust to new environment

- Include in reality orientation group to learn to respond to name, present season of the year, time of day (morning or afternoon)
- Do not show frustration if Mr. B is still not able to recall information given

- Provide consistent caregivers

- Maintain quiet, calm, and nonstressful and predictable environment

- Maintain homelike environment (e.g., bedspread from home, afghan, family photos)
- Encourage family support and involvement

Responds to name when called

Is aware of season and whether it is morning or afternoon

Establishes trusting relationship with at least one nurse

Experiences supportive environment

NURSING DIAGNOSIS: Potential for aggression (violence) directed at others related to cognitive deficits

CLIENT GOAL: Have no violent episodes

- Anticipate escalating behavior and institute measures to deescalate behavior (e.g., quiet room, giving reassurance)
- Maintain a calm, predictable, nonstressful and quiet environment as much as possible
- Spend time with Mr. B; convey caring attitude
- Medicate with haloperidol (Haldol) as ordered when necessary; be aware of side effects such as extrapyramidal symptoms and appropriate interventions
- Set limits in advance and in response to specific situation[37]
- Be consistent
- Encourage to express anger constructively

Aggressive behavior kept to a minimum

NURSING DIAGNOSIS: Potential for injury related to impaired judgment and impaired gait associated with stage-two of Alzheimer's disease

CLIENT GOAL: Will not injure self

- Assess environment for potential hazards (e.g., poisonous plants, hot water, slippery floors, steep stairways) and provide a safe environment, particularly in areas where routine patterns of walking have been established
- Assess for hallucinations and protect from self-injury

Environment is safe and free of potential hazards

Continued

Mental Health and Illness in Special Population Groups

MR. B *Continued*

NURSING INTERVENTIONS	OUTCOME CRITERIA

NURSING DIAGNOSIS: Impaired social interaction related to cognitive deficits in stage two of Alzheimer's disease

CLIENT GOAL: Socializes with at least one client

- Provide activities requiring interaction with other clients, as able to tolerate (e.g., reminiscence group, occupational therapy group, socialization group)
- Relate to Mr. B as a person while assisting with activities of daily living

Interacts with at least one client

NURSING DIAGNOSIS: Altered nutrition, less than body requirements related to lack of appetite and agitation-restlessness

CLIENT GOAL: Consume diet appropriate for age, body size, and nutritional needs and not lose weight

- Obtain dietary consult
- Offer meals in nonstressful and calm place
- Allow ample time to eat; do not rush
- Provide small portions of food
- Keep finger foods available
- Provide foods high in fiber
- Provide adequate fluid intake (2000–3000 mL/day unless contraindicated)
- Assess condition of dentition and obtain consult if needed
- Observe for difficulty chewing, swallowing, or food left in mouth
- Obtain body weight weekly

Maintains adequate nutrition and hydration
Experiences nonstressful meal time
Constipation prevented

NURSING DIAGNOSIS: Dysfunctional family process related to declining health status of Mr. B

FAMILY GOAL: Wife regains physical and emotional balance, resolves guilt over psychiatric placement of husband

- Give Mrs. B positive strokes for being able to care for Mr. B up to this point
- Include in decision making for care of Mr. B
- Teach stress management skills
- Encourage Mrs. B to take time out for herself while Mr. B is hospitalized

Mrs. B is relieved of any guilt feelings she may have because she is not able to care for husband at home

- Provide information about support groups for Alzheimer's disease caregivers, respite care in the home and out of home, adult day care services for Mr. B, and organizations such as Alzheimer's Disease and Related Disorders Association
- Discuss the possibility of nursing home placement for Mr. B
- Refer to social services for financial counseling

Mrs. B experiences a support system that enables her to continue to cope with her husband's illness

SUMMARY

Persons with Alzheimer's disease encounter many problems as the disease progresses. There is no known cure for the disease, but nurses can assume an essential role in decreasing some of the symptoms that accompany the disease. Commitment, caring, understanding, flexibility, and creativity are needed to work successfully with the client who has Alzheimer's disease. Families need resources such as support groups, respite care, and day care, as well as financial assistance to help them in meeting the challenge of caring for their loved ones with a progressive, devastating illness such as Alzheimer's disease.

References

1. Alzheimer's Disease and Related Disorders Association, Inc. Alzheimer's Disease Association of Greater Washington; 1987.
2. Alzheimer's Disease and Related Disorders Association, Inc. Alzheimer's disease, an overview; 1987.
3. American Psychiatric Association. Diagnostic and statistical manual of mental disorders, 3rd ed, revised. Washington, DC: American Psychiatric Association; 1987.
4. Beck C, Heacock P. Nursing interventions for patients with Alzheimer's disease. Nurs Clin North Am. 1988;23:95–123.
5. Blazer D. Psychiatric disorders. In: Raumen I, ed. Clinical geriatrics. Philadelphia: JB Lippincott; 1986.
6. Crapper DR, Krishman SS, Dalton AJ. Brain aluminum distribution, in Alzheimer's disease and experimental neurofibrillary degeneration. Science. 1973;180:511–513.
7. Davis P, Maloney AJF. Selective loss of central cholinergic neurons in Alzheimer's disease [Letter to the Editor]. Lancet. 1976;2:1403.
8. Dorland's illustrated medical dictionary, 25th ed. Philadelphia: WB Saunders; 1985.
9. Evans LK. Sundown syndrome in institutionalized elderly. J Am Geriatr Soc. 1987;35:101–108.
10. Fopmal-Loy J. Wandering: causes. J Psychoso Nurs. 1988; 26:9–18.
11. Geriatrics panel discussion. Practical considerations in managing Alzheimer's disease: I. Geriatrics. 1987;42(Sept):78–98.
12. Geriatrics panel discussion. Practical considerations in managing Alzheimer's disease: II. Geriatrics. 1987;42(Oct):55–65.
13. Given CW, Collins CE, Givens BA. Sources of stress among families caring for relatives with Alzheimer's disease. Nurs Clin North Am. 1988;23:69–81.
14. Group for the advancement of psychiatry: The psychiatric treatment of Alzheimer's disease. New York: Brunner/Mazel; 1988.
15. Gwyther LP, Matteson MA. Care for the caregivers. J Gerontol Nurs. 1983;9:93–110.
16. Gwyther LP. Treating behaviors as a symptom of illness. Provider. 1986;May:18–21.
17. Ihara Y, et al. Antibodies to paired helical filaments in Alzheimer's disease do not recognize normal brain proteins [Letters]. Nature. 1983;304:727–740.
18. Leroux C. Coping and caring. Washington, DC: American Association of Retired Persons; 1986.
19. Liston EH. Delirium in the aged. Psychiatr Clin North Am. 1982;5:49–66.
20. National Institute on Aging. Progress report on Alzheimer's disease, Bethesda, MD: US Department of Health & Human Services; 1987.
21. National Institute on Aging. National Institute on Aging special report on Alzheimer's disease, Unpublished Report to Congress; 1988.
22. Pajk M. Alzheimer's disease: inpatient care. Am J Nurs. 1984;84:215–222.
23. Palmer MH. Alzheimer's disease and critical care. J Gerontol Nurs. 1983;9:86–91.
24. Patrick M. Daily living with cognitive deficits and behavioral problems. In: Carnevali D, Patrick M, eds. Nursing management for the elderly, 2nd ed. Philadelphia: JB Lippincott; 1986.
25. Peck A, Wollach L, Rodstein M. Mortality of the aged with chronic brain syndrome II. In: Katzman R, Terry R, Bick K, eds. Alzheimer's disease: senile dementia and related disorders. New York: Raven Press; 1978.
26. Reubin A, Bierman EL, Hazzard WR. Principles of geriatric medicine. New York: McGraw-Hill; 1985.
27. Roach M. Another name for madness. Boston: Houghton Mifflin; 1984.
28. Rothwell A. Teaching plan for the Alzheimer's Center. Chevy Chase, MD, Neurology Center; 1989.
29. Schneck MK, Reisberg B, Ferris S. An overview of current concepts of Alzheimer's disease. Am J Psychiatry. 1982; 139:165–173.
30. Tomlinson BE, Kitchener D. Granulovacuolar degeneration of hippocampus pyramidal cells. J Pathol. 1972;106:165–185.
31. Tomlinson BE, Blessed G, Rogh M. Observations on the brains of demented old people. J Neurol Sci. 1970;11:205–242.
32. US Department of Health and Human Services, Public Health Service, National Institute of Health. Progress report on Alzheimer's disease, vol II. National Institute on Aging; July 1984.
33. US Department of Health and Human Services, Public Health Service, National Institute of Health. Q&A: Alzheimer's disease. NIH Publication No. 85-1646, Reprinted May, 1985.
34. US Department of Health and Human Services, Public Health Service, National Institute of Health. The dementias. Office of Scientific and Health Reports, National Institute of Neurological and Communicative Disorders and Stroke; March 1981.
35. Wang Z, Sriwatanakul K. Drug used for the treatment of dementia. Rationale Drug Therapy. 1983;17:1–4.
36. Williams L. Alzheimer's: the need for caring. J Gerontol Nurs. 1986;12:20–27.
37. Willis P. Cognitive changes of normal aging and the dementias. In: Carnevali D, Patrick M. eds. Nursing management for the elderly, 2nd ed. Philadelphia: JB Lippincott; 1986.
38. Wlodarczyk DM. Dementia: guidelines for improving tx. Geriatrics. 1985;40:35–45.
39. Woodward JS. Clinicopathologic significance of granulovacuolar degeneration in Alzheimer's disease. J Neuropathol. 1962;21:83–91.

27

Joan Norris

Chronically Mentally Ill Clients

OBJECTIVES

After reading this chapter, the reader will be able to:

1. Describe characteristics of the chronically mentally ill population
2. Categorize community services for the mentally ill
3. Identify problems related to providing funding and accessing community-based services by the chronically mentally ill
4. Discuss client-based problems that pose difficulties in providing aftercare services in the community to chronically mentally ill clients
5. Identify the components of a comprehensive assessment that are basic to provision of effective aftercare services for chronically mentally ill clients
6. Identify significant nursing roles in the care of the chronically mentally ill client
7. Identify common nursing diagnoses related to chronic mental illness
8. Formulate a plan of care for chronically mentally ill clients that incorporates discharge planning, aftercare, and caregiver support
9. Describe selected research findings relevant to patient compliance and aftercare of the chronically mentally ill.

DESCRIPTION

Although many mental disorders may persist and recur over long periods of time, the chronically mentally ill are commonly considered to be those persons with a major mental disorder who continue to experience impaired functioning for a year or more. Based on various data sources available to the National Institutes of Mental Health, Dr. Ronald Manderscheid, Chief of the Survey and Reports Branch, estimates that 2.8 million Americans are chronically mentally ill (telephone communication, July 11, 1988). This population includes persons with schizophrenic or major affective disorders and organic mental disorders secondary to trauma, disease, or substance abuse. Table 27-1 describes the residence settings for the chronically mentally ill, which range from family households to group homes, long-term care settings, residential hotels, and shelters for the homeless.

Population Characteristics

The chronically mentally ill are a diverse group with a number of different conditions, living in a variety of circumstances (see Table 27-1). Elderly individuals with organic mental disorders may live independently with supportive family nearby, may reside with family or friends, or may be in a variety of supervised long-term care arrangements such as foster care or nursing homes. Many people with schizophrenic or affective disorders in remission function effectively as family members and employees, whereas others with residual symptoms and diminished functional capacity may rely on disability income or work only sporadically. These persons may live in group or foster homes or decaying urban hotels or may join the homeless mentally ill on the streets of cities.[2] Some mentally ill persons may be inappropriately placed in prisons. Sub-

stance abuse may be a chronic primary problem or may be used by the emotionally disordered as a form of self-medication to ease the pain of living. The chronically mentally ill range in age from young adults to the very old. Persons with chronic mental illness experience a variety of problems and burdens related to long-term mental and emotional disability and to the stigma of mental illness.

Community-based Services

The dramatic changes in psychiatric care in the 1960s and 1970s resulted in deinstitutionalization of large numbers of the chronically mentally ill, with relocation of mental health care into the community. Federal funding for this relocation of services was designed to decrease gradually as local communities and agencies increased their financing of mental health care. However, this intended shift to local financing did not occur because local agencies were unable or unwilling to increase funding for necessary community mental health programs.[11] The decrease in federal support thus led to reduction and fragmentation of mental health services with, in many cases, more frequent hospitalizations offsetting the shorter length of stay (the revolving door syndrome). In the mid 1980s, there have been efforts on the part of the National Institute of Mental Health and some other agencies to target research and programming funds to address the needs of the chronically mentally ill as an underserved population.

In general, the needs of the chronically mentally ill population for community services can be categorized as services to address basic needs for health and shelter, provision of psychological and emotional support, education and support for caregivers, and case management to promote continuity and coordination of care. The services to meet these needs are not unfamiliar to nurses and social workers; most are available to some extent in every community.

TABLE 27-1
Residential sites of the chronically mentally ill in 1985 according to NIMH data*

APPROXIMATE NUMBERS	SITE	DESCRIPTION
1.1 million	Nursing homes	Private or public long-term care
1.1 million	Households	Includes those who live with their families, foster families, or friends and those who live alone in homes, apartments, or residence hotels that meet US Census definition of a household
100 thousand	Long-term psychiatric care	Institutionalization in a long-term psychiatric facility such as a state hospital for more than 3 months
100 thousand	The "revolving door" phenomenon	Repeated, brief readmissions to inpatient psychiatric care facilities
150–275 thousand	Group living arrangements	Halfway houses or group homes in which supervised transitional living arrangements help people learn social and home management skills. Clients can move on to independent living in the community or may continue in a supervised group home as a long-term placement
125–250 thousand	Homeless	Living on the streets with or without temporary shelter

* Numbers of the chronically ill in each setting provided in a telephone communication by Dr. Ronald Manderscheid, Chief of the Survey and Reports Branch of the National Institute of Mental Health, July 11, 1988.

Problems can arise at any of the several steps necessary to obtain and utilize these services, however. The chronically mentally ill person may be mistrustful and avoidant of others, may deny problems, or may lack the necessary knowledge or communication skills to identify appropriate service agencies and make his or her needs known. Also, many health professionals are not aware of the various agencies providing specific services and their eligibility requirements. Family education and support services may or may not be available. The services that do exist may require contacting several agencies in order to meet comprehensive care needs. Despite the availability of hospitals, mental health centers, and community service agencies, a large percentage of the homeless seen in shelters are chronically mentally ill.[3]

Clearly, there is a need for more acceptable residential options for clients as well as for coordination of services designed to maintain functional capacity and provide vocational and social services appropriate to the client's individual level of functioning. It has been demonstrated consistently that fragmentation and gaps in services for the chronically mentally ill remain a problem. Social workers, community health nurses, and psychiatric nurses who work in discharge planning or as liaison community linkage agents are likely to find themselves in the case management role. The case manager seeks to provide the most cost-effective services available and to coordinate these services in order to foster self-care capacity and to assure comprehensiveness and continuity of care. The case manager may need to serve as a client advocate to obtain necessary services but generally serves to foster self-determination and informed choices by clients and families. Principles of primary nursing are applicable, but nurses are advised to seek advanced education in psychiatric nursing with specialization in chronic illness for the case manager role. Nursing's comprehensive focus on the needs of the total person and on maximizing the client's level of function[7] is particularly relevant to the needs of this population.

Problems in Community-based Care

Problems in meeting the needs of the chronically mentally ill arise because of specific factors associated with the clients themselves, with social factors such as attitudes toward the mentally ill, and with community priorities and resource limitations. Specific client problems related to schizophrenic, organic mental, and substance-abuse disorders are addressed in other chapters of this text. This chapter will focus on common problems of these chronically mentally ill groups in the community.

The problems these individuals have are diverse, as was noted earlier. Some persons will function adequately with the help of supportive family or friends, others will require placement in long-term care facilities, and the rest will need placement in supervised halfway houses, group homes, foster care, residential hotels, or boarding houses. Some of these placements will be unsuccessful, and these residents may find themselves being exploited or neglected or in constant conflict with other residents. Those persons with placements they perceive as unsatisfactory may join the ranks of the homeless or be rehospitalized frequently (the revolving door syndrome). The majority of younger chronically mentally ill persons requiring community services tend to fall into one of the following three categories: (1) the higher functioning, (2) the passively accepting, and (3) those who strongly deny mental illness.[9] Aggressive young adults who deny their illness often have difficulty accepting group or supervised housing and prefer the independence of residential hotels or the streets. Many clients who live independently may withdraw, neglect themselves, and stop taking prescribed antipsychotic drugs and can be exploited by others. However, some programs offering patient, persistent support and intensive case management have helped these clients adapt to group homes despite conflicts with roommates and repeated hospitalizations.[4]

A current legal, ethical, and social dilemma in this country is whether chronically mentally ill clients should receive involuntary treatment for their own good and that of the community (a paternalistic stance) or, whether they should be permitted the autonomy to choose whether to accept care and treatment if they do not pose a clear and present danger to self or others. This latter approach is the current practice and frequently results in distress to both the mentally ill person and concerned family members as suspicion, self-neglect, lack of motivation, and bizarre behavior disrupt relationships and meaningful work or social interactions.

Social Problems

The chronically mentally ill lack higher-level social and interaction skills. Society reinforces social withdrawal and exacerbates the isolation of these people through attitudes based in fear, revulsion, or ridicule. These negative attitudes contribute further to community resistance to locating residential centers and group homes in neighborhoods, as well as to lack of community support for funding of necessary vocational, social, and recreational programs for the mentally ill.

It is more efficient and easier to care for large numbers of the mentally ill in centralized facilities where there can be a high level of environmental structure, staff training, and supervision. However, highly structured environments over a period of time can decrease clients' autonomy and initiative and lead to iatrogenic deterioration of personal and social skills. Staff members in residential care may have to deal with aggression, conflict, and, occasionally, dangerous behavior in a much less structured environment, often with less training and fewer resources. Personnel in these settings need to provide a safe semi-structured environment and promote interpersonal learning and social skills development, while dealing effectively with occasional episodes of aggressive or acutely psychotic behavior. If there are no liaison and consultation services available from competent professionals in mental health centers or clinics, the potential for client disorganization and personnel burnout is increased.[4]

Custodial care can occur in the community as well as in the institution. A Canadian study suggests that long-term undemanding foster home placements can reduce stress and some symptoms of chronic mental illness but are not able to improve social skills and functioning.[4] In other words, reductions in disturbing symptoms are obtained by accepting lower-level functioning and decreasing the stress of active rehabilitation efforts. This tradeoff is probably true of many of the long-term care facilities in which many older chronically mentally ill clients are housed. Residential care in the community requires substantial back-up, programming assistance, and consultation from other agencies in order to identify and provide care appropriate to the needs of various individuals.

There are few people to advocate for the needs of the chronically mentally ill despite their significant numbers in the population. In a time of diminishing resources for health and social programs, this means that an already underserved population is likely to receive even less. The National Alliance for the Mentally Ill is composed of families of the mentally ill and is an advocacy group formed to speak for acceptance and adequate programs to meet the needs of this population. State and local chapters provide information, support, and advocacy for client needs at community levels.

ASSESSMENT

Nursing's comprehensive focus and background in primary care provides an excellent foundation on which to base assessments of emotional needs and behavioral problems as well as physical needs, functional status, living arrangements, social skills, and supports and community resource needs of chronically mentally ill clients.

Psychosocial Needs

Psychosocial assessment involves recognition of individual strengths, behavior patterns, and problems that have the potential to enhance or inhibit success in residential placement, getting along with others, experiencing a sense of belonging, and making some contribution sufficient to bolster client self-esteem. Specific assessment areas include communication skills, level of social interaction and participation, knowledge of social amenities, and responses to frustration or conflict situations. Is the person verbally or physically aggressive? If violent episodes have occurred, how difficult were these to manage, and were other persons the objects of attack? Attacks directed toward people signal

the potential for dangerous behavior and require higher levels of skilled supervision. Awareness of the individual's level of functioning and social participation is important in promoting adaptation and anticipating problems related to living arrangements. It is vital that the chronically mentally ill be accepted at their current level of functioning but that limits be set on behavior that is dangerous to self or others. Only then, in a climate of acceptance, can efforts begin to optimize client potential.

Health Maintenance

Basic physical assessment skills are important. Many chronically mentally ill persons have poor nutrition and dental care. Some lack the cognitive awareness and resources to carry out most health behaviors and may even lack the capacity for some basic activities of living such as hygiene or grooming. They may have specific deficits in fluid and nutrient intake, may have additional acute or chronic medical problems, and may demonstrate inadequate cognition and self-care. The homeless may, in addition, have been exposed to vermin, physical assault, and extremes of heat and cold. Whether the client is seen at home, in a residential care setting, or in a shelter for the homeless, the nurse needs to be alert to physical needs and self-care capacity. On the basis of any identified deviations from normal, the client can be referred to an appropriate health care clinic (see nursing diagnosis entitled Altered Health Maintenance).

Careful assessments are needed to determine the manner and consistency of the client's self-care and therapeutic compliance in the community. Does the person maintain a basic standard of living and self-care to sustain at least a minimum standard of health and personal safety? If medications are prescribed, are they taken consistently and in the appropriate amount? If not, what factors appear to be related to noncompliance? Does the person use alcohol and nonprescription drugs and in what amounts? What is the pattern and duration of substance abuse? Alcoholism and drug dependency may be a primary problem or the individual's way of attempting to cope with mental illness. If referring the client to a substance-abuse treatment center, it is important to chose an agency where the client will be allowed to remain on prescribed antipsychotic drugs. Customary substance-abuse treatment procedures require clients to remain drug free, but without continuation of the antipsychotic drug, the client is likely to decompensate under the stress of confrontational group therapy and social living expectations.

Functional Capacity

Careful assessment of occupational functioning is helpful for decisions on appropriate maintenance and rehabilitation strategies. Occupational and related school history can be useful in identifying the potential to master specific types of skills. In combination with social and communication skills, these factors make it possible to assess the likelihood that the person will be able to hold a particular kind of job. Occupational therapy staff can assist with specific skill assessments for both the schizophrenic and the organically mentally disordered prior to discharge. These assessments can help to identify whether an elderly person, for example, is capable of performing basic self-care independently, or whether a young schizophrenic client has the motivation and attention span to respond to and follow directions. Many clients are capable of functioning in work and family roles on discharge. However, younger clients may not have established job skills or attitudes, and referral to vocational testing and training services often can be a significant factor in establishing and maintaining functional status.

Social Supports and Resources

Assessments of the families of chronically mentally ill clients have two major goals: (1) to determine the family's ability to support the client's specific needs for symptom control, personal maintenance, and growth; and (2) to address the needs of the family as a group for education, support, and respite care as they attempt to cope with the problems of being long-term caregivers. Initially, it is important to determine who constitutes "family" for the client, as this may vary widely from an aged and disabled spouse or parent to a supportive parent or sibling or a residential group in foster or transitional care. For some individuals, the social isolation is sufficiently pronounced that no family or significant others can be found. Other families may be unable or unwilling to provide the necessary care and support. If supportive family is identified, it becomes important to determine their knowledge of the client's condition and their appropriate role as caregivers. Some families may reinforce dependency by doing too much for the client and expecting too little, whereas others may exert pressure to resume social roles faster than the client's current capabilities permit. Clients may be excluded from family decision-making processes and may become scapegoats for family problems. The family will require careful assessment to determine their level of functioning and coping capacity, their interest in and capacity for growth, and their ability to provide long-term support for the client.[8]

To supplement the family's caregiving and support capacity, there will need to be an assessment of available community resources for client and family needs. In general, these needs can be categorized as follows:

1. Education: knowledge of the disorder; early recognition of signs and symptoms of recurrence and need for psychiatric care; and information on antipsychotic drug therapy, pertinent precautions, and those side effects that require reporting vs those that can be managed symptomatically.
2. Social support: awareness of caring others who understand or may have experienced similar problems (i.e., client support and socialization groups and family support groups).
3. Respite services: services that permit caregivers to take time for personal interests and needs such as agencies that provide trained individuals for short-term home-based care or daycare programs that permit regular attendance so that family members may work, attend school, and have time for themselves or other activities.
4. Therapeutic services: partial hospitalization or outpatient care groups and programming that build social and leisure skills for clients.
5. Adult protective services: social services that respond to suspected abuse, neglect, or exploitation of the chronically mentally ill by family members or others in the community.
6. Social welfare: services to identify resources and agencies to help with financial, medical, or other services.
7. Care coordination and advocacy: agencies, social service departments, community health nurses, and self-help groups attempting to pull together knowledge of various services in the community, identify gaps in services, and assist clients and families in matching and accessing services to meet their needs.

TREATMENT MODALITIES AND NURSING ROLES

The nurse has several key roles and functions in relation to the overall treatment of the chronically mentally ill. Medical treatment of chronic mental disorders is oriented toward diagnosis and symptom control. However, symptom control does not necessarily lead to adequate functioning. Rehabilitative care is an interdisciplinary focus with significant roles and functions that are appropriate to nurses.

Discharge Planning

To minimize the revolving door syndrome common in clients with chronic mental disorders and to prevent further deterioration and neglect of the client, discharge planning is vital. The primary goals here are to involve the client, family, or both in selecting an appropriate residential setting, facilitating social adjustment, and planning aftercare that addresses health maintenance and rehabilitation needs of the client and the family.

Residential care settings can range from the very structured to the highly independent. The client's self-care capacity, social interaction skills, and ability to structure free time productively will influence the degree of structure and supervision needed. Newly discharged clients with long-term patterns of nonproductive behaviors frequently require structured transitional living arrangements. Examples include halfway houses for recovering alcoholics or drug abusers and social group homes for chronic schizophrenics to foster social living and self-care capacities. The organically mentally disordered person may require long-term care (i.e., a nursing home) or services to support family care such as daycare, respite care, and home health care.

Facilitating social adjustment requires preparation of the client for the new setting and preparation of the family or other setting for the client. This will require educational programming on both individual and group levels and provision of social support in the form of a consistent, accessible contact person and a support group or consultation services to agencies or personnel who work with chronically ill clients.

Aftercare programs need to be tailored to the client's strengths and needs. Some common aspects include medication education and monitoring, therapeutic or rehabilitation approaches for specific client problems, and social support. Medication monitoring may involve home visits and help in arranging the week's prescription supply into daily time frames for those who have difficulty remembering what pills to take, when, and whether they took them. Weekly pill counts can assist in monitoring whether the correct number of doses is gone from week to week. Chronic schizophrenics who repeatedly stop taking their antipsychotic drugs may be placed on long-acting injectable preparations administered by an outpatient or community nurse every 1 to 4 weeks. The client may still refuse an injection, but at least someone is aware of the noncompliance early, and it can be discussed. In addition to monitoring compliance with prescribed drugs, it is important to assess for use of other substances. Substance abusers' sobriety should be monitored. This is not easy, because the person may deny use even after a return to previous substance-abusing behavior. The nurse may need to rely on secondary cues such as family or work problems and physical signs or symptoms. Social support groups are frequently used to reduce dependency and promote social competencies. There is limited research on aftercare modalities, but in one study, chronically mentally ill clients attending a medication clinic had better socialization and care satisfaction than comparable clients in a social support group. The researchers speculated that the results may reflect the preference of some clients for individual rather than group care.[10]

Therapeutic approaches may include reminiscing, socialization, activity, or remotivation groups for older adults with chronic mental disorders. Socialization and support, coping, communication, social skills, and vocational or leisure skills can all be helpful in meeting specific needs of schizophrenic clients. These can be offered in individual counseling but more frequently are used in groups in daycare or outpatient settings.

Substance abuse therapy aims to facilitate the client's movement from therapy to a halfway house, if needed, to self-help groups such as Alcoholics Anonymous (AA) or Narcotics Anonymous (NA) and community living. The social support component of all of these therapeutic approaches is designed to help the client gain a sense of acceptance and belonging in which social isolation and the stigma of the disorder are reduced.

Families should be included in discharge planning. They need education about the condition and its current treatment and information about community resources that promote family advocacy and support; for example, Al-Anon, the National Alliance for the Mentally Ill, and the Alzheimer's Disease and Related Disorders Association. Many people find groups such as these both informational and a significant source of coping help and emotional support. The discharge plan should address significant aspects of living arrangements, social adjustment, and aftercare. It should be specific and individualized and, if well planned and implemented, can contribute to rehabilitation rather than neglect and deterioration.

Case Coordination

The community health nurse or nurse in the community mental health center will serve as a liaison, with monitoring, support, and advocacy roles to assist the client and the family or residential care group. Principles of primary care nursing apply as the discharge planner and community nurse meet with the client and, if possible, family members to become acquainted and initiate relationships. If the client is to be involved with a new setting in the community, it is important that a trusted person accompany the client on the initial visits and provide introductions to the new people in the setting. As comfort builds, greater independence can be fostered in attendance. Community services should be centered on the unique needs and strengths of clients. They should be flexible, culturally appropriate, and designed to empower clients and families rather than foster dependency.

The client and significant others can be assisted to monitor such aspects as therapeutic compliance, stressors and stress tolerance, symptomatology, and progress in maintaining and building the targeted social, educational, or vocational skills. The nurse should assist with identifying and encouraging use of any needed referral sources. This may involve some preliminary telephone contacts by the nurse or family to facilitate the client's access. Role play, as rehearsal for new contacts and tasks, may help the client feel more prepared and confident in new situations. A good relationship with the family or group home leader will permit the nurse to obtain additional help in monitoring the client's progress and becoming alert to early signs of distress or further withdrawal. The nurse may also be a support to those who live with the client, who have needs of their own. Chronic caregiving is stress-

TABLE 27-2
Common nursing diagnoses in chronically mentally ill clients and their families[6]

SELECTED NURSING DIAGNOSES	RELATED FACTORS	SELECTED DEFINING CHARACTERISTICS
Anxiety	Changes in role functions or environment; unmet needs; threats to perception of self	Increased tension and helplessness Feelings of inadequacy, distress Stimulation of CNS symptoms Expressed concerns
Noncompliance (with antipsychotic drug therapy)	Negative beliefs and attitudes; client–provider relations	Failure to adhere to prescribed schedule; evidence of exacerbation of symptoms Failure to progress
Ineffective individual coping	Personal vulnerability; inadequate support; inadequate coping methods	Inability to cope, ask for help, meet needs, or solve problems Altered social participation Destructive behavior to self or others; inappropriate use of defense mechanisms
Impaired social interaction	Social skills deficit; communication barriers	Social discomfort; inability to communicate or receive a sense of belonging, caring, or interest Dysfunctional pattern of interaction with significant other
Self esteem disturbance	Negative perception of self and capabilities	Inability to accept positive reinforcement; self-neglect or denigration; poor eye contact
Altered health maintenance	Altered ability to communicate and make thoughtful judgments; perceptual or cognitive impairment	Health knowledge deficits Lack of adaptive behavior to cope with changes History of lack of health-seeking or self-care behaviors
Family coping: potential for growth	Family or significant person has need for information on building family strengths and coping with client illness	Family member(s) seek to understand illness's effects on client Family may express interest in contact with others experiencing the problem for mutual support; exhibit readiness to learn and grow

ful, can become a burden, and can distort the family's focus such that family strengths and needs are neglected.

COMMON NURSING DIAGNOSES

Some nursing diagnoses in chronically mentally ill patients and their families are identified in Table 27-2. The client may also have altered perception/cognition, which results in problems with reality testing and daily living activities. The self-concept and self-esteem of both client (self-esteem disturbance) and family may be disturbed by the stigma of chronic mental illness and the difficulties of coping with the problems on a long-term basis. In addition, family coping may be compromised (ineffective family coping: compromised)* or disabled (ineffective family coping: disabling),* and knowledge deficits need to be addressed in order to function effectively as caregivers and as a family.[6] If these problems are not addressed, impaired social interaction and a sense of powerlessness can influence both client and caregivers.

It is also well to remember that homeless mentally ill clients define their problems much more basically than do mental health workers. The homeless may attribute their frequent hospitalizations, not to lack of therapies and social support, but to a lack of the necessary re-

sources to maintain themselves, such as food, clothing, and shelter (impaired resource management). These basics must be considered for those who lack them.

CASE STUDY

Richard A is a 30-year-old man who has been diagnosed as having a schizophrenic disorder since his initial breakdown in college at age 19. He has been hospitalized repeatedly for bizarre and agitated behavior. The current diagnosis is schizophrenia, undifferentiated type, as he exhibits signs of both catatonic excitement and paranoid ideation.[1] He has been living with his 60-year-old widowed mother when not hospitalized. She has had frequent hospitalizations for depression and currently insists that she can no longer cope with his problems and behavior that includes excessive motor activity, posturing, episodic street preaching, cross-dressing in bizarre outfits, a belief that he has been "marked by alien gods," and self-mutilation. He is intelligent but has never held a job and relates to others only by engaging in long, rambling discourses on obscure philosophies and rock music lyrics. Much of his time is spent alone, reading philosophy and listening to music. He is physically healthy, of average weight and height, and eats well. He is on antipsychotic drug therapy but frequently stops taking the medication because, "it is not good for the spirit to be controlled by earthly things." This discontinuance results in acute disorganization and rehospitalization. Richard is currently in remission and ready for discharge. He is very anxious about possibly being assigned to a group home and is ambivalent toward his mother, alternately expressing concern for her depression and veiled anger at "women who cannot care

---

* Other NANDA nursing diagnosis.

NURSING CARE PLAN 27-1

RICHARD A

NURSING INTERVENTIONS	OUTCOME CRITERIA

NURSING DIAGNOSIS: Anxiety related to changes in environment and roles

CLIENT GOAL: Become secure in new group home setting

- Assess level of anxiety
- Promote social transition in adjustment by accompanying him to group home
- Introduce to group home supervisor and acquaint with skills, preferences, and current needs
- Provide strong initial support in adjustment with demands carefully limited as client adjusts to group home
- Encourage client to discuss feelings and concerns about group home

Statements of satisfaction and comfort with new living arrangement

Appearance of security in new setting after adjustment period

NURSING DIAGNOSIS: Ineffective individual coping related to personal vulnerability

CLIENT GOAL: Gain new coping skills to foster social interaction and greater independence

- Gradually introduce and support in group social and task activities
- Provide group activities for social skills and interpersonal learning
- Select (as appropriate) individualized level of task/goal attainment (e.g., carrying out ADL assignments, completing high school equivalency training, or learning a vocational skill)
- Provide appropriate encouragement and assistance to reach goal
- Provide liaison between client and job to assist client in coping with evaluative feedback or interaction with others

Makes personal contribution to group home task accomplishments

Engages in social interactions on at least a daily basis

Develops a skill that promotes self-esteem

NURSING DIAGNOSIS: Noncompliance (antipsychotic medication) related to negative attitudes

CLIENT GOAL: Take prescribed medication consistently as directed

- Identify attitudes and barriers to compliance
- Identify positive attitudes and benefits associated with compliance
- Work to minimize negative side effects
- Collaborate on a mutually acceptable monitoring procedure
- Provide encouragement and feedback when monitoring on a weekly basis
- Promote achievement of independent self-monitoring and compliance if possible

Takes prescribed antipsychotic daily on arising and at HS and records it

---

and hide behind their subservience and frailty." He appears uncertain and preoccupied with his expressed concerns about "this new place and what it might be like." Residual symptoms include withdrawal into intellectualization; vague, rambling, and abstract speech; and dependence. His strengths are intelligence, good grooming and manners, and a sense of humor. Major nursing diagnoses identified for Richard are anxiety related to changes in environment and roles, ineffective individual coping related to personal vulnerability, and potential for noncompliance (antipsychotic medications) (see Nursing Care Plan 27-1 for a sample care plan for Richard A).

Summary

Deinstitutionalization and reduced funding for mental health have resulted in reductions and fragmentation of services for the chronically mentally ill in the community. Difficulties in finding suitable residential placements include problems caused by the client's mental illness and problems caused by community attitudes. Nursing's emphasis on comprehensive care and coordination of services is very appropriate to

Research Highlights

As previously noted, noncompliance is a common problem in the chronically mentally ill, so improving compliance would be a significant nursing achievement. Davidhizar[5] studied attitudes toward taking medication, insight into illness, and whether there was a relationship between attitudes toward medication and insight in a sample of 100 schizophrenic clients. Each client was asked to respond to three instruments in the following order: (1) open-ended items on attitudes toward medication; (2) a fixed-response instrument developed from the literature on compliance; and (3) an instrument addressing five dimensions of insight. These tools were based on a model that defines attitudes as a combination of feelings and beliefs.

The study found that client attitudes were very individual and composed of a mixture of positive and negative beliefs. Of the total beliefs expressed by all clients, 55% were negative and 41% were positive. The largest number of negative attitudes (30%) were in relation to side effects. An additional 9% of responses related to control or power. Positive responses (15%) addressed the ability to think more clearly. Most clients agreed with two statements: (1) giving medication was a way for the doctor to help; and (2) taking it pleased the doctor.

A very modest relationship between attitudes toward medication and insight was suggested by the correlation of scores on the open-ended instrument and the scores on the insight instrument. The basis for this relationship was unclear. Further research is needed to explore this relationship and to follow up on client attitudes, insight, and compliance in the community. The author also suggests a need for further research into various client teaching approaches for medications and their effectiveness.

Implications for nursing practice are based on the researcher's observation that clients' attitudes about taking medication were highly individual and contained both positive and negative beliefs and feelings. Client beliefs about taking prescribed medication should be carefully assessed so that positive attitudes can be reinforced and negative attitudes can be addressed or minimized through appropriate teaching and support.

meeting the needs of this population. Key concepts and principles for care of the chronically mentally ill are based on recognition of the diverse characteristics and needs of this group of clients and thus the need to individualize care to address both deficits and strengths in order to promote improved functioning. Comprehensive assessments of physical, cognitive, and emotional status and individual behavior patterns are the basis for care planning. Fragmentation of services and the presence of chronic and complex problems necessitate liaison and case coordination services. The goal of aftercare is to maintain and improve the functional status of clients despite the frequent absence of a "cure" for their conditions. Supportive services are important to the client and the family or other caregivers in dealing with chronic conditions. Public awareness and involvement is needed to address the gaps in services for this population and for the homeless, many of whom are chronically mentally ill.

References

1. American Psychiatric Association. Diagnostic and statistical manual of mental disorders. 3rd ed, revised. Washington, DC: American Psychiatric Association; 1987.

2. Anonymous. Forcing the mentally ill to get help. Newsweek. November 9, 1987;48.

3. Bachrach LL. The homeless mentally ill and mental health services: an analytical review of the literature. In Lamb HR, ed. The homeless mentally ill. Washington, DC: American Psychiatric Association; 1984.

4. Cutler DL. Community residential options for the chronically mentally ill. Community Ment Health J. 1986;22(1):61–72.

5. Davidhizer RE. Beliefs, feelings and insight of patients with schizophrenia about taking medication. J Adv Nurs. 1987;12:261–73.

6. Kim MJ, McFarland GK, McLane AM. Pocket guide to nursing diagnoses. 3rd ed. St Louis: CV Mosby; 1989.

7. King I. A theory for nursing—systems, concepts, process. New York: John Wiley & Sons; 1981.

8. Neal MT. Partial hospitalization: an alternative to inpatient psychiatric hospitalization. Nurs Clin North Am. 1986;21:461–472.

9. Sheets JL, Prevost JA, Reihman J. Young adult chronic patients: three hypothesized subgroups. Hosp Community Psychiatry. 1982;33:197–203.

10. Slavinsky AT, Krauss JB. Two approaches to the management of long-term psychiatric patients in the community. Nurs Res. 1982;31:284–289.

11. Walgrove NJ. Mental health aftercare. Nurs Clin North Am. 1986;21:473–483.

28

Lois Elaine Smith
Beverly Koehler Lunsford

Mental Health Needs of Homeless Persons

OBJECTIVES

After reading this chapter, the reader will be able to:

1. Identify the scope and trends of the problem of homelessness
2. Identify social, economic, and political factors that contribute to homelessness
3. Discuss the interaction of mental illness and homelessness; i.e., mental illnesses that precipitate homelessness and mental illness that is precipitated by homelessness
4. Identify the most common types of mental illness in the homeless population
5. Discuss the interaction of physical and mental health problems of homeless persons
6. Describe four roles for nurses in working with the homeless
7. List the guidelines for assessing problems related to homelessness
8. Identify common nursing diagnoses found in homeless persons
9. Apply the nursing process considering the uniqueness of each homeless person and family
10. Explain the vital importance of an interdisciplinary approach in working with the homeless
11. Discuss the need for nursing research in regard to persons without shelter.

INTRODUCTION

In 1986, the American Public Health Association assembled nurses, clinicians, researchers, administrators, and educators to grapple with the role of nurses in meeting the physical and mental health needs of the homeless.[1] Many issues were raised, solutions proposed, and differences noted. The common agreement was that nurses, as professionals educated to respond to the whole person, can and must respond meaningfully to the many physical and mental health problems of persons who are without the basic necessity of shelter. By listening, observing, questioning, and, most of all, caring, nurses can make assessments that will help in finding ways to assist clients toward health and wholeness.

SCOPE AND TRENDS OF HOMELESSNESS

The way in which homelessness is defined has a great impact on assessments of its extent in our country. For instance, the US Department of Housing and Urban Development (HUD) says "homeless" refers to people in the "streets" who, in seeking shelter, have no alternative but to obtain it from a private or public agency.[30] The agency excludes those living in overcrowded conditions with relatives or friends, no matter how temporary or inadequate the arrangement. At the opposite end of the spectrum, Hopper discussed a definition of homeless that includes anyone "without an address which assures them of at least the following thirty days' sleeping quarters which meet minimal health and safety standards. This includes those who are sleeping on the floors of friends' or family's apartments, tolerating substandard accommodations, or who are institutionalized on a time-limited basis in hospitals and jails, who upon release will be without a residence" (reference 12, p 104).

Size of Homeless Population

The number of homeless people in the US has increased dramatically over the past few years, and estimates now range from 250,000 to 3 million persons.[30] There is no statistical basis for these estimates, but they continue to be used in the absence of an effective research method for counting the homeless. The wide range is related to the definition of the homeless, to ineffective methods used to identify the homeless, and to the bias of group reporting. While the ranks of the homeless continue to swell, with an average increase of 25% per year, the gap between the need for emergency shelter and the resources to provide it widens.[23]

Characteristics and Trends

In the early 1900s, the homeless were stereotyped as happy hoboes, tramps, or "kings of the road." Later, "skid rows" began to emerge in cities, and the stereotyped homeless were viewed as alcoholic "bums." More recently (since 1960), discharged mentally ill roaming city streets, sleeping on grates or in cardboard boxes, and resistant to help have been the commonly accepted view of the homeless.

Families with children are the fastest growing segment of the nation's homeless population. In Boston, Phoenix, Philadelphia, Chicago, and Washington, DC, families are 50% of the total homeless population. In the early 1980s, the average age of the homeless was in the mid-30s; today, with thousands of young children among the homeless, the average age may be even lower. In New York City, it is estimated that more than half the homeless people are under the age of 16.[27]

The homeless population may be subgrouped in a number of overlapping ways. They include mentally disabled (20%–40%),[27] substance abusers (33%),[27] employed persons (20%–25%),[30] public assistance recipients (30%–35%),[30] families and children (20%–30%),[17] single men (56%),[30] single women (15.5%),[30] elderly (6% over 60, 10%–15% over 50),[30] and minorities (40%–50%).[30] The ethnic characteristics of any homeless population reflect the ethnic make-up of the surrounding community. The point of greatest agreement among those examining current homelessness is that the population is diverse and composed of many subgroups whose homelessness may be attributed to many different factors[4,13,19,27,29] (Fig. 28-1).

FACTORS THAT CONTRIBUTE TO HOMELESSNESS

The social, economic, and political factors that have contributed to the increasing numbers of homeless persons in our society are many and complex. As a result of the information gathered by HUD in their 1984 survey of homeless persons across the US,[30] three categories were identified based on three primary causes: *chronic disability, personal crises,* and *economic conditions.* The chronic disabled include those suffering from alcoholism, substance abuse, and mental illness. The second category (40%–50%) includes persons involved with personal crises. The most common crises cited in the HUD survey were divorce, discharge from jail or hospital with no place to go, being stranded while traveling, domestic violence, and health-related problems. Immigrants who are afraid to use "the system" for fear of being deported and "throwaway" teens may also fall into this category of those with personal crises. The third category includes those persons homeless as a result of economic conditions. Some of these may be persons who were middle-class or skilled workers who were laid off, but probably the greater number were persons "at the margin," such as elderly, single parents, and those employed occasionally.

The numbers of mentally ill homeless have increased in part because of the passage of the 1963 Community Mental Health Act (P.L. 88-164).[2] This policy of "dein-

FIGURE 28–1. Homeless people line up for food in a park across from the White House in Washington, D.C. (Courtesy of Jim Hubbard; used with permission)

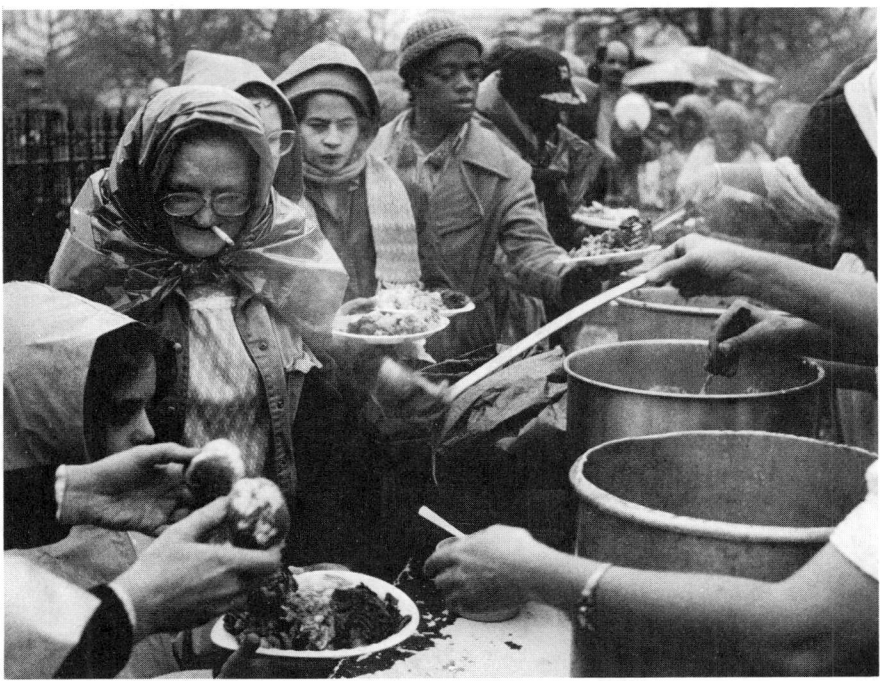

stitutionalization" was intended to create a more humane mental health system by protecting individual rights; i.e., permitting involuntary hospitalization only in cases where a person was either a danger to self or others or gravely disabled, and providing community mental health services to support those who did not need to be hospitalized but did need structure in their community. As a result, large numbers of mentally ill persons were released from or ceased being admitted to mental institutions.

It is important to recognize that most chronic mentally disabled persons who were deinstitutionalized are not homeless. However, there was a failure of the public to provide adequate, accessible, or acceptable community mental health services to meet the needs of many persons who have been discharged. Those mentally disabled persons who are not linked with adequate community services now have the double burden of homelessness and mental illness.[17]

In addition to the deinstitutionalized mentally ill, there are the never-institutionalized and those hospitalized briefly who contribute to the numbers of the mentally ill homeless. With more stringent admission and retention policies, those who need help are discharged back into an inadequately prepared community, only to be readmitted to an emergency unit when they cause some disturbance. They may be kept for perhaps 72 hours and released (often referred to as the "revolving door" mental health system). The cycle then begins again and underscores the need for more comprehensive inpatient and outpatient services in the community that will respond to all needs of those who are mentally ill.

RELATIONSHIP OF MENTAL HEALTH AND HOMELESSNESS

Perhaps no group of disabled people in the US is as impoverished and underserved as the homeless mentally ill. People who are homeless and emotionally ill bear a dual disenfranchisement, both from society and from service providers. Mentally ill persons are often excluded from programs designed to serve the homeless, and homeless individuals are typically screened out from receiving services designed for the long-term, severely mentally ill.[17]

It is not always clear whether some persons are homeless as a result of a mental illness or if emotional instability and even mental illness is secondary to the extreme stress and many losses experienced by homeless individuals and families. The instability of no permanent place to live aggravates any existing mental health problem, and a person who is homeless over time certainly begins to experience high levels of psychological distress.[14] Baxter and Hopper[8] suggest that if mentally ill homeless individuals were to receive several nights of sleep, an adequate diet, and warm social contact, some of their symptoms might subside (Fig. 28-2).

A further complicating factor in assessing the presence of mental illness is determining which behaviors, although seemingly somewhat bizarre, may be good coping mechanisms given the situation of homelessness and life on the streets. This was dramatically demonstrated in the case of a woman in New York who had been taken from her favorite heat grate on the streets

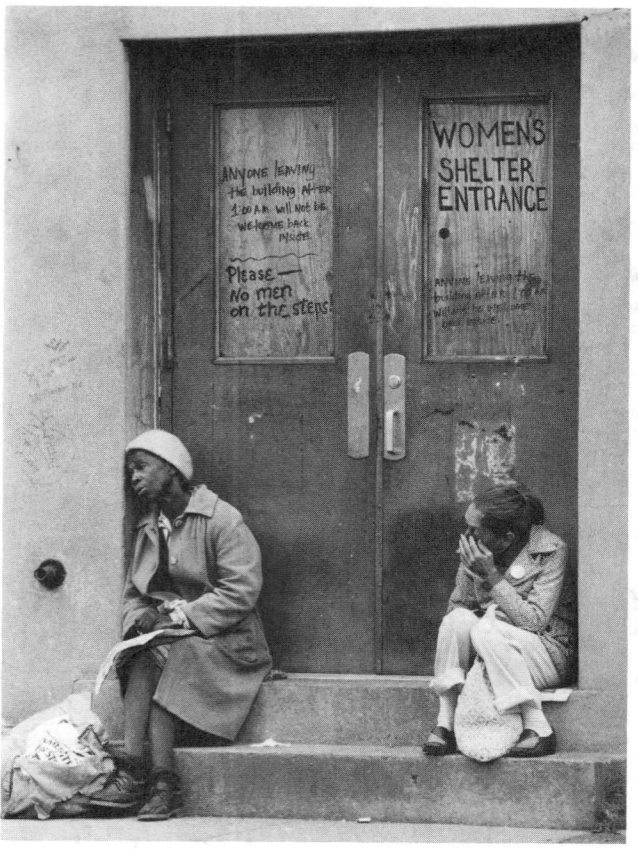

FIGURE 28–2. Two women wait for a shelter to open. Door signs warn entrants that they will not be allowed back in if they leave the building after 1 A.M. (Courtesy of Jim Hubbard; used with permission)

against her will and hospitalized. One of her behaviors, burning money, caused widespread disagreement among the psychiatrists as to her sanity: to some psychiatrists, this was insane behavior; to others, it was appropriate in light of her explanations. "I burn the money if it is given to me with a bad attitude. I also burn all my paper money at night so I won't be robbed."[3]

In a recent study in Phoenix, Arizona, it was discovered that one in every three homeless persons had been robbed or assaulted during the previous 6 months. The more frequently victimized were the chronically mentally ill, who, in the view of their assailants, are the easiest to "take."[28] Even the mentally disabled who survive in such a hostile and dangerous atmosphere have remarkably well-developed skills for survival.

In a study of homeless children in Massachusetts, Bassuk and Rubin[5] found that developmental delays, severe depression and anxiety, and learning difficulties were common. With research screening instruments, about half the children were found in need of psychiatric referral and evaluation. Teens in homeless families exhibit a variety of behaviors: embarrassment, depression, acting out, and hiding from friends. They are reluctant to go to new schools because they do not want to be identified as "homeless" (Fig. 28–3).

Most Common Types of Mental Illness Among the Homeless

Several studies have focused on the prevalence of mental or psychiatric impairment among the homeless population. In Philadelphia in 1981, a psychiatrist in-

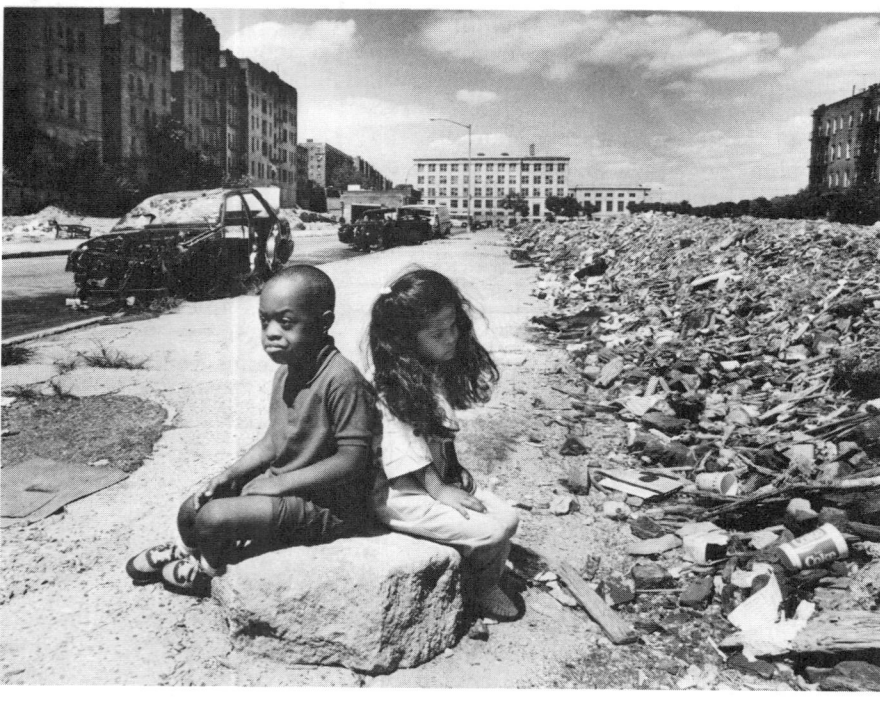

FIGURE 28–3. Homeless children on the streets of New York City amid the destruction of abandoned cars and demolished buildings. (Courtesy of Jim Hubbard; used with permission)

terviewed residents of an emergency shelter and classified 85% as having psychiatric disorders. The most common problem was schizophrenia. Less common problems were personality disorders, affective disorders, organic brain syndrome, and other mental illness.[18] A similar study of shelter guests by Bassuk found a 90% incidence of diagnosable mental illness. Again, psychosis and character disorders were the most common.[4]

A mobile mental health outreach program in New York City was organized to try to meet the heterogenous needs of the homeless. Program workers describe six general psychiatric problem areas: "schizophrenia–chronic and residual (paranoid, undifferentiated, disorganized); bipolar affective disorder (acute manic agitation with psychotic features, manic agitation with history of depression); substance abuse/dependence (alcohol, heroin, cocaine); organic brain syndrome; depression (with or without psychotic features); and adjustment disorder (with disturbances of conduct and mood)" (reference 20, p 63).

It is not easy to differentiate between the homeless who are mentally ill, those who have substance abuse problems, and those who have the dual diagnosis of mental illness and substance abuse. Many of the mentally ill use substances as a form of self-medication. The homeless also drink and use street drugs to relieve chronic pain and to lessen the harsh realities of their existence.

There is probably no group that is less welcome in shelters and places of treatment than those who are homeless, use drugs or alcohol, and are mentally ill. Alcohol and drug treatment centers often feel unprepared to respond to the mental health needs. Likewise, mental health centers feel they cannot care for the mental health needs as long as a drug or alcohol problem exists. There is tremendous need for a concerted effort to respond to those who have the dual diagnosis of mental illness and substance abuse, especially among persons who are homeless.

Interaction of Physical and Mental Health

It is critical to consider the whole person, as mental health can support or hinder one's physical health. Mentally ill persons frequently are impaired in their ability to make judgments regarding self-care, to solve problems, and to understand health care instructions. Uncomplicated health problems thus become life-threatening illnesses because of inappropriate treatment or inability to provide adequate self-care. This problem is exacerbated by fear of large institutions, inability to pay, and perceptions by health care providers of the homeless as undesirable clients (Fig. 28-4).

A homeless lifestyle may precipitate several health problems, such as communicable diseases; i.e., hepatitis and tuberculosis, skin diseases, malnutrition, pneumonia, dental problems, cirrhosis, and ulceration sores, especially of the feet and hands.[18] Cardiovascular diseases may cause increased dependent edema as a result of sleeping upright or constant walking. Compromised vascular conditions coupled with difficulties in personal hygiene and self-care result in edema and cellulitis.

Traumas such as head injury and lacerations from robbery may be common to persons living on the

FIGURE 28–4. The combination of substance abuse and mental illness is worsened by homelessness and often creates physical problems as well. (Courtesy of Jim Hubbard; used with permission)

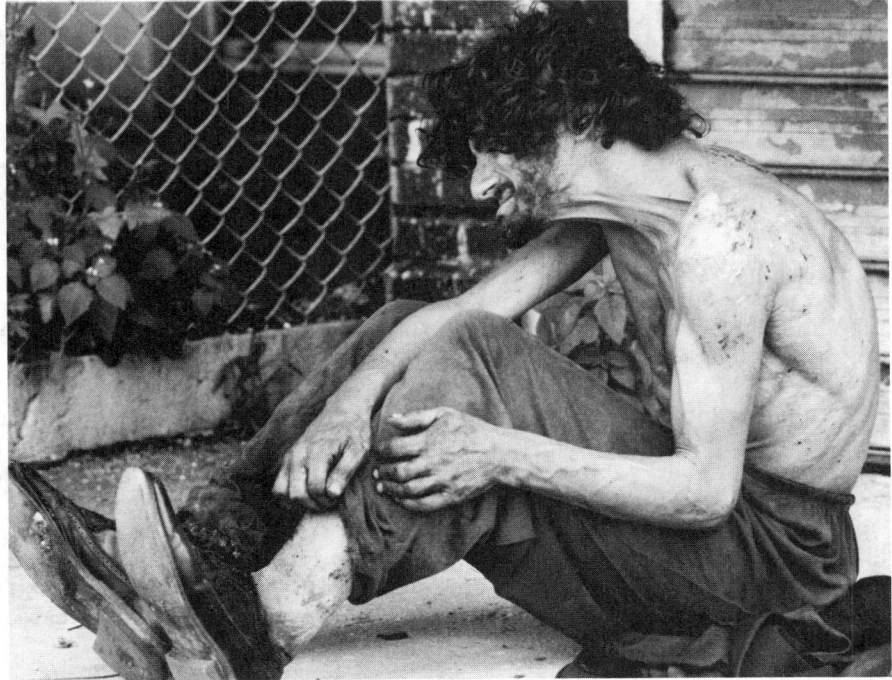

streets. Rape is a frequent assault that may result in further mental and physical injury, as well as infection. Alcohol use impairs judgment and the body's thermoregulatory system, increasing the likelihood of frostbite, leading to gangrene and eventual amputation.[31]

Communicable diseases are common, especially in children. Frequently, parents have been unable to attend to basic immunization programs for their children. More serious communicable diseases, diarrhea and meningitis, are of particular concern.[26]

Just as mental illness, anxiety, depression, and fear can impair one's ability for self-care, so too does inattention to physical health impair one's mental status. After a brief period on the streets seeking any available shelter, many of the homeless become disorganized without becoming psychotic. They may be unable to pass a mental status examination, such as ability to count backwards from 100 by 7, or to recall such information as what day it is or who is president. Thus, persons who previously were functional experience a profound life change and may be unable to cope.[20]

Lack of sleep, lack of food, and fear of the unknown can create tremendous anxiety. Sleep deficit can result in actual psychosis or spouse and child abuse as nervous tension builds. Hartmann[11] discusses the importance of sleep for dealing with emotional stress as well as physical exertion and trauma. His studies suggest a relation between REM sleep and mental functioning. Certainly, homeless persons experience high levels of emotional and physical stress, and research is warranted to determine the full impact of sleeplessness on homeless persons.

For those whose homelessness has been precipitated by a personal crisis such as divorce, death of spouse, illness, or loss of job, there is the dimension of decreased self-esteem, loss, and powerlessness impinging on desperate needs to provide safe shelter, food, and emergency medical care for loved ones (Figs. 28-5 and 28-6). In some families, women and children may be eligible for public assistance if the employable spouse/father is not present. The man therefore may move out to the streets, causing even greater family disruption.

ROLES OF THE NURSE

Four roles have been identified for the nurse to recognize and care effectively for persons without homes: outreach and assessment, clinician, case manager, and advocate. The values inherent in nursing are particularly important in caring for the homeless population: a holistic approach that recognizes the importance of environment on health; ability to respond to the client's perceived need and to proceed at client's rate of speed; supportive care when cure is uncertain; respect for the dignity and worth of each person; recognition of the importance of interfacing with other professionals; and advocacy on an individual and social level.

The nursing role of *outreach and assessment* is most appropriate for nurses as they are most likely to come in direct contact with persons who have no home or are

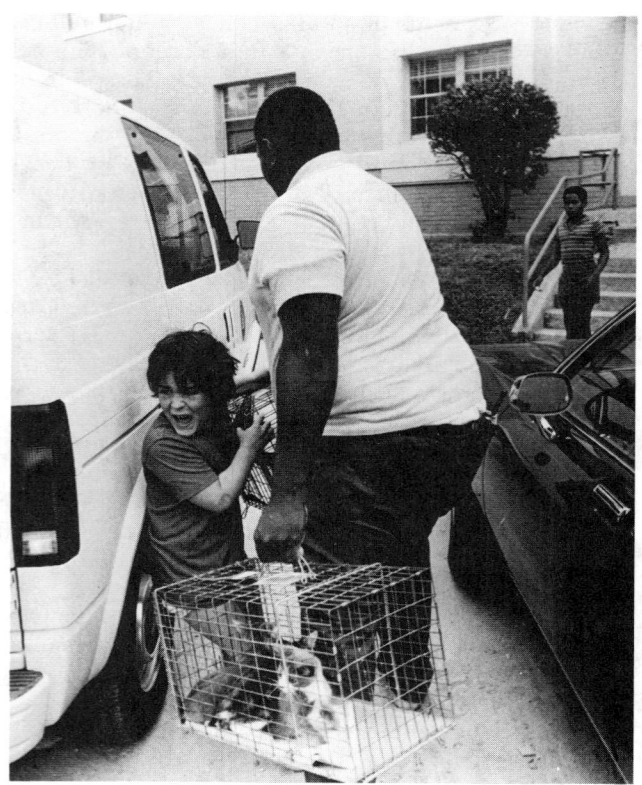

at risk of becoming homeless. It takes time, however, to establish a rapport that promotes disclosure of such highly personal information as surrounds homelessness. There may also be an unconscious desire to avoid asking critical questions because of the overwhelming complexity of tasks that may be required to address the needs.

The second nursing role is that of *clinician.* Crisis intervention, supportive therapy, and family therapy can be provided by traditional and nontraditional methods. Meeting the mental health needs of homeless persons and families requires a flexibility in how one approaches counseling and where one chooses to conduct counseling sessions. Health care workers often insist on rigid appointments at a particular time and place, which may be unreasonable for persons without clocks and ready transportation. The nurse has the ability to "lay on hands" and, in that process, touch patients who generally see themselves as untouchable. Nurses can thereby stretch a moment of assessing blood pressure into a therapeutic encounter. These acts open the door for trust to be established.

Mulkern[22] suggests that the homeless see their needs in fairly concrete terms; that is, jobs, housing, food, and clothing. In fact, dental care ranked higher than physical health care, and mental health care ranked last. Mulkern found that a large majority of homeless persons in Boston had not sought mental health services. Ninety-seven per cent of homeless persons seeking

FIGURE 28–6. *A young family, evicted, joins the homeless population. (Courtesy of Jim Hubbard; used with permission)*

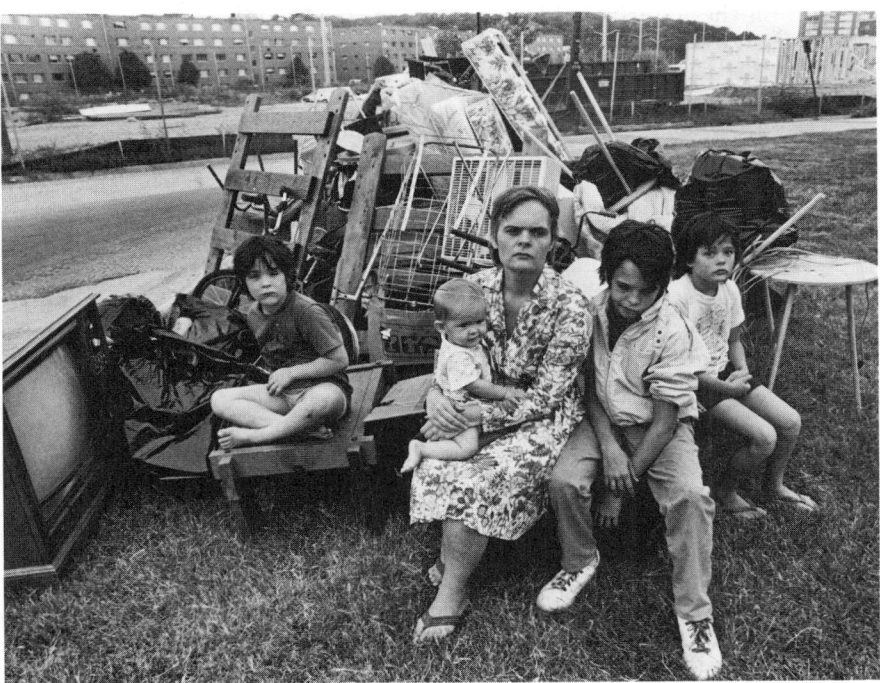

mental health care did indeed find it. Mulkern says that this suggests that, "accessibility to mental health care may not be a barrier for homeless persons, but acceptability may be" (reference 22, p 28).

Thus, the nurse may assume the third role, that of a *case manager*. This role is an aggressive, comprehensive approach to accessing and securing basic physical, mental, and social health services for persons who are most in need.[25] Given the many services available, it is easy for a person to get lost in the system and feel fragmented. A case manager becomes the one person who coordinates all of the services needed by the client.

A nurse functioning as a case manager must utilize a holistic approach that can make sense of the many parts that impinge on the whole. This nurse performs the dual function of providing a one-to-one relationship, which is critical for maintaining trust, and pulling together the services needed to address complex problems. The nurse must be in regular contact with the client and have access to the variety of services and professionals that are essential.

The last nursing role is that of an *advocate*. This role may involve speaking for clients until they are able and willing to speak for themselves. As a trusted member of the community, the nurse has a responsibility to speak out regarding needs and possible community responses to those needs. One of the current problems is that communities are resistant to the placement of residential group homes for persons needing a structured environment. Although there is no documented basis for concern, fear and prejudice abound. Nurses can be important sources of community education and support for such facilities.

There also is need and opportunity for nurses who are knowledgeable about the problems and needs of the homeless to provide information and education to persons who set public policy. An exciting development is that of nurse-run clinics established to meet the needs of persons without shelter.[9,16,18]

GUIDELINES FOR ASSESSING HOMELESS PERSONS

Assessing the physical and mental health needs of persons who are homeless is a challenge. There is insufficient research at this time to identify adequately all the areas of needed assessment in each of the subgroups among the homeless populations. However, as nurses begin to look at problems of homelessness and see the interrelations that homelessness has with other areas of assessment, nurses will begin to develop a broader body of knowledge, which should enable them to give more effective care. As has been stated previously, the broad spectrum of physical and mental illnesses found in the population at large can be found in persons who are homeless, so that assessment tools used with these populations are certainly appropriate if the added stress of homelessness is taken into account. This may be accomplished by collecting the following data:

I. Environmental issues:
    1. Where does the client usually stay? Street, shelter (temporary or long term), abandoned building, or car? Where did the person stay the last three nights and where does he or she plan to stay tonight?
    2. What is the client's degree of comfort or distress with the living situation? What problems does he or she identify?

3. Is there refrigeration and a place to cook available?
4. Are shower and toilet facilities available?

II. Social issues:
1. How long has the client been homeless?
2. How many times homeless?
3. What is the client's perception of the reason for homelessness?
4. What services are available to the client; i.e., food, shelter, health care, school, job training?
5. What services are acceptable to the client?
6. Who are the support people for the client?

III. Physical/mental health issues:
1. Where is the usual source of health care?
2. When was this source last seen?
3. What is the current physical health? Any chronic health problems? Treatments, medications?
4. Sleep pattern?
5. Eating pattern?
6. Mental health history; i.e., previous hospitalizations, medications, mental status, substance abuse?
7. Relationship of homelessness to mental and physical health?

IV. Other:
1. Will client come to health professional, or must health professional go to him or her?
2. What does client perceive as most important need? How can the nurse respond to that need?
3. What are the client's coping strengths that have helped in survival?

A nonjudgmental attitude is vital in assessing the needs of the homeless. They are accustomed to being blamed for their own situation and are highly sensitive to nonaccepting attitudes. Whether the homeless person lives on the streets or is a mother with several children in a shelter, the wariness toward professionals is often high. A warm, accepting attitude and atmosphere and a degree of privacy encourage clients to share more openly.

Because of the diverse causes of homelessness and the many different persons finding themselves without homes, it is essential that the nurse make an adequate assessment before making nursing diagnoses or planning interventions based solely on lack of shelter.

CASE STUDY

Vicky is a 28-year-old woman who entered the community health center on a hot, muggy summer day with her five children. Two of the children, the baby and the 2-year-old, as well as Vicky herself, appeared exhausted and lethargic. Vicky said she just needed a place to rest for awhile, but as a nurse sat beside her, Vicky told her their situation. Vicky was alternately rational and exhibiting bizarre behavior. She denied drug use, but it was difficult to determine what factors contributed to her erratic behavior. Vicky and her family were on the "Open Market," a system in the District of Columbia in which, if there is no room in the intake shelter,

families are assigned to a motel in another area of town on a night-by-night basis. Each day, the mother must check out of the room, take all of her children and belongings, and make the long bus ride across town to the intake shelter to receive meals and then wait, sometimes as late as 1 o'clock in the morning, to find out where she and her children will stay that night. Vicky and her children were homeless as a result of a personal crisis; i.e., the rape of Vicky, which occurred in front of her children. She had been able to escape with her children, but as she walked the streets and rode the bus, she was in constant fear. She had a pelvic infection as a result of the rape, the 3-month-old baby had an ear infection, and the toddler was on medication for an asthma attack several days ago. Each was on special medications, but Vicky's own prescription had gone unfilled because she did not have the 50 cents required to fill a Medicaid prescription. Eventually, the nurse accompanied Vicky to the shelter worker to explain the relationship between sleeplessness and disorientation, and to request that Vicky be placed in one motel room for a long weekend to give the family much-needed rest for emotional and physical healing (see Nursing Care Plan 28-1 for a sample care plan for Vicky and her family).

CASE STUDY

John, a 55-year-old man living in an abandoned building with no heat or hot water, was becoming increasingly disoriented and paranoid. The local community mental health department was unable to see him on a home visit, and John refused to go there because he was afraid he would be hospitalized. Although he had been under psychiatric treatment before, he found it difficult to take the high doses of psychotropic medications prescribed for him, and he disliked the side effects.

As a child, he had lived in foster homes and a center for abandoned and disorderly children and youth. During his adult life, he had been assaulted repeatedly, had been hospitalized at the local psychiatric hospital several times, and had lived in one of the shelters for homeless men.

At the time, John was losing weight and "talking crazy." A friend came to a small general practice clinic for help and talked about her frustrations with her own inability to get a job and then just mentioned John in passing. She was fearful that she would not get help for John until he did something violent, as he would not be seen as a psychiatric emergency unless threatening to hurt himself or others. The community mental health nurse offered to see John. Taking along her blood pressure cuff and stethoscope, often a symbol that generates trust, the nurse entered the rodent-infested building and found John sitting on a chair, rocking back and forth and talking to himself. As the nurse talked gently with John about his health, he slowly raised his head, allowed the nurse to take his blood pressure, and then looked at the nurse with some perception and said, "Are you one of those mental health nurses?" The nurse admitted that she was but said that her immediate concern was John's loss of weight and lack of food. Over several months, trust was built by focusing on John's need for food, shelter, and relationship. In time, the nurse was able to encourage John to begin to take psychotropic medications and to attend a day treatment program.

After taking the medications for a few weeks, John's thought processes cleared, and he no longer had auditory hallucinations. However, he became increasingly de-

Text continued on page 676

VICKY AND HER FAMILY

NURSING INTERVENTIONS	OUTCOME CRITERIA

NURSING DIAGNOSIS (FOR VICKY): Anxiety related to the unknown and sleeplessness

CLIENT GOAL: Experience reduced anxiety

- Provide supportive counseling
- Maintain calm and safe environment
- Problem solve with Vicky to identify manageable problems
- Maintain consistent one-to-one relationship
- Make arrangements so that consistent sleeping quarters will allow sleep recovery

Demonstrates decreased level of anxiety, as evidenced by decreased insomnia and increased ability to solve problems

NURSING DIAGNOSIS (FOR VICKY): Rape trauma syndrome related to lack of follow-up of rape event and inadequate support system

CLIENT GOAL: Cope with cognitive and emotional response to rape and obtain medical intervention

- Provide crisis intervention
- Refer Vicky for immediate gynecologic care, provide transportation, and advocate for support
- Provide respite child care
- Refer to sex offender squad to apprehend rapist
- Provide transportation as needed
- Refer for ongoing therapy

Obtains mental and physical care

NURSING DIAGNOSIS (FOR FAMILY): Noncompliance (with medical regimen) related to lack of refrigeration for drugs, time orientation, and money

CLIENT GOAL: Become more compliant with medical regimen

- Assess interrelations of noncompliance with environmental factors
- Discuss alternative approaches with client
- Solicit free medications, antibiotics, theophylline, decongestant, vaginal cream, clear liquids
- Exchange present medication for one not needing refrigeration
- Negotiate with shelter cafeteria for clear liquid meals
- Obtain 14 disposable vaginal cream applicators
- Develop written schedule for medications during the day
- Obtain large duffle bag for medications and formula

Complies with medical regimen for children and self

NURSING DIAGNOSIS (FOR FAMILY): Dysfunctional family processes related to situational crisis

CLIENT GOAL: Experience improved family functioning

- Provide respite child care while mother rests and attends appointments
- Accompany mother to help with sick children during periods of extreme fatigue and anxiety to establish trust and maintain safety
- Refer for ongoing therapeutic counseling

Family stays together with nurturing and protection from mother

NURSING CARE PLAN 28–2

JOHN

NURSING INTERVENTIONS	OUTCOME CRITERIA

NURSING DIAGNOSIS: Situational crisis related to homelessness

CLIENT GOAL: Obtain safe housing

- Assess available and acceptable shelter options
- Explore long-term housing options with social services

Obtains adequate and acceptable housing

NURSING DIAGNOSIS: Altered resource management (no financial income) related to lack of job or benefits

CLIENT GOAL: Obtain financial resources

- Involve social worker in helping John apply for benefits

Obtains adequate income

NURSING DIAGNOSIS: Self-esteem disturbance related to multiple previous negative experiences

CLIENT GOAL: Experience self-respect, self-worth, and self-confidence

- Use nonjudgmental attitude
- Use active listening
- Treat John with respect and dignity
- Recognize and give feedback regarding strengths
- Help John identify skills
- Give honest and reliable responses
- Establish reachable goals with John
- Recognize long-term chronicity of illness and the risks of relapses

Demonstrates increased trust in self and others

Differentiates trustworthy from nontrustworthy persons

Recognizes and utilizes skills and abilities

CLIENT GOAL: Recognize value of recommended therapies

- Provide individual supportive therapy
- Accompany John to day treatment center
- Allow John to talk about experiences in day treatment program
- Encourage participation in day treatment program as precursor to job skill training program

Participates in recommended therapies

NURSING DIAGNOSIS: Self-care deficit related to mistrust of bureaucracies, paranoia, lack of facilities for personal hygiene and cooking

CLIENT GOAL: Develop self-care skills

- Offer hope by providing facilities to bathe and eat
- Assist in obtaining clothing
- Respect right to choose own clothes
- Emphasize housing, health and personal hygiene, leisure time
- Give honest praise for appearance
- Introduce job skills training program

Demonstrates improved self-care practices

Participates in job training

CLIENT GOAL: Increase use of assertive behaviors and recognize impact on self-worth

- Teach client assertive communication skills by example as well as word
- Serve as advocate for client with mental health and social service system

Speaks on own behalf with personnel within larger systems

Continued

JOHN *Continued*

NURSING INTERVENTIONS	OUTCOME CRITERIA

NURSING DIAGNOSIS: Altered nutrition, less than body requirements, related to lack of resources

CLIENT GOAL: Attain adequate diet

- Assess availability of food
- Assist in obtaining immediate food through local church pantry

Gains weight
Improves sense of well being

CLIENT GOAL: Experience less fatigue and poor health associated with inadequate food

- Assist in continuing to obtain food
- Provide food when John comes to clinic

Establishes trust
Improves health

NURSING DIAGNOSIS: Perception/cognition altered (auditory hallucinations) related to lack of daily life routine and structure and not taking psychotropic medication

CLIENT GOAL: Accept self as valued human being and understand that voices are part of illness

- Assist in describing hallucinatory experience
- Avoid making jokes about voices
- Help to find safe and more structured environment
- Teach voice dismissal for persistent hallucinations
- Assist in recognizing increase in altered perception as part of illness
- Encourage compliance with medication regimen

Experiences freedom from or reduced auditory hallucinations

CLIENT GOAL: Achieve orientation to present reality

- Provide orientation to time, person, and place
- Give simple, clear directions
- Talk about concrete objects in environment (smells, sights, sounds)

Experiences freedom from or reduced auditory hallucinations

CLIENT GOAL: Rely less on voices to cope with anxiety, loneliness, and fear

- Assist in becoming involved in activities in community
- Support John when he begins to tell voices to go away
- Listen to John talk about loneliness without voices

Builds relationships

CLIENT GOAL: Takes medication

- Assist John in understanding use of medication and side effects

Takes medications

NURSING DIAGNOSIS: Noncompliance (clinic appointments and medications) related to mistrust

CLIENT GOAL: Verbalize knowledge of relations among emotional factors, homelessness, and noncompliance

- Provide consistent one-to-one relationship to explore emotional issues
- Encourage John to come to clinic daily to establish contact
- Clarify agency services and roles of caregivers
- Make home visit if John does not come
- As trust builds, establish regular weekly visits at clinic
- Work with John's priorities

Keeps appointments

Continued

JOHN *Continued*

NURSING INTERVENTIONS	OUTCOME CRITERIA
■ Provide transportation as needed to keep appointments	
■ Assist in exploration of mistrust and threats to autonomy based on past experiences as basis for noncompliance	
■ Promote decision-making and control in as many areas as possible	Makes own decisions and follows through
■ Explore factors related to John's distress with side effects of medication	Takes medication appropriately
■ Discuss action/side effects of medication. Simplify instructions	Verbalizes awareness of benefits of medication despite side effects
■ Work with psychiatrist to introduce medication slowly to reduce side effects	
■ Encourage John to talk about side effects	

pressed. In a weekly session with the nurse, at which they shared a sandwich as well as conversation, John confided, "I miss the voices. It's so lonely sometimes." John and the nurse talked about the loneliness and his loss of his "voices." As he was leaving that day, John turned to the nurse and stated, "You know, in other clinics, they always talked about my sick mind. Here, you share a sandwich with me and bring me health."

Many agencies and persons were needed to work with John, but the one person who remained constant was the nurse. After a period in day treatment, individual and group therapy, and job training, John is now working full time as a clerical assistant. Deep wounds from his childhood make him highly vulnerable to relapses as a result of unusual pressures (see Nursing Care Plan 28-2 for a sample care plan for John).

INTERDISCIPLINARY APPROACH

Addressing the complex needs of persons without shelter requires an interdisciplinary approach. Social services are needed for short-term and long-term food, housing, and entitlement services. Formal and informal networks must be developed and utilized by the nurse to access specialty medical services, emergency food pantries, transportation, overnight shelter, and respite care for children while the parent negotiates systems. Churches often provide for emergency needs and long-term support. Legal services are needed to advocate for the rights and entitlements of the disenfranchised. Children who are homeless require interaction with school systems, former health care providers, day

care centers, and, often, child protective services to promote health and prevent further illness or trauma. Many other public and private agencies serve the needs of particular ages and problems.

On a larger scale, nurses need to be involved in public policy and legislation that provides for the immediate needs of homeless individuals and families. Society must provide long-term solutions to change the system that has precipitated such wide-scale homelessness. Any legislation must address the need for emergency shelter and food, physical and mental health care, housing, and educational and vocational programs for adults, children, and youth.

SUMMARY

Physical and mental health problems are intensified by homelessness, and conversely, homelessness precipitates health problems. The subgroups included in the homeless are diverse and heterogeneous. Nursing and other professionals must be aware of differing needs of these subgroups to plan and implement effective care. The numbers of homeless are increasing rapidly because of a number of complex factors, including social, economic, political, and personal. In efforts to respond to the homeless, nurses must play significant roles: outreach and assessment, clinician, case manager, and advocate. Nurses must be involved in an interdisciplinary approach, locally and nationally, to respond to problems of homelessness and to prevent future homelessness.

Research Highlights

There are many knowledge gaps that could be filled by nursing research. Maurin[21] observes that preliminary data must center on defining the universe of subjects and then determine how to draw samples that will permit a reasonable degree of confidence in the results. In addition, she offers questions that nurse researchers are in a unique position to address.

The first area of nursing research that Maurin suggests is to increase our knowledge of factors that support and promote health in individuals and families. Examples are the effects of circadian rhythm disturbance during homelessness, mental and physical health problems of various homeless groups, family and social networks among homeless persons, and insight into the individual's perception of homelessness.

The second area of nursing research would increase our knowledge of the impact of social and physical environments on health. Many of the problems of the homeless are obvious. However, there may be subtle interactions that can exacerbate health problems, such as pharmacologic, psychological, metabolic, and nutritional problems.[21]

Because of the large number of homeless persons who are chronically ill, disabled, or dying, Maurin[21] believes there is a need for research to address how we care for individuals and families during illness. There is a need particularly for new strategies to work with the mentally ill. This study must include families, who frequently become alienated from the chronically disabled person.

The last area suggested for nursing research is identification of the health care delivery systems that are most effective and efficient in providing care. This work must evaluate systems and patient outcomes as well as policies regarding people's health.

References

1. American Public Health Association. The role of nurses in meeting the health/mental health needs of the homeless. Proceedings of the Workshop, March 6–7. Washington, DC: American Public Health Association; 1986.

2. Axelroad S, Toff G. Outreach services for the homeless mentally ill people. Intergovernmental Health Policy Project, George Washington University, No. 278-86-0006. Washington, DC: National Institute for Mental Health; 1987.

3. Barbanel J. Homeless woman sent to hospital under Koch plan is ordered freed. New York Times. November 13, 1987:B2.

4. Bassuk EL. The homeless problem. Sci Am. 1984;251(1):40–45.

5. Bassuk E, Rubin L. Homeless children: a neglected population. Am J Orthopsychiatry. 1986;57:2.

6. Bassuk EL, Rubin L, Lauriat A. Is homelessness a mental health problem? Am J Psychiatry. 1984;141(12):1546–1550.

7. Bassuk EL, Rubin L, Lariat AS. Characteristics of sheltered homeless families. Am J Public Health. 1986;76:9.

8. Baxter E, Hopper K. Troubled on the streets. In: Talbott JA, ed. The chronic mental patient. New York: Grune & Stratton; 1984.

9. Department of Health and Human Services. Innovative homeless and indigent contract: memorandum to all Nurses in the Public Health Service. Rockville, Maryland: US Public Health Service; March 1987.

10. Goldman H, Morrissey J. The alchemy of mental health policy: homelessness and the fourth cycle of reform. Am J Public Health. 1985;75:727–731.

11. Hartmann EL. The functions of sleep. New Haven: Yale University Press; 1973.

12. Hopper K. Homelessness: reducing the distance. N Engl J Hum Serv. Fall 1983;3(4):30–47.

13. Hopper K, Hamberg J. The making of America's homeless: from skid row to new poor. New York: Community Service Society of New York; 1984.

14. Koegel P, Farr R, Burnam M. Heterogeneity in an inner-city homeless population: a comparison between individuals surveyed in traditional skid row locations and in voucher hotel rooms. Psychosoc Rehab J. 1986;10:31–46.

15. Lamb H. The homeless mentally ill. In: Homelessness: Critical Issues for Policy and Practice. Boston: The Boston Foundation; 1987.

16. Lenehan G, McInnis B, O'Donnell D, Hennessey M. A nurses' clinic for the homeless. Am J Nurs. 1985;85:11.

17. Levine IS, Haggard LK. Homelessness as a public health mental health problem. In: Rochefort D, ed. Handbook on Mental Health Policy in the United States. New York: Greenwood Press, 1989.

18. Long M. What are the health needs of the homeless? the homeless: findings from the Ohio study. Presented at special meeting on the homeless with alcohol related problems. Rockville, MD: National Institute on Alcohol Abuse and Alcoholism; 1986.

19. Marin P. Helping and hating the homeless. Harper's. January 1987:39–49.

20. Martin MA. What are the health needs of the homeless? The role of nurses in meeting the health/mental health needs of the homeless. Proceedings of the Workshop, March 6–7. Washington, DC: American Public Health Association; 1986:63–66.

21. Maurin JT. Knowledge gaps which can be addressed through nursing research. The role of nurses in meeting the health/mental health needs of the homeless. Proceedings of the Workshop, March 6–7. Washington, DC: American Public Health Association; 1986:67–76.

22. Mulkern V, Bradley V. Service utilization and service preferences of homeless persons. Psychosoc Rehab J. 1986; 10:23–31.

23. National Coalition for the Homeless: National neglect/national shame: America's homeless: outlook. Washington, DC: National Coalition for the Homeless; Winter 1986–87.

24. Rafferty M. The role of nurses in meeting the needs of the elderly homeless. The role of nurses in meeting the health/mental health needs of the homeless. Proceedings of the workshop, March 6–7. Washington, DC: American Public Health Association; 1986:179–190.

25. Rog D, Andranovich G, Rosenblum S. Intensive case management for persons who are homeless and mentally ill. Washington, DC: COSMOS Corporation; 1987.

26. Smith LE. Excerpts of testimony before the District of Columbia Commission on Homelessness. Washington, DC: Community of Hope; November 20, 1984.

27. Stark LR. Who are the homeless? What are the subgroups? What are the causes of homelessness? The role of nurses in meeting the health/mental health needs of the homeless. Proceedings of the workshop, March 6–7. Washington, DC: American Public Health Association; 1986:51–55.

28. Stark L. Blame the system, not its victims. In: Homelessness: critical issues for policy and practice. Boston: The Boston Foundation; 1987:7–11.

29. Talbott JA, Lamb HR. Summary and recommendations. In: Lamb HR, ed. The homeless mentally ill. Washington, DC: National Institute of Mental Health; 1984.

30. US Department of Housing and Urban Development: A report to the Secretary on the homeless and emergency shelters. Washington, DC: US Government Printing Office; 1984.

31. Wright JD. The Johnson–Pew "Health Care for the Homeless" Program. Paper presented at special meeting on The homeless with alcohol related problems. Rockville, MD: National Institute on Alcohol Abuse and Alcoholism; 1985.

29

Donna R. Baughcum

Abused Persons

DESCRIPTION
ASSESSMENT
TREATMENT MODALITIES AND RELATED NURSING ROLES
Nurse–Client Relationship
Framework for Nursing Intervention
COMMON NURSING DIAGNOSES
CATEGORIES OF ABUSE
Spouse Abuse
   Description
   Assessment, Nursing Diagnoses, and Interventions
   Treatment Modalities
Rape
   Description
   Assessment and Nursing Diagnoses
   Treatment Modalities
Child Abuse and Neglect
   Description
   Assessment and Nursing Diagnoses
   Treatment Modalities
Child Sexual Abuse
   Description
   Assessment and Nursing Diagnoses
   Treatment Modalities
CASE STUDY

OBJECTIVES

After reading this chapter, the reader will be able to:

1. Define the term abuse *and list categories of abuse*
2. Identify assessment measures for four categories of abuse
3. Describe the four principal nursing diagnoses in order of priority for each of the four categories of abuse
4. Conduct an initial interview with victims of abuse
5. Prepare a nursing care plan for a victim of abuse.

DESCRIPTION

The term *abuse*, as defined by Webster, means "to take unfair or undue advantage of; to use or treat so as to injure, hurt or damage." This definition implies the misuse of power by one individual to inflict pain and injury on another who is less powerful. The person who misuses power is the abuser; the recipient or target of this behavior becomes the victim. The abuser–victim relationship can be seen not only between individuals but also between whole groups, countries, societies, or races. In this chapter, the individual victim is the focus of discussion.

Abuse may involve omission: the failure to behave in a reasonable way to avert injury, pain, or damage to another person. This behavior is known as neglect and is seen most often in caregiving relationships in which the caregiver often is the more powerful member. Neglect is most often identified in families between parents and children but can also be found between grown children and their elderly parents or other relatives. Institutional neglect, which is reported in nursing homes, chronic care facilities, and mental institutions, has become a problem in this country's health care delivery system.

Sexually abusive behavior refers to some action such as fondling of the genital area, oral–genital contact, or penetration of a bodily orifice. Sexual abuse of children and adults includes expressions of aggression, cruelty, and misuse of power. This abuse hampers the psychological development of the victim by betraying his or her basic trust of a family member, spouse, or friend. A related concept, specific to the definition of sexual abuse, is the ability of both parties to give free and informed consent to a sexual relationship. A sexual relationship between a child and an adult is wrong— and abusive—because the fundamental condition of informed consent has not been met.

ASSESSMENT

Although definitions of physical and emotional abuse of persons are changing in the legal and health care systems, it is estimated that 8 million to 10 million of the 56 million families in the US are affected by some type of physical violence and abuse.[7] It also has been estimated that three of every four runaway adolescents are involved in some type of abusive family situation.[5] Rape, whether it is random, date, or familial, is still believed to be one of the most underreported crimes against persons;[3] the 1985 figure of 138,490 rapes is considered to be only half the number that actually took place.[11] National Center on Child Abuse and Neglect data indicate that 1,928,000 cases of child abuse were reported to protective services in 1985.[5] Three million to four million women and men are estimated to be subjected to physical battering by their sexual partner.[12] The figures on elder abuse and neglect are difficult to obtain, because most states do not have

mandatory reporting of such abuse. However, it is estimated that 4% of the population over age 65—1 million elderly—are abused each year.[8]

No population or socioeconomic group is immune to abuse or neglect. Whenever any infant, child, adolescent, adult, or elderly person or group is perceived as powerless in a social or professional situation, there is a potential for physical or psychological abuse and neglect. Also, any societal subgroup that can be labelled deviant has an increased risk for abuse. Vulnerable and nonconformist individuals and groups thus are highly susceptible to abuse. Foster infants and children, stepchildren, AIDS clients, the developmentally disabled, and the severely physically handicapped are at particular risk. In general, the less powerful the person within a social structure, the less likely the person is to acknowledge any type of abuse openly or to seek the assistance of others.[8]

Because nurses function in a variety of health care settings, they have a unique opportunity to identify and assess abused persons, consult with and report to the necessary interdisciplinary agencies, and initiate reversal of the victimization. The prepared nurse can provide comprehensive assessment and diagnosis as well as crisis intervention services to victims of abuse and to their families. In certain settings, the nurse acts as client advocate in interpreting and communicating the victim's needs to the family, health care system, and any other agencies involved, i.e., social services, police, and the courts. In a case manager role, the nurse acts as coordinator of interdisciplinary services and as a community liaison to assure quality of services and positive patient outcomes. As a certified practitioner and clinical specialist working with abused persons, the nurse engages in long-term therapeutic interventions with victims and their families and assists in preventing future victimization.

In psychiatric settings, the incidence, prevalence, and negative effects of abuse often are seen in disguised forms, such as marital difficulties, depression with suicidal ideation, borderline personality disorder, and self-destructive alcohol and substance abuse.[4] Obtaining a history of possible victimization can be difficult but is not impossible if the nurse is sensitized to the possibility that abuse has occurred.

TREATMENT MODALITIES AND RELATED NURSING ROLES

The nursing care of abused persons is one of the most difficult tasks facing the nurse today. Unless the nurse is sensitized to the possibility that abuse might exist, she or he may fail to pick up the cues from the client and thus unwittingly contribute further to the abuse.

Nurse–Client Relationship

An effective tool for assisting individuals to regain a sense of power and control over their lives is the therapeutic nurse–client relationship. Abused individuals, whether adults or children, have been robbed of power and control over their own lives and often distrust others who offer assistance. An empathic, sensitive nurse who is knowledgeable about the complex dynamics of abuse can make the difference in determining a positive outcome in the resolution of the trauma inflicted by the abuse.

Unless nurses are comfortable with their own feelings about abuse and victimization, it is difficult to convey comfort and support to the victim of abuse. Instead, nurses will focus on their own reactions and feelings, rather than on the needs and concerns of the client. Also, the nurse can end up judging the victim rather than trying to understand what has happened.

How does the nurse become comfortable with feelings about abuse and develop constructive values regarding victims of abuse? Values clarification is a useful framework through which to work through responses to abuse. The process can be accomplished individually or in a group. It requires that the nurse develop self-awareness skills, which can be useful in the care of victims of all types of abuse. Structured learning activities for values clarification of attitudes and responses to rape[3] can be altered to apply to other categories of abuse.

Developing self-awareness with regard to abuse can be a difficult, growth-producing process. It requires the nurse to examine attitudes regarding being a male or female in contemporary society and the inequality of power between men and women and between adults and children. It requires the nurse to look at the past and present in examining how imbalances of power have impacted on the self. Also, the nurse needs to identify personal feelings about individuals who misuse power to inflict pain on others and then must be able to separate personal feelings toward the abuser from those of the client. Only after going through this process of values clarification is the nurse prepared to enter into a truly therapeutic relationship with the client.

Framework for Nursing Intervention

Crisis intervention theory is a useful framework for providing nursing care to victims of abuse and their families. *Crisis* is defined as an upset in a steady state that results in disequilibrium and disorganization. The disclosure or identification of abuse usually results in a crisis for the victim and the victim's family. Therefore, knowledge of crisis theory and intervention strategies is essential, for the nurse is called on to provide the initial assessment and treatment for the victim, regardless of the setting (see Chapter 35).

As noted earlier, the nurse is capable of providing comprehensive assessment and crisis intervention to victims of abuse and their families and also acts as an advocate for the victim. The nurse also may act as coordinator and case manager to provide interdisciplinary services to the victim and family, so that duplication of effort and further abuse or neglect by the system is avoided.

If, after an initial period of assessment and intervention, it becomes clear that a victim needs specific psychiatric services, the nurse generalist can make an appropriate referral to a mental health clinician. This referral should be based on the needs and wishes of the victim, which can be communicated to an experienced and knowledgeable clinician. The most appropriate referral would be to a masters' or doctorally prepared psychiatric nurse, a psychologist, a social worker, or a psychiatrist who has specialized knowledge of and expertise in the treatment of victims of abuse. Group treatment in lieu of or in conjunction with individual treatment often is recommended for victims of abuse. Support groups composed of victims of similar types of abuse frequently help empower the victims to begin to regain control and direction of their lives. Family members of abuse victims often find support groups helpful also, as they struggle to meet their needs and the needs of the victim.

COMMON NURSING DIAGNOSES

How the victim reacts to an abusive experience depends on the type of abuse, its duration and severity, the relationship of the abuser to the victim, and the victim's age and developmental level. Four primary nursing diagnoses characterize the responses of almost all victims of abuse. These diagnoses, refined by data from the specific situation, provide the basis for the formulation of nursing intervention to victims of abuse and are appropriate within the theoretical model of crisis intervention. The diagnoses are anxiety, powerlessness, guilt, and disturbance in self-concept. These diagnoses are made more specific for the individual client after collecting more data relating to the nature of the abuse, the psychological and emotional developmental level of the client, family history, current functioning abilities, and support systems available to the client.

Anxiety is a common diagnosis for individuals who are experiencing a crisis. Related nursing diagnoses that may be appropriate are post-trauma response and rape trauma syndrome.

Powerlessness occurs in all victims of abuse: the reality that the individual has become a victim implies a loss of power and control. The sense of powerlessness can be terrifying and permeate every aspect of a victim's life to the point that he or she may be unable to function normally. Hospitalization occasionally is required. At the very least, powerlessness heightens anxiety. In addition, the sense of having no control over life can prohibit a victim from being freed from a chronically abusive situation, thus perpetuating a cycle of revictimization.

Guilt is a common reaction to all types of abuse, regardless of the reality of the situation. For example, a woman may be raped under the most random circumstances but still maintain that somehow she was negligent in her vigilance and caused the attack. Guilt can prevent action for self-protection against further abuse and perpetuate the cycle of revictimization.

Self-concept disturbance results when anxiety, powerlessness, and guilt are experienced by the individual for a long period of time. Self-worth becomes devastated, and the victim's sense of competence is altered. Victims frequently have difficulty performing normal roles and tasks of daily living, such as job tasks, parenting, school work, and, in some extremes, daily hygiene. The abuse of one individual by another can be an overpowering blow to the personality and functioning potential of the victim. Thus, it is crucial that the abuse be detected quickly and strategies for intervention be implemented in such a way as to maximize the possibility for a successful, timely outcome.

CATEGORIES OF ABUSE

Although there are many categories of abuse, this chapter will discuss only four major ones: spouse abuse, rape, child physical abuse and neglect, and child sexual abuse.

Spouse Abuse

DESCRIPTION

There is no single definition of spouse abuse. In this chapter, the term *spouses* refers to adults who are married or otherwise involved in an intimate relationship. Spouse abuse means physical violence between members of the same household. Assaults on women are the most common and result in more serious injury.[12] Battering precipitates one in every four suicide attempts by all women and half of all suicide attempts by black women. Half of all rapes of women over the age of 30 are part of the battering syndrome. Battered women comprise a significant percentage, not only of rape and suicide victims, but also of psychiatric patients, alcoholics, and mothers of abused children.[12]

Eighty per cent of battered women report their injuries at least once to medical personnel, and 40% seek medical attention on at least five occasions.[12] Often, the health care professional is the first person these women turn to, if only because the injuries require medical attention. Battered women often are afraid to admit to having been victimized for fear of reprisal from their spouse and because they frequently feel responsible for having caused the beating. This guilt leads to feelings of failure, helplessness, and powerlessness. Thus, they may present to the health care provider in ways that can preclude the recognition of the abuse. For example, they may explain the injuries as being self-inflicted or accidental, or they may present with symptoms that are not directly related to the abuse, such as stress-related complaints (sleeplessness, anxiety, drug overdosage with little actual evidence of ingestion) or complaints associated with the later stages of battering;

i.e., alcoholism and depression. Thus, the battered woman's condition may be misdiagnosed, and she will be treated only for the obvious presenting complaints, being then sent home to await the next episode of violence.

Walker describes a pattern of spouse abuse that consists of three phases: the tension-building phase, the acute beating phase, and finally the loving phase.[13] During the first phase, tension builds, usually over a series of small incidents, such as the wife asking for money or serving a meal that displeases her spouse. What follows is inevitable. The woman becomes the object of assaultive behavior ranging from verbal insults to punches, choking, knifing, or shooting. When the battering is over, the couple moves into the third phase, in which the batterer is remorseful and assures his spouse that he will not harm her again. She desperately wishes to believe him, so they are reconciled, and the cycle continues.

Why do women stay in relationships with men who batter? Women who are involved in an abusive relationship often feel responsible for, and therefore guilty about, the abusive behavior. They believe that their actions within the relationship can stop the abuse. They then become placators who try to please and not to antagonize their husbands. They live in hope that if they try hard enough, the men will love them and not beat them. However, this hope is unlikely to be realized, as the husband continues his pattern of violence and dominance. Ultimately, the wife, having little sense of self-worth, can become immobilized, unable to remove herself from the relationship.[13]

In addition, society's view of women often contributes to the difficulty wives experience in their struggle to free themselves from an abusive partner. Traditionally, women are believed to be responsible for the well-being of the family and to have a duty to be loyal and protective of family members. Until the women's movement began in the 1960s, many women had little status in the relationship and historically were submissive to their husbands. To leave a marriage, whatever the reason, still renders many women vulnerable to financial difficulties, particularly those who have no income or marketable skills and those with responsibility for children. Many women also risk stigmatization by relatives, friends, and churches. Others are fearful of retaliation for attempting to leave the relationship; many battered wives state, "he would find and kill me if I left." This inability to act in the face of repeated physical abuse can be extremely frustrating to the outside professional who is attempting to intervene in the family. Efforts to coerce the wife out of the victim role by well-meaning medical staff, social services, and police can be fruitless, as the wife drops charges against her husband and returns home with him.

ASSESSMENT, NURSING DIAGNOSES, AND INTERVENTIONS

The outlook for a victim of spousal abuse does not have to be bleak, and change is possible. It is important for the health care provider to be sensitive to the subtle cues to the abuse and knowledgeable about intervention skills and the community resources available for these women. Using a nonjudgmental approach, the nurse can treat the victim with respect and as a person who is capable of making decisions. The victim may then be able to gather the necessary strength to take appropriate action. It is especially important to realize that the nurse's timetable for action is not always the client's timetable. The client has the right to change in a manner consistent with experiences, personality, and the present situation. If the necessary information is given about the resources available, and if a choice is made to act, the realization may emerge that there are alternatives that ultimately may be life saving.

The nurse can play a critical role in the initial assessment phase when the victim arrives at a health care facility for treatment of injuries. Persons who have been physically assaulted often suffer from injuries at multiple sites, rather than a discrete injury at a specific site. The sites of these injuries are informative. Nonabusive injuries tend to be on the extremities, whereas abusive injuries tend to be around the head, neck, chest, abdomen, and genitalia.[12] In addition, the extent of the injuries may be inconsistent with the description of how they occurred. For example, a woman may come for treatment of two black eyes and attribute the injury to having "fallen on a wet floor."

If the nurse, after the initial examination, suspects that the client might have been beaten, she should ask, "did someone do this to you?" If clients do not choose to acknowledge that they have been victimized, the nurse still needs to record the assessment that the client's description of the injuries is inconsistent with the extent and pattern of the injury. In this way, there will be a record of suspected abuse, which may be useful during future visits for treatment. With careful tracking of these cases, more factual information will be available to assist these persons to recognize their own victimization and begin to break out of the pattern of violence.

If the client does admit to being battered, it is important that evidence be gathered that will be useful if the victim chooses to prosecute either then or later. With the victim's consent, photographs of the injuries should be taken and kept with any other evidence that validates the abuse, such as torn clothing. These materials should be carefully labeled with the victim's name and date of collection, then sealed and stored in a secure place. Most hospital emergency rooms and health clinics have protocols for the collection of evidence of abuse, as well as designated secure areas for storage. The police should be called if the victim gives permission. If the victim does not give permission to notify police, the evidence should still be saved in the event that there is a later decision to prosecute.

For victims of spouse abuse, the nursing diagnoses that have priority are often powerlessness followed by self-concept disturbance, guilt, and anxiety (Table 29-1) (see Chapter 13). The problem of spouse abuse is usually chronic, with periodic episodes of random violence within a longstanding relationship between the victim and the abuser. Therefore, the loss of power and

TABLE 29-1
Selected common nursing diagnoses in order of priority

CATEGORY OF ABUSE	NURSING DIAGNOSES
Spouse abuse	Powerlessness Self-concept disturbance Guilt Anxiety
Rape	Anxiety Powerlessness Guilt Self-concept disturbance
Physical abuse of children	Anxiety Self-concept disturbance Powerlessness Guilt
Child sexual abuse	Anxiety Powerlessness Guilt Self-concept disturbance

control is pervasive throughout the victim's life, resulting in impairment of self-concept. However, when these women begin to feel empowered, they begin to feel better about themselves, and change is possible. As one former victim stated, "I may have only one dress to wear, but I'm never gonna feel like dirt again." Another nursing diagnosis that can thus be identified is dysfunctional family processes.

Before discharge, the nurse can provide the victim with information that can be useful in helping the victim begin to move away from the battering pattern and possibly to save a life. The victim should be given an emergency hotline number, along with a list of advocacy, police, legal, and welfare services available in the community. Since the 1960s, a number of communities have opened temporary safe shelters for battered women and their children. While there, they receive counseling to decide the best course of action for themselves and their children.

Helping the victim develop a contingency plan for preventing future episodes of beating is also useful. For example, is another set of car keys available? Is there a friend or neighbor on whom to call? And, can money be saved to be used in an emergency? Working with victims around these specific plans can begin to give them the first feelings that, indeed, they can protect themselves and their children.

TREATMENT MODALITIES

Battered women, as well as the men who beat them, need outside psychotherapeutic intervention in order to break the pattern of violence. Individual psychotherapy can help individuals understand the dynamics of abuse and how their own unique history and personality rendered them vulnerable to the establishment of this destructive relationship. Only then can they begin to develop alternatives that are more satisfying and safer as well as ego-enhancing for each individual.

One of the most useful modalities for these women is group treatment: the support of others who have similar difficulties is a powerful tool in assisting individuals to make positive changes in their lives. Group therapy also is effective for male abusers. Usually, they have been ordered by a court to attend and thus come initially because it is preferable to jail. To be a part of a group whose members have experienced similar if not worse patterns of violence in their families of origin is a powerful agent for change. For the women, group therapy often begins in shelters for women, where the battered victim first begins to realize that she is not alone, that others have experienced what she has. With the support of the group, the victim's self-esteem is enhanced and guilt is diminished, so that she begins to feel empowered to take control of her own life. It is then that she can start to utilize the resources available in her community. For example, she may need financial assistance, job training, child care, and legal counsel in order to establish herself and her children in a new and more independent way of life.

Rape

DESCRIPTION

The term *rape* is derived from the Latin word *rapere*, which means to steal or seize. Rape is defined as an assault in which sexual penetration of a body orifice occurs against the victim's will and without the victim's consent. Threats, intimidation, and physical violence may be employed in an effort to exert dominance and control over the victim. In one act, rape is both "a blow to the body and a blow to the mind."[3] It implies a total loss of self, whereby the victim is treated as a mere object to be used by the rapist for the gratification of the need for power and dominance over another.[3] Because rape can be a random event, everyone is vulnerable to the possibility of rape, regardless of sex, age, or race.

Reported rapes in the US are rising at an alarming rate. Rape also is considered to be one of the most underreported crimes. Although men can be raped, women are by far the most frequently reported victims in our society. A total of 138,490 rapes were reported in this country in 1985.[10] However, it is estimated that this figure represents only 50% of the actual number of rapes that year.[10] Men who are raped rarely report the crime, because of the stigma of being victims of a sexual crime, and women often do not report out of fear of reprisal from their attacker, embarrassment at the prospect of public disclosure of the crime, anxiety about the lengthy court process, and the stigma that often attaches to women who have been victims of a sexual attack.

ASSESSMENT AND NURSING DIAGNOSES

As in any crisis, the initial encounter between the helping professional and the client is crucial in either aiding recovery or contributing to the distress. Therefore, it is important for the nurse to have an under-standing of how such an assault can affect the victim, both in terms of the immediate, acute reaction, as well as the effects days, weeks, and months after the attack. The victim should be assessed for the defining characteristics associated with rape trauma syndrome (see Chapter 13).

Nursing diagnoses in order of priority are anxiety, powerlessness, guilt, and self-concept disturbance. Rape by definition is episodic abuse, or at best an isolated event, rather than a chronic pattern of interaction. The degree to which the victim's anxiety can be alleviated and the sense of power restored determines the severity of the guilt and self-concept disturbance. Therefore, the nurse who is planning for the care of the rape victim assesses the level of the client's anxiety and intervenes appropriately and quickly to prevent further symptom development and to restore the client to precrisis functioning. Rape trauma syndrome, as developed in Chapter 13, can also be a useful nursing diagnosis referring to the sequelae of responses following rape.

TREATMENT MODALITIES

A primary treatment model for rape victims is an issue-oriented crisis-intervention model that begins with the first contact with the victim. The client is considered "normal" and therefore managing adequately in the lifestyle prior to this crisis. The focus is on the rape itself, and the goal is to aid victims to return to the precrisis level of functioning as soon as possible. Previous problems not directly associated with the rape are not priority issues. Crisis counseling is not considered psychotherapy. Whenever the victim indicates that other issues are of concern, or if the victim becomes suicidal or psychotic, a referral is made to another treatment program.

Telephone counseling after the initial contact has proved useful in many rape program protocols. It provides quick access to the victim and places the burden on the nurse to seek out the client at a time when she is in crisis and having difficulty with decision-making and reaching out for assistance. Also, intervention via the telephone allows the victim more control than if she has to come to the nurse in a health care setting. This is an important concept for the individual who has been robbed of power and control as a result of being raped. Telephone counseling also encourages the resumption of a normal lifestyle for the victim and can be very cost-effective. As one rape victim stated, "I never would have been able to walk in the door for counseling, after the hospital visit, but I could not have gone on had it not been for that nurse who kept calling me during those weeks after the attack."

Child Abuse and Neglect

DESCRIPTION

For centuries, children were physically abused and neglected by their parents or caretakers, but little was done to provide protection for them, as government and health care providers were reluctant to interfere in family problems. However, in the early 1960s, Dr. C. Henry Kempe coined the term "battered child syndrome," and the American health care community began to concern itself with this difficult manifestation of family violence.[1] Legislation for the protection of children was passed, and federal funds gradually became available to provide research and treatment for the abused child.

The Federal Child Abuse Prevention and Treatment Act (P.L. 100-294 Section 14) defines child abuse and neglect as "physical or mental injury, sexual abuse or exploitation, negligent treatment, or maltreatment of a child by a person who is responsible for the child's welfare, under circumstances which indicate that the child's health or welfare is harmed or threatened."[9] In this chapter, child sexual abuse will be covered as a separate category of abuse.

Most experts in the field believe that there is no one specific cause for child abuse and neglect. Instead, certain risk factors have been identified that make certain families vulnerable to abusing their children. These factors can be derived from three stress areas within the family—the child, the parent, and the situational context. An example of a risk factor produced by the child is a child who is different from the rest of the family by virtue of a handicap, behavior, or temperament. Thus, foster or stepchildren tend to be more vulnerable to abuse. An example of a parent risk factor is a history of having been abused himself or herself in the family of origin or a parent suffering from a psychiatric illness or addiction. Finally, examples of situational risk factors are unemployment, isolation, frequent mobility, and an unstable parental relationship characterized by excessive punitive discipline and assaultive interaction.[1] There are other risk factors in child abuse and neglect, and research continues to attempt to understand what renders families vulnerable to abuse of their children. Each family is different, and each family story is unique. Only by understanding the social, familial, psychological, and physiologic characteristics of the individuals in each situation can one begin to intervene helpfully with the abusive family.

ASSESSMENT AND NURSING DIAGNOSES

When assessing a child for physical abuse or neglect, the nurse should be sensitive to the possibility that abuse exists but should avoid premature conclusions. Because it is repugnant to consider parents inflicting physical pain and damage to their children, health care providers sometimes join the parents in denying the possibility that abuse has occurred. Alternatively, the provider may be so zealous to discover victims of abuse that premature judgments are made and conclusions drawn on less than adequate information. In both cases, neither the child nor the family is provided the services necessary to meet their needs.

Any time a discrepancy is found between the history of how an injury occurred and the actual physical evidence, the possibility of child abuse must be considered. Careful evaluation and history-taking are necessary, as is concrete documentation of injuries by means of photographs and detailed descriptions. Physical evidence of child abuse may include any injury in an infant under 12 months of age, repeated or multiple injuries of a child of any age, and fractures in various stages of healing. Also, intracranial injuries, inability to move certain body parts, undue irritability, and any other neurologic signs of brain damage should alert the nurse to the need for further assessment. Any unexplained cuts, burns, bruises, or rope or strap marks, as well as abdominal distention or bleeding from any body orifice, should be investigated. Poisoning of children may follow a family crisis and should be evaluated further. Behavioral indicators of possible child abuse include extreme fright, blunting of affect, withdrawal, or expressions of helplessness. Helplessness can be demonstrated by actual verbal statements from the child or by behaviors such as silent crying or suicidal ideation. Child abuse should be considered when hearing reports of acting out behaviors, such as running away from home, substance abuse, or truancy from school.

Indicators of parental neglect of children include failure to thrive in infants, unexplained weight loss, malnutrition, and dehydration under unexplained circumstances. In addition, signs of neglect can include severe hunger, poor hygiene, dirty or inappropriate clothing, and abandonment for periods of time that may be unsafe given the child's age and psychological development. Finally, whenever there are delays of days or weeks in seeking health care for injuries, one must consider the possibility of child neglect.[2]

It is important that the interview with the child and family be in a setting allowing privacy and freedom from interruption. The initial interview sets the tone for the evaluation and the outcome of the intervention. Therefore, it is important that the nurse interviewer be familiar with the principles of interviewing for assessment. The goal of the interaction is to establish a level of trust with the parents and child so that sufficient information can be obtained and entry made into the family system. Only then can nursing intervention be effective.

The parents and child should be interviewed separately. In this manner, all members of the family can share their concerns privately, and discrepancies in the stories of the injury can be discerned more easily. Sometimes, very young children have difficulty separating from their parents. However, every effort short of inflicting additional trauma on the child should be made to allow children privacy to tell their version of what happened.

In conducting the interview with the child, the nurse should be as nonthreatening as possible in tone of voice, conduct, and choice of words. The nurse should use language appropriate for the child's chronologic age and development. The use of age-appropriate toys such as puppets and dolls can encourage the child to tell what happened. Drawing materials are useful adjuncts to talking, as many youngsters like to illustrate what they sometimes have difficulty putting into words (Fig. 29-1). Throughout the session with the child, the nurse

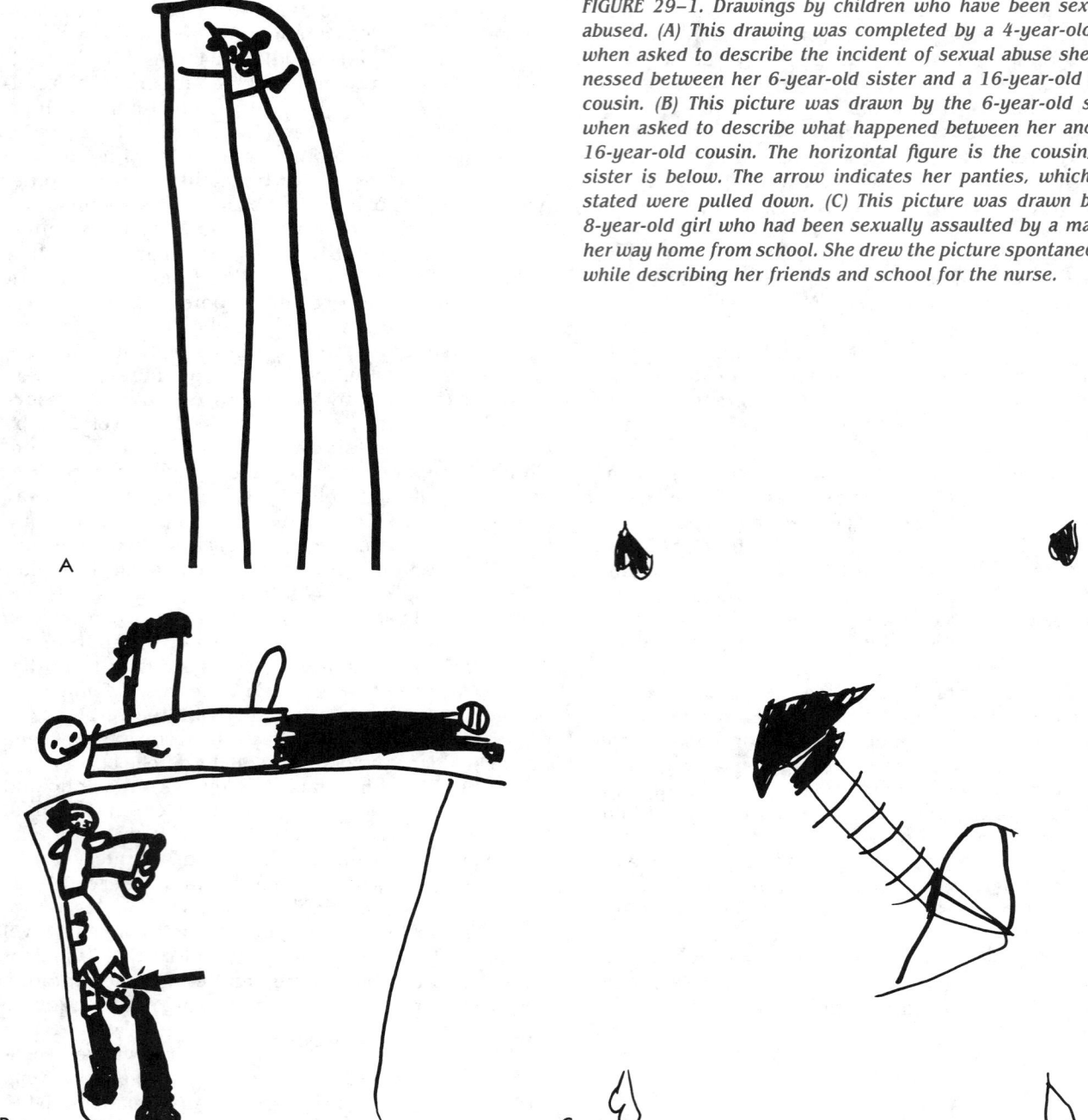

A

B

C

FIGURE 29–1. Drawings by children who have been sexually abused. (A) This drawing was completed by a 4-year-old girl when asked to describe the incident of sexual abuse she witnessed between her 6-year-old sister and a 16-year-old male cousin. (B) This picture was drawn by the 6-year-old sister when asked to describe what happened between her and her 16-year-old cousin. The horizontal figure is the cousin; the sister is below. The arrow indicates her panties, which she stated were pulled down. (C) This picture was drawn by an 8-year-old girl who had been sexually assaulted by a man on her way home from school. She drew the picture spontaneously while describing her friends and school for the nurse.

should be assessing, not only how the child relates to the nurse, but also the child's appearance, mood or affect, coping mechanisms, and concept of self. In other words, a thorough mental status evaluation should be completed. This evaluation will be critical in planning intervention for the child and family.

The problem of physical abuse and neglect is often a longstanding one, with periodic violence. The child frequently knows no other way of life except to be on the receiving end of the parent's violent or neglectful behavior. If one parent inflicts the injuries, usually, the other parent is unable to protect the child and prevent the abuse. This inability to protect is equally damaging to the youngster, who may come to feel that no place is safe and no one is trustworthy. In the initial crisis setting, the most immediate psychological problem is the child's *anxiety*. However, the most difficult nursing diagnosis to deal with is the child's self-concept disturbance resulting from the chronic nature of the abuse, followed by powerlessness and guilt (see Table 29-1). Children feel powerless by virtue of their size or dependence in relation to their parents, but it is especially difficult if those parents exert that power in physically destructive ways. In addition, children are developmentally egocentric: they believe that they are the center of the universe and the cause of all bad things that happen in their immediate environment. Thus, they frequently believe that they caused their parents to act in a violent way toward them and that they deserve the treatment. For example, a 6-year-old boy who had been treated for cigarette burns on his back stated, "I picked up a cigarette butt and my daddy told me not to."

It is important that the nurse keep the child informed about what is going to happen in each step of the evaluation and the treatment of the injuries. In preparation for the physical examination or treatment procedures, anticipatory guidance should be given in terms of what the physical sensations will be. Words such as "wet and cold" or "pricking pressure" should be used rather than "pain" and "hurt." The child should be given an opportunity to express concerns and ask questions. The nurse must not make promises that cannot be kept. For example, it may be a mistake to tell children either that they will be admitted to the hospital or that they will be allowed to return home with the parents before the evaluation and protective service investigation is completed.

Trust is an essential component of the interview with the parents, also. Intimidation and judgments must be avoided if the nurse expects to gather an accurate account of what happened to the child. An alliance of concern and support is necessary in order to gain entry into the family system. It usually is more helpful to discuss the child's history with the parents before discussing the present injury. Important information includes the family composition, the prenatal history of the child, and the child's growth and development. This early history provides data concerning how the child is perceived by the family and his or her role and place within the system. Often, abused children are seen as "different" or "bad" from the moment of their birth or entry into the family. Assessment of the family's current situation also is important. Areas of inquiry include living conditions, financial status, crises within the past year, and kinds of network supports available to the parent. These supports might include extended family, friends, and neighbors who are seen as helpful to the parents in coping with the demands and stresses on them. Another nursing diagnosis that could be considered is dysfunctional family processes.

The child's injury generally will be the most anxiety-producing topic. The nurse's approach needs to be low-key and nonjudgmental, allowing the parents to tell their story in their own words. Ample time should be allowed so that anxiety is reduced for the nurse and the parent. No party should feel rushed or hurried. The following points should be covered: (1) the circumstances of the injury; i.e., what was the child doing prior to the injury, and who was with the child; (2) the nature of the injury; i.e., how did the injury occur, and how was it discovered; (3) events after the injury; i.e., who initiated action, and when was medical assistance sought; and (4) the concerns, fears, and worries of the parents.

When there are sufficient data to suggest the possibility of child abuse, the health care provider is obliged by law to report the case to child protective services. Parents need to be informed of this decision to report. They should be told the reasons for reporting and what to expect. Telling a parent that a report will be filed is not easy but can be a positive step in preventing further abuse and in helping the family gain needed community services. If this information is presented as something that is required by law and as an aid to the family, the outcome can be perceived as helpful to both child and family, as well as to the nurse.

TREATMENT MODALITIES

Treatment of child abuse and neglect is complicated and difficult, requiring the coordination of a variety of community agencies: medical, psychiatric, protective service, and legal. Therefore, it is crucial that each agency have a clear plan of its role in these cases. Each case must be managed in such a way that the family does not get lost or further abused by the very systems that are designed to help. A multidisciplinary team can be a means of coordinating roles and responsibilities in the care of these families. This team might consist of a physician, social worker, psychiatric nurse, and attorney. Working with abusive families is extremely difficult and stressful. The team can provide much-needed support and peer supervision for the caregivers.

Crisis intervention usually is the initial form of treatment for child abuse. The purpose of this intervention is to reduce the stress affecting the family and to protect the child. Occasionally, a child will need to be hospitalized temporarily or placed in foster care until the home can be made a safe place.

Long-term treatment for these families is needed to reverse the patterns of abusive parenting that frequently are inflicted by one generation on the next. Commitment to group and individual treatment for both parents and children is necessary. This treatment may be mandated by the courts if the family is unwilling to participate voluntarily. Programs involve abusive parents in groups whose purpose is to "parent the parents" and teach new ways of dealing with their children. These programs seem to be the most effective and cost-efficient method of treatment.

Child Sexual Abuse

DESCRIPTION

Child sexual abuse can be divided into three components for the purposes of definition: sexual misuse, rape, and incest. *Sexual misuse* refers to any sexual activity that is inappropriate because of that child's immature age and development and because of the child's role in the family.[7] Sexually misused children can be fondled, masturbated, or enticed to stimulate adults sexually without engaging in coital activity. *Rape* is the term when actual penetration of a body orifice occurs as part of the sexual activity. With very young children, oral penetration is the most frequent type of penetration. The term *incest* refers to the relationship between the victim and the abuser and is used when the abuser is a blood relative or is in a caretaking role, such as a stepparent.

Of the almost 2 million children who were reported as victims of abuse in the 1987 Incidence Study, 113,000 were reported because of sexual maltreatment.[5] Sexual abuse tends to be reported in isolation from other types of child abuse, as shown by the fact that 89% of the reported cases were for sexual abuse alone. Again, these statistics are based on reported cases; the actual numbers of abused children would be much higher. Girls are reported more often than boys by a ratio of 4:1.[5]

Sexual abuse differs from other physical abuse in several ways. First, physical abuse is committed equally by men and women, whereas more than three-fourths of all reported perpetrators of sexual abuse are male. Second, sexual abuse can occur both inside and outside the family, whereas physical abuse tends to occur within the family and to be inflicted by the parents. Third, with sexual abuse, there usually is little physical trauma beyond possibly genital irritation or infection. Thus, the scars may be less visible, if just as devastating, as the obvious ones of physical abuse.

ASSESSMENT AND NURSING DIAGNOSES

When assessing a child who may have been sexually abused, the nurse should be sensitive to the needs of the child and the family. Although the child usually is not in a life-threatening situation with physical injuries, the possibility of sexual abuse creates a crisis for the child and the family. These children need to be treated as a priority, because sexual abuse is a devastating form of child abuse. Most hospital emergency rooms that see children have protocols for intervention in cases of physical and sexual abuse. These protocols include procedures for collection of specimens and other evidence of abuse for possible legal action.

The child usually is brought for treatment when the parent or caretaker suspects that something has happened or when the child has disclosed the abuse. Occasionally, there are physical signs and symptoms, but more often, there has been only some type of verbal disclosure of abusive behavior. Disclosure may be intentional, accidental, or reactive. *Intentional disclosure* occurs when the child chooses someone to tell what has happened. Usually, it is someone who can be trusted and who may be able to stop the abuse. *Accidental disclosure* means just that—the disclosure is accidental. For example, a mother returns home earlier than planned and finds her child and the teenage babysitter naked in bed. *Reactive disclosure* occurs when the child is upset or angry about something other than the abuse and discloses out of anger. Reactive disclosure often occurs with adolescent incest victims who reveal the incestuous behavior, often when angry with either parent, perhaps over a curfew or some

other limit. Regardless of the type of disclosure, who the child chooses to tell is important: that person is usually seen as a supportive protector and ally by the child. The person the child tells can play a critical part in the intervention process and can help to create a positive or negative outcome for both the victim and the family.

Physical indicators of sexual abuse include any trauma to the genital area, such as lacerations, chronic irritations, bruising, or presence of foreign bodies. In addition, the presence of venereal disease in children, either in the genital, anal, or throat area, is strongly indicative of possible sexual abuse. Enuresis and encopresis, particularly of sudden onset, can be indicators of sexual abuse. Pregnancy can also be symptomatic of sexual abuse, especially in early-adolescent girls.

Behavioral indicators include any statement by a child that something has happened. Children rarely lie about sexual abuse. Therefore, their statements should be taken seriously. Another frequent indicator, particularly in young children, is sleep disturbance, which can range from difficulty in going to sleep to inability to sleep alone, nightmares, or frequent waking. Another behavioral indicator of sexual abuse in young children is eroticization of behavior, such as sexualized speech and play and compulsive overt masturbatory activity. Sexually abused preschoolers frequently engage in imitative sexual behaviors with other children or with their dolls that display knowledge they are unlikely to possess unless they have been exposed to or engaged in adult sexual activity. Excessive phobias and fears of specific persons or places also are suggestive. For example, a 4-year-old girl was raped by a stranger in a public restroom. Afterward, she was afraid to go to any bathroom, including her own, unless her mother accompanied her. Separation anxiety, expressed as increased clinging behavior, is frequently reported by mothers of sexually abused young children. A sudden decline in school performance is another common indicator of sexual abuse in latency age children. Also, any change in a child's usual behavior or mood, such as increased aggressiveness, acting out, or withdrawal and depression, can be a clue that the child may have been sexually abused. Running away, especially in young adolescents, is often a reaction to sexual abuse within the family.

Many of these behaviors are ways in which all children exhibit symptoms of distress when they are overwhelmed by forces with which they cannot cope. Therefore, it is important that nurses who regularly assess children be sensitized to the possibility that sexual abuse may be one of the stresses the child is attempting to deal with. Questions such as, "has anyone touched you in your private parts?" should be a routine part of any regular physical examination or psychological evaluation.

The principles of interviewing children and their families described in the preceding section on physical abuse also apply to interviewing suspected victims of child sexual abuse and their families. The nurse needs to know that children who have been sexually abused can present in a variety of ways, depending on their basic personalities and on how they react to stressful situations. Some children are cooperative and compliant to the wishes of the health care providers. Others are highly anxious and have difficulty focusing on the interview itself, even when the content is not stressful. Still other children are quiet and withdrawn and have difficulty sharing any information about themselves. They may be unable to separate from their parents. In this case, it is wise to conduct the interview with the protective parent in the room rather than to increase the child's anxiety level by continued insistence on separation.

Talking with children about sexual matters can be anxiety-producing for the nurse, as well as the child. If the nurse can manage to keep personal anxiety under control and learn to be comfortable dealing with discussions of sex, then the interview will be more productive. Using the same terms that the child uses for private parts helps the child to tell the story more easily; i.e., pee-pee, bum, weenie, etc. Dolls and drawing materials can also aid children to tell what happened, especially if they are having difficulty expressing themselves.

The nurse may be the first person outside the family to hear the child relate what happened. It is important that the nurse obtain as many details about the abuse as the child is able to relate without using leading questions or putting words in the child's mouth. Recording verbatim what the child says is important for documentation of the abuse, as there usually are few physical signs of symptoms.

For victims of child sexual abuse, *anxiety* is an important nursing diagnosis followed by powerlessness, guilt, and self-concept disturbance. Anxiety is related to the crisis-producing event surrounding the disclosure. This is true regardless of whether the abuse is chronic or a one-time occurrence. Sexual abuse is a misuse of trust whereby the child is rendered helpless to control the more powerful adult. Children and adolescent victims often feel responsible for what has happened. If the abuse continues over many months or years, the child's self-concept is most certainly impaired (see Chapter 13). An example is often seen in later life when adults who were victims of incest as children seek psychiatric treatment. Many have lives filled with pain and unsatisfying relationships.

Disclosure of sexual abuse causes a crisis within the family. The nurse should know that it is not unusual for a child to recant the story later. Pressures produced by the turmoil within the family, sometimes including the actual break-up of the family unit if the abuse occurred within the family, can result in a child or parent denying that the abuse took place. For example, the father of a 4-year-old girl, upon learning that his daughter had graphically described fellatio with his middle-aged uncle, initially decided that she must have misinterpreted the uncle's behavior when giving her a cough drop for her sore throat. Interviewing the family of the sexually abused child requires a sensitive, supportive approach, because the family usually is in crisis also. Even if the abuse has occurred outside the family, the guilt and rage of the family are acute and must be dealt with in order that the abused child can receive protection and support from the family.

If the abuse has occurred within the family, the question of divided loyalties arises. If the father is the alleged perpetrator, the mother has to choose whether to believe her husband or her child. This dilemma is more difficult if the mother is dependent on her husband for financial and emotional support. How protective the mother can be for the child not only determines with whom the child is placed, but often is the most important factor in the child's resolution of the abusive experience. Assessing the mother's level of protectiveness, then, is a critical aspect of the interview. Questions that might be useful are: does this mother believe her child's account of the sexual abuse? Is this mother prepared to take the steps necessary to protect her child from the abuser, whoever he is? Has she sought the necessary medical care for her child? Does she have a history of sexual abuse in her own growing up, and if so, how was it handled? The mother's answer will shed light on how she views what has happened to her own child and her protective capacity. The nursing diagnosis dysfunctional family processes may be identified.

TREATMENT MODALITIES

Treatment of sexual abuse is multidimensional and requires the coordination of the medical, legal, and psychosocial services. The cases are emotionally laden and require agency cooperation if intervention is to be successful. Often, the nurse is the case manager who advocates for the victim and coordinates the various necessary services. Goals for treatment include the prevention of further sexual abuse for the victim and the prevention of retaliation for disclosure. Other goals are to reduce the symptomatology of the child, as well as to strengthen the protectiveness of the parents.

Individual play therapy is a useful treatment mode for young children who have been sexually abused. Through play, these children can work through the abusive experience by mastering their anxiety, overcoming their feelings of guilt and powerlessness, and thereby reducing their symptoms. Group treatment is helpful for sexually abused children of all ages but is especially useful for working with adolescent victims. Because working with sexually abused children is complex and emotionally laden, two clinicians often work together. One develops a therapeutic relationship with the child, and the other works with the parents, with joint sessions periodically as needed.

Programs for the treatment of victims of incest often include intensive group work. The offenders, generally the fathers or stepfathers, are usually in one group, the mothers in another group, and the children in a third group. The family remains separated during treatment until the abuser is prepared to admit to the abuse and take responsibility for his actions. Such programs are frequently court mandated; the abuser is ordered to treatment in lieu of jail. Following such treatment, the family may or may not reunite and utilize family therapy. However, long-term treatment of the abuser may be required.

CASE STUDY

Heather B is 7 years old. She was brought for treatment after disclosing to her mother that her maternal uncle was "putting his thing between my legs." This occurred periodically over the last 6 months when she was staying at the uncle's house while her mother was out. Mrs. B is divorced and a single parent. She lives alone with her daughter. Her extended family is nearby and helps with child care so that Mrs. B can maintain a full-time job. Upon learning of the alleged sexual abuse from her daughter, the mother was horrified but acted appropriately and protectively. She immediately took Heather to her pediatrician. There was evidence of penetration, but cultures for venereal disease were negative. Mrs. B also stopped taking Heather to the uncle's house and informed him of her reason. The case was reported to child protective services, who investigated the allegations. During the initial interview with the nurse, Heather presented as an intelligent, attractive youngster whose affect was one of sadness. She was anxious and somewhat withdrawn but became more comfortable as the nurse established rapport with her. She utilized the play materials and was then able to talk more easily about herself, her school, friends, and family and, finally, the sexual abuse. She related that her uncle would come into the bedroom where she was sleeping, lie on top of her, and rub his penis between her legs. This behavior frightened her. She stated that he told her not to tell or she would be sorry. She also said that he did not come into her room every time she visited, but that she always stayed awake fearing that he would. She described having "scary dreams" to the point that she was afraid to go to sleep. She also said that she thought about the abuse frequently and could not concentrate on her schoolwork. Her grades had declined from all A's to C's and D's. She referred to herself as being "stupid."

She said that it was her fault that the abuse occurred, because her uncle had probably found out that she did not like him. Mrs. B reported that Heather had become more helpless and clinging in recent months. Heather cried frequently when the mother had to leave her for even a short time. She requested assistance for dressing, tying her shoes, and other activities she had been able to do independently, stating that she was too "dumb." The diagnosis according to the DSM-III-R was post traumatic stress disorder (see Nursing Care Plan 29-1 for a sample care plan for Heather B).

SUMMARY

A framework by which the nurse can understand the dynamics of abuse and its devastating effects on both adult and child victims is presented. Nurses are in key positions to discover abuse and must be knowledgeable about assessment and intervention skills in order to help these victims. Crisis intervention strategies are the most useful tools for the initial care of victims. The nurse's own self-awareness and values clarification regarding abuse are essential components in effective intervention of any abused client.

Four major categories of abuse are spouse abuse, rape, child physical abuse, and child sexual abuse. Nursing diagnoses frequently identified in abused persons are anxiety, powerlessness, guilt, and self-concept disturbance. Caring for victims of abuse is difficult work. The importance of support for the nurse in terms of supervision and peer support is stressed, as well as careful coordination of other multidisciplinary services involved in these cases.

Research Highlights

Limandri's study of abused women's patterns of seeking help and factors in the nurse's response that facilitate or inhibit change demonstrates the importance of research in clinical nursing practice. The study utilized a descriptive–correlational design applied to interviews with 40 abused women in the San Francisco Bay area who responded to the study advertisements. The participants were predominately Caucasian, between 20 and 58 years of age, of at least high school education, and working mostly in clerical positions or as unpaid homemakers. Fifteen per cent were married, and the mean length of the relationships was 7.8 years.

Limandri's findings were that abused women seek help in a wave-like process. Several contacts with different helpers are more likely than continuing contacts with a single helper over a period of time. The principal factors identified as influential in the abused client's seeking of help were the level of self-esteem, the extent to which the woman identified herself as a victim of abuse, and the helper's response to her disclosure of the abuse. The study also identified 13 responses by nurses that facilitate the continued seeking and responding to intervention, as well as eight responses that inhibit further help-seeking behavior. Although the victim's disclosure of violence

may be disguised or concealed, it is critical for the nurse to acknowledge the violence and take an active advocate role with the client. The study also emphasized that working with abused clients arouses intense countertransference reactions in the nurse that must be addressed if the intervention is to be successful.[6]

Another useful area of research would be to attempt to isolate indicators of vulnerability of families to abuse. These indicators would serve as predictors for abuse, thus permitting early intervention or possibly prevention of abusive behavior. Certain family histories, crises, losses, and personality traits have been identified as producing high-risk situations for abuse within families. However, not enough emphasis has been placed on the study of nonabusive families, who may have many of the stated vulnerabilities but do not resort to abusive behavior. Nurses are involved in areas of health maintenance where they have access to families who may experience many of the stresses that can lead to abuse, yet do not abuse. These families would be useful for comparative study in order to understand the differences between abusive and nonabusive families. Through the contributions of nursing research, new approaches to prevention of abuse in our society can become a reality.

NURSING CARE PLAN 29-1

HEATHER B

NURSING INTERVENTIONS	OUTCOME CRITERIA

NURSING DIAGNOSIS: Anxiety related to sexual abuse

CLIENT GOAL: Gain control over anxiety and be able to function at precrisis level

■ Assist Heather to connect present behaviors as a reaction to abuse by uncle ■ Assure Heather that she is safe and physically intact ■ Assist Heather to talk about the abuse, utilizing drawing materials, dolls, etc. in order to gain mastery of the event	Able to sleep Experiences fewer nightmares Improves schoolwork Tolerates separation from mother Able to dress self

NURSING DIAGNOSIS: Powerlessness related to sexual abuse

CLIENT GOAL: Regain power through belief in own ability and competence

■ Allow Heather to make decisions in interview ■ Teach mother to allow Heather to make decisions at home	Makes decisions on own Functions more independently without mother's presence

NURSING DIAGNOSIS: Guilt related to abusive relationship with uncle

CLIENT GOAL: Relinquish belief of responsibility for causing the abuse

■ Tell Heather that she did her best, and the abuse was not her fault ■ Assist mother to reinforce above message at home ■ Support Heather in her decision to disclose the abuse	Makes no statements of self-blame for the abuse

NURSING DIAGNOSIS: Self-concept disturbance related to sexual abuse

CLIENT GOAL: Believe in self again as a competent 7-year-old

■ Reinforce positive age-appropriate behaviors and encourage family to do same at home ■ Treat Heather as a worthwhile, competent 7-year-old ■ Teach parents to reinforce Heather's strivings to resolve the trauma of the abuse ■ Teach principles of abuse prevention	No longer refers to self as "dumb" or "stupid" Makes statements indicating belief in her own competence

References

1. Bittner S, Newberger EH. Pediatric understanding of child abuse and neglect. Pediatr Rev. 1981;2:197–207.
2. Burgess AW. Psychiatric nursing in the hospital and the community. 4th ed. Englewood Cliffs: Prentice-Hall; 1985.
3. Foley T, Davies MA. Rape: nursing care of victims. St Louis: CV Mosby; 1983.
4. Gelinas DJ. The persisting negative effects of incest. Psychiatry. 1983;46:312–332.
5. Highlights of Official Child Abuse and Neglect Reporting 1985. Denver: American Humane Association; 1987.
6. Limandri BJ. The therapeutic relationship with abused women. J Psychosoc Nurs. 1987;25:9–16.
7. Newberger EH, Bourne R, eds. Unhappy families. Littleton, Massachusetts: PSG; 1985.
8. Pillemer K. The dangers of dependency: new findings on domestic violence against the elderly. Presented at Annual Meeting of American Sociological Association, Washington, DC; August 27, 1985.
9. Public Law 100-294 Section 14, signed April 25, 1988.
10. Sonkin DJ, Martin D, Walker LEA. The male batterer. New York: Springer Publishing; 1985.
11. Source Book of Criminal Justice Statistics. Washington, DC: US Department of Justice; 1986.
12. Stark E, Flitcraft A, Zuckerman D, Grey A, Robison J, Frazier W. Wife abuse in the medical setting: an introduction for health personnel. Monograph Series No. 7. Rockville, Maryland: National Clearinghouse on Domestic Violence; 1981.
13. Walker LE. The battered woman syndrome. New York: Springer Publishing; 1984.

30

Sharon L. Bernier

Mental Health Issues and Nursing in Corrections

OBJECTIVES

After reading this chapter, the reader will be able to:
1. Describe psychosocial issues related to incarceration
2. Describe the prison environment and its hazards
3. Discuss the role of the nurse in a correctional setting
4. Describe a practice model for nursing in corrections
5. Utilize the nursing process in formulating a plan of care with an individual in a correctional setting
6. Suggest a health care team approach to improving prison conditions.

THE CORRECTIONAL SYSTEM

Historical Overview

The late 1970s and the 1980s have seen changes in attitudes toward persons who commit a criminal offense. There has been public demand for more effective detention of criminals. The rehabilitation philosophy of the 1960s and early 1970s appears to have been unsuccessful in stopping recidivism. In fact, many critics of the rehabilitation philosophy point to an increase in crime in the United States during this time.[6]

Both the federal prison system and the state and local systems have experienced unprecedented overcrowding. The U.S. Federal Prison population is increasing 15 times faster than the general population.[11] This system, with a capacity to hold 28,000 prisoners, now has at least 45,000.[11] The nation's jail populations, as distinguished from prisons, are also critically overcrowded, with a prisoner population that has increased by 23% in the last three years. The Bureau of Justice Statistics reported that 274,400 people, 90% male, occupied a jail cell in this country on June 30, 1986. Over half of these persons were in jail awaiting arraignment or trial. This rise in the prison population has been historic in this decade. The United States now locks up 210 people per 100,000 population. More blacks are in prison than are enrolled in colleges, and the women's prison population is growing more rapidly than the men's.[11]

Overcrowding in the jails is related to (1) the overload of the court system, (2) the new laws in some jurisdictions requiring that drug offenders be held until trial, and (3) the inefficiency of the present court system. The 1980s have seen an increase in violent crimes that is considered to be directly related to drug trafficking and drug use in the United States. In 1986, 30% of those persons serving time were arrested on drug charges, as compared with 25% in 1980 and 17% in 1970. It is estimated that by 1990 over one-half of all prisoners will be incarcerated on drug-related charges.[11]

The Environment

A prison is a closed system responsible for the control and management of every aspect of a prisoner's life. Prisons are designed to deny a person freedom and to be a punishment. The issue of punishment has created the greatest conflict for the optimistic, compassionate, and idealistic rehabilitation philosophy. The rehabilitation philosophy was influenced by the growth of the social sciences, especially psychology, in the post-World War II era (1949–1970). Social scientists began to study such things as how environmental factors, over which an individual may have little control, contributed to criminal behavior. This led to the belief that a person should be incarcerated not for punishment, but for rehabilitation. At the same time that the rehabilitation model was being evaluated, a rise in crime and an increase in drug sales and use gained the attention of the media, the public, and politicians.

Advocates of building more prisons and giving longer sentences denounced the rehabilitation philosophy.[6] Two landmark decisions of the 1980s reflected this new mood: (1) The omnibus antidrug law of October 1986 demanded tougher measures to deal with drug users and dealers. This has led to increased arrests and subsequent incarceration in an already overcrowded system; and (2) Federal sentencing guidelines, effective November 1, 1987, limited the discretion federal judges have in determining an appropriate sentence for a convicted offender. These guidelines dictate how long a person *must* be incarcerated (minimum) to have paid for the crime.

It is generally accepted that prisons and jails are hostile environments. This hostility permeates the institution and affects all who are there—the inmate, the corrections worker, and health care personnel. There is an overall high level of anxiety, with a pervasive sense of fear, humiliation, and violence. These are the everyday conditions under which the system functions. A major motivating factor for the correctional system is to maintain order.[5] In prisons with severe overcrowding, most prisoners spend the greater part of each day (up to 22 hours) in their cells or barracks. Prison overcrowding has also created a situation referred to as "double or triple bunking" in which cells originally intended for one person may be occupied by two or three persons. The tension within the facility is a breeding ground for lack of trust and feelings of aggression. This is not a safe place for anyone to live by most of society's standards.[3]

The Prison Population

To have a more complete understanding of the mental health issues within a prison, it is necessary to have a picture of the prisoner in today's system. Most inmates are ethnic minority men between the ages of 16 and 30, whose lives have been marked by poverty, aimlessness, illiteracy, and lack of vocational skills.[5] Their crimes are often related to drugs that they sell and/or use. These young men often have grown up in a subculture with different norms than those of the dominant society. A major problem in providing health care to them is noncompliance with health care regimens. This is often the result of ignorance on the part of the health care worker who has differing cultural views of health and illness. Nurses, when assessing a client's needs, must be aware of the cultural components of illness for various ethnic groups, depending on geographic location.[4]

During the 1980s, an increasing number of women have been jailed. These women prisoners are usually young and are often responsible for minor children. They are generally arrested and jailed for victimless crimes, such as prostitution, but are unable to pay (or "make") their bail.[12]

Assessment

In an article in the *California Prisoner,* Weinstein states that "prisons both collect and create people with psychological problems" (reference 13, p 4). A profile of this population reveals a number of considerations for the nurse when carrying out a psychosocial assessment among prisoners.

1. Most are products of juvenile detention facilities or have been involved in some way with the city or state social services.
2. Many are products of homes, families, or institutions where they were sexually, physically, and psychologically abused.
3. They have great difficulty in dealing with authority figures.
4. Low self-esteem, anger, fearfulness, and feelings of hopelessness and helplessness prevail.
5. Intimacy is a little-known experience, probably a result of basic mistrust of the world.
6. Impulse control is limited and causes both the inmate and the corrections staff to be on guard at all times.
7. Attitudes of arrogance, bragging, swaggering, and disdain are usually defenses for the foregoing feelings.

It is currently estimated that 15% to 20% of all incarcerated people in the United States suffer from a significant mental disorder. This psychiatric subpopulation of prisoners may experience any number of psychiatric disorders (e.g., psychoactive substance use disorder, adult antisocial behavior, impulse control disorder, and schizophrenia). The nurse may observe depression, hallucinations, phobic fears, inability to relate to others, withdrawal, and sometimes regressive behaviors—soiling of self, thumb sucking, playing with food, poor hygiene, and impulsive behavior including sexual acting out.[10]

CORRECTIONAL HEALTH NURSING
Health Conditions

Health care in jails and prisons has not always been a major concern of correctional administrations or society in general. A prisoner who became "seriously" ill or injured was sent to the prison infirmary or to a special ward of the city hospital. Before the 1970s, prison infirmaries were miserably inadequate.[5] Health promotion was not a common concept. Government studies and media attention to health conditions within prisons have brought these issues into the open. Judges have issued court orders for prisons or jail systems to show cause for unsanitary conditions and threat to the health and welfare of the inmate. The care and treatment of the emotionally and mentally ill prisoner is grossly inadequate in most systems. The treatment of

choice is medication. Often the mentally ill inmate must be housed in what is described as "protective custody" for reasons of personal safety. This means removing the inmate from the main prison population to provide protection from harm. Such custody increases isolation, labeling of the individual, and concern for safety should the prisoner be returned to the general population.

Recently, two societal issues have had a major impact on the prison population. First, the deinstitutionalization plans of the 1960s led to mental hospitals reducing their census and moving to community-based programs. Jails and prisons now incarcerate some of these mentally ill persons. Second, treatment programs for incarcerated drug abusers and users are nearly nonexistent. When budgets are cut by state legislators, such programs as alcohol and drug rehabilitation are decreased or stopped completely. Correctional staff frequently adopt the attitude that a drug problem is not an addiction but a "cop out." Some drug users die while withdrawing from the abused substance because of absence of medical treatment and nursing care.

A Practice Model

Four special health problem areas that confront the inmate in a correctional system can serve as a basis for a nursing practice model in correctional health.[9]

HAZARDS OF THE INCARCERATION PROCESS

From the moment of arrest until the time of probation or parole, fear, apprehension, and humiliation are overwhelming to the offender and family. Whether the individual is found guilty or not guilty, the process is the same. The following story (which will be expanded on in the later Case Study section) relates an actual occurrence:

A nurse studying for an advanced degree in forensic psychiatric nursing fulfilled a course requirement by participating in a "citizen ride-along" program in a large city in the eastern part of the United States. Upon arrival at the precinct, the nurse was introduced to the officer with whom she would ride. His patrol covered a poor part of the city known for its drug sales, prostitution, and general fear and chaos. The nurse thought that since it was cold and dark people would be inside. But at 10 PM, the streets were crowded with people of all ages, including young children. The officer related that this was a highly stressful job with fear for safety and long hours as major concerns. He chain smoked, ate candy bars, and admitted that his marriage had ended in divorce. There were many frightening and challenging experiences that evening, but one arrest stands out in the nurse's memory. The officer received a call for backup for a suspected robbery. The siren was turned on and the car sped through city streets at a terrifying speed. It arrived at a vacant lot with an adjoining church on one side and the backs of closed stores on the other. Two other cruisers were there with lights flashing and radios blaring. There appeared to be a scuffle, and then, a young man was thrust against one of the police cars to be searched and read his rights. He was handcuffed and roughly put into the car. To the nurse, the young man looked like an animal caught in a trap. He could not have been more than 17 years old, and his eyes were both frantic and belligerent. The nurse observed the arrest with ambivalence. There was concern and empathy for the young man, mixed with relief that he was caught—the issue of guilt before proven innocent nudged at her conscience. Then there was the recognition that she had managed in this short time to identify with the officer and be concerned for his safety too. She began to think about the ambivalence of her feelings toward the would-be criminal and the law enforcer. She was frightened for both of them, they were frightened for themselves. Agitation, anxiety, fear, and impotence were the overriding emotions she identified for herself, the officer, and the prisoner.

The correctional system can be viewed as a subculture of the larger culture. It has its own rules, regulations, language, and formal and informal procedures. It is perceived by the detainee as a hostile environment. The young man in the foregoing case, to be referred to as Mr. B, would have been "booked" at the precinct, which includes a search, fingerprinting, and sometimes an observed urine sample. He would then be detained in a "holding" cell block for arraignment in court the next day. If he were to be held over for trial and could not make bail, he would then be transported to the city jail to await trial. Some overworked courts are so backlogged that Mr. B could be in jail for up to three months before his trial. In jail he would be stripped of all of his belongings, given a prison suit, and placed in a cell. His days would be filled with idle time because jails are not rehabilitation centers. Mr. B would suffer from isolation, humiliation, fear, and anger. He would have to learn the rules of this part of the system to survive. The suicide rate for persons at this point in the process is believed to be high, although statistics are not readily available.

If the crime committed carries a sentence of under one year, the prisoner would usually serve that sentence in a jail. If, however, the crime is a felony and carries a sentence of more than one year, the person would be sentenced to a state prison, unless it is a federal crime, and then he would go to a federal prison. There are exceptions to all of these conditions. To understand the usual process, Mr. B will be followed through the system after his conviction of a felony crime and subsequent imprisonment.

Once at the prison, Mr. B would undergo an orientation process. The thoroughness of this phase varies from facility to facility. The formal orientation may include psychological and vocational testing, planning a specific rehabilitation program, and assignment to living quarters based on special needs. All, some, or none of these may take place, based on the philosophy and resources of the institution.

If the facility employs a psychiatric nurse, he or she would be a member of the evaluation team participat-

ing in the overall plan for Mr. B. The nursing assessment of Mr. B would lead ultimately to a plan of care for him.

Mr. B's informal orientation would be done by the inmates. This is where he learns the "real" rules of the institution: whom to fear, how to stay alive, to whom he must answer. Mr. B's survival depends on how well he learns these rules.

HAZARDS OF THE CORRECTIONAL ENVIRONMENT

In addition to the considerations of the environment within the prisons already cited, there are other more dangerous and more personally threatening issues to be considered.

Sexual Assault. Sexual assault in prisons is occurring at an alarming rate. This may be related to the overcrowding, boredom, racism, frustration, and increased availability of illicit drugs within the system. It is generally not sexually motivated, but instead, serves a number of purposes such as control and power, release of anger, a "get even" strategy, and the degradation of the usually weaker, smaller, and younger inmate. Contrary to societal beliefs, most victims and their assaulters are heterosexual males. Estimates of the numbers of prisoners who are sexually assaulted varies widely. Factors influencing this information are (1) the "rat factor" (the life expectancy of a "snitch" is very short); and (2) denial on the part of prison officials that it exists. In two separate studies, however, the rate of reported assaults was startling. A 1982 study of medium-security prisons reported that 14% of all prisoners had been assaulted.[8] In 1980, a survey of all New York State correctional facilities found that 28% of all inmates had been assaulted.[8]

Victimization. Nursing considerations in working with the victim of sexual assault are many. Consequences for the victim may be physical injury, contraction of a sexually transmitted disease (STD), including the human immunodeficiency virus (HIV), and incidence of post-traumatic stress disorder (PTSD). Psychologically, the victim experiences feelings of humiliation, depression, shame, anger, violent mood swings, flashbacks, nightmares, and an inability to concentrate. Since "real men" do not discuss their emotions, assistance in resolution of these problems often does not occur.

The victim loses any sense of safety in the environment, and there is a disruption of social relations. Usually the nurse will observe an individual who is increasingly more withdrawn and isolated and at a much higher risk for suicide. Humiliation and degradation are intensified by the rape victim's status in the institution as a "sex slave," labeled as "punks" in the California system and as "maytags" in the East. These victims must perform chores for their masters (e.g., wash laundry, wear women's clothing). They may also be pimped to others for drugs, candy, and cigarettes.[8] Because most staff cannot tolerate the idea of male sexual assault, it is difficult to confront the problem and treat the victim. The nurse is a pivotal person in identifying the victim, initiating crisis intervention, giving psychiatric counseling, and acting as the inmate's ombudsman in seeking legal recourse.[8]

SPECIAL PROBLEMS OF PROBATION AND PAROLE

With many of the new laws governing mandatory sentencing now in place, both probation and parole have been seriously affected. If a person is convicted of a particular crime, a minimum mandatory sentence dictates when he can be eligible for parole. There are many movements to establish plans for alternatives to incarceration. These include such things as community payback by the perpetrator of the crime, alternative time served in community service, and cash payback.

There are some prison systems looking at early release policies for persons with acquired immune deficiency syndrome (AIDS). Because the prison population is considered a high-risk group for AIDS, this is a controversial issue that medical staff in corrections will have to address. Currently, AIDS is the leading cause of death of prisoners in the New York State system; intravenous drug abuse is a major problem in New York City, and may account for the large number of HIV-positive prisoners there.[7]

Nurses practicing in prison systems must have a working understanding of AIDS to treat those prisoners infected with HIV in a caring manner. There is a great deal of confusion about the virus and its transmission on the part of prisoners and corrections staff alike. If an individual is known to be infected or becomes ill, he is effectively isolated, psychologically and physically, from the main population. Anonymity in testing procedures within prisons is not considered a right. Persons who receive probation instead of being incarcerated may be assigned to a drug rehabilitation program, a half-way house, or to some other alternative program. The nurse can be the source of community referral and information for the prisoner and the courts. Knowledge of community resources and referral procedures are a must for this aspect of corrections nursing.

When inmates are nearing the time for parole, there is an excellent opportunity for the nurse to hold group meetings specifically focused on reentry into the community. Some ex-offenders have organized support groups in the community to assist those first coming out of prison.

UNIQUE HEALTH CONCERNS OF WOMEN

Women are in the minority within the prison system. Facilities to house them are often inhumane by male prison standards and sometimes are nonexistent. If no separate facilities exist, women may be housed in sections of male facilities or sent to facilities many miles from their homes and families.

Women's Health. Women who enter prisons have generally committed crimes such as prostitution, petty larceny, and drug possession. The crimes are nonviolent, but the women lack the resources to be released on bail. Women in prisons share many of the same concerns and general living conditions as men. However, they are often responsible for minor children for whom they lose custody to the state. Their prisons are overcrowded and unsanitary. They do not have the long history of "working the system" that male inmates have developed, and are less likely to speak out and demand better treatment and conditions. The women are concerned about pregnancy, sexually transmitted diseases, and health and dental care. They had poor health care before incarceration, and low self-esteem does not permit them to expect decent treatment. Acting-out and volatile behavior are common in the women's prisons. Depression is an overriding mental health problem reflecting the anger, fear, frustration, and losses experienced by these women.

Nurses working with women in prisons must have excellent communication skills and have a desire to assist the inmates in learning about their bodies and minds and the health practices they need to know to maintain optimum wellness. This is usually new information for the women who did not have access to health care in the community. They are usually suspicious, apprehensive, and fearful of the unknown with regard to their health status. Working with women can be a rewarding experience if the concept of unconditional positive regard is a major nurse–client component.[12]

COMMON NURSING DIAGNOSES

When considering the diversity of individuals who enter the criminal justice system, it is possible to suggest the application of nearly every nursing diagnosis category. Frequently identified nursing diagnoses are suspiciousness, impaired social interaction, altered health maintenance, self-esteem disturbance, suicide potential, post-trauma response, altered impulse control, aggression, bizarre behavior, depression, and substance abuse (alcohol, drugs).

CASE STUDY

The case of the arrest of Mr. B was related earlier. Mr. B was subsequently tried for assault and robbery, a felony offense. He stated his age as 18 years and was found to have had two prior arrests. Because of these circumstances he received a sentence of not fewer than ten years in the state prison. Upon arrival at the induction and orientation section of the prison, the admitting psychiatric nurse specialist assessed Mr. B. Mr. B was found to be a seemingly healthy black male, aged 18 years, height 6'2", weight 155 lb. He reported that he had been physically healthy all of his life, with the exception of infections related to use of "dirty works" when shooting-up. He was treated with antibiotics at a city clinic. He has never been treated for a STD and has not been tested for HIV. Mr. B is the middle child of five

NURSING CARE PLAN 30–1

MR. B

NURSING INTERVENTIONS	OUTCOME CRITERIA
NURSING DIAGNOSIS: Depression related to loss of freedom	
CLIENT GOAL: Achieve adequate balance of rest, sleep and activity	
■ Promote an adequate balance of rest, sleep, and activity by limits on rest periods, isolation behavior ■ Talk with Mr. B daily for brief periods ■ Encourage involvement in activities	Verbalizes acceptance of loss of freedom Sleeps through the night Participates in exercise program
CLIENT GOAL: Establish and maintain adequate nutrition, hydration, and elimination	
■ Closely observe Mr. B's food and fluid intake ■ Ask Mr. B about his elimination daily	Begins to adapt to the environment by eating his meals, taking in adequate fluids, and having a regular elimination schedule
CLIENT GOAL: Develop and increase feelings of self worth	
■ Encourage good personal grooming and hygiene ■ Give positive feedback for accomplishments ■ Give information on educational and self-help programs in the prison	Shaves and bathes regularly and when permitted wears own clothing Enrolls in a program to obtain additional education Joins a Narcotics Anonymous (NA) group
NURSING DIAGNOSIS: Grieving related to loss of freedom	
CLIENT GOAL: Identify the loss	
■ Encourage verbalization about loss ■ Talk with Mr. B realistically concerning the loss; correct any misinformation ■ Acknowledge similarity of other's responses to loss	Able to discuss feelings about loss of freedom and to look at options for himself during incarceration
CLIENT GOAL: Express feelings both verbally and nonverbally	
■ Meet with Mr. B for specific sessions related to his loss of freedom ■ Encourage Mr. B to express himself in NA meetings ■ Encourage Mr. B to maintain contact with his girlfriend	Verbalizes feelings to nurse Talks in NA meeting and eventually leads a meeting Telephones and writes to his girlfriend *Continued*

Mental Health and Illness in Special Population Groups

MR. B *Continued*

NURSING INTERVENTIONS	OUTCOME CRITERIA
CLIENT GOAL: Progress through the phases of grieving	
■ Facilitate sharing of feelings ■ Encourage group discussion of loss and grief	Demonstrates physical recuperation from the stress of the loss Adheres to the rules of the facility and talks about his future Participates in a group for newly arrived prisoners to help them with their adjustment
NURSING DIAGNOSIS: Suicide potential related to depression	
CLIENT GOAL: Experience no self-inflicted harm	
■ Provide a safe environment	Demonstrates increased impulse control
CLIENT GOAL: Express anger and hostility outwardly in a safe and acceptable manner	
■ Assist in ability to express and deal with feelings in a healthy manner	Verbalizes acceptance of anger toward himself and others

children born to his mother who is presently an inpatient at a local mental hospital suffering from depression. Mr. B's father is unknown to him. Mr. B spent most of his early childhood living with relatives in the South or in foster homes. He related a history of sexual and physical abuse while in these homes. Mr. B presented to the orientation section as a tall, well-built young man, who had apparently lost substantial weight within the last month (possibly as much as 20 lb) since his arrest. He had a dull and despondent look and became teary when spoken to. His transfer report from the jail stated that Mr. B had become quiet, withdrawn, had difficulty sleeping, and has had a loss of appetite. The nursing diagnoses formulated included depression related to loss of freedom, grieving related to loss

Research Highlights

Research in the field of psychiatric correctional nursing is a fertile area for nursing research to be conducted.

Nurses as general health care providers have been major forces in jails and prisons only within the past 10 to 20 years. Because this is largely an untapped research area, the nurse researcher may want to "begin at the beginning." A descriptive study of nurses in corrections —who are they? What do they do? What do they see as areas needing study? How did they choose this field? The inmate population must also be described in terms of nursing needs. Descriptive studies lay the foundation for studies that may quantify the problem, and for studies of treatment methods. The possibilities are infinite in this area of nursing.

of freedom, and suicide potential related to depression (see Nursing Care Plan 30-1 for a sample care plan for Mr. B).

SUMMARY

Inmates in the nation's jails and prisons live in a hostile environment in which personal safety is in constant jeopardy. There has been a dramatic increase in the numbers of inmates because of changes in sentencing laws and increased arrests for drug-related crimes.

The inmate population has many health problems including psychiatric conditions and substance abuse problems. The psychiatric nurse, as a member of the interdisciplinary health team, is in a unique position to assess and assist the inmate to work through emotional problems and to seek treatment for psychotic symptoms.

The psychiatric nurse in a correctional setting must meet challenges to personal values and nursing knowledge. It is important to have awareness of the varying cultural and ethnic issues for the inmate. Women prisoners may have concerns different from males, especially for issues of family and personal health care. The age of the average inmate is young, which demands that issues of late adolescence and young adulthood be addressed. The challenge for the psychiatric nurse is great, and the possibilities for research are many.

References

1. American Nurses' Association Council of Community Health Nurses. Standards of nursing practice in correctional facilities. Kansas City, MO: The American Nurses' Association; 1985.
2. American Psychiatric Association. Diagnostic and statistical manual of mental disorders, 3rd ed, revised. Washington, DC: The American Psychiatric Association; 1987.
3. An anonymous lifer. The new Folsom way. Calif Prisoner. 1988;17(Apr):1,8.
4. Benjamin S. Cross-cultural health care: insuring compliance in minority populations. Correct Care. 1988;2(Apr):3,8.
5. Bernier S. Corrections and mental health. J Psychosoc Nurs. 1986;24(Jun):20–25.
6. Berrigan H. The purpose of punishment. Blueprint Soc Justice. 1987;40(Jun):1–7.
7. Cade J, Elvin J. Prisoners with AIDS in New York live half as long as those on outside. J Natl Prison Proj. 1988;Spring, 7–8.
8. Cahill T. Rape behind bars, a victim's analysis. Calif Prisoner. 1987;16(Sept):5.
9. Freeman R, Heinrich J. Community Health Nursing Practice, 2nd ed. Philadelphia: WB Saunders; 1981.
10. Tauxe R, Patterson C. A word about prisons: "desmoteric." N Engl J Med. 1987;317:1669–1670.
11. Vodika J. U.S. prison population mushrooms. Judgement. 1987;10(Dec):4–5, 12.
12. Walton C. Women in correctional health (inmate: nurse providers). Correct Care. 1988;2(Apr):9,12.
13. Weinstein C. Neglect and death: the sorry state of prison medical services. Calif Prisoner. 1987;16(Sept):4.

31

Mary Kunes-Connell

Clients With Eating Disorders

OBJECTIVES
After reading this chapter, the reader will be able to:
1. *Define anorexia nervosa, bulimia nervosa, and obesity*
2. *Identify the etiologies and characteristics of the individual with anorexia nervosa, bulimia nervosa, or obesity*
3. *Identify possible nursing diagnoses and related factors associated with eating disorders*
4. *Describe general treatment strategies and nursing interventions for individuals displaying behaviors associated with eating disorders.*

INTRODUCTION

Many individuals, particularly in Western cultures, equate thinness with fitness and health. As a result, many people become preoccupied with their physical body image. This preoccupation with bodily appearance is exemplified in two recent studies.[3,21] In a study by Cash and associates[3] data were analyzed to determine attitudes and perceptions about physical appearance and associated eating behaviors. This study surveyed 30,000 men and women concerning thoughts and attitudes toward bodily appearance and related eating behaviors. The findings of the study supported the growing belief that Americans are more dissatisfied with their physical appearance in 1985 than they were in 1972. Most individuals, despite their level of physical fitness, perceive weight as central to body image. Compared with 1972, when 15% of the men surveyed revealed dissatisfaction with overall appearance, 1985 figures identified 34% of surveyed men as dissatisfied with their physical appearance. Thirty-eight percent (38%) of the women surveyed in 1985 indicated dissatisfaction with body appearances, compared with 25% of 1972 female respondents. Furthermore, 29% of the men who were within a normal weight range perceived themselves as overweight, whereas 47% of the women in a normal-weight category saw themselves as overweight.[3] This study also served to support the fact that many individuals are consistently attempting to do something to promote weight loss, even if unnecessary. Weight loss behaviors ranged from crash dieting to binge eating and purging.

Thompson's[21] study focused specifically on the body measurement perceptions of females not exhibiting eating disorders. In this study ($N = 100$) 95% of the females overestimated body proportions by at least 25% over actual proportions. These body image distortions were no different from those exhibited by eating-disordered persons. Both researchers[3,21] believe that this preoccupation with the physical self may serve as a precursor to a wide variety of eating disorders, ranging from anorexia nervosa to obesity. This is not to say that every individual concerned about body weight and physical appearance will develop an eating disorder. Rather, studies such as these serve to alert the professional to the increased vulnerability of an individual who is concerned about weight and body image.[3,7,16,20,21]

Currently, the most common eating disorders include anorexia nervosa, bulimia nervosa, and obesity (Box 31-1). *Anorexia nervosa* is defined as the refusal to maintain a body weight that is appropriate for the height and age of the individual.[1,18] This refusal manifests itself as a self-imposed starvation in response to a distorted body image and fear of being fat. *Bulimia nervosa* is defined as an episodic consumption of a large amount of high-calorie food over short periods, often followed by extreme guilt over the loss of control. The guilt can result in purging episodes to relieve the physical and emotional discomfort associated with the binge eating.[1,19] *Obesity*, although not classified as a DSM-III-

R disorder, is defined as actual body weight exceeding 15% of ideal range of weight for the individual's height and age.[19]

Eating disorders affect primarily the female population.[1,24] Approximately 95% of those with a diagnosis of anorexia are female. Although the number of males manifesting anorexia is on the increase, only 5% to 7% of those with a diagnosis of anorexia are males.[1] The statistics on bulimia nervosa are more vague. It is believed that bulimia nervosa affects approximately 5% of the female population.[1] Obesity occurs in 33% of the female population and 25% of the male population.

ETIOLOGIES OF EATING DISORDERS
Biological Model

Models to explain anorexia nervosa, bulimia nervosa, and obesity can be categorized as biological, intrapersonal, developmental–family, and sociocultural models. Correlation between the physical or biological factors and eating disorders remains nebulous. It is difficult to determine whether or not the physical abnormalities (i.e., hormonal or biochemical imbalances) precipitate the disorders, or whether they are themselves sequelae to the disorders. It is safe to assume that a number of physical abnormalities can create situations remarkably similar to those created by functional eating disorders. Adrenal insufficiency, hypothalamic–pituitary tumors, uremia, gastrointestinal disturbances, and hepatic disorders can result in an anorexic state, whereby the individual exhibits weight loss and all of the sequelae associated with severe weight loss.[22] Bulimic behaviors have been correlated with tumors of the hypothalamus, as well as with severe hypertension.[22]

Recent research has linked both anorexia and bulimia with affective disorders. Herzog,[12] Kirkley,[15] and Larocca[16] summarize a number of studies that have focused on a link between depression and eating disorders. Findings from these studies indicate that (1) many subjects who often experience bulimia correspondingly have abnormal dexamethasone suppression test results; (2) many subjects exhibiting anorexia and bulimia have a corresponding diagnosis of depression; (3) a number of individuals with eating disorders and depression have demonstrated a family history of affective disorders; (4) a number of individuals manifesting bulimic behaviors have been known to show low blood levels of serotonin. Decreased serotonin in the brain is known to increase the need for intake of carbohydrates, but peripheral serotonin, as might be measured in the blood, is not always a reflection of central serotonin. Low levels of serotonin are closely tied to onsets of affective disorders.[12,15,16] These studies support a possible biochemical or genetic link to eating disorders because affective disorders are known to have a strong biochemical or genetic link. However, difficulty in direct correlation relates to an inability to determine if affective disorders lead to eating disorders or vice versa.

BOX 31–1
Characteristics Associated With Anorexia Nervosa, Bulimia Nervosa, and Obesity[1,2,10,24,25]

ANOREXIA NERVOSA	BULIMIA NERVOSA	OBESITY
Underweight, emaciated appearance; bodyweight 15% below weight for height and age	Most are normal weight	Minimum 15% over ideal weight for height and age (based on height, age, weight tables)
Obsessed with thinness	Frequent weight fluctuations of 5–10 lb Obsessed with body image	Guilt and negative self-concept associated with appearance
Starvation is main form of weight control Consuming increasingly fewer calories, attempts to cut out fats, then carbohydrates	Frequent binge eating behavior lasting minutes to hours, (minimum of 2 binges a week)	Sedentary life-styles with excessive food intake
Hides/hoards food but never eats it Obsessed with counting calories	Purging is the weight control method Five methods to purge: vomiting, diuretics, cathartics, fasting, extreme exercise	
Prepares gourmet meals and forces others rather than themselves to eat	"Closet eater": rarely binges in public, binges in private Hoards/hides food	
Constipation	Constipation	Normal bowel movements or constipation
Potential bowel obstruction Potential paralytic ileus	Diarrhea Potential bowel obstruction Potential paralytic ileus	
Amenorrhea Decreased libido Breast atrophy Loss of pubic/axillary hair Confusion/anxiety over sexual role Avoidance of more intimate relationships	Ofen overcompensates for "interpersonal relationship" anxiety by promiscuous behavior	
Alexithymia Food is primary coping mechanism Attempts to "overcontrol" own impulses (starvation)	Alexithymia Food is primary coping mechanism Poor impulse control (binging)	Alexithymia Food is primary coping mechanism Poor impulse control (overeating)
DIAGNOSTIC TESTING OFTEN REVEALS	**DIAGNOSTIC TESTING OFTEN REVEALS**	**DIAGNOSTIC TESTING OFTEN REVEALS**
Hypokalemia Hyponatremia Hypochloremia Anemia Hypovolemia Hypotension Hypothermia (compensates through production of lanugo on arms, legs, lower back)	Hypokalemia Hyponatremia Hypochloremia Hypovolemia Parotid gland swelling	Increased triglyceride levels Increased fasting blood sugar levels Elevated cholesterol levels
Cardiac irregularities Muscle weakness Dehydration	Cardiac irregularities Muscle weakness Dehydration	Coronary artery disease Hypertension Pulmonary insufficiency (depending on severity of obesity)
Oral Manifestations Dental caries Xerostomia Bleeding gums Chapped lips Mouth sores	**Oral manifestations** Dental caries Xerostomia Decayed enamel Mouth sores	

The characteristics associated with interpersonal relations are general tendencies and may not apply to all individuals manifesting eating disorders.

(continued)

BOX 31–1
Characteristics Associated With Anorexia Nervosa, Bulimia Nervosa, and Obesity[1,2,10,24,25] *(continued)*

ANOREXIA NERVOSA	BULIMIA NERVOSA	OBESITY
Distorted body image: perceives self as fat despite emaciation	Dissatisfied with body image, but does not distort image as does the client with anorexia	Dissatisfied with body image, but does not distort image as anorexic
Tends to lack assertiveness; views self as powerless/ineffective	Tends to lack assertiveness; views self as powerless/ineffective	May lack assertiveness; may view self as powerless/ineffective
Low self-esteem	Low self-esteem	Low self-esteem
Overprotective family	Overprotective family	Often has overprotective family
Family sets high, often unrealistic expectations		
Denial/repression of feelings/conflicts	Denial/repression of feelings/conflicts	Denial/repression of feelings/conflicts
Sexuality topics are often "taboo"		
At least one family member is weight conscious	Oftentimes other family members are obese	Oftentimes other members are obese
Role reversal often occurs: the child is forced to nurture parents because of conflicts between parents		

Numerous physical disorders have been associated with the onset and progression of obesity. Localized hypothalamic tumors induce excessive eating that can result in obesity. Hormonal changes associated with hypothyroidism, excessive insulin secretion, or adrenal insufficiencies create situations that severely decrease the basal metabolic rate, resulting in obesity.[4,22]

Biological causes must be taken into consideration with any individual manifesting eating disorders. A knowledge of biological factors is essential if the psychiatric mental health nurse expects to conduct a thorough and accurate assessment, as well as determine the most appropriate modalities for treatment.[4,22]

Intrapersonal Model

Several traits seem to dominate the personality of clients with eating disorders. Regardless of the type of eating disorder exhibited by the individual, three common characteristics exist: (1) a low self-esteem, (2) a sense of powerlessness over the environment, and (3) an inability to adequately identify and assertively express feelings and needs.[4–6,15,16,25] Females are often socialized into believing that their self-worth is dependent on meeting the expectations of others; that is, they can like themselves and feel good about themselves only if they can please others.[10] As a result, a woman may attempt to meet everyone's expectations while her own needs and wishes becoming secondary. If she does not live up to others' expectations, she may begin to perceive herself as a failure resulting in even higher, more unrealistic self-expectations. If this persistent pattern occurs, chronic low self-esteem will result. The person with anorexia responds to these feelings by relentlessly pursuing perfection through thinness. The

belief becomes: "The thinner I am, the more perfect I will be. The more perfect I am, the more others will like me. The more that people like me, the better I will feel about myself." The person with bulimia responds to a low self-esteem in a slightly different manner. Binge eating becomes a way to relieve the negative feelings about oneself; that is, it becomes a self-comforting technique. When the eating is out of control, negative personal feelings become even more exaggerated, resulting in purging behavior.[15] The obese individual can also use food as a self-comforting device to deal with the low self-esteem or other stressors including perceived loss of control over one's environment. Eating temporarily relieves the negative feelings. The positive reinforcement allows the continuance of this type of behavior.

Another personality characteristic common in each of these disorders is the person's belief about being powerless over the environment. Many times, the person with an eating disorder comes from a family that is overprotective, disallowing expressions of personal autonomy. Attempts at independence are sabotaged by the family. As the individual matures, cognitive patterns associated with helplessness and powerlessness emerge. The individual does not sense that decisions and choices have an influence on the environment, and thus attempts to control it in other ways. Therefore, the individual with an eating disorder may use food as the response to this feeling of powerlessness. Persons with anorexia believe that the only controllable thing in the environment is their own body. Therefore, the person begins the ultimate exercise in control; that is, controlling what is put into the mouth. The belief is that starvation is control. Being thin is equated with being in control. The person also discovers that excessive weight control methods have the effect of controlling others. The person finds that the others now alter their behavior to accommodate the individual with anorexia. These effects serve as a secondary gain to the person, thereby making the alleviation of the disorder even more difficult. The individual with bulimia responds to this sense of powerlessness by initially "giving in" to the feeling through uncontrolled eating. However, the person begins to realize that binge eating represents an even further loss of control. This individual attempts to regain this control through purging behaviors. Purging temporarily restores a sense of control over self. However, this feeling is only transient. The obese person basically "gives in" to the feelings. In some ways the obese person begins to take on a defeatist or submissive attitude toward life.

Individuals with eating disorders have difficulty identifying and verbalizing feelings. The phenomenon of being without words for moods has been termed *alexithymia*.[2,4,25] The person has often grown up in an atmosphere in which feelings were actively denied. As a result, feelings, especially negative ones, are considered foreign. Certain emotions (e.g., anger) serve to increase the anxiety level of the individual. First, the person begins to feel "out of control" when confronted by confusing or unacceptable emotions. There is a strong need to regain control. Second, never being taught to verbally work-through feelings, the first response is to act out the anxiety associated with the emotion. The client with an eating disorder uses food as the vehicle for control. The person with anorexia attempts to deal with this anxiety by denying that it exists. The denial is manifested through self-starvation. This individual is saying "see how in control I am—I don't give in to feelings." On the other hand, the individual with bulimia uses food as a comforting device in an attempt to "undo" the feeling. However, this proves quite ineffective because this person develops even stronger negative feelings of guilt that must be alleviated. Purging becomes the method to alleviate these feelings. The obese individual perceives food as the ultimate comforting agent. It becomes so powerful that even the guilt often associated with overeating are overshadowed by the eating behavior.

Family–Developmental Model

The focus of the family–developmental model is on the interplay between dysfunctional family behaviors, communication patterns, and the emotional vulnerability of the developing adolescent. There are certain rigid rules common to many families of individuals with eating disorders. These rules include (1) family members do not acknowledge and honestly confront feelings and conflicts, (2) sexual issues are not topics to be openly discussed, (3) autonomous behavior is not accepted by family members, and (4) perfectionism is the only acceptable behavior in the family.[6,12,13,15,19] These rules may be acceptable to the child, when the individual is a child; however, they become a major

source of conflict as the child enters adolescence. The adolescent needs to be allowed to (1) make decisions, (2) question the family's value system, and (3) make mistakes. In rigid families, the teenager is unable to successfully negotiate these tasks because they are diametrically opposed to the family rules. Eating behaviors are often the adolescent's attempt to cope and gain control over life.[6,19] In essence, in all three eating disorders, the individuals use food as a means to avoid dealing with the issues of adolescence and young adulthood. Starvation eventually brings about emaciation and the "little girl look." The individual begins to believe that through starvation she can remain a little girl. By remaining a "child" there is no need to face responsibilities associated with growing up. On the other hand, the person with bulimic behaviors is attempting to act out much of the anxiety and ambivalence associated with conflicts. This anxiety and ambivalence cannot be overtly expressed because a characteristic of these individuals is their lack of self-esteem and assertiveness.[15,16] Overeating represents the opposite of anorexia, even though it accomplishes the same purpose. The obese adolescent often carries a stereotypical role of being a lazy, nonsexual, nonassertive, asocial person. This role may be readily accepted by the individual who may be seeking a safe way to avoid confronting certain issues.

Sociocultural Model

The sociocultural model has become increasingly associated with an explanation for the increase in both the incidence and prevalence of all types of eating disorders in all age groups. Society's values have tremendous impact on the individual's behavior. The following values influence an individual's self-concept and eating behaviors.

Strong Emphasis on Beauty and Thinness. Television, movies, and magazines emphasize diet and exercise. The media give a message that to have the best clothes, best job, best car, and best looking friends one must be thin. On a more clinical level, the media have been used to convey the message that a high-fat intake will not only cause obesity, but will lead to severe cardiovascular problems. In spite of being barraged with these messages, a great emphasis is also placed on food. There are very few activities that do not revolve around food. These double messages can be very confusing to individuals.[15,16,18,20]

Strong Emphasis on Personal Achievement, Success, and Control. Society equates self-esteem with success and control. Perfect test scores, all A's, awards, and scholarships tend to be measurements of success and self-esteem. Family, teachers, and friends often push adolescents beyond their capacities to achieve. Beauty and thinness also are equated with success and control.[15,16,18,20,21,24] When sexuality, success, and control are perceived solely as physical qualities, and health is perceived as thinness, the individual may resort to extreme starvation attempts to attain this thinness and this perfection.[15,16,18,20,21] On the other hand, the individual who develops bulimia often begins these behaviors in an attempt to lose weight. This individual often begins the maladaptive behaviors as a response to being slightly overweight. The individual begins the cycle by using some form of restrictive diet to lose weight. However, the person begins to feel deprived and wants to eat. The result may be a total loss of control. The person begins to binge. This behavior leads to guilt and a strong desire to maintain the perfect body image. These feelings can lead to eventual purging. Purging allows the person to have the best of both worlds; that is, one can eat while not worrying about gaining weight.[20] At the other end of the continuum, the person who is obese may fear aspects of sexuality, achievement, and control and may attempt to avoid dealing with these issues through overeating. In this sense, overeating may be a coping mechanism for the anxiety associated with certain life issues.[16,24]

ASSESSMENT FOR EATING DISORDERS

The multidimensional nature of eating disorders requires a comprehensive physical, psychosocial, and cognitive assessment. A screening for possible biochemical, neurologic, or other physiologic factors must be considered. Diagnostic tests such as complete blood count, urinalysis, thyroid test, and dexamethasone suppression test, should supplement all other methods of assessment.[2,12,15,16,22] These methods may yield data to facilitate a determination of possible physiologic precipitators to eating disorders. Second, these tests may help to determine the severity of physical effects associated with eating disorders. Effects such as hypokalemia, hyponatremia, and anemia associated with anorexia and bulimia can be verified by diagnostic testing. Furthermore, measuring for weight and total body fat content can serve to discern the severity of an eating disorder. In addition to diagnostic testing, an assessment of dietary habits, weight control methods, attitudes toward food, elimination patterns, activity level, and sexuality attitudes and behaviors can provide a wealth of data about the severity of the eating disorder.

Although it is necessary to do a complete physical and psychosocial evaluation when assessing eating disorders, priority must be given to the following: (1) nutritional patterns, (2) elimination patterns, (3) sexual attitudes and behaviors, (4) activity patterns, (5) self-concept and body image assessments, and (6) coping patterns. Secondary emphasis should be placed on the following: (1) cognitive patterns and (2) family and peer interactions. Box 31-2 identifies the elements under each assessment category. These elements serve as general guidelines for the psychiatric mental health nurses' assessment of eating disorders.

NURSING DIAGNOSES COMMONLY ASSOCIATED WITH EATING DISORDERS

The assessment data often demonstrates that physical, psychosocial, and emotional problems confront the individual with an eating disorder. The psychiatric mental health nurse must be cognizant of the interplay between the physical, emotional, and psychosocial elements of the disorders as the nursing diagnoses and plans of care are formulated. Table 31-1 illustrates a listing of potential nursing diagnoses related to anorexia, bulimia, and obesity.

Not all clients will experience every diagnosis. However, a number of nursing diagnoses tend to occur commonly among the three disorders. The person presenting with anorexic or bulimic behaviors often does not take in the nutrients necessary for a healthy lifestyle. The diagnosis, altered nutrition, less than body requirements, may aptly apply to these individuals. On the other hand some obese persons who eat more of everything in a normal diet than they are able to use, will present with a nursing diagnosis of altered nutrition, more than body requirements.*

Self-esteem disturbance is the psychosocial nursing diagnosis that predominates in all three disorders. Body image disturbance is related to each disorder.

Powerlessness is another nursing diagnosis that must be considered. The nurse must remember that food often becomes the substitute for unexpressed feelings of powerlessness and lack of control over situations.

TREATMENT MODALITIES FOR CLIENTS WITH EATING DISORDERS

Treatment planning for eating disorders center primarily on promoting a weight change (e.g., loss or gain of weight) and ultimate weight stabilization while working through the emotional and psychosocial issues that often lead to or accompany the particular eating disorder.[13,16] Promoting a weight change without concurrently dealing with emotional and psychosocial issues produces only short-term success for the individual. A number of treatment procedures might be used simultaneously in an attempt to meet both goals. No approach should be used in isolation, because no single method has, as yet, proved successful.[16,23]

Treatment Issues in Anorexia Nervosa

A successful weight gain and stabilization process is based on two contentions. First, unless it is a medical emergency, drastic measures should not be attempted to rapidly promote weight gain for an individual with

---

* Other NANDA nursing diagnosis.

BOX 31–2
Key Elements of Assessment for Eating Disorders[1,2,8,9,15,17]

KEY ELEMENTS OF ASSESSMENT	ASSESSMENT METHOD
NUTRITION PATTERNS	
Dietary recall	Ask client to keep diary for one week
Attitudes toward food	Attitudinal surveys (e.g., Eating Disorders Inventory,
Attitudes toward weight	Eating Attitudes Test)[6,9,17]
Weight: actual	Structured interview
History: weight loss/gain	Physical assessment:
Weight control methods:	Vital signs
Vomiting (frequency, methods used, content of vomitus)	Body temperature
Laxatives (frequency of use, types, dose, results)	Hair/skin/mucous membrane assessment
Diuretics (frequency of use, types, dose, results)	Weight
Fasting	Diagnostic testing
Food habits/behaviors/rituals	Complete blood count
Electrolyte levels (especially, K^+, Na^+, Cl^-)	Urinalysis
Body fat percentage	Chemistry profile
Muscle tone	Thyroid tests
Body temperature	Dexamethasone suppression test
ELIMINATION PATTERNS	
Patterns of bowel elimination	Structured interview
Laxative use (frequency of use, type of medication, dose,	Intake and output measures
time used, result of use)	Abdominal assessment
Pain (before/during/after elimination)	Bowel sounds
Bowel sounds	Palpation
Urinary elimination patterns	Distention observation
Diuretic use (frequency of use, type of medication, dose,	Urinalysis
times used, result of use)	
SEXUALITY PATTERNS	
Menstruation patterns (regularity, last menstrual period, quality	Interview: individual
of flow)	Definition of sexuality
Attitude towards own sexuality	
Sex-role identity (feminine versus masculine qualities)	
ACTIVITY LEVEL	
Exercise habits (patterns of exercise)	Interview: individual
Attitudes towards exercise	Interview: family
	Observation of exercise patterns
	Daily log of exercise activities
SELF-CONCEPT	
Body image assessment	Interview
Self-esteem assessment	Assessment of strengths and weaknesses
Perception of locus of control (e.g., decision-making capabilities)	
COPING: STRESS PATTERNS	
Life events and situational stressors	Structured interview
Intrapersonal stressors	Daily journal (discussion of stressors and individual's
Interpersonal stressors	response to stressors)
Environmental stressors	Observation of verbal and nonverbal display of affect
Coping styles	
Use of defense mechanisms	
Impulse control	
Past/present suicide attempts	
Use of food to cope with stress	
Expression of feelings	
Use of defense mechanisms	
Range of moods (restricted, labile)	
Ability to identify and acknowledge feelings	
COGNITIVE PATTERNS	
Coherency/relevance of thought	Mental status examination
Distorted thought patterns	Structural interview
Ability to make decisions/judgments	Observation of verbalization concerning body image

(continued)

BOX 31–2
Key Elements of Assessment for Eating Disorders[1,2,8,9,15,17] *(continued)*

KEY ELEMENTS OF ASSESSMENT	ASSESSMENT METHOD
FAMILY–PEER INTERACTIONS	
Family	
Family structure	Interview: individual
Family rules	Interview: family
Family communication patterns:	
Husband–wife communication	
Parent–child communication	
Decision-making strategies	
Conflict resolution patterns	
Peers	
Patterns of peer relationships	Interview: individual
Dating habits	Interview: family
Social anxiety	

anorexia. Rapid weight gain only serves to exacerbate the person's fears of becoming obese, thereby increasing the underlying behaviors.[13] Furthermore, a rapid weight gain tends to serve as a "quick fix" and often results in a relapse of the anorexic behaviors.[5] Second, the weight gain process must be a mutual endeavor among the nurse, client, and family. By dictating the diet and weight gain goals to the client, the nurse succeeds only in adding to the person's perceived loss of control. Again, this feeling will only exaggerate the self-starvation behaviors because these behaviors serve as coping mechanisms when one feels powerless.[5,19]

The foregoing two assumptions are the foundation for a gradual approach to weight gain and more healthy

eating habits. Because the person with anorexia fails to see the behavior as a problem, entry into treatment is often seen as coercion. The person has little trust in the caregivers themselves. There is a perception that the caregiver is attempting to take away the only control that the individual has known; that is, control over the body. Therefore, the individual enters treatment with a great deal of anger.[4–6,13,16,19,25] Immediately upon admission to the hospital, the nurse seeks to form an alliance with the client in an attempt to establish a climate of trust. The client must be aware that the nurse is concerned about the person versus the disorder. Active listening and encouraging the ventilation of feelings in a nonjudgmental atmosphere promotes a sense of car-

TABLE 31–1
Nursing diagnoses associated with anorexia nervosa, bulimia nervosa, and obesity[11,14]

ANOREXIA NERVOSA	BULIMIA NERVOSA	OBESITY
Nutrition, altered, less than body requirements	Nutrition, altered: more than body requirements* Nutrition, altered, less than body requirements	Nutrition, altered, more than body requirements*
Constipation*	Constipation*, diarrhea*	Potential constipation*
Altered growth and development		
Potential for injury	Potential for injury	
Defensive coping (denial, projection)	Defensive coping (denial, projection)	Defensive coping (denial, projection)
Powerlessness	Powerlessness	Powerlessness
Body image disturbance	Body image disturbance	Body image disturbance
Self-esteem disturbance	Self-esteem disturbance	Self-esteem disturbance
Impaired social interaction	Impaired social interaction	Impaired social interaction
Loneliness	Loneliness	Loneliness
	Boredom	
Sexual dysfunction	Sexual dysfunction	Sexual dysfunction
Altered impulse control	Altered impulse control	Altered impulse control
Ineffective individual coping	Ineffective individual coping	Ineffective individual coping
Emotional lability	Emotional lability	
Manipulation	Manipulation	Manipulation
Dysfunctional family processes	Dysfunctional family processes	Dysfunctional family processes

* Other NANDA nursing diagnosis.

ing for the client. The time spent with the client should not enter solely on a discussion of food, weight, or physical appearance. It becomes vital to get to know the client's strengths, likes and dislikes, fears, emotions, and other aspects of the client as a person. Furthermore, the psychiatric mental health nurse needs to convey to the client a belief in the client's ability to take healthy control over life. This can be accomplished by determining the client's goals in conjunction with the client. The nurse must give the client the message that the client will not be allowed to "get fat," but that some weight gain is healthy and will allow the client the freedom and control that the client has not achieved to this point in life.[5,13,16]

CONTRACTING

Contracting can be used in the one-to-one relationship and in milieu therapy as a technique to promote control while facilitating a healthy weight gain.[19] Contracting uses the principles of behavior modification to positively reinforce goal accomplishment. The contract involves mutual collaboration of realistic weight gain goals, as well as methods to reach these goals. The contract spells out the responsibilities of the nurse, client, and family in accomplishing these goals. It is a positive method in that it provides rewards for follow-through and goal accomplishment. These rewards should be mutually determined to have genuine meaning and positive significance for the client. The contract places the control on the person with anorexia. This is an important aspect of therapy because loss of control is a causal factor to anorexia. It is explained to the client that ultimate control resides in the self. When the client follows the contract, rewards are earned. When the client chooses not to follow the contract, the client chooses not to earn the reward.

GROUP THERAPY

Group therapy is useful because the client is engaged in therapy with individuals experiencing the same eating disorder problems.[16] Group therapy can serve as an effective medium in a number of ways: (1) It can decrease the client's feeling of isolation (i.e., others are experiencing the same problems); (2) it can balance supportive techniques, as well as peer pressure techniques, for changing maladaptive behaviors. Because the client with eating disorders uses excessive denial in dealing with the disorder, a psychoeducational approach may be used in the group. This approach attempts to provide the client with an objective view of the disorder and its effects. It is hoped that when this information is given in an objective, supportive, and nonjudgmental atmosphere, the individual will begin to change patterns of thinking about the disorder. The group approach is also used to assist the client to increase insight into his or her own behavioral patterns by using group members to help each other correlate feelings associated with behaviors. The group also helps the individual analyze whether or not the person's own expectations are real-

istic and how certain behaviors may result from unrealistic self-expectations. Therefore, the group provides a medium for both a cognitive reframing of the problem and insight into the client's own responses to the environment.[13,16,19,25]

FAMILY INTERVENTION

The family often faces numerous problems as a result of the anorexic behavior exhibited by the individual.[23] A multidimensional approach to family treatment is often undertaken. When knowledge deficit has impinged on the family, a psychoeducational approach can be effective.[16] This can include teaching the family about the dynamics of the illness, behavior of the individual, and the reasons for the behavior. Education allows the family members the opportunity to gain insight into "what is happening" with the family.

A supportive approach to family problem solving is always helpful, even essential. The family often experiences a great deal of difficulty coping with a number of issues including: the client's illness, their own presumed "guilt" in "causing the disorder," the individual's hospitalization, and the stigma attached to the disorder. The anxiety of living with the client on a daily basis can be overwhelming. The family is in need of developing adaptive coping mechanisms in an attempt to carry on with their lives. This can be accomplished through family therapy sessions or referral to family support groups.[18] More in-depth family therapy sessions might focus on the identification of family interaction patterns. Emphasis is then placed on a reframing of these interactions to promote a more healthy family communication pattern.[6,7,12,13,16,19,23]

Treatment Issues in Obesity

Conservative forms of treatment for obesity are emphasized unless extreme obesity exists. Usually, the mildly obese client responds well to a weight-loss program that focuses on the restructuring of the diet, eating habits, and exercise regimen. Restructuring the diet involves developing a safe, low-caloric diet that is suited to meet the individualized needs of the client (i.e., life-style, ethnic patterns, family situations, and finances, among other areas of need). No diet will be successful if it is not suited to the client's life-style. If knowledge deficit is identified, then nutrition teaching is an appropriate intervention.

In situations for which overeating is related to boredom or inability to express feelings, cognitive restructuring is appropriate. Cognitive restructuring involves an identification of trigger situations, the thoughts and feelings associated with these situations, and the eating behaviors as a response to these thoughts and feelings. The attempt is then made to alter the situation, feelings, or behavior, or all.[16]

The approach to the obese client is one of sharing concern and being supportive. This involves supporting the client in the development of attainable, desired goals and the practical behaviors to be undertaken to achieve these goals (e.g., how to eat out, how to eat differently from meal companions). When the client, "chooses" to deviate from the plan, the antecedent events to the choice are identified as a basis for developing additional control options.

Severe obesity may require more drastic medical therapy. Often, the client seeks help after numerous failed attempts at diet programs. One method for treating severely obese persons involves a form of fasting, using high-protein liquid supplements. These programs are time-limited and designed to produce quick results. Surgery is a last resort. Bypass and restriction surgeries are designed to produce weight loss through a malabsorption process.[16,22] There are disadvantages to both fasting and surgery. Although they promote a quick weight loss, they do nothing to alter eating behaviors nor the psychosocial factors that contribute to the eating behavior. Therefore, it is important that these methods be accomplished by a psychoeducative–behavioral approach designed to alter eating behaviors. These programs are rarely successful without the concurrent psychosocial approach.

Treatment Issues in Bulimia Nervosa

The individual with bulimia faces slightly different problems from either the client with anorexia or obesity. The therapeutic goal in bulimia is not so much centered on promoting weight loss or weight gain, but on the promotion of more controlled eating. Principles of behavioral contracting and family therapy discussed in the previous sections apply to the treatment of bulimia. In addition to these modalities, cognitive therapy principles are quite effective in promoting change in the client. The client's bulimic behaviors are often the result of distorted patterns of thinking. Therefore, it becomes necessary for the individual to (1) identify the distorted thought patterns and emotions resulting from these thoughts; (2) connect the bulimic behaviors with the thoughts and emotions; (3) restructure the thought patterns; and (4) alter the behaviors in light of the new thought patterns. The cognitive approach can be effectively implemented in individual or group therapy.[12,15,16,18,19] This approach requires a strong commitment on the part of the client, because there must be a willingness to do homework in the form of daily record keeping and diaries.

Medication therapy cannot be discounted. Hsu[13] and Larocca[16] have summarized a number of studies focusing on the correlation between psychotropic administration and decreased bulimic behavior. It has been noted in a number of studies that use of tricyclic antidepressants has been effective in reducing the incidence of bulimic behaviors in clients. It is postulated that this success rate may be due to alleviation of depression that may underly bulimia. If this proves to be

true, then concurrent treatment of depression is essential in alleviating the behaviors.[13,15,16]

CASE STUDY

Jane, a 32-year-old woman, entered the Eating Disorder Center for long-term obesity. Her entry into an eating disorder program was based on her physician's insistence. Jane has a recent diagnosis of severe hypertension related to obesity. During a recent physical examination an electrocardiogram (ECG) revealed a series of cardiac arrythmias. The physician also made a diagnosis of dysthymic disorder related to the recent physical problems as well as to Jane's poor body image. At 5'5", Jane weighed 250 lb. She described trying a number of diets and diet programs over the past 17 years, with little or no success. Furthermore, she described using a number of over-the-counter diet pills and drinks, which were not successful. She stated that she gave thought to intestinal surgery, but had not followed through with this idea. She believed that the center was her last resort, as she expressed being quite depressed over her body image, lack of physical energy, and absence of any social life.

On physical assessment, Jane appeared to be 120 lb overweight (weight should range between 116 and 130 lbs for her height and age). She stated that her physician placed her on a low-sodium, 1200 calorie diet that she sporadically follows. Jane is involved in no formal or informal exercise program. She experiences dyspnea and dizziness on exertion and views herself as too fat to exercise. The physical examination and history revealed no evidence of pituitary, thyroid, or adrenal dysfunction. Currently, her blood pressure is 160/90 (lying and standing). Jane described herself as mostly a loner. Although she has a couple of girlfriends, she does not date and feels uncomfortable in social situations. She feels embarrased by her weight.

After a dietary recall, it was discovered that Jane usually skipped breakfast, but began "snacking" between 10 and 11 AM. She usually ate fast food for lunch. She described not eating a formal dinner. However, she stated that she snacked from 5:00 PM until bedtime. She reported eating even though not hungry. She acknowledged eating when she is bored, sad, happy, angry, or depressed. The following nursing diagnoses were identified: altered nutrition, more than body requirements*; self-esteem disturbance; and ineffective individual coping (emotions). Nursing Care Plan 31-1 illustrates interventions for Jane's care based on these three diagnoses. During hospitalization, Jane was helped to identify alternative outlets to expressing her feelings. Jane was also educated on proper eating behaviors and how to control her eating in situations and events that revolve around food (e.g., parties, picnics).

SUMMARY

Societal obsession with physical appearance has set off warning signals to many mental health professionals. It is believed that this obsession with physical appearance has lead to an increased number of clients with eating disorders in the last ten years. The psychiatric mental health nurse plays a vital role in the preven-

---

* Other NANDA nursing diagonsis.

JANE

NURSING INTERVENTIONS	OUTCOME CRITERIA

NURSING DIAGNOSIS: Altered nutrition (more than body requirements)* related to family patterns, inability to express emotions, boredom, and social isolation

CLIENT GOAL: Attain normal body weight for height, age, and body frame

- Assess present nutritional status
- Refer Jane to nutritionist for mutual planning of a safe, healthy diet that provides variety while being easy to follow
- Reinforce eating all foods on the diet for adequate nutritional intake
- Encourage weekly as opposed to daily weigh-ins
- Give Jane positive reinforcement for follow-through with the diet plan
- Do not belittle when Jane does not lose weight or follow plan; be supportive and accept nonjudgmentally "occasional cheats" or plateaus/weight gain
- Help Jane plan for situations that involve food (e.g., parties)
- Teach Jane how to select foods from menus in restaurants

Demonstrates weekly weight loss of 1–3 lb

Verbalizes own methods of tracking daily dietary intake

Demonstrates accuracy in calorie counting/exchanges on a daily basis

CLIENT GOAL: Develop alternative approaches to present eating behaviors

Facilitate Jane's identification of

- Situations/events/feelings that lead to eating
- Patterns of eating by the following:

  - Negotiate with Jane to enter into a diary the types and amounts of food eaten, situations/events occurring before eating behaviors

  - Review the diary daily or weekly with Jane to identify stimuli provoking certain eating behaviors
  - Identify ways to alter the events or situations or the response (overeating) to certain stimuli
  - Refer Jane to self-help groups for further support through weight loss and maintenance stage

Verbalizes an awareness of situations/events that bring on certain eating behaviors

Verbalizes feeling more in control of herself when confronted by certain situations/events

Verbalizes restructuring home environment to decrease the temptation of overeating

CLIENT GOAL: Increase knowledge of healthy nutritional habits

- Assess Jane's present knowledge level of nutritional concepts
- Teach nutritional concepts (i.e., basic food groups, calorie counts)

- Teach the correlation between exercise, food intake, and weight loss/gain
- Develop a sound exercise program for Jane to be done three to four times per week for 20–30 min
- Identify forms of informal exercise (i.e., stairs versus elevator)

Reports follow-through with some type of exercise program at least three times a week

Verbalizes basic nutritional concepts, related to weight gain

* Other NANDA nursing diagonsis.

Continued

NURSING CARE PLAN 31–1

JANE *Continued*

NURSING INTERVENTIONS

OUTCOME CRITERIA

NURSING DIAGNOSIS: Self esteem disturbance related to being overweight

CLIENT GOAL: Develop a more realistic perception of own body image

- Assess Jane's perception of her strengths and weaknesses

- Reinforce that Jane's physical self represents only one aspect of her personality
- Identify Jane's strengths
- Ignore self-degrading comments made by Jane and redirect to more positive comments
- Reality test Jane's perception of body size and shape

Verbalizes positive
  statements about self
Decreases verbalization of
  negative comments
  concerning body
  image

NURSING DIAGNOSIS: Ineffective individual coping related to inability to express emotions in an assertive manner

CLIENT GOAL: Develop ability to correlate eating behaviors as coping mechanism for dealing with painful emotions

- Assess Jane's ability to express feelings
- Help Jane name feelings through use of techniques such as reflections of content, validation, verbalizing the implied
- Do not tell Jane how she should feel
- Identify relationships between feelings (i.e., anxiety, sadness, boredom) and eating behavior
- Help Jane develop a repertoire of behaviors for expressing feelings in a variety of situations
- Give positive reinforcement for appropriate expression of feelings
- Refer Jane to assertiveness training to facilitate her ability to identify and express emotions
- Teach Jane to structure the environment to decrease stress before mealtimes

Verbalizes relationship
  between feelings and
  eating behavior
Verbalizes feelings
  appropriate to
  situations

Research Highlights

Palmer and coworkers[17] designed a clinical eating disorder rating instrument to be used by clinicians. The purpose of the research study was to establish interrater reliability for this scale. Originally, the tool consisted of 31 possible defining characteristics of anorexia and bulimia. These characteristics were based on the clinical experience of the authors as well as literature reviews. These 31 characteristics were divided into three categories: behavioral patterns, (binge eating habits, purging habits, beliefs about foods, and weight control methods); attitudinal patterns (fantasies about eating and weight, body image perceptions, and appetite); and other symptoms (mood levels, thought patterns, and anxiety levels). Each characteristic was given an operational definition along with a set of interview questions to elicit the mate-

rial. The tool was set up as a rating scale from 0 (absence of symptoms) to 3 (severe symptoms). Two studies were performed to establish reliability of the tool. With use of Kendall's Coefficient of Correlations, the first study concluded that all 31 characteristics were significant at the 0.0001 level. Following this study several interview questions were revised and four new characteristics were added. The second study elicited similar results. A reliable, research-based assessment tool can be quite useful to the clinician as an objective method of quantifying critical indicators of anorexia and bulimia. This leads to a more accurate diagnosis of problems related to the disorders and, ultimately, to more efficient and accurate treatment planning.

tion, identification and treatment of these disorders. If nurses are to be effective in their treatment, it will be imperative for them to have adequate knowledge of the issues related to the etiologies, nursing diagnoses, and treatment of these disorders.

References

1. American Psychiatric Association. Diagnostic and statistical manual of mental disorders, 3rd ed, revised. Washington, DC: American Psychiatric Association; 1987.
2. Bryant SO, Kopeski LM. Psychiatric nursing assessment of the eating disordered client. Adv Nurs Sci. 1986;9:57–65.
3. Cash TF, Winstead BA, Janda LH. The great American shape-up. Psychol Today. 1986;20:30–37.
4. Davis MS, Marsh L. Self-love, self-control, and alexithymia: narcissistic features of two bulimic adolescents. Am J Psychother. 1986;40:224–230.
5. Deering CG. Developing a therapeutic alliance with the anorexia nervosa client. J Psychosoc Nurs Ment Health Serv. 1987;25:10–17.
6. Doyen L. Primary anorexia nervosa: a review and critique of selected papers. J Psychosoc Nurs Ment Health Serv. 1982;20:12–18.
7. French RN, Baker EL. Anorexia nervosa and bulimia. Indiana Med. 1984; pp. 241–245.
8. Garner DM, Garfinkel PE. The eating attitudes test: an index of the symptoms of anorexia nervosa. Psychol Med. 1979;9:273–279.
9. Garner DM, Olmsted MP, Polivy J. Development and validation of a multidimensional eating disorder inventory for anorexia nervosa and bulimia. Int J Eating Disorders. 1983;2:15–33.
10. Gilligan C. In a different voice: psychological theory and women's development. Cambridge: Harvard University Press; 1982.
11. Gordon M. Nursing diagnosis: process and application. New York: McGraw-Hill; 1982.
12. Herzog DB. Bulimia in the adolescent. Am J Dis Child. 1982;136:985–989.
13. Hsu G. The treatment of anorexia nervosa. Am J Psychiatry. 1986;143:573–581.
14. Kim MJ, McFarland GK, McLane AM. Pocket guide to nursing diagnoses, 3rd ed. St Louis: CV Mosby; 1989.
15. Kirkley BG. Bulimia: clinical characteristics, development, and etiology. J Am Diet Assoc. 1986;86:468–472.
16. Larocca FE. Eating disorders: effective care and treatment, vol 1. St Louis: Ishiyaku EuroAmerica; 1986.
17. Palmer R, Christie M, Cordle C, Davis D, Kenrick J. The clinical eating disorder rating instrument (CEDRI): a preliminary description. Int J Eating Disorders. 1987;6:9–16.
18. Reed G, Sech EP. Bulimia: a conceptual model for group treatment. J Psychosoc Nurs Ment Health Serv. 1985;23:16–27.
19. Sanger E, Cassino T. Eating disorders: avoiding the power struggle. Am J Nurs. 1984;84:31–35.
20. Schwartz DM, Thompson MG, Johnson CL. Anorexia nervosa and bulimia: the sociocultural context. Int J Eating Disorders. 1982;1:20–34.
21. Thompson JK. Larger than life. Psychol Today. 1986;20:38–44.
22. Thorn GW, Adams RD, Braunwald E, Isselbacher KJ, Petersdorf RG. Principles of internal medicine, 8th ed. New York: McGraw-Hill; 1977.
23. Vandereycken W. The constructive family approach to eating disorders: critical remarks on the use of family therapy in anorexia nervosa and bulimia. Int J Eating Disorders. 1987;6:455–465.
24. Wergowske GL, Goldenberg K, Barnes HV. Adolescent obesity: intervening at a crucial biologic stage. Consultant. 1986;26:42–49.
25. Zeller CL. Treatment of ego deficits in anorexia nervosa. Am J Orthopsychiatry. 1982;52:356–359.

32

Carol Ann Dunphy

Mental Health Needs of Clients Along the Continuum of Human Immunodeficiency Virus (HIV) Infection

EPIDEMIOLOGY
NURSES CARING FOR CLIENTS WHO ARE HIV-POSITIVE
NURSING ASSESSMENT
THE WORRIED WELL
CLIENTS WHO ARE HIV-NEGATIVE
CLIENTS WHO ARE HIV-POSITIVE
CLIENTS WITH SYMPTOMATIC HIV INFECTION OR AIDS-
    RELATED COMPLEX
CLIENTS WITH AIDS
FAMILIES, PARTNERS, AND FRIENDS OF CLIENTS WITH AIDS
SUBSTANCE ABUSE AND AIDS
WOMEN, CHILDREN, AND AIDS
PEOPLE OF COLOR AND AIDS
VACCINE AND ANTIVIRAL DRUGS

OBJECTIVES
After reading this chapter, the reader will be able to:
1. Discuss epidemiology, risks, transmission, spectrum of disease, and prevention
2. Identify nursing diagnoses for worried well, HIV-positive asymptomatic, and those manifesting HIV disease
3. Describe client goals and nursing interventions for worried well, HIV-positive asymptomatic, and those manifesting HIV disease
4. Describe manifestations of HIV neurologic disease
5. Identify existence of, or need for, resources in the community and the approach to developing the resources needed
6. Discuss the impact of caring for persons with AIDS on health care workers and the means for preventing burnout
7. Assess needs in the following domains: physical, emotional, support, housing, finances, family, lover, and friends.

INTRODUCTION

In the late 1970s, physicians in New York and California were caring for young men who had previously been healthy, but now were having rare infections diagnosed that indicated they had an immune deficiency. More of the same cases occurred; therefore, in 1981 the Centers for Disease Control (CDC) began studying this apparently new disease. Since then the acquired immune deficiency syndrome (AIDS) has grown into a frightening epidemic of disease and fear. Research on the nature of the human immunodeficiency virus (HIV), antiviral drugs, and potential vaccines is ongoing; however, no cure or vaccine is pending. Thus, society can expect a continuing epidemic, touching many individuals in this country. This chapter will address the complex psychosocial issues of AIDS for nurses.

EPIDEMIOLOGY

By the end of the year 1991, the number of diagnosed cases of AIDS in the United States is expected to reach 270,000. The life expectancy after AIDS is diagnosed ranges from several months to two years and up to four years in rare cases; the mean survival time after diagnosis of AIDS is 13.4 months. Approximately 58% of persons with an AIDS diagnosis have died. Ninety-two percent of cases are men; 7% are women. Most cases of AIDS occur between the ages of 30 and 39, and disproportional numbers of cases occur in racial minorities.[11]

Acquired immune deficiency syndrome is caused by the human immunodeficiency virus (HIV). A retrovirus, HIV causes a state of permanent infection in those who have been exposed. The rate of progression from initial HIV infection to HIV-related disease (opportunistic infections) appears to be 25% to 50% within five to ten years.[4] Much has been learned about modes of transmission of HIV. Behaviors associated with transmission include the following:

1. *Sexual Contact:* Vaginal, anal, and oral intercourse can transmit HIV. The most efficient mode of transmission is receptive anal sex; however, vaginal and oral sex are also risky. Currently, most cases (92%) have occurred in men who have sex with men, but HIV can also be transmitted from men to women, women to men, and from women to women.
2. *Blood Exposure:* HIV is found in the highest concentrations in blood. Intravenous drug abuse with needle sharing is the most common blood exposure transmission. Blood transfusions from 1978 to 1985 and clotting factors given to hemophiliacs have also been implicated in transmission. Several health care workers also have become infected with HIV through accidental needlestick injuries or blood contact on nonintact skin or mucous membranes.
3. *Mother to Child:* Prenatal and perinatal transmission of HIV from an infected mother to her infant

occurs in about 50% of infants whose mothers are infected. Transmission of HIV by breast milk has also been documented.[8]

Human immunodeficiency virus is known to cause a spectrum of disease in those infected. The classification of HIV infections is as follows:

Class I: Acute HIV infection
Class II: Asymptomatic HIV infection
Class III: Persistent generalized lymphadenopathy
Class IV: Disease
      A: Constitutional disease
      B: Neurologic disease
      C_1: Infectious diseases
      C_2: Other secondary infectious diseases
      D: Secondary cancers
      E: Other HIV conditions

The primary cell of HIV infection damage is the helper T lymphocyte; HIV also infects macrophages and central nervous system cells. Most individuals with HIV infection appear to be healthy (class II, III). Class IV disease includes both AIDS-related complex (ARC) and AIDS. Subgroup A includes individuals with constitutional symptoms, such as persistent unexplained fever, diarrhea, and weight loss greater than 10% of body weight. This syndrome previously was known as ARC; however, no standard definition of ARC has been established. Subgroup C includes the opportunistic infections included in past definitions of AIDS. The definition of actual AIDS is currently broader, with diagnosis being established through the existence of disabling ARC; neurologic complications; secondary infections, such as *Pneumocystis carinii* pneumonia; or a cancer, such as Kaposi's sarcoma. Thus, categories A, B, C_1, and D are indicative of AIDS. Categories C_2 and E are not diagnostic of AIDS, but occur in clients who are seropositive.

The AIDS epidemic is one of both HIV infection and fear. Education about means of transmission, manifestations of infection, and needs of persons with AIDS is important to stop the epidemic of fear. Prevention of transmission of HIV can be accomplished by avoiding high-risk behaviors through using safer sex practices, disinfection of needles and syringes used to inject street drugs, and, for health care workers, by avoiding body fluid contact on skin and mucous membranes and using care to prevent accidental needle sticks.

The only absolute way to prevent sexual transmission of HIV is to not be sexually active. It is important to assist clients to explore other possible ways to become intimate and to socialize with persons who choose not to be sexually active. Specific safer sexual practices that are unlikely to transmit HIV include mutual masturbation, dry kissing, body-to-body rubbing, and unshared sex toys. Use of condoms for vaginal, anal, and oral sex, and French kissing involve a higher degree of sexual transmission risk. However, if condoms are used correctly, they should offer substantial protection. Sexual practices that are unsafe and likely to transmit

HIV infection are vaginal, anal, and oral sex without a condom.

As sexual desire and needs can change with progression of HIV infection, regular assessment of this aspect of sexuality should be made for persons with HIV infection, as well as for their partners.

The ideal means for prevention in intravenous (IV) drug users is abstinence from drug use, with the support of methadone maintenance or drug-free treatment. For those who are unable or unwilling to abstain from use of drugs, there are other modes of prevention. Disinfection of needles and syringes can be easily accomplished by rinsing twice with household bleach, followed by rinsing twice with tap water. Avoidance of needle-sharing behavior also may be accomplished by the ready availability of needles and syringes in the community (e.g., needle exchange programs).

Health care workers, as well as partners, friends, and family members involved in the care of clients with AIDS should follow the precautions outlined in the Centers for Disease Control (CDC) guidelines for prevention of transmission in health care workers. These precautions are

1. Use barrier (e.g., gloves) to prevent contact of blood, feces, urine, or wound drainage on provider's skin or mucous membranes. These precautions should be used by health workers in the care of all clients because it may not always be known which clients are HIV-positive.
2. Prevent accidental needle sticks by not recapping needles after use; needles should be disposed of in puncture-proof containers after use.[13]

A general rule to use in talking with clients and families is that there need be no changes in social, family, or workplace contact; one should not be able to single out a HIV-infected person by behavior in these settings. Hugging, touching, eating meals together, and use of bathroom facilities may continue as before.

NURSES CARING FOR CLIENTS WHO ARE HIV-POSITIVE

Nurses caring for clients with HIV-related disease need to carefully evaluate and monitor their own values, fears, and feelings concerning sexuality (theirs and others), alternative life-styles, and death. This is important not only in providing good care, but also in preventing burnout. Eight countertransference issues in working with clients with AIDS have been identified[6] and are outlined in Box 32-1.

Awareness that such feelings occur can enable the provider to seek support and a person to talk with about their feelings. This will facilitate empathic regard for clients and will decrease potential for burnout caused by denial or repression of feelings such as anger and helplessness. Fears are normal responses to difficult situations and need not be harmful if dealt with properly.

BOX 32-1
Countertransference Issues in Working With AIDS Clients[6]

1. *Fear of the unknown:* Working with a disease that still has a great number of unknowns can cause detachment and a subjective approach in the provider rather than the more therapeutic approaches of empathy and objectivity.
2. *Fear of contagion:* Much is known about the transmission of HIV. However, fears of contagion can cause intense anxiety and even panic in experienced providers, despite educational programs aimed at reducing this fear.
3. *Fear of death and dying:* Working with clients who are dying challenges providers to think about their own mortality. This process can be exacerbated when working with young clients who are dying.
4. *Denial of helplessness:* Providers can, by denying their own feelings of helplessness, try to gain control of the situation by belief in their own omnipotence. This can lead to provider guilt or sense of personal failure.
5. *Fear of homosexuality:* Continual monitoring of feelings of homophobia needs to occur in both gay and straight providers.
6. *Overidentification:* Homosexual providers may identify too closely with homosexual clients. This may cause lost objectivity and enhance chances of burnout in a provider.
7. *Anger:* Anger can be experienced as a result of feelings of helplessness, fear, and guilt. Anger can also serve to distance the provider from the client, as well as act as a form of self-preservation that can serve to protect the provider from experiencing the pain of loss.
8. *Need for professional omnipotence:* Helping professionals may not be comfortable with a relationship that has both the provider and the client active in the decision-making process

---

Also, providers should be given opportunities to attend educational programs that address these and other AIDS-related issues.

NURSING ASSESSMENT

Dramatic and rapid changes in physical and psychosocial status can occur in persons with HIV infection. Assessments for nursing diagnoses and planning for interventions need to occur frequently and quickly (Box 32-2).

A variety of difficult psychosocial needs and issues confront nurses and the clients for whom they provide care or with whom they interact. The focus of these needs and issues centers not just on clients with AIDS-related disease, but also on persons who are concerned about their actual or perceived risk for having infection. Many persons feel that the issues surrounding AIDS are hopeless. Although there is now no vaccine or cure for AIDS, creative assessment and approach to problem solving can help to redefine hope for persons along the spectrum of HIV infection.

BOX 32–2
Guidelines for Nursing Assessment of Persons With HIV Infection

PHYSICAL STATUS

Symptoms: Fever, Fatigue, Weight Loss, Cough, Dyspnea, Headaches, Diarrhea, Sores in Mouth, Skin Rash, Memory Loss, Personality Change, Paresthesias, Limb Weakness or Paralysis

Medications

Activity

No restrictions
Not well but can care for self
Needs help with cooking, cleaning, shopping, laundry
Lives alone, but needs assistance
Unable to live alone, but can do basic self-care
Needs assistance with all needs

PSYCHOSOCIAL

Demographic Data

Religion (practicing or not)
Education (highest level completed)
Marital status
Children
Living situation

Support Systems

Life-style and Risk Factors

Recent stressors, life changes
Sleep pattern
Smoking
Drinking
Drug use

Mental Status Examination

Specific Concerns (Ask Open-ended Question)

"What is most on your mind?"
"How can I help you?"
"How do your health concerns affect your daily life?"[16]

SEXUAL HISTORY

Sex with men, women, or both
Does client have primary partner, regular partner(s)
Changes in sexual expression due to the infection, disease
Is client using safer sex; what does "safer sex" mean to this client?
Satisfaction with means of sexual expression
How is partner(s) responding to changes around HIV infection, disease
If not sexually active, how does client feel about this?

FINANCIAL

Is the client working? Potential to continue work
Income
Assets: car, savings, investments, home
Debts or loans, credit cards, child support
Insurance: does client have medical insurance, copayments, deductible?
Life or disability insurance
Eligible for public assistance, SSI, Social Security, disability
Plans to live on potentially decreased income

HOUSING

What is client's housing situation? own home, apartment, live alone, roommate?
Can client keep up cleaning, cooking of housing unit?
Is client capable of living alone?
What are potential plans if client cannot live alone? What options does client have, what options are acceptable?

THE WORRIED WELL

The first group of concerned persons on the continuum of HIV infection are persons worried about AIDS who have either no risk, or little risk, for the infection. Often called the "worried well," these individuals experience much anxiety, anger, depression, fears about contagion, and sexual difficulty. Symptomatology similar to that found in clients with HIV disease (e.g., fatigue, weight loss, lymphadenopathy, and diarrhea) can occur. Individuals in this group may include those who have no personal or sexual contact with those at high risk or persons, family members, or friends of those at risk.

To appropriately determine whether or not persons fit in this category, an assessment of risk for HIV infection should be made.

Persons at High Risk for HIV Infection
1. Men who have had sexual contact with other men
2. Persons who use intravenous drugs and share needles

3. Women who are partners of bisexual men
4. Sexual or needle-sharing partners of intravenous drug users
5. Infants born to mothers with HIV infection
6. Sexual partners of persons who are HIV-positive
7. Persons who have had multiple blood transfusions, before 1985, in high AIDS incidence areas (i.e., New York, San Francisco)
8. Hemophiliacs

Persons at Moderate Risk for HIV Infection
1. Heterosexual persons with multiple sexual partners
2. Health care workers with accidental needle sticks, or with substantial blood exposure to HIV positive individuals

Persons at Low Risk or No Risk for HIV Infection
1. Persons in monogamous relationships since 1978
2. Persons who have engaged only in safer sex (i.e., mutual masturbation, sex with condoms)

3. Persons who are not sexually active
4. Household, social, workplace contacts of HIV-positive persons

Nursing diagnoses to consider with the worried well include:

■ Fear related to sexual behavior and death associated with HIV
■ Anxiety related to the unknown elements of HIV
■ Knowledge deficit about risk and need for behavior change
■ Powerlessness related to feeling of lack of choice about change and resources available

CLIENTS WHO ARE HIV-NEGATIVE

Persons who are at high risk for HIV infection have needs that can be specifically examined, with some overlap, by dividing them into two groups according to HIV antibody status. Little has been written in the literature about persons at risk who are HIV antibody-negative. Experience in working with this population has helped the writer to identify some special needs of these individuals.

A negative HIV antibody test result represents, to many persons, freedom from fears of death, infecting others, necessary disclosure of information of risk or test result to health care providers, lover, family, or friends. However, fear of inaccurate test results and fear of future sexual contacts that may again put the person at risk for HIV infection are not eliminated. Also continuing are stigmatization because of sexuality, contagion concerns, issues of loss and grieving for means of sexual expression not recommended for practice anymore, concern about how to bring up safer sex, condom use, slips of unsafe sex, and decisions about issues such as: Is it all right to engage in French kissing? Guilt over past sexual partners, drug use, and fears of disclosure of risk to partners who are not at risk also foster substantial anxiety in these individuals. Especially intense anxiety and fear may be found in at-risk heterosexual or bisexual men who have or are thinking to become fathers. Denial of ongoing risk can also be found in these individuals.

Nursing diagnoses to consider with clients who are HIV-negative include:

■ Anxiety related to unknowns about transmission and infection
■ Impaired communication related to discussion of sexual practices with partners
■ Fear related to being or becoming HIV-positive
■ Fear related to disclosing past sexual practices and drug use to new partners
■ Defensive coping (denial) related to putting self and others at risk for HIV infection
■ Grieving related to losses in sexual expression

CLIENTS WHO ARE HIV-POSITIVE

Individuals who have chosen to determine their HIV infection status and have found that they are infected with HIV have the same needs as those who are HIV-negative, but also have some special psychological needs.

Depression can be a serious problem. Those who are HIV antibody-positive frequently feel helpless and bleak about their future. Profound apathy may also be present. One of the first responses people have when told they are HIV-positive is that they feel they are dying. Potential loss of self-image as a healthy person, loss of attractiveness, loss of opportunity to conceive a child, all generate deep anger and fear in these persons. Guilt over behaviors related to acquiring HIV infection is also a major problem. Suicidal ideation frequently occurs in HIV-positive persons.

Intense anxiety and panic attacks around thoughts of health, risks to loved ones, and death and dying are common. Anxiety and panic attacks may be precipitated by worrisome symptoms that may not even be AIDS related. Somatization, stress-related physical and emotional symptoms, and hypochondriasis also occur. Denial may be a powerful defense mechanism in HIV seropositive persons. Some persons cope with the news of seropositivity by maintaining or reverting to previous behaviors in an attempt to deny that anything has changed. Persons may also discount serious physical and psychological symptoms and avoid needed medical care.

Social isolation can be fostered by unrealistic fears of infecting others or being exposed to infections others have. Many persons fear rejection and stigmatization associated with AIDS, and to deal with this fear, they avoid contact with others as much as possible. Sexual dysfunction expressed by impotence or inhibited sexual desire may be a reaction to known HIV seropositivity. Persons may feel they are sexually undesirable or dangerous. These persons also face possible loss of employment, housing, relationships, family, and friends in response to disclosure of their HIV status.

Nursing diagnoses to consider with clients who are HIV-positive include:

■ Anxiety related to what the future holds with HIV-positive status
■ Defensive coping (denial and intellectualization) related to positive HIV status
■ Depression related to HIV seropositivity
■ Anticipatory grieving related to possible change in appearance, life-style and death with HIV-positive status
■ Fear related to contagion to others
■ Situational crisis related to HIV-positive status
■ Suicide potential related to knowledge of HIV-positive status
■ Sexual dysfunction related to knowledge of HIV seropositivity

CLIENTS WITH SYMPTOMATIC HIV INFECTION OR AIDS-RELATED COMPLEX

Over time, some clients with HIV infection progress to a symptomatic state or are given a diagnosis of AIDS-related complex (ARC). Symptoms such as fatigue, weight loss, diarrhea, and oral candidiasis are common; some symptom complexes are severe enough to cause disability. Depending on the severity of symptoms, many clients in this group will suffer further immune system damage, and AIDS will be diagnosed.

Clients in this group often experience the highest levels of subjective discomfort. Causes of this discomfort are the ambiguity of the diagnosis: Are the symptoms real? What will happen next? Much emotional energy may be spent trying to convince providers that symptoms are real. High levels of anxiety, severe depression, a strong sense of isolation, and preoccupation with death are common. Fears of getting worse, daily uncertainties, stigma, becoming helpless, and pain and suffering occur. Also, clients in this group may be confronted with disclosing risk factors (homosexuality, IV drug abuse) to family members as well as a possible or impending diagnosis of AIDS.

Nursing diagnoses to consider with clients with ARC include:

- Anxiety related to ARC or AIDS status
- Depression related to life-style changes and possible death
- Fear related to loss of control, pain, suffering
- Anticipatory grieving related to possible impending fatal diagnosis of AIDS
- Guilt related to having caused HIV infection through behavior (sexual practices, needle sharing, child born to HIV-positive woman)
- Powerlessness related to feelings of stigmatization
- Impaired social interaction related to ARC

CLIENTS WITH AIDS

When individuals hear the word *AIDS*, a common feeling response is fear; a powerful association with death also occurs. Clients who are aware of their clear risk for HIV infection, or who know they are HIV antibody-positive, experience many intense and powerful emotions. Anger, sorrow, guilt, and hopelessness result. Preoccupation with death and dying is common. For clients who have experienced symptoms or ARC, a diagnosis of AIDS, (established through existence of disabling ARC, neurologic complications, secondary infections such as *Pneumocystis carinii* pneumonia, or a cancer such as Kaposi's sarcoma) can bring a sense of relief and an end to that constant anxiety related to uncertainty of the future.

Psychological concerns for clients with AIDS are numerous. Isolation, peace of mind and spirit, employ-ment, financial status, social support, physical intimacy, role status, stigma, and suicide are issues to be dealt with.[16] Losses in many areas—health, appearance, body function, impending death or death of friends—compound the grieving process. Anxiety and depression may intensify. Many clients with AIDS blame themselves for their illness. Feelings of contamination are common, and fears of disclosure of risk, sexuality, and diagnosis intensify again.

Adding to these psychological concerns are frequent neurologic complications. Clinical involvement of the nervous system occurs in at least 40% of clients with AIDS and may be the initial manifestation of HIV infection in 10% to 30% of patients. Several neuropathologic studies have found evidence of central nervous system HIV infection in as many as 90% of cases.[3] Progressive dementia or AIDS dementia complex is the most common neurologic presentation. Early cognitive signs are forgetfulness, decreased concentration, and confusion. In late-stage dementia, confusion and memory loss occur. Behavioral manifestations are apathy and social withdrawal to indifference, awakeness, wide-eyed stare, and incontinence. Organic psychosis may also occur.[3] Mental status changes warrant careful neurologic evaluation, as these symptoms may also be caused by treatable central nervous system infections, such as *Toxoplasma gondii*-caused encephalitis or cryptococcal meningitis.

Nursing diagnoses to consider for clients with AIDS include:

- Grieving related to diagnosis of AIDS
- Ineffective individual coping related to overwhelming emotions and physical illness
- Confusion related to neurologic infection with HIV
- Self-concept disturbance related to physical and psychological effects of AIDS
- Self-care deficit related to physical illness and neurologic complications of AIDS
- Spiritual distress related to realization of impending death
- Suicide potential related to depression, fear of suffering, actual suffering, or fear of being a burden to others

Basic psychological needs of clients with AIDS can be met by

1. Providing information about AIDS
2. Helping clients develop a plan for living
3. Giving recognition to the person as a valuable, worthwhile human being
4. Reinforcing the sense of legitimacy for symptoms and suffering
5. Advocating for the client with social service, chore service, medical, mental health agencies
6. Listening
7. Facilitating a sense of control
8. Giving permission or support for denial to protect against overwhelming emotions

CLIENTS WITH AIDS

NURSING INTERVENTIONS	OUTCOME CRITERIA

NURSING DIAGNOSIS: Grieving related to diagnosis of AIDS

CLIENT GOAL: Engage in grieving process

- Assess stage of grieving process
- Listen, allow expression of full range of emotions
- Do not confront denial because the client may need denial to cope, deal with overwhelming situation
- Refer to support group
- Assist to accept reality of loss by being accepting, supportive, reassuring
- Explore all potential areas of loss

Engages in grieving process

NURSING DIAGNOSIS: Ineffective individual coping related to overwhelming emotions and physical illness

CLIENT GOAL: Develop coping skills

- Convey trust in client's ability to act and to struggle
- Identify and reinforce what client has already done to assist coping with future situations
- Provide factual information on responses of persons in crisis
- Assist client to identify and make changes in health behaviors necessary because of stressful situation
- Serve as role model, social support for coping behaviors, activities of daily living
- Help to identify areas for which client has little control and areas for which client has control
- Teach decision making, problem solving, assertiveness, goal setting, evaluation, relaxation, and role-play these skills
- Encourage, seek ways to expand social support system
- Support medical care to alleviate physical symptoms

Copes adequately with feelings and physical signs and symptoms

NURSING DIAGNOSIS: Confusion related to neurologic infection with HIV

CLIENT GOAL: Live in supportive, accepting, safe environment to decrease confusion

- Complete mental status examination if change in cognition or behavior
- If person is hospitalized or in a new living situation, include special and personal belongings in room or living area to provide an emotionally secure, independent environment
- Use simple, few-step instructions, reminders, notes for directions, tasks
- Provide caretaking or chore services as needed
- Decrease amount of stimulation in environment
- Be supportive of client's feelings, awareness of confusion, memory loss

Maintains awareness of self and environment as much as possible
Feels supported and accepted

NURSING DIAGNOSIS: Self-concept disturbance related to physical and psychological effects of AIDS

CLIENT GOAL: Improve self-esteem, body image, role performance

- Use nonjudgmental attitude
- Show unconditional positive regard
- Focus on strengths and emphasize success
- Facilitate grieving process

Achieves positive self-concept

Continued

CLIENTS WITH AIDS Continued

NURSING INTERVENTIONS	OUTCOME CRITERIA

- If having difficulty with grooming, provide assistance and teach skill as needed
- Because weight loss is so common, facilitate access to clothes that fit, haircuts; encourage appearance in areas of special importance to client
- Problem solve with client to maintain constructive roles as much as possible

NURSING DIAGNOSIS: Self-care deficit related to physical illness and neurologic complications of AIDS

CLIENT GOAL: Reestablish a pattern of living without total dependence on others as long as possible

<ul><li>Supervise self-care activities</li><li>Provide positive feedback for success</li><li>Offer support as needed, but do not make client dependent on others</li><li>Arrange living environment to facilitate safe, self-care</li><li>Evaluate on ongoing basis as condition may change rapidly</li></ul>	Engages in self-care activities as much as possible

NURSING DIAGNOSIS: Spiritual distress related to realization of impending death

CLIENT GOAL: Obtain support for spiritual needs and relief from spiritual distress

<ul><li>Assess spiritual needs and resources</li><li>Encourage support from others with similar spiritual beliefs</li><li>Assist in developing meaning in life or suffering</li><li>Support client's existing spiritual resources</li></ul>	Draws support from spiritual resources

NURSING DIAGNOSIS: Suicide potential related to depression, fear of suffering, actual suffering, or fear of being a burden to others

CLIENT GOAL: Have reduced potential for suicide

<ul><li>Assess potential for suicide</li><li>Encourage help-seeking behaviors as needed</li><li>Increase social support system to isolation</li></ul>	No suicide attempts

Finally, one of the more difficult issues to deal with is that of maintaining hope in the face of a disease for which there is no known cure. Hope may vary from person to person—to tolerate zidovudine (AZT) therapy, to go home for Christmas, to die at home with lover, friends, and family (see Nursing Care Plan 32-1 for a sample care plan for clients with AIDS).

FAMILIES, PARTNERS, AND FRIENDS OF CLIENTS WITH AIDS

Responses of family members, partners, and friends to knowledge of HIV infection, ARC, or AIDS diagnosis vary, but nurses can expect these individuals to be on a fast, frightening rollercoaster ride with their family member, partner, or friend who is ill. Some responses are similar to reactions of persons who have AIDS—denial, anger, sadness, fear of contagion.

Response of the biologic family will depend on the means by which the family member contracted the disease. Families of hemophiliacs may express much anger at the blood supplier or at infected persons who have unknowingly donated their blood.[12] For situations in which the infection was acquired through sexual contact or needle sharing, a diagnosis of AIDS may also lead to knowledge of drug addiction or homosexuality. In many situations, family members have not previously known their sons were gay. Homophobic responses can occur, but appropriate support can help families deal with this information and continue caring for the sons.

An especially difficult circumstance is that of a married bisexual man's explanation to his unsuspecting spouse. Risk to the spouse's health must be addressed. The nurse can provide resources for HIV antibody testing, physical evaluation, and emotional support for the unsuspecting spouse or partner. Nurses need to listen to each spouse and particularly to each spouse's request for what information may or may not be shared.

Gay couples also have some special issues affecting their relationship. Guilt over possible past or future transmission of HIV to each other occurs. Both partners may be sick, or the caregiving partner may be concerned about his own health. Both may be grieving over the loss of other friends. Also, men may have a difficult time being taken care of.

Nursing diagnoses to consider with the families, partners, and friends of clients with AIDS include:

- Anticipatory grieving related to expected loss of loved one
- Family coping, potential for growth
- Dysfunctional family processes related to disclosure of AIDS diagnosis by family member
- Knowledge deficit (AIDS, homosexuality)

Nurses can meet the needs for family, lover, and friends by providing information about AIDS, facilitating access to the medical team, giving emotional support, and acceptance (see Nursing Care Plan 32-2 for a sample care plan for families, partners, and friends of clients with AIDS).

SUBSTANCE ABUSE AND AIDS

The issue of AIDS and substance abuse raises a number of concerns for both medical and mental health professionals. Answers for these concerns are not simple; however, an impact on these problems can be made in a number of ways.

Intravenous drug abuse is a factor in 25% of all cases of AIDS. The HIV seroprevalence in this population varies from 50% to less than 1%. Once HIV infection becomes established in a geographic area, drug users become a primary source for heterosexual and in utero transmission.[5]

Alcohol and drug abuse are thought to be factors that increase an HIV-infected person's risk for developing AIDS. Poor nutritional habits and lack of sleep result in stress on the immune system. Thus, intervention in areas of alcohol and drug abuse are warranted.

Finally, persons who are under the influence of alcohol and drugs may be less likely, because of reduction in their inhibitions, to practice safer sex.

Three target groups have been identified for HIV and AIDS prevention. These are:

1. Those who have not begun IV drug use
2. Those who use drugs, but are willing to enter treatment
3. Those who use drugs and are not willing to enter treatment to eliminate IV drug use[5]

Important preventive strategies in these areas are education in schools and elsewhere about the dangers of AIDS and IV drug use and increasing the number of available treatment openings in both methadone maintenance and drug-free treatment programs. For those who are not willing to enter treatment programs, prevention may be improved by increasing the legal availability of sterile needles and syringes, by teaching use of bleach to sterilize needles and syringes, and by needle-exchange programs. Because the potential for spread of HIV in IV drug abusers, their sexual partners, and infants will probably account for most new HIV infections, implementation of these strategies is crucial.

Medical and mental health providers need to include substance abuse assessments in evaluation of persons with HIV infection or disease. Not dealing with substance abuse issues can undermine other efforts to cope with the many problems that come with AIDS. In addition to affecting medical and mental health care, projections suggest that substance abuse issues will command even more attention from educators, health care providers, and health policy issues.[7] Health care providers can also intervene effectively by recognizing how their own values and anxieties impact upon treatment. Staying informed about community resources available to help make accurate assessments and develop effective treatment strategies is also important. Lastly, the choice to seek treatment or to remain addicted will be made by the client; this fact is basic to all treatment strategies.

WOMEN, CHILDREN, AND AIDS

Currently, about 8% of cases of AIDS are occurring in women.[11] Pregnant women who have HIV infection have a 50% chance of delivering an HIV-seropositive infant. About 1% of cases of AIDS have occurred in children younger than 13. Also, of women with AIDS, 53% were IV drug abusers themselves, 21% had heterosexual contact with a person at risk (67% in this group had heterosexual contact with an IV drug abuser).[9]

Women who have HIV infection or AIDS have some unique psychological issues to deal with. The first is that women get pregnant. Some information shows that HIV-infected women may undergo an accelerated process of disease if they are pregnant.[15] Pregnant women also need counseling about the risks of HIV infection to themselves and their babies. Discussion of options for continuing or terminating the pregnancy should occur; not all babies born to HIV-infected women are born infected.

Next, when a woman becomes ill with AIDS or ARC, she may not be able to carry out her customary role as mother and caretaker, so children and other adults in the household will be affected. A mother's children may also be directly affected by her diagnosis; for example, the children may be excluded from school. Finally, many women who have a child with AIDS may themselves also be ill. Foster care may be needed. If the

NURSING CARE PLAN 32–2

FAMILIES, PARTNERS, AND FRIENDS OF CLIENTS WITH AIDS

NURSING INTERVENTIONS	OUTCOME CRITERIA

NURSING DIAGNOSIS: Anticipatory grieving related to expected loss of loved one

FAMILY GOAL: Engage in anticipatory grieving

■ Assist through stages of grieving ■ Recognize that client with AIDS and different family members may be in different stages of grieving process concurrently ■ Recognize the multiple AIDS-related losses that may be a part of the life of partner of client with AIDS	Family, lover, friends progressing through the anticipatory grieving process, ideally to stage of acceptance

NURSING DIAGNOSIS: Family coping, potential for growth

FAMILY GOAL: Have increased ability to cope with AIDS

■ Listen to all family members ■ Acknowledge varying concerns and fears of family members ■ Identify family history, means of communication, reactions to previous difficult situations, and use or propose modifications needed ■ Teach steps in problem solving and decision making	Family members interacting and communicating about AIDS and its effect on themselves

NURSING DIAGNOSIS: Dysfunctional family processes related to disclosure of AIDS diagnosis by family member

FAMILY GOAL: Resolve dysfunctional family processes

■ Listen to all family members, assuring each that what they say is confidential ■ Act as mediator and do not take sides ■ Serve as role model for expressing feelings, communicating, problem solving, making suggestions, setting limits ■ Assist in clarifying issues and identifying problems that need to be resolved ■ Teach steps in problem solving and decision making ■ Listen to family members' fear of change ■ Support trials of new behavior	Family process functional for all members

NURSING DIAGNOSIS: Knowledge deficit (AIDS, homosexuality)

FAMILY GOAL: Obtain information about AIDS, homosexuality

■ Listen and acknowledge feelings about situation ■ Teach about transmission, diagnosis, effects, fears, course of disease ■ Talk about homosexuality (many parents feel guilty about son's homosexuality; i.e., that being a bad parent caused it) ■ Refer to support group for family members ■ Serve as role model for expressing feelings about homosexuality ■ Refer to community group such as Parents and Friends of Lesbians and Gays (PFLAG) ■ Acknowledge family members' suffering	Family able to discuss information about AIDS, homosexuality

mother is healthy enough to care for her child, she still must be able to cope with all of the other issues of medical care, finances, school access, family, and friends, identified earlier in this chapter under the headings of ARC and AIDS.

In response to these often extraordinary circumstances, women need specific AIDS services designed to meet their special needs. These resources and services must be designed to also address minority issues. Outreach programs and culturally appropriate health care is needed. Nurses can play an important role in developing and providing access to these services.

Nursing diagnoses to consider for mothers with AIDS include:

- Dysfunctional family processes related to AIDS-related illness of mother
- Altered parenting related to AIDS
- Situational crisis related to illness and AIDS in mother, child, or both

PEOPLE OF COLOR AND AIDS

AIDS has disproportionately affected communities of persons of color, primarily among blacks and Latinos. Twenty-four percent of cases have occurred among blacks, although blacks constitute only 12% of the United States population. Blacks are three times more likely to be infected with HIV than are whites. Fourteen percent of cases have occurred in Latinos, who make up only 6.3% of the United States population. Asian-Americans and Native Americans comprise about 2.4% of the United States population, but account for 1% of cases of AIDS.[2]

These ethnic differences are even more pronounced among women and children with AIDS. Black women account for 52% of cases of AIDS in women; Latino women account for 18%.[9] Fifty-three percent of cases of pediatric AIDS are in black children, and 23% are in Latino children.[1]

Black and Latino persons with AIDS show a broader epidemiologic infection pattern than do white persons with the disease. IV drug use with needle sharing is an important transmission mode for people of color; many heterosexual contact cases result from sexual contact with IV drug users, and pediatric AIDS cases most frequently occur in infants born to women who are IV drug users themselves, or who are sexual partners of IV drug users.

Poverty in urban black and Latino communities is a major contributor to the AIDS epidemic in these persons. Also, cultural and religious values relative to birth control and parenthood are factors. For example, for some ethnic minorities, birth control is viewed as genocidal, depriving individuals as well as the community of the ethnic pride of parenthood.[2]

Elements of successful HIV transmission prevention programs in communities of color must include networking to, and working with, key persons, agencies, churches, and organizations in these communities. Ed-

ucation and counseling for HIV antibody testing for prenatal or prepregnancy care, and intervention around alcohol and drug abuse also needs to be culturally sensitive. Realities of poverty in daily life, means to survive in poverty, and religious and cultural values, all must be taken into account in carrying out AIDS interventions in these communities. A 50% chance of having an infant born with HIV infection is not necessarily a deterrent to childbearing in a woman who is already dealing with high infant mortality in her community. Nursing care planning must be done with such facts in consideration.

VACCINE AND ANTIVIRAL DRUGS

Current HIV primary prevention strategies center on education to prevent transmission of the virus between persons. Special programs to effect change to safer sex practices in persons who are having difficulty changing are being developed. A safe and effective vaccine for prevention of HIV infection is urgently needed because of the seriousness of the disease and the extent to which HIV infection has spread throughout the world. The outlook for an effective vaccine is uncertain, however. The role of HIV antibodies in providing host defense against infection is not yet clear. Lack of an animal model for HIV infection limits ability to do preclinical trials. Other questions yet to be answered are how will efficacy trials in humans be conducted, and for whom should the vaccine be available? Clearly, again, elimination of risk behaviors for transmission will be the primary means of prevention for some time.

Current estimates by the CDC of the number of persons in the United States who are infected with HIV range from 1 to 2 million.[10] Secondary prevention efforts (i.e., preventing progression from HIV infection to AIDS disease), until recently, focused on teaching ways to enhance mental and physical well-being. Research has begun on use of antiviral drugs to prevent further immune system damage by HIV. The life cycle of HIV follows a set pattern of virus attachment, entry into the host cell, virus uncoating, viral replication, virus assembly, and release from the cell. Each of these steps represent a potential target area for antiviral drugs.

The most extensively studied antiviral drug at this time is zidovudine (AZT). The proposed pharmocologic action of this drug is inhibition of reverse transcriptase, an enzyme necessary for viral replication. Studies of this drug in those with AIDS and ARC indicated lower mortality, better physical and mental performance, weight gain, and increased energy.[17] Unfortunately, serious side effects of granulocytopenia and anemia necessitated reduction in dose or discontinuation of the drug. Rash, pruritus, nausea, headache, and mild confusion may also be noted. Studies of zidovudine in persons with asymptomatic HIV infection have begun; however, studies to examine preventing progression from asymptomatic infection to disease will require several years for data gathering.

Clearly, prospects for pharmacologic intervention in

Research Highlights

Major AIDS prevention efforts now focus on people's ability to make changes in sexual practices. Changes to safer sex practices or abstinence will prevent spread of HIV infection. The ability of public health or medical providers to successfully facilitate changes in sexual practices has promoted much change. However, a core of sexually compulsive or addictive persons remain, for information alone is not helping these persons to become safe sexually. A research project is now underway at the University of Washington to develop an intervention to help these persons become safer sexually.[14]

The relapse prevention model has been applied in treatment of a variety of health-risk behaviors that characteristically are highly reinforcing in the short-term, but are detrimental or fatal in the long-term. Clinical strategies used by this model are primarily cognitive/behavioral and aim at identification and modification of activities, cognitive factors, and problem factors that support the problem behavior. Persons wishing to make stable behavior change are helped to develop three kinds of coping skills: anticipatory coping, or learning to identify and avoid triggers or behavioral chains that tend to lead to problem behavior; immediate coping, or developing alternative ways to respond to such triggers; and remedial coping, or learning to respond to any lapses in problem behavior that do occur in a manner such that total relapse is avoided.[14]

The key elements in this treatment approach include motivation enhancement; identification of situational, cognitive, and effective triggers or cues that tend to precipitate the target behavior; training in coping skills; cognitive reframing; development of a healthy and balanced life-style; use of social support; and development of long-term maintenance strategies.

The components of this research are operationally divided into a series of 20 weekly, one-hour sessions, followed by four sessions taking place at four-week intervals. Findings of this study showed a decline in sexual activity over time, with a tendency for safer sexual practices to account for a higher proportion of all sexual contacts. There also was a significant reduction over time in the total number of unsafe and possibly unsafe sexual practices.[14] The research design and the small number of subjects limit generalizability of findings. Further research is needed to document lasting and continued behavior change over time; this model for behavior change offers much promise for persons who seek help and support to become sexually safer.

HIV infection exist. In the meantime, interventions for the spectrum of HIV infection are counseling about risk, risk reduction, facilitating and supporting behavior change, and helping persons who have HIV infection to find optimum physical and mental well being—hope.

SUMMARY

Behaviors associated with transmission of the human immunodeficiency virus are sexual contact, blood exposure, and mother-to-child transmission. The HIV is known to cause a spectrum of disease in those infected. Nurses caring for clients with HIV-related disease need to carefully evaluate and monitor their own values, fears, and feelings about sexuality, alternative lifestyles, and death. Nurses assess, diagnose, and intervene with clients ranging from the worried well to the those who have AIDS. Dramatic and rapid changes in physical and psychosocial status can occur in persons with HIV infection, necessitating frequent and continuing assessment for nursing diagnoses and planning for interventions. There are unique diagnostic issues, depending upon the client's ethnic group, family situation, and substance abuse history.

References

1. Centers for Disease Control. AIDS Weekly Surveillance Report—United States. AIDS Program, Center for Infectious Diseases, CDC. July 25, 1988.
2. Cochran S, Mays V, Roberts V. Ethnic minorities and AIDS. In: Lews A, ed. Nursing care of the person with AIDS/ARC. Rockville, MD: Aspen Publishers; 1988:17–24.
3. Collier A, Gayle T, Bahls F. Clinical manifestations and approach to management of HIV infection and AIDS. In: Motulsky A, ed. AIDS: a guide for the primary physician. Univ Wash Med. 1987;13(1):27–33.
4. Confronting AIDS, update 1988. Institute of Medicine. National Academy of Sciences. Washington, DC: National Academy Press; 1988.
5. Des Jarlais DC, Friedman S. HIV infection among intravenous drug users: epidemiology and risk reduction. AIDS. 1987;1:67–76.
6. Dunkel J, Hatfield S. Countertransference issues in working with persons with AIDS. Social Work. 1986;31(Mar–Apr):114–117.
7. Faltz B, Madover S. AIDS and substance abuse. In: Helquist M, ed. Working with AIDS: a resource guide for mental health professionals. San Francisco: The AIDS Project, University of California; 1987.
8. Friedland G, Klein R. Transmission of the human immunodeficiency virus. N Engl J Med. 1987;317:1125–1135.
9. Guinan M, Hardy A. Epidemiology of AIDS in women in the United States, 1981–1987. JAMA. 1987;257:2039–2042.
10. Handsfield H. Epidemiology of acquired immunodeficiency syndrome and human immunodeficiency virus infection in the United States and Pacific Northwest. In: Motulusky A, ed. AIDS: a guide for the primary physician. Univ Wash Med. 1987;13(1):5–9.
11. Hopkins S, Lafferty W. Washington State/Seattle–King County quarterly AIDS surveillance report. First quarter, 1988.
12. Macks J. People with AIDS. In: Helquist M, ed. Working with

AIDS: a resource guide for mental health professionals. San Francisco: The AIDS Health Project, University of California; 1987.

13. Recommendations for prevention of HIV transmission in health care settings. MMWR. 1987;36(2F):3F–18F.

14. Roffman R. Relapse prevention as a means of AIDS risk reduction. A report to the King County AIDS Prevention Project. University of Washington School of Social Work; 1987.

15. Shaw N. AIDS: special concerns for women. In: Helquist M, ed. Working with AIDS—a resource guide for mental health professionals. San Francisco: The AIDS Health Project, University of California; 1987.

16. Strawn J. The psychosocial consequences of AIDS. In: Durham J, Cohen F, eds. The person with AIDS: a nursing perspective. New York: Springer Publishing; 1987.

17. Tartaglione T, Corey L. Prospects in anti-retroviral chemotherapy for treatment of HIV infection. In: Motulusky A, ed. AIDS: a guide for the primary physician. Univ Wash Med. 1987;13(1):36–41.

Specialized Psychiatric Therapies and Treatment Programs and the Nursing Process

33

Barbara Hyatt Baskerville

Milieu Therapy

OBJECTIVES

After reading this chapter, the reader will be able to:

1. Describe basic theoretical concepts related to milieu therapy
2. Describe historical perspectives in the development of milieu therapy
3. Apply the nursing process in milieu therapy
4. Analyze and use research findings in milieu intervention.

INTRODUCTION

Milieu therapy is a complex approach to the care of clients that can be described from many perspectives. A review of the literature reveals some ambiguity in its definition. Generically, however, milieu therapy is described as any program that uses the environment or aspects of the environment in a health-promoting manner.[13] Visher and O'Sullivan[28] depict milieu therapy in a more specific way.

> Milieu therapy may be described as a careful structuring of the social and physical environment of a psychiatric treatment program so that every interaction and activity is therapeutic for the patient.

In this chapter, *milieu therapy* is defined as the organization of the environment to assist clients to control problematic behavior and to use more adaptive psychosocial skills in coping with self, others, and the environment. The environment is structured as a microcosm of the larger society. More specifically, the focus is on social relationships and occupational and recreational activities. Clients are placed in various therapeutic situations in the environment during all their waking hours. The terms *milieu therapy* and *therapeutic milieu* are often used interchangeably and will be used that way throughout this chapter.

Milieu therapy is an approach to the care of clients in a variety of institutional and community settings, which has changed over time.[9] Some of these changes were produced by a diversity of social and technological forces, including deinstitutionalization, increased use of pharmacologic agents, and widespread attention to the rights of clients. With greater recognition of the effect of the treatment environment on the client, milieu therapy evolved as an alternative to approaches emphasizing psychopathology. Accordingly, the focus of therapy shifted from the individual and therapist to the multidisciplinary team and clients in therapeutic groups in the environment. Furthermore, the client's role changed from that of a passive recipient of care, to that of being a more active participant. Although no two approaches are totally alike, milieu therapy in some form is an inevitable and integral component of the nursing management of clients.

Historical Perspectives

In the early 20th century, psychoanalysts, inspired by Freud and his followers, developed a type of milieu therapy that was based on psychoanalytic theory. According to this method, hospital activities and specific staff interactions were prescribed for each client based on a formulation of the client's unconscious needs.[6] The influences of this practice persist, to some degree, in private inpatient settings. Later Sullivan observed that clients with schizophrenia did not behave in a psychotic manner when they were in a ward staffed by sympathetic people.[27] His work was an early attempt to investigate the nature of the social environment and its use in therapy.[29] Frieda Fromm-Reichman expanded on Sullivan's notion about the therapeutic use of ward personnel as she worked with clients with schizophrenia at the Chestnut Lodge Hospital in Maryland.

The concern for the social environment and its effects on clients continued to flourish during the period between 1940 and 1950. Maxwell Jones developed a therapy that was known as the "therapeutic community." This model by Jones, stressed the clients responsibility for his or her own treatment and for the treatment of others.[23] Clients were expected to participate actively and responsibly in the milieu by sharing feelings and information in meetings, performing individual tasks, sharing assignments, and participating in milieu decisions. In addition, Jones believed that the potential for therapeutic outcome is enhanced when clients understand the motivation underlying their own action, as well as possess an awareness of the effects of their behavior on other people.[10] He initially implemented therapeutic community concepts with groups of neurotic clients receiving long-term care. To accomplish the overall goal of resocialization, various daily discussion groups were employed. These groups were attended by clients and staff and focused on topics ranging from health-related problems to issues related to life on the ward. Although nurses composed the largest component of staff, Jones did not envision their participation as individual therapists. In fact, he noted the nurse's role to be one of interpreting and transmitting the unit culture to clients.

In the United States, the use of milieu therapy has been documented in a variety of general hospital settings. For example, a psychiatric head nurse detailed the application of milieu therapy in the 1950s with a small population of soldiers who were experiencing their first psychotic episode.[25] Clients were responsible for the cleanliness of the ward and also participated in some areas of policy development (e.g., post passes and ward routines). Moreover, the therapeutic community was viewed as one in which the staff influenced the growth, development, and effectiveness of clients, while focusing on the immediate present. The nurse's role was viewed as a communicator, manager, teacher, and effective team member.

In the mid-1960s, a therapeutic community was established in the psychiatric unit of a general hospital, with a central and essential aspect of the program being daily community meetings.[22] Community members legislated policy, developed ideas for the management of behavioral problems, and considered all requests for passes. In addition, clients participated in other activities deemed to be of a therapeutic nature, including acting as volunteers in monitoring peers needing close observation. However, the community's authority was delegated by staff, and medical and nursing staff retained veto over matters involving medicolegal responsibility.

Contemporary use of some aspect of milieu-oriented intervention is found in numerous settings including day care and rehabilitation centers, outpatient departments, group homes, hotels, prisons, as well as acute care settings. A case study depicting the use of milieu-oriented strategies in a contemporary setting is presented later in this chapter. No absolute indications for the use of milieu therapy are found in the literature, and Abrams notes that its use relates more to the kinds of social organization and intervention techniques, rather than the type of population with which it is used.[1]

Characteristics

Despite variations in purpose, target clientele and treatment settings, therapeutic milieus retain some common characteristics.[10,11,14] This section briefly discusses the concepts of democracy, commitment and engagement, communalism, and humanitarianism. These characteristics are diagrammed in Figure 33-1.

- *Democracy* refers to social equality and the sharing of power. In milieu therapy, the extent to which the democratic concept is applied depends on the characteristic of the clientele and the philosophy and objectives of the treatment program. Furthermore, it is guided by the medicolegal responsibilities with which staff are empowered. However, the original concept of milieu therapy strongly embraced the idea of shared governances. Both clients and staff contribute information and share responsibility for decision making, planning, and managing the therapeutic environment.
- *Commitment–engagement* implies a sense of obligation or duty. To the extent that their mental and physical status permits, clients are expected to attend and actively participate in all milieu activities. Active participation involves the sharing of

thoughts and feelings among peers, as well as with staff.
- *Communalism* reflects a sense of family or community. Clients live in close association with peers who have similar concerns or problems. In milieu therapy, the extensive use of groups facilitates the development of a cohesive unit. In addition, the sharing of various physical and psychosocial resources fosters a sense of communalism.
- *Humanitarianism* connotes an emphasis on the good of the whole. In milieu therapy, *each* client is expected to demonstrate concern for the well being of *all* clients. Furthermore, every individual, whether client or staff, is expected to engage in empathic interactions. The general feeling tone communicated in interpersonal relationships is one of acceptance, caring and respect.

Principles

Milieu therapy embraces the idea that client's difficulties in relating to others often contribute to the development of problems in responding and adapting to the environment. Thus, an awareness of basic psychosocial principles in essential.[11,14,26] Selected principles that relate to milieu therapy are discussed in this section.

Human Behavior is a Response to the Environment.[14]
Human beings, as open systems, engage in constant interaction with their surroundings. Thus, humans respond to various environmental stimuli or the lack of stimulation. In milieu therapy, every component of the treatment setting is viewed as potentially therapeutic.

Positive and Negative Reinforcement Affect Human Behavior.[14]
Human behavior is shaped or affected by the esteem that is given to or withheld by others.[14] People have a need for positive self-regard. Furthermore, an individual's self-image develops based on the approval or disapproval that is received from significant others, throughout the life cycle. In milieu therapy, it is believed that clients can be motivated to use more adaptive responses, based on reinforcement received from peers and staff. Methods of reinforcement may include rewards, privileges, isolation, or restriction of social interaction.

Human Beings Have a Need for Social Contact.[14]
It is generally accepted that all human beings have a need for social interaction, to some degree. In addition, it is believed that often a client's problems or concerns stem from difficulties in relating to other people. Thus, the focus of milieu therapy is on the improvement of psychosocial skills. This is accomplished by the extensive use of group interactions.

Every Individual Has a Helping Capacity.[26]
Every individual, regardless of education, specialized skills or

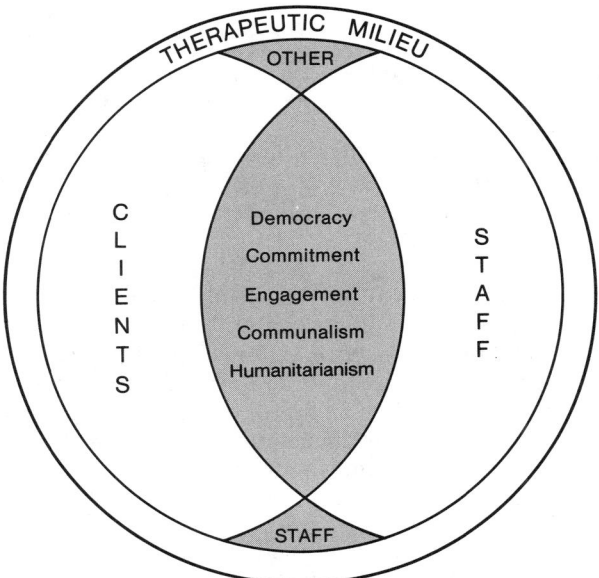

FIGURE 33–1. Characteristics of milieu therapy.

role, possesses the potential to help another person. Thus, with adequate structure and support, clients have the potential to become therapeutic agents. Because clients often spend more time with each other than with staff, they may be able to share information and perspectives previously unknown to staff, during various milieu forums.

Illness and Therapy Are Both Opportunities for Learning About Oneself, Others, and Relationships.[11]
The crisis state of illness can create within individuals increased receptivity to assistance. Appropriate role-modeling by staff can provide opportunities for clients to learn more adaptive responses. In addition, through exploration and analysis, clients can gain an increased awareness of the relationship between thoughts, feelings, and subsequent behavior.

MILIEU THERAPY AND THE NURSING PROCESS
Assessment and Nursing Roles

A multiplicity of physical, social, spiritual, emotional, and educational factors affect the creation of a therapeutic environment. Nursing assessment of these factors is essential to determine whether the milieu meets the needs of individual and groups of clients. Selected questions, roles of the nurse, and illustrations that enhance the assessment process are presented in the following:

Physical
1. Is the environment free of sharp and dangerous objects?
2. Does the environment provide privacy in bathrooms?
3. Are the bedrooms clean, spacious, and personal?
4. Are personal belongings allowed to be displayed?

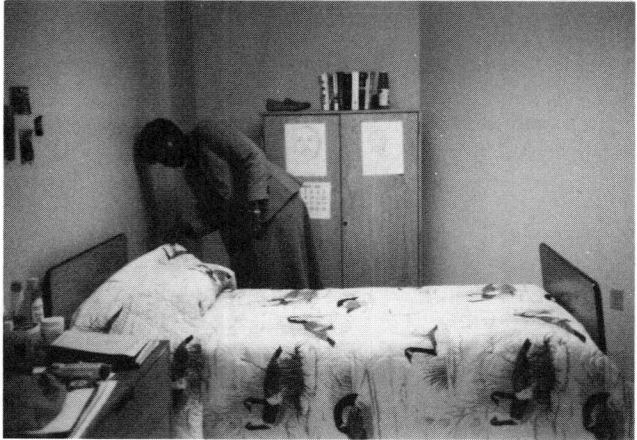

FIGURE 33–2. A client's bedroom can display his or her individuality.

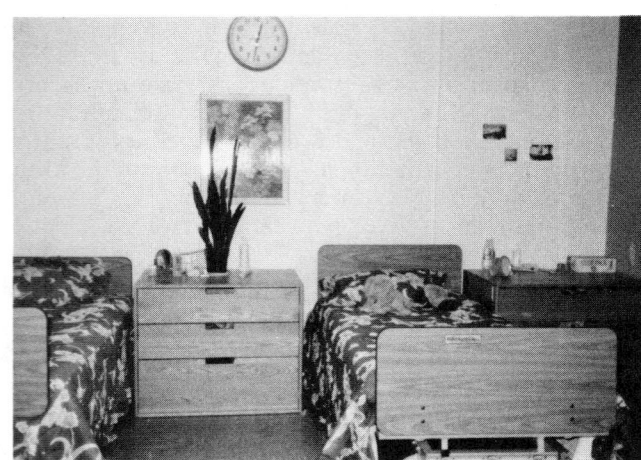

FIGURE 33–3. This double bedroom provides space for clients' belongings and a clock for orientation.

5. Are bedrooms available for single and multioccupancy?

The role of the psychiatric mental health nurse in maintaining a safe environment is particularly important for clients who are psychotic and suicidal. The primary nurse assigned to a group of clients must check their rooms for harmful items or conditions detrimental to their well-being. Nurses can reduce stressors in the environment which may be perceived as disturbing by some clients (i.e., loud radios, television, or client noise). Nurses also provide for clients to participate in decisions on room assignment and evaluates clients' readiness for various arrangements. Therefore, several room options should be available[21] (Figs. 33-2 and 33-3).

Social
1. Are clients oriented to the environment?
2. Are clients aware of the boundaries in the environment (e.g., rules, schedules)?
3. Are areas available to facilitate interaction? (Fig. 33-4)
4. Are clients' rights posted?
5. Are social activities available based on cultural needs?
6. Are activities available for family members or significant others to engage in with clients and/or staff members (e.g., dinners, movies, discussion groups)? (Fig. 33-5)

Roles of psychiatric mental health nurses, in the social dimension of clients' milieu focus on facilitating clients' interaction with others. Socialization is enhanced through various community meetings and structured activities facilitated by nurses. Nurses are primary providers of information to other health team members, families, and significant others.

Spiritual
1. Are worship services available at this institution?
2. Are times available on the unit for meeting spiritual needs?

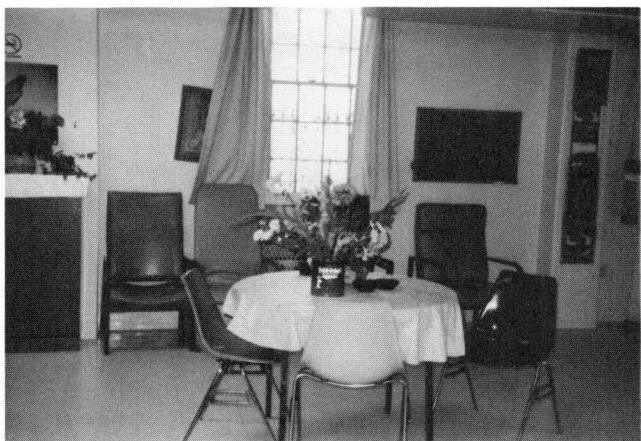

FIGURE 33–4. Space for informal interaction is important in the therapeutic milieu.

3. Are chaplains accessible to clients?
4. Are religious needs addressed in the treatment plan?

The psychiatric mental health nurse has a role in assisting clients to meet their spiritual needs. One strategy is to allow time for clients to have solitude and reflection. This may be accomplished by allocating free time in daily or weekly schedules. In addition, nursing staff facilitate clients' attendance at various religious services and assure that escorts are available as needed (Fig. 33-6).

Emotional
1. Does the environment encourage expression of feelings?
2. Are staff members available to assist clients with specific problems (e.g., grief, family conflicts)?
3. Is a support system available to clients in the environment (e.g., family, peers, staff)?

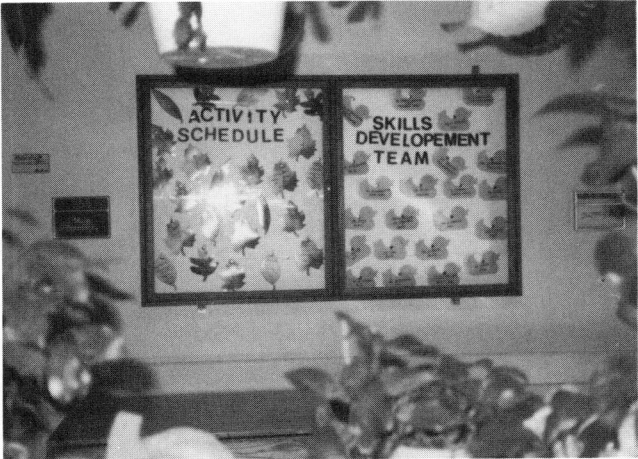

FIGURE 33–5. Team members' names and the schedule of various activities are posted for clients' information.

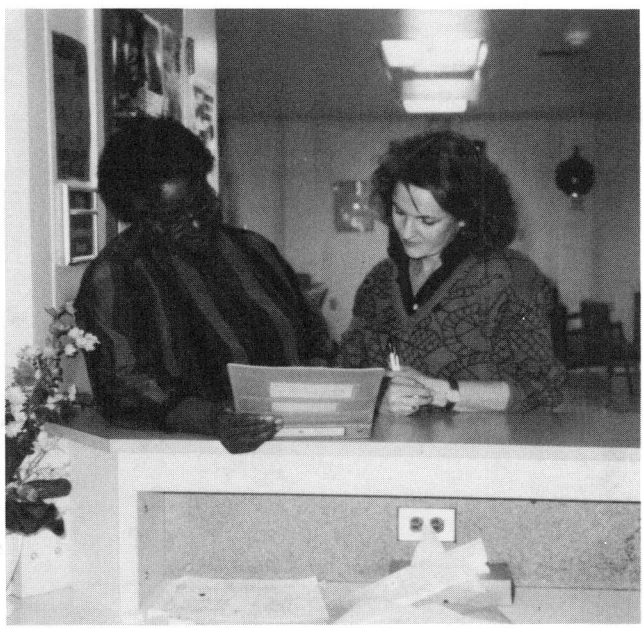

FIGURE 33–6. The hospital chaplain, an active participant in this therapeutic milieu, converses with a client.

4. What is the emotional tone of the environment?
5. Does the environment allow for growth and individual differences (i.e., individualized treatment based on individual client's need versus group's needs)?
6. Is counseling, family, group, or other therapies available to family members or significant others?

The psychiatric mental health nurse plays a major role in creating a therapeutic environment that encourages clients to share their problems and successful and unsuccessful coping skills with their peers. In addition, nurses serve as counselors and/or therapists to individuals, families, and groups of clients in the milieu. Furthermore, the role of the nurse as a member of the mental health team has emerged from one of passivity to one of action (Fig. 33-7).

Educational and Learning
1. Does the environment provide an atmosphere to learn and practice new behaviors?
2. Are clients provided with health education classes?
3. Are self-medication classes provided?
4. Are opportunities available to learn new occupational skills or maintain current job skills?
5. Are classes held to teach clients about symptoms and various aspects of mental illness?

Mental health teaching is an essential role of the psychiatric mental health nurse in a therapeutic milieu. Nurses conduct health education classes that may address medical and psychiatric problems, psychotropic medications, communication and problem solving, stress management, and human sexuality. Family members or significant others are frequently involved

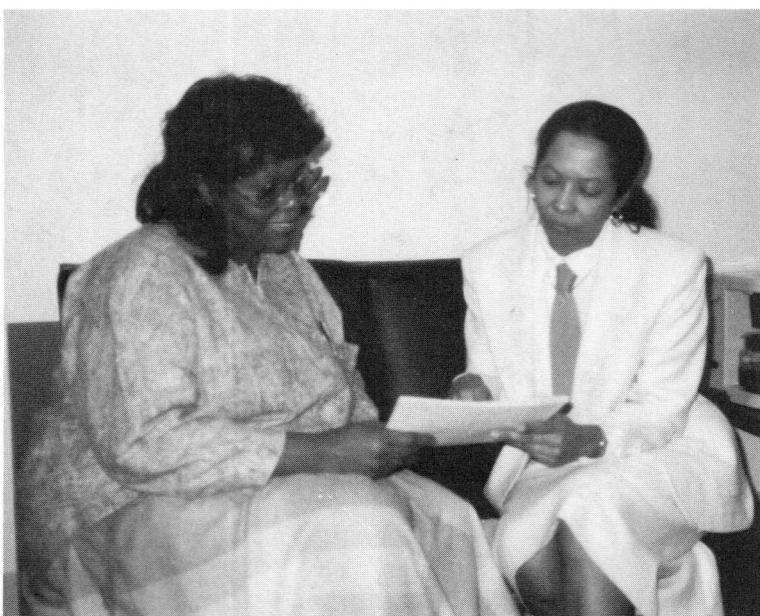

FIGURE 33–7. The primary nurse counsels her client and reviews the client's contract with her in the privacy of the nurse's office.

in health education classes with clients. The multifaceted roles of nurses, creative application of the nursing process, and active client participation greatly influence the achievement of therapeutic outcomes[3] (Figs. 33-8 and 33-9).

Goals and Planning

Milieu goals and strategies evolve from the characteristics of the client population and the needs of individuals and groups of clients. Consequently, the goals described in this section, although not universally appropriate, do reflect themes found in the literature. Visher and O'Sullivan[28] describe the overall goal of milieu therapy as the use of experiences of daily living to correct dysfunctions in communication and interpersonal relations. Abroms[1] identifies limit setting and the teaching of social skills as the main goals of psychiatric treatment, regardless of the therapeutic approach used. Adler[2] delineates control, insulation, social reintegration, client role induction, structure, support, and involvement as functions of the therapeutic milieu. An

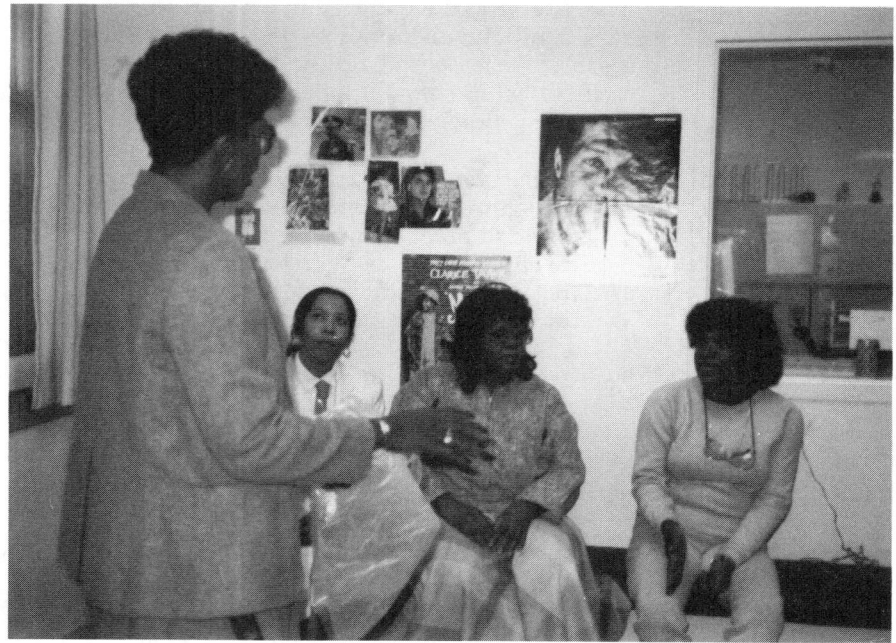

FIGURE 33–8. Health education classes for clients are conducted in a bright meeting room on the unit.

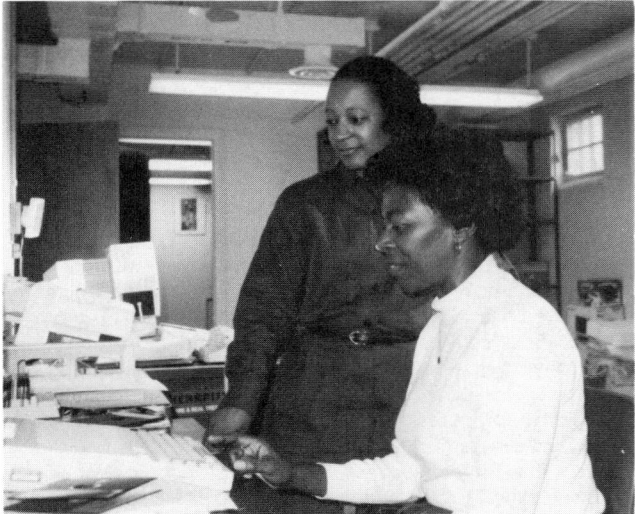

FIGURE 33–9. *An occupational therapist instructs the client in the use of a computer.*

attempt to translate these themes into specific client and interrelated staff goals is outlined as follows:

Client Will
- Recognize self as being ill and accept staff assistance
- Exercise self control in relation to destructive, dependent, or acting-out behavior
- Engage in problem solving with others
- Actively participate in rehabilitative activities.

Staff Will
- Confront client's denial of illness and share observations of current behavior
- Provide a safe environment by employing limit setting with disruptive behavior and removing harmful objects from the environment
- Provide support using praise, encouragement, constructive criticism and problem solving
- Facilitate client's preparation for discharge by assistance with social, occupational and leisure skills.

Milieu Intervention Strategies

The implementation of milieu strategies involves a series of forums in which clients and staff share information about individual and group behavior, define community norms and policies, develop and modify therapeutic plans, and resolve interpersonal conflicts that interfere with the therapeutic process. Prominent among specific milieu strategies are (1) staff premeeting or morning report; (2) community meeting; (3) postmeeting or rehash; (4) client government meeting; (5) small group meetings; (6) multidisciplinary team meeting; and (7) staff meeting. Unless otherwise stated, the meetings last one hour and are held weekly. A brief description of each of the strategies follows.[1]

STAFF PREMEETING OR MORNING REPORT

Staff premeeting or morning report is often the first meeting of the day. The purpose of this meeting is to share information about clients' behavior during the past 24 hours. In the staff premeeting, nurses generally provide information to other staff members. Whereas, in morning report, clients attend and contribute information to the discussion.

COMMUNITY MEETING

Community meeting, an innovation of Maxwell Jones, remains a major tool for fostering collaborations between clients and staff. Typically all clients and staff are seated in a large circle. Discussion may address admissions and discharge, staffing changes, the general atmosphere and participation level in the community, as well as policy issues (e.g., privileges and past requests). However, the final decision-making on medicolegal issues rest with staff. Furthermore, staff, especially nursing staff, provide assistance in the identification of themes of discussion and management of clients with disruptive behavior.

POSTMEETING OR REHASH

Postmeeting or rehash is usually a brief discussion held immediately after community meeting. The purpose of this meeting is to review the content and dynamics of the community meetings. Furthermore, it also provides an opportunity for immediate support to staff or clients about their participation in community meeting. Staff and clients may conduct this forum separately or jointly.

CLIENT GOVERNMENT MEETING

Client government meeting focuses on concerns related to the immediate environment and problems that arise in sharing the same environment. Typical issues might include the cleanliness of the unit, lights-out policy, and the use of the community's funds. This meeting is conducted by a community president. Other officers may include a vice president, secretary, treasurer, and various committee chairs (e.g., pass, housekeeping, recreation). Staff are often represented by nursing personnel and provide consultation on unit and hospital policies.

SMALL GROUP MEETINGS

Small group meetings are usually led or co-led by a psychiatrist or nurse. The group generally consists of ten or fewer clients. Discussion in this forum is on a more intimate level and focuses on factors impinging on clients' illnesses and the identification of more effective coping strategies.

MULTIDISCIPLINARY TEAM MEETING

Multidisciplinary team meeting is attended by all disciplines including nurses, psychiatrists, psychologists, social workers, occupational therapists, as well as students or interns in these professions. Each client's therapeutic program including problems, goals, approaches, and the discipline primarily responsible for implementation is discussed. All team members share observations on the client's behavior and progress.

STAFF MEETING

Staff meeting is limited to staff participation. Central to this forum is the discussion of here-and-now communication and interpersonal conflicts that interfere with a harmonious team approach to therapeutic outcomes.

OTHER ACTIVITIES

Other types of therapeutic activities may include psychodrama, educational activities, industrial therapy, music, art, recreational and exercise therapy, as well as life skills (e.g., cooking groups). After referral by medical staff, nurses often assist clients in scheduling and participating in various therapeutic activities.

Evaluation

Evaluation involves the appraisal of clients' responses to milieu therapy. The establishment of specific outcome criteria is an integral part of this process. Outcome criteria may address the effectiveness of a program, specific characteristics of clients and staff or measures of client progress. Several researchers have attempted to determine the effectiveness of various aspects of milieu therapy programs.[16-20] Reports from these studies reveal mixed results and are described in the section on Research Highlights.

CASE STUDY

Tony, a 40-year-old man, was admitted to the long-term care unit with the diagnosis of schizophrenia, paranoid type. His admission was precipitated by the loss of his job as an accountant and an investment failure. Tony accused office workers of plotting to kill him and saying bad things about him. As his ability to problem solve and make decisions decreased, the employer found it necessary to terminate him. Tony was not known to have any close friends or contact with relatives. Tony severed relationships with his two siblings after the death of his parents 25 years ago. During the admission interview, Tony expressed ideas of reference, delusions, and acknowledged hearing voices that had a hostile tone. His speech was pressured, he seemed preoccupied with his thoughts, he mumbled to himself, and occasionally stared blankly.

At morning report, the head nurse discussed Tony's behavior with the staff and made the following nursing diagnoses: impaired social interaction related to misperceptions, lack of support system, and inadequate social skills; and aggression related to misperceptions and hostility.

An initial care plan was formulated with a plan for his primary nurse to spend time with Tony to provide support and to establish a relationship.

At the community meeting Tony became disruptive, shouting in a loud abusive tone at a female client to shut up. Also, he accused the group of talking about him. Tony's primary nurse sat beside him to assure other clients that Tony would not harm them and to assist him to control his behavior. It was agreed by the community that Tony needed to be removed from the meeting. His primary nurse escorted him to his room and remained with him. The primary nurse conveyed a sense of caring and understanding of Tony's behavior, which is essential in establishing a trustful relationship. The female client he had shouted at was upset by Tony's remarks and expressed her perception that it was deliberately done to upset her. Staff reassured the client that Tony's response was a means of coping with his own feelings. Group members discussed strategies for handling future disruptions in the group and agreed to try out some techniques (e.g., reassuring the person that no group member will be harmed, asking the client to share current feelings).

During the discussion at a nursing staff care planning meeting to update Tony's plan, several members expressed anger and frustration toward Tony. One staff member felt that he was engaged in attention-seeking behavior and not involved in the community. The primary nurse reminded the staff members of how the client's history of failure of relationships in early childhood, death of parents, unresolved conflicts with siblings, lack of social network, and subsequent feelings of worthlessness contributed to the mistrustful, isolative, and passive behavior that he displayed in the milieu. Staff members commented that the information given to them helped them to better understand the dynamics behind the client's behavior. The head nurse encouraged the staff to convey caring and understanding when clients act out, even though limits are set to control behavior.

At the multidisciplinary meeting several activities were recommended (exercise group, gym, and swimming) to assist Tony to deal with anger and hostility. In addition, Tony, who was present, chose to add the walking group to his schedule. Incorporating all the suggestions made, a comprehensive individualized plan was developed (Nursing Care Plan 33-1). An activity schedule for Tony is illustrated in Table 33-1. For clients displaying disturbed behavior related to schizophrenia, a therapeutic environment is needed that is orderly, consistent, and productive. More specifically, Tony needed a structured environment to provide opportunities for him to learn to trust others, maximize his strengths, develop social skills, learn new coping skills, and test out new behaviors. Tony's primary nurse planned to assist him in following the milieu activities and evaluating the effectiveness of the activities in accomplishing his treatment goals.

The case study illustrates the roles that both clients and staff play in the use of resources in the milieu to achieve therapeutic goals. Eventually, Tony became a candidate for community placement in a half-way house or group home. A comprehensive after-care plan was developed prior to discharge which included follow-up in a community mental health center, a job, monitoring of self-medication, community resources (support group, social club, structured group therapy sessions, and health teachers). Tony's potential to

TABLE 33–1
Typical schedule of milieu activities

TIME	MONDAY	TUESDAY	WEDNESDAY	THURSDAY	FRIDAY	SATURDAY	SUNDAY
6–7	Wake up; bathing and grooming	Bathing and grooming 6:45–7 Exercise	Bathing and grooming	Bathing and grooming 6:45–7 Exercise	Bathing and grooming 6:45–7 Exercise	6:30 Bathing and grooming	6:30 Bathing and grooming
7–7:30	Medications	Medications	Medications	Medications	Medications	Medications	Medications
7:30–8:15	Breakfast	Breakfast	Breakfast	Breakfast	Breakfast	Breakfast	Breakfast
8:30–9:30	Care of sleeping area Ward chores	Care of sleeping area Ward chores	Care of sleeping area Ward chores	Care of sleeping area Ward chores	Care of sleeping area Ward chores	Care of sleeping area Ward chores	Care of sleeping area Ward chores
9:30–10:15	Community meeting	Psychodrama	Community meeting	Psychodrama	Community meeting	Current events group	Worship services
10:15–11:30	Health awareness group Medication group	Arts and crafts Skills development group	Health awareness group Medication group	Arts and crafts group Skills development group	Gym Health awareness group	Walking group	Worship services
11:30–12	Free	Free	Free	Free	Free	Free	Free
12–1	Lunch	Lunch	Lunch	Lunch	Lunch	Lunch	Lunch
1–1:30	Medications	Medications	Medications	Medications	Medications	Medications	Medications
1:30–2:30	Free	Free	Free	Free	Free	Free	Free
2:30–3:30	Individual therapy	Swimming	Current events group	Individual therapy	Bowling	Recreational therapy	Social hour
3:30–4:30	Educational group	(Community)	Educational group	Community meeting	(Community)	Games	Social hour
4:30–5	Free	Free	Free	Free	Free	Free	Free
5–6:00	Dinner	Dinner	Dinner	Dinner	Dinner	Dinner	Dinner
6–7:00	Music group	Movie	Music group	Activities of daily living group	Movie	Free	Free
7:00	Medications	Medications	Medications	Medications	Medications	Medications	Medications

NURSING CARE PLAN 33–1

TONY

NURSING INTERVENTIONS	OUTCOME CRITERIA
NURSING DIAGNOSIS: Aggression related to misperceptions and hostility	
CLIENT GOAL: Focus on appropriate responses to the external environment	
■ Help Tony recognize signs of stress and seek help before loss of control	Identifies stressors, reports to primary nurse to seek assistance
■ Demonstrate relaxation techniques to help Tony cope with stress	Uses relaxation techniques in times of increased stress
■ Help Tony dismiss voices by telling the voices to go away; encourage Tony to focus on some aspect of the environment as a technique for dismissing voices	Focuses on activity engaged in, or on person he is interacting with, without interference from voices
■ Reinforce reality thinking by dealing with issues in the here and now and give positive reinforcement to Tony when talks are reality based	Relates to staff and peers realistically
■ Set limits when behavior is inappropriate	
■ Convey caring and understanding to assist Tony to trust	
NURSING DIAGNOSIS: Impaired social interaction related to misperceptions, lack of support system, and inadequate social skills	
CLIENT GOAL: Interact with staff and peers	
■ Establish 1:1 relationship with Tony	Expresses thoughts and feelings spontaneously with staff and peers on a 1 to 1 basis
■ Utilize Tony's strengths (such as reading and math skills) to promote interaction with staff and peers by asking his assistance in planning a budget for a ward program or group trip	Participates in planning the budget for a group trip with a staff member and two peers
■ Observe for clues that Tony cannot tolerate interaction (e.g., pressured speech, shaking of extremity, increased eye movement)	Gives verbal feedback if interactions are not tolerable
■ Support and encourage participation in community and other milieu meetings by giving eye contact, commenting on responses, and giving praise	Participates verbally in small and large group activities
■ Encourage participation in social activities of Tony's choice[12]	Chooses activities of interest within the milieu and other programs
■ Explore dynamics of past relationships	Discusses history of past relationships with primary nurse
■ Encourage Tony to check out his suspicions with staff	

remain in the community is high, providing he complies with his medication regimen, remains employed, and follows other aspects of his prescribed treatment.

SUMMARY

Milieu therapy, with its focus on the immediate environment, evolved from Maxwell Jones's therapeutic community. The contemporary approach stresses clients' responsibility not only in their own care, but in the care of peers as well. The extent to which milieu therapy is used is dependent upon the philosophy, type of client population, length of stay, and resources of the facility. Most milieu programs are characterized by common characteristics: democracy, commitment, engagement, communalism, and humanitarianism. Some aspects of milieu therapy have been documented in a diversity of institutional and community settings.

With a 24-hour presence in the therapeutic environment, nurses have the primary responsibility for structuring and maintaining the therapeutic milieu in collaboration with clients and other health team members. Contemporary nurses function in expanded

Research Highlights

Concepts presented throughout this chapter have delineated the importance of the therapeutic environment in facilitating positive changes in the behavior of clients. Several studies attempt to systematically conceptualize and evaluate various environmental dimensions. Notable among these research studies are investigations by Rudolph H. Moos. Moos, and colleagues[17,19] developed tools that assess environmental factors. Moos and Houts developed the Ward Atmosphere Scale (WAS).[16] The WAS is a 99-item questionnaire that measures a variety of dimensions in the treatment environment. It consists of ten subscales that assess relationships, treatment programs, and administrative variables. The first subscales which are ward involvement, support and spontaneity, are conceptualized as *relationship* variables. They assess (1) clients involvement and support of each other, (2) staff support of clients, and (3) the extent of open expression of feelings by clients.[17] The next subscales are autonomy, practical orientation, personal problem orientation, anger, and aggression, which are conceptualized as being particularly relevant to the *treatment program*. These variables measure the degree of emphasis on independence, open expression of aggressive feelings, understanding one's problems, and the orientation of the environment toward preparing clients for discharge.[17] The subscales of order and organization, program clarity, and staff control are conceptualized as *administrative* variables. These administrative variables measure the extent to which the program is clear and effectively planned, as well as the strictness and determination of rules by staff.[17] The WAS has been used to assess the perceptions of both clients and staff. In addition, it has been standardized on a national reference group of 160 psychiatric wards.[17]

Moos and his colleagues have conducted several investigations that analyze treatment environments.[18–20] Moos and Schwartz described the relationship of the treatment environment to treatment outcomes.[19] Seven large wards in a Veterans Administration hospital were studied. Dimensions of the treatment environment, as perceived by 192 staff members and 292 hospitalized male clients were measured using the Ward Atmosphere Scale. Background characteristics of hospitalized clients were comparable among wards studied. Treatment outcomes were measured for each ward using dropout (elopements and discharges against medical advice) rates, release (discharge)

rates, and length of stay in the community for released, but readmitted clients. A total of 725 clients composed the group of released, but readmitted, clients. These clients were profiled to be unmarried, under 60-year-old men, with a psychiatric diagnosis of schizophrenia.

The findings of this study indicated that the wards that had high dropout rates were perceived by clients as being low in emphasizing practical orientation, order, and organization. Staff presented a different viewpoint. They viewed the wards with high dropout rates as having low emphasis on support, involvement, and program clarity, with high emphasis on anger, aggression, and staff control.[19] Thus, clients tended to leave wards for which they perceived there was little focus on effective planning of activities and for which staff perceived (1) little emphasis on involvement in interpersonal relationships and (2) much emphasis on the encouragement of clients to express aggressive feelings. In addition, wards with high release rates were perceived by clients as being high in the degree of practical orientation and staff control. However, staff perceived the wards with high release rates to have low emphasis on spontaneity.[19] In other words, clients tended to stay until discharge when they perceived the environment to stress strictness, and determination of rules by staff, as well as an orientation toward preparation of clients for discharge. Furthermore, wards that released clients who stayed in the community the longest before readmission were perceived by both clients and staff to have high emphasis on staff control. Thus, the strictness and determination by staff of rules had a positive correlation to longer community tenure of released, but later readmitted, clients.

The findings of this study are consistent with those of Ellsworth in suggesting a relationship between treatment environment and release and community tenure rates.[8] However, it adds the dimension of dropout rates. Moos has cited the potential usefulness of tools, such as the WAS, not only in the analysis of psychiatric wards, but also for institutional and individual self analyses. Moreover, he notes that this type of social systems analysis can help determine the congruency between the perceptions of staff and clients and milieu purposes and goals. Thus, clients who are at risk for dropout or failure could be identified and appropriate interventions instituted. Finally, Moos delineates the possible usefulness of social systems analysis in the maintenance of quality control.

roles including leadership of various group activities, health education, and counseling. Furthermore, nurses are recognized as active members of the multidisciplinary team, rather than passive providers of custodial care. By using knowledge of psychosocial principles and research findings, nurses apply the nursing process in the implementation of various milieu intervention strategies.

References

1. Abroms GM. Defining milieu therapy. Arch Gen Psychiatry. 1969;21:553–560.
2. Adler WN. Milieu therapy. In: Lion J, Adler WN, Webb WL, eds. Modern hospital psychiatry. New York: WW Norton; 1988.
3. American Nurses Association. Standards of psychiatric and mental health nursing practice. Kansas City, MO: American Nurses' Association; 1982.
4. Benfer B, Schroder P. Nursing in the therapeutic milieu. Bull Menninger Clin. 1985;49:451–465.
5. Berry D. A therapeutic approach. Nurs Times. 1984;80:20–21.
6. Bettleheim B, Sylvester E. A therapeutic milieu. Am J Orthopsychiatry. 1948;18:191–206.
7. Brooks A. Role of psychiatric nurse. In: Lion J, Adler WN, Webb WL, eds. Modern hospital psychiatry. New York: WW Norton; 1988.
8. Ellsworth R, Maroney R, Klett W, Gordon H, Gunn R. Milieu characteristics of successful psychiatric programs. Am J Orthopsychiatry. 1971;41:427–441.
9. Gutheil TG. The therapeutic milieu: changing themes and theories. Hosp & Commun Psychiatry. 1985;36:1279–1285.
10. Jones M. The therapeutic community. New York: Basic Books; 1953.
11. Kennard D, Roberts J. An introduction to therapeutic communities. London: Routledge and Kegan Paul; 1983.
12. Kim M, McFarland G, McLane A. Pocket guide to nursing diagnoses, 3rd ed. St Louis: CV Mosby; 1989.
13. Kraft AM. The therapeutic community. In: Arieti S, ed. The american handbook of psychiatry. New York: Basic Books; 1966.
14. Lennard HL, Gralnick A. The psychiatric hospital context,
15. McFarland G, Wasli E. Nursing diagnosis and process in psychiatric nursing. Philadelphia: JB Lippincott; 1986.
16. Moos R. Assessment of the psychosocial environments of community oriented psychiatric treatment programs. J Abnorm Psychol. 1972;79:9–17.
17. Moos R, Houts P. Assessment of social atmosphere of psychiatric wards. J Abnorm Psychol. 1968;73:595–604.
18. Moos R, Houts P. Differential effects of social atmosphere on psychiatric wards. Hum Relat. 1970;23:47–60.
19. Moos R, Schwartz J. Treatment environment and treatment outcome. J Nerv Ment Dis. 1972;154:264–275.
20. Moos R, Shelton R, Petty C. Perceived ward climate and treatment outcome. J Abnorm Psychol. 1973;82:291–298.
21. Proshansky HM, Ittelson WH, Reubin LG. Freedom of choice and behavior in a physical setting. In: Proshansky HM, Ittelson WH, Reubin LG, eds. Environmental psychology: man and his physical setting. New York: Holt, Rinehart & Winston; 1970.
22. Quattlebaum JT. A therapeutic community on a short term psychiatric unit. In: Rossi JJ, Filstead WJ, eds. The therapeutic community. A sourcebook of readings. New York: Behavioral Publications; 1973.
23. Rasinski K, Rozensky R, Pasulka P. Practical implications of the "therapeutic milieu" for psychiatric nursing practice. J Psychiat Nurs Ment Health Serv. 1980;80:16–19.
24. Robertson P. The therapeutic community nurse: a blurring of traditional roles. J Psychiat Nurs Ment Health Serv. 1976;76(4):28–31.
25. Rodeman C. The nursing service in milieu therapy. Washington, DC: WRAMC, WRAIR; 1960.
26. Stubblebine JM. The therapeutic community—a further formulation. In: Rossi JJ, Filstead WJ, eds. The therapeutic community. A sourcebook of readings. New York: Behavioral Publications; 1973.
27. Sullivan HS. Socio-psychiatric research: its implication for the schizophrenia problem and for mental hygiene. Am J Psychiatry. 1931;10:977.
28. Visher JS, O'Sullivan M. Nurse and patient responses to study of milieu therapy. Am J Psychiatry. 1970;127:93–98.
29. Wolf MS. A review of literature on milieu therapy. J Psychiat Nurs Mental Health Serv. 1977;15:26–33.

34

Peggy Ann Hansen
Janet M. Rhode
Vivian Wolf-Wilets

Stress Management

OBJECTIVES

After reading this chapter, the reader will be able to:

1. Discuss the key concepts of stress, including how stress affects the body
2. Describe how stress management therapies assist the client in controlling or preventing a stress reaction
3. Describe nursing roles in stress management
4. List nursing diagnoses commonly found in clients seeking help with stress management
5. Cite case examples of clients with problems of stress
6. Discuss current research related to stress management.

THE STRESS RESPONSE

Stress is prevalent enough and powerful enough to cause health problems and even death. Therefore, it is important that the psychiatric mental health nurse understands the physical and psychological manifestations of stress and ways to manage it.

A stressor is a stimulus for change arising from events in the environment, from interpretations of experiences, or from self-talk. Stress is a conscious and unconscious set of responses involving an alerting response via the reticular activating system and increased sympathetic nervous system activity. It can range in magnitude from simple arousal to serious illness and or death. The principal stress physiology pathways are shown in Figure 34-1. The stress response is a product of learning, cultural experiences, genetics, physiology, and the type, severity, and duration of stressors. A negative experience, such as being involved in an automobile accident, is obviously a stressor. Also, buying a car, even though a positive experience for an individual, is a stressor, as change is involved.

The most immediate general body response to a stressor is brought about by the sympathetic nervous system, as seen on the left of Figure 34-1 (reference 1, p 67). Sympathetic nervous system stimulation leads to dilated pupils, inhibition of the flow of saliva, acceleration of the heartbeat, dilated bronchi, inhibition of gastric peristalsis and secretion, stimulation of the liver to convert glycogen to glucose, stimulation of epinephrine and norepinephrine release, and inhibition of bladder contraction. Epinephrine and norepinephrine (called catecholamines) act in slightly different ways. Epinephrine increases the force of heart muscle contraction, leading to the feeling of the heart pounding; norepinephrine elevates the heart rate and stroke volume and leads to constriction of the blood vessels (reference 1, p 68), which makes the hands feel cold. The combined action of these chemicals increases the blood pressure.

The intermediate effects begin when the adrenal medulla is stimulated by release of acetycholine from sympathetic nerve fibers. Epinephrine and norepinephrine are produced. The catecholamines from the medulla are produced at only one-tenth the rate in the sympathetic nervous system, but their effects last ten times longer (reference 1, pp 69–70).

The long-term effects begin when the endocrine system is activated. Adrenocorticotropic hormone (ACTH) and thyroid-stimulating hormone (TSH) are released from the anterior pituitary gland and vasopressin from the posterior pituitary gland. ACTH stimulates the adrenal cortex, leading to release of "glucocorticoids which stimulate the liver to produce more sugar. More fats and proteins also are released into the blood for more energy. Release of too much protein for energy can reduce protein normally available for construction of white blood cells and other antibodies, thereby weakening the body's immune system over the long run. Release of too much fat in turn can promote atherosclerosis" (reference 19, p 27). Stimulation of aldosterone (mineralocorticoid) release from the cortex of the adrenal increases sodium reabsorption by the kidneys, thereby raising blood pressure (reference 1, p 73).

Thyroxine is released from the thyroid gland. It is responsible for increasing the metabolic rate, for cerebral irritability that can lead to a decrease in concentration and to insomnia, and for gastrointestinal distress such as diarrhea or constipation.

Vasopressin, which is released from the pituitary gland, stimulates constriction of arterial blood vessels, increasing blood pressure.

General Adaptation Syndrome

Selye described stages in the body's response to stressors,[21,22] which he called the General Adaptation Syndrome. These three stages of Alarm, Resistance, and Exhaustion are described on the lower portion of Figure 34-1.[15] In the case of a car accident, an alarm response would be generated immediately. If a high level of stress continued; for example, if the person sustained multiple injuries necessitating hospitalization, then the resistance stage may ensue in which the body fights to maintain itself. If complications developed that could not be controlled, the body might not be able to deal with all the demands placed on it. The result would be a state of exhaustion, with loss of the ability to respond to stress.

Depression or Fight–Flight

There are individual variations in the physiology of emotional responses to stress (Fig. 34-2). Henry and Stephens have presented evidence of two possible reaction pathways to a given stressor.[10] When a stimulus is perceived as stressful and coping patterns are not adequate, a person could feel a sense of helplessness and inability to meet expectations as shown in the right pathway. The hippocampal–pituitary–adrenocortical system becomes more involved in this reaction as the feeling of loss of control and withdrawal predominates. This may be an underlying physiological and emotional reaction pattern characteristic of some depressions.[10,26,20] In the left pathway, when an individual perceives a threat to control, the amygdala and sympathetic adrenomedullary system are activated. The response made in order to control the situation could be one of anger or fear (fight or flight).[10,26] A comparison of the different hormones, bodily responses, and signs and symptoms generated by each type of activation is presented at the bottom of Figure 34-2.[26]

Sources of Stress

People experience stress from three basic sources: events in their environment, their interpretations of

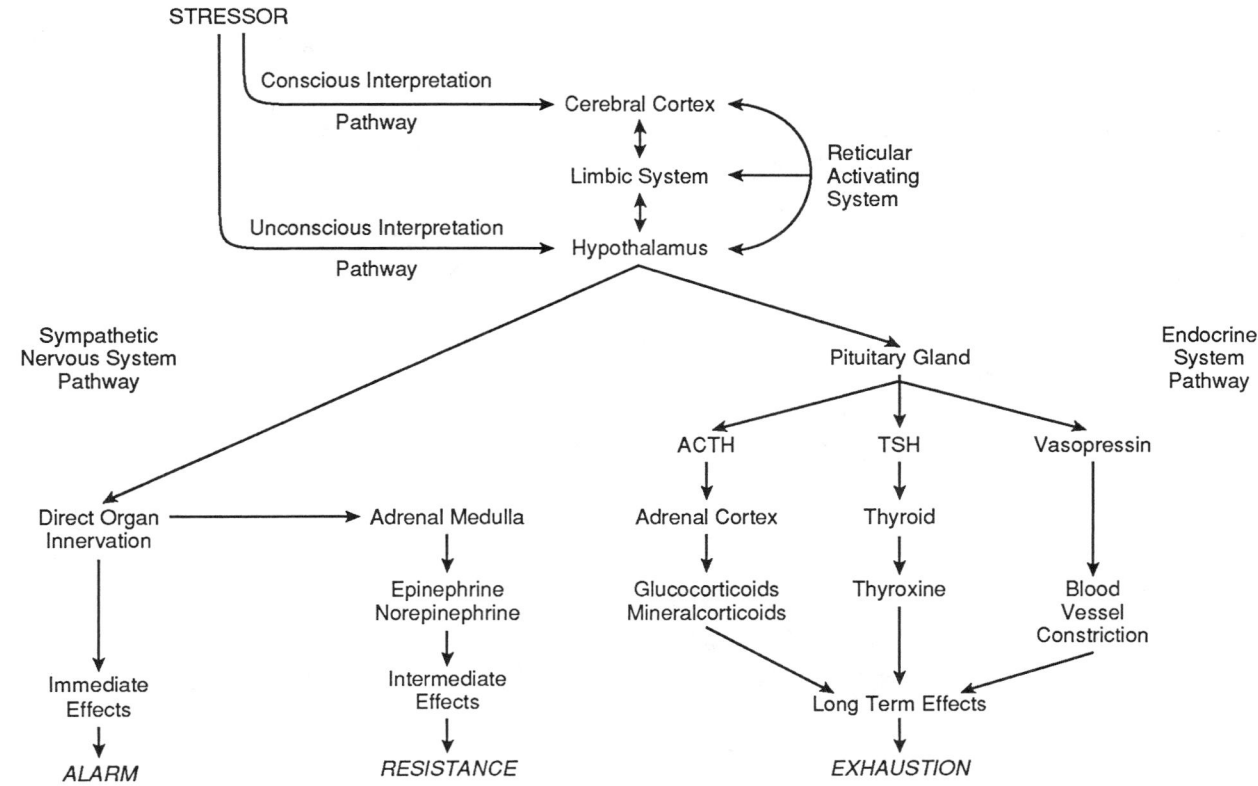

STRESSOR

Conscious Interpretation Pathway → Cerebral Cortex

Unconscious Interpretation Pathway → Hypothalamus

Limbic System

Reticular Activating System

Sympathetic Nervous System Pathway

Pituitary Gland

Endocrine System Pathway

ACTH   TSH   Vasopressin

Direct Organ Innervation → Adrenal Medulla

Adrenal Cortex   Thyroid

Epinephrine Norepinephrine

Glucocorticoids Mineralcorticoids   Thyroxine   Blood Vessel Constriction

Immediate Effects

Intermediate Effects

Long Term Effects

ALARM   *RESISTANCE*   *EXHAUSTION*

GENERAL ADAPTATION SYNDROME

Stage I: Alarm reaction Mobilization of the body's defensive forces and activation of the "fight-or-flight" mechanism	Stage II: Stage of resistance Optimal adaptation to stress within the person's capabilities	Stage III: Stage of exhaustion Loss of ability to resist stress because of depletion of body resources

Physical Change

Release of norepinephrine and epinephrine causing vasoconstriction, increased blood pressure, and increased rate and force of cardiac contraction Increased hormone levels Enlargement of adrenal cortex Marked loss of body weight Shrinkage of thymus, spleen, and lymph nodes Irritation of the gastric mucosa	Hormone levels readjust Reduction in activity and size of cortex Lymph nodes return to normal size Weight returns to normal	Decreased immune response with suppression of T cells and atrophy of thymus Depletion of adrenal glands and hormone production Weight loss Enlargement of lymph nodes and dysfunction of lymphatic system If exposure to the stressor continues, cardiac failure, renal failure, or death may occur

Psychosocial Changes

Increased level of alertness Increased level of anxiety Task-oriented, defense-oriented, inefficient or maladaptive behavior may occur	Increased and intensified use of coping mechanisms Tendency to rely on defense-oriented behavior	Defense-oriented behaviors become exaggerated Disorganization of thinking Disorganization of personality Sensory stimuli may be misperceived with appearance of illusion Reality contact may be reduced with appearance of delusions or hallucinations If exposure to the stressor continues, stupor or violence may occur

FIGURE 34–1. Major stress physiology pathways. (From Shafer W: Stress management for wellness. Holt, Rinehart and Winston, 1987, p 24.[19] General adaptation syndrome from Kneisl, CR, Ames SW: Adult health nursing: a biopsychosocial approach. Addison Wesley, 1986, p 20[15])

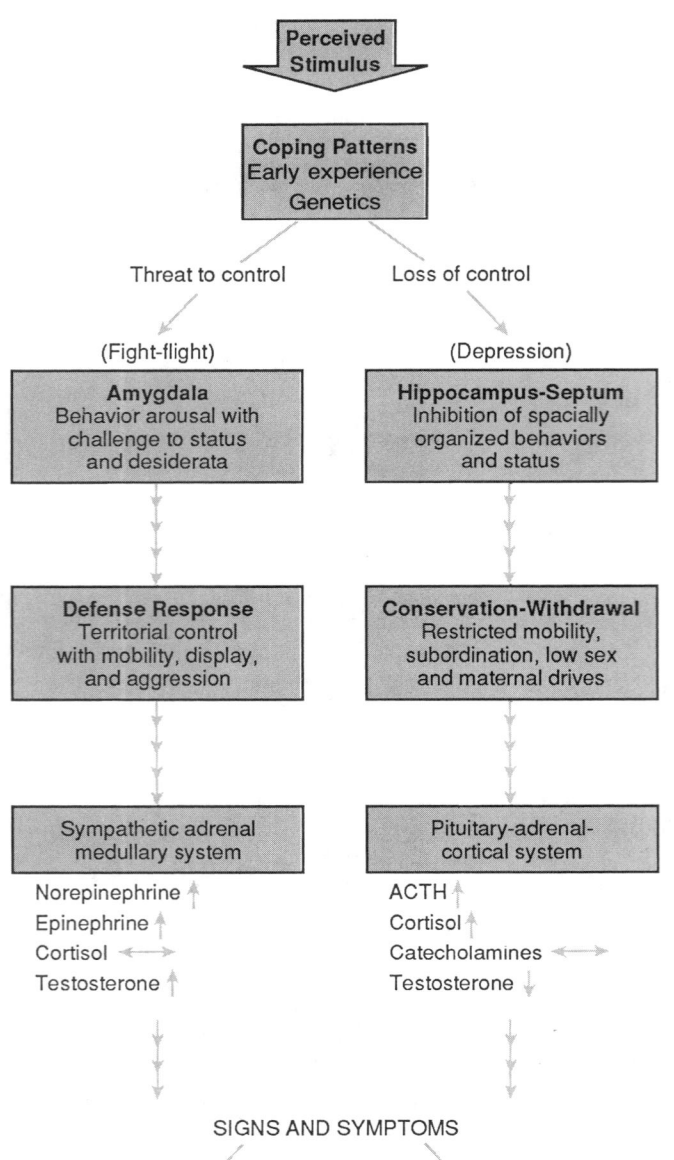

FIGURE 34–2. Fight–flight versus depression coping patterns and the resulting responses. (Adapted from Henry and Stephens[10] and Wolf-Wilets[26])

events, and their self-talk. The effect of a person's adaptation to change is twofold: a physical response and an emotional response.[7] This basic framework is depicted in Figure 34-3.

An *event* is a reality that has entered the consciousness and requires a response. *Interpretations* of events help determine unique and individualized responses:

interpretations act as filters that define how the world is viewed and how an individual defines a sense of control. Some events can be controlled (control of event = mastery and a sense of well-being). Others cannot (lack of control of event = nonmastery and a sense of impending threat).[2] Adaptation to changing events is constant: the degree of stress experienced depends on

FIGURE 34–3. *Interpretation, self-talk, and response as a feedback system.*

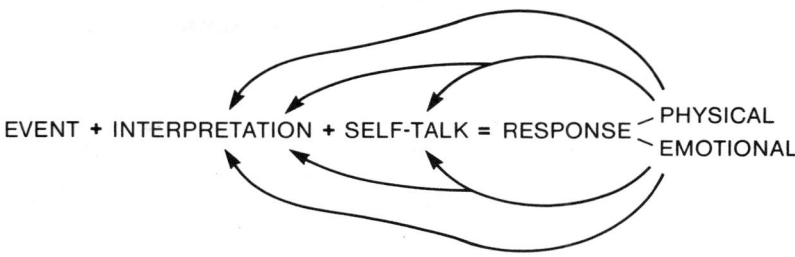

the interpretation of these events. Children learn to interpret the environment very early in life from parents, teachers, and peers. Life experiences and cultural values influence this learning. A small, rural, agricultural community provides different learning opportunities than a large, densely populated urban area. Television, books, newspapers, and magazines also are powerful influences on the way the world is perceived.

Self-talk is unspoken verbal thoughts about the internal and external world. Self-talk further refines meanings and allows for a feedback system of appraisal and reappraisal of the initiating event. A twofold physical and emotional response pattern then develops (the last step in the equation) that joins the feedback loop and alters the chain of reactions with each feedback pass. Thinking about an event can lead to the stress response. For example, reliving a car accident can give rise to the same bodily responses as did the original

situation. Self-talk such as, "I was so stupid not to be driving carefully," can induce the same neuroendocrine responses as being faced with actual dangers.

Life Changes

The effects of stress are cumulative and increase the probability of illness or injury. Table 34-1 details Holmes and Rahe's questionnaire, the Social Readjustment Rating Scale, which asks individuals what types of life changes they have had and how recent these changes were.[12] Some events, such as the death of a spouse, were found to be more stressful than others. Therefore, on the basis of research, each event was given a weighted score.[11] The higher the total score of life changes, the higher the probability of illness or injury. Thus, 37% of the persons having Life Change

TABLE 34–1
Social readjustment rating scale

RANK	LIFE EVENT	MEAN VALUE	RANK	LIFE EVENT	MEAN VALUE
1	Death of spouse	100	24	Trouble with in-laws	29
2	Divorce	73	25	Outstanding personal achievement	28
3	Marital separation	65	26	Wife begins or stops work	26
4	Jail term	63	27	Begin or end school	26
5	Death of close family member	63	28	Change in living conditions	25
6	Personal injury or illness	53	29	Revision of personal habits	24
7	Marriage	50	30	Trouble with boss	23
8	Fired at work	47	31	Change in work hours or conditions	20
9	Marital reconciliation	45	32	Change in residence	20
10	Retirement	45	33	Change in schools	20
11	Change in health of family member	44	34	Change in recreation	19
12	Pregnancy	40	35	Change in church activities	19
13	Sex difficulties	39	36	Change in social activities	18
14	Gain of new family member	39	37	Mortgage or loan less than $10,000	17
15	Business readjustment	39	38	Change in sleeping habits	16
16	Change in financial state	38	39	Change in number of family get-togethers	15
17	Death of close friend	37	40	Change in eating habits	15
18	Change to different line of work	36	41	Vacation	13
19	Change in number of arguments with spouse	35	42	Christmas	12
20	Mortgage over $10,000	31	43	Minor violations of the law	11
21	Foreclosure of mortgage or loan	30			
22	Change in responsibilities at work	29			
23	Son or daughter leaving home	29			

Holmes TH, Rahe RH: The social readjustment scale. Reprinted with permission from J Psychosom Res. 1968;11:213–218. Copyright 1968. Pergamon Press, Ltd.[12]

Unit scores of 150 to 200 had an associated health change within 1 year, 51% of those having Life Change scores of 200 to 299 had health changes, and 79% of the persons with Life Change scores of 300 or higher had health changes.[11] This does not mean that everyone having high life changes became ill, as these are average scores. These results are most likely related to the physiological changes discussed earlier.

Persons with high life changes are more apt to have accidents and injuries. The effects of life changes are cumulative (see Fig. 34-1). The man involved in a car accident may have had other stressful life events preceding the accident that affected his adaptive response at the time of the accident.

Social Support

A lifestyle factor that fosters high performance and personal life satisfaction is building and maintaining a strong social support system. Lack of an adequate system contributes to the intensity of the stress response.[18] Social support can be defined as interactions that lead an individual to feel loved, esteemed, and a member of a network of individuals working for the same end.[4] A social support system does not have to be limited to people: an animal can make an individual feel loved and secure. Social support helps increase resistance and protect people from becoming ill in a wide variety of situations.[18]

A good analogy would be to think of the individual as the hub of a wheel and the social support systems as the spokes that define the shape of that wheel. If the spokes are all on one side, the wheel will not function as designed. Likewise, if individuals have all their supports from one arena of their lives (school, work), the support system is lopsided and will not function correctly.

Benefits of Illness

A benefit of illness refers to a reason an individual may be ill. The reason may be unconscious and not readily apparent. These motivations for illness are called secondary gains and increase the likelihood of the client continuing to be ill or to have symptoms. Common benefits of illness have been identified by Carl Simonton:[23]

1. Receiving permission to get out of dealing with a troublesome problem or situation.
2. Getting attention, care, or nurturing from people around them.
3. Having an opportunity to regroup psychological energy to deal with a problem or to gain a new perspective.
4. Gaining an incentive for personal growth or for modifying undesirable habits.

5. Not having to meet their own or others' high expectations (reference 23, pp 133–34).

It is necessary to help the client develop an awareness of psychological and emotional needs and then help the client learn how to receive support in the areas listed as benefits of illness. It will then no longer be necessary for the client to become sick to fulfill these needs, and the client can learn to respond to stress in a healthier manner.

It becomes apparent that an effective stress management program must deal with all facets of the stress response equation. If the causes of the "disease" (i.e., events, interpretations, and self-talk) are not addressed, and if interventions are aimed only at the response side of the equation, clients will make only a partial recovery.

MANAGEMENT OF STRESS

Stress is managed by increasing awareness of the basis for the stressors being experienced and by building structures to support change behaviors. The goals of comprehensive stress management programs are to assist clients to: (1) identify their needs; (2) understand their response patterns; and (3) choose behaviors that support their highest level of wellness.

Cognitive and Behavioral Strategies

AWARENESS

The first step in stress management is to increase the client's awareness of the events, interpretations, and self-talk that trigger a stress response, along with an awareness of individual response patterns. Common triggers and reactions can be identified using an assessment tool such as the one in Table 34-2.

CONTROL

Once the client is aware of stress triggers and response patterns, he or she can learn control measures. Clients entering stress management programs often are seeking help because they feel out of control with their symptoms. Having a sense of control is essential to any return to equilibrium.[8]

Control of Events. The event (stressor) is the reality that begins the chain of reactions. Control of the event can be approached in three ways: avoiding, altering, or accepting.[25]

A first strategy is to avoid the situation that has been identified as creating stress. Two options are available. The first is to predict the situation and take steps not to encounter it or to become involved. This can be done by defining limits or refusing to participate. When initial avoidance is not possible, an alternative strategy is

TABLE 34-2
Awareness assessment

The first step in stress management is increasing your awareness of the events that trigger your stress reaction; and how you then respond as a unique individual.
Please check the stress triggers and stress reactions that apply to you.

STRESS TRIGGERS	STRESS REACTION
Professional	**Physical**
___ too many responsibilities	___ headaches
___ too high standards for myself	___ fatigue
___ conflicts with coworkers/boss	___ aching muscles
___ I don't like my work duties	___ stomach upset
___ I'm concerned about my future	___ cold hands/cold feet
___ I have difficulty saying no	___ rapid heartbeat
___ I don't get enough recognition	___ rapid breathing
___ I don't have enough time	___ change in sexual relationship
___ my work is unchallenging	___ sleep problems
___ I don't handle problems well	___ hypertension
Personal	___ skin problems
___ too many family responsibilities	___ jaw tension
___ I have problems with my spouse	**Psychological**
___ I have problems with children/parents	___ feeling fearful or frightened
___ I have too many things to do	___ nervousness
___ I am concerned about my health	___ irritability
___ I can't control my eating/drinking	___ become mad or angry easily
___ I smoke/use drugs to an extreme	___ react angrier than event calls for
___ I'm concerned about owing money	___ reduced motivation
___ I have trouble making decisions	___ feeling sad/depressed
___ I feel lonely	___ anxious
___ I feel I have little control	___ feeling drained
___ I'm unable to express myself	___ apathy

Developed by Northwest Stress Management, Rhode and Hansen, Seattle, WA. Copyright 1985.

to remove oneself from the situation physically or emotionally. This can be accomplished by walking away or by delegating responsibility for the situation that is stressful.

Altering the situation is a second strategy. Where disorganization in daily living is a stressor, steps can be taken to prioritize, to deal with procrastination, and to develop acceptable schedules or options. Where inability to communicate is a source of stress, the stressor can be altered by gaining communication skills. Sometimes, stress emerges from lack of assertiveness, and learning assertiveness skills can be beneficial. Validating clients' needs and giving them permission to ask for what they need can help them feel more in control of themselves and their environment.

There are events that cannot be controlled—events that enter lives whether wanted or not. At these times, control is maintained by the choices made. *Acceptance* can be one of these choices. To accept an event as out of control is not a passive technique: it means recognition that action must be taken to preserve equilibrium so that the unwanted reality will not cause additional harm. This means that a strong effort is needed to build and maintain resistance. This is preventive stress management. Protection is developed by physically, mentally, spiritually, and socially building strengths.

A person also can learn how to make educated choices by examining the consequences of choices before reacting. There is not always a choice between a positive and negative consequence. Sometimes, the choice is finding the consequence with the least negative impact, as when a psychiatric nurse is treating a client for anxiety with panic attacks. The treatment plan includes biofeedback training using systematic desensitization. The psychiatric nurse and client have set up a hierarchy of events that the client has identified as triggers for his anxiety reaction. The client becomes anxious each time he thinks of the triggers and has a panic attack during one of the training sessions. He chooses to continue in treatment, even though he fears the possibility of another attack. The client has accepted his anxiety and is learning to alter his response patterns.

Control of Interpretations. By the time the teen years are reached, interpretation habits and well-defined perceptual triggers have been developed that can add to the stress reaction. Control of stress-producing interpretations involves *relabeling*: taking a "second look" to identify the meaning attached to a threatening experience. At this point, it is possible consciously to choose a different, less stressful, interpretation. Each day offers many opportunities to choose labels for what happens: forgetting something important, hearing angry voices, or learning about friends' dieting. Whether these events are stressful depends on the choice of meaning and labels given to experiences.

As people grow and develop, they occupy a variety of roles. These *role definitions* are an identity base that further influences interpretations. For each role assumed, there are expectations of role-related behaviors, and every person with whom there is interaction while in the role also has expectations for that role. Where role expectations are not compatible, there can be conflict for those involved. Where the person is unfamiliar with the role and its expectations, there can be role incompetence, uncertainty, and ambiguity, all of which are sources of stress. Clarification of behavioral expectations for each role assumed can reduce stress related to that role.

Control of Self-Talk. People continually engage in self-talk, which is internal thought language. These are the sentences that describe and interpret the world. If the self-talk is accurate and in touch with reality, there is high function; if it is negative and irrational, it can trigger a stress response. There are times when denial, a kind of irrational self-talk, can serve a protective function that allows the client to adjust to changes and recover from events, such as a heart attack.

A system called *Rational Emotive Therapy* has been developed to help refute irrational ideas and beliefs and replace them with realistic statements about the world.[7] The basic thesis is that between an event and the emotional reaction to that event is realistic or unrealistic self-talk that actually is the stimulus for the emotion. In this view, thoughts, directed and controlled by us, are what create anxiety, anger, depression, a sense of helplessness, or powerlessness.

To dispute and eliminate irrational ideas, the following five steps are helpful:

1. Select a situation that consistently generates stressful emotions, such as speaking in front of an audience.
2. Write down the facts as they occur; e.g., as I prepare for the speech, my mouth gets dry and my hands become clammy.
3. Write down the self-talk about the event ("I probably will make a fool of myself"). Note the emotional response—angry, depressed, feeling worthless.
4. Dispute and change the irrational self-talk; e.g., "Other people do it. There is no evidence that I will make a fool of myself. I had positive feedback from my last talk."
5. Substitute alternative self-talk, such as "I prepared well, and I will do a good job. I have the skill. It doesn't have to be perfect" (reference 6, pp 110–112).

Relaxation Response Strategies

This section focuses on the right side of the stress response equation (see Fig. 34-3)—the physical and emotional responses to stressors; in particular, the strategies for healthy management of those responses. Herbert Benson coined the term "*relaxation response*," the bodily state physiologically opposite to the fight or flight response.[3] The relaxation response is self-induced (controlled), alters the body's response patterns, and leads to a more balanced state. Excess tension threatens the body's well-being; eliciting the relaxation response can decrease or reverse the adverse effects of stress.

The techniques that follow are a sampling of the strategies that can be presented to clients in a stress management program. No one technique is a panacea. Clients are encouraged to explore and understand their own individual need and response patterns and to choose what works best for them at any given time.

BREATHING

Deep, diaphragmatic breathing is a cornerstone for other relaxation exercises. It is important because one of the first changes in the fight or flight response is a holding of the breath or a change to rapid and shallow breathing. A critical part of nursing assessment and observation skills concerns alertness to breathing patterns. An essential step, then, in changing and controlling response patterns is an awareness of the breath. The importance of attention to the breath has been well known in Asia and India for a long time, and breathing control has been practiced extensively. Incorporating this into Western habits for physical, mental, and spiritual development is a powerful and important addition to self-regulation techniques.

Effective breathing entails maintaining loose abdominal muscles so the diaphragm can expand and contract unimpeded. This allows the lungs to fill to capacity, the

---

BOX 34–1
Breathing Exercise

Lie or sit in a comfortable position. Uncross your legs and arms; close your eyes, if comfortable. Place one hand on your chest and the other on your abdomen, below the rib cage. Inhale, allowing the hand on the abdomen to rise. The hand on the chest remains still. Exhale, letting the abdomen fall. Repeat. Notice with each breath that the abdomen rises and the chest remains quiet.
Continue the breathing. In a slow, rhythmic voice, begin to count mentally with each breath saying:

In—Two . . . Hold—Two . . . Out—Two—Three—Four —Relax
In—Two . . . Hold—Two . . . Out—Two—Three—Four —Relax

Repeat this process for 10 minutes. When other thoughts come in to interrupt, say, "back to center—breathe" and begin the count again (In—Two, etc.).

blood to be well oxygenated, and carbon dioxide to be released. This technique interrupts the internal processes of the alarm reaction and, if the lungs are normal, induces marked bodily changes (decreased pulse and blood pressure and more efficient oxygen consumption) (Box 34-1).

QR (QUIETING RESPONSE–REFLEX)

The QR is a quick (6-second) breathing skill developed by Charles Stroebel.[24] This technique prevents the emergency response from being activated inappropriately by creating a pause that allows a person the chance to decide if body activation is necessary. When practiced consistently and consciously over a period of 4 to 6 months, the quieting response becomes automatic; i.e., the quieting reflex.

This self-regulation skill is different from relaxation in that it is a quieting experience, a gear-shifting mechanism, that is accomplished even when the body is active and sensing stress. Because it is practiced throughout the day at times of stress, the potential build-up of arousal is diffused. Busy nurses and active clients are much more willing to use this technique throughout the day instead of taking the 15 to 20 minutes once or twice a day needed to practice other relaxation techniques (Box 34-2).

AFFIRMATIONS

An affirmation is a positive self-statement. When practiced consistently and used with breathing techniques, affirmations can help change negative feeling states to more positive ones, providing an interruption of the stress–tension cycle. Affirmations are stated in a positive framework ("I enjoy eating healthy foods," not "I won't eat sweets"); are stated in the present tense ("I am relaxed," not "I will relax"); and are repeated three to five times during daily relaxation practices or repeated frequently throughout the day, like QR. It is helpful to imagine doing what is said in as much detail and with as much pleasure as possible (Box 34-3). Examples of affirmation statements include: "I can," "I choose peace," "I possess abundant energy and draw upon it at will," "I express my feelings freely, fully, and easily," and "I like myself."

PROGRESSIVE RELAXATION

Edmund Jacobson developed the techniques of progressive relaxation,[13] which have served as an important concept for eliciting the relaxation response. Alternately tensing and relaxing muscles helps increase awareness of muscles and their state of relaxation vs tension. Consciously focusing on early clues to daily tension can help interrupt the build-up of arousal and the consequent responses, such as tension headaches, backaches, jaw tension, and muscle spasms. The exercises progress sequentially through the musculature of the body, hence the term "progressive."

Active Progressive Relaxation. The active technique consists of consciously tensing a muscle group and then consciously relaxing the muscle group, recog-

---

BOX 34–4
Active Progressive Relaxation Exercise

Get yourself into a comfortable position and begin to focus on slow, deep breathing. Allow your eyes to close. Let go of any thoughts from the day. Remember to continue to breathe calmly and regularly throughout the exercise, releasing tension each time you exhale. Follow the instructions below for each muscle group listed in the "sequence of muscle groups" section:

STEPS IN EXERCISE
- Slowly tense the muscle
- Hold the tension
- Focus on the tension, noticing how it feels and where you feel it
- Release the tension
- Notice the difference between tension and no tension
- At each step, check for residual tension in the rest of your body; check your breathing to make sure it is slow and regular; allow the tension to drain out of the body with each exhalation.

SEQUENCE OF MUSCLE GROUPS:
Right toes and foot; left
Right lower leg; left
Right upper leg; left
Buttocks
Lower back
Abdomen
Upper back and shoulders
Right forearm; left
Right upper arm; left
Neck
Forehead
Jaw and mouth (exaggerate a smile)
Eyes (squeeze shut)

VISUALIZATION AND IMAGERY

The use of imagination to change a mental or physiological state is a self-regulation skill that can be used alone or as an adjunct to other relaxation techniques. Creating a positive mental picture can help reduce stress, enhance healing processes, and maintain health. For the best results, it is important to encourage clients to choose images that are important and meaningful to them. It is also important to identify the goal of visualization. For basic stress management, the goal is to elicit the relaxation response. The client picks an image (such as lying on a beach in the warm sand, breathing in harmony with the calming rhythm of the waves—washing in with each inhalation and flowing out with each exhalation) and deepens into a relaxed state.

Another goal of visualization that is being employed in a variety of health care settings is to enhance the body's resistance to disease. The Simontons have pioneered work with cancer patients, helping them develop powerful images of their immune system (such as "Pac-Men" with teeth to gobble cancer cells) to activate and support healing.[23]

The technique of visualization is similar to that of affirmations. The mental image is in the present tense (seeing oneself as healthy and relaxed right now) and positively framed (seeing the healthy self, not the diseased self), and the person has to want the change that is asked for. If there is any secondary gain for the symptom or illness, or if the person is unclear on what is desired, visualization may not be successful (Box 34-5).

---

nizing the difference between tension and relaxation. This technique is helpful for people who have any form of skeletal muscle tension or pain, as some people with chronic pain are cut off from their body sensations. Actively tensing and relaxing muscles can increase awareness of degrees of tension and pain and help such clients feel more able to control or change what they feel. People who are active, such as type A individuals, and individuals who are very concrete thinkers do well with this technique (Box 34-4).

Passive Progressive Relaxation.
In passive relaxation, the muscles are not intentionally tensed. Instead, there is passive release of any tension during a slow progression through the muscle groups. Slow, rhythmic diaphragmatic breathing is used at the same time. This is an excellent technique for anxious clients and those who tend to pick up and hold tension. The same sequence of muscle groups can be used as in the active exercise, with the goal of gently focusing on each group, breathing deeply, and letting any tension flow out with each outgoing breath.

BOX 34–5
Mental Imagery Exercise

Gently close your eyes. Focus on the breath. Air moving in. Air moving out. Release any tension. Slowly begin to imagine a rose. In your mind's eye, imagine a pink rose. Focus the mind on that rose. See the detail of the pink rose. See the color . . . pink . . . the clarity of color . . . the uniformity of color . . . the velvety/vibrancy of color. See the size of the rose flower. See the stage of unfoldment . . . the petals. Note the fragrance. Note the dew drops . . . the leaves . . . the detail of stem . . . thorns.
Become aware of any feelings the rose evokes . . . the mood . . . any soothing feeling . . . any energy.
Take a deep breath in . . . release. Allow the image to fade. Allow the quietness . . . the calm . . . soothing . . . relaxation to stay with you as awareness is returned to the present moment. Know you can create this sense of calm simply by breathing and creating any kind of quieting, positive vision.

Adapted from Cohen A. Setting the Seen: Creative Visualization for Healing. New York: Eden Publishing Co.; 1982:7.[5]

MEDITATION

Meditation is a way of narrowing the attention so as to become wholly involved with a single focus. It is a form of self-discipline and a route into one's interior world of thoughts and feelings. Meditation was developed centuries ago in Eastern cultures. Skilled meditators have a heightened ability to control autonomic functions (decreasing heart rate, blood pressure, oxygen consumption) and fewer stress-related complaints.[9] The necessary components for meditation include a passive, allowing attitude; a quiet environment; a 20-minute block of time; an empty stomach; and an object or subject to focus on such as the breath, a candle flame, or a mantra; e.g., a word such as "one," repeated over and over.

BIOFEEDBACK

Biofeedback has become an important treatment in the field of self-regulation. With the use of machines, clients can interact with and learn to control their physiologic processes. Biofeedback has opened the door to researching the mind–body connections. The machine completes the feedback loop between a client and the system being monitored. The signal can be in the form of an auditory tone, visually integrated numerical data or meter reading, a blinking light or light bar display, and, more recently, computerized graphics.

Clients do not necessarily "feel" the autonomic processes they are learning to control. Rather, through consistent practice with feedback, subtle and complex patterns are identified and used to elicit the desired results. Passive attention, not determined concentration, is an important element of success. Biofeedback, when paired with other relaxation techniques and cognitive strategies, enhances clients' beliefs about the control they can have over their bodies.

Electromyography (EMG). Biofeedback with EMG measures skeletal muscle tension by amplifying the electrical impulses that trigger muscle contractions and converting the impulses into a signal that can be seen or heard. With this information, clients with conditions such as tension headaches, back pain, muscle spasms, or spasticity can learn to reduce muscle tension. Clients who have had strokes or other injuries can use the feedback in rehabilitating their muscles.

Skin Temperature. Skin temperature biofeedback senses changes as the arterial smooth muscles constrict, causing the temperature to fall. The fight or flight response affects blood flow, shifting blood away from the periphery. With relaxation, smooth muscles relax, blood flow increases, and temperature rises. Temperature training is helpful for clients with symptoms

---

BOX 34–6
Autogenics Exercise

Autogenics training is a self-regulation technique often used with EMG and skin temperature biofeedback. The goal is to reverse the alarm response with the use of autosuggestions (self-generated suggestions; hence the term "autogenics") about what one feels when relaxation is experienced. The key elements for successful autogenic training include assuming a comfortable body position, minimal external stimuli, repetition of the verbal formulas, and an attitude of passive concentration (i.e., alert to the experience without analyzing it). Johannes Schultz developed the autogenic training system, in which there are six elements that comprise the self-statements:[6,14]

1. Heaviness (relaxation of skeletal muscles)
   Say: "My right arm is heavy"
   Repeat 3 times each for right arm, left arm, and neck and shoulders
2. Warmth (relaxation of smooth muscles)
   Say: "My right arm is warm"
   Repeat 3 times each for right arm, left arm, and neck and shoulders
3. Heartbeat (normalized cardiac activity)
   Say: "My heartbeat is calm and regular"
   Repeat 3 times
4. Breathing (normalized respiratory system)
   Say: "My breathing is calm and regular"
   Repeat 3 times
5. Abdominal warmth (calm body center)
   Say: "My abdomen is warm and calm"
   Repeat 3 times
   (Caution: If you have bleeding ulcers, abdominal problems, or diabetes or are in third trimester of pregnancy, use the statement: "I am calm and relaxed")
6. Forehead cool (decreased blood flow to head)
   Say: "My forehead is cool and calm"
   Repeat 3 times

Reprinted with permission from Mason L. Guide to Stress Reduction. Berkeley: Celestial Arts; 1980:26–27.[16] Copyright 1980, 1985 by L. John Mason.

---

of vascular system tension such as migraine headaches, hypertension, and Raynaud's syndrome (Box 34-6).

Skin Conductance (Galvanic Skin Response, or GSR). GSR biofeedback measures changes in sweat gland activity. Skin responds to thoughts, emotions, and changes in the environment with either an increase in sweat gland activity, with stimulation and stressors, or a decrease (drier skin), with resting or relaxation. The skin reaction, which occurs with change in catecholamine levels, is immediate and can reflect emotional state and unconscious feelings. This is the principle used in lie detector testing. The GSR helps clients become more aware of stressful situations and emotional reactions to them.

Other Modalities. Blood pressure, pulse rate, and brain wave activity (EEG) are other types of biofeedback helpful in teaching clients self-management strategies.

Success with biofeedback is determined by the ability of clients to duplicate the results outside the health care setting. An increased awareness of body cues, a willingness to take responsibility for practice, a willingness to explore a variety of techniques, and a permissive mental attitude are all important components of success in self-regulation.

NURSING ROLES IN STRESS MANAGEMENT

Stress management is a life-long process for all individuals. As nurses explore and expand their own personal response patterns to stress, they will be better equipped to observe patterns in clients, to understand the dynamics, and to model positive behaviors.

The traditional medical model of illness is being challenged by current integrated mind–body research. Nurses in all settings (hospitals, communities, agencies) essentially assess levels of stress and coping responses and help clients plan and implement measures and evaluate outcomes. Psychiatric nurses are pivotal in making assessments and applying the specific treatment techniques.

Clinical Specialists with master's degrees in psychosocial nursing and with American Nurses' Association certification have moved into private practice, offering stress management programs for clients with acute or chronic physical or emotional symptoms. The focus of treatment ranges from decreasing symptoms to maintaining and supporting clients toward their highest potential for wellness. Doctorally prepared nurses are conducting research to obtain new knowledge and techniques, as well as to validate the rationales of current treatments. As long as the nursing profession espouses the "total person" philosophy of care, stress management will remain an integral part of the caring process.

COMMON NURSING DIAGNOSES

The reasons clients seek treatment and the associated nursing diagnostic categories are summarized in Table 34-3.

CASE STUDY

Sue was a 25-year-old nursing student who had moved to another state to go to school. She worked part time, 30 hours a week, while going to school full time. She ended a relationship with one boyfriend 6 months ago and had recently married. She was given a promotion at her job, and with the extra money, the couple decided to buy a house. Sue developed symptoms of depression. As her daily workload increased and the bills for the new house began

TABLE 34–3
Summary of common nursing diagnoses for clients seeking help in stress management

REASON FOR SEEKING TREATMENT	NURSING DIAGNOSTIC CATEGORY
PHYSICAL	
Headache	*Altered comfort: pain
	*Altered comfort: chronic pain
	Ineffective individual coping
Back pain	*Altered comfort: pain
	*Altered comfort: chronic pain
	Ineffective individual coping
Muscle tension	Anxiety
	*Altered comfort: chronic pain
	Ineffective individual coping
	Fear
	Post-trauma response
Hypertension	Anxiety
	Ineffective individual coping
	Fear
	Noncompliance
	Post-trauma response
Gastrointestinal disorder	Anxiety
	Ineffective individual coping
	Fear
	Self-esteem disturbance
	Impaired social interaction
Temporomandibular joint pain	Anxiety
	*Altered comfort: chronic pain
	Ineffective individual coping
	Fear
	Impaired social interaction
EMOTIONAL	
Anxiety	Anxiety
	Ineffective individual coping
Depression	Depression
	*Altered comfort: chronic pain
	Ineffective individual coping
	*Impaired adjustment
	Dysfunctional grieving
	Hopelessness
	Powerlessness
	Post-trauma response
	Self-esteem disturbance
Anger	*Impaired adjustment
	Anger
	Ineffective individual coping
	Fear
	Dysfunctional grieving
	Hopelessness
	Powerlessness
	Post-trauma response

* Other NANDA nursing diagnosis.

arriving, she felt less and less able to concentrate during the day or to sleep at night. When her husband asked her what she felt, she indicated that things had just gotten out of control. Sue started staying home from work and expressing many complaints to her husband. He did a lot of the housework and gave her more attention and affection when she felt ill. A pattern had developed where Sue thought that she received more attention, affection, and assistance when she felt sick.

Life changes had produced many stressors for Sue. Some may be very positive, such as her new marriage and pro-

NURSING CARE PLAN 34–1

SUE

NURSING INTERVENTIONS	OUTCOME CRITERIA
NURSING DIAGNOSIS: Depression related to multiple life changes	
CLIENT GOAL: Gain pleasure from daily activities	
■ Develop baseline data: assess and evaluate level of depression to include appetite/weight control, fatigue/activity level, sleep patterns, and pleasure gained from activity	Maintains weight Sleeps minimum of 6 hours a night Experiences increased enjoyment in life
■ Encourage physical activity as part of daily schedule	Experiences increased energy from physical activity
■ Teach reversal of negative thinking patterns	Recognizes negative thinking and prevents it
CLIENT GOAL: Learn to meet needs without using illness as coping strategy	
■ Develop baseline data: assess and evaluate level of secondary gains	Identifies her secondary gains of illness Establishes other forms of satisfaction and recognition
■ Teach alternative methods of meeting needs	Identifies alternative methods of meeting needs
■ Establish reward system	Feels motivated to work for reward
CLIENT GOAL: Feel in control of own environment and complete tasks	
■ Develop baseline data: assess and evaluate anxiety level to include sense of control, ability to concentrate, completion of tasks at home and work, areas of major concerns, and distorted thinking patterns	Experiences reduced anxiety with an increased sense of control Demonstrates ability to complete tasks
■ Assess and evaluate present level of coping skills	Has improved coping skills with the generation of several alternatives
■ Teach priority setting, scheduling, and time management	Develops a satisfying set of priorities Finds a sense of control and accomplishment in creating and checking off activities on her "Do" list. Develops a schedule that gives structure and control but has flexibility

Continued

SUE *Continued*

NURSING INTERVENTIONS	OUTCOME CRITERIA
■ Teach relaxation techniques, include EMG/thermal biofeedback	Uses affirmations and deep breathing daily
CLIENT GOAL: Decrease number of life changes	
■ Develop baseline data: assess and evaluate number of life changes by use of Schedule of Recent Events	Shows a decrease of life changes or carefully evaluates each life change and its effect Spaces out life changes when possible
■ Teach client to focus energy on prioritized concerns	Makes appropriate choices for control

motion, whereas others may be negative, such as the ending of the relationship with her former boyfriend. All required Sue to adapt and increased her risk of a health change. During the course of the illness, she discovered rewards for being ill (secondary gains); for Sue, these gains were the release from some tasks and additional attention and affection. The nursing diagnoses identified were depression and anxiety related to multiple life changes (see Nursing Care Plan 34-1 for a sample care plan for Sue).

SUMMARY

Stress management, as explored in this chapter, is a multidimensional process. It involves learning and un-derstanding the stress response and the individual's physiological and emotional reactive patterns. It is important to identify the sources of stress—the events, interpretations, and self-talk—that precipitate those responses. As awareness begins to develop, it is possible to learn control measures. The individual achieves control and balance from using a variety of cognitive, behavioral, and relaxation strategies. As a professional practitioner, the nurse engages with clients as teacher, change agent, problem solver, evaluator, and re-searcher. As a participant, the nurse practices the techniques of stress management, enhancing the quality of her or his own life and serving at the same time as a role model for clients.

Research Highlights

Work stress, hardiness, and burnout in hospital staff nurses was studied by McCranie, Lambert, and Lambert.[17] The central question addressed was, would personal hardiness moderate the impact of job stressors on burnout? A sample of 107 registered staff nurses responded to questionnaires. Hardiness—personal resil-ience—was measured by a 36-item scale developed by Kobasa, Maddi, Donner, Merrick, and White in 1984. Job stressors were measured by the Nursing Stress Scale de-veloped by Gray–Toft and Anderson in 1981. Burnout was measured by the Tedium Scale developed by Pines and Aronson in 1981. The findings were that burnout was significantly related to higher perceived job stress and lower levels of personality hardiness. Although personal-ity hardiness helped reduce burnout, if job stresses were high, personality hardiness did not prevent burnout.[17]

References

1. Allen R. Human Stress Response: Its Nature and Control. Minneapolis: Burgess Publishing Co; 1983.
2. Bandura A. Self-efficacy: toward a unifying theory of behavioral change. Psychol Rev. 1977;84:191–215.
3. Benson H. The Relaxation Response. New York: Avon Press; 1976.
4. Cobb S. Social support as a moderator of life stress. Psychosom Med. 1976;38:300–314.
5. Cohen A. Setting the Seen: Creative Visualization for Healing. New York: Eden Publishing Co; 1982.
6. Davis M, Eshelman E, McKay M. The Relaxation and Stress Reduction Workbook. Oakland: New Harbinger Publications; 1982.
7. Ellis A, Harper R. A New Guide to Rational Living. Englewood Cliffs: Prentice-Hall; 1975.
8. Glasser W. Control Theory. New York: Harper & Row, 1984.
9. Green E, Green A. Beyond Biofeedback. New York: Delacort; 1977.
10. Henry JP, Stephens PM. Stress, Health and the Social Environment. New York: Springer-Verlag, 1977.
11. Holmes T, Masuda M. Life changes and illness susceptibility. ARS. 1973;94:176.
12. Holmes T, Rahe R. The Social Readjustment Rating Scale. J Psychosom Res. 1968;11:213–218.
13. Jacobson E. Progressive Relaxation. Chicago: University of Chicago Press; 1974.
14. Luthe W, Schultz J. Autogenic Training. New York: Grune and Stratton; 1965.
15. Kneisel CR, Ames SW. Adult Health Nursing: A Biopsychosocial Approach. Menlo Park, Calif: 1986.
16. Mason L. Guide to Stress Reduction. Culver City, Calif: Peace Press; 1980.
17. McCranie E, Lambert V, Lambert CE Jr. Work stress, hardiness and burnout among hospital and staff nurses. Nurs Res. 1987; 36(2):374–378.
18. Pelletier K. Healthy People in Unhealthy Places. New York: Delacorte; 1984.
19. Schafer W. Stress Management for Wellness. New York: Holt, Rinehart and Winston; 1987.
20. Seligman M. Helplessness: On Depression, Development and Death. San Francisco: WH Freeman Co; 1975.
21. Selye H. Stress Without Distress. New York: Signet Books; 1974.
22. Selye H. The Stress of Life. New York: McGraw-Hill; 1978.
23. Simonton C, Matthews–Simonton S, Creighton J. Getting Well Again. New York: Bantam Books; 1978.
24. Stroebel C. QR: The Quieting Reflex. New York: GP Putnam's Sons; 1982.
25. Tubesing NL, Tubesing DA, eds. Structured Exercises in Wellness Promotion. Vol 1. Duluth, Minnesota: Whole Person Press; 1982.
26. Wolf–Wilets VC. Stress. In: Patrick M, Craven R, Woods S, Rokowsky J, Bruno P, eds. Medical Surgical Nursing: Pathophysiological Concepts. Philadelphia: JB Lippincott; 1986.

35

Joan M. Cunningham

Crisis Intervention

OBJECTIVES

After reading this chapter, the reader will be able to

1. Discuss the historical development of crisis theory
2. Define a crisis
3. Define types of crises
4. Define crisis intervention
5. Discuss the nurse's role in crisis intervention
6. Discuss nursing diagnoses for the client in crisis
7. Discuss various types of crisis intervention programs.

HISTORICAL PERSPECTIVES

Lindemann[14] studied the behavior of survivors and close relatives of the victims of the Cocoanut Grove fire in Boston, focusing on the symptomatology and management of acute grief reactions. He concluded that when threatening situations arise in an individual's life, either the individual adapts to the situation or, failing to adapt, has impaired functioning. He believed that interventions utilized during bereavement could be applied to other stressful events such as marriage and childbirth and concluded that when crises were properly managed, impaired functioning could be avoided.[6]

Caplan, emphasizing a community approach, developed a conceptual framework for understanding crisis intervention and used the principles of preventive psychiatry (primary, secondary, and tertiary prevention) as a basis for his work. He viewed primary prevention as decreasing the incidence of psychiatric illness while promoting mental health through social and interpersonal interventions, such as working with community and political groups to obtain necessary reforms and helping people deal with stresses such as illness or death. Secondary prevention was defined as reduction of the number of existing cases of mental illness through early diagnosis and treatment. Early referrals, screening programs, and improvements in the use of diagnostic tools are examples of secondary prevention. Tertiary prevention was considered to be the reduction of the rate of chronic disability resulting from mental illness. Here, the focus is rehabilitation. Secondary prevention includes primary prevention; tertiary prevention includes both primary and secondary prevention.[6]

The need for crisis intervention services was identified in a report by the Joint Commission on Mental Illness and Health, which led to making federal funds available for the establishment of community-based mental health centers through P.L. 94-63. Crisis intervention was one of the services required if a comprehensive community mental center was to receive government funding.

CRISIS THEORY

A person in crisis is at a turning point.[1,10,13] Crisis is a danger, because it threatens to overwhelm individuals and their families, but it is also an opportunity, because during a crisis, individuals are more receptive to therapeutic intervention and growth. A crisis is the experience of being confronted with an unfamiliar obstacle in life's path that is perceived as threatening and not manageable by coping mechanisms that have worked before. As a result, the individual experiences an increase in anxiety and tension and is not sure what to do. As anxiety increases, the individual feels less able to solve problems and thus less competent. Feelings such as anxiety, depression, guilt, helplessness, and fear are experienced. The crisis results from a combination of the individual's perceptions of the precipitating event and the individual's inability to cope with it.[13,14]

Phases in the Development of a Crisis

A crisis does not occur instantaneously.[1] Rather, there are identifiable stages leading to a crisis state. The precipitating event can usually be identified as one of loss, threat of a loss, or challenge. The loss may be the death of a spouse, parent, or a child. The threat of a loss may be the illness of a family member. Challenge may be a job promotion, a career change, or more responsibility at work.

Caplan describes four phases in the development of a crisis.[6] In the first phase, a perceived threat or event causes an increase in anxiety. The individual employs the usual problem-solving methods to resolve the crisis. If these do not bring relief, the individual moves on to the second phase, in which anxiety increases and disorganization occurs as a result of the failure of coping mechanisms. The individual cannot think clearly nor determine what to do. Failure to resolve the crisis will result in the individual entering the third phase, in which the anxiety level increases further. The individual then uses every resource available, including new ones, to diminish the anxiety. At this point, attempts may be made to redefine the problem so that old coping mechanisms can work. If resolution does not occur, the individual goes on to the fourth phase, in which, anxiety may escalate to severe or panic levels. Cognitive, emotional, and behavioral disorganization may occur.[6]

Crises are self-limiting. A crisis reaches some type of resolution—either healthy or unhealthy—within a 4- to 6-week period because in most instances, the individual cannot tolerate a crisis state for a longer period of time.

Coping Mechanisms

On a regular basis, individuals encounter experiences that disrupt their usual cognitive and affective equilibrium and create an "emotionally hazardous event."[2] Individuals may experience a change in relationships with others or in expectations of the self in ways perceived to be negative. The rise in tension induces problem-solving behaviors (coping mechanisms) aimed at relieving the tension. These coping mechanisms may be conscious or unconscious and are employed to restore equilibrium after an emotionally hazardous event.[2]

Coping begins at birth and continues until death. Most individuals develop a range of coping mechanisms, some that are adaptive and some that are less so. When individuals feel threatened, they usually revert to maladaptive ways of coping. The emotionally hazardous event leads to a crisis when there is failure to cope effectively.

Types of Crises

As discussed previously in the section on maturational and situational crisis (Chapter 13), crises can be divided into two types: maturational and situational. Maturational crises are experienced in relation to predictable life changes: every individual's life is subject to changes secondary to the process of maturational development and changing situations within the environment.[9] A situational crisis occurs in response to an event or events that threaten a person's biologic, social, and psychological integrity. It is experienced as being beyond the person's control and results in some degree of disequilibrium.

CHARACTERISTICS OF CRISIS INTERVENTION

The goal of crisis intervention is to restore equilibrium, at the same or, ideally, at a better level of functioning than before the crisis. The minimal goal is to avoid catastrophe, suicide, homicide, or family disintegration.

Dealing with Client Feelings

For healthy adjustment to a traumatic event or loss, the feelings aroused need to be experienced and expressed. However, feelings are dealt with in a limited way in crisis intervention. Once the client has released some pressure by discussing feelings in a controlled and receptive situation, the nurse accepts the feelings and moves to a broader understanding of the crisis. This measure avoids ventilation of feelings with escalating emotionality and instead allows for rational exploration and problem solving.

Promoting Self-Reliance

In crises, clients may see themselves as inadequate and helpless failures. The nurse needs to convey to clients that they are capable, normal persons who have temporarily been overwhelmed by extreme stress and therefore can use help to cope with these stressors. The client in crisis may be tempted to let go and become totally dependent, which must be actively discouraged from the beginning. Otherwise, the client's self-esteem may be further lowered, and the situation will be worse because of the client's continuing immobilization. The nurse must avoid magical reassurance as would be implied by statements such as "I know everything will be

fine." Support is given only as indicated, and the client is expected to work at solving the problem. The client's involvement in the plan of action increases the chance of productive outcomes.

Reducing Anxiety

One of the sources of client anxiety is the fear that no one will be in control and that things will get out of hand, resulting in chaos and danger. When the nurse conveys to the client that the nurse is in control of the situation, it reduces anxiety, increases rapport, and facilitates communication.

Focusing on the Here and Now

In crisis intervention, it is important that the here and now be the focus. Tangential materials, such as disagreements of 15 years ago, must be avoided. The focus can be maintained on the present by considering why the client came for help now.

Resolving the Problem

The psychiatric mental health nurse attempts to gain as much collaboration and involvement from the client as possible to outline the chain of events leading to the present crisis, emphasizing the relation of each event to the ones preceding and following in such a way that the sequence makes sense both to the nurse and to the client. This exercise will greatly enhance understanding of the crisis situation, and it will suggest further interventions. The perception of the problem is validated with the client, and any misconceptions are clarified. After exploring with the client the feelings experienced during the crisis situation, new problem-solving methods and more adaptive coping mechanisms are examined. Goals are set, and new problem-solving methods are tested.

Increasing Social Support

For clients in crisis, a social support system is important. Clients may need assistance to identify the presence or absence of important people on whom they can rely for support. The support system may be composed of family members, friends, fellow workers, and clergy. Clients may also utilize self-help groups to provide support and friendship.[15]

Making Referrals

An important aspect of crisis intervention is the process of making referrals. A referral may be made in order to obtain services that will be ancillary to the crisis intervention process or that will be part of the follow-up work after the process. The client should be clear where and for what purpose referrals are being made. It is important that a referral be handled well so that the client does not feel rejected or "sloughed off" or "fall through the cracks."[8]

CRISIS INTERVENTION PROGRAMS

Crisis intervention programs may differ in the population they serve, but the focus for all of these programs is short-term treatment.

Brief Crisis Counseling

Brief crisis counseling generally lasts from one to six sessions, with the emphasis on problem solving and the development of a collaborative relationship with the client. Intervention is geared toward achieving a certain goal and reducing the stress the client is experiencing.[3,4]

Crisis Groups

Crisis groups are short-term groups that emphasize problem solving. Members assist each other in problem resolution and encourage exploration of feelings. The nurse acts as the group leader and as a role model for effective problem solving. Crisis groups are usually scheduled for one and a half hours once a week for 6 weeks.

Family Crisis Counseling

Family crisis counseling involves the entire family for about six sessions. It is a brief therapy model that is problem focused and does not explore general family issues and problems. It is the preferred mode for most children and adolescents in crisis.[17,19]

Mobile Crisis Intervention

The crisis intervention staff on a mobile team responds directly and immediately at the scene of the crisis event. Their role is one of assessment, intervention, and resolution of the problem. The mobility of the crisis intervention team increases the chances of clients not being hospitalized: clients who are seen in psychiatric emergency rooms are admitted more often than clients who are seen at home. The mobile crisis unit is also an effective means of diverting inappropriate referrals to the emergency room.[5]

Crisis Programs for Adolescents

Crisis intervention, because it is short term and focused on the immediate problem, can be especially relevant for adolescents because their motivation for treatment frequently declines rapidly after the symptoms have diminished. There are hospital-based crisis intervention programs that serve adolescents who are experiencing acute psychiatric crises; their primary goal is returning the adolescent to the community as quickly as possible. These programs offer immediate access for any adolescent facing a crisis situation and provide hospitalization if necessary. During hospitalization, extensive liaison work is done with families, referral sources, and community agencies to rebuild or replace the adolescent's support system.[11,18]

Crisis-Oriented Residential Treatment Programs

Many persons experiencing a crisis can be maintained at home if they receive high levels of support. Residential crisis services are utilized when it is necessary to remove individuals in crisis from their own environment. These services should be reserved for clients experiencing the most severe crises, who need intensive support, structure, and supervision during the period of stabilization. The most common type of program is the family-based crisis home, in which carefully selected and trained families provide short-term housing and support. Therapeutic services are provided by case managers, who coordinate all needed services. The homes have access to 24-hour emergency back-up crisis services. Some agencies provide residential crisis services in group residences with professional staff in attendance. The therapeutic tool utilized to encourage more active and functional behavior is an emphasis on the role the client plays in the group and the household. The maximum length of stay in a group crisis residence usually is 2 weeks.[23]

Telephone Crisis Counseling

Suicide prevention and crisis intervention centers utilize telephone counseling, which provides immediate help for the individual in crisis.[21]

Crisis Programs for Rape Victims

Many rape victims call a rape crisis hotline seeking help, and it is often the victim's first step toward seeking professional assistance. In dealing with rape victims, a more directive and educational approach is used than is taken with most clients. The reason for this approach is that the victim has a need for basic information, for answers to questions about what is being experienced, and for a referral to services that can meet immediate needs.

Follow-up telephone contact with the victim is essential. The greatest number of calls need to be made during the impact and acute phases of the crisis. When the victim becomes more able to function independently and has more people in the social network for support, the number of follow-up calls can decrease. Scheduled calls are best continued until 3 months after the rape. After this period, calls can be made periodically to assess the victim's progress.[22]

Family Crisis Intervention Programs in a Medical Intensive Care Unit

When a family member becomes ill, the entire family system may be disrupted. The other members are confronted with a crisis: there are role changes, financial concerns, transportation problems to and from the hospital, and emotional turmoil. The family crisis intervention program is designed to provide information and emotional support during this time. Upon the patient's admission to the unit, the nurse meets with the family to provide them with as much information as possible. A teaching pamphlet is provided that gives general information about the unit and its standard invasive and noninvasive equipment. A specially trained volunteer is in the waiting room during visiting hours to provide support to the family and answer questions as they arise. A daily telephone call is made to one family member per patient to provide information about the patient's condition. A follow-through program was designed to maintain contact with bereaved families and former patients and their families.[12]

NURSING ROLES

The psychiatric nurse generalist is in a unique position of utilizing crisis intervention techniques in a wide variety of settings. Through knowledge of crisis theory, the nurse is able to identify clients who may be experiencing a crisis and to intervene in an appropriate manner. Appropriate and well-timed intervention in a crisis can be instrumental in producing a positive outcome.

The psychiatric clinical nurse specialist provides clinical supervision, short-term brief therapy for selected clients, family therapy, and inservice education programs and acts as a liaison between the crisis team and other agencies. He or she is also a resource person for other team members who need assistance with clients who have medical problems.[7]

NURSING DIAGNOSES AND CRISIS INTERVENTION

Clients who are in crisis would be expected to have a nursing diagnosis of maturational or situational crisis. Other nursing diagnoses typical in this population include anxiety, depression, fear, guilt, ineffective individual coping, grieving, hopelessness, self-concept disturbance, rape trauma syndrome, post-trauma response, suicide potential, and powerlessness.[16]

CASE STUDY

Annette, a 38-year-old woman, was extremely upset when David, a family friend, called the crisis intervention unit. Annette's husband had been badly hurt earlier that day in a fall and had been airlifted to a trauma unit some distance away. David, afraid that Annette would try to kill herself, asked whether the crisis unit could help him. The mobile crisis unit was dispatched to the home immediately. When the unit arrived, David gave the crisis nurse some background information. He said that the previous year, Annette's teenage son had been killed in an automobile accident. At that time, Annette had slashed her wrists and had to be hospitalized. Since then, her ability to function both at work and at home had been somewhat impaired. She and her husband worked together, and he had taken over many of her responsibilities in order to protect her.

Annette was in a state of disbelief, pacing, and very anxious. She kept repeating, "It can't be true. I don't know what I'm going to do." Her two daughters, ages 12 and 14, were sitting quietly with their maternal grandparents. Annette revealed to the crisis team that she and her husband had been experiencing marital problems. The focus had been his depression, which she believed was brought about by his impending retirement and by his taking over many of her responsibilities. Annette said she did not know what she was going to do, that she felt unable to deal with the present situation and the future. The clinical nurse specialist on the crisis team identified the nursing diagnoses suicide potential related to past history and current crisis situation, powerlessness related to crisis and lack of problem-solving skills. (see Nursing Care Plan 35-1 for a sample care plan for Annette).

SUMMARY

A crisis is the experience of being confronted with an unfamiliar obstacle in life's path. When the obstacle is perceived as threatening and not manageable, the client experiences a crisis. A crisis occurs in four phases, and the precipitating event can usually be identified. Crises can be divided into two types: maturational and situational. Maturational crises are predictable and occur in the lives of most people. Situational crises are a response to a sudden event that threatens a person's biologic, social, and psychological integrity and is usually beyond the individual's control. Crisis intervention programs differ in their com-

NURSING CARE PLAN 35–1

ANNETTE

NURSING INTERVENTIONS	OUTCOME CRITERIA

NURSING DIAGNOSIS: Suicide potential related to past history and current crisis situation

CLIENT GOAL: Refrain from engaging in behavior harmful to self

■ Assess Annette for suicidal thoughts, suicide plan, means for carrying out plan, and lethality of plan ■ Institute measures to protect Annette if she becomes suicidal	Does not harm self

NURSING DIAGNOSIS: Powerlessness related to crisis and lack of problem-solving skills

CLIENT GOAL: Experience increased ability to control present situation and future

■ Assist Annette to reduce level of anxiety ■ Help Annette describe her present situation, including her concerns about her husband and her daughters, and her options concerning travel to the site of his hospitalization ■ Help Annette differentiate what can be changed from what cannot	Anxiety lessened to level at which learning can occur Verbalizes realistic understanding of her situation
■ Assist Annette to solve problems according to what can be done in the current situation and which of her friends and family can help ■ Arrange for referrals to appropriate agencies ■ Check with Annette later to assess need for and willingness to participate in family counseling	Solves problems and activates social supports and other resources

---

Research Highlights

Mobile crisis intervention has proved to be an effective alternative to hospitalization in many situations. The most effective emergency psychiatric treatment takes place before the client ever reaches the hospital. Bengelsdorf and Alden found that clients first seen at the hospital are admitted more often, whereas those first seen at home require hospitalization less frequently.[5] According to the study of the 67 clients seen each week by the crisis intervention team, 70% were treated in the community without hospitalization. The mobility of the crisis intervention team increases the chances of treating clients without resorting to hospitalization, and brief intervention by the team is sometimes all that is required.

Mobile crisis intervention can also expedite and facilitate those admissions that are necessary.[5]

Mobile crisis intervention vastly improves the delivery of services, and treatment is brought even to the unwilling client. Other advantages of mobile crisis intervention are that families are engaged, supported, and enlisted as participants in the client's treatment. Also, other mental health agencies are supported and backed up in their work. Referrals can be made quickly and follow-up done to ensure that clients comply. Mobile crisis intervention thus provides a much-needed service to a wide range of clients.[5]

position, but the focus for all of them is short-term treatment. Nurses intervene with clients in crisis in a variety of settings. Through knowledge of crisis theory, the nurse is able to identify the client in crisis and to intervene in an appropriate manner.

References

1. Aguilera DC, Messic JM. Crisis Intervention: Theory and Methodology, 5th ed. St. Louis: CV Mosby; 1986.

2. Baldwin BA. A paradigm for the classification of emotional crises: implication for crisis intervention. Am J Orthopsychiatry. 1978;48(3):538–551.

3. Bellak L, Siegel H. Handbook of Intensive Brief and Emergency Psychotherapy. Larchmont, NY: CPS, Inc; 1983.

4. Bellak L, Faithorn P. Crises and Special Problems in Psychoanalysis and Psychotherapy. New York: Brunner/Mazel; 1981.

5. Bengelsdorf H, Alden D. A mobile crisis unit in the psychiatric emergency room. Hosp Community Psychiatry. 1987; 38:662–665.

6. Caplan G. Principles of Preventive Psychiatry. New York: Basic Books; 1964.

7. Critchley D, Maurin J. The Clinical Specialist in Psychiatric Mental Health Nursing. New York: John Wiley & Sons; 1985.

8. Ellison JM, Wharff EA. More than a gateway: the role of the emergency psychiatric service in the community mental health network. Hosp Community Psychiatry. 1985;36:180–185.

9. Erikson EH. Childhood and Society. New York: WW Norton and Co; 1950.

10. Everstine DS, Everstine L. People in Crisis. New York: Brunner/Mazel; 1983.

11. Gutstein SE, Rudd MD, Graham JC, Rayha LL. Systemic crisis intervention as a response to adolescent crises: an outcome study. Family Process. June 1988;27:201–211.

12. Hodovanic BH, Reardon D, Reese W, Hedges B. Family crisis intervention program in the medical intensive care unit. Heart Lung. May 1984;13(3):243–249.

13. Hoff LA. People in Crisis: Understanding and Helping. Menlo Park, Calif: Addison-Wesley; 1984.

14. Lindemann E. Symptomatology and management of acute grief. Am J Psychiatry. 1944;101:141–148.

15. McGee RF. Hope: a factor influencing crisis resolution. Adv Nurs Sci. 1984;6(4):34–44.

16. McFarland G, Wasli E. Nursing Diagnoses and Process in Psychiatric Mental Health Nursing. Philadelphia: JB Lippincott; 1986.

17. Perlmutter R, Jones R. Assessment of families in psychiatric emergencies. Am J Orthopsychiatry. 1985;55(1):130–139.

18. Piersma HL, Van Winger S. A hospital-based crisis service for adolescents: a program description. Adolescence. Summer 1988;23(90):491–500.

19. Pittman FS. Turning Points: Treating Families in Transition and Crisis. New York: WW Norton and Co; 1987.

20. Schram P, Burti L. Crisis intervention techniques designed to prevent hospitalization. Bull Menninger Clin. 1986; 50(2):194–204.

21. Stein DM, Lambert MJ. Telephone counselling and crisis intervention: a review. Am J Community Psychology. 1984;12(1):101–126.

22. Underwood M, Fiedler N. The crisis of rape: a community response. Community Ment Health J. 1983;19(3):227–30.

23. Walker J. Psychiatric Emergencies: Interventions and Resolutions. Philadelphia: JB Lippincott; 1983.

36

Maxine E. Loomis

Group Therapy

OBJECTIVES
After reading this chapter, the reader will be able to:
1. Identify client needs for group therapy
2. Formulate a health care contract for a specific group of clients
3. Discuss the issues related to selection and preparation of clients for group therapy
4. Discuss the therapeutic factors present in therapy groups
5. Identify interventions for dealing with threats to group cohesiveness
6. Discuss plans for termination of therapy groups.

INTRODUCTION

The assessment and interventions for group therapy presented in this chapter are based in part on the group process concepts and principles explained in Chapter 7. While group process research was being conducted by social psychologists, a number of psychiatrists and clinical psychologists were attempting to extend their ideas about individual psychotherapy to treating patients in groups. During World War II, group psychotherapy was used in the military because of the large number of clients and the relatively small number of psychiatrists available to treat them. The effectiveness and economy of treating psychiatric clients in groups gradually led to the inclusion of group psychotherapy in the education and practice of master's level psychiatric nurses, psychiatrists, clinical psychologists, and social workers.

PURPOSE OF GROUP THERAPY

The purpose of group therapy is closely related to the purpose of nursing care: to diagnose and treat human responses to actual or potential health problems. Human responses are defined as objective and subjective behaviors: physiological, affective, cognitive, or motor activities. In its simplest form, health care involves the maintenance of existing healthy behaviors, the alteration of some existing behaviors, and the learning of new behaviors on the part of the people that nurses help.

Groups are often considered to be a more economical mode of intervention than individual therapy. A greater number of clients can be reached at one time, resulting in a more efficient use of the nurse's time and energy. For example, parents of hyperactive children can be counseled together. In an aftercare clinic where a large number of newly discharged state hospital clients receive treatment, a group of 10 or 12 clients can receive an hour of the nurse's attention rather than the usual 5 minutes per visit.[11] The health care objectives that can be accomplished in groups are much more important, however, than the economical use of the nurse's time and energy or the fact that more clients can be reached in a shorter time.

The primary advantage of a group lies in the composition of the group itself—the fact that a variety of people with similar problems or objectives are working on them together. This experience of the commonality of problems often has therapeutic value in and of itself. It helps the group members break through their barrier of aloneness and isolation and experience a mutual concern with other human beings. The sharing of common concerns may occur in a group of children with alcoholic parents who are discussing their difficulties with maintaining close relationships, in a group of parents whose children are hospitalized for major surgery, or in an aftercare group for former drug addicts. Regardless of the grouping of clients or the problem being solved, the sharing of basic human problems is one of the benefits of group therapy.

GROUP THERAPY GOALS

Psychiatric mental health nurses often refer clients to self-help, community, or social groups because they will have a therapeutic or helpful effect. A choral society may be just the group for a person who is frightened by friendship or intimate relationships yet needs to be around people and learn to share common experiences. Alcoholics Anonymous has a long history of group and individual self-help for clients with alcoholism that has a very therapeutic effect. The groups to be discussed in this chapter, however, are those groups that the psychiatric mental health nurse can organize in inpatient and community settings for the purpose of helping people change. These therapy groups are specifically structured to effect change in the group members.

Activity Groups

Activity groups are used in psychiatric settings to help clients structure time and experience the sense of accomplishment that comes from completing a project or sharing a group activity. Clients who are psychotic or who have poor self-esteem can benefit from participation in a goal-directed activity. For example, a nurse on one inpatient adult psychiatric unit organized a group of clients to redecorate the day room. Utilizing their collective skills, the group decided to break the project down into its component parts and divided tasks among subgroups. With some guidance from the nurse, one subgroup conducted a car wash to raise the necessary funds, while another subgroup purchased the paint and materials needed for redecorating. Another small group of psychotic clients who were not yet ready to deal with the complexities of the outside world remained on the ward repairing and re-covering the worn furniture. Within 3 months, the redecoration was completed, with minimal expense to the hospital and maximum sense of accomplishment on the part of the patients who participated in the group activity.

Clients who participate in such activity groups learn how to plan and structure complex activities and how to work together over time to achieve their goals. The nurse helps all clients contribute to the best of their functional abilities. This type of goal-directed collaborative behavior can contribute to the rehabilitation and recovery of a variety of clients.

In a community health agency, another nurse recognized the need for greater community acceptance and understanding of the needs of the older adult. Instead of mounting such a campaign herself, she enlisted several senior citizen groups to develop and implement the project. Not only were the ideas and information that resulted more relevant to the actual experience of the older adults, but there was a benefit to the older clients from participating in their own public awareness campaign. The project gave these people an outlet for their interests and provided many enjoyable hours of useful activity. Several ongoing projects resulted from the involvement of the older adults in the public awareness campaign. One of these projects was an adopted grandparents service, whereby families in the community who wanted their children to have contact with an older adult "adopted" a "grandparent" who contracted for inclusion in certain family activities. In this manner, the needs of both the older adults and the younger people in the community were satisfied.

There are any number of social and athletic groups that can be used by nurses in the treatment of psychiatric clients. Even the most common activity such as a sewing group, a card group, or a volleyball team can be used to help clients change. At times, the nurse's goal is simply to help clients structure their time and focus their attention on something outside themselves and their problems. More often, however, a skillful psychiatric mental health nurse can use the activity as a vehicle for helping clients solve concrete problems (e.g., how to find the sewing supplies) or cooperate with other people (e.g., setting up a net shot in volleyball) or relate to other people (e.g., coming to a group agreement on which movie to watch). The goal is not merely to complete the task or planned activity: the underlying goal of all activity groups in treatment settings should be to help clients maintain or improve their mental health and ability to function in the real world.

Learning and Behavioral Change Groups

Because nurses are concerned with affecting the health behavior of clients, they are necessarily involved with the alteration of existing unhealthy behaviors and the learning of new, healthier ones. Positive outcomes of a nurse-led medication group on an acute psychiatric unit have been noted by Neizo and Murphy.[10] Clients in the group learned about their medications, shared information about side effects, and discussed their feelings about being on psychotropic medications. Not only did they need information that could be transmitted more efficiently in a group than on a one-to-one basis, but they also needed to alter certain of their pre-illness behaviors to implement their treatment plans.

A study by Lewin during World War II provided one of the earliest demonstrations of the effectiveness of groups in producing behavioral change.[4] Because of the war, pork and beef were scarce, and families were being encouraged to obtain protein through consumption of organ meats. Lewin demonstrated that women who made a commitment as a group to increase the family consumption of organ meats changed their shopping and cooking behaviors at a higher rate than did women who were provided with information and made no such group commitment. Although a high consumption of organ meats would not be encouraged

today, the study does have implications for the teaching of clients who need to alter their diets (because of diabetes, hypertension, renal disease, and the like) by means of a group intervention. If the nurse can transmit information to clients in a group and then obtain a group commitment to behavioral change, the probabilities are greater that the clients will follow through.

There is a need for nursing research to explore the phenomenon of group commitment with various client groups in different settings. It is possible that the clients will need an ongoing group contact to maintain their newly learned behaviors. It has been demonstrated that group instruction is as effective as individual instruction for teaching progressive muscle relaxation techniques to hypertensive patients.[9] Again, there is a need for research to determine the length and extent of group follow-up required for permanent change.

Numerous groups already exist that deal with health care learning and behavioral change. Weight Watchers International is a private corporation with branches in many local communities that makes use of group commitment and group reinforcement to assist people in losing weight and maintaining this weight loss. Lamaze techniques of natural childbirth are usually taught in group classes. Parent Effectiveness Training and Parents Anonymous are two more examples of approaches that make use of group techniques to facilitate learning and behavioral change. Because these groups are basically set up as teaching–learning experiences, it may be useful with certain clients to utilize them as an adjunct to counseling or treatment experiences.

The goal of learning and behavioral change groups in mental health settings is also to help clients learn new behaviors with which they will be able to function more comfortably and effectively in their homes, work settings, and communities. For example, the psychiatric mental health nurse in a community aftercare clinic offered a time-limited, eight-session group to help clients newly discharged from the state hospital learn the skills necessary to obtain a job. She helped the group members read the help wanted ads and select the jobs they would like and be good at; clients then practiced completing job applications. One entire group session was devoted to job interviewing, at which the members practiced being interviewer and interviewee with each other. As the group members actually began applying for work, the group sessions were used to share successes and learn from unsuccessful experiences, and the members supported each other through the difficult and frustrating process of obtaining jobs. In the process of learning new behaviors, the group members also learned to support and care about each other as they shared an experience.

Psychotherapy Groups

The goals of psychotherapy groups are stated differently depending on the theoretical orientation of the therapist and the characteristics of the group members.

The content and process of psychotherapy groups will also vary with the theoretical orientation and educational preparation of the therapist. For example, psychiatric nurses are more likely to take a holistic approach to working with clients because of the integration of biopsychosocial content in their nursing education. In general terms, psychotherapy groups are concerned with the treatment of clients and are conducted by a therapist with the objectives of insight or behavioral change or both.

The origins of group psychotherapy are strongly tied to various theoretical schools of psychotherapy; for example, Sullivan, Rogers, Berne, and Perls. As therapists who had been trained in one of the theories of psychotherapy began to apply their treatment framework in groups, they also began to develop specific concepts and techniques of group therapy, which extended beyond theoretical orientations.

Therapy groups are for people who are dissatisfied or uncomfortable with their lives and want to change something about themselves. Members may be self-referred or be sent by a family member or social agency, but usually, there is some motivating force that defines the need for change. This does not preclude the occasional group member who, once confronted with the possibility of change, decides that he or she is either not ready or not willing to change. The process of change, whether implicit or explicit, in most treatment groups often requires that clients develop some degree of insight regarding personal problems in order to change their feelings and behaviors.

Therapy groups are usually led by therapists who have a graduate degree in nursing, medicine, social work, or psychology as well as supervised experience and training in group psychotherapy. Depending on the theoretical orientation of the therapist, the group will usually focus on the intrapersonal or interpersonal problems of the client. The group is viewed as a social microcosm in which clients demonstrate their problematic feelings and behaviors and in which they can experience the corrective emotional experience of being responded to differently. Within this context, the therapist assumes a facilitator role by helping clients learn new ways of coping.

In summary, a variety of client needs can be met in groups. The general categories of client needs discussed in this chapter are activity, learning and behavioral change, and psychotherapy. The majority of client needs confronted by the nurse can readily be identified as fitting into one of these categories. These categories will be discussed with respect to the structure, process, and outcomes of utilizing groups for health care intervention.

FORMULATING THE GROUP THERAPY CONTRACT

A group therapy contract is an openly negotiated, clearly stated set of mutual expectations that indicates what the nurse and client can expect of each other regarding the client's treatment. (See Chapter 7 for the definition of group contracts.) The contract consists of a set of shared objectives as well as a clear understanding of the structure and process for arriving at mutually determined outcomes.[7] The process of developing a contract for therapy groups begins with the selection and preparation of clients and is refined, altered, or reaffirmed throughout the life of the group. Several specific aspects of the contract for group therapy deserve elaboration.

Selection of Members

Frequently, psychiatric nurses realize that a number of clients with whom they have contact demonstrate a similar need or problem. For example, most clients who have been discharged from the state hospital have difficulty obtaining work, and many mothers who suffer from schizophrenia have trouble setting limits with their school-age children. Even clients who do not have the same diagnosis may share needs that could be met in a group. This heterogeneity of members might be seen in a public health nurse's caseload where a number of clients who live alone would benefit from a weekly activity group.

What criteria should the psychiatric mental health nurse use for selecting group members? A cohesive group is more likely to be successful in meeting member needs and group objectives. As discussed in Chapter 7, group cohesiveness is determined by the extent to which clear goals are defined and there is agreement on means for goal achievement, as well as on the extent to which clear norms are present and there is member conformity to group norms. The objectives and goals for the proposed group must be clear. The nurse must then determine which clients have needs that coincide with the group goals. If the client need is socialization and the group goal is learning and behavioral change, there is a discrepancy between the client need and the group objectives. In contrast, if the client need is weight loss and the group goal is supportive dietary control, weight reduction, and weight-loss maintenance, the client need and the group objectives are compatible. Table 36-1 contains examples of the factors that influence group cohesiveness for each type of therapy group.

There is fairly good consensus among clinicians and researchers that clients with organic mental disorders, substance use disorders, or antisocial personality disorders and those who are acutely psychotic or suicidal should not be included in heterogeneous therapy groups. However, clients with substance use disorders and those with antisocial personality disorders have been treated successfully in homogeneous therapy groups; i.e., groups composed of clients with the same diagnosis. Clients who are acutely psychotic or actively suicidal or who are impaired by organic mental disorders generally require more individual attention than is available in group therapy and are best treated

TABLE 36–1
Factors influencing group cohesiveness

TYPE OF THERAPY GROUP	CLEAR GROUP GOALS	MEANS TO ACHIEVE GOALS	CLEAR GROUP NORMS	CONFORMITY TO GROUP NORMS
Activity	Discuss current events	Daily discussion of previous day's TV news and local newspaper	Daily attendance Watch TV news, read local newspaper	Each member must contribute one current event item per session
Learning/Behavioral change	Help discharged state hospital patients obtain employment	Structured practice Information sharing Support and discussion	Attend all 8 sessions Participate in group practice sessions Apply for job(s)	All members must be committed to finding employment
Psychotherapy	Improved self-esteem and interpersonal relationships	Weekly group therapy sessions to talk about problems	Regular attendance Contract for change Open sharing of personal thoughts, feelings, and experiences	Silence, lying, and emotional withholding are considered deviant behavior and confronted

with structured individual nursing interventions. An approach for group psychotherapy with chronic schizophrenic outpatients, whereby these clients can engage in a moderately intensive insight-oriented therapy, has been proposed by White and Kahn.[12]

Preparation of Members

It is important to prepare clients for their group therapy experience. The primary purpose of this preparation is to develop a set of mutual expectations between the nurse and client. The client should emerge from this discussion with a clear and accurate picture of the objectives, structure, process, and expected outcomes of the therapy group. Both client and nurse should have had the opportunity to share their expectations and arrive at a beginning contract for how they will work together in the group.

It is useful to share information with clients about the structure of the group. Clients need to know the time, place, size, and setting for the group sessions. Often, the time and location will influence whether an interested client can attend the group. It is also important to share any expectations regarding attendance (e.g., "Please call if you are sick or otherwise unable to attend a session") and commitment (e.g., "It is important that you plan to attend all eight weekly classes"). Any fees or expenses involved in group participation should be explained at this time.

Part of the client's preparation for the group involves a beginning introduction to what the group is all about. Just as health professionals have many questions regarding the benefits of group interventions, clients likewise often wonder how they will be helped in a therapy group. If nurses are interested in utilizing the group process as a treatment vehicle, they will need gradually to educate their group members regarding what to expect. What will be the role of the leader? What will be expected of the client, and what can be expected of other group members?

The final step in a good preparatory session is a restatement of the anticipated outcomes from participation in group therapy. By the end of the session, both client and nurse should be able to state clearly what they expect of each other within the context of the group and how they will evaluate success. The nurse will have a beginning relationship with the client that can then be transferred to the group setting. The nurse will also have a plan for how to work with the client within the group.

FACILITATING CHANGE IN THERAPY GROUPS

Therapeutic Factors

What occurs in group therapy that helps clients change? If psychiatric mental health nurses can answer this question, then they will be able to utilize group interventions for maximum benefits to clients. Therapeutic factors that operate within groups have been examined by interviewing and testing 20 long-term group therapy clients identified as being the "most successful" by their therapists (ID Yalom, J Tinklenberg, M Gilula; unpublished data). On the basis of the results of that study and his own professional experience, Yalom identified the therapeutic factors listed in Table 36-2.[14] Although the distinctions between these therapeutic factors are to some degree arbitrary, therapists and clients alike have been able to identify significant events during the course of their groups that correspond with these categories. The high, medium, and low ratings offer some indication of the relative importance of each therapeutic factor in different type groups.

TABLE 36–2
Importance of therapeutic factors

THERAPEUTIC FACTORS	ACTIVITY GROUP	LEARNING/BEHAVIORAL CHANGE GROUP	PSYCHOTHERAPY GROUP
Instillation of hope	Low	Medium	High
Universality	Low	Medium	High
Imparting of information	Medium	High	Low
Altruism	Low	Low	Medium
Corrective recapitulation of the primary family group	Low	Low	High
Development of socializing techniques	High	Medium	Low
Imitative behavior	High	High	Low
Interpersonal learning	Medium	Low	High
Group cohesiveness	High	Medium	High
Catharsis	Low	Low	High
Existential factors	Low	Low	High

INSTILLATION OF HOPE

Instillation of hope is an important element in any type of therapeutic relationship. Often, it is the hope of cure or the hope that things can be different that keeps the client returning for appointments. Some clients will endure even prolonged pain or emotional discomfort because of their hope for relief.

In a group setting, the instillation of hope can be approached even more directly. No matter what the nature of the group, it is a common occurrence to find that other group members have experienced a similar feeling or event and lived through it. For example, in a group of postoperative clients, one woman who had just undergone a radical mastectomy was able to talk directly with others who had experienced the same change in body image and fear of cancer she was experiencing and to learn how they had worked through their feelings. The degree of hope that this type of sharing engenders should not be overlooked. During the initial stages of a group experience, the hope that "because others have been able to endure or change, perhaps I can too" may be all that a client has for comfort.

UNIVERSALITY

Universality is closely related to instillation of hope. As group members share their experiences, they learn that they are not alone. They find that regardless of race, sex, occupation, or any other distinguishing personal attributes, the event or feeling they are experiencing is similar to that of some other human being. They learn that they are not so unique that their problems are beyond solution. Morrow[8] reported such an experience for a recovering group of disabled workers.

Many persons in today's society bear silently and alone the weight of feelings of shame or inadequacy. It is a relief to unload this burden and find that others in the group are open and responsive to sharing a common experience. The author has led groups in which young women reluctantly, yet eagerly, told the secret horrors of paternal rape that were previously too shameful to share. Invariably, there is at least one other woman in the group who was subjected to either incest or the traumas of childhood enemas, which were a more rational, yet equally frightening, substitute. To find that one is not alone—that the carefully guarded secrets of being human are shared—is indeed a healing experience in and of itself.

IMPARTING OF INFORMATION

The imparting of information includes all of the health care teaching that is done by the nurse and other group members. Whether or not this is the primary objective of the group, there is a considerable amount of information shared during the course of a health care group. Normal growth and development, normal and therapeutic diets, good physical and mental health practices, and the various stages in the grieving process are only a few types of information that can be learned in a group. For example, Krumm, Vannata, and Sanders[2] reported their success with a group for teaching chemotherapy to cancer patients.

Very few people will change with just information alone. On the other hand, there is a cognitive element that precedes behavioral change in most health care situations. The renal disease patient must know what the diet is before discussing with the nurse why there is difficulty in following it. Manic depressive clients must learn the side effects of lithium and the management of their nutritional needs and daily activities. When information about physical and mental health practices is shared in a group, there is often benefit to more patients than just the one who asked the question. Perhaps there is also some secondary benefit in the process of sharing and experiencing others' willingness to share information.

ALTRUISM

Altruism is the experience of sharing a part of oneself with others. Within a group setting, there is opportunity for a great deal of sharing of information, support, feelings, experiences, and concrete assistance. If the group is cohesive and the members care about each other, it is not uncommon for group members to offer to call each other, visit, or share material goods to assist another member through a period of crisis or need.

Part of the socialization of clients to a therapy group may involve providing evidence that they can indeed help each other. The prevailing norm in our society is to expect individual service from a health professional when dealing with a health care problem. Some clients doubt that other persons in a similar situation can help them and may regard groups as a second-rate form of assistance. The group leader needs to be convinced about the benefits of group intervention so that the client is given a clear and convincing message before entering the group. Once having experienced the support and assistance of the other group members, most clients readily shed their initial concerns about the group.

CORRECTIVE RECAPITULATION OF PRIMARY FAMILY GROUP

Groups can provide a corrective recapitulation of the primary family group. Because groups are composed of members who can be viewed as symbolic siblings and a leader or leaders who can be viewed as more nurturing, expert, and powerful parent figures, clients are able to act out some of the conflicts they experienced in their primary family group. When group members dominate the conversation, sit quietly unless they are asked a question, set up arguments with the leader or other group members, or present themselves as being helpless, they probably are demonstrating behaviors that were learned and reinforced in their family of origin. This is a general type of transference that most people bring into their everyday relationships.

Different groups will utilize this recapitulation of the primary family experience to various degrees. In a learning and behavioral change group, very little attention may be paid to the genetic origins of some member behaviors. In some psychotherapy groups, a great deal of time and attention is paid to understanding why the client is behaving and feeling a particular way. In other psychotherapy groups, the behavior itself may be the focus of attention, with little concern about its origins. The one common therapeutic benefit, regardless of the nature of the group, appears to reside in the corrective nature of the leader and member responses to the behavior in question. If the client receives a more healthy response from the group than he or she did from the family, the probability is greater that the behaviors will be altered eventually.

DEVELOPMENT OF SOCIALIZING TECHNIQUES

The development of socializing techniques is a process present to one degree or another in all therapy groups. The degree to which relating to other people is an explicit part of the treatment contract may differ from one group to another. For example, an aftercare group for newly discharged state hospital clients may focus primarily on the development of the social skills required for reentry into the community. Increase in client-to-client verbal interactions among members of a resocialization group led by nurses in a nursing home setting has been reported by Gray and Stevenson.[1] On the other hand, a psychotherapy group may not focus directly on developing social skills, although these skills may appear as a secondary benefit of relating directly, honestly, and intimately to other people in the group.

For many people, a therapy group provides a unique opportunity to reflect on themselves and their relationships. The skills that are acquired in this type of atmosphere can be transferred into other intimate or social relationships. For example, a young diabetic mother who learns to be assertive about her own needs in her therapy group is likely to respond differently to her friends and family when they are pressing her to engage in strenuous activity. She has learned that it is acceptable to take care of herself as well as to care about others and to consider the effects of her behavior on both herself and her friends and family.

IMITATIVE BEHAVIOR

The capacity for imitative behavior is developed at a very early age. Small children imitate the behavior of those who care for them and are rewarded for learning to talk and developing motor skills and appropriate interpersonal behavior. In later life, persons still learn by imitation without necessarily being aware of it.

In therapy groups, the other members, as well as the leader, become models of new, healthier behavior. The language and health care value system of the group are learned in part by imitation, just as a child first learns to speak. The new behavior may at first seem awkward and not fully belonging to the person, but imitation may very well be the first step toward internalizing new behavior and values. There are many clients whose initial decisions to give up suicidal behavior were based on the value system of the therapist and the group. Later, these people gradually internalized the feeling that their life was worth living.

INTERPERSONAL LEARNING

Interpersonal learning is a complex process that overlaps several of the process variables already mentioned. Especially in psychotherapy and counseling groups, the process of interpersonal learning is one of the primary therapeutic factors. Because most mental health problems are acquired interpersonally and are manifested in disturbed interpersonal relations, it is reasonable that their treatment should focus on interpersonal learning.

The psychotherapy group provides an excellent medium in which the clients' various interpersonal styles can be readily displayed, explored, and corrected. In time, the group actually becomes a social microcosm in which the clients engage in a range of interpersonal behaviors that closely parallel their lives outside the group. It is a common experience for the members to identify in the group the interpersonal problem for which a client is seeking help in the work, social, or home situation. In a psychotherapy group, the members give each other direct feedback about their behavior and the effect it has on themselves and others. Once the clients assume responsibility for the roles they are playing in creating their own interpersonal dilemma and understand the sequence of events that led to their dissatisfaction, the road is paved for behavioral change.

GROUP COHESIVENESS

Group cohesiveness is not only a process variable, but a necessary condition for the therapeutic functioning and outcomes of most, if not all, health care groups. Cohesiveness in group therapy has been described as the group equivalent of the relationship in individual therapy.[14] Group cohesiveness is a broad concept, encompassing the patient's relations with the group therapist, the other group members, and the group as a whole. A number of group therapy studies illustrate the importance of group cohesiveness. The most common conclusion of these studies is that attraction to the group and the quality of member-to-member interaction is a strong determinant of positive therapeutic outcome in the clients and groups. Group cohesiveness can affect the attendance rate, the quality and quantity of member interaction, and the influence that members have on each other.

Specific information has been given about ways the leader can influence group cohesiveness in Chapter 7. At this point, it is important to emphasize the influence that this particular process variable can have on group outcomes. It seems reasonable that persons who are attracted to the goals and norms of the group will attend group sessions and will be more likely to follow the health care prescriptions of the members and leader. Group cohesiveness is therefore an important method for capturing the attention and commitment of clients in the process of influencing their behavior.

CATHARSIS

Catharsis is a process variable cited by many clients as being an important aspect of their group therapy experience. The expression of emotions previously unexpressed has long been considered of therapeutic value by psychotherapists. However, very few experienced therapists believe that catharsis alone is sufficient to produce longstanding therapeutic change. If anger, sadness, fear, or pleasure are expressed, they must also be integrated into the ongoing experience of the client.

Catharsis is also related to group cohesiveness in a circular cause-and-effect fashion. The expression and mutual working through of strong emotions is likely to increase the feelings of closeness and cohesiveness of the group. On the other hand, group cohesiveness is a prerequisite for group members to share their feelings. This is the reason there is so little sharing of strong emotions during the early phases of a treatment group.

The objectives of the group also will exert a strong influence on the use of catharsis as a group process variable. An activity group may be less tolerant of the expression of feelings that are perceived as interfering with having a good time. Also, feelings may be dealt with in a learning group only insofar as they interfere with the learning objectives of the group. It is primarily in psychotherapy groups that catharsis is viewed as contributing directly to achieving the objectives of the group.

EXISTENTIAL FACTORS

Existential factors are those elements in the process of a group that help members deal with the meaning of their own existence. These factors are more likely to be present in a group that is concerned with thinking, talking, and feeling than in a group whose focus is on accomplishing a task or planning an activity.

When people come together and share the experience of having a terminal illness, of divorce, or of feeling afraid or angry, there is a certain comfort in the sharing and commonality of one's experience. There is also a sobering solitude when people confront the reality that they alone must decide to change. Whether the experience is one of deciding how to confront life or how to deal with death, each person is at once a part of yet separate from all other persons in the environment. A group that is open to acknowledging this fact can utilize such existential factors in helping its members to live their lives differently because of this awareness.

In summary, the eleven therapeutic factors discussed above are important activities for the nurse to foster as group therapist. These factors help to explain how people change in groups and offer ways in which the group leader can utilize the group process to therapeutic advantage.

Role of the Nurse Therapist

In a study of encounter groups conducted by Lieberman, Yalom, and Miles,[5] four basic leadership functions were identified. These four categories accounted for almost 75% of all the activities of the 17 group leaders in the study. The researchers labeled those functions as emotional stimulation, caring, meaning attribution, and executive function.

EMOTIONAL STIMULATION

Emotional stimulation was described as the leader's behaviors that encouraged the group members actively to share their feelings. The leader's role was to confront, challenge, exhort, and model the revelation of personal values and feelings. This meant that the leader was very active with the group. In fact, the leaders who were rated highest on emotional stimulation ran leader-centered groups. Their use of referent power meant that much of the member activity focused on the leader in either a positive or a negative reaction to the leader's personalized style. The primary objective of emotional stimulation is to generate feelings on which the group members can work.

CARING

Caring as a leadership function involved the modeling of warm, accepting, positive feelings to assist the group in developing an accepting and supportive climate in which the members could work on their problems. The focus of the caring was not so much on feeling positively about the leader as on the acceptance of and caring for each other by the group members.

MEANING ATTRIBUTION

Meaning attribution was the leadership function by which the group leaders developed understanding of feelings and behaviors within the group. This function calls on the expert power of the leader to help the group members understand why certain feelings and behaviors were occurring. Meaning attribution recognizes the importance of the cognitive or intellectual element in changing behavior. For many people, it is not enough to have had a certain experience: they want to understand it.

EXECUTIVE FUNCTION

Executive function included all of the organizing, limit-setting, and management activities of the group leader. Starting and stopping the group on time, asking members to speak, and setting rules for member behavior are examples of the executive function of the leader. Leaders who rated highly on executive function acted more as facilitators than as involved members of the group. In many ways, the executive function can be described as the opposite of the emotional stimulation function.

One of the many interacting findings of the Lieberman, Yalom, and Miles[5] study of encounter groups involved the relations of these four basic group leadership functions. The leaders rated as most effective in the study were those who were moderate in their degree of emotional stimulation, high in caring, high in meaning attribution, and moderate in executive function. What emerges from the data in this study is the general profile of the effective group leader contained in Figure 36-1.

The reader is reminded that this study was conducted on encounter and therapy-type groups with "normal" university students as the group members. It is not yet clear how these groups are similar to or different from various types of health care groups. There is a need for clinical validation and nursing research on health care groups. In the meantime, the four leadership functions outlined above provide a useful point of reference for discussing the role of the leader in health care groups.

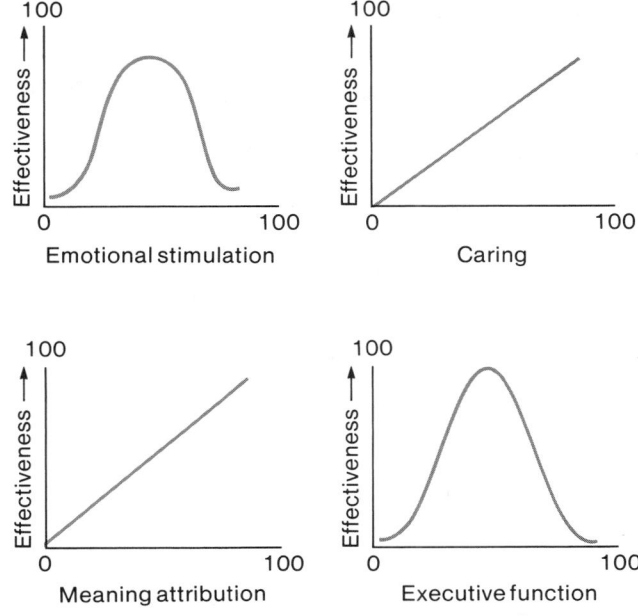

FIGURE 36-1. Effective group leader profile.

Group Cohesiveness

The role of the leader in the development of group cohesiveness relates directly to the goals and norms of the group. In effect, the goals and norms are vehicles the leader can use to develop and nurture group cohesiveness. Reference has already been made to the role of the leader in establishing the goals and beginning norms of the group during the process of structuring the group and selecting and preparing members. Because the leader is often the initial link between a new member and the group, the leader's statement of goals and norms is extremely influential.[13]

A significant portion of the leader's responsibility for executive functioning centers on structuring the goals and norms of the group to maximize its therapeutic potential. Once the group is started, the leader may move gradually toward a posture of sharing executive functions with the group. Less of the leader's energy and time are devoted to the task of structuring the group, and more attention is given to assisting the group to develop norms that will facilitate attainment of its goals and objectives. During the group's initial sessions, the leader may have responded readily to questions as a way of reducing member anxiety and uncertainty. Gradually, however, the leader should encourage group members to ask questions of each other and foster group discussion of relevant issues as a way of developing group cohesiveness. As the group engages in more sharing of feelings and experiences, it is important that the leader comment positively and thereby reinforce increased member interaction. As the group members work collaboratively to develop shared norms and goals, group cohesiveness will increase. Members will assist in the executive functions previously fulfiled by the leader, thus freeing the leader to focus more on the process that is developing within the group.

While group cohesiveness is developing, it is important that the leader increase the stimulation function by paying special attention to any reinforcement of interactions that support the goals and norms of the group. If the goal of the group is a specific change in member behavior, the leader should acknowledge members who have made positive changes. The leader also should encourage the group members to acknowledge each other's progress. Comments such as, "I'm pleased so many of you noticed Joan is less depressed tonight," or, "What do the rest of you think about Joan's recent changes?" are often facilitative.

The stimulation and caring functions of the leader are equally important to the formation of group cohesiveness. As the leader stimulates the expression of feelings, the change of behavior, or other interpersonal risk taking on the part of the members, it is imperative that this be done from a caring position. People are not likely to make interpersonal changes or share themselves with others if they do not feel safe. The leader must offer, not only permission to change, but also a protective environment in which new behaviors can be learned. For example, a young mother who shares her feelings of anger at becoming pregnant for the sixth time is less likely to be that open again with a group that chastises her for not loving her children. A caring group response would consist of acknowledging the validity of her feeling and how difficult it might have been to share it with others. Perhaps other group members have had similar experiences and can share their own feelings and how they dealt with the situation. The young mother can then be assisted to decide what she will do about her own situation in an atmosphere of acceptance and caring. One such event handled well by the group and leader can have a marked effect on the goals, norms, and subsequent cohesiveness of the group.

The leader becomes a role model in the development of group goals and norms. When the leader listens with interest, verbally reinforces, ignores, or actively disapproves of certain group interactions or member behaviors, the rest of the group incorporates what is being modeled. It is in this manner that the leader can influence the formation of enabling rather than restrictive norms. For example, when the leader discourages the expression of negative feelings, the group probably will have difficulty dealing with anger or may even ignore that emotion entirely. The leader's silent acceptance of member lateness and absences will assist the group in ignoring the importance of attendance to the group functioning.

The leader must make clear the interdependence of the members in accomplishing the group goals. In a study by Loomis of group-contingent reinforcement,[6] six chronic patients in a state hospital were offered rewards (money and outings) if the entire group performed certain target behaviors related to work and grooming. Even though this regressed group of men had no commitment to each other prior to this research project, they were readily able to comprehend their interdependence in achieving the group-contingent reinforcement. On their own initiative, the men found ways of helping each other with their cafeteria jobs, assisted each other in obtaining clothing on the designated days, and even taught one group member to shave himself.

The members' caring about each other generalized to behaviors other than those targeted for reinforcement. One day after the men had received their pay for working and achieving the target behaviors for the study, one group member offered to keep John's money for him so that he would not give it away to other patients who regularly approached him for "gifts" on payday. This group member proposed that whenever John wanted to go to the hospital snack bar or store, he would go with John to assist; John readily accepted. Although this type of caring behavior was not a specific goal of the study, it was observed as a healthy spinoff of the group-contingent reinforcement. It stands as striking evidence of the impact that can be achieved when group members are helped to see that they are dependent on each other for accomplishing a shared goal.

Meaning attribution is a leadership function that assumes increased importance in assisting the group to become more cohesive. It is the leader who should have both the perspective and the expertise to help the group members understand what they are doing together. The leader should point out the norm and value positions the group is developing, acknowledge with the group how difficult it is to change one's behavior or share feelings long hidden from others, carefully follow the discussion themes that are developing in the group —whether they are working at avoiding conflict or deciding on restrictive solutions in their problem solving. In short, the leader should help them to make some sense of their experiences in the group. This function of meaning attribution will increase during the life of a healthy group.

TERMINATION IN GROUP THERAPY

Termination is an important event in the life of therapy groups. Depending on the circumstances surrounding individual or group terminations, the event can take on the significance of graduation or a funeral. Indeed, the ending of relations within the group can be viewed as a microcosm of experiences in the larger world.

The leader of a therapy group is responsible for assisting the group members to deal with termination issues. Beginning with the initiation of a group contract, termination should be a clear issue for the group members. If the group is time limited with a set number of sessions, this reality is a part of the initial contract. The knowledge of an ending point serves as a time measure against which the leader and members can pace their work. If the group is open ended with members leaving and entering at irregular intervals, each member's contract for work in the group should include a clear definition of what that person intends to accomplish and how he or she will know when the objectives have been met. This contract can be renegotiated any number of times as members work in the group, but their objectives should always be clear. Ideally, this clarity will help both members and leader know when their work in the group is finished.

In therapy groups, termination can occur in one of two ways: either the entire group terminates, or an individual member or leader leaves the group. With either type of termination, the general approach is the same. Termination of any sort is an extremely important event in health care groups. It should be recognized, explored, and resolved much as any other working issue in the group. Regardless of the type of termination, people need to say goodbye.

Preparation for Termination

Preparation for termination begins the moment the group leader and potential client make contact. Depending on the type of therapy group under consideration, the client will know more or less specifically when termination will occur. If there is a specific contract for behavioral change, the group experience will be over when the desired changes have occurred. When a learning and behavioral change group has a plan for maintaining the new behavior, this should be made clear during the client's preparation for entering the group. For example, an outpatient group for agarophobic women may expect clients to attend group once a month for 6 months once their fear of going out in public has decreased. Clients who require additional assistance after this period can then renegotiate a contract for continuing group participation that meets their specific needs. With most hospital groups, the client's participation in the group is over when the client is discharged. In these instances, discharge from the facility is the criterion for leaving the group, and this should be made clear during the initial interview. Most work within therapy groups is done with a target for completion defined either by time, behavior, or circumstances. It is the leader's responsibility to select clients who are able to work within this context and to share with them the reality of their termination from the group from the initial preparation on. All work that is done within the group can then be planned to fit safely within the time allotted for the individual's participation in the group. For example, a client should not tackle a problem that will take 12 sessions to solve if the group is to meet only two more sessions.

Working Through

Working through the process of termination is not an easy task for groups. Because many people, including group leaders, deny the reality of impending termination, the tendency within health care groups will usually be in the direction of not dealing with the issue adequately. Some clients will "forget" that they are leaving so soon. Others will simply not show up for group and when contacted by the leader will explain why they decided to quit. Still others will write letters of goodbye rather than share their feelings directly with the group.

There also are clients who go to great lengths not to terminate. Some will continue to generate problems on which to work. Others will experience a sudden return of symptoms just prior to leaving in a valiant attempt to remain in the group. Still others will emotionally deny that for them the group is ending. They may arrange to meet with the group members socially and avoid saying goodbye to the group because, "I'll be seeing all of you during the next few weeks anyway."

Working through the process of termination involves activities similar to the working through of other group issues. The issue must be identified and acknowledged, alternative solutions identified and pursued, feelings expressed and dealt with, and a facilitating resolution achieved.

Evaluation of Progress

Evaluation of progress for individual members and the group as a whole can be used to facilitate the termination process. Termination is a good time to review progress and evaluate the usefulness of the group experience. Engaging in this type of evaluation also appears to facilitate the group's dealing with termination issues. When an individual member is leaving the group, the members may engage in a positive form of reminiscing that underscores the person's progress. Comments such as the following are common: "I'll never forget how angry you looked the first night of group. I thought you weren't even going to stay. It's certainly impressive how much you've changed into an open, caring person. I feel safe with you now." "You're thinking so much better now about how to take care of yourself and not be scared."

The group leader can enhance this termination evaluation by asking directly for feedback. What did you like about the way the group was set up? How would you evaluate our work together? Are there things you would have liked changed? What would you suggest we do differently in future groups like this one? In this way, members can be assisted to focus on any unfinished business they have with the group leader as well as provide valuable feedback for future use.

It is important also that the leaders share their perceptions of group functioning during this process. Leaders and members alike need validation of their own perceptions. Both the process and the outcomes of the health care group can be examined to provide a feeling of completeness and closure to the group experience. Planning is an important aspect of the evaluation of the progress of group members. As members review what they have gotten from the group and what, if anything, they still need from the group, they must plan for alternative ways of meeting their needs once the group has terminated.

Research Highlights

Lettieri–Marks D. Research in short-term inpatient group psychotherapy: a critical review. Arch Psychiatr Nurs. 1987;1(6):407–421.

The author presents a critical review of the research literature that specifically addresses short-term inpatient group psychotherapy conducted with adults. The structure, functions, treatment contexts, and research findings reported in published research articles are reviewed, and the author provides a critique of variables that are not addressed in the research literature.

Despite the growing importance and frequent use of short-term inpatient group psychotherapy by psychiatric mental health nurses, there is a paucity of published research on this treatment modality. This means that clinical interventions with inpatient groups are not empirically grounded. The author proposes several reasons for this situation. To begin with, there is a crucial need for the development of conceptual models or maps to identify possible relations between variables involved in the therapeutic process. Second, outcome variables must be identified and valid and reliable instruments developed to measure group outcomes. Then it will be possible for clinical researchers to examine and compare the conditions that facilitate client change in different types of psychotherapy groups.

Group therapy research in clinical settings is difficult to conduct because there are so many variables that cannot be controlled. However, audio and video equipment for observation can be used to provide a valid basis for descriptive research on objectives, structure, process, and outcome variables that are important for therapeutic effectiveness.

Sometimes, members need to leave the group before they are ready. If the group is ending or the person is moving to a new location, it is the leader's responsibility to assist the client in locating an appropriate health care structure for continuing the work. If the client is willing, direct referral to a new group or health care provider is desirable. It is important that all clients, whether they have completed their work in the group or not, know how to find assistance should they need it. The door to continued health care should be left open, and the path for returning should be clear.

In summary, the termination process is an extremely important phase in the life of therapy groups. When this phase is given appropriate attention, the group will enjoy the experience of having completed its work. During this phase, the leader's functions are to provide a high level of caring and meaning attribution with a concomitant decrease in the stimulation of new issues. The group members must be helped to place their experience together in the larger context of the lives they live outside the group. They take with them new learnings, feelings, and behaviors that they must use without the ongoing support of the group. It is hoped that they will carry their group memory with them as a positive experience from which they have benefited.

SUMMARY

The purpose of group therapy is to diagnose and treat human responses to actual or potential health problems. Some clients will benefit from working on their problems together in a group. Psychiatric mental health nurses have specific goals or objectives they hope to accomplish with different types of groups. Activity groups are used in psychiatric settings to help clients structure time and experience the sense of accomplishment that comes from completing a project or sharing a group activity. The goal of learning and behavioral change groups is to help clients learn new behaviors with which they will be able to function more comfortably and effectively in their homes, work settings, and communities. Psychotherapy groups are for the treatment of clients who desire insight and interpersonal change. A group therapy contract consists of a set of shared objectives as well as a clear understanding of the structure and process for arriving at the mutually determined outcomes. Common needs and the development of group cohesiveness are important factors to consider when selecting clients for group therapy. Preparation for group therapy should include a discussion of the objectives, structure, process, and outcomes for the group. There are eleven therapeutic factors the nurse can foster to help clients change through group therapy. The relative importance of these factors will differ depending on the type of therapy group. Emotional stimulation, caring, meaning attribution, and executive function are important leadership functions of the nurse in leading therapy groups. The group leader is responsible for structuring the goals and norms of the treatment group to enhance group cohesiveness and positive outcomes. The leader can help the group deal with termination issues by being clear from the beginning about the time, situational, or outcome criteria for individual and group termination. Working through termination issues is important for individual clients and the entire group.

References

1. Gray P, Stevenson JS. Changes in verbal interaction among members of resocialization groups. J Gerontol Nurs. 1980;6(2):86–90.
2. Krumm S, Vannata P, Sanders J. A group for teaching chemotherapy. Am J Nurs. May 1979;916.
3. Lettieri–Marks D. Research in short-term inpatient group

psychotherapy: a critical review. Arch Psychiatr Nurs. 1987;1:407–421.

4. Lewin K. Forces behind food habits and methods of change. Bull Natl Resource Council. 1943;108:35–65.

5. Lieberman MA, Yalom ID, Miles MB. Encounter Groups: First Facts. New York: Basic Books; 1972.

6. Loomis ME. Use of group contingencies with psychiatric patients. In: ANA Clinical Sessions—1972. New York: Appleton-Century-Crofts; 1973.

7. Loomis ME. Group Process for Nurses. St. Louis: CV Mosby Co; 1979.

8. Morrow ET. Stress and survival of illness: a study of disability-work groups and their effect on employee productivity and well-being. Occup Health Nurs. February 1985:79–85.

9. Nath C, Rinehart J. Effects of individual and group relax-ation therapy on blood pressure in essential hypertensives. Res Nurs Health. 1979;2:119–126.

10. Neizo B, Murphy MK. Medication groups on an acute psychiatric unit. Perspect Psychiatr Care. 1983;21(2):70–73.

11. Rosenthal RH, Thomas NS, Vandiveer CA. Triage, education, and group meetings: efficient use of the interdisciplinary team with chronic psychiatric outpatients. J Psychosoc Nurs Ment Health Serv. April 1979:14–19.

12. White EM, Kahn EM. Use of modifications in group psychotherapy with chronic schizophrenic outpatients. J Psychosoc Nurs Ment Health Serv. 1982;20(2):14–20.

13. White EM. Effective inpatient groups: challenges and rewards. Arch Psychiatr Nurs. 1987;1:422–428.

14. Yalom ID. The Theory and Practice of Group Psychotherapy. New York: Basic Books; 1985.

37

Joan E. Bowers

Family Therapy

OBJECTIVES

After reading this chapter, the reader will be able to:

1. Describe the development of family therapy
2. Identify assumptions that underlie the family approach in psychiatric mental health nursing
3. Discuss selected family therapy models
4. Describe nursing roles in relation to family therapy
5. Identify common nursing diagnoses of families in family therapy
6. Identify issues in family therapy research.

INTRODUCTION

Family therapy is a form of psychotherapeutic intervention that focuses on the family system as a unit. A primary assumption that guided the early practice of family therapy defined the presenting problem of an individual as a symptom of *family level* dysfunction. Much of the early activity, including research in the use of family therapy, was thus focused on families with schizophrenic members or those with acting-out children. An excellent analysis of the early history of family therapy is available to the interested reader.[6]

As the usefulness of family therapy for both family and individual problems was recognized, elaborations on the basic format evolved. Furthermore, as families with members diagnosed with schizophrenia came together and supported each other in their efforts to negotiate the mental health system, they also became critical of the system that labeled their families as dysfunctional.[4] These families and their organization, the National Alliance for the Mentally Ill, have been very effective in changing attitudes and improving the care provided to their members and themselves.

Concurrently, research focused on the biologic substrates of human behavior has resulted in findings that implicate brain function in the development and course of schizophrenia,[20] generally removing the burden of responsibility for *causing* the schizophrenia from the family as a social system. However, families have felt the impact of the schizophrenic process in their affected members. This has brought about the elaboration of therapeutic methods that address the family as a unit, but that move beyond the formalized practice of family therapy. Family-focused interventions that are in use today, therefore, range from the highly structured family therapy models, to the family psychoeducational models used for helping families with members who have severe psychiatric impairments, to models that incorporate many features of a self-management intervention approach. Finally, the use of family interviewing[26] and the elaboration of nursing diagnoses regarding family functioning (see nursing diagnoses entitled Family Coping, Potential for Growth, and Dysfunctional Family Processes) represent yet another approach to family intervention that is gaining ascendance in the health care arena.

Currently, family therapy is used for treating a variety of problems that may be presented either by an individual or by a family as a unit. The former is exemplified by the case of a teenager who is experiencing suicidal fantasies following the breakup of a relationship; the nurse therapist may choose to involve the family in dealing with this crisis. An example of the latter is that of a family responding to the crisis of the loss of their home following a natural catastrophe such as a tornado. As family therapy has gained acceptance, more disciplines have engaged in training students in this clinical modality.

DEVELOPMENT OF FAMILY THERAPY

The movement from the traditional individually focused, psychodynamically based psychotherapy to the focus on the family as the unit of treatment has been described by Jones as a "scientific revolution."[11] In this sense, the development of family therapy, as for other scientific revolutions in modern history, represents a noncumulative developmental movement in which an older paradigm is replaced in whole or in part by an incompatible new one. This sort of paradigm shift requires that one change one's conception of the problem. Integral to this paradigm shift is the need to specify the assumptions that underlie the use of a family model for understanding human behavior and, in particular, human dysfunction. The following is a brief outline of assumptions that may be useful for guiding the clinician who proposes to use a family approach in health care practice:

- Families represent the basic social unit in human functioning.
- Families are multicultural and multidimensional social phenomena. To speak of "the family" as though one set of variables could explain all families is no longer acceptable.
- As primary socializing agents for individuals, families exert the greatest influence of all social systems on both the development and the continuation of a person's behavior.
- As one of the basic social systems, families serve the essential function of transmitting cultural values and traditions through the generations.
- Family systems evolve and increase in organizational complexity by progressing through a series of developmental stages.
- Individuals also proceed through developmental stages and this experience generally occurs within a family context.
- Families experience transitions consequent to developmental events such as birth, death, divorce, and remarriage. These events invoke changes in membership and composition in family systems.
- Families possess and develop internal strengths and resources. Among these resources is the ability to adapt and change in response to internal and external demands.
- Changes in a family system's structure and processes lead to changes in all members.
- Changes in the behavior and functioning of individual family members affect that family system and all of the other family members.
- A family as a system is more than the sum of the functioning of its individual members (nonsummativity).
- Changes in a family's structure and functioning can be facilitated by family therapy (adapted from Lomax & Van Servellen[14]).

FAMILY THERAPY MODELS

In the early years of the family therapy movement, several distinct approaches evolved. These will be briefly summarized; the reader is also encouraged to learn more about these "first-generation" approaches.[6,11]

Bowen Theory

An approach that gained popularity and that continues to be used by a number of nurses who conduct family therapy is the model developed by Bowen. Bowen's[11] early training was in psychoanalysis; his movement into a family focus developed because of his discontent with treating individuals in isolation from their environments, particularly as these environments contributed to the individual's illness. The therapeutic unit in this approach is the family as a system; pathology is viewed as a product of the larger family system, rather than of the individual member. Therapy is conducted with the two adult members who are assessed as being locked in a *triangle*, defined by Bowen as a ". . . three person emotional configuration . . . the smallest relationship system" (reference 15, p 26). The third point of the triangle may be another person, issue, or object that is pulled in to decrease discomfort in the relationship system.[15] Triangles are essentially conservative in that the process maintains family patterns and level of differentiation. Alternatively, therapy may be conducted with that member of the family who is most *differentiated* from the *family emotional system*. The role of the therapist includes four major functions:

1. Define and clarify the relationship between the spouses
2. Keep self de-triangled from the family emotional system
3. Teach about the functioning of emotional systems
4. Demonstrate differentiation by taking the "I" position during the course of therapy[11]

Thus, the therapeutic process consists primarily of "coaching" or supervising one or two individuals within the family. The therapy is basically a cognitive approach to modifying the family emotional system. Major concepts of this theoretic model are presented in Box 37–1.

Structural Family Therapy

The structural family therapy model was initially developed by Minuchin in his work with incarcerated boys and their families in New York.[16] Similar to the work of several other first-generation family therapists, Minuchin's early work was formally organized as a re-

---

BOX 37–1
Bowen Theory Concepts

1. Differentiation of self: determinant of how emotional relationships are established and how they grow (p 7).
2. Triangles are building blocks of any emotional system and are the automatic emotional response in all families used to manage anxiety in relationships (pp 8–9).
3. Multigenerational transmission process defines the family as a dynamic, timeless system that extends for many generations. Issues and problems are passed on from generation to generation and patterns of relationship remain unchanged (pp 38–40).
4. Sibling position is the place a person occupies in the family with respect to other siblings; considered to be an important predictor of behavior (p 48).
5. Nuclear family emotional system refers to patterns of family interaction and degree to which these patterns promote emotional fusion (p 62).
6. Emotional cutoff: process whereby a distanced family style is maintained as a means of dealing with intimacy issues (p 53).
7. Family projection process describes the way anxiety about specific issues is transmitted through the generations (p 67).

Adapted from Miller SR, Winstead-Fry P. Family systems theory in nursing practice. Reston, VA: Reston Publishing; 1982.

---

search project and reported as such, rather than as a new method of therapy.

The family is conceptualized as an *open sociocultural system* that is constantly faced by demands for *adaptation*.[11] Family *functioning* breaks down when the demand for adaptation is met with maladaptive responses, either from an individual member or from the family system itself. These demands may come from *situational factors* in the sociocultural environment or from the *developmental changes* that occur in family members and in the family as a unit. A consequence of the breakdown in family functioning is the emergence of *dysfunctional transactional patterns*, the prototypes of which are *enmeshment* and *disengagement*. These concepts are discussed in detail in the nursing diagnosis entitled Family Coping, Potential for Growth.

The focus of therapy is the structure of the family and its transformation from maladaptive to adaptive or growth-facilitating patterns. Three phases to the therapeutic endeavor include joining the family, evaluating the underlying family structure, and orchestrating circumstances or experiences that permit the structure to change.[11] The outcome of therapy is, thus, both the change in the symptomatic or problem behavior of the identified patient and the structural changes in the family that permit a new and higher level of functioning.

Strategic Family Therapy

Jay Haley's[7] name is most prominently associated with this model of family therapy, although others have contributed importantly to the development of the strategic approach.[24] These authors and others such as Satir[19] are engaged in an approach to family therapy that is based on communication theory.[11]

The basic tenets of communication theory[24] are as follows: All behavior is communication; therefore, it is impossible to *not* communicate. The verbal message is referred to as the digital communication or message, whereas all other behavior is understood to be analogic communication. Thus, the various components of behavior serve to modify and qualify each other. Of particular importance is the tenet that every communication contains two messages: the content (digital) message and the relationship (analogic) message. Behavior is ongoing, rather than discontinuous. In this respect, interpersonal communication is continuously predicated on each other's behavior. In ongoing relationships, communication becomes highly patterned and, thus, *repetitive* or redundant *interactions* evolve.

Strategic or problem-solving therapy[7] has as its primary goal the removal of the presenting symptoms through the use of *directives* that require behavior change to be practiced at home and *paradox*, defined as the delivery of two conflicting messages simultaneously. There is little emphasis placed on the history of the problem or the motivation for it. The strategic therapist does not emphasize the development of insight, which, rather, is seen as counterproductive to the course of therapeutic change.

Therapy can be conducted with one or more members of the family and may or may not include the identified patient. Decisions for this will depend on who sought help, that is, the person who is most uncomfortable with the problem and, thus, most willing to change. A detailed description of the problem and determining the family's minimal goal of treatment constitute the first steps of therapy. The *strategies* of therapy include *reframing*, in which the problem is redefined by the therapist as being needed by the family: for example, *positively connoting* the problem, a type of reframing specifically developed to define the problem as serving a useful purpose in the family; *restraint from change*, in which, for example, the family might be asked to engage in the problem behavior for another week to be able to more fully describe it to the therapist; and use of therapeutic *paradox* or contradictory messages such that the family's "resistance" is heightened and change is brought about as a response.

The strategic therapist is viewed as an active and deliberate change agent. Responsibility for success of the therapeutic endeavor lies squarely with the therapist. Failure of the therapy is never attributed to client or family resistance; rather, the therapist has failed to assess the problem appropriately or to devise an effective strategy that will produce change in the family.

Systemic Family Therapy

In recent years, an approach has evolved that significantly modified the early work of the strategic therapists. In particular, the work of Boscolo and Cecchin[3] has gained precedence. Others who are also involved in developing this approach include Hoffman,[9] Penn[18] and their colleagues at the Ackerman Institute for Family Therapy in New York, and Tomm[23] and his group at the University of Calgary. Working with this latter group are Wright,[26] Leahey,[13] and other nurses who have extended this approach for use by nurses in various types of clinical settings (other than the traditional psychiatric or mental health setting).

The theoretic underpinnings of the systemic model owe much to Bateson's[2] work on cybernetic circularity as a prototype for living systems. An early publication that outlines a dynamic approach based on Bateson's work proposes the following as components of the model:[21] *Hypothesizing* is identified as the basic guideline for the assessment process. The proposed hypothesis must be *systemic*: it must account for all the elements in a problem situation and how these link together.

Circular questioning translates cybernetic circularity into an interviewing technique.[3] The circular questioning grew out of Bateson's proposal that the knowledge we have of external events is based on the use of mechanisms that scan the environment for difference.[21] Living systems are characterized by *loop formations* rather than by linear sequences of cause and effect. Circular questions ask for information about differences: in perceptions about relationships; in degree; regarding now as compared with then; regarding hypothetical and future differences. Questions such as these are constructed in response to cues that the family offers that indicate a fruitful approach for developing or evolving a hypothesis.

The third element, *neutrality,* translates this same concept of cybernetic circularity into a basic therapeutic stance. The neutral therapeutic stance implies a multipositional stance, rather than a nonpositional one. If the therapist has successfully achieved this multipositional stance, family members will be able to say that no member's side in particular was taken by the therapist.

In some respects, the circular questioning is in itself a type of therapeutic intervention. Other approaches that have superficial similarity to the previously described strategic interventions are also used. Positive connotation has been changed to *logical connotation:* instead of telling the family that the problem is useful, good, or functional, the therapist tells the family that they have become used to the problem and that old habits are hard to break.[3] Thus, the family may be freed up to search for an alternative to the symptom that will answer the same need but does so less destructively.

The use of *ritual* or *ceremony* usually addresses the double-binding communication in a family.[3] The ritual is frequently structured to put the double-binding interaction, which by definition is simultaneous, conflicting directives, into a sequential pattern. Specifically, parents who disagree about the discipline of a child may be asked to alternate responsibility for discipline on odd and even days. In the event that the directive for conducting the ritual is ignored, this is not viewed as resistance, but rather, as new information about how the family works and, therefore, is used to develop further hypotheses.

In summary, whatever the intervention(s) used by systemic therapists, these are not directed toward any particular predetermined outcome. Rather, the intervention is believed to "jog the system toward unpredictable outcomes" (reference 3, p 19). This philosophic premise carries an implicit faith in the ability of the family system to produce its own solutions. In the last analysis, this is the collaboration with the client to which nursing has long been devoted.

Family Therapy Variations

A major approach to the use of family therapy that emerged in the 1960s is that of *multiple family therapy*.[12] This approach brought together, in the state hospital setting, families of persons with chronic schizophrenia to engage in the therapeutic endeavor. A structured format was developed, and the benefits of the approach were articulated; however, research to support its effectiveness was not conducted. The approach continues to find adherents and has been used with a variety of populations.[17]

Possibly one of the most extensively researched approaches to a family-based intervention, the *psychoeducational* approach, had its beginnings following the outgrowth of research that investigated expressed emotion in relatives of psychiatrically impaired persons (see nursing diagnosis entitled Family Coping, Potential for Growth for a review of this research). Another impetus for developing this approach was the activism of the families themselves, who responded to what they experienced as victimization from the psychiatric professional community.

The psychoeducational approach[5,10] is based on the premise that the schizophrenic impairment of a family's member brings with it certain demands with which the family must be helped to cope. The approach is highly structured, usually time-limited, and proposes to educate family members about the mental illness and to provide both the primary client and the family caretakers with the skills needed to cope with certain predictable demands and situations. Frequently, the approach is offered by a team of clinicians and may be conducted in an intensive workshop format or in a more extended series of sessions offered over weeks or months. Families may be seen individually or in groups, and some of the models include a psychodynamically based psychotherapy component, as well as the structured educational content. Regardless of for-

mat, the aims of the approach are to (1) influence the course of the illness; (2) reduce relapse rate; (3) improve the client's psychosocial functioning by educating the family about the illness, symptomatic behavior management, treatment approaches (e.g., medication management, side effects); and (4) reduce stress for the family and for the client.[8]

Finally, another approach that is receiving an extensive research focus is that developed by Webster-Stratton[25] and her colleagues. Basically, this is a highly structured *parent-training* approach based on a behavior therapy model for use in families with behavior-disordered preschoolers. A major feature of the approach that is being carefully scrutinized is that parents are provided with videotapes of typical problem situations and the recommended behavioral strategies, which they view and then test out with their child at home. In other words, after diagnosis of the child's behavioral disorder, the parent(s) engage in a self-help intervention program. Not only has this intervention method been very effective when tested against more traditional approaches in a random-assignment experimental research design, but it also is highly cost-effective.

NURSING ROLES

The Standards for Psychiatric and Mental Health Nursing Practice[22] proposes that the role of family therapist is restricted to those nurses with advanced education (i.e., a graduate degree) in psychiatric mental health nursing and special training and supervision in family therapy practice. The training process in a particular model is usually an intensive experience in supervised practice and includes a structured didactic component. How the nurse functions in the role of therapist is, in some measure, dependent on the particular family therapy approach, as indicated in the foregoing descriptions of the various models. The generic aspects of the therapeutic process hold across models and these include (1) initiating the relationship or "joining"; (2) assessment and planning; (3) implementation or "working stage"; and (4) evaluation and termination.

The nurse who is prepared at less than the master's level may function as a member of a team that conducts family interventions, such as those described above (multiple-family therapy or psychoeducational interventions). In these situations, the nurse functions under the guidance and supervision of a qualified professional, such as a psychiatric clinical nurse specialist or other mental health specialist with advanced training and experience in family therapy. This nurse might also function independently to conduct family assessments that contribute to the data base for an individual client. Nurses who work in the field of community health conduct family assessments routinely as part of the family nursing process. These nurses may also carry out family-based interventions that share some aspects of family therapy, but are not considered to be family therapy per se. When nurses prepared at this level assess complex family problems, the appropriate intervention strategy is referral to a professional family therapist.

COMMON NURSING DIAGNOSES

Families for whom family therapy is an appropriate intervention will most likely receive a nursing diagnosis of dysfunctional family processes. Additionally, families who receive a nursing diagnosis of family coping: potential for growth may be appropriate clients for family therapy. As described earlier, families who are in crisis secondary to a disaster, or those families in whom a member is the victim of a major mental disorder, may also be benefited by selected family therapy approaches. Finally, those families in whom a member's illness or behavior problem is either affecting or is influenced by family processes may be appropriate participants in a family therapy approach to treatment.

CASE STUDY

Ethan J, a 20-year-old young man employed as an office supply company clerk, was referred to the clinical nurse specialist by his employer. Ethan's performance had fallen off over the past two weeks. Ethan cried as he explained to his employer that all he could think about was his former girlfriend who broke off with him after a four-month living-together relationship. Ethan was expressing suicidal ideas, and so his employer called for help. The clinical nurse specialist called Ethan to set up contact. Ethan was asked to invite his parents to be present at the first session; an appointment was made for that afternoon.

The family history revealed that Mr. and Ms. J married right after high school and Ethan was conceived shortly thereafter. Mr. J enlisted in the military and was sent overseas in the Korean conflict; his son was 18 months old before they met. After his return, the marriage floundered and a divorce ensued. Both partners remarried quickly. Ms. J remained in close contact with Mr. J's family and Ethan developed close bonds with his father's relatives. Ms. J's second marriage ended in divorce after two years. The following ten years found Ms. J and Ethan on their own with only occasional contact from Mr. J. About a year before Ethan's crisis, Mr. J's mother became critically ill. Ethan's parents met over their concern for her and rediscovered each other; they gradually decided that they wanted to be together again. Eventually Mr. J divorced his second wife and remarried his first wife and moved in with her and their son.

Ethan, at this time, was a late teenager who had no aspirations for college; he hoped to find a job that would allow him freedom to develop his artistic talents. Things got tense at home when his father began expecting that Ethan be more responsible in a variety of ways. Ms. J went along with this, satisfied that her husband was fitting right in and setting limits that she may have been reluctant to exercise over the years that she and Ethan lived together. The tension escalated, never reaching a boiling point, until Ethan met Mindy, with whom he quickly became intensely involved. They dated six weeks when they decided to find an apartment together. Ethan went into considerable debt, but he said that he and Mindy were happy for a couple of months. Then her family began to interfere in their relationship. Things quickly came to a head and she insisted he leave. His only recourse was to move back with his parents. Although his parents were supportive, they also made it clear that this was temporary and that the earlier restrictions and expectations still held. Ethan could not share with them the depth of his grieving, and so he became more obsessed with his pain. When he found himself virtually unable to concentrate at work and, thereby, at risk of losing his job, he felt he had hit bottom; taking his own life seemed the only solution.

The psychosocial assessment revealed a bright young man who gave no evidence of psychosis. Although he was very anxious and desperate enough to be thinking about suicide, he had not formulated any plans about how this might be accomplished. Other symptoms included episodes of crying, difficulty sleeping, and diminished appetite. Ethan had an unremarkable health history and had no physical symptoms of disease. Ethan's parents were eager to know how they might help him recover his equanimity. Mr. J seemed a bit impatient with his son; he advised him to "forget that girl; you're young and you'll meet someone new without any trouble."

Ethan was diagnosed as suffering from adjustment disorder with mixed emotional features.[1] The family was deemed to be in transition, following the parents' remarriage. They were also engaged in a process of family coping with potential for growth, which was formulated as the family diagnosis. Although loss issues were not directly explored in the therapy sessions, all three members were diagnosed as grieving: Mr. J for his recently divorced family and Ethan and his mother for their close relationship, terminated by Mr. J's return.

The family was seen four times within a period of three weeks. In addition, Ethan was seen individually four times over five weeks. Focus in the family sessions was on opening up communications about the distress Ethan was experiencing. The relationship between Ethan and his father needed negotiation: both men had unrealistic expectations of each other and of their relationship. The marital relationship was addressed indirectly by focusing on issues of decision making and limit setting. Ms. J's willingness to let her new husband step into this role too quickly was based, in part, on the premise of his parental right, given his biologic relationship with Ethan. However, his absence over the years placed him now in the role of interloper and "stepfather." Interventions with Ethan alone focused on assisting with his grieving process, sorting out his short-term goals, and making some action plans for his living arrangements, debts, and work situation. Termination of treatment began when Ethan began doing better both at work and in his evening and weekend hours. At the last session, he reported having met a young woman at a fair; he arranged a date with her and was looking forward to exploring their mutual interests in music and art. Mr. and Ms. J were satisfied with Ethan's progress and expressed an interest in his being able to move out on his own again when he demonstrated readiness. Meanwhile, the couple were in agreement about the negotiated expectations for their son and both were involved in reinforcing these in their daily interactions with him (see Nursing Care Plan 37-1 for a sample care plan for the J family).

NURSING CARE PLAN 37-1

THE J FAMILY

NURSING INTERVENTIONS	OUTCOME CRITERIA

NURSING DIAGNOSIS: Family coping, potential for growth

PARENT GOAL: Function more closely as a team in defining and enacting expectations and limits for their son

■ Assist parents to develop a negotiation process with their son on rules and limits	Family members report satisfaction with the results of this process

COUPLE GOAL: Moderate their expectations for Mr. J's rapid reentry into the family system

■ Explore with the couple issues having to do with the transition from a single-parent to a two-parent family	Mr. J demonstrates willingness to go more slowly in his dealings with his son

FAMILY GOAL: Develop open patterns of communication that permit sharing a range of emotions and ideas

■ Role-model open communication in the therapy session ■ Assist members to identify blocks to open communication	Family members engage in freer expression in session; report same at home as well

SUMMARY

Several approaches to family therapy that are commonly used in mental health practice were reviewed. These are primarily based on the assumptions that the family functions as a system and that the event of a psychiatric or behavioral disorder in a member can most effectively be treated by changing some aspect of the system. Different approaches to family therapy propose to effect change in the family system by influencing different aspects of the family, such as structure (Minuchin), family differentiation level (Bowen), the family problem (Haley), or parenting effectiveness (Webster-Stratton). Thus, strategies that form the basis of the therapeutic endeavor differ in each of these approaches, although there can be a great deal of overlap

Research Highlights

Very little research on the effectiveness of family therapy has been systematically conducted over the many years that it has been a mainstream intervention approach. The work of Webster-Stratton[25] and her colleagues is an important exception. Some of the issues that strongly merit investigation are (1) what is the relative effectiveness of family therapy versus individual therapy for selected psychosocial disabilities; (2) does a particular family therapy model work better than others with a given problem; (3) what are the conditions under which family therapy is contraindicated? Design issues that must be considered include comparison of several approaches (rather than testing family therapy against no treatment); use of adequate control group procedures; random assignment of the treatment condition; appropriate length of time over which the subjects are studied; multiple data collection points and respondents; inclusion of objective data, such as the child's school attendance record, as a test of treatment effectiveness.

in the techniques used by the different approaches; that is, the use of directives is a technique that might be used in several approaches. How the directive is phrased and when in the course of the session it is used might differ depending on the therapeutic strategies that evolve from the basic assumptions of the particular approach.

Finally, as with all other interpersonal therapeutic approaches, family therapy comprises stages including (1) the engaging or joining stage, (2) the assessment and planning stage, (3) the working or implementation stage, and (4) the evaluation and termination stage.

References

1. American Psychiatric Association. Diagnostic and statistical manual of mental disorders, 3rd ed, revised. Washington, DC: American Psychiatric Association; 1987.
2. Bateson G. Steps to an ecology of the mind. New York: Ballantine Books; 1972.
3. Boscollo L, Cecchin G, Hoffman L, Penn P. Milan systemic family therapy: conversations in theory and practice. New York: Basic Books; 1987.
4. Francell CG, Conn VS, Gray DP. Families' perceptions of burden of care for chronic mentally ill relatives. Hosp Commun Psychiatry. 1988;39:1296–1300.
5. Greenberg L, Fine SB, Larson K, Michaelson-Baily A, Rubinton P, Glick ID. An interdisciplinary psychoeducation program for schizophrenic patients and their families in an acute care setting. Hosp Commun Psychiatry. 1988;39:277–282.
6. Guerin PJ, ed. Family therapy: theory and practice. New York: Gardner Press; 1976.
7. Haley J. Leaving home, 2nd ed. San Francisco: Jossey-Bass; 1987.
8. Helm PE. Family therapy. In: Stuart GW, Sundeen SJ, eds. Principles and practice of psychiatric nursing, 3rd ed. St. Louis: CV Mosby; 1987.
9. Hoffman L. Beyond power and control: toward a "second order" family systems therapy. Fam Sys Med. 1986;4:381.
10. Hogarty GE, Anderson CM, Reiss DJ, et al. Family psychoeducation, social skills training, and maintenance chemotherapy in the aftercare treatment of schizophrenia. Arch Gen Psychiatry. 1986;43:633–642.
11. Jones SL. Family therapy: a comparison of approaches. Bowie, MD: Robert J Brady; 1980.
12. Laqueur H, Laburt H, Morong E. Multiple family therapy: further developments. In: Haley J, ed. Changing families: a family therapy reader. New York: Grune & Stratton; 1971.
13. Leahey M, Wright LM, eds. Families and psychosocial problems. Springhouse, PA: Springhouse Corp; 1987.
14. Lomax JI, Van Servellen GM. Family therapy. In: Birckhead LM, ed. Psychiatric mental health nursing: the therapeutic use of self. Philadelphia: JB Lippincott; 1989.
15. Miller SR, Winstead-Fry P. Family systems theory in nursing practice. Reston, VA: Reston Publishing; 1982.
16. Minuchin S, Montalvo B, Guerney BG, Rosman BL, Schumer F. Families of the slums: an exploration of their structure and treatment. New York: Basic Books; 1967.
17. O'Shea M, Phelps R. Multiple family therapy: current status and critical appraisal. Fam Process. 1985;24:555–582.
18. Penn P. Feed forward: future questions, future maps. Fam Process. 1985;24:299–310.
19. Satir V. Conjoint family therapy, 3rd ed. Palo Alto, CA: Science and Behavior Books; 1967.
20. Seeman P. Dopamine receptors and the dopamine hypothesis of schizophrenia. Synapse. 1987;1:133–152.
21. Selvini Palazzoli M, Boscolo L, Cecchin G, Prata G. Hypothesizing-circularity-neutrality. Fam Process. 1980;19:3–12.
22. Standards of psychiatric and mental health nursing practice. Kansas City, MO: American Nurses' Association; 1982.
23. Tomm K. Interventive interviewing: Part I. Strategizing as a fourth guideline for the therapist. Fam Process. 1987;26:3–13.
24. Watzlawick P, Beavin J, Jackson D. Pragmatics of human communication. New York: WW Norton; 1967.
25. Webster-Stratton C, Kolpacoff M, Hollinsworth T. Self-administered videotape therapy for families with conduct-problem children. J Consult Clin Psychol. 1988;56:558–566.
26. Wright LM, Leahey M, eds. Nurses and families: a guide to family assessment and intervention. Philadelphia: FA Davis; 1984.

38

Gordon L. Dickman
Carolyn A. Livingston

Sex Therapy

OBJECTIVES

After reading this chapter the reader will be able to:

1. *Describe the varieties of sex therapies including both medical and psychotherapeutic interventions*
2. *Describe treatment models for various sexual disorders*
3. *Discuss nursing roles in relation to sex therapy*
4. *List common nursing diagnoses for individuals in sex therapy.*

DESCRIPTION AND RATIONALE

The World Health Organization (WHO) has called for sexuality education, counseling, and therapy to be available as part of total health care.[16] Sexual disorders and the need for sex counseling or therapy can occur irrespective of cultural, ethnic, or socioeconomic status. People of all sexual orientations and sexual life-styles can experience sexual disorders. Successful sex therapy takes into account differences in life experiences, and sexual life-style. Ideally, sex therapy would be available and practiced in ways that reflect this diversity.

Sexual disorders are described in DSM-III-R as paraphilias or as sexual dysfunctions.[1] *Paraphilias* represent recurrent, intense sexual fantasies or urges toward objects or nonconsenting persons. They may be deeply disturbing to the patient and may be against the law. *Sexual dysfunctions* are described as disruptions of the sexual response cycle.

The pioneering work in modern sex therapy was done by Masters and Johnson. They observed and described the physical responses of females and males to sexual stimulation. They demonstrated that sexual functioning was more than just a "natural" bodily function, rather it was a complex interaction of physical and emotional responses, sexual knowledge and skills, and communication skills. They also provided a common understanding of the physiologic basis of sexual functioning and a shared vocabulary for talking about it.[11]

Masters and Johnson[11] divided sexual response into four phases: excitement, plateau, orgasm, and resolution. The *excitement phase* is described as the body's initial response to sexual stimulation. Females may experience vaginal lubrication and males an erection. The *plateau phase* is defined as the stage of physical arousal just before orgasm. It may last for a short or long period, depending upon the intensity of sexual arousal and interest. *Orgasm*, which is a mental as well as a physical event, is defined as the reversal of myotonia and vasocongestion. The *resolution phase* is defined as the period before another excitement, plateau, orgasm sequence begins. This is a clearly defined period for males and, particularly in elderly males, may last for several days.

Kaplan[6] described an additional phase—sexual desire—that precedes the other four phases described by Masters and Johnson. *Sexual desire* is defined as the wish or appetite for sex.[6] Sexual desire, or "horniness," is influenced by both environment and brain chemistry. Inhibited sexual desire describes those times when a person feels "turned off" to sex. When this becomes chronic and is described by the client as dissatisfying and disruptive, then it is a sexual dysfunction. Females as well as males experience sexual desire, although not necessarily in the same way. Cultural influences seem to play an important role in how females and males experience this desire. A clearer picture of the similarities and differences in female and male sexual experiences will emerge with further research on the role of nature and nurture in sexual development.

The work of John Money is in the forefront of research into the etiology of paraphilic behavior. His work includes describing the role of sex hormones on fetal brain development.[13] An understanding of the neural and hormonal links to paraphilic behaviors strengthens traditional therapies used to control and manage these behaviors.

Just as sexuality is multidimensional, sex therapy may intervene on many levels. A therapist may give brief support and information or may form a long-term counseling relationship. Interventions may be medical or psychotherapeutic. Theoretical orientations of individuals doing sex therapy include psychoanalytic, behavioral, cognitive, and social–interpersonal frameworks.

There is no single best technique or therapy model for all clients. For example, a client who has a sexual dysfunction clearly related to a medical condition may well experience discord in a sexual relationship and emotional distress. Both medical and counseling interventions, involving different health care professionals, may be indicated. Hence, sexual health requires cooperative and informed health care workers.

Medical interventions may assist clients suffering from disruptions of hormonal, vascular, and neurologic systems influencing their sexual functioning. Hormonal therapy may be used to decrease paraphilic urges. Sexual behaviors that are affected by a limited range of motion or pain from disease processes may be enhanced by medical intervention. Great strides have been made in recent years in the understanding of the effect of medications on sexual desire and sexual functioning. Many cases of erectile dysfunction are now being treated pharmacologically or by penile implant surgery.[4] Surgery for breast reconstruction, genital reconstruction or alteration, and cosmetic surgery to improve body image can enhance sexual function.

Sexual disorders can be treated with a wide variety of psychotherapeutic approaches. These approaches include analysis, talk therapies, skills building and education, and interactional therapies involving group or couples therapy.

Psychoanalysis used for the relief of sexual disorders is not as prevalent as it once was. Disorders arising from remote, underlying causes that do not respond to techniques that are based on gaining knowledge, skills, and insights in the present may respond to this kind of long-term analysis. But because of its expense and the length of time required for analysis, it is beyond the reach of many clients.

The behavioral therapy model views sexual disorders as learned over time. From this viewpoint, the dysfunctional behavior is reinforced and maintained by factors in the patient's environment. Anxiety, sexual skills deficits, and lack of sexual information contribute to the dysfunctional behavior. Therapy revolves around learning new information and skills that will replace or assist in adapting the dysfunctional ones to the present situation. Behavioral therapy has been used to relieve such dysfunctions as performance anxiety, conflicts between sex partners, and lack of orgasmic response caused by fear or ignorance. Annon's PLISSIT model for treating sexual dysfunctions is a widely used intervention model. The letters in the model name stand for permission, limited information, specific suggestions, and intensive therapy.[2] Interventions using this model start with validating clients' feelings about the dysfunction. They are given permission to begin to talk about their feelings and issues related to the dysfunction. The next level of intervention may involve giving clients limited information about the dysfunction. A more involved intervention might involve giving specific suggestions for dealing with the dysfunction. Intensive therapy to relieve the dysfunction is the most complex intervention. The model offers clients and therapists a multilevel approach for helping the client deal with anxiety and learn new information and skills.

Social–interpersonal therapy includes approaches that are client centered, focused on the present, and view the client's interactions as part of a system. These therapies include, among others, group work, family-of-origin work, and cognitive insight work. Females participating in a group for preorgasmic women may be invited to look at their past learning experiences, their interactions with a partner for those who have one, and their knowledge and skills as part of their therapy. Males and females experiencing lack of desire because of sexual abuse or incest may be invited to inform their families of their abuse and even to confront their abuser in person or by letter.

PSYCHOSEXUAL DISORDERS AND TREATMENT

The term *psychosexual* is used to describe those disorders that seem to be chiefly psychological in origin. Even when there are clear organic factors behind a sexual disorder, there are often psychological issues as a secondary component of the dysfunction.

The DSM-III-R divides sexual disorders into two major categories: paraphilias and sexual dysfunctions. Any sexual disorder that cannot be classified in the two major categories is placed in a third category called sexual disorder not otherwise specified.[1]

Transsexuality describes the condition in which the client believes that the biologic body does not match the inner sense of sexual identity. Formerly classified along with sexual disorders, transsexuality is now classified as a personality disorder. This does not preclude a transsexual client from experiencing disorders that could be classified as sexual disorders.

Paraphilias

Paraphilias are defined in DSM-III-R as intense and recurrent sexual urges and sexual fantasies directed at nonhuman objects, real (not simulated) suffering, or humiliation of self or partner, or children, or other nonconsenting persons (Table 38–1).[1] For a sexual disorder to meet these criteria the client must have had these urges and fantasized about them for at least six months and be markedly distressed by them or have acted on them. For some persons, the paraphilic behavior may be a necessity for sexual arousal. For others, it may only occur during episodes of stress or not be necessary for sexual arousal. Some persons may not view their paraphilic behavior as problematic. The behaviors take on legal and social implications when the rights of others are violated and when there are children or nonconsenting partners involved.

As described by Money, paraphilic behavior has its genesis in the distortion of what would otherwise have been a normal psychosexual development.[13] In this view, psychosexual development has two components: the influence of sex hormones on fetal brain development and the influence of the social environment on sociosexual learning. Similar to a predisposition for language learning, newborn brains are predisposed to the development of sexual and erotic behaviors. In the process of normative childhood growth and social development, these sexual and erotic behaviors can develop in ways that, after puberty, are normative, satisfying, and reciprocal. Money uses the term *lovemap* to describe these "sexuoerotic" patterns of thought and behavior.[13]

Money views paraphilic behavior as the result of disruptions in the developing lovemap during the childhood years. This may be due to "neglect, suppression, or traumatization" of normal sexuoerotic development.[13] At some point, in some way, normative sexuoerotic growth and development is interfered with.

TABLE 38–1
Summary of DSM-III-R categories of paraphilias[1]

CATEGORY	CHARACTERISTICS
Exhibitionism	Exposure of one's genitals to strangers
Fetishism	Use of nonliving objects
Frotteurism	Touching and rubbing against a nonconsenting person
Pedophilia	Sexual activity with a prepubescent child
Sexual masochism	Acts (real, not simulated) of being humiliated, beaten, bound, or otherwise made to suffer
Sexual sadism	Acts (real, not simulated) that cause the psychological or physical suffering of the partner
Transvestic fetishism	Heterosexual male cross-dressing for sexual arousal
Voyeurism	Acts of observing unsuspecting people, usually strangers, who are naked, undressing, or engaged in sexual activity
Paraphilia, not otherwise specified	Examples: animals, feces, urine, enemas, telephone lewdness, corpses

The child adopts a distorted lovemap to compensate for the disruption. Sexual fantasies and sexual behavior seek out a new path. Objects, such as certain articles of clothing, or body parts, or fantasies of humiliation and degradation, or children or partners who are nonconsenting become the focus of sexual arousal. The paraphilic behavior allows sexual arousal and response to take place, but only in the distorted arousal pattern.[13]

Sexuoerotic lovemaps, as explained by Money, are resistant to change. They have developed over a lifetime. Therapy may involve assisting the client to relieve anxiety about the paraphilia and integrate it more positively into the client's life. When the paraphilic behavior is harmful to the client, to others, and against the law, then the therapy issues emphasize control and change. The treatment of male sex offenders who victimize children (pedophiles) offers a paradigm for this kind of therapy. Motivation for change may come from the client, but more likely it comes from the client's involvement with the legal system. Money advocates administering synthetic progestins (medroxyprogesterone; [Depo-Provera]) to reduce levels of the male sex hormone testosterone. This results in a reduction of sexual urges, allowing the client to focus more fully on the therapy.[13] The goal of therapy is to first reduce the urgent nature of the behavior, then to work toward controlling the behavior itself. Therapy includes examining the underlying beliefs behind the behavior, learning appropriate coping skills for expressing sexual urges, and creating an environment that is supportive of change.

Sexual Dysfunction

The DSM-III-R classification of *sexual dysfunctions* describes dysfunctions in any of the phases of the sexual response cycle: desire phase, arousal phase, orgasm phase, and resolution phase. A dysfunction of sexual appetite affects the desire to be sexual. A dysfunction of sexual excitement affects the sense of sexual pleasure and the physical changes in the body during arousal, such as vaginal lubrication and erection of the penis. A dysfunction of orgasm affects the ability to achieve orgasm. A dysfunction of resolution affects the ability to experience release and a sense of well-being after sexual behavior (Table 38-2).[1]

A woman's desire to have sex may be diminished because of a wide variety of factors. Assessment should include questions about the use of birth control pills, use of alcohol and drugs, any history of sexual abuse or pain associated with sex, discomfort being sexual with her partner, and fear, anxiety, or depression associated with being sexual. The goal of therapy is to increase sexual desire. Each woman is different and intervention needs to be individually designed for the unique characteristics of her presenting concerns. If the woman has a partner, then couples therapy is usually recommended, so that they may begin to communicate about what is pleasing and not pleasing to them sexually. Both partners need to learn about what experi-

TABLE 38-2
Summary of DSM-III-R categories of sexual dysfunctions[1]

CATEGORY	CHARACTERISTICS
Sexual desire disorders	Deficient or absent sexual fantasies and desire for sexual activity; extreme aversion to or avoidance of genital sexual contact with a partner
Sexual arousal disorders	Females: failure to attain vaginal vasocongestion and lubrication; lack of subjective sense of sexual excitement
	Males: failure to attain or maintain erection to completion of sexual activity; lack of subjective sense of sexual excitement
Orgasm disorders	Females: persistent or recurrent delay in or absence of orgasm
	Males: persistent or recurrent delay in or absence of orgasm, or premature ejaculation
Sexual pain disorders	Dyspareunia in females and males: pain before, during, or after intercourse
	Vaginismus: involuntary spasm of musculature of outer third of vagina that interferes with penetration
Other sexual disorders	Marked feelings of inadequacy about body, genitals, or other characteristics related to self-imposed sexual standards; distress about patterns of nonparaphilic sexual addiction behaviors; persistent and marked distress about one's sexual orientation

ences and stimuli trigger their sexual desire. Learning how to ask for what one wants sexually, learning how to deal with anger and resentments, and learning how to accept and refuse sexual advances are major communication skills that need to be taught or reviewed.

Female sexual arousal involves vaginal lubrication and the engorging of the labia and entrance to the vagina with blood. It also involves the subjective sense of being erotically aroused. It is possible for the genitals to respond with vasocongestion and lubrication, but the client does not experience it as erotically arousing. Thus, both elements must be present for it to be defined as arousal. The amount of vaginal lubrication varies from woman to woman. It may also vary within the arousal pattern of an individual woman. Medications, disease processes, and aging can affect lubrication. Sexual trauma, either in childhood or as an adult, can affect the subjective sense of arousal.

Orgasmic dysfunction in women is divided into two categories: primary orgasmic dysfunction and secondary orgasmic dysfunction. The woman with primary orgasmic dysfunction has never experienced an orgasm, whereas the woman with secondary orgasmic dysfunction has been orgasmic in the past, but for some reason is currently unable to be orgasmic. The most common reasons for orgasmic dysfunction are lack of information about sexual functioning; inadequate sexual stimulation, that is, not sufficient for orgasm; and lack of communication skills for telling a partner what types of sexual stimulation are essential for an orgasm. It is important to assess the level of knowledge about sexual functioning, as nonorgasmic women often do not know what type of stimulation they need. Other factors to consider are the woman's own feelings about herself as a sexual person, her feelings about control, independence, and the expectations she has for herself as a sexual person. Intervention for nonorgasmic women usually centers around education and communication. Although individual therapy may be used, a preorgasmic women's group is the treatment of choice if it is available. The group process provides education, peer support, and peer permission to be sexual. Specific homework assignments provide information and experience with relaxation, masturbation, and sexual fantasies. Women are also encouraged to read books such as *For Yourself* by Lonnie Barbach.[3] As the woman learns to be orgasmic through masturbation, communication skills necessary to relate this new-found self-awareness to her partner are added to the therapy. The success rate for women learning how to be orgasmic through group therapy is quite high. Barbach reports a 90% success rate after ten group sessions.[3]

Sexual pain disorders are most likely to have a physiologic rather than psychological cause. A complete pelvic examination is essential to the assessment of dyspareunia or painful penetration. One of the major causes of dyspareunia is lack of adequate vaginal lubrication for comfortable penetration to occur. Physiologic factors that can decrease vaginal lubrication are drugs, such as antihistamines, certain tranquilizers, marijuana, and alcohol. All have a drying effect on the vaginal mucosa. Estrogen deficiencies, vaginal infection, pelvic disease, and pelvic changes caused by surgery, endometriosis, urethritis, and cervicitis, are just a few of the other possible physical reasons for dyspareunia. Psychological problems that sometimes are associated with dyspareunia may stem from intense fear or anxiety. The woman may also be experiencing shame or guilt as a result of not being able to tolerate being sexual with her partner. Medical interventions and behavior modification have a high success rate in treating dyspareunia.[15]

Vaginismus is a relatively rare sexual dysfunction. A woman with vaginismus experiences an involuntary constriction of the outer one-third of her vagina that makes penetration very painful, if not impossible.[15] It is important to assess the severity of this dysfunction because in some women the vagina closes so tightly that neither a finger nor tampon can be inserted. For some women, insertion of a finger is possible, but anything larger causes severe pain. It is not unusual for these women to have had a history of sexual abuse; painful pelvic examinations; severe anxiety or guilt about being sexual; fear of men; or rigid, restrictive sexual attitudes learned as a child. It is important to rule out any physical factors that may be contributing to vaginismus. An educational pelvic examination with a knowledgeable and sensitive practitioner is vital. The nurse and the client go through the pelvic examination step by step. The goal is to give the patient the opportunity to learn about her genital anatomy, to gain comfort in examining herself, and to establish a baseline of what are normal-looking anatomic structures for her. Individual therapy or couples therapy have proven successful with vaginismus. The focus of the therapy centers around teaching the woman a series of exercises that help her to take control of her vaginal musculature. She is taught how to relax her whole body, especially her vaginal opening. Sometimes the woman is given a set of dilators of increasing size for use in the privacy of her home. She is given specific instructions on how to relax her vaginal musculature and insert the dilators. She increases the size of the dilators at a pace that is most comfortable for her. When she feels ready, she invites her partner to join her in the exercises. In the next step, she learns to become comfortable with her partner's finger and, then, if she is heterosexual, her partner's penis in her vagina.[15] In addition to working with her body, the woman is encouraged to share her sexual feelings, resentments, expectations, and fears. Improvement in communication is essential to the overall goal of being able to have penetration without vaginal constriction.

Men, like women, can suffer from lack of sexual desire or loss of interest in being sexual. Such feelings are inconsistent with the cultural expectations that males are always interested in and ready for sex. Lack of desire presents an interesting and sometimes painful contradiction to the traditional male sex role.[10] It is thought that chronic conflict in a relationship often results in lack of sexual desire.[8] Relationship issues that should be assessed include levels of anger and hostility, hidden agendas, poor communication, and level of trust. Depression and drug or alcohol abuse may also be contributing factors in lack of sexual desire. Assessment of mood, anorexia, and sleep disturbance helps differentiate depression and low levels of sexual desire. The depressed client will usually not respond to or even be interested in therapy aimed at sexuality.[8] Alcohol and drug use must be thoroughly assessed because their prolonged abuse can have a detrimental effect on sexual desire. A medication history during therapy is important, because antihypertensive, antidepressant, and some antipsychotic medications can cause differences in levels of desire (Table 38–3). Therapy should include a partner, if there is one. Relationship dynamics are clarified and homework exercises are designed to reduce the levels of tension and anxiety around sex. Self-esteem may be very fragile from the conflict with role expectations. The therapy may include nonsexual, but sensual awareness exercises such as explorations of feelings and responses to other bodily sensations.

Sexual arousal disorders or erectile dysfunctions are divided into two categories: primary and secondary erectile dysfunction. *Primary erectile dysfunction* is fairly rare. It is defined as never having been able to achieve and maintain an erection sufficient for penetration to take place. Men with this dysfunction may be able to achieve or maintain an erection during masturbation, but are never successful with a partner. The

TABLE 38–3
Selected examples of drugs that may effect sexual functioning

MEDICATION (trade name example)	EFFECTS
ANTIANXIETY AND HYPNOTICS	
Benzodiazepines	
Alprazolam (Xanax)	Increased and decreased libido;* impaired ejaculation; galactorrhea;
Chlordiazepoxide (Librium)	amenorrhea; gynecomastia
Diazepam (Valium)	
Lorazepam (Ativan)	
Oxazepam (Serax)	
Temazepam (Restoril)	
Triazolam (Halcion)	
Other	
Chloral hydrate	Changes in libido
ANTIDEPRESSANTS	
Tricyclic, Tetracyclic Compounds	
Amitriptyline (Amitril, Endep, Elavil)	Impaired erection, ejaculation; delayed orgasm; changes in libido
Amoxapine (Asendin)	
Desipramine (Norpramin, Pertofrane)	
Doxepin (Adapin)	
Imipramine (Tofranil)	
Maprotiline (Ludiomil)	
Nortriptyline (Aventyl, Pamelor)	
Protriptyline (Vivactil)	
Other Antidepressant	
Trazodone (Desyrel)	Priapism; retrograde ejaculation; in addition to tricyclic, tetracyclic effects
Monoamine Oxidase Inhibitors	
Isocarboxazid (Marplan)	Impaired erection, ejaculation; difficult orgasm
Phenelzine (Nardil)	
Tranylcypromine sulfate (Parnate)	
ANTIMANICS	
Lithium Carbonate (Eskalith, Lithonate)	Periodic impaired erections; decreased libido
ANTICONVULSANTS	
Carbamazepine (Tegrctol)	Impaired erection, ejaculation; delayed orgasm; changes in libido
Valproic acid (Depakene)	Amenorrhea; galactorrhea
ANTICHOLINERGICS	
Antiparkinsonian	
Benztropine (Cogentin)	Impaired erection
Biperiden (Akineton)	
Procyclidine (Kemadrin)	
Trihexyphenidyl (Artane, Tremin)	
Gastrointestinal Anticholinergics/ Antispasmodics	
Methantheline (Banthine)	Impaired erection
ANTIPSYCHOTICS	
Chlorpromazine (Thorazine)	Galactorrhea, gynecomastia; amenorrhea; increased & decreased
Fluphenazine (Prolixin, Permitil)	libido; impaired erection, ejaculation, priapism; orgasm inhibition
Haloperidol (Haldol)	
Perphenazine (Trilafon)	
Thioridazine (Mellaril)	
Thiothixene (Navane)	
Trifluoperazine (Stelazine)	
ANTIHYPERTENSIVES	
Antiadrenergic— Centrally acting	
Clonidine (Catapres)	Decreased libido; impaired erection, ejaculation; gynecomastia;
Methyldopa (Aldomet)	galactorrhea (Methyldopa; reserpine); amenorrhea (Methyldopa)
Reserpine (Serpasil)	
Antiadrenergic—Peripherally acting	
Guanethidine (Ismelin)	Decreased libido; impaired erection, ejaculation

Continued

TABLE 38-3
Selected examples of drugs that may effect sexual functioning *Continued*

MEDICATION (trade name example)	EFFECTS
ANTIHYPERTENSIVES *Continued*	
Beta-blockers	
Propranolol (Inderal)	Impaired erection; decreased libido
	Impaired erection; decreased emission; retrograde ejaculation; decreased libido
DIURETICS	
Chlorthalidone (Hygroton)	Impaired erection; decreased libido
Hydrochlorothiazide (Hydrodiuril)	Impaired erection; decreased libido
Spironolactone (Aldactone)	Impaired erection; decreased libido; decreased vaginal lubrication; amenorrhea; gynecomastia
HORMONE PREPARATIONS	
Clomiphene citrate (Clomid)	Increased libido
Cyproterone acetate	Loss of libido; impaired erection; ejaculatory delay
NARCOTIC ANALGESICS	
Methadone, morphine, heroin, codeine	Decreased libido, impaired erection, ejaculation; menstrual irregularities
ETHYL ALCOHOL	Acute: increased and decreased libido*; impaired erection; Chronic: (men) decreased libido; impaired erection; gynecomastia; feminization; testicular atrophy; sterility; Chronic: (women) difficulty having orgasm; decreased vaginal lubrication; oligomenorrhea
STIMULANTS	
Amphetamines	Impaired erection, ejaculation
Cocaine	Enhanced sexual desire and orgasm (more research needed); impaired erection, ejaculation
OTHER ILLEGAL DRUGS	
LSD	Alters perception of sexual experience (more research needed)
Marijuana	Acute: increased libido;* Chronic: impaired erection; gynecomastia
MISCELLANEOUS	
Amyl nitrite	Increased orgasmic intensity
Cimetidine (Tagamet)	Impaired erection; decreased libido
Clofibrate (Atromid-S)	Impaired erection; decreased libido

* Increased libido may occur with low doses due to a disinhibiting effect, while increased dose or prolonged use may decrease libido

second category is secondary erectile dysfunction. A man with this diagnosis has experienced penetration for sexual pleasure at some points in his life, but currently, he is not able to do so in most of his sexual encounters. Most men experience this dysfunction as frustrating, humiliating, or devastating. Depression thus often accompanies this dysfunction. On the other hand, depression can sometimes cause erectile dysfunction. A detailed sexual assessment is helpful to determine if the etiology is physiologic or psychological. A complete physical examination to identify or rule out physiologic conditions that might be contributing to sexual dysfunction is essential. Physiologic factors that can cause erectile dysfunction include neurologic disorders, such as spinal cord injury or multiple sclerosis; vascular insufficiency problems; hormonal deficiencies; and genital infections or injuries.[14] Diabetes and alcoholism are the two most common physiologic causes of erectile dysfunction. Some prescription medications such as thioridazine (Mellaril) and "street"

drugs can cause erectile problems. The distinction between physiologic and psychological causes is not always clear.

Psychological factors that may cause erectile dysfunction are fear of failure, performance anxiety, fear of rejection, poor communication skills, anger, power struggles, and unresolved conflict within a relationship. Anticipatory anxiety related to sexual performance can start a self-defeating cycle of fear that escalates from a single failure into a state of serious chronic dysfunction. This "spectatorship" may result in a lack of ability to perform sexually and, thereby, reconfirms a man's anxieties and fear of failure. Fear of rejection by the partner or excessive need to please may also generate anxiety. Poor communication can become a self-defeating cycle in which partners perpetuate ignorance, lack of understanding, and misinformation about their sexual and emotional needs. Men's sex role stereotype has historically been to know all about how to be sexual. The male who has not had the benefits of learning the value of sharing his thoughts and feelings openly and honestly with his partner may find himself withdrawn, angry, and with no erection.

Although the assessment for diagnosis of erectile failure has greatly advanced in the last years, such has not been true for the psychological intervention strategies.[10] Treatment for the physiologic causes of erection problems has centered around penile prothesis implants that cause an artificial erection in the penis. Penile protheses have been inserted in men who, due to permanent physiologic impairment, would otherwise never be able to have erections.[4] Hormone therapy, such as injections of testosterone, has raised questions about the long-term effect of such a treatment. Pharmacologic treatment of certain erectile dysfunctions involves the self-injection of papaverine, a smooth-muscle relaxant, and phentolamine into the corpora cavernosa, which can result in a hard, firm erection that can last two to three hours.[5]

One of the most common orgasm disorders for males, especially for young males, is premature ejaculation. It is defined as the absence of voluntary control over the ejaculatory reflex.[7] Ejaculatory control is assumed to be a learned process. There are several causative factors that trigger the quick response of the ejaculatory reflex. Ejaculatory control may be lacking because the man in his early masturbatory behavior learned to stimulate himself very quickly without understanding what the long-term ramifications would be. Performance anxiety may be a result in a sexual relationship for which the partner's goal is to prolong penetration. Assessment should include a physical examination to rule out any possible genitourinary tract disorders. A sex history will assess for unproductive patterns of sexual behavior that were learned at an early age and carried on to adulthood. Anxiety, guilt, and fear must also be assessed because many men begin to avoid sexual contact to avoid the fear of failure. Therapy for premature ejaculation has two parts. One part involves teaching the male to control or delay ejaculation by recognizing the signs of imminent ejaculation and changing the pattern of stimulation. The other part of therapy involves teaching the man how to reduce performance anxiety when being sexual. Successful methods found to be helpful in delaying ejaculation include using a stop–start method of stimulation, changing sexual positions, and changing the tempo of thrusting during penetration.

Inhibited ejaculation is the inability to ejaculate. A male may have an erection, but he cannot ejaculate, no matter what kind of stimulation is used. The exact etiology for inhibited ejaculation is unknown. It is thought that fear of impregnating a partner, fear of loss of control, or relationship problems are important factors to explore with these men. Organic factors must be ruled out because some neurologic disorders, diseases such as Parkinson, or antiadrenergic drugs may cause impaired ejaculatory response.

Painful intercourse for males can be the result of disease processes, respiratory or cardiac insufficiency, or problems with mobility.[6] Angina and shortness of breath may result from the exertion of sexual activity. Sexual mobility may be painful or restricted because of back pain or joint disease. Penile skin may be hypersensitive because of herpes or shingles. Diseases of the penile anatomy, such as Peyrone's disease, or trauma to the penis may be the source of pain. Internal disease processes such as orchitis, cancer, or prostatic infections may make penetration and ejaculation painful.

NURSING ROLES

Psychiatric mental health nurses can expect to play a role at every level of intervention in sex therapy. At one end of the helping spectrum, the nurse can create a workplace setting that signals to clients an openness to dealing with sexual concerns. At the other end of the helping spectrum is the nurse psychotherapist with graduate education practicing intensive sex therapy. In between are other roles such as sex educator, counselor, therapist, and resource person.

The initial contact with the client is affected by the degree of openness of the nurse to sexual concerns, the ability of the client to convey the concerns, and the atmosphere in which the initial contact occurs. The nurse should not expect the client to bring up sexual issues. Silence on the part of the client does not mean the client has no concern to present. Part of creating an environment open to sexual problems is giving clients an opportunity to talk about any sexual questions or concerns they may have. Nurses with little or no background in interventions for sexual concerns can do much to foster a climate in which the client and the nurse can seek out alternate resources.

Nurses as sex educators may work with the individual client regarding sex education or as an educator in the health care setting or in the community. Sex education emphasizes the clarification of sexual attitudes and beliefs, accurate and honest information about sexuality, and the skills necessary to communicate about sexuality. More and more nurses are serving as public sex educators because of the increased need for education about acquired immune deficiency syndrome (AIDS), sexually transmitted diseases, and contraception.

Nurses as counselors deal with focused, short-term intervention strategies. Not only information, but also specific suggestions, are part of counseling interventions. Intensive sex therapy requires nurses to have training and certification in sex therapy, and it is thus the most specialized of the nursing roles. Sex therapy is appropriate if a client's sexual concerns are not relieved by permission, education, or suggestions for new or different behaviors.

Still another role for the nurse is that of consultant and resource person. It should not be assumed that the health care field is always prepared to deal with clients' sexual concerns. Nurses with specialized training as sex educators, counselors, or therapists can be a valuable asset as consultants to health care professionals. The American Association of Sex Educators, Counselors, and Therapists (ASSECT) has set the training standards for sex education and therapy. It acts as the certifying body for such work. A thorough knowledge of the sexual health resources of the community are a vital part of the total health care network. Clients who have information about, and access to, a variety of sexual health resources are in a better position to participate in maintaining their own sexual health.

COMMON NURSING DIAGNOSES

Sexual dysfunction would be a common nursing diagnosis among clients involved in sex therapy. Other nursing diagnoses that may be identified include: anxiety, fear, guilt, knowledge deficit, rape trauma syndrome, disturbance in self-esteem, and disturbance in body image.

CASE STUDY

Jane, a 24-year-old woman, was seen in a community clinic for a routine physical examination. During the initial assessment, the nurse practitioner asked if she had any concerns about her sexual health. The client acted surprised by the question, saying this was the first time anyone had asked. She went on to say that she had been married for four years, had a very supportive and loving relationship with her husband, but had never had an orgasm. She began to cry and was able to state that this was a major source of tension in her marriage and she did not know what to do about it. She expressed shame, embarrassment, and the thought that something must be wrong with her. The client had never received sex education at home or in school, and the only persons she had confided in were her husband and her older sister. Her sister had talked with her about sex, masturbation, and orgasm, but the client had mixed feelings about touching herself "down there." She had attempted to masturbate on two occasions, but felt guilty doing it. The

nurse practitioner reassured Jane that her questions about sexual health were important and that she was glad that Jane had told her about her concerns.

The following nursing diagnoses were identified: self-esteem disturbance related to sexuality; and sexual dysfunction (primary orgasmic dysfunction) related to lack of knowledge. The nurse practitioner then offered to do an educational pelvic examination as part of the physical examination and said she would talk with her more about her options for treatment after the physical examination. The client was eager to learn all she could about her genital anatomy. The nurse reinforced the fact that she was a healthy woman with normal genitals. The client was pleased, saying she had never realized there was so much to know about herself and was eager to tell her husband. The nurse practitioner then talked with her about primary orgasmic dysfunction and told her about preorgasmic women's groups in terms of focus, content, and time, and gave her the name of a nurse sex therapist who led such groups. The client said she felt much better since someone had understood the importance of her sexual concerns and had given her permission to talk about her sexual feelings. She was relieved to know that she was not alone with this problem and felt reassured and supported in her quest to seek more individualized help for her concerns. At her six-month follow-up appointment, the client said she had been very successful in the preorgasmic therapy group, was now orgasmic, and that it had made a big difference in her marriage, and she now felt like a complete person (see Nursing Care Plan 38–1 for a sample care plan for Jane).

SUMMARY

Sexual health is part of total health. Psychosexual disorders can occur at many points in a client's physical, mental, social, and spiritual life. Sex therapy is multidimensional with medical and psychotherapeutic interventions not being mutually exclusive. The nurse's role in sex therapy includes creating an open environ-

Research Highlights

Sex therapy research is attempting to validate therapy modalities, the outcomes of which reflect successful treatment strategies. Studies of treatments for female sexual dysfunction have attempted to isolate factors most likely to lead to successful resolution of the dysfunctions.

Mathews compared the use of hormone therapy and anxiety reduction in treating lack of sexual interest in two different groups of women.[12] It was hoped that a better understanding of successful treatment strategies would lead to a better understanding of the causes of sexual problems. The study found that, although hormonal factors may be relatively important to sexual functioning, there was insufficient evidence to relate them to sexual dysfunction. Strategies aimed primarily at reducing anxiety were also found to be not generally effective at alleviating sexual dysfunction. The study con-

cludes that neither anxiety nor simple androgen deficiency adequately explain female sexual dysfunction nor lead the way to successful therapy techniques for dealing with the dysfunction.

Libman and her colleagues compared three therapeutic protocols for the treatment of secondary orgasmic dysfunction. The sample of 23 married women had experienced dissatisfaction from low frequency of orgasmic response. The women and their partners were assigned to one of three treatment groups: group therapy, standard couple therapy, or self-help bibliotherapy. The therapy content and the sequence of steps were the same for all three groups. Couples therapy was found to be the most effective. The study also demonstrated the need for assessment procedures and therapy goals that were multidimensional and clearly defined.[9]

NURSING CARE PLAN 38–1

JANE

NURSING INTERVENTIONS	OUTCOME CRITERIA
NURSING DIAGNOSIS: Self-esteem disturbance related to sexuality	
CLIENT GOAL: Communicate more easily about sexual concerns	
■ Explain to Jane that she is not alone with her concerns	Expresses increased sexual self-worth
■ Assure Jane that it is useful to ask questions about her sexual concerns	Is more willing to ask questions about sexuality
■ Explain that skills in communicating about sexuality are learned over time	
■ Assist Jane with ways to discuss her sexual concerns	Expresses confidence in ability to relate details of her sexual wants and needs
NURSING DIAGNOSIS: Sexual dysfunction (primary orgasmic dysfunction) related to lack of knowledge	
CLIENT GOAL: Increase knowledge about genital anatomy and sexual response	
■ Explain purpose of educational pelvic examination	Asks questions and makes comments indicating increased knowledge about genital anatomy and sexual response
■ Explain anatomy and answer questions fully	
■ Teach about genital anatomy and sexual response using charts	
■ Encourage Jane to share her new knowledge with her partner	Expresses interest in sharing new information with partner
CLIENT GOAL: Become orgasmic	
■ Accept Jane's feelings of sadness, anxiety, or depression	Expresses sense of being accepted
■ Assure Jane that it is a realistic goal to want to be orgasmic	
■ Discuss options for preorgasmic treatment	Expresses interest in seeking out treatment
■ Refer Jane to a preorgasmic women's group	

ment where sexual concerns can be discussed, giving permission and validating feelings, teaching information and skills, and doing counseling or therapy. This work may occur in a variety of settings. Psychosexual disorders are divided into two major categories: paraphilias are sexual disorders in which sexual arousal is dependent on nonliving objects, children, nonconsenting partners, or pain and humiliation; sexual dysfunctions are sexual experiences the client describes as unrewarding or inadequate. Common sexual dysfunctions include disorders of sexual desire, sexual arousal disorders, disorders of orgasm and ejaculation, and sexual pain. The assessment and diagnosis process is based on a theoretical knowledge of sexuality and sexual dysfunction, client sex and health history, and peer validation. The nursing process in sexual disorders must consider current sex research to make a positive difference in client sexual health.

References

1. American Psychiatric Association. Diagnostic and Statistical Manual of Mental Disorders, 3rd ed, revised. Washington, DC: American Psychiatric Association; 1987.
2. Annon J. The behavioral treatment of sexual problems, vol 1. Brief therapy. Honolulu: Enabling Systems; 1975.
3. Barbach LG. For yourself. New York: Doubleday & Co; 1975.
4. Beutler LE, Scott FB, Rogers RR et al. Inflatable and noninflatable penile prostheses: comparative follow-up evaluation. Urology. 1986;27:136–143.

5. Gasser TC, Roach RM, Larsen EH et al. Intracavernous self-injection with phentolamine and papaverine for the treatment of impotence. J Urol. 1987;137:678–680.

6. Kaplan HS. Disorders of sexual desire. New York: Simon & Schuster; 1979.

7. Kaplan HS. The new sex therapy. New York: Brunner/Mazel; 1974.

8. LaFerla JJ. Inhibited sexual desire and orgasmic dysfunction in women. Clin Obstet Gynecol. 1984;27:738–749.

9. Libman E, Fichten CS, Brender W. A comparison of three therapeutic formats in the treatment of secondary orgasmic dysfunction. J Sex Marital Ther. 1984;10:147–159.

10. LoPiccolo J. Diagnosis and treatment of male sexual dysfunction. J Sex Marital Ther. 1985;11:215–232.

11. Masters W, Johnson V, Kolodny R. Human sexuality. Boston: Little, Brown & Co; 1982.

12. Mathews A. Progress in the treatment of female sexual dysfunction. J Psychosom Res. 1983;27:165–173.

13. Money J. Lovemaps—clinical concepts of sexual/erotic health and pathology, paraphilia, and gender transposition in childhood, adolescence, and maturity. New York: Irvington Publishers; 1986.

14. Slag MF, Morley JE, Elson MK et al. Impotence in medical clinic outpatients. JAMA. 1983;249:1736–1740.

15. Steege JF. Dyspareunia and vaginismus. Clin Obstet Gynecol. 1984;27:750–759.

16. World Health Organization. Education and treatment in human sexuality: the training of health professionals, report of a WHO meeting. Geneva: WHO Technical Report Series, no. 572; 1975.

17. Zilbergeld B. Male sexuality. Boston: Little, Brown & Co; 1978.

39

Melodie A. Lohr

Psychopharmacology

OBJECTIVES

After reading this chapter, the reader will be able to:

1. *Describe different types of psychotropic medications, including neuroleptics, antiparkinsonian medications, lithium, tricyclic antidepressants, monoamine oxidase inhibitors, and antianxiety medications*
2. *Discuss the indications for these medications and their potential side effects*
3. *Describe the rationale for the use of more than one drug in many instances in psychiatric practice*
4. *Discuss nursing roles in psychopharmacology.*

DESCRIPTION

Psychopharmacology is the field of treatment of mental disorders with medications. As a general class, drugs used to treat psychiatric illnesses are called *psychotropic medications*. There are several major categories of psychotropic drugs, including neuroleptic (or antipsychotic) medications, antiparkinsonian medications, lithium, antidepressants, and antianxiety medications, along with a number of other drugs that have also been shown to be efficacious in certain psychiatric conditions.

NEUROLEPTIC MEDICATIONS

Neuroleptic medications (Table 39-1) are the primary medications used today to treat psychosis, and for this reason, they are sometimes referred to as antipsychotic medications. However, other medications besides neuroleptics are used to treat psychosis. There is currently no good evidence to indicate that any one neuroleptic medication is consistently better than any other in treating psychotic symptoms, although neuroleptics do differ considerably in terms of their side effects.

Neuroleptics are often divided into low-potency, medium-potency, and high-potency groups, depending on how much antipsychotic effect they have on a "per milligram" basis. Thus, neuroleptics that are usually effective when given in the range of 30 mg/day, or less, are called high-potency; those that are usually effective when more than 400 mg/day are given are termed low-potency, and those intermediate in dosage, medium-potency. The side effects of a given neuroleptic can often be tentatively predicted from its potency: the higher the potency, the greater the incidence of extrapyramidal side effects; the lower the potency, the greater the incidence of sedation, hypotension, and cardiovascular side effects.

Indications for Use

Neuroleptics are generally used for psychotic symptoms (e.g., hallucinations, delusions) that occur in schizophrenia, as well as in delusional disorder, mood disorders (with psychosis), and other psychotic states (including drug-induced, toxic, and metabolic). Although some investigators have questioned the effectiveness of neuroleptics for the so-called negative symptoms of schizophrenia, including apathy, anhedonia, and social withdrawal, there is some evidence that neuroleptics may favorably affect these symptoms as well.[47] Neuroleptics are also sometimes used in conditions in which there is marked confusion, agitation, or delirium, although caution should be used because as in anticholinergic delirium, neuroleptics may exacerbate the condition. Because of their ability to block transmission of the neurotransmitter dopamine,[47] neuroleptics have been used in a variety of hyperkinetic movement disorders, such as Tourette's syndrome (a disorder of multiple tics) and Huntington disease (a disorder marked by progressive dementia and choreoathetoid movements). Neuroleptics have been used for behavioral problems associated with autism, mental retardation, and organic behavioral problems (e.g., secondary to brain trauma). In combination with tricyclic antidepressants, neuroleptic medications have been reported to be effective in some clients with psychotic depression. Short-term treatment with neuroleptics has been reported to be of benefit in clients with nausea and vomiting, intractable hiccups, and pruritus. Finally, neuroleptics have been prescribed for other conditions such as stuttering, anxiety, and insomnia, but it is currently recommended that clients with these conditions *not* be treated with neuroleptics because of the possible development of irreversible tardive dyskinesia, which will be discussed later.

Guidelines for Administration

Currently, it is recommended that neuroleptics be used in the lowest dose possible, to minimize the risks of extrapyramidal side effects, including tardive dyskinesia. Although the dose of neuroleptic must be individualized, in general, a dosage of 400 to 800 mg/day of chlorpromazine, or its approximate equivalent (e.g., 8 to 15 mg/day of haloperidol), is adequate for many clients. Some clients require much less than this, especially clients with personality disorders, the elderly, and children. Many schizophrenic clients also require very little maintenance antipsychotic to prevent relapse. Some clients, however, require very high doses —up to 80 mg/day of haloperidol or more—but that is rare. For most neuroleptics, once-a-day dosage is possible, and the sedative effects of the neuroleptics can be used to facilitate sleep in insomnic clients. Sometimes, the doses are divided to reduce the occurrence of extrapyramidal side effects or to spread the calming effect of the medication more evenly across a 24-hour period.

TABLE 39-1
Neuroleptic medications

GENERIC NAME	TRADE NAME	DOSE EQUIVALENT (MG)	DOSE RANGE (MG)	SIDE EFFECTS		
				Sedative	EPS	Hypotensive
PHENOTHIAZINES						
Aliphatics						
Chlorpromazine	Thorazine	100	25–1200	+++	++	++
Trifluopromazine	Vesprin	25–30	50–150	++	+++	++
Piperidines						
Thioridazine	Mellaril	90–100	50–800	+++	+	++
Mesoridazine	Serentil	50	25–500	+++	+	++
Piperazines						
Trifluoperazine	Stelazine	5	2–100	+	+++	+
Perphenazine	Trilafon	10	4–64	++	++	+
Fluphenazine*	Prolixin, Permitil	2	1–100	+	+++	+
Acetophenazine	Tindal	15–20	20–120	++	++	+
THIOXANTHENES						
Aliphatic						
Chlorprothixene	Taractan	70–100	25–600	+++	++	++
Piperazine						
Thiothixene	Navane	3–5	5–100	+	+++	+
BUTYROPHENONES						
Haloperidol*	Haldol	2–3	2–100	+	+++	+
DIHYDROINDOLONES						
Molindone	Moban	8–10	15–225	++	+	+/−
DIBENZOXAPINES						
Loxapine	Loxitane	10–15	20–325	++	++	+
DIBENZODIAZEPINES						
Clozapine†	Leponex	50	50–900	+++	+/−	++
DIPHENYLBUTYLPIPERIDINES						
Pimozide	Orap	1–2	0.5–20	+	+++	+/−
RAUWOLFIA ALKALOIDS						
Reserpine‡	Serpasil	3–10	0.1–5	+++	++	+++

* Available in long-acting depot form for intramuscular injection (as decanoate).
† Clozapine became available in 1990, especially for treatment-resistant clients.[36]
‡ Reserpine causes a depression-like syndrome, limiting its utility as an antipsychotic, although it is used for clients for whom side-effects or allergic reactions limit the use of other neuroleptics.
+/− = questionable, + = mild, ++ = moderate, +++ = severe, gen = generic preparation available.

Neuroleptic medications can be given in a number of different forms. Although all neuroleptics are available in oral preparations, for some there are also intramuscular and intravenous preparations. For intramuscular use, there are both short-acting and long-acting (depot) preparations available for fluphenazine and haloperidol. Some neuroleptics, such as chlorpromazine, may be very irritating when given intramuscularly. Therefore, it is important to vary the site of injection with these drugs. However, the gluteal region is the preferred site of injection, and other sites (triceps, vastus lateralis) should be used only if the amount of injected fluid is small, or if the client has a lot of muscular tissue in those sites. Intravenous neuroleptics (mainly haloperidol) are very rarely given, and are usually restricted to those clients in whom there is agitated psychosis that requires very prompt attention and the intravenous route is readily available, such as acute psychosis occurring in intensive care unit settings.

As mentioned previously, fluphenazine and haloperidol are available in long-acting depot forms that are administered intramuscularly. The most popular of these are fluphenazine decanoate and haloperidol decanoate. Fluphenazine decanoate can usually be given every two to three weeks (occasionally every four weeks), and haloperidol decanoate can usually be given every three to four weeks (rarely, up to every six weeks). A typical dose of fluphenazine decanoate is 25 mg every two weeks, and of haloperidol decanoate, 100 mg every month. There is some evidence that, with the long-acting intramuscular forms, client compliance may increase,[35,45] although it is not clear if the use of long-acting preparations has any effect on relapse rates.[56] Nevertheless, with clients who have difficulty

BOX 39–1
Extrapyramidal Side-Effects (EPS) of Neuroleptic Medications

ACUTE DYSTONIC REACTIONS
Dystonic reactions are long-lasting contractions or spasms of muscles, usually involving the eyes, jaw, tongue, or neck, but may involve any other part of the body. Common dystonic reactions include those of eye muscles, in which the eyes are pulled up or to the side (oculogyric crises), forced eye closure (blepharospasm), forced jaw closure (trismus), pulling the head to the side (torticollis). Dystonic reactions usually appear within 12–36 hr after a client is started on neuroleptic therapy or has the dose increased and are probably the least common of all EPS (occurring in probably 10% or fewer of clients treated with neuroleptics,[41] mainly in young males). Treatment consists of the administration of an anticholinergic or antihistaminergic agent, usually 1–2 mg of oral benztropine or the equivalent dose of some similar anticholinergic agent, repeated after 30 min if response is incomplete. Parenteral routes of administration may be used so that the client will obtain more rapid relief.

NEUROLEPTIC-INDUCED PARKINSONISM (NIP)
NIP shares the major signs of Parkinson disease—hypokinesia, rigidity, tremor, and postural instability. Client with NIP may have any combination of these signs. *Hypokinesia* is a loss of movement, and may present as slowing of movement or difficulty initiating movement, as well as decreased or absent arm-swing when walking, and a decrease in facial expressiveness. *Rigidity* is increased resting tension of muscles, sometimes called "lead-pipe" or "plastic," and there is often an overlying ratcheting upon passive flexion at a joint, called cogwheeling. *Tremor* is typically an alternating or "pill-rolling" resting tremor, usually involving the hands and wrists, but may spread to involve the other areas. Loss of postural reflexes may contribute to falls and injuries in the elderly.

The reported incidence of NIP has varied from 5% to 90%, although it is probably in the range of 15% or so of clients.[41] Although larger doses of neuroleptics generally cause more parkinsonism than smaller doses, this is highly individualized. Women may be more commonly affected than men. NIP often improves spontaneously within 3–6 months although it may last much longer.

Treatment consists of discontinuation or reduction of neuroleptic dose, if possible. Following this, antiparkinsonian drugs are indicated, but again should be used for the shortest possible time.

AKATHISIA
Akathisia is a state of motor restlessness, usually manifested as excessive movement in the lower extremities. A number of behaviors occur, such as fidgeting, frequent changes in posture, and crossing and uncrossing legs. Clients usually complain of vague feelings of discomfort ("anxiety," "nerves," "itchiness,"). When severe, clients may be unable to sit or lie quietly, and must get up, pace, or perform other activities. It may be the most common form of EPS, occurring in as many as half of clients treated.[41] High-potency neuroleptics appear to more commonly cause akathisia than low-potency.

Akathisia is often very difficult to treat. The best approach is to minimize the neuroleptic dosage. After this, anticholinergic medications, benzodiazepines (such as lorazepam, or clonazepam), or propranolol are often used.

NEUROLEPTIC-INDUCED CATATONIA (NIC)
NIC is frequently difficult to distinguish from catatonia emerging as part of the underlying psychiatric condition. The typical signs are cataplexy (waxy flexibility), automatic obedience, stereotypies, mannerisms or grimacing, bizarre behavior, posturing,

(Continued)

taking oral medications regularly, for example, because of memory impairment or paranoia, a trial of depot neuroleptics should be considered.

Extrapyramidal Side Effects

Neurologic side effects of neuroleptics are among the most common ones seen with these medications. In fact, it is partly because of the high frequency of such side effects that the drugs are termed *neuroleptics*. Approximately one-third to one-half of clients will develop distressing neuroleptic side effects, and these are especially common in the elderly.

The neurologic side effects of neuroleptics are often subsumed under the term extrapyramidal side effects or extrapyramidal signs (EPS).[43] This is because many of the neurologic side effects of neuroleptics resemble conditions seen in diseases in which there is known damage to extrapyramidal structures, such as Parkin-

son's and Huntington's diseases. However, it is not clear if all the neurologic side effects described truly relate to the extrapyramidal system. Nevertheless, the term *EPS* is commonly used to describe neurologic side effects of neuroleptics, and this definition is adhered to here.

Neuroleptic-induced EPS may be divided into two forms, depending upon their time of onset. Acute EPS occur within several months of either initiation or increase in neuroleptic medications, and late-onset or *tardive* EPS occur after at least three months of neuroleptic treatment. Acute EPS consist of dystonic reactions, neuroleptic-induced parkinsonism (NIP), akathisia, neuroleptic-induced catatonia (NIC), and neuroleptic malignant syndrome (NMS). The most common tardive EPS is tardive dyskinesia (TD),[33] although other tardive syndromes including tardive dystonia, tardive akathisia, tardive Tourette's (or tardive tic) disorder, and others have also been described. These different forms of EPS are described in Box 39-1.

BOX 39–1
Extrapyramidal Side-Effects (EPS) of Neuroleptic Medications (*continued*)

NEUROLEPTIC-INDUCED CATATONIA (NIC) (continued)
echo phenomena, catatonic rigidity, and mutism and staring. NIC has been reported mainly in schizophrenic clients, but has also been reported in other conditions as well. It may be more common with high-potency neuroleptics.
Because NIC is poorly understood, treatment is difficult. Reduction or discontinuation of the neuroleptic is usually the first step. Although antiparkinsonian medications may be of benefit, there is evidence that amantadine in daily doses of 200–300 mg p.o. may be more rapidly effective than anticholinergic drugs.[41] Benzodiazepines, especially lorazepam, may also help in certain cases.

NEUROLEPTIC MALIGNANT SYNDROME (NMS)
NMS is a condition that occurs days or weeks after the institution of neuroleptics, or after changing the dosage.[41] It occurs in less than 1% of clients treated with neuroleptics, and consists of severe rigidity, often accompanied by dystonia and coarse tremor, fever, tachycardia, diaphoresis, tachypnea, hypertension or hypotension, and urinary incontinence. The clients are frequently confused or mute, and may become stuporous or comatose, rendering mental status testing difficult. A leukocytosis (12,000–30,000 cells/mm³) and elevation of creatine phosphokinase (up to 340,000 U/mL) is also usually found. Complications include renal failure from severe dehydration, myoglobinuria secondary to rhabdomyolysis, respiratory failure, pneumonia, and pulmonary embolism. The untreated syndrome often lasts from 1 to 3 wk, and requires intensive care. The mortality for untreated NMS may be as high as 25%. Although NMS occurs most commoly in schizophrenia (50% of cases), it can occur in almost anyone treated with neuroleptics.
Treatment consists of immediate neuroleptic discontinuation. After this, treatment is largely supportive, involving maintenance of renal, cardiac, and pulmonary function, and suppression of infection.

Other drugs, such as dantrolene and bromocriptine have been reported to be effective in some cases.

TARDIVE DYSKINESIA (TD)
TD consists mainly of choreic (jerky irregular) and athetoid (smooth, sinuous, and somewhat irregular) movements affecting primarily the lower face (tongue, jaw, lips) and the extremities, but other areas can be affected as well. By definition, the movements occur after at least 3 mo of neuroleptic treatment. The prevalence of TD is believed to be around 20%–25%.[33] If neuroleptics are discontinued, the course of the syndrome can vary from fully reversible to persistent. About one-third of cases of TD are reversible, with disappearance of the movements within months of drug-withdrawal.[33] After discontinuation, some clients suffer an initial temporary exacerbation of the movements; other clients show immediate improvement. The administration of anticholinergic medication may uncover latent TD, or exacerbate existing TD, but it is not yet clear whether or not anticholinergic administration represents a risk factor for the development of TD.
Risk factors for TD include old age, female gender, and having a mood disorder. Other risk factors may include high cumulative neuroleptic dose, mental retardation, brain damage, length of neuroleptic exposure, anticholinergic drugs, acute EPS, depot neuroleptics, drug interruptions or holidays, elevated serum neuroleptic concentration, late-onset psychosis, and smoking.
Treatment consists of tapering and discontinuing all antiparkinsonian medications, and reducing the dose of neuroleptic medication as much as possible. Although no drugs have been reported to be generally successful in the treatment of TD, some drugs that may be helpful in certain cases include propranolol, clonidine, and benzodiazepines, including diazepam and lorazepam.

Other Side Effects

SEDATION

Sedation is a particularly common side effect, especially when low-potency neuroleptics are used. When clients are given neuroleptics for acute agitated psychoses, often the sedative effects are not obvious until later when the psychosis begins to abate. As with many of the side effects of neuroleptics, the client usually accommodates to the sedation within several weeks. Clients should be reassured during this time. Occasionally it helps if most of the neuroleptic dosage is given at night.

ORTHOSTATIC HYPOTENSION

Orthostatic hypotension, which is due to the α-adrenergic blocking effects of neuroleptics, is also more common with low-potency than with high-potency neuro-

leptics, although it can occur with high-potency drugs, especially in the elderly. Clients often describe light-headedness, dizziness, or weakness, accompanied by tachycardia or palpitations, especially when arising rapidly from a reclining position. When mild, clients usually accommodate within several weeks.

GALACTORRHEA

Galactorrhea (excessive milk production) and other disturbances in hypothalamic–pituitary functioning occasionally occur following neuroleptic treatment.[9] Galactorrhea is believed to be caused by the dopamine blocking effects of neuroleptics, resulting in increased release of prolactin. When mild, it can usually be controlled by wearing small breast pads in the bra. When this is not practical, switching to another neuroleptic may be helpful. Other hypothalamic disturbances may also occur, including amenorrhea, gynecomastia in men, and increased appetite. Again, when such symptoms are mild, reassurance is usually sufficient, but more severe symptoms may warrant dosage reduction or neuroleptic change.

HYPOSEXUALITY

Hyposexuality is a fairly common side effect of neuroleptics and is one that many clients have difficulty talking about. Therefore, any client who is receiving long-term neuroleptic therapy should be asked about sexual functioning. A variety of sexual disturbances are seen, including impairments in arousal and performance. Thioridazine has been reported to be a common cause of sexual dysfunction, including, in particular, ejaculatory impairment such as retrograde ejaculation.

SEIZURES

Although many neuroleptic medications, especially chlorpromazine, reduce the seizure threshold, most neuroleptics cause seizures only rarely in individuals without epilepsy or organic brain conditions.[49] In clients with epilepsy, however, there may be an increase in seizure frequency.

ANTICHOLINERGIC SIDE EFFECTS

Anticholinergic side effects, which are discussed in detail in the next section on antiparkinsonian medications, are also more common with low-potency neuroleptics, such as chlorpromazine and thioridazine, than with haloperidol and fluphenazine. The risk of anticholinergic toxicity is increased in clients who are given a combination of drugs high in anticholinergic activity, such as certain tricyclic antidepressants and, of course, anticholinergic medications, as well as a number of over-the-counter cold remedies.

PIGMENTARY RETINOPATHY

Pigmentary retinopathy has been reported in clients taking high doses of thioridazine, and may cause blindness. Clients receiving thioridazine should never be treated with more than 800 mg/day. Mesoridazine, an active metabolite of thioridazine and approximately two to three times more potent on a milligram-per-milligram basis, is not as clearly associated with retinopathy as is thioridazine,[24] but nevertheless, should probably be limited to 500 mg/day.

There have been many other side effects reported, mainly with the use of low-potency agents, such as chlorpromazine, including photosensitivity (in which sunburns occur very easily), allergic reactions, cholestatic jaundice, agranulocytosis, skin and eye pigmentation, hyperglycemia, heartburn, nausea, vomiting, and diarrhea, all of which can occur, but are uncommon in clients receiving high-potency neuroleptics; virtually all of these side effects are reversible upon discontinuation of the neuroleptic.

Nursing Roles

Special attention should be given to assessing the client for development of the side effects of neuroleptics. Of critical importance is the development of tardive dyskinesia; hence, all clients should be routinely and carefully monitored for the development of abnormal movements, especially of the face, because the initial signs of tardive dyskinesia can be quite subtle. Other neuroleptic-induced EPS, such as dystonic reactions and NMS, also often require prompt attention. Such reactions are very frightening for clients and reassurance and explanations are important both during and after the episode. Sexual dysfunction related to neuroleptics should be inquired about, because clients are often uncomfortable talking about these issues.

Clients taking lower-potency neuroleptics, and especially chlorpromazine, should be advised to wear a sunscreen and hats when out in the sun; photosensitivity often develops with these drugs. Because of the orthostatic effects of these drugs, clients should be instructed to rise gradually from a recumbent position, first sitting and dangling their legs over the bed for at least one minute before standing. When severe, hypotension is potentially serious, since falls and fractures may occur, especially in the elderly. One particularly dangerous place is the bathroom, because the orthostatic effects of neuroleptics can combine with vagovagal effects of urination or defecation, resulting in falls onto hard bathroom surfaces.

When administering depot intramuscular medications, such as fluphenazine or haloperidol decanoate, it is important to remember to use a Z-track injection method. Patients should be given decanoate preparations only gluteally, and sites should be alternated.

ANTIPARKINSONIAN MEDICATIONS

Antiparkinsonian medications (Table 39-2) are used for side effects that result from the use of neuroleptic med-

TABLE 39-2
Antiparkinsonian medications

GENERIC NAME	TRADE NAME	DOSE RANGE (MG)
ANTICHOLINERGIC MEDICATIONS		
Procyclidine	Kemadrin	6–20
Trihexyphenidyl	Artane, Pipanol	2–15
Biperiden	Akineton	2–10
ANTICHOLINERGIC AND ANTIHISTAMINERGIC MEDICATIONS		
Benztropine	Cogentin	1–6
Diphenhydramine	Benadryl	25–200
Ethopropazine	Parsidol	50
Orphenadrine	Disipal, Norlex	50–250
DOPAMINE AGONISTS		
Amantadine	Symmetryl	100–300
Bromocriptine	Parlodel	5–50

ications. It is believed that neuroleptic medications, by blocking dopamine receptors in the brain, cause an imbalance in dopamine–acetylcholine transmission. In other words, blocking dopamine causes a relative increase in acetylcholine transmission, especially in those areas of the brain involved with the production of movement. This balance, therefore, can be corrected in two ways: (1) by decreasing acetylcholine transmission or (2) by increasing dopamine transmission. The first is accomplished by the use of cholinergic antagonists or anticholinergic medications (such as benztropine or trihexyphenidyl) and, the second, by the use of dopaminergic stimulants (such as amantadine). Both of these types of drugs are useful in the treatment of Parkinson disease, as well as neuroleptic-induced parkinsonism and dystonia, and are collectively called antiparkinsonian medications.

Indications for Use

There are no primary indications for anticholinergic drugs in psychiatry, and they are used to treat only EPS. It is still a matter of some controversy whether or not clients started on a neuroleptic medication regimen should be prophylactically treated with anticholinergic drugs, with proponents stating that prophylaxis decreases the incidence of acute dystonic reactions and, hence, enhances compliance, whereas opponents believe that drugs should be given only when needed, especially when such drugs carry with them adverse side effects. Currently, many researchers recommend that mainly those clients at high risk for developing dystonic reactions (such as young males who are treated with high doses of neuroleptics) be given the prophylactic anticholinergic drugs, but that an attempt should be made to taper and discontinue these drugs after several weeks.[41] Antiparkinsonian drugs can exacerbate tardive dyskinesia, for which they should not be used. All clients with tardive dyskinesia should have anticholinergic medications tapered and discontinued, if possible.

The use of direct dopaminergic agonists, such as amantadine and bromocriptine, is still controversial, with many investigators advocating the use of these drugs in those clients with EPS in whom the use of anticholinergic drugs is either not effective, or may cause delirium or memory impairment, such as in the elderly and the demented.[41] However, dopaminergic agonists should probably be reserved as second-line treatment, because of the possibility that they may exacerbate psychosis.

Guidelines for Administration

For acute dystonic reactions, a single tablet or injection of an anticholinergic agent (such as 1 to 2 mg of benztropine) is usually sufficient to reverse the reaction. Rarely, clients require more than one administration. For more chronic EPS, such as parkinsonism or akathi-

sia, prolonged treatment with anticholinergic drugs is often necessary. However, in any clients treated with these medications, attempts to taper and discontinue them should periodically be made.

Some anticholinergics, such as benztropine, need only to be given once a day, although twice a day may be slightly more effective in controlling EPS. Other drugs, such as trihexyphenidyl, require split-dosing regimens and should be given three times a day, if possible.

Some drugs, such as trihexyphenidyl, are mainly anticholinergic, whereas others, such as diphenhydramine, are both anticholinergic and antihistaminergic. Drugs that are more antihistaminergic are generally more sedating.

Most of the time anticholinergic medications can be given orally, but intramuscular injections may be required, especially if there is difficulty swallowing or the mouth is clamped shut by a dystonic reaction. Less commonly, intravenous administration may be necessary, mainly for life-threatening or extremely frightening dystonic reactions, as the intravenous route works slightly faster than other routes of administration.

Side Effects

Anticholinergic medications have a number of side effects, most of which are minor, and nearly all of which are readily reversible upon discontinuation of the medications. The most common are dry mouth, nasal congestion, and blurring of vision. Other side effects include constipation and, less commonly, urinary retention, which is potentially serious, especially in older clients. Although it is not usually clinically apparent, psychological testing has revealed that many clients who are given anticholinergic drugs have problems with recent memory, even when they are given routine doses of medications.

When anticholinergic side effects, such as development of urinary hesitancy or retention, become severe, a cholinergic stimulant, such as bethanechol, may occasionally be used. However, it usually is used only in those clients for whom anticholinergics cannot be discontinued and direct dopaminergic agonists cannot be prescribed.

Rarely, clients may develop an anticholinergic delirium, marked by disorientation, agitation, tachycardia, and tachypnea; dry, hot, flushed skin; mydriasis (enlarged pupils); hypoactive bowels; and memory impairment. This syndrome is usually reversible upon discontinuation of the drug, or administration of a cholinergic stimulant, such as physostigmine, intramuscularly or intravenously.[30] The syndrome is particularly likely to occur in elderly clients and in clients treated with multiple agents that possess anticholinergic activity, such as low-potency neuroleptics and tricyclic antidepressants.

Amantadine, which is not highly anticholinergic, is also associated with side effects. It can cause delirium or worsen psychosis, especially in the elderly.

Nursing Roles

Anticholinergic drugs are used only to treat the side effects of neuroleptics and, because they carry with them a number of side effects of their own, should be used in minimal doses and only when necessary. Nevertheless, many clients require these drugs, and it is important to continually monitor for EPS.

Because EPS can so frequently mimic other conditions, the use of anticholinergic medications is often helpful from a diagnostic standpoint. For example, subtle forms of akathisia may present as increased agitation and may erroneously be interpreted as an exacerbation of the psychosis. If the akathisia is not correctly identified, the neuroleptic dose may be increased, which may result in a worsening of the condition. Clients may also have subtle dystonic reactions, which they may describe in unusual ways, such as a thickened tongue or muscle ache. In both of these conditions, response to an anticholinergic medication may be very helpful in determining if the problem is related to EPS.

Many clients simply require reassurance for many of the anticholinergic side effects. For example, blurred near vision, which some clients describe as "double vision," (although it is not true diplopia) or difficulty reading or watching television, often causes clients to ask if they can get a new pair of glasses. Reassurance that most of the time these problems will go away with continued treatment is often very helpful. However, it is also important to be aware of serious anticholinergic side effects, such as urinary retention or anticholinergic delirium, both of which may be difficult to identify in psychotic clients.

LITHIUM

Lithium is administered as a salt, usually in the form of lithium carbonate (occasionally lithium citrate) and, within several hours of ingestion, it distributes throughout the body water in the form of lithium ion. It is not metabolized, but is excreted unchanged by the kidneys in which it competes with sodium for reabsorption.

Lithium was used in the 19th century for the treatment of gout because lithium urate is so soluble in water.[34] In the 1940s, an Australian named John Cade was administering lithium salts to guinea pigs when he noticed increased sedation in the animals. He decided to try the substance in some severely agitated manic clients and noted substantial improvement, which he reported in 1949.[16] Many clinical trials have since supported the efficacy of lithium in bipolar disorder and other conditions.[7,57]

Indications for Use

Lithium is an effective treatment for bipolar mood disorder, especially in treating the manic episodes. Unfor-
tunately, it can take up to several weeks for the mood-stabilizing effects to occur, and many manic clients who require more rapid treatment are often given a combination of neuroleptic and lithium, at least initially, until the antimanic effect of the lithium occurs. Some bipolar clients require long-term treatment with both lithium and neuroleptics. Lithium does not appear to be as effective in the treatment of acute depressive phases of the illness and, in some depressed clients, treatment with lithium actually makes them feel more depressed. Lithium has been shown to be effective in the prophylaxis of both bipolar and unipolar disorders.[58]

In addition to mood disorders, lithium has also been used in the treatment of schizoaffective disorder and schizophrenia with some success. Cyclothymic disorder also responds to lithium. Lithium is effective in the treatment of a condition known as periodic catatonia, in which catatonic features come and go, and which may be related to either schizophrenia or bipolar disorder. Some investigators have reported that lithium is effective in the treatment of some clients with violent, aggressive, or self-abusive behavior, especially when the violence consists of repetitive, sudden, impulsive, unpredictable attacks of uncontrollable rage. Lithium may also be of benefit in some clients with labile affect, such as occurs in borderline and histrionic personality disorder.

Guidelines for Administration

The therapeutic index of lithium (i.e., the toxic dose/effective dose ratio) is about 3, which is quite narrow (in comparison the therapeutic index of tricyclic antidepressants is about 10 and that of neuroleptics is about 100). Lithium can be measured in the serum, with the usual therapeutic serum range for lithium being about 0.7 to 1.2 mEq/L. Lithium is rarely effective in doses that result in a blood level below 0.1 mEq/L, and toxicity often occurs at serum levels higher than 1.5 mEq/L, with severe toxicity, coma, and even fatalities occurring above 3.0 mEq/L. Lithium levels should be monitored in the morning, 12 to 14 hours after the last dose.[3] Because of its short half-time, lithium should be given in divided doses, preferably three times daily. There are, however, newer longer-acting forms of lithium that can be more easily given twice daily. Lithium is given only orally.

Side Effects

The side effects of lithium are, to a large extent, dependent on serum concentration. There are many side effects that occur in the therapeutic range of less than 1.5 mEq/L. These include a fine hand tremor, metallic taste in the mouth, polyuria and polydipsia, diarrhea, and muscular weakness.[13] Most of the time these side effects are mild and, except for the tremor, self-limited and do not require treatment. The tremor (which is often most observable by laying a sheet of paper over the outstretched hands) can be treated with propranolol, if necessary, but usually it is not serious enough to warrant treatment.

At serum concentrations of 1.5 to 2.5 mEq/L, tremor, diarrhea, and muscle fatigue may increase and be accompanied by nausea and vomiting, dysarthria, tinnitus, rigidity, ataxia, and blurred vision. Finally, in the toxic range of higher than 2.5 mEq/L, ataxia, nystagmus, dysarthria, and tremor may become quite severe, and dyskinesias, hallucinations, confusion, and delirium can occur. Severe toxicity can result in seizures, stupor, coma, and death. Toxicity can occur on lower lithium doses if the lithium concentration increases secondary to dehydration caused by vomiting, diarrhea, or excessive sweating, or if there is a low-salt diet, an intake of diuretics, or renal disease.

Several endocrinologic problems can result from the use of lithium. The most common is hypothyroidism,[8] which can occur in 5% or more of clients, preponderantly women, and it is frequently accompanied by goiter, although some clients have goiter without hypothyroidism, and some, hypothyroidism without goiter. Sometimes thyroid supplementation is necessary. Lithium has also been reported to cause hyperparathyroidism, with elevated serum calcium concentration, decreased serum phosphate concentration and decreased urinary excretion of calcium.

A very common side effect is a mild leukocytosis and, occasionally, lithium has been used as a treatment for leukopenia. White blood cell counts in the range of 10,000 to 14,000 are not unusual, and are usually benign.

One of the more controversial side effects of lithium concerns renal damage.[5] Although a variety of different forms of renal dysfunction have been observed to occur with lithium, it appears that most of the changes are without consequence, and that clinically significant renal damage with therapeutic lithium concentrations is rare.

There are several important drug interactions, apart from those already discussed. Lithium can potentiate the sedating effects of alcohol, antidepressants, neuroleptics, and antihypertensives. Also, a number of drugs can increase the plasma lithium level, potentially into the toxic range; these include sodium-losing diuretics (thiazides, ethacrynic acid, triamterene, spironolactone), tetracyclines, metronidazole, indomethacin, ibuprofen, naproxin, and piperoxicam. Some drugs can also lower lithium concentration, including low-potency neuroleptics, theophylline, caffeine, and sodium-sparing diuretics (such as acetazolamide).

Nursing Roles

Because it is important to maintain a relatively stable blood level of lithium, and because of the low therapeutic ratio of the drug, it is particularly important that clients receive medications at the correct times and in the correct doses. Thus, strict compliance is of special importance in clients receiving lithium. Sometimes, administration of lithium citrate in liquid form is preferable, especially in those clients who may "cheek" their medications. Blood levels need to be monitored regularly. It is also important to constantly check for side effects of lithium, and especially, lithium toxicity, which is potentially very serious and may occur in the face of "therapeutic" lithium levels.

ANTIDEPRESSANTS

Antidepressant medications (Tables 39-3 and 39-4) can be divided into three groups: tricyclic antidepressants,

TABLE 39–3
Tricyclic and atypical antidepressant medications

GENERIC NAME	TRADE NAME	DOSE EQUIVALENT (MG)	SIDE EFFECTS			
			Sedative	Anticholin.	Hypotensive	Cardiac
TRICYCLIC ANTIDEPRESSANTS						
Amitriptyline	Elavil, Endep	25–250	++++	++++	++++	++++
Nortriptyline*	Pamelor, Aventyl	50–200	++	+++	+	+++
Protriptyline*	Vivactil	10–100	+/−	+++	++	++++
Imipramine	Tofranil	25–250	+++	+++	++++	++++
Desipramine*	Norpramin, Pertofrane	25–250	++	++	++	+++
Trimipramine	Surmontil	25–250	++++	++++	+++	++++
Amoxapine	Asendin	50–600	+++	+++	++	+
Maprotiline	Ludiomil	25–200	+++	+++	++	+++
Doxepin	Sinequan, Adapin	25–300	++++	++++	++	++
ATYPICAL ANTIDEPRESSANTS						
Trazodone	Desyrel	50–600	+++	+/−	++++	+
Fluoxetine*	Prozac	20–80	+/−	+/−	+/−	+
Bupropion*	Wellbutrin	200–450	+/−	+	+	+

* May be mildly stimulating, especially early in the course.
+/− = questionable, + = mild, ++ = moderate, +++ = moderately severe, ++++ = severe.

TABLE 39–4
Monoamine oxidase inhibitors

GENERIC NAME	TRADE NAME	DOSE RANGE (MG)
Phenelzine	Nardil	15–90
Tranylcypromine	Parnate	10–30
Isocarboxazid	Marplan	10–30

monoamine oxidase (MAO) inhibitors, and newer atypical antidepressants. The first antidepressants to be discovered were actually the MAO inhibitors. The drug isoniazid (and the related drug iproniazid) were used in the early 1950s in the treatment of tuberculosis and, in the course of this treatment, it was noticed that many clients had an improvement in mood.[12] Later it was discovered that these drugs inhibited the enzyme monoamine oxidase, which is one of the major enzymes responsible for the metabolism and inactivation of catecholamines, such as norepinephrine and dopamine. In fact, the discovery of the efficacy of these drugs in depression became one of the major pieces of evidence for the catecholamine theory of depression, in which some cases of depression are thought to be due to a hypocatecholaminergic state (involving a decrease in norepinephrine transmission in the brain). Later, in the 1950s, a drug called iminodibenzyl was investigated in schizophrenic clients because it resembled structurally the drug chlorpromazine. This drug was not effective in schizophrenia; but it was noted to have major mood-elevating properties. Shortly thereafter, the drug imipramine was investigated and introduced in Europe in 1958, and in North America in 1959. This was the beginning of the use of tricyclic antidepressants—drugs that structurally resemble phenothiazine neuroleptics. In fact, the tricyclic drug amoxapine, a more recent discovery that is chemically related to loxapine, appears to have both antidepressant and antipsychotic properties.[19]

Although several different terms have been used to describe various antidepressants with a cyclic chemical structure, including the terms *cyclic*, *bicyclic* (for fluoxetine), *tetracyclic* (for maprotiline), and *heterocyclic* (for amoxapine and trazodone), as Baldessarini[7] has pointed out many of these terms are chemically imprecise or are misnomers. Thus, following Baldessarini, the term *tricyclic* is retained for all antidepressants that have a tricyclic or related structure, and the term *atypical* is used for all other non-MAOI antidepressants.

Indications for Use

The primary indication for the use of antidepressants is depression. Although usually reserved for use in severe major depressive illness, these drugs have been used for the treatment of depression secondary to organic causes (such as stroke and tumors) and depression occurring in combination with other psychiatric disorders (such as schizophrenia, anxiety disorders, and personality disorders). It is possible that some forms of depression, such as those associated with personality disorders in which there are often "atypical" features (e.g., hypersomnia and weight gain, rather than hyposomnia and weight loss), may respond better to MAO inhibitors than to tricyclics, but this is not completely clear.[38] Both tricyclic antidepressants and MAO inhibitors have been found to be effective in the treatment of panic disorder,[63,67] for which they are much more effective than most benzodiazepines (except alprazolam[18]). Tricyclic antidepressants, and especially imipramine, have also been useful in the treatment of attention deficit disorder[64] and enuresis in children and adolescents. Interestingly, whereas the clinical efficacy of antidepressants in depression usually takes a week or more to become manifest, in attention deficit disorder and enuresis, the effects are very rapid. The drug clomipramine (Anafranil), available in Canada and Europe, has been shown to be effective in the treatment of obsessive–compulsive disorder and narcolepsy. Antidepressants have also been used to treat clients with chronic pain and eating disorders. Protriptyline has been used in the treatment of sleep apnea.

Guidelines for Administration

Typical tricyclic antidepressants are effective in the range of 50 to 250 mg/day (see Table 39-3 for dose ranges of different antidepressants), although much lower doses are used in the elderly.[53] The usual starting dose for a typical tricyclic antidepressant, such as imipramine, is 50 mg at night (10 to 25 in the elderly), with the dose raised, in divided doses, every several days to approximately 150 mg. Some clients require 250 mg and, rarely, 300 mg for full effect. Although clients may prefer that the entire dose be taken at bedtime, it is usually best to divide the dose if the client is receiving more than 150 mg/day, mainly because of hypotension.

With most tricyclic antidepressants, raising the dosage of medication usually results in either increased response or no change. There is evidence, however, that raising the dose of the drug nortriptyline beyond a certain point may actually result in lessened therapeutic efficacy.[4,14] This therapeutic window for nortriptyline has not been clearly demonstrated for other antidepressants. Thus, to make sure that the dose is in the therapeutic range, monitoring of blood levels is important when nortriptyline is used.

It often takes two to three weeks before the clinical effects of tricyclics are apparent. Clients in their first depressive episode are usually treated for four to eight months. Clients with a history of recurrent depressive episodes may require lifelong treatment with antidepressants. There is some evidence that the combination of lithium with an antidepressant may provide more effective prophylaxis against recurrent depressions than the antidepressant alone.[51]

Because clients with depression are often suicidal and tricyclics are potentially lethal in overdose,[10,48] clients at risk for suicide should be given no more than one week's supply of medication, or no more than 1000 mg of a typical tricyclic, such as amitriptyline or imipramine.

In clients with cardiac disease, antidepressants such as nortriptyline, desipramine, or atypical agents, are used more frequently than the more highly anticholinergic drugs, such as amitriptyline, imipramine, trimipramine, or the longer-acting drug, protriptyline. Drugs are given in small, divided doses to these clients, and special attention should be given to the conduction status of the heart and to the occurrence of orthostatic hypotension.

The use of MAO inhibitors should also follow the guidelines of starting at a low dose and raising the dosage over the next week or two. Typical starting dosages are 10 mg b.i.d. of tranylcypromine and 15 mg b.i.d. of phenelzine. It has been determined that a good clinical response is associated with greater than 85% to 90% inhibition of MAO, so that a determination of the degree of inhibition may be helpful in cases of depression with an apparent lack of response. It has also been determined that phenelzine is only rarely effective if given in dosages less than 45 mg/day. The MAO inhibitors, as do the tricyclics, often require one to three weeks before a clinical response is observed, and they should also be tapered over one to two weeks when discontinued because of the risk of withdrawal symptoms.

The most important feature of the administration of MAO inhibitors is that clients be strongly encouraged to follow the MAO inhibitor diet. Because MAO inhibitors inhibit the action of an enzyme that degrades catecholamines, intake of excess amines can lead to hypertensive crises, described later. Especially important are foods containing the pressor amine *tyramine*, which is a production of bacterial fermentation found in wines and cheeses, and substances containing stimulants, especially over-the-counter cold remedies and diet pills. Substances to avoid are listed in Boxes 39-2 and 39-3.

Because the effect of MAO inhibitors can last for a week or so after discontinuation, the MAOI diet should be continued for at least that period. Also, when switching from an MAO inhibitor to a tricyclic, there should be a period of seven to ten days without drug overlap, because of the risk of toxic reactions occurring with combination treatment, involving excitation, seizures, hyperpyrexia, blood pressure instability, which may rarely be fatal. It should be noted, however, that occasionally clients are treated with a combination of MAO inhibitor and tricyclic,[60,66] and special attention should be devoted to side effects and toxic interactions in such clients.

Often, tricyclics or MAO inhibitors are given in combination with antipsychotic drugs, especially in cases of psychotic depression, schizoaffective disorder, and borderline personality disorder. In these clients, there is often risk of anticholinergic toxicity, especially when

---

BOX 39-2
Foods Containing Tyramine or Other Substances That Can Interact with MAO Inhibitors to Cause Acute Hypertensive Crises

FOOD	CONTENT OF TYRAMINE
CHEESES	
Liederkrantz	Extremely high
Blue, brick, brie, Camembert, cheddar, Edam, Gruyere, Romano, Stilton, Swiss	Very high
Gouda, Limburger, mozzarella, parmesan	Moderately high
American	Moderate
Cottage cheese, cream cheese	Low
FRUITS AND VEGETABLES	
Broad-bean pods, figs, avocados	Moderate
Sauerkraut, raisins	Low
BEVERAGES	
Chianti	Moderate
Red wines, liqueurs	Low (but variable)
White wines	Very low
Distilled spirits	Trace
Caffeinated drinks (in large amounts)	Low
MISCELLANEOUS	
Lunch meats (bologna, pepperoni, salami)	Very high
Yeast products	Very high
Preserved liver, meat, or fish	Very high
Caviar, pickled herring	Very high
Preserved snails	Moderate
Chocolate	Low
Soy sauce	Low

---

anticholinergic drugs are used as well. When the combination of a tricyclic and an antipsychotic is used, it is often possible to decrease the dose of anticholinergic drug (if the client is receiving such) because of the anticholinergic effect of many of the tricyclics.

Antidepressants are virtually always given orally, and some clients with depressions and paranoia may be afraid to take their medications and may "cheek" them. In these cases, liquid forms of medication may be preferable.

Side Effects of Tricyclic Antidepressants

Probably at least one fourth of clients treated with tricyclic antidepressants experience some form of notable side effects, with the incidence of side effects increasing with age. The most common are anticholinergic side effects, including dry mouth, blurred vision, constipation, sweating, erectile dysfunction and, of more concern, urinary retention. Elderly men with prostate enlargement often show a worsening of urinary prob-

BOX 39-3
Medications to be Avoided by Clients Taking MAO Inhibitors

GENERIC NAME	CONTAINED IN MEDICATIONS WITH FOLLOWING TRADE NAMES*
α-Methyldopa	Aldoclor, Aldomet, Aldoril
d-Amphetamine	Dexedrine, Obetrol
Ephedrine	Bronkaid tablets, Quibron, Vicks Nyquil
Epinephrine	Bronkaid mist, Primatene
L-Dopa	Larodopa, Sinemet
Methamphetamine	Desoxyn
Methylphenidate	Ritalin
Oxymetazoline	Afrin, Duration
Pemoline	Cylert
Phenylephrine	Chlor-Trimeton, Congespirin, Coricidin, Coryban-D, Demazin, Dristan decongestants, 4-Way nasal spray, NTZ, Neo-Synephrine, Prefrin liquifilm, Sinex, Rynatan, Rynatuss, Sucrets cold decongestant, Trind
Phenylpropanolamine	A.R.M. allergy relief medicine, Alka-Seltzer Plus, Allerest, Anorexin, Appedrine, Bromphen, C3 cold cough capsules, Children's Hold, Codimal, Comtrex, Congespirin, Contac, Control, Coryban-D, CoTylenol, Cremacoat 3 and 4, Daycare daytime colds medicine, Decontabs, Dex-A-Diet II, Dexatrim, Diadax, Dietec, Dieutrim, Dimetane, Dorcol, Dura Tap, Dura-Vent, E.N.T., Entex, 4-Way cold tablets, Fiogesic, Fluidex-Plus, Formula 44-D, Head & Chest, Histalet, Histaminic, Hungrex Plus, Hycomine, Korigesic, Kronohist, Liqui-Trim diet drops, Naldecon, Nolamine, Novahistine, Ornacol, Ornade, Ornex, P.V.M. appetite control, Permathene-12, Poly-Histine, Pro-Dax 21, Prolamine, Propagest, Quadrahist, Rhindecon, Ru-Tuss, S-T Forte, Sinarest, Sine-Aid, Sine-Off, Sinubid, Sinulin, Sinutab, St. Joseph cold tablets for children, Sucrets cold decongestant formula, Super Odrinex, Tavist-D, Thinolar, Triaminic, Triaminicol, Tussagesic, Tuss-Ornade, Tuss-Ade, Ursinus
Pseudoephedrine	Ambenyl, Chlorafed, Cosanyl, CoTylenol, Deconamine, Detussin, Entuss-D, Fedahist, First Sign, Multi-Symptom, Novahistine, Probahist, Rhinosyn, Rondec, Ryna, Sinufed, Sudafed, Symptom-2, Triafed, Viro-Med

* The list is not exhaustive.

lems with tricyclics. Usually, some degree of tolerance develops to these effects over several weeks, and symptoms, such as dry mouth, are often relieved by chewing sugarless gum or candy, but rarely cholinergic agents are prescribed.

Orthostatic hypotension is a common side effect,[27] occurring in perhaps more than 20% of clients, and this can be especially worrisome in clients with cardiac disease or in clients at risk for stroke or falls and fractures.

Sedation is another relatively common side effect, with amitriptyline, trazodone, and amoxapine causing more sedation than other tricyclics. Occasionally, however, some antidepressants, in particular protriptyline and fluoxetine, may cause excitation. Sometimes, the extra sedation afforded by agents may be clinically useful, although, in cases of severe anergic, hypersomnic depressions, a more activating agent may be preferable.

Confusion and delirium may occur with tricyclics, often accompanied by signs of anticholinergic toxicity, especially in elderly clients treated with tricyclics in combination with low-potency neuroleptics or anticholinergic drugs. Sometimes, however, confusion can occur in the absence of a clear-cut anticholinergic syndrome.

Most tricyclic medications cause weight gain. Often, this may be related to the fact that many depressed clients have lost weight and, with treatment of the depression, gain the weight back. However, some clients may become overweight, and this appears especially true in clients who have weight gain (instead of loss) as a component of the depression. The new antidepressant, fluoxetine, differs from most currently available antidepressants in that it may actually result in weight loss in many clients.

Maprotiline and bupropion have been associated with a greater risk of grand mal seizures and, hence, should be used with care, although most of the tricyclics lower the seizure threshold and should be used cautiously in epileptic clients.[54]

One of the most serious concerns with the use of tricyclic antidepressants is their effect on cardiac function, mentioned earlier.[15,17,23,26] Many tricyclics cause palpitations and tachycardia, and many of them, especially those that are highly anticholinergic, have effects on cardiac conduction and may precipitate arrhythmias, although the likelihood of this is low when the drugs are used in therapeutic doses. Also, tricyclics have been found to possess *antiarrhythmic* action, which in many respects resembles quinidine. Nevertheless, great care should be exercised when any cardiac client receives a tricyclic medication, especially those clients who are already receiving cardiodepressive antiarrhythmics (such as quinidine, procainamide, or disopyramide) and in those clients with known cardiac conduction defects, such as bundle-branch block.

Because of the potential for serious drug interactions, tricyclic antidepressants should be used with care in clients taking a variety of other drugs. Tricyclics can potentiate the effects of other sedatives, especially alcohol, and can increase the respiratory compromise caused by narcotics as well as the excitatory effect of stimulants. They can reduce the effect of antihypertensives and α-adrenergic antagonists. The potentially dangerous interactions of tricyclics with MAO inhibitors and cardiac drugs, as well as with anticholinergic medications, have already been mentioned. The ability of tricyclics to lower the seizure threshold may cause reduced seizure control. Other drugs that interact with tricyclics include L-dopa, thyroid hormones, anticoagulants, insulin and oral hypoglycemics, steroids, and aspirin.

Other side effects of tricyclics include jaundice, hair loss, purpura, agranulocytosis, hypoglycemia, sexual dysfunction, dizziness, light-headedness, insomnia, and fatigue.

A nonspecific withdrawal syndrome, consisting of anxiety and restlessness, has also been described with tricyclics if they are discontinued without tapering.[55,59]

Side Effects of Monoamine Oxidase Inhibitors

The most pronounced side effect of MAO inhibitors is hypotension and, in particular, orthostatic hypotension. This side effect is of special concern in elderly clients or clients at risk for stroke, myocardial infarction, or fractures. Sometimes this problem can be minimized by slowly increasing the dosage of medication.

Although MAO inhibitors possess little in the way of anticholinergic activity (unlike tricyclics), many clients complain of anticholinergic-like effects, including dry mouth, blurred vision, constipation, sexual dysfunction, and urinary retention. The cause of these problems is unknown.

A variety of toxic symptoms involving the central nervous system have been observed, including agitation, insomnia, psychosis, and myoclonus (rapid muscular jerks), especially with overdoses of MAO inhibitors.

The most important complication of MAO inhibitors is their propensity to cause acute hypertensive crises.[11,52,62] These result when sympathomimetic amines are ingested in food or drugs, which then cause increased blood pressure because MAO, an enzyme that degrades these substances, is inhibited. Tyramine, a substance found in well-ripened, veined, or triple-cream cheeses, red wines, and other foods, has been classically associated with the syndrome. Important foods and drugs that interact with MAO inhibitors are listed in Boxes 39-2 and 39-3. Clients with pheochromocytoma or carcinoid syndrome should not be given MAO inhibitors.

MAO inhibitors also interact with a variety of other drugs. They may potentiate the action of sedatives to hypnotics (such as alcohol, barbiturates, general anesthetics, and benzodiazepines), neuroleptics, anticonvulsants, narcotics, anticholinergic and antiparkinsonian medications, L-dopa, hydralazine, α-antagonists, insulin and oral hypoglycemics, clonidine, and anticoagulants. They may produce toxic reactions with meperidine, nitrofuran antibiotics, reserpine, α-meth-

yldopa, and guanethidine. Finally, there are also interactions of an unpredictable nature with β-adrenergic blocking drugs.

Nursing Roles

Clients receiving antidepressants, especially the elderly, require constant monitoring of their blood pressure. Because antidepressants can be very dangerous in overdose, and depressed clients are probably at higher risk for suicidal behavior than any other single group of clients, it is very important to make sure that potentially suicidal clients are prescribed limited amounts of antidepressant medication (usually less than one week's supply). Also, it is important to make sure that clients do not hoard medication for later overdose attempts.

It is crucial for clients taking MAO inhibitors to follow the diet as closely as possible. Some clients try to cheat on the diet and, because the tyramine content of foods is variable, they may at one time be able to eat a prohibited food without problems, but the next time develop a hypertensive reaction. Clients must be told about the risk of these reactions and, especially, the risk of stroke and paralysis and, possibly, even death.

ANTIANXIETY MEDICATIONS

Today, benzodiazepines are the most popular antianxiety drugs in use, and are among the most commonly prescribed of all medications. Recently, another antianxiety drug, buspirone, has been introduced, which may have value in the treatment of clients with chronic anxiety. Table 39-5 lists a variety of commonly used antianxiety agents.

Indications for Use

The primary indication for the use of benzodiazepines is anxiety. Benzodiazepines appear to be more effective for generalized anxiety, but less effective for panic disorder or for phobic anxiety. The benzodiazepine alprazolam appears to be especially useful in the treatment of anxiety accompanying depression.[18] Certain benzodiazepines, such as flurazepam, temazepam, and triazolam, are more sedating than others, and are used for treatment of insomnia. Diazepam and clonazepam possess anticonvulsant activity. Benzodiazepines including diazepam and chlordiazepoxide are frequently used to withdraw clients who are dependent on sedative–hypnotic drugs, particularly alcohol, although lorazepam and oxazepam are being used with increasing frequency for this purpose. Lorazepam also appears to be useful in the treatment of catatonia.

Benzodiazepines are often divided into short-, moderately long-, and long-acting agents. In part, this is because certain benzodiazepines, including diazepam, prazepam, clorazepate, halazepam, and, to a lesser ex-

TABLE 39–5
Antianxiety and hypnotic medications

GENERIC NAME	TRADE NAME	HALF-LIFE (HR)	DOSE RANGE (MG)
ANXIOLYTIC BENZODIAZEPINES			
Short-acting			
Oxazepam	Serax	8	10–60
Alprazolam*	Xanax	12	0.5–4
Lorazepam	Ativan	15	1–6
Moderately Long-acting			
Chlordiazepoxide	Librium, etc.	18	10–60
Long-acting			
Halazepam	Paxipam	50	20–160
Diazepam	Valium	60	2–60
Prazepam	Centrax	100	5–40
Clorazepate	Tranxene	100	7.5–60
ANTICONVULSANT AND ANTIPANIC BENZODIAZEPINE			
Clonazepam*	Klonopin	34	0.5–10
HYPNOTIC BENZODIAZEPINES			
Triazolam	Halcion	2–3	0.125–0.5
Temazepam	Restoril	11	15–30
Flurazepam	Dalmane	2 and 72†	15–30
OTHER ANTIANXIETY MEDICATIONS			
Buspirone‡	Buspar		15–60
Hydroxyzine	Atarax, Vistaril		100–400

* These drugs may also have antidepressant effects.
† Flurazepam has active metabolites with a long half-life.
‡ Buspirone often requires several weeks for the antianxiety effect to become manifest.

tent, chlordiazepoxide, have active metabolites with very long half-lives. Thus, these drugs are much longer acting than are lorazepam, oxazepam, and temazepam. The metabolism of some benzodiazepines, such as diazepam, chlordiazepoxide, and flurazepam, is more dependent on liver function than is that of lorazepam, oxazepam, and temazepam. Thus, there is increasing use of these latter drugs in clients with liver disease and in the elderly.

Guidelines for Administration

In general, it is recommended that benzodiazepines be used for short periods whenever possible, especially in the treatment of acute anxiety states, because of the possibility of developing dependence on the drugs. Some clients, however, require long-term administration of benzodiazepines.[32] If short-acting benzodiazepines are used, then in general the drugs will have to be given more than once-a-day, whereas longer-acting benzodiazepines often require only once-a-day or even once-every-other-day dosing. The dosage of benzodiazepines is often highly individualized; however, some clients require six to eight divided doses of even a long-acting drug, such as diazepam, for adequate control of anxiety. There is often a considerable amount of sedation and mental slowing in the first week or two of

therapy, and clients should be cautioned to postpone important decisions and avoid driving, operating dangerous machinery, or engaging in other activities involving physical risk.

Because of the possibility of tolerance and withdrawal, benzodiazepines should be tapered when they are being discontinued. A tapering schedule of at least two weeks is necessary, and up to six weeks is usually preferable, especially for alprazolam.

Some clients are treated with the combination of a benzodiazepine and a β-adrenergic blocking drug, such as propranolol, for the combined treatment of "psychic" and "somatic" components of anxiety (the somatic components often consisting of tachycardia, palpitations, and diaphoresis).

Benzodiazepines are usually prescribed orally, although occasionally other routes of administration may be employed. In status epilepticus, for instance, intravenous diazepam is often given. In severe catatonic states, intramuscular or intravenous lorazepam has been used with some success. Other benzodiazepines, such as chlordiazepoxide or diazepam, are more erratically absorbed when given intramuscularly, and this route of administration should not be used.

The atypical antianxiety drug buspirone appears to be effective in some clients with chronic anxiety. Unlike benzodiazepines, which often exert an antianxiety effect after a single dose, buspirone resembles antidepressants and neuroleptics in that one to three weeks of treatment may be necessary to achieve a response. Buspirone, so far, does not appear to be associated with dependence or withdrawal symptoms.

Side Effects

The primary side effects of benzodiazepines are fatigue, drowsiness, and mental slowing, although if benzodiazepines are used for insomnia these are the main effects desired. Nevertheless, benzodiazepines potentiate the effects of other sedative–hypnotic medications, and clients should be told to avoid any of these, especially alcohol, when taking benzodiazepines. Although the risk of irreversible morbidity and mortality is exceedingly low when benzodiazepines are taken in overdose alone, when taken in combination with other sedatives, there may be an increased risk. Benzodiazepines by themselves cause little respiratory depression but they may exacerbate respiratory problems in clients with preexisting lung disease, such as emphysema, asthma, or bronchitis.

Apart from other sedatives, benzodiazepines are remarkably free of drug interactions. The only really significant drug interaction is with cimetidine; clients who are taking cimetidine often show increased sedation with benzodiazepines.

Another important side effect involves the occurrence of so-called paradoxical reactions to benzodiazepines.[31] These reactions, which often occur in the elderly and in those with brain damage or mental retardation, consist of unexpected agitation, hostility, agressiveness, and emotional lability. Usually, these reactions are seen in the first two weeks of starting therapy with a benzodiazepine, but they can occur at later times and, although often reversible, occasionally necessitate discontinuing the drug.

Although severe withdrawal symptoms from benzodiazepines are relatively uncommon, considering the large numbers of clients who receive these medications, they can occur, especially in clients who have been taking higher than recommended doses for several months or more.[2,20] These reactions often consist of anxiety, dizziness, nausea, anorexia, and insomnia, but, when more severe, they can progress to tremor, weakness, and orthostatic hypotension and, finally, to hyperthermia, convulsions, and delirium. Anxiety is a cardinal feature of withdrawal, and sometimes is of near-panic proportion, accompanied by headaches, dry mouth, weakness in the legs, a feeling of choking, irritability, sleep disturbance, and generalized aches and pains. Occasionally, there is diaphoresis, hand tremor, depression, hypersensitivity to sensory stimuli, paresthesias, perception of strange or unusual smells, and a metallic taste in the mouth. Rarely, there may be a paranoid psychosis. Any benzodiazepine can produce this syndrome, which usually appears within the first week after discontinuing the drug. Short-acting benzodiazepines produce withdrawal soon after discontin-

uation of the drug, and longer-acting agents produce later-appearing withdrawal symptoms.

Nursing Roles

Unlike many other psychotropic medications in which there is often concern that clients may not be taking their medications, with benzodiazepines there is often concern that clients will abuse the drugs. Although the physical dangers of overdose with benzodiazepines are low, in combination with other sedatives there can be an increased risk of respiratory depression and other problems. Because many benzodiazepines have "street value," some clients, often those with antisocial personality traits, will collect the medications and sell them instead of taking them. Therefore, it is important for the nurse to determine the abuse potential of these drugs in the clients who are taking them, and this is often a complex assessment involving the client's psychopathology, family structure, and social environment.

OTHER PSYCHOTROPIC MEDICATIONS

Propranolol

INDICATIONS FOR USE

Propranolol (Inderal) is a nonselective β-adrenergic antagonist that has been demonstrated to be useful in the treatment of a number of psychiatric conditions. The largest body of evidence concerns the use of propranolol in the treatment of anxiety,[37] especially anxiety accompanied by significant somatic features, such as palpitations, diaphoresis, tachycardia, diarrhea, and trembling. There is also evidence that propranolol may be helpful in the treatment of aggressive behavior, bipolar mood disorder, and psychosis. It has been used in the treatment of essential tremor, tremor secondary to lithium, and neuroleptic-induced akathisia.[40] Propranolol has also been helpful in cases of anxiety caused by the "floppy mitral valve" syndrome.

GUIDELINES FOR ADMINISTRATION

Propranolol should always be given first in a test dose of 10 to 20 mg, to determine whether there is any excessive sensitivity to the drug, determined by monitoring the pulse, which should remain above 60 beats per minute. If no such sensitivity is found, then it is a common practice to start therapy with 20 mg b.i.d., raising the dosage over the course of one to two weeks to 40 mg q.i.d. or until there is symptomatic relief. Although occasional clients require dosages of up to 240 mg/day, these are unusual. For psychiatric purposes, propranolol is administered only orally.

SIDE EFFECTS

Propranolol should be used with extreme caution in clients with asthma or heart disease. It is contraindicated in clients with cardiogenic shock, sinus bradycardia, heart block (greater than first degree), bronchial asthma, and most cases of congestive heart failure. Propranolol causes bradycardia and hypotension and should be used with caution in hypotensive clients or for clients who are taking catecholamine-depleting agents such as reserpine. There is also evidence that propranolol can cause depression in some clients or exacerbate a preexisting depression,[65] and it may rarely cause other psychiatric problems such as insomnia, fatigue, disorientation, or hallucinations.

NURSING ROLES

Care should be taken to monitor the client's blood pressure and pulse during treatment, and the pulse should not fall below 60.

Carbamazepine

INDICATIONS FOR USE

Carbamazepine (Tegretol) is a drug that is structurally related to the tricyclic antidepressants and was initially used in the treatment of tic douloureux (trigeminal neuralgia) and, later, in seizure disorders. It was discovered to be perhaps the drug of choice for partial complex seizures. Over the past decade or so, carbamazepine has been discovered to be a useful treatment for bipolar mood disorder, either used in combination with, or apart from, treatment with lithium.[39] There is also evidence that carbamazepine may be useful in the treatment of aggressive outbursts and rage attacks, depression, and psychosis.

GUIDELINES FOR ADMINISTRATION

It is best to start with low dosages of carbamazepine in psychiatric clients, about 200 to 400 mg/day, raising over the course of a week or so to 200 mg t.i.d. Sometimes as much as 1200 mg/day is required. The blood concentration should be monitored, with the therapeutic range being approximately 6 to 12 μg/mL. Carbamazepine can be used alone in the treatment of bipolar illness, or in combination with lithium or other drugs. Carbamazepine is given orally only.

SIDE EFFECTS

The most important side effect is suppression of bone marrow and aplastic anemia, which is very rare, unpredictable, and often reversible after discontinuation of the medication. Most clients, it should be noted, will develop a mild benign leukopenia when treated with carbamazepine, which is not of clinical significance. Nevertheless, the complete blood count of clients should be followed routinely, especially when instituting carbamazepine therapy or when clients are receiving high doses. Hepatic abnormalities can also occur; therefore, liver function tests also require routine monitoring. Other common side effects include sedation, diplopia, dizziness, ataxia, nystagmus, tremor, depression, diarrhea, and depressed thyroid function.

NURSING ROLES

Carbamazepine is a relatively new drug in psychiatry, and all clients should be observed carefully for the occurrence of side effects. Of special importance is the development of an aplastic anemia, which usually becomes manifest clinically with increased risk for infections and fever. Clients should also be carefully observed for the development of toxicity.

Stimulants

Although stimulants were initially used in the treatment of depression, they have been largely supplanted by the tricyclic antidepressants and MAO inhibitors that were discovered to be effective in the 1950s. Nevertheless, there continue to be indications for the use of these drugs, even today. The main stimulants in use in the United States today are d-amphetamine (Dexedrine), methylphenidate (Ritalin), and pemoline (Cylert).

INDICATIONS FOR USE

The main indication for the use of stimulants is in the treatment of attention deficit disorder in children and adolescents. It is also clear that attention deficit disorder can persist into adulthood, and some of these persons are also responsive to stimulants. Stimulants are also used in the treatment of withdrawn or apathetic states occurring in the elderly[25] and in severely withdrawn schizophrenic clients. Stimulants are helpful in the treatment of narcolepsy, a condition marked by sleep attacks during the day accompanied by cataplexy (sudden loss of muscular tone), hypnogogic and hypnopompic hallucinations (hallucinations upon falling asleep and awakening), and sleep paralysis.

GUIDELINES FOR ADMINISTRATION

Stimulants have relatively short half-lives and thus must be given in divided doses, but usually not at night. The usual dosage range for d-amphetamine is 10 to 30 mg/day, that of methylphenidate, 20 to 40, and pemoline, 37.5 to 75.

SIDE EFFECTS

Common side effects include insomnia, dysphoria, anxiety, agitation, and anorexia. Occasionally, delirium and paranoid psychosis is observed. In children, there is concern over the possibility of growth retardation. Rapid withdrawal from stimulants after prolonged treatment may result in "crashing," with anergia, depression, and sleep disturbance; but pain, seizures, and delirium have not been reported. Stimulants can exacerbate anxiety and withdrawal syndromes secondary to sedative–hypnotic dependence. Stimulants can also cause movement disorders, such as chorea and tics,[21,44] and can cause of worsening of psychotic and manic symptoms.

NURSING ROLES

Stimulants are drugs with considerable abuse potential, and all of the problems associated with benzodiazepine abuse described in that section also apply here.

Other Drugs

The α_2-adrenergic agonist clonidine has been shown to be useful in the treatment of opiate and nicotine withdrawal, and the dopaminergic stimulant bromocriptine has been reported helpful in treating cocaine withdrawal.

Other drugs that may be useful for psychiatric disorders in the future include calcium channel blockers, such as verapamil and nifedipine, the specific MAO inhibitors, clorgyline and deprenyl,[22] and the atypical neuroleptic clozapine.

PSYCHOTROPIC MEDICATIONS IN PREGNANCY

If possible, psychotropic medications should be discontinued during pregnancy. In some clients, because of severe psychosis or mood disorder, this is not possible. In general, neuroleptic medications appear reasonably safe to use in pregnancy and during lactation, and some investigators have advocated the use of higher-potency agents.[7,28,61] The safety of antidepressant and antianxiety medications in this regard is not yet established, however. When used in pregnancy, antidepressants may be associated with neonatal distress, and benzodiazepines with cleft palate, other physical abnormalities, as well as with neonatal intoxication and depression.[7,29] These drugs should be used with care in pregnant or lactating women. Lithium, however, should probably not be used in pregnancy at all, and especially never during the first trimester, for it has been associated with development of cardiovascular malformations and Down syndrome.[1,7,29]

SUMMARY

Psychotropic medications, unlike many drugs in medicine, are often very complicated to use, require highly individualized dosage schedules, and are often administered to clients who are receiving more than one drug at a time. Therefore, special care should be devoted to the clinical symptomatology of clients and to the possibilities of drug interactions. Although many drugs have names that imply one specific function, such as "antidepressant," most psychotropic drugs have more than one function and are used in a variety of situations. Antidepressants, for example, in addition to being used for depression, often are also used for panic attacks, anxiety, enuresis, and even attention deficit disorder.

Neuroleptics are the mainstay of treatment for psychosis, and the extrapyramidal side effects of neuroleptics often warrant the concomitant use of antiparkinsonian medications, although these should generally be used sparingly and only when necessary. Lithium is the primary drug for the treatment of bipolar mood disorder and it may be given in combination with neuroleptics and other drugs. Lithium can be used to prevent recurrence of both unipolar and bipolar mood disorder. Tricyclic antidepressants are the most commonly used antidepressants, although monoamine oxidase inhibitors are growing in popularity, even though these latter drugs require a special diet that is low in substances containing tyramine, because of the risk of hypertensive crises. Benzodiazepines are now the most commonly prescribed antianxiety–hypnotic drugs, since they are far safer than other drugs such as the

Research Highlights

One of the most troublesome problems of clients who develop tardive dyskinesia (TD) after long-term treatment with neuroleptics is that many of them are not aware of having a movement disorder. To investigate this further, Lohr et al.[42] developed a self-rating questionnaire for perception of abnormal involuntary movements and parkinsonism and administered it to a variety of clients with psychiatric and movement disorders. Although most clients with neurologic motor diseases (Huntington's disease and Parkinson's disease) were aware of the movement disorder, approximately one-third of clients with TD were not aware of the abnormal movements. Furthermore, 14 of 26 clients with schizophrenia were unaware of the movement disorder, whereas all clients with schizoaffective disorder were aware of TD. Because many clients with schizophrenia have TD, and may not be aware of it, it is very important for nurses to specifically seek out evidence of the movement disorder in this population of clients.

barbiturates. Stimulants are infrequently used in psychiatry, being reserved mainly for attention deficit disorder, narcolepsy, and withdrawn states associated with schizophrenia. Finally, there are some newer psychiatric uses for currently available drugs, including the use of carbamazepine for mood disorders and propranolol for anxiety disorders.

References

1. Allan LD, Desai G, Tynan MJ. Prenatal echocardiographic screening for Ebstein's anomaly for mothers on lithium therapy. Lancet. 1982;2:875.
2. Allquander C. Dependence on sedative and hypnotic drugs. Acta Psychiatr Scand. Suppl 1978;270:1.
3. Amdisen A. Monitoring of lithium treatment through determination of lithium concentration. Dan Med Bull. 1977;22:277.
4. Asberg M. Plasma nortriptyline levels: relationship to clinical effects. Clin Pharmacol Ther. 1974;16:215.
5. Ayd FJ Jr. Lithium and the kidney. Int Drug Ther Newslett. 1978;14(7):25.
6. Baldessarini RJ. Chemotherapy in psychiatry: principles and practice, revised ed. Cambridge, MA: Harvard University Press; 1985.
7. Baldessarini RJ, Stephens JH. Lithium carbonate for affective disorders: I. Clinical pharmacology and toxicology. Arch Gen Psychiatry. 1970;22:72.
8. Berens SC, Bernstein RS, Robbins J, Wolff J. Antithyroid effects of lithium. J Clin Invest. 1970;49:1357.
9. Beumont PJV, Gelder MG, Friesen HG, et al. The effects of phenothiazines on endocrine function: I. Patients with inappropriate lactation and amenorrhea. Br J Psychiatry. 1974;124:413.
10. Biggs JT, Spiker DC, Petit JM, et al. Tricyclic antidepressant overdose: incidence of symptoms. JAMA. 1977;238:135.
11. Blackwell B, Marley E, Price J, Taylor D. Hypertensive interactions between monoamine-oxidase inhibitors. Br J Psychiatry. 1967;113:349.
12. Bloch R, Dooneieff A, Buchberg A, Spellman S. The clinical effects of isoniazid and iproniazid in the treatment of pulmonary tuberculosis. Ann Intern Med. 1954;40:881.
13. Branchey MH, Charles J, Simpson GM. Extrapyramidal side effects of lithium maintenance therapy. Am J Psychiatry. 1976;133:444.
14. Burrows G, Scoggins BA, Turecek LR, et al. Plasma nortriptyline and clinical response. Clin Pharmacol Ther. 1974;16:639.
15. Burrows GD, Bohra J, Hunt D, et al. Cardiac effects of different tricyclic antidepressant drugs. Br J Psychiatry. 1976;129:335.
16. Cade JFJ. Lithium salts in the treatment of psychotic excitement. Med J Aust. 1949;2:349.
17. Cassem N. Cardiovascular effects of antidepressants. J Clin Psychiatry. 1982;43:22.
18. Chouinard G, Annable L, Fontaine R, Solyom L. Alprazolam in the treatment of generalized anxiety and panic disorders. Psychopharmacology. 1982;77:229.
19. Cohen BT, Harris PQ, Altesman RI, Cole JO. Amoxapine: a neuroleptic as well as an antidepressant? Am J Psychiatry. 1982;139:1165.
20. Covi L, Lipman RS, Pattison JH, et al. Length of treatment with anxiolytic sedatives and response to their sudden withdrawal. Acta Psychiatr Scand. 1971;49:51.

21. Denckla MB, Bemporad JR, MacKay MC. Tics following methylphenidate administration: a report of 20 cases. JAMA. 1976;235:1349.
22. Finberg JPM, Youdim MBH. Selective MAO A and B inhibitors: their mechanism of action and pharmacology. Neuropharmacology. 1983;22(3B):441.
23. Freeman JW, Mundy GR, Beattie RR, Ryan C. Cardiac abnormalities in poisoning with tricyclic antidepressants. Br Med J. 1969;2:610.
24. Gershon S, Sakalis G, Bowers PA. Mesoridazine—a pharmacodynamic and pharmacokinetic profile. J Clin Psychiatry. 1981;42:463.
25. Gilbert J, Donnelly KJ, Zimmer LE, Kubis JF. Effect of magnesium pemoline and methylphenidate on memory improvement and mood in normal aging subjects. Aging Hum Dev. 1973;4:35.
26. Glassman AH, Bigger JT Jr. Cardiovascular effects of therapeutic doses of tricyclic antidepressants. Arch Gen Psychiatry. 1981;38:815.
27. Glassman AH, Bigger JT Jr, Giardina EV, et al. Clinical characteristics of imipramine-induced orthostatic hypotension. Lancet. 1979;1:468.
28. Goldberg HL, DiMascio A. Psychotropic drugs in pregnancy. In: Lipton MA, DiMascio A, Killam KF, eds. Psychopharmacology: a generation of progress. New York: Raven Press; 1978.
29. Goldfield MD, Weinstein MR. Lithium in pregnancy: a review with recommendations. Am J Psychiatry. 1971;127:888.
30. Granacher RP, Baldessarini RJ. Physostigmine: its use in acute anticholinergic syndrome with antidepressant and antiparkinson drugs. Arch Gen Psychiatry. 1975;32:375.
31. Hall RCW, Disook S. Paradoxical reactions to benzodiazepines. Br J Clin Pharmacol. 1981;11(suppl 1):99S.
32. Hollister LE, Conley FK, Britt RH, Shuer L. Long-term use of diazepam. JAMA. 1981;246:1568.
33. Jeste DV, Wyatt RJ. Understanding and treating tardive dyskinesia. New York: Guilford Press; 1982.
34. Johnson FN. The history of lithium therapy. London: Macmillan; 1984.
35. Kane JM. Prevention and treatment of neuroleptic noncompliance. Psychiatr Ann. 1986;16:576.
36. Kane JM, Honigfeld G, Singer J, Meltzer H. Clozapine for the treatment-resistant schizophrenic: a double-blind comparison with chlorpromazine. Arch Gen Psychiatry. 1988;45:789.
37. Kathol RG, Noews R Jr, Sylmen DJ, et al. Propranolol in chronic anxiety disorders. Arch Gen Psychiatry. 1980;37:1361.
38. Liebowitz MR, Quitkin FM, Stewart JW, et al. Phenelzine vs imipramine in atypical depression. Arch Gen Psychiatry. 1984;41:669.
39. Lipinski JF, Pope HG. Possible synergistic action between carbamazepine and lithium carbonate in the treatment of three acutely manic patients. Am J Psychiatry. 1982;139:948.
40. Lipinski JF, Zubenko G, Cohen BM, Barreira P. Propranolol in the treatment of neuroleptic-induced akathisia. Am J Psychiatry. 1984;141:412.
41. Lohr JB, Jeste DV. Neuroleptic-induced movement disorders: acute and subacute disorders. In: Cavenar JO Jr, ed. Psychiatry. Philadelphia: JB Lippincott; 1988.
42. Lohr JB, Lohr MA, Wasli E, et al. Self-perception of tardive dyskinesia and neuroleptic-induced parkinsonism: a study of clinical correlates. Psychopharmacol Bull. 1987;23:211.
43. Lohr JB, Wisniewski A. Movement disorders: a neuropsychiatric approach. New York: Guilford Press; 1987.
44. Lowe TL, Cohen DJ, Detlor J, et al. Stimulant medications precipitate Tourette's syndrome. JAMA. 1982;247:1729.

45. Marder SR. Approaches to maintenance therapy in schizophrenia. Psychiatr Ann. 1983;13:31.

46. Meltzer HY, Sommers AA, Luchins DJ. The effect of neuroleptics and other psychotropic drugs on negative symptoms in schizophrenia. J Clin Psychopharmacol. 1986;6:329.

47. Meltzer HY, Stahl SM. The dopamine hypothesis of schizophrenia: a review. Schizophr Bull. 1976;2:19.

48. Nicotra MB, Rivera M, Pool JL, Noall MW. Tricyclic antidepressant overdoses: clinical and pharmacological observations. Clin Toxicol. 1981;18:599.

49. Oliver AP, Luchins DJ, Wyatt RJ. Neuroleptic-induced seizures: an in vitro technique for assessing relative risk. Arch Gen Psychiatry. 1982;39:206.

50. Petursson H, Lader MH. Withdrawal from long-term benzodiazepine treatment. Br Med J. 1981;283:643.

51. Prien RF, Klett CJ, Caffey EM Jr. Lithium carbonate and imipramine in prevention of affective episodes. Arch Gen Psychiatry. 1973;29:420.

52. Raskin A. Adverse reactions to phenelzine: results of a nine-hospital depression study. J Clin Pharmacol. 1972;12:22.

53. Reynolds CF, Marin RS, Spiker D. Clinical considerations in prescribing antidepressants for geriatric patients. Geriat Med Today. 1983;2:45.

54. Rotblatt MD. Antidepressants and seizures. Drug Int Clin Pharmacol. 1982;16:749.

55. Sathananthan GL, Gershon S. Imipramine withdrawal: an akathisia-like syndrome. Am J Psychiatry. 1973;130:1286.

56. Schooler NR, Levine J, Severe JB, et al. Prevention of relapse in schizophrenia: an evaluation of fluphenazine decanoate. Arch Gen Psychiatry. 1980;37:16.

57. Schou M. Biology and pharmacology of the lithium ion. Pharmacol Rev. 1957;9:17.

58. Schou M. Lithium as a prophylactic agent in unipolar affective illness: comparison with cyclic antidepressants. Arch Gen Psychiatry. 1979;36:849.

59. Shatan C. Withdrawal symptoms after abrupt termination of imipramine. Can Psychiatr Assoc J. 1966;2:150.

60. Spiker DH, Pugh DD. Combining tricyclic and monoamine oxidase inhibitor antidepressants. Arch Gen Psychiatry. 1976;33:828.

61. Sriwatanakul K, Weis O. Using antipsychotic drugs during pregnancy. Drug Ther. 1982;Nov:107.

62. Stockley IH. Monoamine oxidase inhibitors: I. Interactions with sympathomimetic amines. Pharmacol J. 1973;210:590.

63. Tyrer P, Candy J, Kelly D. Phenelzine in phobic anxiety: a controlled trial. Psychol Med. 1973;3:120.

64. Waizer J, Hoffman SP, Polizos P, Engelhardt DM. Outpatient treatment of hyperactive school children with imipramine. Am J Psychiatry. 1974;131:587.

65. Waal HGJ. Propranolol-induced depression. Br Med J. 1967;2:50.

66. White K, Simpson G. Combined MAOI–tricyclic antidepressant treatment: a reevaluation. J Clin Psychopharmacol. 1981;1:264.

67. Zitrin CM, Klein DF, Woerner MG, et al. Treatment of phobias: I. Comparison of imipramine hydrochloride and placebo. Arch Gen Psychiatry. 1983;40:125.

40

Mary T. Bush

Electroconvulsive Therapy and Other Biologic Therapies

OBJECTIVES

After reading this chapter, the reader will be able to:

1. Describe four biologic therapies used in public mental institutions before 1955
2. Identify two trends in psychiatric care that influenced the decline of these therapies
3. Compare early (unmodified) ECT with contemporary (modified) ECT in terms of procedure and safety
4. Outline a nursing protocol for preparation of a client for ECT
5. Identify themes of current medicolegal and ethical controversy over ECT
6. Name three other contemporary biologic therapies
7. List nursing diagnoses common with a client undergoing ECT
8. Suggest client goals, nursing interventions, and outcome criteria for use with these nursing diagnoses
9. Identify possible influences on the nurse's attitudes about ECT.

HISTORICAL PERSPECTIVE

The exciting advances in psychodynamic theory and psychotherapy that were made in the early 1900s did little to immediately influence the care or treatment of most persons suffering from severe mental illness. These patients were housed in large public psychiatric hospitals and were treated with a variety of biologically based techniques as they developed, seemingly by trial and error. The primary goal of treatment was symptom alleviation, which often translated into behavior control for this large group of patients. The modalities that evolved included hydrotherapy, insulin coma therapy, pharmacoconvulsive therapies, psychosurgery, and electroshock or electroconvulsive therapy (ECT).

Other than psychopharmaceuticals, the only biologic therapy remaining in significant use today is ECT. This chapter will focus on ECT, with other less well-known and utilized therapies being presented briefly. First, however, an historical review is in order so the nurse will have an awareness of the experience of some older psychiatric clients and to shed light from the past on current controversy.

Hydrotherapy

Some of the earliest methods for symptom control in psychiatric hospitals involved the use of spas, baths, warm and cold water packs, and sometimes douches and sprays of water.[1,20] The objective of treatment was generally to calm the patient, and a nurse or attendant's role would be to reassure the patient, wrap the patient in sheets if necessary, and periodically check the temperature of the water and the well-being of the patient. An example of this experience can be found in Green's *I Never Promised You a Rose Garden* in which Deborah received the therapy in response to a frightening psychotic interlude, a result of telling her doctor about her secret world and its power. After Deborah had been wrapped in icy wet sheets and restrained for four hours, she, indeed, emerged exhausted—but still with clear perceptions of her colorful, punitive psychotic world.[6]

Insulin Coma Therapy

In 1933, Manfred Sakel observed that schizophrenic patients seemed to improve after experiencing coma, and he began to treat them by inducing coma with insulin injections. The insulin was given early in the morning to a fasting patient. An initial trial dose was increased daily until a light hypoglycemic coma was produced, usually requiring 100 to 200 U of insulin. The first coma was terminated after 15 minutes with orange juice through a nasogastric tube. Later glucagon was used to terminate coma. The length of coma was increased daily until it lasted a maximum of 60 minutes. Most patients required 40 to 60 treatments, and catatonic patients reportedly showed the greatest improvement.[1] The nurse's role in insulin therapy involved monitoring patient progress, reassuring the patient, and involving the patient in other therapies after treatment. Insulin coma therapy was a dangerous procedure, and there were a significant number of deaths caused by the complications of prolonged coma. The treatment was difficult to administer and enjoyed only a brief period of high utilization.

Pharmacoconvulsive Therapies

The Hungarian psychiatrist, Meduna, is credited with the introduction of seizure therapy in 1934. On the basis of a review of the literature and the erroneous observation that schizophrenia and epilepsy were incompatible with one another, Meduna hypothesized that seizures were therapeutic. He produced seizures in psychiatric patients by the intramuscular injection of camphor in oil.[9] Early successes were reported. Patients seemed to be less psychotic after a spontaneous seizure, but there were difficulties in producing the seizure reliably and within a specific time frame. A synthetic derivative, pentylenetetrazol (Metrazol), given intravenously produced more predictable seizures, and soon pharmacoconvulsive therapy was used to treat not only schizophrenia, but also depression and mania. In the 1950s a convulsive gas anesthetic, fluorothyl (Indoklon), was briefly popular as a seizure-producing agent.[9] This treatment was terrifying to patients because of the anticipation of one or more unmodified grand mal seizures. Pharmacoconvulsive therapy is no longer used.

Psychosurgery

While the pharmacoconvulsive therapies were developing in the 1930s, another emerging area of investigation was psychosurgery. A beginning knowledge of the relationship between cortical and subcortical functions was being expanded by the use of encephalograms and stimulation or ablation of areas of animal brains. It was noted that ablation of the frontal lobes in monkeys had a calming effect, but did not seem to impair cognitive function. The first publicized "successful" lobotomy on a human was performed by Egas Moniz, a Portuguese psychiatrist, in 1936. A technique developed by Freeman and Watts was used in this country during the 1940s and 1950s to perform prefrontal lobotomies for a number of psychiatric conditions. The early benefits of psychosurgery were often dramatic: there was elimination of aggressive and assaultive behavior in patients for whom few therapeutic alternatives existed. Many prefrontal lobotomies were performed, and in 1949 Moniz received the Nobel Prize for Medicine for his contribution.[3,20] However, by this time, opposition to the procedure was already mounting. Clinical data indicated a mortality of up to 5% and epilepsy rates of up to 15% because of scar tissue. It became evident that long-term undesirable behavior changes, such as apathy, extreme lability, or vegetative states occurred frequently. This data fueled an emerging moral opposition and, with the development of psychotropic medication and the advances in safety of ECT, few prefrontal lobotomies were performed after 1955.[3] However, psychosurgery did not completely fade away, and neurosurgeons continued to quietly experiment with "targeted" operations that destroyed comparatively smaller areas of the brain.[20]

Electroconvulsive Therapy

The Italian neuropsychiatrists Cerletti and Bini introduced the induction of seizures by electrical current in 1938. They were conducting epilepsy research and tried their experiment of passing an electric current through the brain of an acutely psychotic schizophrenic man, who experienced a remission of symptoms. Their success was widely reported, and the use of electroconvulsive therapy developed and spread rapidly.[10] Early ECT was as frightening as pharmacoconvulsive therapy. It was unmodified, that is, given without benefit of anesthetic, sedation, or muscle relaxant. Staff were required to firmly hold patients during the seizure, but fractures still resulted. Some patients were given treatments forcibly, and reports of misuse and abuse of the therapy in large public mental hospitals abounded. Perhaps the most well-known example of the era of ECT and public mental hospitals is found in Kesey's book, *One Flew Over the Cuckoo's Nest:*

> They try to hush his singing with a piece of rubber hose for him to bite on . . . just as those irons get close enough to the silver on his temples—light arcs across, stiffens him, bridges him off the table till nothing is down but his wrists and ankles and out around that crimped black rubber hose a sound like hooeee! and he's frosted over completely with sparks (reference 11, p 270).

When other less invasive treatment alternatives appeared, the use of ECT declined.

CONTEMPORARY ELECTROCONVULSIVE THERAPY

Electroconvulsive therapy today is a treatment in which a brief application of electrical stimulus is used to produce a generalized seizure. It is administered in private general hospitals, private psychiatric hospitals, and in some university hospital settings. Because it is expensive to administer and because of concern about past abuses, ECT is not offered at most public institutions.[13] More than 100,000 clients may currently be receiving ECT in the United States.[18] The use of ECT is growing because of the increasingly apparent drawbacks of psychotropic medication, continued refinement in treatment techniques, research findings that

support a biochemical theory of action, and more favorable popular media portrayals.

Procedure and Case Example

The modern day ECT treatment has very little resemblance to the ECT of the 1940s. The following case is presented to focus on the specific procedural and technical safeguards and refinements that are a part of contemporary practice.

> Mrs. Anne F, a 62-year-old client with a DSM-III-R diagnosis of major depression, recurrent episode, severe, was admitted to the hospital to receive a course of ECT. The psychiatrist and psychiatric nurse had explained the procedure to Anne and her family, and she gave consent. A pre-ECT workup was done that included a chest x-ray, electrocardiogram, laboratory studies, and physical examination. All findings were negative, and Anne was scheduled for treatment the next morning. That evening, she and her family watched a video recording demonstrating the procedure. A psychiatric nurse was on hand to answer questions. Anne was given nothing by mouth from midnight previous to the treatment.
>
> Approximately one-half hour before her scheduled treatment time, Anne was given 0.6 mg atropine IM to decrease secretions. Reassured by the experienced staff, a monitoring pad was placed on her back, and she was helped onto a stretcher. An automatic blood pressure monitor and a cardiac monitor were attached. The anesthesiologist started a small intravenous catheter in her arm and injected 80 mg of methohexital (Brevitol), a fast, short-acting anesthetic, and 60 mg of succinylcholine (Anectine), a strong muscle relaxant. As Anne fell asleep, a rubber headband with two electrodes was placed on her forehead. An electrical stimulus was given, which lasted 1.5 seconds, and a seizure was induced. There were no visible signs of the seizure, which lasted 45 seconds. A graph from the ECT machine gave the staff a documented picture of the seizure from beginning to end. The anesthesiologist administered 100% oxygen to Anne until she awoke five minutes later.
>
> Anne was moved to a quiet recovery area where a nurse monitored vital signs and provided reassurance and brief, orienting contacts. After an hour she was returned to her room where a light breakfast was offered. [Boblet, JA. Electroconvulsive therapy: barbarism or effective treatment. unpublished manuscript, 1987].

Selection Criteria

Most researchers and clinicians agree that ECT is a treatment alternative for those major depressions that show strong biologic and psychotic features.[7] The clinical picture of a person responsive to ECT would be a severely depressed client with insomnia, weight loss, psychomotor retardation, and guilty, somatic, or persecutory delusions. Electroconvulsive therapy seems as effective as lithium in the treatment of mania, and it has been successful with the schizophrenic client who has a short duration of illness, acute onset, and intense affective symptoms.[2,13] The fast action and relative safety of ECT make it a treatment alternative for the patient who is dangerously suicidal, is debilitated by depression, or who cannot tolerate the side effects of psychotropic medication. Clients who have not responded to trials of psychotropic medications and those who have previously responded to ECT are good candidates.

Contraindications to Electroconvulsive Therapy

Increased intracranial pressure or brain tumor are contraindications because the treatment transiently increases cerebrospinal fluid pressure. A very recent myocardial infarction may be a contraindication because cardiac arrythmias may occur during the seizure. General anesthesia risks—allergies to medication used or poor liver or renal function—need to be kept in mind.[7] However, ECT is not contraindicated for pregnant women and elderly patients. They are far more susceptible to untoward effects from medication than to untoward effects from ECT, and ECT is considered a safe treatment alternative for them.[7]

Theory of Action

Early psychodynamic explanations of the effectiveness of ECT have given way to research supporting a psychobiologic model. Although the definitive explanation for why ECT works has not been accepted, it is likely that important neurochemical changes associated with the seizure activity influence the hypothalamus and limbic regions of the brain.[5,16] Data are emerging almost daily, and some researchers predict that the antidepressants and ECT will be found to have related neurochemical effects.[2]

Safety and Side Effects

Mortality is very low for ECT procedures; the risks are similar to those of using short-acting barbiturate anesthetics. Similarly, complications have been virtually eliminated with present techniques. Clients no longer receive fractures as a result of ECT. There is no evidence that brain damage occurs, and clients are not awake during the procedure so have no memory of it. Transient bradycardia may occur during the seizure because of vagal stimulation. Postseizure headaches or nausea sometimes occur. Rarely, a client may become agitated during the immediate recovery phase and require medication.

Disruption of memory function during ECT treatment is common. Both short-term inability to acquire new information and amnesia for events immediately surrounding the treatment can be observed. Memory dysfunction reaches its peak around the fourth treatment and is proportional to the number of treatments received. It gradually subsides over the weeks or months after treatment. Most studies have demonstrated no long-term effects on cognitive function; but others have demonstrated mild lasting effects.[17,22] Recent research indicates that traditional bilateral ECT (in which electrodes are placed on both sides of the head) results in more memory loss and confusion than does unilateral ECT to the nondominant hemisphere. New developments in medical equipment allow the individual seizure threshold to be determined for each patient and allow titration of "dose" of electrical energy required, thereby diminishing the confusion and amnesia associated with high-powered treatments. Brief-pulse stimulus techniques are also being developed to deliver less electrical energy and, hence, a possible reduction in side effects (Fig. 40-1).[15]

Controversy

Medicolegal and ethical aspects of ECT have been hotly debated. The controversy is apparent in the popular media, in professional journals, and in the courts. Issues involved are right to treatment, right to refuse treatment, competence, and informed consent. Some denounce ECT because of its very nature, and others are strong advocates. There is a fear of the political abuse of psychiatry and the memory of past inhumane treatment. Today, use of ECT is influenced by suggested minimum standards established by the American Psychiatric Association in 1978 and updated in 1985. Its use is controlled from state to state by statute, in varying degrees. In most states, laws address the following areas: medical practice and qualifications of physicians, record keeping, competency, consent, and due process.[23] It is hoped that the current trend toward research and refinement of technique will influence the amount of emotion connected with the evaluation of ECT as a treatment alternative.

Common Nursing Diagnoses

A client undergoing ECT will likely have a number of nursing diagnoses related to a clinical picture of major depression. These might include hopelessness; altered nutrition, less than body requirements; self care deficit; sleep pattern disturbance; and impaired social interaction. Suicide potential must always be assessed. Diagnoses that may relate specifically to the ECT treatment include knowledge deficit, fear, and memory loss.

Nursing Roles

Nursing actions for a client undergoing ECT are similar to those required for clients undergoing other procedures under anesthesia. The teaching and supportive

FIGURE 40–1. Modern ECT requires state-of-the-art equipment and the presence of a prepared nurse, anesthesiologist, and physician. (Courtesy of Media Services, Providence Medical Center, Seattle, Washington)

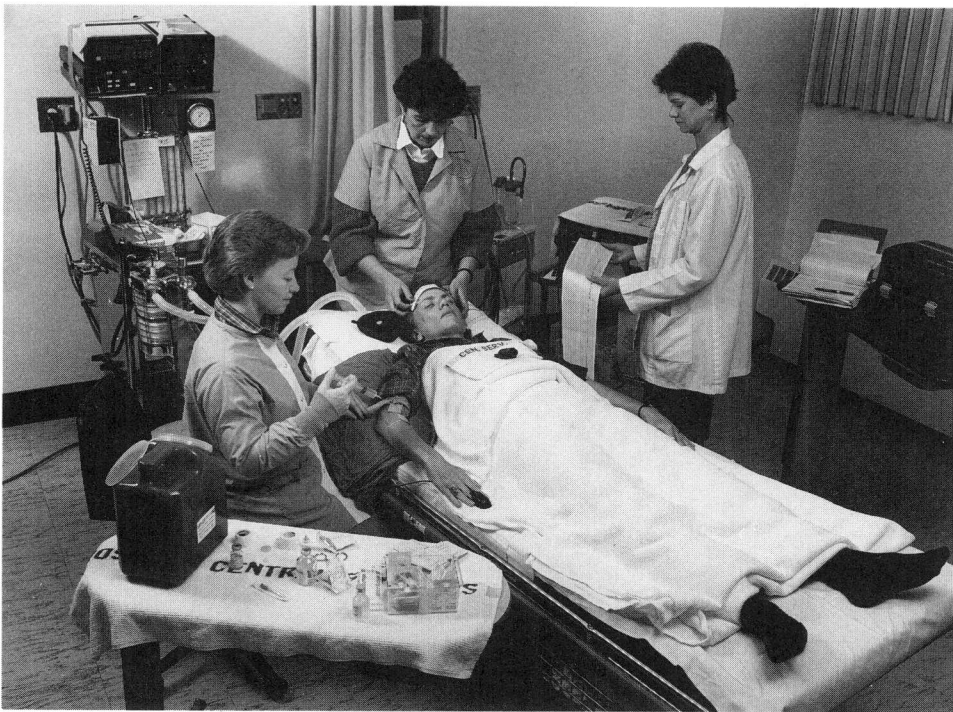

roles of the psychiatric mental health nurse with both the client and family are important to emphasize. In addition, the nurse must assess the effects the treatment is having on the client and monitor for signs of improvement or memory loss. Other important nursing functions in caring for the client receiving ECT include documentation of client response in the patient record, communication with other health team members, and participation in decision making with the treatment team (Fig. 40-2).

OTHER CONTEMPORARY BIOLOGIC THERAPIES

Psychosurgery

Similar to ECT, the psychosurgery performed today has little in common with the procedures of the past. It is now accepted that the limbic system plays a major role in regulating emotions, and psychosurgery is aimed at interrupting microscopic pathways within this system. Operations, such as cingulotomy, do not have most of the adverse effects associated with the prefrontal lobotomies performed before 1955. Psychosurgery is used by some for relieving the symptoms of severe depression not responding to medication or ECT. It has also been used for the treatment of epilepsy and chronic pain. In patients who experience thought disorders, psychosurgery eliminates the affective component, but has no effect on other symptoms.[3] The nursing role in caring for a patient who has undergone psychosurgery includes monitoring neurologic status

and assisting with resocialization in individual and group therapy. Serious questions about the ethics of psychosurgery were raised in the early 1970s over the rumored use of brain surgery as a means of control of convicts and violent patients. Psychosurgery was debated in the popular press, in congressional hearings, in professional meetings, and in legal circles. As a result, legislation restricting or banning the practice of psychosurgery was enacted by most states and, by 1982, fewer than 200 operations a year were being performed in this country.[20] Psychosurgery continues in the United Kingdom, Australia, and some European countries and psychiatric centers abroad are conducting research and publishing guidelines.[3]

Amobarbital (Amytal) Interviews

Narcotherapy, also known as "truth serum" or amobarbital (Amytal) interviews, was first used widely in World War II to treat traumatic neurosis. The terms refer to the use of intravenous barbituates to produce a light trancelike state.[1] Today, amobarbital interviews are used as an adjunct to psychotherapy, to promote freer communication, to overcome resistance, to gain more data for assessment, or to confirm a diagnosis. Occasionally, a videotape of the interview may be used to present "hidden" material to the patient, with supportive guidance, or to convince the patient of a diagnosis. Risks include that of physiologic or psychological dependence on the drug used to produce the desired mental state. The actual procedure needs to be performed in a setting where adequately trained staff and

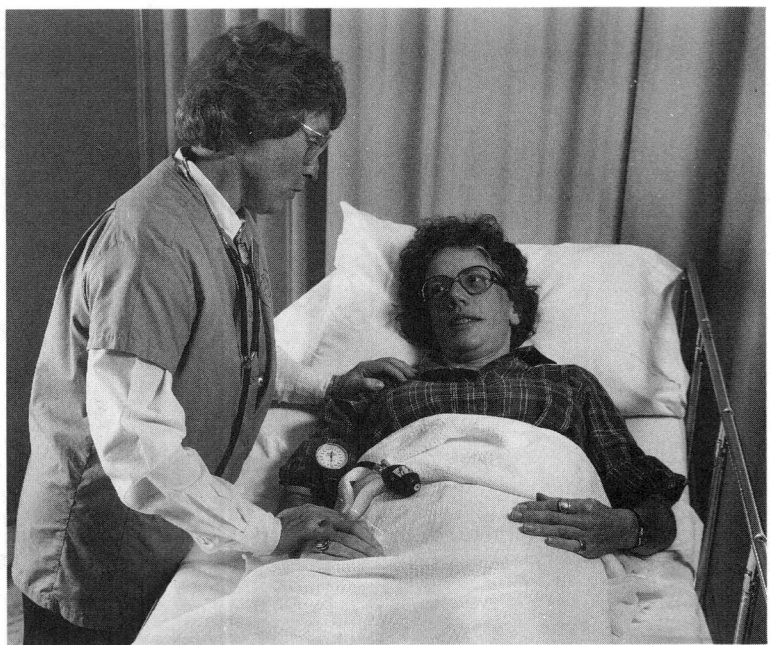

FIGURE 40–2. The nurse offers brief, frequent orienting contacts during the recovery phase. The use of touch is often reassuring. (Courtesy of Media Services, Providence Medical Center, Seattle, Washington)

emergency equipment are available. A patient may awaken from an interview in an agitated, distraught state, and staff members must be prepared to ensure the safety of all concerned.[1]

Detoxification

The belief that a toxin may be the cause of mental illness has recurred throughout history. In 1977, hemodialysis was used in the United States by Wagemaker and Cade to remove a polypeptide believed to cause schizophrenia. There was early enthusiasm for this therapy, but initial positive research findings were not replicated. Today dialysis units in this country are no longer used to treat mental illness. A very real and useful role of dialysis, however, is in the detoxification of patients after potentially lethal overdose ingestions.[1]

Orthomolecular Psychiatry

Orthomolecular refers to the underlying premise that the molecular composition of the brain is corrected in this treatment.

Orthomolecular or megavitamin therapy was first proposed in 1952 when large doses of nicotinic acid were used to detoxify methylated biogenic amines believed to cause schizophrenia. This treatment was reported to be highly effective, but again, attempts at replication were unsuccessful.[1]

In 1967, Pauling proclaimed that deficiency of ascorbic acid was the basis of many illnesses, including mental disorders. His work, combined with the earlier work on biogenic amines, led to an approach in which large doses of vitamins, minerals, hormones, and dietary regimens were prescribed for schizophrenia.

In 1972, an American Psychiatric Association task force concluded that claims of success were based on inadequate research.[1] Patients were often treated with other modalities in addition to the megavitamin therapy, and these modalities seemed more likely to be responsible for improvement. However, there are still clinicians, clients, and families around the country who are convinced that the orthomolecular approach is sound. *The Eden Express* by Mark Vonnegut gives an enlightening account not only of his experience of schizophrenia, but of his positive response to orthomolecular psychiatry.[21]

CASE STUDY

Mr. Stephen O, a 52-year-old successful business executive, was admitted to a private psychiatric hospital because of sudden onset of suicidal ideation and intent. His wife and grown son had been forced to remain with Stephen constantly at home for the previous three days to prevent him from harming himself. Stephen had the delusional belief that he had lost all of the family's resources in a bad business investment and was preoccupied with guilt and worthlessness. Stephen had one previous experience of a moderate depression that resolved untreated, and several previous episodes of extreme energy and productivity. He had a mild heart attack two years before hospitalization, but suffered no permanent damage to the heart muscle and modified his stressful life-style very little. Stephen's father committed suicide at age 60 by gunshot. Stephen's DSM-III-R diagnosis was bipolar disorder, depressed, with mood congruent psychotic features. In the hospital, Stephen's nursing diagnosis of suicide potential related to depression initially required one-to-one nursing care to prevent self-harm. Because of the sudden onset and lethality of his symptoms, the psychiatrist recommended ECT. A consultant psychiatrist was asked to review the case and concurred in this recommendation. Family members were at first reluctant to

STEPHEN O

NURSING INTERVENTIONS	OUTCOME CRITERIA
Initial Plan	
NURSING DIAGNOSIS: Suicide potential related to depression	
CLIENT GOAL: Remain safe and not harm self	
■ Provide for one-to-one care ■ Provide safe environment ■ Establish no suicide contract and verify every shift	Has decreased potential for suicide
NURSING DIAGNOSIS: Fear of ECT related to lack of knowledge	
CLIENT GOAL: Express perceptions and concerns	
■ Help Stephen identify specific perceptions and concerns about ECT	Has decreased fear
CLIENT GOAL: Gain more information about ECT	
■ Provide information appropriate to Stephen's needs and situation ■ Offer teaching resources to family and enlist their support and participation	Has increased knowledge and comfort concerning ECT
Addition After Second ECT Treatment	
NURSING DIAGNOSIS: Memory loss related to ECT	
CLIENT GOAL: Experience less frustration with memory lapse	
■ Encourage sharing of experiences with other clients who have received ECT ■ Post calendar, schedule, and brief biographic summary near bedside stand ■ Offer orienting comments frequently ■ Report significant mental status changes to treatment team and document in patient record	Verbalizes understanding of transient nature of memory problems Uses orienting aids

consider ECT, but were able to support the recommendation after viewing a teaching videotape and discussing their concerns with the psychiatrist and the psychiatric nurse. Stephen agreed to the treatment after a day of fearful and ambivalent dialogue with his family, psychiatrist, and psychiatric mental health nurse, and gave written consent. The pre-ECT workup yielded no contraindications, and a course of treatment was scheduled. He received nine right unilateral brief pulse ECT treatments. After the second treatment he became less concerned about his family's finances and denied intent to harm himself. He was included in the unit community meeting and his status was changed from "suicide precautions" to "close observation." After the fourth treatment, Stephen complained about not remembering what circumstances brought him to the hospital and was observed to be forgetful of new information. A nursing diagnosis of memory loss related to ECT was made. After six treatments Stephen had been included in all unit activities and expressed dismay that he was such a worry to his family. After his final ECT treatment and three weeks in the

hospital, Stephen was eager to return home. Although frustrated by his lapses in memory, he seemed appreciative of the support he received from those around him. He was agreeable to taking maintenance antidepressant medication and keeping regular therapy appointments, and planned to gradually return to his challenging job. Three months after his hospitalization, Stephen was successfully working and interacting with his family. He noted no further problems with memory impairment and, in therapy, was exploring ways to moderate his fast-paced life. He and his family evidenced understanding of the early warning signs of recurrent depression (see Nursing Care Plan 40-1 for a sample care plan for Stephen O).

SUMMARY

This chapter has reviewed the development of the major biologic therapies, other than psychotropic med-

Research Highlights

Attitudes of professionals toward a treatment or procedure can greatly influence therapeutic outcomes, and it follows that nurses' ambivalence or negative feelings about ECT will be communicated to the patient and render the treatment course less than effective. The nursing literature reflects the interest, concern, and polarized viewpoints members of the profession hold regarding the use of ECT.[4,12,14,19]

Janicak and his colleagues reported the results of a study to determine the attitudes of mental health professionals toward ECT and the variables that may affect such attitudes.[8] A questionnaire including an ECT knowledge scale, two ECT attitude scales, a self-evaluation of knowledge, and questions concerning professional background and clinical experience was sent to 200 mental health professionals. Students and practicing professionals in medicine, nursing, social work, and psychology were included. There were 195 respondents. Five separate analyses were made to determine if there were significant relationships among the variables of clinical experience, knowledge, professional training, and attitudes toward ECT.

Results indicated that the more knowledge and clinical experience a mental health professional has, the more positive his or her attitude will be toward ECT as an effective treatment modality. Knowledge scores increased with clinical experience, and physicians and nurses had the highest knowledge scores. The authors recommended that student- and staff-training programs be developed and implemented that provide factual and experiential knowledge about ECT to minimize the possibility of its underutilization.

---

ication, from 1930 until the present day. Initial therapies evolved from trial and error of professionals overwhelmed with caring for hundreds of thousands of institutionalized mentally ill. Hydrotherapy gave way to pharmacoconvulsive therapies, psychosurgery, and unmodified ECT. In retrospect, these treatments seem inhumane, and the period in psychiatric care before the introduction of neuroleptics has a negative public image.

With the introduction of medication, increasing legal and ethical concerns, improved research, and beginning biochemical explanations for mental illness and treatments, most of these therapies have been abandoned. Modern ECT, however, is increasingly being utilized as a safe and effective treatment in certain well-defined situations. The nursing role in the care of patients undergoing ECT is similar to the role in other medical treatments, but it is of primary importance that the nurse examine personal attitudes and beliefs about this treatment.

References

1. Campbell RJ. Miscellaneous organic therapies. In: Kaplan HI, Sadock BJ, eds. Comprehensive textbook of psychiatry, 4th ed. Baltimore: Williams & Wilkins; 1985.
2. Cook KG. Electroconvulsive therapy for the affectively disordered. In: Rogers CA, Ulsafer-Van Lanen J, eds. Nursing interventions in depression. New York: Grune & Stratton; 1985.
3. Donnelly J. Psychosurgery. In: Kaplan HI, Sadock BJ, eds. Comprehensive textbook of psychiatry, 4th ed. Baltimore: Williams & Wilkins, 1985.
4. Fine M, Jenike M. Electroshock—exploding the myths. RN. 1985;48(9):58–66.
5. Fink M. Neuroendocrine aspects of convulsive therapy. In: Abrams R, Essman W, eds. Electroconvulsive therapy, biological foundations and clinical applications. New York: Spectrum Publications; 1982.
6. Green H. I never promised you a rose garden. New York: Holt, Rinehart and Winston; 1964.
7. Hamilton M. Electroconvulsive therapy: indications and contraindications. In: Malitz S, Sackeim H, eds. Electroconvulsive therapy, clinical and basic research issues. Ann NY Acad Sci. 1986;462:7–10.
8. Janicak P, Mask J, Trimakas K, Gibbons R. ECT: an assessment of mental health professionals' knowledge and attitudes. J Clin Psychiatry. 1985;46:262–266.
9. Kalinowski LB. History of convulsive therapy. In: Malitz S, Sackeim H, eds. Electroconvulsive therapy, clinical and basic research issues. Ann NY Acad Sci. 1986.
10. Kalinowski LB. The history of electroconvulsive therapy. In: Abrams R, Essman W, eds. Electroconvulsive therapy, biological foundations and clinical applications. New York: Spectrum Publications; 1982.
11. Kesey K. One flew over the cuckoo's nest. New York: Viking Press; 1962.
12. Mawson D. Shock waves. Nurs Times. 1985;81(46):42–44.
13. National Institute of Mental Health. Consensus conference on electroconvulsive therapy. JAMA. 1985;254:2103–2108.
14. Packham H. A shocking business. Nurs Mirror. 1984;159:19–21.
15. Runck B. ECT: assuring benefits and minimizing risks. Hosp Comm Psychiatry. 1983;34:409–410.
16. Selvin B. Electroconvulsive therapy—1987. Anesthesiology. 1987;67:367–385.
17. Squire LR. Neuropsychological effects of ECT. In: Abrams R, Essman W, eds. Electroconvulsive therapy, biological foundations and clinical applications. New York: Spectrum Publications; 1982.
18. Squire S. Shock therapy's return to respectability. NY Times Magazine. 1987;Nov 22.
19. Talbot K. ECT: exploring myths, examining attitudes. J Psychosoc Nurs Ment Health Serv. 1986;24:6–11.
20. Valenstein E. Great and desperate cures. New York: Basic Books; 1986.
21. Vonnegut M. The Eden express. New York: Praeger Publishers; 1975.
22. Weiner RD, Rogers HJ, Davidson JR, Squire LR. Effect of stimulus parameters on cognitive side effects. In: Malitz S, Sackeim H, eds. Electroconvulsive therapy, clinical and basic research issues. Ann NY Acad Sci. 1986.
23. Winslade WJ, Liston EH, Ross JW, Weber KD. Regulation of ECT in the United States. Am J Psychiatry. 1984;141:1349–1355.

41

Fe Nieves-Khouw

Behavior Therapy

OBJECTIVES
After reading this chapter, the reader will be able to:
1. Discuss the assumptions and key concepts of behavior therapy
2. Define problems and therapeutic goals in behavioral terms
3. Design a behavior therapy based care plan
4. Discuss the applicability of behavior therapy to different target client populations in various therapeutic settings.

BEHAVIOR THERAPY AS A TECHNIQUE

Introduction

Behavior therapy emerged in the 1950s as an alternative approach to psychodynamic theory. It grew out of what was regarded as the lack of specificity and verifiability of the treatment outcomes of intrapsychic approaches. As it is practiced today, behavior therapy connotes an approach, rather than a formal system.[6] But, it is more than a set of techniques. It is a comprehensive orientation and practice that treats behavioral problems and is based primarily on operant conditioning principles and procedures.[3] Behavior therapy differs from psychodynamic therapy and other, more traditional, approaches by focusing on recent antecedents and consequences of behavior and rejecting remote causes, such as unconscious motivation, to explain behavior. Behavior, instead of being seen as a symptom of deeper psychological pathology, is regarded as significant in its own right and is the focus of treatment.

The behavior approach considers normal and dysfunctional behavior to be learned through the same processes.[15] The treatment focuses on behaviors that either have been learned or need to be learned. Because behavior therapy is concerned with the development of adaptive behavior, it strongly emphasizes methodology and objective verification of treatment outcomes. Treatment goals are stated in terms of accurate and detailed descriptions of behavior or behavioral units. Observations and assessments are critical in the design and implementation of treatment.

In behavior therapy, therapists are actively involved with the clients in the role of teacher and model. Contrary to the belief that behavioral techniques are distant, cold, and sometimes inhumane,

> . . . behavior therapy cannot be implemented in a rigid, robot-like fashion. However, the therapeutic relationship assumes a different role in behavior therapy from the role it assumes in many traditional modes of psychotherapy. In behavior therapy, the therapeutic relationship facilitates implementing the primary therapeutic procedures, which directly influence the maintaining conditions of the target behavior. A good therapeutic relationship is necessary but is not a sufficient condition for effective behavior therapy (reference 19, p 328).

Hersen further states ". . . experience has shown that a warm relationship with the client is mandatory for the successful application of the many facets of a given behavioral strategy" (reference 14, p 9).

One major disadvantage of psychodynamic treatment is that clients are often taken out of their natural environment and brought into the office of specially trained professionals for treatment. Behavior therapists believe that behavior of a person removed from the natural environment is not likely to be the same as the problematic behavior in the original natural situation. Moreover, the environmental conditions that contribute to the problem behavior may be present only in the original situation.[15] In behavior therapy, the client's environment and social network are significant in the identification of naturally occurring antecedents and reinforcers. Parents, teachers, spouses, and friends are often important resources in the treatment of behavioral problems. They provide reinforcers within the client's natural environment that encourage generalization of skill and transfer of learning. In behavior therapy, transfer of learning is a significant stage of treatment that encourages self-management and discourages dependence on the therapist.

In summary, Hersen[12] defined *behavior therapy* as ". . . comprising those approaches to treatment of maladaptive behavior that focus on observables and that are derived from experimentally established procedures and principles of behavior" (reference 12, p 34). A more extensive definition was quoted by Franks[6] from the Association for the Advancement of Behavior Therapy. According to this definition

> Behavior therapy involves primarily the application of principles derived from research in experimental and social psychology for the alleviation of human suffering and the advancement of human functioning. Behavior therapy emphasizes a systematic evaluation of the effectiveness of its application. Behavior therapy involves environmental change and social interaction rather than direct alteration of bodily processes by biological procedures. The aim is primarily educational. The techniques facilitate improved self-control. In the conduct of behavior therapy, a contractual agreement is negotiated, in which mutually agreeable goals and procedures are specified. Reasonable practitioners using approaches are guided by generally acceptable ethical principles (reference 6, p 45).

Behavior Therapy Approaches

Behavior therapy is significantly related to learning. Four types of learning theories form the basis for the four approaches to behavior therapy as it is practiced today.[6,13,15,16] (1) Stimulus response theory forms the basis for the classical conditioning approach; (2) operant theory uses reinforcement schedules as the basis for operant conditioning strategies; (3) social learning theory assumes that individuals learn by observing others, and this forms the basis for approaches such as social skill training, assertion training, and participant modeling;[2] (4) cognitive theory assumes the significance of mediational covert activity in the determination of behavior. This theory forms the basis for covert conditioning approaches such as rational–emotive therapy and self-instructional training. Classical and operant conditioning approaches will be described in more detail in this chapter. Cognitive behavioral therapy will be discussed in Chapter 42.

Classical Conditioning

Pavlov theorized that behavior is an involuntary response to the environmental stimuli that precede it.[15] Classical conditioning, therefore, is concerned with stimuli that evoke certain automatic responses. This behavior therapy approach attempts to structure specific responses by pairing stimuli. The main concepts of classical conditioning are the following: (1) Unconditioned stimulus—is any environmental phenomenon that evokes an automatic response—for example, the presentation of food, which stimulates salivation. (2) Unconditioned response usually refers to automatic or involuntary behavior elicited by an unconditioned stimulus, for example, the blinking reflex in response to a jab aimed at an individual's eyes. (3) Classical conditioning is a process by which a predetermined response is gradually structured through pairing of antecedent stimuli. Two unconditioned stimuli occur simultaneously until either of them, occurring alone, produces the same response as was produced by the paired stimuli. (4) Conditioned stimulus is a stimulus which, after being strategically paired with an unconditioned stimulus, produces the same response as the unconditioned stimulus. (5) Conditioned response is a predetermined response brought about by repeated exposures to conditioned stimulus.

The following situation illustrates the process of classical conditioning.

> An adult male was placed in an empty room where there was a blinking yellow light and showed no anxiety reaction. However, when he was exposed to the sounds of sirens and alarm bells ringing, he looked around anxiously, became restless, and fidgeted in his seat. By means of classical conditioning, the response of fear can be structured by repeated exposure of this man to both the sight of a blinking yellow light and the sounds of sirens and alarm bells. His response would be considered conditioned when he reacts with fear and anxiety when exposed solely to the stimulus of the blinking yellow light.

Box 41–1 shows how the fear response was conditioned to the neutral stimulus of the blinking yellow light after it has been paired with the stimulus sounds of sirens and alarm bells.

Behavior techniques derived from the principles of classical conditioning are used in the treatment of a range of behavioral problems ranging from cigarette smoking to deviant sexual behavior and are commonly used with clients with diagnoses of developmental disorders, gender identity disorders, or anxiety disorders (or anxiety and phobic neuroses). Examples of classical conditioning techniques are systematic desensitization, flooding, and implosive therapy.[2] A treatment example is described in Box 41–2.

Operant Conditioning

Operant conditioning is the theory that supports most behavior therapy techniques as they are currently practiced. The concept of operant conditioning, developed by B. F. Skinner, holds that behaviors are learned and are increased or decreased depending on their impact on the environment.[6] The environment responds to the behavior by way of consequences or reinforcers. It is these reinforcers that affect the frequency by which the behavior will be repeated.

Operant conditioning differs from classical conditioning in that it focuses on reinforcers rather than antecedents. Although operant conditioning acknowledges the presence of antecedent stimuli in the causation of behavior, it maintains that whether the behavior is learned or not is a function of the environmental response. The key principles of operant conditioning are the following: (1) Operant behavior—behavior is considered operant when it has impact on the environment and generates consequences that, in turn, affect the frequency by which the behavior is repeated. (2) Reinforcers are consequences or events that follow behavior, strengthening or weakening the behavior. (3) Contingent behavior is behavior that, when performed, results in the delivery of specific consequences or reinforcers. (4) Operant conditioning is the process of altering behavior through the manipulation of the environmental consequences that follow it. In operant conditioning, an antecedent stimulus is considered a cue that sets the stage for the behavior. The probability that the behavior will occur depends on environmental reinforcers. (5) Extinction refers to no longer following behavior with an event that was previously delivered.[15]

In Box 41–3, the behavior is a response to apparent feelings of being left out; the environmental consequence is immediate attention from the nurse. If this chain is not altered by altering the consequences, it is

---

BOX 41–1
Process of Classical Conditioning

	STIMULUS	RESPONSE
Neutral stimulus	Blinking yellow light	No fear
Unconditioned stimulus	Sound of sirens and alarm bells	Fear, anxiety
Classical conditioning	Blinking yellow light and sound of sirens and alarm bells	Fear, anxiety
Conditioned stimuli	Blinking yellow light	Fear, anxiety (conditioned response)

BOX 41–2
Treatment Example Using Classical Conditioning

BACKGROUND
A 32-year-old professional sought treatment for a two-pack-a-day smoking habit. The client had developed decreased cardiac function and was strongly advised to quit smoking.

ASSESSMENT
The client was asked to keep a diary for a week, focusing on antecedents of his smoking behavior. After seven days, the diary revealed a specific pattern of heavy smoking when attending meetings and conferring with colleagues. Smoking was least observed when the client was writing.

CLASSICAL CONDITIONING
Classical conditioning in this case was accomplished through stimulus control. Because the stimulus of meetings led to increased smoking, and the stimulus of writing revealed decreased smoking, pairing the two stimuli—taking minutes (writing) and attending meetings—could structure the response of decreased smoking to the conditioned stimulus, meetings.

OUTCOME
After two months of conscientiously pairing the stimulus of attending meetings with the stimulus of taking minutes, the client was able to sit through meetings without taking minutes and without reaching for a cigarette.

TRANSFER
Once the biggest hurdle of associating meetings with smoking was broken, it was easier for the client to transfer the nonsmoking behavior first to conferences with colleagues, then to other work-oriented situations, and finally to his smoking habit at home.

---

ety disorders, medical conditions, such as hypertension, migraine headaches and pain, schizophrenia, impulse control disorders, and marital problems. A treatment example is described in Box 41–4.

The Process of Operant Conditioning

IDENTIFYING THE PROBLEM

To objectively describe a problem and establish a baseline for intervention, it is necessary to focus on the actual behavior manifested by the client. To operationalize behavior means to describe behavior according to actual observation without interpretation or rater judgment. Some authors have also referred to these descriptions as pinpointed behavior. Examples of pinpointed statements are (1) Johnny eats only a third of his meals, wakes up at 4 AM and is not able to go back to sleep, sits alone crying softly during the day, (2) Don was observed to have slammed the telephone, cursed out loud, and refused to talk to staff members after he finished talking to his mother on the telephone; (3) Linda is prancing up and down the hallway, talking very loudly and touching male peers on the neck, asking for a kiss. Pinpointed behavioral statements facilitate problem identification in that they are more observable and can potentially reduce disagreement among caregivers, allowing consistency in the focus of treatment, not only among nursing professionals, but also others on the multidisciplinary team.

TARGET BEHAVIOR

The target behavior, the behavior that is to be strengthened or weakened through operant conditioning, is defined by establishing what, where, when, how frequently, and in what situation the behavior is to be performed. The target behavior should be within the person's repertoire of responses. If the person is not able to do the expected behavior, it should be taught, modeled, and practiced before it is expected to be demonstrated. The behavior chosen to be subjected to operant conditioning techniques could be any one of the following[1]: (1) an adaptive behavior that needs to be strengthened; (2) maladaptive behavior that needs to be weakened or extinguished; (3) adaptive behavior that is to be taught and reinforced to replace maladaptive be-

likely that this client will maintain or increase this inappropriate behavior to gain attention.

The principles of operant conditioning are frequently applied in residential treatment settings ranging from inpatient units for acute and chronic psychiatric patients to residential facilities for juvenile delinquents. They are also used in classrooms as tools teachers use to motivate their students. Principles of operant conditioning are used in the treatment of a wide variety of problems including psychoactive substance use disorders, disruptive behavior disorders, eating disorders, sexual dysfunctions, organic mental syndromes, anxi-

---

BOX 41–3
How Antecedent, Behavior, and Consequences Are Linked

CUE/ANTECEDENT	BEHAVIOR	CONSEQUENCE
Other clients playing cards and talking together	Crying and yelling, running around in circles	Immediate nurse attention and counseling

BOX 41–4
Treatment Example Using Operant Conditioning

BACKGROUND
Johnny, a nine-year-old third grader, was referred to the clinic for problems of hyperactivity and attention deficit in the classroom. The teacher stated that this boy is intelligent and can easily do third-grade work "if only he would settle down to do this work."

ASSESSMENT
Data were collected over a period of five days. The boy was observed for 45-minute periods and data were collected on (1) how many times he got out of his seat and (2) how long he was able to sit and do work. The observer also recorded the teacher's and the students' responses to the boy every time he got up, as well as when he was concentrating on doing his work.
In a 45-minute period, the boy got up an average of five times. Every time he got up, the teacher was immediately by his side, and the classmates seated around him looked toward his direction. He was able to sit an average of ten minutes to do his work. The teacher helped other students when the boy was quietly attending to his school work.
It was further established that the behavior happened most when Johnny was asked to do a work sheet or read and do work on his own.

OPERANT CONDITIONING
A more detailed discussion of operant conditioning will follow. The following serves only as an illustration of the process.

TARGET BEHAVIOR
Johnny will not get up out of his seat and will be able to attend to his schoolwork for 45 minutes.

Intermediate Goals And Stages

1. Johnny will get up from his seat only four times and be able to attend to his schoolwork for at least 15 minutes.
2. Johnny will get up from his seat only twice and be able to attend to his schoolwork for a 20-minute stretch during a 45-minute school period.
3. Johnny will get up only once during a 45-minute period and be able to concentrate on his schoolwork for 30 minutes.

REINFORCERS
The teacher will ignore Johnny whenever he gets up; she will work with other students instead.
The other students will continue to do their work and not look at him or give him attention. The cooperation of the other students was facilitated by informing them that Johnny will be working on a project of concentrating on finishing his work and discussing with them the importance of their role in helping Johnny reach his goal. The teacher will praise Johnny and stand by his desk when he is doing his work. Every time Johnny is able to complete a 15-minute period without getting up, he will get a gold star by his name on the board.
These reinforcers will be kept all through the different intermediate goals. Every time Johnny is able to spend a full 45-minute period doing his work, he will be given a treat by the teacher, e.g., baseball cards and sticker cards.

OUTCOME
Reinforcement of the incompatible behavior (attending to schoolwork) led to the extinction of the problem behavior (getting up from seat).

GENERALIZATION
Johnny's ability to work through a 45-minute period can be transferred to other school periods.

havior; or (4) adaptive behavior that needs to be generalized to other situations. An example follows:

Identified Problem: Lisa falls asleep in group on Wednesday afternoon.

Target Behavior: Lisa will speak out two times during Mr. Gray's social skills group on Wednesday afternoon.

ASSESSMENT

The assessment phase includes developing baseline data as well as identifying the client's strengths and weaknesses. Identifying the client's strengths and weaknesses helps to determine whether or not the desired behavior is within the client's repertoire of responses. A behavioral history is taken to establish the client's pattern of responses and to reveal specific limitations that deter the client from performing the desired behavior. Baseline data is a measure of the fre-

quency or extent of the identified problem. It serves two purposes[7]: (1) It verifies whether the problem is in fact a problem; and (2) it provides a data base with which the response to the operant-conditioning program can be compared. Baseline data then serve to verify whether treatment or rehabilitation has occurred. The establishment of baseline data involves gathering information about the frequency and duration of the target behavior,[5] as well as its antecedents and consequences. Measuring behavior is accomplished through (1) counting, which is the method of choice for measuring how frequently a behavior is observed, for example, counting the frequency of a client's walking behavior at night. (2) Checking is applicable when the purpose of gathering the information is to establish the presence or absence of behavior by direct observation. A routine procedure in most inpatient units is to conduct rounds at regular intervals during the night between 10 PM and 6 AM to check on each patient's sleeping pattern. Checking on the presence or absence of sleep is important, especially for clients who are suffering from mood disorders, anxiety disorders, and for those who are very psychotic. (3) Timing as a measure of behavior is most applicable to problems of duration and length, for example, timing the length of a tantrum displayed by a preschooler, timing the length of time a client is able to concentrate on a task. (4) When an individual exhibits both positive and negative behaviors, it is helpful to determine the *ratio* of negative behaviors/positive behaviors, for example, a client's self-controlled behavior (not yelling, hitting, or swearing at) can be compared with the number of times when there is loss of control.

The value of the baseline data is dependent on the accuracy of record keeping. Checklists, charts, diaries, and schedules are examples of record-keeping methods. Raw data can then be transformed into graphs (bar or line graphs) to chart a pattern or illustrate the frequency or extent of the identified problem. To be useful, charts should contain the name of the client as well as the name of the rater. Specific instructions on the behavior to be observed, the frequency of observation, the duration of observation, and the codes to be used to record the information should be explicit.

CONSEQUENCES

Assessment of consequences should include an identification of positive and negative reinforcers. Positive reinforcers are consequences that, when delivered, maintain or increase the behavior that precedes them. *Positive reinforcement* is associated with desirable consequences, such as praise, attention, material rewards, or awards. The term *reward* is often used interchangeably with positive reinforcer; but, a reward or an event that immediately follows behavior and may be perceived by the client as positive is not necessarily a positive reinforcer. A positive reinforcer is defined by its effect on behavior.[15] Therefore, a reward, if it does not lead to the increase or maintenance of the behavior that precedes it, cannot be considered positively reinforcing. On the other hand, an event that would normally be considered negative could be perceived as positive by the client. For example, in a facility for adjudicated juvenile delinquents, the staff observed that physically restraining some youths who are out of control does not result in the decrease of the incidents of combative behavior. As more information emerged, it was discovered that for those youths, being physically restrained was not an aversive experience, but rather, an opportunity for human physical contact. For these clients, what would normally constitute an aversive condition was actually positively reinforcing. There are four simple rules to follow to assure effective reinforcement: (1) make reinforcement contingent upon appropriate behavior; (2) reinforce consistently; (3) reinforce immediately; and (4) reinforce genuinely (especially when giving praise and attention).[4]

Negative reinforcement refers to the removal of an aversive event following the performance of a response. A requisite of negative reinforcement is the presence of an aversive condition. An example is the client who has been placed in locked seclusion because of threatening and aggressive behavior. When the client behaves in a cooperative, nonthreatening manner, he or she is allowed out of the seclusion room. The removal of the aversive condition, locked seclusion, is negatively reinforcing if it increases or maintains the client's cooperative and nonhostile demeanor. In contrast, *punishment* is the application of an aversive stimulus, or withholding of positive stimulus, in response to the undesired behavior. Consider the same example, placing the client who presents with threatening and aggressive behavior in locked seclusion is punishment. Its removal after the performance of appropriate behavior on the part of the client is negative reinforcement. Punishment is not an effective and desirable reinforcer when it is not partnered with teaching appropriate behavior. The use of punishment can lead to avoidance of similar situations, sneakiness, or lying behavior. By itself, punishment does not encourage the learning of more adaptive behavior.

Reinforcers are situation- and person-specific. What reinforces one individual may not reinforce another. What reinforces an individual at one time may not reinforce the same individual at another time. Food may be a reinforcer for a hungry individual, but not for an individual who is nauseated or for an individual who has just eaten and is not hungry. Types of reinforcers include (1) material—food, money, clothing; (2) social—praise, attention, achievement awards, recognition; (3) activity—going to the movies, group or individual games, parties.

The *Premack principle* states that when the performance of a preferred or high frequency behavior is made contingent upon the performance of the target behavior, the performance of the target behavior will increase.[4] An example is the client who likes to sit and watch television (high frequency behavior) will be allowed to do so only after he sits with staff and converses for ten minutes every morning (target behavior).

In the token economy treatment approach, specific behaviors are assigned values.[8] Performance of specific appropriate behaviors leads to the accumulation of tokens or points, which can then be exchanged for different backup reinforcers. An essential component of token economies is the presence of a wide array of backup reinforcers. These backup reinforcers are also assigned values. Butler and Rosenthal[4] list the merits of the use of tokens: (1) they are easily recorded; (2) they give the individual a choice of how the token is going to be spent; (3) they are easily carried about by staff; (4) they are tangible; (5) they are durable; (6) there is no satiation because of a wide variety of backup reinforcers; (7) they cannot be stolen; (8) they can be given continuously during treatment; (9) they can be easily controlled; (10) they have an educational value; and (11) they bridge the delay between desired response and a reinforcer. An example of the token economy approach is assigning ten tokens for verbally participating in group therapy; five tokens for eating in the dining room using fork and knife. Tokens earned can be exchanged for material, activity, or social reinforcers: two tokens exchanged for candy, whereas going to the dance on Friday needs ten tokens. Token economies work when they are applied as part of a unit-wide or facility-wide behavior therapy program.

PROGRAM DESIGN

Program design should include input from the client and consideration of what is realistic in the client's environment, specifically the environment in which the target behavior occurs. Program design should include the following steps: (1) Operationally define the target behavior or behaviors. In defining the target behavior, it is important to validate whether the target behavior is part of the client's repertoire of behavior. (2) Establish good baseline data, including cues that occasion the behavior as well as the timing of the behavior. (3) Plan to teach and model the behavior if it is not part of the client's repertoire. (4) Design a reinforcement or consequence plan. This stage of the program design should include choosing the effective reinforcers to use; defining the schedule of reinforcements; and identifying the persons who will provide the reinforcers. Also, in this stage of the program design, other methods of dealing with the problem behavior are identified. The problem behavior can be ignored or not reinforced, whereas positive reinforcers are applied when the appropriate behavior is demonstrated; response cost[11] is when a previously acquired reinforcer is taken away upon the display of inappropriate behavior. The reinforcer that is taken away may or may not have a direct relationship with the offense. Loss of privileges is a common example of response cost. Use of time-out or the imposition of other aversive conditions in response to the display of inappropriate behavior is another way to deal with behavior. Response costs may be planned when designing a conditioning program. Positive reinforcers to be used can be identified in several ways:[4,13] (1) asking a client what is reinforcing; (2) observing a client directly; (3) applying the Premack principle; (4) using reinforcer sampling (i.e., presenting the client with reinforcers with which he is unfamiliar and observing his reactions or asking for his choice); (5) asking the client's family or significant others for ideas of reinforcing events.

PROGRAM IMPLEMENTATION

The program design should be implemented as consistently as possible by all staff members involved in the program. Consistency in the implementation of the program design is necessary to enhance the learning of, or the generalization of, adaptive behavior. In operant conditioning, partial or intermittent reinforcement results in greater resistance to extinction.[16] Butler and Rosenthal[4] discuss the importance of having control over the specified reinforcers. "Where reinforcers are not under the control of the therapist, the possibility of treatment is slight. Lack of reinforcer control occurs mainly under two conditions: (1) where people involved with the patient or program do not cooperate, and (2) where the patient finds ready access to the reinforcer" (reference 4, p 127). In a psychiatric hospital, for example, suspending the smoking privileges of patients caught smoking in designated nonsmoking areas does not improve compliance with this smoking rule because cigarettes and lights are readily available from other patients.

PROGRAM EVALUATION

Program evaluation is an ongoing process accomplished through program monitoring. Strict program monitoring is essential to ascertain the consistency of the program implementation and the accomplishment of specified program outcomes at different stages. Intermittent adjustments and reworking of the program may be necessary at certain points when problems arise in program implementation. The goals of treatment are accomplished when the target behavior has been learned or altered. The end behavior is compared with the baseline data. Successful operant conditioning has occurred when adaptive behavior is increased and is followed by pleasant, positive consequences, whereas maladaptive behavior has decreased or been readily associated with aversive or absent reinforcement.

THE NURSE AND BEHAVIOR THERAPY

The concepts and techniques involved in behavior therapy are naturally compatible, not only with the nurse's role in client care, but also her skills and strengths. Behavior therapy proposes planned intervention based on accurate, objective measures and well documented observations. The nurse's education provides her with skills in these areas. The nurse's role as direct caregiver provides the unique arena to observe clients as they negotiate daily living in the environment. Her frequent contacts with clients provide the opportunity to intervene and promote behavioral change. The nurse's knowledge and expertise in the area of health teaching provide the technical tool to teach and model more adaptive behavior.

The nurse's role as an agent of change focuses on four functions:[1,4] (1) increasing adaptive behavior; (2) decreasing maladaptive behavior; (3) altering maladaptive behavior by teaching alternative coping strategies; and (4) increasing the occurrence of adaptive behavior by generalizing to other situations and environments.

Fuoco and Tyson[10] wrote that dependent and institutionalized behaviors are promoted by traditional residential treatment because the environment provided for the clients often does not correspond to the realities of the world outside the program. Butler and Rosenthal[4] further expounded on the direct role of the nurse in promoting dependent and institutionalized behaviors. These authors identify some of the problem areas: (1) Nurse's attitude—if the nurse believes that chronic psychiatric clients have hopeless prognoses, the nurse's behavior toward the clients will communicate such, and more adaptive behaviors are less likely to be encouraged. To counter these attitudes, it is important to emphasize that the emotionally ill client can learn more adaptive behaviors and that nurses play a primary and significant role in accomplishing such a change. (2) Attending to undesirable behavior—bizarre or inappropriate behavior often stands out and demands immediate attention and intervention from the nurse. Consequently, the client's negative behavior is inadvertently reinforced by the nurse's attention and intervention, whereas the quiet, more positive, more adaptive behaviors receive little or no reinforcement. (3) Lack of interaction—nurses generally give low priority to interacting with clients if the interaction is outside of supplying or seeking information. Attention is a powerful positive reinforcer, and quality client interaction can be made contingent on performance of desirable behavior. (4) Stereotyped interaction—nurse's interaction with clients should focus on motivating and teaching the patient to make independent choices and to perform appropriate behavior independently of the nurse's prompting.

In the context of behavior therapy, every nurse–client contact is a therapeutic opportunity to teach, model, or reinforce adaptive behavior. Principles of behavior therapy can be applied to specific problems such as withdrawn behaviors,[10] delusional verbalization,[10] noncommunicative behavior,[4,10] disruptive behavior,[11] skill training,[10,11] and interaction skills, problem solving, and activities of daily living. The techniques available to the nurse are numerous and varied; some of these are defined in Table 41–1. They range from use of time-out,[2] positive and negative reinforcement,[4,8,10,11,18] contracting,[11,14] shaping,[2] chaining,[2] overcorrection,[10,18] selective ignoring (extinction),[2] role-playing,[4] and selective application of attention.[13]

According to Milne,[17] the role of the nurse in behavior therapy programs ranges in complexity from the "applicator" role to the "nurse therapist role." Beginning psychiatric nurses will perform more in the role of "applicator." This role is defined by Milne[17] as applying simple instructions on how to respond to such psychiatric problems as psychotic talk or violence toward other clients. Other roles identified[17] are "technician," a nurse who may be trained in and apply more than one behavioral technique; the "specialist"—a nurse who has greater expertise, but has a restricted range of competence; the "generalist" has a higher level of therapy sophistication and can respond to a wide array of problems; and the "nurse therapist"—a nurse with at least 18 months of training in behavior therapy, who can treat a wide range of problems independently.

CASE STUDY

Debra H is a 20-year-old single mother who was admitted to the hospital for phencyclidine (PCP) intoxication. She has a long history of repeated hospitalizations and has been diagnosed with schizoaffective disorder, bipolar type. Debra and her son live with her mother, who has always given in to Debra's demands, especially when Debra became loud and threatening. Debra's mother has complained of being emotionally exhausted and indicated that she could no longer manage her daughter. Debra's intoxicated state was only one of her behavioral problems. For two days, she was oppositional and sometimes belligerent, but mostly she complained of being very tired and wanted to be left alone to sleep. After she was detoxified, Debra pre-

TABLE 41–1
Behavioral techniques defined

TECHNIQUE	DEFINITION
Time-out	Temporary removal of positively reinforcing environment after display of specific negative behavior.
Positive reinforcement	Application of rewarding consequence following display of target behavior.
Negative reinforcement	Removal of aversive condition following display of target behavior.
Contracting	A set of rules, reinforcements, and consequences agreed upon by the therapist and the client contingent upon performance or nonperformance of target behavior.
Shaping	A technique applied in complex behaviors in which the target behavior is broken down into intermediate approximations of the behavior. Each approximation is then reinforced until the target behavior is achieved.
Chaining	A technique in which a set of responses is linked together, starting from the last response and working backward to the initial response. In chaining, each response is a discriminative reinforcer to the response that preceeds it as well as a discriminative stimulus to the response that follows it.[15]
Overcorrection	Clients are required to correct the negative effects of their behavior and to intensively practice the corresponding appropriate behavior.[19]
Selective ignoring	Not reinforcing (through attention) negative behavior that was previously reinforced.
Role playing	The client practices with the therapist ways to deal with a problem situation by assuming various roles of the significant people involved in the situation.
Selective application of attention	Making attention contingent on performance of target behavior.

NURSING CARE PLAN 41–1

DEBRA H

NURSING INTERVENTIONS	OUTCOME CRITERIA
NURSING DIAGNOSIS: Impaired social interaction related to need for attention and belonging	
CLIENT GOAL: Learn two more appropriate peer interaction behaviors	
Develop Baseline Data	
■ Identify when, where, and with whom the use of loud tone of voice most occurs	Listens and maintains eye contact with peer who is talking
■ Observe Debra's ability to appropriately interact with peers	Voice tone is appropriate to the level of interaction
■ Increase interaction with Debra to provide opportunities for socialization	Maintains a conversation by asking appropriate follow-up questions
■ Teach such skills as listening, eye contact, appropriate joking, and following-up on a question	Laughs and jokes at appropriate times
Reinforce Appropriate Behavior	
■ Give individual attention and praise when taught skills are practiced by Debra in social settings	
■ Ask peers to ignore Debra when she is being loud and to give attention when she is being appropriate	
■ Give Debra a special treat of her choice when she exhibits three days of continuous appropriate interaction behaviors	
NURSING DIAGNOSIS: Moderate aggression towards perceived authority figures	
CLIENT GOAL: Discuss differences in opinion and thinking without becoming argumentative	
■ Give Debra immediate feedback when she is being argumentative	Able to state differing opinion without being argumentative
■ Limit argumentative interaction to two minutes	Listens to explanation given, thinks about it before responding
■ Be available to resume interaction when Debra is more calm	
■ Teach anger control skills Counting from 1 to 20 Taking a deep breath before responding Asking clarifying questions Restating one's opinion Listening closely to what is being said	Shows self-control when hearing an explanation she does not want to hear
■ Provide direct, concise explanation	
■ Extend interaction with Debra for five minutes whenever she is able to handle differences appropriately	
■ Increase social interaction as more appropriate behavior is achieved	

Continued

DEBRA H *Continued*

NURSING INTERVENTIONS	OUTCOME CRITERIA

NURSING DIAGNOSIS: Regressed behavior related to need frustration

CLIENT GOAL: Express anger and frustration appropriately

- Draw up a contract with Debra for the following:
  Tantrum behavior will result in time-out for 30 minutes

Disappearance of any of the identified tantrum behavior

- The 30-minute time out can be reduced by
  No thumb sucking: time-out reduced by five minutes
  No foot stomping: time-out reduced by five minutes
  No loud crying: time-out reduced by five minutes
  If Debra is quiet in time-out room for ten straight minutes, she may come out
- Teach and encourage use of appropriate skills to handle frustration
  Labeling and expressing feelings
  Expressing one's opinion
  Exercising self-control skills
- Provide immediate feedback and praise whenever Debra is able to reduce time-out time
- Provide 30 minutes of staff time to be used with staff member of Debra's choice to do an activity of her selection after she has refrained from any tantrum behavior following limit setting; activity should be appropriate

Expresses feelings of frustration appropriately
Problem solves situations instead of having a tantrum

---

sented with her more difficult and long-standing problems. She was loud, argumentative, demanding, threw tantrums in which she cried loudly, stomped her feet, and sucked her thumb whenever a limit was set. The most frustrating and difficult behavior for nursing staff to handle was that Debra would demand explanations for intervention, but would not listen to them. It eventually became clear that although Debra demanded explanations, she was not truly interested in those explanations. Rather, this was a way to keep the staff members involved in what very often turned out to be negative and quickly deteriorating interactions. During these times, Debra would also repeatedly call her mother collect on the pay telephone and demand that she be brought home.

A behavior modification program was established to deal with three specific behaviors: loud tone of voice when interacting with peers; argumentativeness with staff; and tantrums when limits were set. The program had another purpose, and that was to provide the nursing staff with a structure in which to respond therapeutically to these most difficult behaviors without getting involved in negative episodes with the client. The care plan developed for Debra identified three nursing diagnoses: (1) impaired social interaction related to need for attention and belonging; (2) moderate aggression towards perceived authority figures; (3)

regressed behavior related to need frustration (see Nursing Care Plan 41–1 for a sample care plan for Debra H).

SUMMARY

Classical and operant conditioning differ in the emphasis each approach gives to the role of antecedent stimulus in the learning or maintenance of behavior. Operant conditioning focuses on the significance of environmental reinforcers. These reinforcers range from positive reinforcers, negative reinforcers, extinction, punishment, and response cost.

Behavior therapy emphasizes the importance of data gathering and the formulation of objectively measured, observable treatment goals. The program design is carefully planned and consistently implemented. Evaluation of treatment outcome is accomplished by comparing specific observed behaviors with the baseline data gathered on those behaviors.

The nurse can implement the principles of behavior therapy in planning for the care of her clients. Specific behavior therapy techniques, such as positive rein-

Research Highlights

A team of investigators led by Frederick Fuoco[9] investigated the efficacy of the use of Daily Living Schedules to increase appropriate behaviors in the areas of (1) ward jobs; (2) interactive activities; (3) involvement in individual or ward-wide treatment programs and to decrease behavior such as isolation and sleeping. The experiment involved seven adult psychiatric patients whose ages ranged from 21 to 43 years old. The mean number of psychiatric hospitalizations was five and ranged from 1 to 13.

The study was conducted in two phases. Both phases involved a baseline and treatment stage. The main strategies used were (1) training in scheduling skills and (2) contingent verbal reinforcement. In phase 1, stage 1, the participants were observed for five consecutive days, but were not required nor prompted to complete the Daily Living Schedule and suffered no consequences for not engaging in target behaviors. In phase 1, stage 2, which is the treatment phase, the use of the Daily Living Schedule was taught and demonstrated by a health care technician. Subsequently, each participant independently completed the Daily Living Schedule and was given feedback on his or her performance. Each participant was then instructed to complete the Daily Living Schedule every day before 8 AM and to engage in behaviors specified in the schedule. The participants were then observed for (1) completing the schedule by 8 AM as required and (2) engaging in behaviors specified. Observations were made by health care technicians and other independent observers. Phase 2 of the study was conducted to ascertain whether the behaviors learned in phase 1, stage 2 (treatment stage), were maintained. Phase 2 began with a baseline stage in which the clients were again observed for five consecutive days, but were not required nor prompted to complete the Daily Living Schedule. To reinforce the maintenance of the learned behaviors, phase 2, stage 2, repeated the techniques and strategies used in the treatment stage of phase 1; that is, training in scheduling techniques and verbal reinforcement.

The study revealed that the use of the Daily Living Schedule procedure produced "increases in appropriate social, ward, and scheduling behavior" (reference 9, p 178) and decreases in isolation and sleeping. However, treatment effects gained in phase 1 were not substantially maintained in phase 2. The investigators attributed the lack of maintenance to the short duration of the treatment stage.

This study demonstrated two simple techniques (training and verbal praise) to increase motivation and active behavior on the part of psychiatric patients. Such techniques are easily used in any setting and do not call for specialized training on the part of the treatment providers.

forcement, extinction, response cost, and teaching specific skills from activities of daily living to interpersonal skills, can be used by the nurse to respond to a wide array of behaviors and problems presented by different psychiatric clients.

References

1. Barker P, Douglas F, eds. The nurse as therapist: a behavioral model. Dover, NH: Croom Helm; 1985.
2. Bellack AS, Hersen M, eds. Dictionary of behavioral therapy techniques. New York: Pergamon Press; 1985.
3. Berkowitz S. Behavior therapy. In: Abt LE, Stuart IR, eds. The newer therapies: a sourcebook. New York: Van Nostrand Reinhold; 1982.
4. Butler R, Rosenthal G. Behavior and rehabilitation: treatment for long stay patients. Bristol: Wright Press; 1985.
5. Cantela JR, Kearney A. The covert conditioning handbook. New York: Springer Publishing; 1986.
6. Franks CM, ed. New developments in behavior therapy: from research to clinical application. New York: Haworth Press; 1984.
7. Fuoco FJ, Christian WP, eds. Behavioral analysis and therapy in residential programs. New York: Van Nostrand Reinhold; 1986.
8. Fuoco F, Naster BJ, et al. Behavioral procedures for a psychiatric unit and halfway house. New York: Van Nostrand Reinhold; 1985.
9. Fuoco F, Naster BJ, Vernon J, Morley R, Smith B, Cancilliere AEB. The use of a resident daily scheduling procedure to increase appropriate social, ward and scheduling behavior in adult psychiatric residents. Behav Resident Treat Interdisc J. 1986;1(Jul):169–182.
10. Fuoco F, Tyson W. Behavior therapy in residential programs for psychiatric clients. In: Fuoco F, Christian WP, eds. Behavioral analysis and therapy in residential programs. New York: Van Nostrand Reinhold; 1986.
11. Gardner W, Cole C. Acting out disorders. In Hersen M, ed. Practice of inpatient behavior therapy: a clinical guide. Orlando, FL: Grune & Stratton; 1985.
12. Hersen M, ed. Pharmacological and behavioral treatment: an integrative approach. New York: John Wiley & Sons; 1986.
13. Hersen M, ed. Practice of inpatient behavior therapy, a clinical guide. Orlando, FL: Grune & Stratton; 1985.
14. Hersen M, Last CG, eds. Behavior therapy casebook. New York: Springer Publishing; 1985.
15. Kazdin A, ed. Behavior modification in applied settings. Homewood, IL: Dorsey Press; 1984.
16. Krug R, Cass AR. Behavioral sciences. New York: Springer-Verlag; 1987.
17. Milne D. Training behavior therapists: methods, evaluation and implication with parents, nurses and teachers. Cambridge, MA: Brookline Books; 1986.
18. Matson JA, DiLorenzo TM. Punishment and its alternatives: a new perspective for behavior modification. New York: Springer Publishing; 1984.
19. Spiegler MD. Contemporary behavioral therapy. Palo Alto, CA: Mayfield Publishing; 1983.

42

Barbara S. Levinson

Cognitive Behavioral Therapy

OBJECTIVES

After reading this chapter, the reader will be able to:
1. *Define cognitive behavioral therapy*
2. *Distinguish between cognitive events, cognitive processes, and cognitive structures*
3. *Describe three different forms of cognitive behavioral therapy and state the theorist associated with each form*
4. *State strategies used in cognitive behavioral therapy*
5. *Identify the nurse's role in using cognitive behavioral therapy*
6. *List the nursing diagnoses commonly found in clients treated with cognitive behavioral therapy*
7. *Prepare a nursing care plan based on this theoretical framework.*

DESCRIPTION

History and Definition

The historical roots of cognitive behavioral therapy are complex. Some theorists such as Mahoney and Kendall see cognitive behavioral therapy as growing out of the behavior modification model. Beck and Ellis, however, credit their early training in the work of Adler and Horney as central to their formulation of a cognitive model of psychotherapy.[4] Cognitive behavioral therapy may be viewed as a mixture of the behavioral and psychodynamic models of therapy. One definition that is offered by Kendall is that *cognitive behavioral therapy* is a ". . . purposeful attempt to preserve the demonstrated efficiencies of behavior modification within a less doctrinaire context and to incorporate the cognitive activities of the client in the effort to produce therapeutic change" (reference 7, p 1). The cognitive behavioral approach "is a combination of the performance-oriented and methodologically rigorous behavioral techniques with the treatment and evaluation of cognitive–mediational phenomena" (reference 7, p 2). In other words, cognitive behavioral therapists borrow from their behavioral colleagues a focus on behavioral change and a variety of behavioral techniques and strategies. From their psychodynamically oriented colleagues, cognitive behavioral therapists have taken the notion of the importance of understanding the internal dialogue and process. The cognitive behavioral therapist helps patients redirect their thinking, attitudes, and behaviors.

Cognitive behavioral therapy is a series of strategies that relieve psychological suffering by correcting distorted and maladaptive thinking.[1] The core of the theory holds that a person's private meanings determine his or her unique emotional responses. Clients' thoughts, feelings, and wishes are used in therapy to understand their emotions and behaviors.

Cognitive Features

In referring to the role of the individual's thoughts, the cognitive behavioral theorist discusses cognitive events, cognitive processes, and cognitive structures.[9]

COGNITIVE EVENTS

Cognitive events refer to conscious, identifiable thoughts and images that occur in an individual's stream of consciousness and can be readily retrieved upon request. They are sometimes referred to as "automatic thoughts"[2] or as "internal dialogue."[9] According to Beck, automatic thoughts are specific and distinct; they occur rapidly, as if by reflex.[1,2] These thoughts are often difficult to stop or shut off. Anxious people regard their automatic thoughts as plausible and worthy of belief. Automatic thoughts are contrary to objective appraisal; those that assert the most influence on behavior are the most idiosyncratic to that person. Cognitive events or automatic thoughts may include attributions

or expectancies and evaluations of self or tasks. Cognitive events are likely to occur when (1) learning a new skill, (2) when an individual has to exercise choice or judgment in uncertain or novel situations, or (3) when an individual anticipates or experiences an intense emotional reaction. For example, when learning a new skill, the person thinks, "This is hard, I'll never be able to do it."

COGNITIVE PROCESSES

Cognitive processes are those processes that shape, transform, or construct mental representations into schemes of experiences and action.[9] They are the way in which external stimuli are appraised and transformed. Subsumed under this construct are such things as distorted interpretations, unwarranted catastrophic anticipations, self-denigrating ideation, and disruptive feelings such as anxiety, depression, or loneliness.[9] These processes may operate in an automatic, scripted fashion, including the events that are attended to, how those events are appraised, and which events are stored and retrieved. For example, the extremely lonely person may automatically feel lonely, even in a group of other people.

COGNITIVE STRUCTURES

Cognitive structures refer to tacit assumptions and beliefs that give rise to habitual ways of construing the self and the world.[9] The individual's personal schema, current concerns, hidden agendas, and personal goals influence the way that information is processed and the way that behavior is organized. Schemata are identified as "organized representations of prior experiences" and as "systems for classifying stimuli." For example, an individual's "dog schema" may contain general knowledge, such as "has fur, is animal, walks on four legs and barks" and may contain information about the relationship among attributes, such as "when angry it barks, runs around on its four legs, and the fur on its back stands up." Thus, schemata are collections of hypotheses, enabling the perceiver to attend to certain stimuli. Schemata enable individuals to identify stimuli quickly, cluster them into manageable events, select strategies for obtaining further information, solve problems, and reach goals.[12] It is also important to note that schemata consist of affective components. Certain stimuli will produce certain affects and vice versa.

A particularly important type of schema is the self-schema. These are collections of "cognitive generalizations about the self, derived from past experiences that organize and guide social experience."[12] Self-schema may guide any experiences that are personally relevant. Self-schema are particularly affect laden. Individuals often will place themselves in situations that influence their self-schema and may be particularly difficult to change. Self-schema can distort one's perception of reality. For example, if an individual sees himself as assertive, he is more likely to selectively choose to obtain feedback about his assertiveness as opposed to his passivity. Another example is the person who possesses a schema of mistrusting others. The person will tend to perceive things in their environment to fit into this mistrustful schema. Self-schema tend to make one resistive to information that contradicts one's schema. Cognitive behavioral therapists intervene at all levels of these cognitive features.

Cognitive Therapy

Cognitive therapy is both active and directive. The goal of therapy is to help clients uncover their dysfunctional and irrational thinking patterns, reality test their thinking and behavior, and build more adaptive and functional techniques for responding.[4] There is a great deal of diversity in the clinical procedures: rational psychotherapies, coping skills therapy, self-instructional training, and problem-solving therapies all are included under the heading of cognitive behavioral therapy. Each of these procedures differ in that they focus on different aspects of the cognitive features and each procedure intervenes at a different point in the affect–thought–behavior continuum.

ALBERT ELLIS

Albert Ellis[3] is commonly credited with being one of the pioneers in the field of cognitive behavioral therapy. His rational emotive therapy (RET) is based on the assumption that humans largely create their own emotional and behavioral disturbances by strongly believing in irrational beliefs. Irrational beliefs can lead to extremely stressful emotional consequences (anxiety, anger, depression) and behavioral reactions (aggression, withdrawal) that make it difficult for a person to improve the situation. This assumption is central to Ellis' *ABCDE* theory of change. Ellis suggests that an event (*A*—activating event) leads to an emotional or behavioral consequence (*C*). However, Ellis believes that *C* does not automatically follow *A*. Rather, the person causes his or her own consequence by strong beliefs (*B*) about *A*. What the person says to himself at *B*, about *A*, determines *C*. *D* (disputation) involves questioning the person's irrational beliefs and helping him to generate new hypotheses that will lead to *E* (new behavioral effects). Rational emotive therapy attempts to change the individual's overall philosophy and assumptions—whereas other forms of cognitive behavioral therapy are more problem-focused or behavior-focused—and defines goals of treatment in terms of specific behavioral changes.

DONALD MEICHENBAUM

Another major contributor to the advancement of cognitive behavioral therapy is Donald Meichenbaum.[9] His contribution is generally associated with self-instructional training (SIT), but over the years, his model of behavior change has evolved toward placing greater emphasis on the role of the client's cognitive structures or belief system. Self-instructional training places emphasis, not only on one's "self-talk," but on the individual's methods of coping with these thoughts. This approach emphasizes practical coping skills for dealing with problematic situations. Meichenbaum's therapy has incorporated three stages. The *first phase* is conceptualization of the problem. In this phase the client recognizes his or her faulty style or belief system that may be causing the presenting problem. The *second phase* helps the client, through self-monitoring and therapist-guided activities, to discover how his or her own thoughts help elicit and maintain the problem. The *third phase* focuses on helping the client modify his or her own cognitions and produce new adaptive behaviors.[10]

AARON BECK

A third therapist associated with cognitive behavioral therapy is Aaron Beck.[2] He is most noted for his cognitive theory of depression. Beck's cognitive therapy consists of (1) monitoring negative automatic thoughts; (2) recognizing the connection between cognition, affect, and behavior; (3) examining the evidence for and against the distorted thoughts; (4) substituting more reality-oriented interpretations; and (5) learning to identify and alter dysfunctional beliefs that predispose to distorted experiences.

Beck's cognitive theory of depression holds that the client presents a "negative triad," which consists of (1) a client having a negative view of self, (2) interpreting ongoing experiences in a negative way, and (3) having a negative view of the future. The cognitive model views other signs and symptoms of depression as consequences of the negative thought processes. Another feature of Beck's theory is that the individual has faulty information processing, examples of which are (1) drawing conclusions in absence of evidence, (2) focusing on details taken out of context, (3) overgeneralization, (4) magnification and minimization, (5) personalization, and (6) placing all experiences in an "either–or" category.[2] Various techniques are used to explore the logic behind and basis for specific thoughts and assumptions. The client is also taught to recognize, monitor, and record negative thoughts. Cognitions and underlying assumptions are examined for logic and validity. The therapy may also focus on specific target symptoms such as suicidal impulses. The thoughts underlying these symptoms, such as "I am worthless and can't change it," are then subjected to logical and empirical investigation.[2]

Clinical Applications

Cognitive behavioral therapy has been utilized with chronic anger, medical crises, control of pain, test anxiety, social anxiety, lack of assertiveness, uncontrollable and impulsive behavior, depression, stress, eating disorders, sexual dysfunction, posttraumatic stress disorder, and panic disorders.

Cognitive behavioral interventions have been used in individual psychotherapy, as well as in group and family therapies. It has been used with children and adolescents as well as adults. When working with clients with anxiety disorders, for example, the therapist can use any number of intervention strategies, such as teaching the client coping skills, problem solving, or cognitive restructuring. The generalist psychiatric mental health nurse can use some of these intervention strategies when working with clients in the hospital setting.

Kendall[5] has reported that cognitive behavioral therapy can be used successfully with children with pervasive developmental disorder, in which impulse control is a major factor. Impulsive children display a behavioral pattern that evidences a lack of forethought. Actions may result in unwarranted effects that could be avoided if forethought were activated. Proper treatment for impulsive disorders may include the teaching of thinking skills. However, a child's affective state (i.e., being angry or depressed) may influence the learning of these skills. Additional treatment, therefore, needs to be focused on the client's feeling and "affective state." Role-playing is often a good technique when dealing with children to help them express their feelings.

Intervention Strategies

Cognitive restructuring refers to a variety of therapeutic procedures that modify the client's self-statements as well as the premises, assumptions, and beliefs underlying these self-statements.[10] Three major forms of cognitive restructuring are Ellis's rational therapy, Meichenbaum's self-instructional training and Beck's cognitive therapy.

Rational therapy emphasizes the content and incidence of irrational beliefs, whereas self-instructional therapy places greater emphasis on teaching the client new coping skills. Both therapies teach the client a host of strategies that can be employed when confronted with an anxiety-provoking situation. The rational therapist teaches clients to monitor their internal dialogue in anxiety-producing situations (e.g., what actual thoughts occurred). The self-instructional therapist teaches clients to use anxiety as a cue for generating a variety of cognitive and behavioral coping strategies. For example, one strategy consists of monitoring maladaptive self-verbalizations actually stated by the person.

Beck's[2] cognitive behavioral approach is the model on which most cognitive therapy is based. The model emphasizes cognitive restructuring, but utilizes behavioral techniques and may include such interventions as scheduling activities, recording of mastery and pleasure of activities, homework assignments, graded task assignments, cognitive rehearsals (imagining steps in a sequence leading to a completion of a task), assertiveness training, and role-playing, to name just a few. The behavioral techniques, however, are a means to an end that, according to Beck, is cognitive change.

Problem-solving training has been used by a number of clinical practitioners in successful treatment packages. One such problem-solving approach is conceptu-

alized as a basic seven-step sequence represented by the mnemonic SCIENCE (Box 42–1).[8]

In the various stages of problem solving the client develops skills, such as self-monitoring, means–ends thinking, evaluation of consequences, and rehearsal of options. The problem solving perspective is extremely valuable and can yield encouraging clinical results.[8] This approach can also be utilized by the nurse in a variety of situations. Clients can be taught specific coping skills as well as more general strategies of assessment and problem definition. This approach may help the client implement adjustment strategies in particular situations. The problem solving therapies also require the active participation of the client and can enhance their independent abilities and offer a sense of accomplishment, so often necessary in the treatment of psychiatric patients.

Kendall and Braswell[6] have modified Meichenbaum's self-instructional training and developed a self-instructional training procedure outlined in Box 42–2 that can be particularly useful with a variety of psychiatric clients. These procedures have been used with children and with adults with schizophrenia. Any content can be taught; however, the content elaborated in Box 42–2 deals with problem solving.

Social skills training, which helps clients with interpersonal deficits related to social withdrawal, lack of spontaneity, and impaired styles of communication, is another extremely useful cognitive behavioral intervention. A variety of programs have been designed to help clients effectively manage typical social interaction situations. A client may have either a skills deficit or a performance deficit or a combination of the two. A performance deficit may occur when clients have interfering thoughts preventing them from performing certain behaviors. Some form of cognitive restructuring is useful in dealing with the maladaptive thoughts. Social skills may be taught by the use of instruction, modeling, discussion, behavioral rehearsal, coaching, feedback, behavioral rehearsal again, and more feedback. This technique is most often employed in group situations from which the client can receive feedback from peers. When teaching specific skills, the client can also be asked what is being thought at the time. Alternatives to maladaptive thoughts may be inserted by the therapist or by asking other members of the group. Role playing may also be used at this time, and others may

---

BOX 42–1
Seven-Step Problem Solving Approach (SCIENCE)[6,8]

S Specify general problem
C Collect information
I Identify causes or patterns
E Examine options
N Narrow options and experiment
C Compare data
E Extend, review, or replace

identify alternative cognitions that can be more adaptive. An initial goal of cognitive behavioral therapy is to help a client restructure thinking by first becoming more aware of thought processes.

The foregoing intervention strategies can be readily learned and used by the generalist psychiatric mental health nurse, since they are within the scope of generalist practice. Additional examples of such strategies are listed in Box 42–3. There are, however, other interventions used by the therapist who specializes in cognitive behavioral therapy that are beyond the scope of this chapter.

ROLE OF THE NURSE

The professional nurse is often the one who makes the initial contact with the client. Communication and the development of this most important therapeutic relationship can be the vehicle for assessing the client's underlying assumptions and distorted beliefs. By asking simple questions, the nurse can ascertain the client's thinking style and begin to see how the client may be processing faulty information. As stated previously, *automatic thoughts* are directly accessible cognitive material that reflect the client's ongoing negative self-evaluation. For example, a depressed client may offer the following, when in a particular situation: "I'm so awful. I can't cope. I can't do anything right." These automatic thoughts can help the nurse to understand the client's core cognitive processes and central beliefs. "Core cognitive processes are related to the definition and experience of the self in some fundamental way."[11]

By understanding the client's automatic thoughts, the nurse can provide opportunities and situations during which these beliefs may be called into question. For instance, the depressed client discussed above may have a core cognitive belief, "If I am not always strong and in control, then others won't respect me." The nurse can help to alter this faulty belief by manipulating the environment in such a way that the client can see that one does not always have to be in control of everything to be well-liked and respected. Such intervention strategies can be implemented while taking the client to meals, going to activities, playing cards and other games, going on outings, or taking the client on trips or to the movies.

On the basis of the self-instructional training model, self-verbalizations by the nurse are very effective for the client. The most effective modeling strategy is a coping model in which the nurse verbalizes "I can handle this," while demonstrating coping behaviors. In this way, behavioral modeling is enhanced by the inclusion of cognitive modeling. The nurse may have several opportunities to model appropriate behaviors for the client that are based on an understanding of the need for self-verbalizations during a particular task or while in a particular situation. For example, if the nurse is working on a child psychiatric unit and sees that a child is isolating himself from the group, by keeping the child's cognitive processes in mind, the nurse, thinking out loud, says "Gee, they're really running around. Is it okay to do that?" (pause) "This is playtime, I guess it's okay to run around, but what if I don't play the game right?" (pause) "But it doesn't look like they really care about the rules very much." (pause) "Maybe I'll play too." (pause) "No, I can't, they are all better players than I am." (pause) "Well look there, someone just made a mistake, and nobody cared, maybe I'll play for a few minutes." In this scenario, the nurse thinks through the process in a manner directly consistent with how the isolated child might interpret the situation. This technique increases the likelihood of the child's participating.

Theorists believe that the cognitive problems associated with adult disorders can be classified as *cognitive errors*. Cognitive errors may be illogical interpretations of the environment, irrational beliefs about personal performance abilities, inaccurate perceptions of everyday demands, and all-or-none categorical thinking. In contrast, the cognitive processing problems related to childhood disorders are typically cognitive *absences*. Often, the child fails to engage in the active information-processing activities of a problem solver and fails to initiate the reflective thinking that can govern behavior. The central role of cognitive absences in problems of childhood is evident in acting-out, conduct disorders, and attentional and hyperactive problems. The likelihood that cognitive errors also play a part in problems of childhood increases with the socially isolated and withdrawn child. Isolative patterns may correspond to self-criticism, inaccurate anticipation of rejection, and elaborate internal standards for success. Knowing this, the psychiatric nurse can utilize the strategies elaborated upon previously, such as social

BOX 42–3
Cognitive Behavioral Strategies

A. Counting automatic thoughts
  1. Help client identify automatic thoughts of a negative, irrational, or counterproductive nature.
  2. Instruct client to count automatic thoughts.
  This procedure allows the client to experience some control and mastery over them, and to recognize their automatic quality, rather than accepting them as an accurate reflection of reality.
B. Asking questions
  1. The nurse can ask the following questions:
    a. What is the evidence for this?
    b. Where is the logic?
    c. Are you thinking in all or none terms?
    d. Are you confusing your version of the facts with the real facts?
  This technique is particularly useful because asking questions often helps the client utilize more adaptive methods of information processing.
C. Acting "as if" or pretending
  1. Clients are asked to identify troublesome situations.
  2. They are then instructed to "act as if" they had no fears.
  This is most useful in a group situation and can be used when teaching social skills or when role-playing.
D. Explaining the connection between thinking, feeling, and behaving
  1. Nurse helps client identify particular behavior to be changed.
  2. Nurse asks client to identify thoughts before occurrence of behavior.
  3. Nurse asks client to identify feelings before or occurring at time of behavior.
  This is particularly useful when helping a client change a particular behavior. The identification of thoughts and feelings occurring before or at the time of the behavior may help the client to connect the particular unwanted behavior with possible dysfunctional or irrational thoughts.
E. Recording of dysfunctional thoughts
  1. Ask the client to record (write down): events, feelings, cognitions, possible alternatives.
    Example: *Event*—"My husband asked me how I felt and when the doctor thought I would be coming home." *Feeling*—Anxious and scared. *Cognitions*—"He doesn't want me home and he doesn't think I will ever get better." *Other possible interpretations*—"He really cares about me. He is concerned and wants me home. He wants to be involved in my treatment. He misses me."
  Having the client record dysfunctional thoughts can be extremely useful and can help the client to see that there are other alternatives to maladaptive thinking.

skills training, problem solving teachings, and role playing. For example, the psychiatric nurse can suggest to a group of children that they should develop a skit on how to make a new friend. Role switching and behavioral rehearsal can be utilized in this strategy. These are seemingly simple interventions, but when done with a specific purpose in mind, constructive behavioral change can result.

Some of the literature on social skills training in adults offers complementary advice. The integration of cognitive and behavioral procedures with depressed clients, socially isolated, or withdrawn patients, for example, makes use of peer-assisted role playing, reflective thinking, rehearsal, and modification of internal thinking processes.

COMMON NURSING DIAGNOSES

Cognitive behavioral therapy is utilized with clients with diagnoses of pervasive developmental disorder, panic disorder, social phobia, simple phobia, obsessive–compulsive disorder, post-traumatic stress disorder, generalized anxiety disorder, major depressive episodes, bipolar disorder, depressed, major depression, schizophrenia, anorexia, and bulimia. There are several nursing diagnoses that can be commonly found

in such clients: anger; anxiety; ineffective individual coping; depression; diversional activity deficit; fear; grieving; anticipatory grieving; dysfunctional grieving; guilt; altered growth and development; hopelessness; altered impulse control; knowledge deficit; manipulation; post-trauma response; powerlessness; impaired resource management; ritualistic behavior; self-concept disturbance; impaired social interaction; substance abuse; and suicide potential.

With any of these diagnoses the psychiatric nurse may find distorted beliefs, irrational thoughts, faulty information processing, impaired cognitive processes, disturbance in thoughts, or lack of skills caused by either skills deficit or performance deficits.

CASE STUDY

Susan, a 15-year-old girl, was admitted to a psychiatric hospital by her mother and stepfather. This was her first hospital admission, which was precipitated by a suicidal attempt. According to the parents, Susan had been having difficulty academically and socially ever since their move from another state.

Susan had become increasingly isolated and was, according to her parent's view, dressing "like a boy." She was sometimes unmanageable at home and would not follow the rules of the house. About two months before her hospi-

SUSAN

NURSING INTERVENTIONS	OUTCOME CRITERIA

NURSING DIAGNOSIS: Depression related to developmental issues and cognitive distortions

CLIENT GOAL: Remain free from self-inflicted harm

- Continually assess Susan's potential for suicide
- Help Susan to structure time on unit

No incidents of self-inflicted injury

CLIENT GOAL: Express feelings of anger and hostility in a safe, acceptable manner

- Provide a safe environment in which to express anger in a controlled manner
- Help Susan recognize feelings of sadness and encourage expression of these in a controlled setting

No incidents of angry, aggressive outbursts

CLIENT GOAL: Identify cognitive distortions and monitor automatic thoughts

- Help Susan to recognize negative thoughts as they occur
- Spend frequent visits with Susan and establish relationship of trust and caring; assign the same staff member to work with Susan

Keeps a record of automatic thoughts and cognitions

CLIENT GOAL: Identify faulty information processing

- Promote Susan's feelings of self-worth
- Give honest praise when applicable
- Ask questions that will help Susan evaluate faulty information processing without direct confrontations to avoid power struggles
- Engage Susan in problem-solving process

Identifies faulty information processing by use of monitoring record

NURSING DIAGNOSIS: Self-esteem disturbance related to unclear role performance and sexual identity issues

CLIENT GOAL: Exhibit increased feelings of self-worth as evidenced by verbal expression of positive aspects about self, past accomplishments, and future prospects

- Help Susan to recognize and focus on strengths and accomplishments
- Minimize attention given to past (real or perceived) failures
- Help Susan identify areas she would like to change and explore alternative methods of coping

Verbalizes positive aspects of self and past and recent accomplishments

CLIENT GOAL: Demonstrate a beginning understanding of role performance and sexual identity

- Encourage Susan to attend all groups, discuss confusion over sexual issues
- Assist Susan in problem-solving technique and setting realistic goals

Verbalizes less confusion and conflict

Demonstrates a decrease in self-derogatory statements

Discusses age-appropriate sexual behaviors and identifies areas of concern

Continued

NURSING CARE PLAN 42-1

SUSAN *Continued*

NURSING INTERVENTIONS	OUTCOME CRITERIA
NURSING DIAGNOSIS: Altered impulse control related to cognitive deficit	
CLIENT GOAL: Experience decreased number of incidents of impulsive behavior	
■ Interrupt any impulsive act and provide opportunity for self-instructional training	Demonstrates having thought about consequences before acting
■ Help Susan explore areas of life wherein she feels out of control; be aware of distorted beliefs	Verbalizes awareness of own limits of control
■ Provide one-to-one interaction for verbalization of feelings; try to ascertain affective state occurring at time of impulsive behavior	Verbalizes tension rather than acting on it
■ Help redirect anger and tension by providing structured activities and new social skills utilizing role-playing, feedback, and behavioral rehearsal	
NURSING DIAGNOSIS: Manipulation related to concern about getting needs met	
CLIENT GOAL: Decrease use of manipulative behavior	
■ Identify Susan's attempts to manipulate and ask Susan to offer alternative coping strategies	Identifies manipulative behaviors and identifies alternatives to manipulation with use of the problem-solving approach
■ Encourage Susan to identify strengths and to use talents in a socially acceptable manner	
■ Encourage the use of the problem-solving approach when confronted with a situation where manipulative behavior has been used	
■ Provide firm, consistent limits	
■ Help Susan to recognize distorted beliefs by keeping monitoring record	
■ Use role-playing and social skills training to enhance learning of new coping skills	

---

talization, Susan had developed a very close relationship with another girl of whom her parents did not approve. At one point, Susan was spending most of her time with this friend, and when she was at home would use the phone hours at a time. One night her parents confronted her with a rumor they had heard about her association with her girlfriend. Apparently her girlfriend's parents had called and said they were concerned about the overly close friendship between the two girls. The parents felt that Susan was very intimidating and possessive of their daughter and perhaps "pushing their daughter to do things she should not." This confrontation precipitated several runaway episodes in the months that followed. Susan's behavior seemed to be out of control, and her parents felt they could not talk to her. Her grades declined even further, and there was suspicion of some drug abuse. Her parents took her to a therapist whom Susan refused to see regularly. Susan began to lose weight, lost interest in any sort of activity, and would often cry at the slightest provocation. The suicide attempt consisted of the ingestion of 20 to 30 aspirin while her parents were at home. Susan was admitted to the hospital with a psychiatric diagnosis of major depressive episode and possible borderline personality disorder.

Upon admission, Susan was uncommunicative and did not make eye contact. She stated that she wanted to die and that her life was not worth living. She was an attractive girl, who appeared to be ashamed of her physical attributes.

During her stay on the unit, Susan was extremely difficult to approach. She was often belligerent with the staff, and they saw her as very manipulative. She was demanding at times, and, when she did not get her way, she would often revert to depressive behavior (i.e., not eating, saying she was going to kill herself, saying that nobody understood her, and everyone hated her). She was, however, very charming when she got what she wanted and would be very skilled at getting her needs met through manipulation of the staff. She would often threaten to "be violent" if she did not get her way. She was very impulsive and would often act before thinking about any consequences. She was becoming increasingly more difficult to deal with on the unit, and a special treatment team meeting was called.

Susan's final psychiatric diagnoses were major depressive disorder and borderline personality disorder. Her psychological testing showed a severe disturbance in her self-concept. She was extremely angry with her parents and had unresolved feelings about her mother's remarriage. She ruminated about her real father, whom her mother had described during the social history as a sociopath, and a wife and child beater. Susan's nursing diagnoses were depression, self esteem disturbance, altered impulse control, and manipulation.

Because Susan needed to develop a trust relationship with a consistent person on the unit, a psychiatric mental health nurse who would not be easily manipulated by Susan decided, with the agreement of the team, to set up regular meetings with Susan. After some trust developed, the nurse learned that many of Susan's problems stemmed from irrational beliefs about herself and her environment. It also became evident that Susan was aware of her manipulative behavior and impulsive acting-out, but said that she generally had little control of her impulsiveness. The nurse believed that Susan had disturbed interpersonal relationships related to her distorted beliefs about herself and others. It was also apparent that Susan lacked the age-appropriate social skills necessary for a teenager. After learning all of this through several interactions with Susan and spending much time with her on the unit, the nurse began to intervene in some of Susan's behaviors.

The nurse explained the connection between thoughts, feelings, and actions and asked Susan if she wanted to work on any particular behavior. The behavior that seemed to get her in trouble the most was her impulsiveness and manipulation. Together the nurse and Susan developed an action plan to deal with this. The nurse utilized the cognitive behavioral strategy often used with impulsive disorders, which is verbal self-instruction procedures. Susan and the nurse chose several problem situations and went through the problem-solving approach. Susan got experience focusing her attention, slowing down, choosing alternatives, and looking at consequences. It was difficult for Susan, as well as the staff, but over several months there was marked improvement in her behavior. Other problems were addressed as well, including her distorted beliefs about her self-image, such as "I am ugly and look like a man"; her distortions about her father, such as "I am just like him and will grow up to be no good"; and her negative view of the world, which was, "Everybody hates me and has it in for me." The nurse addressed these issues through assisting her to monitor her automatic thoughts and asking questions about her faulty information processing. This was all done in a nonjudgmental manner and without direct confrontation, which might have led to power struggles. The nurse also helped other staff members understand the nature of Susan's manipulation, which was distorted beliefs that she would not be able to get her needs met. After the staff was able to understand the underlying motivation, they were

Research Highlights

In 1982, Kendall and Braswell[6] examined cognitive behavioral therapy for self-control. The purpose of the study was to evaluate the usefulness of the cognitive components of the cognitive behavioral treatment and to include classroom observations and parent ratings among the outcome measures. Subjects were 27 teacher-referred children who exhibited non–self-controlled behavior that interfered with academic and social performance. Subjects were third to sixth graders and were homogeneous in problematic impulsive classroom behavior. The presence and extent of learning disability, aggressive behavior, and clinically hyperactive behavior varied.

The 27 subjects were rank ordered according to the Self-Control Rating Scale (SCRS) and randomly assigned to the cognitive behavioral group, the behavior group, and the attention-control group. All subjects received twelve, 45 to 55 minute sessions twice a week. The cognitive behavioral group received training in verbal self-instruction through modeling, social reward for correct performance, response–cost procedures contingent upon errors, and positive reinforcement for certain behaviors. In addition, self-instructional training was used to teach the children five steps in problem solving. Social reinforcement from the therapist also accompanied appropriate performance. Throughout the sessions therapists modeled self-instructions. In the behavior group, the distinguishing feature was the lack of self-instructional training and cognitive modeling in problem resolution. In other ways the interventions were the same for the cognitive behavioral group and the behavior group. In the attention-control condition, children received rewards for cooperation and control. The control condition included neither self-instruction, modeling, nor contingencies.

Outcome measures included the Self-Control Rating Scale (SCRS), the Hyperactivity Scale, the Matching Familiar Figures Test (MFF), the Wide-Range Achievement Scale (WRAT), and the Children's Self-Concept Scale. Hyperactivity ratings and SCRS were completed by both teachers and parents. Results of the MFF latency scores showed significant improvement by the cognitive behavioral and behavioral groups from pretreatment to posttreatment. Only the behavioral group maintained significant changes between pretreatment and ten-week follow-up. All three groups showed significant reduction in MFF errors between pretreatment and posttreatment and ten-week follow-up. On the WRAT, only the cognitive behavioral group showed significant change between pretreatment and posttreatment scores on the reading subtest, although all three groups manifested significant reading score gains between pretreatment and ten-week follow-up. Both the cognitive behavioral and behavior therapy groups showed significant changes from pretreatment to posttreatment and to ten-week follow-up on WRAT spelling and math scores. Teacher ratings of self-control on the SCRS showed that the cognitive behavioral group was significantly more improved than either of the other two groups. On the self concept measure, only the cognitive behavioral group had significantly improved scores from pretreatment to posttreatment and to follow-up. Between-group differences, however, were nonsignificant. The authors note that because of inconsistent effects found on outcome measures, caution must be used in interpreting the data. Although the results of the investigation by Kendall and colleagues on the efficacy of cognitive behavioral treatments for self-control in children are mixed, they do provide some support of cognitive behavioral therapy.

less likely to become angry and were more willing to spend time with her (see Nursing Care Plan 42–1 for a sample care plan for Susan).

SUMMARY

Cognitive behavioral therapy integrates behavioral and psychodynamic models of therapy. Clients' thoughts, feelings and wishes are used in therapy to understand their emotions and behaviors. The goal of cognitive behavioral therapy is to help patients uncover their dysfunctional and irrational thinking patterns, reality test their thinking and behavior, and build more adaptive and functional techniques for responding. Rational psychotherapy, coping skills therapy, self-instructional training, and problem-solving therapies are included in cognitive behavioral therapy. Major contributors to cognitive behavioral therapy are Albert Ellis, Donald Meichenbaum, and Aaron Beck.

Social skills training, problem-solving therapies, and self-instructional training have been used to treat a variety of disorders. There are several strategies that the nurse can employ when working within this framework: questioning, acting as if, role-playing, behavioral rehearsal, and recording of dysfunctional thoughts are just a few.

References

1. Beck A, Emery G. Anxiety disorders and phobias. New York: Basic Books; 1985.
2. Beck A, Rush J, Shaw B, Emery G. Cognitive therapy of depression. New York: Guilford Press; 1979.
3. Ellis A, Bernard M. Rational–emotive approaches to the problems of childhood. New York: Plenum Press; 1983.
4. Freeman A. Cognitive therapy with couples and groups. Plenum Press; 1983.
5. Kendall P. Toward a cognitive behavior model of child psychopathology and a critique of related interventions. J Abnorm Psychol. 1985;13:357–370.
6. Kendall P, Braswell L. Cognitive-behavioral self-control therapy for children: a component analysis. J Counsel Clin Psychol. 1982;50:672–689.
7. Kendall P, Hollon S. Cognitive behavioral interventions, overview and current status. In: Cognitive-behavior interventions, theory research and procedures. New York: Academic Press; 1979.
8. Mahoney M, Arnkoff D. Cognitive and self-control therapies. In: The handbook of psychotherapy and behavior change, 2nd ed. New York: John Wiley & Sons, 1978.
9. Meichenbaum D. A cognitive–behavioral perspective of childhood psychopathology: implications for assessment and training. In: McMahon E, Peters R, eds. Childhood disorders: behavioral developmental approaches. New York: Brunner Mazel; 1984.
10. Reynolds W, Stark K. Cognitive behavior modification: the clinical application of cognitive strategies. In: Lewis J, Presly M, eds. Cognitive strategy training. New York: Spring Valley; 1983.
11. Safron J, Vallis T, Segal Z, Shaw B. Assessment of core cognitive processes in cognitive therapy. Cogn Ther Res. 1986;10:509–526.
12. Turk D, Salovey P. Cognitive structures, cognitive processes, and cognitive behavior modification. Cogn Ther Res. 1985;9:1–17.

43

Ann Knecht-Kirkham

Transactional Therapy

OBJECTIVES

After reading this chapter, the reader will be able to:

1. Identify the major concepts related to transactional analysis
2. Describe how to assess ego states
3. Define the term contaminated ego state and relate delusions and prejudice to contamination
4. Draw a complementary, crossed, and duplex transaction
5. Describe how strokes are the result of one's life position
6. Give examples of games frequently played with psychiatric clients and how to avoid them
7. Discuss the application of transactional analysis in psychiatric nursing.

DESCRIPTION OF TRANSACTIONAL ANALYSIS

Eric Berne was the originator of transactional analysis.[3] Sometimes referred to as TA, transactional analysis is a relatively new therapy, described in 1967 by Thomas A. Harris in the book *I'm OK—You're OK.*[4] All behavior, thinking, feeling, and experience is categorized into three ego states, the Parent, Adult, and Child ego states. These ego states are diagrammed in Figure 43-1 by circles with the letters *P, A, and C* indicating the Parent, Adult, and Child.

These ego states are indicated by nonverbal changes: changes in voice tone, expression, and words. In the Child ego state, it is as if the person feels and thinks as he or she did as a child. The common emotions of the Child ego state are: dependency, fear, anger, rebellion, self-pity, and sadness. People in their Child ego state are frequently impulsive, creative, spontaneous, self-centered, affectionate, fun-loving, or caring. The Child ego state operates on the pleasure principle.

The Adult ego state organizes and processes information in an objective, rational way. Thinking that is clear, objective, based on reality, and without emotion, is said to be a product of the Adult ego state.

A Parent ego state also exists within each person, where memories of actual experiences, unquestioned or imposed thoughts, feelings, injunctions, declarations, and instructions from parent figures, perceived by the person in the early years, are recorded.[5] Sometimes, these rules for living received by the person from their parents are referred to as parent tapes. Everything the child saw the parents do and say is "recorded" in the Parent. These Parent ego state feelings are expressed either in critical, directive, judgmental behavior, or in nurturing behavior. The primary feelings expressed by the behavior of people in the Parent ego state are as follows: being judgmental, being critical, being directive, nurturing, being protective, and wisdom. Some professionals utilizing this theory separate the Parent into "nurturing parent" and "critical parent." The Parent can be life-supporting and nurturing, or can be over-controlling, suffocating, and oppressive.

Because these three ego states are theorized to exist in some proportion in most persons, it is important to remember that all ego states serve a valuable purpose. For example, in decision making it is of critical importance to adopt the rational Adult ego state. On the other hand, the childlike openness to new experiences and willingness to be creative is very valuable. Appropriate nurturing comes from the Parent ego state. There is beauty and appropriateness in each ego state. Theoretically, a person might engage in two ego states at the same time. Some therapists describe guilt as "the Parent beating the Child."[2] Intrapsychic conflicts may be rendered more comprehensible by the transactional model.

Assessing Ego States

A person can readily learn to identify which ego state is in control. There are four ways of determining ego states.

ASSESS BEHAVIOR AND WORDS

Observe the way the person sits, stands, walks, and the voice tone. For example, Parent words might be "cute," "marvelous," "awful," or "filthy." Parent behavior might be finger pointing, hands on hips, tongue clucking, or controlling facial expressions.

Adult words might be "suitable," "practical," and "correct." Adult behavior would be characterized by clear, objective, emotionless messages, with a straightforward affect.

Words such as "gee," "wow," "won't," and "can't" are common Child words. Behavior would be childlike, such as pouting, bashfulness, silliness, and fun-loving. The Child feels and expresses joy as well as despair in an unabashed spontaneous manner. Sometimes the Child demonstrates crafty, deceitful, cunning, or manipulative behavior. Some theorists have subdivided the Child into the natural Child and the adapted Child. The natural Child would express itself very transparently with openness, whereas the adapted Child has learned that openness can sometimes bring trouble; therefore the person would demonstrate learned behaviors that are less open and honest. Herein lies much of the reason for people being misunderstood because they were less than open, honest, and clear in their requests.

ASSESS INTERPERSONAL INTERACTIONS

People may interact with each other in any one of the three ego states; for example, a child in the Adult ego state or an Adult in either the Child or Parent ego state. The Parent ego state in one person will frequently "hook" or catch the Child ego state in the person with whom he or she is interacting. The term *hook* refers to a situation in which a person is impelled to respond in a

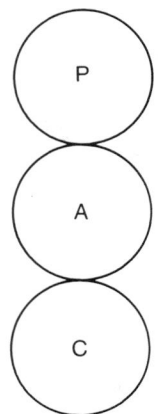

FIGURE 43–1. The three ego states.

particular ego state. For example, if a person is behaving in a fun-loving and gregarious manner from the Child ego state, the Child in others will be elicited. If a person in the Child ego state is defiant, the Parent in others may be "hooked." When the Adult ego state is in operation, there is a better chance that the other person's Adult will be operationalized. This is particularly important to remember when one is attempting to resolve a difference with another person.

ASSESS EARLY YEARS

To assess an ego state, the person should try to remember what words were used in the particular person's home. When the nurse is teaching a client how to identify ego states, encourage the client to remember certain words associated with the client's childhood and with his or her parents.

ASSESS FEELINGS

This is the most important information utilized in the assessment of a person's ego state. Because feelings flow from thoughts, if a client is able to identify either the thoughts or feelings, then needs will be easier to identify. For example, a depressed client may sit all day and not be motivated to participate in any activities. Ask the client to identify what messages are being thought. This is sometimes referred to as self-talk, (i.e., those thoughts that seem to come into consciousness for no particular reason). When a particular client was asked to do this, the thought, "it's not worth it," was perceived each time the client was tempted to try to participate in activities. This thought was commonly used by the client's depressed mother when the client was growing up. Once the client identified the thought and the source of the thought, the unmotivated feelings that went with the thought were more understandable. The client decided to substitute the thought, "it is worth it," each time the client was aware of the previous thought. The client was able to change the depressed feelings, by substituting this positive thought.

A person can actually feel the ego state that is active at any given time. If a client feels like a parent (either nurturing or critical parent), for example, the client is probably in the Parent ego state. If the client feels like a child (left out, unloved, ecstatic, or exuberant), the client is probably in the Child ego state. The Adult is the ego state probably easiest to identify because of the apparent absence of feelings.

Each person is potentially capable of being in any of the three ego states. All three are important. The Child is the most fun and is very important because the unfinished business is in the Child ego state.[5] It is the Adult's job to help meet the Child's needs and to help the Child avoid trouble.[2] The role of the "Parent" is to treat the Child with respect and love. Because of a client's past, this frequently does not happen. Therefore, two important questions to ask the client are as follows:

1. Which ego state is currently dominating your behavior?
2. What are you thinking (self-talk) and what is the source of the message?

This internal dialogue is identified readily when talking to a client experiencing severe feelings of guilt. Statements such as "I'll never be able to show my ugly face in church ever again," indicate the Parent "beating" or belittling the Child. Therapy here is to help the client clarify the rationality of the Parent statements. For example, is whatever the client did considered such a sin that the client will not be able to attend church? Or did the client's parents try to control the client's behavior by frightening the client into acceptable behavior?

Contaminated Ego States

Some people have an Adult that is contaminated by the Parent (Fig. 43-2). This is an example of a prejudice.[3] For example, in some situations a person might believe he or she is speaking from the Adult; however, the Parent in the person is doing the talking. If the person's mother believed that people of another race are no good, the Parent in that person may talk the same way the mother did. If the person's Adult is contaminated by the person's Parent, then the person's Adult may take what the person's mother said as fact, without really verifying it. Some people have an Adult who is contaminated by the Child (Fig. 43-3). This is an example of a delusion, such as "people talk behind my back."

Transactions

Transactions are defined as an exchange between two people. All conversations are a series of transactions. Transactional analysis analyzes transactions to gain insight into the dynamics of interpersonal problems. When the lines of the transaction are parallel, the transaction is said to be *complementary*.[3] These trans-

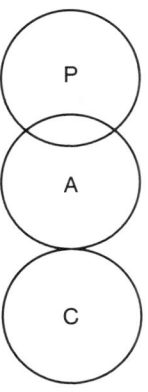

FIGURE 43–2. Adult contaminated by Parent.

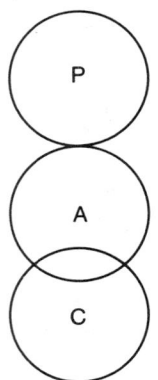

FIGURE 43–3. *Adult contaminated by Child.*

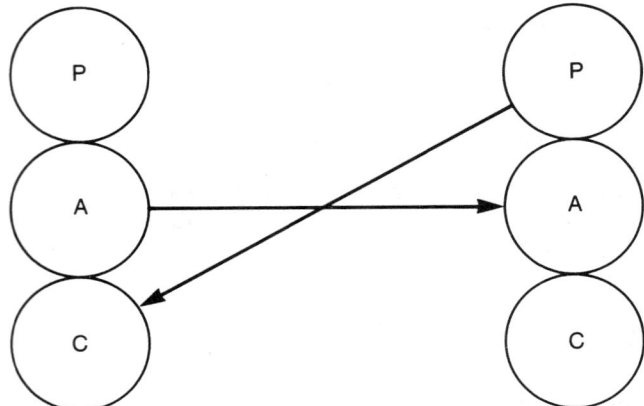

FIGURE 43–5. *Crossed transaction: Adult asks Adult: "What time is it?" Parent responds, "Are you late again?"*

actions are depicted in Figure 43-4. When the lines of the transaction cross, communication stops[4] (Fig. 43-5). Chances are great that the person asking for the correct time will come back defensively with a Child response, "I'm not late very often." One of the principles of transactional analysis is that when transaction lines cross, productive communication ceases. This does not necessarily mean that the communication will cease, but the participants will have a sense that there is a communication breakdown. Berne[2] states that this type of crossed transaction in which the stimulus is directed to the Adult, whereas the response originates from the Child is most likely the most common cause of misunderstandings in marriage and work situations. Clinically, it is referred to as the classic transference transaction.

The reader may wish to diagram the following transactions, rate them as to whether they are complementary or crossed, and then refer to Figures 43-6 through 43-9.

1. Person A "Did you brush your teeth?" Person B "Get off my case."
2. Person A "I have to finish a paper that is due tomorrow." Person B "Why do you always leave things to the last minute?"
3. Person A "She should stay home with her kids." Person B "She obviously has no sense of duty."
4. Person A "That is a nice-looking dress." Person B "Thank you."

A mixed message sent by a person results in a duplex transaction (Fig. 43-10). For example, a husband says to wife, "Where did you hide the can opener?" The question sounds like an objective, information-seeking question. However, there is a covert message in the word "hide," that is, "You are a poor housekeeper, I wish I could just once find something where it belongs." This duplex message is coming from the Parent. The wife then, depending on which ego state is hooked, might respond from the Adult, "It is right next to the measuring cups." or the Child, "Why don't you pitch in and help with this mess, you got a broken leg?" A third option is apparent. The wife could deal with the covert message and ask for clarification from the Adult, "I don't understand why you use the word 'hide.'"

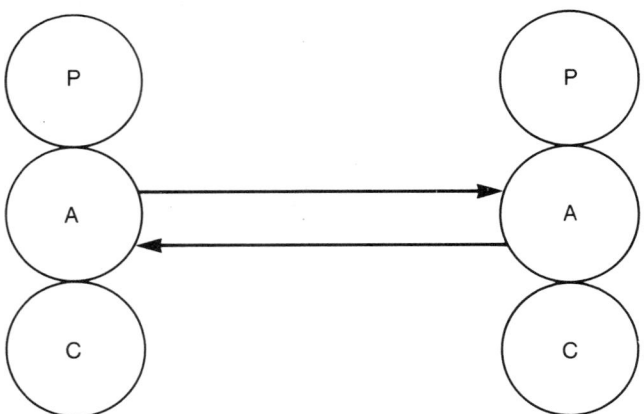

FIGURE 43–4. *Adult–adult complementary transaction. Adult to another adult: "What time is it?" Adult responds to Adult: "It is four o'clock."*

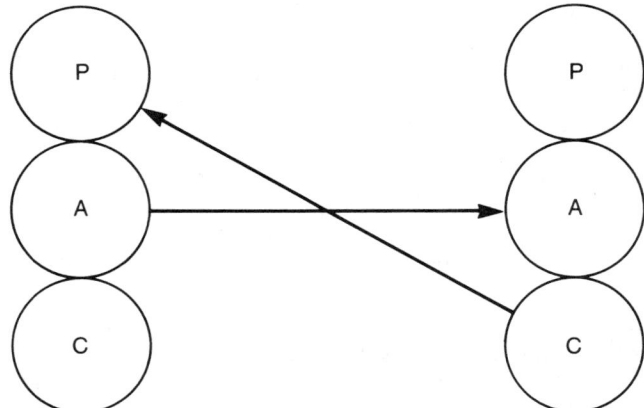

FIGURE 43–6. *Crossed transaction: Adult to Adult: "Did you brush your teeth?" Child responds to Parent: "Get off my case."*

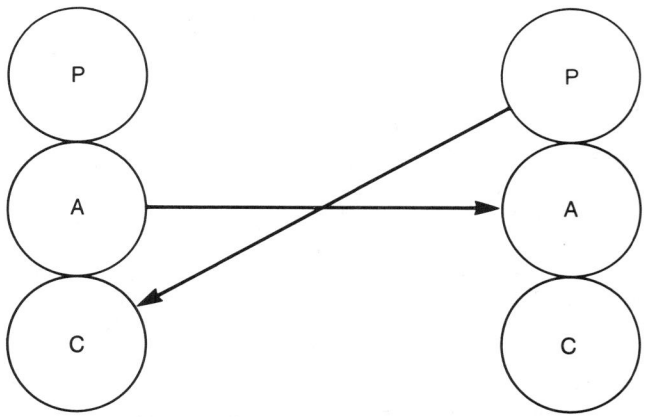

FIGURE 43–7. Crossed transaction: Adult to Adult: "I have to finish a paper that is due tomorrow." Parent responds to child: "Why do you always leave things until the last minute?"

Strokes

The notion of "strokes" is another component of transactional analysis. All people need strokes. A stroke can be a compliment, a pat on the back, or a kick on the shin. There are pleasant and unpleasant strokes. The old saying, "Kick me or kiss me, but don't ignore me," is very appropriate in this discussion of strokes. A negative stroke is one that tells the person, "you are not OK," whereas a positive stroke tells the person "you are OK." A conditional stroke is given for what a person does, not what the person is. For example: "I love you when you make good grades." Some people have trouble asking for strokes. Some people elicit certain types of strokes. What type of strokes does the nurse give? What type does the nurse receive? Is the nurse needing more strokes than are being received and, thus, eliciting strokes from clients? Virginia Satir[7] refers to positive strokes as "warm fuzzies." Some people predominantly seek and elicit positive strokes, whereas others predominantly seek negative strokes. The reason for

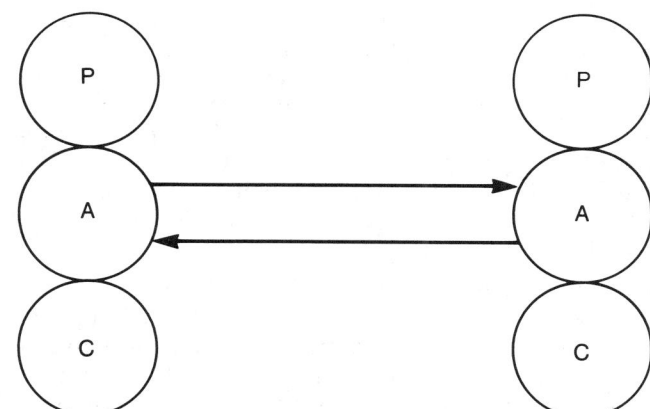

FIGURE 43–9. Complementary transaction: Adult to Adult: "That is a nice dress." Adult responds to Adult: "Thank you."

the differences are believed to be based on the person's basic life position. *Life position* refers to how the person feels about the self and others. There are four basic life positions:[4]

1. *I'm okay; you're okay* (the only healthy position)
2. *I'm okay; you're not okay* (a distrustful position taken by a Child who is suspicious of others)
3. *I'm not okay; you're okay* (a depressed position taken by the Child who usually feels low)
4. *I'm not okay; you're not okay* (a state in which the person has given up on getting any strokes, and simply tries to exist. The person may become regressed or extremely withdrawn.

Games

Games are an important part of transactional analysis. The term *games*, as utilized in transactional analysis, can cause trouble, wreck relationships, and should not be confused with having fun. They are a series of com-

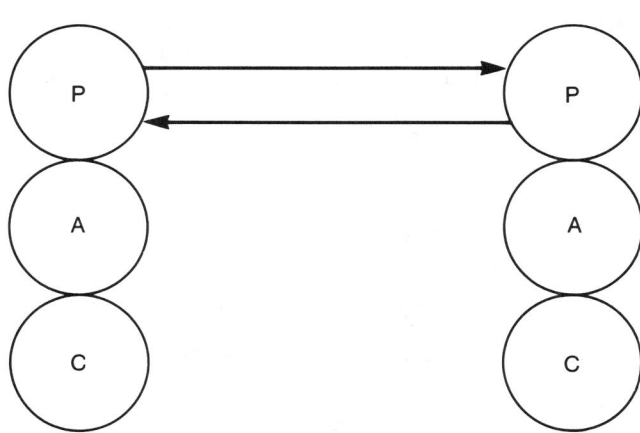

FIGURE 43–8. Complementary transaction: Parent to Parent: "She should stay at home with her kids." Parent responds to Parent: "She obviously has no sense of duty."

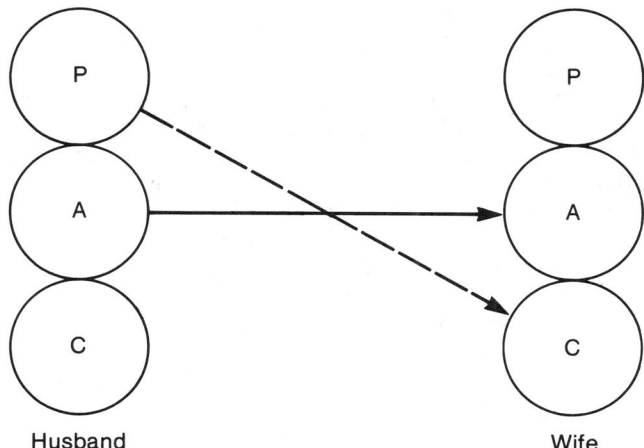

Husband   Wife

FIGURE 43–10. Duplex transaction: Adult to Adult: "Where did you hide the can opener?" Covert message is Parent to Child: "You are a poor housekeeper. I wish I could find things where they belong."

plementary duplex transactions progressing to a well-defined outcome or payoff.[1] This payoff is the feeling the player gets at the game's end. A common game is, "Why don't you, yes but." One player initiates the game by presenting a problem. The second player responds by making a suggestion for resolving the problem. The first player then systematically refutes each suggestion made, as in the example below between a client and the nurse:

CLIENT: "I never get to talk with my doctor."
NURSE: "Why don't you call his office and ask them to remind Dr. P you would like to talk with him?"
CLIENT: "Yes, I tried that, but they forgot to tell him."
NURSE: "Why don't I leave a note on your chart that you wish to talk with him."
CLIENT: "Yes, but I know he'll be upset with me for asking."

This game could continue as long as the nurse provides the "why don't you." The payoff in this game is that the Child in the client has been able to confound the Parent in the nurse and, thereby, prove the nurse impotent and the client's problem insoluble. The way to stop this game is to stop offering suggestions and turn the problem back to the client by saying something like, "I don't have any other ideas, what do you think?" Harris[4] warns that labeling the game in front of the client can be hostile and nontherapeutic. The best way to utilize knowledge of transactional analysis games is to recognize them and avoid playing them. The book *Games People Play* by Berne[1] and *Games Alcoholics Play* by Claude Steiner[8] are recommended for a fuller understanding of games.

Transactional analysis has been used with clients with a wide variety of psychiatric disorders and also with abusive families. Physically abusive parents are treated in a group with other physically abusive parents, without the children present. Because transactional analysis is also considered a communication model, it is used frequently by management teams in an effort to improve communication and increase productivity. Churches use it to increase members' growth in relationships with others. Some addiction treatment programs utilize transactional analysis as part of a multiple therapy approach to increase insight into the motivation of addiction. Depressed clients and very inhibited clients gain much from a transactional analysis approach; it is somewhat less threatening than direct confrontation, and the cognitive understanding of a client's behavior serves to extinguish the behavior. Transactional analysis has been utilized even with psychotic clients, with limited success. To utilize transactional analysis, however, a person must have the capacity to conceptualize abstractly. Thus, transactional analysis is less likely to be useful with clients suffering from schizophrenia.

NURSING IMPLICATIONS

Transactional analysis is helpful in assessing the nurse's own ego state. If the nurse can consciously con-

trol the ego state from which the transactions with clients come, therapeutic relationships will be maintained at a much more consistent level. When interacting with colleagues, knowledge of transactional analysis will enable improved working relationships. Many power struggles between physicians and nurses are instigated by the physician being in a Parent ego state and the nurse being in a Child ego state. If the nurse can move to the Adult, the transaction is crossed; therefore, this unproductive communication ceases and the possibility of Adult to Adult communication exists.

The basic principles of transactional analysis are easily taught to most clients. The nurse then has a means of communication that seems less threatening than using conventional words. For example, telling a client that he or she is acting childish is more threatening than if the transaction is drawn and analyzed together, indicating that the client is responding from the Child ego state. Some group therapists utilize transactional analysis in group sessions. The nurse's role as a cotherapist is to help assess ego states and identify transactions and games that are troublesome for the client. Guarding against countertransference is probably one of the most important uses for transactional analysis in psychiatric nursing. Countertransference is the phenomenon of responding inappropriately to a client as if he or she were an important figure in the nurse's life. For example, when the nurse frequently responds from the Parent ego state with a particular client, this may be a clue that the nurse is experiencing a countertransference reaction. When this happens pathologic client behavior can be reinforced. Minshull[6] warns that "too much involvement with people with problems may cause problems for ourselves" (reference 6, p 1202). Transactional analysis can help the nurse keep an ongoing assessment of child and parental needs so that these needs are met through social and personal time, instead of using the client to meet the nurse's needs.

COMMON NURSING DIAGNOSES

Nursing diagnoses for which transactional analysis could serve as an intervention strategy include aggression, anger, anxiety, impaired communication, ineffective individual coping, depression, fear, guilt, altered impulse control, loneliness, manipulation, altered parenting, regressed behavior, self-concept disturbance, impaired social interaction, and substance abuse.

CASE STUDY

Carolyn D is a 30-year-old married woman with two children, ages eight and ten. She was raised in a very rigid, restrictive family. She was not allowed to be assertive and never went against her parents directives for fear of rejection and abandonment. This total submission carried over into the marriage, even though Carolyn appeared quite autonomous. Her husband is a rigid, domineering executive with a large national corporation. She quit working outside the home when she had their first child, even though she had a college degree in dietetics. She experienced brief

NURSING CARE PLAN 43-1

CAROLYN D

NURSING INTERVENTIONS	OUTCOME CRITERIA

NURSING DIAGNOSIS: Ineffective individual coping related to inability to identify and deal with feelings and needs, articulate them to husband, and predominance of Child ego state

CLIENT GOAL: Gain skill in analyzing transactions as they are occurring as a base for meeting client's own needs more effectively and satisfactorily

■ Teach Carolyn how to diagram interactions with husband and children and explore implications of the diagrammed transactions	Describes openly wants and needs
■ Assist Carolyn in identifying ego states in self, in husband, and in children	
■ Assist Carolyn in identifying her internal dialogue between Parent and Child	
■ Help Carolyn relate this internal dialogue with what happens between herself and her husband	Behaves in ways to achieve what is desired from husband and children
■ Role-play with Carolyn how to clearly communicate desires to husband and to handle his potential responses and discomfort	
■ Encourage Carolyn to allow Child to get needs met	Meets own needs in satisfying ways even when significant others are not supportive or actively reject
■ Encourage Carolyn to discuss fears of abandonment and isolation	
■ Assist Carolyn in establishing the connection between being true to self and being abandoned for behaving in a manner that displeases husband	
■ Enable Carolyn to describe angry feelings related to not being assertive in getting needs met	
■ Encourage Carolyn to ventilate anger and frustration to the nursing staff and other "safe" people	
■ Teach Carolyn the importance of seeking constructive outlets for anger	
■ Teach Carolyn how unresolved dependency issues between parent and child can influence relationships in the present	
■ With marriage counseling, encourage Carolyn to openly and honestly discuss needs and desires with husband	
■ Encourage Carolyn to be independent	
■ Encourage Carolyn to explore the rationality of fear of abandonment as related to being autonomous, i.e., decontaminate the Child/Adult	Verbalizes fear of abandonment and rejection and realistically analyzes risks as well as the rationality of such fears

postpartum depression, but rallied from it after a few short psychotherapy sessions.

When the children were one and three years old, Mr. D was transferred to another state and Carolyn followed with the children. Carolyn speaks of the years before the transfer as "the best years of our marriage." The transfer was never discussed between husband and wife. Mr. D assumed that if his job took him to a different city, they would, of course, move. Carolyn coped with loneliness and was adjusting fairly well after 13 months in the new city. Mr. D was transferred again, to another state. Again Carolyn did not discuss her dislike of moving, but moved for the second time in 13 months. Carolyn never allowed herself to become aware of the intense anger she felt about her life being out of her own control. Once settled in a new home in the new city,

Carolyn became progressively more and more socially isolated. She cried frequently, but when she thought of reaching out, she decided she had to stay home because repairmen were always coming to fix things on the new house, and her husband would be angry if she was not there to supervise the work. Mr. D became engrossed in his new position. Carolyn, on the other hand, felt very sad, discouraged, self-deprecating, and bewildered by her reaction to the move. When Carolyn found that she was not able to even get dressed in the mornings, she decided the situation was desperate and telephoned a psychiatrist whose name she selected from the yellow pages in the phone book. The psychiatrist admitted Carolyn to a psychiatric hospital. On admission, Carolyn displayed the classic signs of depression: anorexia, insomnia, hopelessness, loss of interest in anything, slowed responses, and irritability. She had suicidal thoughts, but no plan. She said, "my religion and the children keep me from being serious about suicide." She had been staying in bed most of the day and was barely able to function as a homemaker. The staff at this psychiatric hospital were educated in and utilized transactional therapy in groups and individually along with other appropriate treatment modalities.

The DSM-III-R diagnoses were:

Axis I Major Depression
Axis II Dependent Personality Disorder
Axis III None known
Axis IV Severity of psychosocial stressors rated 4 (moderate)
Axis V Global assessment of functioning past year rated 5—serious symptoms resulting from situational depression

The primary nurse for Carolyn formulated a nursing diagnosis of ineffective individual coping and a care plan (Nursing Care Plan 43-1). Carolyn responded to transactional analysis and began diagramming transactions with other clients, staff, and her husband. The marriage counseling took place on the hospital unit and the nurses were particularly available to Carolyn after these sessions for ventilating and clarification of marriage dynamics. Carolyn's depression began to lift and weekend passes went well. Much material for further discussion was available to Carolyn and the nursing staff after the weekend passes. Carolyn was discharged three weeks after admission and continued marriage counseling and individual therapy as an outpatient. Carolyn was also informed of the meeting times of an educational class on transactional analysis to enhance her skills and understanding of transactional analysis.

SUMMARY

In transactional analysis all behavior, thinking, feeling, and experience is categorized into three ego states: Parent, Adult, and Child. These ego states can be identified by nonverbal changes, changes in voice tone, expressions, and words. Transactional analysis analyzes transactions to gain insight into the dynamics of interpersonal problems. When the lines of the transaction are parallel, the transaction is complementary. When the lines of the transaction cross, communication stops. Strokes and games are other components of transactional analysis.

Research Highlights

The following brief annotated bibliography describes types of research related to transactional analysis:

Goldson E, Milla PJ, Bentovim A. Failure to thrive: a transactional issue. Fam Sys Med. 1985;3:205–213.

This study describes a form of failure to thrive with both organic and psychological causes in seven children (aged two months to six years). An indepth discussion of a six-month-old child with this form of failure to thrive is included. A transactional systems analysis of the problem is presented that includes the child, family, and professional network. A broader perspective on the diagnosis and treatment of failure to thrive is proposed.

Moses J. Stroking the Child in withdrawn and disoriented elders. Transact Anal J. 1985;14:152–158.

This study investigated the effects of physical and verbal stroking on the social behavior of elderly persons in a nursing home. Nineteen residents, 70 and older, of a skilled-care nursing home participated in group activities that were held twice weekly. Results indicated that physical touch, using the person's name, stimulation through music, and acknowledging the feelings expressed through confused statements and incongruent nonverbal cues had positive effects on the person's behavior. Over a five-month period, the residents in the study became more alert, relaxed, and responsive.

Moses J. Part-time mental health technicians: a special fields study in an intermediate care facility. Transact Anal J. 1984;14:199–204.

The article describes a program in which part-time mental health workers, such as nurses, nursing assistants, recreation therapists, and social workers, led experimental groups using transactional analysis concepts with thirty-four, 34- to 83-year-old residents for six months. The experimental group completed pre- and posttreatment Life Satisfaction Index forms. The residents attending these groups, when compared with those who did not, demonstrated improvement in independence, reduced reliance on staff for attention and emotional support, and less use of psychotropic medications. Also, the number of discharges from the experimental group exceeded staff expectations. The scores on the Life Satisfaction Index were higher after the group experience.

Misawa-Hideo. Ego states of nurses in nursery schools: a study comparing ego state of nurses and mothers as measured by transactional analysis ego state questionnaire. J Child Dev. 1981;17:24–31.

This researcher investigated ego states of 65 nurses (a term used to denote daycare workers who tend children eight hours a day while their mothers work) in nursery schools and 45 mothers of children (aged three to five). A specially constructed ego state questionnaire based on transactional analysis theory was administered to the nurses and mothers. By using cluster analysis in classifying individuals, the subjects were grouped into various subtypes on the basis of their responses to the questionnaire. Findings suggest that nurses appeared to acquire more desirable ego states than do mothers.

References

1. Berne E. Games people play. New York: Grove Press; 1964.
2. Berne E. Principles of group treatment. New York: Grove Press; 1966.
3. Berne E. Transactional analysis in psychotherapy. New York: Grove Press; 1961.
4. Harris T. I'm okay—you're okay a practical guide to transactional analysis. New York: 1967.
5. McCormick P, Campos L. Introduce yourself to transactional analysis, 2nd ed. Berkeley: CA: San Joaquine TA Study Group; 1970.
6. Minshull D. Counselling in psychiatric nursing. Nurs Times. 1982;78:28.
7. Satir V. Conjoint family therapy. Palo Alto: Science and Behavior Books; 1964.
8. Steiner C. Games alcoholics play. New York: Ballantine Books; 1971.

44

Fe Nieves-Khouw

Reality Therapy

OBJECTIVES

After reading this chapter, the reader will be able to:

1. Discuss the concepts of control theory and reality therapy
2. Identify the steps in the process of reality therapy
3. Apply the principles of reality therapy in individual interaction with clients
4. Design a care plan using the methods of reality therapy.

INTRODUCTION

Glasser, who developed the groundwork for reality therapy in the late 1950s through the mid-1960s, was dissatisfied with psychoanalytic theory and was convinced that present behavior and thoughts are much more significant than past experiences.[6,15] He rejected the idea of mental illness and proposed that psychological problems are due to a lack of need satisfaction.[2,14] The success of the application of his theoretical perspective and therapy approaches, which were tested in the Ventura School for Girls in California, provided the impetus for expansion.[10] Currently, reality therapy is practiced by mental health professionals, including nurses, in settings ranging from schools to mental health institutions, correctional facilities, and industrial corporations. At present, the principles and therapy techniques of reality therapy are more commonly implemented in school systems and correctional institutions and have much to offer practitioners in psychiatric nursing, especially in the area of establishing therapeutic relationships and helping the client plan for behavior change.

Reality therapy focuses on teaching clients to improve their ability to fulfill basic needs in ways that are more successful and do not infringe on the rights of others.[3] It emphasizes individual responsibility for behavior by guiding clients to evaluate the effectiveness of their behavior in the light of need fulfillment. Reality therapy encourages active involvement of the therapist with the client, not as a transference object, but as model, teacher, and friend.[1,13]

"Reality therapy is a series of theoretical concepts and principles which can trace its origins to learning theory and existential thought" (reference 3, p 79). Reality therapy is also based on the concepts of control theory. Glasser's control theory is supported by independent research performed by William J. Langer.[12] Langer defines *control* as ". . . the active belief that one has a choice among responses that are differentially effective in achieving the desired outcome" (reference 12, p 20). Glasser believes that ". . . all of our behavior is our attempt to control our lives" (reference 11, p xiii). Glasser's control theory[11] assumes that problems arise from a lack of need satisfaction. A perceptual error is created when a difference exists between what one wants and what one has. This perceptual error triggers the behavioral mechanism that presents the individual with choices of behavior to remedy the error. Once an organized behavior is chosen, the person is completely responsible for it. Control theory further holds that problems are more accurately expressed as verbs instead of nouns or adjectives (i.e., anger is expressed as "angering," depressed as "depressing"). The verbs express the significance of the "doing component," which is more amenable to change. This doing component is the focus of reality therapy, as it attempts to help the individual learn new behaviors to respond to need satisfaction.

Reality therapy differs from conventional psychodynamic therapy in six significant areas:[5] (1) It rejects the concept of mental illness. Reality therapy assumes that a problem, which may be termed mental illness by others, is caused by an irresponsible attempt to meet one's need, and the focus is on increasing the ability for effective need fulfillment in the present and not on analysis of a noxious event in the past. (2) Reality therapy does not deal with the client's past. (3) The reality therapist relates to the client as a person, rather than as a transference object. (4) Reality therapy does not deal with unconscious motivation because that is considered akin to accepting excuses for behavior. (5) It emphasizes the morality of the behavior. Reality therapists guide clients in evaluating their behavior, both in terms of its effectiveness in meeting needs and its effect on others. (6) Finally, reality therapists engage in active teaching and modeling of more effective ways to fulfill felt needs. Reality therapy differs from behavior therapy in that it accepts the concept of basic needs as internal forces that motivate behavior.[6,8,11]

KEY CONCEPTS AND PRINCIPLES OF CONTROL THEORY AND REALITY THERAPY

Basic Needs

Glasser believes that all human beings are driven by internal forces that serve as motivators for behavior.[6,7] These internal forces are basic needs that are "built into our genetic instructions, into the very core of our being . . . [and which] we must satisfy continually" (reference 11, p 5). The basic needs, according to Glasser, share certain characteristics:[7] they (1) do not change with age; (2) do not differ between normal and abnormal people; (3) are not affected by differences in sex, age, color, or race; and (4) do not change in relation to one's contact with reality.

In contrast with Maslow's hierarchy of needs,[17] which classifies needs in ascending order from the most simple to the most complex, Glasser asserts that man's basic needs are in constant conflict and that ". . . our continual struggle to satisfy these disparate forces—and especially to resolve the ever-present conflicts between them—has pushed us to become the most intelligent of life" (reference 11, p 17).

According to reality therapy and control theory, there are universal human needs that can be organized into two groups:[7,9] *physiologic needs*, the most urgent of which is the need for air, but equally important are the needs for food, water, and sex; and *psychologic needs* —the need for love and affection and to be worthwhile to ourselves and others,[6,7] the need for fun,[9,11] the need for power, and the need for freedom.[11] Glasser also suggests that individuals may be able to identify other needs, but what is important is the recognition that to be in control of one's life, one has to fulfill these identified needs in ways that do not frustrate another's fulfillment of basic needs.

Glasser's control theory asserts that human functioning is controlled by two parts of the brain. The part of the brain that is responsible for satisfying physiologic needs and for controlling all involuntary activities that allow a person to live and participate in daily activities is termed *old brain*. Glasser believes that the cerebral cortex, which he referred to as *new brain*, is responsible for all conscious activities. It is in the new brain that activities related to reality testing, needs satisfaction, behavioral reorganization, and redirection occur. It is in the new brain that pictures of what will satisfy a person's needs exist.

According to this theory, the new brain and the old brain work together very closely. The old brain allows behavior to occur, for it controls the physiologic functions of the body. The new brain directs the old brain to satisfy a person's needs and wants through the pictures it has of what is satisfying. The old brain almost never refuses to follow directions from the new brain. It can be taxed to go beyond its normal capacity, and it will deliver the demanded activity by reorganizing and finding other ways to produce the demanded activity (i.e., produce more chemicals to increase the body's energy to accommodate the demand). In Glasser's analysis, psychosomatic illness exemplifies the old brain's struggle to satisfy the new brain's demands.[9,11] For example, in the case of an individual who develops duodenal ulcers because of ineffective control of a chronically stressful job, the old brain reorganizes continuously to deliver the necessary physiologic functions to respond to the individual's need to deal with the chronic stress and overwork. The old brain can be so taxed that it eventually fails to function normally, and then a physical condition is created. Glasser acknowledges that his thinking about psychosomatic illnesses is controversial. However, he is convinced that a significant component of these illnesses is the individual's inability to gain control of some aspect of life. Furthermore, he believes that discovering what the real concern is and identifying ways to be in better control are as important as medical care of the physiologic complaint.

Of the psychological needs, perhaps the most vulnerable to frustration is the need for love and belonging. This need drives individuals to seek friends and establish relationships. In relationships, the need for power often conflicts with the need for love and belonging. Power is defined as the ability to exert influence on another to cause him or her to act in terms of one's own goals. Satisfaction of the need for power increases self-esteem and confidence in one's abilities. However, the wish to control how another should behave may be in direct conflict with the other's self-concept. In relationships, the power struggle that ensues can eventually overshadow the positive relationship that initially characterized the interaction. In another situation, a person's need for power may be pursued through recognition and achievement at work. When this pursuit of power demands high investment of time and energy, it can lead to starvation of other relationships and, particularly, the marital relationship. The time and energy devoted to work is subtracted from the relationship, thereby thwarting the other mate's need for love and belonging. When the balance between the need for power and the need for love and belonging are not negotiated effectively, the relationship may end.

The need for freedom is fundamental. There are prized freedoms that are easily taken for granted—freedom of movement, speech, thought, religion, and freedom to decide how to live one's life. The need for freedom is always somewhat constrained by legal and moral obligations to respect others' rights and freedoms. In addition, the need for freedom sometimes conflicts with the need for love and the need for power. The feeling of belonging comes from commitment to other persons or to systems. These commitments set limits on some freedoms.

According to Glasser's control theory, the need for fun is a basic need because it is inextricably tied with learning. Individuals learn more effectively when learning is fun. Leisure activities are valuable not only because they provide respite from hard work, but because they provide an avenue for learning. Jokes and comedies are often appreciated because of their sharp focus on truth, which otherwise would not be apparent. Playing games and sports is more fun when played with interesting people. The activity becomes an avenue for experiencing, relating, and learning.

Reality, Responsibility, Right and Wrong

REALITY

As has been discussed, a cornerstone concept of reality therapy is effective need fulfillment. Glasser asserts that all psychiatric clients share a common problem with juvenile delinquents and others with emotional problems, in that these individuals deny the reality of the world around them.[6] Denial of reality is manifested through a wide array of behaviors, ranging from delusions to criminal and antisocial behaviors. The object of therapy is not only to help clients face reality, no matter how miserable it is, but also to help the person to find ways to fulfill needs within the reality.

In Glasser's theory, it is the ego's function to test the world of reality and to find the best ways to fulfill needs.[7] This functioning of the ego involves judgment and decision making and, at times, involves frustration and pain. This function of the ego is developed and strengthened within the family. "The more consistent, realistic and loving the family, the better prepared are the children to face the reality of the unprotected (common) world" (reference 7, p 8).

RESPONSIBILITY

Reality therapy works to improve accountability for personal behavior. *Responsibility* is defined as "the ability to fulfill one's needs and to do so in a way that does not deprive others of the ability to fulfill their needs" (reference 6, p 13). Behaviors are evaluated in terms of how effective they are in meeting personal needs. Irresponsible behavior is seen as the best effort, at the moment, to satisfy a need. To learn responsible behavior is to learn more effective need-satisfying behavior. When there is a difference between perceived need and perceived reality, the individual goes through a period of reorganization during which destructive and creative ideas are produced.[11] These ideas are accepted or rejected by the individual, based on their value in satisfying a need. Reality therapy focuses on teaching alternative behaviors that are more effective in maintaining control and satisfying needs on a long-term basis.

RIGHT AND WRONG

The concepts of right and wrong, good and bad, are intrinsic parts of reality therapy. The encouragement of value judgment significantly differentiates reality therapy from conventional psychodynamic therapy. The belief that the client should be guided to evaluate the morality of his or her behavior is based on the premise that all society is based on morality, and encouragement of behavioral evaluation will help the client terminate unsatisfactory behavior and face reality, which includes standards of behavior.[5] Glasser believes that unless the client confronts and judges personal behavior, change will not be achieved.[5] The individual is guided to make an evaluation of behavior in terms of its effectiveness in getting his or her needs met and its fairness to others. Reality therapy asserts that to effectively meet personal needs is dependent upon not depriving others of their need fulfillment. To meet personal needs at the expense of another person usually leads to problems and, eventually, to compromising need fulfillment. A delinquent's quest for power, satisfied by stealing cars and brutalizing others, will eventually lead to incarceration, where personal power is compromised. Although stealing cars may be the best effort to meet the individual's power needs at the moment, in the long run, it is ineffective.

Picture Album

According to Glasser's control theory, individuals are born without knowledge of what basic needs are and how they can be satisfied.[11] However, throughout life, a picture album of need-satisfying events is stored as part of total memory. Glasser prefers the term *picture* to the term *perception*, since he believes that perceptions are mostly visual, and picture, therefore, is more accurate. Glasser assumes that behavior is triggered by the difference between what is wanted and what is possessed.[11] As persons grow, they develop a voluminous picture album of what is need-satisfying. This album is developed through pleasurable experiences and may contain one or up to thousands of pictures to satisfy a need. This picture album does not include everything that the individual knows. It is not the same as mem-

ory, but is a part of it. It contains only need-satisfying pictures, pictures that will bridge what is wanted and what is possessed. These pictures do not have to be rational and, sometimes, can be life-threatening. An example of a life-threatening picture is the one a teenage alcoholic has of drinking to satisfy the need for love and belonging. The power of the picture album to satisfy a need is so strong that the picture can ignore the need for survival. But the pictures in the picture album are not permanent. Replacing pictures, however, is difficult because pictures cannot be erased without being replaced by other need-satisfying pictures. Often, an individual persists in the same behavior because, although the picture is no longer need-satisfying, there is no other picture that is perceived to be more effective.

Behavioral System

There are four components of total behavior that are often considered separate behaviors:[11] (1) the doing component refers to the behavioral component of any behavior. It pertains to the movement of the parts of the body to accomplish a predetermined product (e.g., walk, talk). (2) The thinking component refers to the voluntary or involuntary production of thoughts. (3) Feeling is a component of behavior that is generated in much the same way as doing and thinking; examples are anger, joy, depression, and anxiety; and (4) physiology, which refers to the voluntary or involuntary physical mechanism involved in doing, thinking, and feeling. Consistent with the assumption that all these four components are part of behavior, control theory and reality therapy express every reaction in behavioral terms (e.g., depressed as depressing, phobia as phobicking, anger as angering). Although the feeling component is often the first identified by the individual, the total behavior is more accurately expressed by the doing component. In "depressing," for example, the doing component will be not eating, not talking to anyone, not sleeping well, or crying all the time. It is these doing components that are manifestations of a depressed condition.

In helping others effect change, it is important to remember that total behavior has four components and, of the four, the doing component is most amenable to change. In Glasser's words, "I may not have the ability to change how I feel, separate from what I do and think, but I have almost complete control over what I do and some ability to change what I think, regardless of how I am choosing to feel" (reference 11, p 50). Because behavior is controlled by the individual, once the behavior changes, the thinking and feeling components are also presumed to change.

Glasser refers to all parts of the brain from which behaviors arise as the *behavioral system*.[11] A perceptual error occurs when there is a difference between what is wanted and what is now possessed. Once a perceptual error occurs, the behavioral system presents the individual with one of two things—an organized familiar behavior that results in the correction of the error, or it starts to produce new behaviors randomly, a part of a process called *reorganization*. The new behaviors produced are not necessarily need-satisfying and can be maladaptive.[9] The individual does not have to follow any of the behaviors produced as the behavioral system is reorganizing, but can choose only those that have the most significant chance of correcting the perceptual error. However, once a behavior is chosen, it becomes an organized behavior that can be implemented. At this point, the individual is in full control of his behavior and is responsible for all its repercussions and consequences. This process is referred to as *redirection*.[9,11] Glasser gives the example of John Hinkley, who attempted to assassinate President Reagan. Glasser believes that as part of Hinkley's effort to meet his need for power and belonging, one alternative that his behavioral system created was shooting the President. However, according to Glasser, when Hinkley chose to act on this alternative, he was fully responsible for the decision and, therefore, for the behavior. "He is not responsible for getting the idea—we all get crazy ideas—but he is responsible for putting it into practice" (reference 11, p 99).

Besides reorganization and redirection, another way the behavioral system responds to perceptual error is new information. An example would be Armando, who is lonely and isolated since moving to a new country. His picture of being with his friends and relatives is threatened by his inability to speak the language of the new country and his lack of knowledge of resources. New information about international associations and being introduced to bilingual peers can correct this error and meet his need for belonging.

How the behavioral system works to respond to a need is illustrated in Figure 44-1.

REALITY THERAPY AS A PROCESS

Steps in Reality Therapy and Nursing Roles

Steps involved in the process of reality therapy are identified.[6,9,10]

STEP 1. MAKE FRIENDS

Man's basic needs are fulfilled through involvement with others. It is through involvement with a responsible, loving other that an individual learns responsible, loving behavior. If a person grows up without benefit of this kind of involvement, it is still possible to become responsible and loving through involvement with a therapist who is willing to invest in the person.

Reality therapists are expected to be warm, concerned individuals who want to help the client in every possible way. This sets the atmosphere for a trusting relationship and provides the safe atmosphere in which the nurse and the client can explore what the client really wants. Clients come to therapy usually defending against the real need. This defensiveness makes it difficult to identify what the client's real needs and wants are. In the initial stage of making friends, the psychiatric mental health nurse and the client can talk about anything that is of interest to the client. Although this may not seem to be therapeutic, it helps the client focus on other things besides problems. This is a valuable approach, as it is an avenue to confirm the individual's worth and it helps to provide information on the client's internal world.

For some clients this stage will take the longest time and the most energy investment on the part of the nurse. It may be that having someone communicate to the client that someone cares and finds the client worthwhile is enough to encourage the flow of creativity and energy to engage in active problem solving. The questions "What do you really want, and what do you need?" are questions answered during this stage. These questions are approached gradually depending on the nurse's evaluation of the client's readiness to face his incongruent reality. For some clients, the question "What do you really want?" is hard to grasp or respond to. The alternative question "Are you happy with your present situation?" and "Is there anything you would like to change about your life now?"[16] are alternative ways of getting at the same concerns.

Bassin suggests ways to achieve involvement with the client:[1] (1) Respond to questions as one human being talking to another and be prepared to discuss one's own successes and failures. (2) Use the pronouns "I" and "me" as much as possible. Communication takes place best when the therapist is personal and

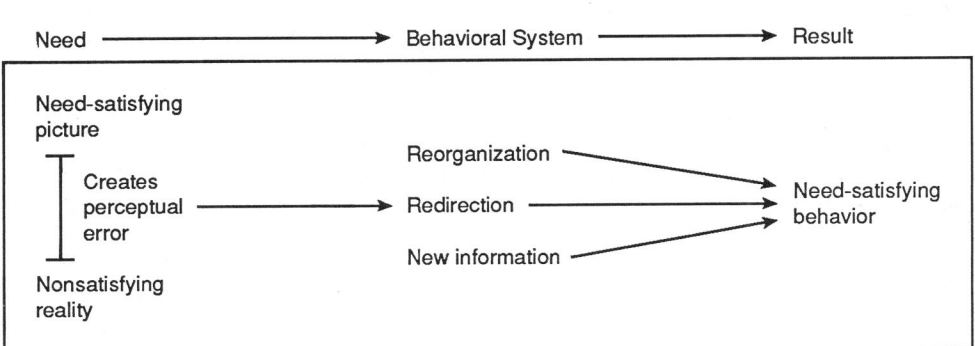

FIGURE 44–1. Behavioral systems at work.

Need ⟶ Behavioral System ⟶ Result

Need-satisfying picture

Creates perceptual error

Nonsatisfying reality

Reorganization

Redirection

New information

Need-satisfying behavior

congruent. (3) Concentrate on the here and now. Bassin asserts that, the more the origins of problems are discussed, the more difficult human involvement becomes.

STEP 2. WHAT ARE YOU DOING NOW?

This second stage focuses on evaluating the doing component of behavior. Although most complaints come in the form of feeling behaviors—"I feel depressed"—or in terms of thinking behaviors—"I cannot concentrate"—it is the doing component that is most tangible and amenable to exploration and change. In the final analysis, it is the doing component that constitutes the problem for the client; for example, "I cannot concentrate so I am not able to complete my work at the office," or "I am so depressed that I cannot take care of my baby."

The nurse, although acknowledging the client's feelings, should guide the client to describe behaviors on a daily basis or in response to an identified problem. Questions such as "What are you doing now?" or "What behaviors have you used to deal with the problem?" emphasize the doing component of behavior and focus the client's attention on planning for action.

STEP 3. IS BEHAVIOR HELPING?

The nurse guides the client to evaluate behavior by asking such questions as "Is what you are doing now getting you what you want?" Using control theory psychology, the nurse guides the client to be aware of an imbalance between identified needs and present reality in terms of whether behavior is need or non–need-satisfying. By introducing this concept of value judgment, the nurse also emphasizes that the client has a choice and can opt for alternative behaviors that better satisfy needs. An aspect of this stage of reality therapy is helping the client assess the different components of total behavior.[18] "Does it help to be depressed about the situation?" How is the client's perception of the problem helping to decide what action to take? "What are the consequences of behavior chosen so far? How effective is the behavior in the long run?" The goal of self-evaluation is to lay the foundation for behavior change. If self-evaluation results in furthering the client's ineffective behavior, it is worthless.

STEP 4. MAKE A PLAN TO DO BETTER

When the client has made a judgment that his behaviors are not effective, the nurse moves quickly to the stage of problem solving. In this stage, the nurse is an active teacher offering choices, alternatives, advice, and encouragement. At the same time, the nurse cautiously guides the client toward plans with the most chance for success. The exploration of alternatives can be initiated by the question, "What could satisfy you right now?" or "What actions can you take to make you feel better?" In helping the client plan realistically, the nurse asks detailed questions and helps the client pre-

pare for contingencies.[1] It is also possible for the nurse to refer the client for advice to a nurse colleague who may have more experience in the specific area that is being planned.[3]

STEP 5. GET A COMMITMENT

For the change to occur, the nurse asks the client for commitment: (1) Is the client committed to change?[4] and (2) is the client committed to the alternatives discussed? It is necessary to get a commitment on the part of the client to try something different, because there are clients who often want to use therapy to complain; however, after evaluating their situation, they conclude that a change is not necessary, but that the opportunity to ventilate was helpful. Being committed to change enhances the possibility that the client will seriously attempt to implement the plan, despite any difficulties the plan may present. Commitment to the plan can be expected only when the plan is specific, understandable, and realistic. A way to enhance commitment to the plan is to use a written contract between the nurse and the client.

STEP 6. NO EXCUSES

When a client fails to execute a plan that has been agreed upon, the nurse is tough in not accepting excuses, because to accept excuses is to accept the person as inadequate and unable. If the plan was reasonable and specific, the client should be allowed to experience the reasonable consequences of its failure. The plan should be reworked, but not explained away. By not accepting excuses, the nurse helps the client develop accountability for his or her behavior and also conveys to the client the nurse's commitment to provide guidance and support to identify an action plan that will eventually lead to need satisfaction. Questions such as "What is the plan now?" "What part of the plan did not work?" and "What kind of help do you need and where can we get that help?" are questions the nurse should persistently ask in an effort to keep the client focused on problem solving, rather than complaining or giving up.

STEP 7. NO PUNISHMENT

When a plan fails or the client gives up, the nurse should not criticize or reject the client for giving up. Punishment in the form of communicating to the client that the nurse has wasted time attempting to help creates only greater loneliness and isolation. At these difficult times, the nurse continues to ask the client whether the need identified is still a need, and if it is, a plan should be identified to help the client achieve need fulfillment. At the same time, the nurse communicates to the client that the choices are his or hers and that no excuses will be accepted, but that the nurse will be there to persist in helping out even when difficulties arise.

STEP 8. DO NOT GIVE UP

It is important to convey hope in the client's ability for more effective behavior. However, it is also appropriate to challenge the client to act as a condition for continuing treatment. Some clients become so complacent with the therapist's accepting involvement that they slump into being help-rejecting complainers who are not committed to action.

The nurse's ability to care for clients is greatly enhanced by her or his involvement with the client in negotiating life on a daily basis. Interaction between the nurse and the client in the context of daily routines allows the nurse to provide corrective emotional experiences to the client. The principles and steps of reality therapy provide a clear guideline and structure for the psychiatric mental health nurse to follow. If the nurse recognizes and encourages clients to make choices, to feel more in control of what happens in their life, at the same time that action orientation and planning is encouraged, both the nurse and the client will achieve specific identifiable results. Reality therapy encourages nurses to get involved with clients. It encourages nurses to get in touch with the patient's internal world through mutual sharing of experiences and interacting on a human level. Although the nurse should never lose sight of the fact that the professional is the helper, this approach to involvement with the client can and does greatly enhance development of a trusting and therapeutic relationship by affirming the client's innate acceptability and worthiness as a human being.

COMMON NURSING DIAGNOSES

Glasser and proponents of reality therapy are greatly opposed to psychiatric diagnoses. Glasser asserts that a specific treatment logically follows a diagnosis, which is true only of medical conditions.[5] In the psychiatric field, the treatment regimen of a client with paranoid schizophrenia may be exactly the same as that of a juvenile delinquent. In reality therapy, specifically, treatment of different psychiatric conditions is the same, based on the premise that all of these conditions arise from lack of need fulfillment. However, to use generally accepted nomenclature, reality therapy has been used to treat clients with schizophrenia, mood disorders, anxiety disorders, impulse control disorders, psychoactive substance use disorders, depressive disorders, and adjustment disorders. Some of the nursing diagnoses commonly occurring in these clients are: aggression, ineffective individual coping, anger, impaired communication, grieving, hopelessness, altered impulse control, and loneliness.

CASE STUDY

Rebecca, an 11-year-old sixth grader, was referred for counseling with the school nurse because of increasing negative behavior and poor grades. Teachers reported that Rebecca, who had been an A student, had become sullen, moody, and usually unprepared for class. Her friends reported that Rebecca is "not the same." She kept to herself and refused to play during recess and after school. At times, she feigned illness in order to go to the nurse's office and avoid tests. Rebecca began using profanity and doodling on the pages of her books—something that the school strictly forbids. Rebecca's mother reported that since her daughter came back from vacationing with her father, she has been a "different girl." She talked back, had tantrums, and sometimes engaged in baby talk to gain attention. Her seclusiveness in school was also observed at home. Rebecca was the only child of divorced parents, both of whom have remarried in the last two years. Her mother

Research Highlights

A study was conducted by Paul Yarish[19] to investigate the effect of reality therapy techniques on the development of an individual's feeling of control over personal fate. It was conducted in a state facility for juvenile offenders, with 60 boys between the ages of 12 and 16 years admitted to the center. Of the 60 boys, 45 completed treatment. These 45 boys also completed the pre- and post–locus of control scale used as an instrument in this research. The other 15 completed the pretest and posttest, but did not complete treatment because they were transferred to more secure facilities. The researcher developed a reality therapy evaluation scale as a measure of whether reality therapy techniques were being applied by the four group leaders. An analysis of variance found that all four group leaders were, in fact, conducting reality therapy. The instrument used to measure the locus of control was the Norwicki-Strickland Locus of Control for Children. In comparing the pretest and posttest results of the juveniles who completed treatment with those who did not, a matched-pairs *T*-test was employed. The study revealed that the juveniles who completed treatment had moved significantly toward an internal direction wherein they believed that they had more control over their own fate because they chose the behavior that better met their needs. However, because the boys who did not complete treatment had been transferred to more secure facilities, a question can be raised about whether they were comparable to those who stayed in the same facility.

Most psychiatric clients, as do juvenile offenders, feel a loss of control over their own experiences and behaviors. A certain helplessness occurs that often leads to dependence on family members, therapists, or the institution. Reality therapy appears to offer an alternative, nonintrusive treatment to give back to the clients a sense of mastery over their environment and their experiences in it.

NURSING CARE PLAN 44-1

REBECCA

NURSING INTERVENTIONS	OUTCOME CRITERIA

NURSING DIAGNOSIS: Anger related to need for love, belonging, and power

CLIENT GOAL: Learn appropriate ways to ask for attention and expressions of love

Identify needs and wants

- Discuss what matters most to Rebecca
- Ask what she wants from school; what she wants from her friends; what she wants from her mother; what she wants from her father; what she wants from her step-parents
- Ask what pictures Rebecca has in her head as satisfying what she wants
- Help Rebecca to develop specific pictures

Discusses specific pictures of what will make her satisfied in school and at home

Evaluate perceptions and behavior

- Discuss with Rebecca what her behaviors are
- Help Rebecca to decide whether these behaviors get her what she wants
- Discuss consequences of behavior
- Discuss how Rebecca thinks others feel because of her behavior
- Discuss whether the pictures in Rebecca's head are attainable

States that her current behaviors do not get her what she wants

Ask Rebecca if she wants to learn more effective behaviors to get her what she wants

- Discuss how hard Rebecca wants to work on it
- Give encouragement that changes can occur
- Discuss how alternative behaviors can help

Commits to change and to try new behaviors

Teach alternative behaviors

- Teach positive attention-getting behavior
- Discuss ways to help Rebecca tell her mother that she wants to spend time with her alone
- Discuss how Rebecca can enjoy the new babies
- Reinforce Rebecca's already organized behaviors: making friends, achieving in school
- Teach behaviors that will help Rebecca feel more in control of her situation; behavior that will help her feel more influential

Talks about how new ways can help her
Suggests some alternative behaviors herself

Help Rebecca to put plan into action

- Provide support and feedback
- Help evaluate and rework plan as needed

No doodling on pages of school books present
Increases interaction with peers
Does not feign illness
Improves school achievement

---

gave birth to a baby girl during the summer; her stepmother, who lives in another state, also gave birth to a baby girl in the fall. Although Rebecca claimed to welcome her two new sisters, her behavior has changed. Rebecca consented to talk to the school nurse three times a week during her lunch period. The school nurse worked with Rebecca until the end of the school year, using reality therapy and focusing on the nursing diagnosis: anger related to need for belonging, love, and power (see Nursing Care Plan 44-1 for a sample care plan for Rebecca).

SUMMARY

Reality therapy is an unconventional approach to helping clients that assumes that emotional and psychiatric conditions originate in a lack of need satisfaction. It emphasizes involvement, responsibility, and value judgments as it guides the client to develop an action-oriented plan to deal with issues and concerns. Although its theoretical framework needs further testing, the strategies of reality therapy offer nurses a different approach to help clients deal effectively with their problems.

References

1. Bassin A. The reality therapy paradigm. In: Bassin A, Bratter TE, Rachin RL, eds. The reality therapy reader. New York: Harper & Row; 1976.

2. Bratter TE. The practice of reality therapy: introduction. In: Bassin A, Bratter TE, Rachin RL, eds. The reality therapy reader. New York: Harper & Row; 1976.

3. Bratter TE. Something old, something new, something borrowed. In: Bassin A, Bratter TE, Rachin RL, eds. The reality therapy reader. New York: Harper & Row; 1976.

4. Buck NS. Are you willing? J Reality Ther. 1987; 6(Spring):37–38.

5. Glasser W. Notes on reality therapy. In: Bassin A, Bratter TE, Rachin RL, eds. The reality therapy reader. New York: Harper & Row; 1976.

6. Glasser W. Reality therapy: a new approach to psychiatry. New York: Harper & Row; 1965.

7. Glasser W. Mental health or mental illness: psychiatry for practical action. New York: Harper & Row; 1960.

8. Glasser W. The identity society. New York: Harper & Row; 1975.

9. Glasser W. Stations of the mind. New York: Harper & Row; 1981.

10. Glasser W. What children need. In: Bassin A, Bratter TE, Rachin RL, eds. The reality therapy reader. New York: Harper & Row; 1976.

11. Glasser W. Control theory: a new explanation of how we control our lives. New York: Harper & Row; 1984.

12. Langer EJ. The psychology of control. Beverly Hills, CA: Saga Publications; 1983.

13. LeBlanc AF. About reality therapy. In: Bassin A, Bratter TE, Rachin RL, eds. The reality therapy reader. New York: Harper & Row; 1976.

14. O'Donnell DJ. History of the growth of the institute for Reality Therapy. J Reality Ther, 1987;7(Fall):2–8.

15. Reilly S. Dr. Glasser without failure. In: Bassin A, Bratter TE, Rachin RL, eds. The reality therapy reader. New York: Harper & Row; 1976.

16. Rosser RL. Reality therapy with the Khmer refugee resettled in the United States. J Reality Ther. 1986;6(Fall):21–29.

17. Silverman RE. Psychology, 5th ed. Englewood Cliffs, NJ: Prentice Hall; 1985.

18. Thatcher JA. Value judgments: a significant aspect of reality therapy. J Reality Ther. 1987;7(Fall).

19. Yarish P. Reality therapy and the locus of control of juvenile offenders. J Reality Ther. 1986;6(Fall):3–10.

45

Helen Palisin

Alternative Therapies

OBJECTIVES
After reading this chapter, the reader will be able to:
1. Describe the traditional biomedical and holistic paradigms
2. Identify the factors contributing to the holistic paradigm
3. List the categories of alternative therapies
4. Identify the framework for evaluating therapies
5. Discuss the limitations of alternative therapies.

INTRODUCTION

A variety of alternative therapies have been introduced in recent years and have been found useful by some clients. Many of these therapies involve a holistic emphasis that challenges the assumptions that mind and body are separate and that the individual can be understood out of the context of the environment in which he or she is functioning. The challenge comes from a shift in perceptions about what constitutes the universe, human nature, and health and illness. To understand the alternative therapies, the paradigm shift that has occurred in society and in health care will be examined.

TWO PARADIGMS

Traditional and alternative therapies represent two different *paradigms* of health and illness. Kuhn describes how scientists will use a paradigm until it becomes clear that it has some limitations, then a shift to a new paradigm begins to take place.[16] However, for some time, both paradigms operate simultaneously, influencing the thought and practice within a profession. That is the current situation, with the traditional biomedical model of health now shifting to a more holistic model.

Traditional Biomedical Model

Capra traces the biomedical model to the 17th century philosopher Descartes, who viewed body and mind, spirit and matter as being separate and unconnected entities.[3] The Cartesian approach was supplemented by Bacon's emphasis on the scientific method, which Newton unified into the methodology of natural science that continues to this day. This scientific approach is based on a view of the universe as a machine or clock full of parts that can be objectified, categorized, and analyzed. Problems can be repaired if necessary—the right cause or broken part need only be found. Disease came to be seen as a breakdown of the body machine that only health professionals could repair, and healing was reduced to a mechanical process. Even though psychiatry was concerned with the mind, rather than the body, psychiatrists extended the scientific method to the treatment of the psyche. This led to a focus on identifying the malfunctioning parts of the psyche, or of the organs, or of bacteria that were causing the problems, and use of organic or chemical treatments to alleviate them.

Holistic Model

A second paradigm is the holistic one, which views all of creation and human nature as integrated, rather than separated into component elements. The term *holism* refers to unified wholes that are greater than the simple sum of their parts. The whole is seen as being so integrated that the properties cannot be reduced to smaller units—there is an interdependence of body, soul, and environment. Some of the dichotomies of body–mind, spirit–matter are being challenged by health professionals who recognize the limitations of such polarities.[3,30]

The rationale for a holistic paradigm has come from several disciplines, including philosophy, religion, psychology, and physics. Philosophers in the mid-19th century began questioning the belief that human experience was divided into subjective–objective components and that abstract truths were more real than immediate human existence.[20] Philosophers, such as Kierkegaard and Nietzsche, attacked these positions as interfering with true Christian beliefs.[14,22] The attacks were on institutionalized religion, which saw God as being external to ordinary human experience and promoted a legalistic approach to true Christian commitment. Their emphasis was on a search for God and spiritual unity, rather than placing God in some external reality. They argued that reality and truth and God were subjective and to be found in the here and now of the human condition.

Theologians and religious historians have also examined the sources of traditional Judeo–Christian teachings about the dualism of human nature.[5,9,23,28] Their research revealed that the beliefs about human nature as having an evil component because of original sin came from a reinterpretation of early scriptures. Teachings in earlier centuries focused on a spirituality that came from a unified and integrated self, with God at the center, rather than external to the individual. These two views of spirituality—a self that is evil and must be suppressed, or a self that is divine—are examples of the views influencing current approaches to spiritual growth.

In psychology there were three forces influencing a new paradigm: Freudian psychology, behaviorism, and existential–gestalt psychology. Although Freud is usually associated with traditional therapies, his original intent was holistic: to integrate body and mind. His theory was influenced by existential philosophy, physiology, and neurology, but he ultimately used the language and concepts from the mechanistic model.[18,20] However, the theory was an assault on the dichotomy of body and psyche and, through techniques such as free association, brought validity to primary subjective processes in human experience. The development of art, music, dance, drama, and poetry as alternative therapies have been directly influenced by psychoanalytic theory.[7] They became an extension of free association to other settings and methods of communication.

The second force in psychology came with behaviorists and their emphasis on the external factors that influenced the organism's behavior.[20] In its own way, behaviorism linked internal human responses with external influences, thereby integrating the individual with the environment. It added the dimension of social interaction to the mechanistic view of human functioning, and it is used extensively in many therapies for reinforcing new behaviors.

A third force came from the influence of existential–gestalt psychology. This was, in part, an extension of Adler and Horney's belief that humans were more integrated than Freud's theory was suggesting. They were looking past the psychic structures of id and ego to the realization of a more unified self and its potential.[11,20] Maslow popularized the term self-actualization as the highest of five levels of need in human beings. This has become identified with the humanist approach and with alternative therapies.[18] Human potential, or self-actualizing psychology, sees the individual as going beyond basic needs or drives to a more spiritual or existential level of functioning. This perspective envisions individuals moving easily between inner and outer reality and between objective and subjective information.

Gestalt psychologists discovered through visual experiments that perceptions begin as a whole, rather than being built up from parts, and how those parts are identified depends on the configuration in which they are viewed. Just as parts have meaning in relation to the whole, the organism's behavior must be viewed in the same context—as moving toward closure on a gestalt or configuration in their lives.[24,28] Maslow's work, along with the influence of Rogers and Perls, provided impetus to the human potential movement and the development of transpersonal psychology.

Physicists, while searching for the piece of matter that would be the building block of a Newtonian universe, were astonished to discover it did not exist. Particles smashed in cyclotrons did not remain in constant form but transformed themselves continuously depending on the environment in which they existed. Even more surprising was the discovery that particles separated by great distances responded to each other as though connected.[3,30] The results cast serious doubt on the whole notion of a mechanistic universe of basic building blocks.

The influence of all these fields have contributed in some way to the holistic paradigm that is the foundation for alternative therapies. It is not unusual to find language from philosophy, religion, psychology, and physics in the descriptions of the therapies. But the continuing influence of the traditional paradigm can also be seen in the alternative therapies.

CLASSIFICATION OF ALTERNATIVE THERAPIES

There are multiple ways of examining the alternative therapies; a useful approach comes from Marmor's classification into five major categories, to which a sixth is added:[19]

1. Emotional release therapies without body manipulation

2. Emotional release therapies with body manipulation
3. Emotional control or self-regulating therapies
4. Religious or inspirational therapies
5. Cognitive–emotional therapies
6. Emotional expression through creative therapies

The categories are not absolute and have considerable overlap among them, but they are a useful approach for making comparisons.

Emotional Release Therapies Without Body Manipulation

Some of the emotional release therapies include encounter groups, gestalt therapy, lifespring, primal therapy, and Erhard seminars training (est).[12,19,24] These can be seen in Table 45-1, which compares them on the dimensions of prime concern; patient variables; mode of change; therapist's task, tools and techniques; cognitive, behavioral, and affective learning; and length of treatment. The major principle involved in the emotional release therapies is catharsis and working through of emotions, by using a variety of methods to achieve that goal. Although the principle comes from Freud, it is not restricted to individual therapy and uses group dynamics for support, feedback, and vicarious learning.

Emotional Release Therapies With Body Manipulation

The interest in emotional release through body contact comes from several sources.[19] Although Freud did not promote body contact, his principle of catharsis is also the underlying mechanism for these therapies. They include Reich's extension of libido to body tension or character armor. Bioenergetic psychotherapy is based on the concept that muscular tension inhibits the capacity for the expression of pleasure—sexual or otherwise. Another therapy, Rolfing, rests on the assumption that problems in human functioning arise from body structure that is misaligned and bound by fascia and must be restored to proper structural integration through deep massage.

Z-Therapy is also known as rage-reduction therapy and is based on the theory that rage reduction is necessary to remove cognitive and sensorimotor deficits. The technique seeks to elicit rage responses through tickling or restraint until the patient is exhausted and stops struggling. A far different approach comes from Arica therapy, which uses body massage as part of a series of nine stages of religious training, aimed at reducing muscle tension, mental stress, and guiding development toward higher consciousness. These different forms of body-contact therapies are shown in Table 45-2.

TABLE 45–1
Emotional release therapies without body manipulation

DIMENSIONS	ENCOUNTER	GESTALT	LIFESPRING	PRIMAL THERAPY	EST
Prime concern	Emotional restriction	Alienation	Self-acceptance and enhancement	"Primal pool" of pain	Self-acceptance
Patient variables	No serious disorders; search for meaning	Exhibitionistic, narcissistic, no serious disorders	No serious disorders; search for self-actualization	Exhibitionistic, all forms of functional psychopathology, repressed anger and hurt, especially at parents	No serious disorders; search for meaning
Mode of change	Communication of spontaneous feelings to others in a group situation with group feedback	Immediate experiencing; sensing or feeling in the immediate moment (i.e., spontaneous expression of experience)	Cognitive learning and spontaneous experiencing in small groups	Discharge of accumulated pain through primal scream experiences	Immediate experiencing with group feedback
Therapist's task	To create an atmosphere in which feelings in the group can be spontaneously and honestly communicated	To interact in a mutually accepting atmosphere for arousal of self-expression (from somatic to spiritual)	To give didactic lectures and also to interact in mutually accepting and empathic manner to encourage self-expression	To encourage release of early painful memories and associated feelings	To give didactic lectures and to create an atmosphere of emotional tension to facilitate abreaction
Tools, techniques	Encounter, exercises to reduce feelings of distance or alienation	Encounter; shared dialogue, experiments or games, dramatization or playing-out of feelings	Didactic lectures, meditation, role-playing, guided fantasies, games, small group discussions	Abreaction	Marathon encounter with authoritarian group leader
Cognitive learning	De-emphasized	De-emphasized	Included	De-emphasized—secondary	Included
Behavior modification	Group reinforcement, rehearsal of behavior	Group reinforcement, rehearsal of behavior	Group reinforcement, role-playing	Powerful suggestion, group reinforcement	Group rehearsal
Affective experience	Explosive catharsis	Explosive catharsis and feeling in touch	Affective experiencing in permissive group setting	Explosive catharsis	Explosive catharsis
Frequency of treatment	Either episodic or may be once a week	Individual and groups, once a week	Three consecutive evenings plus entire weekend	Daily individual session at outset; later weekly group sessions	Daily for nine days

Condensed from Marmor J. Experiential, inspirational, cognitive/emotive, and other therapies. In: Karasu TB, ed. The psychosocial therapies. Washington DC: American Psychiatric Association; 1984, used with permission.

TABLE 45-2
Emotional release therapies with body manipulation

DIMENSIONS	BIOENERGETIC PSYCHOTHERAPY	ROLFING	Z-THERAPY	ARICA
Prime concern	Reduction of muscular tension	Elimination of tensions that are "locked into" muscle, fascia, & tendons	Rage reduction	Total self-realization
Patient variables	Denial of psychological causality; search for answers in somatic changes	Denial of psychological causality; search for answers in somatic changes	Depressed, masochistic, search for quick magical cure	No serious disorders; search for transcendental experience and meaning
Mode of change	Discharge of repressed emotions through postural and muscular movements	Deep, painful massage	Immediate experiencing of repressed rage	Cognitive learning, deep body massage, meditation, guided fantasy, breathing exercise, Tarot cards, and Eastern mystic philosophy
Therapist's task	To diagnose and release patterns of muscular tension to promote emotional abreaction	To diagnose and release areas of myofascial tension	To provoke and elicit violent rage reaction	Didactic, to teach and communicate complex series of ritual tasks
Tools, techniques	One-to-one sessions, client disrobed, communication of feelings, abreaction	One-to-one sessions	Painful body stimulation with patient in restraint	Didactic lectures, meditation, massage, guided fantasy, breathing exercises, Tarot cards, mystic philosophy
Cognitive learning	De-emphasized	De-emphasized	De-emphasized	Emphasized—part of total program
Behavior modification	Relatively slight	Relatively slight	Encouragement of rage expression	Group reinforcement
Affective experience	Strong catharsis in response to body manipulation	Strong catharsis in response to body manipulation.	Explosive catharsis	Affective experiencing in group setting and atmosphere of mysticism
Frequency of treatment	Once or twice a week as a rule	Once or twice a week	Twice a week?	Daily for 40 days, then intermittent

Condensed from Marmor J. Experiential, inspirational, cognitive/emotive, and other therapies. In: Karasu TB ed. The psychosocial therapies. Washington, DC: American Psychiatric Association; 1984, used with permission.

Not shown in the table are simple body manipulation techniques (e.g., Swedish massage), which originated in Eastern traditions and have been integrated into Western cultures.[27] These and variations such as therapeutic touch or acupressure use two principles. The first is the mechanics of improving the physiology of the tissue through increasing circulation, but the second involves the belief that human touch can transmit energy and healing attitudes.

Emotional Control or Self-Regulating Therapies

The emotional control/self-regulating therapies are aimed at control of body processes and are better understood as self-regulatory therapies. They include *imagery*, *meditation*, and *biofeedback*, which are shown in Table 45-3. Although imagery and biofeedback are discussed in Chapter 34, they are included here for comparison purposes. Imagery is a technique that ranges from the guided imagery approach of Leuner for psychoanalytic interpretations, to simple relaxation techniques for personal benefit. Leuner's method uses symbols to elicit psychosexual associations that are communicated verbally to the therapist. With the pure relaxation approach, there is no intent to elicit projections or interpretations.[1,4,17] The distinctions are often confused in practice, especially among lay practitioners. There are many types of meditative techniques, from the prayers of early Judeo–Christian tradition to transcendental meditation shown in Table 45-3. Biofeedback, discussed in an earlier chapter, is

included to show its relationship with the self-regulatory therapies. It is often combined with the other two therapies.[1] There is variation among the techniques in how negative or unwanted thoughts are dealt with. Some therapists simply acknowledge them and proceed, others work through them, whereas still others recommend will power to banish them.

Religious or Inspirational Therapies

The religious and inspirational therapies include healing rituals, such as anointing with oils, faith and miracle healing by television ministries, pilgrimages to shrines, or inspirational messages from charismatic preachers. The basic factors seem to involve the individual's belief and hope for a change or cure, along with faith in the message being conveyed or the practice being undertaken. It is not unusual for the supplicant to experience a profound emotional or spiritual conversion that has a cathartic effect.[19]

Another religious-healing approach is that of Christian Science, which differs from the other religious therapies in its attention to cognitive processes. Illness and disease are seen as being due to an error in thinking, and cure is obtained by recognizing the error and changing the thoughts. Healers and client engage in readings from *Science and Mind*, the text of the founder.[19]

Another form of religious therapy comes from groups, such as the International Society for Krishna Consciousness—or Hare Krishnas. The society promotes the basic belief that each member is an external

TABLE 45-3
Emotional control therapies

DIMENSIONS	RELAXATION/IMAGERY	TRANSCENDENTAL MEDITATION	BIOFEEDBACK
Prime concern	Reduction of tension	Self-enhancement	Self-awareness to regulate biologic dysfunction
Patient variables	Search for awareness of physical and psychological responses	Search for self-fulfillment and transcendental experience	Accept responsibility for physiologic responses
Mode of change	Reduce conscious control of mental processes and repression	Meditation, achievement of transcendental states	Integration of thoughts, emotions, and physiology
Therapist's task	Provide setting, motifs, guide the process of sequential relaxation, interpret symbols	Teaching of techniques, selection of mantra	Teach relaxation, attuning to internal cues and their physiologic consequences
Tools, techniques	Client lying down in dim lighting; music or verbal imagery to produce fantasy	Meditation, mantra	Relaxation, imagery, electrophysiologic monitors
Cognitive learning	Varies—none to moderate depending on therapeutic goals	Minimal	Learn techniques for controlling responses
Behavior modification	Varies from self-reinforcement to therapist's support	Training in relaxation	Extensive—responses shaped through immediate and continuous feedback
Affective experience	Increased awareness, catharsis of repressed feelings, memories	Variable—may be considerable	May be considerable
Length of treatment	Average of 40 hours for psychotherapeutic purpose	20 minutes twice a day	Varies

Transcendental Meditation condensed from Marmor J. Experiential, inspirational, cognitive/emotive, and other therapies. In: Karasu TB, ed. The psychosocial therapies. Washington, DC: American Psychiatric Association; 1984, used with permission.

spirit soul whose purpose is service to God or Krishna. The life-style is rigorous, with much of the day spent in prayer and classes in Vedic teachings. The strong structure and common purpose may provide initial external stability for people who need that kind of support. Cognitive, behavioral, and affective learning are strongly reinforced by the leader and group.[19]

Cognitive–Emotional Therapies

Cognitive–emotional therapies include reality therapy of Glasser discussed in Chapter 44 and rational–emotive therapy of Ellis discussed in Chapter 42. Both are based on the principle that emotions are derived from thought and can be corrected by reeducation.

Ellis believes that humans are capable of reassessing their beliefs, ideas, and values and making necessary changes in their lives. He does not agree with the Freudian view of an instinct-driven organism, and he does not think it is realistic to expect cognitive changes through warm existential encounters.[6,19] In his view, problems arise from false expectations about the need for acceptance, competence, dependency, and perfect solutions to life's problems. The goal of therapy is to help the client become aware of these expectations and abandon them. The therapist is authoritarian in having the correct answers and in pressuring the patient to recognize them. Changes in affect are seen as secondary to changes in thoughts and actions. Behavioral change takes place through the therapist's and group members' responses to the client.

Emotional Expression Through Creative Therapies

The creative arts therapies offer a vehicle for emotional expression through various media.[2,8,21,25] The therapeutic value of creative expression was recognized by ancient cultures, but their application in clinical situations was stimulated by the psychoanalytic focus on the expression of unconscious energy. The creative therapies permit such expression through innovative verbal or nonverbal channels. As can be seen in Table 45-4, the modes of expression are diverse. They range from vicarious emotional experience of audience participation, to active production in one of the creative forms of art, dance, drama, music, or poetry. They also require different levels of physical involvement from fine muscle coordination to gross motor movements, and different levels of vocalizations or verbalizations. Many use imagery and relaxation techniques as part of the warmups to the activity. Other forms of creative media such as film, audio or videotaping are also being used for expression of personal experiences.

NURSING ROLES

It should be evident that not all alternative therapies come from the holistic, humanist, existential, or East-

ern traditions. Some reject the organic or mechanistic model of illness and therapy, but incorporate a mixture of paradigms: this is the source of many problems. There is an assumption that rejection of the medical model or the psychoanalytic approach precludes a need for training. Self-styled therapists sometimes promote catharsis without understanding the principles involved, the role of defenses, the potential for the leader's or group members' use of projection, or recognizing how growth occurs. But knowledge about the mechanism of behavioral change becomes more important as the criteria for expertise shifts from one model to another. Nurses are knowledgeable about both the biomedical and holistic paradigms and are in an excellent position to understand the strengths and limitations of the alternative therapies and of those who conduct them.

One of the most obvious aspects of the alternative approaches is the emphasis on self-development, either through growth, awareness, enlightenment, improved cognition, or spirituality. The goal in most cases is to bring the individual into harmony with some aspect of his or her existence. It is apparent that many of the techniques and approaches have been incorporated into growth or self-awareness movements in the community.[10] The use of imagery, relaxation, and meditative techniques are widespread. So are behaviors and phrases from almost every technique reviewed. As more people have become familiar with the alternative approaches, the practices find their way into many aspects of community life. It is wise for the health professional to sample or investigate the therapies in a community or obtain feedback about the practices before recommending them to patients or clients. Nurses may also choose to become certified as practitioners in some approaches that require such certification.

CASE STUDY

Helen M is a 42-year-old divorced woman who came to the community mental health center for treatment of depression. She obtained a divorce from her husband five years ago, after marital counseling failed to resolve their relationship problems that involved dominating, verbally abusive behavior on his part, and angry withdrawal and depressive episodes on hers. Since the divorce, she has worked as an interviewer for a research institute and has found her work very satisfying. But a new director has been hired who is very aggressive and has been critical of her work and expense account records. During one disagreement she was surprised at her emotional outburst of tears and frustration and she avoided any recurrence by remaining silent. She became alarmed at her progressive withdrawal, weeping, and frequent absences from work because of illness. She felt that she did not even want to see her friends. The clinical nurse specialist who interviewed her at the mental health center made a nursing diagnosis of ineffective individual coping related to difficulty expressing herself in the work setting.

One of the client goals was to discover alternate methods of expressing her beliefs and feelings effectively. One approach that was used was role-playing, a technique that

TABLE 45–4
Emotional expression through creative therapies

DIMENSIONS	ART	DANCE/MOVEMENT	DRAMA/PSYCHODRAMA	MUSIC	POETRY
Prime concern	Self-expression	Release physical restriction	Self-expression and integration of emotional and physical states	Self-expression through sound	Self-expression through creative language
Patient variables	Full spectrum—no serious disorders to severely regressed	Full spectrum—no serious disorders to severely regressed	Full spectrum—no serious disorders to severely regressed	Full spectrum—no serious disorders to severely regressed	Full spectrum—no serious disorders to severely regressed
Mode of change	Nonverbal expression of inner state through use of hands and media	Nonverbal expression of inner state through use of body movement	Reality amplified, clarified and concretized through verbal and nonverbal dramatization	Experience of primitive emotions in safety of structured environment	Communication or experience of inner states through symbols and rhythms
Therapist's task	Assess anxiety level, select goals and media, provide instruction	Create atmosphere for safe expression of body language	Select goals and techniques to meet needs of individuals or group	Identify cultural preferences for music and select materials or instruments	Select poems to reflect feelings of group, or elicit creation of poems
Tools, techniques	All forms of artistic media for free-form expression, and elicit patient associations	Muscle warmups, relaxation, music, self and instructor observation of body mechanics	Theater techniques—scripts, roles in drama; creation of both scripts and roles by protagonist in psychodrama, auxiliary egos, doubles, etc.	Vocal or instrumental participation in group production	Relaxation, imagery, recognition of inner rhythms and responses
Cognitive learning	Minimal—emphasis on process vs product	Varies—may be extensive as in movement analysis	May be extensive	Minimal	Extensive—recognition of universality of experiences
Behavior modification	Extensive—support from group and therapist	Varies from minimal to extensive feedback	Extensive with group and director feedback	Extensive, self-reinforcing also group support	Extensive, self-reinforcing with group and therapist support
Affective experience	Extensive	Extensive	Extensive	Extensive	Extensive
Length of treatment	Varies based on goal	Varies based on goal	Weekend workshops to ongoing groups	Varies based on goal	Varies based on goal

NURSING CARE PLAN 45-1

HELEN M

NURSING INTERVENTIONS	OUTCOME CRITERIA
NURSING DIAGNOSIS: Ineffective individual coping related to difficulty expressing herself in work setting	
CLIENT GOAL: Rehearse alternate behavior and responses to problem interaction through role-playing	
■ Ask Helen to select one situation that has created a problem in the past	Describes problematic situation
■ Bring Helen's reality into here and now for observation	
■ Ask Helen to stage the scene	
■ Elicit details of setting including role nurse is to play in the reenactment, since details facilitate concretization of experience into observable units and also reduces anxiety	
■ Observe body language, affect, verbalizations, and "blocks" in the drama	Understands own part in problematic situation
■ Direct Helen's attention to behaviors involved	
■ Discuss alternate responses and roles and have Helen try them out	Expands range of responses through rehearsal

came from dramatic arts and has since been incorporated in many alternative therapies such as gestalt[24] (see Nursing Care Plan 45-1 for a sample care plan for Helen M).

SUMMARY

Alternative therapies have arisen from several forces operating in the fields of philosophy, religion, psychology, and physics, that promote the view that humans have the potential for functioning in an integrated, holistic manner, in harmony within themselves and with the universe. The first task toward this higher consciousness requires a level of self-development that is less concerned with removing problems than in attaining wholeness. The approaches may be through creative therapies, emotional release, body integration, self-regulation, spiritual inspiration, or cognitive activities. The goal is unity.

Research Highlights

Karasu TB, Conte HR, Plutchik R. Psychotherapy outcome research. In: Karasu TB, ed. The psychosocial therapies. Washington, DC: American Psychiatric Association; 1984.

Reichardt CS, Cook TD. Beyond qualitative versus quantitative methods. In: Cook TD, Reichardt CS, eds. Qualitative and quantitative methods in evaluation research. Beverly Hills: Sage Publication; 1979.

Yin RK. Case study research, design and methods. Beverly Hills: Sage Publications; 1984.

The shift in paradigms discussed in this chapter extends to research evaluating psychotherapy. Karasu et al. systematically identify and discuss the problems in evaluating psychotherapy in any form. Issues such as standardizing diagnoses, therapists, therapy, patients, and ethical considerations about the use of control groups are only some of the difficulties plaguing the methodology of measuring outcomes.

These problems relate to use of experimental designs and group statistics. There is another paradigm emerging, as can be seen in the works of Reichardt and Cook, and Yin. This paradigm recognizes that in some situations qualitative methods may have greater validity than group statistics. Yin examines the features of the case study method in terms of definition of the problem, design of the study, data collection and analysis, and reporting the results. It is a methodology that is gaining respectability and may be the most appropriate to answer questions about individual outcomes.

References

1. Adler CS, Adler SM. Biofeedback. In: Karasu TB, ed. The psychosocial therapies. Washington DC: American Psychiatric Association; 1984.
2. Buchanan DR. Psychodrama. In: Karasu TB, ed. The psychosocial therapies. Washington DC: American Psychiatric Association; 1984.
3. Capra F. The turning point. New York: Bantam Books; 1983.
4. Carrington P, Ephron HS. Meditation as an adjunct to psychotherapy. In: Arieti S, Chrzanowski G, eds. New dimensions in psychiatry: a world view. New York: John Wiley & Sons; 1975.
5. Chardin T. The phenomenon of man. New York: Harper & Row; 1961.
6. Ellis A. Humanistic psychotherapy. New York: McGraw-Hill; 1973.
7. Fink PJ, Levick MR, Hays R, Johnson DR, Dulicai D, Briggs CA. Creative therapies. In: Karasu TB, ed. The psychosocial therapies. Washington DC: American Psychiatric Association; 1984.
8. Fleshman B, Fryrear JL. The arts in therapy. Chicago: Nelson-Hall; 1981.
9. Fox M. Original blessing. Santa Fe: Bear & Co; 1986.
10. Gartner A, Riessman F. The self-help revolution. New York: Human Sciences Press; 1984.
11. Horney K. Neurosis and human growth. New York: WW Norton & Co; 1950, 1970.
12. Janov A. The primal scream. New York: G Putnam & Sons; 1971.
13. Karasu TB, Conte HR, Plutchik R. Psychotherapy outcome research. In: Karasu TB, ed. The psychosocial therapies. Washington DC: American Psychiatric Association; 1984.
14. Kierkegaard S. In: Bretall R, ed. A Kierkegaard anthology. New York: The Modern Library; 1946.
15. Kondo A. Morita therapy. In: Arieti S, Chrzanowski G, eds. New dimensions in psychiatry: a world view. New York: John Wiley & Sons; 1975.
16. Kuhn TS. The structure of scientific revolutions. Chicago: University of Chicago Press; 1970.
17. Leuner H. The role of imagery in psychotherapy. In: Arieti S, Chrzanowski G, eds. New dimensions in psychiatry: a world view. New York: John Wiley & Sons; 1975.
18. Maslow A. Toward a psychology of being. New York: D Van Nostrand; 1968.
19. Marmor J. Experiential, inspirational, cognitive/emotive, and other therapies. In: Karasu TB, ed. The psychosocial therapies. Washington DC: American Psychiatric Association; 1984.
20. May R. The meaning of anxiety. New York: Ronald Press; 1950.
21. Moreno JL. Psychodrama, vol 1. New York: Beacon House; 1946.
22. Nietzsche F. The gay science. In: Kaufmann W, ed. The portable Nietzsche. New York: Viking Press; 1970.
23. Pagels E. Adam, Eve, and the serpent. New York: Random House; 1988.
24. Perls F, Hefferline RE, Goodman P. Gestalt therapy. New York: Dell Publishing; 1951.
25. Pesso A. Movement in psychotherapy. New York: New York University Press; 1969.
26. Reichardt CS, Cook TD. Beyond qualitative versus quantitative methods. In: Cook TD, Reichardt CS, eds. Qualitative and quantitative methods in evaluation research. Beverly Hills: Sage Publications; 1979.
27. Tappan FM. Healing massage techniques. Reston, VA: Reston Publishing; 1978.
28. Walker JL. Body and soul. New York: Abingdon Press; 1971.
29. Yin RK. Case study research, design and methods. Beverly Hills: Sage Publications; 1984.
30. Zukav G. The dancing Wu Li masters. New York: William Morrow & Co; 1979.

Health Care Delivery System: Current and Future Issues

46

Irene Daniels Lewis

The Mental Health Care Delivery System

OBJECTIVES

After reading this chapter, the reader will be able to:

1. Identify selected leaders in the evolution of the psychiatric mental health care delivery system
2. Recognize the impact of legislation on the psychiatric mental health care delivery system
3. Analyze the influence funding has upon a community mental health delivery system
4. Compare the past mental health delivery system with the current mental health delivery system.

INTRODUCTION

This chapter presents a brief history of the mental health care delivery system and a detailed description of its current status. Selected roles and issues in psychiatric mental health nursing will be discussed. Additionally, a discussion of the influence of legislation and funding, especially for community-based service delivery will be addressed. Finally, some unmet needs and problems with today's system of care will be discussed.

PRIMITIVE SOCIETIES: CARE OF MENTALLY ILL

Throughout its history, the mental health care delivery system has been influenced by a lack of scientific knowledge of the etiology of mental illness. For centuries, in primitive societies, care was based on traditions, customs, and myths.[5,11,13] A prevailing belief concerning the cause of mental illness was that it was a result of invasion of the body by evil spirits or evil substances.[5,11,13] As Figures 46-1 and 46-2 indicate, "treatment" included exorcism of the evil spirits by a priest or attempts to bleed the "evil" out of a mentally ill person through the application of leeches. Those behaving in socially unacceptable ways were sometimes labeled as "witches" or "demon possessed" and were ostracized or killed.

EIGHTEENTH AND NINETEENTH CENTURIES

In the mid-18th century, Dr. Phillippe Pinel (Fig. 46-3) advocated a humanitarian approach in the care of mentally ill persons. His "moral treatment" included regular meals; kind, but firm, treatment from attendants; and recreational activities. He and other physicians in Valencia are credited with literally unchaining the insane in hospitals and prisons.[5] Pinel based his humane approach upon "personal notes" taken during regular observation of the insane. The idea of systematically recording behaviors and interactions of the insane was very innovative, if not revolutionary, during this period.[5] About the same time, in 1752, the first hospital in America to admit mentally ill persons opened in Philadelphia. Dr. Benjamin Rush, known as the Father of American Psychiatry, joined the Pennsylvania Hospital staff in 1783. He also instituted a humane approach for the delivery of care to mentally ill persons.[6]

Unfortunately, the aforementioned approaches to care, instituted by Pinel and Rush, were in the minority. Most hospitals for the mentally ill remained places where mass confusion and gross neglect prevailed. Until the 1880s, the St. Mary of Bethlehem Hospital in London allowed the public to view mentally ill persons for entertainment. Tourists paid an admission fee to "gawk" at the insane. This unkindly and inhumane treatment was commonly practiced in many countries throughout Europe (Figs. 46-4 and 46-5).

MENTAL HEALTH LAY MOVEMENT

Significant reforms in the mental health care delivery system in the United States are credited to Dorothea Dix, an energetic school teacher (Fig. 46-6). Shocked by the deplorable way that mentally ill persons were treated in Cambridge, Massachusetts, in 1842, Dorothea Dix became a leader in the reformation of the system. She researched facilities in the United States

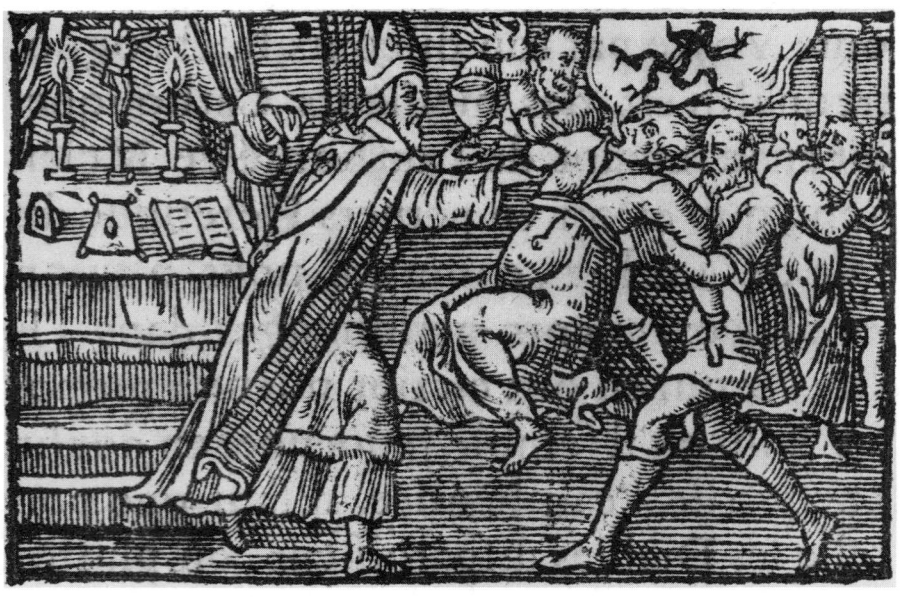

FIGURE 46–1. Demon being exorcised from a woman in front of an altar with a priest in attendance. (Woodcut by Pierre Boaistuau, Histoires prodigieuses et memorables . . . . , Paris, 1598. Used with permission from the National Library of Medicine)

FIGURE 46–2. A woman, seated at a table, applies a leech to her forearm. (Used with permission from the National Library of Medicine)

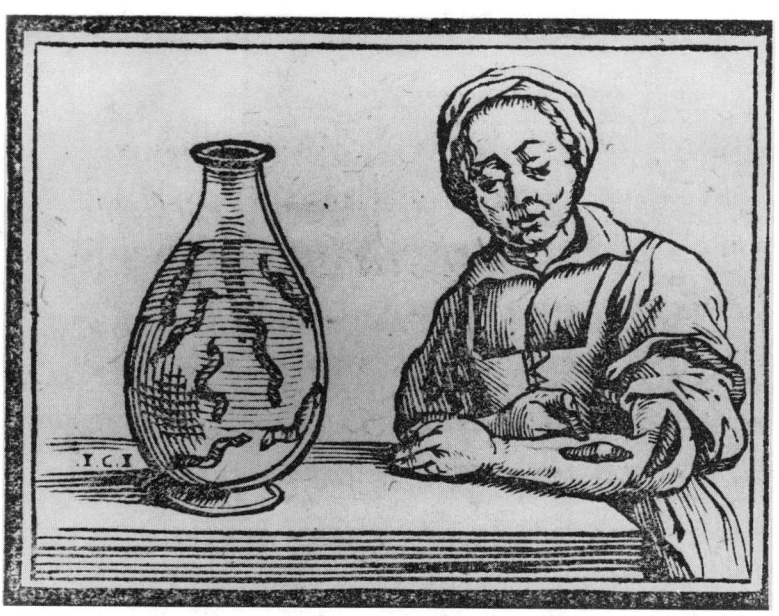

and in Canada and shared her findings with legislators, other key decision makers, and the general public. Finally, in 1844, as a result of increased awareness of grossly inadequate treatment of the mentally ill, the Association of Medical Superintendents of American Institutions of the Insane was formed.[6] The Association of Medical Superintendents achieved some of the economic and sociopolitical changes essential to the demise of a cruel, punishing mental health delivery system. However, spiraling costs made this more humane care unaffordable for most families. Once again, in the 1860s, institutions for the mentally ill, especially indigent chronically mentally ill persons became "snake pits."[6]

Later, in 1894, Clifford W. Beers published, A Mind that Found Itself, an autobiographical account of his life in an American mental institution. His book led to increased public awareness of the mentally ill person's plight in institutions.[3] Although some progress toward an improved mental health delivery system can be credited to Rush, Dix, Beers, and their followers, generally the system remained unchanged and unresponsive to the needs of mentally ill persons. Institutions were not well maintained and were grossly understaffed. Many facilities lacked adequate heat and light. Most employees were untrained or poorly trained. Few facilities had nurses, and those that did, did not have enough for the number of clients.

FIGURE 46–3. Dr. Phillippe Pinel (center left) at the Hospital of Salpetriere. (Used with permission from the National Library of Medicine)

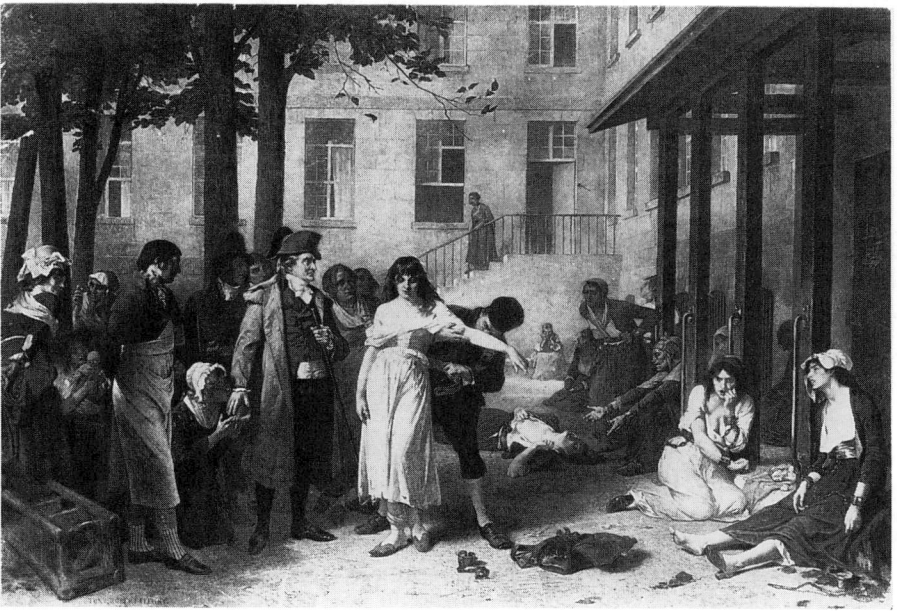

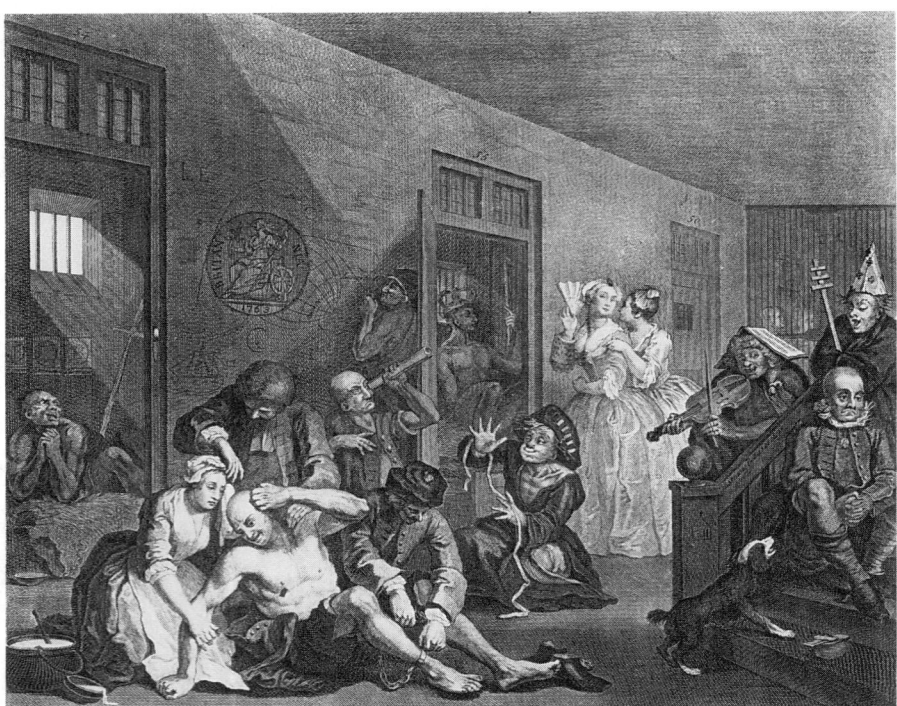

FIGURE 46–4. "Bedlam." (Engraving by William Hogarth, 18th century. Used with permission from the National Library of Medicine)

TWENTIETH CENTURY

The first four decades of the 20th century were characterized by custodial care and physical treatments of symptomatology. The range of treatments included electric shock, cold wet sheet packs, restraints, and prefontal lobotomies. Psychiatric mental health nurses provided physical care including pre- and postoperative care for such treatments as lobotomies.

In the 1950s and 1960s, four factors helped to change the mental health delivery system: introduction of therapeutic milieu; use of psychotropic drugs; increases in the number of mentally ill persons, especially following World War II and the Korean War, and then, later, the Viet Nam War; and deinstitutionalization of psychiatric clients. Drug therapy expanded the role of psychiatric mental health nurses. By this time, the idea of nurse as therapist was developed, accepted, and practiced in most psychiatric settings, except for the more isolated state hospitals or conservative medical communities. A response to the rapid influx of veterans from World War II was group therapy. Deinstitutionalization of clients within the psychiatric mental health delivery system was influenced by federal laws and dollars. The next section will discuss federal laws and federal fundings related to the mental health delivery system.

FEDERAL LEGISLATION

Important federal laws that influenced the mental health delivery system in the 1900s included the Harrison Narcotic Act,[10] which fostered mental health research. Not until after World War II did the government pass more legislation affecting mental health. The National Mental Health Act of 1946 was a giant step for the field. It created the National Institute of Mental Health (NIMH), which provided monies to train professional personnel: psychiatrists, psychiatric nurses, psychologists, and psychiatric social workers. Additionally, the act allocated funds for both research and direct aid to states to establish new treatment facilities.[7]

Later, the 1963 Mental Retardation Facilities and Community Mental Health Centers Act and its subsequent amendments were passed. These combined laws mandated that psychiatric clinics and centers be located within communities as contrasted with the remoteness of many state hospitals. The Community Mental Health Centers Act and its amendments gave rise to the decentralization movement. Four other key factors that contributed to the deinstitutionalization movement were: (1) the confluence of psychotropic drugs and the therapeutic milieu (both appeared to have eradicated a need for indefinite hospitalization for mentally ill persons); (2) state government costs, which were expected to decrease because of matching federal dollars; (3) public opinion and mass media, which in the context of increased awareness of human rights, were advocating more legal rights for mentally ill persons; and (4) concerns about the long-term state hospital residents who became institutionalized, that is, those who had lost the social and interpersonal skills needed for reentry into society.[30]

Community Mental Health Centers

The Mental Retardation Facilities and Community Mental Health Centers Act of 1963 sanctioned the es-

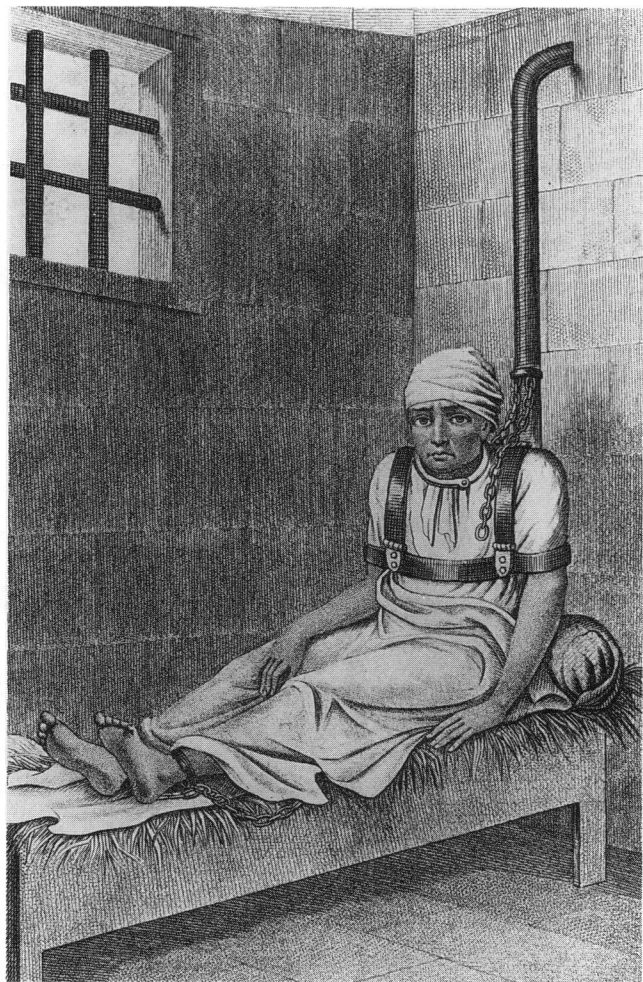

FIGURE 46–5. Mental patient. (From Esquirol E. Les maladies mentales. Paris, 1838. Used with permission from the National Library of Medicine)

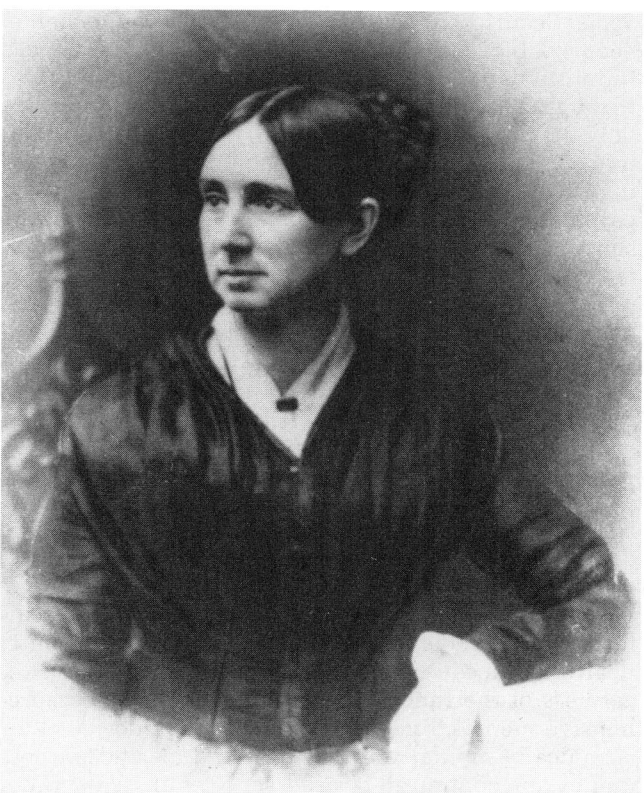

FIGURE 46–6. Dorothea Lynde Dix, 1802–1887. (Used with permission from the National Library of Medicine)

tablishment of, and funding for, local community mental health centers (CMHCs) to provide outpatient mental health treatment. President John F. Kennedy, who was sensitive to the need, perhaps because a family member was mentally retarded, was persuasive in his encouragement for this legislative action. Passage of the 1975 Community Mental Health Centers Act and, subsequently, the 1978 amendments, enabled mentally ill persons to be treated in their communities. These centers were staffed by psychiatrists, psychologists, psychiatric nurses, psychiatric social workers, community outreach workers, and ancilliary workers. Initially, passage of the aforementioned federal laws seemed to give the community-based mental health delivery system more clout. However, upon closer review, serious gaps in funding and delivery services (i.e., supportive services) became evident. In 1980, the Mental Health Systems Act expanded upon existing delivery services, yet inadequate funding and insufficient supportive services continued. A fatal blow for the community-based delivery system was the 1981 Omnibus Budget Reconciliation Act, because it repealed

the 1975 and 1980 acts. Accountability and allocations for community-based mental health delivery services shifted from governmental control under the National Institutes of Mental Health, to the Alcohol, Drug Abuse, and Mental Health (ADAMHA) Block Grant Programs, giving control to individual states.[8] Thus, attempts by the federal government to devise an improved mental health delivery system began to erode.

Funding

Today, in the United States, funding for mental health services is limited. Basically there are only three sources of payment for mental health services: federal, state, and private. The Community Mental Health Centers Acts provided seed monies that were designed to decrease over time. However, many states failed to respond adequately to this plan, and consequently, a piecemeal funding system resulted. Now, community-based mental health services are fragmented.

PUBLIC FUNDING

Federal dollars are allocated to categorical programs[18] with limited parameters (i.e., programs focused toward a particular mission). Mental health services are funded through Social Services (formerly Title XX),

Social Security Disability Income (SSDI), Supplemental Security Income (SSI), and Medicare and Medicaid.[24] Individuals may need to qualify for such programs through a means eligibility test. Medicare provides only 250 dollars per person each year with a prohibitive 50% coinsurance rate that many people frequenting CMHCs cannot afford. Medicaid covers inpatient psychiatric care in nursing homes that precipitated the substitution of nursing homes for state mental hospitals, because costs for treating chronically mentally ill persons are less in nursing homes than in state hospitals.[25,26] States have discretionary powers for administering Medicaid funds; therefore, CMHCs are under the fiscal umbrella of Medicaid in some states, but not in others.[29]

PRIVATE FUNDING

Historically, persons with financial means have had no difficulty obtaining mental health services, regardless of setting. However, problems exist for middle income individuals with private insurance carriers. Fiscal intermediaries have clauses that severely limit mental health services owing to their prohibitive costs. Regardless of the funding source, none support comprehensive mental illness services, none are designed for chronically mentally ill persons, and all allocate less money for community-based services than for inpatient care.[19,26,28]

Types of Services

Unquestionably, funding influences the range of mental health care. Although limited, inpatient treatment far exceeds community-based care in breadth of supportive services. Both state and acute hospitals can provide social services, psychiatric nursing, x-ray examinations, laboratory work, and occupational and physical therapy. The CMHCs have varied access to limited supportive services. Access depends upon funding arrangements, available transportation, and manpower. If an individual mental health care recipient elects not to follow up a referral, that may be the fatal flaw in receiving care, since mental health care providers, with overextended case loads, are not able to monitor all clients effectively.

GAPS IN COMMUNITY MENTAL HEALTH DELIVERY SYSTEM

What is occurring today is an ever-growing, unplanned community-based residential mental health delivery system. Direction and focus are urgently needed. A task force was established by the American Psychiatric Association in the early 1970s to review and evaluate the current status of these settings and to develop a typology and a uniform nomenclature that would decrease conceptual confusion. This task was required before any research could be conducted on the process and outcome of various mental health treatment programs. The task was completed and a report presented to the professional association in 1980. A summary of the nomenclature they devised is reported here.

TYPOLOGY: COMMUNITY-BASED RESIDENTIAL CARE

Nursing Homes

There are two types of community nursing facilities that provide 24-hour nursing care to mentally or physically ill clients.

1. *Skilled nursing facility* (SNF) clients require skilled nursing observations and medical actions. Either licensed registered nurses or licensed vocational nurses must be employed by the owner, depending upon the facility's licensed bed capacity.
2. *Intermediate care facility* (ICF) clients require less care than a SNF; however, clients need a planned program of health care.

Clients in either SNFs or ICFs may be young or old, and their stay may be brief or indefinite. Federal and state laws regulate these facilities. They are licensed as either for-profit or nonprofit by state health departments and are subject to regular, unannounced evaluative visits by state health officials to determine whether or not minimal requirements are being observed. Neither SNFs or ICFs require psychiatric mental health professional staff or consultation. The task force recommended regular, intermittent psychiatric mental health professional supervision for mentally ill residents.

Group Homes

Group homes are residences for groups of clients (8 to 10 adolescents or 8 to 15 adults). Their focus is psychosocial rehabilitation through structured activities. Psychiatric mental health professional and paraprofessional staff are required. Programmatic goals, structured activities, and length of stay vary according to the needs of the residents. A license is required, and these homes should have contractual agreements with CMHCs and local acute hospitals.

Personal Care Homes

Personal care homes are residences for four or more adults who require some assistance with personal hygiene and activities of daily living. A license is required as well as regular, unannounced evaluative visits, usually by state officials. Their population is usually chronically mentally ill and retarded individuals who may be young or old. Length of stay varies from short-term to indefinite.

Foster Homes

An intact family provides a temporary to lifelong foster home for from one to four children, adolescents, or adults. Ideally, residents are incorporated into the family structure as "members." Psychiatric mental health support is given to the residents and to members of the foster family. Formal arrangements with CMHCs, hospitals, and providers are mandatory. Foster homes are monitored by the placement agency on a regular basis.

Natural Family Placement

Clients live with their own families. The length of stay is variable. Obviously, no contract or license is required. The optimum goal is health maintenance and reintegration of the client into the family and the community. Psychiatric mental health services are available for both client and family.

Satellite Housing

Satellite housing placements accommodate from one to four clients who are capable of semi-independent living. Homes are leased or co-leased by an agency. Agency professionals assist clients in resocialization techniques. Clients perform independent activities of daily living. Formal arrangements are suggested with CMHCs and with hospital emergency psychiatric care units. The client's length of stay varies. No license is required.

Independent Living

Clients live independently in either their own homes or apartments. Frequently, many stay in inexpensive hotels otherwise known as single-room occupancies (SROs).[1,21]

The typology that resulted from the task force's work is summarized in Table 46-1. Note examples of facilities in each classification and the definition of each classification. The need still exists for comprehensive investigations of mental health program offerings, processes, and outcomes stemming from community-based residential setting.

Klerman[14] perceives the shift to community-based residential care from state institutions as a far cry from substantive change. Delivery of mental health services merely changed from single-purpose custodian care in state hospitals to multipurpose custodian care in varied community homes. Talbott[27] coined a new term, *trans-institutionalization*, which is more befitting of the process called *deinstitutionalization*, because many clients are literally transferred from state hospitals to residential care settings in the community. A valid question to raise is: Are mentally ill persons better off now than before, or are they worse off?[4]

MANPOWER

Traditionally there has been a shortage of personnel in mental health care. The missing linkages between the community-based mental health delivery services and professional psychiatric mental health nursing highlights that shortage.[23] Except for a few types of homes, psychiatric mental health nurses do not usually interface with the untrained or undertrained professionals or paraprofessionals serving as administrators or owners of the varied community-based facilities depicted in the summary of the American Psychiatric Association Task Force Report cited earlier. Psychiatric mental health nursing leaders, as well as selected governmental agency administrators, have been concerned about the dearth of psychiatric mental health nurses who were conducting research about the efficacy of treatments and other interventions in the field.[20] The next section will discuss the topic of research in nursing in more detail.

REPORT OF NATIONAL INSTITUTE OF MENTAL HEALTH TASK FORCE ON NURSING

Decision makers at the National Institute of Mental Health (NIMH) have been increasingly concerned about (1) the limited participation by psychiatric mental health nurses in the extramural activities of NIMH; (2) the need for research on strategies to influence care of chronically mentally ill persons; and (3) the growing population at risk for mental illness.[20] In 1986, in response to these concerns, the NIMH Director appointed a Task Force on Nursing from leaders in psychiatric mental health nursing, nursing research, and related disciplines, to study the matter. The task force presented its report to the National Mental Health Advisory Council in 1987. The report includes descriptions of psychiatric mental health nursing research conducted for mentally ill persons.[20] Some research findings cited in that report are summarized here.

Turner[20] studied the extent of disability in a sample of former mental clients living in a rural community. The investigation showed that social support networks in the community were correlated significantly with measured functional capacity of the former clients.

In Phillip's investigation[20] of caregivers and frail elderly homebound clients, two dichotomous groups were identified. One group was labeled abusive, and the other group was labeled nonabusive. These two groups differed in terms of perceived social support, expectations of their caregivers, and perceptions of their caregivers. Motives, attitudes, family structure,

TABLE 46–1
Typology of community residences

TYPE OF RESIDENCE	PSYCHIATRIC TIME ON SITE	ON SITE STAFF FULL-TIME 24 HRS	ON SITE STAFF PART-TIME	CLINICAL LINKAGES REQUIRED
NURSING FACILITY SNF ICF	Part-time on site for evaluations, consultations, emergencies, staff supervision and treatment plng	Nursing staff constant	Medical and mental health professionals and paraprofessional support staff	24-hr ER and medical care
GROUP HOME	Part-time on site for emergency intervention; staff consultation, supervision and training	Mental health professionals and paraprofessionals trained in group process and rehabilitation techniques	Support staff appropriate to treatment goals	Full range mental health and social services; CMHC; hospital; private practitioner; formal
Personal Care Home	X	Manager Proprietor and staff appropriate to program	Home visits and consultations by mental health professional or MHW	Formal with faciliation of referrals and linkages
Foster Home	X	Foster parents and family living in own home	Home visits by mental health professional or mental health dependent or client or parent needs	Formal CMHC, and social service agency
Natural Family Placement	X	X	As above	Informal and prn at option of family
Satellite Housing	X	X	Supervision prn from sponsoring agency	Formal with sponsoring agency

Reprinted with permission from A typology of community residential services: report on the Task Force on Community Residential Service. Copyright 1982, American Psychiatric Association.

and nature of the lifelong family relationships all contributed to differences between the two groups.

Hirschfeld[12] studied families living with an elderly person who had senile brain disease and found that the lower the tension, the greater the quality of the dyadic relationship and management ability and the lesser the need for institutionalization owing to family exhaustion.

Fox and colleagues[20] studied the impact of diagnostic related groups (DRGs) on community and family care services for the elderly. They explored how selected care providers, area agencies on aging, acute care hospital discharge planners, nursing home directors, home health care agency directors, home health care nurses, and family caregivers experienced the impact of DRGs during a three-year period. They found significant patterns of correlations between increased cost, burden for community and family caregivers, and decreased hospital costs associated with DRGs. Family and client stress involving increased mental dysfunction were commonly reported.

And lastly, findings from a study by Chafetz,[20] which examined the homeless and their use of psychiatric emergency centers, indicated that of those clients seen in a psychiatric emergency center, about 40% were residentially unstable, 17% were without any form of shelter, and 29% reported episodic loss of shelter. From these studies, it is clear that psychiatric mental health

nurse researchers are examining important topics and that they are studying important populations in the field. The task force also found that psychiatric mental health nurses were involved in a very limited way in NIMH extramural activities. Nurses submitted few research applications. Successful funding of proposals correlated positively with academic research career development applications but not with pure research applications. Additionally, the task force affirmed that more individuals were at risk for mental illness and that there is a need for more research on effective strategies to influence the delivery of services to the chronically mentally ill. Specific recommendations were offered.[20]

ISSUES

As professional nursing evolves and as clinicians in speciality areas continue to develop and refine their standards of practice, concerns and issues will confront those committed to excellence.[22] Among some of the many pressing questions being discussed by psychiatric mental health nursing leaders are the following:

1. How can the problems created by the unplanned proliferation of community-based residential care

PROGRAM FOCUS	LEVEL OF DISABILITY	SIZE OF POPULATION	LENGTH OF STAY	LICENSE REQUIRED
Medical, nursing, protection	Severe	Variable	Long-term, but can be used for short-term	Yes
Psychosocial rehabilitation through group process and milieu	Moderate to mild	Adult 8–15; adolescents 8–10	Variable depending on program	Yes
Maintain level of functioning and support improvement	Moderate to mild	Variable (depending on size of facility and staff)	Variable (short term to lifelong)	Yes
Treatment based on family model	Severe to mild depending on family skills	Child 1–4; adolescent: 1–2; adults: 1–4; mentally retarded: 1–2	Variable (as above)	Placing agency evaluation and approval
Reintegration and maintenance: support for family	As above	X	X	X
Independent living	Moderate to mild	1–4 per unit	Variable	No

settings for chronically mentally ill clients be most effectively addressed?

2. What effective roles can psychiatric mental health nurses play in raising the standards in community-based residential settings (i.e., nursing homes and CMHCs)?

3. What is the impact of DRGs on the mental health delivery system (community-based and hospital-based)?

4. How can the needs of older persons who suffer from chronic mental illness be met when few professional psychiatric personnel are interested in geropsychiatric practice?

5. How can adequate, comprehensive funding for chronically mentally ill clients be acquired?

6. How can research on routine psychiatric mental health nursing interventions and their effectiveness be encouraged?

7. Is the management of chronically mentally ill clients by nonphysicians (e.g., psychiatric mental health nurse therapists) going to expand? If not, why not? If so, why will it?[9,17]

Considering that the number of chronically mentally ill persons will continue to grow commensurate with the population growth, the absence of a comprehensive mental health delivery system that allows, or encourages, adequate supportive services and, thus, continuity of care, will be an increasingly key public policy issue.[15,16]

Research Highlights

There is an urgent need for more investigations on the most effective ways to deliver care to chronically mentally ill persons. Of particular importance to the field is research about therapeutic actions and environmental modifications that can minimize the effects of illness and improve the coping abilities of individuals and their families to actual or potential mental health problems.[1,20,22]

SUMMARY

In the distant past, people believed that mental illness was caused by evil spirits, and possessed individuals were treated with traditional methods, ostracized, or killed. Scientific developments have led to an understanding that mental illness is treatable. With sustained treatment and monitoring by psychiatric professionals and paraprofessionals, even chronic mental illnesses can be controlled and satisfactorily managed.

Legislation and its subsequent allocations of resources have a direct influence upon the mental health care delivery system. Also, public awareness and public opinions can effect public policy.

Confronting psychiatric mental health nurses today is a decentralized mental health care delivery system fraught with fragmented services, unresolved problems, and unmet client needs.

References

1. American Psychiatric Association. Task Force Report 21. Washington, DC: American Psychiatric Association; 1975.
2. Anthony WA, Kennard WA, O'Brien WF, Forbess R. Psychiatric rehabilitation: past myths and current realities. Commun Ment Health J. 1986;22:(4):249–264.
3. Beers CW. A mind that found itself: an autobiography. New York: Doubleday & Co; 1948.
4. Bellack AS, Mueser KT. A comprehensive treatment program for schizophrenia and chronic mental illness. Commun Ment Health J. 1986;22(3):175–189.
5. Chessick RD. Great ideas in psychotherapy. New York: J Aronson; 1977.
6. Deutsch A. The mentally ill in america: a history of their care from colonial times. Garden City: Doubleday; 1938.
7. English JT, Kritzler ZA, Scherl DJ. Historical trends in the financing of psychiatric services. Psychiatr Ann. 1984; 14:321.
8. Estes CL, Wood JB. A preliminary assessment of the impact of block grants on community mental health centers. Hosp Commun Psychiatry. 1984;35:1125.
9. Fagin CM. Psychiatric nursing at the crossroads: quo vadis. Perspect Psychiatr Care. 1981;19:99.
10. Foley HA, Sharfstein SS. Madness and government: who cares for the mentally ill? Washington, DC: American Psychiatric Association; 1983.
11. Graham TF. Medieval minds: mental health in the middle ages. London: G Allen & Unwin; 1967.
12. Hirschfeld M. Homecare versus institutionalization: family caregiving and senile brain disease. Int J Nurs Stud. 1983;20:1.
13. Horwitz EL. Madness, magic, and medicine: the treatment and mistreatment of the mentally ill. Philadelphia: JB Lippincott; 1977.
14. Klerman GL. National trends in hospitalization. J Hosp Commun Psychiatry. 1979;30:2.
15. Lamb HR. An empirical typology of the chronically mentally ill. Commun Ment Health J. 1986;22:(1):21.
16. Maricle RA, Hoffman WF, Bloom JD, Faulkner LR, Keepers GA. The prevalence and significance of medical illness among chronically mentally ill outpatients. Commun Ment Health J. 1987;23:(2):81–90.
17. Martin EJ. A speciality in decline? Psychiatric-mental health nursing, past, present, and future. J Prof Nurs. 1985;1:48.
18. McLaughlin CP, Zelman WN. Entrepreneurship and state/ mental health center relationships. Commun Ment Health J. 1987;23:1.
19. Morrissey JP, Goldman HH. Cycles of reform in the care of the chronically mentally ill. Hosp Commun Psychiatry. 1984;35:785.
20. National Institute of Mental Health Task Force on Nursing Summary Report. Washington, DC: NIMH; 1987.
21. New York Department of Mental Hygiene Report of Task Force. The development of community residential and rehabilitation programs. New York; 1975.
22. Peplau HE. American Nurses Association's social policy statement: Part 1. Arch Psychiatr Nurs. 1987;1:5.
23. Richie F, Lusky K. Psychiatric home health nursing: a new role in community mental health. Commun Ment Health J. 1987;23:(3):229–235.
24. Rubin J. The national plan for the chronically mentally ill: a review of financing proposals. Hosp Commun Psychiatry. 1981;32:704.
25. Swan JH, Fox PJ, Estes CL. Community mental health services and the elderly: retrenchment or expansion? Commun Ment Health J. 1986;22:(4):275–285.
26. Swan JH. The substitution of nursing homes for inpatient psychiatric care. Commun Ment Health J. 1987;23:(1):3–18.
27. Talbott J. Deinstitutionalization: avoiding the disasters of the past. J Hosp Commun Psychiatry. 1979;30:9.
28. Talbott JA. The fate of the public psychiatric system. J Hosp Commun Psychiatry. 1985;36:46.
29. US General Accounting Office (GAO). The elderly remain in need of mental health services. Gaithersbury, MD: Publication No. GAO/HRD-82; 1982.
30. Wilson HS. Deinstitutionalized residential care for the mentally disordered: the Soteria house approach. New York: Grune & Stratton; 1982.

47

Kathleen C. Buckwalter

Community Mental Health and Home Care

OBJECTIVES

After reading this chapter, the reader will be able to:

1. Describe five outcomes of the deinstitutionalization movement
2. Identify six areas of concern to psychiatric nurses practicing in community settings
3. Discuss nursing diagnoses related to these areas of concern
4. Identify four nursing goals for community-based mental health practice
5. Discuss the value of systematic identification of community mental health needs and strategies to do so
6. Understand the role of the family in community mental health care
7. Describe the key components of a home health care program for the mentally ill
8. Identify areas for nursing research in community mental health.

INTRODUCTION AND HISTORICAL OVERVIEW

Treatment of the more than 2.4 million severely mentally ill in this country has evolved from an era of criminal confinement, through a period characterized by custodial care and management, to a more recent focus on intensive treatment and rapid rehabilitation. Thirty years ago the state hospital system cared for over half of all psychiatric clients and, today, that figure is under 10%.[57] Modern mental health care consists of brief hospitalization during the acute illness phase, with clients returning to the community as early as possible. This emphasis on discharge from mental hospitals and the subsequent influx of mentally ill clients into the community, general hospitals, and nursing homes[18,19] have proliferated health, social, and vocational problems for clients, their families, and those health professionals concerned with care of the mentally ill.[7]

Outcomes of Deinstitutionalization

Passage of the Community Mental Health Centers Act (P.L. 88-164), in 1963, was the first federal initiative to develop community-based mental health services. By 1975 (P.L. 94-63), 12 services were required to be available to quality for federal staffing funds.[65] These services included outpatient, inpatient, emergency, partial hospitalization, specialized services for children and the elderly, screening, aftercare, transitional housing, consultation–education, drug abuse services, and alcoholism treatment.

Although intended to develop new, more effective, and less costly treatment programs that would improve the overall quality of life for the severely mentally ill and to counteract the isolation and social disabilities stemming from institutionalization itself, the community mental health movement has many times resulted in inappropriate discharge, sporadic and fragmented services to severely mentally ill clients, enormous burdens to their families,[48] little if any cost savings,[30] homelessness and abandonment, and an increased likelihood of readmission.[18,32,37,54,57]

Community tenure after hospitalization is determined by a variety of factors, including the extent to which clients perceive aftercare services as accessible or necessary.[17,29,37,68] A number of client behaviors and associated determinants have been identified as well. The stress imposed upon caregivers in the posthospital environment by the following determinants has been found to influence community tenure: severity and duration of mental illness, bizarre and disruptive behav-

ior,[23,36] social maladjustment,[66] a negative family environment, and medication-related problems.[44,50]

A major criticism of community-based treatment has been that medication is often the only treatment offered to long-term clients.[2] Although medication is often a necessary part of the treatment regimen of mentally ill clients, not all clients benefit from neuroleptics, and a significant number (10%–20%) develop adverse side effects such as akinesia and tardive dyskinesia.[28,58] The monitoring of clients taking neuroleptic medications and evaluating the effectiveness of adjunctive treatment strategies in decreasing neuroleptic use in this population is an important role for community-based psychiatric nurses.

The quality of life of many chronic clients living in the community is severely compromised,[29,38] and many former state psychiatric hospital residents are now homeless,[53] unemployed, neglected or abused, in poor health, and dependent upon the social service system for the necessities of life once provided by the state hospitals[5,11] (see also Chapter 28). It has been argued that in many respects the severely mentally ill were better off before the deinstitutionalization movement.[21] In the community, they are often stigmatized by the label of mental illness and have difficulties responding to demands for social and vocational skills.[22,33,42]

Furthermore, the comprehensive array of services needed to keep severely mentally ill clients functioning in the community is often simply not available, particularly in rural areas. Components of such a comprehensive treatment program identified in the literature include medication treatment, family therapy, social skills training, crisis intervention, medical care, rehabilitation in terms of self-maintenance skills, job training, and social services related to income and housing, social support, transportation, and recreational activities.[4,5,59,64] Moreover, there must be active coordination of the variety of services such that existing services are accessible and that continuity of care is achieved.[3] The severely mentally ill experience problems in dealing with ordinary demands of life; coping with the maze of potential services that could assist them can be a difficult task.[34]

To paraphrase the 1981 White House Conference on Aging Report on Long-Term Care[67] and apply it to mental health: There is widespread agreement that the mental health system should promote the independence of the person in making decisions and in performing everyday activities. It should encourage support services in the least restrictive environment, preferably at home or in other community settings. It should try to make available appropriate, cost-effective, accessible, and humane care to all persons who need it at the same time, supporting the care provided by family and friends. For chronically impaired individuals who must receive care in nursing homes and institutional settings, it should ensure the quality of their care and seek to maximize their quality of life. At present, these are but ideals. The nurse's role in operationalizing these ideals in the community is discussed next.

The author acknowledges the contributions of Sharon Trimborn, R.N., M.S.N., to the section on home care; Geraldene Felton, Ed.D., R.N., F.A.A.N., for assistance in conceptualizing the role of the psychiatric nurse in the community; and Joan Crowe for providing invaluable assistance in manuscript preparation.

ROLE OF THE PSYCHIATRIC NURSE IN COMMUNITY SETTINGS

Areas of Concern and Related Nursing Diagnoses

Six major areas of concern to psychiatric nurses in the community related to care of mentally ill clients are (1) material welfare, (2) coping, (3) psychological functioning, (4) social support, (5) sustained motivation, and (6) health maintenance.[16] Each of these areas and related nursing diagnoses will be discussed briefly.

MATERIAL WELFARE AND RELATED NURSING DIAGNOSES

Adequate care for mentally ill clients depends on the knowledge and ability to take advantage of varying categorical programs at federal, state, and local levels that pay for such needs as housing, food, subsistence, and medical care. Mental health nurses who are familiar with how to "utilize" existing entitlements legally can do a great deal for their clients.

Many community mental health center clients require assistance with basic needs that are dependent on material resources. At the most basic level, they require adequate shelter and nutrition. In many communities, the mentally ill are viewed as undesirable neighbors and, therefore, have difficulty locating suitable housing. As communities resist new board-and-care facilities, halfway houses, and other housing arrangements for the chronically mentally ill, mental health programs have often followed the line of least resistance, locating housing for clients in the most ecologically undesirable areas where clients are at high risk of victimization and other indignities. Successful community care requires not only an awareness of clients' material needs, but a knowledge of community organization and welfare arrangements that allows the effective use of public resources. This includes planning for the location of client residences in good proximity to needed mental health services and other community facilities.

Nursing diagnoses common in this area of concern, material welfare, include altered nutrition, less than body requirements; impaired social interaction; knowledge deficit (skills to negotiate the mental health and social welfare systems to obtain needed goods and services); potential for injury; powerlessness; and impaired resource management (inability to obtain or manage housing and finances).

COPING AND RELATED NURSING DIAGNOSES

The adequacy of functioning in the community depends, in part, on problem-solving capacities acquired in the process of social development. Community-dwelling, chronically mentally ill clients commonly lack the basic skills and knowledge essential for every-day living, and the absence of such skills, or their erosion by chronic illness, exacerbates problems of adjustment. Such deficiencies make it difficult for clients to obtain and retain employment, establish interpersonal relations, get around their community, maintain adequate living quarters, and avoid difficulties with authorities. Moreover, because such clients are dependent, they have continuing contacts with services and official bureaucracies, and their skills in managing such relationships have important bearing on their well-being. Recently, demonstration programs have documented that teaching mentally ill clients such simple skills as budgeting, use of public transportation, house maintenance, and self-presentation can contribute a great deal to their effective community adjustment.[48] Nurses need to organize, teach, and monitor such living skills in community care programs and to do so in a context that takes into account clients' disabilities, drug regimen, and overall physical needs.

Nursing diagnoses common in this area of concern, coping, include decisional conflict; family coping, potential for growth; ineffective individual coping; and self-care deficit (bathing/hygiene, dressing/grooming, feeding, toileting).

PSYCHOLOGICAL FUNCTIONING AND RELATED NURSING DIAGNOSES

Improving the psychological functioning of mentally ill clients in the community may be both the most difficult and most uncertain aspect of care provided by psychiatric nurses. It is well established that long-term clients, in particular, have major psychological difficulties, and psychodynamic efforts have not been impressive in modifying or ameliorating the deficiencies commonly found in this population.

Mental health nurses need to be educated in therapeutic methods and techniques of behavior control; these strategies constitute part of a larger approach to the multifaceted needs of the chronically impaired client. Obviously, clients have various individual needs relative to their personalities and particular disabilities. Clients with schizophrenia, for example, may have difficulties with intense personal relationships and are more vulnerable in these circumstances, whereas clients with chronic depression are unusually susceptible to feelings of helplessness and despair in situations in which they perceive a sense of loss. Existing evidence and experience suggest that a pragmatic nursing approach that sets tangible goals and is supportive of the client's efforts offers more promise than more diffuse or insight-oriented psychotherapies.[43] Perhaps the most substantial therapeutic efforts are achieved indirectly by developing networks of social support that enhance the clients' coping efforts and sense of self-esteem.

Nursing diagnoses common in this area of concern, psychological functioning, include aggression, agitation, altered impulse control, altered perception/cognition, anger, anxiety, bizarre behavior, defensive coping, depression, fear, guilt, hopelessness, emotional lability, manipulation, regressed behavior, somatization, suicide potential, and suspiciousness.

SOCIAL SUPPORT AND RELATED NURSING DIAGNOSES

Recent research substantiates that the absence of social support makes people vulnerable to interpersonal and environmental assaults and other adversities.[55,56] Often the simple knowledge that help will be available if needed gives people the confidence to cope successfully. Social supports are important not only for the instrumental assistance they provide but also for the reinforcement and self-affirmation that come from the sympathetic and empathetic interests of others. Research has confirmed the "buffering" effects of social support;[8,10] that is, the finding that persons with high levels of social support suffer fewer negative health consequences after stressful events than those with low levels of support.

Mentally ill clients in the community are particularly vulnerable because social support networks are often unavailable, and such clients are thus isolated from usual community associations. These clients may either have no close relatives or, over the course of time, have alienated family and significant others by their bizarre behavior and personal difficulties. Moreover, many clients have difficulty maintaining close personal relationships, and such relationships depend on an awareness and understanding by significant others of the problems associated with mental illness. Effective community care requires careful attention to the development and maintenance of community, family, and interpersonal supports. An important role for nurses is to coach clients in their roles and responsibilities by providing information and support to relatives and friends and maintaining sympathetic but assertive contact with clients. This is especially true for chronic clients who typically lack supports, but are also less likely to seek them out and maintain them. Thus, community-based service systems must be both well organized and assertive in their outreach efforts. In a very practical article, Manderino and Bzdek[43] describe for psychiatric nurses the planning and implementation of social skills-building groups for chronic clients. They note that research has documented that social skill deficits in psychiatric clients can be partially, and in some cases completely, overcome by appropriate skills-building programs, such as the one they outline.

Nursing diagnoses common in this area of concern, social support, include altered parenting, dysfunctional family processes, impaired social interaction, and loneliness.

SUSTAINED MOTIVATION AND RELATED NURSING DIAGNOSES

Successful social adaptation depends on a continuing willingness to remain engaged and committed to ongo-

ing treatment and social activities. Most chronically disturbed clients have a history of failure and disappointment, and this creates an incentive to withdraw and reduces hopes, expectations, and engagement in everyday tasks. As a consequence, what few skills and social contacts they have may erode, and clients' confidence in their ability to perform ordinary life tasks may diminish. Withdrawal is a natural, and often an effective, means of reducing the psychiatric client's sense of threat or disappointment, and psychiatric nurses must often intervene aggressively to make sure that clients do not "disappear" from the community service system.

Withdrawal and inactivity among community-dwelling mentally ill clients can result in personal deterioration and an incapacity to continue or regain important social roles. The specific activities clients perform are less important than their continued involvement, contact with other people, and exposure to the expectations and constraints of social demands.

Nursing diagnoses common in this area of concern, sustained motivation, include boredom, diversional activity deficit, self-esteem disturbance, role performance disturbance, impaired social interaction, emotional lability, and noncompliance.

HEALTH MAINTENANCE AND RELATED NURSING DIAGNOSES

Mentally ill clients require not only excellent mental health care but also careful attention to their physical health needs. Poor nutrition, neglect, and other conditions associated with both mental impairment and deprived circumstances create many health problems in this population. In addition, the long-term use of high doses of powerful psychoactive drugs, often combined, as well as used with alcohol, creates a serious potential threat to health. Nurses must see that community-dwelling mentally ill clients receive a range of medically related services, such as contraception, optometric, and dental services.

Drug monitoring itself requires a thoughtful, sensitive, but assertive, approach on the part of the nurse. Many chronic clients, such as clients with schizophrenia, require different levels of medication over their lifecourse if episodes of psychosis are to be minimized. Furthermore, clients in crisis commonly discontinue their medication, which can result in even more serious functional problems. The adverse side effects of the antipsychotic medications are often sufficiently unpleasant to induce clients to attempt to function without them. Only through assertive monitoring and encouragement is it possible to achieve high levels of compliance and safety for medication requirements of community-dwelling clients.

Nursing diagnoses common in this area of concern, health maintenance, include altered health maintenance; altered nutrition, less than body requirements; noncompliance; and substance abuse (alcohol and drugs).

Nursing Goals

Nursing goals related to these six areas of concern, material welfare, coping, psychological functioning, social support, sustaining motivation, and health maintenance, can be summarized as follows:

1. Establish rapport with community-based clients
2. Assist community-based clients to develop or maintain an optimal level of independence
3. Help reduce psychiatric symptomatology and increase feelings of self-confidence and control
4. Decrease feelings of hopelessness and withdrawal by enhancing clients' ability to effectively use community-based systems of service and support.

Identification of Community Mental Health Needs

Identification of mental health needs in the community is another important nursing role. Psychiatric nurses must be aware of "information gaps" in the health care delivery systems within their communities. Creative and effective ways of dealing with mental health problems can be developed through the sharing of knowledge and resources; however, the problem areas must first be identified.

A three-stage assessment approach to identification and provision of needed health services within a community includes (1) description of the size and nature of the problem, (2) description of the community, and (3) identification of available services to meet the identified needs.[60] Psychiatric nurses may find this framework useful for systematically assessing the need for mental health services in their community. For example, with support and funding from their workplace, local foundations, or academic centers, nurses may wish to conduct surveys to identify the mental health needs of the community in general, as well as the specialized needs of particular target groups, such as the elderly, impoverished, or chronically mentally ill persons. In community mental health, the emphasis is on prevention, and one way to focus on the community, while at the same time retaining a prevention orientation, is to identify populations who are at particular risk for mental health problems.[35] Community surveys enable the nurse to gather a variety of sociodemographic data and assess community knowledge about the counseling and treatment services provided by mental health centers. Respondents can also be asked to identify additional services they feel are needed in the community, as well as reasons why people do not seek help from the mental health center when confronted with a problem. Development of new programs, and even marketing strategies, can then proceed based upon identified community needs and concerns and available financing.

Role of the Nurse With Families

Although most mentally ill clients return to family settings after hospitalization, the literature is controversial about the role of the family in the development of, and response to, severe mental illness in a relative.[25] Moroney[47] has concluded that the family can play a variety of roles, ranging from creating problems to serving as a resource to the mentally ill person and mental health professionals. These roles may shift over the lifecourse and duration of an unpredictable, fluctuating illness,[26] requiring that families of persons with mental illness confront many adaptive tasks.[62] The work of Falloon and colleagues[14,15] suggests that everyday problem behaviors (e.g., demanding, disruptive, uncooperative) are the most difficult for families of mentally ill clients to deal with. Thus, family members may require professional intervention and services to optimally maintain their caregiving role and to counteract the negative effects caring for a severely ill relative may have on outside relationships and activities; i.e., decreased social support networks for the severely mentally ill person and their family members.[1,6,27,31]

Because the impact of psychiatric illness is multifaceted and affects family members as well as individual clients, the psychiatric nurse who includes family-centered home-based care in a repertoire of community activities provides a much-needed service. In-home assessments often provide a more comprehensive data base for the development of nursing diagnoses than those conducted in the more artificial environment of a mental health center or hospital. Nurses are in an ideal position to help families reorganize roles and relationships; to assist them in developing realistic and attainable goals to meet the challenge of mental illness in a family member; and to be prepared for future crises and social, emotional, and financial burdens.

HOME CARE FOR THE MENTALLY ILL

Program Description

Decreased inpatient lengths of stay (LOS) have prompted the development of alternative home care programs to meet the ongoing needs of psychiatric clients discharged to the community. Psychiatric nursing home care is designed to smooth the transition from hospital to community, to promote the highest level of functioning possible in the community setting, and to decrease recidivism—all in a cost-effective manner.

To this end, psychiatric nurses are collaborating with their colleagues in home health care to develop, implement, and evaluate innovative home care programs, such as the one proposed by Trimborn[63] at the University of Rochester Medical Center Department of Psychiatric Nursing. Highlights of this home care model are presented next, beginning with a list of objectives for the psychiatric home care program.

PROGRAM OBJECTIVES[63]

1. Promote early detection of exacerbation of symptoms by client and family
2. Promote client independence and rehabilitation within family and community settings
3. Provide care specific to the needs of the client or family relative to their social environment
4. Promote client and family education aimed at self-care and early intervention and treatment of new and recurring conditions
5. Ensure the transfer of learned behaviors from the hospital to the home and community setting
6. Evaluate, within the scope of nursing practice, client and family progress relative to the overall interdisciplinary treatment plan.

TARGET POPULATION[63]

The target population includes those psychiatric clients with one or more of the following characteristics: a high rate of readmission; previous noncompliance with prescribed treatment regimens, such as medications, day treatment program, outpatient therapy, community agencies; at risk for suicide; living alone; and having complex medical and psychiatric problems, as is frequently the case with the older adult.

SERVICES[63]

All services related to the home care treatment plan are explained and negotiated with the client and their family and may include the following:
A. Psychiatric evaluation and treatment planning home, provided by psychiatric team (psychiatrist, psychiatric nurse, and home care social worker)
B. Psychiatric nursing visits
   1. Client and family assessment
   2. Client and family education
   3. Client and family support and counseling
C. Mental health aide or case manager
   1. Targeted to clients living alone at high risk because of severity of illness; poor family system
   2. Crisis intervention—personal care, companionship, suicide prevention
   3. Resocialization—structure visits to assist with activities of daily living, shopping, reintegration into activities in home and community
D. Social work visits
   1. Assessment of social and financial problems
   2. Long-term planning to assure continuity of care
   3. Discharge planning
   4. Supportive guidance and counseling
E. Rehabilitative therapies: occupational, speech, and physical therapies
   1. Targeted to clients (particularly elderly) with medical rehabilitation as well as psychiatric needs

F. Other home care services as needed
   1. Laboratory
   2. Pharmacy
   3. Transportation
   4. Equipment and supplies

NURSING ACTIVITIES[63]

Nursing activities focus on the following three domains:

Client and Family Assessment
- Evaluate client's and family's ability to carry out plan of care
- Assess client's overall condition including physical and mental status, compliance with treatment regimens, and medication prescriptions
- Evaluate home environment and community networks

Client and Family Education
- Teach client and family about client's psychiatric illness, signs and symptoms, recommended treatments, and suggested actions for preventing relapse
- Teach client and family about effective communication, problem-solving, and decision-making processes
- Teach client and family strategies to cope effectively with stress and conflict

Client and Family Support and Counseling
- Review and revise care plan to ensure transfer of learned behaviors from hospital or other treatment programs to home
- Assist the client and family to identify current problems and to resolve them through the problem-solving approach
- Assist the client and family to identify and to utilize available supports; initiate referrals when necessary
- Assist the family to identify and to share their feelings toward one another in constructive ways

The psychiatric home care team includes the following five professionals, plus clerical support staff:

1. Psychiatrist
2. Psychiatric nurse, B.S. degree and two years experience
3. Psychiatric nurse specialist (master's or doctorate degree)
4. Home care social worker
5. Mental health aide

PROGRAM EVALUATION[63]

Key questions addressed by analysis of outcomes of the home care program include the following:

1. Does psychiatric nursing home care reduce the LOS, prevent recidivism, and improve compliance with treatment protocols?

2. Which clients benefit most from the home care program in terms of their diagnosis, age, sex, employment status, and family role?
3. Does psychiatric home care reduce total health care costs for this population?

A comprehensive client, family, and service data base is expected to be developed by the Rochester project. This data base can be used to retrieve information related to LOS, client characteristics, rate of readmissions, characteristics of services, utilization patterns, and cost of services. Quality assurance measures such as achievement of client and family care outcomes, efficiency, effectiveness of service delivery systems, client and family satisfaction, and utilization review are also carefully monitored. Attending psychiatrists provide written and signed plans of care.

IMPLICATIONS FOR PSYCHIATRIC MENTAL HEALTH NURSING PRACTICE AND RESEARCH

At present, adequate information on the availability, accessibility, utilization, and costs of community-based services for the mentally ill, especially in rural environments, is lacking. As research and demonstration efforts suggest, ". . . the cost effectiveness of community care is a major public policy concern."[9] There are few comprehensive cost-effectiveness studies of services for the severely mentally ill. Nor is the effectiveness of these services in deterring rehospitalization and long-term institutionalization fully understood. In fact, the disappointing outcomes associated with deinstitutionalization of the severely mentally ill has led researchers, clinicians, and policy makers to call for a reconceptualization of the philosophy of care of the severely mentally ill over the life span.[5,24] Early studies[49] demonstrated that home care of the severely mentally ill, when supplemented by supportive services, could be effective in decreasing hospitalization. More recent research on the quality-of-life experiences of chronically mentally ill clients in a state hospital suggests that compared with community-based clients, those in state hospitals were more dysfunctional and less satisfied.[39]

The question of whether or not community-based treatment is indeed the most efficacious approach to caring for this population, in terms of treatment outcomes and social costs, remains unanswered. Psychiatric nurses must address these and other issues such as the extent to which services are provided to families, the relationship between type and duration of mental illness, the ability of families to provide care for their severely mentally ill relative, and the use of professional services, especially in rural settings. Community-based psychiatric nurses must also determine which interventions best complement informal caregiving efforts.

Thus, it is critical that psychiatric nurses and other mental health professionals explore the determinants, effectiveness, and costs of care for mentally ill clients with different psychiatric diagnoses and in different treatment settings, in a systematic effort to attune the mental health delivery system and policy makers to the needs of this underserved population. The current system of service delivery focuses more on the facilities and settings within which services are provided rather than on the individual needs of persons with severe mental illness.[52] Research is needed so that services, settings, and living arrangements can be tailored to the individual needs of persons with severe mental illness. In keeping with the suggestions of the National Plan for the Chronically Mentally Ill, research is needed that will help to answer the critical questions, "Who uses what services, for what purposes, and at what cost?"[61]

QUALITY-OF-LIFE ISSUES

For many years, evaluation of treatment effectiveness was determined using specific illness-oriented outcome measures such as recidivism rates.[17] Recently, and more in keeping with the nursing perspective, efforts to determine treatment outcomes have included measures focusing on life satisfaction and quality-of-life (QOL) measures.[12,41] Lehman[40] has noted that QOL measures can help us to evaluate different treatment approaches and policies. He further asserts that current understanding of QOL issues and the well-being of chronically mentally ill clients in different treatment settings is very inadequate.

Bachrach[4] has emphasized that the human elements of service provisions are critical to enhancing QOL for the severely mentally ill, although distinctions between QOL and course of the disorder are often blurred. Gurland[24] suggests that the history of the severely mentally ill client's QOL has been characterized by the history of his or her mental illness. Certainly QOL measures "have an intuitive appeal" that captures the "ultimate concern of all health and human services," that is, the well-being of the severely mentally ill.[39] Community mental health services must prevent institutionalization and reduce symptomatology. In sum, psychiatric mental health nursing research on the severely mentally ill living in the community must incorporate multiple assessment and outcome parameters, including, but not limited to, measurement of QOL issues, client functioning, institutionalization rates, and economic and social costs to caregivers and communities.

CURRENT AND FUTURE DIRECTIONS

The mental health field continues to be plagued by competing and conflicting models of care; by lack of an adequate knowledge base of the cause, prevention, and treatment of mental illness; and by the force of traditional practice. Despite these constraints, care of the mentally ill has undergone a remarkable transformation, relocating the provision of treatment, in a large part, from inpatient services to ambulatory and community settings. With federal and state support, there has been a substantial increase in access to mental health services, growing acceptability of care for psychiatric disorders, and increased respect for the needs and rights of the mentally ill.[16]

Research Highlights

A discharge planning study was conducted by Buckwalter and Abraham.[7] The research focused on the reintegration of depressed clients into the community after psychiatric hospitalization.

By using a randomized two-group (e.g., experimental and control) repeated measures design, the researchers tested family-centered predischarge interventions with a cognitive behavioral orientation to help depressed clients adjust to their posthospital environment with its demands for social, vocational, and psychological skills. Results are summarized by the following outcome categories:

Depression

No statistically significant differences were found between experimental and control subjects in self-reported levels of depressive symptomatology in the aftercare period, although families of experimental subjects reported significant improvements in symptomatology.

Social Functioning

Although experimental and control subjects did not differ during the aftercare period in their self-reports on this variable, experimental subjects were perceived as functioning better socially than their control counterparts by family members throughout the aftercare period.

Satisfaction With Social Roles

Experimental subjects reported more satisfaction with their social roles at the end of the study period (three months postdischarge) than immediately after discharge, although no significant differences were detected at each measurement time point (2, 4, 6, 8 weeks postdischarge) between experimental and control subjects. Family members of experimental subjects confirmed that they adjusted better over time, and they reported more satisfaction with the social role adaptation of the client than families of control subjects.

Expectation Levels

Expectation levels for social activities held by experimental and control subjects and their families did not differ significantly during the aftercare period studied. Congruence was found in the ratings of subjects and families in both conditions.

Free-Time Activities

Although experimental and control subjects did not differ in their free-time activities or satisfaction with those activities over the postdischarge period, the family members of experimental subjects were significantly more satisfied with client free-time activities.

Stressors

The stress levels of experimental subjects decreased significantly over the aftercare period, and, by three months postdischarge, experimental subjects reported significantly lower stress levels than control subjects.

Overall Adjustment

A pattern of improvement in the experimental subjects was observed for overall social, vocational, and psychological adjustment of subjects in the aftercare period, with experimental subjects improving over the entire course of the aftercare period and demonstrating better adjustment than control subjects at the end of the three-month postdischarge study period.

Compliance

Experimental subjects were significantly more compliant with their medication regimens and scheduled aftercare appointments than controls.

Recidivism Rates

During the three-month aftercare period, significantly fewer experimental subjects were rehospitalized than were control subjects.

Postdischarge Occupational Status

A greater percentage (40%) of experimental subjects than of control subjects (20%) had returned to work by the end of the study period. However, the large proportion of clients in both groups for whom occupational status was unknown makes these findings inconclusive. As the aftercare period progressed, experimental subjects reported fewer employment related problems and less occupational stress than control subjects.

Results of this study suggest that inclusion of the family of severely mentally ill clients in predischarge planning is of particular benefit to family members in terms of their satisfaction with client behavior during the aftercare period. The findings suggest that the quality of social, family, and community readjustment were influenced in a positive manner. The literature suggests that success in the aftercare period is the result of interactions in and between a variety of personal and environmental factors that influence severely mentally ill clients and their families after discharge. The predischarge intervention tested in this longitudinal field experiment appears to have influenced the clients' families more than the clients themselves or the clinical course of their illness. Because the probability of successful discharge for severely mentally ill clients often depends on strong family and social relationships, the predischarge cognitive behavioral intervention tested in this study has potential for strengthening family relationships in the aftercare period. As discussed in the previous section, these findings lend support to other aftercare research that suggests that successful discharge can be facilitated by procedures that maintain or restore social relationships.

Most mental health care is now provided in psychiatric outpatient settings and mental health centers; clients are living in community housing, board-and-care facilities, nursing homes, and in their own homes. These changes reflect new social attitudes, changing social policies and administrative practices, the availability of more effective psychoactive drugs, and new sources of financing for community maintenance and treatment of the mentally ill. Despite these advances, it is clear that the mentally ill—particularly those with more severe disorders—remain a neglected population, who are outside the mainstream of responsible and effective treatment and rehabilitative services.[16]

Psychiatric nurses play a pivotal role in providing care for the community-dwelling mentally ill client. Their efforts must be persistent and skilled to deal with the vast array of psychological and medical disabilities commonly found in this population. Interventions must be broad based, and incorporate strategies to bolster the self esteem, coping capacities, and social support networks of mentally ill clients residing in the community. Nurses must also be knowledgeable about pharmacologic issues and work with psychiatrists to achieve sensible and effective drug programs that limit adverse side effects.

Similar needs for sophisticated care exist in nursing homes, sheltered care facilities, and in client homes, for there are now more chronically mentally ill persons in such settings than in mental hospitals. These clients require sophisticated drug management and monitoring, social programs of active involvement, and significant interpersonal support, including attention to material welfare, coping, psychological functioning, social support, sustained motivation, and health maintenance.

SUMMARY

Although based on laudable ideals, the deinstitutionalization movement, in many ways, has created more problems than it has solved. Most community mental health systems now lack the comprehensive array of services necessary to keep mentally ill persons functioning at an optimal level in the community. Nurses play a pivotal role in community mental health, and their broad-based practice should target six primary areas of concern: (1) material welfare, (2) coping, (3) psychological functioning, (4) social supports, (5) sustaining motivation, and (6) health maintenance.[16] It is critical for nurses to work closely with family members to achieve their goals of increased client rapport, independence, self-confidence and decreased symptomatology, hopelessness, and withdrawal. Home health care and outreach programs are two important service delivery systems in community mental health, especially in underserved rural areas. Nurses must be involved in systematic efforts to evaluate these and other innovative programs, as well as other areas of research related to improving the quality of life of community-dwelling mentally ill persons.

References

1. Anthony JE. The impact of mental and physical illness on family life. Am J Psychiatry. 1970;127:138–146.
2. Bachrach LL. A conceptual approach to deinstitutionalization. Hosp Commun Psychiatry. 1978;29:573–578.
3. Bachrach LL. Continuity of care for chronic mental patients: a conceptual analysis. Am Psychiatry. 1981;138:1449–1456.
4. Bachrach LL. The challenge of a service planning for chronic mental patients. Commun Ment Health J. 1986;22:170–174.
5. Bellack AS, Mueser KT. A comprehensive treatment program for schizophrenia and chronic mental illness. Commun Ment Health J. 1986;22:175–189.
6. Berkman LF. The assessment of social networks and social support in the elderly. J Am Geriatr Soc. 1983;31:743–749.
7. Buckwalter KC, Abraham IL. Alleviating the discharge crisis: the effects of a cognitive-behavioral nursing intervention for depressed patients and their families. Arch Psychiatr Nurs. 1987;1:350–358.
8. Cassel J. The contribution of the social environment to host resistance. Am J Epidemiol. 1976;104:107–123.
9. Clark RF. The costs and benefits of community care: a perspective from the channeling demonstration. Pride Inst J. 1987;6(2):3–12.
10. Cobb S. Social support as a moderator of life stress. Psychosom Med. 1976;38:300–314.
11. Cordes C. The plight of the homeless mentally ill. APA Monitor 1984;15:1–13.
12. Dickey B, Gudeman J, Hellman S, et al. A follow-up of deinstitutionalized chronic patients four years after discharge. Hosp Commun Psychiatry. 1981;5:326–330.
13. Erickson RC. Outcome studies in mental hospitals: a review. Psychol Bull. 1975;82:519–540.
14. Falloon IRH, Boyd JL, McGill CW, Razani J, Moss HB, Gilderman AM. Family management in the prevention of exacerbations of schizophrenia: a controlled study. N Engl J Med. 1982;306:1437–1441.
15. Falloon IRH, Boyd JL, McGill CW, et al. Family management in the prevention of morbidity of schizophrenia. Arch Gen Psychiatry. 1985;42:887–896.
16. Felton G. Unpublished manuscript. University of Iowa College of Nursing. Iowa City, Iowa; 1988.
17. Friedman I, Von Mering O, Hinks EN. Intermittent patienthood. Arch Gen Psychiatry. 1966;14:386–392.
18. Goldman HH. Epidemiology. In: Talbott JA, ed. The chronic mental patient: five years later. Orlando, FL: Grune & Stratton; 1984.
19. Goldman HH, Adams NH, Taube CA. Deinstitutionalization: the data demythologized. Hosp Commun Psychiatry. 1983;34:129–134.
20. Goldstrom ID, Manderscheid RW. The chronic mentally ill: a descriptive analysis from the uniform client data instrument. Commun Support Serv J. 1981;11:4–9.
21. Gralnick A. Build a better state hospital. Deinstitutionalization has failed. Hosp Commun Psychiatry. 1985;36:738–741.
22. Gruenberg EM. The social breakdown syndrome: some origins. Am J Psychiatry. 1967;123:1481–1489.
23. Gubman GD, Tessler RC. The impact of mental illness on families. J Fam Issues. 1987;8:226–245.
24. Gurland B. Epidemiology of chronically mentally ill elderly. Presented at the NIMH conference Research on the CMI Elderly, Orlando, Florida; December, 1987.
25. Hatfield AB. The family. In: Talbott JA, ed. The chronic mental patient: five years later. Orlando, FL: Grune & Stratton; 1984.
26. Hatfield AB. Coping and adaptation: a conceptual framework for understanding families. In: Hatfield AB, Lefley HP,

eds. Families of the mentally ill: coping and adaptation. New York: Guilford Press; 1987.

27. Hoenig J, Hamilton MW. The schizophrenic patient in the community and his effect on the household. Int J Soc Psychiatry. 1966;12(Sum):165–176.

28. Johnson DAW. Antipsychotic medication: clinical guidelines for maintenance therapy. J Clin Psychiatry. 1985;46:6–15.

29. Jonas A. Health care delivery in the United States. New York: Springer; 1977.

30. Kirk SA, Therrien ME. Community mental health myths and the fate of former hospitalized patients. Psychiatry. 1975;38:209–217.

31. Kreisman DE, Joy VD. Family response to the mental illness of a relative: a review of the literature. Schizophr Bull. 1974;11:34–57.

32. Kubie LS. Pitfalls of community psychiatry. Arch Gen Psychiatry. 1968;18:257–266.

33. Lamb HR. Community survival of long-term patients. San Francisco: Jossey-Bass; 1976.

34. Lamb HR. Therapist-case managers: more than brokers. Hosp Commun Psychiatry. 1980;31:762.

35. Lancaster J, Lancaster IW. The psychiatric nurse's role in community mental health. In: Stuart G, Sundeen S, eds. Principles and practice of psychiatric nursing, 2nd ed. St. Louis: CV Mosby; 1983.

36. Lefley HP. Behavioral manifestations of mental illness. In: Hatfield AB, Lefley HP, eds. Families of the mentally ill: coping and adaptation. New York: Guilford Press; 1987.

37. Lego S. The community mental health system: is it an improvement over the old system? Perspect Psychiatr Care. 1975;13:119.

38. Lehman A. The well-being of chronic mental patients. Arch Gen Psychiatry. 1983;40:369–373.

39. Lehman AF. The effects of psychiatric symptoms on quality of life assessment among the chronically mentally ill. Eval prog plan. 1983;6:143–151.

40. Lehman AF, Possidente A, Hawker F. The well-being of chronic mental patients in a state hospital and community residences. 1986;(unpublished manuscript).

41. Lehman AF, Ward NC, Linn LS. Chronic mental patients: the quality of life issues. Am J Psychiatry. 1982;139:1271–1276.

42. Ludwig AM. Treating the treatment failures. Orlando, FL: Grune & Stratton; 1971.

43. Manderino MA, Bzdek VM. Social skill building with chronic patients. J Psychosoc Nurs Ment Health Serv. 1987;25(9):18–23.

44. McElroy EM. The beat of a different drummer. In: Hatfield AB, Lefley HP, eds. Families of the mentally ill: coping and adaptation. New York: Guilford Press; 1987.

45. Mechanic D. Mental health and social policy, 2nd ed. Englewood Cliffs, NJ: Prentice Hall; 1980.

46. Moon LE, Patton RE. First admissions and readmissions to New York State mental hospitals: a statistical evaluation. Psychiatr Q. 1965;39:476–487.

47. Moroney RM. Families, social services, and social policy: the issue of shared responsibility. Rockville, MD: U.S. Department of Health and Human Services Publication No. (ADM) 80-846; 1980.

48. National Institute of Mental Health, demonstration services projects conference, Seattle, WA; March, 1988.

49. Pasamanick B, Scarpitti FR, Dinitz S. Schizophrenics in the community: an experimental study in the prevention of hospitalization. New York: Appleton-Century-Crofts; 1970.

50. Paul GP. Chronic mental patient: current status—future directions. Psychol Bull. 1972;78:447–456.

51. President's Commission on Mental Health Task Panel on Rural Mental Health, vol. 3, Appendix. Washington DC: US Government Printing Office; 1978:1164.

52. Report on the Bill of Rights for Persons with Mental Retardation, Developmental Disabilities, or Chronic Mental Illness. April [Submitted to the Iowa Legislature by the Iowa Department of Human Services]; 1987.

53. Roth D, Bean GJ Jr, Hyde PS. Homelessness and mental health policy: developing an appropriate role for the 1980s. Commun Ment Health J. 1986;22:203–214.

54. Rouslin S. Commentary on the community mental health approach. Perspect Psychiatr Care. 1975;13:119.

55. Russell D. Stress, social support, and physical and mental health among the elderly: a longitudinal causal model. Presented at the annual meeting of the Gerontological Society of America, Chicago, IL; 1986.

56. Russell D, Cutrona CE. The provisions of social relationships and adaptation to stress. Presented at the American Psychological Association convention, Toronto, Canada; 1984.

57. Sharfstein SS. Sociopolitical issues affecting patients with chronic schizophrenia. In: Bellack AS, ed. Schizophrenia: treatment, management, and rehabilitation. Orlando, FL: Grune & Stratton; 1984.

58. Scrak BM, Greenstein RA. Tardive dyskinesia. J Psychosoc Nurs Ment Health Serv. 1987;25(9):24–28.

59. Stein LI, Test MA. Alternative to mental hospital treatment. I. Conceptual model, treatment program and clinical evaluation. Arch Gen Psychiatry. 1980;37:392–397.

60. Stewart E. The nature of needs assessment in community mental health. Commun Ment Health J. 1979;15:287.

61. Talbott JA. The national plan for the chronically mentally ill: a programmatic analysis. Hosp Commun Psychiatry. 1981;32:699–704.

62. Terkelsen KG. The evolution of family responses to mental illness through time. In: Hatfield AM, Lefley HP, eds. Families of the mentally ill: Coping and adaptation. New York: Guilford Press; 1987.

63. Trimborn S. Home care proposal. University of Rochester Medical Center, Strong Memorial Hospital, Psychiatric Nursing Practice; 1987.

64. Turner JEC, Shifren I. Community support systems: how comprehensive? N Dir Ment Health Serv; 1979;2:1–13.

65. United States Congress: Public Law 94-63, Title 3, Community Mental Health Centers Amendments. Part A, Section 201(b)(1)(c). July 29, 1975.

66. Wallace CJ, Lieberman RP. Social skills training for patients with schizophrenia: a controlled clinical trial. Psychiatr Res. 1985;15:239–247.

67. White House Conference on Aging Final Report, vol 3. Washington DC; 1981.

68. Wilner DM, Walkey RP, O'Neill EJ. Introduction to public health. New York: Macmillan; 1978.

48

Kathleen C. Buckwalter

Rural Mental Health Care

OBJECTIVES

After reading this chapter, the reader will be able to:

1. *Discuss differences between mental health care in rural and urban settings*
2. *Identify barriers and challenges faced by mental health professionals practicing in rural areas*
3. *Describe how legislative trends and issues have influenced the delivery of mental health care in rural environments*
4. *Understand current stresses associated with rural life and their impact upon mental health*
5. *Discuss the role of the psychiatric mental health nurse practicing in rural areas*
6. *Understand the importance of innovative service delivery programs for the mentally ill in rural settings.*

INTRODUCTION AND HISTORICAL OVERVIEW

For many of the more than 59.5 million rural residents of this country, the romanticized vision of a tranquil and prosperous rural life-style has been replaced by the realities of economic deprivation, inadequate housing, and unaddressed physical and mental health problems. Approximately 25% of the people in the United States live in rural areas, and they constitute about 40% of the nation's poor.[27] The mental health status of the rural poor is a complex and multidimensional problem, compounded by lack of education and by fragmented, uncoordinated, frequently inaccessible health and social services.[41]

The first large mental hospitals in this country were built in isolated rural areas to provide both work and sustenance for their residents and employees. But it was not until after World War II that more comprehensive, community-based mental health centers were developed, with a focus on preventive mental health care. During the Kennedy administration, the need for access to mental health care in rural areas became apparent, and an effort to decrease distances rural clients had to travel for care and follow-up treatment was initiated. As a result, mental health services, in the form of satellite clinics, support groups, public education campaigns, and the establishment of communication networks, have become more available in nonmetropolitan areas over the last two decades. However, the current situation is still less than ideal. The 1978 Commission on Mental Health report[37] paid particular attention to the poor distribution of mental health services to rural regions. It contended that the rural elderly population is vastly underserved by the mental health system and emphasized that rural areas have unique mental health service needs.

> Rural communities tend to be characterized by higher than average rates of psychiatric disorders, particularly depression, by severe intergenerational conflicts, by restricted opportunities for developing adequate coping mechanisms for facing stress and for problem solving, by an exodus of individuals who might serve as effective role models for coping, by an acceptance of conditions as being beyond individual control, and by acceptance of fatalistic attitudes and minimal subscription to the idea that change is possible (reference 37, p 1164).

At present, both the number of professionals (including psychiatric mental health nurses) providing mental health services in rural settings and the services, themselves, are inadequate. Geographic and cost factors associated with accessibility of mental health services, and issues related to the stigma of mental illness, cultural norms, and the attitudes of some service providers, make delivery of mental health services in rural areas problematic. Because there are too few mental health services available in rural America, and because many rural Americans are reluctant to accept such services, even where they are available, care alternatives are often restricted to crisis intervention or long-term institutionalization. The farm crisis of the 1980s has finally brought the need for more comprehensive mental health care to the attention of the public, service providers, educational institutions, and policy makers. Yet, many barriers that impede the effective delivery of mental health services for persons experiencing loss as a result of the depressed agricultural economy still exist. These include unavailable and limited mental health services for persons in rural areas; inadequate numbers of staff knowledgeable in the multiple and complex difficulties of rural life; and lack of formalized coordination among mental health services, agriculture, cooperative extension services, job retraining, health care practitioners, and other providers whose services all have been affected by the rural economy.

This chapter highlights factors associated with the development, implementation, and evaluation of rural mental health programs, including rural and urban differences, characteristics of service providers, legislative trends, models for mental health services programs, and research issues. The role of the psychiatric nurse in providing mental health care in rural environments is discussed, and nursing diagnoses, particularly those related to the recent farm crisis and "rural stress," are examined.

DIFFERENCES BETWEEN MENTAL HEALTH CARE IN RURAL AND URBAN SETTINGS

Bachrach[4] classified rural and urban differences in human service delivery according to five factors: nonsocial (e.g., transportation), demographic and ecologic, socioeconomic, interpersonal, and ideologic. These factors suggest that the geography, tax and resource base, power structure, and value systems of rural areas differ markedly from urban regions and affect the delivery of mental health services. Although many of the problems faced by the rural mentally ill are also confronted in urban environments, the following compilation from the literature highlights some of the differences between the mentally ill residing in rural areas and those in urban settings. Compared with their urban counterparts, the rural mentally ill:

- Have lower average incomes:[42] Rural residents constitute 40% of all Americans living below the poverty level, and yet they receive only about 20% of what the government spends on the poor.[28]
- Live in more substandard and dilapidated housing: Sixty percent of the nation's substandard housing is in rural areas.[48]
- Have more health problems.[36]
- Do *not* have their health and mental impairments as readily treated: Only 7% of rural counties have a general hospital with psychiatric facilities, versus 33% of urban counties.[13]

- Receive less abundant, less accessible, and more costly services: The National Institute of Mental Health (NIMH) reports[33] that only 17.5% of mental health services in rural areas are adequate, compared with 49% of the services in urban areas.
- Have less available public transportation: Furthermore, long distances to services increases coordination and communication difficulties.
- Do not enjoy kinship networks that are significantly stronger than kinship networks in urban settings: Moreover, kinship networks and networks among neighbors in rural settings may, in fact, work against the delivery of mental health services in that "everyone knows everybody else's business."[37]
- Have less access to psychiatrists and, therefore, rely on general practitioners, public health nurses, and social service workers for mental health care: Sixty-eight percent fewer staff hours and 93% fewer psychiatric hours were budgeted per capita in rural areas versus those in urban slums.[31]
- Receive only 8% of federal grant monies.[19]

Although persons living in rural areas differ from those in urban settings in a number of ways, they clearly are *not* a homogeneous group that enjoys a common culture. However, several values and themes seem to predominate in rural settings. These include subjugation to nature, individualism, an emphasis on primary relationships and family ties, traditionalism, fatalism, the Protestant work ethic, conservative beliefs, and strong religious values.[4,13] These values influence the identification of certain behaviors as pathologic and affect the type of treatment sought.

Youmans[48] has further identified three value systems that affect mental health services in rural areas: identification with the community and a sense of belonging; a work or "doing" orientation; and fatalistic attitude toward aging. These beliefs may explain why, especially among the rural elderly, decreased ability to perform activities of daily living is correlated with decreased morale, and why supportive social service and health care programs may be viewed with suspicion and contempt.[16]

To be successful, rural mental health services must mesh with other services and informal helping networks. Service providers and researchers must understand and be sensitive to the rural value system and social ecology of the area. Otherwise, mental health workers, including psychiatric nurses, may find themselves addressing assumed rather than real needs. Because of the nature of rural values, borrowing successful urban techniques and imposing them without modification in a rural setting may not be appropriate or effective.

Brown has noted, "An even greater disparity between city and country lies in the ability of these areas to handle problems of mental health; while the shortage of mental health personnel is nationwide, it is particularly severe in our rural areas" (reference 6, pp iii, iv). The next section discusses characteristics of mental health professionals working in rural areas and highlights some of the unique problems they may face.

MENTAL HEALTH PROFESSIONALS IN RURAL SETTINGS

The rural community is not rich with professional human service options, and the role of mental health professionals in rural areas is a demanding one. Psychiatric mental health nurses practicing in rural settings can expect fewer resources, increased job responsibilities, and more loneliness than their urban counterparts.[14,40] It is not surprising that recruitment and retention problems abound in rural settings.

Sidwell[43] identified the following eight functional abilities of "generalists" serving the mental health needs of rural communities:

1. To gather relevant and pertinent data to make rapid, accurate assessments of individual pathology and individual and family functioning
2. To develop relevant interventions for both individuals and families and to systematically evaluate them
3. To intervene in a positive manner with individuals and their family systems to promote independence
4. To use the personal–professional self in a variety of community settings to promote quality of life
5. To conduct professional responsibilities as a member of an interdisciplinary team
6. To become a significant and contributing member of the lay community
7. To practice concepts important in operating a viable business within the human service environment
8. To demonstrate commitment through reasonable community tenure.

This generalist perspective, from which the psychiatric nurse views clients within the context of their total environment,[11] is essential in rural areas. To be effective, the mental health nurse must be acquainted with, and understand, the resources, dynamics, culture, power structure, and politics of the rural community, requiring a broad range of skills and the ability to work autonomously.

The emphasis in rural mental health programs is on family and community systems, with more informal, nonbureaucratic modes of operation.[20] In a national study of community mental health centers, Jones and associates[21] investigated the attitudes of mental health workers in both urban and rural settings. They found rural workers endorsed community mental health ideology, and organizational and personal activism more than urban workers, and they also perceived their centers more as social, rather than medical, agencies. Rural service providers experience less supervision, peer support, privacy, and structure. The resulting lack of referral resources, professional isolation, and narrow community attitudes can become sources of stress for psychiatric mental health nurses in rural environments. These stresses may be further compounded by ethical and legal constraints upon practice.

Hargrove[17] outlined several ethical and legal issues related to mental health practice in rural settings, including confidentiality, limits of practice, multiple levels of relationships, and the impact of professional licensure and certification on rural practice. Hargrove suggests that rural practitioners may experience conflict between prevailing community standards and professional ethical codes, that is, professional guidelines may not "adequately consider the political and cultural realities of rural environments."[17] For example, psychiatric mental health nurses practicing in rural settings may have difficulty meeting state-mandated continuing education requirements because such classes are often offered by academic settings or large clinical facilities that are not in close proximity. Similarly, they may have problems in obtaining the quantity and quality of supervision necessary to meet requirements for American Nursing Association (ANA) certification because such supervision may not be readily available.

LEGISLATIVE TRENDS AND ISSUES

Passage of the Community Mental Health Centers Act (P.L. 88-164) in 1963 was the first federal initiative to develop community-based mental health services. By 1975 (P.L. 94-63), 12 services were required to be available to qualify for federal staffing funds: outpatient, inpatient, emergency, partial hospitalization, specialized services for children and the elderly, screening, aftercare, transitional housing, consultation–education, drug abuse, and alcoholism. Such a comprehensive array of services are not available in most rural areas. Longest and associates[26] noted that comprehensive mental health services were available in only 18% of rural catchment areas, versus in 26% of the urban areas studied. For instance, in many rural areas there are no aftercare services available, and clients are discharged from mental hospitals without provision for mental health services. Similarly, outpatient services are frequently nonexistent or inaccessible.

President Carter appointed the Commission on Mental Health in 1977 to review the country's mental health system. The Commission's 1978 report[37] led to the passage of the Mental Health Systems Act (P.L. 96-398), which would have provided more money for mental health services in rural areas. Regrettably, the Budget Reconciliation Act (P.L. 97-35) of 1981 repealed the Systems Act before it could be implemented. P.L. 97-35, combining as it did mental health service funds with block grants allocated for drug abuse and alcoholism, effectively eliminated money for innovative rural mental health demonstration projects in the area of service delivery.[45] Community mental health services previously funded by categorical grants are now funded by block grants at between 50% to 80% of the prior funding level. On the larger scale, a federal policy

commitment to building mental health programs in rural areas is sorely needed, particularly in light of the recent farm crisis.

CURRENT STRESSES ASSOCIATED WITH RURAL LIFE AND RELATED NURSING DIAGNOSES

With changes in the agribusiness economy, many rural traditions are being threatened, and hard times are tearing at the social fabric of many rural states, especially those in the North Central Region. For example, a recent Iowa poll indicated that three out of five adults believed the economy significantly contributed to problems in their community, ranging from vandalism to suicide.[10] Since the beginning of the current farm crisis in 1980–1981, bankruptcy and foreclosure have become common household words, an outgrowth of foreign grain embargos and weakened export demands, low commodity prices, crippling interest rates, droughts, diminished value of farmland, and the financial collapse of grain elevators and rural railway systems.[7,8,32,47] Mental health professionals working in rural communities have documented the devastating emotional and social impact that forced liquidation and foreclosure have on attachments and values associated with a rural ideology. Difficulties ensue with the severing of these intense ties to the land and nature, the collective effort of several generations working together, and the opportunity for husbands and wives to share a common profession.[12] As research conducted by Molnar[30] has shown, the subjective well-being of many rural inhabitants is intimately linked to their commitment to farming as a way of life. For example, one despondent Minnesota man phoned a mental health center hotline and stated, "I'm afraid of what I'm going to do. I won't be able to face not being a farmer. My grandfather homesteaded this farm, my father kept it together during the depression, and now I'm losing it." Farmer[12] has described similar difficulties among rural families, including the ongoing stresses associated with the lengthy process of the threatened or actual loss of a farm, the sense of rural belonging and distrust for city life, and the loss of independence when forced to work for others. A recent study of farmers by Bultena[7] demonstrated the impact of financial problems on hopefulness and quality-of-life issues. Not surprisingly, personal and familial stress were most prevalent among those in more precarious financial circumstances. Ninety-four percent of the respondents most at risk perceived increased familial stress over the past three years, and two-thirds of the subjects were affected by day-to-day stress related to farm activities, as compared with only 41% of the more financially secure respondents in Bultena's sample.[7] And farmers are not the only ones affected by the rural economic crisis. Implement dealerships have closed, and mainstreet businesses struggle to stay afloat as their longtime customers reduce expenditures and use their savings for living expenses. Administrators of public programs, including mental health programs, grapple with decreased budgets and forced cutbacks in personnel and resources. Furthermore, the frail and vulnerable elderly, who constitute a high proportion of rural residents, have been left alone by the outmigration of youth leaving rural areas for the promise of employment in cities.

Psychiatric nurses who practice in rural settings encounter many symptoms of stress that are directly or indirectly related to the economic crisis of the past decade. These include increases in substance abuse; child, spouse, and elder abuse or neglect; divorce rates; suicide and homocide; and emotional problems related to serious farm accidents. Clinicians practicing in rural areas have noted increased somatic complaints, depression, and a diminished sense of self-worth and loss of dignity among their clientele.[5,12] The most common related nursing diagnoses include anxiety, depression, self-concept disturbance, dysfunctional family processes, fear, guilt, hopelessness, impaired resource management (finances), ineffective individual coping, suicide potential, powerlessness, situational crises, spiritual distress, substance abuse (alcohol), and substance abuse (drugs).[29] Indeed, assessment and treatment of these symptoms and diagnoses, in the face of limited resources, great distances to travel, and a clientele often reluctant to seek or accept help from others, makes the role of the psychiatric nurse in rural environments complex and challenging.

ROLE OF THE PSYCHIATRIC NURSE

Psychiatric nurses play an integral role in the delivery of mental health services in rural communities. They are increasingly called upon to educate and counsel those suffering from stress and its sequelae and to coordinate innovative services in the community. As such, they are pivotal members of the multidisciplinary mental health team and provide many forms of crisis intervention in a variety of settings. Nurses are in an ideal position to establish and lead support groups, such as those that deal with the farm crisis or stress-related problems (e.g., substance abuse, child abuse). Nurses can also provide leadership in the identification, training, and appropriate use of community support, such as church groups that sponsor a farm crisis hotline, or provide food and shelter for those in need. Working with social, political, religious, and other health care leaders in the rural community, nurses can enhance communication networks and heighten community awareness of those most at risk for the development of mental health problems (e.g., the socially isolated, frail elderly). Furthermore, nurses can educate persons living in rural areas about stress reduction; provide skills-training classes on assertiveness, problem solving, and self-esteem; and serve as both a resource and conduit for other community-based services (e.g., respite care, nutritional programs). No longer can psychiatric nurses be bound by the tradi-

tional constraints of role or setting. The farm crisis of the 1980s has provided the impetus for psychiatric nurses to develop, implement, and evaluate innovative and effective delivery services and to take a leadership role in the care of persons experiencing mental health problems who reside in rural environments.

INNOVATIVE SERVICE DELIVERY PROGRAMS FOR THE MENTALLY ILL IN RURAL ENVIRONMENTS

Effective mental health service delivery in rural America requires innovative approaches that include coordination and cooperation among mental health, medical, and social service providers. Two such multi-professional strategies, outreach models and rural adult day-care programs, are highlighted at the conclusion of this section. To be successful, rural mental health service delivery systems must maximize limited resources, address community needs, provide continuity of care, and use professional, paraprofessional, and lay personnel appropriately.[35]

An integrated service structure (combining elements of both direct and indirect service models) has been proposed as the best way to meet these challenges.[4,9] In rural settings, direct mental health services have traditionally been provided by community mental health centers and their satellite offices.[34] This model may be augmented by an indirect service model that offers four mental health features important for rural environments: (1) consultative and educational services to community groups, (2) community guidance for mental health service planning, (3) information sharing on mental health services, and (4) development and coordination of community resources.[9] The integrated service system approach offers several advantages, including staffing flexibility, maximum use of resources, emphasis on preventive mental health services, and decreased "turfdom" among providers.[35]

Mosher[31] describes five models for integrating medical and mental health programs and discusses the concept of the *boundary worker* (persons skilled in the process of relating one system to another) as one way to forge these linkages in rural settings. Briefly, these five models include (1) the linking of a medical clinic with a mental health center in a nearby community; (2) providing psychiatric consultation to general and family practice physicians by telephone; (3) a medical clinic contracting with a mental health center to provide services; (4) a mental health and medical clinic in close proximity, sharing a board of directors and administrative structure and conducting joint staff meetings; and (5) holistic medical centers, in which a variety of practitioners share offices to treat illness and promote wellness through education.[31]

Whatever model is employed, to be successful the agencies involved must share fundamental goals and communication patterns. Too often, collaborative efforts are doomed by misperceptions of goals and poor working relationships among professionals. Lack of centralization, inadequate coordination of agency efforts, and poor relationship skills can also subvert the development of community treatment networks and interfere with continuity of treatment.[1] Ambrosius[2] details three additional deterrents to a coordinated system of services, including loss of agency control, turf battles, and lack of time. Unfortunately, the literature contains primarily descriptive reports and case histories, or describes programs developed for particular groups of clients in particular settings.

Clearly, community mental health center services need to reach a greater percentage of the rural population to identify and attract those persons in need of mental health services. Outreach programs have been suggested as one effective approach in delivering services to the rural mentally ill, because those most at risk do not present themselves to mental health and social services agencies.[44]

Outreach Models

On the basis of sociological studies, Heffernan[18] recommended the development and funding of mental health outreach programs as an important approach to counteracting stresses and depression associated with the farm crisis. Such programs teach professionals and the general public how to identify and refer persons who may need mental health services. Psychiatric nurses play a critical role in the multidisciplinary outreach team, which can overcome some of the limitations of rural mental health services by providing coordinated assessment, treatment, and aftercare to rural residents in their own homes.[25] Outreach can also provide diagnosis and treatment for homebound persons who have physical limitations or major psychiatric illnesses, who are socially isolated, or who are experiencing a combination of problems.

Outreach approaches have proved helpful in treating urban mentally ill persons who might not otherwise enter mental health programs, until a crisis necessitates hospitalization.[46] Evaluations of these urban outreach efforts suggest that they provide rapid and effective mental health assessment and treatment, and minimize disruptions caused by premature institutionalization of clients.[22,38,39] However, the effectiveness of these programs in providing a viable alternative to hospitalization and long-term institutionalization in rural environments is only now being adequately tested.

Rural Adult Day-Care Programs

Adult day-care programs have grown steadily in this country over the past decade, but mostly in major metropolitan areas. These programs provide a structured program of coordinated social, physical health, and mental health services in a protective group setting for some portion of the day. Such programs are oriented toward disease prevention, health maintenance, and rehabilitation of elderly persons, many of whom suffer from some type of mental impairment. Initial efforts to establish adult day-care centers in more rural areas were largely unsuccessful because of geographic distance, lack of transportation, and difficulty identifying and reaching potential clients.[15] Essentially, a few high-cost services were provided to a limited number of clients. Recently, in an effort to overcome these barriers, innovative service delivery systems have been developed and tested. Adult day-care services are being provided to sparsely populated rural areas by means of a mobile team of skilled workers, including psychiatric nurses, utilizing the satellite concept that integrates formal and informal social support systems.[15]

SUMMARY

Persons in rural environments have traditionally been underserved by the mental health system. Barriers to care have included greater distances to travel, fewer

Research Highlights

There are insufficient empirical data documenting the mental health needs of persons in rural settings. There is a dearth of baseline data on which to base planning, and little attention has been paid to regional, cultural, and linguistic differences in this country.

One basic research problem centers on the definition of the term "rural." The U.S. Census Bureau defines *rural* as any community with a population of 2500 or fewer that is located in open country. However, at least seven other quantitative definitions of the term can be found in the literature.[23] Thus, it is not surprising that statistics related to the rural populations vary greatly, often as a function of the definitions used by the researcher.

Babich[3] notes that researchers have approached the problem of ascertaining the prevalence of psychiatric problems in rural areas by measuring the "treated prevalence" (i.e., those already using the mental health system) or by extrapolating prevalence rates from survey findings. Furthermore, mental health survey instruments may be "normed" on urban populations, thus increasing the likelihood that the poor and ethnically diverse rural populations will be judged as deviant.[3] More methodologically rigorous research is needed on the characteristics and mental health problems of the rural persons so that public policy and treatment programs can be more relevant and beneficial.[24]

professionals, and the stigma associated with mental illness in rural settings. The farm economic crisis of the 1980s focused increasing attention on the mental health needs of rural residents, and psychiatric mental health nurses have responded to this challenge. As pivotal members of the mental health care team, psychiatric nurses have helped to resolve some of the stress associated with the farm crisis by providing crisis intervention, leading support groups, developing educational programs, and working with state and local authorities to provide better access to mental health care and services through innovative service delivery mechanisms.

References

1. Allness D, Field G. Principles of inter agency coordination among mental health services. In: Jacobsen M., Kelly P., eds. Issues in rural mental health practice. Iowa City: University of Iowa. Monograph; 1983.

2. Ambrosius GR. To dream the impossible dream: delivering coordinated services to the rural elderly. In: Kim PKH, Wilson CP, eds. Toward mental health of the rural elderly. Washington DC: University Press of America; 1981.

3. Babich KS. Rural mental health care: a summary of the research. In: Mental health issues in rural nursing. Boulder, CO: WICHE; 1982.

4. Bachrach LL. Human services in rural areas: an analytical review. Hum Serv Monogr Ser, Number 22. Project SHARE. Washington, DC: US Department of Health and Human Services; July, 1981.

5. Blundell J. Personal communication. Northwest Iowa Community Mental Health Center, Spencer, IA; August 26, 1988.

6. Brown B. The mental health of rural America, the rural programs of the National Institute of Mental Health, Rockville, MD: US Department of Health, Education and Welfare; 1978.

7. Bultena G. The farm crisis: patterns and impacts of financial stress among Iowa farm families. Journal Paper No. (J-12157) of the Iowa Agriculture and Home Economics Experiment Station. Ames, IA: Project No. 2726; 1986.

8. Business Week. The credit blight down on the farm. Business Week 1981; August 10, 1974.

9. Daniels DN. The community mental health center in the rural area: is the present model appropriate? Am J Psychiatry. 1967;124(suppl):32–37.

10. Des Moines Register, Sunday, February 2, 1986.

11. Dunbar E. Educating social workers for rural mental health settings. In: Dengerink H, ed. Symposium on training for rural mental health. Lincoln, NE: University of Nebraska Press; 1982.

12. Farmer V. Broken heartland. Psychol Today. 1986; Apr:54–62.

13. Flax JW, Wagenfeld MO, Ivens RE, Weiss RJ. Mental health and rural America: an overview and annotated bibliography. Washington DC: National Institute of Mental Health; 1979.

14. Ginsberg L. An overview of social work education for rural areas. Social work in rural communities: a book of readings. New York: Council on Social Work Education; 1976.

15. Gunter PL. A mobile model handbook for developing a rural adult day care program, vol 2. Illinois Department of Aging; 1984.

16. Harbert AS, Wilkinson CW. Growing old in rural America. Aging. January–February, 1979, No. 291–293, 36–40.

17. Hargrove DS. Ethical and legal issues in rural mental health practice. In: Jacobsen M, Kelley P, eds. Issues in rural mental health practice. Iowa City: University of Iowa, Monograph; 1983:55–64.

18. Heffernan WD. Testimony prepared for a hearing of the Joint Economic Committee of the Congress of the United States, Washington, DC; September 19, 1985.

19. Hooyman NR. Mutual help organizations for rural older women. Educ Gerontol Int Q. 1980;5:429–447.

20. Jacobsen M, Kelley P. Reflections on a rural training project. In: Jacobsen M, Kelley P, eds. Issues in rural mental health practice. Iowa City: University of Iowa Monograph; 1983:47–54.

21. Jones JD, Wagenfeld MD, Robins SS. A profile of the rural community health center. Commun Ment Health J. 1976;12:176–181.

22. Kahn R, Tobin S. Community measures for aged persons with altered brain functions. In: Miller NE, Cohen GD, eds. Clinical aspects of Alzheimer's disease and senile dementia. 1981.

23. Kim PKH. The low income rural elderly: underserved victims of public inequity. In: Kim PKH, Wilson CP, eds. Toward mental health of the rural elderly. Washington, DC: University Press of America; 1981:15–27.

24. Kim PKH. Toward rural gerontological education: rationale and model. In: Kim PKH, Wilson CP, eds. Toward mental health of the rural elderly. Washington, DC: University Press of America; 1981:395–403.

25. Lazarus LW, Weinberg J. Psychosocial intervention with the aged. Psychiatr Clin North Am. 1982;5:215–227.

26. Longest J, Konan M, Tweed D. A study of deficiencies in the distribution of mental health resources in facilities. Series BN 15, DHEW Publication No. (ADM): Washington, DC: Superintendent of Documents, US Government Printing Office; 1977:79–517.

27. McAtie P. Rural health care. Pediatr Nurs. 1978;4(4):14–19.

28. McCormick J. America's Third World. Newsweek 1988; Aug 8,20–24.

29. McFarland G, Wasli EL. Nursing diagnoses and process in psychiatric mental health nursing. Philadelphia: JB Lippincott; 1986.

30. Molnar J. Determinants of subjective well-being among farm operators: characteristics of the individual and the farm. Rural Sociol. 1985;50:141–162.

31. Mosher C. Linking medical and mental health services: social workers in rural doctors' offices. In: Jacobsen M, Kelley P, eds. Issues in rural mental health practice. Iowa City: University of Iowa Monograph; 1983.

32. National Geographic. Iowa, America's middle earth, Nat Geogr. 1981;159:603–629.

33. National Institute of Mental Health. Staffing differences between federally funded CMHCs located in metropolitan and nonmetropolitan catchment areas. Memorandum #21. Rockville, MD: Division of Biometry and Epidemiology; October 21, 1977.

34. Ozarin LD. Mental health services in rural areas. In: Day SB, ed. A companion to the life sciences, vol 1. New York: Van Nostrand Reinhold; 1979.

35. Palmer CM, Cunningham ST. Rural mental health delivery: an imperative for creativity. In: Jacobsen M, Kelley P, eds. Iowa City: University of Iowa Monograph; 1983.

36. Pickard L. Long-term care and the rural aged. In: Kim PKH, Wilson CP, eds. Toward mental health of the rural elderly. Washington DC: University Press of America; 1981.

37. President's Commission on Mental Health Task Panel on Rural Mental Health. volume 3, Appendix. Washington DC: US Government Printing Office; 1978.

38. Raskind M, Alvarez C, Petrzyk M, Westerlund K, Herlin S. Helping the elderly psychiatric patient in crisis. Geriatrics 1976;32:51–56.

39. Reifler BV, Kethley A, O'Neill P, Hanley R, Lewis S, Stenchever D. Five year experience of a community outreach program for the elderly. Am J Psychiatry. 1982;139:220–223.

40. Riggs RT, Kugel LF. Transition from urban to rural mental health practice. Soc Casework 1976;57:562–567.

41. Robertson H. Removing barriers to health care. In: Spradley BW, ed. Contemporary community nursing. Boston: Little Brown & Co; 1975.

42. Rural America. Rural America fact sheet: the elderly (RAF #5). Washington DC; 1978.

43. Sidwell LH. Rural mental health practice: the new generalist orientation in services delivery. In: Jacobsen M, Kelley P, eds. Issues in rural mental health practice. Iowa City: University of Iowa Monograph; 1983.

44. Toseland RW, Decker J, Bliesner J. A community outreach program for socially isolated persons. J Gerontol Soc Work. 1979;1:211–224.

45. Walters KS. The changing mental health scene: implications for Iowa. In: Jacobsen M, Kelley P, eds. Issues in rural mental health practice. Iowa City: University of Iowa Monograph; 1983.

46. Wasson W, Ripeckyj A, Lazarus LW, Kupferer S, Barry S, Force F. Home evaluation of psychiatrically impaired elderly: process and outcome. Gerontologist 1984;24:238–242.

47. Westphal D. Riches to rags. Six articles in Des Moines Register. Des Moines Register; June 16–21, 1985.

48. Youmans EG. The rural aged. Ann Am Acad Polit Soc Sci. 1977;419:81–90.

49

Elizabeth Kelchner Gerety

Psychiatric Consultation–Liaison Nursing

OBJECTIVES

After reading this chapter, the reader will be able to:

1. *Define the role of the psychiatric consultation–liaison nurse*
2. *Discuss specific functions of the psychiatric consultation–liaison nurse in the health care delivery system*
3. *Differentiate between client-centered and consultation-centered consultations in psychiatric consultation–liaison nursing practice*
4. *Discuss the application of nursing diagnosis as a component of the nursing process in psychiatric consultation–liaison nursing*
5. *Cite examples of current issues and trends in psychiatric consultation–liaison nursing.*

DEFINITION AND DESCRIPTION OF PSYCHIATRIC CONSULTATION–LIAISON NURSING

Psychiatric consultation–liaison nursing is a subspecialty in psychiatric mental health nursing.[30,38] The scope of practice for this subspecialty includes primary prevention, intervention, and rehabilitation[35] (Box 49-1). Psychiatric consultation–liaison nurses (PCLNs) diagnose and treat the "emotional, spiritual, developmental, and cognitive responses of clients and families who enter the health care system with actual or potential physical dysfunction" (reference 35, p 244). PCLNs work with clients, families, and staff in critical care, obstetrical, pediatric, geriatric and medical-surgical units, as well as in emergency rooms in the general hospital. Nursing homes, long-term care facilities, hospice programs, outpatient and home care, and occupational health are additional settings for psychiatric consultation–liaison nursing practice.[1,2,13,20,21,44] Consultation and liaison activities are mutually complementary.[23] PCLNs provide psychiatric consultation to nurses and other health professionals to ". . . influence and enhance their knowledge of and skill in addressing the biopsychosocial aspects of the care of clients/families, and promote their capacity to function optimally in the practice setting," (reference 35, p 244). Liaison activities are directed toward maintaining clinical contacts with nurses and other health professionals to help interpret psychiatric and psychological problems of clients who have actual or potential physical problems.

Psychiatric consultation–liaison nurses are expected to be clinically self-directed and to accept accountability for their clinical judgments and decisions. They function autonomously as role models and change agents and need to have a high tolerance for ambiguity and frustration in the clinical area. Respect for confidentiality of information that is shared with them by clients, families, nurses, and other professionals is important. PCLNs need to be assertive and willing to take risks in their advocacy for maximizing the coping abilities of clients and families as part of an overall commitment to the delivery of quality client care.[1,2,5,11,21]

BOX 49–1

Direct Client Consultation: Examples of Psychiatric Consultation–Liaison Nursing Diagnoses, Related Factors, and Categories of Interventions and Recommendations

DIAGNOSIS AND RELATED FACTORS

Anticipatory Grieving related to (1) potential loss of own life, (2) potential loss of significant other, (3) potential loss of function, or (4) potential loss of body part

Grieving related to (1) loss of significant other, (2) loss of function or body part, body image change, (3) role change, or (4) losses encountered during aging process

Dysfunctional Grieving related to (1) multiple losses, (2) chronic fatal illness, or (3) losses encountered during aging process

Anxiety related to threats to (1) biological integrity, (2) surgical procedures, (3) diagnostic studies, (4) invasive procedures, (5) pathophysiological processes, or (6) potential or actual loss of significant other

Powerlessness related to threats to (1) biological integrity, (2) surgical procedures, (3) diagnostic studies, (4) invasive procedures, (5) pathophysiological processes, or (6) potential or actual loss of significant other

*Acute Pain** related to (1) cancer, (2) cardiac disease, (3) surgery, (4) fractures, or (5) pancreatitis

Suicide Potential related to (1) acute pain, (2) chronic pain, (3) delirium, (4) alcohol abuse, or (5) drug abuse

Fear related to (1) surgery, (2) invasive procedures, (3) disabling illness, (4) loss of function or body part, or (5) therapies, e.g., radiation, chemotherapy, dialysis

Confusion related to (1) delirium, (2) alcohol or drug abuse, (3) metastatic processes, or (5) loss of familiar surroundings

*Impaired Adjustment** related to (1) chronic illness, (2) altered locus of control, (3) disability requiring change in life-style, or (5) treatment side effects and discomforts

INTERVENTIONS/RECOMMENDATIONS[6]

Crisis intervention; client/family counseling; presence; stress management; instilling hope; advocacy; discharge planning

Crisis intervention; active listening; stress management; presence; client/family counseling; client/family teaching

Client/family counseling; stress management; instilling hope

Crisis intervention; active listening; preparatory sensory information; presence; stress management; client/family teaching; client/family counseling

Crisis intervention; client/family teaching; advocacy; stress management; preparatory sensory information; client/family counseling

Client/family teaching; surveillance; advocacy; stress management; preparatory sensory information

Crisis intervention; surveillance; advocacy; active listening; patient contracting

Crisis intervention; active listening; preparatory sensory information; client/family counseling

Monitoring; advocacy; presence; client/family teaching

Active listening; client/family teaching; instilling hope; stress management; client/family counseling; discharge planning

---

* Other NANDA nursing diagnosis.

DEFINITION AND DESCRIPTION OF CONSULTATION–LIAISON PSYCHIATRY

Consultation-liaison psychiatry is a subspecialty of psychiatry with three major functions: clinical, teaching, and research.[23,29] The focus of consultation–liaison psychiatry is on diagnosing, treating, studying, and preventing psychiatric complications among physically ill clients who are experiencing and communicating emotional distress in a variety of nonpsychiatric health care settings.[25] This subspecialty of psychiatry goes beyond the traditional biomedical model of client evaluation and emphasizes the significance of psychological and social factors, as well as the client's milieu. The term *consultation–liaison* (C–L) reflects the two interrelated roles of this subspecialty. *Consultation* refers to the provision of an expert diagnostic opinion and recommendations by a specialist, for the management of a client's mental state and behavior, in response to a request from a consultee who is another health professional.[23] The term *liaison*, which is frequently synonymous with "teaching," is used to connote the linking up of groups of health professionals to promote effective communication and collaboration and to decrease conflicts between clients and caregivers.[19,24,33,34] Liaison psychiatry is the process for sharing the interrelationships of psychological and social factors within the context of physical illness and its treatment. The use of the term liaison in C–L psychiatry has become somewhat controversial in recent years.[12,19,23] There are some members of the mental health profession who believe that the term is confusing and unnecessary and that the term consultation psychiatry is adequate for conveying the concurrent liaison activities. There are others, however, who believe that liaison continues to be a viable designation to emphasize the integration of the knowledge of psychological and social factors within a psychosomatic model, as opposed to a biomedical model. Although the major portion of C–L psychiatry practice is in general hospitals that are associated with an academic medical center, the scope of this subspecialty encompasses other health care settings, such as nursing homes, community health clinics, rehabilitation centers, and the private offices of physicians; and it extends to stressful work environments, such as air traffic control towers and ship docks.[12,24,29]

EDUCATION AND PREPARATION OF THE PSYCHIATRIC CONSULTATION–LIAISON NURSE

Psychiatric consultation–liaison nurses are clinical nurse specialists who have become experts in the area of psychiatric C–L nursing practice. They are generalists in nursing, who hold baccalaureate degrees in nursing and are masters- or doctorally-prepared in psychiatric mental health nursing. Ideally, they have had a course of study, at the graduate level, that includes supervised practice in psychiatric C–L nursing. They are expected to be proficient in psychiatric assessment and intervention and skilled in group process and teaching. They should be able to synthesize theories from nursing, psychiatry, sociology, consultation, systems, organizational behavior, change, stress and crisis, as well as psychophysiology. Clinical experience in medical–surgical nursing, as well as in psychiatric mental health nursing, is helpful. It is important for the PCLN to have a working knowledge of medical specialties and to have current information on pharmacology. Certification as a clinical nurse specialist in psychiatric mental health nursing is recommended.[4,5,11,15,21,32,38,41]

HISTORICAL REVIEW

The development of C–L psychiatry began in 1902 when Albany Hospital became the first general hospital in the United States to have an inpatient psychiatry unit. The availability of psychiatrists for collaboration and consultation with nonpsychiatric physicians increased as other general hospitals opened inpatient psychiatric units. Funding from the Rockefeller Foundation in 1934 led to the establishment of the first five psychiatric liaison departments in university hospitals. Medicine and psychiatry collaborated during World War II to provide treatment for war-related mental health problems. The development and expansion of the field of psychopharmacology and the use of psychotropic medications in the 1950s and 1960s increased the impact of C–L services in the general hospital. From 1970 until the present time, C–L psychiatry has undergone a transformation from a marginal special interest area into a full-fledged growing and complex subspecialty.[21,23,24,31,37,41]

Psychiatric C–L nursing emerged as a subspecialty of psychiatric nursing during the early 1960s. Betty Sue Johnson provided the first written report of nursing consultations by psychiatric nurses in a 1963 publication that described the development and implementation of a program at Duke University that was designed to address multiple nursing care problems in specific clinical areas. Psychiatric C–L nursing evolved from this early work, as specialists in psychiatric nursing continued to consult with staff nurses on medical–surgical units to help them strengthen their interpersonal relationships with clients by gaining a better understanding of the emotional component of client concerns. The scope of consultation activity expanded to direct assessment of, and interventions with, clients and families. The growth of psychiatric units in general hospitals increased the visibility and availability of psychiatric nurse consultants. Preparation at the graduate level became possible in the early 1970s, when the University of Maryland and Yale University offered graduate programs in C–L nursing.[15,16,21,30,31,37] The first publication of C–L nursing research was during the 1970s.[37] In 1974, the first text, *Liaison Nursing, Psychological Approach to Patient Care,* by Lisa Robinson, was published. Although there were other texts between 1974 and 1982 that addressed relevant C–L nursing themes and concepts, it was not until 1982 that a second text, *Psychiatric Liaison Nursing: The Theory and Clinical Practice,* by Anita Lewis and Joyce Sasson Levy, was published.[39] The First Annual Conference for Psychiatric Liaison Nurses was held in April 1987, in Chicago, the same year that a task force with regional representatives developed the initial proposed Standards of Psychiatric Consultation Liaison Nursing Practice.[35]

ORGANIZATIONAL PLACEMENT AND MODELS OF PRACTICE

The PCLN position is usually in the department of nursing or the department of psychiatry. PCLNs who are in private practice contract with agencies on a fee-for-service basis. Successful clinical relationships and working alliances are more easily established when the PCLN is in a staff position, rather than a line position, within the department of nursing with administrative freedom to respond to clinical problems and issues and when the position is one with no authority over consultees or influence over staff evaluations.[15,21,39,41]

Psychiatric C–L literature describes several models of practice that are based on variations of collaborative practice with an interdisciplinary C–L team or of C–L nursing practice in which there is no formal structure for team collaboration outside of the department of nursing.[3,4,21,38,39,42] The model for C–L practice in many medical centers is an interdisciplinary team headed by a psychiatrist, with additional mental health professionals, for example, psychiatric clinical nurse specialists (PCLNs), clinical psychologists, and psychiatric social workers (Figure 49-1). The interdisciplinary team in a teaching facility may include graduate nursing students, psychiatry residents, psychology interns, and graduate social work students. A collaborative team approach maximizes individual strengths and is based on the philosophy that professionals work together as equals who recognize and value the uniqueness of each other's professional preparation, skills, and specific areas of interest. The interdisciplinary C–L team uses clinical tasks as the foundation for consultation decision making as opposed to a specific discipline. There are mutual benefits for the team with a PCLN. The PCLN has direct access to C–L team members for clinical consultation and back up for nurse- and physician-initiated consultations. The PCLN's accessibility to nursing staff contributes to an expanded referral base for the entire consultation team. Nurse-to-nurse consultations often generate requests for further evaluation by other members of the C–L team. The PCLN's affiliation with nursing staff as well as the C–L team increases staff and client acceptance of a psychiatric consultation. The team with a PCLN is more aware of the emotional impact of illness on the client's family. The visibility of the PCLN during routine clinical rounds, case finding, or direct clinical intervention increases the perception of visibility and ability of the entire consultation team.[5,14,18,31]

ROLES AND FUNCTIONS

Four major categories, which form the acronym, CARE, delineate the roles and functions of the PCLN: clinical, administrative, research, and education. Al-

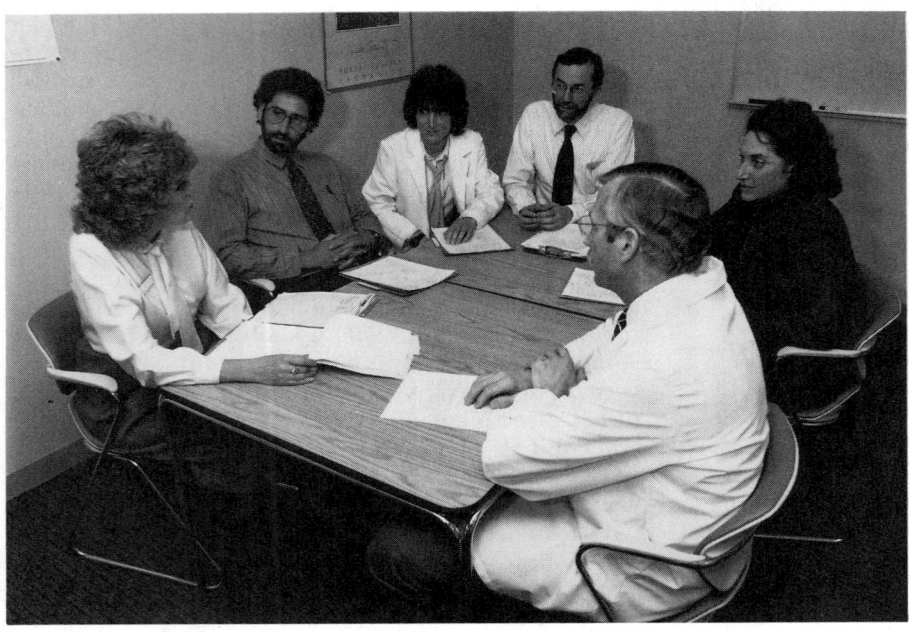

FIGURE 49–1. The psychiatric consultation–liaison nurse discusses a case with the consultation–liaison interdisciplinary team.

though there is overlap among these categories, there are also discrete aspects that characterize each of them. The *clinical role* includes client-centered and consultee-centered consultations. The PCLN in the *administrative role* uses knowledge of organizational and departmental priorities, goals, and constraints in representing administration to the staff and staff to the administration. The *research role* focuses on identification of problems for research, systematic collection of data, analysis of data to answer research questions, and communication of research findings. The *role of educator* includes identifying educational needs, developing teaching modules, and presenting formal and informal educational programs to staff and clients.[2,11,15]

The emphasis on specific clinical, administrative, research, and educational functions within a given C–L role is influenced by variables such as the expectations, philosophy, and goals of administration; the clinical setting (inpatient, outpatient, community); the needs of staff and clients; and the needs, expectations, philosophy, goals, and clinical expertise of the PCLN.

Clinical Role

Clinical functions focus on client-centered and consultee-centered consultations (Figs. 49-2 and 49-3). Most client-centered consultations are initiated by nurses, physicians, or other health professionals for assistance in the evaluation and management of specific client

behaviors. Two additional sources for client-centered consultations are case-finding by the PCLN during routine clinical rounds or specific requests from a client or family.[5] A consultee-centered consultation is provided when the PCLN attends specific unit nursing rounds, interdisciplinary, or multidisciplinary team conferences by request, to give input for the evaluation and management of the health care of clients with complex physiologic and psychosocial problems. Advocacy issues for clients and families that arise during these consultee–consultation clinical discussions sometimes lead to client-centered consultations for the PCLN to evaluate the client's or family's ability to comprehend and cope with ongoing treatment plans or the client's and family's motivation for participating in recommended therapies. Consultee-centered clinical functions also include helping staff to design and to implement a plan of care that is based, in part, on the PCLNs clinical assessment of the presenting consultation problem. Collaboration is an integral function of clinical practice in both client-centered and consultee-centered consultations. For example, a PCLN who was asked by a primary nurse to evaluate "depression" in a 76-year-old client with a recent laryngectomy, formulated the nursing diagnosis of grieving related to loss of voice, change in body image, and hospitalization during Christmas time. The client emphatically denied giving up, and he stressed he had hope for the future. The PCLN recognized that the antidepressant medication that had been prescribed earlier in the week was

FIGURE 49–2. Process: Client-centered consultation.

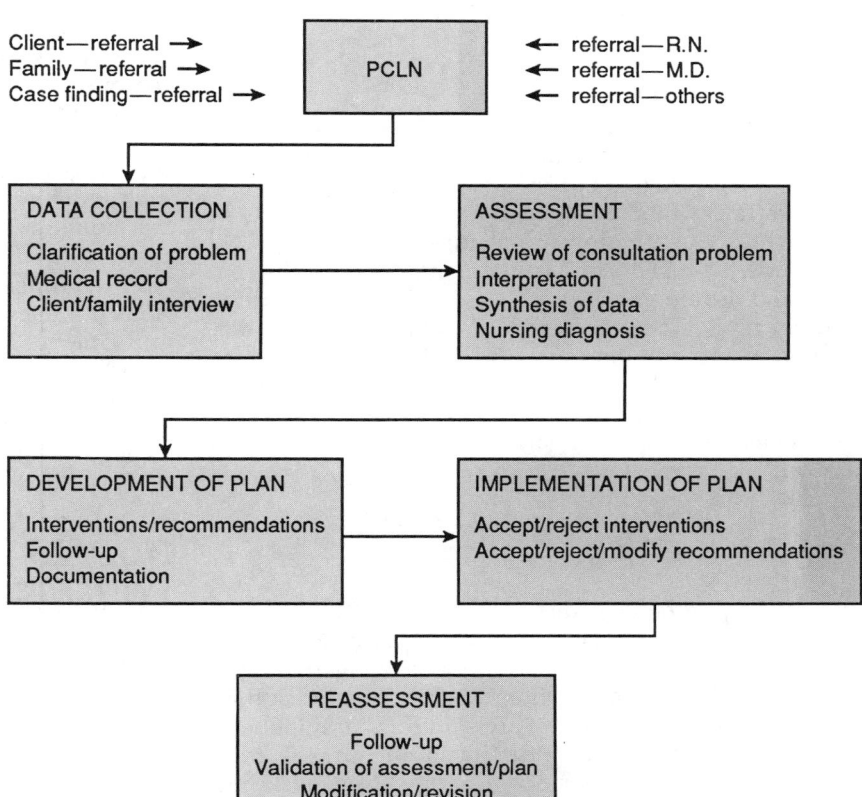

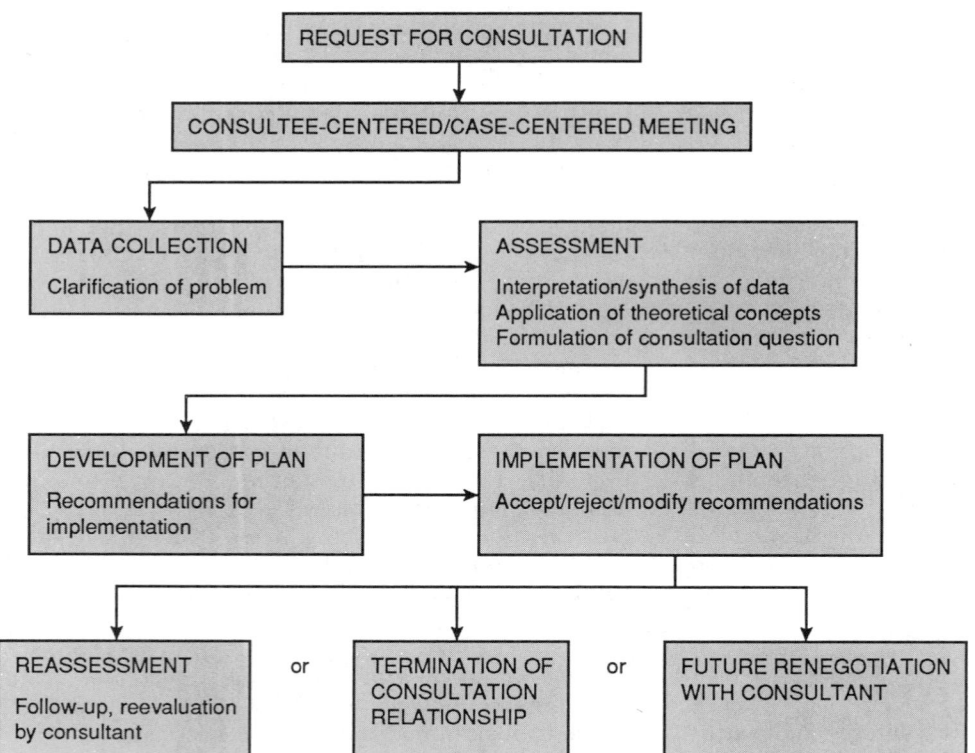

FIGURE 49–3. Process: Consultee-centered consultation.

contraindicated in this situation. Collaboration with the surgery resident and the primary nurse to discuss the consultation findings, resulted in discontinuation of the antidepressant medication and reinforcement of interventions that emphasized hope.

Administrative Role

Membership on policy-making programs and committees at an organizational or departmental level is an administrative function, which provides opportunities for the PCLN to function as a change agent. The PCLN offers critical insights and recommendations for the review and development of policies and procedures that address suicide, violence, and ethical issues to be considered in withholding and withdrawing life-sustaining procedures. Other administrative activities are conducting staff support groups or promoting programs that focus on conflict management and team building for staff.[10,11,45]

Research Role

The research process is incorporated into PCL nursing practice. Accurate and detailed record keeping of C–L activities to provide information for investigating and validating clinical practice is a research function of the PCLN. Current relevant research findings are applied to ongoing practice. The PCLN also encourages and supports research efforts by nursing colleagues and other health professionals.[10,11,41]

Educational Role

Staff and client consultations provide opportunities for informal staff teaching and client education. The PCLN who attends routine nursing rounds uses opportunities to discuss appropriate nursing diagnoses, nursing interventions, nursing responsibilities in pharmacologic management, and the need for ongoing collaboration with other members of the health team. The PCLN in a teaching medical center works closely with graduate and undergraduate nursing students, as well as medical students, interns, and residents to interpret and teach C–L content and issues. Analysis of difficult-to-resolve clinical problems may lead to formal presentations of topics such as pain, grieving, anxiety, suicide, and violence, to nurses and other health professionals. Some PCLNs teach communication and assertiveness skills to staff as well as clients. There is collaboration with staff development and client education personnel to plan specific programs.[10,11,38,45]

MODELS FOR MENTAL HEALTH CONSULTATION

Caplan's theory and models for mental health consultation provide much of the framework for C–L psychiatry and C–L nursing. Caplan identifies four types of consultation: client-centered, consultee-centered, program-centered administrative, and consultee-centered administrative[8] (Boxes 49-2, 49-3, 49-4, and 49-5).

BOX 49–2
Client-Centered Consultation

GOAL
To communicate ways in which the client can be helped

PROCESS
PCLN makes a direct assessment and evaluation of the client and reports findings and recommendations

CASE ILLUSTRATION
The primary nurse on a hematology–oncology unit initiated a request for the PCLN to evaluate the suicide potential in a 63-year-old client diagnosed with lung cancer and bone metastasis. The client's daughter informed the primary nurse that her father had spoken of wanting to take matters into his own hands and "end it all." Although the primary nurse stated that Mr. W rarely asked for pain medication, based on past observations with other clients, the PCLN suspected pain control as a contributor to the problem. After reviewing Mr. W's chart and nursing care plan, the PCLN arranged to meet with Mr. W and his daughter. The interview with Mr. W, which included a suicide and pain assessment, confirmed the nursing diagnosis of acute pain in lower back and ribs related to bone metastasis. Mr. W, a widower for ten years, denied a past history of depression and stated that he had had suicidal ideation with no formulation of a plan, since the recent onset of intolerable pain in his back and ribs. He was hesitant to request pain medication, because "I don't want to get hooked on the stuff." However, he saw himself as being unable to tolerate increasing bone pain until his death. The PCLNs initial interventions with Mr. W and his daughter focused on client and family education of pain assessment and control in coping with cancer. The verbal and written consultation report recommended: (1) negotiate with the client to provide prn pain medication on a regularly scheduled basis; (2) implement a pain flow sheet to monitor client's responses; (3) monitor for recurrence of suicidal ideation and recognize that it could be indicative of inadequate pain control; (4) collaborate with physicians and pharmacists if dosage adjustments are needed. The PCLN provided the staff nurse with information on conducting a suicide assessment to increase her confidence and proficiency in future evaluations. Follow-up contacts by the PCLN with the client, his daughter, and staff validated the assessment that improved pain control would lead to an absence of suicidal ideation.

BOX 49–3
Consultee-Centered Consultation

GOAL
To improve the consultee's ability to manage the client's current situation as well as future similar clinical problems

PROCESS
PCLN assesses and evaluates possible reasons for difficulties and assists consultee to remedy the contributors to the problem

CASE ILLUSTRATION
Nurses at an extended care facility asked the PCLN to attend their weekly nursing rounds to discuss a specific client with whom they were having difficulties. The client was demanding and turned on his call light frequently. Nurses were feeling increasingly frustrated and recognized they were hesitant to get within view of the client. They recognized that there were other clients in the facility who posed similar problems for the staff. The PCLN helped the nurses explore possible dynamics that contributed to their perceptions of "demanding behavior" and their subsequent feelings of helplessness and resentment toward the client. A revision of the client's nursing care plan, which included the nursing diagnosis of powerlessness related to declining physical health and institutional limitations, was discussed. The PCLN suggested specific outcomes and interventions that could be incorporated in the plan of care. Nurses recognized that they had been overlooking the possibility of this diagnosis with other "demanding" clients, and they planned to apply the information to that population.

BOX 49–4
Program-Centered Administrative Consultation

GOAL
To prescribe a course of action for planning or improving a program

PROCESS
PCLN makes short-term and long-term recommendations to an administrator or a designated representative, based on collection and analysis of relevant data

CASE ILLUSTRATION
A PCLN in independent practice was asked by a data-processing company to consult with their occupational health nurse who was developing an Employee Wellness Program with an emphasis on stress management. The PCLN met with the occupational health nurse and representatives from the employee health committee to discuss their concerns and interests. Recommendations were made to the occupational health nurse for initial stress management content that could be developed, as well as for future groups and workshops.

BOX 49–5
Consultee-Centered Administrative Consultation

GOAL
To help the consultees independently develop and implement effective plans for accomplishing the mission of their organization

PROCESS
PCLN assists the consultees to identify, understand, and remedy factors that interfere with their tasks of program development and organization

CASE ILLUSTRATION
The staff development coordinator of a nursing home for extended care contracted with a PCLN to work with the staff development team who recognized a serious morale and potential retention problem among their nursing employees. The PCLN helped the team to identify and to explore specific factors that contributed to the nurses' dissatisfaction. The team formulated an initial strategy to implement for the resolution of the morale and retention problems. The staff development coordinator requested that the PCLN meet with the team in three months to evaluate the effectiveness of the program.

THE CONSULTATION PROCESS IN CLIENT-CENTERED CONSULTATION

The five steps in client-centered consultations are data collection, assessment, development of a plan of action, implementation of the plan, and reassessment[21,41,44] (see Fig. 49-2).

Data Collection

A request for help is conveyed to the PCLN, who determines the urgency of the request, clarifies and defines the problem for which the consultee is seeking help, and gathers as much information as possible within the time constraints of the clinical situation.[19,21,44] The client's chart and previous records are reviewed with a focus on the medical and nursing plan of care, current and past medications, history of substance abuse, laboratory reports, and diagnostic tests and procedures. Brief discussions with other members of the client's treatment team can provide useful information (see Fig. 49-1). Ideally, the client has been informed of the plan for the nurse consultant to visit. In the actual clinical situation, the client may learn of the plan when the consultant arrives. The consultant makes a brief introduction and provides brief, factual information about the purpose for the interview. "I am Carol J, a Registered Nurse. I am a clinical nurse specialist who talks with clients and families about the stress associated with being in the hospital. My clinical specialty is mental health nursing. Your primary nurse, Jim B, has told me a bit about your situation; and he has asked me to try to help him and other nurses with your

nursing plan of care." The length of the interview varies according to the client's physical and emotional status. Medical data are incorporated with psychological data as the PCLN encourages the client to share information about what led to the hospitalization, understanding of current health status, and perceptions of coping with the current situation. The interview is directed toward learning about the client's support system, past hospitalizations (including psychiatric), history of suicide and violence, and substance abuse. The PCLN observes for cultural beliefs that might be manifested as psychiatric problems and determines the need for a culturologic assessment.[7,17] The mental status examination, an important component of data collection, is integrated throughout the interview. Adaptation and modification of the interview and evaluation process are based upon the urgency of the consultation and the client's physical and mental ability to tolerate the consultation. For example, the PCLN may assess the orientation of a ventilator-dependent client, who is unable to write, by asking brief questions that can be answered with hand squeezes or head nods. "Have you given up?" is a useful question for an initial assessment of hopelessness in clients who are unable to speak or write. Direct or telephone interviews with the client's family are additional sources for information. The PCLN observes the client's environment and the manner with which the client interacts with it. How well does the client use the call light to ask for help? Is the client able to articulate requests to nurses? Are there reading materials or cards and letters around to indicate outside interests and supportive contacts?

Assessment

Objectivity and clarification are tasks during the examination of the data that will be compiled in a format for others to review.[19] "What is the consultation question?" is kept in mind as clinical findings are interpreted and synthesized. Defining characteristics and related factors are identified, and a nursing diagnosis is formulated at this time.

Development of a Plan

The development of a pragmatic plan for specific nursing action is based on the assessment. The plan may include direct interventions by the PCLN as well as recommendations for interventions by others (Figure 49-4). The PCLN documents the assessment, nursing diagnosis, recommendations, and any plans for follow-up evaluation on a formal written consultation report for the client's record (see Box 49-1). Some or all of the recommendations may be discussed with the client.

Implementation of the Plan

The PCLN may initiate selected nursing interventions during the first or subsequent consultation contacts

FIGURE 49–4. A psychiatric consultation–liaison nurse discusses relaxation techniques with a cardiac client and his wife.

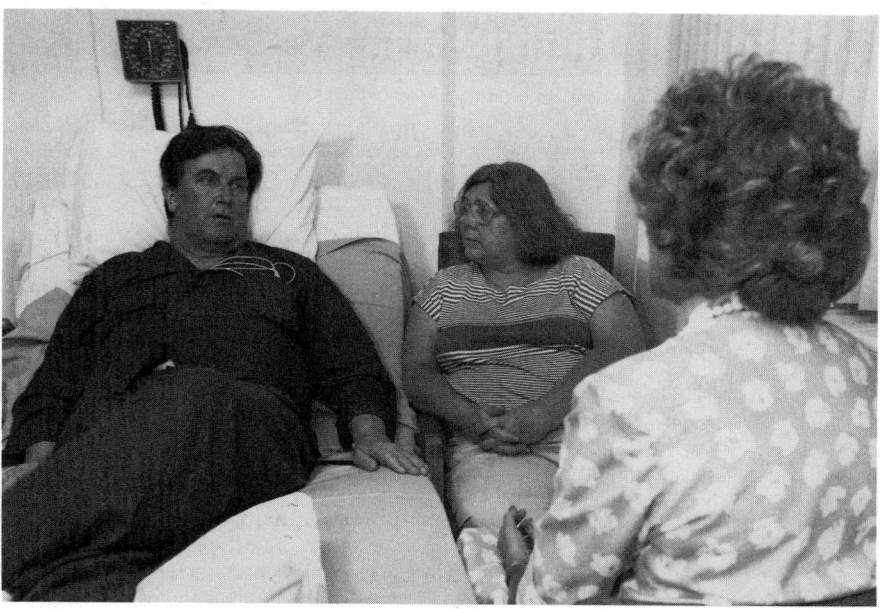

with the client. Interventions and recommendations for staff are specific, relevant, and brief; and they are communicated in a manner that conveys respect and competence to the consultee. The consultee and client may choose to use, modify, or reject all or part of the recommendations.[21]

Reassessment

Reassessment is necessary to achieve closure. The PCLN initiates follow-up to obtain additional data to validate the initial assessment, plan, and interventions and to determine the need for modification and revision of recommendations and interventions. A follow-up interview with the client, as well as the consultee, may be arranged to obtain further insights and to emphasize the value that is placed on the consultation. The collaborative relationship between the PCLN and the consultee is strengthened by the visibility of this activity.[21]

ISSUES AND TRENDS

Consultation–liaison nursing faces the related issues of marketing and research. Documentation of C–L nursing practice is one mechanism for maintaining visibility and credibility in the clinical arena. Literature in C–L cites examples of the limitations of DSM-III-R and DSM-III-R for C–L practice.[9,28,36,40] There is the lack of reliability and the lack of adequate and well-validated diagnostic guidelines for the use of the DSM-III classification system in the medical setting. The PCLN who uses nursing diagnosis as a component of documentation describes client problems in nursing terms as opposed to medical terms, thereby, communicating the value of nursing services that address health problems from a perspective different from that of medicine.[27]

The documentation of C–L practice, which includes nursing diagnosis, is a subtle marketing technique for conveying the PCLN's unique clinical contributions, because it increases collaboration with other health professionals as they learn more about the domain of C–L nursing. These collaborative relationships enhance the power of the PCLN who is in possession of clinical skills that are desired by clients, nurses, physicians, and other health professionals.

The PCLN who uses nursing diagnosis to articulate and document clinical phenomena of concern contributes to the development of knowledge for theory-based research in C–L nursing. Research is a professional responsibility of the PCLN.[21] Research activities that identify and evaluate interventions and outcomes for C–L nursing phenomena of concern add to the body of knowledge of C–L nursing practice. The publication of clinical findings that describe the impact and cost-effectiveness of C–L activities with clients and consultees is a significant marketing technique to demonstrate the value of this subspecialty of psychiatric nursing.

Epidemiologic studies show a significant correlation between psychiatric and physical morbidity.[22] These statistical data support the need for continued focus on the integration of mental health and medical care. Although there are more than 1300 general hospital psychiatric units in the United States, there are only 870 psychiatric consultation-liaison services. Additional C–L services that include PCLNs are needed. The scope of psychiatric C–L nursing practice continues to expand to meet the needs of clients in the community, as well as those who are in long-term, geriatric and rehabilitation care facilities. Individual independent practice, or independent practice that is in conjunction with other clinical nurse specialists or interdisciplinary groups who provide consultation services to private physicians, other disciplines, or agencies, is becoming a more attractive and viable option for some PCLNs.[1,13,20,21]

Research Highlights

Consultation–liaison research cites changes in referral patterns for psychiatric consultations when a C–L team includes a PCLN.[25,26] A comparison of referral patterns of two client samples of 1000 each before and after the arrival of a PCLN identified fewer requests for client disposition and assistance with staff–client conflicts after the PCLN joined the team. Fewer requests for transferring clients to the inpatient psychiatry unit were attributed to the PCLN's availability and skill in decreasing staff–client conflicts. There were increased requests for help with diagnostic and therapeutic problems. These findings, and other observations over a five-year period, led to the recommendation that at least one PCLN be assigned to every C–L team, to enhance the quality of psychosocial care.

Psychiatric C–L nursing research is shifting from a focus on models of practice, role definition, and implementation, to research that examines services provided by the PCLN.[3,18,39,43] The psychiatric C–L component in the department of nursing at a university teaching facility and the psychiatric C–L service within the department of psychiatry of the university's medical school designed a study to delineate the variables that led to a request for formal psychiatric consultation.[42,43] One hundred consecutive psychiatric C–L nursing referrals were compared with 100 consecutive referrals to the consultation service. Demographic data, the clinical area in which the request originated, the reason for referral, and the medical diagnostic category of the client for whom the consultation was requested were evaluated. The data from this study clearly showed that the PCLN saw a client population different from those of the psychiatrist. The PCLN received three times as many consultations from the oncology unit and four times as many requests as the psychiatrist for help in situations in which the client's diagnosis was cancer. Twenty-four percent of the nursing referrals focused on the need for assistance with issues surrounding dying and death; the psychiatrists received no referrals for help with those issues. The PCLN received fewer requests for consultation with clients in the critical care areas and did not receive requests for assistance in clinical areas that had formal ongoing contact with social workers or psychiatrists. The informal availability of the PCLN for consultation requests, compared with the requirement of a formal request from the client's attending physician, was a system variable that affected the source and initiation of a consultation request. The PCLN's accessibility generated additional referrals. Findings from this investigation supported the use of a PCLN in the general hospital setting and contributed to the implementation of programs that addressed the needs of family members and the need for staff support groups.

SUMMARY

Psychiatric C–L nursing, a subspecialty of psychiatric nursing, evolved from the application of the consultative process in psychiatric nursing. Clinical, administrative, research, and educational functions of psychiatric C–L nursing are influenced by organizational and clinical needs, as well as the needs, philosophy, goals, and clinical expertise of the PCLN. Psychiatric C–L nursing practice has expanded from the delivery of psychological health care in the general hospital to include a variety of health care settings in the community that recognize and use the expertise of the psychiatric C–L nurse.[21]

References

1. Alexander S. The consultation role of the psychiatric nurse clinician: from general health care to the industrial setting. Occup Health Nurs. 1985;33:569–571.
2. Barron AM. The CNS as consultant. In: Hamric AB, Spross J, eds. The clinical nurse specialist in theory and practice. New York: Grune & Stratton; 1983.
3. Barton D, Kelso MT. The nurse as a psychiatric consultation team member. Psychiatry Med. 1971;2:108–115.
4. Berarducci M, Blandford K, Garant CA. The psychiatric liaison nurse in the general hospital: three models of practice. Gen Hosp Psychiatry. 1979;1:66–72.
5. Bilodeau CB, O'Connor SO. Role of nurse clinicians in liaison psychiatry. In: Hackett TP, Cassem NH, eds. Massachusetts General Hospital handbook of general hospital psychiatry, 2nd ed. Littleton, MA: PSG Publishing; 1987.
6. Bulechek GM, McCloskey JC. Nursing interventions: treatments for nursing diagnoses. Philadelphia: WB Saunders; 1985.
7. Campinha-Bacote J. Culturological assessment: an important factor in psychiatric consultation–liaison nursing. Arch Psychiatr Nurs. 1988;2:244–250.
8. Caplan G. The theory and practice of mental health consultation. New York: Basic Books; 1970.
9. Cohen-Cole SA, Pincus HA, Stoudemire A, et al. Recent research developments in consultation–liaison psychiatry. Gen Hosp Psychiatry. 1986;8:316–329.
10. Fife B. The challenge of the medical setting for the clinical specialist in psychiatric nursing. J Psychosoc Nurs Ment Health Serv. 1983;23(1):8–13.
11. Fife B, Lemler S. The psychiatric nurse specialist: a valuable asset in the general hospital. J Nurs Admin. 1983;13(4):14–17.
12. Hacket T. Beginnings: consultation psychiatry in a general hospital. In: Hacket TP, Cassem NH, eds. Massachusetts General Hospital handbook of general hospital psychiatry, 2nd ed. Littleton, MA: PSG Publishing; 1987.
13. Hathaway GL. The need for psychiatric nurse clinical specialists in geriatric long-term-care facilities. Nurs Homes. 1987;36(4):32–33.
14. Herrera HR. Interpersonal dimensions of illness. J Psychosoc Nurs Ment Health Serv. 1986;24(9):33–35.
15. Jimerson SS. Expanded practice in psychiatric nursing. Nurs Clin North Am. 1986;21:527–535.
16. Johnson BS. Psychiatric nurse consultant in a general hospital. Nurs Outlook. 1963;2:728–729.
17. Johnson TM, Kleinman A. Cultural concerns in consultation psychiatry. In: Guggenheim FG, Weiner MF, eds. Manual of psychiatric consultation and emergency care. New York: Jason Aronson; 1984.

18. Kaltreider NB, Martens W, Monterrosa S, Sachs L. The integration of psychosocial care in a general hospital: development of an interdisciplinary consultation program. Int J Psychiatry Med. 1974;5:125–134.

19. Kimball CP. Liaison psychiatry approaches and ways of thinking about behavior. Psychiatr Clin North Am. 1979;2:201–210.

20. Klebanoff NA, Casler CB. The psychosocial clinical nurse specialist: an untapped resource for home care. Home Healthcare Nur. 1986;4(6):36–40.

21. Lewis A, Levy J. Psychiatric liaison nursing: the theory and clinical practice. Reston, Va: Reston Publishing; 1982.

22. Lipowski ZJ. Linking mental and medical health care: an unfinished task. Psychosomatics. 1988;29:249–252.

23. Lipowski ZJ. Consultation–liaison psychiatry, an overview. In: Lipowski ZJ, ed. Psychosomatic medicine and liaison psychiatry: selected papers. New York: Plenum Medical; 1985.

24. Lipowski ZJ. Current trends in consultation–liaison psychiatry. In: Lipowski ZJ, ed. Psychosomatic medicine and liaison psychiatry: selected papers. New York: Plenum Medical; 1985.

25. Lipowski ZJ. Liaison psychiatry, liaison nursing, and behavioral medicine. In: Lipkowski ZJ, ed. Psychosomatic medicine and liaison psychiatry: selected papers. New York: Plenum Medical; 1985.

26. Lipowski ZJ, Wolston EJ. Liaison psychiatry referral patterns and their stability over time. In: Lipowski ZJ, ed. Psychosomatic medicine and liaison psychiatry: selected papers. New York: Plenum Medical; 1985.

27. Maas ML. Nursing diagnoses in a professional model of nursing: keystone for effective nursing administration. J Nurs Admin. 1986;16(12):39–42.

28. Mackenzie TB, Popkin MK, Callies Al. Clinical application of DSM-III in consultation–liaison psychiatry. Hosp Commun Psychiatry. 1983;34:628–633.

29. McKegney FP. Consultation–liaison psychiatry. In: Kaplan HI, Sadock BJ, eds. Comprehensive textbook of psychiatry/1V, V2, 4th ed. Baltimore: Williams & Wilkins; 1985.

30. Murphy SA, Hoeffer B. The evolution of subspecialties in psychiatric mental health nursing. Arch Psychiatr Nurs. 1987;1:145–154.

31. Nelson JKN, Schilke DA. The evolution of psychiatric liaison nursing. Perspect Psychiatr Care. 1976;14:61–65.

32. Nursing: a social policy statement. Report of the task force on the nature and scope of nursing practice and characteristics of specialization in nursing. Kansas City: American Nurses' Association publication no. NP-63 35m12 80; 1980.

33. Oken D. Preface. Psychiatr Clin North Am. 1987;10:xi–xiv.

34. Pasnau RO. Consultation–liaison psychiatry: progress, problems, and prospects. Psychosomatics. 1988;29:4–15.

35. Proposed standards of psychiatric consultation–liaison nursing (1987). Draft #3, presented at the 9th southeastern conference of clinical specialists in psychiatric–mental health nursing, Norfolk, VA, Sept 30–Oct 2, 1987. Cited in: Campinha-Bacote J. Culturological assessment: an important factor in psychiatric consultation–liaison nursing. Arch Psychiatr Nurs. 1988;2:244–250.

36. Rait DS, Jacobson PB, Lederberg MS, et al. Characteristics of psychiatric consultations in a pediatric cancer center. Am J Psychiatry. 1988;145:363–364.

37. Robinson L. Psychiatric consultation liaison nursing and psychiatric consultation liaison doctoring: similarities and differences. Arch Psychiatr Nurs. 1987;1:73–80.

38. Robinson L. Designing a psychiatric nursing liaison program in a general hospital. In: Lego S, ed. The American handbook of psychiatric nursing. Philadelphia: JB Lippincott; 1984.

39. Robinson L. Psychiatric liaison nursing 1962–1982: a review and update of the literature. Gen Hosp Psychiatry. 1982;4:139–145.

40. Rosen DH, Gregory RJ, Pollock D, et al. Depression in patients referred for psychiatric consultation a need for a new diagnosis. Gen Hosp Psychiatry. 1987;9:391–397.

41. Simmons MK. Psychiatric consultation and liaison. In: Critchley DL, Maurin JT, eds. The clinical specialist in psychiatric mental health nursing: theory, research, and practice. New York: John Wiley & Sons; 1985.

42. Stickney SK, Hall CW. The role of the nurse on a consultation–liaison team. Psychosomatics. 1981;22:224–235.

43. Stickney SK, Moir G, Gardner ER. Psychiatric nurse consultation: who calls and why. J Psychosoc Nurs Ment Health Serv. 1981;19(10):22–26.

44. Termini M, Ciechoski MA. The consultation process. Issues Ment Health Nurs. 1981;3:77–89.

45. White CL. The psychiatric clinical specialist as mental health consultant. Nurs Manag. 1988;19(6):80, 82.

50

James C. McCann

Impact of the Medicare Prospective Payment System on Psychiatric Care

OBJECTIVES
After reading this chapter, the reader will be able to:
1. *Discuss the two principal types of reimbursement mechanisms utilized by hospitals*
2. *Describe the historical and legislative aspects that led to the development of a prospective payment system (PPS) for Medicare reimbursement*
3. *Define the principles and concepts on which the PPS is based for Medicare reimbursement*
4. *Identify the problem areas that have evolved as a result of hospitals utilizing a PPS with a diagnosis-related group (DRG) methodology*
5. *Identify nursing strategies that can prevent or minimize problems associated with a PPS*
6. *List the essential components for a PPS to work effectively in a psychiatric setting*
7. *Discuss the steps psychiatric hospitals are taking to enhance their potential for profit in an environment of cost containment*
8. *Discuss the implications of cost containment for the profession of nursing in the areas of clinical practice, education, administration, and research.*

OVERVIEW

The funding of mental health services has increased steadily over the past decade with ineffective mechanisms to control costs. Implementing cost-containment strategies can adversely affect the quality of care and treatment clients receive in psychiatric hospitals, and the emergence of cost-containment and reimbursement initiatives has had a profound economic impact on how psychiatric hospitals, psychiatric units in general hospitals, and more importantly, departments of psychiatric nursing provide care to clients. In view of variables such as increased client acuity and life expectancy, decreased lengths of stay, and the nurse shortage, the psychiatric nursing profession must keep abreast of the mechanisms in use to contain nursing costs.

This chapter will focus on the most recent initiative mandated by the federal government, namely, the prospective payment system (PPS) for Medicare reimbursement. The historical aspects of this powerful legislation will be outlined, along with problems that have evolved as a result of using a diagnosis-related group (DRG) classification system for Medicare reimbursement. The challenges and criteria of using a PPS in a psychiatric hospital will be discussed. Current measures being utilized by psychiatric hospitals in a climate of cost containment will be highlighted. Finally, the implications of cost containment and present reimbursement mechanisms on the profession of psychiatric nursing will be addressed. Throughout the chapter, an effort will be made to discuss the impact of cost containment in the area of nursing diagnoses and the nursing process.

HISTORICAL PERSPECTIVES ON COST CONTAINMENT

Types of Reimbursement

There are two principal types of reimbursement for client care: retrospective and prospective. Retrospective reimbursement is based on charges and costs determined after services have been rendered.[23] This type of reimbursement was long the dominant one used by Medicare and third-party payers for the financing of mental health services. The chief problem with retrospective reimbursement is that it has led to increased hospital costs: the hospital had little incentive to control the utilization of its services and its costs because a substantial portion of them will be reimbursed. Prospective reimbursement, in contrast, is based on rates established in advance of service delivery on the basis of a specific unit of payment.[23] This form of reimbursement can use a variety of mechanisms: per service, per diem, per capital, per discharge, and per case.[5] Each of these mechanisms bases hospital reimbursement rates on a specific criterion with a corresponding dollar amount, and all were enacted to help control, even

reduce, costs for reimbursable services. Prospective cost-based reimbursement has served as the framework for the development of the PPS.

Prospective Payment System (PPS) for Medicare

LEGISLATIVE HISTORY

To help control the soaring costs of health care for Medicare beneficiaries, Congress enacted P.L. 97-248, Tax Equity and Fiscal Responsibility Act (TEFRA), in 1982. This act established the foundation for a PPS for Medicare. The principal components of this law include:

Setting new limits on hospital costs that covered total inpatient operating costs;

Establishment of limits on costs on a per-case rather than a per-diem basis;

Adjustment of each hospital's reimbursement limit to reflect its case mix of clinical problems;

Establishment of an overall target rate of increase for each hospital's growth in total costs per discharge;

Establishment of a financial incentive payment when a hospital spends less than its established rate for reimbursement;

Requirement that the federal government develop legislation for a PPS for Medicare.

MEDICARE PROSPECTIVE PAYMENT LAW

In response to TEFRA, the Health Care Financing Administration (HCFA) sent to Congress in 1982 a report outlining a prospective payment approach for hospital reimbursement for Medicare.[5] The principal thrust of this legislation (P.L. 98-21) recommended that hospitals be reimbursed by a per-case method based on the principal diagnosis of a patient after evaluation and treatment. The report recommended that patients be classified using a system of diagnosis-related groups (DRGs) developed by researchers at Yale University.[9] The DRG scheme is based on the concept that patients can be classified into clinically meaningful groups who will consume similar hospital resources. The scheme is patient-centered rather than facility-centered in that DRGs are based on patient characteristics and treatment processes rather than on the number of beds in a hospital or its service speciality.[11]

Under prospective payment, Medicare reimburses hospitals at a fixed rate for routine (room and board and nursing care) and ancillary (medical measures that are either diagnostic or therapeutic) services that is established in advance of a patient's hospitalization. Physicians' professional services are *not* part of this DRG rate; payment for these services is based on "reasonable costs" (what physicians usually and customarily charge). At discharge, a hospitalization is assigned to a specific DRG based on the patient's age, sex, and primary diagnosis after evaluation; and a payment specific to that DRG is made.[16] Each DRG has an assigned value (relative weight) that reflects the relative cost for routine and ancillary services, across all hospitals, of treating patients classified in that DRG. The arithmetic mean identifies the maximum length of stay (LOS) Medicare will reimburse for that particular DRG.

Additional reimbursement can be paid to hospitals for atypical cases known as "outliers;" i.e., care that was extraordinary. Outlier cases are of two types: day outliers and cost outliers. Day outliers are those cases involving unusually long stays and result in additional per-diem payments *beyond* the DRG fixed rate of reimbursement for each day *exceeding* the day outlier threshold criteria for that DRG. An example of a day outlier is a client admitted for viral pneumonia who, during hospitalization, suffers respiratory distress necessitating ventilator assistance. Cost outliers are recognized only if a hospital is not eligible for payment on a day outlier basis. In these cases, payment can be made *beyond* the fixed DRG rate because extraordinary costs were incurred in a short time in treating a patient. However, payment is not made until a hospital reaches a certain threshold of "excess" costs above the fixed DRG rate. Medicare then pays only a certain percentage of costs incurred beyond that threshold point.[3]

Hospital costs that are not restricted under PPS rates include: (1) capital-related costs (e.g., depreciation, property taxes); (2) costs incurred from approved intern and residence training programs; (3) other medical education programs (e.g., laboratory and radiology technician schools); (4) nursing schools operated by hospitals; (5) costs incurred from services provided by certified registered nurse anesthetists; (6) costs incurred by qualifying urban and rural hospitals of a particular bed size who treat a certain percentage of low-income patients; and (7) costs incurred by hospitals if 10% or more of their Medicare discharges are of patients who qualified under the end-stage renal disease program and were admitted for a nondialysis condition.

The DRG classification scheme groups patients into 23 major diagnostic categories (MDCs) with 475 corresponding DRGs. The DRGs relating to mental illness and substance abuse are classified under MDC19 (Mental Diseases and Disorders) and MDC20 (Alcohol/Drug Use and Alcohol/Drug Induced Organic Mental Disorders).[1] Table 50-1 lists the specific DRGs relating to MDC19 and MDC20, along with their relative weights, the arithmetic mean LOS, and the day outlier thresholds.

CURRENT SYSTEM FOR PSYCHIATRIC REIMBURSEMENT UNDER PPS

The HCFA implemented the PPS in general hospitals on October 1, 1984. This mechanism of reimbursement was phased in over a 3-year period to allow hospitals time to adapt to the new system. As of October 1, 1987, all general hospitals were under the PPS for Medicare reimbursement. All third-party payers probably will eventually implement some type of DRG/PPS scheme as their form of reimbursement.

Private and public (state-owned) psychiatric hospitals are currently exempt from PPS to allow further study of the feasibility of using DRGs for inpatient psychiatric hospital reimbursement. Alcohol and drug

TABLE 50-1
Diagnosis-related groups under MDC19 and MDC20*

No.	Title	RELATIVE WEIGHTS	ARITHMETIC MEAN LOS	DAY OUTLIER THRESHOLD
MDC19: MENTAL DISEASE AND DISORDERS				
424	Operating Room Procedure With Principal Diagnoses of Mental Illness	2.2176	21.6	30
425	Acute Adjustment Reaction and Disturbances of Psychosocial Dysfunction	.6004	6.0	21
426	Depressive Neurosis	.6580	8.3	24
427	Neuroses Except Depressive	.6315	8.2	24
428	Disorders of Personality and Impulse Control	.7305	9.8	24
429	Organic Disturbances and Mental Retardation	.8868	10.6	25
430	Psychoses	.9329	13.6	27
431	Childhood Mental Disorders	.7134	8.3	24
432	Other Mental Disorder Diagnoses	.7097	7.0	22
MDC 20: ALCOHOL/DRUG AND ALCOHOL/DRUG INDUCED ORGANIC MENTAL DISORDERS				
433	Alcohol/Drug Abuse or Dependence Left AMA	.4232	5.0	20
434	Alcohol/Drug Abuse or Dependence, Detoxification or Other Systematic Treatment (Tx), with Complication or Comorbidity (C.C.)	.8149	8.3	24
435	Alcohol/Drug Abuse or Dependence, Detoxification or Other Symptomatic Tx, without C.C.	.5903	7.5	23
436	Alcohol/Drug Dependence With Rehabilitation Therapy	.9788	13.6	27
437	Alcohol/Drug Dependence, Combined Rehabilitation and Detoxification Therapy	1.3306	17.6	32

* Federal Register. September 1, 1987;52:33113.

abuse hospitals and units within general hospitals have not been exempt since October 1, 1987.

PROBLEMATIC ISSUES IN PROSPECTIVE PAYMENT SYSTEMS

As the PPS has been implemented, a number of concerns have been identified that can influence the financial and quality of care within a hospital.[21,23]

Client Skimming

Skimming is the process of choosing to admit only clients who have "profitable" DRG rates of reimbursement, whereas other, less profitable, clients are refused admission. This problem has ramifications for the chronically mentally ill person who sometimes requires longer hospital stays and, as a result, puts a hospital (e.g., public facility) at greater financial risk. As Widem and associates stated: "although the DRG system developed in the Medicare program was designed to permit hospitals to specialize in treating those patients it feels best equipped to care for efficiently, hence reducing or eliminating ineffective services and departments, the use of skimming strategies may create overall systems problems" (reference 23, p 450).

Cost Shifting

There also has been concern about hospitals shifting costs to non-Medicare, third-party payers (clients), because the PPS currently relates only to Medicare beneficiaries. This approach then places a greater financial burden on private insurance payers, with an eventual increase in health insurance premiums. In addressing this problem, health economists have argued that in order to prevent cost shifting, an "all-payers system" should be developed in which all hospital costs (Medicare and other insurers) are under the same reimbursement system.

DRG Creeping

It has been suggested that hospitals may resort to *up-coding* a client's diagnosis to obtain a higher rate of reimbursement. This concern has applicability to mental health in that psychiatric hospitals may attempt to mislabel psychiatric clients in order to obtain a higher rate of reimbursement; i.e., give clients diagnoses under DRG 430: Psychosis, rather than DRG 428: Disorders of Personality and Impulse Control, because the principal diagnoses under DRG 428 generally have a lower arithmetic mean LOS than diagnoses under DRG 430.

Diagnosis and Resource Utilization

Professional mental health groups have expressed concern over whether the current DRG classification system, i.e., fixed rates of reimbursement per DRG code in correlation with an established LOS, accurately reflects the severity of psychiatric illnesses. For this reason, psychiatric hospitals were not placed under prospective payments until this issue could be evaluated. This exemption was based on two concerns. First the initial psychiatric DRGs developed by Yale University were based on data obtained only from psychiatric units in general hospitals, not from freestanding psychiatric hospitals (private and public). Second and more importantly, there was concern about a lack of correlation between DRGs and resource utilization; i.e., the acuity level and treatment needs of clients.[6] In granting this exemption, Congress mandated studies concerning the feasibility of psychiatric DRGs and the formulation of alternative classification schemes for reimbursement. Such studies have not produced any definitive results, however, and at present, no decision has been made by the HCFA about when a PPS utilizing DRGs will be implemented.

Quality of Care

The issue of quality of care has raised the most concern among health professionals. The question asked is: "Will the quality of care suffer as a result of containing and reducing hospital costs?" The HCFA has addressed this concern by mandating legislatively that hospitals that are under a PPS be evaluated through peer review organizations, who will closely monitor the quality of care provided as well as the pattern of admissions and discharges. Prospective payment as a major strategy for reimbursement has significant ramifications for nursing. The importance of implementing the nursing process in conjunction with nursing diagnoses, and the appropriate DRG coding of clients based on their symptomatology, can influence the quality of care a client receives. By correctly diagnosing the condition of a client, nurses will be better able to plan care based on the client's needs and problems incorporating the concepts of both efficiency, because of the predetermined LOS, and quality of care.

CHALLENGES IN USING A PPS FOR PSYCHIATRIC SERVICES

As noted, all psychiatric hospitals currently are exempt from prospective payment for Medicare hospital costs. The current system allows psychiatric services to be reimbursed under reasonable costs. Jencks, Goldman, and McGuire identified several criteria that will promote a successful psychiatric PPS. They stated: "A successful psychiatric PPS must promote efficiency, it must be compatible with the rest of Medicare's payment system. It should also minimize risk from random variation, minimize administrative costs, and be clinically credible" (reference 16, p 765).

The criterion of efficiency has relevance to psychiatric nursing. The PPS provides hospitals with a strong incentive to make care more efficient because hospitals receive a fixed rate of reimbursement based on a preestablished LOS. If hospitals discharge patients prior to LOS, they receive the same fixed rate of reimbursement as they would if the patient remained for the established LOS, yet presumably, their costs would be lower. If psychiatric hospitals provide quality-of-care services to clients (e.g., psychiatric nursing care rendered in an organized and timely manner based on client assessment, nursing diagnoses, and planning, implementing, and evaluating strategies), they may shorten clients' hospital stays and minimize costs without compromising quality of care.

The criterion of fairness is also important in that a PPS must be fair both to hospitals and to clients. That is, the system must not discriminate against certain types of clients, nor promote client skimming, cost shifting, or premature discharge (dumping). Psychiatric nurses can promote fairness by acting as a client's advocate when clinically indicated. They can minimize dumping by making sure the client is physically and psychologically ready for discharge and that they have well-formulated discharge plans. Medical and nursing record documentation becomes essential in justifying the statement that a client might need to remain in the hospital longer.

TRENDS IN PSYCHIATRIC CARE AND THEIR RELATION TO REIMBURSEMENT

Epidemiological studies conducted by the National Institute of Mental Health (NIMH) show that 19% of adult Americans (29.4 million) suffer from mental illness, yet fewer than one-fifth of these persons seek mental health services.[17] Despite this need, psychiatric providers are cautious in developing services because of the decrease in the overall utilization of acute-care hospital beds; the fiscal uncertainties associated with Medicare reimbursement; the new financial restrictions other health insurers are imposing; and the number of corporations opening competitive psychiatric hospitals.

To provide needed mental health services in a climate of cost containment, many psychiatric providers are developing specialty services within hospitals such as anorexia and bulimia nervosa units; Alzheimer's disease units; a continuum of psychogeriatric, child, and adolescent services; specialty units that provide psychiatric services solely for women; and evening and night crisis programs sponsored by health maintenance organizations. These initiatives are being developed to help hospitals survive in an increasingly competitive financial environment. The trend is toward offering short-term specialty inpatient treatment in high-growth service areas that attract a specific client population.[20]

Child and Adolescent Services

Despite the increasing need for child and adolescent services, problematic reimbursement issues have emerged. For example, because many of these clients require longer stays, hospitals run the risk of financial loss, because health insurers are restricting the amount of reimbursement for inpatient stays. In response to this concern, providers are beginning to offer a continuum of services such as inpatient, outpatient, residential, and partial-day hospital treatment. However, hospital insurance reimbursement levels vary for these services. In some instances, no reimbursement is available for partial-day hospitalization. As a result, despite the need for services in a least-restrictive setting, development of these services may be deterred.

Psychogeriatric Services

The demand for geriatric psychiatric services is increasing despite limited Medicare coverage; i.e., Medicare beneficiaries can receive a lifetime maximum of 190 days of inpatient psychiatric hospitalization,[2] Medicare reimbursement or its absence does not appear to be a deterrent to the development of psychiatric programs for the elderly,[20] because many senior citizens have supplemental health insurance plans (outside of Medicare) that include psychiatric benefits. The concern relates to supply and demand: as the senior citizen population increases, will there be enough services to meet their mental health needs? Possibly, these individuals will not require inpatient psychiatric hospitalization or a nursing home, but instead an alternative, less costly, service such as geriatric day care, home-based psychogeriatric services, or specialty units that treat both the acute medical and psychiatric needs of this population. It has been suggested by the American Psychiatric Association that general hospitals need to take the lead in meeting the psychiatric needs of senior citizens within reasonable cost-containment strategies by working with nursing homes and other community agencies to develop cost-effective programs in the areas of home-based care, geriatric day care, and respite care services.[20]

Future Directions for Psychiatric Nursing

If many of the programs described earlier become revenue generating, the role of psychiatric nursing can be expanded. Many of these speciality programs would require specific psychiatric clinical nurse expertise. Reimbursement strategies could be developed in which psychiatric nurses would serve as primary caregivers. This approach would be cost effective to hospitals, would expand the role of nursing in the area of third-party payment reimbursement, and would meet the psychiatric needs of the population.

IMPLICATIONS OF COST CONTAINMENT FOR PSYCHIATRIC NURSING

Clinical Practice

Despite the increased emphasis on cost containment, the quality of nursing care clients receive need not deteriorate. Nurses in clinical practice can help curtail hospital costs without sacrificing quality of care by doing the following:

Becoming knowledgeable about the principles on which the PPS is operationalized and the way in which DRGs are organized. Having this expertise, nurses will be better able to assist hospitals in maximizing their reimbursement and in assuring that clients are receiving treatment based on their needs and diagnosis(es). This knowledge will also help to minimize client DRG upcoding, which in the end leads only to increased hospital costs;

Assuring that required services for clients are performed in a timely manner so that unnecessary days of hospitalization are avoided. For example, if a client needs to have certain laboratory studies completed prior to the implementation of a special treatment procedure, these studies should be completed without undue delays caused by administrative problems (e.g., lack of laboratory staff in the evenings). It is important that nurses closely monitor and anticipate client needs and plan accordingly, so that no unnecessary delays in care occur to increase costs for both the hospital and the client;

Becoming more aware of, accountable for, and sensitive to the usage and costs of client supplies. However, quality of care should not be sacrificed because of concern about the costs of client supplies;

Implementing the nursing process immediately upon a client's admission to the hospital. If needs are assessed and problems are treated in a vigorous and therapeutic manner based on principles of active psychiatric nursing diagnosis and treatment, the potential benefit of a client's stay becomes maximized with limited days of hospitalization and costs to hospitals; and

Becoming more involved in the discharge planning components of a patient's hospitalization. In doing so, nurses can help prevent premature discharges by alerting appropriate staff when clients are experiencing difficulties that could decrease their potential for remaining outside the hospital. If nurses

can intervene early in this area, they can sometimes delay a client's discharge by a few days and thereby increase the client's chances of remaining clinically stable and symptom free longer after discharge. This will also help lessen hospital costs by reducing recidivism.

Nursing Education

Schools of nursing should consider integrating the concept of health care economics into their curricula. Possibly, nurses could be educated earlier in their academic preparation about the impact cost containment can have on the delivery and quality of nursing services to clients. Specifically, nursing curricula might address such things as: (1) the legislative, historical, social, and economic implications of various cost-reducing and cost-controlling strategies for health care; (2) current methods of reimbursement available to patients and hospitals, most importantly the PPS; and (3) principles of budget and fiscal management. Students should also be taught good physical assessment, clinical reasoning, and diagnostic skills as well as an appreciation for the importance of documentation, as both can help to support a nurse's rationale for carrying out specific treatment interventions that may have cost-bearing implications for a client or hospital. Lastly, nursing students need to develop an understanding of computers and management information systems, which will facilitate their functioning in both executive and research roles.

Nursing Administration

The emergence of cost-reducing strategies within hospitals has had a profound economic impact on nursing departments. Nurse executives are being challenged to develop methods that will ensure quality of care to clients in an environment of economic constraints. Currently, nursing is only beginning to generate data concerning the impact of nursing care costs on a hospital's fiscal operations. To facilitate nursing impact on the financial operations of a hospital, the following must be done:

Nurse administrators need to participate in all phases of a hospital's budgetary process;

Nurse administrators should develop management information systems that will analyze the impact of nursing care costs in relation to other general hospital care costs; and

Nurse administrators must generate cost reports that define and measure nursing costs based on client acuity levels, nursing diagnosis, and staff time (resource allocation and consumption).

If the above-mentioned strategies are implemented, nurse executives will be able to anticipate the financial worth of nursing services based on cost analysis.

Research Highlights

Essock–Vitale S. Patient characteristics predictive of treatment costs on inpatient psychiatric wards. H&CP 1987;38:263–269.

Essock–Vitale addressed the adequacy of the LOS as the sole measure of hospital costs relating to psychiatric DRG reimbursement. Using nursing care time based on client acuity and LOS as measures of resource consumption, the study identified age and the presence of medical comorbidities (a condition that coexisted with the principal diagnosis at admission) as predictors of increased costs in delivering care to psychiatric clients. Concern was expressed that medical comorbidities have not been considered in the calculation of reimbursement for psychiatric DRGs and, as a result, place psychiatric providers at greater financial risk. The study underscored the poor performance of psychiatric DRGs in predicting costs and the crudeness of LOS as a measure of costs.

Sharfstein SS, Eist H, Sack L, Kaiser IH, Shadoan RA. The impact of third-party payment cutbacks on the private practice of psychiatry: three surveys. H&CP 1984;35: 478–481.

Three surveys were conducted to assess the impact of threatened or actual reductions in third-party payments on the treatment provided to psychiatric clients by private practitioners. One survey found that more than 50% of psychiatrists in Northern California treat severely disturbed outpatient Medicaid clients at lower cost than public clinics. Two surveys conducted in Washington, DC, found that both clients and psychiatrists have suffered from insurance cutbacks, with fewer clients being able to afford intensive private treatment. The most significant adverse effect on clients secondary to cuts in private insurance has been the decreased availability of intensive psychotherapy for adults and children. There is anecdotal evidence of increases in psychiatric hospitalization, premature termination of treatment, and shifts in treatment strategies from potentially curative to more palliative.

Fenton FR, Tessier L, Struening EL, et al. A two-year follow-up of a comparative trial of the cost-effectiveness of home and hospital psychiatric treatment. Can J Psychiatry 1984;29:205–210.

This Montreal study evaluated the cost effectiveness of home-based vs hospital-based treatment of psychiatric clients using manpower and operating costs as measurement indices. The sample consisted of 155 clients who were destined to receive inpatient treatment. Of these, 76 were randomly assigned to home-based treatment and 72 to hospital-based treatment. The two groups were similar in social, demographic, and clinical characteristics, including psychiatric diagnoses. During the entire two-year period of the study, the manpower and operating cost of treatment was higher for hospital-based care. In the second year of the study, the manpower and operating cost of treatment was similar for home- and hospital-based care. Finally, regardless of the setting, the cost of treating schizophrenics was higher than the cost of treating manic-depressives, with the least cost incurred in the treatment of individuals with depressive neurosis. The authors contend that home-based treatment appears to be a more clinically effective and cost-efficient alternative to the hospital treatment of schizophrenics, manic-depressives, and depressive neurotics.

Schumacher DN, Namerow MJ, Parker B, Fox P, Kofie V. Prospective payment for psychiatry: feasibility and impact. N Engl J Med 1986;315:1331–1336.

The authors investigated the ability of psychiatric DRGs to predict hospital LOS and costs by analyzing the charts of 8816 randomly selected clients from 32 private psychiatric hospitals throughout the United States. Grouping clients under the psychiatric DRGs reduced the total variance in LOS by only 3.6%. Grouping clients on the basis of major diagnostic categories, whether the client was transferred from another facility, age, and psychiatric complications and comorbidities reduced the variance by only 7.8%. The study found that DRGs do not adequately predict LOS or costs in psychiatric hospitals. Concern was expressed that if psychiatric DRGs are implemented, systematic bias may be introduced into the payment system, with hospitals "skimming" for patients who will produce "financial wins." This type of payment system will discriminate against clients who require a longer LOS and, as a result, cause this type of client to receive inadequate treatment.

Panniers TL, Tomkiewicz ZM: The ICD-9-CM DRGs: increased homogeneity through use of AS-SCORE. QRB 1985;11(2):47–52.

This study highlighted the benefits of using the AS-SCORE severity-of-illness classification system as a way of increasing the homogeneity of Medicare DRGs. The AS-SCORE system is based on the variables of client age, bodily systems involved with the particular illness, the stage of the disease, complications, and the response to therapy. In this study, the AS-SCORE system was applied to a random sample of 30 medical records of clients who had Medicare DRGs 121 (myocardial infarction [MI] with cardiovascular complications, discharged alive) and 122 (MI without cardiovascular complications, discharged alive). When the AS-SCORE system was added to these two DRGs, the level of homogeneity in terms of LOS and resource consumption was increased. Although the sample was small, nursing costs correlated positively with the level of severity exhibited by these patients, demonstrating that the AS-SCORE system may be a sensitive predictor of variations in the cost of nursing care for patients within a single DRG. The authors contend that the AS-SCORE, when applied to DRGs, has the potential for providing a system of case-mix measurement that will be more meaningful to hospital personnel as they attempt to predict their clients' use of hospital resources, including nursing care requirements. The authors stress that further studies need to be conducted to determine the applicability of AS-SCORE to other medical–surgical DRGs.

The AS-SCORE system may have applicability to psychiatric DRGs as well.

Despite the fact that psychiatric hospitals are currently exempt from the Medicare PPS, nurse administrators must begin to develop a standard nursing cost system for psychiatric DRGs as well as to define the volume of nursing services that might be required under each DRG.[10] If nurse executives develop cost data analyzers relating to nursing care costs under psychiatric DRGs, they will be in a better position to maximize reimbursement under the PPS.

Nursing Research

In order for the profession of psychiatric nursing to justify its financial worth in dollars and cents, it must be able to verify, via nursing research, what nursing services cost in various types of psychiatric health settings (e.g., inpatient, outpatient, day hospital, community–residential care). Research needs to be conducted that substantiates the cost of nursing services based on client acuity, nursing diagnosis, and the utilization of nursing resources (time allocation and consumption). Nurse researchers also need to study which variables (e.g., age, sex, diagnosis, premorbid health, ethnicity, severity of illness, legal status, treatment setting, education) have the greatest potential for influencing a client's LOS. This is particularly important because the LOS will influence the costs incurred by both hospitals and clients.

Studies conducted by Halloran and collaborators have addressed the impact of DRGs, nursing diagnosis, and clients' LOS in acute general hospital settings.[12–15] These studies have shown that nursing diagnoses are generally more effective than DRGs in predicting quality of nursing care and nursing workload and in explaining variations in client LOS. A paucity of studies exists regarding the impact of psychiatric DRGs, psychiatric nursing diagnoses, and LOS in psychiatric hospitals.

Clinical studies need to be conducted that verify which nursing interventions produce the most desired outcomes of care with the least cost. These data must then be disseminated to nursing administrators for use in the development of client classification systems based on nursing diagnoses that correlate with nursing interventions.

Nursing research should be conducted regarding the feasibility and cost impact of psychiatric DRGs in the delivery of psychiatric nursing care. Because the PPS has not yet been implemented in freestanding psychiatric hospitals, psychiatric nurse researchers should seize the opportunity to investigate this area so that client care problems can be minimized once the PPS is implemented in psychiatric hospitals.

SUMMARY

The principal thrust of the Medicare prospective payment system is that hospitals are reimbursed by a per-case method based on the principal diagnosis(es) after

evaluation and treatment. Diagnoses are coded utilizing a scheme, called diagnosis-related groups (DRGs), based on the concept that patients can be classified into clinically meaningful groups who will consume similar hospital resources. Problems that have occurred under the PPS include: (1) patient skimming—admitting only patients who have profitable DRG rates of reimbursement; (2) cost shifting—shifting cost to non-Medicare clients; (3) DRG creeping—upcoding a diagnosis so that a hospital can receive a higher rate of reimbursement; (4) diagnosis vs resource utilization—concern over whether the DRG methodology, i.e., preestablished rates of reimbursement per DRG code in correlation with an established LOS, accurately reflects the severity of psychiatric illness; and (5) quality of care—concern over whether it will be lessened secondary to the PPS and hospitals' interests in implementing cost-containment strategies.

For the profession of nursing cost containment has several implications: (1) clinical practice—nurses need to assess clients and implement the nursing process without unnecessary delays; (2) education—nurses must learn health care economics and become sensitive to the ramifications of costs in their delivery of nursing services; (3) administration—nurse executives have to be able to justify in their budgets the cost of professional nursing services; and (4) research—investigators should verify what nursing interventions produce the most desired outcomes of care for clients with the least cost.

References

1. Averill RF, Mullin RL, Giardi PA, Elia ED. Diagnosis Related Groups. 4th ed. New Haven, Conn: Health Systems International; 1987.
2. Department of Health and Human Services. Code of Federal Regulations. Washington, DC: Part 409.62, 1987;458.
3. Department of Health and Human Services, Health Care Financing Administration. Medicare program: prospective payment for Medicare inpatient hospital services. Federal Register. September 1, 1983;48:39746–890.
4. Department of Health and Human Services, Health Care Financing Administration: Medicare program: changes to the inpatient hospital prospective payment system and fiscal year 1988 rates; final rule. Medicare program: changes to the DRG classification system; final notice. Federal Register. September 1, 1987;52:33034–165.
5. Department of Health and Human Services Report to Congress: Hospital prospective payment for Medicare. Washington, DC; 1982.
6. English JT, Sharfstein SS, Scheril DJ, Astrachan B, Muszynski IL. Diagnosis-related groups and general hospital psychiatry: the APA study. Am J Psychiatry. 1986;143:131–9.
7. Essock–Vitale S. Patient characteristics predictive of treatment costs on inpatient psychiatric ward. H&CP. 1987;38:263–9.
8. Fenton FR, Tessier L, Struening EL, Smith FA, Benoit C, Contandriopoulos AP, Nguyen H. A two-year follow-up of a comparative trial of the cost-effectiveness of home and hospital psychiatric treatment. Can J Psychiatry. 1984;29:205–10.
9. Fetter RB, Shin Y, Freedman JL, Averill RF, Thompson JD.

Case mix definition by diagnosis-related groups. Med Care. 1980;18(1):1–53.

10. Gardner K. Managing under prospective payment. QRB. 1984;10:174.

11. Grimaldi PL. DRGs and long term care. Am Health Care Assoc J. 1985;11(1):6–9.

12. Halloran EH. Nursing workload, medical diagnosis related groups, and nursing diagnoses. Res Nurs Health. 1985;8:421–33.

13. Halloran EH, Halloran DC. Exploring the DRG/nursing equation. Am J Nursing. 1985;85:1093–1095.

14. Halloran EH, Kiley ML. Nursing diagnosis, diagnosis related groups and length of stay. Health Care Financing Rev. 1987;8:27–36.

15. Halloran EH, Kiley ML, England, M. Nursing diagnosis, DRG's and length of stay. Appl Nurs Res. 1988;1(1):22–6.

16. Jencks SF, Goldman HH, McGuire TG. Challenges in bringing exempt psychiatric services under a prospective payment system. H&CP. 1985;36:764–9.

17. National Association of Private Psychiatric Hospitals: Using inpatient psychiatric benefits wisely. Washington, DC: The Association; 1986.

18. Panniers TL, Tomkiewicz ZM. The ICD-9-CM DRGs: increased homogeneity through use of AS-SCORE. QRB. 1985;11:47–52.

19. Schumacher DN, Namerow MJ, Parker B, Fox P, Kofie V. Prospective payment for psychiatry: feasibility and impact. N Engl J Med. 1986;315:1331–6.

20. Shahoda T. Specialty services boost psy providers. Hospitals. 1986;9(20):56–61.

21. Sharfstein SS, Frank RG, Kessler LG. State Medicaid limitations for mental health services. H&CP. 1984;35:213–5.

22. Sharfstein SS, Eist H, Sack L, Kaiser IH, Shadoan RA. The impact of third-party payment cutbacks on the private practice of psychiatry: three surveys. H&CP. 1984;35:478–81.

23. Widem P, Pincus HA, Goldman HH, Jencks S. Prospective payment for psychiatric hospitalization: context and background. H&CP. 1984;35:447–51.

51

S. Robin Shanks

Legal Issues in Psychiatric Mental Health Nursing

OBJECTIVES
After reading this chapter, the reader will be able to:
1. Differentiate the types of hospitalization
2. Discuss the concept of competency and the related need for a guardian
3. List the rights guaranteed to psychiatric clients
4. Distinguish between confidentiality and privilege
5. Identify special legal considerations of minors
6. Discuss evaluations of competency to stand trial, insanity defense, and post-trial commitability
7. Identify the elements of malpractice
8. Discuss the importance of documentation to accountability
9. Identify the types of lawsuits that a psychiatric nurse could become involved in.

ENTERING AND LEAVING THE HOSPITAL

Admission

Individuals requiring psychiatric care are hospitalized and obtain treatment through either a voluntary or an involuntary admission. An individual can sign into a treatment resource voluntarily and may remain hospitalized as long as treatment is needed. A voluntary client has the absolute right to refuse any type of treatment that is prescribed and may sign out of the facility at any time. With involuntary admissions, the court system becomes involved in order to protect the rights of these individuals whose liberty interests are at stake. The authority of the government to intervene with the mentally ill is based on two principles. *Parens patriae power* authorizes the state to care for individuals in need, and *police power* allows the state (government) to place controls on certain groups of individuals so that society, as a whole, can be protected. Historically, these principles have provided the support and legal basis for the laws governing the care and protection of the rights of the mentally ill.

Involuntary admissions include detainment or observational admission, emergency admission, and judicial commitment. The *detainment or observational admission* allows the person to be admitted for a limited time to be evaluated for the need for involuntary hospitalization. The laws are strict and allow detainment only for a certain number of hours. This type of admission is useful when an individual is unwilling to see a clinician so that the need for hospitalization can be assessed. The detainment statutes allow law enforcement officials to take the individual to a clinician so that an evaluation can be performed.

The *emergency admission* occurs when an individual is brought to a psychiatric facility and detained because certain legal requirements have been met, usually imminence of harm to self or others. During this period, a client will be evaluated and a hearing will be scheduled within a statutorily defined period, usually only a few days. At the hearing, the client may be released, or, if the client is still in need of involuntary treatment, the court will make a decision ordering an additional period of commitment. Most states require another hearing at a fixed time, usually one to six months later.

When a client is *involuntarily committed,* even more legal protections are sanctioned because of the possible length of time that liberty interests are restricted. For example, the standard of proof required of the person seeking commitment is higher than that required in other civil hearings. This is one of the results of the case of *Addington v Texas* (441 US 418 [1979]), in which the United States Supreme Court identified the "clear and convincing evidence" standard as the proof to be used in commitment hearings. The Court went on to direct each state to reflect this standard in its statutes.

Discharge

As with admissions, the discharge of a client can take many forms. When a client no longer meets the statutory criteria for an involuntary admission, a discharge must be arranged. In most states, in order to be discharged, the client must be viewed as no longer being a danger to self or others. Dangerousness is defined differently in various state statutes. Some clients, upon discharge from an inpatient facility, may be legally mandated to seek outpatient treatment, and some statutes require recommitment if the client fails to follow through with treatment.[12]

A client who leaves the hospital without the knowledge, consent, or permission of the staff is said to have *eloped* or to be AWOL (away without leave). Several statutes require that the committing judge and the police department be notified of the elopement and also allow law enforcement personnel to detain the individual without a warrant and transport the individual back to the treating facility.[12]

COMPETENCE AND GUARDIANSHIP

An individual is said to be legally competent if he/she possesses the requisite natural or legal qualifications, is capable, and legally fit.[2] An individual who is not competent to make decisions is in need of a guardian to make those decisions. However, it is important to keep in mind that a mentally ill individual is not necessarily in need of a guardian, since a mental illness may result in signs and symptoms that do not interfere with an individual's decision-making ability.

An individual's need for a guardian is an important, and sometimes difficult, determination to make. In order for a treatment or procedure to be performed, an individual must be capable of giving *informed* consent. If, for whatever reason, the individual cannot be educated to the extent of being able to make an informed decision, a court will appoint a guardian. In a guardianship proceeding, the court must determine if the individual is, indeed, incapable of making decisions and, if so, will appoint a guardian who will make decisions for the incompetent individual. *Substituted consent* is the authorization that is given by a court-appointed guardian on behalf of the incompetent individual.

CLIENTS' RIGHTS

The Protection and Advocacy Bill for Mentally Ill Individuals Act of 1986 (42 USC §10801), which covers such areas as access to records and protection from abuse and neglect, contains a restatement of the Bill of Rights of the Mentally Ill (Box 51-1). The Joint Commission on Accreditation of Hospitals also publishes the Patients' Bill of Rights,[6] which applies to all types of hospitalizations but is not to be considered all inclusive (Box 51-2).

BOX 51-1
Restatement of Bill of Rights For Mental Health Patients

Right to appropriate treatment and related services
Right to an individualized, written treatment plan and periodic review and reassessment
Right to participation in planning of mental health services
Right not to receive a mode or course of treatment in the absence of informed, voluntary, written consent, except during an emergency situation or as permitted under applicable law
Right not to participate in experimentation in absence of informed, voluntary, written consent
Right to freedom from restraint or seclusion except during an emergency situation
Right to a humane treatment environment, reasonable protection from harm, and appropriate privacy
Right to confidentiality of records
Right to access of own records
Right to converse with others privately, to have access to telephone and mails, to see visitors
Right to be informed promptly after admission and periodically thereafter of rights described here
Right to assert grievances
Right to access to rights protection services within the facility, the state mental health system, and under Title I to protect and advocate for their rights
Right to exercise these rights without reprisal
Right to referral to other mental health services upon discharge

From Protection and Advocacy For Mentally Ill Individuals Act of 1986, 42 USC §10801.

Civil Rights

Many state laws define the rights that a psychiatric client retains while hospitalized. The only right that an involuntarily committed client loses is the right to liberty. Some examples of civil rights that are guaranteed are the right to dispose of property, the right to execute instruments such as wills and deeds to property, the right to make purchases, the right to enter into contracts, the right to vote, and the right to retain a driver's license and a professional license. Of course, under certain circumstances, a licensing profession can suspend or revoke a license if the holder suffers from a mental condition that renders him/her incapable of practicing the profession. In this situation, due process rights would be afforded the individual before the license could be suspended or revoked.

Right to Visitors, Mail, and Telephone Calls

Clients in psychiatric settings have the right to have visitors and to communicate by mail or telephone. However, there may be situations in which exceptions are permissible. For example, if a client receives a package that contains a weapon or drugs, the treatment plan should reflect this incident and the appropriate procedure instituted to restrict this client from receiving uncensored mail.

Right to Personal Security and Freedom From Undue Bodily Restraint

This right is supported by several mandates, such as the guarantee by the US Constitution's Fourteenth Amendment of the right to privacy, which supports an individual's freedom to do with his/her mind and body as he/she sees fit. The right to be treated in a humane way and in a safe environment is guaranteed by the Protection and Advocacy Bill and the case of *Wyatt v Stickney* (325 F Supp 781 [1971]). The Constitution's Eighth Amendment guarantees protection from cruel and unusual punishment, which applies to the nontherapeutic use of restraints, seclusion, or electroconvulsive therapy. The use of restraints, for example, whether chemical or mechanical, should be carefully assessed and integrated into a plan of treatment. Such therapeutic interventions must be addressed in the nursing care plan and utilized only under strictly prescribed circumstances.

BOX 51-2
Rights and Responsibilities of Patients

PATIENT RIGHTS

Access to care
Respect and dignity
Privacy and confidentiality
Personal safety
Identity
Information
Communication with people outside hospital
Consent
Consultation
Refusal of treatment
Transfer and continuity of care
Explanation of cost of services
Hospital rules and regulations information

PATIENT RESPONSIBILITIES

Provision of information about self
Compliance with instructions
Refusal of treatment—responsible for own actions
Hospital charges
Hospital rules and regulations
Respect and consideration of others

From Joint Commission on Accreditation of Hospitals, Chicago: Bill of Rights Manual; 1987.

Right to Treatment in the Least Restrictive Setting

Clients have the right to treatment, as defined in the 1971 case of *Wyatt v Stickney*. This case was a class action suit filed in Alabama on behalf of the employees and clients of Bryce Hospital, with the plaintiffs alleging that the dismissal of hospital employees would result in a lower standard of care and that the clients had a constitutional right to treatment. In addition to the right to an individualized treatment plan, the court also specifically mentioned a right to privacy, the right to a humane environment, the right to the least restrictive conditions, the right to visitation and communication, the right of clients to wear their own clothes and keep their own personal effects, and the right to a comprehensive physical and mental examination.

One of the leading cases that mandates the least restrictive environment is *O'Conner v Donaldson* (422 US 563 [1975]). The court rejected the contention that the client was in a therapeutic milieu and held that a mentally ill person who is not dangerous cannot be involuntarily committed if capable of surviving in the community alone or with the assistance of family or friends. The concept of the least restrictive environment can also apply to a client who can function safely if hospitalized on an open ward as opposed to a locked ward or who can be discharged with outpatient treatment as opposed to being hospitalized on an open ward with day passes.

Right to Refuse Treatment

Along with the right to treatment, psychiatric clients also have the right to refuse treatment. *Rennie v Klein* (653 F2nd 836 [1981]) was a landmark case that defined this right, with the court ruling that a psychiatric client could refuse treatment in certain circumstances. In 1979, Rennie filed another lawsuit (in which other individuals joined him in pursuing) asking that certain hospitals and the staff be prevented from forcible administration of drugs. The court held that all clients have the right to refuse psychotropic medication and that they must be educated to the extent necessary to make an informed decision about the medication.

Other decisions have been rendered by many courts in other states surrounding this issue of the right to refuse psychotropic medications. The Massachusetts Supreme Judicial Court in *Rogers v Mills* (formerly *Rogers v Okin*)* held that the ultimate authority to make treatment decisions should be left to the court system. However, this court also held that the state could override a client's refusal to take psychotropic medications in the event of a psychiatric emergency,

---

* *Rogers v Okin* (478 F Supp 1342 [D Mass 1979]); *aff'd in part, rev'd in part* in *Rogers v Okin* (634 F2nd 650 (1st Cir 1980P) *vacated and remanded* subnomine *Mills v Rogers* (457 US 291 [1982]); *on remand Rogers v Okin* (738 F2nd [1st Cir 1984]).

and that the attending physician would define the emergency.

It is too early to tell whether this reasoning is universally changing, but some courts may be considering the fact that the attending physician should have more influence in determining whether the client should be allowed to refuse medications.[11] *Stensvad v Reivitz* (84C-3835 slip op WD Wis, January 11, 1985) was such a case, in which a United States District Court in Wisconsin upheld a statute that allowed the forcible administration of medications to committed clients against the clients' will.

Right to Give Informed Consent

Closely related to the right to refuse treatment is the concept of informed consent, which is one of the most widely recognized professional responsibilities in health care today. It is classified under tort or negligence law.[14] Informed consent is defined by Black as "a person's agreement to allow something to happen . . . that is based on a full disclosure of facts needed to make the decision intelligently" (reference 2, p. 701). *Kaimowitz v Michigan Department of Mental Hygiene*[7] identified the elements of informed consent: (1) adequate and accurate knowledge and information given to client; (2) client has legal capacity to consent; i.e., the court has not appointed a guardian to make decisions for the client; and (3) consent is voluntarily given; i.e., the client is not coerced or threatened into making an involuntary decision. In order for a lawsuit to be successful, the plaintiff must prove that the injury sustained resulted from a risk which, prior to the procedure, was not disclosed to the client.[14]

Assuring that an individual with a mental illness has the mental capacity to consent to medication or treatment and is able to comprehend sufficient information to make an informed decision is a very difficult for a clinician. Weisstub quotes several studies that have indicated that even individuals with no mental illness have trouble comprehending medical information.[14] Therefore, it is essential that careful steps be taken in the process of assessing capacity and that the interviews and observations be clearly documented in the medical record.

CONSENT REQUIRED FOR ELECTROCONVULSIVE THERAPY AND PSYCHOSURGERY

Even though electroconvulsive therapy is a controversial treatment, it is accepted in some therapeutic communities as beneficial for certain types of mental disorders. The nurse must be aware that in some states, there are specific laws and regulations concerning the consent required in order to administer electroconvulsive therapy.[12]

Psychosurgery is rarely performed and is, of course, the most intrusive mode of therapy. Therefore, many states have passed legislation to control or even limit or forbid its use.[12] In *Kaimowitz v Michigan Department of Mental Hygiene,*[7] an individual who was charged with rape and murder and identified as a "sexual psychopath" was asked to undergo psychosurgery, to which he agreed. However, the court found that because this was not a routine surgical procedure, this involuntarily detained individual was incapable of giving consent. This ruling implies that the court recognized the controversial and intrusive nature of this procedure.

Nurses are frequently involved in the process of assessing a client's capacity to consent simply because of the nurse's accessibility. Even though the physician holds the ultimate responsibility to obtain informed consent, the nurse is likely to be involved in educating and informing the client and may also be the clinician present should the client revoke a previously given consent. Assessing capacity is an ongoing process that involves careful documentation.

Right to Privacy

The right to privacy is constitutionally protected. In *Rogers v Okin* and *Rennie v Klein,* the courts held that the due process clause of the Fourteenth Amendment, which identifies the right to privacy as an inalienable right, is a legal basis for an individual's freedom to do with his/her mind and body what he/she sees fit. In *Rogers v Okin,* the court held that the clients should be secluded only in emergency situations. More importantly, the court also held that a client had the right to refuse medication unless he/she had been adjudicated incompetent to make this decision. The court stated, "Whatever powers the constitution has granted our government, involuntary mind control is not one of them, absent extraordinary circumstances," referring to the effects of psychotropic medication on a patient's mood, attitude, and thinking. The court based its ruling on the First Amendment, holding that an individual has the right to protection of the communication of ideas, which stems from the freedom of speech.

Other courts, such as previously discussed in *Wyatt v Stickney,* have guaranteed another type of privacy, this right referring to the physical environment, which should allow for a client to enjoy a certain degree of privacy.

Confidentiality and Privilege

Closely related to the right to privacy are the right to confidentiality and the legal concept of privilege. These two terms are often used interchangeably but clearly differ. Confidentiality is the duty to keep certain information from disclosure. This duty is generally governed by state law but is also mentioned in health care disciplines' codes of ethics. Confidentiality ensures that client information is not used for personal gain, curiosity, or gossip, but that it is shared only among those individuals who are responsible for the care of the client.

Privileged communication is defined by Black as statements between certain individuals that the law protects from disclosure.[2] These individuals may include husband–wife, priest–penitent, psychiatrist-client, and nurse–client. Some states have a stricter confidentiality law pertaining to psychiatric hospitalizations than to other types of hospitalization. Some states recognize a nurse–client privilege, whereas others do not. It is imperative that nurses familiarize themselves with law governing these concepts in the state where they work, because psychiatric nurses are frequently asked to disclose information to other facilities for follow-up care of the client, to family members, and to the court system.

EXCEPTIONS

Exceptions to both confidentiality and professional privilege include child abuse allegations, threats voiced by a client to a therapist against a third person, court proceedings in which the issue is the commitability of the client, and a client's waiver of confidentiality and privileges by the filing of a lawsuit.

Child Abuse Allegations. Many states have enacted laws that not only require that any information regarding possible child abuse be disclosed to the proper authorities, but may also mandate criminal prosecution of anyone who fails to disclose. This would include information that is communicated to a nurse by a client relevant to the client's own family or acquaintances, and also observations that a nurse might make from gathering a nursing assessment or history from the client, the client's family, or acquaintances.

Threats Against a Third Party. In *Tarasoff v Board of Regents of the University of California* (592 P2nd 533 [1974]), the court held that a therapist is obligated to use reasonable care to protect intended victims, which could include the duty to warn the intended victim, inform the police, or any other necessary steps. However, in the 1983 case of *Jablonski By Pahls v US* (712 F2d 391 [1983]), the court did not require the presence of an expressed threat against an identifiable third party in order to hold the psychiatrist liable for violence committed by a client with a history of violence documented in records from earlier hospitalizations. Not only do nurses, like other clinicians, have the duty to obtain records from previous hospitalizations, but they have the related duty to document client behavior clearly in the record to ensure that knowledge of dangerous acts or threats is communicated to the appropriate individuals. Hospitals and other agencies should have policies that define the responsibilities and the procedures to be used when obtaining these records.

Court Proceedings. When a client is before the court in an involuntary commitment proceeding or a guardianship hearing, the psychiatrist or any other clinician who testifies is not under a duty to protect information. Clinical information can and must be disclosed.

When an individual brings a lawsuit that puts his/her mental condition in issue, that individual waives any privilege or confidentiality protection that the state law allows. If this exception were not allowed, an individual would be allowed to succeed in court without full disclosure of pertinent information to the court.

Sexual Misconduct by a Therapist. This issue is not technically an exception to confidentiality and privilege, but it is worthy of mentioning here. At present, there are no statutes or professional codes of ethics that clearly define sexual misconduct by a therapist as an exception, nor is there any legal protection provided to the therapist who discloses the otherwise confidential information about the sexual activity that occurred in the other therapist–client relationship. This is not to say that there will not be changes in the near future. However, psychiatrists have been criminally prosecuted because courts view sexual relations in a therapist–client relationship as equivalent to rape.[9] This issue is being pursued more and more by clients in the court system. It is both an ethical and a legal dilemma for a nurse who is informed by a client that the client has been sexually involved with a therapist when the client is not willing to consent to disclosure of this information.

The foregoing list of clients' rights is not all inclusive. A psychiatric nurse is legally responsible to be not only familiar with but well versed in the rights a client possesses.

SPECIAL LEGAL ISSUES IN THE CARE OF MINORS

In the past, minors were regarded as having no rights, legal or otherwise. Parents or guardians were allowed to make decisions about minors' admissions to psychiatric facilities and commitment for treatment. By state, federal, and common law, minors are legally incapable of engaging in certain activities, such as entering into a contract or executing a will. Some states have recognized exceptions as far as a minor's incapacity is concerned that do not require a parent's or guardian's consent, such as the right to consent to an abortion or the right to seek treatment for drug and alcohol abuse. Other states' laws extend the age of minority in some circumstances, as in the case of the legal drinking age being extended to 21.

The care of a mentally ill minor has been greatly impacted by law with the past few decades. In the 1979 case of *Parham v J.R. et al.* (442 US 584), children who were being treated in a Georgia state mental hospital brought suit contending that the state's procedures for involuntary commitment of persons under the age of 18 violated the due process clause of the Fourteenth Amendment. The procedure allowed a parent or guardian to apply for admission of the child to a state mental hospital for "observation and diagnosis." The statute also allowed for an additional period of hospitalization

if there was "evidence of mental illness." The US Supreme Court held that even though the general scheme of the statute was not unconstitutional, "the risk of error inherent in the parental decision to have a child institutionalized for mental health care is sufficiently great that some kind of inquiry should be made by a 'neutral fact finder.' " The court went on to say that this fact finder has the authority to refuse admission of the child and that the need for continuing commitment must be reviewed periodically. A nurse who works with this very special population must recognize their special needs and, very frequently, the more stringent mandates of the law in the psychiatric care of a minor.

CRIMINAL RESPONSIBILITY AND THE PSYCHIATRIC CLIENT

A group of individuals of special concern to the mental health profession, the legal system, and the public as a whole are those who not only have mental illness but who also have become involved in the criminal justice system. This specialized area of mental health care is called forensic psychiatry. These clients' treatment plans include, along with psychiatric care, goals and objectives dealing with security and legal issues, such as an evaluation of competency or insanity. These clients may be hospitalized in a maximum security facility or may be in the general psychiatric population in a state-operated facility. A court may order a pretrial evaluation to determine such issues as competency to stand trial, mental condition at the time of the alleged crime, and commitability.

Competency to Stand Trial

Competency to stand trial refers to the mental condition of a defendant at the time of the criminal trial. Assessment of competency differs from state to state but a widely used assessment is the following: (1) the defendant's ability to assist his/her attorney with the defense; (2) the defendant's ability to understand the nature and consequences of the charge; and (3) the defendant's ability to understand courtroom procedures. In some states, outpatient mental health facilities send a team of clinicians to the jail to evaluate the defendant. On the basis of this evaluation, the defendant may be sent to an inpatient facility for an extended period of evaluation.

If the defendant is assessed as being incompetent to stand trial, treatment is immediately instituted, the main goal being that of achievement or restoration of competency. The treatment regimen may include medication, individual and group psychotherapy, and modalities to educate the defendant about courtroom proceedings and the legal defense. Even when a defendant achieves the state of competency, he or she may still be exhibiting signs and symptoms of a mental illness.

Jackson v Indiana (406 US 715 [1972]) greatly impacted the treatment that an incompetent individual receives. Jackson was a mentally defective deaf–mute who was charged with two robberies, one involving $4 and the other involving $5. He was evaluated as being unlikely ever to become competent to stand trial. The court held that incompetent individuals cannot be detained for an indefinite period without the benefit of the same type of civil commitment hearing to which all civilly committed clients have a right.

The Insanity Defense

The pretrial evaluation order may also require that an assessment be completed regarding the defendant's mental condition at the time he or she allegedly committed the crime. If the defendant meets certain legally prescribed criteria, then the legal defense at trial will be "insanity."

Several tests are used to determine whether an insanity defense exists (Table 51-1). The most widely used today is that promulgated by the American Law Institute, which has been included in many state laws.

Post-Trial Evaluation

When an individual is found to be not guilty by reason of insanity, the court will order another evaluation to determine the individual's need for hospitalization. The statutorily prescribed time period for the evaluation ranges from 30 days to 90 days. During this evaluation, the mental health team assesses the client's need for commitment and appropriate disposition. The court is notified of the recommendations and may choose to have a hearing, during which time the mental health experts will testify as to the assessment.

TABLE 51–1
Tests to determine "insanity"

THE DEFENDANT IS DETERMINED BY THE COURT TO BE INSANE IF:	
He suffered from a disease of the mind which so affected his reason that he was unaware of the nature and quality of his act or that his act was wrong	M'Naughten Rule
He either met the M'Naughten test or in response to an irresistible impulse, he also lacked criminal responsibility even though he knew the wrongfulness of his act	Irresistible Impulse Rule
His acts were the product of a mental disease or defect	Durham Rule
He was suffering from a mental illness at the time of the act, and he was unable to appreciate the wrongfulness of his act, or he was unable to conform his behavior to the requirements of the law	American Law Institute

Guilty but Mentally Ill Verdict

As one result of the controversy over the John Hinkley acquittal in the assassination attempt on President Ronald Reagan, some states have passed "a guilty but mentally ill" plea. This plea is recognized in about 20% of all states but is still the subject of constitutional controversy. This disposition is, ideally, supposed to result in the care and treatment of mentally ill individuals in a correctional setting.[3] However, some states have realized that mental health care is not easily provided under these circumstances.

Nurses are a vital part of a forensic team. Forensic clients are evaluated zealously, and the assessments and documentations are essential for a valid court report. Nurses are also frequently called on to testify on these cases, and in some states, nurses with master's degrees are considered to be expert witnesses on competency issues. Forensic nursing is a specialized area of psychiatric nursing and is an exciting and challenging career opportunity.

LEGAL ROLE OF THE PSYCHIATRIC NURSE
Nurse Practice Acts

Nurse practice acts regulate the practice of nursing and differ from state to state. Most such statutes contain language that expands the role of nursing practice, and some specifically mention the role of the clinical nurse specialist even though the American Nurses' Association has stated that "the law should not provide for identifying clinical specialists in nursing or require certification or other recognition for practice beyond the minimum qualifications," (reference 1, p 3) indicating that this should be left up to the profession. The court in *Sermchief v Gonzalez* (660 SW2nd 683 [Mo banc 1983]) respected the American Nurses' Association's stance in this suit, which was a civil action wherein the medical licensing board petitioned the court to declare that certain acts that nurses were engaging in at a family planning clinic were the practice of medicine and should be enjoined. The court upheld the broad statutory definition of nursing as authorizing a broad scope of practice and found specifically that additional legislation was unnecessary. One nurse-attorney-author wrote, in response to this case, that nurses have more influence over the legislature and other agencies than over a court's decision. Therefore, she argues the importance of professional nursing influencing the lawmaking process, rather than waiting for a suit to be brought. At least one other author sees the *Sermchief* case as expanding nursing's perimeters while barring statutory constraints.[15]

Along with the fact that many nurse practice acts do mention the expanded role of nursing, some states' acts specifically mention the nursing process. The use of the nursing process is essential to the planning and delivery of client care. More legislatures are going to be including the nursing process and nursing diagnoses as legally accountable practices of nursing.[13]

Nursing Malpractice

Nursing malpractice occurs when a nurse deviates from the acceptable standard of care.[4] When a nurse is sued, the case will be heard in a civil court, with the plaintiff (the injured individual who brings the suit) seeking an award of monetary damages. Although not occurring frequently at present, in the past if a court of law did not recognize nursing as a profession, a nurse was sued for simple negligence, which plaintiffs prefer, because the standard of proof required of the plaintiff is much lower, making the plaintiff's case easier to win. In a malpractice suit, on the other hand, the legal duty that the nurse-defendant has toward the client-plaintiff is defined and testified to by nurse expert witnesses and not by unqualified "lay" witnesses.

Each element of a malpractice suit must be proved by the plaintiff in order to prevail in court. When a nurse is sued for malpractice, the plaintiff must prove the following: (1) that the nurse owed a professional nursing duty to the plaintiff; (2) that the nurse breached the duty that was owed the plaintiff; (3) that the nurse's act or omission was the "proximate" or "legal" cause of the injury; and (4) that the act or omission resulted in "damages," which is defined as a pecuniary compensation for the injury that was caused by the nurse. The "duty" that is referred to above is defined by the standard of care under which all nurses are expected to perform. This standard is defined as the nursing practice legally expected from a reasonable, prudent nurse under similar circumstances while practicing with similar expertise.

A nurse can find that standard or duty expected of him/her in documents published by the Joint Commission of American Hospitals; the American Hospital Association; the American Nurses' Association, such as in the Standards of Psychiatric Nursing; and the individual states' nurse practice statutes, along with case law and the policies and procedures of the facility or agency in which the nurse is employed. The following is a list of acts or omissions that have been identified as being frequent sources of injury leading to negligence or malpractice:

1. Failure to provide physical protection;
2. Failure in some aspect of administration of medication;
3. Failure to observe;
4. Failure to intervene appropriately;
5. Failure to advise proper authorities of improper care by another nurse or physician.[10]

As nursing becomes more broadly recognized as an independent profession both by other professions and the legal system, the individual nurse becomes more and more responsible for his or her own practice,

which necessitates becoming familiar with the laws governing nursing, along with the state rules, regulations, and policies under which a nurse is held accountable.

Documentation and Responsible Record Keeping

How is reasonably accepted nursing care tracked, and how do nurses prove their accountability (the assurance that the standard of care is being met)? Avenues of tracking and accountability include quality assurance, peer reviews, and risk management. The mechanism by which these groups function is through documentation. Documentation is important in professional accountability and is the best legal defense that a nurse has. Complete and accurate documentation not only is essential to any legal document, but, more importantly, it is the means of communication by health care providers so that client care is implemented and evaluated.

Medical records are often subpoenaed to court. If a nurse is involved in a malpractice case in which the standard of nursing care is at issue, the medical record will either prove that the nursing care was reasonable and adequate, or it will prove that the duty owed was breached and, therefore, that the nurse is liable.

A nurse should chart as if every record will be subpoenaed to court. Documentation should be objective, clear, concise, and progressive. Progressive charting means that all aspects of client care should be documented, from assessments and the care actually rendered to the benefits and the outcome. The facility that provided the care is the legal owner of the record. However, frequently, clients are granted access to their own records, the degree of accessibility being determined by state law. Many states have laws that define even more stringently the requirements surrounding the accessibility of medical records maintained by a psychiatric facility. A nurse should familiarize herself or himself with both the legal requirements and the facility's policy and procedures that delineate the process involved in releasing the record to the client.

Lawsuits Involving Psychiatric Nurses

Nurses may find themselves involved in or parties to many types of legal actions, including assault and battery, false imprisonment, and invasion of privacy. These actions differ from malpractice or negligence action in that "intent" is required for the plaintiff to prevail; i.e., the nurse's action must have been intentional. Assault and battery can occur when a client is admitted to a hospital for a procedure and the client alleges that he or she did not consent to being touched by the clinician who is being sued. Therefore, the client can sue the clinician, the hospital, or both for assault and bat-

Research Highlights

Seclusion is a controversial treatment method that has legal implications. As mentioned previously, the right to personal security and freedom from undue bodily restraint is guaranteed by the Fourteenth Amendment of the Constitution.

A study entitled "Psychiatric Inpatients' Perceptions of the Seclusion-Room Experience"[8] was conducted to gather information on the clients' perceptions of seclusion, their experiences before and after seclusion, and how they thought these experiences affected them or others. Opponents of the use of seclusion argue the rights of clients, such as the right to the least restrictive environment. Proponents argue the theoretical benefits of isolation and reduction of external stimuli.

In this study, 52 voluntarily admitted adults in a state hospital were interviewed within three days of seclusion. Findings implied that some clients thought that seclusion was unnecessary, but others thought it was beneficial. In many cases, the client's perception of the reason for seclusion was quite different from the staff's. Clients described situations that resulted in the seclusion, whereas the staff described behaviors of that particular client.

The study identifies the necessity of detailed observations and comprehensive documentation of the events both prior to seclusion and during the seclusion period. A formal review of each seclusion was also mentioned in order to help the staff avoid unnecessary seclusions. The psychiatric nurse must be mindful of the impact of seclusion on an individual. All avenues of a less restrictive nature must be explored prior to the choice of seclusion.

Also of great importance in avoiding negligence and false imprisonment suits is objective documentation that reflects the nursing process and the utilization of clear decision making when choosing the mode of treatment.

---

tery, which is defined as the "unlawful touching of another which is without justification or excuse" (reference 2, p 105). This cause of action could accrue during the restraining of a psychiatric client if the force that was used was not reasonable, or during the administration of electroconvulsive treatments if consent was not obtained. If it is proved that the health care provider committed assault and battery with malicious or reckless disregard for the client, criminal liability could attach.

False imprisonment is the intentional and unjustifiable detention of a person against his or her will.[4] This cause of action could arise from the use of restraints and seclusion or merely from the threat of doing so if the client does not remain in his or her room or in another designated area.

Invasion of privacy is the unwarranted exploitation of one's personality or private affairs.[4] This might occur if a nurse who was conducting research used, without permission, in a research publication, photographs of clients who were restrained or secluded. As in a malpractice or negligence lawsuit, these plaintiffs could also sue for monetary damages.

SUMMARY

Both the admission and the discharge process were discussed, with emphasis on the involvement of the legal system arising from the fact that commitments result in a restriction of an individual's liberty interests. The competency of a mentally ill individual is sometimes very difficult to assess. However, all members of a health care team may be involved in this process and must know how, if necessary, to initiate guardianship proceedings.

Clients' rights have been very well attended to by the legal system. This discussion included a list of rights and the legal basis for each.

Minors are a population of psychiatric clients who are recognized by law as requiring special protection, simply because of their recognized legal incapacity to perform certain acts and render certain decisions. The forensic client also demands a special type of attention from health care providers. Nurses may find themselves involved in competency evaluations, insanity evaluations, post-trial evaluations, treatment of these individuals, or even in the trial phase as expert witnesses.

In the section on the legal role of the nurse, nursing practice and malpractice were discussed, along with intentional tort actions that a psychiatric nurse could be involved in. Documentation was identified as important in professional accountability and is the best legal defense that a nurse has. A research study of the use of room seclusion and its legal implications was discussed.

In summation, as the nurse's role expands, so does professional independence and accountability, which are the reasons a nurse must stay informed of the legal requirements and the resulting "duty" owed to the client. Nowhere has the law impacted health care more than in psychiatry, and with consumers becoming more aware of the standard of care that is required, the legal system will continue to be involved in the psychiatric nursing profession.

References

1. American Nurses' Association. The Nursing Practice Act: Suggested State Legislation. Kansas City, Mo.; 1981.
2. Black's Law Dictionary. 5th ed. St. Paul: West Publishing Co; 1979.

3. Brakel SJ, Parry J, Waner BA. The Mentally Disabled and the Law. 3rd ed. Chicago: American Bar Foundation; 1985.

4. Calloway SD. Nursing and the Law. 2nd ed. Eau Claire, Wis: Professional Education System; 1987.

5. Greenlaw J. *Sermchief v Gonzalez* and the debate over advanced nursing practice legislation Law Med Health Care. 1984;12:30–31.

6. Joint Commission on Accreditation of Hospitals. Bill of Rights Manual, Chicago; 1987.

7. *Kaimowitz v Michigan Department of Mental Hygiene.* 2 Prison Law Reporter 433; 1973.

8. Richardson BK. Psychiatric inpatients' perceptions of the seclusion-room experience. Nursing Res. 1987;36:234–238.

9. Riskin L. Sexual relations between psychotherapists and their patients: towards research and restraint. Cal Law Rev. 1979;67:1000–1027.

10. Rocerto LR, Maleski C. The Legal Dimensions of Nursing Practice. New York: Springer Publishing Company; 1982.

11. Simon JT. Clinical Psychiatry and the Law. Washington, DC: American Psychiatric Press; 1987.

12. Tenn Code Annotated 33-3-105; 33-3-106; 33-6-203.

13. Townsend MC. Nursing Diagnoses in Psychiatric Nursing: A Pocket Guide for Care Plan Construction. Philadelphia: FA Davis Company; 1988.

14. Weisstub DN, ed. Law and Mental Health International Perspectives. Toronto: Pergamon Press; 1986.

15. Wolff MA. Court upholds expanded practice roles for nurses. Law Med Health Care. 1971;17(1 Fed Supp 781).

52

Sandra C. Sellin

Ethical Issues in Psychiatric Mental Health Nursing

OBJECTIVES

After reading this chapter, the reader will be able to:

1. Define ethical dilemma
2. State the basic philosophies underlying the utilitarian and deontological theories of ethics
3. Identify three ethical issues common in psychosocial nursing
4. List the steps of the ethical decision-making model
5. Apply the ethical decision model to an ethical dilemma in a clinical situation.

THE BASICS OF ETHICS

Ethics, the branch of philosophy that deals with morality and moral problems and judgments, addresses issues of human conduct that include those actions considered right and good as opposed to immoral and unethical.[7] Ethics as a body of knowledge is generally divided into metaethics and normative ethics. *Metaethics* defines the extent to which moral judgments are justifiable and constitutes the theory of ethical thought. *Normative ethics* explores what is right or what ought to be done in any situation that calls for a moral decision, thus providing the application of ethical theory.[3,6]

ETHICAL DILEMMAS

Ethical dilemmas generally involve relations where there is tension and conflict between two or more people. In health care arenas, ethical dilemmas can occur in relations between clients, nurses, physicians, families, and institutions such as hospitals and community outpatient care facilities.

A situation with an ethical dilemma is one that presents a difficult problem involving a choice between two or more equally unsatisfactory alternatives. There may indeed be no satisfactory solution to the problem. Because ethical dilemmas entail conflicting moral claims, they give rise to questions such as, what is the right thing to do? what ought I do? and what benefit or harm might result if this decision or action were carried out? In most ethical dilemmas, an action that one considers good may not necessarily be right.[2,4,6,8] For example, although forcibly administering an antipsychotic drug to a mildly psychotic client who refuses the medication may diminish delusions and hallucinations, it is not right because forcing the client to take the medication violates the client's right to refuse.

In order to unravel and understand the often uncertain and ambiguous issues that constitute ethical dilemmas in clinical practice, it often is helpful to examine those issues from multiple perspectives.

ETHICAL THEORIES

Although ethical theories do not provide clearcut, definitive answers to ethical questions, they do provide some structure for clarifying and examining the moral basis for judgments, actions, duties, and obligations. Three traditional ethical perspectives, specifically egoism, utilitarianism, and deontology, offer ways to reason through ethical dilemmas.

Ethical Egoism

Ethical egoism involves actions in which a person considers only what is to his or her own advantage. That is, the right action is the one that is best for oneself: the action may or may not be best for the client, the family, or anyone else.[7] From this perspective, there are no conflicting moral claims and thus no real ethical dilemmas.

Utilitarianism

Utilitarianism, or *consequentialist ethics*, reflects the view that the ethically correct action is the one that promotes the greatest good for the greatest number of persons. In utilitarian ethics, each person involved in a situation counts equally. A given situation can involve the client, the psychiatrist(s) or other physician(s), the nurse(s), every member of the client's family, the institution, and society; and consideration of the positive and negative consequences of a moral action must be given to each of these parties. The action that produces the most benefits and the least harm is the ethically correct choice based on the principle of utility.[3,7]

Deontology

Deontology, also known as *formalism*, is an ethical theory that looks neither at a personal position nor at the consequences of an ethical action. Rather, deontology looks at the inherent moral significance of an act and considers the rightness or wrongness of the act itself. Deontological principles and rules of conduct guide ethical action; therefore, judgments about what to do in particular cases should always be determined in light of these principles and rules.[7] This theory uses the principles discussed below.

ETHICAL PRINCIPLES

The ethical principles most important to ethical decision making in health care settings are autonomy, beneficence, nonmaleficence, and justice.

Autonomy

The principle of autonomy is built on the broader principle of respect for persons and means that every human being has a right to be respected for his or her own individuality and to have control over his or her life. The word "autonomy" comes from the Greek words meaning self-rule. The autonomous person delineates his or her own course of action in accordance with a self-chosen plan.[3] Living with the principles of autonomy and respect for persons means accepting individuals' own choices, whether or not those choices are in their best interests.[16]

The principle of autonomy presumes that human beings are capable of making choices based on the principles by which they live. However, not all persons are capable of making autonomous choices. Children, the mentally retarded, and the mentally ill are groups of individuals often thought to be incompetent to make autonomous choices. Judgments of competence and incompetence do not apply to all decisions made by individuals, however. Because some people are judged incompetent to make certain decisions does not mean they are incompetent to make all decisions. Thus, judgments of competence always require a context. In addition, a person's ability to make decisions may vary depending on the person's condition and circumstances. A person who at one time is incompetent to make choices because of mental illness may, at some later time, be clear thinking and competent to make reasoned choices. The concepts of limited competence and intermittent competence can have significant implications and can be of great practical value in many clinical settings, eliminating all-or-none conceptions of competence and incompetence. Autonomy can thereby be preserved because the concepts of limited and intermittent competence justify interference only in those areas where a person is significantly incompetent.[3]

Beneficence and Nonmaleficence

Beneficence, according to Beauchamp and Childress,[3] is the duty to help others further their important and legitimate interests by preventing and removing harms and by promoting good. Implicit in the principle of beneficence is the duty to balance the possible goods against the possible harms of an action. *Nonmaleficence,* on the other hand, is the duty to do no harm. Many philosophers suggest that the principle of nonmaleficence takes precedence over beneficence; that it is more important to avoid doing harm than it is to do good.[8]

Individual interpretations of what constitutes good and harm often lead to conflicts between a person's rights and a person's best interests. When one person decides for another what is best for that person, it is known as *paternalism.* People who morally justify forcing competent people to act for their own good exercise *strong* paternalism, whereas people who believe it is morally justifiable only to force mentally compromised or incompetent people to take care of themselves are said to exercise *weak* paternalism. Sometimes, people are so cognitively compromised that making paternalistic decisions for them is unavoidable, as with individuals in coma or those in a severe psychotic state.[8]

Sometimes, the duty to do no harm can be interpreted as a duty to prevent a person from harming a third person. In cases such as the involuntary hospitalization of violent or mentally ill persons, the duty to prevent harm to others may be considered sufficient reason to limit the person's autonomy.[12]

The principles of beneficence, nonmaleficence, and autonomy and the concept of paternalism are interrelated and are all intimately linked to the concept of competence. According to Mill,[10] one person cannot advance the interests of a competent other by compulsion or coercion. If such is attempted, the harms (physi-

cal, psychological, social, moral) involved outweigh any good done. In Mill's view, paternalism is rarely justified. Others justify paternalism only if: (1) the harms (physical, psychological, social, moral) prevented outweigh the loss of autonomy; (2) a person's physical or mental condition limits his or her ability to choose autonomously; and (3) such paternalistic treatment is universally justified under similar circumstances.[3]

Justice

Justice, specifically *distributive justice,* involves the distribution of limited resources, benefits, and burdens among members of a society. Simply put, distributive justice is a matter of the comparative treatment of individuals within a society. Individual need is commonly used to justify the ways in which a society's resources are distributed, particularly in the area of health care.[6]

An important aspect of the principle of justice involves the duty to treat all people fairly. According to John Rawls,[13] the distribution of the benefits and burdens of society should be considered from the point of view of the least advantaged: the poor and disadvantaged should share in the benefits of society equally with all others.

ETHICAL DILEMMAS COMMON IN PSYCHOSOCIAL NURSING

Most discussions of ethical dilemmas in psychosocial nursing focus on two significant issues: the rights of those involuntarily committed to psychiatric facilities, and the issue of restrictiveness, including chemical and physical restraints and the least restrictive alternative. Each issue is complex and intricately linked to the other. It is difficult to separate the ethical aspects from the legal aspects of these issues, but this discussion focuses on only the ethical aspects.

Rights

Before discussing clients rights, it will be useful briefly to consider rights in general. When most people think of rights, they usually think of entitlements to have or to do something. Beauchamp and Childress define rights as "justified claims that individuals and groups can make upon others or upon society" (reference 3, p 50). Those authors differentiate legal rights, justified by legal principles, and moral rights, justified by moral principles, particularly the principle of autonomy. For each right claimed by one person, there exists a corresponding duty or obligation on the part of another person or of society. And yet, rights are not absolute: any right can be exercised legitimately and create duties for others only when the right outweighs other rights that compete with it.[3]

Clients' Rights

During the 1960s and 1970s, society underwent a social–legal revolution that brought human rights to social consciousness and that challenged the status quo. In response to this social introspection, mental health professionals began to focus on clients' rights and on least restrictive alternatives.[14] Clients' rights and advocacy groups gained changes in mental health policy and the law. Now, individuals, even though mentally ill and perhaps involuntarily committed, maintain the right to make choices and to be involved in determining the course of their own treatment.[11,15] Generally, involuntarily committed clients who are competent have a right to choose between the symptoms of mental illness and the potentially harmful side effects of antipsychotic medications unless they are considered a clear and present danger to themselves or others.[11,17]

The Least Restrictive Alternative

Mentally ill clients have a right to treatment that least restricts their liberty. This right is based on the idea that infringement of one's liberty is unacceptable according to traditional societal standards and that the restriction of personal freedom is clinically harmful. Therefore, the treatment team should use the least restrictive alternative to help the client learn to cope with the level of freedom found outside the hospital.[17]

Discussions of least restrictive alternatives include not only treatment environments, but also the use of physical restraints such as seclusion, four-point leather restraints, and chemical restraints such as antipsychotic drugs, tranquilizers, and other sedatives. Generally, clients have a right to be free from physical and chemical restraints unless those restraints are part of their treatment plan or such restraints are necessary for the safety of the clients themselves or of others.[14,17] Thus, it is ethically justifiable to restrict a client's autonomy in order to protect that client or others from serious harm. However, the means of behavior control the treatment team chooses to protect clients must be the one that offers the least restrictive alternative. Mentally ill clients have basic human rights that must be respected within the limits of safety.

THE ETHICAL DECISION-MAKING PROCESS

Generally, decision making is a reasoning process consisting of a series of steps designed to bring about a workable solution. The process used to make ethical decisions in psychosocial nursing is similar to the decision-making model known to most nurses as the nursing process.

There are many ways to reason through ethical problems. The following decision-making model is based on one outlined by Jameton.[8] As with any decision model, accurate assessment, thoughtful reflection, and constant evaluation are required, and all decisions reached must remain open to new information and reevaluation.

Values Clarification

Because ethical judgments are inextricably tied to personal and professional values, it is important that individuals clearly understand their own values and the ways in which those values influence their decisions. It has been said that values are much like breathing in that individuals are not really aware of them until they are troubling. People make value judgments every day about the worth of objects, thoughts, attitudes, behaviors, and individuals. Every person has values that influence daily decisions.[6] The challenge of ethical reflection is to bring to conscious awareness the values, beliefs, and attitudes that influence not only personal life but also professional life and the kind of nursing care delivered.

The Model

Successful critical inquiry and resolution of an ethical dilemma may be accomplished by moving through the steps diagrammed in Figure 52-1 and outlined as follows.

IDENTIFY THE PROBLEM

Is the problem an *ethical* problem? Is there something about the situation that just does not feel right? Is something going on to which there are *ethical* objections? If the problem is one of poor communication or poor planning, it may not be an ethical problem.

GATHER ALL POSSIBLE RELEVANT INFORMATION

What is the client's diagnosis and prognosis? What is the situation that brought on the problem? What information is available? What additional information is needed? Who is involved in the problem situation (client? psychiatrist or psychologist? family? psychiatric mental health nurse)? List all parties involved in the situation. Who are they, and how do they relate to one another?

Then consider the issues in the situation. What are the client's wishes? What are the views and interests of the other people involved? Consider also issues such as the effects of treatment on the client and the allocation of scarce health care resources. What societal or legal issues may be involved?

LIST OPTIONS, OUTCOMES, AND CONSEQUENCES

On the basis of the information available, list all possible options. Then list all the possible outcomes and consequences for each option. How likely is each possi-

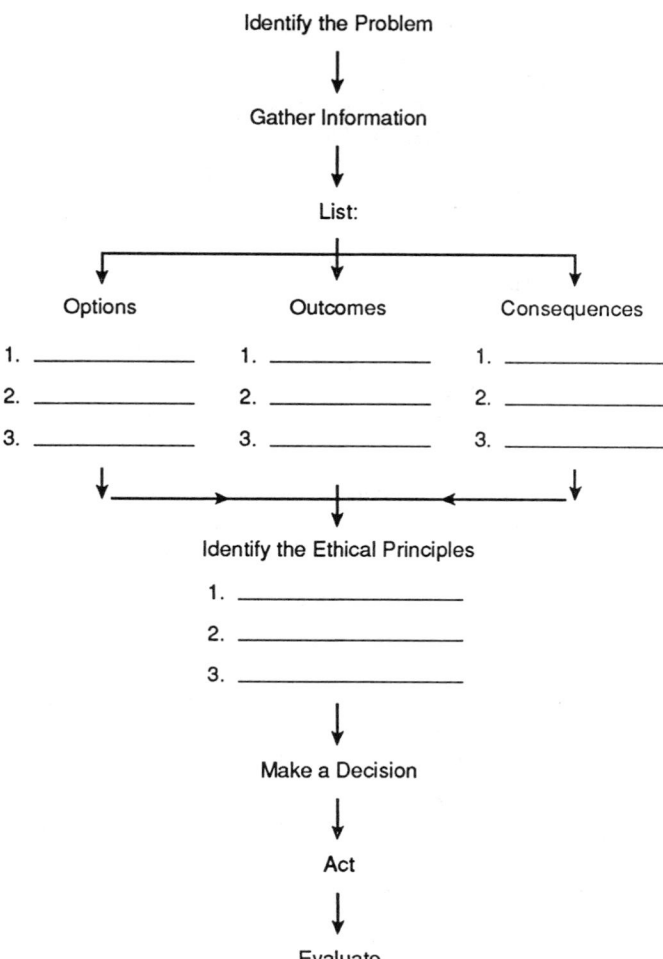

Identify the Problem

↓

Gather Information

↓

List:

Options | Outcomes | Consequences
1. _____ | 1. _____ | 1. _____
2. _____ | 2. _____ | 2. _____
3. _____ | 3. _____ | 3. _____

Identify the Ethical Principles

1. _____
2. _____
3. _____

↓

Make a Decision

↓

Act

↓

Evaluate

FIGURE 52–1. Ethical decision-making model.

ble outcome? How will each possible outcome help or hurt the parties involved? How will the institution or society be affected by the long-term results of each outcome? Project thinking to see all the possible consequences that might result from each option listed.

IDENTIFY THE ETHICAL PRINCIPLES

What ethical principles are involved in the problem situation? Do the wishes and concerns of the client, the family, the psychiatrist, the psychiatric nursing staff, or the institution seem to be of some overriding importance in the case? Or does the futility of further treatment, the maintenance of professional competence, a professional ideal, or some other consideration seem more important?

In situations in which the ethical issues are not so clear, thoughtful reflection on the principles of respect for persons, autonomy, beneficence, nonmaleficence, justice, and utility and on basic values such as health, personal liberty, and those things that give meaning to life can help clarify the ethical issues involved. Rely on those principles that seem most certain and that can be judged most important to the situation. In each case,

the ethical issues will be slightly different, but the basic ethical principles will remain constant.

MAKE A DECISION

On the basis of the best information, the list of possible options and outcomes, and careful consideration of the ethical issues involved, choose a course of action that reflects the best judgment.

Rarely does ethical decision making occur in a vacuum. Therefore, it is advisable to discuss these issues with other health care team members. Ethics rounds and case conferences can be useful for this purpose.[5]

Given the time constraints of most clinical decisions, nurses rarely have time to consider every minute detail of an ethical problem. Thus, at some point, they must stop thinking and assessing and come to a decision.

ACT

Once the decision is made, act.

EVALUATE

After implementing the option of choice, compare the actual outcomes with the outcomes projected earlier. If the results of the decision are acceptable, continue with the chosen course. If the results are not satisfactory, go back to step two: reexamine the problem and the list of options and work out a different solution. Always assess and remember the results of decisions so that future cases can be approached in a more efficient, sensitive, and sophisticated way.

CASE STUDY

RJ is a 28-year-old man with one previous hospitalization for delusional disorder. During his previous hospitalization, RJ was tried on high doses of several antipsychotic drugs before his psychiatrist finally found one that controlled his delusional symptoms. After discharge, RJ's delusions were well controlled with medication; however, he suffered akathisia, which made him unable to sleep. RJ found that he felt better if he reduced his medication intake, and he eventually stopped taking the drug altogether. After several months, RJ's delusional thought patterns returned with paranoid components.

Now RJ is brought in involuntarily by his father who states that RJ has become increasingly suspicious of others and that his delusional, paranoid behavior has been upsetting other family members. The father says he believes RJ is a danger to himself and others because he has been irritable and unpredictable in recent weeks. He therefore wants RJ admitted to the hospital as soon as possible. After a short consultation with RJ and his father, the psychiatrist agrees that immediate hospitalization is advisable.

RJ is admitted to the hospital involuntarily with a DSM-III-R diagnosis of delusional disorder. During the admission interview, RJ appears in control of himself when he tells the nurse that he will not take any drugs because they make him sick. He also tells the nurse that his family and doctor are trying to poison him. The nurse realizes that RJ is experiencing delusional thinking. She also knows that the only way to control RJ's delusional thought pattern is to begin antipsychotic drug treatment as soon as possible. The nurse thus makes a nursing diagnosis of potential for noncompliance (medications) related to concerns about akathisia and to a delusion of being poisoned.

The dilemma: Should the nurse respect the client's refusal to take any drugs? Or should she ignore the client's refusal and forcibly administer the prescribed antipsychotic medication? And on what ethical grounds would the nurse justify either action?

The resolution:

Step 1: *the problem.* The client needs the antipsychotic medication. He refuses to take any drugs voluntarily out of the belief that his family and his psychiatrist are trying to poison him and because of his realistic concern about side effects.

Step 2: *relevant information.* Past use of antipsychotic medications controlled the client's delusional thinking but had side effects. The client has become increasingly paranoid, irritable, and unpredictable. There is uncertainty about whether his behavior has included violence. The client's father believes RJ is a danger to himself and to others, which implies a potential for violence. People directly involved in the situation include the client, the client's family, the psychiatrist, the nurses, and the other clients on the unit. The client refuses the medication and seems in control of himself at the time of the admission interview. However, because of the client's delusional thoughts, there is some question about his competence to make such a decision. The family, psychiatrist, and the nurses all want the client to take the medication. The other clients on the unit want, and are entitled to, a safe therapeutic environment.

Step 3: *options.*

1. The nurse allows the client to refuse. This option allows the client's delusional thinking to continue and possibly worsen, thus allowing potential physical harm to come to the client as well as to those near him.

2. The nurse forcibly administers the prescribed medication with the intent of doing good for the client and

of removing the client and others from harms that might result if treatment is not given. This option restricts the client's autonomy and runs the risk of a short-term aggressive response that might briefly compromise the safety of the client, the staff, and the other clients on the unit. It should be noted here that legal considerations may restrict use of this option without benefit of a court hearing. Under such circumstances, other means such as physical restraints may be more appropriate until legal approval for the administration of medication without the client's consent can be obtained.

3. The nurse suggests that the psychiatrist and the client negotiate a drug treatment regimen that would satisfy both the concerns of the client regarding side effects of the drugs and the needs of the others in the situation who want to remain safe from the client's delusional thinking. The appropriateness of this option depends on the perceived competence of the client to engage in such a negotiation. The demeanor of the client during the admission interview suggests capability to negotiate.

Step 4: *the ethical principles.* The ethical principles involved are autonomy, which protects the client's right to make choices about his treatment plan; beneficence, which involves doing good for the client; and nonmaleficence, which embodies the duty of the staff to do no harm to the client and those around him. If the principles conflict, nonmaleficence takes precedence, because the welfare of one client should not be considered above the welfare of a group of clients.

Step 5: *the decision.* The least restrictive alternative in this case is option 3. From a deontological perspective, this option respects the client's autonomy and the needs of others for safety. From a utilitarian perspective, this option provides the greatest good for the greatest number. The success of this option depends on the client's competence to negotiate and follow through with a treatment plan.

Step 6: *action.* Action means advocating for the client by talking with the psychiatrist about negotiating a drug treatment plan with the client.

Research Highlights

In recent years, ethical decision making and moral behavior in nursing have been the subjects of research. In 1985, Ketefian[9] published a study designed to explore the relations between registered nurses' professional and bureaucratic role conceptions and their moral behavior. Role conceptions were defined as nurses' value orientations toward their nursing role. Professional role orientations espouse principles that deal with loyalty to the nursing profession, specifically involvement in professional organizations, commitment to practice standards, and the exercise of professional judgment in decision making. Bureaucratic role orientations, on the other hand, espouse loyalties to employing institutions and to those in authority and following of administrative rules and routines. Because ethics involves critical and rational analysis of morality, moral behavior was defined as the nurses' assessment of the extent to which the ANA

Code-prescribed nursing actions[1] in simulated ethical dilemmas were likely to be implemented in practice. The sample consisted of 217 registered nurses from all levels of nursing education and from all levels of the hospital hierarchy. The Judgments about Nursing Decisions Test (JAND) measured moral behavior, whereas moral reasoning was measured by the Defining Issues Test (DIT).

The results indicated that a high professional role orientation is a good predictor of moral behavior in congruence with the ANA Code. Ketefian also noted that nurses with high professional role orientations seem to experience more ethical conflict because many consider the values of such an orientation to be nonfunctional within the realities of most bureaucratic work environments. Ketefian suggests that nurses need to cultivate loyalties to both professional and bureaucratic values.

Step 7: *evaluate.* Fortunately, the client in this case is competent to negotiate a treatment plan with the psychiatrist, so option 3 is the ethically correct choice. If he were not competent to negotiate his treatment plan, option 2 would have been the ethically correct choice, because nonmaleficence, the duty to do no harm, takes precedence over a client's right to refuse treatment because the refusal is not an autonomous choice. Option 2 would then provide the greatest good for the greatest number of people.

SUMMARY

The ethical theories of egoism, utilitarianism, and deontology and the ethical principles of autonomy, beneficence, nonmaleficence, justice, and utility are all used in the process of ethical decision making in nursing. The concepts of rights, clients' rights, and least restrictive alternatives are useful with respect to psychosocial nursing problems. The steps of the ethical decision-making model are: (1) identify the problem; (2) gather all possible relevant information; (3) list options, outcomes, and consequences; (4) identify the ethical principles; (5) make a decision; (6) act; and (7) evaluate.

References

1. American Nurses' Association. Code for Nurses, Kansas City, Mo: The Association; 1976.
2. Aroskar M. Anatomy of an ethical dilemma: the theory. Am J Nurs. 1980;80:658–60.
3. Beauchamp TL, Childress JF. Principles of biomedical ethics. 2nd ed. New York: Oxford University Press; 1983.
4. Curtin L, Flaherty MJ. Nursing ethics: theories and pragmatics. Bowie, Md: RJ Brady Co; 1982.
5. Davis AJ. Helping your staff address ethical dilemmas. J Nurs Admin. Feb 1982;9–13.
6. Davis AJ, Aroskar M. Ethical dilemmas and nursing practice. 2nd ed. Norwalk, Conn: Appleton-Century-Crofts; 1983.
7. Frankena WK. Ethics. 2nd ed. Englewood Cliffs, NJ: Prentice-Hall, Inc; 1973.
8. Jameton A. Nursing practice: the ethical issues. Englewood Cliffs, NJ: Prentice-Hall, Inc; 1984.
9. Ketefian S. Professional and bureaucratic role conceptions and moral behavior among nurses. Nurs Res. 1985;34:248–53.
10. Mill JS. Utilitarianism—on liberty—essay on Bentham. New York: New American Library; 1974.
11. Oriol MD, Oriol DO. Involuntary commitment and the right to refuse medication. J Psychosoc Nurs Ment Health Serv 1986;24(11):15–20.
12. Quinn CA, Smith MD. The professional commitment: issues and ethics in nursing. Philadelphia, WB Saunders Co; 1987.
13. Rawls J. Theory of justice. Cambridge: Harvard University Press; 1971.
14. Sclafani M. Violence and behavior control. J Psychosoc Nurs Ment Health Serv 1986;24(11):8–14.
15. Smoyak SA. Ethical perspectives. J Psychosoc Nurs Ment Health Serv 1986;24(11):7.
16. Veatch RM, Fry ST. Case studies in nursing ethics. Philadelphia: JB Lippincott; 1987.
17. Ziegenfuss JT. Patients' rights and professional practice. New York: Van Nostrand Reinhold Co; 1983.

Status and Directions of Psychiatric Mental Health Nursing

53

Christina L. S. Evans

The Future Practice Environment and the Psychiatric Nurse Administrator

ROLE OF THE NURSE MANAGER OR ADMINISTRATOR
ADMINISTRATION OF PSYCHIATRIC MENTAL HEALTH
    NURSING CARE
STATUS OF THE PRACTICE ENVIRONMENT
TRENDS IN PSYCHIATRIC MENTAL HEALTH NURSING CARE
Changes in Client Populations
Demand for Increased Information Processing
Shortages of Nurses
Relationships With Other Health Care Providers
Increased Emphasis on Planning

OBJECTIVES
After reading this chapter, the reader will be able to:
1. Identify the unique administrative components of psychiatric mental health nursing departments
2. Discuss trends that will impact delivery systems for psychiatric mental health nursing care
3. Identify programmatic changes that will be needed if nursing departments are to meet the challenges presented by the identified trends
4. Identify strategies for achieving the programmatic changes.

INTRODUCTION

The future practice environment will present many challenges and much satisfaction to psychiatric mental health nurses. Change will become the routine as psychiatric mental health nursing departments seek to continue to provide high-quality care in a constantly changing health care environment. However, to be successful in the future, psychiatric mental health nursing must begin to plan for that future. This chapter will review both trends that will impact psychiatric mental health nursing care and programmatic changes that will assist a psychiatric nursing department in keeping pace with these trends.

ROLE OF THE NURSE MANAGER OR ADMINISTRATOR

Within any psychiatric mental health care agency, the role of a nurse manager or administrator is to facilitate a professional practice environment in which high-quality nursing care can be delivered in a cost-effective manner.[16] The nursing management team achieves this by planning and implementing programs within the practice environment (such as client classification systems, continuing education programming) that foster the nursing staff's delivery of care and collaboration with the interdisciplinary team.

ADMINISTRATION OF PSYCHIATRIC MENTAL HEALTH NURSING CARE

Administration of psychiatric mental health nursing care requires an approach different from the administration of other nursing specialities because of the characteristics of the client population. Psychiatric mental health clients differ from other nursing clients in several ways. First, the average stay for a psychiatric illness in an acute care setting is generally longer than the average stay for other illnesses.[16] Second, the symptoms presented by psychiatric clients may be more difficult to link to measurable indicators. Third, despite the more enlightened views of modern society, clients with mental illness may still be stigmatized. Persons seeking health care for a psychiatric illness may be dissuaded by those around them and may be perceived differently by family and friends after their treatment.

In addition to the challenges presented by the client population, the psychiatric nursing interventions emphasize the nurse's therapeutic use of self[9] to support and assist clients as they progress. Knowledge, guidelines, and protocols can be taught, but it is the therapeutic use of the self, and the skill and patience with which this tool is utilized, that is the focus of psychiatric mental health nursing. Psychiatric nurses require performance evaluations that are not based primarily on direct observation, as close observation could have a detrimental effect on the client and could handicap the staff's ability to implement the therapeutic use of self. Objective measureable criteria are monitored and measured but not in a manner that could hinder a nurse's ability to practice to the maximum potential.

Because little nursing administration research has been published,[30] both in general and in relation to psychiatric mental health nursing, theory-based administrative practice is difficult to achieve. Thus, nurse administrators and managers often utilize concepts from business administration and general management. This can lead to challenges in establishing a professional practice environment, since these concepts may not be directly applicable to the psychiatric nursing practice environment. However, more information is beginning to be published in texts and journals that can serve as resources for a psychiatric mental health nurse administrator. As programs and tools are adapted to psychiatric agencies, these should be published and publicized to facilitate their use by other psychiatric nursing departments.

STATUS OF THE PRACTICE ENVIRONMENT

Currently, the principal setting for the delivery of psychiatric mental health nursing care is within inpatient agencies, with a secondary emphasis on outpatient settings. Minimal psychiatric mental health nursing is being provided through home care agencies. Public facilities continue to deinstitutionalize and increase their contracts for the delivery of psychiatric mental health nursing care with private agencies. The client population is beginning to contain more children, adolescents, and older adults.

Psychiatric mental health practice environments utilize a variety of delivery systems (team, module/miniteam, primary), and the majority of agencies are experiencing some effects of the nursing shortage. Computer technology is just beginning to be developed for psychiatric settings. Nursing diagnoses are beginning to be utilized more frequently, but standardized classifications are not yet common throughout the country, and the provision of psychiatric mental health nursing is, in some settings, still based on psychiatric diagnoses. Relationships with other health care providers are often characterized by the blurring of roles, with lack of clarity as to specific practice boundaries of each discipline.

TRENDS IN PSYCHIATRIC MENTAL HEALTH NURSING CARE

Various trends have been identified that will impact the future of nursing and health care.[8,15] These trends are grouped into five larger trends important to the future delivery of psychiatric mental health nursing care: (1) changes in the client population; (2) demands for increased information processing; (3) cyclical shortages in available nurses; (4) changes in relationships between nurses and other health care providers; and (5) an increased emphasis on planning.

Changes in Client Populations

Changes in client populations have been predicted[8,15,22,27] that will affect psychiatric mental health agencies. A larger percentage of clients will be elderly,[2,16] with an associated increase in the physical illnesses presented by these clients. The number of chronic mentally ill clients also will increase.[15,17] An increase in clients experiencing depression or eating disorders and in adolescents attempting suicide has already been noted (G McFarland; personal communication), and additional agencies will be needed to provide all levels of psychiatric mental health nursing to infants and children as well as to senior citizens.

As the result of increased cost-containment efforts by health insurers, only the most acutely ill clients will continue to be hospitalized,[14,27] with the approved length of stay for these clients being reduced from current levels. In psychiatric mental health agencies, inpatient clients will tend to be individuals who currently would be identified as dangerous to themselves or others or who are unable to provide for their own basic needs. In addition, the trend for deinstitutionalization of clients will continue.[23] State inpatient settings will continue downsizing or will close, with psychiatric mental health nursing being provided to public clients through contracts with private or local public agencies.

Clients who are less acutely ill will receive treatment in outpatient or homecare agencies, with the number of clients in these settings increasing dramatically. Outpatient or home care agencies will see an increase in the number of clients involved in self-help activities,[26] and all clients will seek a more active role in the treatment process.[21]

New mental illnesses will be differentiated[8] as medical research continues. Additional research will focus on the biochemical causes of mental and emotional illnesses and symptom complexes not previously labeled. Nursing research will continue to focus on nursing diagnoses and the most effective interventions for clients demonstrating specific diagnoses.

Inpatient psychiatric mental health care agencies will seek highly qualified and skilled nurses to plan, provide, and evaluate the nursing care needed. Orientation programs will need to be intensive and focus on both psychiatric mental health and physical problems. Considering the nature of psychiatric nursing content in some integrated nursing curricula,[9,11,20] the orientation program will be critical in facilitating the nurse's transition into psychiatric mental health nursing. Inservice programs will need to address not only the maintenance of current knowledge and skills but also nursing skills that will be needed in the future.

More agency resources will support the delivery of direct psychiatric mental health nursing care.[6] These resources could include computers, references, or clinical nurse specialists. Without such support, the direct care staff could be overwhelmed quickly by the complex care demands of clients and resort to mediocre, rather than effective, approaches to the delivery of care.

Clients will require much more intensive teaching regarding their responses to illnesses and medications and strategies to cope better with their individual stressors.[12] Client education can be considered one of the most valuable assets the psychiatric mental health nurse can provide.[29] Educational programs will need to be reviewed and revised continually in order to meet the changing needs of client populations.

Discharge planning will also be critical[6] and will ideally begin upon initiation of treatment, particularly in cases in which further placements will be needed. Such planning will include contacts by nurses with agencies for follow-up care.

In order to assure that a psychiatric mental health nursing department is able to cope with the changing client population, a nurse administrator will utilize skills in finance, staff assessment, and the facilitation of change. Financial skills are needed to coordinate the objective data used to substantiate budgetary requests. Each nurse administrator should know the cost of providing nursing care in her or his department.[15] These skills are particularly critical in the area of staff education. As client populations and their needs change, the direct care staff will require resources to assist them to individualize nursing care more efficiently. The nurse administrator must be able to demonstrate that the "increased cost of better educated, better prepared staff results in an increased rate of return for the [agency]" (reference 29, p 31). Higher-quality nursing staff enables lengths of stay to be decreased and thus reduces costs for the agency.

Staff assessment skills are particularly important as a psychiatric mental health nurse administrator encourages professional growth of the nursing staff.[23] To do this requires an objective assessment of the current functioning of the staff. Once assessment is complete, mechanisms could be developed to facilitate professional growth for a variety of functional levels. Psychiatric nursing staff will have difficulty in improving unless relevant learning resources are provided. Such resources might include staff development programs, self-learning modules, attendance at conferences, tuition reimbursement, and self-evaluation tools.

The ability to assess potential growth effectively is acquired through knowing the psychiatric nursing staff, not only the educational and experiential levels of each employee, but also the attitudes, feelings, and values that predominate in key nurses. This awareness of skill levels enables the nurse administrator to facilitate professional growth in order to keep pace with the clients' changing needs. More skilled nursing staff can then serve as role models for those less motivated, who will experience peer pressure to improve their level of functioning.

If a psychiatric mental health nursing department is to keep pace with, or anticipate, changes in the client population, continuous planned change will be needed.[21] The delivery of psychiatric mental health nursing care is a continually evolving process that requires regular departmental adjustments. There may be a more efficient or more effective way to deliver care if one only widens the possibilities.

To evaluate a psychiatric mental health nursing department's successful anticipation of, and adjustment to, changes in the client population, a nurse administrator annually reviews the programming. Programs reflect current client needs but, at the same time, need to begin anticipating changes necessitated by population shifts. Ineffective programs can be eliminated or revised to be more effective.

Demand for Increased Information Processing

Because the acutely ill psychiatric mental health clients of the future will have increasingly complex health care needs, there will be a need for more information for care planning. Thus, "tomorrow's nurses must be prepared to work [within an] information society" (reference 3, p 377). In 1985, the amount of general information was doubling every five years; by the year 2000, the amount of information will be doubling every year.[24] It will be crucial for nurses to "learn how to learn and to learn not to be intimidated by change" (reference 24, p 39) as more emphasis is placed on learning "concepts and problem solving" (reference 24, p 39) rather than on the acquisition of facts. The previous agency recruitment emphasis on attracting a certain number of personnel will be replaced by an emphasis on recruiting competence and quality.[12] Nurses need to acquire a broad knowledge base in order to deliver comprehensive care but also need specialized knowledge to cope with changes in client conditions.[8]

"There will be a critical need for nursing practice to be based on empirically tested data [with nurses] expected to demonstrate expertise responsive to the changing environment" (reference 6, p 16). "The clinical management of each and every [client] will take the form of a mini-research design" (reference 12, p 6), with the resulting information being utilized to improve further the nursing care delivered to clients with similar emotional–mental responses. "Thinking and behavior will be integrated into complex levels of sophistication in each practitioner" (reference 12, p 6). The "role of the nurse . . . [will] become increasingly complex [as] will requirements and procedures for licensure" (reference 27, p 58).

In the future, a psychiatric mental health nurse will plan with a client, and assist that person in implementing, a plan of care in the time that previously was provided for initial observation and evaluation.[13,19] One nurse will be more likely to provide care from the client's entry into the agency until discharge, necessi-

tating the quick processing of information, continuous review of the literature, and anticipation of clients' needs. A nurse will function more autonomously in the delivery of nursing care to acutely ill clients. Most likely, inpatient psychiatric agencies will require baccalaureate-prepared nurses or experienced associate degree or diploma graduates.

The role for paraprofessionals in the future will decrease because of the increasing acuity of clients requiring nursing care. Paraprofessionals may assist in the monitoring of the less acutely ill clients, escorting clients, and helping clients in the completion of their activities of daily living. The baccalaureate prepared nurse will develop the plan of care for each client and may delegate selected implementation aspects of that plan to less experienced or less educated nurses and paraprofessionals.

A psychiatric mental health nurse administrator is instrumental in enabling nurses to "establish [a] new level of professionalism" (reference 7, p vii) with the client. The nursing department will need to have a larger budget because of the increased need for professional nurses. However, the psychiatric mental health nursing department will also need to measure client acuity, staff productivity, and departmental cost effectiveness. The nurse administrator will measure the financial impact of increasing the number of professional nurses required by the increasing client acuity.[15]

The evaluation of the department's handling of the processing of increased information also requires a review of current functioning and plans in this area. Increased demands for more efficient methods of processing information within the department involves technological elements as well as human components and budgetary adjustments.

Shortages of Nurses

A shortage of nurses has existed during various times in nursing's history. Psychiatric mental health settings have traditionally attracted only a minority of active nurses: at one point, only 2% of the nursing population was identified as interested in this specialty.

Other events will further reduce the number of nurses entering psychiatric mental health. The number of individuals entering college as well as nursing programs has decreased as career opportunities for women have increased.[22] Hence, fewer nurses are graduating who could enter psychiatric mental health nursing. In addition, psychiatric mental health nursing content is integrated into many nursing school curricula rather than being taught as a separate course.[9,11,20] Yet without an identifiable emphasis on psychiatric nursing and the therapeutic use of self by the nurse,[9] graduating nurses may be uncomfortable delivering care within psychiatric mental health agencies. The number of nurses applying to psychiatric mental health agencies can be adversely affected.

As outpatient agencies increase as a result of the decreasing length of inpatient stay, psychiatric mental health nurses have additional choices for practice sites. Agencies that require weekend and shift work may find fewer applicants as nurses are able to obtain weekday-only positions.

As psychiatric mental health nurses become better educated through continuing and graduate studies and develop a more autonomous level of functioning, they seek, and demand, practice environments that encourage and support a professional level of practice. Participative management styles and shared governance will be expected.[23] Improvements in salary and benefit packages (commensurate with education, experience, and responsibility) are likely to result from increased competition between agencies for employees.

A psychiatric mental health nurse administrator of the future will develop highly competitive and marketable recruitment programs. Components of such programs include a highly competitive salary structure reviewed on a annual basis, a competitive cafeteria-style benefits system, and child care provided by the employing agency alone or in conjunction with other agencies. Nursing certification will be expected and will be facilitated through study groups, resources, and fee reimbursements. Tuition reimbursement will enable nurses to pursue additional education. Again, all aspects of a psychiatric mental health nursing department's recruitment program will need to be reviewed at least annually and modified as indicated.

The practice environment will have been professionalized and will serve as an effective retention tool. Career ladders reward, financially and professionally, all competent nurses who remain in a direct care capacity.[2] Increased flexibility in work hours enables a nurse to better balance work, home, family, and self in order to reduce or to prevent burnout.

A system for flexible budgeting also aids the psychiatric mental health nurse administrator in reducing burnout by maintaining a balanced caseload within the department. Systems will adjust staffing levels as client needs dictate. Contingent staffing groups will aid when there are increases in caseloads. Staff will also be involved in the development of mechanisms to provide additional educational or conference time when caseloads decrease.

Quality circles (groups of nursing staff meeting to plan and implement ways to improve the quality of nursing) will provide a mechanism for open communications between nursing administration and the direct care staff. Both groups will work as a team to provide high-quality nursing care in a cost-effective manner.

Nursing committees (practice, research, quality assurance, library, continuing education, and so on) must exist as needed to expand and maintain a professional environment. Peer review can replace standard performance evaluations.[27] The nurse can experience increased autonomy in the decision-making process and in setting of priorities with clients. As a result, nurses will experience a greater sense of control over their lives, and retention rates will improve.[1]

To facilitate this sense of control in the staff, a psychiatric mental health nurse administrator personally confronts the issue of control. If a nurse administrator cannot delegate, she or he becomes mired in the day-to-day conducting of the department's routine activities. In this situation, a future vision will be a luxury that cannot be afforded, and all nurse managers will be stifled in their growth as they function under the direction of the nurse administrator. Instead, nurse managers should be free to handle the routines of the department creatively, leaving the nurse administrator free to lead the department into the future.

In addition, if a psychiatric mental health nurse administrator is to professionalize the practice environment for nurses, she or he must have sufficient power to be effective. "Political savvy and effectiveness will be indispensable nursing skills. . . . Nurses must learn to influence the political machinery, become politically assertive, and influence, develop, and implement health policy." (reference 2, p 49). These ideas are also relevant in influencing, developing, and implementing policy within an agency. As psychiatric mental health nurse administrators become comfortable with this process, they accept that it is appropriate to care for oneself and one's own interests. In order to prevent burnout while providing high-quality nursing care, nurses must care for themselves and their profession. Without this self-caring, energy is only given and not replaced, eventually resulting in a crisis. A psychiatric mental health nurse administrator, by developing and exercising influence, serves as a role model in replacing the energy needed personally and by the department. Such influence frees an administrator to administer the department in a collaborative, rather than a hierarchical, manner. This influence, once developed, enables a smaller amount of energy to be utilized in the daily management of departmental activities.

The ability to influence, as with other skills, is achieved through a variety of mechanisms. Initially, a psychiatric mental health nurse administrator analyzes her or his level of comfort with the development and use of influence. A nurse administrator who is uncomfortable with the influence process is less effective in achieving a satisfactory level of influence. Through discussions with colleagues and the use of consultants and seminars, a nurse administrator can identify internal areas of resistance to the use of influence and decrease them.

Negotiation skills are crucial[2] in meeting the challenge of the nursing shortage. These skills are needed for a nurse administrator to coordinate the needs of a psychiatric mental health nursing department with the needs of other departments as well as those of the agency as a whole. Through this coordination, a nurse administrator demonstrates the ability to collaborate and to faciliate the movement of potentially conflictual projects, such as budget development. The ability to negotiate is also important for the nurse administrator's role modeling. The psychiatric mental health nurse administrator should be perceived, within both the department and the agency, as someone who listens to both sides of a conflict and acts to produce enabling results for both parties.

Finally, a communication style that includes openness to criticism and the critical analysis of ideas and comments needs to be cultivated.[4] In the process of developing influence and a professional practice environment, a nurse administrator needs to be open to criticism and complaints. Through processing both, a nurse administrator more realistically analyzes the actions of individuals and the overall department. Criticism and complaints, although often not valid, frequently present a point of view not previously considered. To ignore or discount these views isolates the nurse administrator from important information and fosters the development of a "we vs they" climate. Cultivation and analysis of these views demonstrates desirable behavior and fosters the growth of these behaviors within the department and the agency.

Relationships With Other Health Care Providers

The increased demand for nurses, coupled with nursing shortages, will foster a change in the relations between nurses and other health care providers. Nurses will be functioning on a more professional level as a result of changes in the practice environment and will expect to be treated as colleagues rather than the subordinate of the past.[5] Nurses focus on implementing protocols based on nursing diagnoses rather than on dependent functions such as medication administration.[5] It is projected that nursing diagnoses will be utilized more consistently to guide the planning of care and to communicate the focus of nursing care to other nurses and professionals. "The knowledge gap between nurses and physicians will decrease," (reference 12, p 6), and professionals will be grouped in treatment teams based on client needs rather than on traditional roles within a health care agency.[4]

An increasing need for nurses to articulate nursing's role in the delivery of psychiatric mental health care more clearly will support this new collaborative level of relationships. "Commonly understood descriptions of what nurses do for [clients] are essential if nursing is to be recognized as a principal contributor to [health care]" (reference 4, p 73). The collaborative and complementary aspects of the profession in relation to other mental health disciplines may be emphasized in the future rather than focusing on the substitutability of services. Without a clear definition of nursing, "nursing cannot deal effectively in multidisciplinary efforts to obtain scarce resources" (reference 4, p 76). Nurses need to work in collaboration, not in competition, with other health care providers to increase the effectiveness of a jointly derived treatment plan. Such collaboration can shorten the client's stay, and thereby increase the hospital's financial stability.

Initially, some further blurring of roles may occur, but this conflict could be resolved through the use of a peer-to-peer communication style.[3] This style emerges as health care providers recognize that all must work together to treat the client effectively in the most cost-effective manner. Ideally, a psychiatric mental health nurse administrator will anticipate these problems and include extensive communication skills training in both orientation and inservice programming. Assertiveness and conflict resolution could also be stressed through role-playing activities. Nurses will work with physicians to "negotiate policies that provide for shared decision-making, autonomy, improved staffing, career ladders, adequate equipment and resources" (reference 2, p 50).

With the decreasing length of stay, nursing activities that increase the client's ability to cope more quickly and efficiently must be clearly documented. Such documentation includes nursing diagnoses, type of nursing care given, client education, discharge planning, utilization of resources, and an evaluation of nursing care given. These data demonstrate the unique cost-effective role nursing plays within the agency.

Furthermore, the nurse administrator must work to establish, and facilitate the efforts of, joint practice committees. These committees should include representatives from nursing, medicine, occupational–recreational therapy, psychology, social work, and other professions involved in the delivery of direct care. These committees can address generic clinical problems that hinder the efficient delivery of good care. Through these committees, dialogue begins that enhances the collaborative efforts of all disciplines.

In order to accomplish these activities, a psychiatric mental health nurse administrator will need to be effective in conflict resolution.[4] Communication skills and related assertiveness techniques are critical if the nurse administrator is to maintain or improve relations between the nursing department and other departments within the agency. A psychiatric nursing administrator serves as the leader within the department and, as such, a role model within both the department and the agency. If the nursing staff view this individual as assertively communicating issues regarding client concerns and nursing care, they are more likely to be assertive regarding nursing and client issues. If other departments view a nurse administrator as articulating communicating concerns while retaining a perspective of the interests of the overall agency, they will be more likely to perceive clearly the importance of nursing's contributions to client care.

Networking efforts also facilitate collaboration between nursing and other departments.[25] Networking enables the nurse administrator to demonstrate the expertise of nursing to other departments. The contacts made through networking efforts provide a nurse administrator with opportunities to facilitate group movement during group projects. This ability assists in establishing the nurse administrator's image as a leader and improves the overall image of nursing within the setting.

A psychiatric mental health nurse administrator should closely monitor the changing relations between the department and other health care providers. Problem areas should be identified as soon as possible, and corrective actions taken to improve or facilitate collegial relations.

Increased Emphasis on Planning

To assure a professional practice environment for the delivery of psychiatric mental health nursing care, a nurse administrator consistently develops and implements both short- and long-range plans. Competition may increase, i.e., competition for both clients and staff. In addition, this competition may no longer be solely from the health care agency a few miles away. Even today, US hospitals are competing with European agencies to recruit nurses. Furthermore, as nurses' employment opportunities increase, traditional settings compete with businesses, pharmaceutical and health care supply companies, and private practice groups. Psychiatric mental health nurses are particularly qualified for positions in these areas as a result of their broad knowledge, experience, and expertise in communication skills.

To compete effectively in this environment, a psychiatric mental health nurse administrator "should not simply respond to the changes in the health care system, [they] should be involved in making them" (reference 10, p 496). The "potential is unlimited for the willing and able" (reference 4, p 72). The future vision for the department can be communicated through short- and long-term plans,[23] which are reviewed on an annual basis. Such plans encompass, not only mechanisms for coping with the competitive market, but also strategies to anticipate future health care trends. This planning incorporates the development of long-range plans (10 years), medium-range plans (3–5 years), and short-term plans (1 year). Each year, new objectives are developed that will provide the foundation for further implementation of the medium- and long-range plans. Hence, each year's objectives build on the work of previous years until the long-range plans are achieved. In addition, each year, the medium- and long-range plans should be reviewed and revised to ensure their relevancy.

Initially, these plans can be developed by incorporating feedback from quality circle meetings that address the vision of the department's future. An original set of plans is developed and then reviewed by nursing staff for feedback. Thereafter, on a yearly basis, all plans are reviewed by the nursing staff in order to assure that programmatic, and shift-specific, plans support the overall department goals.

In order to complete the planning process effectively, a psychiatric mental health nurse administrator should cultivate the ability to anticipate the future, gather data, and process information analytically. Without the ability to anticipate, planning efforts achieve only a medium-range capability, since long-range goals cannot be conceptualized.

Data gathering skills will also become more crucial. A nurse administrator identifies the data needed, the sources of data, and the individuals best qualified to obtain those data. Without these skills, a nurse administrator spends unnecessary time in this phase of planning.

A logical and analytical approach to planning enables a psychiatric mental health nurse administrator to realistically and specifically detail systematic objectives needed to attain the defined long-term goals. A nurse administrator needs to develop the ability to divide broader concepts and ideas into small components, which are in turn subdivided until division is no longer possible. Through such processing of information, a nurse administrator assists the department in attaining long-range goals through the development of small, realistically attainable objectives.

Interactive planning can be used throughout the department. This is a process "which is directed at gaining control of the future. Interactive planning designs a desirable future and identifies how to bring about a future as close as possible to the desired one" (reference 28, p 3). Part of this process utilizes the "law of the situation" in which an agency regularly "reconceptualizes its purpose in light of the changing world" (reference 29, p 3). A psychiatric mental health nursing department regularly redefines its purpose in order to ensure a realistic appraisal of the future. The resulting future vision is subdivided into smaller components that can be achieved in 1 to 5 years and that are assigned to relevant plans.[4]

"To continue to be effective, nursing cannot stabilize its practice, but must continue . . . to develop new insights into ways to help patients" (reference 4, p 79). There needs to be an increased emphasis on research and other departmental mechanisms to assist the direct care staff in maintaining productivity while caring for more acutely ill clients. Cost containment continues to be emphasized in the planning process as each health care setting seeks to maintain its market share while also maintaining financial stability and growth. This will become increasingly difficult as the economic situation continues to shift and countries move toward more global economies.[3]

Each of the departmental plans should be reviewed annually to ensure that its content is still relevant. The short-term plan needs to be reviewed quarterly, because its objectives may have been accomplished during the previous quarter.

SUMMARY

Clients "are hospitalized because they need nursing care" (reference 18, p 307). In the future, psychiatric mental health agencies will more clearly recognize the central role the nursing department plays in their financial stability. Psychiatric mental health nurse administrators need to act now to prepare the department to meet the challenges presented by the changing health care environment. Five major trends have been discussed from the perspective of a nurse administrator's role and the trend's impact on the psychiatric mental health nursing practice environment. A nurse

Research Highlights

In the past, research on nursing administration has not kept pace with the needs of nurse administrators,[30] particularly in psychiatric mental health nursing. Research is needed that focuses on the development of knowledge that is useful in the creation and facilitation of a professional practice environment.

Additional research is needed in many areas of nursing administration. Research, both initial and replicative, is needed to answer the following questions:

- What are the elements of a professional nursing practice environment?
- How can these elements best be facilitated?
- Does nursing curriculum content direct nurses' selection of a practice area? What influences a nurse's choice of a specialty area?
- What knowledge, skills, and attributes are needed by a nurse executive to enable her or him to lead a nursing department effectively and efficiently? Where

should these attributes, knowledge, and skills be acquired? How can they be acquired most efficiently?
- What model of staff assignment provides for the delivery of high-quality nursing care to a changing psychiatric client population? What model will be needed in the future?
- What role does nursing care play in the financial stability of a health care agency?
- What is the most effective system for evaluating the delivery of psychiatric mental health nursing care and the nursing staff?
- What facilitates collegial relations with other health care providers?

The answers to these and other research questions will aid in the development of a theoretical base for the administration of a psychiatric mental health nursing practice. This base will enable a nurse administrator to maintain a practice environment that facilitates the delivery of high-quality psychiatric mental health nursing care.

---

administrator, by serving as a role model with a vision for the department, will lead the the department into the future in a systematic and progressive fashion.

References

1. American Hospital Association. The nursing shortage: facts, figures and feelings—research report. Chicago: The Association; 1987.
2. Andreoli KG, Musser LA. Trends that may affect nursing's future. Nurs & Health Care. 1985;6:47–51.
3. Bartkowski JJ, Swandby JM. Charting nursing's course through megatrends. Nurs & Health Care. 1985;6:375–7.
4. Beyers M. Future of nursing care delivery. Nurs Admin Q. 1987;11(2):71–80.
5. Bille DA, Wright JE. Year 2000: committed, conscious colleagues. Nurs Admin Q. 1987;11(2):13–6.
6. Boston CM. The changing nursing practice environment: future employment opportunities. Imprint. 1985;32(5):14–7.
7. Brown B. From the Editor. Nurs Admin Q. 1987;11(2):vi–viii.
8. Cabinet on Nursing Research. Directions for nursing research: toward the twenty first century. Kansas City, Mo: American Nurses' Association; 1985.
9. Carter EW. Psychiatric nursing: 1986. J Psychosoc Nurs. 1986;24(6):26–30.
10. Carty R, Bednash G. Insights from the past portray nurses of the future. Nurs & Health Care. 1985;6:492–6.
11. Chamberlain JG. The role of the federal government in development of psychiatric nursing. J Psychosoc Nurs. 1983;21(4):11–8.
12. Christman L. The future of the nursing profession. Nurs Admin Q. 1987;11(2):1–8.
13. Curtin L. Nursing in the Year 2000: learning from the future. J Nurs Manage. 1986;17(6):7.
14. Daria J, Moran S. Nursing in the 90's. Nursing 85. 1985;15(12):26–9.
15. Editors. Ten trends to watch. Nurs & Health Care. 1986;7:17–9.
16. Evans C, Lewis S. Nursing administration of psychiatric-mental health care. Rockville, Md: Aspen Systems Corporation; 1985.
17. Ghiselli WB, Frances PS. The impact of the baby boom on the mental health system. Hosp & Community Psychiatry. 1985;36:536–7.
18. Kirby KK. Issues in nursing resource management: past and present. Nurs Econ. 1986;4:305–8.
19. LaBar C, McKibbin RC. New organizational models and financial arrangements for nursing services. Kansas City, Mo: American Nurses' Association; 1986.
20. McBride AB. Present issues and future perspectives of psychosocial nursing: theory and research. J Psychosoc Nurs. 1986;24(9):27–32.
21. McFarland GK, Leonard HS, Morris MM. Nursing leadership and management: contemporary strategies. New York: John Wiley & Sons; 1984.
22. Pothier P. The future of psychiatric nursing—revisited. Arch Psychiatr Nurs. 1987;1:299–300.
23. Porter–O'Grady T. Creative nursing administration: participative management into the 21st century. Rockville, Md: Aspen Systems Corporation; 1986.
24. Schoolcraft V. The future of nursing education and nursing practice. Imprint. 1985;32(3):38–42.
25. Schull PD. How to survive the coming changes in nursing: 5 things you can do. Nurs Life. 1986;6(4):18–23.
26. Simms LM, Price SA, Ervin NE. The professional practice of nursing administration. New York: John Wiley & Sons; 1985.
27. Spitzer R, Davivier M. Nursing in the 1990's: expanding opportunities. Nurs Admin Q. 1987;11(2):55–61.
28. Vestal K. Futurist executives. Aspen's Advisor for Nurse Executives. 1987;2(8):3.
29. Williams P. Economic responsibility and viability of the nursing department in the prospective pay environment. Nurs Admin Q. 1987;11(2):30–4.
30. Young LC, Hayne AN. Nursing administration: from concepts to practice. Philadelphia: WB Saunders Co; 1988.

54

Gail J. Ray

Quality Assurance in Psychiatric Nursing

OBJECTIVES
After reading this chapter, the reader will be able to:
1. Discuss the status of quality assurance in health care and psychiatric nursing
2. Describe the evolution of quality assurance and factors that have shaped it
3. Identify the components of quality assurance and explain how they relate to each other and to the umbrella concept of quality assurance
4. Describe the principal elements of the quality assurance process
5. Discuss factors to consider in developing a quality assurance plan and in conducting monitoring and evaluation activities.

DEFINITION AND OVERVIEW

Quality assurance is a program of systematic evaluation and action to ensure excellence in health care. Thus, there are three key elements in the quality assurance process: a value system, an appraisal system, and a response system. The focus of appraisal is the quality and appropriateness of important aspects of client care, the operation of systems to provide client care or support its delivery, and staff performance.[7,23,24,28] The aim is to provide meaningful organized information as the basis for guiding actions to maintain or improve the efficiency and effectiveness of practice.[5,27,35]

The five principal components of a comprehensive quality assurance program are client management, program implementation, resource utilization, risk management, and staff preparation[5,12,26,32] (Figure 54-1).

Client management focuses on the direct care and services provided to individual clients.

Program implementation targets the operation of systems and procedures for program and service delivery, including the accomplishment of goals and objectives.

Resource utilization considers the necessity for services as well as the allocation and use of resources.

Risk management examines measures to protect clients, visitors, and staff from injury or personal, material, or economic loss and to protect the organization from operational, human, material, or economic loss.

Staff preparation concentrates on the credentials, qualifications, and competence of personnel.

These five components, with their primary questions, provide a framework for conceptualizing the many factors affecting the quality of health care and of psychiatric nursing in particular (Table 54-1). These components are not mutually exclusive, and more than one may be addressed in a given activity. In fact, the information provided by the monitoring and evaluation activities from multiple perspectives provides a comprehensive view of the state of affairs within an organization.

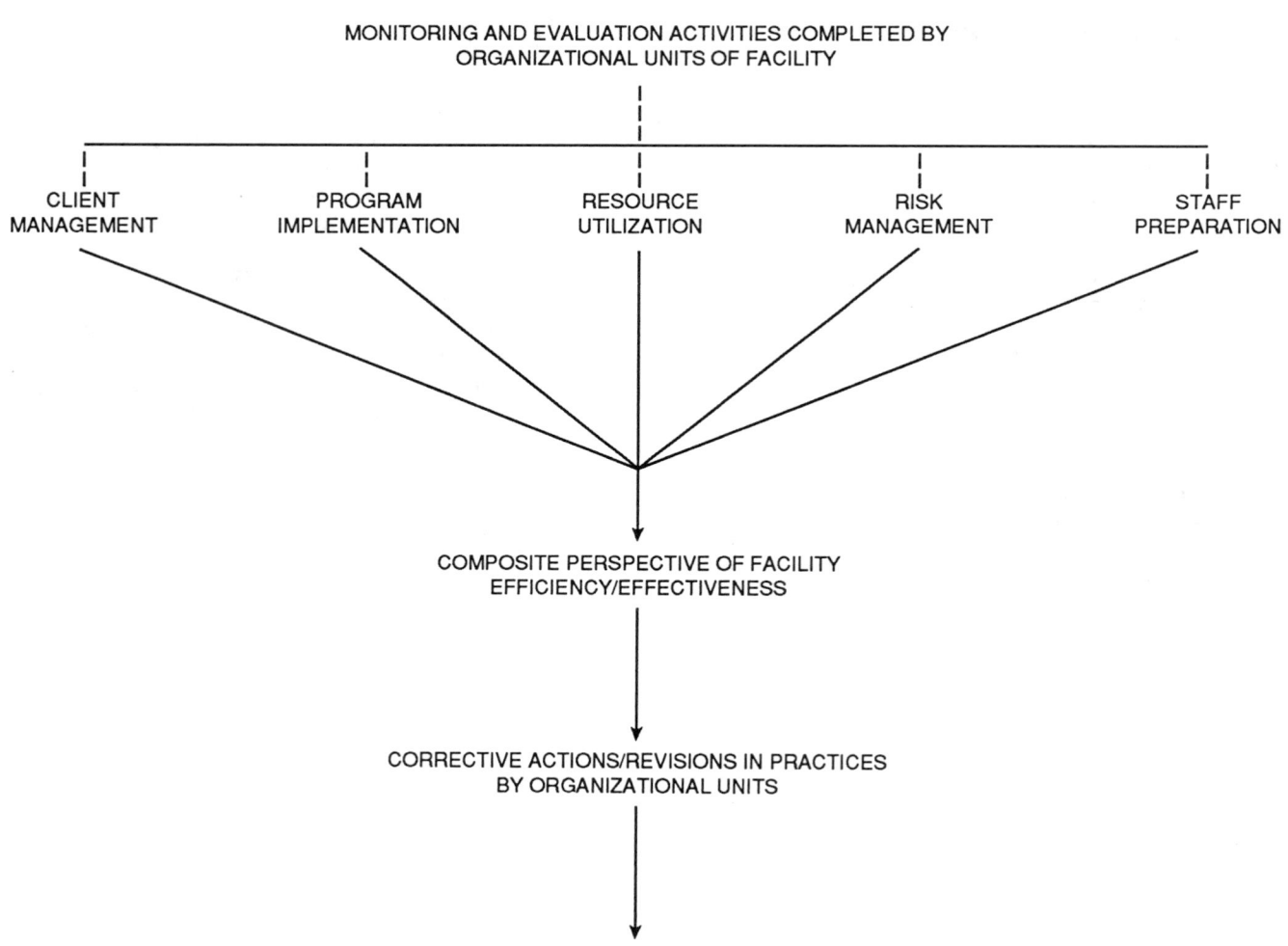

MONITORING AND EVALUATION ACTIVITIES COMPLETED BY
ORGANIZATIONAL UNITS OF FACILITY

CLIENT MANAGEMENT   PROGRAM IMPLEMENTATION   RESOURCE UTILIZATION   RISK MANAGEMENT   STAFF PREPARATION

COMPOSITE PERSPECTIVE OF FACILITY
EFFICIENCY/EFFECTIVENESS

CORRECTIVE ACTIONS/REVISIONS IN PRACTICES
BY ORGANIZATIONAL UNITS

ASSURANCE OF QUALITY CARE AND SERVICES

FIGURE 54–1. System for quality assurance. (© Gail J. Ray, 1988. Used with permission)

TABLE 54-1
Primary questions and potential inquiry areas for quality assurance components

COMPONENT	PRIMARY QUESTIONS	POTENTIAL INQUIRIES
Client management	Is the care provided to individual psychiatric clients appropriate to their clinical needs and provided according to professional standards?	Correctness of nursing diagnoses Appropriate selection of nursing interventions Effective nursing strategies to achieve specific client outcome(s)
Program evaluation	Is the care provided to groups of psychiatric clients through programmed activities appropriate to their clinical needs and provided according to professional standards? Are the systems and procedures that support psychiatric client care and agency operation appropriate to the needs of the recipients of the service or the agency and managed according to standards of good practice? Are goals and objectives appropriate and achieved to the extent necessary?	Appropriateness of selected activities for target group of psychiatric clients Appropriateness/achievement of client/unit/facility goals in selected areas Level of client/family satisfaction Appropriate utilization of volunteers Adequacy of interdisciplinary planning Adequacy of communication systems
Resource utilization	Are psychiatric clients, staff, or units receiving services if and when they are needed? Are human, material, and financial resources utilized efficiently, effectively, and to the extent required?	Necessity for delivering select services Appropriate distribution of personnel Availability of adequate equipment and supplies
Risk management	Are the measures taken to eliminate risks or reduce them to a minimum appropriate and sufficient to protect psychiatric clients, staff, and facility?	Adequacy of safety measures in handling HIV-positive clients and others Adequacy of measures to identify or confine infections within unit/agency Appropriateness of measures to minimize incidence of assault
Staff preparation	Are staff appropriately qualified for and competent in performing their assigned duties?	Sufficient credentials/current competence for providing selected services Appropriateness of staff assignments for meeting clinical needs of clients or units Effectiveness of inservices to enable staff to meet job expectations

FACTORS SHAPING QUALITY ASSURANCE

Quality assurance has been an increasing concern, particularly in the last two decades.[2,9] Psychiatric settings and psychiatric nursing have been affected by the same interplay of forces as other fields of nursing and health care.

The principal forces stimulating quality assurance endeavors are professional accountability; societal changes; demands by consumers, third-party payers (i.e., entities paying health care expenses on behalf of individual clients), and fourth-party payers (i.e., review organizations making determinations about client care on behalf of third parties); legal and political pressures; and technology.[24,25,32] As health care costs have continued to rise, emphasis on efficiency has increased. Simultaneously, and often through litigation, the expectations and rights of consumers have achieved greater prominence. The explosions in knowledge and technology have increased the complexity of nursing and health care delivery. This has contributed to the proliferation of a variety of delivery systems and health care providers. These factors have created external pressures for regulation and for evidence of professional accountability for services of sound quality delivered cost effectively. Concurrently, nursing has internal pressures for expanding and verifying its body of knowledge in order to gain full professional stature. These factors combine to necessitate a systematic method for constructing an organized data base for decisions and actions pertaining to the delivery of services and the performance of individual practitioners.[9,18,24,26,32,45]

Quality assurance practice for all specialties and practice settings has experienced significant changes in focus and advances in methodology through the years (Table 54-2). Efforts to integrate the five components are greater. Demands for increased research rigor and statistical analyses are growing as computers become more available and regulatory demands expand.[13,35,36,42] Nursing's ability to meet these demands in every practice setting is enhanced by the increasing number of nurses prepared with advanced degrees, the familiarity of more nurses at all levels of practice with research and evaluation techniques, and the growing volume of periodical literature within nursing.[36,42]

THE PSYCHIATRIC NURSING QUALITY ASSURANCE PLAN

Psychiatric care agencies are required to conduct comprehensive quality assurance programs and to have

TABLE 54-2
Summary of changes in evolution of quality assurance

PRE-1985	PRESENT
Professionally imposed regulations and definitions of quality	Externally imposed regulations and definitions plus professionally imposed regulations
Joint Commission mandate	Joint Commission and Health Care Financing Administration mandates; also, some states have legislated requirements
Focus on direct client care; mostly retrospective	Focus on all aspects of client care, system operation, and staff performance, including individual practice patterns; mostly concurrent
Problem focus	Routine monitoring for compliance or noncompliance plus problem appraisal
Sporadic reporting of a few problems solved	Systematic and continuous collection and periodic evaluation of data with routine reporting of all findings and activities
Individual departmental programs with few facility-wide concerns	Facility coordinated and integrated programs
Procedures and process focus	Quality/appropriateness and outcome of all major aspects of care/service/performance
Implicit or agency procedure criteria	Explicit criteria based on professional literature/standards and requiring expert judgment to apply/evaluate
Criteria applied by medical records or other select staff	Criteria applied by practitioners providing care or service plus others
Involvement by and concern of a few	Involvement by and concern of many: increased emphasis on peer review and distribution of information to more levels
Simple analyses	Simple and complex analyses

detailed written plans of how the programs operate. The agency's quality assurance plan describes the scope of the program; the responsibilities and authority of key participants, including the relations between organizational units within the agency; and the processes used to implement the program.

The psychiatric mental health nursing quality assurance program is a part of, but apart from, the organization's plan. It is a part of the plan because it is congruent with the mission, philosophy, goals, and objectives of the agency and takes direction from the agency plan. It is apart from the plan because it addresses specific nursing service needs.[10,31]

The requirements of a quality assurance plan and the quality assurance process are the same regardless of the setting, the size of agency, or the psychiatric nursing specialty. Thus, in this discussion, *nursing service* refers to the nursing component of an agency whether it comprises part or all of the organization. *Agency* or *facility* refers to any psychiatric care setting.

Scope

The scope of the nursing quality assurance plan must be sufficiently broad to include the range of care, services, or activities provided by the nursing service.[33,34] The scope differs depending on the size of the psychiatric nursing service and the diversity of practice areas within it. For example, the scope of the plan for a 20-bed adult psychiatric unit in a general hospital will differ from that of a walk-in crisis clinic or a 400-bed psychiatric facility with a range of services for child, adolescent, adult, and geriatric populations who have acute and chronic disorders and enter voluntarily as well as through civil and criminal commitment procedures.

The quality assurance plan specifies the basis for identifying the important aspects of the care, services, and activities provided and the indicators for evaluating them. Three considerations often provide direction for delimiting the important aspects: frequency of occurrence or volume of people/services affected, risk potential, and potential for problems or errors. Therefore, the aspects generally selected are either high frequency or volume, high risk, or problem prone.[1,39] The overriding determinant, however, is the selection of those dimensions or activities that are of greatest significance to the quality of psychiatric nursing and that provide valuable information on which to base decisions.

Roles and Responsibilities

Delineation of roles and responsibilities for ensuring implementation of the nursing quality assurance program is essential. Whether one person or a group is designated to direct and oversee the program depends on the size and complexity of the nursing service or the agency. Supervisory personnel within the agency or nursing service also play key roles in ensuring that the program operates. In addition, those responsible for setting nursing standards, identifying nursing indicators and criteria, completing review activities, analyzing and interpreting the findings, and completing reports are identified. Finally, how articulation occurs with other disciplines and key participants in the facility system is specified.[10,39]

The involvement of nurses throughout the organization in the quality assurance process, especially the review activities, is sometimes debated; however, the trend is toward increasing involvement. Peer review, although only one mechanism in a quality assurance program, is an important component of the quality assurance process and has many advantages. Among these are increased accountability of individual professionals; greater credibility and utility of review findings; increased awareness of standards, with subsequent incorporation into practice; greater integration of quality assurance into daily operations, with increased valuing of activities and findings; more realistic expectations, study of relevant issues, and action plans; and division of workload.[9,11,20,21,37,38,43] Opponents of staff nurse peer review argue that it is too time consuming, that nurses are resistant to evaluating each other, that liability is increased because of confidentiality and expert opinion issues, and that the validity of the findings is contaminated if individuals know the criteria by which they are evaluated or if there are several reviewers.[4,11,21,38,40] However, in one agency where three reviewer assignment options were used—nurse managers only, a few nurses selected by the managers, and multiple nursing staff—there was no difference in the quality of the evaluations.[4] This finding supports the contention that if principles of data collection are observed and interreliability testing mechanisms are used, quality assurance data can be valid, objective, and reliable even though many individuals are involved.[38]

Implementation

Procedures for collecting, tracking, reporting, and managing data are organized and articulated with the organization's total system. Consideration must be given to protecting the privacy and confidentiality of individual clients and care or service providers while ensuring that information is available for analyses and use by those needing the data to make decisions and to secure action when required. Internal systems are needed for scheduling and assigning the monitoring and evaluation activities; forwarding findings of reviews to those whose care, service, or performance was assessed, as well as to those needing the data for compilation and evaluation; writing reports; sharing results with appropriate parties at various levels within the facility; and ensuring that action plans are implemented. Calendars outlining the monitoring and evaluation schedule, flow charts depicting the dissemination of information, and organizational diagrams detailing functions and accountability are useful to supplement the written plan.[10,28,45]

The written plan includes the approaches for monitoring and evaluation such as case reviews and evaluation studies; the methods for data collection and the data sources; the sampling expectations; and the methods for analyzing and reporting data. Standardized formats for developing criteria sheets and data compilation forms or reporting case reviews, evaluation studies, and analyses are often required. These are useful for merging data from a variety of units within nursing or departments and services within the facility

and ensuring a coherent data bank for complex analyses.

A manual system for recording and analyzing data may be adequate for certain types of quality assurance activities or at the unit level. However, as activities increase in complexity and frequency, as more statistical analyses are required, and as the demand for manipulation of data increases, the need for computers increases. Although some software packages designed for quality assurance programs are available, none is comprehensive nor suited to the specific needs of individual facilities or units.[15] Software packages such as Systat and Ethnograph provide the most flexibility for quantitative and qualitative analyses of the variables determined essential for the organization's database. Ideally, information from all five quality assurance components is integrated to prevent errors and to increase efficiency. Coordinating and integrating the psychiatric nursing service analysis plan, including manual or automated aspects, with that of the facility is vital. Issues of confidentiality and liability must be addressed regardless of the data management system. For most agencies, a combination of manual and automated approaches will continue for some time.[6,15,46]

THE QUALITY ASSURANCE PROCESS IN PSYCHIATRIC SETTINGS
Value System

The value system of the quality assurance process is articulated in the standards, indicators, criteria, and compliance levels chosen by an organization and nursing service. These usually are reflected in the tools used for data collection and evaluation rather than the written plan.[33]

STANDARDS

Generic standards that fit the setting often form a practical basis for the quality assurance process. These standards are written universal organization or nursing service values that guide the activities of the agency. Standards express goals for practice. Ideally, they are based on research, but more often, they are based on expert opinion, empiric experience, and the professional literature.[7,11,17,33,41]

INDICATORS

Indicators—elements that reflect the overall quality of the important aspects of psychiatric nursing care, services, or activities—are selected as gauges for performance. The important aspects may differ in different practice settings; e.g., community mental health centers, state hospitals, nurse-operated clinics, research centers, and private practices. Regardless, the indicators encompass the five quality assurance components. They are monitored systematically and evaluated periodically to determine the degree of compliance with the expected level of quality and to make decisions regarding practice.

Two types of indicators are used:[19,29]

Volume indicators provide information regarding how much activity is taking place; e.g., the number of client assaults or the number of clients per nurse therapist. They provide a context for interpreting quality and appropriateness or warn that something may be amiss.

Quality/appropriateness indicators indicate how well the nursing provider or service is performing; e.g., accuracy and precision of nursing diagnoses, adequacy of articulation of services with those of another discipline. These indicators are the heart of the quality assurance program, because they provide information regarding the strengths of the care or service and actual or potential problem areas.[19,29]

Depending on the size and diversity of the nursing service within an organization, some indicators may apply throughout the service, whereas others are unit specific. Both are essential if units within the nursing service have unique features.[7,16]

CRITERIA

Explicit criteria that define compliance with the quality/appropriateness indicators are established before undertaking review activities. All criteria reflect current practice as described in the professional literature and are pertinent for the purpose of the review. Criteria emanate from the agency or nursing service generic standards and define acceptable practice at the case level.[11,34] Rather than focusing on behaviors related to procedures or tasks, the best criteria target sound judgments, pertinent observations, and significant actions that contribute to client welfare or high-quality services. Such criteria accommodate the unique features of each case and provide more relevant information.[22,43] Criteria are developed from three points of view: structure, process, and outcome.

Structure criteria describe conditions that allow or contribute to quality; e.g., complete staff orientation prior to assignment in a new area.

Process criteria describe practices that should take place in the care or service delivery process; e.g., alternative interventions to defuse escalating behavior precede seclusion.

Outcome criteria describe results; e.g., clients completing sessions on thought-stopping techniques identify and interrupt negative self-talk.

Unless the need for information is restricted to one view, relations between structure, process, and outcome are examined rather than considering each separately.[3,43,44] Once criteria are written, they are used repeatedly until the indicator changes. Sometimes,

multiple criteria sets may be established for one indicator. Although used repeatedly, multiple sets provide variety for reviewers and broader perspectives in reviewing key issues.[16,22,33]

COMPLIANCE LEVELS

Because each criterion considers performance at the case level, it is expected the criterion will be met in every case. However, perfect compliance is difficult to achieve and often unrealistic; therefore, an acceptable standard of compliance is established for an aggregate of cases; e.g., 95% of clients have a comprehensive nursing assessment within 24 hours of admission. The level of accepted compliance is based on the degree of adverse effect if the criterion is not met, as well as what is realistic according to expert opinion, experience, and the literature. Compliance levels are established for each criterion, defining compliance with an indicator as well as the indicator as a whole. The individual criteria may all be the same as the indicator or differ depending upon the nature of the criterion.[1,7,22,30]

Sometimes, the compliance level is written as a relative change in performance; e.g., the number of falls resulting from orthostatic hypotension will decline 2% in the next quarter. The factors used for establishing the level of accepted compliance also apply for change levels.[7]

NURSING DIAGNOSES

Nursing diagnoses are traditionally associated with direct care; however, they may be used to develop quality assurance activities for all five components (Table 54-3). Using nursing diagnoses to direct quality assurance activities has important advantages. First, it allows nurses to conceptualize and assess practice from nursing's perspective. Second, systematic evaluation promotes data-based refinement of existing diagnoses and development of new ones. Finally, study of nursing diagnoses in multiple and diverse settings, with sharing through publication, contributes to a scientific knowledge base for clinical nursing practice.

Appraisal System

The appraisal system is the second major element of the quality assurance process. It includes the procedures for gathering information and the systems for evaluating it.

TYPES OF REVIEW

Two primary approaches are used to monitor quality/appropriateness indicators and to evaluate compliance with standards. These are case reviews and evaluation studies.

Case reviews collect data regarding the care or service provided to or by one or a few individuals at a given time, and each review considers one individual

TABLE 54–3
Nursing diagnosis example: suicide potential

COMPONENT	POTENTIAL INDICATORS
Client management	Changes in levels of suicidal ideation and risk are assessed precisely
	Goals for reducing or eliminating suicidal ideation are appropriate for individual
Program evaluation	Therapies assist suicidal clients to learn and use alternative behaviors to manage stress
	Clients can describe community resources and when and how to access them
Risk management	Suicidal clients are identified and correct protective measures instituted
	Environmental hazards are controlled to the extent necessary to protect suicidal clients
Resource utilization	Sufficient staff are assigned to ensure procedures for monitoring suicidal clients are enforced
	Continuous observation is used only to the extent indicated by clients' assessed risk
Staff preparation	Nurses know elements of comprehensive suicide assessment
	Staff are oriented to agency's procedures for handling suicidal clients
Combination Indicator:	Adequacy of Care Compliance: 95%
Criteria:	1. Complete assessment at admission and regular intervals as indicated 95%
	2. Appropriate precautions based on assessed level of risk 95%
	3. Assignment of appropriate therapies 90%
	4. Progress in using alternative behaviors 100%
Approach:	Evaluation study: 40 discharged clients

or event as the unit of analysis. For example, every month, two cases per nurse are reviewed for the quality of documentation regarding client progress toward treatment goals. Such reviews have several advantages. They allow a spot check of care, service, or performance so that problems may be detected early. There is potential to improve staff performance or the care or services being provided to one or a few individuals because the feedback is timely. Reviews can be integrated into the workload with a minimum of disruption, and they are an excellent way to involve staff in quality assurance, maintain their awareness of standards, and improve their performance.

At intervals, when the sample is sufficient, the data can be collated and analyzed for patterns or trends. This approach captures the reality of care, services, or performance over time under varied circumstances and presents opportunities to revise practices if needed to improve care or services for future recipients.[7,11,22,29]

Evaluation studies consider a group of events or individuals as the unit of analysis and collect the data for the group in a reasonably short period of time. That is, the sample is sufficiently large to reflect the status of the whole event or population during one time period so that general conclusions can be drawn about the whole.[22] For example, staffing patterns covering a 1- or 2-month period are analyzed to determine if they meet client nursing care needs adequately. Evaluation studies can be completed at routine intervals to determine compliance with standards and to ascertain patterns or trends. This approach is sometimes preferable to case reviews because of the nature of the indicator or the resources available to complete the activity. In addition, evaluation studies are necessary in order to deter-

mine the scope, cause, or resolution of known or suspected problems.[1,33]

DATA COLLECTION

Data sources and retrieval methods are selected to ensure collection of the most relevant information in the most efficient manner. These methods are dictated by the indicators and criteria. Multiple data sources and retrieval methods are encouraged for flexibility and increased validity. The potential sources of information include client or personnel records; client, visitor, or personnel comments or complaints; logs; oral or written reports; memoranda; minutes of meetings; findings from outside reviewing bodies; program statistics; client–staff interactions; staff–staff interactions; skill demonstrations; and staffing sheets. Common methods include content analysis, observation, interviews, questionnaires, and tests.[22,36,44]

Quality assurance data are collected on a concurrent, retrospective, or prospective basis.

Concurrent reviews consider clients currently being treated or events, activities, or actions occurring in the present; e.g., updating of treatment plans based on ongoing assessment.

Retrospective reviews consider clients who are no longer being treated or past events, activities, or actions; e.g., the care preceding the commission of suicide by a client.

Prospective reviews consider future clients, activities, or events, often with a designated starting point; e.g., the first 20 clients assigned to continuous ob-

CHART 54–1
Considerations in Monitoring and Evaluation Activities

FOCUS OF ACTIVITY

Is the central concern related to important aspect(s) of psychiatric nursing care/service/staff performance?
Does the central concern fall within or target the scope or domain of psychiatric nursing?
Will the results provide useful information for decision making in the psychiatric nursing unit(s) *and* the facility?
Is the evaluation focused on the "quality" and "appropriateness" of the psychiatric nursing care/service/performance?
Is the expert knowledge and judgment of nurses required to conduct the evaluation?

OBJECTIVE MEASURABLE INDICATORS AND CRITERIA

Do they target sound professional judgments, pertinent observations, and significant actions in psychiatric nursing?
Do they focus on valid or important considerations?
Are they current, correct, and consistent with accepted standards for psychiatric nursing practice?
Are they specific and retrievable?
Are they realistic?
Are they relevant to the purpose of the review?
Do they reflect the source of data if several sources are used in the review?

TOOLS

Criteria sheet: individual review
  Is there one per case?
  Are there sufficient identifying data to
    Provide individual performance data for care/service provider if applicable and reviewer?
    Allow quick retrieval of record/data source if there is a need to review again?
    Fix the time of review?
  Is there a compliance rating method to identify achievement of each criterion; e.g., scale, yes/no, points?
  Is the rating method appropriate for the review consideration?
  Is there space for comments to support or explain rating?
  Is it easy to use and limited to one sheet?
Data retrieval tools: Necessity depends on focus of the review activity. If more than a criteria sheet is needed, tools may be developed or selected to gather data against which to apply criteria. Examples are questionnaires, interview guides, and tests.
  Are these constructed according to research or educational principles?
  Do they provide information relevant to the review activity?
Data compilation form: aggregate review
  Does it allow flexibility to look at various sample sizes?
  Does it reflect the criteria used?
  Does it include the level of compliance achieved and the accepted standard for each criterion *and* the indicator composite?
  Does it display information in manner that facilitates identification of patterns?
  Is it easy to use and limited to one sheet?

METHODS

Is there assigned responsibility for collecting data?
Is the frequency of data collection specified?
Does the methodology ensure an adequate sample based on:
  Frequency of occurrence?
  Degree of risk?
  Cases necessary to identify deviations (effect size)?
  Provision of data for each care/service provider if indicated?
Is there assigned responsibility for evaluating data?
Is the frequency for data analysis (evaluation) specified and appropriate to the review activity?
Is there a mechanism for taking action if necessary to correct or improve psychiatric nursing practice?
Are there mechanisms to ensure protection (confidentiality/privacy) of sensitive information and individuals?

EVALUATION OF DATA

Is there an acceptable standard of compliance or relative change in performance established for each criterion?
Is the level of accepted compliance or change appropriate to the focus of the indicator or criterion and the sample size?
Is there identification of criteria with achievement within accepted compliance or change levels?
Is there identification of criteria with achievement below accepted compliance or change levels?
Is there justification for failure to comply with criterion?
Does the noncompliance or lack of change indicate
  More data are needed through intensified monitoring or problem appraisal study?
  Something is wrong?
Are mechanisms in place to handle deviations from accepted compliance or change levels?
What patterns or trends exist in the aggregate analyses?
What patterns or trends exist in the individual analyses; e.g., caregiver, criterion, justified exceptions?
What conclusions may be drawn regarding patterns and trends?

COMMUNICATIONS

Is there assigned responsibility for developing summary reports?
Is the frequency and format for reporting to nursing or facility QA committees or department specified?
Are there mechanisms for providing information to care/service providers regarding
  Nursing unit(s) performance?
  Individual performance if applicable?

servation beginning June 1 for nursing care needs on that status.

Most reviews are concurrent because they allow timely feedback and provide the opportunity to effect any needed change when it will be most helpful. All three types provide opportunities to effect change for the future.[24]

The sampling procedures depend on the purposes of the review. The sample must be adequate to provide the necessary information and representative of the population being monitored, e.g., clients, care or service providers, or services. Considerations include the importance of the indicator; frequency of occurrence; whether the phenomenon being studied has a small, medium, or large effect (small effects require a larger sample to identify variations); number of data collectors; time available; and analysis techniques.[1,36]

ANALYSIS AND INTERPRETATION

The frequency of and sample size for data collection are specified in the monitoring plan or unit calendar. Depending on whether the approach is evaluation study or case review, there may be one or multiple data collection periods to gather a sufficient volume of data for evaluation; i.e., analysis and interpretation. Analysis and interpretation is completed for various levels: individual provider, unit, service, facility. The plan specifies the responsibilities for evaluation and the focus of evaluation at the various levels. The complexity of analysis increases as the level increases.

Analysis and interpretation of the data entails several activities. The data must be displayed in a manner that facilitates identification of patterns. Tabulations are completed to determine the fit between the actual performance and the established standard of compliance or change for each criterion and the indicator. Themes of criteria with high and low compliance are identified, and patterns are examined in relation to elements such as client ages or diagnoses, shifts (if appropriate), units, comments related to compliance or noncompliance, and individual care or service providers. Whether data are submitted to additional statistical analyses is determined by the type of data, level for analysis within the facility, computer support, and preparation and skills of the personnel. Compliance levels and patterns are compared with earlier findings, applicable volume indicators, and findings from other areas to determine the existence of trends. Finally, the findings are interpreted. Compliance levels, patterns, or trends are neither positive nor negative until they are explained or given meaning by an individual or group with the expertise to interpret them. Strengths, as well as areas to improve or correct, must be addressed.[1,8,16]

Response System

The final element in the quality assurance process is the response system. If the needed action exceeds the authority of the nursing service, recommendations are forwarded to the body with the authority to act.

On the basis of the interpretations of the findings,

Research Highlights

As quality assurance expectations have changed through the years, debate has continued regarding the need for and desirability of involving individuals of all levels of practice in quality assurance activities. Yet, familiarity with as well as positive valuing and incorporation of quality assurance activities into everyday practice is essential if quality assurance goals are to be achieved.[4,14,40]

Edwardson and Anderson reported the findings of a study designed to test whether positive attitudes and quality assurance experience are related.[9] Three hundred eight nurses from ten hospitals (76% of a random stratified sample) were surveyed regarding their attitudes toward quality assurance, involvement in various aspects of the hospital nurse's role, and general satisfaction in employment. Nurses who had quality assurance experience were more likely to believe quality assurance was a responsibility of all levels of nursing personnel and part of the nurse's daily activities. They were also more likely to want to participate, especially in activities related to direct client care; i.e., writing standards and reviewing care provided by other nurses. They were less likely to view quality assurance only as a means for achieving accreditation. All quality assurance activities ranked lower than direct client care activities in prefer-

ence for involvement regardless of whether nurses had quality assurance experience.

Smeltzer, Hinshaw, and Feltman also found a positive relation between attitudes and experience when they compared two groups of nurses randomly selected at one hospital: those who had participated in the quality assurance program (N = 82) and those who had not (N = 71).[38] Most of the involved nurses indicated that their participation had an impact on their nursing care. Also, they said they would continue involvement in quality assurance in new positions if they terminated their current employment.

Both studies lend support to the belief that direct involvement in the quality assurance process improves practice, develops more positive attitudes toward participation, increases nurses' perceived value of the quality assurance process, and increases professionalism among nurses through standard setting and peer review. An important implication of these findings is that for the purpose of quality assurance to be achieved, quality assurance activities must be directly linked by job design to the activities that provide internal rewards for nurses and for which they are accountable.

action plans are developed at each level of analysis for implementation within nursing.[41] The action may be to praise high-quality performance and continue current practices. If changes in practice are necessary to improve efficiency or correct deficiencies, the plan contains the following: who or what is expected to change, who is responsible for implementing action, what action is appropriate, and when change is expected.[39] A record is maintained of actions taken, and if necessary, progress reports are made. The effectiveness of the action plan is assessed with the ongoing monitoring and the next evaluation.

Three common causes of problems are insufficient knowledge, defective systems, and deficient behavior or performance. Knowledge deficits may be addressed by providing classes or special educational activities, increasing reference sources, or restructuring inservice and staff development requirements or procedures. System defects may be addressed by adding or revising policies or procedures, redistributing staff, altering the use of equipment or supplies, changing types of equipment or supplies, or modifying communication mechanisms or channels. Staff performance problems may be addressed through counseling or disciplinary procedures, modifications in privileges or staff status, reassignments, or increased supervision.[1,45]

SUMMARY

Quality assurance is assuming an increasingly important position in psychiatric mental health nursing and health care practice. It is a process applicable to any setting (Chart 54-1). Although its fundamental purpose is to improve the care or services within a given organization, quality assurance has the potential to expedite nursing's progress in the quest for professional stature.

References

1. Accreditation for residential treatment centers. Chicago: Joint Commission on Accreditation of Healthcare Organizations; 1988.
2. Barhyte DY. Computer-generated quality assurance: nontraditional uses of data. J Nurs Qual Assur. 1987;1(4):43–9.
3. Beckman JS. What is a standard of practice? J Nurs Qual Assur. 1987;1(2):1–6.
4. Brubakken K, Cheney AM: The nursing care plan: monitoring for quality. J Nurs Qual Assur. 1987;1(3):79–80.
5. Clemenhagen C, Champagne F. Quality assurance as part of program evaluation: guidelines for managers and clinical department heads. QRB. 1986;12(11):383–7.
6. Conroy LL. Integration of manual and computerized components in nursing quality assurance. J Nurs Qual Assur. 1987;1(4):15–22.
7. Coyne C, Killien M. A system for unit based monitors of quality of nursing care. J Nurs Admin. 1987;17(1):26–32.
8. Driever MJ. Interpretation: a critical component of the quality assurance process. J Nurs Qual Assur. 1988;2(2):55–8.
9. Edwardson SR, Anderson DI. Hospital nurses' valuation of quality assurance. J Nurs Admin. 1983;13(7–8):33–9.
10. Evans CLS, Lewis SK. Nursing administration of psychiat-

ric–mental health care. Rockville, Md: Aspen Systems Corporation; 1985.
11. Evans E, Heggie J. Implementing a continuous unit-specific quality assurance monitor. J Nurs Qual Assur. 1988;2(2):16–23.
12. Fifer WR. Risk management and quality assurance. QRB Special Edition: Spring 1980;35–9.
13. Fifer WR. Quality assurance in the computer era. QRB. 1987;13:266–70.
14. Fine RB. Conceptual perspectives on the organization design task and the quality assurance function. Nurs Health Care. 1985;6(2):101–4.
15. Greer J, Hexum J. Dimensions of computerized quality assurance systems. J Nurs Qual Assur. 1987;1(4):9–14.
16. Hexum JM. Monitoring standards instead of problems. J Nurs Qual Assur. 1987;1(3):8–13.
17. Kanar RJ. Standards of nursing practice assessed through the application of the nursing process. J Nurs Qual Assur. 1987;1(4):72–8.
18. Kennedy JR. Risk management for allied health departments. QRB. 1984;10(6):175–80.
19. Kibbee P. Methods of monitoring quality in a psychiatric setting. J Nurs Qual Assur. 1987;1(3):64–70.
20. Maciorowski LF, Beckman JS. QA forum: how do peer review and quality assurance relate? J Nurs Qual Assur. 1987;1(4):77–8.
21. Macioroski L, Beckman J, Schroeder P. QA forum: how can we prepare staff nurses for participation? J Nurs Qual Assur. 1986;1(1):82–4.
22. Marker CGS. Practical tools for quality assurance: criteria development sheet and data retrieval form. J Nurs Qual Assur. 1988;2(2):43–54.
23. Marker CGS. The Marker model: a hierarchy for nursing standards. J Nurs Qual Assur. 1987;1(2):7–20.
24. Meisenheimer CG. Quality assurance: a complete guide to effective programs. Rockville, Md: Aspen Systems Corporation; 1985.
25. Melnick SD, Lyter LL. The negative impacts of increased concurrent review of psychiatric inpatient care. Hosp Community Psychiatry. 1987;38:300–3.
26. Monagle JF. Risk management: a guide for health care professionals. Rockville, Md: Aspen Systems Corporation; 1985.
27. Mottet EA. Monitoring is only the beginning. J Nurs Qual Assur. 1987;1(3):23–7.
28. Nadzam DM, Akins M. The pyramid for quality assurance. J Nurs Qual Assur. 1987;2(1):13–20.
29. Neubauer JA, Begley B, Jankowski BZ, Keller K. Development and implementation of unit-based monitors. J Nurs Qual Assur. 1988;2(2):1–8.
30. Ortega TS, Agbayani FP. Compliance with standards of nursing practice: use of a peer review system. J Nurs Qual Assur. 1987;1(2):59–65.
31. Pelle D. An integrative approach to quality assurance. J Nurs Qual Assur. 1986;1(1):8–16.
32. Pena JJ, Haffner AN, Rosen B, Light DW, eds. Hospital quality assurance. Rockville, Md: Aspen Systems Corporation; 1984.
33. Peters DA, Poe SS. Using monitoring in a home care quality assurance program. J Nurs Qual Assur. 1988;2(2):32–7.
34. Quality assurance in hospital-based psychiatric settings. Chicago: Joint Commission on Accreditation of Hospitals; 1986.
35. Roberts JS, Walczak RM. Toward effective quality assurance: the evolution and current status of the JCAH QA standard. QRB. 1984;10(1):11–5.
36. Schroeder PS, Maibusch RM, eds. Nursing quality assur-

ance: a unit-based approach. Rockville, Md: Aspen Systems Corporation; 1984.

37. Simons S. Monitoring practice: simplifying and strengthening the process. J Nurs Qual Assur. 1987;1(3):71–7.

38. Smeltzer CH, Hinshaw AS, Feltman B. The benefits of staff nurse involvement in monitoring the quality of patient care. J Nurs Qual Assur. 1987;1(3):1–7.

39. Staff of the Division of Education and the Division of Accreditation, Joint Commission on Accreditation of Hospitals. Monitoring and evaluation of the quality and appropriateness of care: a hospital example. QRB. 1986;12(9):326–30.

40. Stahler GJ, Rappaport H. Do therapists bias their ratings of patient functioning under peer review? Community Ment Health J. 1986;22(4):265–74.

41. Thompson MW, Hylka SC, Shaw CF. Systematic monitoring of generic standards of patient care. J Nurs Qual Assur. 1988;2(2):9–15.

42. Watson CA, Bulechek GM, McCloskey JC. QAMUR: a quality assurance model using research. J Nurs Qual Assur. 1987;2(1):21–7.

43. Weinberg N. Creating a culture of quality practice among physicians. QRB. 1987;13(12):405–10.

44. Westfall UE. Nursing diagnosis: its use in quality assurance. Top Clin Nurs. 1984;5(4):78–88.

45. Whittaker A, McCanless L. Nursing peer review: monitoring the appropriateness and outcome of nursing care. J Nurs Qual Assur. 1988;2(2):24–31.

46. Wilson CK. Quality assurance: should you computerize? J Nurs Qual Assur. 1987;1(4):1–8.

55

Irene Daniels Lewis

Education

CURRICULUM DEVELOPMENT
SUBSPECIALITIES
ADVANCED GENERALISTS VS SPECIALISTS
RECRUITMENT
DEVELOPMENT OF RESEARCH CAREER: NIMH ROLE
MARKETPLACE TRENDS
Home Health Agencies
Psychotherapist and Other Roles
Nursing Diagnosis
Case Management

OBJECTIVES
After reading this chapter, the reader will be able to:
1. Compare and contrast the past education of psychiatric mental health nurses with that in the present
2. Describe the present transitional state of psychiatric mental health nursing programs
3. Describe the influence of funding on psychiatric mental health nursing curriculum development
4. Analyze the relation between trends in the marketplace and graduate nursing program development.

INTRODUCTION

In this chapter, past and current trends in psychiatric mental health nursing education will be discussed, as well as selected social and environmental factors that influence this education. Currently, psychiatric mental health nursing education is in a state of flux. A brief look at the history of this field will enable the reader to understand the present situation better.

The first formal programs for student nurses preparing for general medical–surgical client care in the United States were started at the Hospital for Women and Children in Massachusetts and the Women's Hospital in Philadelphia in 1872. Ten years later, a separate training program for psychiatric client care emerged at McLean Hospital in Waverly, Massachusetts. Initially, the training program was for attendants; however, it evolved into a program for nurses.[24] This parallel approach of educating nurses in separate apprenticeship programs continued into the 1900s.

CURRICULUM DEVELOPMENT

From the beginning of psychiatric mental health nursing education in 1882 until the 1930s and early 1940s, theoretical or scientific concepts, with the exception of psychoanalytic theory, played a minimal role. Later, as content developed around somatic and environmental concepts, physicians, who were the nursing instructors at the time, taught psychiatric nurses how to give safe, comforting measures to mentally ill clients.

The National Institute of Mental Health (NIMH) was created in 1946, and one of its mandates from Congress was to increase psychiatric nursing personnel.[6,13] Initially, NIMH awarded six training grants to support graduate education, and as in other nursing graduate programs, the emphasis was on such functional areas as teaching, administration, and consultation. Later, NIMH funded undergraduate programs, and the emphasis was on the integration of mental health and behavioral concepts into undergraduate curricula. By the end of the 1950s, NIMH monies resulted in four significant changes in psychiatric mental health nursing:

1. Master's degree programs in psychiatric mental health nursing ranged from 1 to 2½ years;
2. Psychiatric mental health and behavioral concepts were integrated into undergraduate curricula;
3. The role of psychiatric mental health nurses had expanded and graduates were known as specialists;
4. There was an increase in the use of theoretical and scientific concepts from the social and behavioral sciences as well as an increase in the use of psychoanalytic theory.[6]

By this time, advanced nursing education had moved to universities, and in the 1960s, all post-basic preparation for specialization in nursing was found in graduate programs. Master's degreed psychiatric mental health nurses were sought for deanships, top-ranking professional organizations, and government positions.[10] The speciality was on the "cutting edge of change in nursing" and "was considered avant garde."[10] During this period, the research and theoretical contributions of Dumas, Peplau, and Diers did much to influence psychiatric mental health nursing curricula. At the same time, NIMH's funding priorities emphasized clinical training and research, replacing teaching, administration, and consultation.

Another concurrent change that influenced psychiatric mental health nursing curriculum development was the emergence of community mental health legislation. The 1963, Community Mental Health Centers Act promoted additional changes in psychiatric mental health education in order to incorporate content and skills for another emerging role, that of the community mental health nurse. Information about group dynamics, community organization systems, family and group therapies, health care delivery systems, and the politics of health care were introduced into graduate programs.[6] Concurrent with the 1963 Community Mental Health Centers Act, cultural upheavals, including the civil rights movement and the Vietnam war, had a significant impact on psychiatric mental health nursing education. For the first time, concern about underrepresented population groups and their mental health needs surfaced.[13] The focus in psychiatric theories shifted from psychoanalytic to crisis intervention, reality orientation, psychodrama, and behavior modification. An important change in therapeutic interventions was the popularity of group work with clients, in particular, group work involving psychiatric mental health nurses, in which nurses could apply skills and concepts they had learned in graduate programs.

As nurses worked more closely with clients, the need for coursework in another area became evident. To prepare graduates for the real world of politics in the health care delivery system, information about payment systems was integrated into the curriculum.

SUBSPECIALITIES

The psychiatric mental health nursing speciality has a number of subspecialities. Community mental health and psychiatric liaison nursing are examples. The child psychiatric nursing subspeciality was the first to establish and disseminate standards for practice: in 1985, under the auspices of the Council of Psychiatric and Mental Health Nursing.[3] In the 1970s, three new subspecialities emerged: geropsychiatric nursing,[9] chronically mentally ill care,[17] and substance abuse nursing.[22] This trend toward subspecialities in psychiatric mental health nursing education developed primarily because of new knowledge in the field, public concerns, and funding priorities.

Psychiatric mental health nurse educators and researchers have expressed concerns about the trend toward subspecialization and the need for theory-based practice and whether the former issue is compatible with psychiatric mental health nursing graduate education goals.[11,21] For example, a critical curriculum issue raised by data in the Murphy and Hoeffer article is that because "49% of . . . graduate programs in this survey do not require a theory-and/or research-based core course in psychiatric-mental health nursing . . . the foundation of the speciality is unclear."[21] There were 68 programs in the aforementioned survey, and 18% of the program directors were concerned that core content would be diluted by subspeciality courses in light of the current pressure to shorten programs.

Today, in spite of the American Nurses' Association Council on Psychiatric and Mental Health Nursing Standards of Practice, there continues to be ambiguity among leaders in the field about what constitutes core curriculum content for the speciality.[11,21] In addition, the optimal length for graduate programs is as yet undecided. As early as 1949, the National Organization for Public Health Nursing vigorously debated the optimal and minimal number of required graduate hours in psychiatric mental health nursing education. At that time, recommendations included 12 months, 15 months, and 24 months.[6,13] The debate has continued in spite of current pressure to shorten programs.[21] There are two major reasons for supporting a shortened program. The first is related to the proliferation of doctoral programs in nursing. If a student desires further knowledge, content is available at the advanced level. Second, although most leaders in the field agree that some programs do not allow enough time for course work, clinical experience, and the completion of a master's thesis or comprehensive examination, justification for the funding of programs of 2½ years is becoming more difficult. This lack of consistency in content and indecisiveness about the minimal length of master's degree education is reflected in the final product of psychiatric mental health nursing programs. The author suggests that the aforementioned curriculum trends and concerns be debated, studied, and resolved as soon as possible. It is too early to draw conclusions. However, as new knowledge emerges from targeted research on phenomena related to psychiatric mental health, and as interventions are tested and theory develops, today's issues can and will be resolved.

ADVANCED GENERALISTS VS SPECIALISTS

Another debate in the field poses the question: are programs producing advanced generalists or specialists? According to the American Nurses' Association Statement on Graduate Education, a generalist has a comprehensive approach to health care and can assess, diagnose, plan, intervene, and evaluate health needs of diverse individuals, groups, and communities and has expert knowledge and skills. On the other hand, a specialist can apply a broad range of theories to a population at risk; can draw on scientific knowledge and ex-

tensive experience; and is an expert in a specific area.[8] Some leaders believe that all psychiatric mental health nurses are specialists, whereas others believe that some are specialists but others are more properly described as advanced generalists. Reed and Hoffman stated that both specialists and advanced generalists are produced today,[27] but on the basis of program outcomes, course descriptions, learner objectives, and indepth clinical experiences with age groups across the life span, many graduates of psychiatric mental health nursing programs could be viewed as advanced generalists. On the frontier are those programs that respond to society's changing demographic needs. One such subspeciality is geropsychiatric mental health nursing.

Undergraduates who find psychiatric mental health nursing exciting and challenging and who want to know more about mental health nursing are encouraged to pursue advanced knowledge and skills at the graduate level. For a comprehensive, up-to-date, succinct description of graduate psychiatric mental health nursing programs, the author recommends reviewing the *Journal of Psychosocial Nursing and Mental Health Services* Volume 26, Number 11 (Supplement) 1988: Graduate education survey.[14] A total of 91 programs across the nation are included in the survey.

Thus, society's rapid changes in demographics, growth, and social upheavals have led to changes in the prevalence of psychiatric illnesses and have altered trajectories of the well and at-risk population, including chronically mentally ill clients. These changes are reflected in graduate program offerings today. There are courses on chemical abuse, teenage abuse and suicide, elder abuse and suicide, stress management, cost containment and budgeting, to name only a few. At present, psychiatric mental health nursing curricula are in transition.

RECRUITMENT

The current nursing shortage has serious consequences for psychiatric mental health nursing, as the speciality has experienced dwindling enrollment for 10 years.[26] The 1960s and 1970s were an exciting time for the field as federal support peaked in 1969. At that time, $12 million was budgeted for psychiatric nursing education; then the amount began to decrease.[6] By 1973, only $7.5 million was budgeted, and for some years now it has been completely phased out of the budget.[6,7] Enrollment in graduate psychiatric mental health nursing programs in 1974–75 was 20% of total graduate nursing enrollment. That figure dropped to 13.5% about 10 years later and has continued its downhill trajectory.[23] Clearly, there is a relation between decreases in federal support and graduate psychiatric mental health nursing enrollment.

Recruitment is crucial. Two effective approaches reported in the literature are mentioned here. Knowlton, Ramona, and Klevay[15] offered an intensive psychiatric nursing senior elective with field work and seminars. Two years later, 40% of those involved planned to attend graduate psychiatric nursing programs. Claire Fagin[12] suggested getting expert psychiatric mental health nursing role models more involved in undergraduate psychiatric teaching and planning more positive experiences for undergraduate students. Such students are more likely to select graduate psychiatric programs if they have had positive experiences at that level.[12,15,20]

DEVELOPMENT OF RESEARCH CAREER: NIMH ROLE

As psychiatric mental health nursing educators ponder what constitutes core curricula and what content to include in subspeciality programs, the specialty gained high visibility within NIMH. A 12-member National Task Force, which included the author, was appointed to examine ways of increasing nursing participation in the extramural activities of the Institute. This was very timely, because it gave the field an opportunity to examine the relations and gaps between practice and research and between theory and research. The task force found that psychiatric mental health nurse researchers were submitting small numbers of applications and that academic research career development applications were more successful than regular research project applications. On the basis of these and other findings and the state of the field, the following recommendations were made: (1) more researchers in psychiatric mental health nursing should be prepared; (2) current researchers need research career development; (3) new programs are needed; e.g., Psychiatric Mental Health Nurse Scientist Awards and Multi-Site Awards (for planned program research); (4) the number of nurses serving on Initial Review Groups needs to be increased; and (5) periodic technical assistance workshops should be conducted.[29]

Psychiatric nursing research contributions can be of particular relevance in the area of advancing knowledge on therapeutic actions and environmental changes that alter the effects of illness and that increase the coping behaviors of families and individuals as they respond to actual or potential mental illnesses. Such research can promote stronger interrelations between research, theory, and clinical practice in the speciality. Leaders in the field are convinced that this is necessary if mental health care for clients is to be improved.

MARKETPLACE TRENDS

As stated earlier, the demand for psychiatric mental health nurses is greater than programs can supply. McKevitt[18] studied graduate nursing education program trends between 1979 and 1984. In 1979, there were 81 National League for Nursing accredited master's programs (including psychiatric mental health nursing programs), and by 1984, there were 118 pro-

grams, an increase of 46%. The study revealed these trends: (1) speciality majors were on the rise, especially in the areas of psychiatric mental health and medical–surgical nursing; and (2) prior to admission, more programs were requiring prospective students to have some experience in nursing, to have health (physical) assessment skills, and to have had an undergraduate statistics course. From the author's review of the literature, there seems to have been no additional increase in speciality majors or in preadmission requirements. There is a public demand for psychiatric mental health nurses in the marketplace. Table 55-1 describes the employment settings in which such nurses hold positions and notes the diversity of settings. Psychiatric mental health nursing programs are preparing graduates for more diversified agencies. Also, graduates are carving out positions related to the newer subspecialties. Specialists in psychiatric mental health nursing can attain some wonderful, rewarding, and challenging positions.

Home Health Agencies

Richie and Lusky,[28] psychiatric nurse specialists, reported the services they provided for three different client groups in a home health setting for which they received third-party reimbursement. This had never been done in this agency, because home health agencies had generally hired medical–surgical nurses, not psychiatric nurses.

Psychotherapist and Other Roles

Prospective payment, cost-containment, and long-term community care, especially for the new chemical

TABLE 55–1
Specialists in psychiatric mental health nursing and their employment settings

PRIMARY EMPLOYMENT SETTING	NUMBER
General hospital	244
Veterans Administration hospital	108
Psychiatric hospital	50
State or county hospital	93
Psychiatric clinic	47
Community mental health center	105
Military or federal position	27
Private practice	154
Public health agency	18
College or university	412
Hospital school of nursing	18
Other (psychiatric related)	58
Other	44
Total	1378

Adapted from American Nurses' Association. Psychiatric and mental health clinical nurse specialists: distribution and utilization. 1986; Table 55, p. 43, with permission from the publisher, ANA, Kansas City, Mo.

abusers and for the older frail mentally ill clients, have created a positive climate and an opportunity for the expansion of the psychiatric mental health nursing role of psychotherapist. Many clients with these profiles receive care in community settings; i.e., day care centers, group homes, and halfway houses. This author believes the marketplace is going to have an increasing number of positions for psychiatric nurses in these settings in the next 5 to 10 years. The author also believes that skilled nursing facilities, intermediate care facilities where care is rendered to young and old mentally ill clients, will have an increasing number of positions for psychiatric liaison nurses in the next 5 to 10 years. Finally, the marketplace has many positions for psychiatric mental health nurses as administrators or researchers.

Nursing Diagnosis

Psychiatric mental health nurses can communicate their roles and functions to consumers and other health care providers alike by carefully assessing data and formulating nursing diagnoses. Nurses can diagnose human responses to actual or potential health problems.[25] Clearly, such responses are within the scope of nursing practice rather than medical practice. As the role of psychiatric mental health nursing continues to evolve, nursing diagnosis will become even more important. Nursing diagnosis is an approach to client care that further delineates the scope of nursing practice and the functions of nursing in the mental health care delivery system. Currently, many nursing programs teach nursing diagnosis, and many health facilities have integrated nursing diagnoses into their systems of care.

Case Management

Case management is one of the newest approaches in the health care delivery system growing out of a need for cost containment and accountability.[4] Case management is complex, and there are two primary types.[1] The rehabilitative case management model focuses on mental health services provided as part of a private benefit plan with the goal of rehabilitation and returning the client to a productive role in society. Case management, here, is time limited.[2] In contrast, the supportive case management model focuses on client advocacy in a fragmented public entitlement program. The goal is supportive, and case management has an indefinite time frame.

SUMMARY

Ambiguity exists regarding the core curricula for the specialty of psychiatric mental health nursing and for its subspecialties. Also at issue are the minimal length of the specialty's graduate education program, the role of federal funding and its influence on program directions, and course offerings. Recruitment into the specialty is important, and NIMH has been active in the

Research Highlights

Mian P, Tracey K, Tulchin S. Expanded roles for mental health nurses within an HMO. H&CP. 1981;32:727–9.

Psychiatric mental health nurses with 2 years of experience participated on an interdisciplinary mental health team. These nurse psychotherapists were readily accepted by primary care physicians and nurses. However, clients and other staff members had difficulty with their expanded role. High-quality care was provided at reduced costs.

Koldjeski D. Mental health and psychiatric nursing and primary health care: issues and prospects. In: Proceedings of the Conference on Graduate Education in Psychiatric and Mental Health Nursing. Pittsburgh, April 2–4, 1979. Kansas City, Mo: American Nurses' Association; 1979.

Data were from two pilot studies, review of the literature, and professional observations. The population groups were low socioeconomic people who frequented neighborhood health centers. Fifteen per cent of the population had known and identified mental problems, and 25% had some "emotional problems." Most mental health services were given in non-mental health settings. Data suggested that mental health workers need primary health care concepts and skills integrated into mental health training.

Anderson MD. Care for the worried well. Iss Ment Health Nurs. 1980;2:152–63.

In this literature review, the author found that 50% of emergency room visits and 60% of clinic visits were for psychological distress. Proposed interventions included crisis intervention and assessment of prior and current coping strategies. If problems arose from discontinuing psychotropic medications, it was important to assess symptoms and side effects of the drugs as well as to diagnose and treat client symptoms.

Adams GL, Cheney CC, Gomez E, Stafford L, Tristan MP. Primary mental health care: an innovative model. J Psychiatr Nurs Ment Health Serv. 1980;18(1):26–30.

The model was an interinstitutional consortium formed in Houston primarily to meet the needs of underserved populations. Mental health trainees, psychiatric student nurses, took histories and assisted with client management and evaluation of care. They also participated in planning care for clients.

development of research careers in the field. Finally, trends and issues in the marketplace are impacting new roles for the psychiatric mental health nurse, including the new case management approach.

References

1. Adams GL, Cheney CC, Gomez E, Stafford L, Tristan MP. Primary mental health care: an innovative model. J Psychiatr Nurs Ment Health Serv. 1980;18(1):26–30.

2. American Nurses' Association. Psychiatric and mental health clinical nurse specialists: distribution and utilization. Kansas City, Mo: The Association; 1986.

3. American Nurses' Association. Standards of child and adolescent psychiatric and mental health nursing practice. Kansas City, Mo: The Association; 1985.

4. American Nurses' Association. Case management: a challenge for nurses: task force report. Kansas City, Mo: The Association; 1988.

5. Anderson MD. Care for the worried well. Iss Ment Health Nurs. 1980;2(2)152–63.

6. Chamberlain J. The role of the federal government in development of psychiatric nursing. J Psychosoc Nurs Ment Health Serv. 1983;21(4)11–7.

7. Chamberlain J. Psychiatric nursing education branch, budget allocation & stipends awarded for fiscal years 1976–1986. Washington, DC: National Institute of Mental Health; 1986.

8. Commission on Nursing Education. Statement on graduate education in nursing. Kansas City, Mo: The Association; 1978.

9. Davis BA. The gerontological nurse's role in implementing geropsychiatric primary nursing. In: New Directions for Nursing in the 80s. Kansas City, Mo: The Association; 1980.

10. Dumas RG. Social, economic, and political factors and mental illness. J Psychosoc Nurs Ment Health Serv. 1983; 21(3)31–5.

11. Evans BL. Should we educate for service priorities? In: Fourth National Conference Proceedings on Graduate Education in Psychiatric and Mental Health Nursing. Kansas City, Mo: The Association; 1979;17–9.

12. Fagin CM. Concepts for the future: competition and substitution. J Psychosoc Nurs Ment Health Serv. 1983;21(3)36–40.

13. Garrison E. National mental health training programs in nursing. In: Smoyak SA, Rouslin S, eds. A collection of classics in psychiatric nursing literature. Thorofare, NJ: Charles B Slack, Inc; 1982.

14. Graduate education survey. J Psychosoc Nurs Ment Health Serv. 1988;26(11)6–13.

15. Knowlton CN, Romano EL, Klevay AM. Training student nurses to care for chronic mental patients. Hosp Community Psychiatry. 1987;38(7)770–1.

16. Koldjeski D. Mental health and psychiatric nursing and primary health care: issues and prospects. In: Proceedings of the Conference on Graduate Education in Psychiatric and Mental Health Nursing. Pittsburgh, April 2–4, 1979. Kansas City, Mo: The Association; 1979.

17. Krauss JB, Slavensky A. A model for advanced nursing preparation in chronic psychiatric care. Perspect Psychiatr Care. 1981;19(1)11–20.

18. McKevitt RK. Trends in master's education in nursing. J Professional Nurs. July–August 1986:225–32.

19. Mian P, Tracey K, Tulchin S. Expanded roles for mental health nurses within an HMO. Hosp Community Psychiatry. 1981;32:727–9.

20. Mitsunaga BK. Designing psychiatric and mental health nursing for the future: problems and prospects. J Psychosoc Nurs Ment Health Serv. 1982;20(12)15–21.

21. Murphy SA, Hoeffer B. The evolution of subspecialities in psychiatric and mental health nursing. Arch Psychiatr Nurs. 1987;1:145–54.

22. Naegle MA. The nurse and the alcoholic: redefining an historically ambivalent relationship. J Psychosoc Nurs Ment Health Serv. 1983;21(6):17–24.

23. National League for Nursing. Nursing Data Review. Washington, DC: The League; 1985.

24. Peplau H. Historical development of psychiatric nursing: a preliminary state of some facts and trends. In: Smoyak SA, Rouslin S, eds. A collection of classics in psychiatric nursing literature. Thorofare, NJ: Charles B Slack, Inc; 1982.

25. Peplau H. American Nurses Association's social policy statement 1. Arch Psychiatr Nurs. 1987;1:301–7.

26. Pothier P. The future of psychiatric nursing—revisited. Arch Psychiatr Nurs. 1987;1:299–300.

27. Reed SB, Hoffman SE. The enigma of graduate nursing education: advanced generalist? specialist? Nurs Health Care. 1984;4(1):43–9.

28. Richie R, Lusky K. Psychiatric home health nursing: a new role in community mental health. Community Ment Health J. 1987;23:229–35.

29. US Department of Health and Human Service, Public Health Service, HRSA: National Institute of Mental Health (NIMH) Task Force on Nursing Revised Report. Washington, DC: USDHHS; 1986.

30. US Department of Health and Human Services, Public Health Service, HRSA: National Institute of Mental Health (NIMH) Task Force on Nursing Summary Report. Washington, DC: USDHHS; 1987.

Appendices

APPENDIX I
North American Nursing Diagnosis Association (NANDA)
List of Approved Nursing Diagnostic Categories and Taxonomy I Revised

North American Nursing Diagnosis Association (NANDA)
List of Approved Nursing Diagnostic Categories

PATTERN 1: EXCHANGING

1.1.2.1.	Altered nutrition: More than body requirements	1.4.1.1.	Altered (specify) tissue perfusion (renal, cerebral, cardiopulmonary, gastrointestinal, peripheral)
1.1.2.2.	Altered nutrition: Less than body requirements	1.4.1.2.1.	Fluid volume excess
1.1.2.3.	Altered nutrition: Potential for more than body requirements	1.4.1.2.2.1.	Fluid volume deficit (1)
1.2.1.1.	Potential for infection	1.4.1.2.2.1.	Fluid volume deficit (2)
1.2.2.1.	Potential altered body temperature	1.4.1.2.2.2.	Potential fluid volume deficit
1.2.2.2.	Hypothermia	1.4.2.1.	Decreased cardiac output
1.2.2.3.	Hyperthermia	1.5.1.1.	Impaired gas exchange
1.2.2.4.	Ineffective thermoregulation	1.5.1.2.	Ineffective airway clearance
1.2.3.1.	Dysreflexia	1.5.1.3.	Ineffective breathing pattern
1.3.1.1.	Constipation	1.6.1.	Potential for injury
1.3.1.1.1.	Perceived constipation	1.6.1.1.	Potential for suffocation
1.3.1.1.2.	Colonic constipation	1.6.1.2.	Potential for poisoning
1.3.1.2.	Diarrhea	1.6.1.3.	Potential for trauma
1.3.1.3.	Bowel incontinence	1.6.1.4.	Potential for aspiration
1.3.2.	Altered patterns of urinary elimination	1.6.1.5.	Potential for disuse syndrome
1.3.2.1.1.	Stress incontinence	1.6.2.1.	Impaired tissue integrity
1.3.2.1.2.	Reflex incontinence	1.6.2.1.1.	Altered oral mucous membrane
1.3.2.1.3.	Urge incontinence	1.6.2.1.2.1.	Impaired skin integrity
1.3.2.1.4.	Functional incontinence	1.6.2.1.2.2.	Potential impaired skin integrity
1.3.2.1.5	Total incontinence		
1.3.2.2.	Urinary retention		

PATTERN 2: COMMUNICATING

2.1.1.1.	Impaired verbal communication

PATTERN 3: RELATING

3.1.1.	Impaired social interaction	3.2.1.2.1	Sexual dysfunction
3.1.2.	Social isolation	3.2.2.	Altered family processes
3.2.1.	Altered role performance	3.2.3.1.	Parental role conflict
3.2.1.1.1.	Altered parenting	3.3.	Altered sexuality patterns
3.2.1.1.2.	Potential altered parenting		

PATTERN 4: VALUING

4.1.1.	Spiritual distress (distress of the human spirit)

PATTERN 5: CHOOSING

5.1.1.1.	Ineffective individual coping	5.1.2.1.2.	Ineffective family coping: Compromised
5.1.1.1.1.	Impaired adjustment	5.1.2.2.	Family coping: Potential for growth
5.1.1.1.2.	Defensive coping	5.2.1.1.	Noncompliance (specify)
5.1.1.1.3.	Ineffective denial	5.3.1.1.	Decisional conflict (specify)
5.1.2.1.1.	Ineffective family coping: Disabling	5.4.	Health seeking behaviors (specify)

PATTERN 6: MOVING

6.1.1.1.	Impaired physical mobility	6.5.1.	Feeding self-care deficit
6.1.1.2.	Activity intolerance	6.5.1.1.	Impaired swallowing
6.1.1.2.1.	Fatigue	6.5.1.2.	Ineffective breastfeeding
6.1.1.3.	Potential activity intolerance	6.5.2.	Bathing/hygiene self-care deficit
6.2.1.	Sleep pattern disturbance	6.5.3.	Dressing/grooming self-care deficit
6.3.1.1.	Diversional activity deficit	6.5.4.	Toileting self-care deficit
6.4.1.1.	Impaired home maintenance management	6.6.	Altered growth and development
6.4.2.	Altered health maintenance		

PATTERN 7: PERCEIVING

7.1.1.	Body image disturbance	7.2.	Sensory/perceptual alterations (specify: visual, auditory, kinesthetic, gustatory, tactile, olfactory)
7.1.2.	Self-esteem disturbance	7.2.1.1.	Unilateral neglect
7.1.2.1.	Chronic low self-esteem	7.3.1.	Hopelessness
7.1.2.2.	Situational low self-esteem	7.3.2.	Powerlessness
7.1.3.	Personal identity disturbance		

PATTERN 8: KNOWING

8.1.1.	Knowledge deficit (specify)	8.3.	Altered thought processes

(continued)

North American Nursing Diagnosis Association (NANDA)
List of Approved Nursing Diagnostic Categories (*continued*)

PATTERN 9: FEELING

9.1.1.	Pain	9.2.3.	Posttrauma response
9.1.1.1.	Chronic pain	9.2.3.1.	Rape trauma syndrome
9.2.1.1.	Dysfunctional grieving	9.2.3.1.1.	Rape trauma syndrome: Compound reaction
9.2.1.2.	Anticipatory grieving	9.2.3.1.2.	Rape trauma syndrome: Silent reaction
9.2.2.	Potential for violence: Self-directed or directed at others	9.3.1.	Anxiety
		9.3.2.	Fear

From North American Nursing Diagnosis Association Classification of Nursing Diagnoses. Proceedings of the Eighth Conference. Philadelphia: JB Lippincott; 1989.

Taxonomy I Revised (June 1988)

INTRODUCTION

This version of the NANDA taxonomy represents only a portion of the work carried out by the Taxonomy Committee. It should not be construed as a new taxonomy. It differs from Taxonomy I, in large measure, only by the addition of the nursing diagnoses accepted for clinical testing and use following the seventh and eighth conferences. As before, the bracketed items and blank spaces found within the Taxonomy represent areas that are yet to be named, described, or voted on.

Approved nursing diagnoses were placed within Taxonomy I

by the Taxonomy Committee based on the following considerations:

1. Level of abstraction
2. Consistency with current theoretic views in nursing
3. Consistency with basic definitions within each pattern area
4. The order of numbers within one level was by the order in which the diagnoses were received, not by priority or importance.

1. EXCHANGING

1.1.	Altered nutrition
1.1.1	
1.1.2.	[Systemic]
1.1.2.1.	More than body requirements
1.1.2.2.	Less than body requirements
1.1.2.3.	Potential for more than body requirements
1.2.	[Altered physical regulation]
1.2.1.	[Immunologic]
1.2.1.1.	Potential for infection
1.2.2.	[Temperature]
1.2.2.1.	Potential altered body temperature
1.2.2.2.	Hypothermia
1.2.2.3.	Hyperthermia
1.2.2.4.	Ineffective thermoregulation
1.2.3.	[Neurologic]
1.2.3.1.	Dysreflexia
1.3.	Altered elimination
1.3.1.	Bowel
1.3.1.1.	Constipation
1.3.1.1.1.	Perceived
1.3.1.1.2.	Colonic
1.3.1.2.	Diarrhea
1.3.1.3.	Bowel incontinence
1.3.2.	Urinary
1.3.2.1.	Incontinence
1.3.2.1.1.	Stress
1.3.2.1.2.	Reflex
1.3.2.1.3.	Urge
1.3.2.1.4.	Functional
1.3.2.1.5.	Total
1.3.2.2.	Retention
1.4.	[Altered circulation]

1.4.1.	[Vascular]
1.4.1.1.	Tissue perfusion
1.4.1.1.1.	Renal
1.4.1.1.2.	Cerebral
1.4.1.1.3.	Cardiopulmonary
1.4.1.1.4.	Gastrointestinal
1.4.1.1.5.	Peripheral
1.4.1.2.	Fluid volume
1.4.1.2.1.	Excess
1.4.1.2.2.	Deficit
1.4.1.2.2.1.	Actual (1) Actual (2)
1.4.1.2.2.2.	Potential
1.4.2.	[Cardiac]
1.4.2.1.	Decreased cardiac output
1.5.	[Altered oxygenation]
1.5.1.	[Respiration]
1.5.1.1.	Impaired gas exchange
1.5.1.2.	Ineffective airway clearance
1.5.1.3.	Ineffective breathing pattern
1.6.	[Altered physical integrity]
1.6.1.	Potential for injury
1.6.1.1.	Potential for suffocation
1.6.1.2.	Potential for poisoning
1.6.1.3.	Potential for trauma
1.6.1.4.	Potential for aspiration
1.6.1.5.	Potential for disuse syndrome
1.6.2.	Impairment
1.6.2.1.	Tissue integrity
1.6.2.1.1.	Oral mucous membranes
1.6.2.1.2.	Skin integrity
1.6.2.1.2.1.	Actual
1.6.2.1.2.2.	Potential

2. COMMUNICATION

2.1.	Altered communication
2.1.1.	Verbal

2.1.1.1.	Impaired

3. RELATING

3.1.	[Altered socialization]
3.1.1.	Impaired social interaction
3.1.2.	Social isolation
3.2.	[Altered role]
3.2.1.	Altered role performance
3.2.1.1.	Parenting
3.2.1.1.1.	Actual

3.2.1.1.2.	Potential
3.2.1.2.	Sexual
3.2.1.2.1.	Dysfunction
3.2.2.	Altered family processes
3.2.3.	[Altered role conflict]
3.2.3.1.	Parental role conflict
3.3.	Altered sexuality patterns

4. VALUING

4.1.	[Altered spiritual state]

4.1.1.	Spiritual distress

5. CHOOSING

5.1.	Altered coping
5.1.1.	Individual coping
5.1.1.1.	Ineffective
5.1.1.1.1.	Impaired adjustment
5.1.1.1.2.	Defensive coping
5.1.1.1.3.	Ineffective denial
5.1.2.	Family coping
5.1.2.1.	Ineffective
5.1.2.1.1.	Disabled

5.1.2.1.2.	Compromised
5.1.2.2.	Potential for growth
5.2.	[Altered participation]
5.2.1.	[Individual]
5.2.1.1.	Noncompliance
5.3.	[Altered judgment]
5.3.1.	[Individual]
5.3.1.1	Decisional conflict
5.4.	Health seeking behaviors (specify)

(continued)

Taxonomy I Revised (June 1988) (*continued*)

6. MOVING

6.1.	[Altered activity]
6.1.1.	Physical mobility
6.1.1.1.	Impaired
6.1.1.2.	Activity intolerance
6.1.1.2.1.	Fatigue
6.1.1.3.	Potential activity intolerance
6.2.	[Altered rest]
6.2.1.	Sleep pattern disturbance
6.3.	[Altered recreation]
6.3.1.	Diversional activity
6.3.1.1.	Deficit
6.4.	[Altered ADL]

6.4.1.	Home maintenance management
6.4.1.1.	Impaired
6.4.2.	Health maintenance
6.5.	Self care deficit
6.5.1.	Feeding
6.5.1.1.	Impaired swallowing
6.5.1.2.	Impaired breastfeeding
6.5.2.	Bathing/hygiene
6.5.3.	Dressing/grooming
6.5.4.	Toileting
6.6.	Altered growth and development

7. PERCEIVING

7.1.	Altered self concept
7.1.1.	Body image disturbance
7.1.2.	Self esteem disturbance
7.1.2.1.	Chronic low self esteem
7.1.2.2.	Situational low self esteem
7.1.3.	Personal identity disturbance
7.2.	Altered sensory/perception
7.2.1.	Visual
7.2.1.1.	Unilateral neglect

7.2.2.	Auditory
7.2.3.	Kinesthetic
7.2.4.	Gustatory
7.2.5.	Tactile
7.2.6.	Olfactory
7.3.	[Altered meaningfulness]
7.3.1.	Hopelessness
7.3.2.	Powerlessness

8. KNOWING

8.1.	[Altered knowing]
8.1.1.	Knowledge deficit (specify)

8.2.	[xxxxxxxxxx]
8.3.	Altered thought processes

9. FEELING

9.1.	Altered comfort
9.1.1.	Pain
9.1.1.1.	Chronic
9.2.	[Altered emotional integrity]
9.2.1.	Grieving
9.2.1.1.	Dysfunctional
9.2.1.2.	Anticipatory
9.2.2.	Potential for violence

9.2.3.	Post-trauma response
9.2.3.1.	Rape-trauma syndrome
9.2.3.1.1.	Compound reaction
9.2.3.1.2.	Silent reaction
9.3.	[Altered emotional state]
9.3.1.	Anxiety
9.3.2.	Fear

DIAGNOSIS QUALIFIERS

CATEGORY 1

Actual:	Existing at the present moment; existing in reality.

Potential:	Can, but has not as yet, come into being; possible.

CATEGORY 2

Ineffective:	Not producing the desired effect; not capable of performing satisfactorily.
Decreased:	Smaller; lessened; diminished; lesser in size, amount, or degree.
Increased:	Greater in size, amount, or degree; larger, enlarged.
Impaired:	Made worse, weakened; damaged, reduced; deteriorated.
Depleted:	Emptied wholly or partially; exhausted of.
Deficient:	Inadequate in amount, quality, or degree; defective; not sufficient; incomplete.

Excessive:	Characterized by an amount or quantity that is greater than is necessary, desirable, or usable.
Dysfunctional:	Abnormal; impaired or incompletely functioning.
Disturbed:	Agitated; interrupted; interfered with.
Acute:	Severe but of short duration.
Chronic:	Lasting a long time; recurring; habitual; constant.
Intermittent:	Stopping and starting again at intervals; periodic; cyclic.

From North American Nursing Diagnosis Association Classification of Nursing Diagnoses. Proceedings of the Eighth Conference. Philadelphia: JB Lippincott; 1989.

APPENDIX II
Classification of Human Responses of Concern for Psychiatric Mental Health Nursing Practice

1. HUMAN RESPONSE PATTERNS IN ACTIVITY PROCESSES

1.1	*Motor Behavior*
1.1.1	Potential for Alteration
1.1.1.1*	Activity Intolerance
1.1.1.2	
1.1.2	Altered Motor Behavior
1.1.2.1*	Activity Intolerance
1.1.2.2	Bizarre Motor Behavior
1.1.2.3	Catatonia
1.1.2.4	Disorganized Motor Behavior
1.1.2.5*	Fatigue
1.1.2.6	Hyperactivity
1.1.2.7	Hypoactivity
1.1.2.8	Psychomotor Agitation
1.1.2.9	Psychomotor Retardation
1.1.2.10	Restlessness
1.1.99	Motor Behavior Not Otherwise Specified (NOS)
1.2	*Recreation Patterns*
1.2.1	Potential for Alteration
1.2.1.1	
1.2.1.2	
1.2.2	Altered Recreation Patterns
1.2.2.1	Age Inappropriate Recreation
1.2.2.2	Anti-Social Recreation
1.2.2.3	Bizarre Recreation
1.2.2.4*	Diversional Activity Deficit
1.2.99	Recreation Patterns NOS
1.3	*Self Care*
1.3.1	Potential for Alteration in Self Care
1.3.2*	Potential for Altered Health Maintenance
1.3.3	Altered Self Care
1.3.3.1*	Altered Eating

1.3.3.1.1	Binge-Purge Syndrome
1.3.3.1.2	Non-nutritive Ingestion
1.3.3.1.3	Pica
1.3.3.1.4	Unusual Food Ingestion
1.3.3.1.5	Refusal to Eat
1.3.3.1.6	Rumination
1.3.3.2*	Altered Feeding
1.3.3.2.1*	Ineffective Breast Feeding
1.3.3.3*	Altered Grooming
1.3.3.4*	Altered Health Maintenance
1.3.3.5*	Altered Health Seeking Behaviors
1.3.3.5.1*	Knowledge Deficit
1.3.3.5.2*	Noncompliance
1.3.3.6*	Altered Hygiene
1.3.3.7	Altered Participation in Health Care
1.3.3.8*	Altered Toileting
1.3.4*	Impaired Adjustment
1.3.5*	Knowledge Deficit
1.3.6*	Noncompliance
1.3.99	Self Care Patterns NOS
1.4.	*Sleep/Arousal Patterns*
1.4.1	Potential for Alteration
1.4.2*	Altered Sleep/Arousal Patterns
1.4.2.1	Decreased Need for Sleep
1.4.2.2	Hypersomnia
1.4.2.3	Insomnia
1.4.2.4	Nightmares/Terrors
1.4.2.5	Somnolence
1.4.2.6	Somnambulism
1.4.99	Sleep/Arousal Patterns NOS

2. HUMAN RESPONSE PATTERNS IN COGNITION PROCESSES

2.1	*Decision Making*
2.1.1	Potential for Alteration
2.1.2	Altered Decision Making
2.1.3	Decisional Conflict
2.1.99	Decision Making Patterns NOS
2.2	*Judgment*
2.2.1	Potential for Alteration
2.2.2	Altered Judgment
2.2.99	Judgment Patterns NOS
2.3	*Knowledge*
2.3.1	Potential for Alteration
2.3.2*	Altered Knowledge Processes
2.3.2.1	Agnosia
2.3.2.2	Altered Intellectual Functioning
2.3.99	Knowledge Patterns NOS
2.4	*Learning*
2.4.1	Potential for Alteration
2.4.2	Altered Learning Processes
2.4.99	Learning Patterns NOS
2.5	*Memory*
2.5.1	Potential for Alteration

2.5.2	Altered Memory
2.5.2.1	Amnesia
2.5.2.2	Distorted Memory
2.5.2.3	Long-Term Memory Loss
2.5.2.4	Memory Deficit
2.5.2.5	Short-Term Memory Loss
2.5.99	Memory Patterns NOS
2.6	*Thought Processes*
2.6.1	Potential for Alteration
2.6.2*	Altered Thought Processes
2.6.2.1	Altered Abstract Thinking
2.6.2.2	Altered Concentration
2.6.2.3	Altered Problem Solving
2.6.2.4	Confusion/Disorientation
2.6.2.5	Delirium
2.6.2.6	Delusions
2.6.2.7	Ideas of Reference
2.6.2.8	Magical Thinking
2.6.2.9	Obsessions
2.6.2.10	Suspiciousness
2.6.2.11	Thought Insertion
2.6.99	Thought Processes NOS

3. HUMAN RESPONSE PATTERNS IN ECOLOGICAL PROCESSES

3.1	*Community Maintenance*
3.1.1	Potential for Alteration
3.1.2	Altered Community Maintenance
3.1.2.1	Community Safety Hazards

3.1.2.2	Community Sanitation Hazards
3.1.99	Community Maintenance Patterns NOS
3.2	*Environmental Integrity*

(continued)

Classification of Human Responses of Concern for Psychiatric Mental Health Nursing Practice (continued)

3. HUMAN RESPONSE PATTERNS IN ECOLOGICAL PROCESSES (continued)

3.2.1	Potential for Alteration	3.3.2*	Altered Home Maintenance
3.2.2	Altered Environmental Integrity	3.3.2.1	Home Safety Hazards
3.2.99	Environmental Integrity Patterns NOS	3.3.2.2	Home Sanitation Hazards
		3.3.99	Home Maintenance Patterns NOS
3.3	*Home Maintenance*		
3.3.1	Potential for Alteration		

4. HUMAN RESPONSE PATTERNS IN EMOTIONAL PROCESSES

4.1	*Feeling States*	4.1.2.9	Shame
4.1.1	Potential for Alteration	4.1.3	Affect Incongruous in Situation
4.1.1.1	Anticipatory Grieving	4.1.4	Flat Affect
4.1.2	Altered Feeling State	4.1.99	Feeling States NOS
4.1.2.1	Anger		
4.1.2.2*	Anxiety	*4.2*	*Feeling Processes*
4.1.2.3	Elation	4.2.1	Potential for Alteration
4.1.2.4	Envy	4.2.2	Altered Feeling Processes
4.1.2.5*	Fear	4.2.2.1	Lability
4.1.2.6*	Grief	4.2.2.2	Mood Swings
4.1.2.7	Guilt	4.2.99	Feeling Processes NOS
4.1.2.8	Sadness		

5. HUMAN RESPONSE PATTERNS IN INTERPERSONAL PROCESSES

5.1	*Abuse Response Patterns*	*5.4*	*Family Processes*
5.1.1	Potential for Alteration	5.4.1	Potential for Alteration
5.1.2	Altered Abuse Response	5.4.1.1*	Potential for Altered Parenting
5.1.2.1*	Post-trauma Response	5.4.1.2*	Potential for Family Growth
5.1.2.2*	Rape Trauma Syndrome	5.4.2*	Altered Family Processes
5.1.2.3*	Compound Reaction	5.4.2.1	Ineffective Family Coping
5.1.2.4*	Silent Reaction	5.4.2.1.1*	Compromised
5.1.99	Abuse Response Patterns NOS	5.4.2.1.2*	Disabled
		5.4.99	Family Processes NOS
5.2	*Communication Processes*		
5.2.1	Potential for Alteration	*5.5*	*Role Performance*
5.2.2*	Altered Communication Processes	5.5.1	Potential for Alteration
5.2.2.1	Altered Nonverbal Communication	5.5.2*	Altered Role Performance
5.2.2.2*	Altered Verbal Communication	5.5.2.1	Altered Family Role
5.2.2.2.1	Aphasia	5.5.2.1.1	Parental Role Conflict
5.2.2.2.2	Bizarre Content	5.5.2.1.2	Parental Role Deficit
5.2.2.2.3	Confabulation	5.5.2.2	Altered Play Role
5.2.2.2.4	Ecolalia	5.5.2.3	Altered Student Role
5.2.2.2.5	Incoherent	5.5.2.4	Altered Work Role
5.2.2.2.6	Mute	5.5.3*	Ineffective Individual Coping
5.2.2.2.7	Neologisms	5.5.3.1*	Defensive Coping
5.2.2.2.8	Nonsense/Word Salad	5.5.3.2*	Ineffective Denial
5.2.2.2.9	Stuttering	5.5.99	Role Performance Patterns NOS
5.2.99	Communication Processes NOS		
		5.6	*Sexuality*
5.3	*Conduct/Impulse Processes*	5.6.1	Potential for Alteration
5.3.1	Potential for Alteration	5.6.2	Altered Sexual Behavior Leading to Intercourse
5.3.1.1*	Potential for Violence	5.6.3	Altered Sexual Conception Actions
5.3.1.2	Suicidal Ideation	5.6.4	Altered Sexual Development
5.3.2	Altered Conduct/Impulse Processes	5.6.5	Altered Sexual Intercourse
5.3.2.1	Accident Prone	5.6.6	Altered Sexual Relationships
5.3.2.2	Aggressive/Violent Behavior Toward Environment	5.6.7*	Altered Sexuality Patterns
		5.6.8	Altered Variation of Sexual Expression
5.3.2.3	Delinquency	5.6.9*	Sexual Dysfunction
5.3.2.4	Lying	5.6.99	Sexuality Processes NOS
5.3.2.5	Physical Aggression Toward Others		
5.3.2.6	Physical Aggression Toward Self	*5.7*	*Social Interaction*
5.3.2.6.1	Suicide Attempt(s)	5.7.1	Potential for Alteration
5.3.2.7	Promiscuity	5.7.2*	Altered Social Interaction
5.3.2.8	Running Away	5.7.2.1	Bizarre Behaviors
5.3.2.9	Substance Abuse	5.7.2.2	Compulsive Behaviors
5.3.2.10	Truancy	5.7.2.3	Disorganized Social Behaviors
5.3.2.11	Vandalism	5.7.2.4	Social Intrusiveness
5.3.2.12	Verbal Aggression Toward Others	5.7.2.5*	Social Isolation/Withdrawal
5.3.99	Conduct/Impulse Processes NOS	5.7.2.6	Unpredictable Behaviors
		5.7.99	Social Interaction Patterns NOS

(continued)

Classification of Human Responses of Concern for Psychiatric Mental Health Nursing Practice (*continued*)

6. HUMAN RESPONSE PATTERNS IN PERCEPTION PROCESSES

6.1	*Attention*
6.1.1	Potential for Alteration
6.1.2	Altered Attention
6.1.2.1	Hyperalertness
6.1.2.2	Inattention
6.1.2.3	Selective Attention
6.1.99	Attention Patterns NOS
6.2	*Comfort*
6.2.1	Potential for Alteration
6.2.2*	Altered Comfort Patterns
6.2.2.1	Discomfort
6.2.2.2	Distress
6.2.2.3*	Pain
6.2.2.3.1	Acute Pain
6.2.2.3.2*	Chronic Pain
6.2.99	Comfort Patterns NOS
6.3	*Self Concept*
6.3.1	Potential for Alteration
6.3.2	Altered Self Concept
6.3.2.1*	Altered Body Image

6.3.2.2*	Altered Personal Identity
6.3.2.3*	Altered Self Esteem
6.3.2.3.1*	Chronic Low Self Esteem
6.3.2.3.2*	Situational Low Self Esteem
6.3.2.4	Altered Sexual Identity
6.3.2.4.1	Altered Gender Identity
6.3.3	Undeveloped Self Concept
6.3.99	Self Concept Patterns NOS
6.4	*Sensory Perception*
6.4.1	Potential for Alteration
6.4.2*	Altered Sensory Perception
6.4.2.1	Hallucinations
6.4.2.1.1*	Auditory
6.4.2.1.2*	Gustatory
6.4.2.1.3*	Kinesthetic
6.4.2.1.4*	Olfactory
6.4.2.1.5*	Tactile
6.4.2.1.6*	Visual
6.4.2.2	Illusions
6.4.99	Sensory Perception Processes NOS

7. HUMAN RESPONSE PATTERNS IN PHYSIOLOGICAL PROCESSES

7.1	*Circulation*
7.1.1	Potential for Alteration
7.1.1.1	Fluid Volume Deficit
7.1.2	Altered Circulation
7.1.2.1	Altered Cardiac Circulation
7.1.2.1.1*	Decreased Cardiac Output
7.1.2.2	Altered Vascular Circulation
7.1.2.2.1*	Altered Fluid Volume
7.1.2.2.2*	Fluid Volume Excess
7.1.2.2.3*	Tissue Perfusion
7.1.2.2.3.1*	Peripheral
7.1.2.2.3.2*	Renal
7.1.99	Altered Circulation Processes NOS
7.2	*Elimination*
7.2.1	Potential for Alteration
7.2.2	Altered Elimination Processes
7.2.2.1*	Altered Bowel Elimination
7.2.2.1.1*	Constipation
7.2.2.1.1.1*	Colonic
7.2.2.1.1.2*	Perceived
7.2.2.1.2*	Diarrhea
7.2.2.1.3	Encopresis
7.2.2.1.4*	Incontinence
7.2.2.2*	Altered Urinary Elimination
7.2.2.2.1	Enuresis
7.2.2.2.2*	Incontinence
7.2.2.2.2.1*	Functional
7.2.2.2.2.2.*	Reflex
7.2.2.2.2.3*	Stress
7.2.2.2.2.4*	Total
7.2.2.2.2.5*	Urge
7.2.2.2.3*	Retention
7.2.2.3	Altered Skin Elimination
7.2.99	Elimination Processes NOS
7.3	*Endocrine/Metabolic Processes*
7.3.1	Potential for Alteration
7.3.2	Altered Endocrine/Metabolic Processes
7.3.2.1*	Altered Growth and Development
7.3.2.2	Altered Hormone Regulation
7.3.2.2.1	Premenstrual Stress Syndrome
7.3.99	Endocrine/Metabolic Processes NOS
7.4	*Gastrointestinal Processes*
7.4.1	Potential for Alteration

7.4.2	Altered Gastrointestinal Processes
7.4.2.1	Altered Absorption
7.4.2.2	Altered Digestion
7.4.2.3*	Tissue Perfusion
7.4.99	Gastrointestinal Processes NOS
7.5	*Musculoskeletal Processes*
7.5.1	Potential for Alteration
7.5.1.1*	Potential for Disuse Syndrome
7.5.1.2*	Potential for Injury
7.5.2	Altered Musculoskeletal Processes
7.5.2.1	Altered Coordination
7.5.2.2	Altered Equilibrium
7.5.2.3	Altered Mobility
7.5.2.4	Altered Motor Planning
7.5.2.5	Altered Muscle Strength
7.5.2.6	Altered Muscle Tone
7.5.2.7	Altered Posture
7.5.2.8	Altered Range of Motion
7.5.2.9	Altered Reflex Patterns
7.5.2.10	Altered Physical Mobility
7.5.2.11	Muscle Twitching
7.5.99	Musculoskeletal Processes NOS
7.6	*Neuro/Sensory Processes*
7.6.1	Potential for Alteration
7.6.2	Altered Neuro/Sensory Processes
7.6.2.1	Altered Level of Consciousness
7.6.2.2	Altered Sensory Acuity
7.6.2.2.1	Auditory
7.6.2.2.2*	Dysreflexia
7.6.2.2.3	Gustatory
7.6.2.2.4	Olfactory
7.6.2.2.5	Tactile
7.6.2.2.6	Visual
7.6.2.3	Altered Sensory Integration
7.6.2.4	Altered Sensory Processing
7.6.2.4.1	Auditory
7.6.2.4.2	Gustatory
7.6.2.4.3	Olfactory
7.6.2.4.4	Tactile
7.6.2.4.5	Visual
7.6.2.5*	Cerebral Tissue Perfusion
7.6.2.6*	Unilateral Neglect
7.6.2.7	Seizures
7.6.99	Neuro/Sensory Processes NOS

(*continued*)

Classification of Human Responses of Concern for Psychiatric Mental Health Nursing Practice (*continued*)

7. HUMAN RESPONSE PATTERNS IN PHYSIOLOGICAL PROCESSES (*continued*)

7.7	*Nutrition*
7.7.1	Potential for Alteration
7.7.1.1*	Potential for More Than Body Requirements
7.7.1.2*	Potential for Poisoning
7.7.2	Altered Nutrition Processes
7.7.2.1	Altered Cellular Processes
7.7.2.2	Altered Eating Processes
7.7.2.2.1	Anorexia
7.7.2.2.2*	Altered Oral Mucous Membrane
7.7.2.3	Altered Systemic Processes
7.7.2.3.1*	Less Than Body Requirements
7.7.2.3.2*	More Than Body Requirements
7.7.2.4	Impaired Swallowing
7.7.99	Nutrition Processes NOS

7.8	*Oxygenation*
7.8.1	Potential for Alteration
7.8.1.1*	Potential for Aspiration
7.8.1.2*	Potential for Suffocating
7.8.2	Altered Oxygenation Processes
7.8.2.1	Altered Respiration
7.8.2.1.1*	Altered Gas Exchange
7.8.2.1.2*	Ineffective Airway Clearance
7.8.2.1.3*	Ineffective Breathing Pattern

7.8.2.2*	Tissue Perfusion
7.8.99	Oxygenation Processes NOS

7.9	*Physical Integrity*
7.9.1	Potential for Alteration
7.9.1.1*	Potential for Altered Skin Integrity
7.9.1.2*	Potential for Trauma
7.9.2	Altered Oral Mucous Membrane
7.9.2.2*	Altered Skin Integrity
7.9.2.3*	Altered Tissue Integrity
7.9.99	Physical Integrity Processes NOS

7.10	*Physical Regulation Processes*
7.10.1	Potential for Alteration
7.10.1.1*	Potential for Altered Body Temperature
7.10.1.2*	Potential for Infection
7.10.2	Altered Physical Regulation Processes
7.10.2.1	Altered Immune Response
7.10.2.1.1	Infection
7.10.2.2	Altered Body Temperature
7.10.2.2.1*	Hyperthermia
7.10.2.2.2*	Hypothermia
7.10.2.2.3*	Ineffective Thermoregulation
7.10.99	Physical Regulation Processes NOS

8. HUMAN RESPONSE PATTERNS IN VALUATION PROCESSES

8.1	*Meaningfulness*
8.1.1	Potential for Alteration
8.1.2*	Altered Meaningfulness
8.1.2.1	Helplessness
8.1.2.2*	Hopelessness
8.1.2.3	Loneliness
8.1.2.4*	Powerlessness
8.1.99	Meaningfulness Patterns NOS

8.2	*Spirituality*
8.2.1	Potential for Alteration
8.2.2	Altered Spirituality

8.2.2.1	Spiritual Despair
8.2.2.2*	Spiritual Distress
8.2.99	Spirituality Patterns NOS

8.3	*Values*
8.3.1	Potential for Alteration
8.3.2	Altered Values
8.3.2.1	Conflict With Social Order
8.3.2.2	Inability to Internalize Values
8.3.2.3	Unclear Values
8.3.99	Value Patterns NOS

---

* Approved NANDA Diagnoses
Developed by Loomis M, O'Toole A, Pothier P, West P, and Wilson H
O'Toole AW, Loomis ME. Revision of phenomena of concern for psychiatric mental health nursing. *Arch Psych Nurs.* Oct 1989; III:5, 292–299.

APPENDIX III
DSM-III-R Classification

Multiaxial System

Axis I   Clinical Syndromes   Axis III   Physical Disorders and Conditions
         V Codes   Axis IV   Severity of Psychosocial Stressors
Axis II Developmental Disorders   Axis V   Global Assessment of Functioning
         Personality Disorders

AXES I AND II CATEGORIES AND CODES

DISORDERS USUALLY FIRST EVIDENT IN INFANCY, CHILDHOOD, OR ADOLESCENCE

Developmental Disorders
Note: These are coded on Axis II.

Mental Retardation

317.00	Mild mental retardation	318.20	Profound mental retardation
318.00	Moderate mental retardation	319.00	Unspecified mental retardation
318.10	Severe mental retardation		

Pervasive Developmental Disorders

299.00   Autistic disorder   299.80   Pervasive developmental disorder NOS
         Specify if childhood onset

Specific Developmental Disorders

Academic skills disorders
315.10   Developmental arithmetic disorder   315.31   Developmental expressive language disorder
315.80   Developmental expressive writing disorder   315.31   Developmental receptive language disorder
315.00   Developmental reading disorder   Motor skills disorder
Language and speech disorders   315.40   Developmental coordination disorder
315.39   Developmental articulation disorder   315.90   Specific developmental disorder NOS

Other Developmental Disorders

315.90   Developmental disorder NOS

Disruptive Behavior Disorders

314.01	Attention-deficit hyperactivity disorder	312.00	solitary aggressive type
	Conduct disorder	312.90	undifferentiated type
312.20	group type	313.81	Oppositional defiant disorder

Anxiety Disorders of Childhood or Adolescence

309.21	Separation anxiety disorder	313.00	Overanxious disorder
313.21	Avoidant disorder of childhood or adolescence		

Eating Disorders

307.10	Anorexia nervosa	307.53	Rumination disorder of infancy
307.51	Bulimia nervosa	307.50	Eating disorder NOS
307.52	Pica		

(continued)

Axes I and II Categories and Codes (*continued*)

Gender Identity Disorders

302.60	Gender identity disorder of childhood		*Specify* sexual history: asexual, homosexual, heterosexual, unspecified
302.50	Transsexualism		
	Specify sexual history: asexual, homosexual, heterosexual, unspecified	302.85	Gender identity disorder NOS
302.85	Gender identity disorder of adolescence or adulthood, nontranssexual type		

Tic Disorders

307.23	Tourette's disorder	307.20	Tic disorder NOS
307.22	Chronic motor or vocal tic disorder		
307.21	Transient tic disorder		
	Specify: single episode or recurrent		

Elimination Disorders

307.70	Functional encopresis		*Specify:* nocturnal only, diurnal only, nocturnal and diurnal
	Specify: primary or secondary type		
307.60	Functional enuresis		
	Specify: primary or secondary type		

Speech Disorders Not Elsewhere Classified

307.00	Cluttering	307.00	Stuttering

Other Disorders of Infancy, Childhood, or Adolescence

313.23	Elective mutism	307.30	Stereotypy/habit disorder
313.82	Identity disorder	314.00	Undifferentiated attention-deficit disorder
313.89	Reactive attachment disorder of infancy or early childhood		

ORGANIC MENTAL DISORDERS

Dementias Arising in the Senium and Presenium

	Primary degenerative dementia of the Alzheimer type, senile onset,	290.1x	Primary degenerative dementia of the Alzheimer type, presenile onset, _____
290.30	with delirium		(Note: code 331.00 Alzheimer's disease on Axis III)
290.20	with delusions		
290.21	with depression	290.4x	Multi-infarct dementia, _____
290.00	uncomplicated	290.00	Senile dementia NOS
	(Note: code 331.00 Alzheimer's disease on Axis III)		*Specify* etiology on Axis III if known
		290.10	Presenile dementia NOS

Code in fifth digit:
1 = with delirium, 2 = with delusions, 3 = with depression, 0 = uncomplicated

Specify etiology on Axis III if known (e.g., Pick's disease, Jakob-Creutzfeldt disease)

Psychoactive Substance-Induced Organic Mental Disorders

	Alcohol	292.81	delirium
303.00	intoxication	292.11	delusional disorder
291.40	idiosyncratic intoxication		Caffeine
291.80	uncomplicated alcohol withdrawal	305.90	intoxication
291.00	withdrawal delirium		Cannabis
291.30	hallucinosis	305.20	intoxication
291.10	amnestic disorder	292.11	delusional disorder
291.20	dementia associated with alcoholism		Cocaine
	Amphetamine or similarly acting sympathomimetic	305.60	intoxication
		292.00	withdrawal
305.70	intoxication	292.81	delirium
292.00	withdrawal	292.11	delusional disorder

(*continued*)

Axes I and II Categories and Codes (continued)

Psychoactive Substance-Induced Organic Mental Disorders (continued)

Hallucinogen
305.30	hallucinosis
292.11	delusional disorder
292.84	mood disorder
292.89	posthallucinogen perception disorder

Inhalant
305.90	intoxication

Nicotine
292.00	withdrawal

Opioid
305.50	intoxication
292.00	withdrawal

Phencyclidine (PCP) or similarly acting arylcyclohexylamine
305.90	intoxication
292.81	delirium
292.11	delusional disorder
292.84	mood disorder
292.90	organic mental disorder NOS

Sedative, hypnotic, or anxiolytic
305.40	intoxication
292.00	uncomplicated sedative, hypnotic, or anxiolytic withdrawal
292.00	withdrawal delirium
292.83	amnestic disorder

Other or unspecified psychoactive substance
305.90	intoxication
292.00	withdrawal
292.81	delirium
292.82	dementia
292.83	amnestic disorder
292.11	delusional disorder
292.12	hallucinosis
292.84	mood disorder
292.89	anxiety disorder
292.89	personality disorder
292.90	organic mental disorder NOS

Organic Mental Disorders Associated with Axis III Physical Disorders or Conditions, or Whose Etiology Is Unknown

293.00	Delirium
294.10	Dementia
294.00	Amnestic disorder
293.81	Organic delusional disorder
293.82	Organic hallucinosis
293.83	Organic mood disorder
	Specify: manic, depressed, mixed
294.80	Organic anxiety disorder
310.10	Organic personality disorder
	Specify if explosive type
294.80	Organic mental disorder NOS

PSYCHOACTIVE SUBSTANCE USE DISORDERS

Alcohol
303.90	dependence
305.00	abuse

Amphetamine or similarly acting sympathomimetic
304.40	dependence
305.70	abuse

Cannabis
304.30	dependence
305.20	abuse

Cocaine
304.20	dependence
305.60	abuse

Hallucinogen
304.50	dependence
305.30	abuse

Inhalant
304.60	dependence
305.90	abuse

Nicotine
305.10	dependence

Opioid
304.00	dependence
305.50	abuse

Phencyclidine (PCP) or similarly acting arylcyclohexylamine
304.50	dependence
305.90	abuse

Sedative, hypnotic, or anxiolytic
304.10	dependence
305.40	abuse
304.90	Polysubstance dependence
304.90	Psychoactive substance dependence NOS
305.90	Psychoactive substance abuse NOS

(continued)

Axes I and II Categories and Codes (*continued*)

SCHIZOPHRENIA

Code in fifth digit: 1 = subchronic, 2 = chronic, 3 = subchronic with acute exacerbation, 4 = chronic with acute exacerbation, 5 = in remission, 0 = unspecified.

Schizophrenia,

295.2x	catatonic, _____

295.1x	disorganized, _____
295.3x	paranoid, _____
	Specify if stable type
295.9x	undifferentiated, _____
295.6x	residual, _____
	Specify if late onset

DELUSIONAL (PARANOID) DISORDER

297.10   Delusional (paranoid) disorder
          Specify type: erotomanic
                         grandiose
                         jealous

persecutory
somatic
unspecified

PSYCHOTIC DISORDERS NOT ELSEWHERE CLASSIFIED

298.80   Brief reactive psychosis
295.40   Schizophreniform disorder
          Specify: without good prognostic features or with good prognostic features
295.70   Schizoaffective disorder
          Specify: bipolar type or depressive type

297.30   Induced psychotic disorder
298.90   Psychotic disorder NOS (atypical psychosis)

MOOD DISORDERS

Code current state of Major Depression and Bipolar Disorder in fifth digit:

1 = mild, 2 = moderate, 3 = severe, without psychotic features, 4 = with psychotic features (*specify* mood-congruent or mood-incongruent), 5 = in partial remission, 6 = in full remission, 0 = unspecified.

For major depressive episodes, *specify* if chronic and *specify* if melancholic type.

For Bipolar Disorder, Bipolar Disorder NOS, Recurrent Major Depression, and Depressive Disorder NOS, *specify* if seasonal pattern.

Bipolar Disorders

Bipolar disorder,

296.6x	mixed, _____
296.4x	manic, _____

296.5x	depressed, _____
301.13	Cyclothymia
296.70	Bipolar disorder NOS

Depressive Disorders

Major Depression,

296.2x	single episode, _____
296.3x	recurrent, _____
300.40	Dysthymia (or Depressive neurosis)

Specify: primary or secondary type
Specify: early or late onset
311.00   Depressive disorder NOS

ANXIETY DISORDERS (or Anxiety and Phobic Neuroses)

Panic disorder

300.21	with agoraphobia
	Specify current severity of agoraphobic avoidance
	Specify current severity of panic attacks
300.01	without agoraphobia
	Specify current severity of panic attacks
300.22	Agoraphobia without history of panic disorder

Specify with or without limited symptom attacks

300.23	Social phobia
	Specify if generalized type
300.29	Simple phobia
300.30	Obsessive–compulsive disorder (or Obsessive–compulsive neurosis)
309.89	Post–traumatic stress disorder
	Specify if delayed onset
300.02	Generalized anxiety disorder
300.00	Anxiety disorder NOS

(*continued*)

Axes I and II Categories and Codes (*continued*)

SOMATOFORM DISORDERS

300.70	Body dysmorphic disorder	300.81	Somatization disorder
300.11	Conversion disorder (or Hysterical neurosis, conversion type)	307.80	Somatoform pain disorder
		300.70	Undifferentiated somatoform disorder
	Specify: single episode or recurrent	300.70	Somatoform disorder NOS
300.70	Hypochondriasis (or Hypochondriacal neurosis)		

DISSOCIATIVE DISORDERS (or Hysterical Neuroses, Dissociative Type)

300.14	Multiple personality disorder	300.60	Depersonalization disorder (or Depersonalization neurosis)
300.13	Psychogenic fugue		
300.12	Psychogenic amnesia	300.15	Dissociative disorder NOS

SEXUAL DISORDERS

Paraphilias

302.40	Exhibitionism		*Specify:* exclusive type or nonexclusive type
302.81	Fetishism		
302.89	Frotteurism	302.83	Sexual masochism
302.20	Pedophilia	302.84	Sexual sadism
	Specify: same sex, opposite sex, same and opposite sex	302.30	Transvestic fetishism
		302.82	Voyeurism
	Specify if limited to incest	302.90	Paraphilia NOS

Sexual Dysfunctions

Specify: psychogenic only, or psychogenic and biogenic (Note: If biogenic only, code on Axis III)		302.72	Male erectile disorder
			Orgasm disorders
Specify: lifelong or acquired		302.73	Inhibited female orgasm
Specify: generalized or situational		302.74	Inhibited male orgasm
	Sexual desire disorders	302.75	Premature ejaculation
302.71	Hypoactive sexual desire disorder		Sexual pain disorders
302.79	Sexual aversion disorder	302.76	Dyspareunia
	Sexual arousal disorders	306.51	Vaginismus
302.72	Female sexual arousal disorder	302.70	Sexual dysfunction NOS

Other Sexual Disorders

302.90	Sexual disorder NOS

SLEEP DISORDERS

Dyssomnias

	Insomnia disorder	780.50	related to a known organic factor
307.42	related to another mental disorder (nonorganic)	780.54	Primary hypersomnia
		307.45	Sleep–wake schedule disorder
780.50	related to known organic factor		*Specify:* advanced or delayed phase type, disorganized type, frequently changing type
307.42	Primary insomnia		
	Hypersomnia disorder		Other dyssomnias
307.44	related to another mental disorder (nonorganic)	307.40	Dyssomnia NOS

Parasomnias

307.47	Dream anxiety disorder (Nightmare disorder)	307.46	Sleepwalking disorder
		307.40	Parasomnia NOS
307.46	Sleep terror disorder		

(*continued*)

Axes I and II Categories and Codes (continued)

FACTITIOUS DISORDERS

| | Factitious disorder | 300.16 | with psychological symptoms |
| 301.51 | with physical symptoms | 300.19 | Factitious disorder NOS |

IMPULSE CONTROL DISORDERS NOT ELSEWHERE CLASSIFIED

312.34	Intermittent explosive disorder	312.33	Pyromania
312.32	Kleptomania	312.39	Trichotillomania
312.31	Pathological gambling	312.39	Impulse control disorder NOS

ADJUSTMENT DISORDER

	Adjustment disorder	309.28	with mixed emotional features
309.24	with anxious mood	309.82	with physical complaints
309.00	with depressed mood	309.83	with withdrawal
309.30	with disturbance of conduct	309.23	with work (or academic) inhibition
309.40	with mixed disturbance of emotions and conduct	309.90	Adjustment disorder NOS

PSYCHOLOGICAL FACTORS AFFECTING PHYSICAL CONDITION

316.00 Psychological factors affecting physical condition
        Specify physical condition on Axis III

PERSONALITY DISORDERS
Note: These are coded on Axis II.

Cluster A

301.00	Paranoid
301.20	Schizoid
301.22	Schizotypal

Cluster B

| 301.70 | Antisocial |
| 301.83 | Borderline |

| 301.50 | Histrionic |
| 301.81 | Narcissistic |

Cluster C

301.82	Avoidant
301.60	Dependent
301.40	Obsessive compulsive
301.84	Passive aggressive
301.90	Personality disorder NOS

V CODES FOR CONDITIONS NOT ATTRIBUTABLE TO A MENTAL DISORDER THAT ARE A FOCUS OF ATTENTION OR TREATMENT

| V62.30 | Academic problem |
| V71.01 | Adult antisocial behavior |

| V40.00 | Borderline intellectual functioning (Note: This is coded on Axis II.) |

| V71.02 | Childhood or adolescent antisocial behavior |

V65.20	Malingering
V61.10	Marital problem
V15.81	Noncompliance with medical treatment
V62.20	Occupational problem
V61.20	Parent–child problem
V62.81	Other interpersonal problem
V61.80	Other specified family circumstances
V62.89	Phase of life problem or other life circumstance problem
V62.82	Uncomplicated bereavement

(continued)

Axes I and II Categories and Codes (*continued*)

ADDITIONAL CODES

300.90	Unspecified mental disorder (nonpsychotic)
V71.09	No diagnosis or condition on Axis I
799.90	Diagnosis or condition deferred on Axis I

V71.09	No diagnosis or condition on Axis II
799.90	Diagnosis or condition deferred on Axis II

All official DSM-III-R codes are included in ICD-9-CM. A long dash following a diagnostic term indicates the need for a fifth digit subtype or other qualifying term.

The term *specify* following the name of some diagnostic categories indicates qualifying terms that clinicians may wish to add in parentheses after the name of the disorder.

NOS, not otherwise specified.

AXIS IV
Severity of psychosocial stressors scale: adults

CODE	TERM	EXAMPLES OF STRESSORS	
		Acute Events	**Enduring Circumstances**
1	None	No acute events that may be relevant to the disorder	No enduring circumstances that may be relevant to the disorder
2	Mild	Broke up with boyfriend or girlfriend; started or graduated from school; child left home	Family arguments; job dissatisfaction; residence in high-crime neighborhood
3	Moderate	Marriage; marital separation; loss of job; retirement; miscarriage	Marital discord; serious financial problems; trouble with boss; being a single parent
4	Severe	Divorce; birth of first child	Unemployment; poverty
5	Extreme	Death of spouse; serious physical illness diagnosed; victim of rape	Serious chronic illness in self or child; ongoing physical or sexual abuse
6	Catastrophic	Death of child; suicide of spouse; devastating natural disaster	Captivity as hostage; concentration camp experience
0	Inadequate information, or no change in condition		

Severity of psychosocial stressors scale: children and adolescents

CODE	TERM	EXAMPLES OF STRESSORS	
		Acute Events	**Enduring Circumstances**
1	None	No acute events that may be relevant to the disorder	No enduring circumstances that may be relevant to the disorder
2	Mild	Broke up with boyfriend or girlfriend; change of school	Overcrowded living quarters; family arguments
3	Moderate	Expelled from school; birth of sibling	Chronic disabling illness in parent; chronic parental discord
4	Severe	Divorce of parents; unwanted pregnancy; arrest	Harsh or rejecting parents; chronic life-threatening illness in parent; multiple foster home placements
5	Extreme	Sexual or physical abuse; death of a parent	Recurrent sexual or physical abuse
6	Catastrophic	Death of both parents	Chronic life-threatening illness
0	Inadequate information, or no change in condition		

AXIS V
Global assessment of functioning scale (GAF scale)

Consider psychological, social, and occupational functioning on a hypothetical continuum of mental health-illness. Do not include impairment in functioning due to physical (or environmental) limitations.

Note: Use intermediate codes when appropriate, e.g., 45, 68, 72.

CODE

90 ⎮ 81	**Absent or minimal symptoms** (e.g., mild anxiety before an exam), **good functioning in all areas, interested and involved in a wide range of activities, socially effective, generally satisfied with life, no more than everyday problems or concerns** (e.g., an occasional argument with family members).
80 ⎮ 71	**If symptoms are present, they are transient and expectable reactions to psychosocial stressors** (e.g., difficulty concentrating after family argument); **no more than slight impairment in social, occupational, or school functioning** (e.g., temporarily falling behind in school work).
70 ⎮ 61	**Some mild symptoms** (e.g., depressed mood and mild insomnia) *or some difficulty in social, occupational, or school functioning* (e.g., occasional truancy, or theft within the household), **but generally functioning pretty well, has some meaningful interpersonal relationships.**
60 ⎮ 51	**Moderate symptoms** (e.g., flat affect and circumstantial speech, occasional panic attacks) *or moderate difficulty in social, occupational, or school functioning* (e.g., few friends, conflicts with coworkers).
50 ⎮ 41	**Serious symptoms** (e.g., suicidal ideation, severe obsessional rituals, frequent shoplifting) *or any serious impairment in social, occupational, or school functioning* (e.g., no friends, unable to keep a job).
40 ⎮ 31	**Some impairment in reality testing or communication** (e.g., speech is at times illogical, obscure, or irrelevant) *or major impairment in several areas, such as work or school, family relations, judgment, thinking, or mood* (e.g., depressed man avoids friends, neglects family, and is unable to work; child frequently beats up younger children, is defiant at home, and is failing at school).
30 ⎮ 21	**Behavior is considerably influenced by delusions or hallucinations** *or serious impairment in communication or judgment* (e.g., sometimes incoherent, acts grossly inappropriately, suicidal preoccupation) *or inability to function in almost all areas* (e.g., stays in bed all day; no job, home, or friends).
20 ⎮ 11	**Some danger of hurting self or others** (e.g., suicide attempts without clear expectation of death, frequently violent, manic excitement) *or occasionally fails to maintain minimal personal hygiene* (e.g., smears feces) *or gross impairment in communication* (e.g., largely incoherent or mute).
10 ⎮ 1	**Persistent danger of severely hurting self or others** (e.g., recurrent violence) *or persistent inability to maintain minimal personal hygiene or serious suicidal act with clear expectation of death.*

APPENDIX IV
Laboratory Values

Mary T. Bush

Laboratory tests are used in psychiatry to rule out underlying medical illness or organic causes for psychiatric problems, to aid in making a diagnosis, to monitor a therapeutic regimen, and to assess toxicity in cases of overdose.

   I. Tests used to rule out medical illness

        A. An initial screening for medical illness usually consists of a complete blood count, urinalysis, electrolytes and blood chemistry profile. (Tests included in a screening profile will vary with the institution). If dementia is being considered several other tests will be done, and when test results are abnormal a more detailed work-up is in order.

TEST AND SPECIMEN	NORMAL ADULT VALUES*	RECOMMENDED SI UNITS*
Complete Blood Count (whole blood)		
WBC	5,000–10,000 mm	$5.0–10.0 \times 10^9/L$
RBC	Males 4,600,000–6,200,000/mm	$4.6–6.2 \times 10^{12}/L$
	Females 4,200,000–5,400,000/mm	$4.2–5.4 \times 10^{12}/L$
Hgb	Males 13.5–17.3 g/dL	2.09–2.71 mmol/L
	Females 12.0–16.0 g/dL	1.86–2.48 mmol/L
Hct	Males 41–53%	0.41–0.53 } volume fraction
	Females 36–46%	0.36–0.46
MCV	80–94 μm/red blood cell	80–96 fL
MCH	27–32 pg/red blood cell	0.40–0.53 fmol/cell
MCHC	31–37% Hb/red blood cell	4.81–5.74 mmol Hb/L RBC
platelets	200,000–350,000/mm³	$0.20–0.35 \times 10^{12}/L$
Differential		
Granulocytes	60–70%	0.60–0.70
Lymphocytes	20–30%	0.20–0.30
Monocytes	2–6%	0.02–0.06 } mean number fraction
Eosinophils	1–4%	0.01–0.04
Basophils	0–0.5%	0.00–0.005
Urinalysis (urine)		
pH	4.3–8	Microscopic:
Specific gravity	1.001–1.040	
Protein	Negative	Casts none
Glucose	Negative	WBC <4–5 high-powered field
Ketones	Negative	RBC <2–3 per high-powered field
Blood	Negative	
Electrolytes (serum)		
Na	136–146 mEq/L	136–146 mmol/L
K	3.5–5.1 mEq/L	3.5–5.1 mmol/L
Cl	98–106 mEq/L	98–106 mmol/L
CO_2	23–29 mEq/L	23–29 mmol/L
Random glucose (serum)	70–105 mg/dL	3.89–5.83 mmol/L
Sedimentation rate (whole blood)	Males 0–9 mm/hr	Same
	Females 0–20 mm/hr	Same
B_{12} RIA (serum)	220–940 pg/mL	162–694 pmol/L
Folic acid level by RIA (serum)	>2.3 ng/mL	>5.2 nmol/L
Amylase (serum)	60–160 units/dL	111–296 U/L

        B. Psychotropic medications are detoxified in the liver and excreted by the kidneys; hence, organ function should be assessed before drug therapy is initiated.

TEST AND SPECIMEN	NORMAL ADULT VALUES	RECOMMENDED SI UNITS
Liver Function Tests (serum)		
Total protein	6.0–8.0 g/dL	60–80 g/L
Albumin	3.5–5.0 g/dL	35–50 g/L
SGOT	10–30 U/L	Same
SGPT	<30 U/L	Same
Alkaline phosphatase	25–100 U/L	Same
Bilirubin (direct)	0.0–0.2 mg/dL	0.0–3.4 μmol/L
total bilirubin	<0.2–1.0 mg/dL	<3.4–17.1 μmol/L
γ-Glutamyltransferase	5–40 IU/L	Same
Renal Function Tests (serum)		
BUN	7–18 mg/dL	2.5–6.4 mmol/L
Creatinine	0.6–1.2 mg/dL	53–106 μmol/L
Uric acid	3.0–8.2 mg/dL	0.18–0.48 mmol/L
Calcium	8.4–10.2 mg/dL	2.10–2.55 mmol/L
Phosphorus	2.7–4.5 mg/dL	0.87–1.45 mmol/L

(continued)

Laboratory Values (*continued*)

II. Tests used to aid in diagnosis

A. Thyroid function tests are used to evaluate the hypothalamic–pituitary–thyroid axis. Signs and symptoms of hypothyroidism are similar to vegetative signs of depression. Hyperthyroidism produces generalized anxiety and some manic and schizophrenic symptoms. Acutely psychotic clients may have abnormal thyroid function with no organic explanation.

TEST AND SPECIMEN	ADULT NORMAL VALUES	RECOMMENDED SI UNITS	COMMENTS
TSH (thyroid-stimulating hormone) (serum), RIA (radioimmunoassay)	$<10\ \mu U/mL$	$<10\ mIU/L$	TSH controls production of T_4 and T_3; is sensitive to hypothalamic response to stress; evaluates pituitary function
T_4 (thyroxine), free (serum)	0.8–2.4 ng/dL	10.3–31.0 pmol/L	Most abundant of thyroid hormones
T_4 (thyroxine), RIA (serum)	5–12 μg/dL	65–155 nmol/L	Drugs such as propranolol and birth control pills may interfere with test results. Higher in children, with pregnancy, with liver disease
T_3 uptake	25–35%	0.25–0.35 relevant uptake fraction	May be elevated in thyrotoxicosis when T_4 is normal
T_3, RIA (serum)	60–160 ng/dL	0.92–2.46 nmol/L	

The *TRH stimulation test* or *protirelin test* is used by some as a more refined measure of thyroid function. The fasting client has baseline thyroid function studies drawn and is then given a 500-mg bolus of protirelin. Blood is drawn for serum TSH levels at intervals of 15, 30, 60, and 90 min. Baseline TSH is subtracted from peak TSH to give ΔTSH. Normal change is 7–15 μIU/ml. Hypothyroid patients have elevated ΔTSH; hyperthyroid clients have decreased ΔTSH.[4]

B. Cortisol levels are measured to give information about the function of the adrenal cortex. Elevated levels indicate Cushing's syndrome which may include hyperactivity and psychosis. Subnormal levels occur in Addison's disease or as a complication of AIDS.

TEST AND SPECIMEN	NORMAL ADULT VALUE	RECOMMENDED SI UNITS	COMMENTS
Serum cortisol RIA	8 AM: 5–23 μg/dL 4 PM: 3–15 μg/dL	0.14–0.64 μmol/L 0.084–0.42 μmol/L	Levels higher in AM Patients should be at rest for 2 hr before test and fasting for 3 hr Estrogens increase cortisol level
Urine cortisol	10–100 μg/d for 24 h	27.6–276.0 nmol/d	Have patient void upon awakening then begin collection at time of next void Specimen kept cold to prevent bacterial growth

The *dexamethasone suppression test (DST)* is used to determine if a client has the normal ability to suppress cortisol production. It is seen as an index of the hypothalamic–pituitary–adrenal axis. Dexamethasone 1–2 mg po is given at bedtime. Serum samples are assayed for cortisol levels at 4 PM and 11 PM the following day. With the stimulus of dexamethasone, a person will normally suppress cortisol production, and a value of $<5\ \mu$g/dL will be seen. A value of plasma cortisol $>5\ \mu$g/dL is positive for nonsuppression. It is hypothesized that the inability to suppress cortisol is predictive of a depression that will respond well to somatic intervention. Some clinicians also use DST results to make decisions about when to discontinue antidepressant medication.[3]

III. Tests used to monitor drug therapy

A. Blood levels of medications should be routinely monitored when the patient is in a steady state. Serum level monitoring of the following antimania drugs is *routinely* done.

(*continued*)

Laboratory Values (*continued*)

DRUG	THERAPEUTIC RANGE	RECOMMENDED SI UNITS	COMMENTS
Lithium	0.6–1.2 mEq/L	0.6–1.2 mmol/L	Laboratory draw should be 12 hr after last dose
Carbamazepine (Tegratol)	8–12 μg/mL	34–51 μmol/L	Check CBC and platelet counts regularly because bone marrow depression is possible

B. The monitoring of tricyclic antidepressants is sometimes done,[1,2] although there is great variation in plasma levels and response. These data are most useful in supplementing the individual patient's clinical picture and experience of side effects. Plasma assays are expensive.

DRUG	TRADE NAME	THERAPEUTIC RANGE*	RECOMMENDED SI UNITS
Imipramine	Tofranil	75–250 ng/ml	267–892 nmol/L
Desipramine	Norpramine	150–300 ng/ml	562–1125 nmol/L
Amitriptyline	Elavil	125–250 ng/ml	440–903 nmol/L
Nortriptyline	Aventyl	50–150 ng/ml	190–570 nmol/L
Doxepin	Sinequan	75–300 ng/ml	268–1074 nmol/L

Monitoring of therapeutic ranges of antipsychotic medication is still in the research stage.

IV. Toxicology

A. In a known or suspected overdose, blood, urine, and/or gastric toxicology studies may be ordered. Screening procedures can detect a broad spectrum of compounds in blood including barbiturate and nonbarbiturate hypnotics, narcotic and nonnarcotic analgesics, tranquilizers, CNS stimulants and depressants; and most psychotropic medications. LSD cannot be detected.

Some drugs may be detected in urine through their metabolites. For a broad-spectrum screen, 50–100 mL of urine is required. Less is needed if evidence of a specific drug is sought.

To confirm and quantify the amount of toxin that has been discovered in a sample, both blood and urine or gastric contents will be needed. Individual laboratories have specific procedures. Broad-spectrum toxicology screens are costly and time-consuming.

Drug testing requires informed consent, and legal specimens require special handling. This is an area of current controversy, and laws are constantly changing and being challenged. The nurse must be knowledgeable about her responsibilities.

B. Reference values for commonly misused drugs

DRUG	VALUES	SI UNITS	COMMENTS
Salicyclic acid	<100 μg/mL	<724 μmol/L	Analgesia,
	150–300 μg/mL	1086–2172 μmol/L	anti-inflammatory tinnitus
	>500 μg/mL	>3620 μmol/L	intoxication
Ethyl alcohol	Legal intoxication >100 mg/dL (varies by state)	>21.7 mmol/L	
	Alcoholic stupor; coma; death 250–400 mg/dL	54.3–86.8 mmol/L	
Short-acting barbiturates (pentobarbital, [Nembutal]; secobarbital,[Seconal])	Coma >5 μg/mL	>21.0 μmol/L	
Long-acting barbiturates (phenobarbital; [Luminol])	Coma >100 μg/mL	>430 μmol/L	
Carbon monoxide (hemoglobin saturation)		*FRACTION HEMOGLOBIN SATURATED:*	
	5–10% normal in heavy smokers	0.05–0.10	Cherry red color of lips sometimes occurs
	30–40% marked toxicity, headache nausea, confusion	0.30–0.40	
	40–50% disorientation, hallucination, collapse	0.40–0.50	

(*continued*)

Laboratory Values (*continued*)

DRUG	VALUES	SI UNITS	COMMENTS
Acetaminophen (serum)	Toxic >120 μg/mL	>794 μmol/L	Usually no liver damage
	Hepatotoxic >200 μg/mL	>1324 μmol/L	SGOT and SGPT will rise in 2–4 days after ingestion
	Hepatic necrosis >300 μg/mL or half-life >4 hr	>1986 μmol/L	Half-life is estimated by measuring serial acetaminophen levels 4 hr apart to determine how much of the drug has been eliminated. With liver damage, the half-life is increased.[1]
	Hepatic coma half-life >12 hr		

---

* Laboratory values and norms vary greatly according to laboratory technique. Norms for children and pregnant women often differ from indicated values.

All values from Tietz unless otherwise noted.

References

1. Corbet JV. Laboratory tests and diagnostic procedures with nursing diagnoses. 2nd ed. Norwalk, CT: Appleton & Lange; 1987.
2. Davis JM. Clinical utility of biochemical assays in psychiatry. Ann Rev Med. 1987;38:149–156.
3. Gitlin MJ, Gerner RH. The dexamethasone suppression test and response to somatic treatment: a review. J Clin Psychiatry. 1986;47:16–21.
4. Hall RC, Beresford TP, eds. Handbook of psychiatric diagnostic procedures, 2 vol. New York: Spectrum Publications; 1985.
5. Tietz NW, ed. Clinical guide to laboratory tests. Philadelphia: WB Saunders; 1983.

Index

Page numbers in *italics* indicate figures; those followed by *t* indicate tabular material; those followed by *b* indicate boxed material; those followed by *c* indicate charts.

The Rise and Fall
of the Great Powers

THE
RISE AND FALL
OF THE
GREAT POWERS

Economic Change
and Military Conflict
from 1500 to 2000

BY PAUL KENNEDY

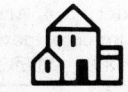

Random House
New York

Grateful acknowledgment is made to the following
for permission to reprint previously published material:

Lexington Books, D. C. Heath and Company: An illustration from *American
Defense Annual 1987–1988*, edited by Joseph Kruzel. Copyright © 1987, D. C.
Heath and Company (Lexington, Mass.: Lexington Books, D. C. Heath and
Company). Reprinted by permission of the publisher.

Library of Congress Cataloging-in-Publication Data

Kennedy, Paul M., 1945-
The rise and fall of the great powers.

Includes index.
1. History, Modern.   2. Economic history.
3. Military history, Modern.   4. Armaments—Economic
aspects.   5. Balance of power.   I. Title.
D210.K46   1988   909.82   87-9690

Book design by Charlotte Staub
Maps by Jean Paul Tremblay

Manufactured in the United States of America

To Cath

Acknowledgments

Whatever the weaknesses of this book, they would have been far greater without the kind help of friends. J. R. Jones and Gordon Lee went through the entire manuscript, asking questions all the way. My colleague Jonathan Spence endeavored (I fear with only partial success) to curb the cultural assumptions which emerged in the first two chapters. John Elliott was encouraging about Chapter 2, despite its being very evidently "not my period." Paddy O'Brien and John Bosher sought to make my comments on eighteenth-century British and French finance a little less crude. Nick Rizopoulos and Michael Mandelbaum not only scrutinized the later chapters, but also invited me to present my ideas at a series of meetings at the Lehrman Institute in New York. Many, many scholars have heard me give papers on subthemes in this book, and have provided references, much-needed criticism, and encouragement.

The libraries and staffs at the universities of East Anglia and Yale were of great assistance. My graduate student Kevin Smith helped me in the search for historical statistics. My son Jim Kennedy prepared the maps. Sheila Klein and Sue McClain came to the rescue with typing and word processing, as did Maarten Pereboom with the bibliography. I am extremely grateful for the sustained support and encouragement which my literary agent, Bruce Hunter, has provided over the years. Jason Epstein has been a firm and patient editor, repeatedly getting me to think of the general reader—and also recognizing earlier than the author did how demanding it would be to deal with themes of this magnitude.

My family has provided support and, more important still, light relief. The book is dedicated to my wife, to whom I owe so much.

Paul Kennedy
Hamden, Connecticut, 1986

CONTENTS

MAPS

TABLES & CHARTS

TABLES

CHARTS

Introduction

This is a book about national and international power in the "modern"—that is, post-Renaissance—period. It seeks to trace and to explain how the various Great Powers have risen and fallen, relative to each other, over the five centuries since the formation of the "new monarchies" of western Europe and the beginnings of the transoceanic, global system of states. Inevitably, it concerns itself a great deal with wars, especially those major, drawn-out conflicts fought by coalitions of Great Powers which had such an impact upon the international order; but it is not strictly a book about military history. It also concerns itself with tracing the changes which have occurred in the global economic balances since 1500; and yet it is not, at least directly, a work of economic history. What it concentrates upon is the *interaction* between economics and strategy, as each of the leading states in the international system strove to enhance its wealth and its power, to become (or to remain) both rich and strong.

The "military conflict" referred to in the book's subtitle is therefore always examined in the context of "economic change." The triumph of any one Great Power in this period, or the collapse of another, has usually been the consequence of lengthy fighting by its armed forces; but it has also been the consequence of the more or less efficient utilization of the state's productive economic resources in wartime, and, further in the background, of the way in which that state's economy had been rising or falling, *relative* to the other leading nations, in the decades preceding the actual conflict. For that reason, how a Great Power's position steadily alters in peacetime is as important to this study as how it fights in wartime.

The argument being offered here will receive much more elaborate analysis in the text itself, but can be summarized very briefly:

The relative strengths of the leading nations in world affairs never remain constant, principally because of the uneven rate of growth among different societies and of the technological and organizational breakthroughs which bring a greater advantage to one society than to another. For example, the coming of the long-range gunned sailing ship and the rise of the Atlantic trades after 1500 was not *uniformly* beneficial to all the states of Europe—it boosted some much more than others. In the same way, the later development of steam power and of the coal and metal resources upon which it relied massively increased the relative power of certain nations, and thereby decreased the relative power of others. Once their productive capacity was enhanced, countries would normally find it easier to sustain the burdens of paying for large-scale armaments in peacetime and of maintaining and supplying large armies and fleets in wartime. It sounds crudely mercantilistic to express it this way, but wealth is usually needed to underpin military power, and military power is usually needed to acquire and protect wealth. If, however, too large a proportion of the state's resources is diverted from wealth creation and allocated instead to military purposes, then that is likely to lead to a weakening of national power over the longer term. In the same way, if a state overextends itself strategically—by, say, the conquest of extensive territories or the waging of costly wars—it runs the risk that the potential benefits from external expansion may be outweighed by the great expense of it all—a dilemma which becomes acute if the nation concerned has entered a period of relative economic decline. The history of the rise and later fall of the leading countries in the Great Power system since the advance of western Europe in the sixteenth century—that is, of nations such as Spain, the Netherlands, France, the British Empire, and currently the United States—shows a very significant correlation *over the longer term* between productive and revenue-raising capacities on the one hand and military strength on the other.

The story of "the rise and fall of the Great Powers" which is presented in these chapters may be briefly summarized here. The first chapter sets the scene for all that follows by examining the world around 1500 and by analyzing the strengths and weaknesses of each of the "power centers" of that time—Ming China; the Ottoman Empire and its Muslim offshoot in India, the Mogul Empire; Muscovy; Tokugawa Japan; and the cluster of states in west-central Europe. At the beginning of the sixteenth century it was by no means apparent that the last-named region was destined to rise above all the rest. But however imposing and organized some of those oriental empires appeared by comparison with Europe, they all suffered from the consequences of having a centralized authority which insisted upon a uniformity of belief and practice, not only in official state religion but also in such areas as commercial activities and weapons development. The lack of any such supreme authority in Europe and the warlike rivalries among its various kingdoms and city-states stimulated a constant search for military improvements, which interacted fruitfully with the newer technological and commercial advances that were also being thrown up in this competitive, entrepreneurial environment. Possessing fewer obstacles to change, European societies entered into a constantly upward spiral of economic growth and enhanced military effectiveness which, over time, was to carry them ahead of all other regions of the globe.

While this dynamic of technological change and military competitiveness drove Europe forward in its usual jostling, pluralistic way, there still remained the possibility that one of the contending states might acquire sufficient resources to surpass the others, and then to dominate the continent. For about 150 years after 1500, a dynastic-religious bloc under the Spanish and Austrian Habsburgs seemed to threaten to do just that, and the efforts of the other major European states to check this "Habsburg bid for mastery" occupy the whole of Chapter 2. As is done throughout this book, the strengths and weaknesses of each of the leading Powers are analyzed *relatively,* and in the light of the broader economic and technological changes affecting western society as a whole, in order that the reader can understand better the outcome of the many wars of this period. The chief theme of this chapter is that despite the great resources possessed by the Habsburg monarchs, they steadily overextended themselves in the course of repeated conflicts and became militarily top-heavy for their weakening economic base. If the other European Great Powers also suffered immensely in these prolonged wars, they managed—though narrowly—to maintain the balance between their material resources and their military power better than their Habsburg enemies.

The Great Power struggles which took place between 1660 and 1815, and are covered in Chapter 3, cannot be so easily summarized as a contest between one large bloc and its many rivals. It was in this complicated period that while certain former Great Powers like Spain and the Netherlands were falling into the second rank, there steadily emerged five major states (France, Britain, Russia, Austria, and Prussia) which came to dominate the diplomacy and warfare of eighteenth-century Europe, and to engage in a series of lengthy coalition wars punctuated by swiftly changing alliances. This was an age in which France, first under Louis XIV and then later under Napoleon, came closer to controlling Europe than at any time before or since; but its endeavors were always held in check, in the last resort at least, by a combination of the other Great Powers. Since the cost of standing armies and national fleets had become horrendously great by the early eighteenth century, a country which could create an advanced system of banking and credit (as Britain did) enjoyed many advantages over financially backward rivals. But the factor of geographical position was also of great importance in deciding the fate of the Powers in their many, and frequently changing, contests—which helps to explain why the two "flank" nations of Russia and Britain had become much more important by 1815. Both retained the capacity to intervene in the struggles of west-central Europe while being geographically sheltered from them; and both expanded into the *extra*-European world as the eighteenth century unfolded, even as they were ensuring that the continental balance of power was upheld. Finally, by the later decades of the century, the Industrial Revolution was under way in Britain, which was to give that state an enhanced capacity both to colonize overseas and to frustrate the Napoleonic bid for European mastery.

For an entire century after 1815, by contrast, there was a remarkable absence of lengthy coalition wars. A strategic equilibrium existed, supported by all of the leading Powers in the Concert of Europe, so that no single nation was either able or willing to make a bid for dominance. The prime concerns of government in these post-1815 decades were with domestic instability and (in the case of Russia and the United States) with further expansion across their continental landmasses. This relatively stable international scene allowed the British Empire to rise to its zenith as a global power, in naval and colonial and commercial terms, and also interacted favorably with its virtual monopoly of steam-driven industrial production. By the second half of the nineteenth century, however, industrialization was spreading to certain other regions, and was beginning to tilt the international power balances away from the older leading nations and toward those countries with both the resources and organization to exploit the newer means of production and technology. Already, the few major conflicts of this era—the Crimean War to some degree but more especially the American Civil War and the Franco-Prussian War—were bringing defeat upon those societies which failed to modernize their military systems, and which lacked the broad-based industrial infrastructure to support the vast armies and much more expensive and complicated weaponry now transforming the nature of war.

As the twentieth century approached, therefore, the pace of technological change and uneven growth rates made the international system much more unstable and complex than it had been fifty years earlier. This was manifested in the frantic post-1880 jostling by the Great Powers for additional colonial territories in Africa, Asia, and the Pacific, partly for gain, partly out of a fear of being eclipsed. It also manifested itself in the increasing number of arms races, both on land and at sea, and in the creation of fixed military alliances, even in peacetime, as the various governments sought out partners for a possible future war. Behind the frequent colonial quarrels and international crises of the pre-1914 period, however, the decade-by-decade indices of economic power were pointing to even more fundamental shifts in the global balances—indeed, to the eclipse of what had been, for over three centuries, essentially a *Eurocentric* world system. Despite their best efforts, traditional European Great Powers like France and Austria-Hungary, and a recently united one like Italy, were falling out of the race. By contrast, the enormous, continent-wide states of the United States and Russia were moving to the forefront, and this despite the inefficiencies of the czarist state. Among the western European nations only Germany, possibly, had the muscle to force its way into the select league of the future world Powers. Japan, on the other hand, was intent upon being dominant in East Asia, but not farther afield. Inevitably, then, all these changes posed considerable, and ultimately insuperable, problems for a British Empire which now found it much more difficult to defend its global interests than it had a half-century earlier.

Although the major development of the fifty years after 1900 can thus be seen as the coming of a bipolar world, with its consequent crisis for the "middle" Powers (as referred in the titles of Chapters 5 and 6), this metamorphosis of the entire system was by no means a smooth one. On the contrary, the grinding, bloody mass battles of the First World War, by placing a premium upon industrial organization and national efficiency, gave imperial Germany certain advantages over the swiftly modernizing but still backward czarist Russia. Within a few months of Germany's victory on the eastern front, however, it found itself facing defeat in the west, while its allies were similarly collapsing in the Italian, Balkan, and Near Eastern theaters of the war. Because of the late addition of American military and especially economic aid, the western alliance finally had the resources to prevail over its rival coalition. But it had been an exhausting struggle for all the original belligerents. Austria-Hungary was gone, Russia in revolution, Germany defeated; yet France, Italy, and even Britain itself had also suffered heavily in their victory. The only exceptions were Japan, which further augmented its position in the Pacific; and, of course, the United States, which by 1918 was indisputably the strongest Power in the world.

The swift post-1919 American withdrawal from foreign engagements, and the parallel Russian isolationism under the Bolshevik regime, left an international system which was more out of joint with the fundamental economic realities than perhaps at any time in the five centuries covered in this book. Britain and France, although weakened, were still at the center of the diplomatic stage, but by the 1930s their position was being challenged by the militarized, revisionist states of Italy, Japan, and Germany—the last intent upon a much more deliberate bid for European hegemony than even in 1914. In the background, however, the United States remained by far the mightiest manufacturing nation in the world, and Stalin's Russia was quickly transforming itself into an industrial superpower. Consequently, the dilemma for the *revisionist* "middle" Powers was that they had to expand soon if they were not to be overshadowed by the two continental giants. The dilemma for the status quo middle Powers was that in fighting off the German and Japanese challenges, they would most likely weaken themselves as well. The Second World War, for all its ups and downs, essentially confirmed those apprehensions of decline. Despite spectacular early victories, the Axis nations could not in the end succeed against an imbalance of productive resources which was far greater than that of the 1914–1918 war. What they did achieve was the eclipse of France and the irretrievable weakening of Britain— before they themselves were overwhelmed by superior force. By 1943, the bipolar world forecast decades earlier had finally arrived, and the military balance had once again caught up with the global distribution of economic resources.

The last two chapters of this book examine the years in which a bipolar world did indeed seem to exist, economically, militarily, and ideologically—and was reflected at the political level by the many crises of the Cold War. The position of the United States and the USSR as Powers in a class of their own also appeared to be reinforced by the arrival of nuclear weapons and long-distance delivery systems, which suggested that the strategic as well as the diplomatic landscape was now entirely different from that of 1900, let alone 1800.

And yet the process of rise and fall among the Great Powers—of differentials in growth rates and technological change, leading to shifts in the global economic balances, which in turn gradually impinge upon the political and military balances—had not ceased. Militarily, the United States and the USSR stayed in the forefront as the 1960s gave way to the 1970s and 1980s. Indeed, because they both interpreted international problems in bipolar, and often Manichean, terms, their rivalry has driven them into an ever-escalating arms race which no other Powers feel capable of matching. Over the same few decades, however, the global productive balances have been altering faster than ever before. The Third World's share of total manufacturing output and GNP, depressed to an all-time low in the decade after 1945, has steadily expanded since that time. Europe has recovered from its wartime batterings and, in the form of the European Economic Community, has become the world's largest trading unit. The People's Republic of China is leaping forward at an impressive rate. Japan's postwar economic growth has been so phenomenal that, according to some measures, it recently overtook Russia in total GNP. By contrast, both the American and Russian growth rates have become more sluggish, and their shares of global production and wealth have shrunk dramatically since the 1960s. Leaving aside all the smaller nations, therefore, it is plain that there already exists a *multi*polar world once more, if one measures the economic indices alone. Given this book's concern with the interaction between strategy and economics, it seemed appropriate to offer a final (if necessarily speculative) chapter to explore the present disjuncture between the military balances and the productive balances among the Great Powers; and to point to the problems and opportunities facing today's five large politico-economic "power centers"—China, Japan, the EEC, the Soviet Union, and the United States itself—as they grapple with the age-old task of relating national means to national ends. The history of the rise and fall of the Great Powers has in no way come to a full stop.

Since the scope of this book is so large, it is clear that it will be read by different people for different purposes. Some readers will find here what they had hoped for: a broad and yet reasonably detailed survey of Great Power politics over the past five centuries, of the way in which the relative position of each of the leading states has been affected by economic and technological change, and of the constant interaction between strategy and economics, both in periods of peace and in the tests of war. By definition, it does not deal with *small* Powers, nor (usually) with small, bilateral wars. By definition also, the book is heavily Eurocentric, especially in its middle chapters. But that is only natural with such a topic.

To other readers, perhaps especially those political scientists who are now so interested in drawing general rules about "world systems" or the recurrent pattern of wars, this study may offer less than what they desire. To avoid misunderstanding, it ought to be made clear at this point that the book is not dealing with, for example, the theory that major (or "systemic") wars can be related to Kondratieff cycles of economic upturn and downturn. In addition, it is not centrally concerned with general theories about the *causes* of war, and whether they are likely to be brought about by "rising" or "falling" Great Powers. It is also not a book about theories of empire, and about how imperial control is effected (as is dealt with in Michael Doyle's recent book *Empires*), or whether empires contribute to national strength. Finally, it does not propose any general theory about which sorts of society and social/governmental organizations are the most efficient in extracting resources in time of war.

On the other hand, there obviously is a wealth of material in this book for those scholars who wish to make such generalizations (and one of the reasons why there is such an extensive array of notes is to indicate more detailed sources for those readers interested in, say, the financing of wars). But the problem which historians—as opposed to political scientists—have in grappling with general theories is that the evidence of the past is almost always too varied to allow for "hard" scientific conclusions. Thus, while it is true that some wars (e.g., 1939) can be linked to decision-makers' fears about shifts taking place in the overall power balances, that would not be so useful in explaining the struggles which began in 1776 (American Revolutionary War) or 1792 (French Revolutionary) or 1854 (Crimean War). In the same way, while one could point to Austria-Hungary in 1914 as a good example of a "falling" Great Power helping to trigger off a major war, that still leaves the theorist to deal with the equally critical roles played then by those "rising" Great Powers Germany and Russia. Similarly, any general theory about whether empires pay, or whether imperial control is affected by a measurable "power-distance" ratio, is likely—from the conflicting evidence available—to produce the banal answer sometimes yes, sometimes no.

Nevertheless, if one sets aside *a priori* theories and simply looks at the historical record of "the rise and fall of the Great Powers" over the past five hundred years, it is clear that some generally valid conclusions can be drawn—while admitting all the time that there may be individual exceptions. For example, there is detectable a causal relationship between the shifts which have occurred over time in the general economic and productive balances and the position occupied by individual Powers in the international system. The move in trade flows from the Mediterranean to the Atlantic and northwestern Europe from the sixteenth century onward, or the redistribution in the shares of world manufacturing output away from western Europe in the decades after 1890, are good examples here. In both cases, the economic shifts heralded the rise of new Great Powers which would one day have a decisive impact upon the military/territorial order. This is why the move in the global productive balances toward the "Pacific rim" which has taken place over the past few decades cannot be of interest merely to economists alone.

Similarly, the historical record suggests that there is a very clear connection *in the long run* between an individual Great Power's economic rise and fall and its growth and decline as an important military power (or world empire). This, too, is hardly surprising, since it flows from two related facts. The first is that economic resources are necessary to support a large-scale military establishment. The second is that, so far as the international system is concerned, both wealth and power are always *relative* and should be seen as such. Three hundred years ago, the German mercantilist writer von Hornigk observed that

> whether a nation be today mighty and rich or not depends not on
> the abundance or security of its power and riches, but principally
> on whether its neighbors possess more or less of it.

In the chapters which follow, this observation will be borne out time and again. The Netherlands in the mid-eighteenth century was richer in *absolute* terms than a hundred years earlier, but by that stage was much less of a Great Power because neighbors like France and Britain had "more . . . of it" (that is, more power and riches). The France of 1914 was, absolutely, more powerful than that of 1850—but this was little consolation when France was being eclipsed by a much stronger Germany. Britain today has far greater wealth, and its armed forces possess far more powerful weapons, than in its mid-Victorian prime; that avails it little when its share of world product has shrunk from about 25 percent to about 3 percent. If a nation has "more . . . of it," things are fine; if "less of it," there are problems.

This does not mean, however, that a nation's relative economic and military power will rise and fall *in parallel*. Most of the historical examples covered here suggest that there is a noticeable "lag time" between the trajectory of a state's relative economic strength and the trajectory of its military/territorial influence. Once again, the reason for this is not difficult to grasp. An economically expanding Power— Britain in the 1860s, the United States in the 1890s, Japan today—may well prefer to become rich rather than to spend heavily on armaments. A half-century later, priorities may well have altered. The earlier economic expansion has brought with it overseas obligations (dependence upon foreign markets and raw materials, military alliances, perhaps bases and colonies). Other, rival Powers are now economically expanding at a faster rate, and wish in their turn to extend their influence abroad. The world has become a more competitive place, and market shares are being eroded. Pessimistic observers talk of decline; patriotic statesmen call for "renewal."

In these more troubled circumstances, the Great Power is likely to find itself spending much *more* on defense than it did two generations earlier, and yet still discover that the world is a less secure environment—simply because other Powers have grown faster, and are becoming stronger. Imperial Spain spent much more on its army in the troubled 1630s and 1640s than it did in the 1580s, when the Castilian economy was healthier. Edwardian Britain's defense expenditures were far greater in 1910 than they were at, say, the time of Palmerston's death in 1865, when the British economy was relatively at its peak; but which Britons by the later date felt more secure? The same problem, it will be argued below, appears to be facing both the United States and the USSR today. Great Powers in relative decline instinctively respond by spending more on "security," and thereby divert potential resources from "investment" and compound their long-term dilemma.

Another general conclusion which can be drawn from the five-hundred-year record presented here is that there is a very strong correlation between the eventual outcome of the *major coalition wars* for

European or global mastery, and the amount of productive resources mobilized by each side. This was true of the struggles waged against the Spanish-Austrian Habsburgs; of the great eighteenth-century contests like the War of Spanish Succession, the Seven Years War, and the Napoleonic War; and of the two world wars of this century. A lengthy, grinding war eventually turns into a test of the relative capacities of each coalition. Whether one side has "more . . . of it" or "less of it" becomes increasingly significant as the struggle lengthens.

One can make these generalizations, however, without falling into the trap of crude economic determinism. Despite this book's abiding interest in tracing the "larger tendencies" in world affairs over the past five centuries, it is *not* arguing that economics determines every event, or is the sole reason for the success and failure of each nation. There simply is too much evidence pointing to other things: geography, military organization, national morale, the alliance system, and many other factors can all affect the relative power of the members of the states system. In the eighteenth century, for example, the United Provinces were the richest parts of Europe, and Russia the poorest—yet the Dutch fell, and the Russians rose. Individual folly (like Hitler's) and extremely high battlefield competence (whether of the Spanish regiments in the sixteenth century or of the German infantry in this century) also go a long way to explain individual victories and defeats. What does seem incontestable, however, is that in a long-drawn-out Great Power (and usually coalition) war, victory has repeatedly gone to the side with the more flourishing productive base—or, as the Spanish captains used to say, to him who has the last escudo. Much of what follows will confirm that cynical but essentially correct judgment. And it is precisely because the power position of the leading nations has closely paralleled their relative economic position over the past five centuries that it seems worthwhile asking what the implications of today's economic and technological trends might be for the current balance of power. This does not deny that men make their own history, but they do make it within a historical circumstance which can restrict (as well as open up) possibilities.

An early model for the present book was the 1833 essay of the famous Prussian historian Leopold von Ranke upon *die grossen Mächte* ("the great powers"), in which he surveyed the ups and downs of the international power balances since the decline of Spain, and tried to show why certain countries had risen to prominence and then fallen away. Ranke concluded his essay with an analysis of his contemporary world, and what was happening in it following the defeat of the French bid for supremacy in the Napoleonic War. In examining the "prospects" of each of the Great Powers, he, too, was tempted from the historian's profession into the uncertain world of speculating upon the future.

To write an essay upon "the Great Powers" is one thing; to tell the story in book form is quite another. My original intention was to produce a brief, "essayistic" book, presuming that the readers knew (however vaguely) the background details about the changing growth rates, or the particular geostrategical problems facing this or that Great Power. As I began sending out the early chapters of this book for comments, or giving trial-run talks about some of its themes, it became increasingly clear to me that that was a false presumption: what most readers and listeners wanted was *more* detail, *more* coverage of the background, simply because there was no study available which told the story of the shifts that occurred in the economic and strategical power balances. Precisely because neither economic historians nor military historians had entered this field, the story itself had simply suffered from neglect. If the abundant detail in both the text and notes which follow has any justification, it is to fill that critical gap in the history of the rise and fall of the Great Powers.

STRATEGY & ECONOMICS
IN THE
PREINDUSTRIAL
WORLD

1
The Rise of
the Western World

In the year 1500, the date chosen by numerous scholars to mark the divide between modern and pre-modern times,[1] it was by no means obvious to the inhabitants of Europe that their continent was poised to dominate much of the rest of the earth. The knowledge which contemporaries possessed about the great civilizations of the Orient was fragmentary and all too often erroneous, based as it was upon travelers' tales which had lost nothing in their retelling. Nevertheless, the widely held image of extensive eastern empires possessing fabulous wealth and vast armies was a reasonably accurate one, and on first acquaintance those societies must have seemed far more favorably endowed than the peoples and states of western Europe. Indeed, placed alongside these other great centers of cultural and economic activity, Europe's relative weaknesses *were* more apparent than its strengths. It was, for a start, neither the most fertile nor the most populous area in the world; India and China took pride of place in each respect. Geopolitically, the "continent" of Europe was an awkward shape, bounded by ice and water to the north and west, being open to frequent landward invasion from the east, and vulnerable to strategic circumvention in the south. In 1500, and for a long time before and after that, these were not abstract considerations. It was only eight years earlier that Granada, the last Muslim region of Spain, had succumbed to the armies of Ferdinand and Isabella; but that signified the end of a regional campaign, not of the far larger struggle between Christendom and the forces of the Prophet. Over much of the western world there still hung the shock of the fall of Constantinople in 1453, an event which seemed the more pregnant because it by no means marked the limits of the Ottoman Turks' advance. By the end of the century they had taken Greece and the Ionian Islands, Bosnia, Albania, and much of the rest of the Balkans; and worse was to come in the 1520s when their formidable janissary armies pressed toward Budapest and Vienna. In the south, where Ottoman galleys raided Italian ports, the popes were coming to fear that Rome's fate would soon match that of Constantinople.[2]

Whereas these threats seemed part of a coherent grand strategy directed by Sultan Mehmet II and his successors, the response of the Europeans was disjointed and sporadic. Unlike the Ottoman and Chinese empires, unlike the rule which the Moguls were soon to establish in India, there never was a united Europe in which all parts acknowledged one secular or religious leader. Instead, Europe was a hodgepodge of petty kingdoms and principalities, marcher lordships and city-states. Some more powerful monarchies were arising in the west, notably Spain, France, and England, but none was to be free of internal tensions and all regarded the others as rivals, rather than allies in the struggle against Islam.

Nor could it be said that Europe had pronounced advantages in the realms of culture, mathematics, engineering, or navigational and other technologies when compared with the great civilizations of Asia. A considerable part of the European cultural and scientific heritage was, in any case, "borrowed" from Islam, just as Muslim societies had borrowed for centuries from China through the media of mutual trade, conquest, and settlement. In retrospect, one can see that Europe was accelerating both commercially and technologically by the late fifteenth century; but perhaps the fairest general comment would be that each of the great centers of world civilization about that time was at a roughly similar stage of development, some more advanced in one area, but less so in others. Technologically and, therefore, militarily, the Ottoman Empire, China under the Ming dynasty, a little later northern India under the Moguls, and the European states system with its Muscovite offshoot were all far superior to the scattered societies of Africa, America, and Oceania. While this does imply that Europe in 1500 was one of the most important cultural power centers, it was not at all obvious that it would one day emerge at the very top. Before investigating the causes of its rise, therefore, it is necessary to examine the strengths and the weaknesses of the other contenders.

Ming China

Of all the civilizations of premodern times, none appeared more advanced, none felt more superior, than that of China.[3] Its considerable population, 100–130 million compared with Europe's 50–55 million in the fifteenth century; its remarkable culture; its exceedingly fertile and irrigated plains, linked by a splendid canal system since the eleventh century; and its unified, hierarchic administration run by a well-educated Confucian bureaucracy had given a coherence and sophistication to Chinese society which was the envy of foreign visi-

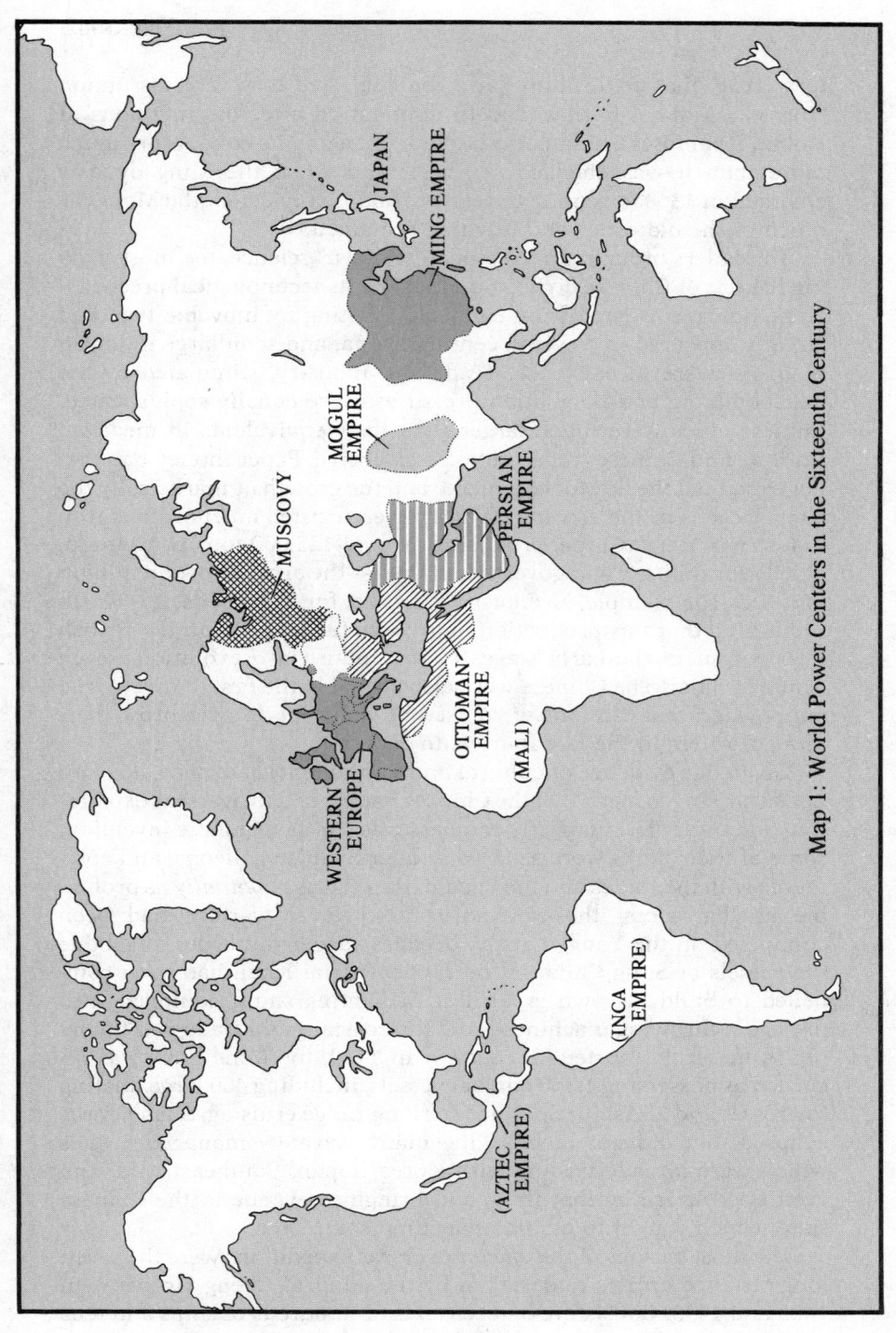

Map 1: World Power Centers in the Sixteenth Century

tors. True, that civilization had been subjected to severe disruption from the Mongol hordes, and to domination after the invasions of Kublai Khan. But China had a habit of changing its conquerors much more than it was changed by them, and when the Ming dynasty emerged in 1368 to reunite the empire and finally defeat the Mongols, much of the old order and learning remained.

To readers brought up to respect "western" science, the most striking feature of Chinese civilization must be its technological precocity. Huge libraries existed from early on. Printing by movable type had already appeared in eleventh-century China, and soon large numbers of books were in existence. Trade and industry, stimulated by the canal-building and population pressures, were equally sophisticated. Chinese cities were much larger than their equivalents in medieval Europe, and Chinese trade routes as extensive. Paper money had earlier expedited the flow of commerce and the growth of markets. By the later decades of the eleventh century there existed an enormous iron industry in north China, producing around 125,000 tons per annum, chiefly for military and governmental use—the army of over a million men was, for example, an enormous market for iron goods. It is worth remarking that this production figure was far larger than the British iron output in the early stages of the Industrial Revolution, seven centuries later! The Chinese were also probably the first to invent true gunpowder; and cannons were used by the Ming to overthrow their Mongol rulers in the late fourteenth century.[4]

Given this evidence of cultural and technological advance, it is also not surprising to learn that the Chinese had turned to overseas exploration and trade. The magnetic compass was another Chinese invention, some of their junks were as large as later Spanish galleons, and commerce with the Indies and the Pacific islands was *potentially* as profitable as that along the caravan routes. Naval warfare had been conducted on the Yangtze many decades earlier—in order to subdue the vessels of Sung China in the 1260s, Kublai Khan had been compelled to build his own great fleet of fighting ships, equipped with projectile-throwing machines—and the coastal grain trade was booming in the early fourteenth century. In 1420, the Ming navy was recorded as possessing 1,350 combat vessels, including 400 large floating fortresses and 250 ships designed for long-range cruising. Such a force eclipsed, but did not include, the many privately managed vessels which were already trading with Korea, Japan, Southeast Asia, and even East Africa by that time, and bringing revenue to the Chinese state, which sought to tax this maritime commerce.

The most famous of the *official* overseas expeditions were the seven long-distance cruises undertaken by the admiral Cheng Ho between 1405 and 1433. Consisting on occasions of hundreds of ships and tens of thousands of men, these fleets visited ports from Malacca and Cey-

lon to the Red Sea entrances and Zanzibar. Bestowing gifts upon deferential local rulers on the one hand, they compelled the recalcitrant to
acknowledge Peking on the other. One ship returned with giraffes from
East Africa to entertain the Chinese emperor; another with a Ceylonese
chief who had been unwise enough not to acknowledge the supremacy
of the Son of Heaven. (It must be noted, however, that the Chinese
apparently never plundered nor murdered—unlike the Portuguese,
Dutch, and other European invaders of the Indian Ocean.) From what
historians and archaeologists can tell us of the size, power, and seawor-
thiness of Cheng Ho's navy—some of the great treasure ships appear
to have been around 400 feet long and displaced over 1,500 tons—they
might well have been able to sail around Africa and "discover" Portugal several decades before Henry the Navigator's expeditions began
earnestly to push south of Ceuta.[5]

But the Chinese expedition of 1433 was the last of the line, and three
years later an imperial edict banned the construction of seagoing
ships; later still, a specific order forbade the existence of ships with
more than two masts. Naval personnel would henceforth be employed
on smaller vessels on the Grand Canal. Cheng Ho's great warships were
laid up and rotted away. Despite all the opportunities which beckoned
overseas, China had decided to turn its back on the world.

There was, to be sure, a plausible strategical reason for this decision. The northern frontiers of the empire were again under some
pressure from the Mongols, and it may have seemed prudent to concentrate military resources in this more vulnerable area. Under such
circumstances a large navy was an expensive luxury, and in any case,
the attempted Chinese expansion southward into Annam (Vietnam)
was proving fruitless and costly. Yet this quite valid reasoning does not
appear to have been reconsidered when the disadvantages of naval
retrenchment later became clear: within a century or so, the Chinese
coastline and even cities on the Yangtze were being attacked by Japanese pirates, but there was no serious rebuilding of an imperial navy.
Even the repeated appearance of Portuguese vessels off the China coast
did not force a reassessment.* Defense on land was all that was required, the mandarins reasoned, for had not all maritime trade by
Chinese subjects been forbidden in any case?

Apart from the costs and other disincentives involved, therefore, a
key element in China's retreat was the sheer conservatism of the Confucian bureaucracy[6]—a conservatism heightened in the Ming period
by resentment at the changes earlier forced upon them by the Mongols.
In this "Restoration" atmosphere, the all-important officialdom was
concerned to preserve and recapture the past, not to create a brighter

*For a brief while, in the 1590s, a somewhat revived Chinese coastal fleet helped the
Koreans to resist two Japanese invasion attempts; but even this rump of the Ming navy declined
thereafter.

future based upon overseas expansion and commerce. According to the Confucian code, warfare itself was a deplorable activity and armed forces were made necessary only by the fear of barbarian attacks or internal revolts. The mandarins' dislike of the army (and the navy) was accompanied by a suspicion of the trader. The accumulation of private capital, the practice of buying cheap and selling dear, the ostentation of the *nouveau riche* merchant, all offended the elite, scholarly bureaucrats—almost as much as they aroused the resentments of the toiling masses. While not wishing to bring the entire market economy to a halt, the mandarins often intervened against individual merchants by confiscating their property or banning their business. *Foreign* trade by Chinese subjects must have seemed even more dubious to mandarin eyes, simply because it was less under their control.

This dislike of commerce and private capital does not conflict with the enormous technological achievements mentioned above. The Ming rebuilding of the Great Wall of China and the development of the canal system, the ironworks, and the imperial navy were for *state* purposes, because the bureaucracy had advised the emperor that they were necessary. But just as these enterprises could be started, so also could they be neglected. The canals were permitted to decay, the army was periodically starved of new equipment, the astronomical clocks (built c. 1090) were disregarded, the ironworks gradually fell into desuetude. These were not the only disincentives to economic growth. Printing was restricted to scholarly works and not employed for the widespread dissemination of practical knowledge, much less for social criticism. The use of paper currency was discontinued. Chinese cities were never allowed the autonomy of those in the West; there were no Chinese burghers, with all that that term implied; when the location of the emperor's court was altered, the capital city had to move as well. Yet without official encouragement, merchants and other entrepreneurs could not thrive; and even those who did acquire wealth tended to spend it on land and education, rather than investing in protoindustrial development. Similarly, the banning of overseas trade and fishing took away another potential stimulus to sustained economic expansion; such foreign trade as did occur with the Portuguese and Dutch in the following centuries was in luxury goods and (although there were doubtless many evasions) controlled by officials.

In consequence, Ming China was a much less vigorous and enterprising land than it had been under the Sung dynasty four centuries earlier. There were improved agricultural techniques in the Ming period, to be sure, but after a while even this more intensive farming and the use of marginal lands found it harder to keep pace with the burgeoning population; and the latter was only to be checked by those Malthusian instruments of plague, floods, and war, all of which were very difficult to handle. Even the replacement of the Mings by the more vigorous Manchus after 1644 could not halt the steady relative decline.

One final detail can summarize this tale. In 1736—just as Abraham Darby's ironworks at Coalbrookdale were beginning to boom—the blast furnaces and coke ovens of Honan and Hopei were abandoned entirely. They had been great before the Conqueror had landed at Hastings. Now they would not resume production until the twentieth century.

The Muslim World

Even the first of the European sailors to visit China in the early sixteenth century, although impressed by its size, population, and riches, might have observed that this was a country which had turned in on itself. That remark certainly could not then have been made of the Ottoman Empire, which was then in the middle stages of its expansion and, being nearer home, was correspondingly much more threatening to Christendom. Viewed from the larger historical and geographical perspective, in fact, it would be fair to claim that it was the Muslim states which formed the most rapidly expanding forces in world affairs during the sixteenth century. Not only were the Ottoman Turks pushing westward, but the Safavid dynasty in Persia was also enjoying a resurgence of power, prosperity, and high culture, especially in the reigns of Ismail I (1500–1524) and Abbas I (1587–1629); a chain of strong Muslim khanates still controlled the ancient Silk Road via Kashgar and Turfan to China, not unlike the chain of West African Islamic states such as Bornu, Sokoto, and Timbuktu; the Hindu Empire in Java was overthrown by Muslim forces early in the sixteenth century; and the king of Kabul, Babur, entering India by the conqueror's route from the northwest, established the Mogul Empire in 1526. Although this hold on India was shaky at first, it was successfully consolidated by Babur's grandson Akbar (1556–1605), who carved out a northern Indian empire stretching from Baluchistan in the west to Bengal in the east. Throughout the seventeenth century, Akbar's successors pushed farther south against the Hindu Marathas, just at the same time as the Dutch, British, and French were entering the Indian peninsula from the sea, and of course in a much less substantial form. To these secular signs of Muslim growth one must add the vast increase in numbers of the faithful in Africa and the Indies, against which the proselytization by Christian missions paled in comparison.

But the greatest Muslim challenge to early modern Europe lay, of course, with the Ottoman Turks, or, rather, with their formidable army and the finest siege train of the age. Already by the beginning of the sixteenth century their domains stretched from the Crimea (where they had overrun Genoese trading posts) and the Aegean (where they were dismantling the Venetian Empire) to the Levant. By 1516, Ottoman forces had seized Damascus, and in the following year they entered Egypt, shattering the Mamluk forces by the use of Turkish cannon. Having thus closed the spice route from the Indies, they moved up the Nile and pushed through the Red Sea to the Indian Ocean, countering the Portuguese incursions there. If this perturbed Iberian sailors, it was nothing to the fright which the Turkish armies were giving the princes and peoples of eastern and southern Europe. Already the Turks held Bulgaria and Serbia, and were the predominant influence in Wallachia and all around the Black Sea; but, following the southern drive against Egypt and Arabia, the pressure against Europe was resumed under Suleiman (1520–1566). Hungary, the great eastern bastion of Christendom in these years, could no longer hold off the superior Turkish armies and was overrun following the battle of Mohacs in 1526—the same year, coincidentally, as Babur gained the victory at Panipat by which the Mughal Empire was established. Would all of Europe soon go the way of northern India? By 1529, with the Turks besieging Vienna, this must have appeared a distinct possibility to some. In actual fact, the line then stabilized in northern Hungary and the Holy Roman Empire was preserved; but thereafter the Turks presented a constant danger and exerted a military pressure which could never be fully ignored. Even as late as 1683, they were again besieging Vienna.[7]

Almost as alarming, in many ways, was the expansion of Ottoman naval power. Like Kublai Khan in China, the Turks had developed a navy only in order to reduce a seagirt enemy fortress—in this case, Constantinople, which Sultan Mehmet blockaded with large galleys and hundreds of smaller craft to assist the assault of 1453. Thereafter, formidable galley fleets were used in operations across the Black Sea, in the southward push toward Syria and Egypt, and in a whole series of clashes with Venice for control of the Aegean islands, Rhodes, Crete, and Cyprus. For some decades of the early sixteenth century Ottoman sea power was kept at arm's length by Venetian, Genoese, and Habsburg fleets; but by midcentury, Muslim naval forces were active all the way along the North African coast, were raiding ports in Italy, Spain, and the Balearics, and finally managed to take Cyprus in 1570–1571, before being checked at the battle of Lepanto.[8]

The Ottoman Empire was, of course, much more than a military machine. A conquering elite (like the Manchus in China), the Ottomans had established a unity of *official* faith, culture, and language over an area greater than the Roman Empire, and over vast numbers of subject peoples. For centuries before 1500 the world of Islam had been culturally and technologically ahead of Europe. Its cities were large, well-lit, and drained, and some of them possessed universities and libraries and stunningly beautiful mosques. In mathematics, cartography, medicine, and many other aspects of science and industry—in mills, guncasting, lighthouses, horsebreeding—the Muslims had enjoyed a lead. The Ottoman system of recruiting future janissaries from Christian youth in the Balkans had produced a dedicated, uniform corps of troops. Tolerance of other races had brought many a talented Greek, Jew, and Gentile into the sultan's service—a Hungarian was Mehmet's chief gun-caster in the Siege of Constantinople. Under a successful leader like Suleiman I, a strong bureaucracy supervised fourteen million subjects—this at a time when Spain had five million and England a mere two and a half million inhabitants. Constantinople in its heyday was bigger than any European city, possessing over 500,000 inhabitants in 1600.

Yet the Ottoman Turks, too, were to falter, to turn inward, and to lose the chance of world domination, although this became clear only a century after the strikingly similar Ming decline. To a certain extent it could be argued that this process was the natural consequence of earlier Turkish successes: the Ottoman army, however well administered, might be able to maintain the lengthy frontiers but could hardly expand farther without enormous cost in men and money; and Ottoman imperialism, unlike that of the Spanish, Dutch, and English later, did not bring much in the way of economic benefit. By the second half of the sixteenth century the empire was showing signs of strategical overextension, with a large army stationed in central Europe, an expensive navy operating in the Mediterranean, troops engaged in North Africa, the Aegean, Cyprus, and the Red Sea, and reinforcements needed to hold the Crimea against a rising Russian power. Even in the Near East there was no quiet flank, thanks to a disastrous religious split in the Muslim world which occurred when the Shi'ite branch, based in Iraq and then in Persia, challenged the prevailing Sunni practices and teachings. At times, the situation was not unlike that of the contemporary religious struggles in Germany, and the sultan could maintain his dominance only by crushing Shi'ite dissidents with force. However, across the border the Shi'ite kingdom of Persia under Abbas the Great was quite prepared to ally with European states against the Ottomans, just as France had worked with the "infidel" Turk against the Holy Roman Empire. With this array of adversaries, the Ottoman Empire would have needed remarkable leadership to have maintained its growth; but after 1566 there reigned thirteen incompetent sultans in succession.

External enemies and personal failings do not, however, provide the full explanation. The system as a whole, like that of Ming China, increasingly suffered from some of the defects of being centralized, despotic, and severely orthodox in its attitude toward initiative, dissent, and commerce. An idiot sultan could paralyze the Ottoman Empire in the way that a pope or Holy Roman emperor could never do for all Europe. Without clear directives from above, the arteries of the bureaucracy hardened, preferring conservatism to change, and stifling innovation. The lack of territorial expansion and accompanying booty after 1550, together with the vast rise in prices, caused discontented janissaries to turn to internal plunder. Merchants and entrepreneurs (nearly all of whom were foreigners), who earlier had been encouraged, now found themselves subject to unpredictable taxes and outright seizures of property. Ever higher dues ruined trade and depopulated towns. Perhaps worst affected of all were the peasants, whose lands and stock were preyed upon by the soldiers. As the situation deteriorated, civilian officials also turned to plunder, demanding bribes and confiscating stocks of goods. The costs of war and the loss of Asiatic trade during the struggle with Persia intensified the government's desperate search for new revenues, which in turn gave greater powers to unscrupulous tax farmers.[9]

To a distinct degree, the fierce response to the Shi'ite religious challenge reflected and anticipated a hardening of official attitudes toward all forms of free thought. The printing press was forbidden because it might disseminate dangerous opinions. Economic notions remained primitive: imports of western wares were desired, but exports were forbidden; the guilds were supported in their efforts to check innovation and the rise of "capitalist" producers; religious criticism of traders intensified. Contemptuous of European ideas and practices, the Turks declined to adopt newer methods for containing plagues; consequently, their populations suffered more from severe epidemics. In one truly amazing fit of obscurantism, a force of janissaries destroyed a state observatory in 1580, alleging that it had caused a plague.[10] The armed services had become, indeed, a bastion of conservatism. Despite noting, and occasionally suffering from, the newer weaponry of European forces, the janissaries were slow to modernize themselves. Their bulky cannons were not replaced by the lighter cast-iron guns. After the defeat at Lepanto, they did not build the larger European type of vessels. In the south, the Muslim fleets were simply ordered to remain in the calmer waters of the Red Sea and Persian Gulf, thus obviating the need to construct oceangoing vessels on the Portuguese model. Perhaps technical reasons help to explain these decisions, but cultural and technological conservatism also played a role (by contrast, the irregular Barbary corsairs swiftly adopted the frigate type of warship).

The above remarks about conservatism could be made with equal or even greater force about the Mogul Empire. Despite the sheer size of the kingdom at its height and the military genius of some of its emperors, despite the brilliance of its courts and the craftsmanship of its luxury products, despite even a sophisticated banking and credit network, the system was weak at the core. A conquering Muslim elite lay on top of a vast mass of poverty-stricken peasants chiefly adhering to Hinduism. In the towns themselves there were very considerable numbers of merchants, bustling markets, and an attitude toward manufacture, trade, and credit among Hindu business families which would make them excellent examples of Weber's Protestant ethic. As against this picture of an entrepreneurial society just ready for economic "takeoff" before it became a victim of British imperialism, there are the gloomier portrayals of the many indigenous retarding factors in Indian life. The sheer rigidity of Hindu religious taboos militated against modernization: rodents and insects could not be killed, so vast amounts of foodstuffs were lost; social mores about handling refuse and excreta led to permanently insanitary conditions, a breeding ground for bubonic plagues; the caste system throttled initiative, instilled ritual, and restricted the market; and the influence wielded over Indian local rulers by the Brahman priests meant that this obscurantism was effective at the highest level. Here were social checks of the deepest sort to any attempts at radical change. Small wonder that later many Britons, having first plundered and then tried to govern India in accordance with Utilitarian principles, finally left with the feeling that the country was still a mystery to them.[11]

But the Mogul rule could scarcely be compared with administration by the Indian Civil Service. The brilliant courts were centers of conspicuous consumption on a scale which the Sun King at Versailles might have thought excessive. Thousands of servants and hangers-on, extravagant clothes and jewels and harems and menageries, vast arrays of bodyguards, could be paid for only by the creation of a systematic plunder machine. Tax collectors, required to provide fixed sums for their masters, preyed mercilessly upon peasant and merchant alike; whatever the state of the harvest or trade, the money had to come in. There being no constitutional or other checks—apart from rebellion—upon such depredations, it was not surprising that taxation was known as "eating." For this colossal annual tribute, the population received next to nothing. There was little improvement in communications, and no machinery for assistance in the event of famine, flood, and plague—which were, of course, fairly regular occurrences. All this makes the Ming dynasty appear benign, almost progressive, by comparison. Technically, the Mogul Empire was to decline because it became increasingly difficult to maintain itself against the Marathas in the south, the Afghanis in the north, and, finally, the East India Company. In reality, the causes of its decay were much more internal than external.

Two Outsiders—Japan and Russia

By the sixteenth century there were two other states which, although nowhere near the size and population of the Ming, Ottoman, and Mogul empires, were demonstrating signs of political consolidation and economic growth. In the Far East, Japan was taking forward steps just as its large Chinese neighbor was beginning to atrophy. Geography gave a prime strategical asset to the Japanese (as it did to the British), for insularity offered a protection from overland invasion which China did not possess. The gap between the islands of Japan and the Asiatic mainland was by no means a complete one, however, and a great deal of Japanese culture and religion had been adapted from the older civilization. But whereas China was run by a unified bureaucracy, power in Japan lay in the hands of clan-based feudal lordships and the emperor was but a cipher. The centralized rule which had existed in the fourteenth century had been replaced by a constant feuding between the clans—akin, as it were, to the strife among their equivalents in Scotland. This was not the ideal circumstance for traders and merchants, but it did not check a very considerable amount of economic activity. At sea, as on land, entrepreneurs jostled with warlords and military adventurers, each of whom detected profit in the East Asian maritime trade. Japanese pirates scoured the coasts of China and Korea for plunder, while simultaneously other Japanese welcomed the chance to exchange goods with the Portuguese and Dutch visitors from the West. Christian missions and European wares penetrated Japanese society far more easily than they did an aloof, self-contained Ming Empire.[12]

This lively if turbulent scene was soon to be altered by the growing use of imported European armaments. As was happening elsewhere in the world, power gravitated toward those individuals or groups who possessed the resources to commandeer a large musket-bearing army and, most important of all, cannon. In Japan the result was the consolidation of authority under the great warlord Hideyoshi, whose aspirations ultimately led him twice to attempt the conquest of Korea. When these failed, and Hideyoshi died in 1598, civil strife again threatened Japan; but within a few years all power had been consolidated in the hands of Ieyasu and fellow shoguns of the Tokugawa clan. This time the centralized military rule could not be shaken.

In many respects, Tokugawa Japan possessed the characteristics of the "new monarchies" which had arisen in the West during the preceding century. The great difference was the shogunate's abjuration of overseas expansion, indeed of virtually all contact with the outside world. In 1636, construction of oceangoing vessels was stopped and Japanese subjects were forbidden to sail the high seas. Trade with

Europeans was restricted to the permitted Dutch ship calling at De-shima in Nagasaki harbor; the others were tumbled out. Even earlier, virtually all Christians (foreign and native) were ruthlessly murdered at the behest of the shogunate. Clearly, the chief motive behind these drastic measures was the Tokugawa clan's determination to achieve unchallenged control; foreigners and Christians were thus regarded as potentially subversive. But so, too, were the other feudal lords, which is why they were required to spend half the year in the capital; and why, during the six months they were allowed to reside on their estates, their families had to remain at Yedo (Tokyo), virtually hostages.

This imposed uniformity did not, of itself, throttle economic devel-opment—nor, for that matter, did it prevent outstanding artistic achievements. Nationwide peace was good for trade, the towns and overall population were growing, and the increasing use of cash pay-ments made merchants and bankers more important. The latter, how-ever, were never permitted the social and political prominence they gained in Italy, the Netherlands, and Britain, and the Japanese were obviously unable to learn about, and adopt, new technological and industrial developments that were occurring elsewhere. Like the Ming dynasty, the Tokugawa shogunate deliberately chose, with a few excep-tions, to cut itself off from the rest of the world. This may not have retarded economic activities in Japan itself, but it did harm the relative power of the Japanese state. Disdaining to engage in trade, and forbid-den to travel or to display their weapons except on ceremonial occa-sions, the samurai warriors attached to their lords lived a life of ritual and boredom. The entire military system ossified for two centuries, so that when Commodore Perry's famous "black ships" arrived in 1853, there was little that an overawed Japanese government could do except grant the American request for coaling and other facilities.

At the beginning of its period of political consolidation and growth, Russia appeared similar to Japan in certain respects. Geographically far removed from the West—partly on account of poor communica-tions, and partly because periodic clashes with Lithuania, Poland, Swe-den, and the Ottoman Empire interrupted those routes which did exist—the Kingdom of Muscovy was nevertheless deeply influenced by its European inheritance, not least through the Russian Orthodox Church. It was from the West, moreover, that there came the lasting solution to Russia's vulnerability to the horsemen of the Asian plains: muskets and cannon. With these new weapons, Moscow could now establish itself as one of the "gunpowder empires" and thus expand. A westward drive was difficult, given that the Swedes and Poles also possessed such armaments, but colonial expansion against the tribes and khanates to the south and east was made much easier by this military-technological advantage. By 1556, for example, Russian troops had reached the Caspian Sea. This military expansionism was accompanied, and often eclipsed, by the explorers and pioneers who steadily pushed east of the Urals, through Siberia, and had actually reached the Pacific coast by 1638.[13] Despite its hard-won military superiority over Mongol horsemen, there was nothing easy or inevitable about the growth of the Russian Empire. The more peoples that were conquered, the greater was the likelihood of internal dissension and revolt. The nobles at home were often restive, even after the purge of their numbers by Ivan the Terrible. The Tartar khanate of the Crimea remained a powerful foe; its troops sacked Moscow in 1571, and it remained independent until the late eighteenth century. Challenges from the West were even more threatening; the Poles, for example, occupied Moscow between 1608 and 1613.

A further weakness was that despite certain borrowings from the West, Russia remained technologically backward and economically underdeveloped. Extremes of climate and the enormous distances and poor communications partly accounted for this, but so also did severe social defects: the military absolutism of the czars, the monopoly of education in the hands of the Orthodox Church, the venality and unpredictability of the bureaucracy, and the institution of serfdom, which made agriculture feudal and static. Yet despite this relative backwardness, and despite the setbacks, Russia continued to expand, imposing upon its new territories the same military force and autocratic rule which was used to command the obedience of the Muscovites. Enough had been borrowed from Europe to give the regime the armed strength to preserve itself, while all possibility of western social and political "modernization" was firmly resisted; foreigners in Russia, for example, were segregated from the natives in order to prevent subversive influences. Unlike the other despotisms mentioned in this chapter, the empire of the czars would manage to survive and Russia would one day grow to be a world power. Yet in 1500, and even as late as 1650, this was scarcely obvious to many Frenchmen, Dutchmen, and Englishmen, who probably knew as much about the Russian ruler as they did about the legendary Prester John.[14]

The "European Miracle"[15]

Why was it among the scattered and relatively unsophisticated peoples inhabiting the western parts of the Eurasian landmass that there occurred an unstoppable process of economic development and technological innovation which would steadily make it the commercial and military leader in world affairs? This is a question which has exercised scholars and other observers for centuries, and all that the following paragraphs can do is to present a synthesis of the existing knowledge. Yet however crude such a summary must be, it possesses the incidental advantage of exposing the main strands of the argument which permeate this entire work: namely, that there was a *dynamic* involved, driven chiefly by economic and technological advances, although always interacting with other variables such as social structure, geography, and the occasional accident; that to understand the course of world politics, it is necessary to focus attention upon the material and long-term elements rather than the vagaries of personality or the week-by-week shifts of diplomacy and politics; and that power is a relative thing, which can only be described and measured by frequent comparisons between various states and societies.

The one feature of Europe which immediately strikes the eye when looking at a map of the world's "power centers" in the sixteenth century is its political fragmentation (see Maps 1 and 2). This was not an accidental or short-lived state of affairs, such as occurred briefly in China after the collapse of one empire and before its successor dynasty could gather up again the strings of centralized power. Europe had *always* been politically fragmented, despite even the best efforts of the Romans, who had not managed to conquer much farther north of the Rhine and the Danube; and for a thousand years after the fall of Rome, the basic political power unit had been small and localized, in contrast to the steady expansion of the Christian religion and culture. Occasional concentrations of authority, like that of Charlemagne in the West or of Kievan Russia in the East, were but temporary affairs, terminated by a change of ruler, internal rebellion, or external invasions.

For this political diversity Europe had largely to thank its geography. There were no enormous plains over which an empire of horsemen could impose its swift dominion; nor were there broad and fertile river zones like those around the Ganges, Nile, Tigris and Euphrates, Yellow, and Yangtze, providing the food for masses of toiling and easily conquerable peasants. Europe's landscape was much more fractured, with mountain ranges and large forests separating the scattered population centers in the valleys; and its climate altered considerably from north to south and west to east. This had a number of important consequences. For a start, it both made difficult the establishment of unified control, even by a powerful and determined warlord, and minimized the possibility that the continent could be overrun by an external force like the Mongol hordes. Conversely, this variegated landscape encouraged the growth, and the continued existence, of decentralized power, with local kingdoms and marcher lordships and highland clans and lowland town confederations making a political map of Europe drawn at any time after the fall of Rome look like a patchwork quilt. The patterns on that quilt might vary from century to century, but no single color could ever be used to denote a unified empire.[16]

Europe's differentiated climate led to differentiated products, suit-

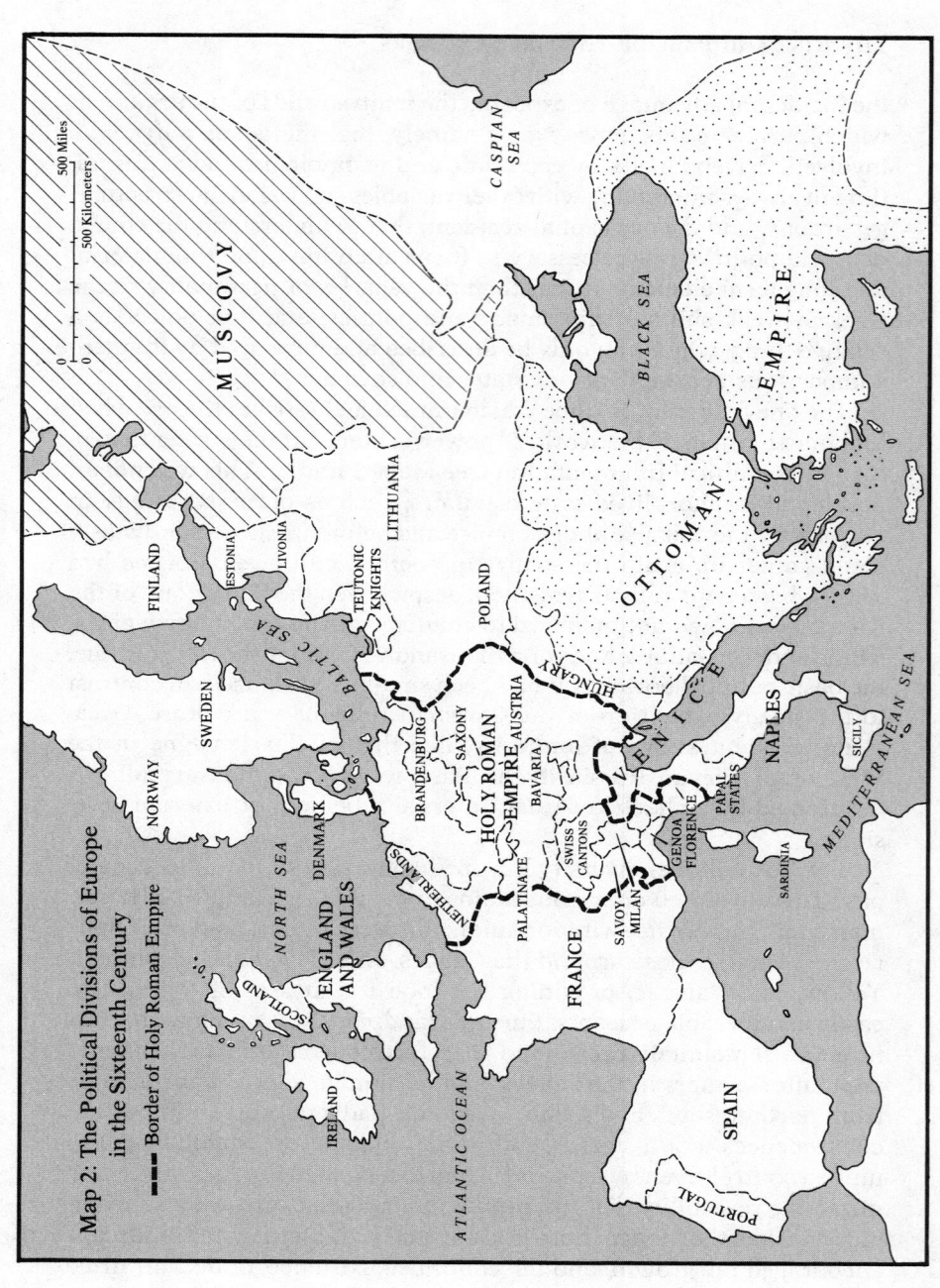

Map 2: The Political Divisions of Europe in the Sixteenth Century

▪▪▪ Border of Holy Roman Empire

500 Miles

500 Kilometers

MUSCOVY

CASPIAN SEA

BLACK SEA

OTTOMAN EMPIRE

FINLAND

ESTONIA

LIVONIA

TEUTONIC KNIGHTS

LITHUANIA

POLAND

HUNGARY

BALTIC SEA

NORWAY

SWEDEN

DENMARK

NORTH SEA

NETHERLANDS

BRANDENBURG

SAXONY

HOLY ROMAN EMPIRE

AUSTRIA

BAVARIA

VENICE

PAPAL STATES

NAPLES

SICILY

MEDITERRANEAN SEA

ENGLAND AND WALES

SCOTLAND

IRELAND

ATLANTIC OCEAN

PALATINATE

SWISS CANTONS

SAVOY

MILAN

GENOA

FLORENCE

SARDINIA

FRANCE

SPAIN

PORTUGAL

able for exchange; and in time, as market relations developed, they were transported along the rivers or the pathways which cut through the forests between one area of settlement and the next. Probably the most important characteristic of this commerce was that it consisted primarily of *bulk* products—timber, grain, wine, wool, herrings, and so on, catering to the rising population of fifteenth-century Europe, rather than the luxuries carried on the oriental caravans. Here again geography played a crucial role, for water transport of these goods was so much more economical and Europe possessed many navigable rivers. Being surrounded by seas was a further incentive to the vital shipbuilding industry, and by the later Middle Ages a flourishing maritime commerce was being carried out between the Baltic, the North Sea, the Mediterranean, and the Black Sea. This trade was, predictably, interrupted in part by war and affected by local disasters such as crop failures and plagues; but in general it continued to expand, increasing Europe's prosperity and enriching its diet, and leading to the creation of new centers of wealth like the Hansa towns or the Italian cities. Regular long-distance exchanges of wares in turn encouraged the growth of bills of exchange, a credit system, and banking on an international scale. The very existence of mercantile credit, and then of bills of insurance, pointed to a basic *predictability* of economic conditions which private traders had hitherto rarely, if ever, enjoyed anywhere in the world.[17]

In addition, because much of this trade was carried through the rougher waters of the North Sea and Bay of Biscay—and also because long-range fishing became an important source of nutrient and wealth—shipwrights were forced to build tough (if rather slow and inelegant) vessels capable of carrying large loads and finding their motive power in the winds alone. Although over time they developed more sail and masts, and stern rudders, and therefore became more maneuverable, North Sea "cogs" and their successors may not have appeared as impressive as the lighter craft which plied the shores of the eastern Mediterranean and the Indian Ocean; but, as we shall see below, they were going to possess distinct advantages in the long run.[18]

The political and social consequences of this decentralized, largely unsupervised growth of commerce and merchants and ports and markets were of the greatest significance. In the first place, there was no way in which such economic developments could be fully suppressed. This is not to say that the rise of market forces did not disturb many in authority. Feudal lords, suspicious of towns as centers of dissidence and sanctuaries of serfs, often tried to curtail their privileges. As elsewhere, merchants were frequently preyed upon, their goods stolen, their property seized. Papal pronouncements upon usury echo in many ways the Confucian dislike of profit-making middlemen and moneylenders. But the basic fact was that there existed no uniform authority

in Europe which could effectively halt this or that commercial development; no central government whose changes in priorities could cause
the rise and fall of a particular industry; no systematic and universal
plundering of businessmen and entrepreneurs by tax gatherers, which
so retarded the economy of Mogul India. To take one specific and
obvious instance, it was inconceivable in the fractured political circumstances of Reformation Europe that everyone would acknowledge
the pope's 1494 division of the overseas world into Spanish and Portuguese spheres—and even less conceivable that an order banning
overseas trade (akin to those promulgated in Ming China and
Tokugawa Japan) would have had any effect.

The fact was that in Europe there were always some princes and
local lords willing to tolerate merchants and their ways even when
others plundered and expelled them; and, as the record shows, op-
pressed Jewish traders, ruined Flemish textile workers, persecuted
Huguenots, moved on and took their expertise with them. A Rhineland
baron who overtaxed commercial travelers would find that the trade
routes had gone elsewhere, and with it his revenues. A monarch who
repudiated his debts would have immense difficulties raising a loan
when the next war threatened and funds were quickly needed to equip
his armies and fleets. Bankers and arms dealers and artisans were
essential, not peripheral, members of society. Gradually, unevenly,
most of the regimes of Europe entered into a symbiotic relationship
with the market economy, providing for it domestic order and a nonar-
bitrary legal system (even for foreigners), and receiving in taxes a
share of the growing profits from trade. Long before Adam Smith had
coined the exact words, the rulers of certain societies of western
Europe were tacitly recognizing that "little else is requisite to carry a
state to the highest degree of opulence from the lowest barbarism, but
peace, easy taxes, and tolerable administration of justice. . . ."[19] From
time to time the less percipient leaders—like the Spanish administrators of Castile, or an occasional Bourbon king of France—would virtually kill the goose that laid the golden eggs; but the consequent decline
in wealth, and thus in military power, was soon obvious to all but the
most purblind.

Probably the only factor which might have led to a centralization
of authority would have been such a breakthrough in firearms technology by one state that all opponents were crushed or overawed. In the
quickening pace of economic and technical development which occurred in fifteenth-century Europe as the continent's population recovered from the Black Death and the Italian Renaissance blossomed, this
was by no means impossible. It was, as noted above, in this broad
period from 1450 to 1600 that "gunpowder empires" were established
elsewhere. Muscovy, Tokugawa Japan, and Mogul India provide excellent examples of how great states could be fashioned by leaders who

secured the firearms and the cannon with which to compel all rivals to obedience.

Since, furthermore, it was in late-medieval and early modern Europe that new techniques of warfare occurred more frequently than elsewhere, it was not implausible that one such breakthrough could enable a certain nation to dominate its rivals. Already the signs pointed to an increasing concentration of military power.[20] In Italy the use of companies of crossbowmen, protected when necessary by soldiers using pikes, had brought to a close the age of the knight on horseback and his accompanying ill-trained feudal levy; but it was also clear that only the wealthier states like Venice and Milan could pay for the new armies officered by the famous *condottieri*. By around 1500, moreover, the kings of France and England had gained an artillery monopoly at home and were thus able, if the need arose, to crush an overmighty subject even if the latter sheltered behind castle walls. But would not this tendency finally lead to a larger transnational monopoly, stretching across Europe? This must have been a question many asked around 1550, as they observed the vast concentration of lands and armies under the Emperor Charles V.

A fuller discussion of that specific Habsburg attempt, and failure, to gain the mastery of Europe will be presented in the next chapter. But the more general reason why it was impossible to impose unity across the continent can briefly be stated here. Once again, the existence of a *variety* of economic and military centers of power was fundamental. No one Italian city-state could strive to enhance itself without the others intervening to preserve the equilibrium; no "new monarchy" could increase its dominions without stirring rivals to seek compensation. By the time the Reformation was well and truly under way, religious antagonisms were added to the traditional balance-of-power rivalries, thus making the prospects of political centralization even more remote. Yet the real explanation lies a little deeper; after all, the simple existence of competitors, and of bitter feelings between warring groups, was evident in Japan, India, and elsewhere, but that of itself had not prevented eventual unification. Europe was different in that each of the rival forces was able to gain access to the new military techniques, so that no single power ever possessed the decisive edge. The services of the Swiss and other mercenaries, for example, were on offer to anyone who was able to pay for them. There was no single center for the production of crossbows, nor for that of cannon— whether of the earlier bronze guns or of the later, cheaper cast-iron artillery; instead, such armaments were being made close to the ore deposits on the Weald, in central Europe, in Málaga, in Milan, in Liège, and later in Sweden. Similarly, the proliferation of shipbuilding skills in various ports ranging from the Baltic to the Black Sea made it extremely difficult for any one country to monopolize maritime power, which in turn helped to prevent the conquest and elimination of rival centers of armaments production lying across the sea.

To say that Europe's decentralized states system was the great obstacle to centralization is not, then, a tautology. Because there existed a number of competing political entities, *most of which possessed or were able to buy the military means to preserve their independence,* no single one could ever achieve the breakthrough to the mastery of the continent.

While this competitive interaction between the European states seems to explain the absence of a unified "gunpowder empire" there, it does not at first sight provide the reason for Europe's steady rise to global leadership. After all, would not the forces possessed by the new monarchies in 1500 have seemed puny if they had been deployed against the enormous armies of the sultan and the massed troops of the Ming Empire? This was true in the early sixteenth century and, in some respects, even in the seventeenth century; but by the latter period the balance of military strength was tilting rapidly in favor of the West. For the explanation of this shift one must again point to the decentralization of power in Europe. What it did, above all else, was to engender a primitive form of arms race among the city-states and then the larger kingdoms. To some extent, this probably had socioeconomic roots. Once the contending armies in Italy no longer consisted of feudal knights and their retainers but of pikemen, crossbowmen, and (flanking) cavalry paid for by the merchants and supervised by the magistrates of a particular city, it was almost inevitable that the latter would demand value for money—despite all the best maneuvers of *condottieri* not to make themselves redundant; the cities would require, in other words, the sort of arms and tactics which might produce a swift victory, so that the expenses of war could then be reduced. Similarly, once the French monarchs of the late fifteenth century had a "national" army under their direct control and pay, they were anxious to see this force produce decisive results.[21]

By the same token, this free-market system not only forced the numerous *condottieri* to compete for contracts but also encouraged artisans and inventors to improve their wares, so as to obtain new orders. While this armaments spiral could already be seen in the manufacture of crossbows and armor plate in the early fifteenth century, the principle spread to experimentation with gunpowder weapons in the following fifty years. It is important to recall here that when cannon were first employed, there was little difference between the West and Asia in their design and effectiveness. Gigantic wrought-iron tubes that fired a stone ball and made an immense noise obviously looked impressive and at times had results; it was that type which was used by the Turks to bombard the walls of Constantinople in 1453. Yet it seems to have been only in Europe that the impetus existed for constant improvements: in the gunpowder grains, in casting much smaller (yet equally powerful) cannon from bronze and tin alloys, in the shape and texture of the barrel and the missile, in the gun mountings and carriages. All of this enhanced to an enormous degree the power and the mobility of artillery and gave the owner of such weapons the means to reduce the strongest fortresses—as the Italian city-states found to their alarm when a French army equipped with formidable bronze guns invaded Italy in 1494. It was scarcely surprising, therefore, that inventors and men of letters were being urged to design some counter to these cannon (and scarcely less surprising that Leonardo's notebooks for this time contain sketches for a machine gun, a primitive tank, and a steam-powered cannon).[22]

This is not to say that other civilizations did not improve their armaments from the early, crude designs; some of them did, usually by copying from European models or persuading European visitors (like the Jesuits in China) to lend their expertise. But because the Ming government had a monopoly of cannon, and the thrusting leaders of Russia, Japan, and Mogul India soon acquired a monopoly, there was much less incentive to improve such weapons once their authority had been established. Turning in upon themselves, the Chinese and the Japanese neglected to develop armaments production. Clinging to their traditional fighting ways, the janissaries of Islam scorned taking much interest in artillery until it was too late to catch up to Europe's lead. Facing less-advanced peoples, Russian and Mogul army commanders had no compelling need for improved weaponry, since what they already possessed overawed their opponents. Just as in the general economic field, so also in this specific area of military technology, Europe, fueled by a flourishing arms trade, took a decisive lead over the other civilizations and power centers.

Two further consequences of this armaments spiral need to be mentioned here. One ensured the political plurality of Europe, the other its eventual maritime mastery. The first is a simple enough story and can be dealt with briefly.[23] Within a quarter-century of the French invasion of 1494, and in certain respects even before then, some Italians had discovered that raised earthworks inside the city walls could greatly reduce the effects of artillery bombardment; when crashing into the compacted mounds of earth, cannonballs lost the devastating impact they had upon the outer walls. If these varied earthworks also had a steep ditch in front of them (and, later, a sophisticated series of protected bastions from which muskets and cannon could pour a crossfire), they constituted a near-insuperable obstacle to the besieging infantry. This restored the security of the Italian city-states, or at least of those which had not fallen to a foreign conqueror and which possessed the vast amounts of manpower needed to build and garrison such complex fortifications. It also gave an advantage to the armies engaged in holding off the Turks, as the Christian garrisons in Malta and in northern Hungary soon discovered. Above all, it hindered the easy conquest of rebels and rivals by one overweening power in Europe, as the protracted siege warfare which accompanied the Revolt of the Netherlands attested. Victories attained in the open field by, say, the formidable Spanish infantry could not be made decisive if the foe possessed heavily fortified bases into which he could retreat. The authority acquired through gunpowder by the Tokugawa shogunate, or by Akbar in India, was not replicated in the West, which continued to be characterized by political pluralism and its deadly concomitant, the arms race.

The impact of the "gunpowder revolution" at sea was even more wide-ranging.[24] As before, one is struck by the relative similarity of shipbuilding and naval power that existed during the later Middle Ages in northwest Europe, in the Islamic world, and in the Far East. If anything, the great voyages of Cheng Ho and the rapid advance of the Turkish fleets in the Black Sea and eastern Mediterranean might well have suggested to an observer around 1400 and 1450 that the future of maritime development lay with those two powers. There was also little difference, one suspects, between all three regions in regard to cartography, astronomy, and the use of instruments like the compass, astrolabe, and quadrant. What was different was *sustained organization.* Or, as Professor Jones observes, "given the distances covered by other seafarers, the Polynesians for example, the [Iberian] voyages are less impressive than Europe's ability to rationalize them and to develop the resources within her reach."[25] The systematic collection of geographical data by the Portuguese, the repeated willingness of Genoese merchant houses to fund Atlantic ventures which might ultimately compensate for their loss of Black Sea trade, and—farther north—the methodical development of the Newfoundland cod fisheries all signified a sustained readiness to reach outward which was not evident in other societies at that time.

But perhaps the most important act of "rationalization" was the steady improvement in ships' armaments. The siting of cannon on sailing vessels was a natural enough development at a time when sea warfare so resembled that on land; just as medieval castles contained archers along the walls and towers in order to drive off a besieging army, so the massive Genoese and Venetian and Aragonese trading vessels used men, armed with crossbows and sited in the fore and aft "castles," to defend themselves against Muslim pirates in the Mediterranean. This could cause severe losses among galley crews, although not necessarily enough to save a becalmed merchantman if its attackers were really determined. However, once sailors perceived the advances which had been made in gun design on land—that is, that the newer bronze cannon were much smaller, more powerful, and less dangerous to the gun crew than the enormous wrought-iron bombards—it was predictable that such armaments would be placed on board. After all, catapults, trebuchets, and other sorts of missile-throwing instruments had already been mounted on warships in China and the West. Even when cannon became less volatile and dangerous to their crews, they still posed considerable problems; given the more effective gunpowder, the recoil could be tremendous, sending a gun backward right across the deck if not restrained, and these weapons were still weighty enough to unbalance a vessel if sufficient numbers of them were placed on board (especially on the castles). This was where the stoutly built, rounder-hulled, all-weather three-masted sailing vessel had an inherent advantage over the slim oared galleys of the inland waters of the Mediterranean, Baltic, and Black seas, and over the Arab dhow and even the Chinese junk. It could in any event fire a larger broadside while remaining stable, although of course disasters also occurred from time to time; but once it was realized that the siting of such weapons amidships rather than on the castles provided a much safer gun platform, the *potential power* of these caravels and galleons was formidable. By comparison, lighter craft suffered from the twin disadvantage of less gun-carrying capacity and greater vulnerability to cannonballs.

One is obliged to stress the words "potential power" because the evolution of the gunned long-range sailing ship was a slow, often uneven development. Many hybrid types were constructed, some carrying multiple masts, guns, *and* rows of oars. Galley-type vessels were still to be seen in the English Channel in the sixteenth century. Moreover, there were considerable arguments in favor of continuing to deploy galleys in the Mediterranean and the Black Sea; they were swifter on many occasions, more maneuverable in inshore waters, and thus easier to use in conjunction with land operations along the coast— which, for the Turks, outweighed the disadvantages of their being short-ranged and unable to act in heavy seas.[26]

In just the same way, we should not imagine that as soon as the first Portuguese vessels rounded the Cape of Good Hope, the age of unchallenged western dominance had begun. What historians refer to as the "Vasco da Gama epoch" and the "Columbian era"—that is, the three or four centuries of European hegemony after 1500—was a very gradual process. Portuguese explorers might have reached the shores of India by the 1490s, but their vessels were still small (often only 300 tons) and not all that well armed—certainly not compared with the powerful Dutch East Indiamen which sailed in those waters a century later. In fact, the Portuguese could not penetrate the Red Sea for a long while, and then only precariously, nor could they gain much of a footing in China; and in the late sixteenth century they lost some of their East African stations to an Arab counteroffensive.[27]

It would be erroneous, too, to assume that the non-European powers simply collapsed like a pack of cards at the first signs of western
expansionism. This was precisely what did happen in Mexico, Peru,
and other less developed societies of the New World when the Spanish
adventurers landed. Elsewhere, the story was very different. Since the
Chinese government had voluntarily turned its back upon maritime
trade, it did not really care if that commerce fell into the hands of the
barbarians; even the quasi-official trading post which the Portuguese
set up at Macao in 1557, lucrative though it must have been to the local
silk merchants and conniving administrators, does not seem to have
disturbed Peking's equanimity. The Japanese, for their part, were
much more blunt. When the Portuguese sent a mission in 1640 to
protest against the expulsion of foreigners, almost all its members
were killed; there could be no attempt at retribution from Lisbon.
Finally, Ottoman sea power was holding its own in the eastern Mediterranean, and Ottoman land power remained a massive threat to central
Europe. In the sixteenth century, indeed, "to most European statesmen
the loss of Hungary was of far greater import than the establishment
of factories in the Orient, and the threat to Vienna more significant
than their own challenges at Aden, Goa and Malacca; only governments bordering the Atlantic could, like their later historians, ignore
this fact."[28]

Yet when all these reservations are made, there is no doubt that
the development of the long-range armed sailing ship heralded a fundamental advance in Europe's place in the world. With these vessels,
the naval powers of the West were in a position to control the oceanic trade routes and to overawe all societies vulnerable to the workings of sea power. Even the first great clashes between the Portuguese
and their Muslim foes in the Indian Ocean made this clear. No doubt
they exaggerated in retrospect, but to read the journals and reports of
da Gama and Albuquerque, describing how their warships blasted
their way through the massed fleets of Arab dhows and other light
craft which they encountered off the Malabar coast and in the Ormuz
and Malacca roads, is to gain the impression that an extraterrestrial,
superhuman force had descended upon their unfortunate opponents.
Following the new tactic that "they were by no means to board, but
to fight with the artillery," the Portuguese crews were virtually invin-
cible at sea.[29] On land it was quite a different matter, as the fierce
battles (and occasional defeats) at Aden, Jiddah, Goa, and elsewhere
demonstrated; yet so determined and brutal were these western invaders that by the mid-sixteenth century they had carved out for
themselves a chain of forts from the Gulf of Guinea to the South
China Sea. Although never able to monopolize the spice trade from
the Indies—much of which continued to flow via the traditional
channels to Venice—the Portuguese certainly cornered considerable

portions of that commerce and profited greatly from their early lead in the race for empire.[30]

The evidence of profit was even greater, of course, in the vast land empire which the conquistadores swiftly established in the western hemisphere. From the early settlements in Hispaniola and Cuba, Spanish expeditions pushed toward the mainland, conquering Mexico in the 1520s and Peru in the 1530s. Within a few decades this dominion extended from the River Plate in the south to the Rio Grande in the north. Spanish galleons, plying along the western coast, linked up with vessels coming from the Philippines, bearing Chinese silks in exchange for Peruvian silver. In their "New World" the Spaniards made it clear that they were there to stay, setting up an imperial administration, building churches, and engaging in ranching and mining. Exploiting the natural resources—and, still more, the native labor—of these territories, the conquerors sent home a steady flow of sugar, cochineal, hides, and other wares. Above all, they sent home silver from the Potosí mine, which for over a century was the biggest single deposit of that metal in the world. All this led to "a lightning growth of transatlantic trade, the volume increasing eightfold between 1510 and 1550, and threefold again between 1550 and 1610."[31]

All the signs were, therefore, that this imperialism was intended to be permanent. Unlike the fleeting visits paid by Cheng Ho, the actions of the Portuguese and Spanish explorers symbolized a commitment to alter the world's political and economic balances. With their ship-borne cannon and musket-bearing soldier, they did precisely that. In retrospect it sometimes seems difficult to grasp that a country with the limited population and resources of Portugal could reach so far and acquire so much. In the special circumstances of European military and naval superiority described above, this was by no means impossible. Once it was done, the evident profits of empire, and the desire for more, simply accelerated the process of aggrandizement.

There are elements in this story of "the expansion of Europe" which have been ignored, or but briefly mentioned so far. The personal aspect has not been examined, and yet—as in all great endeavors—it was there in abundance: in the encouragements of men like Henry the Navigator; in the ingenuity of ship craftsmen and armorers and men of letters; in the enterprise of merchants; above all, in the sheer courage of those who partook in the overseas voyages and endured all that the mighty seas, hostile climates, wild landscapes, and fierce opponents could place in their way. For a complex mixture of motives—personal gain, national glory, religious zeal, perhaps a sense of adventure—men were willing to risk everything, as indeed they did in many cases. Nor has there been much dwelling upon the awful cruelties inflicted by these European conquerors upon their many victims in Africa, Asia, and America. If these features are hardly mentioned

here, it is because many societies in their time have thrown up individuals and groups willing to dare all and do anything in order to
make the world their oyster. What distinguished the captains, crews,
and explorers of Europe was that they possessed the ships and the
firepower with which to achieve their ambitions, and that they came
from a political environment in which competition, risk, and entrepreneurship were prevalent.

The benefits accruing from the expansion of Europe were widespread and permanent, and—most important of all—they helped to
accelerate an already-existing dynamic. The emphasis upon the acquisition of gold, silver, precious metals, and spices, important though
such valuables were, ought not to obscure the worth of the less glamor-
ous items which flooded into Europe's ports once its sailors had
breached the oceanic frontier. Access to the Newfoundland fisheries
brought an apparently inexhaustible supply of food, and the Atlantic
Ocean also provided the whale oil and seal oil vital for illumination,
lubrication, and many other purposes. Sugar, indigo, tobacco, rice,
furs, timber, and new plants like the potato and maize were all to boost
the total wealth and well-being of the continent; later on, of course,
there was to come the flow of grain and meats and cotton. But one does
not need to anticipate the cosmopolitan world economy of the later
nineteenth century to understand that the Portuguese and Spanish
discoveries were, within decades, of great and ever-growing importance in enhancing the prosperity and power of the western portions
of the continent. Bulk trades like the fisheries employed a large number of hands, both in catching and in distribution, which further
boosted the market economy. And all of this gave the greatest stimulus
to the European shipbuilding industry, attracting around the ports of
London, Bristol, Antwerp, Amsterdam, and many others a vast array
of craftsmen, suppliers, dealers, insurers. The net effect was to give to
a considerable proportion of western Europe's population—and not
just to the elite few—an abiding material interest in the fruits of overseas trade.

When one adds to this list of commodities the commerce which
attended the landward expansion of Russia—the furs, hides, wood,
hemp, salt, and grain which came from there to western Europe—then
scholars have some cause in describing this as the beginnings of a
"modern world system."[32] What had started as a number of separate
expansions was steadily turning into an interlocking whole: the gold
of the Guinea coast and the silver of Peru were used by the Portuguese,
Spaniards, and Italians to pay for spices and silks from the Orient; the
firs and timber of Russia helped in the purchase of iron guns from
England; grain from the Baltic passed through Amsterdam on its way
to the Mediterranean. All this generated a continual interaction—of
further European expansion, bringing fresh discoveries and thus trade

opportunities, resulting in additional gains, which stimulated still more expansion. This was not necessarily a smooth upward progression: a great war in Europe or civil unrest could sharply reduce activities overseas. But the colonizing powers rarely if ever gave up their acquisitions, and within a short while a fresh wave of expansion and exploration would begin. After all, if the established imperial nations did not exploit their positions, others were willing to do it instead.

This, finally, was the greatest reason why the dynamic continued to operate as it did: the manifold rivalries of the European states, already acute, were spilling over into transoceanic spheres. Try as they might, Spain and Portugal simply could not keep their papally assigned monopoly of the outside world to themselves, the more especially when men realized that there was no northeast or northwest passage from Europe to Cathay. Already by the 1560s, Dutch, French, and English vessels were venturing across the Atlantic, and a little later into the Indian and Pacific oceans—a process quickened by the decline of the English cloth trade and the Revolt of the Netherlands. With royal and aristocratic patrons, with funding from the great merchants of Amsterdam and London, and with all the religious and nationalist zeal which the Reformation and Counter-Reformation had produced, new trading and plundering expeditions set out from northwest Europe to secure a share of the spoils. There was the prospect of gaining glory and riches, of striking at a rival and boosting the resources of one's own country, and of converting new souls to the one true faith; what possible counterarguments could hold out against the launching of such ventures?[33]

The fairer aspect of this increasing commercial and colonial rivalry was the parallel upward spiral in knowledge—in science and technology.[34] No doubt many of the advances of this time were spinoffs from the arms race and the scramble for overseas trade; but the eventual benefits transcended their inglorious origins. Improved cartography, navigational tables, new instruments like the telescope, barometer, backstaff, and gimbaled compass, and better methods of shipbuilding helped to make maritime travel a less unpredictable form of travel. New crops and plants not only brought better nutrition but also were a stimulus to botany and agricultural science. Metallurgical skills, and indeed the whole iron industry, made rapid progress; deep-mining techniques did the same. Astronomy, medicine, physics, and engineering also benefited from the quickening economic pace and the enhanced value of science. The inquiring, rationalist mind was observing more, and experimenting more; and the printing presses, apart from producing vernacular Bibles and political treatises, were spreading these findings. The cumulative effect of this explosion of knowledge was to buttress Europe's technological—and therefore military—superiority still further. Even the powerful Ottomans, or at least their front-line soldiers and sailors, were feeling some of the consequences of this by the end of the sixteenth century. On other, less active societies, the effects were to be far more serious. Whether or not certain states in Asia would have taken off into a self-driven commercial and industrial revolution had they been left undisturbed seems open to considerable doubt;[35] but what was clear was that it was going to be extremely difficult for other societies to ascend the ladder of world power when the more advanced European states occupied all the top rungs.

This difficulty would be compounded, it seems fair to argue, because moving up that ladder would have involved not merely the acquisition of European equipment or even of European techniques: it would also have implied a wholesale borrowing of those general features which distinguished the societies of the West from all the others. It would have meant the existence of a market economy, if not to the extent proposed by Adam Smith then at least to the extent that merchants and entrepreneurs would not be consistently deterred, obstructed, and preyed upon. It would also have meant the existence of a plurality of power centers, each if possible with its own economic base, so that there was no prospect of the imposed centralization of a despotic oriental-style regime—and every prospect of the progressive, if turbulent and occasionally brutal, stimulus of competition. By extension, this lack of economic and political rigidity would imply a similar lack of cultural and ideological orthodoxy—that is, a freedom to inquire, to dispute, to experiment, a belief in the possibilities of improvement, a concern for the practical rather than the abstract, a rationalism which defied mandarin codes, religious dogma, and traditional folklore.[36] In most cases, what was involved was not so much positive elements, but rather the reduction in the number of *hindrances* which checked economic growth and political diversity. Europe's greatest advantage was that it had fewer *dis*advantages than the other civilizations.

Although it is impossible to prove it, one suspects that these various general features related to one another, by some inner logic as it were, and that all were necessary. It was a combination of economic laissez-faire, political and military pluralism, and intellectual liberty—however rudimentary each factor was compared with later ages—which had been in constant interaction to produce the "European miracle." Since the miracle was historically unique, it seems plausible to assume that only a replication of all its component parts could have produced a similar result elsewhere. Because that mix of critical ingredients did not exist in Ming China, or in the Muslim empires of the Middle East and Asia, or in any other of the societies examined above, they appeared to stand still while Europe advanced to the center of the world stage.

2
The Habsburg Bid
for Mastery, 1519–1659

By the sixteenth century, then, the power struggles within Europe were also helping it to rise, economically and militarily, above the other regions of the globe. What was not yet decided, however, was whether any one of the rival European states could accumulate sufficient resources to surpass the rest, and then dominate them. For about a century and a half after 1500, a continent-wide combination of kingdoms, duchies, and provinces ruled by the Spanish and Austrian members of the Habsburg family threatened to become the predominant political and religious influence in Europe. The story of this prolonged struggle and of the ultimate defeat of these Habsburg ambitions by a coalition of other European states forms the core of this chapter. By 1659, when Spain finally acknowledged defeat in the Treaty of the Pyrenees, the political *plurality* of Europe—containing five or six major states, and various smaller ones—was an indisputable fact. Which of those leading states was going to benefit most from further shifts within the Great Power system can be left to the following chapter; what at least was clear, by the mid-seventeenth century, was that no single dynastic-military bloc was capable of becoming the master of Europe, as had appeared probable on various occasions over the previous decades.

The interlocking campaigns for European predominance which characterize this century and a half differ both in degree and kind, therefore, from the wars of the pre-1500 period. The struggles which had disturbed the peace of Europe over the previous hundred years had been *localized* ones; the clashes between the various Italian states, the rivalry between the English and French crowns, and the wars of the Teutonic Knights against the Lithuanians and the Poles were typical examples.[1] As the sixteenth century unfolded, however, these traditional regional struggles in Europe were either subsumed into or eclipsed by what seemed to contemporaries to be a far larger contest for the mastery of the continent.

The Meaning and Chronology of the Struggle

Although there were always specific reasons why any particular state was drawn into this larger context, two more general causes were chiefly responsible for the transformation in both the intensity and geographical scope of European warfare. The first of these was the coming of the Reformation—sparked off by Martin Luther's personal revolt against papal indulgences in 1517—which swiftly added a fierce new dimension to the traditional dynastic rivalries of the continent. For particular socioeconomic reasons, the advent of the Protestant Reformation—and its response, in the form of the Catholic Counter-Reformation against heresy—also tended to divide the southern half of Europe from the north, and the rising, city-based middle classes from the feudal orders, although there were, of course, many exceptions to such general alignments.[2] But the basic point was that "Christendom" had fractured, and that the continent now contained large numbers of individuals drawn into a *transnational* struggle over religious doctrine. Only in the mid-seventeenth century, when men recoiled at the excesses and futility of religious wars, would there arrive a general, if grudging, acknowledgment of the confessional division of Europe.

The second reason for the much more widespread and interlinked pattern of warfare after 1500 was the creation of a dynastic combination, that of the Habsburgs, to form a network of territories which stretched from Gibraltar to Hungary and from Sicily to Amsterdam, exceeding in size anything which had been seen in Europe since the time of Charlemagne seven hundred years earlier. Stemming originally from Austria, Habsburg rulers had managed to get themselves regularly elected to the position of Holy Roman emperor—a title much diminished in real power since the high Middle Ages but still sought after by princes eager to play a larger role in German and general European affairs.

More practically, the Habsburgs were without equal in augmenting their territories through marriage and inheritance. One such move, by Maximilian I of Austria (1493–1519, and Holy Roman emperor 1508–1519), had brought in the rich hereditary lands of Burgundy and, with them, the Netherlands in 1477. Another, consequent upon a marriage compact of 1515, was to add the important territories of Hungary and Bohemia; although the former was not within the Holy Roman Empire and possessed many liberties, this gave the Habsburgs a great bloc of lands across central Europe. But the most far-reaching of Maximilian's dynastic link-ups was the marriage of his son Philip to Joan, daughter of Ferdinand and Isabella of Spain, whose own earlier union had brought together the possessions of Castile and Aragon (which included Naples and Sicily). The "residuary legatee"[3] to all these marriage compacts was Charles, the eldest son of Philip and Joan. Born in 1500, he became Duke of Burgundy at the age of fifteen and Charles I of Spain a year later, and then—in 1519—he succeeded his paternal grandfather Maximilian I both as Holy Roman emperor and as ruler of the hereditary Habsburg lands in Austria. As the Emperor Charles V, therefore, he embodied all four inheritances until his abdications of 1555–1556 (see Map 3). Only a few years later, in 1526, the death of the childless King Louis of Hungary in the battle of Mohacs against the Turks allowed Charles to claim the crowns of both Hungary and Bohemia.

The sheer heterogeneity and diffusion of these lands, which will be examined further below, might suggest that the Habsburg imperium could never be a real equivalent to the uniform, centralized empires of Asia. Even in the 1520s, Charles was handing over to his younger brother Ferdinand the administration and princely sovereignty of the Austrian hereditary lands, and also of the new acquisitions of Hungary and Bohemia—a recognition, well before Charles's own abdication, that the Spanish and Austrian inheritances could not be effectively ruled by the same person. Nonetheless, that was *not* how the other princes and states viewed this mighty agglomeration of Habsburg power. To the Valois kings of France, fresh from consolidating their own authority internally and eager to expand into the rich Italian peninsula, Charles V's possessions seemed to encircle the French state—and it is hardly an exaggeration to say that the chief aim of the French in Europe over the next two centuries would be to break the influence of the Habsburgs. Similarly, the German princes and electors, who had long struggled against the emperor's having any real authority within Germany itself, could not but be alarmed when they saw Charles V's position was buttressed by so many additional territories, which might now give him the resources to impose his will. Many of the popes, too, disliked this accumulation of Habsburg power, even if it was often needed to combat the Turks, the Lutherans, and other foes.

Given the rivalries endemic to the European states system, therefore, it was hardly likely that the Habsburgs would remain unchallenged. What turned this potential for conflict into a bitter and prolonged reality was its conjunction with the religious disputes engendered by the Reformation. For the fact was that the most prominent and powerful Habsburg monarchs over this century and a half—the Emperor Charles V himself and his later successor, Ferdinand II (1619–1637), and the Spanish kings Philip II (1556–1598) and Philip IV (1621–1665)—were also the most militant in the defense of Catholicism. As a consequence, it became virtually impossible to separate the power-political from the religious strands of the European rivalries which racked the continent in this period. As any contempo-

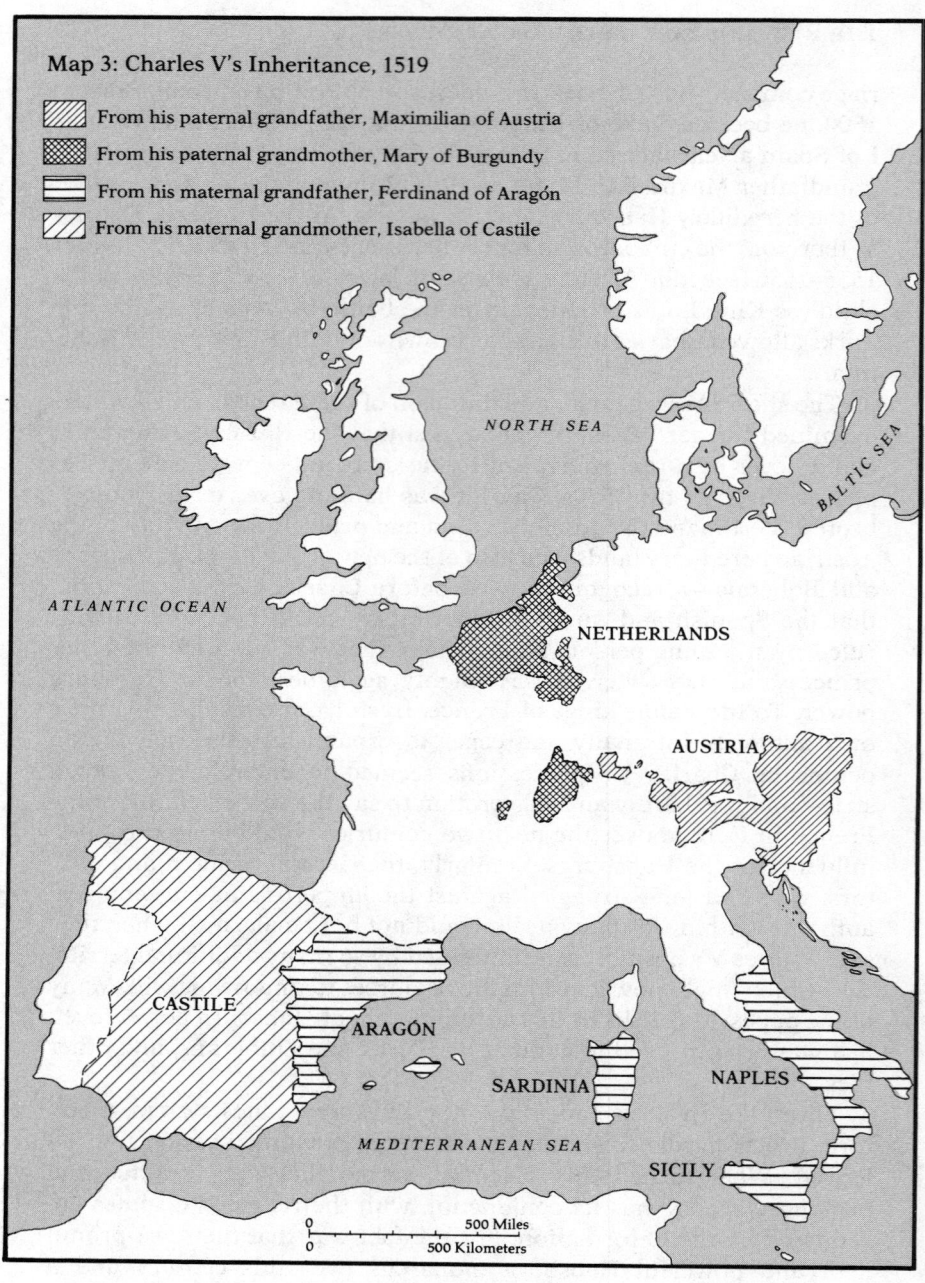

Map 3: Charles V's Inheritance, 1519

- From his paternal grandfather, Maximilian of Austria
- From his paternal grandmother, Mary of Burgundy
- From his maternal grandfather, Ferdinand of Aragón
- From his maternal grandmother, Isabella of Castile

NORTH SEA

BALTIC SEA

ATLANTIC OCEAN

NETHERLANDS

AUSTRIA

CASTILE

ARAGÓN

SARDINIA

NAPLES

MEDITERRANEAN SEA

SICILY

500 Miles

500 Kilometers

rary could appreciate, had Charles V succeeded in crushing the Protestant princes of Germany in the 1540s, it would have been a victory not
only for the Catholic faith but also for Habsburg influence—and the
same was true of Philip II's efforts to suppress the religious unrest in
the Netherlands after 1566; and true, for that matter, of the dispatch
of the Spanish Armada to invade England in 1588. In sum, national
and dynastic rivalries had now fused with religious zeal to make men
fight on where earlier they might have been inclined to compromise.

Even so, it may appear a little forced to use the title "The Habsburg
Bid for Mastery" to describe the entire period from the accession of
Charles V as Holy Roman emperor in 1519 to the Spanish acknowledg-
ment of defeat at the Treaty of the Pyrenees in 1659. Obviously, their
enemies *did* firmly believe that the Habsburg monarchs were bent
upon absolute domination. Thus, the Elizabethan writer Francis
Bacon could in 1595 luridly describe the "ambition and oppression of
Spain":

> France is turned upside down. . . . Portugal usurped. . . . The Low
> Countries warred upon. . . . The like at this day attempted upon
> Aragon. . . . The poor Indians are brought from free men to be
> slaves.[4]

But despite the occasional rhetoric of some Habsburg ministers about
a "world monarchy,"[5] there was no conscious plan to dominate Europe
in the manner of Napoleon or Hitler. Some of the Habsburg dynastic
marriages and successions were fortuitous, at the most inspired, rather
than evidence of a long-term scheme of territorial aggrandizement. In
certain cases—for example, the frequent French invasions of northern
Italy—Habsburg rulers were more provoked than provoking. In the
Mediterranean after the 1540s, Spanish and imperial forces were repeatedly placed on the defensive by the operations of a revived Islam.

Nevertheless, the fact remains that had the Habsburg rulers
achieved all of their limited, regional aims—even their *defensive*
aims—the mastery of Europe would virtually have been theirs. The
Ottoman Empire would have been pushed back, along the North African coast and out of eastern Mediterranean waters. Heresy would have
been suppressed within Germany. The revolt of the Netherlands would
have been crushed. Friendly regimes would have been maintained in
France and England. Only Scandinavia, Poland, Muscovy, and the
lands still under Ottoman rule would not have been subject to Habsburg power and influence—and the concomitant triumph of the
Counter-Reformation. Although Europe even then would not have approached the unity enjoyed by Ming China, the political and religious
principles favored by the twin Habsburg centers of Madrid and Vienna

would have greatly eroded the pluralism that had so long been the continent's most important feature.

The chronology of this century and a half of warfare can be summarized briefly in a work of analysis like this. What probably strikes the eye of the modern reader much more than the names and outcome of various battles (Pavia, Lützen, etc.) is the sheer length of these conflicts. The struggle against the Turks went on decade after decade; Spain's attempt to crush the Revolt of the Netherlands lasted from the 1560s until 1648, with only a brief intermission, and is referred to in some books as the Eighty Years War; while the great multidimensional conflict undertaken by both Austrian and Spanish Habsburgs against successive coalitions of enemy states from 1618 until the 1648 Peace of Westphalia has always been known as the Thirty Years War. This obviously placed a great emphasis upon the relative *capacities* of the different states to bear the burdens of war, year after year, decade after decade. And the significance of the material and financial underpinnings of war was made the more critical by the fact that it was in this period that there took place a "military revolution" which transformed the nature of fighting and made it much more expensive than hitherto. The reasons for that change, and the chief features of it, will be discussed shortly. But even before going into a brief outline of events, it is as well to know that the military encounters of (say) the 1520s would appear very small-scale, in terms of both men and money deployed, compared with those of the 1630s.

The first series of major wars focused upon Italy, whose rich and vulnerable city-states had tempted the French monarchs to invade as early as 1494—and, with equal predictability, had produced various coalitions of rival powers (Spain, the Austrian Habsburgs, even England) to force the French to withdraw.[6] In 1519, Spain and France were still quarreling over the latter's claim to Milan when the news arrived of Charles V's election as Holy Roman emperor and of his combined inheritance of the Spanish and Austrian territories of the Habsburg family. This accumulation of titles by his archrival drove the ambitious French king, Francis I (1515–1547), to instigate a whole series of countermoves, not just in Italy itself, but also along the borders of Burgundy, the southern Netherlands, and Spain. Francis I's own plunge into Italy ended in his defeat and capture at the battle of Pavia (1525), but within another four years the French monarch was again leading an army into Italy—and was again checked by Habsburg forces. Although Francis once more renounced his claims to Italy at the 1529 Treaty of Cambrai, he was at war with Charles V over those possessions both in the 1530s and in the 1540s.

Given the imbalance in forces between France and the Habsburg territories at this time, it was probably not too difficult for Charles V to keep blocking these French attempts at expansion. The task became the harder, however, because as Holy Roman emperor he had inherited many other foes. Much the most formidable of these were the Turks, who not only had expanded across the Hungarian plain in the 1520s (and were besieging Vienna in 1529), but also posed a naval threat against Italy and, in conjunction with the Barbary corsairs of North Africa, against the coasts of Spain itself.[7] What also aggravated this situation was the tacit and unholy alliance which existed in these decades between the Ottoman sultan and Francis I against the Habsburgs: in 1542, French and Ottoman fleets actually combined in an assault upon Nice.

Charles V's other great area of difficulty lay in Germany, which had been torn asunder by the Reformation and where Luther's challenge to the old order was now being supported by a league of Protestant princely states. In view of his other problems, it was scarcely surprising that Charles V could not concentrate his energies upon the Lutheran challenge in Germany until after the mid-1540s. When he did so, he was at first quite successful, especially by defeating the armies of the leading Protestant princes at the battle of Mühlberg (1547). But any enhancement of Habsburg and imperial authority always alarmed Charles V's rivals, so that the northern German princes, the Turks, Henry II of France (1547–1559), and even the papacy all strove to weaken his position. By 1552, French armies had moved into Germany, in support of the Protestant states, who were thereby able to resist the centralizing tendencies of the emperor. This was acknowledged by the Peace of Augsburg (1555), which brought the religious wars in Germany to a temporary end, and by the Treaty of Cateau-Cambresis (1559), which brought the Franco-Spanish conflict to a close. It was also acknowledged, in its way, by Charles V's own abdications—in 1555 as Holy Roman emperor to his brother Ferdinand I (emperor, 1555–1564), and in 1556 as king of Spain in favor of his son Philip II (1556–1598). If the Austrian and Spanish branches remained closely related after this time, it now was the case (as the historian Mamatey puts it) that "henceforth, like the doubleheaded black eagle in the imperial coat of arms, the Habsburgs had two heads at Vienna and at Madrid, looking east and west."[8]

While the eastern branch under Ferdinand I and his successor Maximilian II (emperor, 1564–1576) enjoyed relative peace in their possession (save for a Turkish assault of 1566–1567), the western branch under Philip II of Spain was far less fortunate. The Barbary corsairs were attacking the coasts of Portugal and Castile, and behind them the Turks were resuming their struggle for the Mediterranean. In consequence, Spain found itself repeatedly committed to major new wars against the powerful Ottoman Empire, from the 1560 expedition to Djerba, through the tussle over Malta in 1565, the Lepanto campaign of 1571, and the dingdong battle over Tunis, until the eventual truce of 1581.[9] At virtually the same time, however, Philip's policies of religious intolerance and increased taxation had kindled the discontents in the Habsburg-owned Netherlands into an open revolt. The breakdown of Spanish authority there by the mid-1560s was answered by the dispatch northward of an army under the Duke of Alba and by the imposition of a military despotism—in turn provoking full-scale resistance in the seagirt, defensible Dutch provinces of Holland and Zeeland, and causing alarm in England, France, and northern Germany about Spanish intentions. The English were even more perturbed when, in 1580, Philip II annexed neighboring Portugal, with its colonies and its fleet. Yet, as with all other attempts of the Habsburgs to assert (or extend) their authority, the predictable result was that their many rivals felt obliged to come in, to prevent the balance of power becoming too deranged. By the 1580s, what had earlier been a local rebellion by Dutch Protestants against Spanish rule had widened into a new international struggle.[10] In the Netherlands itself, the warfare of siege and countersiege continued, without spectacular results. Across the Channel, in England, Elizabeth I had checked any internal (whether Spanish or papal-backed) threats to her authority and was lending military support to the Dutch rebels. In France, the weakening of the monarchy had led to the outbreak of a bitter religious civil war, with the Catholic League (supported by Spain) and their rivals the Huguenots (supported by Elizabeth and the Dutch) struggling for supremacy. At sea, Dutch and English privateers interrupted the Spanish supply route to the Netherlands, and took the fight farther afield, to West Africa and the Caribbean.

At some periods in the struggle, especially in the late 1580s and early 1590s, it looked as if the powerful Spanish campaign would succeed; in September 1590, for example, Spanish armies were operating in Languedoc and Britanny, and another army under the outstanding commander the Duke of Parma was marching upon Paris from the north. Nevertheless, the lines of the anti-Spanish forces held, even under that sort of pressure. The charismatic French Huguenot claimant to the crown of France, Henry of Navarre, was flexible enough to switch from Protestantism to Catholicism to boost his claims—and then to lead an ever-increasing part of the French nation against the invading Spaniards and the discredited Catholic League. By the 1598 Peace of Vervins—the year of the death of Philip II of Spain—Madrid agreed to abandon all interference in France. By that time, too, the England of Elizabeth was also secure. The great Armada of 1588, and two later Spanish invasion attempts, had failed miserably—as had the effort to exploit a Catholic rebellion in Ireland, which Elizabeth's armies were steadily reconquering. In 1604, with both Philip II and Elizabeth dead, Spain and England came to a compromise peace. It

would take another five years, until the truce of 1609, before Madrid
negotiated with the Dutch rebels for peace; but well before then it had
become clear that Spanish power was insufficient to crush the Netherlands, either by sea or through the strongly held land (and watery)
defenses manned by Maurice of Nassau's efficient Dutch army. The
continued existence of all three states, France, England, and the United
Provinces of the Netherlands, each with the potential to dispute Habsburg pretensions in the future, again confirmed that the Europe of
1600 would consist of many nations, and not of one hegemony.

The third great spasm of wars which convulsed Europe in this
period occurred after 1618, and fell very heavily upon Germany. That
land had been spared an all-out confessional struggle in the late sixteenth century, but only because of the weakening authority and intellect of Rudolf II (Holy Roman emperor, 1576–1612) and a renewal of
a Turkish threat in the Danube basin (1593–1606). Behind the facade
of German unity, however, the rival Catholic and Protestant forces
were maneuvering to strengthen their own position and to weaken that
of their foes. As the seventeenth century unfolded, the rivalry between
the Evangelical Union (founded in 1608) and the Catholic League
(1609) intensified. Moreover, because the Spanish Habsburgs strongly
supported their Austrian cousins, and because the head of the Evangelical Union, the Elector Palatine Frederick IV, had ties with both England and the Netherlands, it appeared as if most of the states of
Europe were lining up for a final settlement of their political-religious
antagonisms.[11]

The 1618 revolt of the Protestant estates of Bohemia against their
new Catholic ruler, Ferdinand II (emperor 1619–1637), therefore provided the spark needed to begin another round of ferocious religious
struggles: the Thirty Years War of 1618–1648. In the early stages of this
contest, the emperor's forces fared well, ably assisted by a Spanish-
Habsburg army under General Spinola. But, in consequence, a heterogeneous combination of religious and worldly forces entered the
conflict, once again eager to adjust the balances in the opposite direction. The Dutch, who ended their 1609 truce with Spain in 1621, moved
into the Rhineland to counter Spinola's army. In 1626, a Danish force
under its monarch Christian IV invaded Germany from the north.
Behind the scenes, the influential French statesman Cardinal Richelieu
sought to stir up trouble for the Habsburgs wherever he could. However, none of these military or diplomatic countermoves were very
successful, and by the late 1620s the Emperor Ferdinand's powerful
lieutenant, Wallenstein, seemed well on the way to imposing an all-
embracing, centralized authority on Germany, even as far north as the
Baltic shores.[12]

Yet this rapid accumulation of imperial power merely provoked the
House of Habsburg's many enemies to strive the harder. In the early

1630s by far the most decisive of them was the attractive and influential Swedish king, Gustavus Adolphus II (1611–1632), whose well-trained army moved into northern Germany in 1630 and then burst southward to the Rhineland and Bavaria in the following year. Although Gustavus himself was killed at the battle of Lützen in 1632, this in no way diminished the considerable Swedish role in Germany—or, indeed, the overall dimensions of the war. On the contrary, by 1634 the Spaniards under Philip IV (1621–1665) and his accomplished first minister, the Count-Duke of Olivares, had decided to aid their Austrian cousins much more thoroughly than before; but their dispatch into the Rhineland of a powerful Spanish army under its general, Cardinal-Infante, in turn forced Richelieu to decide upon direct French involvement, ordering troops across various frontiers in 1535. For years beforehand, France had been the tacit, indirect leader of the anti-Habsburg coalition, sending subsidies to all who would fight the imperial and Spanish forces. Now the conflict was out in the open, and each coalition began to mobilize even more troops, arms, and money. The language correspondingly became stiffer. "Either all is lost, or else Castile will be head of the world," wrote Olivares in 1635, as he planned the triple invasion of France in the following year.[13]

The conquest of an area as large as France was, however, beyond the military capacities of the Habsburg forces, which briefly approached Paris but were soon hard stretched across Europe. Swedish and German troops were pressing the imperial armies in the north. The Dutch and the French were "pincering" the Spanish Netherlands. Moreover, a revolt by the Portuguese in 1640 diverted a steady flow of Spanish troops and resources from northern Europe to much nearer home, although they were never enough to achieve the reunification of the peninsula. Indeed, with the parallel rebellion of the Catalans—which the French gladly aided—there was some danger of a disintegration of the Spanish heartland by the early 1640s. Overseas, Dutch maritime expeditions struck at Brazil, Angola, and Ceylon, turning the conflict into what some historians describe as the first global war.[14] If the latter actions brought gains to the Netherlands, most of the other belligerents were by this time suffering heavily from the long years of military effort; the armies of the 1640s were becoming smaller than those of the 1630s, the financial expedients of governments were the more desperate, the patience of the people was much thinner and their protests much more violent. Yet precisely because of the interlinked nature of the struggle, it was difficult for any one participant to withdraw. Many of the Protestant German states would have done just that, had they been certain that the Swedish armies would also cease fighting and go home; and Olivares and other Spanish statesmen would have negotiated a truce with France, but the latter would not desert the Dutch. Secret peace negotiations at various levels were carried out in parallel with military campaigns on various fronts, and each power consoled itself with the thought that another victory would buttress its claims in the general settlement.

The end of the Thirty Years War was, in consequence, an untidy affair. Spain suddenly made peace with the Dutch early in 1648, finally recognizing their full independence; but this was done to deprive France of an ally, and the Franco-Habsburg struggle continued. It became purely a Franco-Spanish one later in the year when the Peace of Westphalia (1648) at last brought tranquillity to Germany, and allowed the Austrian Habsburgs to retire from the conflict. While individual states and rulers made certain gains (and suffered certain losses), the essence of the Westphalian settlement was to acknowledge the religious and political *balance* within the Holy Roman Empire, and thus to confirm the limitations upon imperial authority. This left France and Spain engaged in a war which was all to do with national rivalries and nothing to do with religion—as Richelieu's successor, the French minister, Mazarin, clearly demonstrated in 1655 by allying with Cromwell's Protestant England to deliver the blows which finally caused the Spaniards to agree to a peace. The conditions of the Treaty of the Pyrenees (1659) were not particularly harsh, but in forcing Spain to come to terms with its great archenemy, they revealed that the age of Habsburg predominance in Europe was over. All that was left as a "war aim" for Philip IV's government then was the preservation of Iberian unity, and even this had to be abandoned in 1668, when Portugal's independence was formally recognized.[15] The continent's political fragmentation thus remained in much the same state as had existed at Charles V's accession in 1519, although Spain itself was to suffer from further rebellions and losses of territory as the seventeenth century moved to its close (see Map 4)—paying the price, as it were, for its original strategical overextension.

Strengths and Weaknesses of the Habsburg Bloc

Why did the Habsburgs fail?[16] This issue is so large and the process was so lengthy that there seems little point in looking for personal reasons like the madness of the Emperor Rudolf II, or the incompetence of Philip III of Spain. It is also difficult to argue that the Habsburg dynasty and its higher officers were especially deficient when one considers the failings of many a contemporary French and English monarch, and the venality or idiocy of some of the German princes. The puzzle appears the greater when one recalls the vast accumulation of material power available to the Habsburgs:

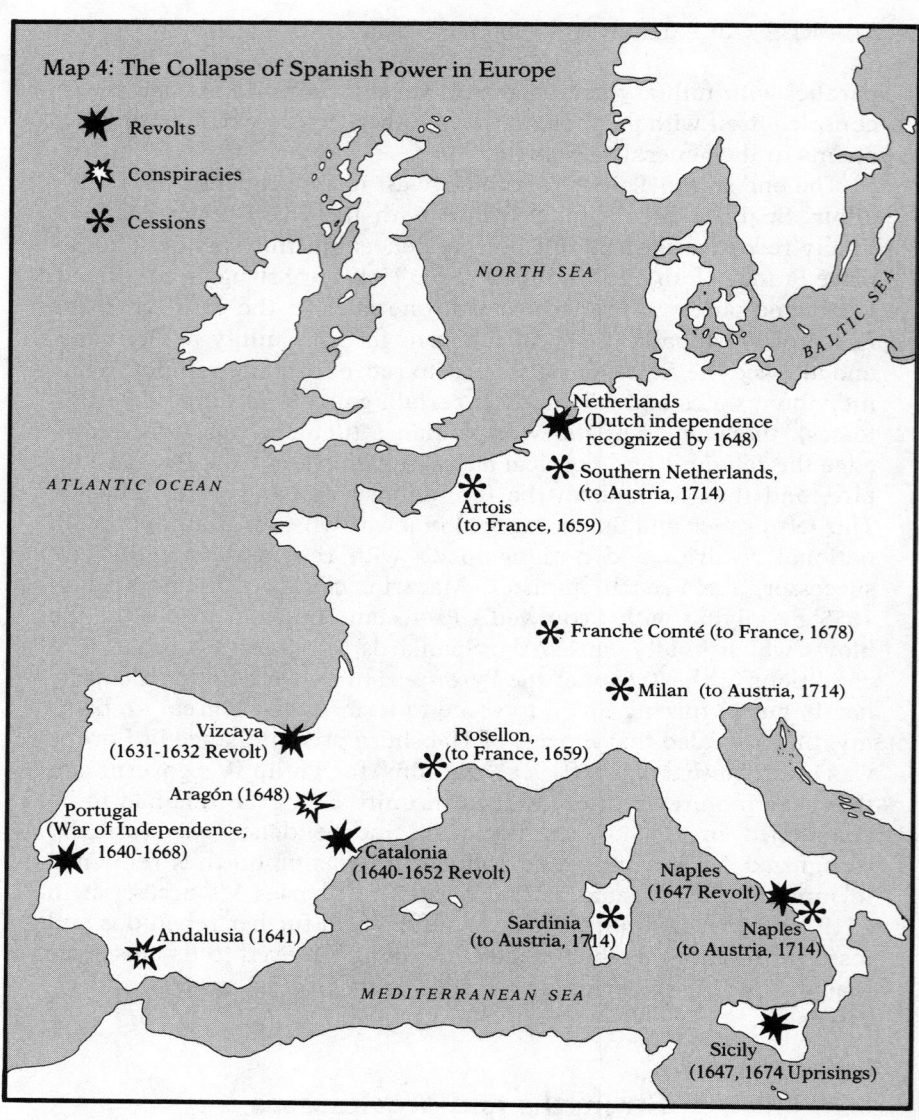

Map 4: The Collapse of Spanish Power in Europe

Revolts

Conspiracies

Cessions

NORTH SEA

BALTIC SEA

ATLANTIC OCEAN

Netherlands
(Dutch independence
recognized by 1648)

Southern Netherlands,
(to Austria, 1714)

Artois
(to France, 1659)

Franche Comté (to France, 1678)

Milan (to Austria, 1714)

Vizcaya
(1631-1632 Revolt)

Rosellon,
(to France, 1659)

Aragón (1648)

Portugal
(War of Independence,
1640-1668)

Catalonia
(1640-1652 Revolt)

Naples
(1647 Revolt)

Andalusia (1641)

Sardinia
(to Austria, 1714)

Naples
(to Austria, 1714)

MEDITERRANEAN SEA

Sicily
(1647, 1674 Uprisings)

Charles V's inheritance of the crowns of four major dynasties, Castile, Aragon, Burgundy, and Austria, the later acquisitions by his house of the crowns of Bohemia, Hungary, Portugal, and, for a short time, even of England, and the coincidence of these dynastic events with the Spanish conquest and exploitation of the New World— these provided the house of Habsburg with a wealth of resources that no other European power could match.[17]

Given the many gaps and inaccuracies in available statistics, one should not place too much reliance upon the population figures of this time; but it would be fair to assume that about one-quarter of the peoples of early modern Europe were living in Habsburg-ruled territory. However, such crude totals* were less important than the wealth of the regions in question, and here the dynastic inheritance seemed to have been blessed with riches.

There were five chief sources of Habsburg finance, and several smaller ones. By far the most important was the Spanish inheritance of Castile, since it was directly ruled and regular taxes of various sorts (the sales tax, the "crusade" tax on religious property) had been conceded to the crown by the Cortes and the church. In addition, there were the two richest trading areas of Europe—the Italian states and the Low Countries—which could provide comparatively large funds from their mercantile wealth and mobile capital. The fourth source, increasingly important as time went on, was the revenue from the American empire. The "royal fifth" of the silver and gold mined there, together with the sales tax, customs duties, and church levies in the New World, provided a vast bonus to the kings of Spain, not only directly but also indirectly, for the American treasures which went into private hands, whether Spanish or Flemish or Italian, helped those individuals and concerns to pay the increasing state taxes levied upon them, and in times of emergency, the monarch could always borrow heavily from the bankers in the expectation of paying off his debts when the silver fleet arrived. The fact that the Habsburg territories contained the leading financial and mercantile houses—those of southern Germany, of certain of the Italian cities, and of Antwerp—must be counted as an additional advantage, and as the fifth major source of income.[18] It was certainly more readily accessible than, say, revenues from Germany, where the princes and free cities represented in the Reichstag voted money to the emperor only if the Turks were at the door.[19]

In the postfeudal age, when knights were no longer expected to perform individual military service (at least in most countries) nor coastal towns to provide a ship, the availability of ready cash and the possession of good credit were absolutely essential to any state en-

---

*As a rough figure, this would mean about 25 million out of the total European population of 105 million in 1600.

gaged in war. Only by direct payment (or promise of payment) could the necessary ships and naval stores and armaments and foodstuffs be mobilized within the market economy to furnish a fleet ready for combat; only by the supply of provisions and wages on a reasonably frequent basis could one's own troops be steered away from mutiny and their energies directed toward the foe. Moreover, although this is commonly regarded as the age when the "nation-state" came into its own in western Europe, all governments relied heavily upon foreign mercenaries to augment their armies. Here the Habsburgs were again blessed, in that they could easily recruit in Italy and the Low Countries as well as in Spain and Germany; the famous Army of Flanders, for example, was composed of six main nationalities, reasonably loyal to the Catholic cause but still requiring regular pay. In naval terms, the Habsburg inheritance could produce an imposing conglomeration of fighting vessels: in Philip II's later years, for example, Mediterranean galleys, great carracks from Genoa and Naples, and the extensive Portuguese fleet could reinforce the armadas of Castile and Aragon.

But perhaps the greatest military advantage possessed by the Habsburgs during these 140 years was the Spanish-trained infantry. The social structure and the climate of ideas made Castile an ideal recruiting ground; there, notes Lynch, "soldiering had become a fashionable and profitable occupation not only for the gentry but for the whole population."[20] In addition, Gonzalo de Córdoba, the "Great Captain," had introduced changes in the organization of infantry early in the sixteenth century, and from then until the middle of the Thirty Years War the Spanish *tercio* was the most effective unit on the battlefields of Europe. With these integrated regiments of up to 3,000 pikemen, swordsmen, and arquebusiers, trained to give mutual support, the Spanish army swept aside innumerable foes and greatly reduced the reputation—and effectiveness—of French cavalry and Swiss pike phalanxes. As late as the battle of Nördlingen (1634), Cardinal-Infante's infantry resisted fifteen charges by the formidable Swedish army and then, like Wellington's troops at Waterloo, grimly moved forward to crush their enemy. At Rocroi (1643), although surrounded by the French, the Spaniards fought to the death. Here, indeed, was one of the strongest pillars in the Habsburg edifice; and it is significant that Spanish power *visibly* cracked only in the mid-seventeenth century, when its army consisted chiefly of German, Italian, and Irish mercenaries with far fewer warriors from Castile.

Yet, for all these advantages, the Spanish-Austrian dynastic alliance could never prevail. Enormous though its financial and military resources appeared to contemporaries, there was never sufficient to meet requirements. This critical deficiency was itself due to three factors which interacted with each other over the entire period—and which, by extension, provide major lessons for the study of armed conflict.

The first of these factors, mentioned briefly above, was the "military revolution" of early modern Europe: that is to say, the massive increase in the scale, costs and organization of war which occurred in the 150 years roughly following the 1520s.[21] This change was itself the result of various intertwined elements, tactical, political, and demographic. The blows dealt to the battlefield dominance of cavalry—first by the Swiss pikemen and then by mixed formations of men bearing pikes, swords, crossbows, and arquebuses—meant that the largest and most important part of an army was now its infantry. This conclusion was reinforced by the development of the *trace italienne,* that sophisticated system of city fortifications and bastions mentioned in the previous chapter. To man such defensive systems, or to besiege them, required a very large number of troops. Of course, in a major campaign a well-organized commander would be successfully employing considerable numbers of cavalry and artillery as well, but those two arms were much less ubiquitous than regiments of foot soldiers. It was not the case, then, that nations scrapped their cavalry forces, but that the infantry proportion in their armies rose markedly; being cheaper to equip and feed, foot soldiers could be recruited in larger numbers, especially since Europe's population was rising. Naturally, all this placed immense organizational strains upon governments, but not so great that they would necessarily overwhelm the bureaucracies of the "new monarchies" of the West—just as the vast increase in the size of the armies would not inevitably make a general's task impossible, provided that his forces had a good command structure and were well drilled.

The Spanish Empire's army probably provides the best example of the "military revolution" in action. As its historian notes, "there is no evidence that any one state fielded more than 30,000 effectives" in the Franco-Spanish struggle for Italy before 1529; but:

In 1536–7 the Emperor Charles V mobilized 60,000 men in Lombardy alone for the defense of his recent conquest, Milan, and for the invasion of French Provence. In 1552, assailed on all fronts at once—in Italy, Germany, the Netherlands and Spain, in the Atlantic and the Mediterranean—Charles V raised 109,000 men in Germany and the Netherlands, 24,000 more in Lombardy and yet more in Sicily, Naples and Spain. The emperor must have had at his command, and therefore at his cost, about 150,000 men. The upward trend continued. In 1574 the Spanish Army of Flanders alone numbered 86,000 men, while only half a century later Philip IV could proudly proclaim that the armed forces at his command in 1625 amounted to no less than 300,000 men. In all these armies the real increase in numbers took place among the infantry, especially among the pikemen.[22]

What was happening on land was to a large extent paralleled at sea. The expansion in maritime (especially transoceanic) commerce, the rivalries among the contending fleets in the Channel, the Indian Ocean, or off the Spanish Main, the threats posed by the Barbary corsairs and the Ottoman galley fleets, all interacted with the new technology of shipbuilding to make vessels bigger and much better armed. In those days there was no strict division between a warship and a merchant-men; virtually all fair-sized trading vessels would carry guns, in order to beat off pirates and other predators. But there was a trend toward the creation of *royal* navies, so that the monarch would at least possess a number of regular warships to form the core around which a great fleet of armed merchantmen, galleasses, and pinnaces could gather in time of war. Henry VIII of England gave considerable support to this scheme, whereas Charles V tended to commandeer the privately owned galleons and galleys of his Spanish and Italian possessions rather than to build his own navy. Philip II, under far heavier pressure in the Mediterranean and then in the Atlantic, could not enjoy that luxury. He had to organize, and pay for, a massive program of galley construction, in Barcelona, Naples, and Sicily; by 1574 he was support-ing a total of 146 galleys, nearly three times the number a dozen years before.[23] The explosion of warfare in the Atlantic during the following decade necessitated an even greater effort there: oceangoing warships were needed to protect the routes to the West Indies and (after Portugal was absorbed in 1580) to the East, to defend the Spanish coastline from English raids, and, ultimately, to convey an invading army to the Brit-ish Isles. After the Anglo-Spanish peace of 1604, a large fleet was still required by Spain to ward off Dutch attacks on the high seas and to maintain communications with Flanders. And, decade by decade, such warships became heavier-armed and much more expensive.

It was these spiraling costs of war which exposed the real weakness of the Habsburg system. The general inflation, which saw food prices rise fivefold and industrial prices threefold between 1500 and 1630, was a heavy enough blow to government finances; but this was com-pounded by the doubling and redoubling in the size of armies and navies. In consequence, the Habsburgs were involved in an almost continual struggle for solvency. Following his various campaigns in the 1540s against Algiers, the French, and the German Protestants, Charles V found that his ordinary *and* extraordinary income could in no way match expenditures, and his revenues were pledged to the bankers for years ahead. Only by the desperate measure of confiscating the treasure from the Indies and seizing all specie in Spain could the monies be found to support the war against the Protestant princes. His 1552 campaign at Metz cost 2.5 million ducats alone—about ten times the emperor's normal income from the Americas at that time. Not surprisingly, he was driven repeatedly to raise fresh loans, but always on worse terms: as the crown's credit tumbled, the interest rates charged by the bankers spiraled upward, so that much of the ordinary revenue had to be used simply to pay the interest on past debts.[24] When Charles abdicated, he bequeathed to Philip II an official Spanish debt of some 20 million ducats.

Philip also inherited a state of war with France, but one which was so expensive that in 1557 the Spanish crown had to declare itself bankrupt. At this, great banking houses like the Fuggers were also brought to their knees. It was a poor consolation that France had been forced to admit its own bankruptcy in the same year—the major reason for each side agreeing to negotiate at Cateau-Cambresis in 1559—for Philip had then immediately to meet the powerful Turkish foe. The twenty-year Mediterranean war, the campaign against the Moriscos of Granada, and then the interconnected military effort in the Netherlands, northern France, and the English Channel drove the crown to search for all possible sources of income. Charles V's revenues had tripled during his reign, but Philip II's "doubled in the period 1556–73 alone, and more than redoubled by the end of the reign."[25]

His outgoings, however, were far larger. In the Lepanto campaign (1571), it was reckoned that the maintenance of the Christian fleets and soldiers would cost over 4 million ducats annually, although a fair part of this burden was shared by Venice and the papacy.[26] The payments to the Army of Flanders were already enormous by the 1570s, and nearly always overdue: this in turn provoking the revolts of the troops, particularly after Philip's 1575 suspension of payments of interest to his Genoese bankers.[27] The much larger flow of income from American mines—around 2 million ducats a year by the 1580s compared with one-tenth of that four decades earlier—rescued the crown's finances, and credit, temporarily; but the armada of 1588 cost 10 million ducats and its sad fate represented a financial as well as a naval disaster. By 1596, after floating loans at an epic rate, Philip again defaulted. At his death two years later his debts totaled the enormous sum of 100 million ducats, and interest payments on this sum equaled about two-thirds of all revenues.[28] Although peace with France and England soon followed, the war against the Dutch ground away until the truce of 1609, which itself had been precipitated by Spanish army mutinies and a further bankruptcy in 1607.

During the few years of peace which followed, there was no substantial reduction in Spanish governmental expenditures. Quite apart from the massive interest payments, there was still tension in the Mediterranean (necessitating a grandiose scheme for constructing coastal fortifications), and the far-flung Spanish empire was still subject to the depredations of privateers (necessitating considerable defense outlays in the Philippines and the Caribbean as well as on the high seas fleet).[29] The state of armed truce in Europe which existed after 1610 hardly suggested to Spain's proud leaders that they could reduce arms expenditures. All that the outbreak of the Thirty Years

War in 1618 did, therefore, was to convert a cold war into a hot one, and to produce an increased flow of Spanish troops and money into Flanders and Germany. It is interesting to note that the run of early Habsburg victories in Europe and the successful defense of the Americas in this period largely coincided with—and was aided by—significant increases in bullion deliveries from the New World. But by the same token, the reduction in treasure receipts after 1626, the bankruptcy declaration of the following year, and the stupendous Dutch success in seizing the silver fleet in 1628 (costing Spain and its inhabitants as much as 10 million ducats) caused the war effort to peter out for a while. And despite the alliance with the emperor, there was no way (except under Wallenstein's brief period of control) that German revenues could make up for this Spanish deficiency.

This, then, was to be the Spanish pattern for the next thirty years of war. By scraping together fresh loans, imposing new taxes, and utilizing any windfall from the Americas, a major military effort like, say, Cardinal-Infante's intervention in Germany in 1634–1635 could be supported; but the grinding costs of war always eventually eroded these short-term gains, and within a few more years the financial position was worse than ever. By the 1640s, in the aftermath of the Catalan and Portuguese revolts, and with the American treasure flow much reduced, a long, slow decline was inevitable.[30] What other fate was due to a nation which, although providing formidable fighters, was directed by governments which consistently spent two or three times more than the ordinary revenues provided?

The second chief cause of the Spanish and Austrian failure must be evident from the narrative account given above: the Habsburgs simply had too much to do, too many enemies to fight, too many fronts to defend. The stalwartness of the Spanish troops in battle could not compensate for the fact that these forces had to be dispersed, in homeland garrisons, in North Africa, in Sicily and Italy, and in the New World, as well as in the Netherlands. Like the British Empire three centuries later, the Habsburg bloc was a conglomeration of widely scattered territories, a political-dynastic *tour de force* which required enormous sustained resources of material and ingenuity to keep going. As such, it provides one of the greatest examples of strategical overstretch in history; for the price of possessing so many territories was the existence of numerous foes, a burden also carried by the contemporaneous Ottoman Empire.[31]

Related to this is the very significant issue of the chronology of the Habsburg wars. European conflicts in this period were frequent, to be sure, and their costs were a terrible burden upon all societies. But all the other states—France, England, Sweden, even the Ottoman Empire—enjoyed certain periods of peace and recovery. It was the Habsburg's, and more especially Spain's, fate to have to turn immediately from a struggle against one enemy to a new conflict against another; peace with France was succeeded by war with the Turks; a truce in the Mediterranean was followed by extended conflict in the Atlantic, and that by the struggle for northwestern Europe. During some awful periods, imperial Spain was fighting on three fronts simultaneously, and with her enemies consciously aiding each other, diplomatically and commercially if not militarily.[32] In contemporary terms, Spain resembled a large bear in the pit: more powerful than any of the dogs attacking it, but never able to deal with all of its opponents and growing gradually exhausted in the process.

Yet how could the Habsburgs escape from this vicious circle? Historians have pointed to the chronic dispersion of energies, and suggested that Charles V and his successors should have formulated a clear set of defense priorities.[33] The implication of this is that some areas were expendable; but which ones?

In retrospect, one can argue that the Austrian Habsburgs, and Ferdinand II in particular, would have been wiser to have refrained from pushing forward with the Counter-Reformation in northern Germany, for that brought heavy losses and few gains. Yet the emperor would still have needed to keep a considerable army in Germany to check princely particularism, French intrigues, and Swedish ambition; and there could also be no reduction in this Habsburg armed strength so long as the Turks stood athwart Hungary, only 150 miles from Vienna. The Spanish government, for its part, could allow the demise of their Austrian cousins neither at the hands of the French and Lutherans nor at the hands of the Turks, because of what it might imply for Spain's own position in Europe. This calculation, however, did not seem to have applied in reverse. After Charles V's retirement in 1556 the empire did not usually feel bound to aid Madrid in the latter's wars in western Europe and overseas; but Spain, conscious of the higher stakes, *would* commit itself to the empire.[34] The long-term consequences of this disparity of feeling and commitment are interesting. The failure of Habsburg Spain's European aims by the mid-seventeenth century was clearly related to its internal problems and relative economic decline; having overstrained itself in all directions, it was now weak at heart. In Habsburg Austria's case, on the other hand, although it failed to defeat Protestantism in Germany, it did achieve a *consolidation* of powers in the dynastic lands (Austria, Bohemia, and so on)—so much so that on this large territorial base and with the later creation of a professional standing army,[35] the Habsburg Empire would be able to reemerge as a European Great Power in the later decades of the seventeenth century, just as Spain was entering a period of even steeper decline.[36] By that stage, however, Austria's recuperation can hardly have been much of a consolation to the statesmen in Madrid, who felt they had to look elsewhere for allies.

It is easy to see why the possessions in the New World were an area of vital importance to Spain. For well over a century, they provided that regular addition to Spain's wealth, and thus to its military power, without which the Habsburg effort could not have been so extensively maintained. Even when the English and Dutch attacks upon the His- pano-Portuguese colonial empire necessitated an ever-increasing ex- penditure on fleets and fortifications overseas, the direct and indirect gains to the Spanish crown from those territories remained considera- ble. To abandon such assets was unthinkable.

This left for consideration the Habsburg possessions in Italy and those in Flanders. Of the two, a withdrawal from Italy had less to recommend itself. In the first half of the sixteenth century, the French would have filled the Great Power vacuum there, and used the wealth of Italy for their own purposes—and to Habsburg detriment. In the second half of that century Italy was, quite literally, the outer bulwark of Spain's own security in the face of Ottoman expansion westward. Quite apart from the blow to Spanish prestige and to the Christian religion which would have accompanied a Turkish assault upon Sicily, Naples, and Rome, the loss of this bulwark would have been a grave strategical setback. Spain would then have had to pour more and more money into coastal fortifications and galley fleets, which in any case were consuming the greater part of the arms budget in the early decades of Philip II's reign. So it made good military sense to commit these existing forces to the active defense of the central Mediterranean, for that kept the Turkish enemy at a distance; and it had the further advantage that the costs of such campaigning were shared by the Habs- burg possessions in Italy, by the papacy, and, on occasions, by Venice. Withdrawal from this front brought no advantages and many potential dangers.

By elimination, then, the Netherlands was the only area in which Habsburg losses might be cut; and, after all, the costs of the Army of Flanders in the "Eighty Years War" against the Dutch were, thanks to the difficulties of the terrain and the advances in fortifications,[37] quite stupendous and greatly exceeded those on any other front. Even at the height of the Thirty Years War, five or six times as much money was allocated to the Flanders garrison as to forces in Germany. "The war in the Netherlands," observed one Spanish councillor, "has been the total ruin of this monarchy." In fact, between 1566 and 1654 Spain sent at least 218 million ducats to the Military Treasury in the Netherlands, considerably more than the sum total (121 million ducats) of the crown's receipts from the Indies.[38] Strategically, too, Flanders was much more difficult to defend: the sea route was often at the mercy of the French, the English, and the Dutch—as was most plainly shown when the Dutch admiral Tromp smashed a Spanish fleet carrying troop reinforcements in 1639—but the "Spanish Road" from Lombardy via the Swiss valleys or Savoy and Franche-Comté up the eastern frontiers of France to the lower Rhine also contained a number of very vulnerable choke points.[39] Was it really worthwhile to keep attempting to control a couple of million recalcitrant Netherlanders at the far end of an extensive line of communications, and at such horrendous cost? Why not, as the representatives of the overtaxed Cortes of Castile slyly put it, let the rebels rot in their heresy? Divine punishment was assured them, and Spain would not have to carry the burden any longer.[40]

The reasons given against an imperial retreat from that theater would not have convinced those complaining of the waste of resources, but they have a certain plausibility. In the first place, if Spain no longer possessed Flanders, it would fall either to France or to the United Provinces, thereby enhancing the power and prestige of one of those inveterate Habsburg enemies; the very idea was repellent to the directors of Spanish policy, to whom "reputation" mattered more than anything else. Secondly, there was the argument advanced by Philip IV and his advisers that a confrontation in that region at least took hostile forces away from more sensitive places: "Although the war which we have fought in the Netherlands has exhausted our treasury and forced us into the debts that we have incurred, it has also diverted our enemies in those parts so that, had we not done so, it is certain that we would have had war in Spain or somewhere nearer."[41] Finally, there was the "domino theory"—if the Netherlands were lost, so also would be the Habsburg cause in Germany, smaller possessions like Franche-Comté, perhaps even Italy. These were, of course, hypothetical arguments; but what is interesting is that the statesmen in Madrid, and their army commanders in Brussels, perceived an interconnected strategical whole, which would be shattered if any one of the parts fell:

> The first and greatest dangers [so the reasoning went in the critical year of 1635] are those that threaten Lombardy, the Netherlands and Germany. A defeat in any of these three is fatal for this Monarchy, so much so that if the defeat in those parts is a great one, the rest of the monarchy will collapse; for Germany will be followed by Italy and the Netherlands, and the Netherlands will be followed by America; and Lombardy will be followed by Naples and Sicily, without the possibility of being able to defend either.[42]

In accepting this logic, the Spanish crown had committed itself to a widespread war of attrition, which would last until victory was secured, or a compromise peace was effected, or the entire system was exhausted.

Perhaps it is sufficient to show that the sheer costs of continuous war and the determination not to abandon any of the four major fronts were bound to undermine Spanish-Imperial ambitions in any case. Yet the evidence suggests that there was a third, related cause: namely, that the Spanish government in particular failed to mobilize available resources in the most efficient way and, by acts of economic folly, helped to erode its own power.

Although foreigners frequently regarded the empire of Charles V or that of Philip II as monolithic and disciplined, it was in fact a congeries of territories, each of which possessed its own privileges and was proud of its own distinctiveness.[43] There was no central administration (let alone legislature or judiciary), and the only real connecting link was the monarch himself. The absence of such institutions which might have encouraged a sense of unity, and the fact that the ruler might never visit the country, made it difficult for the king to raise funds in one part of his dominions in order to fight in another. The taxpayers of Sicily and Naples would willingly pay for the construction of a fleet to resist the Turks, but they complained bitterly at the idea of financing the Spanish struggle in the Netherlands; the Portuguese saw the sense of supporting the defense of the New World, but had no enthusiasm for German wars. This intense localism had contributed to, and was reflected by, jealously held fiscal rights. In Sicily, for example, the estates resisted early Habsburg efforts to increase taxation and had risen against the Spanish viceroy in 1516 and 1517; being poor, anarchical, and possessing a parliament, Sicily was highly unlikely to provide much for the general defense of Habsburg interests.[44] In the kingdom of Naples and in the newer acquisition of Milan, there were fewer legislative obstacles to Spanish administrators under pressure from Madrid to find fresh funds. Both therefore *could* provide considerable financial aid during Charles V's reign; but in practice the struggle to retain Milan, and the wars against the Turks, meant that this flow was usually reversed. To hold its Mediterranean "bulwark," Spain had to send millions of ducats to Italy, to add to those raised there. During the Thirty Years War the pattern was reversed again, and Italian taxes helped to pay for the wars in Germany and the Netherlands; but, taking this period 1519–1659 as a whole, it is hard to believe that the Habsburg possessions in Italy contributed substantially more—if at all—to the common fund than they themselves took out for their own defense.[45]

The Netherlands became, of course, an even greater drain upon general imperial revenues. In the early part of Charles V's reign, the States General provided a growing amount of taxes, although always haggling over the amount and insisting upon recognition of their privileges. By the emperor's later years, the anger at the frequent extraordinary grants which were demanded for wars in Italy and Germany had fused with religious discontents and commercial difficulties to produce a widespread feeling against Spanish rule. By 1565 the state debt of the Low Countries reached 10 million florins, and debt payments plus the costs of normal administration exceeded revenues, so that the deficit had to be made up by Spain.[46] When, after a further decade of mishandling from Madrid, these local resentments burst into open revolt, the

Netherlands became a colossal drain upon imperial resources, with the 65,000 or more troops of the Army of Flanders consuming one-quarter of the total outgoings of the Spanish government for decade after decade.

But the most disastrous failure to mobilize resources lay in Spain itself, where the crown's fiscal rights were in fact very limited. The three realms of the crown of Aragon (that is, Aragon, Catalonia, and Valencia) had their own laws and tax systems, which gave them a quite remarkable autonomy. In effect, the only guaranteed revenue for the monarch came from royal properties; additional grants were made rarely and grudgingly. When, for example, a desperate ruler like Philip IV sought in 1640 to make Catalonia pay for the troops sent there to defend the Spanish frontier, all this did was to provoke a lengthy and famous revolt. Portugal, although taken over from 1580 until its own 1640 rebellion, was completely autonomous in fiscal matters and contributed no regular funds to the general Habsburg cause. This left Castile as the real "milch cow" in the Spanish taxation system, although even here the Basque provinces were immune. The landed gentry, strongly represented in the Castilian Cortes, was usually willing to vote taxes from which they were exempt. Furthermore, taxes such as the *alcabala* (a 10 percent sales tax) and the customs duties, which were the ordinary revenues, together with the *servicios* (grants by the Cortes), *millones* (a tax on foodstuffs, also granted by the Cortes), and the various church allocations, which were the main extraordinary revenues, all tended to hit at trade, the exchange of goods, and the poor, thus spreading impoverishment and discontent, and contributing to depopulation (by emigration).[47]

Until the flow of American silver brought massive additional revenues to the Spanish crown (roughly from the 1560s to the late 1630s), the Habsburg war effort principally rested upon the backs of Castilian peasants and merchants; and even at its height, the royal income from sources in the New World was only about one-quarter to one-third of that derived from Castile and its six million inhabitants. Unless and until the tax burdens could be shared more equitably within that kingdom and indeed across the entirety of the Habsburg territories, this was virtually bound to be too small a base on which to sustain the staggering military expenditures of the age.

What made this inadequacy absolutely certain was the retrograde economic measures attending the exploitation of the Castilian taxpayers.[48] The social ethos of the kingdom had never been very encouraging to trade, but in the early sixteenth century the country was relatively prosperous, boasting a growing population and some significant industries. However, the coming of the Counter-Reformation and of the Habsburgs' many wars stimulated the religious and military elements in Spanish society while weakening the commercial ones. The economic incentives which existed in this society all suggested the wisdom of acquiring a church benefice or purchasing a patent of minor nobility. There was a chronic lack of skilled craftsmen—for example, in the armaments industry—and mobility of labor and flexibility of practice were obstructed by the guilds.[49] Even the development of agriculture was retarded by the privileges of the Mesta, the famous guild of sheep owners whose stock were permitted to graze widely over the kingdom; with Spain's population growing in the first half of the sixteenth century, this simply led to an increasing need for imports of grain. Since the Mesta's payments for these grazing rights went into the royal treasury, and a revocation of this practice would have enraged some of the crown's strongest supporters, there was no prospect of amending the system. Finally, although there were some notable exceptions —the merchants involved in the wool trade, the financier Simon Ruiz, the region around Seville—the Castilian economy on the whole was also heavily dependent upon imports of foreign manufactures and upon the services provided by non-Spaniards, in particular Genoese, Portuguese, and Flemish entrepreneurs. It was dependent, too, upon the Dutch, even during hostilities; "by 1640 three-quarters of the goods in Spanish ports were delivered in Dutch ships,"[50] to the profit of the nation's greatest foes. Not surprisingly, Spain suffered from a constant trade imbalance, which could be made good only by the re-export of American gold and silver.

The horrendous costs of 140 years of war were, therefore, imposed upon a society which was economically ill-equipped to carry them. Unable to raise revenues by the most efficacious means, Habsburg monarchs resorted to a variety of expedients, easy in the short term but disastrous for the long-term good of the country. Taxes were steadily increased by all manner of means, but rarely fell upon the shoulders of those who could bear them most easily, and always tended to hurt commerce. Various privileges, monopolies, and honors were sold off by a government desperate for ready cash. A crude form of deficit financing was evolved, in part by borrowing heavily from the bankers on the credit of future Castilian taxes or American treasure, in part by selling interest-bearing government bonds (juros), which in turn drew in funds that might otherwise have been invested in trade and industry. But the government's debt policy was always done in a hand-to-mouth fashion, without regard for prudent limitations and without the control which a central bank arguably might have imposed. Even by the later stages of Charles V's reign, therefore, government revenues had been mortgaged for years in advance; in 1543, 65 percent of ordinary revenue had to be spent paying interest on the juros already issued. The more the crown's "ordinary" income became alienated, the more desperate was its search for extraordinary revenues and new taxes. The silver coinage, for example, was repeatedly debased with copper vellon. On occasions, the government simply seized incoming American silver destined for private individuals and forced the latter to accept *juros* in compensation; on other occasions, as has been mentioned above, Spanish kings suspended interest repayments and declared themselves temporarily bankrupt. If this latter action did not always ruin the financial houses themselves, it certainly reduced Madrid's credit rating for the future.

Even if some of the blows which buffeted the Castilian economy in these years were not man-made, their impact was the greater because of human folly. The plagues which depopulated much of the country-side around the beginning of the seventeenth century were unpredictable, but they added to the other causes—extortionate rents, the actions of the Mesta, military service—which were already hurting agriculture. The flow of American silver was bound to cause economic problems (especially price inflation) which no society of the time had the experience to handle, but the conditions prevailing in Spain meant that this phenomenon hurt the productive classes more than the unproductive, that the silver tended to flow swiftly out of Seville into the hands of foreign bankers and military provision merchants, and that these new transatlantic sources of wealth were exploited by the crown in a way which worked against rather than for the creation of "sound finance." The flood of precious metals from the Indies, it was said, was to Spain as water on a roof—it poured on and then was drained away.

At the center of the Spanish decline, therefore, was the failure to recognize the importance of preserving the economic underpinnings of a powerful military machine. Time and again the wrong measures were adopted. The expulsion of the Jews, and later the Moriscos; the closing of contacts with foreign universities; the government directive that the Biscayan shipyards should concentrate upon large warships to the near exclusion of smaller, more useful trading vessels; the sale of monopolies which restricted trade; the heavy taxes upon wool exports, which made them uncompetitive in foreign markets; the *internal* customs barriers between the various Spanish kingdoms, which hurt commerce and drove up prices—these were just some of the ill-considered decisions which, in the long term, seriously affected Spain's capacity to carry out the great military role which it had allocated to itself in European (and extra-European) affairs. Although the decline of Spanish power did not fully reveal itself until the 1640s, the causes had existed for decades beforehand.

International Comparisons

Yet this Habsburg failure, it is important to emphasize, was a *relative* one. To abandon the story here without examination of the experiences of the other European powers would leave an incomplete analysis. War, as one historian has argued, "was by far the severest test

that faced the sixteenth-century state."⁵¹ The changes in military techniques which permitted the great rise in the size of armies and the
almost simultaneous evolution of large-scale naval conflict placed
enormous new pressures upon the organized societies of the West.
Each belligerent had to learn how to create a satisfactory administrative structure to meet the "military revolution"; and, of equal importance, it also had to devise new means of paying for the spiraling costs
of war. The strains which were placed upon the Habsburg rulers and
their subjects may, because of the sheer number of years in which their
armies were fighting, have been unusual; but, as Table 1 shows, the
challenge of supervising and financing bigger military forces was common to all states, many of which seemed to possess far fewer resources
than did imperial Spain. How did they meet the test?

Table 1. Increase in Military Manpower, 1470–1660⁵²

Date	Spain	United Provinces	France	England	Sweden
1470s	20,000		40,000	25,000	
1550s	150,000		50,000	20,000	
1590s	200,000	20,000	80,000	30,000	15,000
1630s	300,000	50,000	150,000		45,000
1650s	100,000		100,000	70,000	70,000

Omitted from this brief survey is one of the most persistent and
threatening foes of the Habsburgs, the Ottoman Empire, chiefly because its strengths and weaknesses were discussed in the previous
chapter; but it is worth recalling that many of the problems and deficiencies with which Turkish administrators had to contend—strategical
overextension, failure to tap resources efficiently, the crushing of commercial entrepreneurship in the cause of religious orthodoxy or military prestige—appear similar to those which troubled Philip II and his
successors. Also omitted will be Russia and Prussia, as nations whose
period as great powers in European politics had not yet arrived; and,
further, Poland-Lithuania, which despite its territorial extent was too
hampered by ethnic diversity and the fetters of feudalism (serfdom, a
backward economy, an elective monarchy, "an aristocratic anarchy
which was to make it a byword for political ineptitude"⁵³) to commence its own takeoff to becoming a modern nation-state. Instead, the
countries to be examined are the "new monarchies" of France, England, and Sweden and the "bourgeois republic" of the United Provinces.

Because France was the state which ultimately replaced Spain as
the greatest military power, it has been natural for historians to focus
upon the former's many advantages. It would be wrong, however, to
antedate the period of French predominance; throughout most of the

years covered in this chapter, France looked—and was—decidedly weaker than its southern neighbor. In the few decades which followed the Hundred Years War, the consolidation of the crown's territories vis-à-vis England, Burgundy, and Britanny, the habit of levying direct taxation (especially the *taille*, a poll tax), without application to the States General, the steady administrative work of the new secretaries of state, and the existence of a "royal" army with a powerful artillery train made France appear to be a successful, unified, postfeudal monarchy.[54] Yet the very fragility of this structure was soon to be made clear. The Italian wars, besides repeatedly showing how short-lived and disastrous were the French efforts to gain influence in that peninsula (even when allied with Venice or the Turks), were also very expensive: it was not only the Habsburgs but also the French crown which had to declare bankruptcy in the fateful year of 1557. Well before that crash, and despite all the increase in the *taille* and in indirect taxes like the *gabelle* and customs, the French monarchy was already resorting to heavy borrowings from financiers at high rates of interest (10–16 percent), and to dubious expedients like selling offices. Worse still, it was in France rather than Spain or England that religious rivalries interacted with the ambitions of the great noble houses to produce a bloody and long-lasting civil war. Far from being a great force in international affairs, France after 1560 threatened to become the new cockpit of Europe, perhaps to be divided permanently along religious borders as was to be the fate of the Netherlands and Germany.[55]

Only after the accession of Henry of Navarre to the French throne as Henry IV (1589–1610), with his policies of internal compromise and external military actions against Spain, did matters improve; and the peace which he secured with Madrid in 1598 had the great advantage of maintaining France as an independent power. But it was a country severely weakened by civil war, brigandage, high prices, and interrupted trade and agriculture, and its fiscal system was in pieces. In 1596 the national debt was almost 300 million livres, and four-fifths of that year's revenue of 31 million livres had already been assigned and alienated.[56] For a long time thereafter, France was a recuperating society. Yet its natural resources were, comparatively, immense. Its population of around sixteen million inhabitants was twice that of Spain and four times that of England. While it may not have been as advanced as the Netherlands, northern Italy, and the London region in urbanization, commerce, and finance, its agriculture was diversified and healthy, and the country normally enjoyed a food surplus. The latent wealth of France was clearly demonstrated in the early seventeenth century, when Henry IV's great minister Sully was supervising the economy and state finances. Apart from the *paulette* (which was the sale of, and tax on, hereditary offices), Sully introduced no new fiscal devices; what he did do was to overhaul the tax-collecting machinery, flush out thousands of individuals illegally claiming exemption, recover crown lands and income, and renegotiate the interest rates on the national debt. Within a few years after 1600, the state's budget was in balance. In addition, Sully—anticipating Louis XIV's minister, Colbert—tried to aid industry and agriculture by various means: reducing the *taille*, building bridges, roads, and canals to assist the transport of goods, encouraging cloth production, setting up royal factories to produce luxury wares which would replace imports, and so on. Not all of these measures worked to the extent hoped for, but the contrast with Philip III's Spain was a marked one.[57]

It is difficult to say whether this work of recovery would have continued had not Henry IV been assassinated in 1610. What was clear was that none of the "new monarchies" could properly function without adequate leadership, and between the time of Henry IV's death and Richelieu's consolidation of royal power in the 1630s, the internal politics of France, the disaffection of the Huguenots, and the nobility's inclination toward intrigue once again weakened the country's capacity to act as a European Great Power. Furthermore, when France eventually did engage openly in the Thirty Years War it was not, as some historians have tended to portray it, a unified, healthy power but a country still suffering from many of the old ailments. Aristocratic intrigue remained strong and was only to reach its peak in 1648–1653; uprisings by the peasantry, by the unemployed urban workers, and by the Huguenots, together with the obstructionism of local officeholders, all interrupted the proper functioning of government; and the economy, affected by the general population decline, harsher climate, reduced agricultural output, and higher incidence of plagues which seems to have troubled much of Europe at this time,[58] was hardly in a position to finance a great war.

From 1635 onward, therefore, French taxes had to be increased by a variety of means: the sale of offices was accelerated; and the *taille*, having been reduced in earlier years, was raised so much that the annual yield from it had doubled by 1643. But even this could not cover the costs of the struggle against the Habsburgs, both the direct military burden of supporting an army of 150,000 men and the subsidies to allies. In 1643, the year of the great French military victory over Spain at Rocroi, government expenditure was almost double its income and Mazarin, Richelieu's successor, had been reduced to even more desperate sales of government offices and an even stricter control of the *taille*, both of which were highly unpopular. It was no coincidence that the rebellion of 1648 began with a tax strike against Mazarin's new fiscal measures, and that such unrest swiftly led to a loss in the government's credit and to its reluctant declaration of bankruptcy.[59]

Consequently, in the eleven years of Franco-Spanish warfare which remained after the general Peace of Westphalia in 1648, the two con-

testants resembled punch-drunk boxers, clinging to each other in a
state of near-exhaustion and unable to finish the other off. Each was
suffering from domestic rebellion, widespread impoverishment, and
dislike of the war, and was on the brink of financial collapse. It was
true that, with generals like d'Enghien and Turenne and military reformers like Le Tellier, the French army was slowly emerging to be the
greatest in Europe; but its naval power, built up by Richelieu, had
swiftly disintegrated because of the demands of land warfare;[60] and the
country still needed a solid economic base. In the event, it was France's
good fortune that England, resurgent in its naval and military power
under Cromwell, elected to join the conflict, thereby finally tilting the
balance against a distressed Spain. The Treaty of the Pyrenees which
followed was symbolic less of the greatness of France than of the
relative decline of its overstretched southern neighbor, which had
fought on with remarkable tenacity.[61]

In other words, each of the European powers possessed a mixture
of strengths and weaknesses, and the real need was to prevent the latter
from outweighing the former. This was certainly true of the "flank"
powers in the west and north, England and Sweden, whose interventions helped to check Habsburg ambitions on several critical occasions. It was hardly the case, for example, that England stood poised
and well prepared for a continental conflict during these 140 years. The
key to the English recovery following the Wars of the Roses had been
Henry VII's concentration upon domestic stability and financial prudence, at least after the peace with France in 1492. By cutting down on
his own expenses, paying off his debts, and encouraging the wool trade,
fishing, and commerce in general, the first Tudor monarch provided
a much-needed breathing space for a country hit by civil war and
unrest; the natural productivity of agriculture, the flourishing cloth
trade to the Low Countries, the increasing use of the rich offshore
fishing grounds, and the general bustle of coastal trade did the rest. In
the area of national finances, the king's recovery of crown lands and
seizure of those belonging to rebels and rival contenders to the throne,
the customs yield from growing trade, and the profits from the Star
Chamber and other courts all combined to produce a healthy balance.[62]

But political and fiscal stability did not necessarily equal *power*.
Compared with the far greater populations of France and Spain, the
three to four million inhabitants of England and Wales did not seem
much. The country's financial institutions and commercial infrastructures were crude, compared with those in Italy, southern Germany,
and the Low Countries, although considerable industrial growth was
to occur in the course of the "Tudor century."[63] At the military level,
the gap was much wider. Once he was secure upon the throne, Henry

VII had dissolved much of his own army and forbade (with a few
exceptions) the private armies of the great magnates; apart from the
"Yeomen of the Guard" and certain garrison troops, there was no
regular standing army in England during this period when Franco-
Habsburg wars in Italy were changing the nature and dimensions of
military conflict. Consequently, such forces as did exist under the early
Tudors were still equipped with traditional weapons (longbow, bill)
and raised in the traditional way (county militia, volunteer "companies," and so on). However, this backwardness did not keep his successor, Henry VIII, from campaigning against the Scots or even deter his
interventions of 1513 and 1522–1523 against France, since the English
king could hire large numbers of "modern" troops—pikemen, arquebusiers, heavy cavalry—from Germany.[64]

If neither these early English operations in France nor the two later
invasions in 1528 and 1544 ended in military disaster—if, indeed, they
often forced the French monarch to buy off the troublesome English
raiders—they certainly had devastating financial consequences. Of the
total expenditures of £700,000 by the Treasury of the Chamber in 1513,
for example, £632,000 was allocated toward soldiers' pay, ordnance,
warships, and other military outgoings.* Soon, Henry VII's accumulated reserves were all spent by his ambitious heir, and Henry
VIII's chief minister, Wolsey, was provoking widespread complaints
by his efforts to gain money from forced loans, "benevolences," and
other arbitrary means. Only with Thomas Cromwell's assault upon
church lands in the 1530s was the financial position eased; in fact, the
English Reformation doubled the royal revenues and permitted large-
scale spending upon defensive military projects—fortresses along the
Channel coast and Scottish border, new and powerful warships for the
Royal Navy, the suppression of rebellions in Ireland. But the disastrous wars against France and Scotland in the 1540s cost an enormous
£2,135,000, which was about ten times the normal income of the
crown. This forced the king's ministers into the most desperate of
expedients: the sale of religious properties at low rates, the seizure of
the estates of nobles on trumped-up charges, repeated forced loans, the
great debasement of the coinage, and finally the recourse to the Fuggers and other foreign bankers.[65] Settling England's differences with
France in 1550 was thus a welcome relief to a near-bankrupt government.

What this all indicated, therefore, was the very real limits upon
England's power in the first half of the sixteenth century. It was a

*My colleague Prof. Robert Ashton warns me that any stated figures of English (and pre-
sumably other) state revenues and expenditures in this entire period must be regarded as
nominal; the amounts deducted by officeholders, bribery, corruption, and inefficient bookkeep-
ing drastically reduced the stated "allocations" to the army and navy. In much the same way,
only a portion of the king's "income" ever reached the monarch. The statistics given here are,
therefore, indicative and not authoritative.

centralized and relatively homogeneous state, although much less so in the border areas and in Ireland, which could always distract royal resources and attention. Thanks chiefly to the interest of Henry VIII, it was defensively strong, with some modern forts, artillery, dockyards, a considerable armaments industry, and a well-equipped navy. But it was militarily backward in the quality of its army, and its finances could not fund a large-scale war. When Elizabeth I became monarch in 1558, she was prudent enough to recognize these limitations and to achieve her ends without breaching them. In the dangerous post-1570 years, when the Counter-Reformation was at its height and Spanish troops were active in the Netherlands, this was a difficult task to fulfill. Since her country was no match for any of the real "superpowers" of Europe, Elizabeth sought to maintain England's independence by diplomacy and, even when Anglo-Spanish relations worsened, to allow the "cold war" against Philip II to be conducted at sea, which was at least economical and occasionally profitable.[66] Although needing to provide monies to secure her Scottish and Irish flanks and to give aid to the Dutch rebels in the late 1570s, Elizabeth and her ministers succeeded in building up a healthy surplus during the first twenty-five years of her reign—which was just as well, since the queen sorely needed a "war chest" once the decision was taken in 1585 to dispatch an expeditionary force under Leicester to the Netherlands.

The post-1585 conflict with Spain placed both strategical and financial demands upon Elizabeth's government. In considering the strategy which England should best employ, naval leaders like Hawkins, Raleigh, Drake, and others urged upon the queen a policy of intercepting the Spanish silver trade, raiding the enemy's coasts and colonies, and in general exploiting the advantages of sea power to wage war on the cheap—an attractive proposition in theory, although often difficult to implement in practice. But there was also the need to send troops to the Netherlands and northern France to assist those fighting the Spanish army—a strategy adopted not out of any great love of Dutch rebels or the French Protestants but simply because, as Elizabeth argued, "whenever the last day of France came it would also be the eve of the destruction of England."[67] It was therefore vital to preserve the European balance, if need be by active intervention; and this "continental commitment" continued until the early seventeenth century, at least in a personal form, for many English troops stayed on when the expeditionary force was merged into the army of the United Provinces in 1594.

In performing the twin function of checking Philip II's designs on land and harassing his empire at sea, the English made their own contribution to the maintenance of Europe's political plurality. But the strain of supporting 8,000 men abroad was immense. In 1586 monies sent to the Netherlands totaled over £100,000, in 1587 £175,000, each being about half of the entire outgoings for the year; in the Armada year, allocations to the fleet exceeded £150,000. Consequently, Elizabeth's annual expenditures in the late 1580s were between two and three times those of the early 1580s. During the next decade the crown spent over £350,000 each year, and the Irish campaign brought the annual average to over £500,000 in the queen's last four years.[68] Try as it might to raise funds from other sources—such as the selling of crown lands, and of monopolies—the government had no alternative but to summon the Commons on repeated occasions and plead for extra grants. That these (totaling some £2 million) were given, and that the English government neither declared itself bankrupt nor failed to pay its troops, was testimony to the skill and prudence of the monarch and her councillors; but the war years had tested the entire system, left debts to the first Stuart king, and placed him and his successor in a position of dependence upon a mistrustful Commons and a cautious London money market.[69]

There is no space in this story to examine the spiraling conflict between crown and Parliament which was to dominate English politics for the four decades after 1603, in which finance was to play the central part.[70] The inept and occasional interventions by English forces in the great European struggle during the 1620s, although very expensive to mount, had little effect upon the course of the Thirty Years War. The population, trade, overseas colonies, and general wealth of England grew in this period, but none of this could provide a sure basis for state power without domestic harmony; indeed, the quarrels over such taxes as Ship Money—which in theory could have enhanced the nation's armed strength—were soon to lead crown and Parliament into a civil war which would cripple England as a factor in European politics for much of the 1640s. When England did reemerge, it was to challenge the Dutch in a fierce commercial war (1652–1654), which, whatever the aims of each belligerent, had little to do with the general European balance.

Cromwell's England of the 1650s could, however, play a Great Power role more successfully than any previous government. His New Model Army, which emerged from the civil war, had at last closed the gap that traditionally existed between English troops and their European counterparts. Organized and trained on modern lines established by Maurice of Nassau and Gustavus Adolphus, hardened by years of conflict, well disciplined, and (usually) paid regularly, the English army could be thrown into the European balance with some effect, as was evident in its defeat of Spanish forces at the battle of the Dunes in 1658. Furthermore, the Commonwealth navy was, if anything, even more advanced for the age. Favored by the Commons because it had generally declared against Charles I during the civil war, the fleet underwent a renaissance in the late 1640s: its size was more than doubled from thirty-nine vessels (1649) to eighty (1651), wages and conditions were improved, dockyard and logistical support were bettered, and the funds for all this regularly voted by a House of Commons which believed that profit and power went hand in hand.[71] This was just as well, because in its first war against the Dutch the navy was taking on an equally formidable force commanded by leaders—Tromp and de Ruyter—who were as good as Blake and Monk. When the service was unleashed upon the Spanish Empire after 1655, it was not surprising that it scored successes: taking Acadia (Nova Scotia) and, after a fiasco at Hispaniola, Jamaica; seizing part of the Spanish treasure fleet in 1656; blockading Cádiz and destroying the *flota* in Santa Cruz in 1657.

Yet, while these English actions finally tilted the balance and forced Spain to end its war with France in 1659, this was not achieved without domestic strains. The profitable Spanish trade was lost to the neutral Dutch in these years after 1655, and enemy privateers reaped a rich harvest of English merchant ships along the Atlantic and Mediterranean routes. Above all, paying for an army of up to 70,000 men and a large navy was a costly business; one estimate suggests that out of a total government expenditure of £2,878,000 in 1657, over £1,900,000 went on the army and £742,000 on the navy.[72] Taxes were imposed, and efficiently extorted, at an unprecedented level, yet they were never enough for a government which was spending "four times as much as had been thought intolerable under Charles I" before the English Revolution.[73] Debts steadily rose, and the pay of soldiers and sailors was in arrears. These few years of the Spanish war undoubtedly increased the public dislike of Cromwell's rule and caused the majority of the merchant classes to plead for peace. It was scarcely the case, of course, that England was altogether ruined by this conflict—although it no doubt would have been had it engaged in Great Power struggles as long as Spain. The growth of England's inland and overseas commerce, plus the profits from the colonies and shipping, were starting to provide a solid economic foundation upon which governments in London could rely in the event of another war; and precisely because England— together with the United Provinces of the Netherlands—had developed an efficient market economy, it achieved the rare feat of combining a rising standard of living with a growing population.[74] Yet it still remained vital to preserve the proper balance between the country's military and naval effort on the one hand and the encouragement of the national wealth on the other; by the end of the Protectorate, that balance had become a little too precarious.

This crucial lesson in statecraft emerges the more clearly if one compares England's rise with that of the other "flank" power, Sweden.[75] Throughout the sixteenth century, the prospects for the northern kingdom looked poor. Hemmed in by Lübeck and (especially) by Denmark from free egress to western Europe, engaged in a succession of struggles on its eastern flank with Russia, and repeatedly distracted by its relationship with Poland, Sweden had enough to do simply to maintain itself; indeed, its severe defeat by Denmark in the war of 1611–1613 hinted that decline rather than expansion would be the country's fate. In addition, it had suffered from internal fissures, which were constitutional rather than religious, and had resulted in confirming the extensive privileges of the nobility. But Sweden's greatest weakness was its economic base. Much of its extensive territory was Arctic waste, or forest. The scattered peasantry, largely self-sufficient, formed 95 percent of a total population of some 900,000; with Finland, about a million and a quarter—less than many of the Italian states. There were few towns and little industry; a "middle class" was hardly to be detected; and the barter of goods and services was still the major form of exchange. Militarily and economically, therefore, Sweden was a mere pigmy when the youthful Gustavus Adolphus succeeded to the throne in 1611.

Two factors, one external, one internal, aided Sweden's swift growth from these unpromising foundations. The first was foreign entrepreneurs, in particular the Dutch but also Germans and Walloons, for whom Sweden was a promising "undeveloped" land, rich in raw materials such as timber and iron and copper ores. The most famous of these foreign entrepreneurs, Louis de Geer, not only sold finished products to the Swedes and bought the raw ores from them; he also, over time, created timber mills, foundries, and factories, made loans to the king, and drew Sweden into the mercantile "world system" based chiefly upon Amsterdam. Soon the country became the greatest producer of iron and copper in Europe, and these exports brought in the foreign currency which would soon help to pay for the armed forces. In addition, Sweden became self-sufficient in armaments, a rare feat, thanks again to foreign investment and expertise.[76]

The internal factor was the well-known series of reforms instituted by Gustavus Adolphus and his aides. The courts, the treasury, the tax system, the central administration of the chancery, and education were but some of the areas made more efficient and productive in this period. The nobility was led away from faction into state service. Religious solidarity was assured. Local as well as central government seemed to work. On these firm foundations, Gustavus could build a Swedish navy so as to protect the coasts from Danish and Polish rivals and to ensure the safe passage of Swedish troops across the Baltic. Above all, however, the king's fame rested upon his great military reforms: in developing the national standing army based upon a form of conscription, in training his troops in new battlefield tactics, in his improvements of the cavalry and introduction of mobile, light artillery, and finally in the discipline and high morale which his leadership gave to the army, Gustavus had at his command perhaps the best fighting force in the world when he moved into northern Germany to aid the Protestant cause during the summer of 1630.[77]

Such advantages were all necessary, since the dimensions of the European conflict were far larger, and the costs far heavier, than anything experienced in the earlier local wars against Sweden's neighbors. By the end of 1630 Gustavus commanded over 42,000 men; twelve months later, double that number; and just before the fateful battle of Lützen, his force had swollen to almost 150,000. While Swedish troops formed a *corps d'élite* in all the major battles and were also used to garrison strategic strongpoints, they were insufficient in number to form an army of that size; indeed, four-fifths of that "Swedish" army of 150,000 consisted of foreign mercenaries, Scots, English, and Germans, who were fearfully expensive. Even the struggles against Poland in the 1620s had strained Swedish public finance, but the German war threatened to be far more costly. Remarkably, however, the Swedes managed to make others pay for it. The foreign subsidies, particularly those paid by France, are well known but they covered only a fraction of the costs. The real source was Germany itself: the various princely states, and the free cities, were required to contribute to the cause, if they were friendly; if they were hostile, they had to pay ransoms to avoid plunder. In addition, this vast Swedish-controlled army exacted quarter, food, and fodder from the territories on which it was encamped. To be sure, this system had already been perfected by the emperor's lieutenant, Wallenstein, whose policy of exacting "contributions" had financed an imperial army of over 100,000 men;[78] but the point here is that it was *not* the Swedes who paid for the great force which helped to check the Habsburgs from 1630 until 1648. In the very month of the Peace of Westphalia itself, the Swedish army was looting in Bohemia; and it was entirely appropriate that it withdrew only upon the payment of a large "compensation."

Although this was a remarkable achievement by the Swedes, in many ways it gave a false picture of the country's real standing in Europe. Its formidable war machine had been to a large degree *parasitic;* the Swedish army in Germany had to plunder in order to live— otherwise the troops mutinied, which hurt the Germans more. Naturally, the Swedes themselves had had to pay for their navy, for home defenses, and for forces employed elsewhere than in Germany; and, as in all other states, this had strained governmental finances, which led to desperate sales of crown lands and revenues to the nobility, thus reducing long-term income. The Thirty Years War had also taken a heavy toll in human life, and the extraordinary taxes burdened the peasantry. Furthermore, Sweden's military successes had given it a variety of trans-Baltic possessions—Estonia, Livonia, Bremen, most of Pomerania—which admittedly brought commercial and fiscal benefits, but the costs of maintaining them in peacetime or defending them in wartime from jealous rivals was to bring a far higher charge upon the Swedish state than had the great campaigning across Germany in the 1630s and 1640s.

Sweden was to remain a considerable power, even after 1648, but only at the regional level. Indeed, under Charles X (1654–1660) and Charles XI (1660–1697), it was arguably at its height in the Baltic arena, where it successively checked the Danes and held its own against Poland, Russia, and the rising power of Prussia. The turn toward absolutism under Charles XI augmented the royal finances and thus permitted the upkeep of a large peacetime standing army. Nonetheless, these were measures to strengthen Sweden as it slowly declined from the first ranks. In Professor Roberts's words:

> For a generation Sweden had been drunk with victory and bloated with booty: Charles XI led her back into the grey light of everyday existence, gave her policies appropriate to her resources and her real interests, equipped her to carry them out, and prepared for her a future of weight and dignity as a second-class power.[79]

These were not mean achievements, but in the larger European context they had limited significance. And it is interesting to note the extent to which the balance of power in the Baltic, upon which Sweden no less than Denmark, Poland, and Brandenburg depended, was being influenced and "manipulated" in the second half of the seventeenth century by the French, the Dutch, and even the English, for their own purposes, by subsidies, diplomatic interventions, and, in 1644 and 1659, a Dutch fleet.[80] Finally, while Sweden could never be called a "puppet" state in this great diplomatic game, it remained an economic midget compared with the rising powers of the West, and tended to become dependent upon their subsidies. Its foreign trade around 1700 was but a small fraction of that possessed by the United Provinces or England; its state expenditure was perhaps only one-fiftieth that of France.[81] On this inadequate material base, and without the possibility of access to overseas colonies, Sweden had little chance—despite its admirable social and administrative stability—of maintaining the military predominance that it had briefly held under Gustavus Adolphus. In the coming decades, in fact, it would have its work cut out merely seeking to arrest the advances of Prussia in the south and Russia in the east.

The final example, that of Dutch power in this period, offers a remarkable contrast to the Swedish case. Here was a nation created in

the confused circumstances of revolution, a cluster of seven heterogenous provinces separated by irregular borders from the rest of the
Habsburg-owned Netherlands, a mere part of a part of a vast dynastic
empire, restricted in population and territorial extent, which swiftly
became a great power inside and *outside* Europe for almost a century.
It differed from the other states—although not from its Italian forerunner, Venice—in possessing a republican, oligarchic form of government; but its most distinctive characteristic was that the foundations
of its strength were firmly anchored in the world of trade, industry,
and finance. It was, to be sure, a formidable military power, at least
in defense; and it was the most effective naval power until eclipsed by
England in the later seventeenth century. But those manifestations of
armed might were the consequences, rather than the essence, of Dutch
strength and influence.

It was hardly the case, of course, that in the early years of their
revolt the 70,000 or so Dutch rebels counted for much in European
affairs; indeed, it was not for some decades that they regarded themselves as a separate nation at all, and not until the early seventeenth
century that the boundaries were in any way formed. The so-called
Revolt of the Netherlands was in the beginning a sporadic affair, during which different social groups and regions fought against each other
as well as opposing—and sometimes compromising with—their Habsburg rulers; and there were various moments in the 1580s when the
Duke of Parma's superbly conducted policy of recovering the territories for Spain looked on the verge of success. But for the subsidies and
military aid from England and other Protestant states, the importation
of large numbers of English guns, and the frequent diversion of the
Spanish armies into France, the rebellion then might have been
brought to an end. Yet since the ports and shipyards of the Netherlands
were nearly all in rebel hands, and Spain found it impossible to gain
control of the sea, Parma could reconquer only by slow, landward
siege operations which lost their momentum whenever he was ordered
to march his armies into France.[82]

By the 1590s, then, the United Provinces had survived and could, in
fact, reconquer most of the provinces and towns which had been lost
in the east. Its army was by that stage well trained and led by Maurice
of Nassau, whose tactical innovations and exploitation of the watery
terrain made him one of the great captains of the age. To call it a Dutch
army would be a misnomer: in 1600 it consisted of forty-three English,
thirty-two French, twenty Scots, eleven Walloon, and nine German
companies, and only seventeen Dutch companies.[83] Despite this large
(but by no means untypical) variety of nationalities, Maurice molded
his forces into a coherent, standardized whole. He was undoubtedly
aided in this, however, by the financial underpinning provided by the
Dutch government; and his army, more than most in Europe, was

regularly paid, just as the government continually provided for the maintenance of its substantial navy.

It would be unwise to exaggerate the wealth and financial stability of the Dutch republic or to suggest that it found it easy to pay for the prolonged conflict, especially in its early stages. In the eastern and southern parts of the United Provinces, the war caused considerable damage, loss of trade, and decline in population. Even the prosperous province of Holland found the tax burdens enormous; in 1579 it had to provide 960,000 florins for the war, in 1599 almost 5.5 million florins. By the early seventeenth century, with the annual costs of the war against Spain rising to 10 million florins, many wondered how much longer the struggle could be maintained without financial strain. Fortunately for the Dutch, Spain's economy—and its corresponding ability to pay the mutiny-prone Army of Flanders—had suffered even more, and at last caused Madrid to agree to the truce of 1609.

Yet if the conflict had tested Dutch resources, it had not exhausted them; and the fact was that from the 1590s onward, its economy was growing fast, thus providing a solid foundation of "credit" when the government turned—as all belligerent states had to turn—to the money market. One obvious reason for this prosperity was the interaction of a growing population with a more entrepreneurial spirit, once the Habsburg rule had been cast off. In addition to the natural increase in numbers, there were tens (perhaps hundreds) of thousands of refugees from the south, and many others from elsewhere in Europe. It seems clear that many of these immigrants were skilled workers, teachers, craftsmen, and capitalists, with much to offer. The sack of Antwerp by Spanish troops in 1576 gave a boost to Amsterdam's chances in the international trading system, yet it was also true that the Dutch took every opportunity offered them for commercial advancement. Their domination of the rich herring trade and their reclamation of land from the sea provided additional sources of wealth. Their vast mercantile marine, and in particular their *fluyts* (simple, robust freighters), earned them the carrying trade of much of Europe by 1600: timber, grain, cloth, salt, herrings were transported by Dutch vessels along every waterway. To the disgust of their English allies, and of many Dutch Calvinist divines, Amsterdam traders would willingly supply such goods to their mortal enemy, Spain, if the profits outweighed the risks. At home, raw materials were imported in vast quantities and then "finished" by the various trades of Amsterdam, Delft, Leyden, and so on. With "sugar refining, melting, distilling, brewing, tobacco cutting, silk throwing, pottery, glass, armament manufacture, printing, paper making"[84] among the chief industries, it was hardly surprising that by 1622 around 56 percent of Holland's population of 670,000 lived in medium-sized towns. Every other region in the world must have seemed economically backward by comparison.

Two further aspects of the Dutch economy enhanced its military power. The first was its overseas expansion. Although this commerce did not compare with the humbler but vaster bulk trade in European waters, it was another addition to the republic's resources. "Between 1598 and 1605, on average twenty-five ships sailed to West Africa, twenty to Brazil, ten to the East Indies, and 150 to the Caribbean every year. Sovereign colonies were founded at Amboina in 1605 and Ternate in 1607; factories and trading posts were established around the Indian Ocean, near the mouth of the Amazon and (in 1609) in Japan."[85] Like England, the United Provinces were now benefiting from that slow shift in the economic balances from the Mediterranean to the Atlantic world which was one of the main secular trends of the period 1500–1700; and which, while working at first to the advantage of Portugal and Spain, was later galvanizing societies better prepared to extract the profits of global commerce.[86]

The second feature was Amsterdam's growing role as the center of international finance, a natural corollary to the republic's function as the shipper, exchanger, and commodity dealer of Europe. What its financiers and institutions offered (receiving deposits at interest, transferring monies, crediting and clearing bills of exchange, floating loans) was not different from practices already established in, say, Venice and Genoa; but, reflecting the United Provinces' trading wealth, it was on a larger scale and conducted with a greater degree of certainty—the more so since the chief investors were a part of the government, and wished to see the principles of sound money, secure credit, and regular repayment of debt upheld. In consequence of all this, there was usually money available for government loans, which gave the Dutch Republic an inestimable advantage over its rivals; and since its credit rating was firm because it promptly repaid debts, it could borrow more cheaply than any other government—a major advantage in the seventeenth century and, indeed, at all times!

This ability to raise loans easily was the more important after the resumption of hostilities with Spain in 1621, for the cost of the armed forces rose steadily, from 13.4 million florins (1622) to 18.8 million florins (1640). These were large sums even for a rich population to bear, and the more particularly since Dutch overseas trade was being hurt by the war, either through direct losses or by the diversion of commerce into neutral hands. It was therefore politically easier to permit as large a part of the war as possible to be financed from public loans. Although this led to a massive increase in the official debt—the Province of Holland's debt was 153 million florins in 1651—the economic strength of the country and the care with which interest was repaid meant that the credit system was never in danger of collapse.[87] While this demonstrates that even wealthy states winced at the cost of military expenditures, it also confirmed that as long as success in war depended upon the length of one's purse, the Dutch were always likely to outstay the others.

War, Money, and the Nation-State

Let us now summarize the chief conclusions of this chapter. The post-1450 waging of war was intimately connected with "the birth of the nation-state."[88] Between the late fifteenth and the late seventeenth centuries, most European countries witnessed a centralization of political and military authority, usually under the monarch (but in some places under the local prince or a mercantile oligarchy), accompanied by increased powers and methods of state taxation, and carried out by a much more elaborate bureaucratic machinery than had existed when kings were supposed to "live of their own" and national armies were provided by a feudal levy.

There were various causes for this evolution of the European nation-state. Economic change had already undermined much of the old feudal order, and different social groups had to relate to each other through newer forms of contract and obligation. The Reformation, in dividing Christendom on the basis *cuius regio, eius religio,* that is, of the rulers' religious preferences, merged civil and religious authority, and thus extended secularism on a national basis. The decline of Latin and the growing use of vernacular language by politicians, lawyers, bureaucrats, and poets accentuated this secular trend. Improved means of communication, the more widespread exchange of goods, the invention of printing, and the oceanic discoveries made man more aware not only of other peoples but also of differences in language, taste, cultural habits, and religion. In such circumstances, it was no wonder that many philosophers and other writers of the time held the nation-state to be the natural and best form of civic society, that its powers should be enhanced and its interests defended, and that its rulers and ruled needed—whatever the specific constitutional form they enjoyed—to work harmoniously for the common, national good.[89]

But it was war, and the consequences of war, that provided a much more urgent and continuous pressure toward "nation-building" than these philosophical considerations and slowly evolving social tendencies. Military power permitted many of Europe's dynasties to keep above the great magnates of their land, and to secure political uniformity and authority (albeit often by concessions to the nobility). Military factors—or better, geostrategical factors—helped to shape the territorial boundaries of these new nation-states, while the frequent wars induced national consciousness, in a negative fashion at least, in that Englishmen learned to hate Spaniards, Swedes to hate Danes, Dutch rebels to hate their former Habsburg overlords. Above all, it was war—

and especially the new techniques which favored the growth of infantry armies and expensive fortifications and fleets—which impelled belligerent states to spend more money than ever before, and to seek out a corresponding amount in revenues. All remarks about the general rise in government spending, or about new organizations for revenue-collecting, or about the changing relationship between kings and estates in early-modern Europe, remain *abstract* until the central importance of military conflict is recalled.[90] In the last few years of Elizabeth's England, or in Philip II's Spain, as much as three-quarters of all government expenditures was devoted to war or to debt repayments for previous wars. Military and naval endeavors may not always have been the *raison d'être* of the new nation-states, but it certainly was their most expensive and pressing activity.

Yet it would be wrong to assume that the functions of raising revenues, supporting armies, equipping fleets, sending instructions, and directing military campaigns in the sixteenth and seventeenth centuries were carried out in the manner which characterized, say, the Normandy invasion of 1944. As the preceding analysis should have demonstrated, the military machines of early-modern Europe were cumbersome and inefficient. Raising and controlling an army in this period was a frighteningly difficult enterprise: ragtag troops, potentially disloyal mercenaries, inadequate supplies, transport problems, unstandardized weapons, were the despair of most commanders. Even when sufficient monies were allocated to military purposes, corruption and waste took their toll.

Armed forces were not, therefore, predictable and reliable instruments of state. Time and again, large bands of men drifted out of control because of supply shortages or, more serious, lack of pay. The Army of Flanders mutinied no less than forty-six times between 1572 and 1607; but so also, if less frequently, did equally formidable forces, like the Swedes in Germany or Cromwell's New Model Army. It was Richelieu who sourly observed, in his *Testament Politique*:

> History knows many more armies ruined by want and disorder than by the efforts of their enemies; and I have witnessed how all the enterprises which were embarked on in my day were lacking for that reason alone.[91]

This problem of pay and supply affected military performance in all sorts of ways: one historian has demonstrated that Gustavus Adolphus's stunningly mobile campaigns in Germany, rather than being dictated by military-strategic planning in the Clausewitzian sense, reflected a simple but compelling search for food and fodder for his enormous force.[92] Well before Napoleon's aphorism, commanders knew that an army marched upon its stomach.

But these physical restrictions applied at the national level, too, especially in raising funds for war. No state in this period, however prosperous, could pay immediately for the costs of a prolonged conflict; no matter what fresh taxes were raised, there was always a gap between governmental income and expenditure which could only be closed by loans—either from private bankers like the Fuggers or, later, through a formally organized money market dealing in government bonds. Again and again, however, the spiraling costs of war forced monarchs to default upon debt repayments, to debase the coinage, or to attempt some other measure of despair, which brought short-term relief but long-term disadvantage. Like their commanders frantically seeking to keep troops in order and horses fed, early-modern governments were engaged in a precarious hand-to-mouth living. Badgering estates to grant further extraordinary taxes, pressing rich men and the churches for "benevolences," haggling with bankers and munitions suppliers, seizing foreign treasure ships, and keeping at arm's length one's many creditors were more or less permanent activities forced upon rulers and their officials in these years.

The argument in this chapter is *not*, therefore, that the Habsburgs failed utterly to do what other powers achieved so brilliantly. There are no stunning contrasts in evidence here; success and failure are to be measured by very narrow differences.[93] All states, even the United Provinces, were placed under severe strain by the constant drain of resources for military and naval campaigns. All states experienced financial difficulties, mutinies of troops, inadequacies of supply, domestic opposition to higher taxes. As in the First World War, these years also witnessed struggles of endurance, driving the belligerents closer and closer to exhaustion. By the final decade of the Thirty Years War, it was noticeable that neither alliance could field armies as large as those commanded by Gustavus and Wallenstein, for each side was, literally, running out of men and money. The victory of the anti-Habsburg forces was, then, a marginal and relative one. They had managed, but only just, to maintain the balance between their material base and their military power better than their Habsburg opponents. At least some of the victors had seen that the sources of national wealth needed to be exploited carefully, and not recklessly, during a lengthy conflict. They may also have admitted, however reluctantly, that the trader and the manufacturer and the farmer were as important as the cavalry officer and the pikeman. But the margin of their appreciation, and of their better handling of the economic elements, was slight. It had been, to borrow the later words of the Duke of Wellington, a "damned close-run thing." Most great contests are.

3
Finance, Geography, and the Winning of Wars, 1660–1815

The signing of the Treaty of the Pyrenees did not, of course, bring to an end the rivalries of the European Great Powers, or their habit of settling these rivalries through war. But the century and a half of international struggle which occurred after 1660 was different, in some very important respects, from that which had taken place in the preceding hundred years; and, as such, these changes reflected a further stage in the evolution of international politics.

The most significant feature of the Great Power scene after 1660 was the maturing of a genuinely *multipolar* system of European states, each one of which increasingly tended to make decisions about war and peace on the basis of "national interests" rather than for transnational, religious causes. This was not, to be sure, an instant or absolute change: the European states prior to 1660 had certainly maneuvered with their secular interests in mind, and religious prejudice still fueled many international quarrels of the eighteenth century. Nevertheless, the chief characteristic of the 1519–1659 era—that is, an Austro-Spanish axis of Habsburg powers fighting a coalition of Protestant states, plus France—now disappeared, and was replaced by a much looser system of short-term, shifting alliances. Countries which had been foes in one war were often to find themselves partners in the next, which placed an emphasis upon calculated *Realpolitik* rather than deeply held religious conviction in the determination of policy.

The fluctuations in both diplomacy and war that were natural to this volatile, multipolar system were complicated by something which was not new, but was common to all ages: the rise of certain states and the decline of others. During this century and a half of international rivalry between Louis XIV's assumption of full authority in France in 1660–1661 and Napoleon Bonaparte's surrender after Waterloo in 1815, certain leading nations of the previous period (the Ottoman Empire, Spain, the Netherlands, Sweden) fell back into the second rank, and Poland was eclipsed altogether. The Austrian Habsburgs, by various territorial and structural adjustments in their hereditary lands, managed to remain in the first order; and in the north of Germany, Brandenburg-Prussia pulled itself up to that status from unpromising beginnings. In the west, France after 1660 swiftly expanded its military might to become the most powerful of the European states—to many observers, almost as overwhelming as the Habsburg forces had appeared a half-century earlier. France's capacity to dominate west-central Europe was held in check only by a combination of maritime and continental neighbors during a series of prolonged wars (1689–1697; 1702–1714; 1739–1748; 1756–1763); but it was then refashioned in the Napoleonic era to produce a long line of Gallic military victories which were brought to an end only by a coalition of four other Great Powers. Even in its defeat in 1815, France remained one of the leading states. Between it in the west and the two Germanic countries of Prussia and the Habsburg Empire in the east, therefore, a crude trilateral equilibrium slowly emerged within the European core as the eighteenth century unfolded.

But the really significant alterations in the Great Power system during that century occurred on the *flanks* of Europe, and even farther afield. Certain of the western European states steadily converted their small, precarious enclaves in the tropics into much more extensive domains, especially in India but also in the East Indies, southern Africa, and as far away as Australia. The most successful of these colonizing nations was Britain, which, domestically "stabilized" after James II was replaced by William and Mary in 1688, steadily fulfilled its Elizabethan potential as the greatest of the European maritime empires. Even its loss of control over the prosperous North American colonies in the 1770s—from which there emerged an independent United States of formidable defensive strength and considerable economic power—only temporarily checked this growth of British global influence. Equally remarkable were the achievements of the Russian state, which expanded eastward and southward, across the steppes of Asia, throughout the eighteenth century. Moreover, although sited on the western and eastern margins of Europe, both Britain and Russia had an interest in the fate of the center—with Britain being involved in German affairs because of its dynastic links to Hanover (following George I's accession in 1714) and Russia being determined to have the chief voice in the fate of neighboring Poland. More generally, the governments in London and St. Petersburg wanted a balance of power on the European continent, and were willing to intervene repeatedly in order to secure an equilibrium which accorded with their interests. In other words, the European states system was becoming one of *five* Great Powers—France, the Habsburg Empire, Prussia, Britain, and Russia—as well as lesser countries like Savoy and declining states such as Spain.[1]

Why was it that those five Powers in particular—while obviously not possessing exactly the same strengths—were able to remain in (or to enter) the "major league" of states? Purely military explanations are not going to get us very far. It is hard to believe, for example, that the rise and fall of Great Powers in this period was caused chiefly by changes in military and naval technology, such as might benefit one country more than another.* There were, of course, many small-scale improvements in weaponry: the flintlock rifle (with ring bayonet) eliminated the pikeman from the battlefield; artillery became much more mobile, especially after the newer types designed by Gribeauval in France during the 1760s; and the stubby, shorter-ranged naval gun known as the carronade (first built by the Carron Company, of Scotland, in the late 1770s) enhanced the destructive power of warships. There were also improvements in tactical thought and, in the background, steady increases in population and in agricultural output which would permit the organization of far larger military units (the division; the corps) and their easier sustenance upon rich farmlands by the end of the eighteenth century. Nonetheless, it is fair to say that Wellington's army in 1815 was not significantly different from Marlborough's in 1710, nor Nelson's fleet much more advanced technologically than that which had faced Louis XIV's warships.[2]

Indeed, the most significant changes occurring in the military and naval fields during the eighteenth century were probably in *organization,* because of the enhanced activity of the state. The exemplar of this shift was undoubtedly the France of Louis XIV (1661–1715), where ministers such as Colbert, Le Tellier, and others were intent upon increasing the king's powers at home as well as his glories abroad. The creation of a French war ministry, with intendants checking upon the financing, supply, and organization of troops while Martinet as inspector general imposed new standards of training and discipline; the erection of barracks, hospitals, parade grounds, and depots of every sort on land, to sustain the Sun King's enormous army, together with the creation of a centrally organized, enormous fleet at sea—all this forced the other powers to follow suit, if they did not wish to be eclipsed. The monopolization and bureaucratization of military power by the state is clearly a central part of the story of "nation-building"; and the process was a reciprocal one, since the enhanced authority and resources of the state in turn gave to their armed forces a degree of *permanence* which had often not existed a century earlier. Not only were there "professional," "standing" armies and "royal" navies, but there was also a much more developed infrastructure of war academies, barracks, ship-repair yards, and the like, with administrators to run them.

---

*For example, in the way in which the coming of steam-driven warships after 1860 benefited Britain (which had plenty of coal) over France (which had little).

Power was now *national* power, whether expressed through the enlightened despotisms of eastern Europe, the parliamentary controls of Britain, or the later demogogic forces of revolutionary France.[3] On the other hand, such organizational improvements could be swiftly copied by other states (the most dramatic example being Peter the Great's transformation of Russia's army in the space of a couple of decades after 1698), and by themselves provided no guarantee of maintaining a country's Great Power position.

Much more important than any of these strictly military developments in explaining the relative position occupied by the Great Powers in the years 1660–1815 were two other factors, *finance* and *geography*. Taken together—for the two elements frequently interacted—it is possible to gain some larger sense of what at first sight appears as a bewildering pattern of successes and failures produced by the many wars of this period.

The "Financial Revolution"

The importance of finance and of a productive economic base which created revenues for the state was already clear to Renaissance princes, as the previous chapter has illustrated. The rise of the *ancien régime* monarchies of the eighteenth century, with their large military establishments and fleets of warships, simply increased the government's need to nurture the economy and to create financial institutions which could raise and manage the monies concerned.[4] Moreover, like the First World War, conflicts such as the seven major Anglo-French wars fought between 1689 and 1815 were struggles of endurance. Victory therefore went to the Power—or better, since both Britain and France usually had allies, to the Great Power coalition—with the greater capacity to maintain credit and to keep on raising supplies. The mere fact that these were *coalition* wars increased their duration, since a belligerent whose resources were fading would look to a more powerful ally for loans and reinforcements in order to keep itself in the fight. Given such expensive and exhausting conflicts, what each side desperately required was—to use the old aphorism—"money, money, and yet more money." It was this need which formed the background to what has been termed the "financial revolution" of the late seventeenth and early eighteenth centuries,[5] when certain western European states evolved a relatively sophisticated system of banking and credit in order to pay for their wars.

There was, it is true, a second and nonmilitary reason for the financial changes of this time. That was the chronic shortage of specie, particularly in the years before the gold discoveries in Portuguese Brazil in 1693. The more European commerce with the Orient devel-

oped in the seventeenth and eighteenth centuries, the greater the outflow of silver to cover the trade imbalances, causing merchants and
dealers everywhere complain of the scarcity of coin. In addition, the
steady increases in European commerce, especially in essential products such as cloth and naval stores, together with the tendency for the
seasonal fairs of medieval Europe to be replaced by permanent centers
of exchange, led to a growing regularity and predictability of financial
settlements and thus to the greater use of bills of exchange and notes
of credit. In Amsterdam especially, but also in London, Lyons, Frankfurt, and other cities, there arose a whole cluster of moneylenders,
commodity dealers, goldsmiths (who often dealt in loans), bill merchants, and jobbers in the shares of the growing number of joint-stock
companies. Adopting banking practices which were already in evidence in Renaissance Italy, these individuals and financial houses
steadily created a structure of national and international credit to
underpin the early modern world economy.

Nevertheless, by far the largest and most sustained boost to the
"financial revolution" in Europe was given by war. If the difference
between the financial burdens of the age of the Philip II and that of
Napoleon was one of degree, it still was remarkable enough. The cost
of a sixteenth-century war could be measured in millions of pounds;
by the late-seventeenth century, it had risen to *tens* of millions of
pounds; and at the close of the Napoleonic War the outgoings of the
major combatants occasionally reached a hundred million pounds *a
year*. Whether these prolonged and frequent clashes between the Great
Powers, when translated into economic terms, were more of a benefit
to than a brake upon the commercial and industrial rise of the West
can never be satisfactorily resolved. The answer depends, to a great
extent, upon whether one is trying to assess the *absolute* growth of a
country as opposed to its *relative* prosperity and strength before and
after a lengthy conflict.[6] What is clear is that even the most thriving and
"modern" of the eighteenth-century states could not immediately pay
for the wars of this period out of their ordinary revenue. Moreover,
vast rises in taxes, even if the machinery existed to collect them, could
well provoke domestic unrest, which all regimes feared—especially
when facing foreign challengers at the same time.

Consequently, the only way a government could finance a war adequately was by borrowing: by selling bonds and offices, or better, nego-
tiable long-term stock paying interest to all who advanced monies to
the state. Assured of an inflow of funds, officials could then authorize
payments to army contractors, provision merchants, shipbuilders, and
the armed services themselves. In many respects, this two-way system
of raising and *simultaneously* spending vast sums of money acted like
a bellows, fanning the development of western capitalism and of the
nation-state itself.

Yet however natural all this may appear to later eyes, it is important to stress that the success of such a system depended on two critical factors: reasonably efficient machinery for raising loans, and the maintenance of a government's "credit" in the financial markets. In both respects, the United Provinces led the way—not surprisingly, since the merchants there were part of the government and desired to see the affairs of state managed according to the same principles of financial rectitude as applied in, say, a joint-stock company. It was therefore appropriate that the States General of the Netherlands, which efficiently and regularly raised the taxes to cover governmental expenditures, was able to set interest rates very low, thus keeping down debt repayments. This system, superbly reinforced by the many financial activities of the city of Amsterdam, soon gave the United Provinces an international reputation for clearing bills, exchanging currency, and providing credit, which naturally created a structure—and an atmosphere—within which long-term funded state debt could be regarded as perfectly normal. So successfully did Amsterdam become a center of Dutch "surplus capital" that it soon was able to invest in the stock of foreign companies and, most important of all, to subscribe to a whole variety of loans floated by foreign governments, especially in wartime.[7]

The impact of these activities upon the economy of the United Provinces need not be examined here, although it is clear that Amsterdam would not have become the financial capital of the continent had it not been supported by a flourishing commercial and productive base in the first place. Furthermore, the very long-term consequence was probably disadvantageous, since the steady returns from government loans turned the United Provinces more and more away from a manufacturing economy and into a *rentier* economy, whose bankers were somewhat disinclined to risk capital in large-scale industrial ventures by the late eighteenth century; while the ease with which loans could be raised eventually saddled the Dutch government with an enormous burden of debt, paid for by excise duties which increased both wages and prices to uncompetitive levels.[8]

What is more important for the purposes of our argument is that in subscribing to *foreign* government loans, the Dutch were much less concerned about the religion or ideology of their clients than about their financial stability and reliability. Accordingly, the terms set for loans to European powers like Russia, Spain, Austria, Poland, and Sweden can be seen as a measure of their respective economic potential, the collateral they offered to the bankers, their record in repaying interest and premiums, and ultimately their prospects of emerging successfully from a Great Power war. Thus, the plummeting of Polish governmental stock in the late eighteenth century and, conversely, the remarkable—and frequently overlooked—strength of Austria's credit for decade after decade mirrored the relative durability of those states.[9]

But the best example of this critical relationship between financial strength and power politics concerns the two greatest rivals of this period, Britain and France. Since the result of their conflict affected the entire European balance, it is worth examining their experiences at some length. The older notion that eighteenth-century Great Britain exhibited adamantine and inexorably growing commercial and industrial strength, unshakable fiscal credit, and a flexible, upwardly mobile social structure—as compared with an *ancien régime* France founded upon the precarious sands of military hubris, economic backwardness, and a rigid class system—seems no longer tenable. In some ways, the French taxation system was less regressive than the British. In some ways, too, France's economy in the eighteenth century was showing signs of movement toward "takeoff" into an industrial revolution, even though it had only limited stocks of such a critical item as coal. Its armaments production was considerable, and it possessed many skilled artisans and some impressive entrepreneurs.[10] With its far larger population and more extensive agriculture, France was much wealthier than its island neighbor; the revenues of its government and the size of its army dwarfed those of any western European rival; and its *dirigiste* regime, as compared with the party-based politics of Westminster, seemed to give it a greater coherence and predictability. In consequence, eighteenth-century Britons were much more aware of their own country's relative weaknesses than its strengths when they gazed across the Channel.

For all this, the English system possessed key advantages in the financial realm which enhanced the country's power in wartime and buttressed its political stability and economic growth in peacetime. While it is true that its *general* taxation system was more regressive than that of France—that is, it relied far more upon indirect than direct taxes—particular features seem to have made it much less resented by the public. For example, there was in Britain nothing like the vast array of French tax farmers, collectors, and other middlemen; many of the British duties were "invisible" (the excise duty on a few basic products), or appeared to hurt the foreigner (customs); there were no *internal* tolls, which so irritated French merchants and were a disincentive to domestic commerce; the British land tax—the chief direct tax for so much of the eighteenth century—allowed for no privileged exceptions and was also "invisible" to the greater part of society; and these various taxes were discussed and then authorized by an elective assembly, which for all its defects appeared more representative than the *ancien régime* in France. When one adds to this the important point that per capita income was already somewhat higher in Britain than in France even by 1700, it is not altogether surprising that the population of the island state was willing and able to pay proportionately larger taxes. Finally, it is possible to argue—although more difficult to prove statistically—that the comparatively light burden of direct taxation in Britain not only increased the propensity to save among the better-off in society (and thus allowed the accumulation of investment capital during years of peace), but also produced a vast reserve of taxable wealth in *wartime*, when higher land taxes and, in 1799, direct income tax were introduced to meet the national emergency. Thus, by the period of the Napoleonic War, despite a population less than half that of France, Britain was for the first time ever raising more revenue from taxes each year in *absolute* terms than its larger neighbor.[11]

Yet however remarkable that achievement, it is eclipsed in importance by the even more significant difference between the British and French systems of public credit. For the fact was that during most of the eighteenth-century conflicts, almost three-quarters of the *extra* finance raised to support the additional wartime expenditures came from loans. Here, more than anywhere else, the British advantages were decisive. The first was the evolution of an institutional framework which permitted the raising of long-term loans in an efficient fashion and simultaneously arranged for the regular repayment of the interest on (and principal of) the debts accrued. The creation of the Bank of England in 1694 (at first as a wartime expedient) and the slightly later regularization of the national debt on the one hand and the flourishing of the stock exchange and growth of the "country banks" on the other boosted the supply of money available to both governments and businessmen. This growth of paper money in various forms *without* severe inflation or the loss of credit brought many advantages in an age starved of coin. Yet the "financial revolution" itself would scarcely have succeeded had not the obligations of the state been guaranteed by successive Parliaments with their powers to raise additional taxes; had not the ministries—from Walpole to the younger Pitt—worked hard to convince their bankers in particular and the public in general that they, too, were actuated by the principles of financial rectitude and "economical" government; and had not the steady and in some trades remarkable expansion of commerce and industry provided concomitant increases in revenue from customs and excise. Even the onset of war did not check such increases, provided the Royal Navy protected the nation's overseas trade while throttling that of its foes. It was upon these solid foundations that Britain's "credit" rested, despite early uncertainties, considerable political opposition, and a financial near-disaster like the collapse of the famous South Seas Bubble of 1720. "Despite all defects in the handling of English public finance," its historian has noted, "for the rest of the century it remained more honest, as well as more efficient, than that of any other in Europe."[12]

The result of all this was not only that interest rates steadily dropped,* but also that British government stock was increasingly attractive to foreign, and particularly Dutch, investors. Regular dealings in these securities on the Amsterdam market thus became an important part of the nexus of Anglo-Dutch commercial and financial relationships, with important effects upon the economies of both countries.[13] In *power-political* terms, its value lay in the way in which the resources of the United Provinces repeatedly came to the aid of the British war effort, even when the Dutch alliance in the struggle against France had been replaced by an uneasy neutrality. Only at the time of the American Revolutionary War—significantly, the one conflict in which British military, naval, diplomatic, and trading weaknesses were most evident, and therefore its credit-worthiness was the lowest—did the flow of Dutch funds tend to dry up, despite the higher interest rates which London was prepared to offer. By 1780, however, when the Dutch entered the war on France's side, the British government found that the strength of its own economy and the availability of domestic capital were such that its loans could be almost completely taken up by domestic investors.

The sheer dimensions—and ultimate success—of Britain's capacity to raise war loans can be summarized as in Table 2.

Table 2. British Wartime Expenditure and Revenue, 1688–1815
(pounds)

Inclusive Years	Total Expenditure	Total Income	Balance Raised by Loans	Loans as % of Expenditure
1688–97	49,320,145	32,766,754	16,553,391	33.6
1702–13	93,644,560	64,239,477	29,405,083	31.4
1739–48	95,628,159	65,903,964	29,724,195	31.1
1756–63	160,573,366	100,555,123	60,018,243	37.4
1776–83	236,462,689	141,902,620	94,560,069	39.9
1793–1815	1,657,854,518	1,217,556,439	440,298,079	26.6
Totals	2,293,483,437	1,622,924,377	670,559,060	33.3

And the strategical consequence of these figures was that the country was thereby enabled "to spend on war out of all proportion to its tax revenue, and thus to throw into the struggle with France and its allies the decisive margin of ships and men without which the resources previously committed might have been committed in vain."[14] Although many British commentators throughout the eighteenth century trembled at the sheer size of the national debt and its possible consequences, the fact remained that (in Bishop Berkeley's words) credit

*By the time of the War of Austrian Succession (1739–1747), the government was able to borrow large sums at 3 or 4 percent, half the rate of interest which had prevailed in Marlborough's time.

was "the principal advantage that England hath over France." Finally, the great growth in state expenditures and the enormous, sustained demand which Admiralty contracts in particular created for iron, wood, cloth, and other wares produced a "feedback loop" which assisted British industrial production and stimulated the series of technological breakthroughs that gave the country yet another advantage over the French.[15]

Why the French failed to match these British habits is now easy to see.[16] There was, to begin with, no proper system of *public* finance. From the Middle Ages onward, the French monarchy's financial operations had been "managed" by a cluster of bodies—municipal governments, the clergy, provincial estates, and, increasingly, tax farmers—which collected the revenues and supervised the monopolies of the crown in return for a portion of the proceeds, and which simultaneously advanced monies to the French government—at handsome rates of interest—on the expected income from these operations. The venality of this system applied not only to the farmers general who gathered in the tobacco and salt dues; it was also true of that hierarchy of parish collectors, district receivers, and regional receivers general responsible for direct taxes like the *taille.* Each of them took his "cut" before passing the monies on to a higher level; each of them also received 5 percent interest on the price he had paid for office in the first place; and many of the more senior officials were charged with paying out sums directly to government contractors or as wages, without first handing their takings in to the royal treasury. These men, too, loaned funds—at interest—to the crown.

Such a lax and haphazard organization was inherently corrupt, and much of the taxpayers' monies ended in private hands. On occasions, especially after wars, investigations would be launched against financiers, many of whom were induced to pay "compensations" or accept lower interest rates; but such actions were mere gestures. "The real culprit," one historian has argued, "was the system itself."[17] The second consequence of this inefficiency was that at least until Necker's reforms of the 1770s, there existed no overall sense of national accounting; annual tallies of revenue and expenditure, and the problem of deficits, were rarely thought to be of significance. Provided the monarchy could raise funds for the immediate needs of the military and the court, the steady escalation of the national debt was of little import.

While a similar sort of irresponsibility had earlier been shown by the Stuarts, the fact was that by the eighteenth century Britain had evolved a parliamentary-controlled form of public finance which gave it numerous advantages in the duel for primacy. Not the least of these seems to have been that while the rise in government spending and in the national debt did not hurt (and may indeed have boosted) British investment in commerce and industry, the prevailing conditions in

France seem to have encouraged those with surplus capital to purchase
an office or an annuity rather than to invest in business. On some
occasions, it was true, there were attempts to provide France with a
national bank, so that the debt could be properly managed and cheap
credit provided; but such schemes were always resisted by those with
an interest in the existing system. The French government's financial
policy, if indeed it deserves that name, was therefore always a hand-to-
mouth affair.

France's commercial development also suffered in a number of
ways. It is interesting to note, for example, the disadvantages under
which a French port like La Rochelle operated compared with Liverpool or Glasgow. All three were poised to exploit the booming "Atlantic
economy" of the eighteenth century, and La Rochelle was particularly
well sited for the triangular trade to West Africa and the West Indies.
Alas for such mercantile aspirations, the French port suffered from the
repeated depredations of the crown, "insatiable in its fiscal demands,
unrelenting in its search for new and larger sources of revenue." A vast
array of "heavy, inequitable and arbitrarily levied direct and indirect
taxes on commerce" retarded economic growth; the sale of offices
diverted local capital from investment in trade, and the fees levied by
those venal officeholders intensified that trend; monopolistic companies restricted free enterprise. Moreover, although the crown compelled the Rochelais to build a large and expensive arsenal in the 1760s
(or have the city's entire revenues seized!), it did not offer a *quid pro
quo* when wars occurred. Because the French government usually
concentrated upon military rather than maritime aims, the frequent
conflicts with a superior Royal Navy were a disaster for La Rochelle,
which saw its merchant ships seized, its profitable slave trade interrupted, and its overseas markets in Canada and Louisiana eliminated—all at a time when marine insurance rates were rocketing and
emergency taxes were being imposed. As a final blow, the French
government often felt compelled to allow its overseas colonists to trade
with neutral shipping in wartime, but this made those markets ever
more difficult to recover when peace was concluded. By comparison,
the Atlantic sector of the British economy grew steadily throughout the
eighteenth century, and if anything benefited in wartime (despite the
attacks of French privateers) from the policies of a government which
held that profit and power, trade and dominion, were inseparable.[18]

The worst consequence of France's financial immaturity was that
in time of war its military and naval effort was eroded, in a number
of ways.[19] Because of the inefficiency and unreliability of the system,
it took longer to secure the supply of (say) naval stores, while contractors usually needed to charge more than would be the case with the
British or Dutch admiralties. Raising large sums in wartime was always more of a problem for the French monarchy, even when it drew

increasingly upon Dutch money in the 1770s and 1780s, for its long history of currency revaluations, its partial repudiations of debt, and its other arbitrary actions against the holders of short-term and long-term bills caused bankers to demand—and a desperate French state to agree to—rates of interest far above those charged to the British and many other European governments.* Yet even this willingness to pay over the odds did not permit the Bourbon monarchs to secure the sums which were necessary to sustain an all-out military effort in a lengthy war.

The best illustration of this relative French weakness occurred in the years following the American Revolutionary War. It had hardly been a glorious conflict for the British, who had lost their largest colony and seen their national debt rise to about £220 million; but since those sums had chiefly been borrowed at a mere 3 percent interest, the annual repayments totaled only £7.33 million. The actual costs of the war to France were considerably smaller; after all, it had entered the conflict at the halfway stage, following Necker's efforts to balance the budget, and for once it had not needed to deploy a massive army. Nonetheless, the war cost the French government at least a billion livres, virtually all of which was paid by floating loans at rates of interest at least double that available to the British government. In both countries, servicing the debt consumed half the state's annual expenditures, but after 1783 the British immediately embarked upon a series of measures (the Sinking Fund, a consolidated revenue fund, improved public accounts) in order to stabilize that total and strengthen its credit—the greatest, perhaps, of the younger Pitt's achievements. On the French side, by contrast, large new loans were floated each year, since "normal" revenues could never match even peacetime expenditures; and with yearly deficits growing, the government's credit weakened still further.

The startling statistical consequence was that by the late 1780s France's national debt may have been almost the same as Britain's—around £215 million—but the interest payments each year were nearly double, at £14 million. Still worse, the efforts of succeeding finance ministers to raise fresh taxes met with stiffening public resistance. It was, after all, Calonne's proposed tax reforms, leading to the Assembly of Notables, the moves against the *parlements,* the suspension of payments by the treasury, and then (for the first since 1614) the calling of the States General in 1789 which triggered off the final collapse of the *ancien régime* in France.[20] The link between national bankruptcy and revolution was all too clear. In the desperate circumstances which followed, the government issued ever more notes (to the value of 100

---

*In the early years of Louis XIV, by contrast, France had been able to borrow at cheaper rates of interest than the Stuarts, or even William III.

million livres in 1789, and 200 million in 1790), a device replaced by the Constituent Assembly's own expedient of seizing church lands and issuing paper money on their estimated worth. All this led to further inflation, which the 1792 decision for war only exacerbated. And while it is true that later administrative reforms within the treasury itself and the revolutionary regime's determination to know the true state of affairs steadily produced a unified, bureaucratic, revenue-collecting structure akin to those existing in Britain and elsewhere, the internal convulsions and external overextension that were to last until 1815 caused the French economy to fall even further behind that of its greatest rival.

This problem of raising revenue to pay for current—and previous—wars preoccupied *all* regimes and their statesmen. Even in peacetime, the upkeep of the armed services consumed 40 or 50 percent of a country's expenditures; in wartime, it could rise to 80 or even 90 percent of the far larger whole! Whatever their internal constitutions, therefore, autocratic empires, limited monarchies, and bourgeois republics throughout Europe faced the same difficulty. After each bout of fighting (and especially after 1714 and 1763), most countries desperately needed to draw breath, to recover from their economic exhaustion, and to grapple with the internal discontents which war and higher taxation had all too often provoked; but the competitive, egoistic nature of the European states system meant that *prolonged* peace was unusual and that within another few years preparations were being made for further campaigning. Yet if the financial burdens could hardly be carried by the French, Dutch, and British, the three richest peoples of Europe, how could they be borne by far poorer states?

The simple answer to this question was that they couldn't. Even Frederick the Great's Prussia, which drew much of its revenues from the extensive, well-husbanded royal domains and monopolies, could not meet the vast demands of the war of the Austrian Succession and Seven Years War without recourse to three "extraordinary" sources of income: profits from debasement of the coinage; plunder from neighboring states such as Saxony and Mecklenburg; and, after 1757, considerable subsidies from its richer ally, Britain. For the less efficient and more decentralized Habsburg Empire, the problems of paying for war were immense; but it is difficult to believe that the situation was any better in Russia or in Spain, where the prospects for raising monies—other than by further squeezes upon the peasantry and the underdeveloped middle classes—were not promising. With so many orders (e.g., Hungarian nobility, Spanish clergy) claiming exemptions under the *anciennes régimes,* even the invention of elaborate indirect taxes, debasements of the currency, and the printing of paper money were hardly sufficient to maintain the elaborate armies and courts in peacetime; and while the onset of war led to extraordinary fiscal measures for the national emergency, it also meant that increasing reliance had to be placed upon the western European money markets or, better still, direct subsidies from London, Amsterdam, or Paris which could then be used to buy mercenaries and supplies. *Pas d'argent, pas de Suisses* may have been a slogan for Renaissance princes, but it was still an unavoidable fact of life even in Frederician and Napoleonic times.[21]

This is not to say, however, that the financial element *always* determined the fate of nations in these eighteenth-century wars. Amsterdam was for much of this period the greatest financial center of the world, yet that alone could not prevent the United Provinces' demise as a leading Power; conversely, Russia was economically backward and its government relatively starved of capital, yet the country's influence and might in European affairs grew steadily. To explain that seeming discrepancy, it is necessary to give equal attention to the second important conditioning factor, the influence of geography upon national strategy.

Geopolitics

Because of the inherently competitive nature of European power politics and the volatility of alliance relationships throughout the eighteenth century, rival states often encountered remarkably different circumstances—and sometimes extreme variations of fortune—from one major conflict to the next. Secret treaties and "diplomatic revolutions" produced changing conglomerations of powers, and in consequence fairly frequent shifts in the European equilibrium, both military and naval. While this naturally caused great reliance to be placed upon the expertise of a nation's diplomats, not to mention the efficiency of its armed forces, it also pointed to the significance of the geographical factor. What is meant by that term here is not merely such elements as a country's climate, raw materials, fertility of agriculture, and access to trade routes—important though they all were to its overall prosperity—but rather the critical issue of strategical *location* during these multilateral wars. Was a particular nation able to concentrate its energies upon one front, or did it have to fight on several? Did it share common borders with weak states, or powerful ones? Was it chiefly a land power, a sea power, or a hybrid—and what advantages and disadvantages did that bring? Could it easily pull out of a great war in Central Europe if it wished to? Could it secure additional resources from overseas?

The fate of the United Provinces in this period provides a good example of the influences of geography upon politics. In the early seventeenth century it possessed many of the domestic ingredients for national growth—a flourishing economy, social stability, a well-trained army, and a powerful navy; and it had not then seemed disadvantaged by geography. On the contrary, its river network provided a barrier (at least to some extent) against Spanish forces, and its North Sea position gave it easy access to the rich herring fisheries. But a century later, the Dutch were struggling to hold their own against a number of rivals. The adoption of mercantilist policies by Cromwell's England and Colbert's France hurt Dutch commerce and shipping. For all the tactical brilliance of commanders like Tromp and de Ruyter, Dutch merchantmen in the naval wars against England had either to run the gauntlet of the Channel route or to take the longer and stormier route around Scotland, which (like their herring fisheries) was still open to attack in the North Sea; the prevailing westerly winds gave the battle advantage to the English admirals; and the shallow waters off Holland restricted the draft—and ultimately the size and power—of the Dutch warships.[22] In the same way as its trade with the Americas and Indies became increasingly exposed to the workings of British sea power, so, too, was its Baltic *entrepôt* commerce—one of the very foundations of its early prosperity—eroded by the Swedes and other local rivals. Although the Dutch might temporarily reassert themselves by the dispatch of a large battle fleet to a threatened point, there was no way in which they could permanently preserve their extended and vulnerable interests in distant seas.

This dilemma was made worse by Dutch vulnerability to the landward threat from Louis XIV's France from the late 1660s onwards. Since this danger was even greater than that posed by Spain a century earlier, the Dutch were forced to expand their own army (it was 93,000 strong by 1693) and to devote ever more resources to garrisoning the southern border fortresses. This drain upon Dutch energies was twofold: it diverted vast amounts of money into military expenditures, producing the upward spiral in war debts, interest repayments, increased excise duties, and high wages that undercut the nation's commercial competitiveness in the long term; and it caused a severe loss of life during wartime to a population which, at about two million, was curiously static throughout this entire period. Hence the justifiable alarm, during the fierce toe-to-toe battles of the War of Spanish Succession (1702–1713), at the heavy losses caused by Marlborough's willingness to launch the Anglo-Dutch armies into bloody frontal assaults against the French.[23]

The English alliance which William III had cemented in 1689 was simultaneously the saving of the United Provinces and a substantial contributory factor in its decline as an independent great power—in rather the same way in which, over two hundred years later, Lend-Lease and the United States alliance would both rescue and help undermine a British Empire which was fighting for survival under

Marlborough's distant relative Winston Churchill. The inadequacy of Dutch resources in the various wars against France between 1688 and 1748 meant that they needed to concentrate about three-quarters of defense expenditures upon the military, thus neglecting their fleet—whereas the British assumed an increasing share of the maritime and colonial campaigns, and of the commercial benefits therefrom. As London and Bristol merchants flourished, so, to put it crudely, Amsterdam traders suffered. This was exacerbated by the frequent British efforts to prevent *all* trade with France in wartime, in contrast to the Dutch wish to maintain such profitable links—a reflection of how much more involved with (and therefore dependent upon) *external* commerce and finance the United Provinces were throughout this period, whereas the British economy was still relatively self-sufficient. Even when, by the Seven Years War, the United Provinces had escaped into neutrality, it availed them little, for an overweening Royal Navy, refusing to accept the doctrine of "free ships, free goods," was determined to block France's overseas commerce from being carried in neutral bottoms.[24] The Anglo-Dutch diplomatic quarrel of 1758–1759 over this question was repeated during the early years of the American Revolutionary War and eventually led to open hostilities after 1780, which did nothing to help the seaborne commerce of either Britain or the United Provinces. By the time of the French Revolutionary and Napoleonic struggles, the Dutch found themselves ground ever more between Britain and France, suffering from widespread debt repudiations, affected by domestic fissures, and losing colonies and overseas trade in a global contest which they could neither avoid nor take advantage of. In such circumstances, financial expertise and reliance upon "surplus capital" was simply not enough.[25]

In much the same way, albeit on a grander scale, France also suffered from being a hybrid power during the eighteenth century, with its energies diverted between continental aims on the one hand and maritime and colonial ambitions on the other. In the early part of Louis XIV's reign, this strategical ambivalence was not so marked. France's strength rested firmly upon *indigenous* materials: its large and relatively homogeneous territory, its agricultural self-sufficiency, and its population of about twenty million, which permitted Louis XIV to increase his army from 30,000 in 1659 to 97,000 in 1666 to a colossal 350,000 by 1710.[26] The Sun King's foreign-policy aims, too, were land-based and traditional: to erode still further the Habsburg positions, by moves in the south against Spain and in the east and north against that vulnerable string of Spanish-Habsburg and German territories Franche Comté, Lorraine, Alsace, Luxembourg, and the southern Netherlands. With Spain exhausted, the Austrians distracted by the Turkish threat, and the English at first neutral or friendly, Louis enjoyed two decades of diplomatic success; but then the very hubris of French claims alarmed the other powers.

The chief strategical problem for France was that although massively strong in defensive terms, she was less well placed to carry out a decisive campaign of conquest: in each direction she was hemmed in, partly by geographical barriers, partly by the existing claims and interests of a number of great powers. An attack on the southern (that is, Habsburg-held) Netherlands, for example, involved grinding campaigns through territory riddled with fortresses and waterways, and provoked a response not merely from the Habsburg powers themselves but also from the United Provinces and England. French military efforts into Germany were also troublesome: the border was more easily breached, but the lines of communication were much longer, and once again there was an inevitable coalition to face—the Austrians, the Dutch, the British (especially after the 1714 Hanoverian succession), and then the Prussians. Even when, by the mid-eighteenth century, France was willing to seek out a strong German partner—that is, either Austria or Prussia—the natural consequence of any such alliance was that the *other* German power went into opposition and, more important, strove to obtain support from Britain and Russia to neutralize French ambitions.

Furthermore, every war against the maritime powers involved a certain division of French energies and attention from the continent, and thus made a successful land campaign less likely. Torn between fighting in Flanders, Germany, and northern Italy on the one hand and in the Channel, West Indies, Lower Canada, and the Indian Ocean on the other, French strategy led repeatedly to a "falling between stools." While never willing to make the all-out financial effort necessary to challenge the Royal Navy's supremacy,* successive French governments allocated funds to the marine which—had France been *solely* a land power—might have been used to reinforce the army. Only in the war of 1778–1783, by supporting the American rebels in the western hemisphere but abstaining from any moves into Germany, did France manage to humiliate its British foe. In all its other wars, the French never enjoyed the luxury of strategical concentration—and suffered as a result.

In sum, the France of the *ancien régime* remained, by its size and population and wealth, always the greatest of the European states; but it was not big enough or efficiently organized enough to be a "superpower," and, restricted on land and diverted by sea, it could not prevail

---

*During the 1689–1697 and 1702–1714 conflicts, for example, France allocated less than 10 percent of total expenditure to its navy, and between 57 percent and 65 percent to its army. (The corresponding British figures were 35 percent to the navy and 40 percent to the army. In 1760 the French navy received only one-quarter of the sums allocated to the army. Even when monies were forthcoming, France's geographical position meant that it was often extremely difficult to get naval stores from the Baltic in wartime, to keep the fleet in good order.

against the coalition which its ambitions inevitably aroused. French actions confirmed, rather than upset, the plurality of power in Europe. Only when its national energies were transformed by the Revolution, and then brilliantly deployed by Napoleon, could it impose its ideas upon the continent—for a while. But even there its success was temporary, and no amount of military genius could ensure permanent French control of Germany, Italy, and Spain, let alone of Russia and Britain.

France's geostrategical problem of having to face potential foes on a variety of fronts was not unique, even if that country had made matters worse for itself by a repeated aggressiveness and a chronic lack of direction. The two great German powers of this period—the Habsburg Empire and Brandenburg-Prussia—were also destined by their geographical position to grapple with the same problem. To the Austrian Habsburgs, this was nothing new. The awkwardly shaped conglomeration of territories they ruled (Austria, Bohemia, Silesia, Moravia, Hungary, Milan, Naples, Sicily, and, after 1714, the southern Netherlands—see Map 5) and the position of other powers in relation to those lands required a nightmarish diplomatic and military juggling act merely to retain the inheritance; increasing it demanded either genius or good luck, and probably both.

Thus, while the various wars against the Turks (1663–1664, 1683–1699, 1716–1718, 1737–1739, 1788–1791) showed the Habsburg armies generally enhancing their position in the Balkans, this struggle against a declining Ottoman Empire consumed most of Vienna's energies in those selected periods.[27] With the Turks at the gates of his imperial capital in 1683, for example, Leopold I was bound to stay neutral toward France despite the provocations of Louis XIV's "reunions" of Alsace and Luxembourg in that very year. This Austrian ambivalence was somewhat less marked during the Nine Years War (1689–1697) and the subsequent War of the Spanish Succession (1702–1713), since Vienna had by that time become part of a gigantic anti-French alliance; but it never completely disappeared even then. The course of many later eighteenth-century wars seemed still more volatile and unpredictable, both for the defense of general Habsburg interests in Europe and for the specific preservation of those interests within Germany itself following the rise of Prussia. From at least the Prussian seizure of the province of Silesia in 1740 onward, Vienna always had to conduct its foreign and military policies with one eye firmly on Berlin. This in turn made Habsburg diplomacy more elaborate than ever: to check a rising Prussia within Germany, the Austrians needed to call upon the assistance of France in the west and, more frequently, Russia in the east; but France itself was unreliable and needed in turn to be checked by an Anglo-Austrian alliance at times (e.g., 1744–1748). Furthermore,

Russia's own steady growth was a further cause of concern, particularly when czarist expansionism threatened the Ottoman hold upon Balkan lands desired by Vienna. Finally, when Napoleonic imperialism challenged the independence of *all* other powers in Europe, the Habsburg Empire had no choice but to join any available grand coalition to contest French hegemony.

The coalition war against Louis XIV at the beginning of the eighteenth century and those against Bonaparte at its end probably give us less of an insight into Austrian weakness than do the conflicts in between. The lengthy struggle against Prussia after 1740 was particularly revealing: it demonstrated that for all the military, fiscal, and administrative reforms undertaken in the Habsburg lands in this period, Vienna could not prevail against another, smaller German state which was considerably more efficient in its army, revenue collection, and bureaucracy. Furthermore, it became increasingly clear that the non-German powers, France, Britain, and Russia, desired neither the Austrian elimination of Prussia nor the Prussian elimination of Austria. In the larger European context, the Habsburg Empire had already become a *marginal* first-class power, and was to remain such until 1918. It certainly did not slip as far down the list as Spain and Sweden, and it avoided the fate which befell Poland; but, because of its decentralized, ethnically diverse, and economically backward condition, it defied attempts by succeeding administrations in Vienna to turn it into the greatest of the European states. Nevertheless, there is a danger in anticipating this decline. As Olwen Hufton observes, "the Austrian Empire's persistent, to some eyes perverse, refusal conveniently to disintegrate" is a reminder that it possessed hidden strengths. Disasters were often followed by bouts of reform—the *rétablissements*—which revealed the empire's very considerable resources even if they also demonstrated the great difficulty Vienna always had in getting its hands upon them. And every historian of Habsburg decline has somehow to explain its remarkably stubborn and, occasionally, very impressive military resistance to the dynamic force of French imperialism for almost fourteen years of the period 1792–1815.[28]

Prussia's situation was very similar to Austria's in geostrategical terms, although quite different internally. The reasons for that country's swift rise to become the most powerful northern German kingdom are well known, and need only be listed here: the organizing and military genius of three leaders, the Great Elector (1640–1688), Frederick William I (1713–1740), and Frederick "the Great" (1740–1786), the efficiency of the Junker-officered Prussian army, into which as much as four-fifths of the state's taxable resources were poured; the (relative) fiscal stability, based upon extensive royal domains and encouragement of trade and industry; the willing use of foreign soldiers and entrepreneurs; and the famous Prussian bureaucrats operating under the General War Commissariat.[29] Yet it was also true that Prussia's rise coincided with the collapse of Swedish power, with the disintegration of the chaotic, weakened Polish kingdom, and with the distractions which the many wars and uncertain succession of the Habsburg Empire imposed upon Vienna in the early decades of the eighteenth century. If Prussian monarchs seized their opportunities, therefore, the fact was that the opportunities were there to be seized. Moreover, in filling the "power vacuum" which had opened up in north-central Europe after 1770, the Prussian state also benefited from its position vis-à-vis the other Great Powers. Russia's own rise was helping to distract (and erode) Sweden, Poland, and the Ottoman Empire. And France was far enough away in the west to be not usually a mortal danger; indeed, it could sometimes function as a useful ally against Austria. If, on the other hand, France pushed aggressively into Germany, it was likely to be opposed by Habsburg forces, Hanover (and therefore Britain), and perhaps the Dutch, as well as by Prussia itself. Finally, if that coalition failed, Prussia could more easily sue for peace with Paris than could the other powers; an anti-French alliance was sometimes useful, but not imperative, for Berlin.

Within this advantageous diplomatic and geographical context, the early kings of Prussia played the game well. The acquisition of Silesia—described by some as *the* industrial zone in the east—was in particular a great boost to the state's military-economic capacity. But the limitations of Prussia's real power in European affairs, limitations of size and population, were cruelly exposed in the Seven Years War of 1756–1763, when the diplomatic circumstances were no longer so favorable and Frederick the Great's powerful neighbors were determined to punish him for his deviousness. Only the stupendous efforts of the Prussian monarch and his well-trained troops—assisted by the lack of coordination among his foes—enabled Frederick to avoid defeat in the face of such a frightening "encirclement." Yet the costs of that war in men and material were enormous, and with the Prussian army steadily ossifying from the 1770s onward, Berlin was in no position to withstand later diplomatic pressure from Russia, let alone the bold assault of Napoleon in 1806. Even the later recovery led by Scharnhorst, Gneisenau, and the other military reformers could not conceal the still inadequate bases of Prussian strength by 1813–1815.[30] It was by then overshadowed, militarily, by Russia; it relied heavily upon subsidies from Britain, paymaster to the coalition; and it still could not have taken on France alone. The kingdom of Frederick William III (1797–1840) was, like Austria, among the least of the Great Powers and would remain so until its industrial and military transformation in the 1860s.

*   *   *

By contrast, two more distant powers, Russia and the United States, enjoyed a relative invulnerability and a freedom from the strategical ambivalences which plagued the central European states in the eighteenth century. Both of these future superpowers had, to be sure, "a crumbling frontier" which required watching; but neither in the American expansion across the Alleghenies and the great plains nor in the Russian expansion across the steppes did they encounter militarily advanced societies posing a danger to the home base.[31] In their respective dealings with occidental Europe, therefore, they had the advantage of a relatively homogeneous "front." They could each pose a challenge—or, at least, a distraction—to some of the established Great Powers, while still enjoying the invulnerability conferred by their distance from the main European battle zones.

Of course, in dealing with a period as lengthy as 1660 to 1815, it is important to stress that the impact of the United States and Russia was much more in evidence by the end of that era than at the beginning. Indeed, in the 1660s and 1670s, European "America" was no more than a string of isolated coastal settlements, while Muscovy before the reign of Peter the Great (1689–1725) was almost equally remote and even more backward; in commercial terms, each was "underdeveloped," a producer of timber, hemp, and other raw materials and a purchaser of manufactured wares from Britain and the United Provinces. The American continent was, for much of this time, an object to be fought over rather than a power factor in its own right. What changed that situation was the overwhelming British success at the end of the Seven Years War (1763), which saw France expelled from Canada and Nova Scotia, and Spain excluded from West Florida. Freed from the foreign threats which hitherto had induced loyalty to Westminster, American colonists could now insist upon a merely nominal link with Britain and, if denied that by an imperial government with different ideas, engage in rebellion. By 1776, moreover, the North American colonies had grown enormously: the population of two million was by then doubling every thirty years, was spreading out westward, was economically prosperous, and was self-sufficient in foodstuffs and many other commodities. This meant, as the British found to their cost over the next seven years, that the rebel states were virtually invulnerable to merely naval operations and were also too extensive to be subjected by land forces drawn from a home island 3,000 miles away.

The existence of an independent United States was, *over time,* to have two major consequences for this story of the changing pattern of world power. The first was that from 1783 onward there existed an important extra-European center of production, wealth, and—ultimately—military might which would exert long-term influences upon the global power balance in ways which other extra-European (but economically declining) societies like China and India would not.

Already by the mid-eighteenth century the American colonies occupied a significant place in the pattern of maritime commerce and were beginning the first hesitant stages of industrialization. According to some accounts, the emergent nation produced more pig iron and bar iron in 1776 than the whole of Great Britain; and thereafter, "manufacturing output increased by a factor of nearly 50 so that by 1830 the country had become the 6th industrial power of the developed world."[32] Given that pace of growth, it was not surprising that even in the 1790s observers were predicting a great role for the United States within another century. The second consequence was to be felt much more swiftly, especially by Britain, whose role as a "flank" power in European politics was affected by the emergence of a potentially hostile state on its own Atlantic front, threatening its Canadian and West Indian possessions. This was not a constant problem, of course, and the sheer distance involved, together with the United States isolationism, meant that London did not need to consider the Americans in the same serious light as that in which, say, Vienna regarded the Turks or later the Russians. Nevertheless, the experiences of the wars of 1779–1783 and of 1812–1814 demonstrated all too clearly how difficult it would be for Britain to engage fully in European struggles if a hostile United States was at her back.

The rise of czarist Russia had a much more immediate impact upon the international power balance. Russia's stunning defeat of the Swedes at Poltava (1709) altered the other powers to the fact that the hitherto distant and somewhat barbarous Muscovite state was intent upon playing a role in European affairs. With the ambitious first czar, Peter the Great, quickly establishing a navy to complement his new footholds on the Baltic (Karelia, Estonia, Livonia), the Swedes were soon appealing for the Royal Navy's aid to prevent being overrun by this eastern colossus. But it was, in fact, the Poles and the Turks who were to suffer most from the rise of Russia, and by the time Catherine the Great had died in 1796 she had added another 200,000 square miles to an already enormous empire. Even more impressive seemed the temporary incursions which Russian military forces made to the west. The ferocity and frightening doggedness of the Russian troops during the Seven Years War, and their temporary occupation of Berlin in 1760, quite changed Frederick the Great's view of his neighbor. Four decades later, Russian forces under their general, Suvorov, were active in both Italian and Alpine campaigning during the War of the Second Coalition (1798–1802)—a distant operation that was a harbinger of the relentless Russian military advance from Moscow to Paris which took place between 1812 and 1814.[33]

It is difficult to measure Russia's rank accurately by the eighteenth century. Its army was often larger than France's; and in important manufactures (textiles, iron) it was also making great advances. It was a dreadfully difficult, perhaps impossible country for any of its rivals to conquer—at least from the west; and its status as a "gunpowder empire" enabled it to defeat the horsed tribes of the east, and thus to acquire additional resources of manpower, raw materials, and arable land, which in turn would enhance its place among the Great Powers. Under governmental direction, the country was evidently bent upon modernization in a whole variety of ways, although the pace and success of this policy have often been exaggerated. There still remained the manifold signs of backwardness: appalling poverty and brutality, exceedingly low per capita income, poor communications, harsh climate, and technological and educational retardation, not to mention the reactionary, feckless character of so many of the Romanovs. Even the formidable Catherine was unimpressive when it came to economic and financial matters.

Still, the relative stability of European military organization and technique in the eighteenth century allowed Russia (by borrowing foreign expertise) to catch up and then outstrip countries with fewer resources; and this brute advantage of superior numbers was not really going to be eroded until the Industrial Revolution transformed the scale and speed of warfare during the following century. In the period before the 1840s and despite the many defects listed above, Russia's army could occasionally be a formidable offensive force. So much (perhaps three-quarters) of the state's finances were devoted to the military and the average soldier stoically endured so many hardships that Russian regiments could mount long-range operations which were beyond most other eighteenth-century armies. It is true that the Russian logistical base was often inadequate (with poor horses, an inefficient supply system, and incompetent officials) to sustain a massive campaign on its own—the 1813–1814 march upon France was across "friendly" territory and aided by large British subsidies; but these infrequent operations were enough to give Russia a formidable reputation and a leading place in the councils of Europe even by the time of the Seven Years War. In grand-strategical terms, here was yet another power which could be brought into the balance, thus helping to ensure that French efforts to dominate the continent during this period would ultimately fail.

It was, nonetheless, to the *distant* future that early-nineteenth-century writers such as de Tocqueville usually referred when they argued that Russia and the United States seemed "marked out by the will of Heaven to sway the destinies of half the globe."[34] In the period between 1660 and 1815 it was a maritime nation, Great Britain, rather than these continental giants, which made the most decisive advances, finally dislodging France from its position as the greatest of the powers. Here, too, geography played a vital, though not exclusive, part. This British advantage of location was described nearly a century ago in Mahan's classic work *The Influence of Sea Power upon History* (1890):

> ... if a nation be so situated that it is neither forced to defend itself by land nor induced to seek extension of its territory by way of land, it has, by the very unity of its aim directed upon the sea, an advantage as compared with a people one of whose boundaries is continental.[35]

Mahan's statement presumes, of course, a number of further points. The first is that the British government would not have distractions on *its* flanks—which after the conquest of Ireland and the Act of Union with Scotland (1707), was essentially correct, though it is interesting to note those occasional later French attempts to embarrass Britain along the Celtic fringes, something which London took very seriously indeed. An Irish uprising was much closer to home than the strategical embarrassment offered by the American rebels. Fortunately for the British, this vulnerability was never properly exploited by foes.

The second assumption in Mahan's statement is the superior status of sea warfare and of sea power over their equivalents on land. This was a deeply held belief of what has been termed the "navalist" school of strategy,[36] and seemed well justified by post-1500 economic and political trends. The steady shift in the main trade routes from the Mediterranean to the Atlantic and the great profits which could be made from colonial and commercial ventures in the West Indies, North America, the Indian subcontinent, and the Far East naturally benefited a country situated off the western flank of the European continent. To be sure, it also required a government aware of the importance of maritime trade and ready to pay for a large war fleet. Subject to that precondition, the British political elite seemed by the eighteenth century to have discovered a happy recipe for the continuous growth of national wealth and power. Flourishing overseas trade aided the British economy, encouraged seamanship and shipbuilding, provided funds for the national Exchequer, and was the lifeline to the colonies. The colonies not only offered outlets for British products but also supplied many raw materials, from the valuable sugar, tobacco, and calicoes to the increasingly important North American naval stores. And the Royal Navy ensured respect for British merchants in times of peace and protected their trade and garnered further colonial territories in war, to the country's political and economic benefit. Trade, colonies, and the navy thus formed a "virtuous triangle," reciprocally interacting to Britain's long-term advantage.

While this explanation of Britain's rise was partly valid, it was not the whole truth. Like so many mercantilist works, Mahan's tended to emphasize the importance of Britain's external commerce as opposed to domestic production, and in particular to exaggerate the importance of the "colonial" trades. Agriculture remained the fundament of British wealth throughout the eighteenth century, and exports (whose ratio to total national income was probably less than 10 percent until the 1780s) were often subject to strong foreign competition and to tariffs, for which no amount of naval power could compensate.[37] The navalist viewpoint also inclined to forget the further fact that British trade with the Baltic, Germany, and the Mediterranean lands was—although growing less swiftly than those in sugar, spices, and slaves—still of great economic importance;* so that a France permanently dominant in Europe might, as the events of 1806–1812 showed, be able to deliver a dreadful blow to British manufacturing industry. Under such circumstances, isolationism from European power politics could be economic folly.

There was also a critically important "continental" dimension to British grand strategy, overlooked by those whose gaze was turned outward to the West Indies, Canada, and India. Fighting a purely maritime war was perfectly logical during the Anglo-Dutch struggles of 1652–1654, 1665–1667, and 1672–1674, since commercial rivalry between the two sea powers was at the root of that antagonism. After the Glorious Revolution of 1688, however, when William of Orange secured the English throne, the strategical situation was quite transformed. The challenge to British interests during the seven wars which were to occur between 1689 and 1815 was posed by an essentially *land-based* power, France. True, the French would take this fight to the western hemisphere, to the Indian Ocean, to Egypt, and elsewhere; but those campaigns, although important to London and Liverpool traders, never posed a direct threat to British national security. The latter would arise only with the prospect of French military victories over the Dutch, the Hanoverians, and the Prussians, thereby leaving France supreme in west-central Europe long enough to amass shipbuilding resources capable of eroding British naval mastery. It was therefore not merely William III's personal union with the United Provinces, or the later Hanoverian ties, which caused successive British governments to intervene militarily on the continent of Europe in these decades. There was also the compelling argument—echoing Elizabeth I's fears about Spain—that France's enemies had to be given assistance *inside* Europe, to contain Bourbon (and Napoleonic) ambitions and thus to preserve Britain's own long-term interests. A "maritime" and a

*Not to mention the *strategic* importance of Baltic naval stores, upon which both the Royal Navy and the mercantile marine relied—a dependency reflected in the frequent dispatch of a British fleet into the Baltic to preserve the balance of power and the free flow of timber and masts.

"continental" strategy were, according to this viewpoint, complementary rather than antagonistic.

The essence of this strategic calculation was nicely expressed by the
Duke of Newcastle in 1742:

> France will outdo us at sea when they have nothing to fear on land.
> I have always maintained that our marine should protect our al-
> liances on the Continent, and so, by diverting the expense of France,
> enable us to maintain our superiority at sea.[38]

This British support to countries willing to "divert the expense of
France" came in two chief forms. The first was direct military operations, either by peripheral raids to distract the French army or by the
dispatch of a more substantial expeditionary force to fight alongside
whatever allies Britain might possess at the time. The raiding strategy
seemed cheaper and was much beloved by certain ministers, but it
usually had negligible effects and occasionally ended in disaster (like
the expedition to Walcheren of 1809). The provision of a continental
army was more expensive in terms of men and money, but, as the
campaigns of Marlborough and Wellington demonstrated, was also
much more likely to assist in the preservation of the European balance.

The second form of British aid was financial, whether by directly
buying Hessian and other mercenaries to fight against France, or by
giving subsidies to the allies. Frederick the Great, for example, received from the British the substantial sum of £675,000 each year from
1757 to 1760; and in the closing stages of the Napoleonic War the flow
of British funds reached far greater proportions (e.g., £11 million to
various allies in 1813 alone, and £65 million for the war as a whole).
But all this had been possible only because the expansion of British
trade and commerce, particularly in the lucrative overseas markets,
allowed the government to raise loans and taxes of unprecedented
amounts without suffering national bankruptcy. Thus, while diverting
"the expense of France" inside Europe was a costly business, it usually
ensured that the French could neither mount a sustained campaign
against maritime trade nor so dominate the European continent that
they would be free to threaten an invasion of the home islands—which
in turn permitted London to finance its wars and to subsidize its allies.
Geographical advantage and economic benefit were thus merged to
enable the British brilliantly to pursue a Janus-faced strategy: "with
one face turned towards the Continent to trim the balance of power
and the other directed at sea to strengthen her maritime dominance."[39]

Only after one grasps the importance of the financial and geographical factors described above can one make full sense of the statistics
of the growing populations and military/naval strengths of the powers
in this period (see Tables 3–5).

Table 3. Populations of the Powers, 1700–1800[40]
(millions)

	1700	1750	1800
British Isles	9.0	10.5	16.0
France	19.0	21.5	28.0
Habsburg Empire	8.0	18.0	28.0
Prussia	2.0	6.0	9.5
Russia	17.5	20.0	37.0
Spain	6.0	9.0	11.0
Sweden		1.7	2.3
United Provinces	1.8	1.9	2.0
United States	—	2.0	4.0

Table 4. Size of Armies, 1690–1814[41]
(men)

	1690	1710	1756/60	1778	1789	1812/14
Britain	70,000	75,000	200,000		40,000	250,000
France	400,000	350,000	330,000	170,000	180,000	600,000
Habsburg Empire	50,000	100,000	200,000	200,000	300,000	250,000
Prussia	30,000	39,000	195,000	160,000	190,000	270,000
Russia	170,000	220,000	330,000		300,000	500,000
Spain		30,000			50,000	
Sweden		110,000				
United Provinces	73,000	130,000	40,000			
United States	—	—	—	35,000	—	—

Table 5. Size of Navies, 1689–1815[42]
(ships of the line)

	1689	1739	1756	1779	1790	1815
Britain	100	124	105	90	195	214
Denmark	29	—	—	—	38	—
France	120	50	70	63	81	80
Russia	—	30	—	40	67	40
Spain	—	34	—	48	72	25
Sweden	40	—	—	—	27	—
United Provinces	66	49	—	20	44	—

As readers familiar with statistics will be aware, such crude figures have to be treated with extreme care. Population totals, especially in the early period, are merely guesses (and in Russia's case the margin for error could be several millions). Army sizes fluctuated widely, depending upon whether the date chosen is at the outset, the midpoint, or the culmination of a particular war; and the total figures often include substantial mercenary units and (in Napoleon's case) even the troops of reluctantly co-opted allies. The number of ships of the line indicated neither their readiness for battle nor, necessarily, the availability of trained crews to man them. Moreover, statistics take no account of generalship or seamanship, of competence or neglect, of national fervor or faintheartedness. Even so, it might appear that the above figures at least *roughly* reflect the chief power-political trends of the age: France and, increasingly, Russia lead in population and military terms; Britain is usually unchallenged at sea; Prussia overtakes Spain, Sweden, and the United Provinces; and France comes closer to dominating Europe with the enormous armies of Louis XIV and Napoleon than at any time in the intervening century.

Aware of the financial and geographical dimensions of these 150 years of Great Power struggles, however, one can see that further refinements have to be made to the picture suggested in these three tables. For example, the swift decline of the United Provinces relative to other nations in respect to army size was not repeated in the area of war finance, where its role was crucial for a very long while. The nonmilitary character of the United States conceals the fact that it could pose a considerable strategical distraction. The figures also understate the military contribution of Britain, since it might be subsidizing 100,000 allied troops (in 1813, 450,000!) as well as providing for its own army, and naval personnel of 140,000 in 1813–1814;[43] conversely, the true strength of Prussia and the Habsburg Empire, dependent on subsidies during most wars, would be exaggerated if one merely considered the size of their armies. As noted above, the enormous military establishments of France were rendered less effective through financial weaknesses and geostrategical obstacles, while those of Russia were eroded by economic backwardness and sheer distance. The strengths and weaknesses of each of these Powers ought to be borne in mind as we turn to a more detailed examination of the wars themselves.

The Winning of Wars, 1660–1763

When Louis XIV took over full direction of the French government in March 1661, the European scene was particularly favorable to a monarch determined to impose his views upon it.[44] To the south, Spain was still exhausting itself in the futile attempt to recover Portugal. Across the Channel, a restored monarchy under Charles II was trying to find its feet, and in English commercial circles great jealousy of the Dutch existed. In the north, a recent war had left both Denmark and Sweden weakened. In Germany, the Protestant princes watched suspiciously for any fresh Habsburg attempt to improve its position, but the imperial government in Vienna had problems enough in Hungary and Transylvania, and slightly later with a revival of Ottoman power. Poland was already wilting under the effort of fending off Swedish and Muscovite predators. Thus French diplomacy, in the best traditions of Richelieu, could easily take advantage of these circumstances, playing off the Portuguese against Spain, the Magyars, Turks, and German princes against Austria, and the English against the Dutch—while buttressing France's own geographical (and army-recruitment) position by its important 1663 treaty with the Swiss cantons. All this gave Louis XIV time enough to establish himself as absolute monarch, secure from the internal challenges which had afflicted French governments during the preceding century. More important still, it gave Colbert, Le Tellier, and the other key ministers the chance to overhaul the administration and to lavish resources upon the army and the navy in anticipation of the Sun King's pursuit of glory.[45]

It was therefore all too easy for Louis to try to "round off" the borders of France in the early stages of his reign, the more especially since Anglo-Dutch relations had deteriorated into open hostilities by 1665 (the Second Anglo-Dutch War). Although France was pledged to support the United Provinces, it actually played little part in the campaigns at sea and instead prepared itself for an invasion of the southern Netherlands, which were still owned by a weakened Spain. When the French finally launched their invasion, in May 1667, town after town quickly fell into their hands. What then followed was an early example of the rapid diplomatic shifts of this period. The English and the Dutch, wearying of their mutually unprofitable war and fearing French ambitions, made peace at Breda in July and, joined by Sweden, sought to "mediate" in the Franco-Spanish dispute in order to limit Louis's gains. The 1668 Treaty of Aix-la-Chapelle achieved just that, but at the cost of infuriating the French king, who eventually made up his mind to be revenged upon the United Provinces, which he perceived to be the chief obstacle to his ambitions. For the next few years, while Colbert waged his tariff war against the Dutch, the French army and navy were further built up. Secret diplomacy seduced England and Sweden from their alliance with the United Provinces and quieted the fears of the Austrians and the German states. By 1672 the French war machine, aided by the English at sea, was ready to strike.

Although it was London which first declared war upon the United Provinces, the dismal English effort in the third Anglo-Dutch conflict of 1672–1674 requires minimal space here. Checked by the brilliant efforts of de Ruyter at sea, and therefore unable to achieve anything on land, Charles II's government came under increasing domestic criticism: evidence of political duplicity and financial mismanagement, and a strong dislike of being allied to an autocratic, Catholic power like France, made the war unpopular and forced the government to pull out of it by 1674. In retrospect, it is a reminder of how immature and uncertain the political, financial, and administrative bases of English power still were under the later Stuarts.[46] London's change of policy was of *international* importance, however, in that it partly reflected the widespread alarm which Louis XIV's designs were now arousing throughout Europe. Within another year, Dutch diplomacy and subsidies found many allies willing to throw their weight against the French. German principalities, Brandenburg (which defeated France's only remaining partner, Sweden, at Fehrbellin in 1675), Denmark, Spain, and the Habsburg Empire all entered the issue. It was not that this coalition of states was strong enough to *overwhelm* France; most of them had smallish armies, and distractions on their own flanks; and the core of the anti-French alliance remained the United Provinces under their new leader, William of Orange. But the watery barrier in the north and the vulnerability of the French army's lines against various foes in the Rhineland meant that Louis himself could make no dramatic gains. A similar sort of stalemate existed at sea; the French navy controlled the Mediterranean, Dutch and Danish fleets held the Baltic, and neither side could prevail in the West Indies. Both French and Dutch commerce were badly affected in this war, to the indirect benefit of neutrals like the British. By 1678, in fact, the Amsterdam merchant classes had pushed their own government into a separate peace with France, which in turn meant that the German states (reliant upon Dutch subsidies) could not continue to fight on their own.

Although the Nymegen peace treaties of 1678–1679 brought the open fighting to an end, Louis XIV's evident desire to round off France's northern borders, his claim to be "the arbiter of Europe," and the alarming fact that he was maintaining an army of 200,000 troops in peacetime disquieted Germans, Dutchmen, Spaniards, and Englishmen alike.[47] This did not mean an immediate return to war. The Dutch merchants preferred to trade in peace; the German princes, like Charles II of England, were tied to Paris by subsidies; and the Habsburg Empire was engaged in a desperate struggle with the Turks. When Spain endeavored to protect its Luxembourg territories from France in 1683, therefore, it had to fight alone and suffer inevitable defeat.

From 1685, however, things began to swing against France. The persecution of the Huguenots shocked Protestant Europe. Within another two years, the Turks had been soundly defeated and driven away from Vienna; and the Emperor Leopold, with enhanced prestige and military strength, could at last turn some of his attention to the west. By September 1688, a now-nervous French king decided to invade Germany, finally turning this European "cold" war into a hot one. Not only did France's action provoke its continental rivals into declaring hostilities, it also gave William of Orange the opportunity to slip across the Channel and replace the discredited James II on the English throne.

By the end of 1689, therefore, France stood alone against the United Provinces, England, the Habsburg Empire, Spain, Savoy, and the major German states.[48] This was not as alarming a combination as it seemed, and the "hard core" of the Grand Alliance really consisted of the Anglo-Dutch forces and the German states. Although a disparate grouping in certain respects, they possessed sufficient determination, financial resources, armies, and fleets to balance the Sun King's France. Ten years earlier, Louis might possibly have prevailed, but French finances and trade were now much less satisfactory after Colbert's death, and neither the army nor the navy—although numerically daunting—was equipped for sustained and distant fighting. A swift defeat of one of the major allies could break the deadlock, but where should that thrust be directed, and had Louis the will to order bold measures? For three years he dithered; and when in 1692 he finally assembled an invasion force of 24,000 troops to dispatch across the Channel, the "maritime powers" were simply too strong, smashing up the French warships and barges at Barfleur–La Hogue.[49]

From 1692 onward, the conflict at sea became a slow, grinding, mutually ruinous war against trade. Adopting a commerce-raiding strategy, the French government encouraged its privateers to prey upon Anglo-Dutch shipping while it reduced its own allocations to the battle fleet. The allied navies, for their part, endeavored to increase the pressures on the French economy by instituting a commercial blockade, thus abandoning the Dutch habit of trading with the enemy. Neither measure brought the opponent to his knees; each increased the economic burdens of the war, making it unpopular with merchants as well as peasants, who were already suffering from a succession of poor harvests. The land campaigns were also expensive, slow struggles against fortresses and across waterways: Vauban's fortifications made France virtually impregnable, but the same sort of obstacles prevented an easy French advance into Holland or the Palatinate. With each side maintaining over 250,000 men in the field, the costs were horrendous, even to these rich countries.[50] While there were also extra-European campaigns (West Indies, Newfoundland, Acadia, Pondicherry), none was of sufficient importance to swing the basic continental or maritime balance. Thus by 1696, with Tory squires and Amsterdam burghers complaining about excessive taxes, and with France afflicted by famine, both William and Louis had cause enough to compromise.

In consequence, the Treaty of Ryswick (1697), while allowing Louis some of his earlier border gains, saw a general return to the status quo ante. Nonetheless, the results of the Nine Years War of 1689–1697 were not as insignificant as contemporary critics alleged. French ambitions had certainly been blunted on land, and its naval power eroded at sea. The Glorious Revolution of 1688 had been upheld, and England had secured its Irish flank, strengthened its financial institutions, and rebuilt its army and navy. And an Anglo-Dutch-German tradition of keeping France out of Flanders and the Rhineland was established. Albeit at great cost, the political plurality of Europe had been reasserted.

Given the war-weary mood in most capitals, a renewal of the conflict scarcely seemed possible. However, when Louis's grandson was offered the succession to the Spanish throne in 1700, the Sun King saw in this an ideal opportunity to enhance France's power. Instead of compromising with his potential rivals, he swiftly occupied the southern Netherlands on his grandson's behalf, and also secured *exclusive* commercial concessions for French traders in Spain's large empire in the western hemisphere. By these and various other provocations, he alarmed the British and Dutch sufficiently to cause them to join Austria in 1701 in another coalition struggle to check Louis's ambitions: the War of the Spanish Succession.

Once again, the general balance of forces and taxable resources suggested that each alliance could seriously hurt, but not overwhelm, the other.[51] In some respects, Louis was in a stronger position than in the 1689–1697 war. The Spaniards readily took to his grandson, now their Philip V, and the "Bourbon powers" could work together in many theaters; French finances certainly benefited from the import of Spanish silver. Moreover, France had been geared up militarily—to the level, at one period, of supporting nearly half a million troops. However, the Austrians, less troubled on their Balkan flank, were playing a greater role in this war than they had in the previous one. Most important of all, a determined British government was to commit its considerable national resources, in the form of hefty subsidies to German allies, an overpowering fleet, and, unusually, a large-scale continental army under the brilliant Marlborough. The latter, with between 40,000 and 70,000 British and mercenary troops, could join an excellent Dutch army of over 100,000 men and a Habsburg army of a similar size to frustrate Louis's attempt to impose his wishes upon Europe.

This did not mean, however, that the Grand Alliance could impose *its* wishes upon France, or, for that matter, upon Spain. Outside those two kingdoms, it is true, events turned steadily in favor of the allies. Marlborough's decisive victory at Blenheim (1704) severely hurt the Franco-Bavarian armies and freed Austria from a French invasion threat. The later battle of Ramillies (1706) gave the Anglo-Dutch forces most of the southern Netherlands, and that at Oudenarde (1708) brutally stopped the French effort to regain ground there.[52]

At sea, with no enemy main fleet to deal with after the inconclusive battle of Malaga (1704), the Royal Navy and its declining Dutch equivalent could demonstrate the flexibility of superior naval power. The new ally, Portugal, could be sustained from the sea, while Lisbon in turn provided a forward fleet base and Brazil a source of gold. Troops could be dispatched to the western hemisphere to attack French possessions in the West Indies and North America, and raiding squadrons could hunt for Spanish bullion fleets. The seizure of Gibraltar not only gave the Royal Navy a base controlling the exit from that sea, but divided the Franco-Spanish bases—and fleets. British fleets ensured the capture of Minorca and Sardinia; they covered Savoy and the Italian coasts from French attack; and when the allies went onto the offensive, they shepherded and supplied the imperial armies' invasion of Spain and supported the assault upon Toulon.[53]

This general Allied maritime superiority could not, however, prevent a resumption of French commerce-raiding, and by 1708 the Royal Navy had been forced to institute a convoying system in order to limit the losses to the merchant marine. And just as British frigates could not keep French privateers from slipping in and out of Dunkirk or the Gironde, so also were they unable to effect a commercial blockade, for that would have meant patrolling the entire Franco-Spanish coastline; even the seizure of corn ships off French ports during the dreadful winter of 1709 could not bring Louis's largely self-sufficient empire to its knees.

This allied capacity to wound but not kill was even more evident in the military campaigns against France and Spain. By 1709 the allied invasion army was falling back from a brief occupation of Madrid, unable to hold the country in the face of increasing Spanish assault. In northern France, the Anglo-Dutch armies found no further opportunity for victories like Blenheim; instead, the war was grinding, bloody, and expensive. Moreover, by 1710 a Tory ministry had come into office at Westminster, eager for a peace which secured Britain's maritime and imperial interests and reduced its expenses in a continental war. Finally, the Archduke Charles, who had been the allies' candidate for the Spanish throne, unexpectedly succeeded as emperor, and thus caused his partners to lose any remaining enthusiasm for placing him in control of Spain as well. With Britain's unilateral defection from the war in early 1712, followed later by that of the Dutch, even the Emperor Charles, so eager to be "Carlos III" of Spain, accepted the need for peace after another fruitless year of campaigning.

The peace terms which brought the War of the Spanish Succession to an end were fixed in the treaties of Utrecht (1713) and Rastadt (1714). Considering the settlement as a whole, there was no doubt that the great beneficiary was Britain.[54] Although it had gained Gibraltar, Minorca, Nova Scotia, Newfoundland, and Hudson Bay and trade concessions in the Spanish New World, it did not ignore the European balance. Indeed, the complex of eleven separate treaties which made up the settlement of 1713–1714 produced a satisfying, sophisticated reinforcement of the equilibrium. The French and the Spanish kingdoms were to remain forever separated, whereas the Protestant Succession in Britain was formally recognized. The Habsburg Empire, having failed in Spain, was given the southern Netherlands and Milan (thus building in further checks to France), plus Naples and Sardinia. Dutch independence had been preserved, but the United Provinces were no longer such a formidable naval and commercial power and were now compelled to devote the greater part of their energies to garrisoning their southern borders. Above all, Louis XIV had been finally and decisively checked in his dynastic and territorial ambitions, and the French nation had been chastened by the horrific costs of war, which had, among other consequences, increased total government debts *sevenfold*. The balance of power was secure on land, while at sea Britain was unchallenged. Small wonder that the Whigs, who returned to office on George I's accession in 1714, were soon anxious to preserve the Utrecht settlement and were even willing to embrace a French *entente* once their archenemy Louis died in the following year.

The redistribution of power among the western European states which had occurred in this half-century of war was less dramatic than the changes which took place in the east. The borders there were more fluid than in the west, and enormous tracts of land were controlled by marcher lords, Croatian irregulars, and Cossack hosts rather than by the professional armies of an enlightened monarch. Even when the nation-states went to war against each other, their campaigning would frequently be over great distances and involve the use of irregular troops, hussars, and so on in order to implement some grand strategical stroke. Unlike the campaigning in the Low Countries, success or failure here brought with it tremendous transfers of land, and thus emphasized the more spectacular rises and falls among the Powers. For example, these few decades alone saw the Turks pose their final large-scale military threat to Vienna, but then suffer swift defeat and decline. The remarkable initial response by Austrian, German, and Polish forces not only rescued the imperial city from a Turkish investing army in 1683 but also led to much more extensive campaigning by an enlarged Holy League.[55] After a great battle near Homacs (1687), Turkish power in the Hungarian plain was destroyed forever; if the lines then stabilized because of repeated calls upon German and Habsburg troops against France during the 1689–1697 War, the further defeats of the Turkish army at Zalankemen (1691) and Zenta (1697) confirmed the trend. Provided it could concentrate its resources on the Balkan front and possessed generals of the caliber of Prince Eugene, the Habsburg Empire could now more than hold its own against the Turks. While it could not organize its heterogeneous lands as efficiently as the western monarchies, nonetheless its future as one of the European great states was assured.

Measured by that criterion, Sweden was far less lucky. Once the young Charles XII came to the Swedish throne in 1697, the predatory instincts of the neighboring states were aroused; Denmark, Poland, and Russia each desired parts of Sweden's exposed Baltic empire and agreed in autumn 1699 to combine against it. Yet when the fighting commenced, Sweden's apparent vulnerability was at first more than compensated for by its own very considerable army, a monarch of great military brilliance, and Anglo-Dutch naval support. A combination of all three factors allowed Charles to threaten Copenhagen and force the Danes out of the war by August 1700, following which he transported his army across the Baltic and routed the Russians in a stunning victory at Narva three months later. Having savored the heady joys of battle and conquest, Charles then spent the following years overrunning Poland and moving into Saxony.

With the wisdom of retrospect, historians have suggested that Charles XII's unwise concentration upon Poland and Saxony turned his gaze from the reforms which Peter the Great was forcing upon Russia after the defeat at Narva.[56] Aided by numerous foreign advisers and willing to borrow widely from the military expertise of the west, Peter built up a massive army and navy in the same energetic way in which he created St. Petersburg from the swamps. By the time Charles with a force of 40,000 troops turned to deal with Peter in 1708, it was probably already too late. Although the Swedish army generally performed better in battle, it suffered considerable losses, was never able to crush the main Russian army, and was hampered by inadequate logistics—such difficulties intensifying as Charles's force moved south into the Ukraine and endured the bitter winter of 1708–1709. When the great battle finally occurred, at Poltava in July 1709, the Russian army was vastly superior in numbers and in good defensive positions. Not only did this encounter wipe out the Swedish force, but Charles's subsequent flight into Turkish territory and lengthy exile there gave Sweden's foes nearer home their opportunity. By the time Charles finally returned to Sweden, in December 1715, all his trans-Baltic possessions had gone and parts of Finland were in Russian hands.

After further years of fighting (in which Charles XII was killed in yet another clash with the Danes in 1718), an exhausted, isolated Sweden finally had to admit to the loss of most of its Baltic provinces in the 1721 Peace of Nystad. It had now fallen to the second order of the powers, while Russia was in the first. Appropriately enough, to mark the 1721 victory over Sweden, Peter assumed the title Imperator. Despite the later decline of the czarist fleet, despite the great backwardness of the country, Russia had clearly shown that it, like France and Britain, "had the strength to act independently as a great power without depending on outside support."[57] In the east as in the west of Europe there was now, in Dehio's phrase, a "counterweight to a concentration at the center."[58]

This general balance of political, military, and economic force in Europe was underwritten by an Anglo-French *détente* lasting nearly two decades after 1715.[59] France in particular needed to recuperate after a war which had dreadfully hurt its foreign commerce and so increased the state's debt that the interest payments on it alone equaled the normal revenue. Furthermore, the monarchies in London and Paris, not a little fearful of their own succession, frowned upon any attempts to upset the status quo and found it mutually profitable to cooperate on many issues.[60] In 1719, for example, both powers were using force to prevent Spain from pursuing an expansionist policy in Italy. By the 1730s, however, the pattern of international relations was again changing. By this stage, the French themselves were less enthusiastic about the British link and were instead looking to recover their old position as the leading nation of Europe. The succession in France was now secure, and the years of peace had aided prosperity—and also led to a large expansion in overseas trade, challenging the maritime powers. While France under its minister Fleury rapidly improved its relations with Spain and expanded its diplomatic activities in eastern Europe, Britain under the cautious and isolationist Walpole was endeavoring to keep out of continental affairs. Even a French attack upon the Austrian possessions of Lorraine and Milan in 1733, and a French move into the Rhineland, failed to provoke a British reaction. Unable to obtain any support from the isolationist Walpole and the frightened Dutch, Vienna was forced to negotiate with Paris for the compromise peace of 1738. Bolstered by military and diplomatic successes in western Europe, by the alliance of Spain, the deference of the United Provinces, and the increasing compliance of Sweden and even Austria, France now enjoyed a prestige unequaled since the early decades of Louis XIV. This was made even more evident in the following year, when French diplomacy negotiated an end to an Austro-Russian war against the Ottoman Empire (1735–1739), thereby returning to Turkish possession many of the territories seized by the two eastern monarchies.

While the British under Walpole had tended to ignore these events within Europe, commercial interests and opposition politicians were much more concerned at the rising number of clashes with France's ally, Spain, in the western hemisphere. There the rich colonial trades and conflicting settler expansionisms offered ample materials for a quarrel.[61] The resultant Anglo-Spanish war, which Walpole reluctantly agreed to in October 1739, might merely have remained one of that series of smaller regional conflicts fought between those two countries in the eighteenth century but for France's decision to give all sorts of aid to Spain, especially "beyond the line" in the Caribbean. Compared with the 1702–1713 War of the Spanish Succession, the Bourbon powers were in a far better position to compete overseas, particularly since neither Britain's army nor its navy was equipped to carry out the conquest of Spanish colonies so favored by the pundits at home.

The death of the Emperor Charles VI, followed by Maria Theresa's

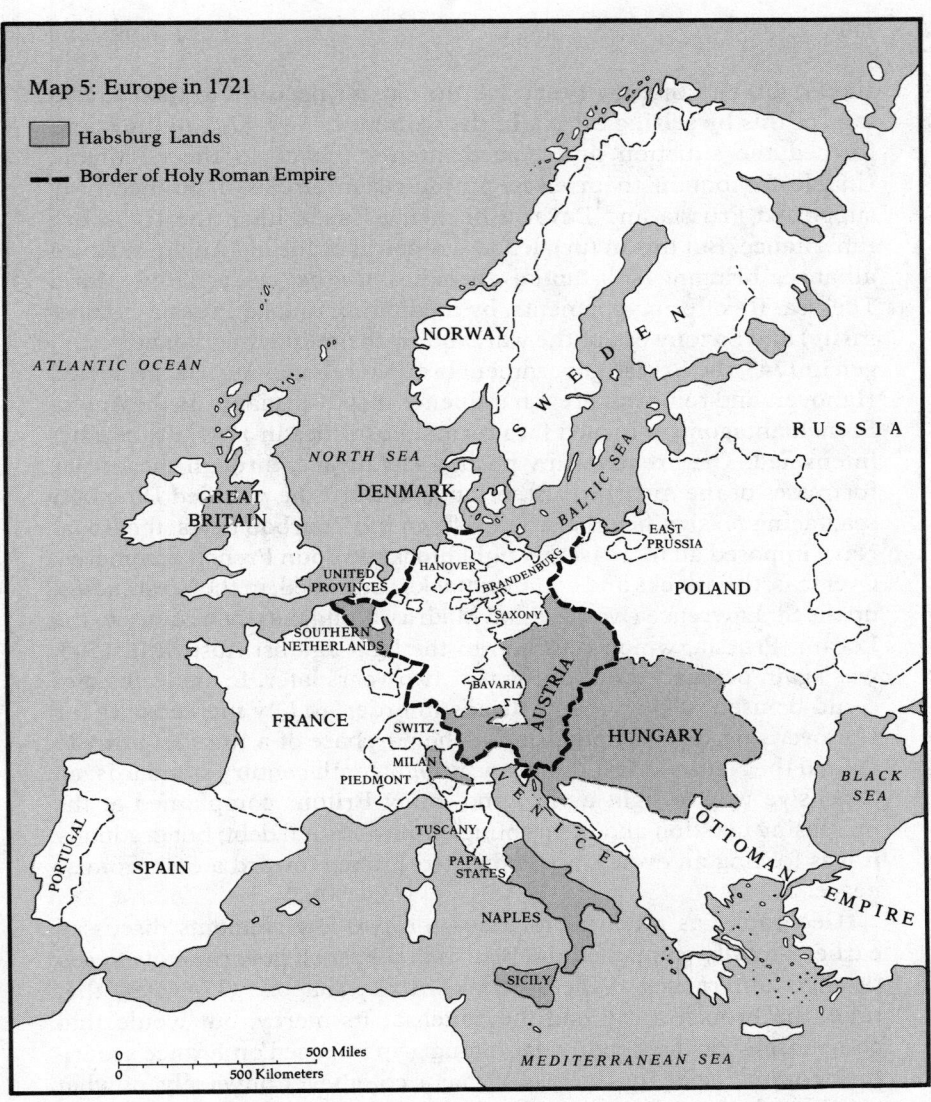

Map 5: Europe in 1721

▨ Habsburg Lands

▬ ▬ Border of Holy Roman Empire

ATLANTIC OCEAN

NORWAY

S W E D E N

RUSSIA

NORTH SEA

DENMARK

BALTIC SEA

GREAT
BRITAIN

EAST
PRUSSIA

HANOVER

BRANDENBURG

POLAND

UNITED
PROVINCES

SAXONY

SOUTHERN
NETHERLANDS

BAVARIA

AUSTRIA

HUNGARY

FRANCE

SWITZ.

MILAN

BLACK
SEA

PIEDMONT

VENICE

PORTUGAL

TUSCANY

OTTOMAN

SPAIN

PAPAL
STATES

EMPIRE

NAPLES

SICILY

500 Miles

500 Kilometers

MEDITERRANEAN SEA

succession and then by Frederick the Great's decision to take advantage of this by seizing Silesia in the winter of 1740–1741, quite transformed the situation and turned attention back to the continent. Unable to contain themselves, anti-Austrian circles in France fully supported Prussia and Bavaria in their assaults upon the Habsburg inheritance. But this in turn led to a renewal of the old Anglo-Austrian alliance, bringing substantial subsidies to the beleaguered Maria Theresa. By offering payments, by meditating to take Prussia (temporarily) and Saxony out of the war, and by the military action at Dettingen in 1743, the British government brought relief to Austria, protected Hanover, and removed French influence from Germany. As the Anglo-French antagonism turned into formal hostilities in 1744, the conflict intensified. The French army pushed northward, through the border fortresses of the Austrian Netherlands, toward the petrified Dutch. At sea, facing no significant challenge from the Bourbon fleets, the Royal Navy imposed an increasingly tight blockade upon French commerce. Overseas, the attacks and counterattacks continued, in the West Indies, up the St. Lawrence river, around Madras, along the trade routes to the Levant. Prussia, which returned to the fight against Austria in 1743, was again persuaded out of the war two years later. British subsidies could be used to keep the Austrians in order, to buy mercenaries for Hanover's protection and even for the purchase of a Russian army to defend the Netherlands. This was, by eighteenth-century standards, an expensive way to fight a war, and many Britons complained at the increasing taxation and the trebling of the national debt; but gradually it was forcing an even more exhausted France toward a compromise peace.

Geography as much as finance—the two key elements discussed earlier—finally compelled the British and French governments to settle their differences at the Treaty of Aix-la-Chapelle (1748). By that time, the French army had the Dutch at its mercy; but would that compensate for the steadily tightening grip imposed on France's maritime commerce or for the loss of major colonies? Conversely, of what use were the British seizure of Louisburg on the St. Lawrence and the naval victories of Anson and Hawke if France conquered the Low Countries? In consequence, diplomatic talks arranged for a general return to the status quo ante, with the significant exception of Frederick's conquest of Silesia. Both at the time and in retrospect, Aix-la-Chapelle was seen more in the nature of a truce than a lasting settlement. It left Maria Theresa keen to be revenged upon Prussia, France wondering how to be victorious overseas as well as on land, and Britain anxious to ensure that its great enemy would next time be defeated as soundly in continental warfare as it could be in a maritime/colonial struggle.

*   *   *

In the North American colonies, where British and French settlers (each aided by Indians and some local military garrisons) were repeatedly clashing in the early 1750s, even the word "truce" was a misnomer. There the forces involved were almost impossible to control by home governments, the more especially since a "patriot lobby" in each country pressed for support for their colonists and encouraged the view that a fundamental struggle—not merely for the Ohio and Mississippi valley regions, but for Canada, the Caribbean, India, nay, the entire extra-European world—was underway.[62] With each side dispatching further reinforcements and putting its navy on a war footing by 1755, the other states began to adjust to the prospect of another Anglo-French conflict. For Spain and the United Provinces, now plainly in the second rank and fearing that they would be ground down between these two colossi in the west, neutrality was the only solution—despite the inherent difficulties for traders like the Dutch.[63]

For the eastern monarchies of Austria, Prussia, and Russia, however, abstention from an Anglo-French war in the mid-1750s was impossible. The first reason was that although some Frenchmen argued that the conflict should be fought at sea and in the colonies, the natural tendency in Paris was to attack Britain via Hanover, the strategical Achilles' heel of the islanders. This, though, would not only alarm the German states but also compel the British to search for and subsidize military allies to check the French on the continent. The second reason was altogether more important: the Austrians were determined to recover Silesia from Prussia; and the Russians under their Czarina Elizabeth were also looking for a chance to punish the disrespectful, ambitious Frederick. Each of these powers had built up a considerable army (Prussia over 150,000 men, Austria almost 200,000, and Russia perhaps 330,000) and was calculating when to strike; but all of them were going to need subsidies from the west to keep their armies at that size. Finally, it was in the logic of things that if any of these eastern rivals found a "partner" in Paris or London, the others would be impelled to join the opposing side.

Thus, the famous "diplomatic revolution" of 1756 seemed, strategically, merely a reshuffling of the cards. France now buried its ancient differences with the Habsburgs and joined Austria and Russia in their war against Prussia, while Berlin replaced Vienna as London's continental ally. At first sight, the Franco-Austro-Russian coalition looked the better deal. It was decidedly bigger in military terms, and by 1757 Frederick had lost all his early territorial gains and the Duke of Cumberland's Anglo-German army had surrendered, leaving the future of Hanover—and Prussia itself—in doubt. Minorca had fallen to the French, and in the more distant theaters France and its native allies were also making gains. Overturning the treaty of Utrecht, and in Austria's case that of Aix-la-Chapelle, now appeared distinctly possible.

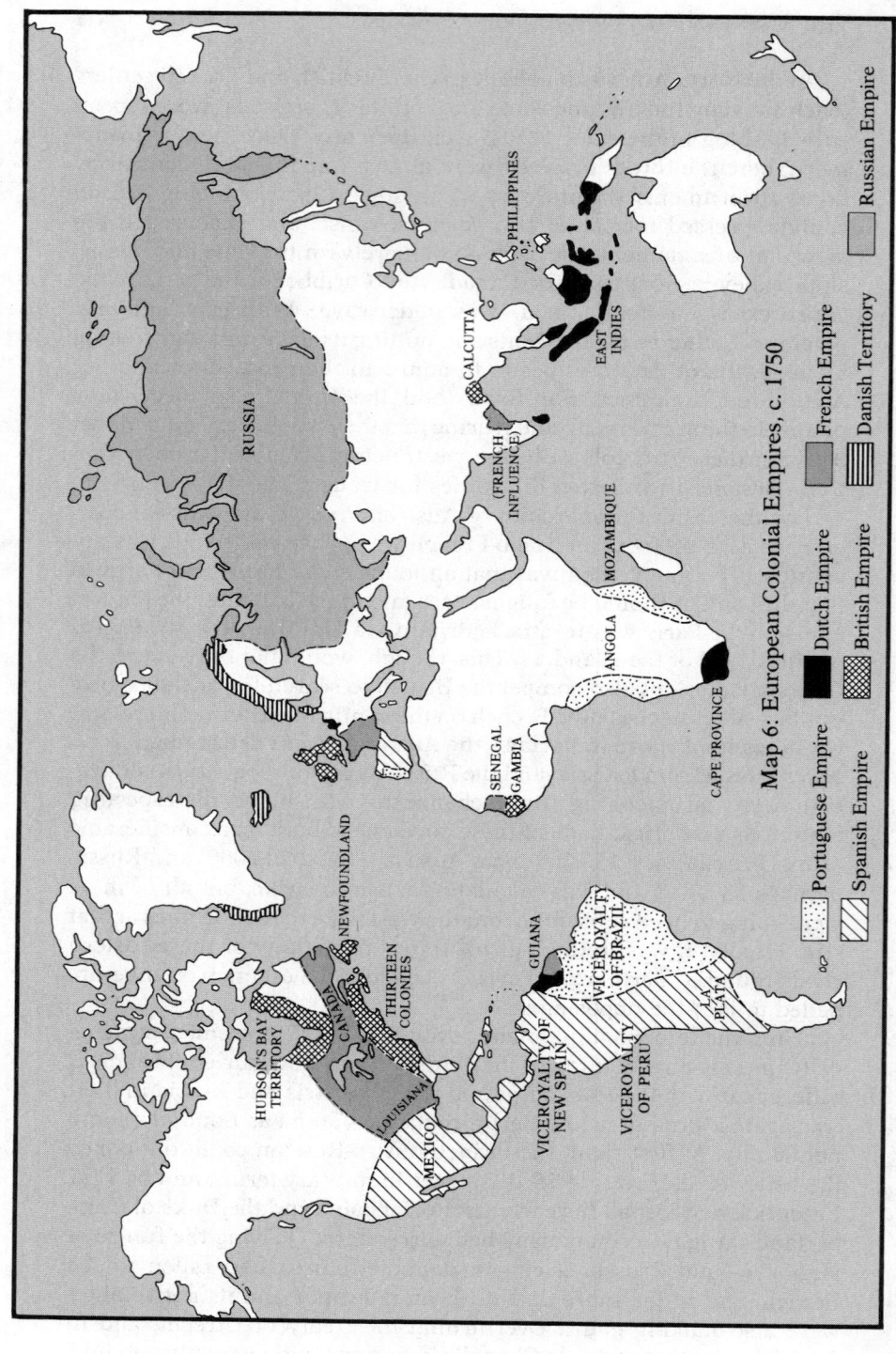

Map 6: European Colonial Empires, c. 1750

RUSSIA

PHILIPPINES

CALCUTTA

EAST
INDIES

(FRENCH
INFLUENCE)

MOZAMBIQUE

ANGOLA

SENEGAL

GAMBIA

CAPE PROVINCE

HUDSON'S BAY
TERRITORY

NEWFOUNDLAND

CANADA

THIRTEEN
COLONIES

LOUISIANA

MEXICO

VICEROYALTY OF
NEW SPAIN

GUIANA

VICEROYALTY
OF BRAZIL

LA
PLATA

VICEROYALTY
OF PERU

Portuguese Empire

Spanish Empire

Dutch Empire

British Empire

French Empire

Danish Territory

Russian Empire

The reason this did not happen was that the Anglo-Prussian combination remained superior in three vital aspects: leadership, financial staying power, and military/naval expertise.[64] Of Frederick's achievement in harnessing the full energies of Prussia to the pursuit of victory and of his generalship on the field of battle there can be no doubt. But the prize goes, perhaps, to Pitt, who after all was not an absolute monarch but merely one of a number of politicians, who had to juggle with touchy and jealous colleagues, a volatile public, and then a new king, and simultaneously pursue an effective grand strategy. And the measure of that effectiveness could not simply be in sugar islands seized or French-backed nabobs toppled, because all these colonial gains, however valuable, would be only temporary if the foe occupied Hanover and eliminated Prussia. The correct way to a decisive victory, as Pitt gradually realized, was to complement the popular "maritime" strategy with a "continental" one, providing large-scale subsidies to Frederick's own forces and paying for a considerable "Army of Observation" in Germany, to protect Hanover and help contain the French.

But such a policy was in turn very dependent upon having sufficient resources to survive year after year of grinding warfare. Frederick and his tax officials used every device to raise monies in Prussia, but Prussia's capacity paled by comparison with Britain's, which at the height of the struggle possessed a fleet of over 120 ships of the line, had more than 200,000 soldiers (including German mercenaries) on its pay lists, and was also subsidizing Prussia. In fact, the Seven Years War cost the Exchequer over £160 million, of which £60 million (37 percent) was raised on the money markets. While this further great rise in the national debt was to alarm Pitt's colleagues and contribute to his downfall in October 1761, nevertheless the overseas trade of the country increased in every year, bringing enhanced customs receipts and prosperity. Here was an excellent example of profit being converted into power, and of British sea power being used (e.g., in the West Indies) for national profit. As the British ambassador to Prussia was informed, "we must be merchants before we are soldiers. . . . trade and maritime force depend upon each other, and . . . the riches which are the true resources of this country depend upon its commerce."[65] By contrast, the economies of all the other combatants suffered heavily in this war, and even inside France the minister Choiseul had ruefully to admit that

> in the present state of Europe it is colonies, trade and in consequence sea power, which must determine the balance of power upon the continent. The House of Austria, Russia, the King of Prussia are only powers of the second rank, as are all those which cannot go to war unless subsidized by the trading powers.[66]

The military and naval expertise displayed by the Anglo-Prussian alliance, at least after the early setbacks, worked in the following way. At sea an enormous Royal Navy under Anson's direction steadily imposed a blockade upon France's Atlantic ports, and had sufficient surplus of force to mask Toulon and regain maritime supremacy in the Mediterranean as well. When fleet actions did occur—at Cartagena, off Lagos, and in Hawke's incomparable gale-battered pursuit of Conflans's fleet into Quiberon Bay—the superiority of British seamanship was made manifest time and again. What was more, this blockading policy—maintained now in all weathers, with the squadrons supplied by a comprehensive provisioning system—not only throttled much of France's maritime trade and thus protected Britain's commerce and its territorial security, but also prevented adequate reinforcements of French troops being sent to the West Indies, Canada, and India. In 1759, the *annus mirabilis*, French colonies were falling into British hands right across the globe, nicely complementing the considerable victory of the Anglo-German troops over two French armies at Minden. When Spain foolishly entered the war in 1762, the same fate befell its colonies in the Caribbean and Philippines.

Meanwhile, the House of Brandenburg had already seen its share of "miracles," and in the battles of Rossbach and Leuthen, Frederick not only ruined a French and an Austrian army respectively, but also blunted the eagerness of those two nations to press into northern Germany; after Frederick caught the Austrians again, at Liegnitz and Torgau in 1760, Vienna was virtually bankrupt. Nevertheless, the sheer costs of all this campaigning were slowly grinding down Prussian power (60,000 soldiers lost in 1759 alone), and the Russian foe proved much more formidable—partly because of Czarina Elizabeth's hatred of Frederick but chiefly because each encounter with the Russian army was such a bloody affair. Yet with the other combatants feeling the pace as well, and France keen to come to terms with a British government now also disposed to peace, Prussia found that it still had enough strength to keep the Austrians and Russians at bay until rescued by Elizabeth's death in 1762. After this, and the new Czar Peter's swift withdrawal from the war, neither Austria nor France could expect anything better than a peace settlement on the basis of a return to the prewar status in Europe—which was, in effect, a defeat for those who had sought to bring Prussia down.

In the 1762–1763 settlements the one obvious beneficiary was again Great Britain. Even after returning various captured territories to France and Spain, it had made advances in the West Indies and West Africa, had virtually eliminated French influence from India, and, most important of all, was now supreme in most of the North American continent. Britain thus had access to lands of far greater extent and potential wealth than Lorraine, Silesia, and those other regions over which the continental states fought so bitterly. In addition, it had helped to check France's diplomatic and military ambitions inside Europe and thereby had preserved the general balance of power. France, by comparison, had not only lost disastrously overseas but had also—unlike in 1748—failed in Europe; indeed, its lackluster military performance suggested that the center of gravity had shifted from western Europe to the east, a fact confirmed by the general disregard of France's wishes during the first partition of Poland in 1772. All this nicely suited British circles, satisfied with their own primacy outside Europe and not eager to be drawn into obligations on the continent.

The Winning of Wars, 1763–1815

The "breathing space" of well over a decade which occurred before the next stage in the Anglo-French struggle gave only a few hints of the turnaround which would occur in British fortunes. The Seven Years War had so overstrained the taxable capacity and social fabric of the Great Powers that most leaders frowned upon a bold foreign policy; introspection and reform tended to be the order of the day. The cost of the war to Prussia (half a million dead, including 180,000 soldiers) had shocked Frederick, who now preferred a quieter life. Although it had lost 300,000 men, the Habsburg Empire's army itself had not done too badly; but the overall governmental system was obviously in need of changes which would doubtless arouse local resentments (especially among the Hungarians) and consume the attentions of Maria Theresa's ministers. In Russia, Catherine II had to grapple with legislative and administrative reforms and then suppress the Pugachev revolt (1773–1775). This did not prevent further Russian expansion in the south or the maneuvers to reduce Poland's independence; but those could still be classed as local issues, and quite distinct from the great *European* combinations which had preoccupied the powers during the Seven Years War. Links with the western monarchies were now less important.

In Britain and France, too, domestic affairs held the center of the stage. The horrendous rise in the national debts of both countries led to a search for fresh sources of revenue and for administrative reform, producing controversies which fueled the already poor relations between George III and the opposition, and between the crown and *parlements* in France. These preoccupations inevitably made British foreign policy in Europe more haphazard and introspective than in Pitt's day, a tendency increased by the rising quarrel with the American colonists over taxation and enforcement of the Acts of Trade and Navigation. On the French side, however, foreign-policy matters were not so fully eclipsed by domestic concerns. Indeed, Choiseul and his successors, smarting from the defeat of 1763, were taking measures to strengthen France's position for the future. The French navy was steadily built up, despite the pressing need to economize; and the "family compact" with Spain was deepened. It is true that Louis XV frowned upon Choiseul's strong encouragement of Spain against Britain in the 1770 clash over the Falkland Islands, since a Great Power war at that point would have been financially disastrous. Nonetheless, French policy remained distinctly anti-British and committed to extracting advantages from any problems which Britain might encounter overseas.[67]

All this meant that when London's quarrel with the American colonists turned into open hostilities, Britain was in a much weaker position, in so many respects, than in 1739 or 1756.[68] A great deal of this was due to personalities. Neither North, nor Shelburne, nor any of the other politicians could offer national leadership and a coherent grand strategy. Political faction, heightened by George III's own interventions and by a fierce debate on the merits of the American colonists' case, divided the nation. In addition, the twin props of British power—the economy and the navy—were eroded in these years. Exports, which had stagnated following the boom period of the Seven Years War, actually declined throughout the 1770s, in part because of the colonists' boycott and then because of the growing conflict with France, Spain, and the Netherlands. The Royal Navy had been systematically weakened during fifteen years of peace, and some of its flag officers were as unseasoned as the timbers which had gone into the building of the ships of the line. The decision to abandon the close blockade strategy when France entered the war in 1778 may have saved wear and tear on British vessels, but it was, in effect, surrendering command of the sea: relief expeditions to Gibraltar, the West Indies, and the North American coast were no real substitute for the effective control of the Western Approaches off the French coast, which would have prevented the dispatch of enemy fleets to those distant theaters in any case. By the time the Royal Navy's strength had been rebuilt and its dominance reasserted, by Rodney's victory at the Saints and Howe's relief of Gibraltar in 1782, the war in America was virtually over.

Yet even if the navy had been better equipped and the nation better led, the 1776–1783 conflict contained two strategical problems which simply did not exist in any of the other eighteenth-century wars fought by Britain. The first of these was that once the American rebellion spread, its suppression involved large-scale *continental* fighting by British forces at a distance of 3,000 miles from the home base. Contrary to London's early hopes, maritime superiority alone could not bring the largely self-sufficient colonists to their knees (though obviously it might have reduced the flow of weapons and recruits from Europe). To conquer and hold the entire eastern territories of America

would have been a difficult task for Napoleon's Grand Army, let alone
the British-led troops of the 1770s. The distances involved and the
consequent delay in communications not only hampered the strategical direction of the war from London or even from New York, but also
exacerbated the logistical problem: "every biscuit, man, and bullet
required by the British forces in America had to be transported across
3,000 miles of ocean."[69] Despite significant improvements by the British war ministry, the shortages of shipping and the difficulties of procurement were simply too much. Moreover, colonial society was so
decentralized that the capture of a city or large town meant little. Only
when regular troops were in occupation of the territory in question
could British authority prevail; whenever they were withdrawn, the
rebels reasserted themselves over the loyalists. If it had taken 50,000
British soldiers, *with substantial colonial support,* to conquer French
Canada two decades earlier, how many were needed now to reimpose
imperial rule—150,000, perhaps 250,000? "It is probable," one historian has argued, "that to restore British authority in America was a
problem beyond the power of military means to solve, however perfectly applied."[70]

The second unprecedented difficulty in the realm of grand strategy
was that Britain fought alone, unaided by European partners who
would distract the French. To a large degree, of course, this was a
diplomatic rather than a military problem. The British were now paying for their break with Prussia after 1762, their arrogance toward
Spain, their heavy-handed treatment of the shipping of neutral states
like Denmark and the United Provinces, and their failure to secure
Russian support. Thus London found itself not only friendless in
Europe but also, by 1780, facing a suspicious League of Armed Neutrality (Russia, Denmark, Portugal) and a hostile United Provinces, while
it was already overstretched in dealing with American rebels and the
Franco-Spanish fleets. But there is more to this story than British
diplomatic ineptitude. As noted above, during the 1760s and 1770s the
interests of the eastern monarchies had become somewhat detached
from those in the West, and were concentrated upon the future of
Poland, the Bavarian succession, and relations with the Turks. A
France intent upon becoming "arbiter of Europe," as in Louis XIV's
day, might have made such detachment impossible; but the relative
decline of its army after the Seven Years War and its lack of political
engagement in the east meant that London's acute concern about
French designs from 1779 onward was not shared by former allies. The
Russians under Catherine II were probably the most sympathetic, but
even they would not intervene unless there was a real prospect that
Britain would be eliminated altogether.

Finally, there was the significant fact that for once France had
adopted Choiseul's former argument and now resisted the temptation

to attack Hanover or to bully the Dutch. The war against Britain would be fought *only* overseas, thus dislocating the "continental" from the "maritime" arm of traditional British strategy. For the first time ever, the French would concentrate their resources upon a naval and colonial war.

The results were remarkable, and quite confounded the argument of the British isolationists that such a conflict, unencumbered by continental allies and campaigns, was best for the island state. During the Seven Years War, the French navy had been allocated only 30 million livres a year, one-quarter of the French army's allocation and only one-fifth of the monies provided to the Royal Navy each year. From the mid-1770s onward, the French naval budget steadily rose; by 1780 it totaled about 150 million livres, and by 1782 it had reached a staggering 200 million livres.[71] At the time France entered the war, it possessed fifty-two ships of the line, many of them being larger than their British equivalents, and the number was soon increased to sixty-six. To this could be added the Spanish fleet of fifty-eight ships of the line and, in 1780, a Dutch fleet of not more than twenty effectives. While the Royal Navy remained superior to any one maritime rival (in 1778 it had sixty-six ships of the line; in 1779, ninety), it now found itself repeatedly outnumbered. In 1779 it even lost control of the Channel, and a Franco-Spanish invasion looked possible; and in the 1781 encountered between Graves's and de Grasse's fleets off the Chesapeake, French numerical superiority kept the British force at bay and thus led to Cornwallis's surrender at Yorktown and to the effective end of the American campaign. Even when the Royal Navy's size increased and that of its foes fell away (in 1782 it had ninety-four ships of the line to France's seventy-three, Spain's fifty-four, and the United Provinces' nineteen), the margin was still too narrow to do *all* the tasks required: protect the North Atlantic convoys, periodically relieve Gibraltar, guard the exit from the Baltic, send squadrons to the Indian Ocean, and support the military operations in the Caribbean. British naval power was temporary and regional and not, as in previous wars, overwhelming. The fact that the French army was not fighting in Europe had a lot to do with the islanders' unhappy condition.

By 1782, it is true, the financial strain of maintaining such a large navy was hitting the French economy and compelling some retrenchment. Naval stores were now more difficult to obtain, and the shortage of sailors was even more serious. In addition, some of the French ministers feared that the war was unduly diverting attention and resources to areas outside Europe, and thus making it impossible to play any role on the continent. This political calculation, and the parallel fear that the British and Americans might soon settle their differences, caused Paris to hope for an early end to hostilities. Economically, their Dutch and Spanish allies were in an equally bad plight. Nevertheless,

Britain's greater financial stamina, the marked rise in exports from 1782 onward, and the steady improvements in the Royal Navy could not now rescue victory from defeat, nor convince the political factions at home to support the war once America was clearly seen to be lost. Although Britain's concessions at the 1783 Peace of Versailles (Minorca, Florida, Tobago) were hardly a reversal of the great imperial gains of 1763, the French could proclaim themselves well satisfied at the creation of an independent United States and at the blow dealt to Britain's world position. From Paris's perspective, the strategical balance which had been upset by the Seven Years War had now been sensibly restored, albeit at enormous cost.

In eastern Europe, by contrast, the strategical balances were not greatly distorted by the maneuvers of the three great monarchies during the decades after 1763.[72] This was chiefly due to the triangular nature of that relationship: neither Berlin nor Vienna in particular, nor even the more assertive St. Petersburg, wished to provoke the other two into a hostile alliance or to be involved in fighting of the dimensions of the Seven Years War. The brief and ultracautious campaigning in the War of Bavarian Succession (1778–1779), when Prussia opposed Austria's attempt at expansion, merely confirmed this widespread wish to avoid the costs of a Great Power struggle. Further acquisitions of territory could therefore take place only as a result of diplomatic "deals" at the expense of weaker powers, most notably Poland, which was successively carved up in 1772–1773, 1793, and 1795. By the later stages, Poland's fate was increasingly influenced by the French Revolution, that is, by Catherine II's determination to crush the "Jacobins" of Warsaw, and Prussia and Austria's desire to gain compensation in the east for their failures in the west against France; but even this new concern with the French Revolution did not fundamentally change the policies of mutual antagonism and reluctant compromise which the three eastern monarchies pursued toward one another in these years.

Given the geographical and diplomatic confines of this triangular relationship, it was not surprising that Russia's position continued to improve, relative to both Austria and Prussia. Despite Russia's backwardness, it was still far less vulnerable than its western neighbors, both of which strove to placate the formidable Catherine. This fact, and the traditional Russian claims to influence in Poland, ensured that by far the largest portion of that unfortunate state fell to St. Petersburg during the partition. Moreover, Russia possessed an open, "crumbling" frontier to the south, so that during the early 1770s great advances were made at Turkey's expense; the Crimea was formally annexed in 1783, and a fresh round of gains was secured along the northern coast of the Black Sea in 1792. All this confirmed the decline of Ottoman fighting power, and secretly worried both Austria and Prussia almost as much as those states (Sweden in 1788, Britain under the younger Pitt in 1791) which more actively sought to blunt this Russian expansionism. But with Vienna and Berlin eager to keep St. Petersburg's goodwill, and with the western Powers too distracted to play a lasting and effective role in eastern Europe, the growth of the Czarist Empire proceeded apace.

The structure of international relations in the decade or so prior to 1792 therefore gave little sign of the transformation bearing down upon it. For the main part, the occasional quarrels between the major powers had been unconnected regional affairs, and there seemed to exist no threat to the general balance of power. If the future of Poland and the Ottoman Empire preoccupied the great nations of the east, traditional maneuvering over the fate of the Low Countries and over "rival empires of trade" consumed the attention of the western Powers. An Anglo-Spanish clash over Nookta Sound (1790) brought both countries to the brink of war, until Spain reluctantly gave way. While relations between Britain and France were more subdued because of mutual exhaustion after 1783, their commercial rivalry continued apace. Their mutual suspicions also swiftly showed themselves during an internal crisis in the Netherlands in 1787–1788, when the pro-French "Patriot" party was forced out of power by Prussian troops, urged on by the assertive younger Pitt.

Pitt's much more active diplomacy reflected not merely his own personality, but also the significant general recovery which Britain had made in the ranks of the Powers since the setback of 1783. The loss of America had not damaged the country's transatlantic trade; indeed, exports to the United States were booming, and both that market and India's were much more substantial than those in which France had the lead. In the six years 1782–1788 British merchant shipping more than doubled. The Industrial Revolution was under way, fired by consumer demand at home and abroad and facilitated by a spate of new inventions; and the productivity of British agriculture was keeping pace with the food needs of an expanding population. Pitt's fiscal reforms improved the state's finances and restored its credit, yet considerable monies were always voted to the navy, which was numerically strong and well administered. On these firm foundations, the British government felt it could play a more active role abroad when national interests demanded it. On the whole, however, political leaders in Whitehall and Westminster did not envisage a Great Power war occurring in Europe in the foreseeable future.[73]

But the clearest reason why Europe would not be convulsed by a general conflict seemed to lie in the worsening condition of France. For some years after the victory of 1783, its diplomatic position had appeared as strong as ever; the domestic economy, as well as foreign trade with the West Indies and the Levant, was growing rapidly.

Nonetheless, the sheer costs of the 1778–1783 war—totaling more than France's three previous wars together—and the failure to reform national finances interacted with the growing political discontents, economic distress, and social malaise to discredit the *ancien régime*. From 1787 onward, as the internal crisis worsened, France seemed ever less capable of playing a decisive role in foreign affairs. The diplomatic defeat in the Netherlands was caused primarily by the French government's recognition that it simply could not afford to finance a war against Britain and Prussia, while the withdrawal of support for Spain in the Nootka Sound controversy was due to the French assembly's challenge to Louis XVI's right to declare war. All this hardly suggested that France would soon be seeking to overturn the entire "old order" of Europe.

The conflict which was to absorb the energies of much of the continent for over two decades therefore began slowly and unevenly. The French were concerned only with domestic struggles in the period which followed the fall of the Bastille; and although the increasing radicalization of French politics worried some foreign governments, the resultant turmoil in Paris and the provinces suggested that France was of little account in European power politics. For that reason, Pitt was seeking reductions in British military expenditures as late as February 1792, while in the east the three great monarchies were much more interested in the carving up of Poland. Only with the growing rumors about émigré plots to restore the monarchy and the French revolutionaries' own move toward a more aggressive policy on the borders did external and internal events produce an escalation into war. The slow and uncertain maneuvers of the allied armies as they moved across the French frontiers showed how ill prepared they were for this contest, which in turn allowed the revolutionaries to claim victory after the desultory encounter at Valmy (September 1792). It was only in the following year, when the successes of the French armies seemed to threaten the Rhineland, the Low Countries, and Italy and the execution of Louis XVI demonstrated the radical republicanism of the new regime in Paris, that the struggle assumed its full strategical and ideological dimensions. Prussia and the Habsburg Empire, the original combatants, were now joined by an enormous array of other states headed by Britain and Russia and including all of France's neighbors.

Although it is easy in retrospect to see why this First Coalition (1793–1795) against France failed so miserably, the outcome was a surprise and bitter disappointment at the time; after all, the odds were more uneven than in *any* preceding war. In the event, the sheer impetus of the French Revolution led to the adoption of desperate measures—the *levée en masse* and the mobilization of all seizable national resources to fight France's many foes. Moreover, as many writers have pointed out, a very important period of reform had occurred in the French army—in matters of organization, staff planning, artillery, and battle tactics—during the two or three decades before 1789; and what the Revolution did was to sweep aside the aristocratic hindrances to these new ideas and to give the reformers the opportunity (and the weight of numbers) to put their concepts into practice when war broke out. The "total war" methods employed on the home front and the newer tactics on the battlefield seemed as much a reflection of the newly released demagogic energies of the French as the cautious, half-hearted maneuvers of the Coalition armies were symbolic of the habits of the old order.[74] With an army of about 650,000 (July 1793), fired by enthusiasm and willing to take the risks involved in lengthy marches and aggressive tactics, the French were soon overrunning neighboring territories—which meant that from this time onward, the costs of maintaining such an enormous force fell largely upon the populations *outside* France's borders, which in its turn permitted a certain recovery of the French economy.

Any power seeking to blunt this heady expansionism would therefore have to devise the proper means for containing such a new and upsetting form of warfare. This was not an impossible task. The French army's operations under its early leader Dumouriez, and even the much larger and more elaborate campaigns of Napoleon, revealed deficiencies in organization and training and weaknesses in supply and communications, of which a well-trained foe could take great advantage. But where was that well-trained opponent? It was not merely that the elderly generals and slow-moving, baggage-laden troops of the Coalition were tactically inadequate in the face of swarms of skirmishers and hard-hitting columns of the French. The real point was that the necessary political commitment and strategical clarity were also missing among France's enemies. There was, obviously, no transcendent political ideology to fire the soldiers and citizens of the *ancien régime;* indeed, many of them were attracted to the intoxicating ideas of the Revolution, and only when, much later, Napoleon's armies turned "liberation" into conquest and plunder could local patriotism be used to blunt the French hegemony.

Furthermore, at this early stage few members of the Coalition took the French threat seriously. There was no overall agreement as to aims and strategy between the various members of the alliance, whose precarious unity manifested itself in their increasing demands for British subsidies but in not much else. Above all, the first years of the Revolutionary War overlapped with, and were overshadowed by, the demise of Poland. Despite her vitriolic denunciations of the French Revolution, Catherine II was more concerned with eliminating Polish independence than in sending troops to the Rhineland. This caused an anxious Prussian government, already disenchanted by the early campaigns in the west, to switch more and more of its troops from the Rhine to the Vistula, which in turn compelled Austria to keep 60,000 men on its northern frontier in case Russia and Prussia moved against the remaining Polish territories. When the third and final partition did occur, in 1795, it was all too evident that Poland had been a more effective ally to France in its death throes than as a living, functioning state. By that time, Prussia had already sued for peace and abandoned the left bank of the Rhine to the French, leaving Germany in a state of uneasy neutrality and thus permitting France to turn its attention elsewhere; most of the smaller German states had followed this Prussian lead; the Netherlands had been overrun, and converted into the Batavian Republic; and Spain, too, deserting the Coalition, had returned to its early anti-British alignment with France.

This left only Sardinia-Piedmont, which in early 1796 was crushed by Napoleon; the luckless Habsburg Empire, which was driven out of much of Italy and forced into the Peace of Campo Formio (October 1797); and Britain. Despite the younger Pitt's wish to imitate his father in checking French expansionism, the British government also failed to pursue the war with the necessary determination and strategical clarity.[75] The expeditionary force sent to Flanders and Holland under the Duke of York in 1793–1795 had neither the strength nor the expertise to deal with the French army, and its remnants eventually came home via Bremen. Moreover, as so often happened before and since, ministers (such as Dundas and Pitt) preferred the "British way in warfare"—colonial operations, maritime blockade, and raids upon the enemy's coast—to any large-scale continental operation. Given the overwhelming superiority of the Royal Navy and the disintegration of its French equivalent, this looked like an attractive and easy option. But the British troop losses caused by disease in the West Indies operations of 1793–1796 meant that London paid dearly for these strategical diversions: 40,000 men were killed, another 40,000 rendered unfit for service—more than all the casualties in the Spanish Peninsular War—and the campaigns cost at least £16 million. Yet it is doubtful whether Britain's steadily augmented domination of the extra-European theaters or its peripheral operations against Dunkirk and Toulon compensated for France's growing power within Europe. Finally, the subsidies demanded by Prussia and Austria to maintain their armies in the field soared alarmingly, and were impossible to provide. In other words, British strategy had been simultaneously inefficient *and* expensive, and in 1797 the foundations of the entire system were shaken—at least temporarily—by the Bank of England's suspension of cash payments and by the naval mutinies at Spithead and the Nore. During that troubled period, the exhausted Austrians sued for peace and joined all the other states which admitted French primacy in western Europe.

If the British could not defeat France, the revolutionary govern-

ment could not in its turn undermine the enemy's naval mastery. Early
attempts to invade Ireland and to raid the western coasts of England
had come to little, although that was due as much to the weather as to
local defenses. Despite the temporary fright over the 1797 suspension
of cash payments, the British credit system held firm. The entry of
Spain and the Netherlands into the war on France's side led to the
smashing of the Spanish fleet off Cape St. Vincent (February 1797) and
to the heavy blows inflicted upon the Dutch at Camperdown (October
1797). France's new allies also had to endure the progressive loss of
their colonies overseas—in the East and West Indies, and at Colombo,
Malacca, and the Cape of Good Hope, all of which provided new markets for British commerce and additional bases for its naval squadrons. Unwilling to pay the high price demanded by the French
government for peace, Pitt and his fellow ministers resolved to fight
on, introducing income tax as well as raising fresh loans to pay for
what—with French troops assembling along the Channel coast—had
become a struggle as much for national survival as for imperial security.

Here, then, was the fundamental strategical dilemma which faced
both France and Britain for the next two decades of war. Like the
whale and the elephant, each was by far the largest creature in its own
domain. But British control of the sea routes could not by itself destroy
the French hegemony in Europe, nor could Napoleon's military mastery reduce the islanders to surrender. Furthermore, because France's
territorial acquisitions and political browbeating of its neighbors
aroused considerable resentment, the government in Paris could never
be certain that the other continental powers would permanently accept
the French imperium so long as Britain—offering subsidies, munitions, and possibly even troops—remained independent. This, evidently, was also Napoleon's view when he argued in 1797: "Let us
concentrate our efforts on building up our fleet and on destroying
England. Once that is done Europe is at our feet."[76] Yet that French
goal could be achieved only by waging a successful maritime and
commercial strategy against Britain, since military gains on land were
not enough; just as the British needed to challenge Napoleon's continental domination—by direct intervention and securing allies—since
the Royal Navy's mastery at sea was also not enough. As long as the
one combatant was supreme on land and the other at sea, each felt
threatened and insecure; and each therefore cast around for fresh
means, and allies, with which to tilt the balance.

Napoleon's attempt to alter that balance was characteristically
bold—and risky: taking advantage of Britain's weak position in the
Mediterranean in the summer of 1798, he invaded Egypt with 31,000
troops and thus placed himself in a position to dominate the Levant,
the Ottoman Empire, and the route to India. At almost the same time,

the British were distracted by yet another French expedition to Ireland. Each of those strokes, had they been fully successful, would have dealt a dreadful blow to Britain's shaky position. But the Irish invasion was small-scale and belated, and was contained in early September, by which time all of Europe was learning of Nelson's defeat of the French fleet at Aboukir and of Napoleon's consequent "bondage" in Egypt. Just as Paris had suspected, such a setback encouraged all who resented French predominance to abandon their neutrality and to join in the war of the Second Coalition (1798–1800). Besides the smaller states of Portugal and Naples, Russia, Austria, and Turkey were now on the British side, assembling their armies and negotiating for subsidies. Losing Minorca and Malta, defeated in Switzerland and Italy by Austro-Russian forces, and with Napoleon himself unable to achieve victory in the Levant, France appeared to be in serious trouble.

Yet the second coalition, like the first, rested upon shaky political and strategical foundations.[77] Prussia was noticeably absent, so that no northern German front could be opened. A premature campaign by the king of Naples led to disaster, and an ill-prepared Anglo-Russian expedition to Holland failed to arouse the local population and eventually had to retire. Far from drawing the conclusion that continental operations needed to be more substantial, and acutely conscious of the financial and political difficulties of raising a large army, the British government fell back upon its traditional policy of "descents" upon the enemy's coastline; but their small-scale attacks upon Belle-Isle, Ferrol, Cádiz, and elsewhere served no useful strategical purpose. Worse still, the Austrians and Russians failed to cooperate in their defense of Switzerland, and the Russians were driven eastward through the mountains; at that, the czar's disenchantment with his allies intensified into a deep suspicion of British policy and a willingness to negotiate with Napoleon, who had slipped back into France from Egypt. The withdrawal of Russia left the Austrians to receive the full weight of the French fury, at Marengo and Hochstadt (both in June 1800), and six months later at Hohenlinden, compelling Vienna once again to sue for peace. With Prussia and Denmark taking advantage of this turn of events to overrun Hanover, and with Spain launching an invasion of Portugal, the British stood virtually alone in 1801, just as they had been three years earlier. In northern Europe, Russia, Denmark, Sweden, and Prussia had come together in a new Armed Neutrality League.

In the maritime and extra-European campaigning, on the other hand, the British had again done rather well. Malta had been captured from the French, providing the Royal Navy with a vital strategical base. The Danish fleet, the first line of the new Armed Neutrality League's scheme to exclude British trade from the Baltic, was smashed off Copenhagen (although the assassination of Czar Paul a few days earlier spelled the end of the league in any case). In that same month of March 1801 a British expedition defeated the French army at Alexandria, which afterward led to a complete French withdrawal from Egypt. Farther afield, British forces in India overwhelmed the French-backed Tipu in Mysore and continued to make additional gains in the north. French, Dutch, Danish, and Swedish possessions in the West Indies also fell into British hands.

Yet the lack of a solid continental ally by 1801 and the inconclusive nature of the Anglo-French campaigning caused many politicians in England to think of peace; and those sentiments were reinforced by the urgings of mercantile circles whose commerce was suffering in the Mediterranean and, to a lesser extent, in the Baltic. Pitt's resignation over Catholic emancipation hastened the move toward negotiations. In Napoleon's calculation, there was little to be lost from a period of peace: the consolidation of French influence in the satellite states would continue, while the British would certainly not be allowed their former commercial and diplomatic privileges in those areas; the French navy, dispersed in various ports, could be concentrated and rebuilt; and the economy could be rested before the next round of the struggle. In consequence of this, British opinion—which did not offer much criticism of the government at the conclusion of the Peace of Amiens (March 1802)—steadily swung in the other direction when it was observed that France was continuing the struggle by other means. British trade was denied entry into much of Europe. London was firmly told to keep out of Dutch, Swiss, and Italian matters. And French intrigues and aggressions were reported from Muscat to the West Indies and from Turkey to Piedmont. These reports, and the evidence of a large-scale French warship-building program, caused the British government under Addington to refuse to hand back Malta and, in May 1803, to turn a cold war into a hot one.[78]

This final round of the seven major Anglo-French wars fought between 1689 and 1815 was to last twelve years, and was the most severely testing of them all. Just as before, each combatant had different strengths and weaknesses. Despite certain retrenchments in the fleet, the Royal Navy was in a very strong position when hostilities recommenced. While powerful squadrons blockaded the French coast, the overseas empires of France and its satellites were systematically recaptured. St. Pierre et Miquelon, St. Lucia, Tobago, and Dutch Guiana were taken before Trafalgar, and further advances were made in India; the Cape fell in 1806; Curaçao and the Danish West Indies in 1807; several of the Moluccas in 1808; Cayenne, French Guiana, San Domingo, Senegal, and Martinique in 1809; Guadeloupe, Mauritius, Amboina, and Banda in 1810; Java in 1811. Once again, this had no *direct* impact upon the European equilibrium, but it did buttress Britain's dominance overseas and provide new "vents" for exports denied their traditional access into Antwerp and Leghorn; and, even in its early stages, it prompted Napoleon to contemplate the invasion of southern England more seriously than ever before. With the Grand Army assembling before Boulogne and a grimly determined Pitt returned to office in 1804, each side looked forward to one final, decisive clash.

In actual fact, the naval and military campaigns of 1805 to 1808, despite containing several famous battles, revealed yet again the strategical constraints of the war. The French army was at least three times larger and much more experienced than its British equivalent, but command of the sea was required before it could safely land in England. Numerically, the French navy was considerable (about seventy ships of the line), a testimony to the resources which Napoleon could command; and it was reinforced by the Spanish navy (over twenty ships of the line) when that country entered the war late in 1804. However, the Franco-Spanish fleets were dispersed in half a dozen harbors, and their juncture could not be effected without running the risk of encountering a Royal Navy of vastly greater battle experience. The smashing defeat of those fleets at Trafalgar in October 1805 illustrated the "quality gap" between the rival navies in the most devastating way. Yet if that dramatic victory secured the British Isles, it could not undermine Napoleon's position on land. For this reason, Pitt had striven to tempt Russia and Austria into a third coalition, paying £1.75 million for every 100,000 men they could put into the field against the French. Even before Trafalgar, however, Napoleon had rushed his army from Boulogne to the upper Danube, annihilating the Austrians at Ulm, and then proceeded eastward to crush an Austro-Russian force of 85,000 men at Austerlitz in December. With a dispirited Vienna suing for peace for the third time, the French could once again assert control in the Italian peninsula and compel a hasty withdrawal of the Anglo-Russian forces there.[79]

Whether or not the news of these great blows caused Pitt's death in early 1806, they revealed once more the difficulty of bringing down a military genius like Napoleon. Indeed, the following few years ushered in the zenith of French predominance in Europe. (See Map 7.) Prussia, whose earlier abstention had weakened the coalition, rashly declared war upon France in October 1806 and was crushed within the month. The large and stubborn Russian armies were an altogether different matter, but after several battles they, too, were badly hurt at the battle of Friedland (June 1807). At the peace treaties of Tilsit, Prussia was turned into a virtual satellite and Russia, while escaping lightly, agreed to ban British trade and promised eventually to join a French alliance. With southern and much of western Germany merged into the Confederation of the Rhine, with western Poland turned into the grand duchy of Warsaw, with Spain, Italy, and the Low Countries subservient, with

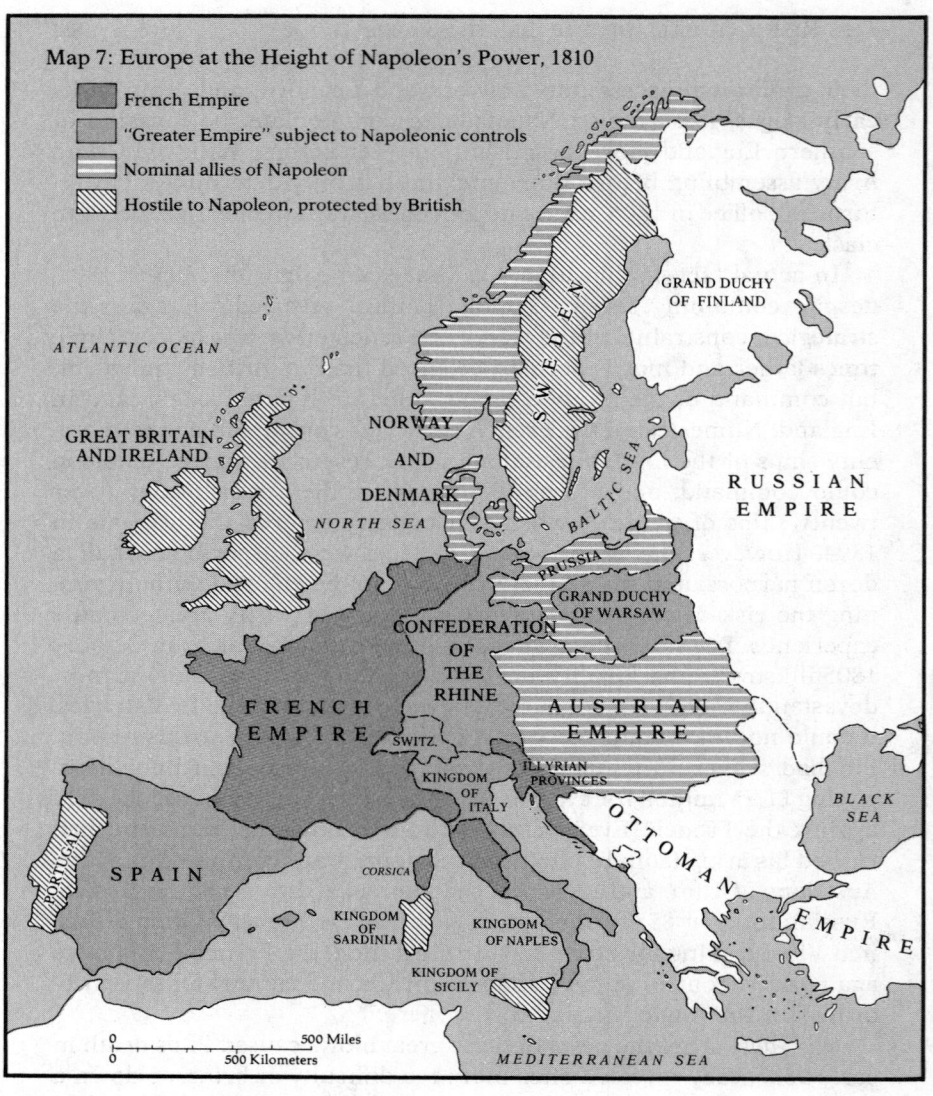

Map 7: Europe at the Height of Napoleon's Power, 1810

French Empire

"Greater Empire" subject to Napoleonic controls

Nominal allies of Napoleon

Hostile to Napoleon, protected by British

ATLANTIC OCEAN

GRAND DUCHY OF FINLAND

NORWAY AND DENMARK

SWEDEN

BALTIC SEA

RUSSIAN EMPIRE

GREAT BRITAIN AND IRELAND

NORTH SEA

PRUSSIA

GRAND DUCHY OF WARSAW

CONFEDERATION OF THE RHINE

FRENCH EMPIRE

SWITZ.

KINGDOM OF ITALY

AUSTRIAN EMPIRE

ILLYRIAN PROVINCES

BLACK SEA

PORTUGAL

SPAIN

CORSICA

KINGDOM OF SARDINIA

KINGDOM OF NAPLES

OTTOMAN EMPIRE

KINGDOM OF SICILY

0   500 Miles
0   500 Kilometers

MEDITERRANEAN SEA

the Holy Roman Empire at an end, there was no independent state—and no ally for the British—between Portugal and Sweden. This, in its turn, gave Napoleon his opportunity to ruin the "nation of shopkeepers" in the most telling fashion: by banning their exports to Europe and hurting their economy, while accumulating for his own purposes the timber, masts, and other shipbuilding resources now denied to the Royal Navy. Indirectly, the British would be weakened before a further direct assault was mounted. Given Britain's dependence upon European markets for its export industries and upon Baltic masts and Dalmatian oak for its fleet, the threat was immense. Finally, reduced earnings from exports would deny London the currency needed to pay subsidies to any allies and to purchase goods for its own expeditionary armies.

More than ever before, in this war, therefore, economic factors intermeshed with strategy. At this central stage in the Anglo-French duel for supremacy, between Napoleon's Berlin/Milan decrees banning trade with Britain (1806–1807) and the French retreat from Moscow in 1812, the relative merits of the two opposing systems deserve further analysis. With each seeking to ruin the other economically, any significant weaknesses would sooner or later emerge—and have dire power-political consequences.

There is no doubt that Britain's unusually large dependence upon foreign commerce by this time made it very vulnerable to the trading ban imposed under Napoleon's "Continental System."[80] In 1808, and again in 1811–1812, the commercial warfare waged by the French and their more compliant satellites (e.g., the Danes) was producing a crisis in British export trades. Vast stocks of manufactures were piled in warehouses, and the London docks were full to overflowing with colonial produce. Unemployment in the towns and unrest in the counties increased businessmen's fears and caused many economists to call for peace; so, too, did the staggering rise in the national debt. When relations with the United States worsened and exports to that important market tumbled after 1811, the economic pressures seemed almost unbearable.

And yet, in fact, those pressures were borne, chiefly because they were never applied long or consistently enough to take full effect. The revolution in Spain against French hegemony eased the 1808 economic crisis in Britain, just as Russia's break with Napoleon brought relief to the 1811–1812 slump, allowing British goods to pour into the Baltic and northern Europe. Moreover, throughout the entire period large amounts of British manufactures and colonial re-exports were smuggled into the continent, at vast profits and usually with the connivance of bribed local officials; from Heligoland to Salonika, the banned produce traveled in circuitous ways to its eager customers—as it later traveled between Canada and New England during the Anglo-American War of 1812. Finally, the British export economy could also be sustained by the great rise in trade with regions untouched by the Continental System or the American "nonintercourse" policy: Asia, Africa, the West Indies, Latin America (despite all the efforts of local Spanish governors), and the Near East. For all these reasons, and despite serious disruption to British trade in *some* markets for *some* of the time, the overall trend was clear: total exports of British produce rose from £21.7 million (1794–1796) to £37.5 million (1804–1806) to £44.4 million (1814–1816).

The other main reason that the British economy did not crumble in the face of external pressures was that, unfortunately for Napoleon, it was now well into the Industrial Revolution. That these two major historical events interacted with each other in many singular ways is clear: government orders for armaments stimulated the iron, steel, coal, and timber trades, the enormous state spending (estimated at 29 percent of gross national product) affected financial practices, and new export markets boosted production of some factories just as the French "counterblockade" depressed it. Exactly how the Revolutionary and Napoleonic wars affected the growth of the British economy *as a whole* is a complex and controversial topic, still being investigated by historians, many of whom now feel that the earlier notions of the swift pace of British industrialization in these decades are exaggerated. What *is* clear, however, is that the economy grew throughout this period. Pig-iron output, a mere 68,000 tons in 1788, had already soared to 244,000 tons in 1806 and rose further to 325,000 tons in 1811. Cotton, virtually a new industry before the war, expanded stupendously in the next two decades, absorbing ever more machinery, steam power, coal, and labor; by 1815, cotton goods had become Britain's greatest export by far. A vast array of new docks and, inland, new canals, turnpikes, and iron rail tracks improved communications and stimulated further production. Regardless of whether this "boom" would have been even greater without the military and naval struggle against France, the fact remains that British productivity and wealth were still rising fast—and could help to bear the burdens which Pitt and his successors imposed in order to pay for the war. Customs and excise receipts, for example, jumped from £13.5 million (1793) to £44.8 million (1815), while the yield from the new income and property taxes rose from £1.67 in 1799 to £14.6 million in the final year of the war. In fact, between 1793 and 1815 the British government secured the staggering sum of £1.217 billion from direct and indirect taxes, and proceeded to raise a further £440 million in loans from the money markets without exhausting its credit—to the amazement of the more fiscally conservative Napoleon. In the critical final few years of the war, the government was borrowing more than £25 million annually, giving itself that decisive extra margin.[81] To be sure, the British were taxed way beyond the limits conceived of by eighteenth-century bureaucrats, and the national debt almost trebled; but the new wealth made such burdens easier to bear— and permitted them, despite their smaller size and population, to endure the costs of war better than the imposing Napoleonic Empire.

The story of France's economy between 1789 and 1815, and of its capacity to sustain large-scale war, is an even more complicated one for historians to unravel.[82] The collapse of the *ancien régime* and the turmoil which followed undoubtedly caused a reduction in French economic activity for a while. On the other hand, the outpouring of public enthusiasm for the Revolution and the mobilization of national resources to meet foreign enemies led to a staggering increase in the output of cannon, small arms, and other military equipment, which in turn stimulated the iron and textile trades. In addition, some of the economic obstacles of the old order such as internal tariffs were swept away, and Napoleon's own legal and administrative reforms aided the prospects for modernization. Even if the coming of the Consulate and the Empire led to the return of many of the features of the monarchical regime (e.g., reliance upon private bankers), this did not check a steady economic growth fueled naturally by population increases, the stimulus of state spending, enhanced tariff protection, and the introduction of certain new technologies.

Nevertheless, there seems no doubt that the rate of growth in the French economy was much slower than in Britain's. The most profound reason for this was that the agricultural sector, the largest by far, changed very little: for the replacement of the seigneur by his peasants was not, of itself, an *agricultural* revolution; and such widely proclaimed policies as the development of sugar beets (in substitution for British colonial cane sugar) had limited results. Poor communications meant that farmers were still tied to local markets, and little stimulus existed for radical innovations. This conservative frame of mind could also be seen in the nascent industrial sector, where new machinery and large-scale enterprises in, say, iron production were the exception rather than the rule. Significant advances were made, of course, but many of them were under the distorting influence of the war and the British naval blockade. Thus, the cotton industry benefited from the Continental System to the extent that it was protected from superior British competition (not to mention the competition from neutral or satellite states, whose goods were excluded by the high French tariffs); and it also benefited from the enhanced domestic market, since Napoleon's conquests of bordering lands increased the number of "Frenchmen" from 25 million in 1789 to 44 million in 1810. But this was offset by the shortage and high price of raw cotton, and by the slowdown in the introduction of new techniques from England. On the whole,

French industry emerged from the war in a distinctly *less competitive* state because of this protection from foreign rivals.

The impact of the naval blockade increased this turning inward of the French economy.[83] Its Atlantic sector, the fastest-growing in the eighteenth century and (as had been the case in Britain) potentially a key catalyst for industrialization, was increasingly cut off by the Royal Navy. The loss of Santa Domingo in particular was a heavy blow to French Atlantic trade. Other overseas colonies and investments were also lost, and after 1806, even trade via neutral bottoms was halted. Bordeaux was dreadfully hurt. Nantes had its profitable French slave trade reduced to nothing. Even Marseilles, with alternative trading partners in the hinterland and northern Italy, saw its industrial output fall to one-quarter between 1789 and 1813. By contrast, regions in the north and east of France, such as Alsace, enjoyed the comparative security of land-based trade. Yet even if those areas, and people within them like winegrowers and cotton-spinners, profited in their protected environment, the *overall* impact upon the French economy was much less satisfactory. "Deindustrialized" in its Atlantic sector, cut off from much of the outside world, it turned inward to its peasants, its small-town commerce, and its localized, uncompetitive, and relatively small-scale industries.

Given this economic conservatism—and, in some cases, definite evidence of retardation—the ability of the French to finance decades of Great Power war seems all the more remarkable.[84] While the popular mobilization in the early to middle 1790s offers a ready reason, it cannot explain the Napoleonic era proper, when a long-service army of over 500,000 men (needing probably 150,000 new recruits each year) had to be paid for. Military expenditures, already costing at least 462 million francs in 1807, had soared to 817 million francs in 1813. Not surprisingly, the normal revenues could never manage to pay for such outlays. Direct taxes were unpopular at home and therefore could not be substantially raised—which chiefly explains Napoleon's return to duties on tobacco, salt, and the other indirect taxes of the *ancien régime;* but neither they nor the various stamp duties and customs fees could prevent an annual deficit of hundreds of millions of francs. It is true that the creation of the Bank of France, together with a whole variety of other financial devices and institutions, allowed the state to conduct a disguised policy of paper money and thus to keep itself afloat on credit—despite the emperor's proclaimed hostility to raising loans. Yet even that was not enough. The gap could only be filled elsewhere.

To a large if incalculable degree, in fact, Napoleonic imperialism was paid for by plunder. This process had begun internally, with the confiscation and sale of the property of the proclaimed "enemies of the Revolution."[85] When the military campaigns in defense of that revolution had carried the French armies into neighboring lands, it seemed altogether natural that the foreigner should pay for it. War, to put it bluntly, would support war. By confiscations of crown and feudal properties in defeated countries; by spoils taken directly from the enemy's armies, garrisons, museums, and treasuries; by imposing war indemnities in money or in kind; and by quartering French regiments upon satellite states and requiring the latter to supply contingents, Napoleon not only covered his enormous military expenditures, he actually produced considerable profits for France—and himself. The sums acquired by the administrators of this *domaine extraordinaire* in the period of France's zenith were quite remarkable and in some ways foreshadow Nazi Germany's plunder of its satellites and conquered foes during the Second World War. Prussia, for example, had to pay a penalty of 311 million francs after Jena, which was equal to half of the French government's ordinary revenue. At each defeat, the Habsburg Empire was forced to cede territories *and* to pay a large indemnity. In Italy between 1805 and 1812 about half of the taxes raised went to the French. All this had the twin advantage of keeping much of the colossal French army *outside* the homeland, and of protecting the French taxpayer from the full costs of the war. Provided that army under its brilliant leader remained successful, the system seemed invulnerable. It was not surprising, therefore, to hear the emperor frequently asserting:

> My power depends on my glory and my glories on the victories I have won. My power will fail if I do not feed it on new glories and new victories. Conquest has made me what I am and only conquest can enable me to hold my position.[86]

How, then, *could* Napoleon be brought down? Britain alone, lacking the military manpower, could not do it. And an attack upon France by any single continental opponent was always doomed to failure. Prussia's ill-timed entry into the war in 1806 proved that point, although it did not stop the frustrated Austrians from renewing hostilities with France once again, early in 1809; yet while Austria fought with great spirit at the battles of Eckmühl and Aspern, its further losses at Wagram once more compelled Vienna to sue for peace and to cede additional lands to France and its allies. The French successes against Austria had, moreover, followed closely upon Napoleon's drive into Spain to crush the revolt there. Thus it seemed that wherever opposition to the emperor's will arose, it was swiftly dealt with. And although at sea the British showed a similar ruthlessness toward enemies, actual or potential, as in their Copenhagen attack (August 1807), they still tended to fritter away military resources in small-scale raids off southern Italy, in an inept attack upon Buenos Aires, and in the disastrous Walcheren operation in the summer of 1809.[87]

Yet it was precisely when Napoleon's system seemed unbeatable that the first significant cracks in the imperial edifice began to appear. Despite the successive military victories, French casualties in these battles had been large—15,000 lost at Eylau and 12,000 at Friedland, 23,000 killed or surrendered at Bailen, a massive 44,000 casualties at Aspern, and another 30,000 at Wagram. Experienced troops were becoming rare, at least outside the exclusive Guard regiments; for example, of the 148,000 men of the Armée de l'Allemagne (exclusive of the Guard) in 1809, 47,000 were underage conscripts.[88] Although Napoleon's army, like Hitler's included many from the conquered territories and the satellites, French manpower stocks were clearly being eroded; whereas the unpredictable czar still had enormous reserves and, even after Wagram, the stubborn and resentful Austrians possessed a very considerable "army in being." All this would have meaning in the near future.

Furthermore, Napoleon's drive into Spain in late 1808 had not "decided" that campaign, as he fondly imagined. In dispersing the formal Spanish armies, he had inadvertently encouraged the local populace to resort to guerrilla warfare, which was altogether more difficult to suppress and which multiplied the logistical problems for the French forces. Denied foodstuffs by the local population, the French army was critically dependent upon its own precarious supply lines. Moreover, in making a battlefield of Spain and, still more, of Portugal, Napoleon had unintentionally chosen one of the few areas in which the still-cautious British could be induced to commit themselves, at first tentatively but then with growing confidence as they saw how Wellington exploited local sympathies, the geography of the peninsula, command of the sea, and—last but not least—his own increasingly professional regiments to contain and erode French élan. The 25,000 casualties suffered by Massena's army in his fruitless march against Lisbon in 1810–1811 were an early sign that "the Spanish ulcer" could not be lanced, even when some 300,000 French troops had been dispatched south of the Pyrenees.[89]

Besides weakening France, the Spanish business simultaneously relieved the strain upon Britain, strategically as well as commercially. After all, during most of the preceding Anglo-French wars, Spain had fought on France's side—which not only had posed a landward threat to Gibraltar and a seaward threat (in the form of the Franco-Spanish combined fleets) to British naval mastery, but had also affected export markets in the Peninsula, Latin America, and the Mediterranean generally. A friendly rather than a hostile Spain meant an end to all those pressures. The damage done to British trade by the Continental System was now greatly eased, as the products of Lancashire and the Midlands returned to old markets; by 1810, total British exports had soared to a record £48 million (from £37 million in 1808). Although this relief was but temporary, and was increasingly overshadowed by the closure of the Baltic and by the Anglo-American dispute over impressment and blockade, it was enough. It sustained Napoleon's great *extra*-continental foe, and just at the time when the European continent itself was breaking into revolt.

In effect, the Napoleonic system in Europe rested upon a contradiction. Whatever the merits or demerits of the Revolution within France itself, a nation proclaiming liberty, fraternity, and equality was now—at the direction of its emperor—conquering non-French populations, stationing armies upon them, sequestering their goods, distorting their trade, raising enormous indemnities and taxes, and conscripting their youth.[90] Resentment was also felt at the controls being increasingly imposed under the Continental System, since it was not only Nantes and Bordeaux but also Amsterdam, Hamburg, and Trieste which were being hurt by the economic warfare Napoleon was waging against Britain. Few would openly rise in arms, like the Spaniards, or decide to pull out of the ruinous Continental System, as the Russians did in December 1810.[91] However, once Napoleon's Grand Army was devastated in the Moscow campaigns and the Armée de l'Espagne was being pushed back to the Pyrenees, the opportunity at last beckoned to throw off the French hegemony. What the Prussians, Russians, Swedes, Austrians, and others then needed was a ready supply of the rifles, boots, and clothing—not to mention the money—which the British were already providing to their Portuguese and Spanish allies. Thus, the security of the British Isles and its *relative* prosperity on the one hand, and the overstretched and increasingly grasping nature of French rule on the other, at last interacted to begin to bring down Napoleon's empire.

Such a sweeping analysis of economic and geopolitical factors tends, inevitably, to downplay the more personal aspects of this story, such as Napoleon's own increasing lethargy and self-delusion. It also may underemphasize the very precarious nature of the military equilibrium until almost the final year of the war—for the French even then possessed the resources to build an enormous navy, had they persisted in that course. The British export economy was to receive its severest test only in 1812; and until the battle of Leipzig (October 1813) there appeared good prospects that Napoleon could smash one of his eastern enemies and thus dissolve the coalition against him.

Nonetheless, the French "overstretch," reflecting Napoleon's own hubris, was by this time extreme, and any major setback was bound to affect other parts of the system—simply because these parts had to be drained of troops in order to repair the broken front. By 1811, there were some 353,000 French troops in Spain, and yet, as Wellington observed, they had no authority beyond the spot where they stood; defending their lines of communication consumed most of their efforts, and left them vulnerable to the Anglo-Portuguese-Spanish advance. When, in the year following, Napoleon decided to reduce Russia's independence, a mere 27,000 men could be withdrawn from Spain to join the march upon Moscow. Of the more than 600,000 men in the Grand Army, only 270,000 of that total were Frenchmen, the same number as remained in the Peninsula. Furthermore, since "native" Frenchmen now included the Belgians, Dutch, and many Italians in the annexed territories, troops raised from within the *pre*-1789 French borders were in a decided minority during the Russian campaign. This may not have mattered in the early, successful stages, but it did become important during the retreat, when men were desperate to escape from the bitter weather and marauding Cossacks and to return to their own homes.[92]

The Grand Army's casualties in the Russian campaign were enormous: perhaps as many as 270,000 men were killed and 200,000 captured, and about 1,000 guns and 200,000 horses were lost. The eastern front, more than any other factor, weakened the morale of the French army. Nonetheless, it is important to understand how the eastern European and peninsular campaigns interacted from 1813 onward to produce the eventual downfall: for by then the Russian army had little capacity (and many of its generals little enthusiasm) for pursuing the French across Germany; the British were somewhat distracted by their American war; and Napoleon had raised a fresh force of 145,000 men in the early summer of 1813, which enabled him to hold the line in Saxony and to negotiate an armistice. Although Prussia had prudently switched to the Russian side and Metternich was threatening to intervene with an Austrian army of a quarter of a million men, the eastern powers were still divided and uncertain. Thus, the news that Wellington's troops had smashed Joseph Bonaparte's army at Vitoria (June 1813) and were driving it back to the Pyrenees was important in encouraging the Austrians to declare war and to combine with the Russian, Swedish, and Prussian forces in order to expel the French from Germany. The subsequent battle of Leipzig in October was fought on a scale unknown to the British army—195,000 Frenchmen were overwhelmed in four days of fighting by 365,000 allied troops; but the latter were being economically underpinned by vast British subsidies, as well as being provided with 125,000 muskets, 218 artillery pieces, and much other equipment from the island state.[93]

In turn, the French defeat at Leipzig encouraged Wellington, now north of the Pyrenees, to advance upon Bayonne and Toulouse. As the armies of Prussia and Austria poured across the Rhine and the Cossacks invaded Holland, Napoleon conducted a brilliant tactical defense of northeastern France early in 1814; but his army was drained in strength and contained too many raw recruits. Moreover, the French populace, now that the fighting was on its soil, was (as Wellington had foretold) less than enthusiastic. Stiffened by British urgings to reduce France to its former size and by the pledge of a further £5 million in British subsidies at the Chaumont treaty of March 9, the allied governments kept up their pressure to the end. By March 30, 1814, even Napoleon's marshals had had enough, and within another week the emperor had abdicated.

Compared with these epic events, the Anglo-American war of 1812–1814 was a strategical sideshow.[94] Economically, it might have been far more serious to British interests had it not coincided with the collapse of the Continental System, and had not the New England states, largely dependent upon Anglo-American trade, remained luke-warm (and often neutral) in the conflict. The proclaimed "march on Canada" by American forces soon petered out, and both on land and at sea—despite the raids upon York (Toronto) and Washington, and some impressive single-ship frigate actions—each side demonstrated that it could hurt but not defeat the other. To the British in particular, it showed the importance of the American trades and it revealed the difficulties of maintaining large military and naval establishments overseas at the same time as the armed services were desperately required in the European theater. As was the case in India, trans-oceanic possessions and commerce were simultaneously a strengthen-ing of Britain's power position and a strategical distraction.[95]

Napoleon's final campaign of March to June 1815, while certainly not a sideshow, was a strategical footnote to the great war in Europe.[96] His sudden return to France from exile interrupted the quarrels of the victors over the future of Poland, Saxony, and other lands, but it did not shake the alliance. Even if the hastily assembled French force had not been defeated by Wellington and Blücher at Waterloo, it is difficult to see how it could have resisted the other armies which were being diverted toward Belgium, and still more difficult to see how France could have economically sustained a long war thereafter. Neverthe-less, Napoleon's last escapade was important politically. It reinforced Britain's position in Europe and strengthened the argument that France needed to be surrounded by an array of strong "buffer states" in the future. It demonstrated Prussia's military recovery after Jena, and thus partly readjusted the balances in eastern Europe. And it com-pelled all the powers at Vienna to bury their remaining differences in order to achieve a peace which would enshrine the principles of the balance of power.[97] After two decades of near-constant war and well over a century of Great Power tensions and conflict, the European states system was at last being fashioned along lines which ensured a rough equilibrium.

The final Vienna settlement of 1815 did not, as the Prussians had once suggested, partition France. It did, however, surround Louis XVIII's domain with substantial territorial units—the Kingdom of the Netherlands to the north, an enlarged Kingdom of Sardinia (Piedmont) to the southeast, and Prussia in the Rhineland; while Spain, returned to the Bourbons, was guaranteed in its integrity by the powers. Farther east, the idea of a *balance* of power was also implemented, after heated quarrels between the victors. Because of Austrian objections, Prussia was not permitted to swallow Saxony and instead accepted compensation in Posen and the Rhineland, just as Austria was compensated in Italy and in parts of southeastern Germany for the fact that it retained only the Galician region of Poland. Even Russia, whose claims to the lion's share of Polish territories had finally to be conceded, was considerably shaken at the beginning of 1815 by the threat of an Anglo-French-Austrian alliance to resist dictation over the future of Saxony, and quickly backed down from a confrontation. No power, it appeared, would not be permitted to impose its wishes upon the rest of Europe in the way Napoleon had done. The egoism of the leading states had in no way been evaporated by the events of 1793–1815, but the twin principles of "containment and reciprocal compensation"[98] meant that a unilateral grasp for domination of Europe was now unlikely; and that even small-scale territorial changes would need the approval of a majority of the members of the Concert.

For all the talk about a European "Pentarchy," however, it is important to recall that the five Great Powers were not in the same relationship to one another as they had been in 1750 or even in 1789. Despite Russia's growth, it was fair to say that a rough balance of power existed on land after Napoleon's fall. On the other hand, there was no equivalent at sea, where the British enjoyed a near-monopoly of naval power, which simultaneously reinforced and was underpinned by the economic lead which they had gained over all their rivals. In some cases, like India, this was the result of steady military expansionism and plunder, so that war and profit-seeking had interacted to draw the subcontinent into a purely British orbit by the end of the eighteenth century.[99] Similarly, the seizure of Santo Domingo—which had been responsible for a remarkable three-quarters of France's colonial trade before the Revolution—was by the late 1790s a valuable market for *British* goods and a great source of *British* re-exports. In addition, not only were these overseas markets in North America, the West Indies, Latin America, India, and the Orient growing faster than those in Europe, but such long-haul trades were also usually more profitable and a greater stimulus to the shipping, commodity-dealing, marine insurance, bill-clearing, and banking activities which so enhanced London's position as the new financial center of the world.[100] Despite recent writings which have questioned the rate of growth of the British economy in the eighteenth century and the role of foreign trade in that growth,[101] the fact remains that overseas expansion had given the country unchallenged access to vast new wealth which its rivals did not enjoy. Controlling most of Europe's colonies by 1815, dominating the maritime routes and the profitable re-export trades, and well ahead of other societies in the process of industrialization, the British were now the richest nation in per capita terms. During the next half-century—as will be seen in the following chapter—they would become even richer, as Britain grew to be the "superdominant economy" in the world's trading structure.[102] The principle of equilibrium which Pitt and Castlereagh held so high was one which applied to European territorial arrangements, not to the colonial and commercial spheres.

Little of this can have surprised intelligent early-nineteenth-century observers. Despite his own assumptions of grandeur, Napoleon seems to have become obsessed with Britain at times—with its invulnerability, its maritime dominance, its banks and credit system—and to have yearned to see it all tumble in the dust. Such feelings of envy and dislike doubtless existed, if in a less extreme form, among the Spaniards, Dutch, and others who saw the British monopolizing the outside world. The Russian general Kutusov, wishing to halt his army's westward advance in 1812, once the Grand Army had been driven from the homeland, may have spoken for more than himself when he doubted the wisdom of totally destroying Napoleon, since the "succession would not fall to Russia or to any other continental power, but to the power which already commands the sea, and whose domination would be intolerable."[103] At the end of the day, however, that result was unavoidable: Napoleon's hubris and refusal to compromise ensured not only his downfall, but his greatest enemy's supreme victory. As Gneisenau, another general with a sense of the larger issues, wryly concluded:

> Great Britain has no greater obligation than to this ruffian [Napoleon]. For through the events which he has brought about, England's greatness, prosperity, and wealth have risen high. She is mistress of the sea and neither in this dominion nor in world trade has she now a single rival to fear.[104]

STRATEGY &
ECONOMICS
IN THE
INDUSTRIAL ERA

4

Industrialization and the Shifting Global Balances, 1815–1885

The international system which developed in the half-century and more following Napoleon's downfall possessed an unusual set of characteristics, some merely temporary, while others became permanent features of the modern age.

The first was the steady and then (after the 1840s) spectacular growth of an integrated global economy, which drew ever more regions into a transoceanic and transcontinental trading and financial network centered upon western Europe, and in particular upon Great Britain. These decades of British economic hegemony were accompanied by large-scale improvements in transport and communications, by the increasingly rapid transfer of industrial technology from one region to another, and by an immense spurt in manufacturing output, which in turn stimulated the opening of new areas of agricultural land and raw-materials sources. The erosion of tariff barriers and other mercantilist devices, together with the widespread propagation of ideas about free trade and international harmony, suggested that a new international order had arisen, quite different from the eighteenth-century world of repeated Great Power conflict. The turbulence and costs of the 1793–1815 struggle—known to the nineteenth century as "the Great War"—caused conservatives and liberals alike to opt as far as possible for peace and stability, underpinned by devices as varied as the Concert of Europe or free-trade treaties. These conditions naturally encouraged long-term commercial and industrial investment, thereby stimulating the growth of a global economy.

Secondly, this absence of prolonged Great Power wars did not mean that all interstate conflict came to an end. If anything, the European and North American wars of conquest against less developed peoples intensified, and were in many ways the military concomitant to the economic penetration of the overseas world and to the swift decline in its share of manufacturing output. In addition, there still were regional and individual conflicts among the European powers, especially over questions of nationality and territorial borders; but, as we shall see, open struggles such as the Franco-Austrian War of 1859 or the wars of German unification in the 1860s were limited both in duration and area, and even the Crimean War could hardly be called a major conflict. Only the American Civil War was an exception to this rule, and deserves to be examined as such.

Thirdly, technology deriving from the Industrial Revolution began to make its impact upon military and naval warfare. But the changes were much slower than has sometimes been represented, and it was only in the second half of the century that railways, telegraphs, quick-firing guns, steam propulsion, and armored warships really became decisive indicators of military strength. While the new technology increased the lead in firepower and mobility which the Great Powers enjoyed in the overseas world, it was going to be many decades before military and naval commanders revised their ideas of how to fight a European war. Nevertheless, the twin forces of technical change and industrial development were steadily having an impact, on land and at sea, and also affecting the relative strengths of the Powers.

Although it is difficult to generalize, the shifts in the Great Power balances caused by the uneven pattern of industrial and technological change probably affected the outcome of mid-nineteenth-century wars more than did finance and credit. This was partly because the massive expansion of national and international banking in the nineteenth century and the growth of governmental bureaucracies (treasuries, inspectors, tax collectors) made it easier for most regimes to raise funds from the money markets, unless their credit rating was appallingly bad or there was a temporary liquidity crisis in the international banking system. But it was chiefly due to the fact that most of the wars which occurred were relatively short, so that the emphasis was upon a speedy victory in the field using existing military strength, rather than the long-term mobilization of national resources and the raising of fresh revenues. No amount of newly available funds could, for example, have saved Austria after its battlefield defeats of 1859 and 1866, or a very wealthy France after its armies had been crushed in the war of 1870. It was true that superior finances aided the North in its Civil War victory over the South, and that Britain and France were better able to afford the Crimean War than a near-bankrupt Russia— but that reflected the general superiority of their economies rather than the singular advantage they had in respect of credit and finance. For this reason, there is less to say about the role of war finance in the nineteenth century than there was about the previous period.

This cluster of factors—the growth of the international economy, the productive forces unleashed by the Industrial Revolution, the relative stability of Europe, the modernization of military and naval technology over time, and the occurrence of merely localized and short-term wars—naturally favored some of the Great Powers more than others. Indeed, one of those countries, Britain, benefited so much from the general economic and geopolitical trends of the post-1815 era that it became a different type of Power from the rest. All the other countries were affected, often very seriously, in their relative strength. By the 1860s, however, the further spread of industrialization was beginning to change the balance of world forces once again.

One further feature of this period is worth mentioning. From the early nineteenth century onward, historical statistics (especially of economic indicators) help to trace the shifts in the power balances and to measure more accurately the dynamics of the system. It is important to realize, however, that many of the data are very approximate, particularly for countries lacking an adequate bureaucracy; that certain of the calculations (e.g., shares of world manufacturing output) are merely estimates made by statisticians many years later; and that—the most important caveat of all—economic wealth did not immediately, or always, translate into military power. All that the statistics can do is give rough indications of a country's material potential and of its position in the relative rankings of the leading states.

The "Industrial Revolution," most economic historians are at pains to stress, did not happen overnight. It was, compared with the political "revolutions" of 1776, 1789, and 1917, a gradual, slow-moving process; it affected only certain manufactures and certain means of production; and it occurred region by region, rather than involving an entire country.[1] Yet all these caveats cannot avoid the fact that a fundamentally important transformation in man's economic circumstances began to occur sometime around 1780—not less significant, in the view of one authority, than the (admittedly far slower) transformation of savage Paleolithic hunting man to domesticated Neolithic farming man.[2] What industrialization, and in particular the steam engine, did was to substitute inanimate for animate sources of power; by converting heat into work through the use of machines—"rapid, regular, precise, tireless" machines[3]—mankind was thus able to exploit vast new sources of energy. The consequences of introducing this novel machinery were simply stupendous: by the 1820s someone operating several power-driven looms could produce twenty times the output of a hand worker, while a power-driven "mule" (or spinning machine) had two hundred times the capacity of a spinning wheel. A single railway engine could transport goods which would have required hundreds of packhorses, and do it far more quickly. To be sure, there were many other important aspects to the Industrial Revolution—the factory system, for example, or the division of labor. But the vital point for our purposes was the massive increase in productivity, especially in the textile industries, which in turn stimulated a demand for more machines, more raw materials (above all, cotton), more iron, more shipping, better communications, and so on.

Moreover, as Professor Landes has observed, this unprecedented increase in man's productivity was self-sustaining:

> Where previously an amelioration of the conditions of existence, hence of survival, and an increase in economic opportunity had always been followed by a rise in population that eventually consumed the gains achieved, now for the first time in history, both the economy and the knowledge were growing fast enough to generate a continuing flow of investment and technological innovation, a flow that lifted beyond visible limits the ceiling of Malthus's positive checks.[4]

The latter remark is also vitally important. From the eighteenth century onward, the growth in world population had begun to accelerate: Europe's numbers rose from 140 million in 1750 to 187 million in 1800 to 266 million in 1850; Asia's exploded from over 400 million in 1750 to around 700 million a century later.[5] Whatever the reasons— better climatic conditions, improved fecundity, decline in diseases— increases of that size were alarming; and although agricultural output both in Europe and Asia also expanded in the eighteenth century and was in fact another general reason for the rise in population, the sheer number of new heads (and stomachs) threatened over time to cancel out the benefits of all such additions in agricultural output. Pressure upon marginal lands, rural unemployment, and a vast drift of families into the already overcrowded cities of Europe in the late eighteenth century were but some of the symptoms of this population surge.[6]

What the Industrial Revolution in Britain did (in very crude macroeconomic terms) was to so increase productivity on a sustained basis that the consequent expansion both in national wealth and in the population's purchasing power constantly outweighed the rise in numbers. While the country's population rose from 10.5 million in 1801 to 41.8 million in 1911—an annual increase of 1.26 percent—its national product rose much faster, perhaps as much as fourteenfold over the nineteenth century. Depending upon the area covered by the statistics,* there was an annual average rise in gross national product of between 2 and 2.25 percent. In Queen Victoria's reign alone, product per capita rose two and a half times.

Compared with the growth rates achieved by many nations after 1945, these were not spectacular figures. It was also true, as social historians remind us, that the Industrial Revolution inflicted awful costs upon the new proletariat which labored in the factories and mines and lived in the unhealthy, crowded, jerry-built cities. Yet the fundamental point remains that the sustained increases in productiv-

---

*That is to say, some of the historical statistics refer to Great Britain (minus Ireland), some to the United Kingdom (with Ireland), and some include only northern but not southern Ireland.

ity of the Machine Age brought widespread benefits over time: average real wages in Britain rose between 15 and 25 percent in the years 1815–1850, and by an impressive 80 percent in the next half-century. "The central problem of the age," Ashton has reminded those critics who believe that industrialization was a disaster, "was how to feed and clothe and employ generations of children outnumbering by far those of any earlier time."[7] The new machines not only employed an increasingly large share of the burgeoning population, but also boosted the nation's overall per capita income; and the rising demand of urban workers for foodstuffs and essential goods was soon to be met by a steam-driven communications revolution, with railways and steamships bringing the agricultural surpluses of the New World to satisfy the requirements of the Old.

We can grasp this point in a different way by using Professor Landes's calculations. In 1870, he notes, the United Kingdom was using 100 million tons of coal, which was "equivalent to 800 million million Calories of energy, enough to feed a population of 850 million adult males for a year (actual population was then about 31 million)." Again, the capacity of Britain's steam engines in 1870, some 4 million horsepower, was equivalent to the power which could be generated by 40 million men; but "this many men would have eaten some 320 million bushels of wheat a year—more than three times the annual output of the entire United Kingdom in 1867–71."[8] The use of inanimate sources of power allowed industrial man to transcend the limitations of biology and to create spectacular increases in production and wealth without succumbing to the weight of a fast-growing population. By contrast, Ashton soberly noted (as late as 1947):

> There are today on the plains of India and China men and women, plague-ridden and hungry, living lives little better, to outward appearance, than those of the cattle that toil with them by day and share their places of sleep by night. Such Asiatic standards, and such unmechanised horrors, are the lot of those who increase their numbers without passing through an industrial revolution.[9]

The Eclipse of the Non-European World

Before discussing the effects of the Industrial Revolution upon the Great Power system, it will be as well to understand its impacts farther afield, especially upon China, India, and other non-European societies. The losses they suffered were twofold, both relative and absolute. It was not the case, as was once fancied, that the peoples of Asia, Africa, and Latin America lived a happy, ideal existence prior to the impact of western man. "The elemental truth must be stressed that the charac-

teristic of any country before its industrial revolution and modernization is poverty. . . . with low productivity, low output per head, in
traditional agriculture, any economy which has agriculture as the
main constituent of its national income does not produce much of a
surplus above the immediate requirements of consumption. . . ."[10] On
the other hand, in view of the fact that in 1800 agricultural production
formed the basis of both European and non-European societies, and
of the further fact that in countries such as India and China there also
existed many traders, textile producers, and craftsmen, the differences
in per capita income were not enormous; an Indian handloom weaver,
for example, may have earned perhaps as much as half of his European
equivalent prior to industrialization. What this also meant was that,
given the sheer numbers of Asiatic peasants and craftsmen, Asia still
contained a far larger share of world manufacturing output* than did
the much less populous Europe before the steam engine and the power
loom transformed the world's balances.

Just how dramatically those balances shifted in consequence of
European industrialization and expansion can be seen in Bairoch's two
ingenious calculations (see Tables 6–7).[11]

The root cause of these transformations, it is clear, lay in the staggering increases in productivity emanating from the Industrial Revolution. Between, say, the 1750s and the 1830s the mechanization of
spinning in Britain had increased productivity in that sector alone by a
factor of 300 to 400, so it is not surprising that the British share of total
world manufacturing rose dramatically—and continued to rise as it
turned itself into the "first industrial nation."[12] When other European
states and the United States followed the path to industrialization, their
shares also rose steadily, as did their per capita levels of industrialization and their national wealth. But the story for China and India was
quite a different one. Not only did their shares of total world manufacturing shrink relatively, simply because the West's output was rising so
swiftly; but in some cases their economies declined absolutely, that is,
they de-industrialized, because of the penetration of their traditional
markets by the far cheaper and better products of the Lancashire textile
factories. After 1813 (when the East India Company's trade monopoly
ended), imports of cotton fabrics into India rose spectacularly, from 1
million yards (1814) to 51 million (1830) to 995 million (1870), driving
out many of the traditional domestic producers in the process. Finally—
and this returns us to Ashton's point about the grinding poverty of
"those who increase their numbers without passing through an industrial revolution"—the large rise in the populations of China, India, and
other Third World countries probably reduced their general per capita
income from one generation to the next. Hence Bairoch's remarkable—

*Following, at least, the definition of "manufactures" that Bairoch employs (see note 11).

Table 6. Relative Shares of World Manufacturing Output, 1750–1900

	1750	1800	1830	1860	1880	1900
(Europe as a whole)	23.2	28.1	34.2	53.2	61.3	62.0
United Kingdom	1.9	4.3	9.5	19.9	22.9	18.5
Habsburg Empire	2.9	3.2	3.2	4.2	4.4	4.7
France	4.0	4.2	5.2	7.9	7.8	6.8
German States/Germany	2.9	3.5	3.5	4.9	8.5	13.2
Italian States/Italy	2.4	2.5	2.3	2.5	2.5	2.5
Russia	5.0	5.6	5.6	7.0	7.6	8.8
United States	0.1	0.8	2.4	7.2	14.7	23.6
Japan	3.8	3.5	2.8	2.6	2.4	2.4
Third World	73.0	67.7	60.5	36.6	20.9	11.0
China	32.8	33.3	29.8	19.7	12.5	6.2
India/Pakistan	24.5	19.7	17.6	8.6	2.8	1.7

Table 7. Per Capita Levels of Industrialization, 1750–1900
(relative to U.K. in 1900 = 100)

	1750	1800	1830	1860	1880	1900
(Europe as a whole)	8	8	11	16	24	35
United Kingdom	10	16	25	64	87	[100]
Habsburg Empire	7	7	8	11	15	23
France	9	9	12	20	28	39
German States/Germany	8	8	9	15	25	52
Italian States/Italy	8	8	8	10	12	17
Russia	6	6	7	8	10	15
United States	4	9	14	21	38	69
Japan	7	7	7	7	9	12
Third World	7	6	6	4	3	2
China	8	6	6	4	4	3
India	7	6	6	3	2	1

and horrifying—suggestion that whereas the per capita levels of industrialization in Europe and the Third World may have been not too far apart from each other in 1750, the latter's was only one-eighteenth of the former's (2 percent to 35 percent) by 1900, and only one-fiftieth of the United Kingdom's (2 percent to 100 percent).

The "impact of western man" was, in all sorts of ways, one of the most noticeable aspects of the dynamics of world power in the nineteenth century. It manifested itself not only in a variety of economic relationships—ranging from the "informal influence" of coastal traders, shippers, and consuls to the more direct controls of planters, railway builders, and mining companies[13]—but also in the penetrations of explorers, adventurers, and missionaries, in the introduction of western diseases, and in the proselytization of western faiths. It occurred as much in the centers of continents—westward from the Missouri, southward from the Aral Sea—as it did up the mouths of African rivers and around the coasts of Pacific archipelagoes. If it eventually had its impressive monuments in the roads, railway networks, telegraphs, harbors, and civic buildings which (for example) the British created in India, its more horrific side was the bloodshed, rapine, and plunder which attended so many of the colonial wars of the period.[14] To be sure, the same traits of force and conquest had existed since the days of Cortez, but now the pace was accelerating. In the year 1800, Europeans occupied or controlled 35 percent of the land surface of the world; by 1878 this figure had risen to 67 percent, and by 1914 to over 84 percent.[15]

The advanced technology of steam engines and machine-made tools gave Europe decisive economic and military advantages. The improvements in the muzzle-loading gun (percussion caps, rifling, etc.) were ominous enough; the coming of the breechloader, vastly increasing the rate of fire, was an even greater advance; and the Gatling guns, Maxims, and light field artillery put the final touches to a new "firepower revolution" which quite eradicated the chances of a successful resistance by indigenous peoples reliant upon older weaponry. Furthermore, the steam-driven gunboat meant that European sea power, already supreme in open waters, could be extended inland, via major waterways like the Niger, the Indus, and the Yangtze: thus the mobility and firepower of the ironclad *Nemesis* during the Opium War actions of 1841 and 1842 was a disaster for the defending Chinese forces, which were easily brushed aside.[16] It was true, of course, that physically difficult terrain (e.g., Afghanistan) blunted the drives of western military imperialism, and that among non-European forces which adopted the newer weapons and tactics—like the Sikhs and the Algerians in the 1840s—the resistance was far greater. But whenever the struggle took place in open country where the West could deploy its machine guns and heavier weapons, the issue was never in doubt. Perhaps the greatest disparity of all was seen at the very end of the century, during the battle of Omdurman (1898), when in one half-morning the Maxims and Lee-Enfield rifles of Kitchener's army destroyed 11,000 Dervishes for the loss of only forty-eight of their own troops. In consequence, the firepower gap, like that which had opened up in industrial productivity, meant that the leading nations possessed resources fifty or a hundred times greater than those at the bottom. The global dominance of the West, implicit since da Gama's day, now knew few limits.

Britain as Hegemon?

If the Punjabis and Annamese and Sioux and Bantu were the "losers" (to use Eric Hobsbawm's term)[17] in this early-nineteenth-century expansion, the British were undoubtedly the "winners." As noted in the previous chapter, they had already achieved a remarkable degree of global preeminence by 1815, thanks to their adroit combination of naval mastery, financial credit, commercial expertise, and alliance diplomacy. What the Industrial Revolution did was to enhance the position of a country already made supremely successful in the preindustrial, mercantilist struggles of the eighteenth century, and then to transform it into a different sort of power. If (to repeat) the pace of change was gradual rather than revolutionary, the results were nonetheless highly impressive. Between 1760 and 1830, the United Kingdom was responsible for around "two-thirds of Europe's industrial growth of output,"[18] and its share of world manufacturing production leaped from 1.9 to 9.5 percent; in the next thirty years, British industrial expansion pushed that figure to 19.9 percent, despite the spread of the new technology to other countries in the West. Around 1860, which was probably when the country reached its zenith in relative terms, the United Kingdom produced 53 percent of the world's iron and 50 percent of its coal and lignite, and consumed just under half of the raw cotton output of the globe. "With 2 percent of the world's population and 10 percent of Europe's, the United Kingdom would seem to have had a capacity in modern industries equal to 40–45 percent of the world's potential and 55–60 percent of that in Europe."[19] Its energy consumption from modern sources (coal, lignite, oil) in 1860 was five times that of either the United States or Prussia/Germany, six times that of France, and 155 times that of Russia! It alone was responsible for one-fifth of the world's commerce, but for two-fifths of the trade in manufactured goods. Over one-third of the world's merchant marine flew under the British flag, and that share was steadily increasing. It was no surprise that the mid-Victorians exulted at their unique state, being now (as the economist Jevons put it in 1865) the trading center of the universe:

> The plains of North America and Russia are our corn fields; Chicago and Odessa our granaries; Canada and the Baltic are our timber forests; Australasia contains our sheep farms, and in Argentina and on the western prairies of North America are our herds of oxen; Peru sends her silver, and the gold of South Africa and Australia flows to London; the Hindus and the Chinese grow tea for us, and our coffee, sugar and spice plantations are in all the Indies. Spain and France are our vineyards and the Mediterranean our fruit garden; and our cotton grounds, which for long have occupied the

Southern United States, are now being extended everywhere in the warm regions of the earth.[20]

Since such manifestations of self-confidence, and the industrial and commercial statistics upon which they rested, seemed to suggest a position of unequaled dominance on Britain's part, it is fair to make several other points which put this all in a better context. First—although it is a somewhat pedantic matter—it is unlikely that the country's gross national product (GNP) was ever the largest in the world during the decades following 1815. Given the sheer size of China's population (and, later, Russia's) and the obvious fact that agricultural production and distribution formed the basis of national wealth everywhere, even in Britain prior to 1850, the latter's overall GNP never looked as impressive as its per capita product or its stage of industrialization. Still, "by itself the volume of total GNP has no important significance";[21] the physical product of hundreds of millions of peasants may dwarf that of five million factory workers, but since most of it is immediately consumed, it is far less likely to lead to surplus wealth or decisive military striking power. Where Britain was strong, indeed unchallenged, in 1850 was in modern, wealth-producing industry, with all the benefits which flowed from it.

On the other hand—and this second point is not a pedantic one—Britain's growing industrial muscle was not organized in the post-1815 decades to give the state swift access to military hardware and manpower as, say, Wallenstein's domains did in the 1630s or the Nazi economy was to do. On the contrary, the ideology of laissez-faire political economy, which flourished alongside this early industrialization, preached the causes of eternal peace, low government expenditures (especially on defense), and the reduction of state controls over the economy and the individual. It might be necessary, Adam Smith had conceded in *The Wealth of Nations* (1776), to tolerate the upkeep of an army and a navy in order to protect British society "from the violence and invasion of other independent societies"; but since armed forces *per se* were "unproductive" and did not add value to the national wealth in the way that a factory or a farm did, they ought to be reduced to the lowest possible level commensurate with national safety.[22] Assuming (or, at least, hoping) that war was a last resort, and ever less likely to occur in the future, the disciples of Smith and even more of Richard Cobden would have been appalled at the idea of organizing the state for war. As a consequence, the "modernization" which occurred in British industry and communications was not paralleled by improvements in the army, which (with some exceptions)[23] stagnated in the post-1815 decades.

However preeminent the British economy in the mid-Victorian period, therefore, it was probably less "mobilized" for conflict than at any time since the early Stuarts. Mercantilist measures, with their emphasis upon the links between national security and national wealth, were steadily eliminated: protective tariffs were abolished; the ban on the export of advanced technology (e.g., textile machinery) was lifted; the Navigation Acts, designed among other things to preserve a large stock of British merchant ships and seamen for the event of war, were repealed; imperial "preferences" were ended. By contrast, defense expenditures were held to an absolute minimum, averaging around £15 million a year in the 1840s and not above £27 million in the more troubled 1860s; yet in the latter period Britain's GNP totaled about £1 billion. Indeed, for fifty years and more following 1815 the armed services consumed only about 2–3 percent of GNP, and central government expenditures as a whole took much less than 10 percent—proportions which were far less than in either the eighteenth or the twentieth century.[24] These would have been impressively low figures for a country of modest means and ambitions. For a state which managed to "rule the waves," which possessed an enormous, far-flung empire, and which still claimed a large interest in preserving the European balance of power, they were truly remarkable.

Like that of the United States in, say, the early 1920s, therefore, the size of the British economy in the world was not reflected in the country's fighting power; nor could its laissez-faire institutional structures, with a minuscule bureaucracy increasingly divorced from trade and industry, have been able to mobilize British resources for an all-out war without a great upheaval. As we shall see below, even the more limited Crimean War shook the system severely, yet the concern which that exposure aroused soon faded away. Not only did the mid-Victorians show ever less enthusiasm for military interventions in Europe, which would always be expensive, and perhaps immoral, but they reasoned that the equilibrium between the continental Great Powers which generally prevailed during the six decades after 1815 made any full-scale commitment on Britain's part unnecessary. While it did strive, through diplomacy and the movement of naval squadrons, to influence political events along the vital peripheries of Europe (Portugal, Belgium, the Dardanelles), it tended to abstain from intervention elsewhere. By the late 1850s and early 1860s, even the Crimean campaign was widely regarded as a mistake. Because of this lack of inclination and effectiveness, Britain did not play a major role in the fate of Piedmont in the critical year of 1859, it disapproved of Palmerston and Russell's "meddling" in the Schleswig-Holstein affair of 1864, and it watched from the sidelines when Prussia defeated Austria in 1866 and France four years later. It is not surprising to see that Britain's military capacity was reflected in the relatively modest size of its army during this period (see Table 8), little of which could, in any case, be mobilized for a European theater.

Table 8. Military Personnel of the Powers, 1816–1880[25]

	1816	1830	1860	1880
United Kingdom	255,000	140,000	347,000	248,000
France	132,000	259,000	608,000	544,000
Russia	800,000	826,000	862,000	909,000
Prussia/Germany	130,000	130,000	201,000	430,000
Habsburg Empire	220,000	273,000	306,000	273,000
United States	16,000	11,000	26,000	36,000

Even in the extra-European world, where Britain preferred to deploy its regiments, military and political officials in places such as India were almost always complaining of the *inadequacy* of the forces they commanded, given the sheer magnitude of the territories they controlled. However imposing the empire may have appeared on a world map, district officers knew that it was being run on a shoestring. But all this is merely saying that Britain was a different sort of Great Power by the early to middle nineteenth century, and that its influence could not be measured by the traditional criteria of military hegemony. Where it *was* strong was in certain other realms, each of which was regarded by the British as far more valuable than a large and expensive standing army.

The first of these was in the naval realm. For over a century before 1815, of course, the Royal Navy had usually been the largest in the world. But that maritime mastery had frequently been contested, especially by the Bourbon powers. The salient feature of the eighty years which followed Trafalgar was that no other country, or combination of countries, seriously challenged Britain's control of the seas. There was, it is true, the occasional French "scare"; and the Admiralty also kept a wary eye upon Russian shipbuilding programs and upon the American construction of large frigates. But each of those perceived challenges faded swiftly, leaving British sea power to exercise (in Professor Lloyd's words) "a wider influence than has ever been seen in the history of maritime empires."[26] Despite a steady reduction in its own numbers after 1815, the Royal Navy was at some times probably as powerful as the next three or four navies in actual fighting power. And its major fleets *were* a factor in European politics, at least on the periphery. The squadron anchored in the Tagus to protect the Porguguese monarchy against internal or external dangers; the decisive use of naval force in the Mediterranean (against the Algiers pirates in 1816; smashing the Turkish fleet at Navarino in 1827; checking Mehemet Ali at Acre in 1840); and the calculated dispatch of the fleet to anchor before the Dardanelles whenever the "Eastern Question" became acute: these were manifestations of British sea power which, although geographically restricted, nonetheless weighed in the minds of European governments. Outside Europe, where smaller Royal Navy fleets or even individual warships engaged in a whole host of activities—suppressing piracy, intercepting slaving ships, landing marines, and overawing local potentates from Canton to Zanzibar—the impact seemed perhaps even more decisive.[27]

The second significant realm of British influence lay in its expanding colonial empire. Here again, the overall situation was a far less competitive one than in the preceding two centuries, where Britain had had to fight repeatedly for empire against Spain, France, and other European states. Now, apart from the occasional alarm about French moves in the Pacific or Russian encroachments in Turkestan, no serious rivals remained. It is therefore hardly an exaggeration to suggest that between 1815 and 1880 much of the British Empire existed in a power-political vacuum, which is why its colonial army could be kept relatively low. There were, it is true, limits to British imperialism—and certain problems, with the expanding American republic in the western hemisphere as well as with France and Russia in the eastern. But in many parts of the tropics, and for long periods of time, British interests (traders, planters, explorers, missionaries) encountered no foreigners other than the indigenous peoples.

This relative lack of external pressure, together with the rise of laissez-faire liberalism at home, caused many a commentator to argue that colonial acquisitions were unnecessary, being merely a set of "millstones" around the neck of the overburdened British taxpayer. Yet whatever the rhetoric of anti-imperialism within Britain, the fact was that the empire continued to grow, expanding (according to one calculation) at an average annual pace of about 100,000 square miles between 1815 and 1865.[28] Some were strategical/commercial acquisitions, like Singapore, Aden, the Falkland Islands, Hong Kong, Lagos; others were the consequence of land-hungry white settlers, moving across the South African veldt, the Canadian prairies, and the Australian outback—whose expansion usually provoked a native resistance that often had to be suppressed by troops from Britain or British India. And even when formal annexations were resisted by a home government perturbed at this growing list of new responsibilities, the "informal influence" of an expanding British society was felt from Uruguay to the Levant and from the Congo to the Yangtze. Compared with the sporadic colonizing efforts of the French and the more localized internal colonization by the Americans and the Russians, the British as imperialists were in a class of their own for most of the nineteenth century.

The third area of British distinctiveness and strength lay in the realm of finance. To be sure, this element can scarcely be separated from the country's general industrial and commercial progress; money had been necessary to fuel the Industrial Revolution, which in turn produced much more money, in the form of returns upon capital invested. And, as the preceding chapter showed, the British government had long known how to exploit its credit in the banking and stock markets. But developments in the financial realm by the mid-nineteenth century were both qualitatively and quantitatively different from what had gone before. At first sight, it is the quantitative difference which catches the eye. The long peace and the easy availability of capital in the United Kingdom, together with the improvements in the country's financial institutions, stimulated Britons to invest abroad as never before: the £6 million or so which was annually exported in the decade following Waterloo had risen to over £30 million a year by midcentury, and to a staggering £75 million a year between 1870 and 1875. The resultant income to Britain from such interest and dividends, which had totaled a handy £8 million each year in the late 1830s, was over £50 million a year by the 1870s; but most of that was promptly reinvested overseas, in a sort of virtuous upward spiral which not only made Britain ever wealthier but gave a continual stimulus to global trade and communications.

The consequences of this vast export of capital were several, and important. The first was that the returns on overseas investments significantly reduced the annual trade gap on visible goods which Britain always incurred. In this respect, investment income added to the already considerable invisible earnings which came from shipping, insurance, bankers' fees, commodity dealing, and so on. Together, they ensured that not only was there never a balance-of-payments crisis, but Britain became steadily richer, at home and abroad. The second point was that the British economy acted as a vast bellows, sucking in enormous amounts of raw materials and foodstuffs and sending out vast quantities of textiles, iron goods, and other manufactures; and this pattern of visible trade was paralleled, and complemented, by the network of shipping lines, insurance arrangements, and banking links which spread outward from London (especially), Liverpool, Glasgow, and most other cities in the course of the nineteenth century.

Given the openness of the British home market and London's willingness to reinvest overseas income in new railways, ports, utilities, and agricultural enterprises from Georgia to Queensland, there was a general complementarity between visible trade flows and investment patterns.* Add to this the growing acceptance of the gold standard and the development of an international exchange and payments mechanism based upon bills drawn on London, and it was scarcely surprising that the mid-Victorians were convinced that by following the principles of classical political economy, they had discovered the secret

*Argentina, for example, would be able to find a ready market in the U.K. for its exports of beef and grain, thereby allowing it not only to pay for imported British manufactures and for the various service fees but also to repay the long-term loans floated in London, and thus to keep its own credit high for further borrowing. The contrast with U.S. loans to Latin America in the twentieth century—lending at short term, and not allowing the importation of agricultural produce—is striking.

which guaranteed both increasing prosperity and world harmony. Although many individuals—Tory protectionists, oriental despots, new-fangled socialists—still seemed too purblind to admit this truth, over time everyone would surely recognize the fundamental validity of laissez-faire economics and utilitarian codes of government.[29]

While all this made Britons wealthier than ever in the short term, did it not also contain elements of strategic danger in the longer term? With the wisdom of retrospect, one can detect at least two consequences of these structural economic changes which would later affect Britain's relative power in the world. The first was the way in which the country was contributing to the long-term expansion of other nations, both by establishing and developing foreign industries and agriculture with repeated financial injections and by building railways, harbors, and steamships which would enable overseas producers to rival its own production in future decades. In this connection, it is worth noting that while the coming of steam power, the factory system, railways, and later electricity enabled the British to overcome natural, physical obstacles to higher productivity, and thus increased the nation's wealth and strength, such inventions helped the United States, Russia, and central Europe even more, because the natural, physical obstacles to the development of their landlocked potential were much greater. Put crudely, what industrialization did was to equalize the chances to exploit one's own indigenous resources and thus to take away some of the advantages hitherto enjoyed by smaller, peripheral, naval-cum-commercial states and to give them to the great land-based states.[30]

The second potential strategical weakness lay in the increasing dependence of the British economy upon international trade and, more important, international finance. By the middle decades of the nineteenth century, exports composed as much as one-fifth of total national income,[31] a far higher proportion than in Walpole's or Pitt's time; for the enormous cotton-textile industry in particular, overseas markets were vital. But foreign imports, both of raw materials and (increasingly) of foodstuffs, were also becoming vital as Britain moved from being a predominantly agricultural to being a predominantly urban/industrial society. And in the fastest-growing sector of all, the "invisible" services of banking, insurance, commodity-dealing, and overseas investment, the reliance upon a world market was even more critical. The world was the City of London's oyster, which was all very well in peacetime; but what would the situation be if ever it came to another Great Power war? Would Britain's export markets be even more badly affected than in 1809 and 1811–1812? Was not the entire economy, and domestic population, becoming too dependent upon imported goods, which might easily be cut off or suspended in periods of conflict? And would not the London-based global banking and financial system collapse at the onset of another world war, since the markets might be closed, insurances suspended, international capital transfers retarded, and credit ruined? In such circumstances, ironically, the advanced British economy might be more severely hurt than a state which was less "mature" but also less dependent upon international trade and finance.

Given the Liberal assumptions about interstate harmony and constantly increasing prosperity, these seemed idle fears; all that was required was for statesmen to act rationally and to avoid the ancient folly of quarreling with other peoples. And, indeed, the laissez-faire Liberals argued, the more British industry and commerce became integrated with, and dependent upon, the global economy, the greater would be the disincentive to pursue policies which might lead to conflict. In the same way, the growth of the financial sector was to be welcomed, since it was not only fueling the midcentury "boom," but demonstrating how advanced and progressive Britain had become; even if other countries followed her lead and did industrialize, she could switch her efforts to servicing that development, and gaining even more profits thereby. In Bernard Porter's words, she was the first frogspawn egg to grow legs, the first tadpole to change into a frog, the first frog to hop out of the pond. She was economically different from the others, but that was only because she was so far ahead of them.[32] Given these auspicious circumstances, fears of strategical weakness appeared groundless; and most mid-Victorians preferred, like Kingsley as he cried tears of pride during the Great Exhibition at the Crystal Palace in 1851, to believe that a cosmic destiny was at work:

> The spinning jenny and the railroad, Cunard's liners and the electric telegraph, are to me . . . signs that we are, on some points at least, in harmony with the universe; that there is a mighty spirit working among us . . . the Ordering and Creating God.[33]

Like all other civilizations at the top of the wheel of fortune, therefore, the British could believe that their position was both "natural" and destined to continue. And just like all those other civilizations, they were in for a rude shock. But that was still some way into the future, and in the age of Palmerston and Macaulay, it was British strengths rather than weaknesses which were mostly in evidence.

The "Middle Powers"

The impact of economic and technological change upon the relative position of the Great Powers of continental Europe was much less dramatic in the half-century or so following 1815, chiefly because the industrialization which did occur started off from a much lower base than in Britain. The farther east one went, the more feudal and agricultural the local economy tended to be; but even in western Europe, which had been close to Britain in many aspects of commercial and technological development prior to 1790, two decades of war had left a heavy mark: population losses, changed customs barriers, higher taxes, the "pastoralization" of the Atlantic sector, the loss of overseas markets and raw materials, the difficulties of acquiring the latest British inventions, were all setbacks to general economic growth, even when (for special reasons) certain trades and regions had flourished during the Napoleonic wars.[34] If the coming of peace meant a resumption of normal trade and also allowed continental entrepreneurs to see how far behind Great Britain they had fallen, it did not produce a sudden burst of modernization. There simply was not enough capital, or local demand, or official enthusiasm, to produce a transformation; and many a European merchant, craftsman, and handloom weaver would bitterly oppose the adoption of English techniques, seeing in them (quite correctly) a threat to their older way of life.[35] In consequence, although the steam engine, the power loom, and the railway made some headway in continental Europe,

> between 1815 and 1848 the traditional features of the economy remained preeminent: the superiority of agriculture over industrial production, the absence of cheap and rapid means of transport, and the priority given to consumer goods over heavy industry.[36]

As Table 7 above shows, the relative increases in per capita levels of industrialization for the century after 1750 were not very impressive; and only in the 1850s and 1860s did the picture begin to change.

The prevailing political and diplomatic conditions of "Restoration Europe" also combined to freeze the international status quo, or at least to permit only small-scale alterations in the existing order. Precisely because the French Revolution had been such a frightening challenge both to the internal social arrangements and to the traditional states system of Europe, Metternich and fellow conservatives now regarded any new developments with suspicion. An adventurist diplomacy, running the risk of a general war, was as much to be frowned upon as a campaign for national self-determination or for constitutional reform. On the whole, political leaders felt that they had enough on their hands simply dealing with domestic turbulences and the agitation of sectional interests, many of which were beginning to feel threatened by even the early appearances of new machinery, the growth of urbanization, and other incipient challenges to the guilds, the crafts, and the protective regulations of a preindustrial society. What one historian has described as an "endemic civil war that produced the great outbreaks of insurrection in 1830, as well as a host of intermediate revolts,"[37] meant that statesmen generally possessed neither the energies nor the desires to engage in foreign conflicts which might well weaken their own regimes.

In this connection, it is worth nothing that many of the military actions which did occur were initiated precisely to defend the existing sociopolitical order from revolutionary threat—for example, the Austrian army's crushing of resistance in Piedmont in 1823, the French military's move into Spain in the same year to restore to King Ferdinand his former powers, and, the most notable cause of all, the use of Russian troops to suppress the Hungarian revolution of 1848. If these reactionary measures grew increasingly unpopular to British opinion, that country's insularity meant that it would not intervene to rescue the liberal forces from suppression. As for territorial changes within Europe, they could occur only after the agreement of the "Concert" of the Great Powers, some of which might need to be compensated in one way or another. Unlike either the age of Napoleon preceding it or the age of Bismarck following it, therefore, the period 1815–1865 internationalized most of its tricky political problems (Belgium, Greece), and frowned upon unilateral actions. All this gave a basic, if precarious, stability to the existing states system.

The international position of Prussia in the decades after 1815 was clearly affected by these general political and social conditions.[38] Although greatly augmented territorially by the acquisition of the Rhineland, the Hohenzollern state now seemed much less impressive than it had been under Frederick the Great. It was, after all, only in the 1850s and 1860s that economic expansion took place on Prussian soil faster than virtually anywhere else in Europe. In the first half of the century, by contrast, the country seemed an industrial pigmy, its annual iron production of 50,000 tons being eclipsed by that not only of Britain, France, and Russia but also of the Habsburg Empire. Furthermore, the acquisition of the Rhineland not only split Prussia geographically but also exacerbated the political divisions between the state's more "liberal" western and more "feudal" eastern provinces. For the greater part of this period, domestic tensions were at the forefront of politics; and while the forces of reaction usually prevailed, they were alarmed at the reformist tendencies of 1810–1819, and quite panicked by the revolution of 1848–1849. Even when the military reimposed a profoundly illiberal regime, fear of domestic unrest made the Prussian elite reluctant to contemplate foreign-policy adventures; on the contrary, conservatives felt, they needed to identify as closely as possible with the forces of stability elsewhere in Europe, especially Russia and even Austria.

Prussia's internal-politics disputes were complicated still further by the debate about the "German question," that is to say, about the possibility of an eventual union of the thirty-nine German states, and the means by which that goal could be secured. For not only did the issue predictably divide the liberal-nationalist bourgeoisie of Prussia from most of the conservatives, but it also involved delicate negotiations with the middle- and south-German states and—most important of all—revived the rivalry with the Habsburg Empire that had last been seen in the heated disputes over Saxony in 1814. Although Prussia was the undisputed leader of the increasingly important German Customs Union (Zollverein) which developed from the 1830s onward, and which the Austrians could not join because of the protectionist pressures of their own industrialists, the balance of political advantage generally lay in Vienna's favor during these decades. In the first place, both Frederick William III (1797–1840) and Frederick William IV (1840–1861) feared the results of a clash with the Habsburg Empire more than Metternich and his successor Schwarzenberg did with their northern neighbor. In addition, Austria presided over the German Federation's meetings at Frankfurt; it had the sympathy of many of the smaller German states, not to mention the Prussian old conservatives; and it seemed indisputably a European power, whereas Prussia was little more than a German one. The most noticeable sign of Vienna's greater weight came in the 1850 agreement at Oelmuetz, which temporarily ended their jockeying for advantage in the German question when Prussia agreed to demobilize its army and to abandon its own schemes for unification. A diplomatic humiliation, in Frederick William IV's view, was preferable to a risky war so shortly after the 1848 revolution. And even those Prussian nationalists like Bismarck, smarting at such a retreat before Austrian demands, felt that little could be done elsewhere until "the struggle for mastery in Germany" was finally settled.

One quite vital factor in Frederick William's submission at Oelmuetz had been the knowledge that the Russian czar supported Austria's case in the "German question." Throughout the entire period from 1812 until 1871, in fact, Berlin took pains to avoid provoking the military colossus to the east. Ideological and dynastic reasons certainly helped to justify such obsequiousness, but they did not fully conceal Prussia's continued sense of inferiority, which the Russian acquisition of most of Congress Poland in 1814 had simply accentuated. Expressions of disapproval by St. Petersburg over any moves toward liberalization in Prussia, Czar Nicholas I's well-known conviction that German unification was utopian nonsense (especially if it was to come about, as was attempted in 1848, by a radical Frankfurt assembly offering an emperor's crown to the Prussian king!), and Russia's support of Austria before Oelmuetz were all manifestations of this overshadowing foreign influence. It was scarcely surprising, therefore, that the outbreak of the Crimean War in 1854 found the Prussian government desperately eager to stay neutral, fearing the consequences of going to war against Russia even while it worried at losing the respect of Austria and the western powers. Given its circumstances, Prussia's position was logical, but, because the British and Austrians disliked Berlin's "wavering" policy, Prussian diplomats were not allowed to join the other delegates at the Congress of Paris (1856) until some way into the proceedings. Symbolically, then, it was still being treated as a marginal participant.

In other areas, too—although less persistently—Prussia found itself constrained by foreign powers. Palmerston's denunciations of the Prussian army's move into Schleswig-Holstein in 1848 was the least worrying. Much more disturbing was the potential French threat to the Rhineland, in 1830, again in 1840, and finally in the 1860s. All those periods of tension merely confirmed what the quarrels with Vienna and occasional growls from St. Petersburg already suggested: that Prussia in the first half of the nineteenth century was the least of the Great Powers, disadvantaged by geography, overshadowed by powerful neighbors, distracted by internal and inner-German problems, and quite incapable of playing a larger role in international affairs. This seems, perhaps, too harsh a judgment in the light of Prussia's various strengths: its educational system, from the parish schools to the universities, was second to none in Europe; its administrative system was reasonably efficient; and its army and its formidable general staff were early in studying reforms in both tactics and strategy, especially in the military implications of "railways and rifles."[39] But the point was that this potential could not be utilized until the internal-political crisis between liberals and conservatives was overcome, until there was firm leadership at the top, in place of Frederick William IV's vacillations, and until Prussia's industrial base had been developed. Only after 1860, therefore, could the Hohenzollern state emerge from its near-second-class status.

Yet, as with many other things in life, strategical weakness is relative; and, compared with the Habsburg Empire to the south, Prussia's problems were perhaps not so daunting. If the period 1648–1815 had seen the empire "rising" and "asserting itself,"[40] that expansion had not eliminated the difficulties under which Vienna labored as it strove to carry out a Great Power role. On the contrary, the settlement of 1815 compounded these difficulties, at least in the longer term. For example, the very fact that the Austrians had fought so frequently against Napoleon and emerged on the winning side meant that they required "compensations" in the general shuffling of boundaries which occurred during the negotiations of 1814–1815; and although the Habsburgs wisely agreed to withdraw from the southern Netherlands, southwestern Germany (the Vorlande), and parts of Poland, this was balanced by their large-scale expansion in Italy and by the assertion of their leading role in the newly created German Federation.

Given the general theory of the European equilibrium and especially those versions preferred by British commentators as well as by Metternich himself—this reestablishment of Austrian power was commendable. The Habsburg Empire, sprawled across Europe from the northern-Italian plain to Galicia, would act as the central fulcrum to the balance, checking French ambitions in western Europe and in Italy, preserving the status quo in Germany against both the "greater-German" nationalists and the Prussian expansionists, and posing a barrier to Russian penetration of the Balkans. It was true that each of these tasks was supported by one or more of the other Great Powers, depending upon the context; but the Habsburg Empire was vital to the functioning of this complex five-sided checkmate, if only because it seemed to have the greatest interest of all in freezing the 1815 settlement—whereas France, Prussia, and Russia, sooner or later, wanted some changes, while the British, seeing fewer and fewer strategical and ideological reasons to support Metternich after the 1820s, were consequently less willing to aid Austria's efforts to maintain all aspects of the existing order. In the view of certain historians, indeed, the general peace which prevailed in Europe for decades after 1815 was due chiefly to the position and functions of the Habsburg Empire. When, therefore, it could gain no military support from the other powers to preserve the status quo in Italy and Germany in the 1860s, it was driven out of those two theaters; and when, after 1900, its own survival was in doubt, a great war of succession—with fateful implications for the European balance—was inevitable.[41]

So long as the conservative powers in Europe were united in preserving the status quo—against French resurgence, or the "revolution" generally—this Habsburg weakness was concealed. By appealing to the ideological solidarity of the Holy Alliance, Metternich could usually be assured of the support of Russia and Prussia, which in turn allowed him a free hand to arrange the interventions against any liberal stirrings—whether by sending Austrian troops to put down the Naples insurrection of 1821, or by permitting the French military action in Spain to support the Bourbon regime, or by orchestrating the imposition of the reactionary Carlsbad Decrees (1819) upon the members of the German Federation. In much the same way, the Habsburg Empire's relations with St. Petersburg and Berlin benefited from their shared interest in suppressing Polish nationalism, which for the Russian government was a far more vital issue than the occasional disagreements over Greece or the Straits; the joint suppression of the Polish revolt in Galicia and Austria's incorporation of the Free City of Kracow in 1846 with the concurrence of Russia and Prussia showed the advantages which could be gained from such monarchical solidarity.

Over the longer term, however, this Metternichian strategy was deeply flawed. A radical *social* revolution could fairly easily be kept in check in nineteenth-century Europe; whenever one occurred (1830, 1848, the 1871 Commune), the frightened middle classes defected to the side of "law and order." But the widespread ideas and movements in favor of national self-determination, stimulated by the French Revolution and the various wars of liberation earlier in the century, could not be suppressed forever; and Metternich's attempts to crush independence movements steadily exhausted the Habsburg Empire. By resolutely opposing any stirrings of national independence, Austria quickly lost the sympathy of its old ally, Britain. Its repeated use of military force in Italy provoked a reaction among all classes against their Habsburg "jailor," which in turn was to play into the hands of Napoleon III a few decades later, when that ambitious French monarch was able to help Cavour in driving the Austrians out of northern Italy. In the same way, the Habsburg Empire's unwillingness to join the Zollverein for economic reasons and the constitutional-geographical impossibility of its becoming part of a "greater Germany" disappointed many German nationalists, who then began to look to Prussia for leadership. Even the czarist regime, which generally supported Vienna's efforts to crush revolutions, occasionally found it easier than Austria to deal with national questions: witness Alexander I's policy, in cooperation with the British, of supporting Greek independence during the late 1820s despite all Metternich's counterarguments.

The fact was that in an age of increasing national consciousness, the Habsburg Empire looked ever more of an anachronism. In each of the other Great Powers, it has been pointed out,

> a majority of the citizenry shared a common language and religion. At least 90 percent of Frenchmen spoke French and the same proportion belonged at least nominally to the Catholic Church. More than eight in every ten Prussians were German (the rest were mostly Poles) and of the Germans 70 percent were Protestant. The Tsar's seventy million subjects included some notable minorities (five million Poles, three and a half million Finns, Ests, Letts and Latvians, and three million assorted Caucasians), but that still left fifty millions who were both Russian and Orthodox. And the inhabitants of the British Isles were 90 percent English-speaking and 70 percent Protestant. Countries like this needed little holding together; they had an intrinsic cohesion. By contrast the Austrian Emperor ruled an ethnic mishmash that must have made him groan every time he thought about it. He and eight million of his subjects were German, but twice as many were Slavs of one sort or another (Czechs, Slovaks, Poles, Ruthenians, Slovenes, Croats and Serbs), five million

were Hungarians, five million Italians and two million Romanians. What sort of nation did that make?

The answer is none at all.[42]

The Habsburg army, regarded as "one of the most important, if not the most important, single institutions" in the empire, reflected this ethnic diversity. "In 1865 [that is, the year before the decisive clash with Prussia for mastery of Germany], the army had 128,286 Germans, 96,300 Czechs and Slovaks, 52,700 Italians, 22,700 Slovenes, 20,700 Rumanians, 19,000 Serbs, 50,100 Ruthenes, 37,700 Poles, 32,500 Magyars, 27,600 Croats, and 5,100 men of other nationalities on its muster roles."[43] Although this made the army almost as colorful and variegated as the British-Indian regiments under the Raj, it also created all sorts of disadvantages when compared with the much more homogeneous French or Prussian armies.

This potential military weakness was compounded by the lack of adequate funding, which was due partly to the difficulties of raising taxes in the empire, but chiefly caused by the meagerness of its commercial and industrial base. Although historians now speak of "the economic rise of the Habsburg Empire"[44] in the period 1760–1914, the fact is that during the first half of the nineteenth century industrialization occurred only in certain western regions, such as Bohemia, the Alpine lands, and around Vienna itself, whereas the greater part of the empire remained relatively untouched. While Austria itself advanced, therefore, the empire *as a whole* fell behind Britain, France, and Prussia in terms of per capita industrialization, iron and steel production, steam-power capacities, and so on.

What was more, the costs of the French wars "had left the empire financially exhausted, burdened with a heavy public debt and a mass of depreciated paper money,"[45] which virtually compelled the government to keep military spending to a minimum. In 1830 the army was allocated the equivalent of only 23 percent of the total revenues (down from 50 percent in 1817), and by 1848 that share had sunk to 20 percent. When crises occurred, as in 1848–1849, 1854–1855, 1859–1860, and 1864, extraordinary increases in military spending were authorized; but they were never enough to bring the army up to anywhere like full strength, and they were just as swiftly reduced when the crisis was perceived to be over. For example, the military budget was 179 million florins in 1860, dropped to 118 million by 1863, rose to 155 million in the 1864 conflict with Denmark, and was drastically cut back to 96 million in 1865—again, just a year before the war with Prussia. None of these totals kept pace with the military budgets of France, Britain, and Russia, or (a little later) that of Prussia; and since the Austrian military administration was regarded as corrupt and inefficient even by mid-nineteenth-century standards, the monies which *were* allocated were not very well spent. In sum, the armed strength of the Habsburg Empire in no way corresponded to the wars it might be called upon to fight.[46]

All this is not to antedate the demise of the empire. Its staying power, as many historians have remarked, was quite extraordinary: having survived the Reformation, the Turks, and the French Revolution, it also proved capable of weathering the events of 1848–1849, the defeat of 1866, and, until the very last stages, the strains of the First World War. While its weaknesses were evident, it also possessed strengths. The monarchy commanded the loyalty not only of the ethnic German subjects but also of many aristocrats and "service" families in the non-German lands; its rule, say, in Poland was fairly benign compared with the Russian and Prussian administrations. Furthermore, the complex, multinational character of the empire, with its array of local rivalries, permitted a certain amount of *divide et impera* from the center, as its careful use of the army demonstrated: Hungarian regiments were stationed chiefly in Italy and Austria and Italian regiments in Hungary, half of the Hussar regiments were stationed abroad, and so on.[47]

Finally, it possessed the negative advantage that none of the other Great Powers—even when engaged in hostilities with the Habsburg Empire—knew what to put in its place. Czar Nicholas I might resent Austrian pretensions in the Balkans, but he was willing enough to lend an army to help crush the Hungarian revolution of 1848; France might intrigue to drive the Habsburgs out of Italy, but Napoleon III also knew that Vienna could be a useful future ally against Prussia or Russia; and Bismarck, though determined to expel all Austrian influence from Germany, was keen to preserve the Habsburg Empire as soon as it capitulated in 1866. As long as that situation existed, the Empire would survive—on sufferance.

Despite its losses during the Napoleonic War, the position of France in the half-century following 1815 was significantly better than that of either Prussia or the Habsburg Empire in many respects.[48] Its national income was much larger, and capital was more readily available; its population was far bigger than Prussia's and more homogeneous than the Habsburg Empire's; it could more easily afford a large army, and could pay for a considerable navy as well. Nonetheless, it is treated here as a "middle power" simply because strategical, diplomatic, and economic circumstances all combined to prevent France from concentrating its resources and gaining a decisive lead in any particular sphere.

The overriding fact about the years 1814–1815, at the power-political level, was that all of the other great states had shown themselves determined to prevent French attempts to maintain a hegemony over

Europe; and not only were London, Vienna, Berlin, and St. Petersburg willing to compose their quarrels on other issues (e.g., Saxony) in order to defeat Napoleon's final bid, but they were also intent upon erecting a postwar system to block France off in the future from its traditional routes of expansion. Thus, while Prussia acted as guardian to the Rhineland, Austria strengthened its position in northern Italy, and British influence was expanded in the Iberian peninsula; behind all this lay a large Russian army, ready to move across Europe in defense of the 1815 settlement. In consequence, however, much Frenchmen of all parties might urge a policy of "recovery,"[49] it was plain that no dramatic improvement was possible. The best that could be achieved was, on the one hand, the recognition that France was an equal partner in the European Concert, and on the other, the restoration of French political influence in neighboring regions *alongside* that of the existing powers. Yet even when the French could achieve parity with, say, the British in the Iberian Peninsula and return to playing a major role in the Levant, they always had to be wary of provoking another coalition against them. Any move by France into the Low Countries, as it became clear in the 1820s and 1830s, instinctively produced an Anglo-Prussian alliance which was too strong to combat.

The other card available to Paris was to establish close relations with *one* of the Great Powers, which could then be exploited to secure French aims.[50] Given the latent rivalries between the other states and the considerable advantages a French alliance could offer (money, troops, weapons), this was a plausible assumption; yet it was flawed in three respects. First, the other power might be able to exploit the French more than France could exploit it—as Metternich did in the mid-1830s, when he entertained French overtures simply to divide London and Paris. Secondly, the changes of regime which occurred in France in these decades inevitably affected diplomatic relations in a period where ideology played so large a role. For example, the long-felt hopes of an alliance with Russia crashed with the coming of the 1830 revolution in France. Finally, there remained the insuperable problem that while several of the other powers wanted to cooperate with France at certain times, none of them in this period desired a change in the status quo: that is, they offered the French only diplomatic friendship, not the promise of territorial gain. Not until after the Crimean War was there any widespread sentiment outside France for a reordering of the 1815 boundaries.

These obstacles might have appeared less formidable had France been as strong vis-à-vis the rest of Europe as it had been under Louis XIV at the height of his power, or under Napoleon at the height of his. But the fact was that France after 1815 was not a particularly dynamic country. Perhaps as many as 1.5 million Frenchmen had died in the wars of 1793–1815,[51] and, more significant still, the French population increase was slower than that of any other Great Power throughout the nineteenth century. Not only had that lengthy conflict distorted the French economy in the various ways mentioned above (see pp. 131–33 above), but the coming of peace exposed it to the commercial challenge of its great British rival. "The cardinal fact for most French producers after 1815 was the existence of an overwhelmingly dominant and powerful industrial producer not only as their nearest neighbor but as a mighty force in all foreign markets and sometimes even in their own heavily protected domestic market."[52] This lack of competitiveness, the existing disincentives within France to modernize (e.g., small size of agricultural holdings, poor communications, essentially local markets, absence of cheap, readily available coal), and the loss of any stimulus from overseas markets meant that between 1815 and 1850 its rate of industrial growth was considerably less than Britain's. At the beginning of the century, the latter's manufacturing output was level with France's; by 1830 it was 182.5 percent of France's; and by 1860 that had risen to 251 percent.[53] Moreover, even when France's rate of railway construction and general industrialization began to quicken in the second half of the nineteenth century, it found to its alarm that Germany was growing even faster.

Yet it is now no longer so clear to historians that France's economy during this century should be airily dismissed as "backward" or "disappointing"; in many respects, the path taken by Frenchmen toward national prosperity was just as logical as the quite different route taken by the British.[54] The social horrors of the Industrial Revolution were less widespread in France; yet by concentration upon high-quality rather than mass-produced goods, the value per capita added to each manufacture was substantially greater. If the French on the whole did not invest domestically in large-scale industrial enterprises, this was often a matter of calculation rather than a sign of poverty or retardation. There was, in fact, considerable surplus capital in the country, much of which went into industrial investments elsewhere in Europe.[55] French governments were not likely to be embarrassed by a shortage of funds, and there *was* investment in munitions and in metallurgical processes related to the armed forces. It was French inventors who produced the shell gun under General Paixhans, the "epoch-making ship designs" of the *Napoleon* and *La Gloire*, and the Minié bullet and rifling.[56]

Nevertheless, the fact remains that France's *relative* power was being eroded in economic terms as well as in other respects. While France was, to repeat, greater than Prussia or the Habsburg Empire, there was no sphere in which it was the decisive leader, as it had been a century earlier. Its army was large, but second in numbers to Russia's. Its fleet, erratically supported by successive French administrations, was usually second in size to the Royal Navy—but the gap between them was enormous. In terms of manufacturing output and national product, France was falling behind its trail-blazing neighbor. Its launching of *La Gloire* was swiftly eclipsed by the Royal Navy's H.M.S. *Warrior*, just as its field artillery fell behind Krupp's newer designs. It did play a role outside Europe, but again its possessions and influence were far less extensive than Britain's.

All this points to another acute problem which made difficult the measurement—and often the deployment—of France's undoubted strength. It remained a classic *hybrid* power,[57] frequently torn between its European and its non-European interests; and this in turn affected its diplomacy, which was already complicated enough by ideological and balance-of-power considerations. Was it more important to check Russia's advance upon Constantinople than to block British pretensions in the Levant? Should it be trying to prize Austria out of Italy, or to challenge the Royal Navy in the English Channel? Should it encourage or oppose the early moves toward German unification? Given the pros and cons attached to each of these policies, it is not surprising that the French were often found ambivalent and hesitating, even when they were regarded as a full member of the Concert.

On the other hand, it must not be forgotten that the general circumstances which constrained France also enabled it to act as a check upon the other Great Powers. If this was especially the case under Napoleon III, it was also true, incipiently, even in the late 1820s. Simply because of its size, France's recovery had implications in the Iberian and Italian peninsulas, in the Low Countries, and farther afield. Both the British and the Russian attempts to influence events in the Ottoman Empire needed to take France into account. It was France, much more than the wavering Habsburg Empire or even Britain, which posed the chief military check to Russia during the Crimean War. It was France which undermined the Austrian position in Italy, and it was chiefly France which, less dramatically, ensured that the British Empire did not have a complete monopoly of influence along the African and Chinese coasts. Finally, when the Austro-Prussian "struggle for mastery in Germany" rose to a peak, both rivals revealed their deep concern over what Napoleon III might or might not do. In sum, following its recovery after 1815 France during the decades following remained a considerable power, very active diplomatically, reasonably strong militarily, and better to have as a friend than as a rival—even if its own leaders were aware that it was no longer so dominant as in the previous two centuries.

The Crimean War and the Erosion
of Russian Power

Russia's *relative* power was to decline the most during the post-1815 decades of international peace and industrialization—although that was not fully evident until the Crimean War (1854–1856) itself. In 1814 Europe had been awed as the Russian army advanced to the west, and the Paris crowds had prudently shouted "Vive l'empéreur Alexandre!" as the czar entered their city behind his brigades of cossacks. The peace settlement itself, with its archconservative emphasis against future territorial and political change, was underwritten by a Russian army of 800,000 men—as far superior to any rivals on land as the Royal Navy was to other fleets at sea. Both Austria and Prussia were overshadowed by this eastern colossus, fearing its strength even as they proclaimed monarchical solidarity with it. If anything, Russia's role as the gendarme of Europe increased when the messianic Alexander I was succeeded by the autocratic Nicholas I (1825–1855); and the latter's position was further enhanced by the revolutionary events of 1848–1849, when, as Palmerston noted, Russia and Britain were the only powers that were "standing upright."[58] The desperate appeals of the Habsburg government for aid in suppressing the Hungarian revolt were rewarded by the dispatch of three Russian armies. By contrast, the waverings of Frederick William IV of Prussia toward internal reform movements, together with the proposals for changes in the German Federation, provoked unrelenting Russian pressure until the court at Berlin accepted policies of domestic reaction and the diplomatic retreat at Oelmuetz. As for the "forces of change" themselves after 1848, all elements, whether defeated Polish and Hungarian nationalists, or frustrated bourgeois liberals, or Marxists, were agreed that the chief bulwark against progress in Europe would long remain the empire of the czars.

Yet at the economic and technological level, Russia was losing ground in an alarming way between 1815 and 1880, at least relative to other powers. This is not to say that there was no economic improvement, even under Nicholas I, many of whose officials had been hostile to market forces or to any signs of modernization. The population grew rapidly (from 51 million in 1816, to 76 million in 1860, to 100 million in 1880), and that of the towns grew the fastest of all. Iron production increased, and the textile industry multiplied in size. Between 1804 and 1860, it was claimed, the number of factories or industrial enterprises rose from 2,400 to over 15,000. Steam engines and modern machinery were imported from the west; and from the 1830s onward a railway network began to emerge. The very fact that historians have quarreled over whether an "industrial revolution" occurred in Russia during these decades confirms that things were on the move.[59]

But the blunt point was that the rest of Europe was moving far faster and that Russia was losing ground. Because of its far bigger population, it had easily possessed the largest *total* GNP in the early nineteenth century. Two generations later, that was no longer the case, as shown in Table 9.

Table 9. GNP of the European Great Powers, 1830–1890[60]
(at market prices, in 1960 U.S. dollars and prices; in billions)

	1830	1840	1850	1860	1870	1880	1890
Russia	10.5	11.2	12.7	14.4	22.9	23.2	21.1
France	8.5	10.3	11.8	13.3	16.8	17.3	19.7
Britain	8.2	10.4	12.5	16.0	19.6	23.5	29.4
Germany	7.2	8.3	10.3	12.7	16.6	19.9	26.4
Habsburg Empire	7.2	8.3	9.1	9.9	11.3	12.2	15.3
Italy	5.5	5.9	6.6	7.4	8.2	8.7	9.4

But these figures were even more alarming when the per capita amount of GNP is studied (see Table 10).

Table 10. Per Capita GNP of the European Great Powers, 1830–1890[61]
(in 1960 U.S. dollars and prices)

	1830	1840	1850	1860	1870	1880	1890
Britain	346	394	458	558	628	680	785
Italy	265	270	277	301	312	311	311
France	264	302	333	365	437	464	515
Germany	245	267	308	354	426	443	537
Habsburg Empire	250	266	283	288	305	315	361
Russia	170	170	175	178	250	224	182

The figures show that the increase in Russia's *total* GNP which occurred during these years was overwhelmingly due to the rise in its population, whether by births or by conquests in Turkestan and elsewhere, and had little to do with real increases in productivity (especially industrial productivity). Russia's per capita income, and national product, had always been behind that of western Europe; but it now fell even further behind, from (for example) one-half of Britain's per capita income in 1830 to one-quarter of that figure sixty years later.

In the same way, the doubling of Russia's iron production in the early nineteenth century compared badly with Britain's *thirtyfold* increase;[62] within two generations, Russia had changed from being Europe's largest producer and exporter of iron into a country increasingly dependent upon imports of western manufactures. Even the improvements in rail and steamship communications need to be put in perspective. By 1850 Russia had little over 500 miles of railroad, compared with the United States' 8,500 miles; and much of the increase in steamship trade, on the great rivers or out of the Baltic and Black seas, revolved around the carriage of grains needed for the burgeoning home population and to pay for imported manufactured goods by the dispatch of wheat to Britain. What new developments occurred were all too frequently in the hands of foreign merchants and entrepreneurs (the export trade certainly was), and turned Russia ever more into a supplier of *primary* materials for advanced economies. On closer examination of the evidence, it appears that most of the new "factories" and "industrial enterprises" employed fewer than sixteen people, and were scarcely mechanized at all. A general lack of capital, low consumer demand, a minuscule middle class, vast distances and extreme climates, and the heavy hand of an autocratic, suspicious state made the prospects for industrial "takeoff" in Russia more difficult than in virtually anywhere else in Europe.[63]

For a long while, these ominous economic trends did not translate into a noticeable Russian military weakness. On the contrary, the post-1815 preference shown by the Great Powers for *ancien régime* structures in general could nowhere be more clearly seen than in the social composition, weaponry, and tactics of their armies. Still in the shadows cast by the French Revolution, governments were more concerned about the political and social reliability of their armed forces than about military reforms; and the generals themselves, no longer facing the test of a great war, emphasized hierarchy, obedience, and caution—traits reinforced by Nicholas I's obsession with formal parades and grand marches. Given these general circumstances, the sheer size of the Russian army and the steadiness of its mass conscripts appeared more impressive to outside observers than such arcane matters as military logistics or the general level of education among the officer corps. What was more, the Russian army *was* active and often successful in its frequent campaigns of expansion into the Caucasus and across Turkestan—thrusts which were already beginning to worry the British in India, and to make Anglo-Russian relations in the nineteenth century much more strained than they had been in the eighteenth.[64] Equally impressive to outside eyes was the Russian suppression of the Hungarian rebellion of 1848–1849, and the czar's claim that he stood ready to dispatch 400,000 troops to quell the contemporaneous revolt in Paris. What those observers failed to note was the less imposing fact that the greater part of the Russian army was always pinned down by internal garrison duties, by "police" actions in Poland and Finland, and by other activities, such as border patrols and the Military Colonies; and that what was left was not particularly efficient—of the 11,000 casualties incurred in the Hungarian campaign, for example, all but

1,000 were caused by diseases, because of the inefficiency of the army's logistical and medical services.[65]

The campaigning in the Crimea from 1854 until 1855 provided an all too shocking confirmation of Russia's backwardness. Czarist forces could not be concentrated. Allied operations in the Baltic (while never very serious), together with the threat of Swedish intervention, pinned down as many as 200,000 Russian troops in the north. The early campaigning in the Danubian principalities, and the far greater danger that Austria would turn its threats of intervention into reality, posed a danger to Bessarabia, the western Ukraine, and Russian Poland. The fighting against the Turks in the Caucasus placed immense demands upon both troops and supply systems, as did the defense of Russian territories in the Far East.[66] When the Anglo-French assault on the Crimea brought the war to a highly sensitive region of Russian territory, the armed forces of the czar were incapable of repudiating such an invasion.

At sea, Russia possessed a fair-sized navy, with competent admirals, and it was able to destroy completely the weaker Turkish fleet at Sinope in November 1853; but as soon as the Anglo-French fleets entered the fray, the positions were reversed.[67] Many Russian vessels were fir-built and unseaworthy, their firepower was inadequate, and their crews were half-trained. The allies had many more steam-driven warships, some of them armed with shrapnel shells and Congreve rockets. Above all, Russia's enemies had the industrial capacity to build newer vessels (including dozens of steam-driven gunboats), so that their advantage became greater as the war lengthened.

But the Russian army was even worse off. The ordinary infantryman fought well, and, under the inspired leadership of Admiral Nakhimov and the engineering genius of Colonel Todtleben, Russia's prolonged defense of Sevastopol was a remarkable feat. But in all other respects the army was woefully inadequate. The cavalry regiments were unadventurous and their parade-ground horses incapable of strenuous campaigning (here the irregular cossack forces were better). Worse still, the Russian soldiers were wretchedly armed. Their old-fashioned flintlock muskets had a range of 200 yards, whereas the rifles of the Allied troops could fire effectively up to 1,000 yards; thus Russian casualties were far heavier.

Worst of all, even when the hugeness of the task was known, the Russian system *as a whole* was incapable of responding to it. Army leadership was poor, ridden with personal rivalries, and never able to produce a coherent grand strategy—here it simply reflected the general incompetence of the czar's government. There were very few trained and educated officers of the middle rank, such as the Prussian army possessed in abundance, and initiative was totally frowned upon. Astonishingly, there were also very few reservists to call up in the event of a national emergency, since the adoption of a mass short-service system would have involved the demise of serfdom.* One consequence of this system was that Russia's long-service army included many *over-aged* troopers; another even more fatal consequence was that some 400,000 of the new recruits hastily enrolled at the beginning of the war were totally untrained—for there were insufficient officers to do the job—and the withdrawal of that many men from the serf labor market hurt the Russian economy.

Finally, there were the logistical and economic weaknesses. Since there were no railways south of Moscow (!), the horse-drawn supply wagons had to cross hundreds of miles of steppes, which were a sea of mud during the spring thaw and the autumn rains. Furthermore, the horses themselves required so much fodder (which in turn had to be carried by other packhorses, and so on) that an enormous logistical effort produced disproportionately small results: allied troops and reinforcements could be sent from France and England by sea to the Crimea in three weeks, whereas Russian troops from Moscow sometimes took three months to reach the front. More alarming still was the collapse of the Russian army's equipment stocks. "At the beginning of the war 1 million guns had been stockpiled; [at the end of 1855] only 90,000 were left. Of the 1,656 field guns, only 253 were available. . . . Stocks of powder and shot were in even worse shape."[68] The longer the war lasted, the greater the allied superiority became, while the British blockade stifled the importation of new weapons.

But the blockade did more than that: it cut off Russia's flow of grain and other exports (except for those going overland to Prussia) and made it impossible for the Russian government to pay for the war other than by heavy borrowing. Military expenditures, which even in peacetime took four-fifths of the state revenue, rose from about 220 million rubles in 1853 to about 500 million in both war years 1854 and 1855. To cover part of the alarming deficit, the Russian treasury borrowed in Berlin and Amsterdam, but then the ruble's international value tumbled; to cover the rest, it resorted to printing paper money, which led to large-scale price inflation and increasing peasant unrest. The earlier, brave attempts of the finance ministry to create a silver-based ruble and to ban all promissory notes—which had been the ruination of "sound finance" during the Napoleonic War and the campaigns against Persia, Turkey, and the Polish rebels—were now completely wrecked by the war in the Crimea. If Russia persisted in its fruitless struggle, the Crown Council was warned on January 15, 1856, the state would go bankrupt.[69] Negotiations with the Great Powers offered the only way to avoid catastrophe.

---

*It being argued that any man who had competed two or three years in the army could no longer be a serf; and that it was safer to recruit a small proportion of each year's males as *long-service* troops.

All this is not to say that the allies found the Crimean War easy; for them, too, the campaigning involved strain and unpleasant shocks. The least badly affected, interestingly enough, was France, which for once benefited from being a hybrid power—it was less backward industrially and economically than Russia, and less "unmilitarized" than Britain. The armed forces sent eastward under General Saint-Arnaud were well equipped, well trained because of their North African operations, and reasonably experienced in overseas campaigning; their logistical and medical-support systems were as efficient as any which a midcentury administration could produce; and the French officers showed justified bemusement at their amateur British opposite numbers with their overloaded baggage. The French expeditionary force was by far the largest and made most of the major breakthroughs in the war. To some degree, then, the nation recovered its Napoleonic heritage in this fighting.

By the later stages of the campaign, however, France was beginning to reveal signs of strain. Although it was a rich country, its government had to compete for ready funds with railway constructors and others seeking money from the Crédit Mobilier and other bankers. Gold was being drained away to the Crimea and Constantinople, sending up prices at home; and poor grain harvests didn't help. Although the full war losses (100,000) were not known, early French enthusiasm for the conflict quickly evaporated. Popular riots over inflation reinforced the argument, widespread after the news of Sevastopol's fall, that the war was being prolonged only for selfish and ambitious British purposes.[70] By that time, too, Napoleon III was eager to bring the fighting to an end: Russia had been chastised, France's prestige had been boosted (and would rise further following a great international peace conference in Paris), and it was important not to get too distracted from German and Italian matters by escalating the conflict around the Black Sea. Even if he could not substantially redraw the map of Europe in 1856, Napoleon could certainly feel that France's prospects were rosier than at any time since Waterloo. For another decade, the post–Crimean War fissures in the old Concert of Europe would allow that illusion to continue.

The British, by contrast, were far from satisfied with the Crimean War. Despite certain efforts at reform, the army was still in the Wellingtonian mold, and its commander, Raglan, had actually been Wellington's military secretary in the Peninsular War. The cavalry was adequate—as cavalry forces go—but often misused (not just at Balaclava), and could scarcely be deployed in the Sevastopol siegeworks. While the soldiers were toughened old sweats who fought hard, the appalling lack of warm shelter in Crimean rains and winter, the incapacity of the army's primitive medical services to handle large-scale outbreaks of dysentery and cholera, and the paucity of land transport caused needless losses and setbacks which infuriated the British nation. More embarrassing still, since the British army, like the Russian, was a long-service force chiefly useful for garrison duties, there was no trained reserve which could be drawn upon in wartime; but while the Russians could at least forcibly conscript hundreds of thousands of raw recruits, laissez-faire Britain could not, leaving the government in the embarrassing position of advertising for foreign mercenaries with which to fill the shortfall of troops in the Crimea. Yet while its army always remained a junior partner to the French, Britain's navy had no real chance to secure a Nelsonic victory against a foe who prudently withdrew his fleet into fortified harbors.[71]

The explosion of public discontent in Britain at the London *Times'* notorious revelations of military incompetence and of the sufferings of the sick and wounded troops can only be mentioned in passing here; it not only led to a change of ministry, but also provoked an earnest debate upon the difficulties inherent in being "a liberal state at war."[72] More than that, the whole affair revealed that what had seemed to be Britain's peculiar strengths—a low degree of government, a small imperial army, a heavy reliance upon sea power, an emphasis upon individual freedoms and an unfettered press, the powers of Parliament and of individual ministers—quite easily turned into weaknesses when the country was called upon to carry out an extensive military operation throughout all seasons against a major foe.

The British response to this test was (rather like the American response to wars in the twentieth century) to allocate vast amounts of money to the armed forces in order to make up for past neglect; and, once again, the crude figures of the military expenditures of the combatants go a long way toward explaining the eventual outcome of the conflict (see Table 11).

Table 11. Military Expenditures of the Powers in the Crimean War[73]
(millions of pounds)

	1852	1853	1854	1855	1856
Russia	15.6	19.9	31.3	39.8	37.9
France	17.2	17.5	30.3	43.8	36.3
Britain	10.1	9.1	76.3	36.5	32.3
Turkey	2.8	?	?	3.0	?
Sardinia	1.4	1.4	1.4	2.2	2.5

But even when Britain bestirred itself, it could not swiftly create the proper instruments of power: military spending might multiply, hundreds of steam-driven vessels might be ordered, the expeditionary force might enjoy a *surplus* of tents and blankets and ammunition by 1855, and a belligerent Palmerston might assert the need to break up the Russian Empire; yet Britain's small army could do little if France moved toward peace and Austria stayed neutral—which was precisely what happened in the months after the fall of Sevastopol. Only if the British nation and political economy became much more "militarized" could it sustain the war alone against Russia in any meaningful way; but the likely costs were far too high to a political leadership already made uneasy at the strategical, constitutional, and economic difficulties which the Crimean campaign had thrown up.[74] While feeling cheated of a proper victory, therefore, the British also were willing to compromise. What all this did was to make many Europeans (Frenchmen and Austrians as well as Russians) suspicious of London's aims and reliability, just as it made the British public ever more disgusted at being entangled in continental affairs. While Napoleon's France moved to the center of the European stage of 1856, therefore, Britain steadily moved to the edge—a drift which the Indian Mutiny (1857) and domestic reform movements could only intensify.

If the Crimean War had shocked the British, that was nothing compared to the blow which had been delivered to Russia's power and self-esteem—not to mention the losses caused by the 480,000 deaths. "We cannot deceive ourselves any longer," Grand Duke Konstantin Nikolayevich flatly stated. ". . . we are both weaker and poorer than the first-class powers, and furthermore poorer not only in material but also in mental resources, especially in matters of administration."[75] This knowledge drove the reformers in the Russian state toward a whole series of radical changes, most notably the abolition of serfdom. In addition, railway-building and industrialization were given far greater encouragement under Alexander II than under his father. Coal production, iron and steel production, large-scale utilities, and far bigger industrial enterprises were more in evidence from the 1860s onward, and the statistics provided in the economic histories of Russia are impressive enough at first sight.[76]

As ever, however, a change of perspective affects one's judgment. Could this modernization keep pace with, let alone draw ahead of, the vast annual increases in the numbers of poor, uneducated peasants? Could it match the explosive increases in iron and steel production, and manufactures, taking place in the West Midlands, the Ruhr, Silesia, and Pittsburgh during the following two decades? Could it, even with its reorganized army, keep pace with the "military revolution" which the Prussians were about to reveal to the world, and which would emphasize again the *qualitative* over the *quantitative* elements of national strength? The answers to all those questions would disappoint a Russian nationalist, all too aware that his country's place in Europe was substantially reduced from the position of eminence it had occupied in 1815 and 1848.

The United States and the Civil War

As mentioned previously, observers of global politics from de Tocqueville onward felt that the rise of the Russian Empire went in parallel with that of the United States. To be sure, everyone admitted that there were fundamental differences in the political culture and constitutions of those two states, but in World Power terms they seemed very much alike in respect to their geographical size, their "open" and ever-moving frontiers, their fast-growing populations, and their scarcely tapped resources.[77] While much of that is true, the fact remains that throughout the nineteenth century there were important economic discrepancies between the United States and Russia which would have an increasing impact upon their national power. The first of these was in terms of total population, although the gap significantly narrowed between 1816 (Russia 51.2 million, United States 8.5 million) and 1860 (Russia 76 million, United States 31.4 million). What was more pertinent was the character of that population: whereas Russia consisted overwhelmingly of serfs, with low income and low production, Americans on their homesteads or in the swiftly growing cities generally* enjoyed a high standard of living, and of national output, relative to other countries. Already in 1800, wages had been about one-third higher than those in western Europe, and that superiority was to be preserved, if not increased, throughout the century. Despite the vast inflow of European immigrants by the 1850s, the ready availability of land in the west, together with constant industrial growth, caused labor to be relatively scarce and wages to be high, which in turn induced manufacturers to invest in labor-saving machinery, further stimulating national productivity. The young republic's isolation from European power struggles, and the *cordon sanitaire* which the Royal Navy (rather than the Monroe Doctrine) imposed to separate the Old World from the New, meant that the only threat to the United States' future prosperity could come from Britain itself. Yet despite sore memories of 1776 and 1812, and border disputes in the northwest,[78] an Anglo-American war was unlikely; the flow of British capital and manufactures toward the United States and the return flow of American raw materials (especially cotton) tied the two economies ever closer together and further stimulated American economic growth. Instead of having to divert financial resources into large-scale defense expenditures, therefore, a strategically secure United States could concentrate its own (and British) funds upon developing its vast economic potential. Neither conflict with the Indians nor the 1846 war with Mexico was a substantial drain upon such productive investment.

The result of all this was that even before the outbreak of the Civil

---

*Except the black slaves, and the still relatively populous Indians.

War in April 1861, the United States had become an economic giant, although its own distance from Europe, its concentration upon internal development (rather than foreign trade), and the rugged nature of the countryside partly disguised that fact. While its share of world manufacturing output in 1860 was well behind that of Great Britain, it had already surged past Germany and Russia and was on the point of overtaking France. The United States, with only 40 percent of Russia's population in 1860, had an urban population more than twice as large, produced 830,000 tons of iron to Russia's 350,000 tons, had an energy consumption from modern fuel sources fifteen times as large, and a railway mileage thirty times greater (and even three times greater than Britain's). By contrast, the United States possessed a regular army of a mere 26,000 men compared with Russia's gigantic force of 862,000.[79] The disparity between the economic indices and the military indices of the two continent-wide states was perhaps never greater than at this point.

Within another year, of course, the Civil War had begun to transform the amount of national resources which Americans devoted to military purposes. The origins and causes of that conflict are not for discussion here; but since the leadership of both sides had determined upon a fight to the finish, and since each side could call upon hundreds of thousands of men, the struggle was likely to be prolonged. What made it more so was the distances involved, with the "front" ranging from the Virginia coast to the Mississippi, and even farther westward into Missouri and Arkansas—much of this being forest, mountain range, and swamplands. Similarly, the North's naval blockade of its foes' ports involved patrolling a coastline as extensive as that between Hamburg and Genoa. Crushing the South, in other words, would be an extraordinarily difficult logistical and military task, especially for a people which had kept its armed forces to a minimum and had no experience of large-scale war.

Yet while the four years of conflict were exhausting and fearfully bloody—the Union losing about 360,000 men to the Confederacy's 258,000*—they also catalyzed the latent national power which the United States possessed, transforming it (at least for a short while) into the greatest military nation on earth before its post-1865 demobilization. From amateur beginnings, the armed forces of each side turned themselves into mass conscript armies, employing modern rifled artillery and small arms, grinding away in the siege warfare of northern Virginia or being shuttled en masse by rail to the western theaters, communicating by telegraph to army headquarters, and drawing upon the resources of a mobilized war economy; the naval campaigns, more-

---

*About one-third in battle, the rest chiefly through diseases. The grand total of around 620,000 was more than the American losses in World War I, World War II, and the Korean War put together, and was suffered by a much smaller population.

over, witnessed the first use of ironclads, of rotating turrets, of early torpedos and mines, and of swift, steam-driven commerce raiders. Since this conflict much more than either the Crimean struggle or Prussia's wars of unification lays claim to being the first real industrialized "total war" on proto-twentieth-century lines, it is worth noting why the North won.

The first and most obvious reason—assuming that willpower would remain equal on each side—was the disproportion in resources and population. It may have been true that the South enjoyed the morale advantage of fighting for its very existence and (usually) on its own soil; that it could call upon a higher proportion of white males who were used to riding and shooting; that it possessed determined and good-quality generals and that, for a long while, it could import munitions and other supplies to make up for its matériel deficiencies.[80] But none of these could fully compensate for the great numerical imbalance between the North and the South. While the former contained a population of approximately twenty million whites, the Confederacy had only six million. What was more, the Union's total was steadily enhanced by immigrants (more than 800,000 arrived between 1861 and 1865) and by the 1862 decision to enlist black troops—something which the South avoided, predictably enough, until the last few months of the war. Around two million men served in the Union Army, which reached a peak strength of about one million in 1864–1865, whereas only about 900,000 men fought for the Confederate Army, whose maximum strength was never more than 464,500—from which "peak," reached in late 1863, it slowly declined.

But there was, as usual, more to war than sheer numbers. Even to reach the army size it did, the South ran the risk of taking too many men away from agriculture, mines, and foundries, thus weakening its already questionable capacity to fight a prolonged war. From the very beginning, in fact, the Confederates found themselves disadvantaged economically. In 1860 the North possessed 110,000 manufacturing establishments to the South's 18,000 (and many of the latter relied upon Northern technological expertise and skilled laborers); the Confederacy produced only 36,700 tons of pig iron, whereas Pennsylvania's total alone was 580,000 tons; New York State manufactured almost $300 million worth of goods—well over four times the production of Virginia, Alabama, Louisiana, and Mississippi combined. This staggering disparity in the economic base of each belligerent steadily transformed itself into real military effectiveness.

For example, whereas the South could make very few rifles (chiefly from the machinery captured at Harper's Ferry) and heavily relied upon imports, the North massively expanded its home manufactures of rifles, of which nearly 1.7 million were produced. The North's railway system (some 22,000 miles in length, and fanning out from the east to the southwest) could be maintained, and even expanded, during the war; the South's mere 9,000 miles of track, and inadequate supplies of locomotives and rolling stock, was gradually worn out. Similarly, while neither side possessed much of a navy at the outset of the conflict, the South was disadvantaged by having no machine shop which could build marine engines, whereas the North possessed several dozen such establishments. Although it took time for the Union's maritime supremacy to make itself felt—during which period blockade runners brought European-made munitions to the Confederate Army, and Southern commerce raiders inflicted heavy losses upon the North's merchant marine—the net slowly and inexorably tightened around the South's ports. By December 1864 the Union's navy totaled some 671 warships, including 236 steam vessels built since the war's beginning. Northern sea power was also vital in giving its armed forces control of the great inland rivers, especially in the Mississippi-Tennessee region; it was the successful use of *combined* rail and water transport which aided the Union's offensives in the western theater.

Finally, the Confederates found it impossible to pay for the war. Their chief income in peacetime came from the export of cotton; when that trade dried up and when—to the South's disappointment—the European powers did not intervene in the struggle, there was no way to compensate for the loss. There were few banks in the South, and little liquid capital; and taxing land and slaves brought little revenue when the productivity of both was being hard hit by the war. Borrowing from abroad produced little, yet without foreign currency or specie it was difficult to pay for vital imports. Inevitably, perhaps, the Confederate treasury turned to the printing press, but "overabundant paper money combined with severe commodity shortages to create rampant inflation"[81]—which in turn dealt a severe blow to the populace's will to continue the fight. By contrast, the North could always raise enough money, from taxation and loans, to pay for the conflict; and its printing of "greenbacks" in some ways stimulated further industrial and economic growth. Impressively, the Union's productivity surged again during the war, not only in munitions, railway-building, and ironclad construction, but also in agricultural output. By the end of the war, Northern soldiers were probably better fed and supplied than any army in history. If there was going to be a particularly American approach to military conflict—an "American way of war," to use Professor Weigley's phrase[82]—then it was first forged here, in the Union's mobilization and deployment of its massive industrial-technological potential to crush its foe.

If all the above sounds too deterministic an explanation for the outcome of a conflict which seemed to sway backward and forward for nearly four years, then it may be worth stressing the fundamental strategical problem which faced the South. Given the imbalances in size and population, there was no way in which it could overrun the North; the best that could be achieved was to so blunt the enemy's armies, and willpower, that he would abandon his policy of coercion and admit the South's claims (to slavery, or to secede, or both). This strategy would have been greatly aided if the border states like Maryland and Kentucky had overwhelmingly voted to join the Confederacy, which simply didn't happen; and it would have been helped beyond measure if a foreign power like Britain had intervened, but to suppose that was likely was a staggering misreading of British political priorities in the early 1860s.[83] With the exclusion of those two possibilities of swinging the *overall* military balance in favor of the South, the Confederates were simply left with the strategy of resisting the Union's pressures and hoping that a majority of Northerners would tire of the war. But that meant, unavoidably, a long-drawn-out conflict—and the lengthier the war was, the more the Union could mobilize its greater resources, boost its munitions production, lay down hundreds of warships, and inexorably squeeze the South, by naval blockade, by unrelenting military pressure in northern Virginia, by long-range campaigning in the west, and by Sherman's devastating drives through enemy territories. As the South's economy, morale, and front-line forces waned—by the beginning of 1865 its "present for duty" troop total was down to 155,000 men—surrender was the only realistic choice left.

The Wars of German Unification

Although the American Civil War was studied by a number of European military observers,[84] its special features (of distance, of the wilderness, of being a civil conflict) made it appear less of a pointer to general military developments than the armed struggles which were to occur in Europe during the 1860s. There the Crimean War had not only undermined the old-style Concert diplomacy but had also caused each of the "flank" powers to feel less committed to intervention in the center: Russia needed many years to recover from its humiliating defeat; and Britain preferred to concentrate upon imperial and domestic issues. This therefore left European affairs dominated, artificially as it turned out, by France. Prussia, having occupied a seemingly inglorious place under Frederick William IV during the Crimean War, was now convulsed by the constitutional quarrels between his successor William I and the Prussian parliament, especially over the issue of army reform. The Habsburg Empire, for its part, was still juggling with the interrelated problem of preserving its Italian interests against Piedmont and its German interests against Prussia, while at the same time endeavoring to contain Hungarian discontents at home.

France, by contrast, seemed strong and confident under Napoleon III. Banking, railway, and industrial development had all advanced since the early 1850s. Its colonial empire was extended in West Africa, Indochina, and the Pacific. Its fleet was expanded so that at times (e.g., 1859) it caused alarm on the other side of the English Channel. Militarily and diplomatically, it seemed to be the decisive third force in any solution of either the German or the Italian question—as was amply shown in 1859, when France swiftly intervened on Piedmont's behalf in the short-lived war against Austria.[85]

Yet however important the battles of Magenta and Solferino were in compelling the Habsburg Empire to surrender its hold upon Lombardy, acute observers in 1859 would have noticed that it was Austrian military incompetence, not French military brilliance (and certainly not Piedmontese military brilliance!), which decided the outcome. France's army did have the advantage of possessing many more rifles than Austria—this being responsible for the numerous casualties which so unnerved the Emperor Francis Joseph—but French deficiencies were also remarkable: medical and ammunition supplies were sorely lacking, mobilization schedules were haphazard, and Napoleon III's own leadership was less than brilliant. This did not matter so much at the time, since the Habsburg army was weaker and the leadership of General Gyulai was even more dithering.[86] Military effectiveness is, after all, *relative*—which was later demonstrated by the fact that Habsburg forces could still deal easily with the Italians on land (at Custozza, in 1866) and at sea (at Lissa) even when they were incapable of taking on France, or Prussia, or Russia. But this meant, by extension, that France itself would not be automatically superior in a future conflict against a *different* foe. The outcome of that war would depend upon the varying levels of military leadership, weapons systems, and productive base possessed by each side.

Since it was precisely in the era of the 1850s and 1860s that the technological explosion caused by the Industrial Revolution made its first real impacts upon warfare, it is not surprising that armed services everywhere were now found grappling with unprecedented operational problems. What would be the more important arm in battle—the infantry with its new breech-loading rifles, or the artillery with its new steel-barreled, mobile guns? What was the impact of railways and telegraphs upon command in the field? Did the new technology of war give the advantage to the advancing army, or the defending one?[87] The proper answer to such questions was, of course, that it all depends on the circumstances. That is, the outcome would be affected not only by newer weaponry but also by the terrain in which it was used, the morale and tactical competence of the troops, the efficacy of the supply systems, and all of the other myriad factors which help to decide the fate of battles. Since knowing beforehand how everything would work out was an impossibility, the key factor was the possession of a military-political leadership adept at juggling the various elements and a military instrument flexible enough to respond to new circumstances. And in these vital respects, neither the Habsburg Empire nor even France were going to be as successful as Prussia.

The Prussian "military revolution" of the 1860s, soon to produce what Disraeli would grandly term the "German revolution" in European affairs, was based upon a number of interrelated elements. The first of these was a unique short-service system, pushed through by the new King Wilhelm I and his war minister against their Liberal opponents, which involved three years' obligatory service in the regular army and then another four in the reserve before each man passed into the Landwehr—which meant that the fully mobilized Prussian army had seven annual intakes.* Since no substitutes were permitted, and the Landwehr could take over most garrison and "rear area" duties, such a system gave Prussia a far larger front-line army relative to its population than any other Great Power had. This depended, in turn, upon a relatively high level of at least primary education among the people—a rapidly expandable, short-service system, in the opinion of most experts, would be difficult to work in a nation of uneducated peasants—and it depended also upon a superb organization simply to handle such great numbers. There was, after all, little use in raising a force of half a million or a million men if they could not be adequately trained, clothed, armed, and fed, and transported to the decisive battle zone; and it would be even more of a waste of manpower and resources if the army commander could not communicate with and control the sheer masses involved.

The body imparting control to this force was the Prussian General Staff, which rose from obscurity in the early 1860s to be "the brains of the army" under the elder Moltke's genius. Hitherto, most armies in peacetime had consisted of combat units, supported by quartermaster, personnel, engineering, and other branches; actual military staffs were scrambled together only when campaigning began and a command was established. In the Prussian case, however, Moltke had recruited the brightest products of the War Academy and taught them to plan and prepare for possible future conflicts. Operations plans had to be made, and frequently revised, well before the outbreak of hostilities; war games and maneuvers bore careful study, as did historical campaigns and operations carried out by other powers. A special department was created to supervise the Prussian railway system and make sure that troops and supplies could be speeded to their destinations. Above all, Moltke's staff system attempted to inculcate in the officer corps the operational practice of dealing with large bodies of men

*And, exceptionally, the first Landwehr annual intake as well.

(army corps or full armies) which would move and fight independently but always be ready to converge upon the scene of the decisive battle. If communication could not be maintained with Moltke's headquarters in the rear, generals at the front were permitted to use their initiative and to act according to a few basic ground rules.

The above is, of course, an idealized model. The Prussian army was not perfect and was to suffer from many teething troubles in actual battle even after the reforms of the early to middle 1860s. Many of the field commanders ignored Moltke's advice and crashed blindly ahead in premature attacks or in the wrong direction—the Austrian campaign of 1866 was full of such blunders.[88] At the tactical level, too, the frontal assault (and heavy loses) of the Prussian Guards at Gravelotte-St. Privat in 1870 demonstrated a crass stupidity. The railway supply system by itself did not guarantee success; often it merely built up a vast stockpile of stores at the frontier, while the armies which needed those stocks had moved away from any nearby lines. Nor could it be said that Prussian scientific planning had ensured that their forces always possessed the best weapons: Austrian artillery was clearly superior in 1866, and the French Chassepot bolt-action rifle was stupendously better in 1870.

The real point about the Prussian system was not that it was free of errors, but that the general staff carefully studied its past mistakes and readjusted training, organization, and weapons accordingly. When the weakness of its artillery was demonstrated in 1866, the Prussian army swiftly turned to the new Krupp breechloader which was going to be so impressive in 1870. When delays occurred in the railway supply arrangements, a new organization was established to improve matters. Finally, Moltke's emphasis upon the deployment of several full armies which could operate independently yet also come to one another's aid meant that even if one such force was badly mauled in detail—as actually occurred in both the Austro-Prussian and Franco-Prussian wars—the overall campaign was not ruined.[89]

It was therefore a combination of factors which gave the Prussians the swift victory over the Austrians in the summer of 1866 that few observers had anticipated. Although Hanover, Saxony, and other northern German states joined the Habsburg side, Bismarck's diplomacy had ensured that none of the Great Powers would intervene in the initial stages of the struggle; and this in turn gave Moltke the opportunity to dispatch three armies through separate mountain routes to converge on the Bohemian plain and assault the Austrians at Sadowa (Koeniggratz). In retrospect, the outcome seems all too predictable. Over one-quarter of the Habsburg forces were needed in Italy (where they were victorious); and the Prussian recruitment system meant that despite Prussia's population being less than half that of its various foes, Moltke could deploy almost as many front-line troops.

The Habsburg army had been underfinanced, had no real staff system, and was ineptly led by Benedek; and however bravely individual units fought, they were slaughtered in open clashes by the far superior Prussian rifles. By October 1866, the Habsburgs had been forced to cede Venetia and to withdraw from any interest in Germany—which was by then well on its way to being reorganized under Bismarck's North German Federation.[90]

The "struggle for mastery in Germany" was almost complete; but the clash over who was supreme in western Europe, Prussia or an increasingly nervous and suspicious France, had been brought much closer, and by the late 1860s each side was calculating its chances. Ostensibly, France still appeared the stronger. Its population was much larger than Prussia's (although the total number of *German-speakers* in Europe was greater). The French army had gained experience in the Crimea, Italy, and overseas. It possessed the best rifle in the world, the Chassepot, which far outranged the Prussian needlegun; and it had a new secret weapon, the *mitrailleuse,* a machine gun which could fire 150 rounds a minute. Its navy was far superior; and help was expected from Austria-Hungary and Italy. When the time came in July 1870 to chastise the Prussians for their effrontery (i.e., Bismarck's devious diplomacy over the future of Luxembourg, and over a possible Hohenzollern candidate to the Spanish throne), few Frenchmen had doubts about the outcome.

The magnitude and swiftness of the French collapse—by September 4 its battered army had surrendered at Sedan, Napoleon III was a prisoner, and the imperial regime had been overthrown in Paris—was a devastating blow to such rosy assumptions. As it turned out, neither Austria-Hungary nor Italy came to France's aid, and French sea power proved totally ineffective. All therefore had depended upon the rival armies, and here the Prussians proved indisputably superior. Although both sides used their railway networks to dispatch large forces to the frontier, the French mobilization was much less efficient. Called-up reservists had to catch up with their regiments, which had already gone to the front. Artillery batteries were scattered all over France, and could not be easily concentrated. By contrast, within fifteen days of the declaration of war, three German armies (of well over 300,000 men) were advancing into the Saarland and Alsace. The Chassepot rifle's advantage was all too frequently neutralized by the Prussian tactic of pushing forward their mobile, quick-firing artillery. The *mitrailleuse* was kept in the rear, and never employed effectively. Marshal Bazaine's lethargy and ineptness were indescribable, and Napoleon himself was little better. By contrast, while individual Prussian units blundered and suffered heavy losses in "the fog of war," Moltke's distant supervision of the various armies and his willingness to rearrange his plans to exploit unexpected circumstances kept up the momentum of the invasion until the French cracked. Although republican forces were to maintain a resistance for another few months, the German grip around Paris and upon northeastern France inexorably tightened; the fruitless counterattacks of the Army of the Loire and the irritations offered by *francs-tireurs* could not conceal the fact that France had been smashed as an independent Great Power.[91]

The triumph of Prussia-Germany was, quite clearly, a triumph of its military system; but, as Michael Howard acutely notes, "the military system of a nation is not an independent section of the social system but an aspect of it in its entirety."[92] Behind the sweeping advances of the German columns and the controlled orchestration of the general staff there lay a nation much better equipped and prepared for the conditions of modern warfare than any other in Europe. In 1870, the German states combined already possessed a larger population than France, and only disunity had disguised that fact. Germany had more miles of railway lines, better arranged for military purposes. Its gross national product and its iron and steel production were just then overtaking the French totals. Its coal production was two and a half times as great, and its consumption from modern energy sources was 50 percent larger. The Industrial Revolution in Germany was creating many more large-scale firms, such as the Krupp steel and armaments combine, which gave the Prusso-German state both military and industrial muscle. The army's short-service system was offensive to liberals inside and outside the country—and criticism of "Prussian militarism" was widespread in these years—but it mobilized the manpower of the nation for warlike purposes more effectively than the laissez-faire west or the backward, agrarian east. And behind all this was a people possessing a far higher level of primary and technical education, an unrivaled university and scientific establishment, and chemical laboratories and research institutes without an equal.[93]

Europe, to repeat the quip of the day, had lost a mistress and gained a master. Under Bismarck's astonishingly adroit handling, the Great Power system was going to be dominated by Germany for two whole decades after 1870; all roads, diplomats remarked, now led to Berlin. Yet as most people could see, it was not merely the cleverness and ruthlessness of the imperial chancellor which made Germany the most important power on the European continent. It was also German industry and technology, which boomed still faster once national unification had been accomplished; it was German science and education and local administration; and it was the impressive Prussian army. That the Second German Reich possessed major internal flaws, over which Bismarck constantly fretted, was scarcely noticed by outside observers. Every nation in Europe, even the isolationist British to some degree, felt affected by this new colossus. The Russians, although staying benevolently neutral during the 1870–1871 war and taking advantage of the crisis in western Europe to improve their own position in the Black Sea,[94] resented the fact that the European center of gravity was now located in Berlin and secretly worried about what Germany might do next. The Italians, who had occupied Rome in 1870 while the French (the pope's protectors) were being crushed in Lorraine, steadily gravitated toward Berlin. So, too, did the Austro-Hungarian Empire (as it became known after Vienna's 1867 compromise with the Hungarians), which hoped to find in the Balkans compensation for its loss of place in Germany and Italy—but was well aware that such an ambition might provoke a Russian reaction. Finally, the shocked and embittered French felt it necessary to reexamine and reform vast areas of government and society (education, science, railways, the armed forces, the economy) in what was to be a fruitless attempt to regain parity with their powerful neighbor across the Rhine.[95] Both at the time and even more in retrospect, the year 1870 was viewed as a decisive watershed in European history.

On the other hand, perhaps because most countries felt the need to draw breath after the turbulences of the 1860s, and because statesmen operated cautiously under the new order, the *diplomatic* history of the Great Powers for the decade or so after 1871 was one of a search for stability. Being concerned respectively with the post–Civil War reconstruction and with the aftermath of the Meiji Revolution, neither the United States nor Japan were part of the "system," which if anything was more Eurocentric than before. While there now existed a recast version of the "European pentarchy," the balances were considerably altered from those which pertained after 1815. Prussia-Germany, under Bismarck's direction, was now the most powerful and influential of the European states, in place of a Prussia which had always been the weakest. There was also another new power, united Italy, but its desperate condition of economic backwardness (especially the lack of coal) meant that it was never properly accepted into the major league of powers, even though it was obviously more important in European diplomacy than countries such as Spain or Sweden.[96] What it did do, because of its pretensions in the Mediterranean and North Africa, was to move into a state of increasing rivalry with France, distracting the latter power and offering a useful future ally to Germany; secondly, because of its legacy of liberation wars against Vienna and its own ambitions in the western Balkans, Italy also disconcerted Austria-Hungary (at least until Bismarck had cemented over those tensions in the Austro-German-Italian "Triple Alliance" of 1882). This meant that neither Austria-Hungary nor France, the two chief "victims" of Germany's rise, could concentrate its energies fully upon Berlin, since both now possessed a vigorous (if not too muscular) Italy in their rear. And whereas this fact simply added to the Austrian reasons for reconciling themselves to Germany, and becoming a quasi-satellite in consequence, it also meant that even France's greater degree of national strength and alliance worthiness[97] was compromised in any future struggle against Berlin by the existence of a hostile and unpredictable Italy to the south.

With France isolated, Austria-Hungary cowed, and the intermediate "buffer states" of southern Germany and Italy now merged into their larger national units,[98] the only substantial checks to the further aggrandizement of Germany seemed to lie with the independent "flank" powers of Russia and Great Britain. To British administrations oscillating between a Gladstonian emphasis upon internal reforms (1868–1874) and a Disraelian stress upon the country's "imperial" and "Asian" destinies (1874–1880), this issue of the European equilibrium rarely seemed very pressing. This was probably not the case in Russia, where Chancellor Gorchakov and others resented the transformation of their Prussian client-state into a powerful Germany; but such feelings were mingled with the close dynastic and ideological sympathies that existed between the courts of St. Petersburg and Potsdam after 1871, by the still-pressing Russian need to recover from the Crimean War disasters, by the hope of obtaining Berlin's support for Russian interests in the Balkans, and by the renewal of interest in central Asia. On the whole, however, the flank powers' likelihood of intervening in the affairs of west-central Europe would depend heavily upon what Germany itself did; there was certainly no need to become involved if it could be assumed that the second German Reich was now a satiated power.[99]

This assurance Bismarck himself was all too willing to give after 1871, since he had no wish to create a *gross-deutscher* ("Greater German") state which incorporated millions of Austrian Catholics, destroyed the Austro-Hungarian Empire, and left Germany isolated between a vengeful France and a suspicious Russia.[100] It therefore seemed to him far safer to go along with the creation of the Three Emperors' League (1873), a quasi-alliance which stressed the ideological solidarity of the eastern monarchies (as against "republican" France) and simultaneously cemented over some of the Austro-Russian clashes of interest in the Balkans. And when, during the "war-in-sight" crisis of 1875, indications arose that the German government might be contemplating a preventive war against France, the warnings from both London and (especially) St. Petersburg convinced Bismarck that there would be strong opposition to any further alterations in the European balance.[101] For internal-political as well as external-diplomatic reasons, therefore, Germany remained within the boundaries established in 1871—a "half-hegemonial power," as some historians have termed it—until its military-industrial growth and the political ambitions of a post-Bismarckian leadership would once again place it in a position to question the existing territorial order.[102]

However, to pursue that transformation would take us well into the next chapter. For the period of the 1870s and into the 1880s, Bismarck's own diplomacy ensured the preservation of the status quo which he now deemed essential to German interests. The chancellor was partially helped in this endeavor by the flaring-up, in 1876, of another acute phase in the age-old "eastern question" when Turkey's massacre of the Bulgarian Christians and Russia's military response to it turned all attention from the Rhine to Constantinople and the Black Sea.[103] It was true that the outbreak of hostilities on the lower Danube or the Dardanelles could be dangerous even to Germany, if the crisis was allowed to escalate into a full-scale Great Power war, as seemed quite possible by early 1878. However, Bismarck's diplomatic skills in acting as "honest broker" to bring all the Powers to a compromise at the Congress of Berlin reinforced the pressures for a peaceful solution of the crisis and emphasized again the central—and stabilizing—position in European affairs which Germany now occupied.

But the great Eastern Crisis of 1876–1878 also did a great deal for Germany's *relative* position. While the small Russian fleet in the Black Sea performed brilliantly against the Turks, the Russian army's 1877 campaigning revealed that its post–Crimean War reforms had not really taken effect. Although bravery and sheer numbers produced an eventual Russian victory over the Turks in both the Bulgarian and the Caucasian theaters of operation, there were far too many examples of "extremely inadequate reconnaissance of the enemy positions, lack of coordination between the units, and confusion in the high command";[104] and the threat of British and Austrian intervention on Turkey's behalf compelled the Russian government, once again aware of a looming bankruptcy, to agree to compromise on its demands by late 1877. If the Pan-Slavs in Russia were later to blame Bismarck for supervising the Berlin Conference which formalized those humiliating concessions, the fact remained that many among the St. Petersburg elite were more than ever aware of the need to maintain good relations with Berlin—and even to reenter, in a revised form, another Three Emperors' understanding in 1881. Similarly, although Vienna had threatened to break away from Bismarck's controls at the peak of the crisis in 1879, the secret Austro-German alliance of the following year tied it again to German strings, as did the later Three Emperors' alliance of 1881, and the Triple Alliance between Berlin, Vienna, and Italy of 1882. All of these agreements, moreover, had the effect of drawing the signatories away from France and placing them in some degree of dependence upon Germany.[105]

Finally, the events of the late 1870s had reemphasized the long-standing Anglo-Russian rivalry in the Near East and Asia, which inclined both of those powers to look toward Berlin for benevolent neutrality, and turned public attention even further away from Alsace-

Lorraine and central Europe. This tendency was to become even stronger in the 1880s, when a whole series of events—the French acquisition of Tunis (1881), the British intervention in Egypt (1882), the wholesale "scramble" for tropical Africa (1884 onward), and the renewed threat of an Anglo-Russian war over Afghanistan (1885)— marked the beginnings of the age of the "New Imperialism."[106] Although the longer-term effects of this renewed burst of western colonialism were going to profoundly alter the position of many of the Great Powers, the short-term consequence was to emphasize Germany's diplomatic influence within Europe and thus aid Bismarck's endeavors to preserve the status quo. If the peculiarly tortuous system of treaties and countertreaties which he devised during the 1880s was not likely to produce lasting stability, it nonetheless seemed to ensure that peace prevailed among the European powers at least in the near future.

Conclusions

With the important exception of the American Civil War, the period 1815–1885 had not witnessed any lengthy, mutually exhausting military struggles. The lesser campaigns of this age, like the Franco-Austrian clash in 1859 or the Russian attack upon Turkey in 1877, did little to affect the Great Power system. Even the more important wars were limited in some significant ways: the Crimean War was chiefly a regional one, and concluded before Britain had fully harnessed its resources; and the Austro-Prussian and Franco-Prussian wars were over in one season's campaigning—a remarkable contrast to the far lengthier conflicts of the eighteenth century. No wonder, then, that the vision which military leaders and strategic pundits entertained of Great Power struggles in the future was one of swift knockout victories *à la Prusse* in 1870—of railways and mobilization schedules, of general staff plans for a speedy offensive, of quick-firing guns and mass, short-service armies, all of which would be brought together to overwhelm the foe within a matter of weeks. That the newer, quick-firing weapons might, if used properly, benefit defensive rather than offensive warfare was not appreciated at the time; nor, alas, were the portents of the American Civil War, where a combination of irreconcilable popular principles and extensive terrain had made for a far lengthier and deadlier conflict than any short, sharp European conflict of this period.

Yet all of these wars—whether fought in the Tennessee Valley or the Bohemian plain, in the Crimean Peninsula or the fields of Lorraine— pointed to one general conclusion: the powers which were defeated were those that had failed to adopt to the "military revolution" of the mid-nineteenth century, the acquisition of new weapons, the mobilizing and equipping of large armies, the use of improved communications offered by the railway, the steamship, and the telegraph, and a productive industrial base to sustain the armed forces. In all of these conflicts, grievous blunders were to be committed on the battlefield by the generals and armies of the winning side from time to time—but they were never enough to cancel out the advantages which that belligerent possessed in terms of trained manpower, supply, organization, and economic base.

This leads to a final and more general set of remarks about the period after about 1860. As noted at the beginning of this chapter, the half-century which followed the battle of Waterloo had been characterized by the steady growth of an international economy, by large-scale productive increases caused by industrial development and technical change, by the relative stability of the Great Power system and the occurrence of only localized and short-term wars. In addition, while there had been some modernization of military and naval weaponry, new developments within the armed forces were far less than those occurring in civilian spheres exposed both to the Industrial Revolution and to constitutional-political transformation. The prime beneficiary of this half-century of change had been Britain; in terms both of productive power and of world influence, it probably reached its peak in the late 1860s (even if the policies of the first Gladstone ministry tended to conceal that fact). The prime losers had been the nonindustrialized peasant societies of the extra-European world, which were able to withstand neither the industrial manufactures nor the military incursions of the West. For the same fundamental reason, the less industrialized of the European Great Powers—Russia, the Habsburg Empire—began to lose their earlier place, and a newly united nation, Italy, never really made it into the first rank.

From the 1860s, moreover, these trends were to intensify. The volume of world trade and, even more important, the growth of manufacturing output increased swiftly. Industrialization, formerly confined to Britain and certain parts of continental Europe and North America, was beginning to transform other regions. In particular, it was boosting the positions of Germany, which in 1870 already possessed 13 percent of world *industrial* production, and of the United States, which even then had 23 percent of the total.[107] Thus the chief features of the international system which was emerging by the end of the nineteenth century were already detectable, even if few observers could fully recognize them. On the other hand, the relatively stable Pentarchy of the post-1815 Concert system was dissolving, not merely because its members were more willing to fight against each other by the 1860s than a few decades earlier, but also because some of those states were two or three times more powerful than others. On the other hand, Europe's own monopoly of modern industrial production was being broken across the Atlantic. Steam power, railways, electricity, and other instruments of modernization could benefit any society which had both the will and the freedom to adopt them.

The absence of major conflicts during that post-1871 period in which Bismarck dominated European diplomacy may have suggested that a new equilibrium had been established, following the fissures of the 1850s and 1860s. Yet away from the world of armies and navies and foreign offices, far-reaching industrial and technological developments were under way, changing the global economic balances more swiftly than ever before. And it would not be too long before those alterations in the productive/industrial base would have their impacts upon the military capacities and external policies of the Great Powers.

5

The Coming of a Bipolar World and the Crisis of the "Middle Powers": Part One, 1885-1918

In the winter of 1884–1885, the Great Powers of the world, joined by a few smaller states, met in Berlin in an attempt to reach an agreement over trade, navigation, and boundaries in West Africa and the Congo and the principles of effective occupation in Africa more generally.[1] In so many ways, the Berlin West Africa Conference can be seen, symbolically, as the zenith of Old Europe's period of predominance in global affairs. Japan was not a member of the conference; although modernizing swiftly, it was still regarded by the West as a quaint, backward state. The United States, by contrast, *was* at the Berlin Conference, since the issues of trade and navigation discussed there were seen by Washington as relevant to American interests abroad;[2] but in most other respects the United States remained off the international scene, and it was not until 1892 that the European Great Powers upgraded the rank of their diplomatic representatives to Washington from minister to ambassador—the mark of a first-division nation. Russia, too, was at the conference; but while its interests in Asia were considerable, in Africa it possessed little of note. It was, in fact, in the second list of states to be invited to the conference,[3] and played no role other than generally giving support for France against Britain. The center of affairs was therefore the triangular relationship between London, Paris, and Berlin, with Bismarck in the all-important middle position. The fate of the planet still appeared to rest where it had seemed to rest for the preceding century or more: in the chancelleries of Europe. To be sure, if the conference had been deciding the future of the Ottoman Empire instead of the Congo basin, then countries such as Austria-Hungary and Russia would have played a larger role. But that still would not gainsay what was reckoned at the time to be an incontrovertible truth: that Europe was the center of the world. It was in this same period that the Russian general Dragimirov would declare that "Far Eastern affairs are decided in Europe."[4]

Within another three decades—a short time indeed in the course of the Great Power system—that same continent of Europe would be tearing itself apart and several of its members would be close to collapse. Three decades further, and the end would be complete; much of the continent would be economically devastated, parts of it would be in ruins, and its very future would be in the hands of decision-makers in Washington and Moscow.

While it is obvious that no one in 1885 could accurately forecast the ruin and desolation which prevailed in Europe sixty years later, it *was* the case that many acute observers in the late nineteenth century sensed the direction in which the dynamics of world power were driving. Intellectuals and journalists in particular, but also day-to-day politicians, talked and wrote in terms of a vulgar Darwinistic world of struggle, of success and failure, of growth and decline. What was more, the future world order was already seen to have a certain shape, at least by 1895 or 1900.[5]

The most noticeable feature of these prognostications was the revival of de Tocqueville's idea that the United States and Russia would be the two great World Powers of the future. Not surprisingly, this view had lost ground at the time of Russia's Crimean disaster and its mediocre showing in the 1877 war against Turkey, and during the American Civil War and then in the introspective decades of reconstruction and westward expansion. By the late nineteenth century, however, the industrial and agricultural expansion of the United States and the military expansion of Russia in Asia were causing various European observers to worry about a twentieth-century world order which would, as the saying went, be dominated by the Russian knout and American moneybags.[6] Perhaps because neomercantilist commercial ideas were again prevailing over those of a peaceful, Cobdenite, free-trading global system, there was a much greater tendency than earlier to argue that changing economic power would lead to political and territorial changes as well. Even the usually cautious British prime minister Lord Salisbury admitted in 1898 that the world was divided into the "living" and "dying" powers.[7] The recent Chinese defeat in their 1894–1895 war with Japan, the humiliation of Spain by the United States in their brief 1898 conflict, and the French retreat before Britain over the Fashoda incident on the Upper Nile (1898–1899) were all interpreted as evidence that the "survival of the fittest" dictated the fates of nations as well as animal species. The Great Power struggles were no longer merely over European issues—as they had been in 1830 or even 1860—but over markets and territories that ranged across the globe.

But if the United States and Russia seemed destined by size and population to be among the future Great Powers, who would accompany them? The "theory of the Three World Empires"—that is, the popular belief that only the three (or, in some accounts, four) largest and most powerful nation-states would remain independent—exercised many an imperial statesman.[8] "It seems to me," the British minister for the colonies, Joseph Chamberlain, informed an 1897 audience, "that the tendency of the time is to throw all power into the hands of the greater empires, and the minor kingdoms—those which are non-progressive—seem to fall into a secondary and subordinate place. . . ."[9] It was vital for Germany, Admiral Tirpitz urged Kaiser Wilhelm, to build a big navy, so that it would be one of the "four World Powers: Russia, England, America and Germany."[10] France, too, must be up there, warned a Monsieur Darcy, for "those who do not advance, go backwards and who goes back goes under."[11] For the long-established powers, Britain, France, and Austria-Hungary, the issue was whether they could maintain themselves in the face of these new challenges to the international status quo. For the new powers, Germany, Italy, and Japan, the problem was whether they could break through to what Berlin termed a "world-political freedom" before it was too late.

It need hardly be said that not every member of the human race was obsessed with such ideas as the nineteenth century came to a close. Many were much more concerned about domestic, social issues. Many clung to the liberal, laissez-faire ideals of peaceful cooperation.[12] Nonetheless there existed in governing elites, military circles, and imperialist organizations a prevailing view of the world order which stressed struggle, change, competition, the use of force, and the organization of national resources to enhance state power. The less-developed regions of the globe were being swiftly carved up, but that was only the beginning of the story; with few more territories to annex, the geopolitician Sir Halford Mackinder argued, efficiency and internal development would have to replace expansionism as the main aim of modern states. There would be a far closer correlation than hitherto "between the larger geographical and the larger historical generalizations,"[13] that is, size and numbers would be more accurately reflected in the international balances, provided that those resources were properly exploited. A country with hundreds of millions of peasants would count for little. On the other hand, even a modern state would be eclipsed also if it did not rest upon a large enough industrial, productive foundation. "The successful powers will be those who have the greatest industrial base," warned the British imperialist Leo Amery. "Those people who have the industrial power and the power of invention and science will be able to defeat all others."[14]

*   *   *

Much of the history of international affairs during the following half-century turned out to be a fulfillment of such forecasts. Dramatic changes occurred in the power balances, both inside Europe and without. Old empires collapsed, and new ones arose. The *multipolar* world of 1885 was replaced by a *bipolar* world as early as 1943. The international struggle intensified, and broke into wars totally different from the limited clashes of nineteenth-century Europe. Industrial productivity, with science and technology, became an ever more vital component of national strength. Alterations in the international shares of manufacturing production were reflected in the changing international shares of military power and diplomatic influence. Individuals still counted—who, in the century of Lenin, Hitler, and Stalin, could say they did not?—but they counted in power politics only because they were able to control and reorganize the productive forces of a great state. And, as Nazi Germany's own fate revealed, the test of world power by war was ruthlessly uncaring to any nation which lacked the industrial-technical strength, and thus the military weaponry, to achieve its leader's ambitions.

If the broad outlines of these six decades of Great Power struggles were already being suggested in the 1890s, the success or failure of *individual* countries was still to be determined. Obviously, much depended upon whether a country could keep up or increase its manufacturing output. But much also depended, as always, upon the immutable facts of geography. Was a country near the center of international crises, or at the periphery? Was it safe from invasion? Did it have to face two or three ways simultaneously? National cohesion, patriotism, and the controls exercised by the state over its inhabitants were also important; whether a society withstood the strains of war would very much depend upon its internal makeup. It might also depend upon alliance politics and decision-making. Was one fighting as part of a large alliance bloc, or in isolation? Did one enter the war at the beginning, or halfway through? Did other powers, formerly neutral, enter the war on the opposite side?

Such questions suggest that any proper analysis of "the coming of a bipolar world, and the crisis of the 'middle powers'" needs to consider three separate but interacting levels of causality: first, the changes in the military-industrial productive base, as certain states became materially more (or less) powerful; second, the geopolitical, strategical, and sociocultural factors which influenced the responses of each *individual* state to these broader shifts in the world balances; and third, the diplomatic and political changes which also affected chances of success or failure in the great coalition wars of the early twentieth century.

The Shifting Balance of World Forces

Those *fin de siècle* observers of world affairs agreed that the pace of economic and political change was quickening, and thus likely to make the international order more precarious than before. Alterations had always occurred in the power balances to produce instability and often war. "What made war inevitable," Thucydides wrote in *The Peleponnesian War,* "was the growth of Athenian power and the fear which this caused in Sparta."[15] But by the final quarter of the nineteenth century, the changes affecting the Great Power system were more widespread, and usually swifter, than ever before. The global trading and communications network—telegraphs, steamships, railways, modern printing presses—meant that breakthroughs in science and technology, or new advances in manufacturing production, could be transmitted and transferred from one *continent* to another within a matter of years. Within five years of Gilcrist and Thomas's 1879 invention of a way to turn cheap phosphoric ores into basic steel, there were eighty-four basic converters in operation in western and central Europe,[16] and the process had also crossed the Atlantic. The result was *more* than a shift in the respective national shares of steel output; it also implied a significant shift in military potential.

Military potential is, as we have seen, not the same as military power. An economic giant could prefer, for reasons of its political culture or geographical security, to be a military pigmy, while a state without great economic resources could nonetheless so organize its society as to be a formidable military power. Exceptions to the simplistic equation "economic strength = military strength" exist in this period, as in others, and will need to be discussed below. Yet in an era of modern, industrialized warfare, the link between economics and strategy was becoming tighter. To understand the long-term shifts affecting the international power balances between the 1880s and the Second World War, it is necessary to look at the economic data. These data have been selected with a view to assessing a nation's potential for war, and therefore do not include some well-known economic indices* which are less helpful in that respect.

Population size by itself is never a reliable indicator of power, but Table 12 does suggest how, at least demographically, Russia and the United States could be viewed as a different sort of Great Power from

*E.g., shares of world trade, which disproportionately boost the position of maritime, trading nations, and underemphasize the economic power of states with a large degree of self-sufficiency.

the others, with Germany and (later) Japan beginning to draw a little away from the remainder.

Table 12. Total Population of the Powers, 1890–1938[17]
(millions)

		1890	1900	1910	1913	1920	1928	1938	
1	Russia	116.8	135.6	159.3	175.1	126.6	150.4	180.6	1
2	United States	62.6	75.9	91.9	97.3	105.7	119.1	138.3	2
3	Germany	49.2	56.0	64.5	66.9	42.8	55.4	68.5	4
4	Austria-Hungary	42.6	46.7	50.8	52.1	—	—	—	
5	Japan	39.9	43.8	49.1	51.3	55.9	62.1	72.2	3
6	France	38.3	38.9	39.5	39.7	39.0	41.0	41.9	7
7	Britain	37.4	41.1	44.9	45.6	44.4	45.7	47.6	5
8	Italy	30.0	32.2	34.4	35.1	37.7	40.3	43.8	6

There are, however, two ways of "controlling" the raw data of Table 12. The first is to compare the total population of a country with the part of it that is living in urban areas (Table 13), for that is usually a significant indicator of industrial/commercial modernization; the second is to correlate those findings with the per capita levels of industrialization, as measured against the "benchmark" country of Great Britain (Table 14). Both exercises are enormously instructive, and tend to reinforce each other.

Without getting into too detailed an analysis of the figures in Tables 13 and 14 at this stage, several broad generalizations can be made. Once such measures of "modernization" as the size of urban population and the extent of industrialization are introduced, the positions of most of the powers are significantly altered from those in Table 12: Russia drops from first to last, at least until its 1930s industrial expansion, Britain and Germany gain in position, and the United States' unique combination of having both a populous *and* a highly industrialized society stands out. Even at the beginning of this period, the gap between the strongest and the weakest of the Great Powers is large, both absolutely and relatively; by the eve of the Second World War, there still remain enormous differences. The process of modernization might involve all these countries going through the same "phases";[18] it did not mean that, in *power* terms, each would benefit to the same degree.

The important *differences* between the Great Powers emerge yet more clearly when one examines detailed data about industrial productivity. Since iron and steel output has often been taken as an indicator of potential military strength in this period, as well as of industrialization *per se*, the relevant figures are reproduced in Table 15.

But perhaps the best measure of a nation's industrialization is its

Table 13. Urban Population of the Powers (in millions) and as Percentage of the Total Population, 1890–1938[19]

	1890	1900	1910	1913	1920	1928	1938	
1 Britain	11.2	13.5	15.3	15.8	16.6	17.5	18.7	5
(1)	(29.9%)	(32.8%)	(34.9%)	(34.6%)	(37.3%)	(38.2%)	(39.2%)	(1)
2 United States	9.6	14.2	20.3	22.5	27.4	34.3	45.1	1
(2)	(15.3%)	(18.7%)	(22.0)	(23.1%)	(25.9%)	(28.7%)	(32.8%)	(2)
3 Germany	5.6	8.7	12.9	14.1	15.3	19.1	20.7	3
(4)	(11.3%)	(15.5%)	(20.0%)	(21.0%)	(35.7%)	(34.4%)	(30.2%)	(3)
4 France	4.5	5.2	5.7	5.9	5.9	6.3	6.3	7
(3)	(11.7%)	(13.3%)	(14.4%)	(14.8%)	(15.1%)	(15.3%)	(15.0%)	(7)
5 Russia	4.3	6.6	10.2	12.3	4.0	10.7	36.5	2
(8)	(3.6%)	(4.8%)	(6.4%)	(7.0%)	(3.1%)	(7.1%)	(20.2%)	(5)
6 Italy	2.7	3.1	3.8	4.1	5.0	6.5	8.0	6
(5)	(9.0%)	(9.6%)	(11.0%)	(11.6%)	(13.2%)	(16.1%)	(18.2%)	(6)
7 Japan	2.5	3.8	5.8	6.6	6.4	9.7	20.7	3
(6)	(6.3%)	(8.6%)	(10.3%)	(12.8%)	(11.6%)	(15.6%)	(28.6%)	(4)
8 Austria-Hungary	2.4	3.1	4.2	4.6	—	—	—	
(7)	(5.6%)	(6.6%)	(8.2%)	(8.8%)				

Table 14. Per Capita Levels of Industrialization, 1880–1938[20]

(relative to G.B. in 1900 = 100)

	1880	1900	1913	1928	1938	
1 Great Britain	87	[100]	115	122	157	2
2 United States	38	69	126	182	167	1
3 France	28	39	59	82	73	4
4 Germany	25	52	85	128	144	3
5 Italy	12	17	26	44	61	5
6 Austria	15	23	32	—	—	
7 Russia	10	15	20	20	38	7
8 Japan	9	12	20	30	51	6

Table 15. Iron/Steel Production of the Powers, 1890–1938[21]

(millions of tons; pig-iron production for 1890, steel thereafter)

	1890	1900	1910	1913	1920	1930	1938
United States	9.3	10.3	26.5	31.8	42.3	41.3	28.8
Britain	8.0	5.0	6.5	7.7	9.2	7.4	10.5
Germany	4.1	6.3	13.6	17.6	7.6	11.3	23.2
France	1.9	1.5	3.4	4.6	2.7	9.4	6.1
Austria-Hungary	0.97	1.1	2.1	2.6	—	—	—
Russia	0.95	2.2	3.5	4.8	0.16	5.7	18.0
Japan	0.02	—	0.16	0.25	0.84	2.3	7.0
Italy	0.01	0.11	0.73	0.93	0.73	1.7	2.3

energy consumption from modern forms (that is, coal, petroleum, natural gas, and hydroelectricity, but not wood), since it is an indication both of a country's technical capacity to exploit inanimate forms of energy and of its economic pulse rate; these figures are given in Table 16.

Table 16. Energy Consumption of the Powers, 1890–1938[22]
(in millions of metric tons of coal equivalent)

	1890	1900	1910	1913	1920	1930	1938
United States	147	248	483	541	694	762	697
Britain	145	171	185	195	212	184	196
Germany	71	112	158	187	159	177	228
France	36	47.9	55	62.5	65	97.5	84
Austria-Hungary	19.7	29	40	49.4	—	—	—
Russia	10.9	30	41	54	14.3	65	177
Japan	4.6	4.6	15.4	23	34	55.8	96.5
Italy	4.5	5	9.6	11	14.3	24	27.8

Tables 15 and 16 both confirm the swift industrial changes which occurred in *absolute* terms to some of the powers in particular periods—Germany before 1914, Russia and Japan in the 1930s—as well as indicating the slower rates of growth in Britain, France and Italy. This can also be represented in *relative terms* to indicate a country's comparative industrial position over time (Table 17).

Table 17. Total Industrial Potential of the Powers in Relative Perspective, 1880–1938[23]
(U.K. in 1900 = 100)

	1880	1900	1913	1928	1938
Britain	73.3	[100]	127.2	135	181
United States	46.9	127.8	298.1	533	528
Germany	27.4	71.2	137.7	158	214
France	25.1	36.8	57.3	82	74
Russia	24.5	47.5	76.6	72	152
Austria-Hungary	14	25.6	40.7	—	—
Italy	8.1	13.6	22.5	37	46
Japan	7.6	13	25.1	45	88

Finally, it is useful to return in Table 18 to Bairoch's figures on shares of world manufacturing production to show the changes which occurred since the earlier analysis of the nineteenth-century balances in the preceding chapter.

**Table 18. Relative Shares of World Manufacturing
Output, 1880–1938[24]**
(percent)

	1880	1900	1913	1928	1938
Britain	22.9	18.5	13.6	9.9	10.7
United States	14.7	23.6	32.0	39.3	31.4
Germany	8.5	13.2	14.8	11.6	12.7
France	7.8	6.8	6.1	6.0	4.4
Russia	7.6	8.8	8.2	5.3	9.0
Austria-Hungary	4.4	4.7	4.4	—	—
Italy	2.5	2.5	2.4	2.7	2.8

The Position of the Powers, 1885–1914

In the face of such unnervingly specific figures, that a certain power possessed 2.7 percent of world manufacturing production in 1913, or that another had an industrial potential in 1928 which was only 45 percent of Britain's in 1900, it is worth reemphasizing that all these statistics are abstract until placed within a specific historical and geopolitical context. Countries with virtually identical industrial output might nonetheless merit substantially different ratings in terms of Great Power effectiveness, because of such factors as the internal cohesion of the society in question, its ability to mobilize resources for state action, its geopolitical position, and its diplomatic capacities. Given the limitations of space, it will not be possible in this chapter to do for all the Great Powers what Correlli Barnett sought to do in his large-scale study of Britain some years ago. But what follows will try to remain close to Barnett's larger framework, in which he argues that

> the power of a nation-state by no means consists only in its armed forces, but also in its economic and technological resources; in the dexterity, foresight and resolution with which its foreign policy is conducted; in the efficiency of its social and political organization. It consists most of all in the nation itself, the people; their skills, energy, ambition, discipline, initiative; their beliefs, myths and illusions. And it consists, further, in the way all these factors are related to one another. Moreover national power has to be considered not only in itself, in its absolute extent, but relative to the state's foreign or imperial obligations; it has to be considered relative to the power of other states.[25]

There is perhaps no better way of illustrating the diversity of grand-strategical effectiveness than by looking in the first instance at the three relative newcomers to the international system, Italy, Germany, and Japan. The first two had become united states only in 1870–1871;

the third began to emerge from its self-imposed isolation after the Meiji Restoration of 1868. In all three societies there were impulses to emulate the established powers. By the 1880s and 1890s each was acquiring overseas territories; each, too, began to build a modern fleet to complement its standing army. Each was a significant element in the diplomatic calculus of the age and, at the latest by 1902, had become an alliance-partner to an older power. Yet all these similarities can hardly outweigh the fundamental differences in real strength which each possessed.

Italy

At first sight, the coming of a united Italian nation represented a major shift in the European balances. Instead of being a cluster of rivaling small states, partly under foreign sovereignty and always under the threat of foreign intervention, there was now a solid block of thirty million people growing so swiftly that it was coming close to France's total population by 1914. Its army and its navy in this period were not especially large, but as Tables 19 and 20 show, they were still very respectable.

Table 19. Military and Naval Personnel of the Powers, 1880–1914[26]

	1880	1890	1900	1910	1914
Russia	791,000	677,000	1,162,000	1,285,000	1,352,000
France	543,000	542,000	715,000	769,000	910,000
Germany	426,000	504,000	524,000	694,000	891,000
Britain	367,000	420,000	624,000	571,000	532,000
Austria-Hungary	246,000	346,000	385,000	425,000	444,000
Italy	216,000	284,000	255,000	322,000	345,000
Japan	71,000	84,000	234,000	271,000	306,000
United States	34,000	39,000	96,000	127,000	164,000

Table 20. Warship Tonnage of the Powers, 1880–1914[27]

	1880	1890	1900	1910	1914
Britain	650,000	679,000	1,065,000	2,174,000	2,714,000
France	271,000	319,000	499,000	725,000	900,000
Russia	200,000	180,000	383,000	401,000	679,000
United States	169,000	?240,000	333,000	824,000	985,000
Italy	100,000	242,000	245,000	327,000	498,000
Germany	88,000	190,000	285,000	964,000	1,305,000
Austria-Hungary	60,000	66,000	87,000	210,000	372,000
Japan	15,000	41,000	187,000	496,000	700,000

In diplomatic terms, as was noted above,[28] the rise of Italy certainly impinged upon its two Great Power neighbors, France and Austria-Hungary; and while its entry into the Triple Alliance in 1882 ostensibly "resolved" the Italo-Austrian rivalry, it confirmed that an isolated France faced foes on two fronts. Within just over a decade from its unification, therefore, Italy seemed a full member of the European Great Power system, and Rome ranked alongside the other major capitals (London, Paris, Berlin, St. Petersburg, Vienna, Constantinople) as a place to which full embassies were accredited.

But the appearance of Italy's Great Power status covered some stupendous weaknesses, above all the country's economic retardation, particularly in the rural south. Its illiteracy rate—37.6 percent overall and again far greater in the south—was much higher than in any other western or northern European state, a reflection of the backwardness of much of Italian agriculture—smallholdings, poor soil, little investment, sharecropping, inadequate transport. Italy's total output and per capita national wealth were comparable to those of the peasant societies of Spain and eastern Europe rather than those of the Netherlands or Westphalia. Italy had no coal; yet, despite its turn to hydroelectricity, about 88 percent of Italy's energy continued to come from British coal, a drain upon its balance of payments and an appalling strategical weakness. In these circumstances, Italy's rise in population without significant industrial expansion was a mixed blessing, since it slowed its industrial growth in per capita terms relative to the other western Powers,[29] and the comparison would have been even more unfavorable had not hundreds of thousands of Italians (usually the more mobile and able) emigrated across the Atlantic each year. All this made it, in Kemp's phrase, "the disadvantaged latecomer."[30]

This is not to say that there was no modernization. Indeed, it is precisely about this period that many historians have referred to "the industrial revolution of the Giolittian era" and to "a decisive change in the economic life of our country."[31] At least in the north, there was a considerable shift to heavy industry—iron and steel, shipbuilding, automobile manufacturing, as well as textiles. In Gerschrenkon's view, the years 1896–1908 witnessed Italy's "big push" toward industrialization; indeed, Italian industrial growth rose faster than anywhere else in Europe, the population shift from the countryside to the towns intensified, the banking system readjusted itself in order to provide industrial credit, and real national income moved sharply upward.[32] Piedmontese agriculture showed similar steps forward.

However, once the Italian statistics are placed in comparative prospective, the gloss begins to fade. It *did* create an iron and steel industry, but in 1913 its output was one-eighth that of Britain, one-seventeenth that of Germany, and only two-fifths that of Belgium.[33] It did achieve swift rates of industrial growth, but that was from such a very low beginning level that the real results were not impressive. At the outset of the First World War, it had not achieved even one-quarter of the industrial strength which Great Britain possessed in 1900, and its share of world manufacturing production actually dropped, from a mere 2.5 percent in 1900 to 2.4 percent in 1913. Although Italy marginally entered the listings of Great Powers, it is worth noting that—Japan excluded—every other of these powers had two or three times its industrial muscle; some (Germany and Britain) had sixfold the amount, and one (the United States) over thirteen times.

This might have been compensated for somewhat by a relatively greater degree of national cohesion and resolve on the part of the Italian population, but such elements were absent. The loyalties which existed in the Italian body politic were familial and local, perhaps regional, but not national. The chronic gap between north and south, which the industrialization of the former only exacerbated, and the lack of any great contact with the world outside the village community in so many parts of the peninsula were not helped by the hostility between the Italian government and the Catholic Church, which forbade its members to serve the state. The ideals of *risorgimento,* hailed by native and admiring foreign liberals, did not penetrate very far down Italian society. Recruitment for the armed services was difficult, and the actual location of army units according to strategical principles, rather than regional political calculations, was impossible. Civilmilitary relationships at the top were characterized by a mutual miscomprehension and distrust. The general antimilitarism of Italian society, the poor quality of the officer corps, and the lack of adequate funding for modern weaponry raised doubts about Italian military effectiveness long before the disastrous 1917 battle of Caporetto or the 1940 Egyptian campaign.[34] Its unification wars had relied upon the intervention of France, and then the threat to Austria-Hungary from Prussia. The 1896 catastrophe at Adowa (in Abyssinia) gave Italy the awful reputation of having the only European army defeated by an African society without means of effective response. The Italian government decision to make war in Libya in 1911–1912, which took the Italian general staff itself by surprise, was a financial disaster of the first order. The navy, looking very large in 1890, steadily declined in relative size and was always of questionable efficiency. Successive Mediterranean commander in chiefs of the Royal Navy always hoped that the Italian fleet would be neutral, not allied, if it ever came to a war with France in this period.[35]

The consequences of all this upon Italy's strategical and diplomatic position were depressing. Not only was the Italian general staff acutely aware of its numerical and technical inferiority compared with the French (especially) and the Austro-Hungarians, but it also knew that Italy's inadequate railway network and the deep-rooted regionalism made impossible large-scale, flexible troop deployments in the Prussian manner. And not only was the Italian navy aware of its deficiencies, but Italy's vulnerable and lengthy coastline made its alliance politics extremely ambivalent, and thus made strategic planning more chaotic than ever. The alliance treaty that Italy signed in 1882 with Berlin was comforting at first, particularly when Bismarck seemed to paralyze the French; but even then the Italian government kept pressing for closer ties with Britain, which alone could neutralize the French fleet. When, in the years after 1900, Britain and France moved closer together and Britain and Germany moved from cooperation to antagonism, the Italians felt that they had little alternative but to tack toward the new Anglo-French combination. The residual dislike of Austria-Hungary strengthened this move, just as the respect for Germany and the importance of German industrial finance in Italy checked it from being an open break. Thus by 1914, Italy occupied a position like that of 1871. It was "the least of the Great Powers,"[36] frustratingly unpredictable and unscrupulous in the eyes of its neighbors, and possessing commercial and expansionist ambitions in the Alps, the Balkans, North Africa, and farther afield which conflicted with the interests of both friends and rivals. Economic and social circumstances continued to weaken its power to influence events, and yet it remained a player in the game. In sum, the judgment of most other governments seems to have been that it was better to have Italy as a partner than as a foe; but the margin of benefit was not great.[37]

Japan

Italy was a marginal member of the Great Power system in 1890, but Japan wasn't even in the club. For centuries it had been ruled by a decentralized feudal oligarchy consisting of territorial lords (daimyo) and an aristocratic caste of warriors (samurai). Hampered by the absence of natural resources and by a mountainous terrain that left only 20 percent of its land suitable for cultivation, Japan lacked all of the customary prerequisites for economic development. Isolated from the rest of the world by a complex language with no close relatives and an intense consciousness of cultural uniqueness, the Japanese people remained inward-looking and resistant to foreign influences well into the second half of the nineteenth century. For all these reasons, Japan seemed destined to remain politically immature, economically backward, and militarily impotent in World Power terms.[38] Yet within two generations it had become a major player in the international politics of the Far East.

The cause of this transformation, effected by the Meiji Restoration from 1868 onward, was the determination of influential members of the Japanese elite to avoid being dominated and colonized by the West, as seemed to be happening elsewhere in Asia, even if the reform measures to be taken involved the scrapping of the feudal order and the bitter opposition of the samurai clans.[39] Japan had to be modernized not because individual entrepreneurs wished it, but because the "state" needed it. After the early opposition had been crushed, modernization proceeded with a *dirigisme* and commitment which makes the efforts of Colbert or Frederick the Great pale by comparison. A new constitution, based upon the Prusso-German model, was established. The legal system was reformed. The educational system was vastly expanded, so that the country achieved an exceptionally high literacy rate. The calendar was changed. Dressed was changed. A modern banking system was evolved. Experts were brought in from Britain's Royal Navy to advise upon the creation of an up-to-date Japanese fleet, and from the Prussian general staff to assist in the modernization of the army. Japanese officers were sent to western military and naval academies; modern weapons were purchased from abroad, although a native armaments industry was also established. The state encouraged the creation of a railway network, telegraphs, and shipping lines; it worked in conjunction with emerging Japanese entrepreneurs to develop heavy industry, iron, steel, and shipbuilding, as well as to modernize textile production. Government subsidies were employed to benefit exporters, to encourage shipping, to get a new industry set up. Japanese exports, especially of silk and textiles, soared. Behind all this lay the impressive political commitment to realize the national slogan *fukoken kyohei* ("rich country, with strong army"). For the Japanese, economic power and military/naval power went hand in hand.

But all this took time, and the handicaps remained severe.[40] Although the urban population more than doubled between 1890 and 1913, numbers engaged on the land remained about the same. Even on the eve of the First World War, over three-fifths of the Japanese population was engaged in agriculture, forestry, and fishing; and despite all the many improvements in farming techniques, the mountainous countryside and the small size of most holdings prevented an "agricultural revolution" on, say, the British model. With such a "bottom-heavy" agricultural base, all comparisons of Japan's industrial potential or of per capita levels of industrialization were bound to show it at or close to the lower end of the Great Power lists (see Tables 14 and 17 above). While its pre-1914 industrial spurt can clearly be detected in the large rise of its energy consumption from modern fuels and in the increase in its share of world manufacturing production, it was still deficient in many other areas. Its iron and steel output was small, and it relied heavily upon imports. In the same way, although its shipbuilding industry was greatly expanded, it still ordered some warships elsewhere. It also was very short of capital, needing to borrow increasing amounts from abroad but never having enough to invest in industry, in infrastructure, and in the armed services. Economically, it had performed miracles to become the only nonwestern state to go through an industrial revolution in the age of high imperialism; yet it still remained, compared to Britain, the United States, and Germany, an industrial and financial lightweight.

Two further factors, however, aided Japan's rise to Great Power status and help to explain why it surpassed, for example, Italy. The first was its geographical isolation. The nearby continental shore was held by nothing more threating than the decaying Chinese Empire. And while China, Manchuria, and (even more alarming) Korea might fall into the hands of another Great Power, geography had placed Japan far closer to those lands than any one of the other imperialist states—as Russia was to find to its discomfort when it tried to supply an army along six thousand miles of railway in 1904–1905, and as the British and American navies were to discover several decades later as they wrestled with the logistical problems involved in the relief of the Philippines, Hong Kong, and Malaya. Assuming a steady Japanese growth in East Asia, it would only be by the most extreme endeavors that any other major state could prevent Japan from becoming the predominant power there in the course of time.

The second factor was *moral.* It seems indisputable that the strong Japanese sense of cultural uniqueness, the traditions of emperor worship and veneration of the state, the samurai ethos of military honor and valor, the emphasis upon discipline and fortitude, produced a political culture at once fiercely patriotic and unlikely to be deterred by sacrifices and reinforced the Japanese impulses to expand into "Greater East Asia," for strategical security as well as markets and raw materials. This was reflected in the successful military and naval campaigning against China in 1894, when those two countries quarreled over their claims in Korea.[41] On land and sea, the better-equipped Japanese forces seemed driven by a will to succeed. At the end of that war, the threats of the "triple intervention" by Russia, France, and Germany compelled an embittered Japanese government to withdraw its claims to Port Arthur and the Liaotung Peninsula, but that merely increased Tokyo's determination to try again later. Few, if any, in the government dissented from Baron Hayashi's grim conclusion:

> If new warships are considered necessary we must, at any cost, build them: if the organization of our army is inadequate we must start rectifying it from now; if need be, our entire military system must be changed. . . .
>
> At present Japan must keep calm and sit tight, so as to lull suspicions nurtured against her; during this time the foundations of national power must be consolidated; and we must watch and wait for the opportunity in the Orient that will surely come one day. When this day arrives, Japan will decide her own fate. . . .[42]

Its time for revenge came ten years later, when its Korean and Manchurian ambitions clashed with those of czarist Russia.[43] While naval experts were impressed by Admiral Togo's fleet when it destroyed the Russian ships at the decisive battle of Tsushima, it was the general bearing of Japanese society which struck other observers. The surprise strike at Port Arthur (a habit begun in the 1894 China conflict, and revived in 1941) was applauded in the West, as was the enthusiasm of Japanese nationalist opinion for an outright victory, whatever the cost. More remarkable still seemed the performance of Japan's officers and men in the land battles around Port Arthur and Mukden, where tens of thousands of soldiers were lost as they charged across minefields, over barbed wire, and through a hail of machine-gun fire before conquering the Russian trenches. The samurai spirit, it seemed, could secure battlefield victories with the bayonet even in the age of mass industrialized warfare. If, as all the contemporary military experts concluded, morale and discipline were still vital prerequisites of national power, Japan was rich in those resources.

Even then, however, Japan was not a full-fledged Great Power. Japan had been fortunate to have fought an even more backward China and a czarist Russia which was militarily top-heavy and disadvantaged by the immense distance between St. Petersburg and the Far East. Furthermore, the Anglo-Japanese Alliance of 1902 had allowed it to fight on its home ground without interference from third powers. Its navy had relied upon British-built battleships, its army upon Krupp guns. Most important of all, it had found the immense costs of the war impossible to finance from its own resources and yet had been able to rely upon loans floated in the United States and Britain.[44] As it turned out, Japan was close to bankruptcy by the end of 1905, when the peace negotiations with Russia got under way. That may not have been obvious to the Tokyo public, which reacted furiously to the relatively light terms with which Russia escaped in the final settlement. Nevertheless, with victory confirmed, Japan's armed forces glorified and admired, its economy able to recover, and its status as a Great Power (albeit a regional one) admitted by all, Japan had come of age. No one could do anything significant in the Far East without considering its response; but whether it could expand further without provoking reaction from the more established Great Powers was not at all clear.

Germany

Two factors ensured that the rise of imperial Germany would have a more immediate and substantial impact upon the Great Power balances than either of its fellow "newcomer" states. The first was that, far from emerging in geopolitical isolation, like Japan, Germany had arisen right in the center of the old European states system; its very creation had directly impinged upon the interests of Austria-Hungary and France, and its existence had altered the relative position of *all* of the existing Great Powers of Europe. The second factor was the sheer speed and extent of Germany's further growth, in industrial, commercial, and military/naval terms. By the eve of the First World War its national power was not only three or four times Italy's and Japan's, it was well ahead of either France or Russia and had probably overtaken Britain as well. In June 1914 the octogenarian Lord Welby recalled that "the Germany they remembered in the fifties was a cluster of insignificant states under insignificant princelings";[45] now, in one man's lifetime, it was the most powerful state in Europe, and still growing. This alone was to make "the German question" the epicenter of so much of world politics for more than half a century after 1890.

Only a few details of Germany's explosive economic growth can be offered here.[46] Its population had soared from 49 million in 1890 to 66 million in 1913, second only in Europe to Russia's—but since Germans enjoyed far higher levels of education, social provision, and per capita income than Russians, the nation was strong both in the quantity and the quality of its population. Whereas, according to an Italian source, 330 out of 1,000 recruits entering its army were illiterate, the corresponding ratios were 220/1,000 in Austria-Hungary, 68/1,000 in France, and an astonishing 1/1,000 in Germany.[47] The beneficiaries were not only the Prussian army, but also the factories requiring skilled workers, the enterprises needing well-trained engineers, the laboratories seeking chemists, the firms looking for managers and salesmen—all of which the German school system, polytechnical institutes, and universities produced in abundance. By applying the fruits of this knowledge to agriculture, German farmers used chemical fertilizers and large-scale modernization to increase their crop yields, which were much higher per hectare than in any of the other Great Powers.[48] To appease the Junkers and the peasants' leagues, German farming was given considerable tariff protection in the face of more cheaply produced American and Russian foodstuffs; yet because of its relative efficiency, the large agricultural sector did not drag down per capita national income and output to anything like the degree it did in all the other continental Great Powers.

But it was in its industrial expansion that Germany really distinguished itself in these years. Its coal production grew from 89 million tons in 1890 to 277 million tons in 1914, just behind Britain's 292 million and far ahead of Austria-Hungary's 47 million, France's 40 million, and Russia's 36 million. In steel, the increases had been even more spectacular, and the 1914 German output of 17.6 million tons was larger than that of Britain, France, and Russia combined. More impressive still was the German performance in the newer, twentieth-century industries of electrics, optics, and chemicals. Giant firms like Siemens and AEG, employing 142,000 people between them, dominated the European electrical industry. German chemical firms, led by Bayer and Hoechst, produced 90 percent of the world's industrial dyes. This success story was naturally reflected in Germany's foreign-trade figures, with exports tripling between 1890 and 1913, bringing the country close to Britain as the leading world exporter; not surprisingly, its merchant marine also expanded, to be the second-largest in the world by the eve of the war. By then, its share of world manufacturing production (14.8 percent) was higher than Britain's (13.6 percent) and two and a half times that of France (6.1 percent). It had become the economic powerhouse of Europe, and even its much-publicized lack of capital did not seem to be slowing it down. Little wonder that nationalists like Friedrich Naumann exulted at these manifestations of growth and their implications for Germany's place in the world. "The German race brings it," he wrote. "It brings army, navy, money and power. . . . Modern, gigantic instruments of power are possible only when an active people feels the spring-time juices in its organs."[49]

That publicists such as Naumann and, even more, such rabidly expansionist pressure groups as the Pan-German League and the German Navy League should have welcomed and urged the rise of German influence in Europe and overseas is hardly surprising. In this age of the "new imperialism," similar calls could be heard in every other Great Power; as Gilbert Murray wickedly observed in 1900, *each* country seemed to be asserting, "We are the pick and flower of nations . . . above all things qualified for governing others."[50] It was perhaps more significant that the German ruling elite after 1895 also seemed convinced of the need for large-scale territorial expansion when the time was ripe, with Admiral Tirpitz arguing that Germany's industrialization and overseas conquests were "as irresistible as a natural law"; with the Chancellor Bülow declaring, "The question is not whether we want to colonize or not, but that we *must* colonize, whether we want it or not"; and with Kaiser Wilhelm himself airily announcing that Germany "had great tasks to accomplish outside the narrow boundaries of old Europe" although he also envisaged it exercising a sort of "Napoleonic supremacy," in a peaceful sense, over the continent.[51] All this was quite a change of tone from Bismarck's repeated insistence that Germany was a "saturated" power, keen to preserve the status quo in Europe and unenthused (despite the colonial bids of 1884–1885) about territories overseas. Even here it may be unwise to exaggerate the particularly aggressive nature of this German "ideological consensus"[52] for expansion; statesmen in France and Russia, Britain and Japan, the United States and Italy were also announcing *their* country's manifest destiny, although perhaps in a less deterministic and frenetic tone.

What *was* significant about German expansionism was that the country either already possessed the instruments of power to alter the status quo or had the material resources to create such instruments.

The most impressive demonstration of this capacity was the rapid buildup of the German navy after 1898, which under Tirpitz was transformed from being the sixth-largest fleet in the world to being second only to the Royal Navy. By the eve of war, the High Seas Fleet consisted of thirteen dreadnought-type battleships, sixteen older ones, and five battlecruisers, a force so big that it had compelled the British Admiralty gradually to withdraw almost all its capital-ship squadrons from overseas stations into the North Sea; while there were to be indications (better internal construction, shells, optical equipment, gunnery control, night training, etc.) that the German vessels were pound for pound superior.[53] Although Tirpitz could never secure the enormous funds to achieve his real goal of creating a navy "equally strong as England's,"[54] he nonetheless had built a force which quite overawed the rival fleets of France or Russia.

Germany's capacity to fight successfully on land seemed to some observers less impressive; indeed, at first sight, the Prussian army in the decade before 1914 appeared eclipsed by the far larger forces of czarist Russia, and matched by those of France. But such appearances were deceptive. For complex domestic-political reasons, the German government had opted to keep the army to a certain size and to allow Tirpitz's fleet substantially to increase its share of the total defense budget.[55] When the tense international circumstances of 1911 and 1912 caused Berlin to decide upon a large-scale expansion of the army, the swift change of gear was imposing. Between 1910 and 1914, its army budget rose from $204 million to $442 million, whereas France's grew only from $188 million to $197 million—and yet France was conscripting 89 percent of its eligible youth compared with Germany's 53 percent to achieve that buildup. It was true that Russia was spending some $324 million on its army by 1914, but at stupendous strain: defense expenditures consumed 6.3 percent of Russia's national income, but only 4.6 percent of Germany's.[56] With the exception of Britain, Germany bore the "burden of armaments" more easily than any other European state. Furthermore, while the Prussian army could mobilize and equip millions of reservists and—because of their better education and training—actually deploy them in front-line operations, France and Russia could not. The French general staff held that their reservists could only be used behind the lines;[57] and Russia possessed neither the weapons, boots, and uniforms to equip its theoretical reserve army of millions nor the officers to supervise them. But even this does not probe the full depths of the German military capacity, which was also reflected in such unquantifiable factors as good internal lines of communication, faster mobilization schedules, superior staff training, advanced technology, and so on.

But the German Empire was weakened by its geography and its diplomacy. Because it lay in the center of the continent, its growth appeared to threaten a number of other Great Powers simultaneously. The efficiency of its military machine, coupled with Pan-German calls for a reordering of Europe's boundaries, alarmed both the French and the Russians and drove them closer to each other. The swift expansion of the German navy upset Britain, as did the latent German threat to the Low Countries and northern France. Germany, in one scholar's phrase, was "born encircled."[58] Even if German expansionism was directed overseas, where could it go without trespassing upon the spheres of influence of other Great Powers? A venture into Latin America could only be pursued at the cost of war with the United States. Expansion in China had been frowned upon by Russia and Britain in the 1890s and was out of the question after the Japanese victory over Russia in 1905. Attempts to develop the Baghdad Railway alarmed both London and St. Petersburg. Efforts to secure the Portuguese colonies were checked by the British. While the United States could apparently expand its influence in the western hemisphere, Japan encroach upon China, Russia and Britain penetrate into the Middle East, and France "round off" its holdings in northwestern Africa, Germany was to go empty-handed. When Bülow, in his famous "hammer or anvil" speech of 1899, angrily declared, "We cannot allow any foreign power, any foreign Jupiter to tell us: 'What can be done? The world is already partitioned,'" he was expressing a widely held resentment. Little wonder that German publicists called for a redivision of the globe.[59]

To be sure, all rising powers call for changes in an international order which has been fixed to the advantage of the older, established powers.[60] From a *Realpolitik* viewpoint, the question was whether this particular challenger could secure changes without provoking too much opposition. And while geography played an important role here, diplomacy was also significant; because Germany did not enjoy, say, Japan's geopolitical position, its statecraft had to be of an extraordinarily high order. Realizing the unease and jealousy which the Second Reich's sudden emergence had caused, Bismarck strove after 1871 to convince the other Great Powers (especially the flank powers of Russia and Britain) that Germany had no further territorial ambitions. Wilhelm and his advisers, eager to show their mettle, were much less careful. Not only did they convey their dissatisfaction with the existing order, but—and this was the greatest failure of all—the decision-making process in Berlin concealed, behind a facade of high imperial purpose, a chaos and instability which amazed all who witnessed it in close action. Much of this was due to the character weaknesses of Wilhelm II himself, but it was exacerbated by institutional flaws in the Bismarckian constitution; with no body (like a cabinet) collectively possessing responsibility for overall government policy, different departments and interest groups pursued their aims without any check from above or ordering of priorities.[61] The navy thought almost solely of a future war with England; the army planned to eliminate France; financiers and businessmen wished to move into the Balkans, Turkey, and the Near East, eliminating Russian influence in the process. The result, moaned Chancellor Bethmann Hollweg in July 1914, was to "challenge everybody, get in everyone's way and actually, in the course of all this, weaken nobody."[62] This was not a recipe for success in a world full of egoistic and suspicious nation-states.

Finally, there remained the danger that failure to achieve diplomatic or territorial successes would affect the delicate internal politics of Wilhelmine Germany, whose Junker elite worried about the (relative) decline of the agricultural interest, the rise of organized labor, and the growing influence of Social Democracy in a period of industrial boom. It was true that after 1897 the pursuit of *Weltpolitik* was motivated to a considerable extent by the calculation that this would be politically popular and divert attention from Germany's domestic-political fissures.[63] But the regime in Berlin always ran the dual risk that if it backed down from a confrontation with a "foreign Jupiter," German nationalist opinion might revile and denounce the Kaiser and his aides; whereas, if the country became engaged in an all-out war, it was not clear whether the natural patriotism of the masses of workers, soldiers, and sailors would outweigh their dislike of the archconservative Prusso-German state. While some observers felt that a war would unite the nation behind the emperor, others feared it would further strain the German sociopolitical fabric. Again, this needs to be placed in context—for example, German internal weaknesses were hardly as serious as those in Russia or Austria-Hungary, but they did exist, and they certainly could affect the country's ability to engage in a lengthy "total" war.

It has been argued by many historians that imperial Germany was a "special case," following a *Sonderweg* ("special path") which would one day culminate in the excesses of National Socialism. Viewed solely in terms of political culture and rhetoric around 1900, this is a hard claim to detect: Russian and Austrian anti-Semitism was at least as strong as German, French chauvinism as marked as the German, Japan's sense of cultural uniqueness and destiny as broadly held as Germany's. Each of the powers examined here was "special," and in an age of imperialism was all too eager to assert its specialness. From the criterion of power politics, however, Germany did possess unique features which were of great import. It was the one Great Power which combined the modern, industrialized strength of the western democracies with the autocratic (one is tempted to say irresponsible) decision-making features of the eastern monarchies.[64] It was the one "newcomer" Great Power, with the exception of the United States, which really had the strength to challenge the existing order. And it was the one rising Great Power which, if it expanded its borders farther to the east or to the west, could only do so at the expense of powerful neighbors: the one country whose future growth, in Calleo's words, "directly" rather than "indirectly" undermined the European balance.[65] This was an explosive combination for a nation which felt, in Tirpitz's phrase, that it was "a life-and-death question . . . to make up the lost ground."[66]

It seemed a vital matter to the rising states to break through, but it was even more urgent for those established Great Powers now under pressure to try to hold their own. Here again, it will be necessary to point to the very significant differences between the three Powers in question, Austria-Hungary, France, and Britain—and perhaps especially between the first-named and the last. Nonetheless, the charts of their relative power in world affairs would show all of them distinctly weaker by the end of the nineteenth century than they had been fifty or sixty years earlier,[67] even if their defense budgets were larger and their colonial empires more extensive, and if (in the case of France and Austria-Hungary) they still had territorial ambitions in Europe. Furthermore, it seems fair to claim that the leaderships within these nations *knew* the international scene had become more complicated and threatening than that which their predecessors had faced, and that such knowledge was forcing them to consider radical changes of policy in an effort to meet the new circumstances.

Austria-Hungary

Although the Austro-Hungarian Empire was by far the weakest of the established Great Powers—and, in Taylor's words, slipping out of their ranks[68]—this is not obvious from a glance at the macroeconomic statistics. Despite considerable emigration, its population rose from 41 million in 1890 to 52 million in 1914, to go well clear of France and Italy, and some way ahead of Britain. The empire also underwent much industrialization in these decades, though the pace of change was perhaps swifter before 1900 than after. Its coal production by 1914 was a respectable 47 million tons, higher than either France's or Russia's, and even in its steel production and energy consumption it was not significantly inferior to either of the Dual Alliance powers. Its textile industry experienced a surge in output, brewing and sugar-beet production rose, the oilfields of Galicia were exploited, mechanization occurred on the estates of Hungary, the Skoda armaments works multiplied in size, electrification occurred in the major cities, and the state vigorously promoted railway construction.[69] According to one of Bairoch's calculations, the Austro-Hungarian Empire's GNP in 1913 was virtually the same as France's,[70] which looks a little suspect—as does Farrar's claim that its share of "European power" rose from 4.0 percent in 1890 to 7.2 percent in 1910.[71] Nonetheless, it is clear that the empire's growth rates from 1870 to 1913 were among the highest in Europe, and that its "industrial potential" was growing faster even than Russia's.[72]

Once one examines Austria-Hungary's economy and society in more detail, however, significant flaws appear. Perhaps the most fundamental of these was the enormous regional differences in per capita income and output, which to a large degree mirrored socioeconomic and ethnic diversities in a territory stretching from the Swiss Alps to the Bukovina. It was not merely the fact that in 1910 73 percent of the population of Galicia and Bukovina were employed in agriculture compared with 55 percent for the empire as a whole; much more significant and alarming was the enormous disparity of wealth, with per capita income in Lower Austria (850 crowns) and Bohemia (761 crowns) being far in excess of those in Galicia (316 crowns), Bukovina (310 crowns), and Dalmatia (264 crowns).[73] Yet while it was in the Austrian provinces and Czech lands that industrial "takeoff" was occurring, and in Hungary that agricultural improvements were under way, it was in those poverty-stricken Slavic regions that the population was increasing the fastest. In consequence, Austria-Hungary's per capita level of industrialization remained well below that of the leading Great Powers, and despite all the absolute increases in output, its share of world manufacturing production hovered around a mere 4.5 percent in those decades. This was not a strong economic base on which a country with Austria-Hungary's strategical tasks could rest.

This relative backwardness might have been compensated for by a high degree of national-cultural cohesion, such as existed in Japan or France; but, alas, Vienna controlled the most ethnically diverse cluster of peoples in Europe[74]—when war came in 1914, for example, the mobilization order was given in fifteen different languages. The age-old tension between German speakers and Czech speakers in Bohemia was not the most serious of the problems facing Emperor Francis Joseph and his advisers, even if the "Young Czech" movement was making it sound so. The strained relations with Hungary, which despite its post-1867 status as an equal partner clashed with Vienna again and again over such issues as tariffs, treatment of ethnic minorities, "Magyarization" of the army, and so on, were such that by 1899, western observers feared the breakup of the entire empire and the French foreign minister, Delcassé, secretly renegotiated the terms of the Dual Alliance with Russia in order to prevent Germany from succeeding to the Austrian lands and access to the Adriatic coast. By 1905, indeed, the general staff in Vienna was quietly preparing a contingency plan for the military occupation of Hungary should the crisis worsen.[75] Vienna's list of nationality problems did not stop with the Czechs and the Magyars. The Italians in the south resented the stiff Germanization in their territories, and looked over the border for help from Rome—as

the captive Rumanians, to a lesser degree, looked eastward to Bucharest. The Poles, by contrast, were quiescent, in part because the rights
they enjoyed under the Habsburg Empire were superior to those obtaining in the German- and Russian-dominated territories. But by far
the largest danger to the unity of the empire came from the South
Slavs, since dissident groups within seemed to be looking toward
Serbia and, more distantly, toward Russia. Compromises with South
Slav aspirations were urged from time to time, by more liberal circles
in Vienna, but they were fiercely resisted by the Magyar gentry, who
both opposed any diminution of Hungary's special status and also kept
up their strong discrimination of ethnic minorities within Hungary
itself. Since a political solution of this issue was denied to the moder-
ates, the door was open for Austro-German nationalists like the chief
of staff, General Conrad, to argue that the Serbs and their sympathizers
should be dealt with by force. Despite the restraint exercised by Emperor Francis Joseph himself, this always remained a last resort if the
Empire's survival did really seem to be threatened.

All of this undoubtedly effected Austria-Hungary's power, and in a
whole number of ways. It was not that multi-ethnicity inevitably meant
military weakness. The army remained a unifying institution, and
extraordinarily adept at using a whole array of languages of command;
nor had its old skills of divide and rule been forgotten when it came
to garrisons and deployments. But it was increasingly difficult to rely
upon the wholehearted cooperation of the Czech or Hungarian regiments in certain circumstances, and even the traditional loyalty of the
Croats (used for centuries along the "military border") was eroded by
Hungarian persecution. What was more, Vienna's classic answer to all
of these particularist grievances was to smother them with committees, with new jobs, tax concessions, additional railway branch lines,
and so on. "There were, in 1914, well over 3,000,000 civil servants,
running things as diverse as schools, hospitals, welfare, taxation, railways, posts, etc. . . . so . . . that there was not much money left for the
army itself."[76] According to Wright's figures, defense appropriations
took a far smaller share of "national (i.e., central government) appropriations" in the Austria-Hungarian Empire than in any of the other
Great Powers.[77] In consequence, while its fleet never had enough funds
to match even the Italian, let alone the French, navy in the Mediterranean, allocations to the army were between one-third and one-half of
those which the Russian and Prussian armies enjoyed. The army's
weapons, especially artillery, were out-of-date and far too few. Because
of lack of funds, only about 30 percent of the available manpower was
conscripted, and many of them were sent on "permanent leave" or
received only eight weeks training. It was not a system geared to produce masses of competent reserves in wartime.[78]

As the international tensions built up in the decade or so after 1900,

the Austro-Hungarian Empire's strategical position appeared parlous
indeed. Its internal divisions threatened to split the country asunder,
and complicated relations with most of its neighbors. Its economic
growth, although marked, was not allowing it to catch up with leading
Great Powers such as Britain and Germany. It spent less per capita on
defense than many of the other powers, and it conscripted a far smaller
ratio of its eligible youth into the army than any of the continental
nations. To cap it all, it seemed to have so many possible foes that its
general staff had to plan for a whole variety of campaigns—a complication which very few of the other Great Powers were distracted with.

That the Austro-Hungarian Empire had so many potential enemies
was itself due to its unique geographical and multinational situation.
Despite the Triple Alliance, the tensions with Italy became greater after
1900, and on several occasions Conrad advocated a military blow
against this southern neighbor; even if his proposal was firmly rejected
by both the foreign ministry and the emperor, the garrisons and fortresses along the Italian frontier were steadily built up. Much farther
afield, Vienna had to worry about Rumania, which by 1912 became a
distinct threat as it moved into the opposite camp. But the country
which attracted the most venom was Serbia, which, with Montenegro,
seemed a magnet to the South Slavs within the empire and thus a
cancerous growth which had to be eliminated. The only problem with
that agreeable solution was that an attack upon Serbia could well
provoke a military response from Austria-Hungary's most formidable
rival, czarist Russia, which would invade the northeastern front just as
the bulk of the Austro-Hungarian army was pushing southward, past
Belgrade. Although even the hyperbelligerent Conrad asserted that it
was "up to the diplomats"[79] to keep the empire from having to fight all
these foes at once, his own pre-1914 war plans reveal the fantastic
military juggling act for which the army had to prepare. While a main
force (A-Staffel) of nine army corps would be prepared for deployment
against either (!) Italy or Russia, a smaller group of three army corps
would be mobilized against Serbia-Montenegro (Minimalgruppe Balkan). In addition, a strategic reserve of four army corps (B-Staffel)
would hold itself ready "either to reinforce A-Staffel and make it into
a powerful offensive force, or, if there were no danger from either Italy
or Russia, to join Minimalgruppe Balkan for an offensive against
Serbia."[80]

"The heart of the matter," it has been said, "was simply that Austria-
Hungary was trying to act the part of a great power with the resources
of a second-rank one."[81] The desperate efforts to be strong on all fronts
ran a serious risk of making the empire weak everywhere; at the very
least, they placed superhuman demands upon the empire's railway
system, and upon the staff officers who would control it. More than
that, these operational dilemmas confirmed what most observers in

Vienna had reluctantly accepted since 1870: that in the event of a Great Power war, Austria-Hungary needed German support. This would not be the case in a purely Austro-Italian war (although that, despite Conrad's frequent fears, was the least likely contingency); but German military assistance certainly would be required if Austria-Hungary became embroiled in a war with Serbia, and the latter was then aided by Russia; hence the repeated attempts by Conrad prior to 1914 to secure Berlin's assurances on this point. Finally, the baroque nature of this operational planning reflects once again what many contemporaries could see but some later historians have declined to admit:[82] that if the nationalist explosions of discontent in the Balkans, and in the empire itself, continued to go off, the chances of preserving Kaiser Joseph's unique but anachronistic inheritance were well-nigh impossible. And when that happened, the European equilibrium was bound to be undermined.

France

France in 1914 possessed considerable advantages over Austria-Hungary. Perhaps the most important was that it had only one enemy, Germany, against which its entire national resources could be concentrated. This had not been the case in the late 1880s, when France was challenging Britain in Egypt and West Africa and engaged in a determined naval race against the Royal Navy, quarreling with Italy almost to the point of blows, and girding itself for the *revanche* against Germany.[83] Even when more cautious politicians drew the country back from the brink and then moved into the early stages of their alliance with Russia, the French strategical dilemma was still an acute one. Its most formidable foe, clearly, was the German Empire, now more powerful than ever. But the Italian naval and colonial challenge (as the French viewed it) was also disturbing, not only for its own sake, but because a war with Italy would almost certainly involve its German ally. For the army, this meant that a considerable number of divisions would have to be stationed in the southeast; for the navy, it exacerbated the age-old strategical problem of whether to concentrate the fleet in Mediterranean or Atlantic ports or to run the risk of dividing it into two smaller forces.[84]

All this was compounded by the swift deterioration in Anglo-French relations which followed the British occupation of Egypt in 1882. From 1884, the two countries were locked into an escalating naval race, which on the British side was associated with the possible loss of their Mediterranean line of communications and (occasionally) with fears of a French cross-Channel invasion.[85] Even more persistent and threatening were the frequent Anglo-French colonial clashes. Britain and France had quarreled over the Congo in 1884–1885 and over West Africa throughout the entire 1880s and 1890s. In 1893 they seemed to be on the brink of war over Siam. The greatest crisis of all came in 1898, when their sixteen-year rivalry over control of the Nile Valley climaxed in the confrontation between Kitchener's army and Marchand's small expedition at Fashoda. Although the French backed down on that occasion, they were energetic and bold imperialists. Neither the inhabitants of Timbuktu nor those of Tonkin would have regarded France as a power in decline, far from it. Between 1871 and 1900, France had added 3.5 million square miles to its existing colonial territories, and it possessed indisputably the largest overseas empire after Britain's. Although the commerce of those lands was not great, France had built up a considerable colonial army and an array of prime naval bases from Dakar to Saigon. Even in places which France had not colonized, such as the Levant and South China, its influence was large.[86]

France had been able to carry out such a dynamic colonial policy, it has been argued, because the structures of government had permitted a small group of bureaucrats, colonial governors, and *parti colonial* enthusiasts to effect "forward" strategies which the fast-changing ministries of the Third Republic had little chance to control.[87] But if the volatile state of French parliamentary politics had inadvertently given a strength and consistency to its imperial policy—by placing it in the hands of permanent officials and their friends in the colonial "lobby"— it had a far less happy impact upon naval and military affairs. For example, the swift changes of regime brought with them new ministers of marine, some of whom were mere "placemen," others of whom had strongly held (but always varying) opinions on naval strategy. In consequence, although large sums were allocated to the French navy in these decades, the money was not well spent: the building programs reflected the frequent changes from one administration's preference for a *guerre de course* (commerce-raiding) strategy to another's firm support for battleships, leaving the navy itself with a heterogeneous collection of ships which were no match for those of the British or, later, the Germans.[88] But the impact of politics upon the French navy paled by comparison with the effect upon the army, where the strong dislike shown by the officer corps toward republican politicians and a whole host of civil-military clashes (of which the Dreyfus affair was merely the most notorious) weakened the fabric of France and placed in question both the loyalty and the efficiency of the army. Only with the remarkable post-1911 nationalist revival could these civil-military disputes be set aside in the common crusade against the German enemy; but there were many who wondered whether too heavy a dose of politics had not done irreparable damage to the French armed forces.[89]

The other obvious internal constraint upon French power was the state of its economy.[90] The position here is a complex one, and has been made the more so by economic historians' predilections for different indices. On the positive side:

> This period saw a great development in banking and financial institutions participating in industrial investment and in foreign lending. The iron and steel industry was established on modern lines and great new plants were built, especially on the Lorraine orefield. On the coalfields of northern France the familiar, ugly landscape of an industrial society took place. Important strides were made in engineering and the newer industries. . . . France had its notable entrepreneurs and innovators who won a leading place in the late nineteenth and early twentieth century in steel, engineering, motor cars and aircraft. Firms like Schneider, Peugeot, Michelin and Renault were in the vanguard.[91]

Until Henry Ford's mass-production methods were developed, indeed, France was the leading automobile producer in the world. There was a further burst of railway-building in the 1880s, which together with improved telegraphs, postal systems, and inland waterways, increased the trend toward a national market. Agriculture had been protected by the Méline tariff of 1892, and there remained a focus upon producing high-quality goods, with a large per capita added value. Given these indices of absolute economic expansion and the small increase in the number of Frenchmen during these decades, measurement of output which are related to France's population look impressive—e.g., per capita growth rates, per capita value of exports, etc.

Finally, there was the undeniable fact that France was immensely rich in terms of mobile capital, which could be (and systematically was) applied to serve the interests of the country's diplomacy and strategy. The most impressive sign of this had been the very rapid paying off the German indemnity of 1871, which, in Bismarck's erroneous calculation, was supposed to cripple France's strength for many years to come. But in the period following, French capital was also poured out to various countries inside Europe and without. By 1914, France's foreign investments totaled $9 billion, second only to Britain's. While these investments had helped to industrialize considerable parts of Europe, including Spain and Italy, they had also brought large political and diplomatic benefits to France itself. The slow weaning of Italy away from the Triple Alliance at the turn of the century was attended, if not fully caused, by the Italian need for capital. Franco-Russian loans to China, in exchange for railway rights and other concessions, were nearly always raised in Paris and funneled through St. Petersburg. France's massive investments in Turkey and the Balkans—which the frustrated Germans could never manage to match prior to 1914—gave it an edge, not only in politico-cultural terms, but also in securing contracts for French rather than German armaments. Above all, the French poured money into the modernization of their Russian ally, from the floating of the first loan on the Paris market in October 1888 to the critical 1913 offer of lending 500 million francs—on condition that the Russian strategic railway system in the Polish provinces be greatly extended, so that the "Russian steamroller" could be mobilized the faster to crush Germany.[92] This was the clearest demonstration yet of France's ability to use its financial muscle to bolster its own strategic power (although the irony was that the more efficient the Russian military machine became, the more the Germans had to prepare to strike quickly against France).

Yet once again, as soon as comparative economic data are used, this positive image of France's growth fades away. While it was certainly a large-scale investor abroad, there is little evidence that this capital brought the country the optimal return, either in terms of interest earned[93] or in a rise in foreign orders for French products: all too often, even in Russia, German merchants grabbed the lion's share of the import trade. Germany's proportion of exported European manufacturers had already overtaken France's in the early 1880s; by 1911, it was almost twice as high. But this in turn reflected the awkward fact that whereas the French economy had suffered from vigorous British industrial competition a generation or two earlier, it was now being affected by the rise of the German industrial giant. With truly rare exceptions like the automobile industry, the comparative statistics time and time again measure this eclipse. By the eve of war, its total industrial potential was only about 40 percent of Germany's, its steel production was little over one-sixth, its coal production hardly one-seventh. What coal, steel, and iron were produced was usually more expensive, coming from smaller plants and poorer mines. Similarly, for all the alleged advances of the French chemical industry, the country was massively dependent upon German imports. Given its small plants, out-of-date practices, and heavy reliance upon protected local markets, it is not surprising that France's industrial growth in the nineteenth century had been coldly described as "arthritic . . . hesitant, spasmodic, and slow."[94]

Nor were its bucolic charms any consolation, at least in terms of relative power and wealth. The blows dealt by disease to silk and wine production were never fully recovered from; and what the Méline tariff did, in its effort to protect farm incomes and preserve social stability, was to slow down the drift from the land and to support inefficient producers. With agriculture still accounting for 40 percent of the active population around 1910 and still overwhelmingly composed of smallholdings, this was an obvious drag upon both French productivity and overall wealth. Bairoch's data show the French GNP in 1913 only 55 percent of Germany's and its share of world manufacturing production around 40 percent of Germany's; Wright has its national income as being $6 billion in 1914 to Germany's $12 billion.[95] Another war with its eastern neighbor, should France stand alone, could only repeat the result of 1870–1871.

On many of these comparative indices, France had also slipped well behind the United States, Britain, and Russia as well as Germany, so that by the early twentieth century it was only the fifth among the Great Powers. Yet it was the erosion of French power vis-à-vis Germany which mattered, simply because of the bitter relations between the two countries. In this respect, the trends were ominous. Whereas Germany's population rose by nearly eighteen million between 1890 and 1914, France's increased by little over one million. This, together with Germany's greater national wealth, meant that however much the French strained to keep up militarily, they were always outdistanced. By conscripting over 80 percent of its eligible youth, France had produced a staggeringly large army for its size, at least according to certain measurements: for instance, the eighty divisions it could mobilize from a population of 40 million compared favorably with the Austrians' forty-eight divisions from a population of 52 million. But this was to little avail against imperial Germany. Not only could the Prussian general staff, employing its better-trained reserves, mobilize somewhat over one hundred divisions, but it had a vast manpower potential to draw upon—almost ten million men in the requisite age group, compared with France's five million; and it possessed the fantastic figure of 112,000 well-trained NCOs—the key element in an expanding army—compared with France's 48,000. Moreover, although Germany allocated a smaller proportion of its national income to military spending, it devoted much more in absolute terms. Throughout the 1870s and 1880s the French high command had struggled in vain against "a condition of unacceptable inferiority";[96] on the eve of the First World War, the confidential memoranda about the German material superiority were equally alarming: "4,500 machine guns to 2,500 in France, 6,000 77-millimeter cannon to 3,800 French 75s, and an almost total monopoly in heavy artillery."[97] The last aspect in particular showed French weaknesses at their worst.

And yet the French army went into battle in 1914 confident of victory, having dropped its defensive strategy in favor of an all-out offensive, reflecting the heightened emphasis upon morale which Grandmaison and others attempted to inculcate into the army—psychologically, one suspects, as compensation for these very material weaknesses. "Neither numbers nor miraculous machines will determine victory," General Messing preached. "This will go to soldiers with valor and quality—and by this I mean superior physical and moral endurance, offensive strength."[98] This assertiveness was associated with the "patriotic revival" in France which took place after the 1911

Moroccan crisis and which suggested the country would fight far better than it had in 1870, despite the class and political divisions which had made it appear so vulnerable during the Dreyfus affair. Most military experts assumed that the war to come would be short. What mattered, therefore, was the number of divisions which could immediately be put into the field, not the size of the German steel and chemical industries nor the millions of potential recruits Germany possessed.[99]

This revival of national confidence was perhaps most strongly affected by the improvement in France's international position secured by the foreign minister, Delcassé, and his diplomats after the turn of the century.[100] Not only had they nursed and maintained the vital link to St. Petersburg despite all the diplomatic efforts of the Kaiser's government to weaken it, but they had steadily improved relations with Italy, virtually detaching it from the Triple Alliance (and thus easing the strategical problem of having to fight in Savoy as well as Lorraine). Most important of all, the French had been able to compose their colonial differences with Britain in the 1904 *entente*, and then to convince leading members of the Liberal government in London that France's security was a British national interest. Although domestic-political reasons in Britain precluded a fixed alliance, the chances of France obtaining future British support improved with each addition to Germany's High Seas Fleet and with every indication that a German strike westward would go through neutral Belgium. If Britain did come in, the Germans would have to worry not only about Russia but about the effect of the Royal Navy on its High Seas Fleet, the destruction of its overseas trade, and a small but significant British expeditionary force deployed in northern France. Fighting the Boches with Russia and Britain as one's allies had been the French dream since 1871; now it seemed a distinct reality.

France was not strong enough to oppose Germany in a one-to-one struggle, something which all French governments were determined to avoid. If the mark of a Great Power is a country which is willing and able to take on any other, then France (like Austria-Hungary) had slipped to a lower position. But that definition seemed too abstract in 1914 to a nation which felt psychologically geared up for war,[101] militarily stronger than ever, wealthy, and, above all, endowed with powerful allies. Whether even a combination of all those features would enable France to withstand Germany was an open question; but most Frenchmen seemed to think it would.

Great Britain

At first sight, Britain was imposing. In 1900 it possessed the largest empire the world had ever seen, some twelve million square miles of land and perhaps a quarter of the population of the globe. In the preceding three decades alone, it had added 4.25 million square miles

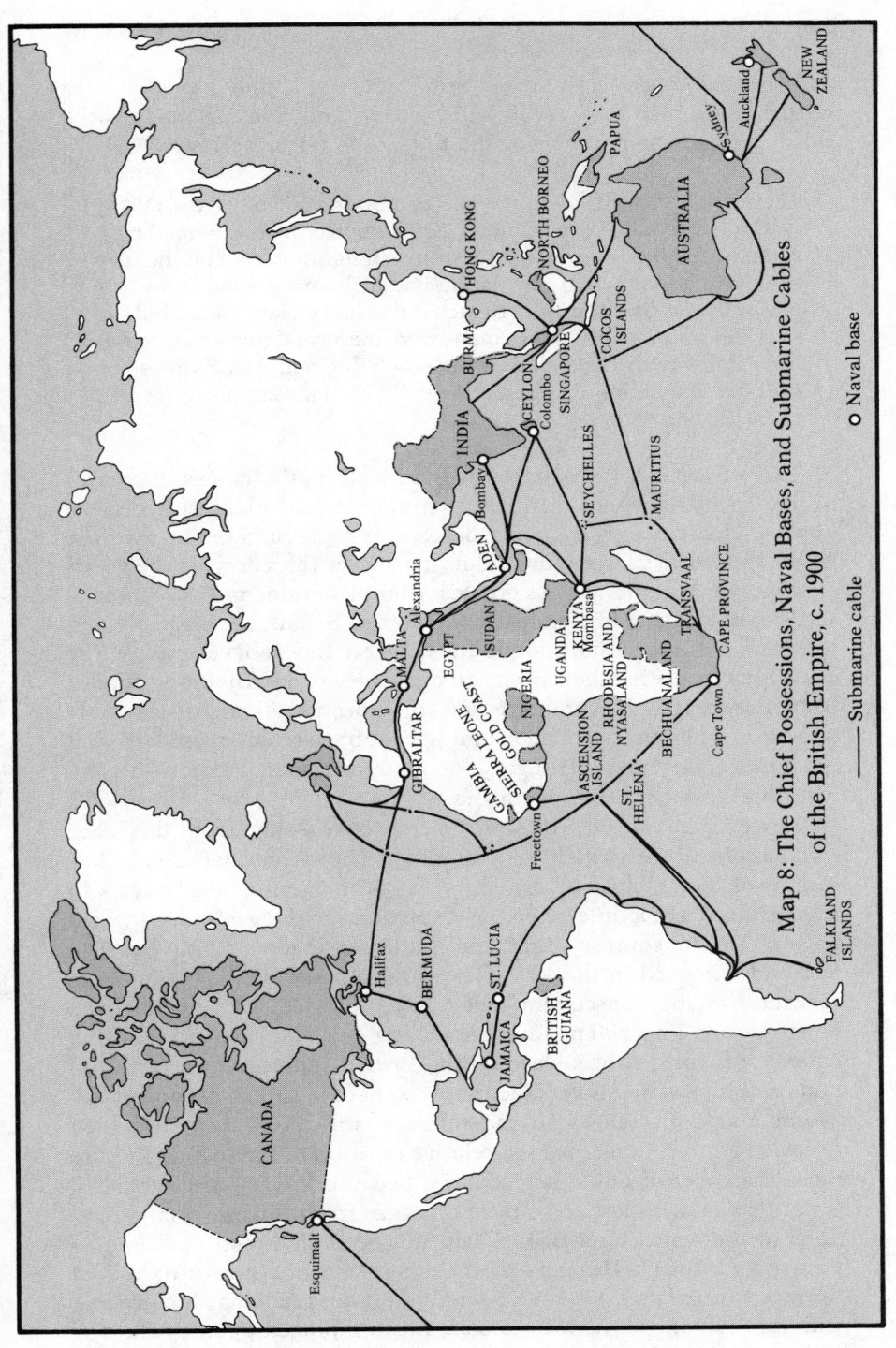

Map 8: The Chief Possessions, Naval Bases, and Submarine Cables
of the British Empire, c. 1900

○ Naval base

—— Submarine cable

NEW ZEALAND

Auckland

Sydney

AUSTRALIA

PAPUA

NORTH BORNEO

HONG KONG

BURMA

COCOS ISLANDS

SINGAPORE

CEYLON

Colombo

INDIA

Bombay

SEYCHELLES

MAURITIUS

ADEN

Alexandria

MALTA

EGYPT

SUDAN

KENYA

Mombasa

UGANDA

TRANSVAAL

CAPE PROVINCE

GIBRALTAR

GAMBIA

SIERRA LEONE

GOLD COAST

NIGERIA

RHODESIA AND NYASALAND

BECHUANALAND

Cape Town

ASCENSION ISLAND

ST. HELENA

Freetown

FALKLAND ISLANDS

Halifax

BERMUDA

ST. LUCIA

JAMAICA

BRITISH GUIANA

CANADA

Esquimalt

and 66 million people to the empire. It was not simply a critical later historian but also the French and the Germans, the Ashanti and the Burmese, and many others at the time, who felt as follows:

> There had taken place, in the half-century or so before the [1914] war, a tremendous expansion of British power, accompanied by a pronounced lack of sympathy for any similar ambition on the part of other nations. . . . If any nation had truly made a bid for world power, it was Great Britain. In fact, it had more than made a bid for it. It had achieved it. The Germans were merely talking about building a railway to Bagdad. The Queen of England was Empress of India. If any nation had upset the world's balance of power, it was Great Britain.[102]

There were other indicators of British strength: the vast increases in the Royal Navy, equal in power to the next two largest fleets; the unparalleled network of naval bases and cable stations around the globe; the world's largest merchant marine by far, carrying the goods of what was still the world's greatest trading nation; and the financial services of the City of London, which made Britain the biggest investor, banker, insurer, and commodity dealer in the global economy. The crowds who cheered their heads off during Victoria's Diamond Jubilee festivities in 1897 had some reason to be proud. Whenever the three or four world empires of the coming century were discussed, it—but not France, or Austria-Hungary, or many other candidates—was always on the short list of members.

However, if viewed from other perspectives—say, from the sober calculations of the British "official mind,"[103] or from that of later historians of the collapse of British power—the late nineteenth century was certainly not a time when the empire was making a "bid for world power." On the contrary, that "bid" had been made a century earlier and had climaxed in the 1815 victory, which allowed the country to luxuriate in the consequent half-century of virtually unchallenged maritime and imperial preeminence. After 1870, however, the shifting balance of world forces was eroding British supremacy in two ominous and interacting ways. The first was that the spread of industrialization and the changes in the military and naval weights which followed from it weakened the relative position of the British Empire more than that of any other country, because it was *the* established Great Power, with less to gain than to lose from fundamental alterations in the status quo. Britain had not been as directly affected as France and Austria-Hungary by the emergence of a powerful, united Germany (only after 1904–1905 would London really have to grapple with that issue). But it was *the* state most impinged upon by the rise of American power, since British interests (Canada, naval bases in the

Caribbean, trade and investment in Latin America) were much more prominent in the western hemisphere than those of any other European country;[104] it was *the* country most affected by the expansion of Russian borders and strategic railways in Turkestan, since everyone could see the threat which that posed to British influence in the Near East and Persian Gulf, and ultimately perhaps to its control of the Indian subcontinent;[105] it was *the* country which, by enjoying the greatest share of China's foreign trade, was likely to have its commercial interests the most seriously damaged by a carving up of the Celestial Empire or by the emergence of a new force in that region;[106] similarly, it was *the* power whose relative position in Africa and the Pacific was affected the most by the post-1880 scramble for colonies, since it had (in Hobsbawm's phrase) "exchanged the informal empire over most of the underdeveloped world for the formal empire of a quarter of it"[107]—which was not a good bargain, despite the continued array of fresh acquisitions to Queen Victoria's dominions.

While some of these problems (in Africa or China) were fairly new, others (the rivalry with Russia in Asia, and with the United States in the western hemisphere) had exercised many earlier British administrations. What was different now was that the relative power of the various challenger states was much greater, while the threats seemed to be developing almost simultaneously. Just as the Austro-Hungarian Empire was distracted by having to grapple with a number of enemies within Europe, so British statesmen had to engage in a diplomatic and strategical juggling act that was literally worldwide in its dimensions. In the critical year of 1895, for example, the Cabinet found itself worrying about the possible breakup of China following the Sino-Japanese War, about the collapse of the Ottoman Empire as a result of the Armenian crisis, about the looming clash with Germany over southern Africa at almost exactly the same time as the quarrel with the United States over the Venezuela–British Guiana borders, about French military expeditions in equatorial Africa, and about a Russian drive toward the Hindu Kush.[108] It was a juggling act which had to be carried out in naval terms as well; for no matter how regularly the Royal Navy's budget was increased, it could no longer "rule the waves" in the face of the five or six foreign fleets which were building in the 1890s, as it had been able to do in midcentury. As the Admiralty repeatedly pointed out, it *could* meet the American challenge in the western hemisphere, but only by diverting warships from European waters, just as it *could* increase the size of the Royal Navy in the Far East, but only by weakening its squadrons in the Mediterranean. It could not be strong everywhere. Finally, it was a juggling act which had to be carried out in military terms, by the transfer of battalions from Aldershot to Cairo, or from India to Hong Kong, to meet the latest emergencies— and yet all this had to be done by a small-scale volunteer force that had been completely eclipsed by mass armies on the Prussian model.[109]

The second, interacting weakness was less immediate and dramatic, but perhaps even more serious. It was the erosion of Britain's industrial and commercial preeminence, upon which, in the last resort, its naval, military, and imperial strength rested. Established British industries such as coal, textiles, and ironware increased their output in absolute terms in these decades, but their relative share of world production steadily diminished; and in the newer and increasingly more important industries such as steel, chemicals, machine tools, and electrical goods, Britain soon lost what early lead it possessed. Industrial production, which had grown at an annual rule of about 4 percent in the period 1820 to 1840 and about 3 percent between 1840 and 1870, became more sluggish; between 1875 and 1894 it grew at just over 1.5 percent annually, far less than that of the country's chief rivals. This loss of industrial supremacy was soon felt in the cutthroat competition for customers. At first, British exports were priced out of their favorable position in the industrialized European and North American markets, often protected by high tariff barriers, and then out of certain colonial markets, where other powers competed both commercially and by placing tariffs around their new annexations; and, finally, British industry found itself weakened by an ever-rising tide of imported foreign manufacturers into the unprotected home market— the clearest sign that the country was becoming uncompetitive.

The slowdown of British productivity and the decrease in competitiveness in the late nineteenth century has been one of the most investigated issues in economic history.[110] It involved such complex issues as national character, generational differences, the social ethos, and the educational system as well as more specific economic reasons like low investment, out-of-date plant, bad labor relations, poor salesmanship, and the rest. For the student of grand strategy, concerned with the *relative* picture, these explanations are less important than the fact that the country as a whole was steadily losing ground. Whereas in 1880 the United Kingdom still contained 22.9 percent of total world manufacturing output, that figure had shrunk to 13.6 percent by 1913; and while its share of world trade was 23.2 percent in 1880, it was only 14.1 percent in 1911–1913. In terms of industrial muscle, both the United States and imperial Germany had moved ahead. The "workshop of the world" was now in third place, not because it wasn't growing, but because others were growing faster.

Nothing frightened the thinking British imperialists more than this relative economic decline, simply because of its impact upon British *power.* "Suppose an industry which is threatened [by foreign competition] is one which lies at the very root of your system of National defence, where are you then?" asked Professor W.A.S. Hewins in 1904. "You could not get on without an iron industry, a great Engineering trade, because in modern warfare you would not have the means of producing, and maintaining in a state of efficiency, your fleets and armies."[111] Compared with this development, quarrels over colonial borders in West Africa or over the future of the Samoan Islands were trivial. Hence the imperialists' interests in tariff reform—abandoning the precepts of free trade in order to protect British industries—and in closer ties with the white dominions, in order to secure both defense contributions and an exclusive imperial market. Britain had now become, in Joseph Chamberlain's frightening phrase, "the weary Titan, [staggering] under the too vast orb of its fate."[112] In the years to come, the First Lord of the Admiralty warned, "the United Kingdom by itself will not be strong enough to hold its proper place alongside of the U.S., or Russia, and probably not Germany. We shall be thrust aside by sheer weight."[113]

Yet if the imperialists were undoubtedly right *in the long term*— "will the Empire which is celebrating one centenary of Trafalgar survive for the next?" the influential journalist Garvin asked gloomily in 1905[114]—they nearly all tended to exaggerate the contemporary perils. The iron and steel trades and the machine-tool industry had been overtaken in various markets, but were certainly not wiped out. The textile industry was enjoying an export boom in the years prior to 1914, which only in retrospect would be seen as an Indian summer. The British shipbuilding industry—vital for both the Royal Navy and the flourishing merchant marine—was still in a class of its own, launching over 60 percent of the world's merchant tonnage and 33 percent of its warships in these decades, which offered some consolation to those who feared that Britain had become too dependent upon imported foodstuffs and raw materials in wartime. It *was* true that if Britain became involved in a lengthy, mass-industrialized conflict between the Great Powers, it would find that much of its armaments industry (e.g., shells, artillery, aircraft, ball bearings, optical equipment, magnetos, dyestuffs) was inadequate, reflecting the traditional assumption that the British army was to be deployed and equipped for small colonial wars and not gigantic continental struggles. But for the greater part of this period, those were exactly the sort of conflicts in which the army was involved. And if the exhausting, lengthy "modern" warfare of trenches and machine guns which at least some pundits were already forecasting in 1898 did come to pass, then the British would not be alone in wanting the correct matériel.

That Britain also possessed economic *strengths* in this period ought to be a warning, therefore, against too gloomy and sweeping a portrayal of the country's problems. In retrospect one can assert, "From 1870 to 1970 the history of Britain was one of steady and almost unbroken decline, economically, militarily and politically, relative to other nations, from the peak of prosperity and power which her industrial revolution had achieved for her in the middle of the nineteenth century";[115] but there is also a danger of exaggerating and anticipating the pace of that decline and of ignoring the country's very considerable assets, even in the nonindustrial sphere. It was, in the first place, immensely wealthy, both at home and abroad, though the British Treasury felt itself under heavy pressure in the two decades before 1914 as the newer technology more than doubled the price of an individual battleship. Moreover, the increases in the size of the electorate were leading to considerable "social" spending for the first time. Yet if the increases in payments for "guns and butter" looked alarming in absolute terms, this was because the night-watchman state had been taking so little of an individual's income in taxes, and spending so little of the national income for government purposes. Even in 1913, total central *and* local government expenditure equaled only 12.3 percent of GNP. Thus, although Britain was one of the heaviest spenders on defense prior to 1914, it needed to allocate a smaller share of its national income to that purpose than any other Great Power in Europe;[116] and if archimperialists tended to disparage Britain's *financial* strength as opposed to *industrial* power, it did have the quite fantastic sum of around $19.5 *billion* invested overseas by then, equaling some 43 percent of the world's foreign investments,[117] which were an undoubted source of national wealth. There was no question that it could pay for even a large-scale, expensive war if the need arose; what was more doubtful was whether it could preserve its liberal political culture—of free trade, low government expenditures, lack of conscription, reliance chiefly upon the navy—if it was forced to devote more and more of its national resources to armaments and to modern, industrialized war.[118] But that it had a deep enough purse was indisputable.

Certain other factors also enhanced Britain's position among the Great Powers. Although it was increasingly difficult to think of defending the *landward* borders of the empire in an age when strategic railways and mass armies were undermining the geopolitical security of India and other possessions,[119] the insularity of the British Isles remained as great an advantage as ever—freeing its population from the fears of a sudden invasion by neighboring armies, allowing the emphasis upon sea power rather than land power, and giving its statesmen a much greater freedom of action over issues of war and peace than those enjoyed by the continental states. In addition, although the possession of an extensive and hard-to-defend colonial empire implied immense strategical problems, it also brought with it considerable strategical advantages. The great array of imperial garrisons, coaling stations, and fleet bases, readily reinforceable by sea, placed it in an extremely strong position against European powers in any conflict fought outside the continent. Just as Britain could send aid to its overseas possessions, so they (especially the self-governing dominions and

India) could assist the imperial power with troops, ships, raw materials, and money—and this was an age when politicians in Whitehall were carefully cultivating their kinsmen overseas in the cause of a more organized "imperial defense."[120] Finally, it might cynically be argued that because British power and influence had been extended so much in earlier times, Britain now possessed lots of buffer zones, lots of less-than-vital areas of interest, and therefore lots of room for *compromise*, especially in its spheres of so-called "informal empire."

Much of the public rhetoric of British imperialism does not suggest that concessions and withdrawals were the order of the day. But the careful assessment of British strategic priorities—which the system of interdepartmental consultation and Cabinet decision-making allowed[121]—went on, year after year, examining each problem in the *context* of the country's global commitments, and fixing upon a policy of compromise or firmness. Thus, since an Anglo-American war would be economically disastrous, politically unpopular, and strategically very difficult, it seemed preferable to make concessions over the Venezuela dispute, the isthmian canal, the Alaska boundary, and so on. By contrast, while Britain would be willing to bargain with France in the 1890s over colonial disputes in West Africa, southeast Asia, and the Pacific, it would fight to preserve its hold on the Nile Valley. A decade later, it would make attempts to defuse the Anglo-German antagonism (by proposing agreements over naval ratios, the Portuguese colonies, and the Baghdad Railway); but it was much more suspicious of offering promises concerning neutrality if a continental war should arise. While Foreign Secretary Grey's efforts toward Berlin prior to 1914 were about as successful as Salisbury's earlier bids to reach Asian accords with St. Petersburg, they both revealed a common assumption that diplomacy could solve most problems that arose in world affairs. To suggest, on the one hand, that Britain's global position around 1900 was as weakened as it was to be in the late 1930s, and to argue, on the other, that there had been "a tremendous expansion of British power" prior to 1914, upsetting the world's balances,[122] are equally one-sided portraits of what was a much more complex position.

In the several decades before the First World War, then, Great Britain had found itself overtaken industrially by both the United States and Germany, and subjected to intense competition in commercial, colonial, and maritime spheres. Nonetheless, its combination of financial resources, productive capacity, imperial possessions, and naval strength meant that it was still probably the "number-one" world power, even if its lead was much less marked than in 1850. But this position as number one was also the essential British problem. Britain was now a *mature* state, with a built-in interest in preserving existing arrangements or, at least, in ensuring that things altered slowly and peacefully. It would fight for certain obvious aims—the defense of

India, the maintenance of naval superiority especially in home waters, probably also the preservation of the European balance of power—but each issue had to be set in its larger context and measured against Britain's other interests. It was for this reason that Salisbury opposed a fixed military commitment *with* Germany in 1889 and 1898–1901, and that Grey strove to avoid a fixed military commitment *against* Germany in 1906–1914. While this made Britain's future policy frustratingly ambiguous and uncertain to decision-makers in Paris and Berlin, it reflected Palmerston's still widely held claim that the country had permanent interests but not permanent allies. If the circumstances which allowed such freedom of action were diminishing as the nineteenth century ended, nevertheless the traditional juggling act between Britain's various interests—imperial versus continental,[123] strategic versus financial[124]—continued in the same old fashion.

Russia

The empire of the czars was also, by most people's reckonings, an automatic member of the select club of "world powers" in the coming twentieth century. Its sheer size, stretching from Finland to Vladivostok, ensured that—as did its gigantic and fast-growing population, which was nearly three times that of Germany and nearly four times that of Britain. For four centuries it had been expanding, westward, southward, eastward, and despite setbacks it showed no signs of wanting to stop. Its standing army had been the largest in Europe throughout the nineteenth century, and it was still much bigger than anybody else's in the approach to the First World War, with 1.3 million frontline troops and, it was claimed, up to 5 million reserves. Russia's military expenditures, too, were extremely high and with the "extraordinary" capital grants on top of the fast-rising "normal" expenditures may well have equaled Germany's total. Railway construction was proceeding at enormous speed prior to 1914—threatening within a short time to undermine the German plan (i.e., the so-called Schlieffen Plan) to strike westward first—and money was also being poured into a new Russian fleet after the war with Japan. Even the Prussian General Staff claimed to be alarmed at this expansion of Russian might, with the younger Moltke asserting that by 1916 and 1917 Prussia's "enemies' military power would then be so great that he did not know how he could deal with it."[125] Some of the French observers, by contrast, looked forward with great glee to the day when the Russian "steamroller" would roll westward and flatten Berlin. And a certain number of Britons, especially those connected with the St. Petersburg embassy, were urging their political chiefs that "Russia is rapidly becoming so powerful that we must retain her friendship at almost any cost."[126] From Galicia to Persia to Peking, there was a widespread concern at the growth of Russian might.

Was Russia really on the point of becoming the gendarme of Europe once more, as these statements might suggest? Assessing that country's effective strength has been a problem for western observers from the eighteenth century to the present, and it has always been made the harder by the paucity of reliable runs of comparative data, by the differences between what the Russians said to foreigners and said to themselves, and by the dangers of relying upon sweeping subjective statements in the place of objective fact. Surveys, however thorough, of "how Europe judged Russia before 1914" are *not* the same as an exact analysis of "the power of Russia" itself.[127]

From the plausible evidence which does exist, however, it seems that Russia in the decades prior to 1914 was simultaneously powerful *and* weak—depending, as ever, upon which end of the telescope one peered down. To begin with, it was now much stronger industrially than it had been at the time of the Crimean War.[128] Between 1860 and 1913—a very lengthy period—Russian industrial output grew at the impressive annual average rate of 5 percent, and in the 1890s the rate was closer to 8 percent. Its steel production on the eve of the First World War had overtaken France's and Austria-Hungary's, and was well ahead of Italy's and Japan's. Its coal output was rising even faster, from 6 million tons in 1890 to 36 million tons in 1914. It was the world's second-largest oil producer. While its long-established textile industry also increased—again, it had many more cotton spindles than France or Austria-Hungary—there was also a late development of chemical and electrical industries, not to mention armaments works. Enormous factories, frequently employing thousands of workers, sprang up around St. Petersburg, Moscow, and other major cities. The Russian railway network, already some 31,000 miles in 1900, was constantly augmented, so that by 1914 it was close to 46,000 miles. Foreign trade, stabilized by Russia's going onto the gold standard in 1892, nearly tripled between 1890 and 1914, when Russia became the world's sixth-largest trading nation. Foreign investment, attracted not only by Russian government and railway bonds but also by the potentialities of Russian business, brought enormous amounts of capital for the modernization of the economy. This great stream of funds joined the torrents of money which the state (flushed from increased customs receipts and taxes on vodka and other items of consumption) also poured into economic infrastructure. By 1914, as many histories have pointed out, Russia had become the fourth industrial power in the world. If these trends continued, might it not at last possess the industrial muscle concomitant with its extent of territory and population?

A look through the telescope from the other end, however, produces a quite different picture. Even if there were approximately three million workers in Russian factories by 1914, that represented the appallingly low level of 1.75 percent of the population; and while firms which employed ten thousand workers in one textile factory looked impressive on paper, most experts now agree that those figures may be deceptive, since the spindles were used through the night by fresh "shifts" of men and women in this labor-rich but technology-poor society.[129] What was perhaps even more significant was the extent to which Russian industrialization, despite some indigenous entrepreneurs, was carried out by foreigners—a successful international firm like Singer, for example, or the large numbers of British engineers—or had at the least been created by foreign investors. "By 1914, 90 percent of mining, almost 100 percent of oil extraction, 40 percent of the metallurgical industry, 50 percent of the chemical industry and even 28 percent of the textile industry were foreign-owned."[130] This was not in itself an unusual thing—Italy's position was somewhat similar—but it does show an extremely heavy reliance upon foreign entrepreneurship and capital, which might or might not (as in 1899 and 1905) keep up its interest, rather than upon indigenous resources for industrial growth. By the early twentieth century, Russia had incurred the largest foreign debt in the world and, to keep the funds flowing in, needed to offer above-average market rates to investors; yet the outward payments of interest were increasingly larger than the "visible" trade balances: in sum, a precarious situation.

That was, perhaps, just one more sign of an "immature" economy, as was the fact that the largest part of Russian industry was devoted to textiles and food processing (rather than, say, engineering and chemicals). Its tariffs were the highest in Europe, to protect industries which were simultaneously immature and inefficient, yet the flood of imported manufactures was rising with every increase in the defense budget and railway building. But perhaps the best indication of its underdeveloped status was the fact that as late as 1913, 63 percent of Russian exports consisted of agricultural produce and 11 percent of timber,[131] both desperately needed to pay for the American farm equipment, German machine tools, and the interest on the country's vast foreign debt—which, however, they did not quite manage to do.

Yet the assessment of Russian strength is worse when it comes to *comparative* output. Although Russia was the fourth-largest industrial power before 1914, it was a long way behind the United States, Britain, and Germany. In the indices of its steel production, energy consumption, share of world manufacturing production, and total industrial potential, it was eclipsed by Britain and Germany; and when these figures are related to population size and calculated on a per capita basis, the gap was a truly enormous one. In 1913 Russia's per capita level of industrialization was less than one-quarter of Germany's and less than one-sixth of Britain's.[132]

At base, the Russia which in 1914 overawed the younger Moltke and the British ambassador to St. Petersburg was a peasant society. Some

80 percent of the population derived its livelihood from agriculture, and a good part of the remainder continued to have ties to the village and the commune. This deadening fact needs to be linked to two others. The first is that most of Russia's enormous increase in population—61 million new mouths between 1890 and 1914 alone—occurred in the villages, and in the most backward (and non-Russian) regions, where poor soil, little fertilizer, and wooden plows were common. Secondly, all the comparative international data of this period show how inefficient Russian agriculture was overall—its crop yield for wheat being less than a third of Britain's and Germany's, for potatoes being about half.[133] Although there were modern estates and farms in the Baltic region, in so many other areas the effect of the communal possession of land and the medieval habit of strip-farming was to take away the incentive for individual enterprise. So too did the periodic redistribution of the lands. The best way to increase one's family share of land was simply to breed more and more sons before the next redistribution. This structural problem was not aided by the poor communications, the unpredictable but dreadful impact of the climate upon the crops, and the great disparity between the "surplus" provinces in the south and the overcrowded, less fertile "importing" provinces in old Russia proper. In consequence, while agricultural output did steadily increase over these decades (at about 2 percent annually), its gains were greatly eroded by the rise in population (1.5 percent annually). And because this enormous agricultural sector was increasing its *per capita* output by a mere 0.5 percent annually, the *real national product of Russia* was only expanding at about 1 percent per head[134]—much less than those of Germany, the United States, Japan, Canada, and Sweden, and of course, a quite different figure from the much-quoted annual *industrial* increases of 5 or 8 percent.

The social consequences of all this are also a factor in any assessment of Russian *power*. Professor Grossman observes that "the extraordinarily swift growth of industry tended to be associated with great sluggishness—and even significant reverses—in other sectors, especially in agriculture and personal consumption; it also tended to outpace the modernization of society, if one may be permitted the phrase."[135] It is, in fact, a most seeming phrase. For what was happening was that a country of extreme economic backwardness was being propelled into the modern age by political authorities obsessed by the need "to acquire and retain the status of a European Great Power."[136] Thus, although one certainly can detect considerable self-driven entrepreneurial activities, the great *thrust* toward modernization was state-inspired and related to military needs—railways, iron and steel, armaments, and so on. But in order to afford the vast flow of imported foreign manufactures and to pay interest on the enormous foreign debt, the Russian state had to ensure that agricultural exports (especially wheat) were steadily increased, even in period of great famine, like 1891; the slow increase in farm output did not, in many years, imply a better standard of living for the deprived and undernourished peasantry. By the same token, in order to pay for the state's own extremely heavy capital investments in industrialization and in defense expenditures, high (chiefly indirect) taxes had to be repeatedly raised and personal consumption squeezed. To use an expression of the economic historians, the czarist government was securing "forced" savings from its helpless populace. Hence the staggering fact that "by 1913 the average Russian had 50 percent more of his income appropriated by the state for current defense than did the average Englishman, even though the Russian's income was only 27 percent of that of his British contemporary."[137]

The larger social costs of this unhealthy combination of agrarian backwardness, industrialization, and top-heavy military expenditures are easy to imagine. In 1913, while 970 million rubles were allocated by the Russian government to the armed forces, a mere 154 million rubles were spent upon health and education; and since the administrative structure did not give the localities the fiscal powers of the American states or English local government, that inadequacy could not be made up elsewhere. In the fast-growing cities, the workers had to contend with no sewerage, health hazards, appalling housing conditions, and high rents. There were fantastic levels of drunkenness—a short-term escape from brute reality. The mortality rate was the highest in Europe. Such conditions, the discipline enforced within the factories, and the lack of any appreciable real rise in living standards produced a sullen resentment of the system which in turn offered an ideal breeding ground for the populists, Bolsheviks, anarchosyndicalists, radicals—indeed, for anybody who (despite the censorship) argued for drastic changes. After the epic 1905 unrest, things cooled off for a while; but in the three years 1912–1914 the incidence of strikes, mass protests, police arrests, and killings was spiraling to an alarming degree.[138] Yet that sort of ferment paled by comparison with the issue which has frightened all Russian leaders from Catherine the Great to the present regime—the "peasant question." When bad harvests and high prices occurred, they interacted with the deep resentments against high rents and grim working conditions to produce vast outbreaks of agrarian unrest. After 1900, the historian Norman Stone records:

> The provinces of Poltyra and Tambov were, for the greater part, devastated; manor houses burned down, animals mutilated. In 1901 there were 155 interventions by troops (as against 36 in 1898) and in 1903, 322, involving 295 squadrons of cavalry and 300 battalions of infantry, some with artillery. 1902 was the high point of the whole

thing. Troops were used to crush the peasantry on 365 occasions. In 1903, for internal order, a force far greater than the army of 1812 was mustered. . . . In sixty-eight of the seventy-five districts of the central Black Earth there were "troubles"—fifty-four estates wrecked. The worst area was Saratov.[139]

Yet when the minister for the interior, Stolypin, tried to reduce this discontent by breaking up the peasant communes after 1908, he simply provoked fresh unrest—whether from villages determined to keep their communal system or from newly independent farmers who swiftly went bankrupt. Thus, "Troops were needed on 13,507 occasions in January 1909, and 114,108 occasions that [whole] year. By 1913, there were 100,000 arrests for 'attacks on State power.' "[140] Needless to say, all this strained a reluctant army, which was also busy crushing the resentful ethnic minorities—Poles, Finns, Georgians, Latvians, Estonians, Armenians—who were seeking to preserve the grudging concessions over "Russification" which they had obtained during the regime's weakness in 1905–1906.[141] Any further military defeat would once again see such groups striving to escape Muscovy's domination. Although we do not have the exact breakdown, there was doubtless a heavy proportion of such groups in the staggering total of two million Russians who got married in August 1914—in order to avoid being drafted into the army.

In short, it is not simply from the perspective of the post–Bolshevik Revolution that one can see that Russia before 1914 was a sociopolitical tinderbox, and very likely to produce large conflagrations in the event of further bad harvests, or reductions in the factory workers' standards of living, or—possibly—a great war. One is bound to use the words "very likely" here, since there also existed (alongside these discontents) a deep loyalty to czar and country in many areas, an increasingly nationalistic assembly, broad Pan-Slavic sympathies, and a corresponding hatred of the foreigner. Indeed, there was many a feckless publicist and courtier, in 1914 as in 1904, who argued that the regime could not afford to appear reticent in great international issues. If it came to war, they urged, the nation would firmly support the pursuit of victory.[142]

But could such a victory be assured, given Russia's likely antagonists in 1914? In the war against Japan, the Russian soldier had fought bravely and stolidly enough—as he had in the Crimea and in the 1877 war against Turkey—but incompetent staffwork, poor logistical support, and unimaginative tactics all had had their effect. Could the armed services now take on Austria-Hungary—and, more particularly, the military-industrial powerhouse of imperial Germany—with any better result? Despite all of its own absolute increases in industrial output in this period, the awful fact was that Russia's productive strength was actually *decreasing* relative to Germany's. Between 1900 and 1913, for example, its own steel production rose from 2.2 to 4.8 million tons, but Germany's leaped forward from 6.3 to 17.6 million tons. In the same way, the increases in Russia's energy consumption and total industrial potential were not as large, either absolutely or relatively, as Germany's. Finally, it will be noticed that in the years 1900–1913 Russia's share of world manufacturing production *sank,* from 8.8 percent to 8.2 percent, because of the expansion of the German and (especially) the American shares.[143] There were not encouraging trends.

But, it has been argued, "by the yardstick with which armies were measured in 1914," Russia *was* powerful, since "a war which tested economics and state bureaucratic structures as well as armies" was not anticipated by the military experts.[144] If so, one is left wondering why contemporary references to German military power drew attention to Krupp steel, the shipyards, the dyestuffs industry, and the efficiency of German railways *as well as* front-line forces.[145] Nonetheless, if it is simply the military figures which matter, then the fact that Russia was creating ever more divisions, artillery batteries, strategic railways, and warships did impress. Assuming that a war would be a short one, these sorts of general statistics all pointed to Russia's growing strength.

Once this superficial level of number-counting is discarded, however, even the military issue becomes altogether more problematical. Once again, the decisive factor was Russia's socioeconomic and technical backwardness. The sheer size of its vast peasant population meant that only one-fifth of each annual cohort was actually conscripted into the armed forces; to have taken in every able-bodied man would have caused the system to collapse in chaos. But those peasants who were recruited could hardly be regarded as ideal material for a modern industrialized war. Thanks to the crude and overheavy concentration upon armaments rather than the broader, more subtle areas of national strength (e.g., general levels of education, technological expertise, bureaucratic efficiency), Russia was frightfully backward at the *personnel* level. As late as 1913 its literacy rate was only 30 percent, which, as one expert has tartly remarked, "was a much lower rate than for mid-eighteenth-century England."[146] And while it was all very well to vote vast sums of money for new recruits, would they be of much use if the army possessed too few trained NCOs? The experts in the Russian general staff, looking with "feelings of inferiority and envy" at Germany's strength in that respect, thought not. They were also aware (as were some foreign observers) of the desperate shortages of good officers.[147] Indeed, from the evidence now available, it appears that in almost all respects—heavy artillery, machine guns, handling of large numbers of infantry, levels of technical training, communications, and even its large fleet of aircraft—the Russian military was acutely conscious of its weaknesses.[148]

The same sort of gloomy conclusions arose when Russia's planned mobilization and strategic-railway system were examined in detail. Although the *overall* mileage of the railway network by 1914 seemed impressive, once it was set against the immense distances of the Russian Empire—or compared with the much denser systems of western Europe—its inadequacy became clear. In any case, since many of these lines were built on the cheap, the rails were often too light and the bedding for the track too weak, and there were too few water tanks and crossings. Some locomotives burned coal, others oil, others wood, which further complicated things—but that was a small problem compared with the awkward fact that the army's peacetime locations were quite different from its wartime deployment areas and affected by its deliberate dispersion policy (Poles serving in Asia, Caucasians in the Baltic provinces, etc.). Yet if a great war came, the masses of troops had somehow to be efficiently transported by the inadequate staff of the railway battalions, of whom "over a third were wholly or partly illiterate, while three-quarters of the officers had no technical training."[149]

The mobilization and deployment problem was exacerbated by the almost insuperable difficulty caused by Russia's commitments to France and Serbia. Given the country's less efficient railway system and the vulnerability of the forces deployed in the Polish salient to a possible "pincer" attack from East Prussia and Galicia, it had seemed prudent prior to 1900 for the Russian high command to stay on the defensive at the outset of war and steadily to build up its military strength; and, indeed, some strategists still argued that case in 1912. Many more generals, however, were keen to smash Austria-Hungary (against which they were confident of victory) and, as the tension between Vienna and Belgrade mounted, to help the latter in the event of an Austro-Hungarian invasion of Serbia. Yet for Russia to concentrate its forces on the southern front was made impossible by the fear of what Germany might do. For decades after 1871, the planners had assumed that a Russo-German war would begin with a massive and swift German assault eastward. But when the outlines of the Schlieffen Plan became clear, St. Petersburg came under enormous French pressure to launch offensives against Germany *as soon as it could,* in order to relieve its western ally. Fear of having France eliminated, together with Paris's tough insistence that further loans be tied to improvements in Russia's *offensive* capabilities, compelled the Russian planners to agree to strike westward as quickly as possible. All this had caused enormous wrangles within the general staff in the few years before 1914, with the various schools of thought disagreeing over the number of army corps to be deployed on the northern as opposed to

the southern front, over the razing of the old defensive fortresses in
Poland (in which, absurdly, so much of the new artillery was sited),
and over the feasibility of ordering a partial rather than a complete
mobilization. Given Russia's diplomatic obligations, the ambivalence
was perhaps understandable; but it did not help the cause of producing
a smoothly run military machine which would secure swift victories
against its foes.[150]

This catalogue of problems could be extended almost ad nauseam.
The fifty divisions of Russian cavalry, thought vital in a country with
few modern roads, required so much fodder—there were about one
million horses!—that they alone would probably produce a breakdown
in the railway system; supplying hay would certainly slow down any
sustained offensive operation, or even the movement of reserves. Because of the backwardness of its transport system and the internal-
policing roles of the military, literally millions of its soldiers in
wartime would not be considered front-line troops at all. And although
the sums of money allocated to the army prior to 1914 seemed enormous, much of it was consumed by the basic needs of food, clothing,
and fodder. Similarily, despite the large-scale increases in the fleet and
the fact that many of the new designs have been described as "excellent,"[151] the navy required a much higher level of technical training as
well as more frequent tactical practice among its personnel to be truly
effective; since it had neither (the crews were still based mainly on
shore) and was forced to divide its fleet between the Baltic and the
Black Sea, the prospects for Russian sea power were not good—unless
it fought only the Turks.

Finally, no assessment of Russia's overall capacities in this period
can avoid some comments upon the regime itself. Although certain
foreign conservatives admired its autocratic and centralized system,
arguing that it gave a greater consistency and strength to national
policies than the western democracies were capable of, a closer examination would have revealed innumerable flaws. Czar Nicholas II was
a Potemkin village in person, simple-minded, reclusive, disliking difficult decisions, and blindly convinced of his sacred relationship with
the Russian people (in whose real welfare, of course, he showed no
interest). The methods of governmental decision-making at the higher
levels were enough to give "Byzantinism" a bad name: irresponsible
grand dukes, the emotionally unbalanced empress, reactionary generals, and corrupt speculators, outweighing by far the number of diligent
and intelligent ministers whom the regime could recruit and who, only
occasionally, could reach the czar's ear. The lack of consultation and
understanding between, say, the foreign ministry and the military was
at times frightening. The court's attitude to the assembly (the Duma)
was one of unconcealed contempt. Achieving radical reforms in this
atmosphere was impossible, when the aristocracy cared only for its

privileges and the czar cared only for his peace of mind. Here was an elite in constant fear of workers' and peasants' unrest, and yet, although government spending was by far the largest in the world in absolute terms, it kept direct taxes on the rich to a minimum (6 percent of the state's revenue) and placed massive burdens upon foodstuffs and vodka (about 40 percent). Here was a country with a delicate balance of payments, but with no chance of preventing (or taxing) the vast outflow of monies which Russian aristocrats spent abroad. Partly because of the traditions of heavy-handed autocracy, partly because of the inordinately flawed class system, and partly because of the low levels of education and pay, Russia lacked those cadres of competent civil servants who made, for example, the German, British, and Japanese administrative systems *work*. Russia was not, in reality, a strong state; and it was still one which, given the drift in leadership, was capable of blundering unprepared into foreign complications, notwithstanding the lessons of 1904.

How then, are we to assess the real power of Russia in these years? That it was growing in both industrial and military terms year by year was undoubted. That it possessed many other strengths—the size of its army, the patriotism and sense of destiny in certain classes of society, the near-invulnerability of its Muscovite heartland—was also true. Against Austria-Hungary, against Turkey, perhaps now even against Japan, it had good prospects of fighting and winning. But the awful thing was that its looming clash with Germany was coming too early for Russia to deal with. "Give the state twenty years of internal and external peace," boasted Stolypin in 1909, "and you will not recognize Russia." That *may* have been true, even if Germany's strength was also likely to increase over the same period. Yet according to the data produced by Professors Doran and Parsons (see Chart 1), the "relative power" of Russia in these decades was just rising from its low point after 1894 whereas Germany's was close to its peak.[152]

And while that may be too schematized a presentation to most readers, it had indeed been true (as mentioned previously) that Russia's power and influence had declined throughout much of the nineteenth century in rough proportion to her increasing economic backwardness. Every major exposure to battle (the Crimean War, the Russo-Japanese War) had revealed both new and old military weaknesses, and compelled the regime to endeavor to close the gap which had opened up between Russia and the western nations. In the years before 1914, it seemed to some observers that the gap was again being closed, although to others manifold weaknesses still remained. Since it could not have Stolypin's required two decades of peace, it would once again have to pass through the test of war to see if it had recovered the position in European power politics which it possessed in 1815 and 1848.

Chart 1. The Relative Power of Russia and Germany

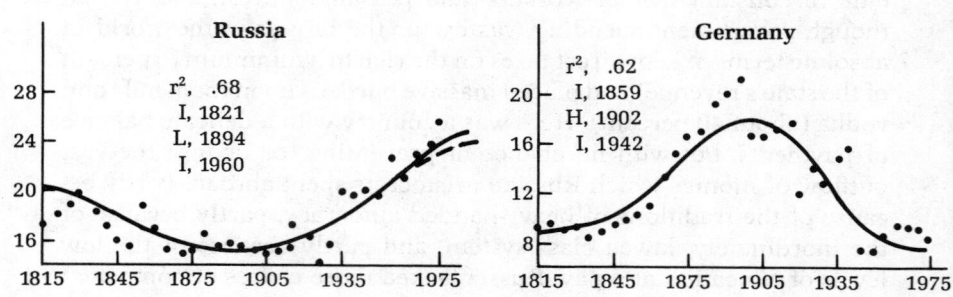

Key:
L = year of low point
H = year of high point
I = year of inflection point

Source: Doran and Parsons

United States

Of all the changes which were taking place in the global power balances during the late nineteenth and early twentieth centuries, there can be no doubt that the most decisive one for the future was the growth of the United States. With the Civil War over, the United States was able to exploit the many advantages mentioned previously—rich agricultural land, vast raw materials, and the marvelously convenient evolution of modern technology (railways, the steam engine, mining equipment) to develop such resources; the lack of social and geographical constraints; the absence of significant foreign dangers; the flow of foreign and, increasingly, domestic investment capital—to transform itself at a stunning pace. Between the ending of the Civil War in 1865 and the outbreak of the Spanish-American War in 1898, for example, American wheat production increased by 256 percent, corn by 222 percent, refined sugar by 460 percent, coal by 800 percent, steel rails by 523 percent, and the miles of railway track in operation by over 567 percent. "In newer industries the growth, starting from near zero, was so great as to make percentages meaningless. Thus the production of crude petroleum rose from about 3,000,000 barrels in 1865 to over 55,000,000 barrels in 1898 and that of steel ingots and castings from less than 20,000 long tons to nearly 9,000,000 long tons."[153] This was not a growth which stopped with the war against Spain; on the contrary, it rose upward at the same meteoric pace throughout the early twentieth century. Indeed, given the advantages listed above, there was a virtual inevitability to the whole process. That is to say, only persistent human ineptitude, or near-constant civil war, or a climatic disaster could have checked this expansion—or deterred the millions of immigrants who flowed across the Atlantic to get their share of the pot of gold and to swell the productive labor force.

The United States seemed to have *all* the economic advantages which *some* of the other powers possessed *in part,* but *none* of their disadvantages. It was immense, but the vast distances were shortened by some 250,000 miles of railway in 1914 (compared with Russia's 46,000 miles, spread over an area two and a half times as large). Its agricultural yields per acre were always superior to Russia's; and if they were never as large as those of the intensively farmed regions of western Europe, the sheer size of the area under cultivation, the efficiency of its farm machinery, and the decreasing costs of transport (because of railways and steamships) made American wheat, corn, pork, beef, and other products cheaper than any in Europe. Technologically, leading American firms like International Harvester, Singer, Du Pont, Bell, Colt, and Standard Oil were equal to, or often better than, any in the world; and they enjoyed an enormous domestic market and economies of scale, which their German, British, and Swiss rivals did not. "Gigantism" in Russia was not a good indicator of industrial efficiency;[154] in the United States, it usually was. For example, "Andrew Carnegie was producing more steel than the whole of England put together when he sold out in 1901 to J. P. Morgan's colossal organization, the United States Steel Corporation."[155] When the famous British warship designer Sir William White made a tour of the United States in 1904, he was shaken to discover fourteen battleships and thirteen armored cruisers being built simultaneously in American yards (although, curiously, the U.S. merchant marine remained small). In industry *and* agriculture *and* communications, there was both efficiency and size. It was therefore not surprising that U.S. national income, in absolute figures and per capita, was so far above everybody else's by 1914.[156]

Table 21. National Income, Population, and per Capita Income of the Powers in 1914

	National Income	Population	Per Capita Income
United States	$37 billion	98 million	$377
Britain	11	45	244
France	6	39	153
Japan	2	55	36
Germany	12	65	184
Italy	4	37	108
Russia	7	171	41
Austria-Hungary	3	52	57

The consequences of this rapid expansion are reflected in Table 21, and in the pertinent comparative statistics. In 1914, the United States was producing 455 million tons of coal, well ahead of Britain's 292 million and Germany's 277 million. It was the largest oil producer in the world, and the greatest consumer of copper. Its pig-iron production was larger than those of the next three countries (Germany, Britain, France) combined, and its steel production almost equal[157] to the next four countries (Germany, Britain, Russia, and France). Its energy consumption from modern fuels in 1913 was equal to that of Britain, Germany, France, Russia, and Austria-Hungary together. It produced, and possessed, more motor vehicles than the rest of the world together. It was, in fact an entire rival continent and growing so fast that it was coming close to the point of overtaking all of Europe. According to one calculation, indeed, had these growth rates continued and a world war been avoided, the United States would have overtaken Europe as the region possessing the greatest economic output in the world by 1925.[158] What the First World War did, through the economic losses and dislocations suffered by the older Great Powers, was to bring that time forward, by six years, to 1919.[159] The "Vasco da Gama era"—the four centuries of European dominance in the world—was coming to an end even before the calaclysm of 1914.

The role of foreign trade in the United States' economic growth was small indeed (around 8 percent of its GNP derived from foreign trade in 1913, compared with Britain's 26 percent),[160] but its economic impact upon other countries was considerable. Traditionally, the United States had exported raw materials (especially cotton), imported finished manufactures, and made up the usual deficit in "visible" trade by the export of gold. But the post–Civil War boom in industrialization quite transformed that pattern. Swiftly becoming the world's largest producer of manufactures, the United States began to pour its farm machinery, iron and steel wares, machine tools, electrical equipment, and other products onto the world market. At the same time, the Northern industrialists' lobby was so powerful that it ensured that foreign products would be kept out of the home market by higher and higher tariffs; raw materials, by contrast, or specialized goods (like German dyestuffs) were imported in ever-larger quantities to supply American industry. But while the surge in the country's industrial exports was the most significant change, the "transportation revolution" also boosted American farm exports. With the cost of carrying a bushel of wheat from Chicago to London plummeting from 40 cents to 10 cents in the half-century before 1900, American agricultural produce streamed across the Atlantic. Corn exports peaked in 1897 at 212 million bushels, wheat exports in 1901 at 239 million bushels; this tidal wave also included grain and flour, meat and meat products.[161]

The consequences of this commercial transformation were, of course, chiefly economic, but they also began to affect international relations. The hyperproductivity of American factories and farms caused a widespread fear that even its enormous domestic market might soon be unable to absorb these goods, and led powerful interest groups (midwestern farmers as well as Pittsburgh steel producers) to press the government to give all sorts of aid to opening up, or at least keeping open, markets overseas. The agitation to preserve an "open door" in China and the massive interest shown in making the United States the dominant economic force in Latin America were only two of the manifestations of this concern to expand the country's share of world trade.[162] Between 1860 and 1914 the United States increased its exports more than sevenfold (from $334 million to $2.365 billion), yet because it was so protective of its own market, imports increased only fivefold (from $356 million to $1.896 billion). Faced with this avalanche of cheap American food, continental European farmers agitated for higher tariffs—which they usually got; in Britain, which had already sacrificed its grain farmers for the cause of free trade, it was the flood of American machines, and iron and steel, which produced alarm. While the journalist W. T. Stead wrote luridly of "the Americanization of the world"—the phrase was the title of his book of 1902— Kaiser Wilhelm and other European leaders hinted at the need to combine against the "unfair" American trading colossus.[163]

Perhaps even more destabilizing, although less well understood, was the impact of the United States upon the world's financial system and monetary flows. Because it had such a vast surplus in its trade with Europe, the latter's deficit had to be met by capital transfers—joining the enormous stream of direct European investments into U.S. industry, utilities, and services (which totaled around $7 billion by 1914). Although some of this westward flow of bullion was reversed by the returns on European investments and by American payments for services such as shipping and insurance, the drain was a large one, and constantly growing larger; and it was exacerbated by the U.S. Treasury's policy of accumulating (and then just sitting on) nearly one-third of the world's gold stock. Moreover, although the United States had by now become an integral part of a complete global trading system—running a deficit with raw-materials-supplying countries, and a vast surplus with Europe—its own financial structure was underdeveloped. Most of its foreign trade was done in sterling, for example, and London acted as the lender of last resort for gold. With no central bank able to control the financial markets, with a stupendous seasonal outflow and inflow of funds between New York and the prairie states conditioned solely by the grain harvest and that by a volatile climate, and with speculators able to derange not merely the domestic monetary system but also the frequent calls upon gold in London, the United States in the years before 1914 was already becoming a vast but unpredictable bellows, fanning but also on occasions dramatically cooling the world's trading system. The American banking crisis of 1907 (originally provoked by an attempt by speculators to corner the market in copper), with consequent impacts on London, Amsterdam, and Hamburg, was merely one example of the way the United States was impinging upon the economic life of the other Great Powers, even before the First World War.[164]

This growth of American industrial power and overseas trade was accompanied, perhaps inevitably, by a more assertive diplomacy and by an American-style rhetoric of *Weltpolitik*.[165] Claims to a special moral endowment among the peoples of the earth which made American foreign policy superior to those of the Old World were intermingled with Social Darwinistic and racial arguments, and with the urging of industrial and agricultural pressure groups for secure overseas markets. The traditional, if always exaggerated, alarm about threats to the Monroe Doctrine was accompanied by calls for the United States to fulfill its "Manifest Destiny" across the Pacific. While entangling alliances still had to be avoided, the United States was now being urged by many groups at home into a much more activist diplomacy—which, under the administrations of McKinley and (especially) Theodore Roosevelt, was exactly what took place. The 1895 quarrel with Britain over the Venezuelan border dispute—justified in terms of the Monroe Doctrine—was followed three years later by the much more dramatic war with Spain over the Cuban issue. Washington's demand to have sole control of an isthmian canal (instead of the older fifty-fifty arrangement with Britain), the redefinition of the Alaskan border despite Canadian protests, and the 1902–1903 battlefleet preparations in the Caribbean following the German actions against Venezuela were all indications of U.S. determination to be unchallenged by any other Great Power in the western hemisphere. As a "corollary" of this, however, American administrations showed themselves willing to intervene by diplomatic pressure *and* military means in Latin American countries such as Nicaragua, Haiti, Mexico, and the Dominican Republic when their behavior did not accord with United States norms.

But the really novel feature of American external policy in this period were its interventions and participation in events *outside* the western hemisphere. Its attendance at the Berlin West Africa Conference in 1884–1885 had been anomalous and confused: after grandiose speeches by the U.S. delegation in favor of free trade and open doors, the subsequent treaty was never ratified. Even as late as 1892 the *New York Herald* was proposing the abolition of the State Department, since it had so little business to conduct overseas.[166] The war with Spain in 1898 changed all that, not only by giving the United States a position in the western Pacific (the Philippines) which made it, too, a sort of Asiatic colonial power, but also by boosting the political fortunes of those who had favored an assertive policy. Secretary of State Hay's "Open Door" note in the following year was an early indication that the United States wished to have a say in China, as was the commitment of 2,500 American troops to the international army sent to restore order in China in 1900. Roosevelt showed an even greater willingness to engage in *grosse Politik*, acting as mediator in the talks which brought an end to the Russo-Japanese War, insisting upon American participation in the 1906 conference over Morocco, and negotiating with Japan and the other Powers in an attempt to maintain the "Open Door" in China.[167] Much of this has been seen by later scholars less as being based upon a sober calculation of the country's real interests in the world than as reflecting an immaturity of foreign-policy style, an ethnocentric naïveté, and a wish to impress audiences both at home and abroad—traits which would complicate a "realistic" American foreign policy in the future;[168] but even if that is true, the United States was hardly alone in this age of imperialist bombast and nationalist pride. In any case, except in Chinese affairs, such diplomatic activism was not maintained by Roosevelt's successors, who preferred to keep the United States free from international events occurring outside the western hemisphere.

Along with these diplomatic actions went increases in arms expenditures. Of the two services, the navy got the most, since it was the front line of the nation's defenses in the event of a foreign attack (or a challenge to the Monroe Doctrine) and also the most useful instrument to support American diplomacy and commerce in Latin America, the Pacific, and elsewhere. Already in the late 1880s, the rebuilding of the fleet had commenced, but the greatest boost came at the time of the Spanish-American War. Since the easy naval victories in that conflict seemed to justify the arguments of Admiral Mahan and the "big navy" lobby, and since the strategists worried about the possibility of a war with Britain and then, from 1898 onward, with Germany, the battle fleet was steadily built up. The acquisition of bases in Hawaii, Samoa, the Philippines, and the Caribbean, the use of naval vessels to act as "policemen" in Latin America, and Roosevelt's dramatic gesture of sending his "great white fleet" around the world in 1907 all seemed to emphasize the importance of sea power.

Consequently, while the naval expenditures of $22 million in 1890 represented only 6.9 percent of total federal spending, the $139 million allocated to the navy by 1914 represented 19 percent.[169] Not all of this was well spent—there were too many home fleet bases (the result of local political pressures) and too few escort vessels—but the result was still impressive. Although considerably smaller than the Royal Navy, and with fewer *Dreadnought*-type battleships than Germany, the U.S. Navy was the third largest in the world in 1914. Even the construction of a U.S.-controlled Panama Canal did not stop American planners from agonizing over the strategical dilemma of dividing the fleet, or leaving one of the country's coastlines exposed: and the records of some officers in these years reveal a somewhat paranoid suspicion of foreign powers.[170] In fact, given its turn-of-the-century *rapprochement* with Great Britain, the United States was immensely secure, and even if it feared the rise of German sea power, it really had far less to worry about than any of the other major powers.[171]

The small size of the U.S. military was in many ways a reflection of that state of security. The army, too, had been boosted by the war with Spain, at least to the extent that the public realized how minuscule it actually was, how disorganized the National Guard was, and how close to disaster the early campaigning in Cuba had come.[172] But the tripling of the size of the regular army after 1900 and the additional garrisoning tasks it acquired in the Philippines and elsewhere still left the service looking insignificant compared with that of even a middle-sized European country like Serbia or Bulgaria. Even more than Britain, the United States clung to a laissez-faire dislike of mass standing armies and avoided fixed military obligations to allies. Less than 1 percent of its GNP went to defense. Despite its imperialist activities in the period 1898–1914, therefore, it remained what the sociologist Herbert Spencer termed an "industrial" society rather than a "military" society like Russia. Since many historians have suggested that "the rise of the superpowers" began in this period, it is worth noting the staggering *differences* between Russia and the United States by the eve of the First World War. The former possessed a front-line army about ten times as large as the latter's; but the United States produced six times as much steel, consumed ten times as much energy, and was four times larger in total industrial output (in per capita terms, it was six times more productive).[173] No doubt Russia seemed the more powerful to all those European general staffs thinking of swiftly fought wars involving masses of available troops; but by all other criteria, the United States was strong and Russia weak.

The United States had definitely become a Great Power. But it was not part of the Great Power system. Not only did the division of powers between the presidency and the Congress made an active alliance policy virtually impossible, but it was also clear that no one was in favor of abandoning the existing state of very comfortable isolation. Separated from other strong nations by thousands of miles of ocean, possessing a negligible army, content to have achieved hemispheric dominance and, at least after Roosevelt's departure, less eager to engage in worldwide diplomacy, the United States in 1913 still stood on the edges of the Great Power system. And since most of the other countries after 1906 were turning their attention from Asia and Africa to developments in the Balkans and North Sea, it was perhaps not surprising that they tended to see the United States as less a factor in the international power balances than had been the case around the turn of the century. That was yet another of the common pre-1914 assumptions which the Great War itself would prove wrong.

Alliances and the Drift to War, 1890–1914

The third and final element in understanding the way the Great Power system was changing in these decades is to examine the volatile alliance diplomacy from Bismarck's demise to the outbreak of the First World War. For although the 1890s saw some relatively small-scale conflicts (the Sino-Japanese War, the Spanish-American War, the Boer War), and later one large if still localized encounter in the Russo-Japanese War, the general tendency after that time was for what Felix Gilbert has termed the "rigidification" of the alliance blocs.[174] This was accompanied by the expectation on the part of most governments that if and when the next great war occurred, they would be members of a coalition. This would enhance and complicate assessments of relative national power, since allies brought disadvantages as well as benefits.

The tendency toward alliance diplomacy did not, of course, affect the distant United States at this time, and it impinged upon Japan only in a regional way, through the Anglo-Japanese alliances of 1902 and 1905. But alliance diplomacy increasingly affected all the European Great Powers, even the insular British, because of the mutual fears and rivalries which arose in these years. This creation of fixed military alliances in peacetime—rarely if ever seen before—was begun by Bismarck in 1879, when he sought to "control" Vienna's foreign policy, and to warn off St. Petersburg, by establishing the Austro-German alliance. In the German chancellor's secret calculations, this move was also intended to induce the Russians to abandon their "erratic policy"[175] and to return to the Three Emperor's League—which, for a time, they did; but the longer-lasting legacy of Bismarck's action was that Germany bound itself to come to Austria-Hungary's aid in the event of a Russian attack. By 1882, Berlin had also concluded a similar mutual treaty with Rome in the event of a French attack, and within another year, both Germany and Austria-Hungary had offered another secret alliance, to aid Rumania against Russian aggression. Scholars of this diplomacy insist that Bismarck had chiefly short-term and defensive aims in view—to give comfort to nervous friends in Vienna, Rome, and Bucharest, to keep France diplomatically isolated, to prepare "fallback" positions should the Russians invade the Balkans. No doubt that is true; but the fact is that he *had* given pledges, and further, that even if the exact nature of these secret treaties was not publicly known, it caused both France and Russia to worry about their own isolation and to suspect that the great wire-puller in Berlin had built up a formidable coalition to overwhelm them in wartime.

Although Bismarck's own "secret wire" to St. Petersburg (the so-called Reinsurance Treaty of 1887) prevented a formal break between Germany and Russia, there was something artificial and desperate in these baroque, double-crossing efforts by the chancellor to prevent the steady drift toward a Franco-Russian alliance in the late 1880s. The respective aspirations of France to recover Alsace-Lorraine and Russia to expand in eastern Europe were chiefly deterred by fear of Germany. There was no other *continental* alliance partner of note for either of them; and there beckoned the mutual benefits of French loans and weaponry for Russia, and Russian military aid for France. While ideological differences between the bourgeois French and the reactionary czarist regime slowed this drift for a while, the retirement of Bismarck in 1890 and the more threatening movements of Wilhelm II's government clinched the issue. By 1894, the Triple Alliance of Germany, Austria-Hungary, and Italy had been balanced by the Franco-Russian Dual Alliance, a political *and* military commitment which would last as long as the Triple Alliance did.[176]

In more ways than one, this new development appeared to stabilize the European scene. A rough equilibrium existed between the two alliance blocs, making the results of a Great Power conflict more incalculable, and thus less likely, than before. Having escaped from their isolation, France and Russia turned away to African and Asian concerns. This was aided, too, by the lessening of tensions in Alsace and in Bulgaria; by 1897, indeed, Vienna and St. Petersburg had agreed to put the Balkans on ice.[177] Furthermore, Germany was also turning toward *Weltpolitik*, while Italy, in its inimitable fashion, was becoming embroiled in Abyssinia. South Africa, the Far East, the Nile Valley, and Persia held people's attention by the mid-1890s. It was also the age of the "new navalism,"[178] with all the powers endeavoring to build up their fleets in the belief that navies and colonies naturally went hand in hand. Not surprisingly, therefore, this was the decade when the British Empire, although generally aloof from European entanglements, felt itself under the heaviest pressure, from old rivals like France and Russia, and then newer challengers like Germany, Japan, and the United States. In such circumstances, the importance of the military clauses of the European alliance blocks seemed less and less relevant, since a general war there would not be triggered off by happenings such as the Anglo-French clash at Fashoda (1898), the Boer War, or the scramble for concessions in China.

Yet, over the slightly longer term, these imperial rivalries were to affect the relations of the Great Powers, even in their European context. By the turn of the century, the pressures upon the British Empire were such that some circles around Colonial Secretary Joseph Chamberlain called for an end to "splendid isolation" and an alliance with Berlin, while fellow ministers such as Balfour and Lansdowne were beginning to accept the need for diplomatic compromises. A whole series of concessions to the United States over the isthmian canal, the Alaska boundary, seal fisheries, etc.—disguised under the term "the Anglo-American *rapprochement*"—took Britain out of a strategically untenable position in the western hemisphere and, more important still, drastically altered what nineteenth-century statesmen had taken for granted: that Anglo-American relations would always be cool, grudging, and occasionally hostile.[179] In forging the Anglo-Japanese Alliance of 1902, British statesmen also hoped to ease a difficult strategical burden in China, albeit at the cost of supporting Japan under certain circumstances.[180] And by 1902–1903, there were influential British circles who thought it possible to compromise over colonial issues with France, which had shown at the earlier Fashoda crisis that it would not go to war over the Nile.

While all these arrangements seemed at first to concern only extra-European affairs, they bore indirectly upon the standing of the Great Powers in Europe. The resolution of Britain's strategical dilemmas in the western hemisphere, plus the support it would gain from the Japanese fleet in the Far East, eased some of the pressures upon the Royal Navy's maritime dispositions and enhanced its prospects of consolidating in wartime; and settling Anglo-French rivalries would mean an even greater boost to Britain's naval security. All this also affected Italy, whose coastlines were simply far too vulnerable to allow itself to be placed in a camp opposite to an Anglo-French combination; in any case, by the early years of the twentieth century, France and Italy had their own good (financial and North African) reasons for improving relations.[181] However, if Italy was drifting away from the Triple Alliance, that was bound to affect its half-submerged quarrels with Austria-Hungary. Finally, even the distant Anglo-Japanese alliance was to have repercussions upon the European states system, since it made it unlikely that any third power would intervene when Japan decided in 1904 to challenge Russia over the future of Korea and Manchuria; moreover, when that war broke out, the specific clauses* of the Anglo-Japanese treaty *and* the Franco-Russian alliance strongly induced the two "seconds," Britain and France respectively, to work with each other to avoid being drawn openly into the conflict. It was not surprising, therefore, that the outbreak of hostilities in the Far East swiftly caused London and Paris to bring their colonial hagglings to an end and to conclude the *entente* of April 1904.[182] The years of Anglo-French rivalry, originally provoked by the British occupation of Egypt in 1882, were now over.

*Britain would be "benevolently neutral" to Japan if the latter was fighting one foe, but had to render military aid if it was fighting more than one; France's agreement to assist Russia was similarly phrased. Unless London and Paris both agreed to stay out, therefore, their new found friendship would be ruined.

Even this might not have caused the famous "diplomatic revolution"[183] of 1904–1905 if not for two other factors. The first was the growing suspicion held by the British and French toward Germany, whose aims, although unclear, looked ambitious and dangerous, as Chancellor Bülow and his imperial master Wilhelm II proclaimed the coming of the "German century." By 1902–1903 the High Seas Fleet, with a range and construction which suggested that it was being built chiefly with Britain in mind, was causing the British Admiralty to contemplate countermoves. In addition, while German aims toward Austria-Hungary were regarded with unease by Paris, its ambitions in Mesopotamia were disliked by British imperialists. Both countries observed with increasing anger Bülow's diplomatic efforts to encourage a Far East war in 1904 and to get them entangled in it—from which event Berlin would be the principal beneficiary.[184]

An even greater influence upon the European balances and relationships resulted from the impressive Japanese naval and military victories during the war, coinciding with the widespread unrest in Russia during 1905. With Russia unexpectedly reduced to a second-class power for some years to come, the military equilibrium in Europe swung decisively in favor of Berlin—against which France would now have worse prospects than in 1870. If ever there was a favorable time for Germany to strike westward, it probably would have been in the summer of 1905. But the Kaiser's concern over social unrest at home, his desire to improve relations with Russia, and his uncertainty about the British, who were redeploying their battleships from China to home waters and considering French pleas for aid if Germany did attack, all had their effect. Rather than plunge into war, Berlin opted instead for diplomatic victories, forcing its archfoe French Foreign Minister Delcassé from office, and insisting upon an international conference to check French pretensions in Morocco. Yet the results of the Algeciras meeting, which saw most of the conference participants supporting France's claim to a special position in Morocco, were a devastating confirmation of just how far Germany's diplomatic influence had declined since Bismarck's day, even as its industrial, naval, and military power had grown.[185]

The first Moroccan crisis returned international rivalries from Africa to the continent of Europe. This trend was soon reinforced by three more important events. The first was the 1907 Anglo-Russian *entente* over Persia, Tibet, and Afghanistan, in itself a regional affair but with wider implications for not only did it eliminate those Asian quarrels between London and St. Petersburg which all powers had taken for granted throughout the nineteenth century, and so ease Britain's defense of India, but it also caused nervous Germans to talk about being "encircled" in Europe. And while there were still many Britons, especially in the Liberal government, who did *not* see themselves as part of an anti-German coalition, their cause was weakened by the second event: the heated Anglo-German "naval race" of 1908–1909, following a further increase in Tirpitz's shipbuilding program and British fears that they would lose their naval lead even in the North Sea. When British efforts over the next three years to try to reduce this competition met with a German demand for London's neutrality in the event of a European war, the suspicious British backed away. They and the French had been nervously watching the Balkan crisis of 1908–1909, in which Russian indignation at Austria-Hungary's formal annexation of the provinces of Bosnia-Herzegovina led to a German demand that Russia accept the *fait accompli* or suffer the consequences.[186] Weakened by their recent war with Japan, the Russians submitted. But this diplomatic bullying produced in Russia a patriotic reaction, an increase in defense expenditures, and a determination to cling closer to one's allies.

Despite occasional attempts at a *détente* between one capital and another after 1909, therefore, the tendency toward "rigidification" increased. The second crisis over Morocco in 1911, when the British strongly intervened for France and against Germany, produced an upsurge of patriotic emotion in both of the latter countries and enormous increases in their army sizes as nationalists talked openly of the coming conflict, while in Britain the crisis had caused the government to confront its divergent military and naval plans in the event of joining a European war.[187] One year later, the failure of the diplomatic mission to Berlin by the British minister, Lord Haldane, and the further increases in the German fleet had driven London into the compromising November 1912 Anglo-French naval agreement. By that time, too, an opportunistic attack upon Turkey by Italian forces had been imitated by the states of the Balkan League, which virtually drove the Ottoman Empire out of Europe before its members then fell out over the spoils. This revival of the age-old "Eastern Question" was the most serious event of all, partly because the passionate strivings for advantage by the rivaling Balkan states could not really be controlled by the Great Powers, and partly because certain of the newer developments seemed to threaten the vital interests of some of those Powers: the rise of Serbia alarmed Vienna, the prospect of increasing German military influence over Turkey terrified St. Petersburg. When the assassination of Archduke Ferdinand in June 1914 provoked Austria-Hungary's actions against Serbia, and then the Russian countermoves, there was indeed much truth in the old cliché that the archduke's death was merely the spark which lit the tinderbox.[188]

The July 1914 assassination is one of the best-known examples in history of a particular event triggering a general crisis, and then a world war. Austria-Hungary's demands upon Serbia, its rejection of the conciliatory Serbian reply, and its attack upon Belgrade led to the

Russian mobilization in aid of its Serbian ally. But that, in turn, led the Prussian General Staff to press for the immediate implementation of the Schlieffen Plan, that is, its preemptive westward strike, via Belgium, against France—which had the further effect of bringing in the British.

While each of the Great Powers in this crisis acted according to its perceived national interests, it was also true that their decision to go to war had been affected by the existing operations plans. From 1909 onward the Germans committed themselves to Austria-Hungary, not just diplomatically but militarily, to a degree which Bismarck had never contemplated. Furthermore, the German operations plan now involved an immediate and massive assault upon France, via Belgium, whatever the specific cause of the war. By contrast, Vienna's military planners still dithered between the various fronts, but the determination to get a first blow in at Serbia was growing. Boosted by French funds, Russia pledged itself to an ever-swifter mobilization and westward strike should war come; while, with even less cause, the French in 1911 adopted the famous Plan XVII, involving a headlong rush into Alsace-Lorraine. And whereas the likelihood that Italy would fight alongside its Triple Alliance partners was now much decreased, a British military intervention in Europe had become the more probable in the event of a German attack upon Belgium and France. Needless to say, in each of the general staffs there was the unquestioned assumption that *speed* was of the essence; that is, as soon as a clash seemed likely, it was vital to mobilize one's own forces and to get them up to and over the border before the foe had a chance to do the same. If this was especially true in Berlin, where the army had committed itself to delivering a knockout blow in the west and then returning to the east to meet the slower-moving Russians, the same sort of thinking prevailed elsewhere. If and when a really great crisis occurred, the diplomats were not going to have much time before the strategic planners took over.[189]

The point about all of these war plans was not merely that they appear, in retrospect, like a line of dominoes which would tumble when the first one fell. What was also important was that since a coalition war was much more likely than in, say, 1859 or 1870, the prospects that the conflict would be prolonged were also that much greater, although few contemporaries appear to have realized it. The notorious miscalculation that the war begun in July/August 1914 would be "over by Christmas" has usually been explained away by the failure to anticipate that quick-firing artillery and machine guns made a *guerre de manœuvre* impossible and forced the masses of troops into trenches, from where they could rarely be dislodged; and that the later resort to prolonged artillery bombardments and enormous infantry offensives provided no solution, since the shelling merely churned up

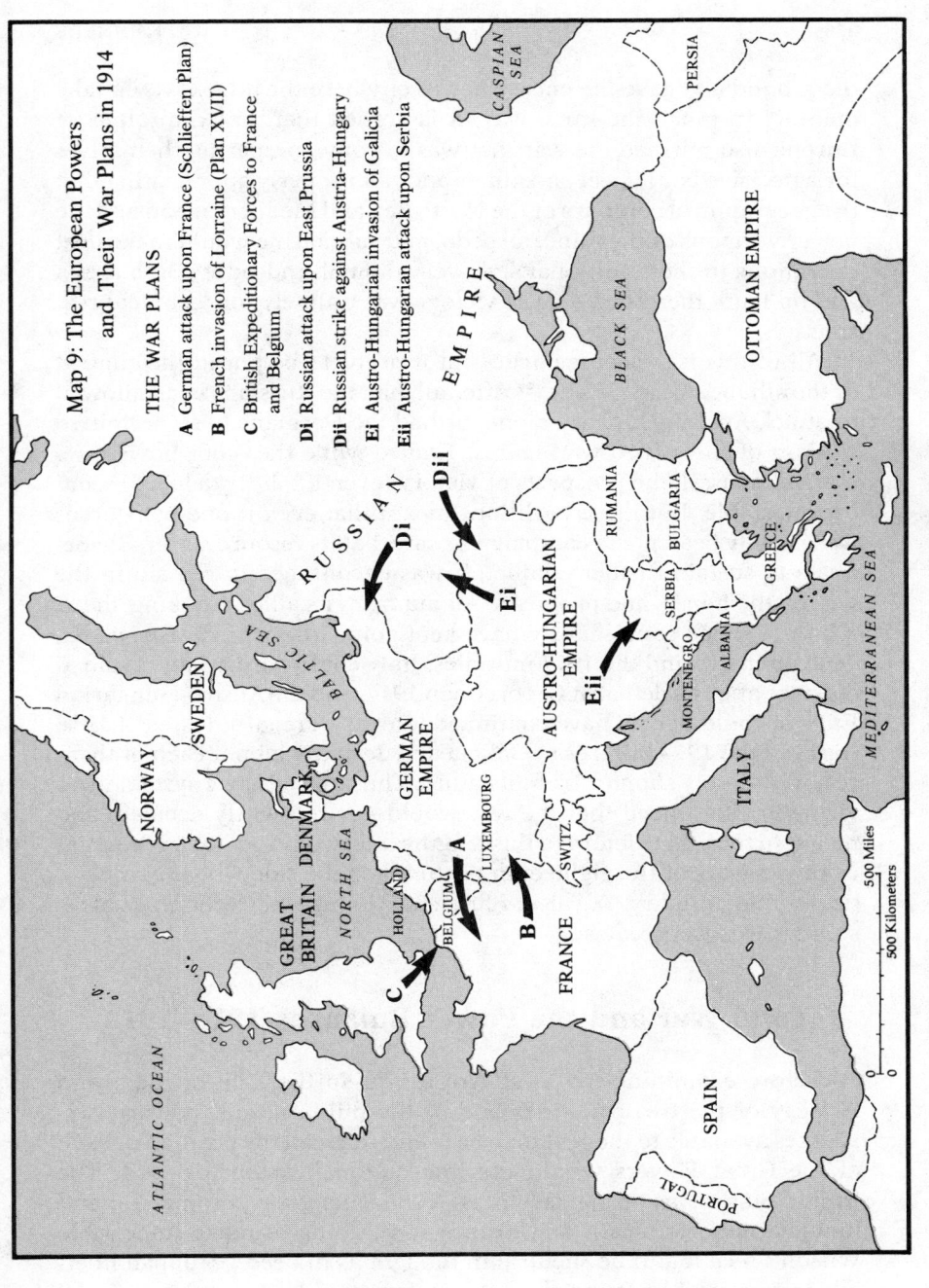

Map 9: The European Powers
and Their War Plans in 1914

THE WAR PLANS

A German attack upon France (Schlieffen Plan)

B French invasion of Lorraine (Plan XVII)

C British Expeditionary Forces to France
and Belgium

Di Russian attack upon East Prussia

Dii Russian strike against Austria-Hungary

Ei Austro-Hungarian invasion of Galicia

Eii Austro-Hungarian attack upon Serbia

the ground and gave the enemy notice of where the attack would take place.[190] In much the same way, it is argued that the admiralties of Europe also misread the war that was to come, preparing themselves for a decisive battle-fleet encounter and not properly appreciating that the geographical contours of the North Sea and Mediterranean and the newer weapons of the mine, torpedo, and submarine would make fleet operations in the traditional style very difficult indeed.[191] Both at sea and on land, therefore, a swift victory was unlikely for technical reasons.

All of this is, of course, true, but it needs to be put in the context of the alliance system itself.[192] After all, had the Russians been allowed to attack Austria-Hungary alone, or had the Germans been permitted a rerun of their 1870 war against France while the other powers remained neutral, the prospects of victory (even if a little delayed) seem incontestable. But these coalitions meant that even if one belligerent was heavily beaten in a campaign or saw that its resources were inadequate to sustain further conflict, it was encouraged to remain in the war by the hope—and promises—of aid from its allies. Looking ahead a little, France could hardly have kept going after the disastrous Nivelle offensive and the 1917 mutinies, Italy could hardly have avoided collapse after its defeat at Caporetto in 1917, and the Austro-Hungarian Empire could hardly have continued after the dreadful losses of 1916 (or even the 1914 failures in Galicia and Serbia) had not each of them received timely support from its allies. Thus, the alliance system itself virtually guaranteed that the war would *not* be swiftly decided, and meant in turn that victory in this lengthy duel would go—as in the great coalition wars of the eighteenth century—to the side whose combination of both military/naval *and* financial/industrial/technological resources was the greatest.

Total War and the Power Balances, 1914–1918

Before examining the First World War in the light of the grand strategy of the two coalitions and of the military and industrial resources available to them, it may be useful to recall the position of each of the Great Powers within the international system of 1914. The United States was on the sidelines—even if its great commercial and financial ties to Britain and France were going to make impossible Wilson's plea that it be "neutral in thought as in deed."[193] Japan liberally interpreted the terms of the Anglo-Japanese Alliance to occupy the German possessions in China and in the central Pacific; neither this nor its naval-escort duties further afield would be decisive, but for the Allies it was obviously far better to have a friendly Japan than a hostile one. Italy, by contrast, chose neutrality in 1914 and in view of its

military and socioeconomic fragility would have been wise to maintain that policy: if its 1915 decision to enter the war *against* the Central
Powers was a blow to Austria-Hungary, it is difficult to say that it was
the significant benefit to Britain, France, and Russia that Allied diplomats had hoped for.[194] In much the same way, it was difficult to say
who benefited most from the Turkish decision to enter the war on
Berlin's side in November 1914. True, it blocked the Straits, and thus
Russia's grain exports and arms imports; but by 1915 it would have
been difficult to transport Russian wheat *anywhere,* and there were no
"spare" munitions in the west. On the other hand, Turkey's decision
opened the Near East to French and (especially) British imperial expansion—though it also distracted the imperialists in India and Whitehall from full concentration along the western front.[195]

The really critical positions, therefore, were those occupied by the
"Big Five" powers in Europe. By this stage, it is artificial to treat
Austria-Hungary as something entirely separate from Germany, for
while Vienna's aims often diverged from Berlin's on many issues, it
could make war or peace—and probably survive as a quasi-indepen-
dent Great Power—only at the behest of its powerful ally.[196] The Austro-German combination was formidable. Its front-line armies were
considerably smaller than those of the French and Russian, but they
operated on efficient internal lines and could be supplemented by a
swelling number of recruits. As can be seen from Table 22 below, they
also enjoyed a considerable superiority in industrial and technological
strength over the Dual Alliance.

The position of France and Russia was, of course, exactly the converse. Separated from each other by more than half of Europe, France
and Russia would find it difficult (to say the least) to coordinate their
military strategy. And while they appeared to enjoy a large lead in
army strengths at the outset of the war, this was reduced by the clever
German use of trained reservists in the front-line fighting, and this lead
declined still further after the reckless Franco-Russian offensives in
the autumn of 1914. With victory no longer going to the swift, it was
more and more likely that it would go to the strong; and the industrial
indices were not encouraging. Had the Franco-Russe alone been involved in a lengthy, "total" war against the Central Powers, it is hard
to think how it could have won.

But the fact was, of course, that the German decision to launch a
preemptive strike upon France by way of Belgium gave the upper hand
to British interventionists.[197] Whether it was for the traditional reasons
of the "balance of power" or in defense of "poor little Belgium," the
British decision to declare war upon Germany was critical, though
Britain's small, long-service army could affect the overall military
equilibrium only marginally—at least until that force had transformed
itself into a mass conscript army on continental lines. But since the

war *was* going to last longer than a few months, Britain's strengths were considerable. Its navy could neutralize the German fleet and blockade the Central Powers—which would not bring the latter to their knees, but would deny them access to sources of supply outside continental Europe. Conversely, it ensured free access to supply sources for the Allied Powers (except when later interrupted by the U-boat campaign); and this advantage was compounded by the fact that Britain was such a wealthy trading country, with extensive links across the globe and enormous overseas investments, some of which at least could be liquidated to pay for dollar purchases. Diplomatically, these overseas ties meant that Britain's decision to intervene influenced Japan's action in the Far East, Italy's declaration of neutrality (and later switch), and the generally benevolent stance of the United States. More direct overseas support was provided, naturally enough, by the self-governing dominions and by India, whose troops moved swiftly into Germany's colonial empire and then against Turkey.

In addition, Britain's still-enormous industrial and financial resources could be deployed in Europe, both in raising loans and sending munitions to France, Belgium, Russia, and Italy, and in supplying and paying for the large army to be employed by Haig on the western front. The economic indices in Table 22 show the significance of Britain's intervention in power terms.

Table 22. Industrial/Technological Comparisons of the 1914 Alliances (taken from Tables 15–18 above)

	Germany/Austria-Hungary	France/Russia	+	Britain		
Percentages of world manufacturing production (1913)	19.2%	14.3%	+	13.6%	=	27.9%
Energy consumption (1913), metric million tons of coal equivalent	236.4	116.8	+	195.0	=	311.8
Steel production (1913), in million tons	20.2	9.4	+	7.7	=	17.1
Total industrial potential (U.K. in 1900=100)	178.4	133.9	+	127.2	=	261.1

To be sure, this made a significant rather than an overwhelming superiority in matériel possessed by the Allies, and the addition of Italy in 1915 would not weigh the scales much further in their favor. Yet if victory in a prolonged Great Power war usually went to the coalition with the largest productive base, the obvious questions arise as to why the Allies were failing to prevail even after two or three years of fighting—and by 1917 were in some danger of losing—and why they then found it vital to secure American entry into the conflict.

One part of the answer must be that the areas in which the Allies were strong were unlikely to produce a swift or decisive victory over the Central Powers. The German colonial empire in 1914 was economically so insignificant that (apart from Nauru phosphates) its loss meant very little. The elimination of German overseas trade was certainly more damaging, but not to the extent that British devotees of "the influence of sea power" imagined; for the German export trades were redeployed for war production, the Central Powers bloc was virtually self-sufficient in foodstuffs provided its transport system was maintained, military conquests (e.g., of Luxembourg ores, Rumanian wheat and oil) canceled out many raw-materials shortages, and other supplies came via neutral neighbors. The maritime blockade had an effect, but only when it was applied in conjunction with military pressures on all fronts, and even then it worked very slowly. Finally, the other traditional weapon in the British armory, peripheral operations on the lines of the Peninsular War of 1808–1814, could not be used against the German coast, since its sea-based and land-based defenses were too formidable; and when it was employed against weaker powers—at Gallipoli, for example, or Salonika—operational failures on the Allied side and newer weapons (mine fields, quick-firing shore batteries) on the defender's side, blunted their hoped-for impact. As in the Second World War, every search for the "soft underbelly" of the enemy coalition took Allied troops away from fighting in France.[198]

The same points can be made about the overwhelming Allied naval superiority. The geography of the North Sea and the Mediterranean meant that the main Allied lines of communication were secure *without* needing to seek out their enemies' vessels in harbor or to mount a risky close blockade of their shores. On the contrary, it was incumbent upon the German and Austro-Hungarian fleets to come out and challenge the Anglo-French-Italian navies if they wanted to gain "command of the sea"; for if they remained in port, they were useless. Yet neither of the navies of the Central Powers wished to send its battle fleets on a virtual suicide mission against vastly superior forces. Thus, the few surface naval clashes which did occur were chance encounters (e.g., Dogger Bank, Jutland), and were strategically unimportant except insofar as they confirmed the Allied control of the seaways. The prospect of further encounters was reduced by the threat posed to warships by mines, submarines, and scouting aircraft or Zeppelins, which made the commanders of each side increasingly wary of sending out their fleets unless (a highly unlikely condition) the enemy's ships were known to be approaching one's own shoreline. Given this impotence in surface warfare, the Central Powers gradually turned to U-boat attacks upon Allied merchantmen, which was a much more serious threat; but by its very nature, a submarine campaign against trade was a slow, grinding affair, the real success of which could be measured only by setting the tonnage of merchant ships lost against the tonnage being launched in Allied shipyards—and that against the number of U-boats destroyed. It was not a form of war which promised swift victories.[199]

A second reason for the relative impotence of the Allies' numerical and industrial superiority lay in the nature of the military struggle itself. When each side possessed millions of troops sprawling across hundreds of miles of territory, it was difficult (in western Europe, impossible) to achieve a single decisive victory in the manner of Jena or Sadowa; even a "big push," methodically plotted and prepared for months ahead, usually disintegrated into hundreds of small-scale battlefield actions, and was usually also accompanied by a near-total breakdown in communications. While the front line might sway back and forth in certain sections, the absence of the means to achieve a real breakthrough allowed each side to mobilize and bring up reserves, fresh stocks of shells, barbed wire, and artillery in time for the next stalemated clash. Until late in the war, no army was able to discover how to get its own troops through enemy-held defenses often *four miles deep,* without either exposing them to withering counterfire or so churning up the ground by earlier bombardments that it was difficult to advance. Even when an occasional surprise assault overran the first few lines of enemy trenches, there was no special equipment to exploit that advantage; the railway lines were miles in the rear, the cavalry was too vulnerable (and tied to fodder supplies), heavily laden infantrymen could not move far, and the vital artillery arm was restricted by its long train of horse-drawn supply wagons.[200]

In addition to this general problem of achieving a swift battlefield victory, there was the fact that Germany enjoyed two more specific advantages. The first was that by its sweeping advances in France and Belgium in August/September 1914, it had seized the ridges of high ground which overlooked the line of the western front. From that time onward, and with a rare exception like Verdun, it stayed on the defensive in the west, compelling the Anglo-French armies to attack under unfavorable conditions and with forces which, although numerically superior, were not sufficient to outweigh this basic disadvantage. Secondly, the geographical benefits of Germany's position, with good internal means of communication between east and west, to some degree compensated for its "encirclement" by the Allies, by permitting generals such as Falkenhayn and Ludendorff to switch divisions from one front to the next, and, on one occasion, to send a whole army across central Europe in a week.[201]

Consequently, in 1914, even as the bulk of the army was attacking in the west, the Prussian General Staff was nervously redeploying two corps to reinforce its exposed eastern front. This action was not a fatal blow to the westward strike, which was logistically unsound in any case;[202] and it did help the Germans to counter the premature Russian offensive into East Prussia by launching their own operation around the Masurian Lakes. When the bloody fighting at Ypres in November 1914 convinced Falkenhayn of the hopelessness of achieving a swift victory in the west, a further eight German divisions were transferred to the eastern command. Since the Austro-Hungarian forces had suffered a humiliating blow in their Serbian campaign, and since the unreal French Plan XVII of 1914 had ground to a halt in Lorraine with losses of over 600,000 men, it appeared that only in the open lands of Russian Poland and Galicia could a breakthrough be effected—although whether that would be a Russian repeat of their victory over Austria-Hungary at Lemberg or a German repeat of Tannenberg/Masurian Lakes was not at all clear. As the Anglo-French armies were battering away in the west throughout 1915 (where the French lost a further 1.5 million men and the British 300,000), the Germans prepared for a series of ambitious strikes along the eastern front, partly to rescue the beleaguered Austro-Hungarians in Carpathia, but chiefly to destroy the Russian army in the field. In fact, the latter was still so large (and growing) that its destruction was impossible; but by the end of 1915 the Russians had suffered a series of devastating blows at the hands of the tactically and logistically superior Germans, and had been driven from Lithuania, Poland, and Galicia. In the south, German reinforcements had joined the Austrian forces, and the opportunistic Bulgarians, in finally overrunning Serbia. Nothing that the western Allies attempted in 1915—from the operationally mishandled Gallipoli campaign, to the fruitless landing at Salonika, to inducing Italy into the war—really aided the Russians or seemed to challenge the consolidated bloc of the Central Powers.[203]

In 1916, Falkenhayn's unwise reversal of German strategy—shifting units westward in order to bleed the French to death by the repeated assaults upon Verdun—merely confirmed the correctness of the older policy. While large numbers of German divisions were being ruined by the Verdun campaign, the Russians were able to mount their last great offensive under General Brusilov in the east, in June 1916, driving the disorganized Habsburg army all the way back to the Carpathian mountains and threatening its collapse. At almost the same time, the British army under Haig launched its massive offensive at the Somme, pressing for months against the well-held German ridges. As soon as these twin Allied operations had led to the winding-down of the Verdun campaign (and the replacement of Falkenhayn by Hindenburg and Ludendorff in late August 1916), the German strategical position improved. German losses on the Somme were heavy, but were less than Haig's; and the switch to a defensive stance in the West once again permitted the Germans to transfer troops to the east, stiffening the

Austro-Hungarian forces, then overrunning Rumania, and later giving aid to the Bulgarians in the south.[204]

Apart from these German advantages of inner lines, efficient railways, and good defensive positions, there was also the related question of *timing*. The larger total resources which the Allies possessed could not be instantly mobilized in 1914 in the pursuit of victory. The Russian army administration could always draft fresh waves of recruits to make up for the repeated battlefield losses, but it had neither the weapons nor the staff to expand that force beyond a certain limit. In the west, it was not until 1916 that Haig's army totaled more than a million men, and even then the British were tempted to divert their troops into extra-European campaigns, thus reducing the potential pressure upon Germany. This meant that during the first two years of the conflict, Russia and France took the main burden of checking the German military machine. Each had fought magnificently, but by the beginning of 1917 the strain was clearly showing; Verdun had taken the French army close to its limits, as Nivelle's rash assaults in 1917 revealed; and although the Brusilov offensive had virtually ruined the Habsburg army as a fighting force, it had done no damage to Germany itself and had placed even more strains upon Russian railways, food stocks, and state finances as well as expending much of the existing trained Russian manpower. While Haig's new armies made up for the increasing weariness of the French, they did not portend an Allied victory in the west; and if they also were squandered in frontal offensives, Germany might still be able to hold its own in Flanders while indulging in further sweeping actions in the east. Finally, no help could be expected south of the Alps, where the Italians were now desperately calling for assistance.

This pattern of ever-larger military sacrifices made by each side was paralleled, inevitably, in the financial-industrial sphere—but (at least until 1917) with the same stalemated results. Much has been made in recent studies of the way in which the First World War galvanized national economies, bringing modern industries for the first time to many regions and leading to stupendous increases in armaments output.[205] Yet on reflection, this surely is not surprising. For all the laments of liberals and others about the costs of the pre-1914 arms race, only a very small proportion (slightly over 4 percent on average) of national income was being devoted to armaments. When the advent of "total war" caused that figure to rise to 25 or 33 percent—that is, when governments at war took decisive command of industry, labor, and finance—it was inevitable that the output of armaments would soar. And since the generals of *every* army were bitterly complaining by late 1914 and early 1915 of a chronic "shell shortage," it was also inevitable that politicians, fearing the effects of being found wanting, entered into an alliance with business and labor to produce the desired goods.[206] Given the powers of the modern bureaucratic state to float loans and raise taxes, there were no longer the fiscal impediments to sustaining a lengthy war that had crippled eighteenth-century states. Inevitably, then, after an early period of readjustment to these new conditions, armaments production soared in all countries.

It is therefore important to ask where the wartime economies of the various combatants showed weaknesses, since it was most likely that this would lead to collapse, unless aid came from better-endowed allies. In this respect, little space will be given to the two weakest of the Great Powers, Austria-Hungary and Italy, since it is clear that the former, although holding up remarkably well in its extended campaigning (especially on the Italian front), would have collapsed in its war with Russia had it not been for repeated German military interventions which turned the Habsburg Empire ever more into a satellite of Berlin;[207] while Italy, which did not need anywhere like that degree of direct military assistance until the Caporetto disaster, was increasingly dependent upon its richer and more powerful allies for vital supplies of foodstuffs, coal, and raw materials, for shipping, and for the $2.96 billion of loans with which it could pay for munitions and other produce.[208] Its eventual "victory" in 1918, like the eventual defeat and dissolution of the Habsburg Empire, essentially depended upon actions and decisions taken elsewhere.

By 1917, it has been argued,[209] Italy, Austria-Hungary, and Russia were racing each other to collapse. That Russia should actually be the first to go was due, in large part, to two problems from which Rome and Vienna were spared; the first was that it was exposed, along hundreds of miles of border, to the slashing attacks of the much more efficient German army; the second was that even in August 1914 and certainly after Turkey's entry into the war, it was strategically isolated and thus never able to secure the degree of either military or economic aid from its allies necessary to sustain the enormous efforts of its fighting machine. When Russia, like the other combatants, swiftly learned that it was using up its ammunition stocks about ten times faster than the prewar estimates, it had massively to expand its home production—which turned out to be far more reliable than waiting for the greatly delayed overseas orders, even if it also implied diverting resources into the self-interested hands of the Moscow industrialists. But the impressive rise in Russian arms output, and indeed in overall industrial and agricultural production, during the first two and a half years of the war greatly strained the inadequate transport system, which in any case was finding it hard to cope with the shipment of troops, fodder for the cavalry, and so on. Shell stocks therefore accumulated miles from the front; foodstuffs could not be transported to the deficit areas, especially in the cities; Allied supplies lay for months on the harborsides at Murmansk and Archangel. These infrastructural inadequacies could not be overcome by Russia's minuscule and inefficient bureaucracy, and little help came from the squabbling and paralyzed political leadership at the top. On the contrary, the czarist regime helped to dig its own grave by its recklessly unbalanced fiscal policies; having abolished the trade in spirits (which produced one-third of its revenue), losing heavily on the railways (its other great peacetime source of income), and—unlike Lloyd George—declining to raise the income tax upon the better-off classes, the state resorted to floating ever more loans and printing ever more paper in order to pay for the war. The price index spiraled, from a nominal 100 in June 1914 to 398 in December 1916, to 702 in June 1917, by which time an awful combination of inadequate food supplies and excessive inflation triggered off strike after strike.[210]

As in industrial production, Russia's military performance was creditable during the first two or three years of the war—even if it was nothing like those fatuous prewar images of the "Russian steamroller" grinding its way across Europe. Its troops fought in their usual dogged, tough manner, enduring hardships and discipline unknown in the west; and the Russian record against the Austro-Hungarian army, from the September 1914 victory at Lemberg to the brilliantly executed Brusilov offensive, was one of constant success, akin to its Caucasus campaign against the Turks. Against the better-equipped and faster-moving Germans, however, the record was quite the reverse; but even that needs to be put into perspective, since the losses of one campaign (say, Tannenberg/Masurian Lakes in 1914, or the Carpathian fighting in 1915) were made up by drafting a fresh annual intake of recruits, which were then readied for the next season's operations. Over time, of course, the quality and morale of the army was bound to be affected by these heavy losses—250,000 at Tannenberg/Masurian Lakes, 1 million in the early 1915 Carpathian battles, another 400,000 when Mackensen struck at the central Polish salient, as many as 1 million in the 1916 fighting which started with the Brusilov offensive and ended with the debacle in Rumania. By the end of 1916, the Russian army had suffered casualties of some 3.6 million dead, seriously sick, and wounded, and another 2.1 million had been captured by the Central Powers. By that time, too, it had decided to call up the second-category recruits (males who were the sole breadwinners in the family), which not only produced tremendous peasant unrest in the villages, but also brought into the army hundreds of thousands of bitterly discontented conscripts. Almost as important were the dwindling numbers of trained NCOs, the inadequate supplies of weapons, ammunition, and food at the front, and the growing sense of inferiority against the German war machine, which seemed to know in advance all of

Russia's intentions,* to have overwhelming artillery fire, and to move faster than anyone else. By the beginning of 1917 these repeated defeats in the field interacted with the unrest in the cities and the rumors of the distribution of land, to produce a widespread disintegration in the army. Kerensky's July 1917 offensive—once again, initially successful against the Austrians, and then slashed to pieces by Mackensen's counterattack—was the final blow. The army, *Stavka* concluded, "is simply a huge, weary, shabby, and ill-fed mob of angry men united by their common thirst for peace and by common disappointment."[211] All that Russia could look forward to now was defeat and an internal revolution far more serious than that of 1905.

It is idle to speculate how close France, too, came to a similar fate by mid-1917, when hundreds of thousands of soldiers mutinied following Nivelle's senseless offensive;[212] for the fact was that despite the superficial similarities with Russian conditions, the French possessed key advantages which kept them in the fight. The first was the far greater degree of national unity and commitment to drive the German invaders back to the Rhine—although even those feelings might have faded away had France been fighting on its own. The second, and probably crucial, difference was that the French could benefit from fighting a *coalition* war in the way that Russia could not. Since 1871, they had known that they could not stand alone against Germany; the 1914–1918 conflict simply confirmed that judgment. This is not to downgrade the French contribution to the war, either in military or economic items, but merely to put it in context. Given that 64 percent of the nation's pig-iron capacity, 24 percent of its steel capacity, and 40 percent of its coal capacity fell swiftly into German hands, the French industrial renaissance after 1914 was remarkable (suggesting, incidentally, what *could* have been done in the nineteenth century had the political commitment been there). Factories, large and small, were set up across France, and employed women, children, and veterans, and even conscripted skilled workers who were transferred back from the trenches. Technocratic planners, businessmen, and unions combined in a national effort to produce as many shells, heavy guns, aircraft, trucks, and tanks as possible. The resultant surge in output has caused one scholar to argue that "France, more than Britain and far more than America, became the arsenal of democracy in World War I."[213]

Yet this top-heavy concentration upon armaments output—increasing machine-gun production 170-fold, and rifle production 290-fold— could never have been achieved had France not been able to rely upon British and American aid, which came in the form of a steady flow of imported coal, coke, pig iron, steel, and machine tools so vital for the

---

*Not surprisingly, since the Russians were incredibly careless with their wireless transmissions.

new munitions industry; in the Anglo-American loans of over $3.6
billion, so that France could pay for raw materials from overseas; in
the allocation of increasing amounts of British shipping, without
which most of this movement of goods could not have been carried
out; and in the supply of foodstuffs. This last-named category seems a
curious defect in a country which in peacetime always produced an
agricultural surplus; but the fact was that the French, like the other
European belligerents (except Britain), hurt their own agriculture by
taking too many men from the land, diverting horses to the cavalry or
to army-transport duties, and investing in explosives and artillery to
the detriment of fertilizer and farm machinery. In 1917, a bad harvest
year, food was scarce, prices were spiraling ominously upward, and
the French army's own stock of grain was reduced to a two-day supply—a potentially revolutionary situation (especially following the
mutinies), which was only averted by the emergency allocation of
British ships to bring in American grain.[214]

In rather the same way, France needed to rely upon increasing
amounts of British and, later, American *military* assistance along the
western front. For the first two to three years of the war, it bore the
brunt of that fighting and took appalling casualties—over 3 million
even before Nivelle's offensive of 1917; and since it had not the vast
reserves of untrained manpower which Germany, Russia, and the British Empire possessed, it was far harder to replace such losses. By
1916–1917, however, Haig's army on the western front had been expanded to two-thirds the size of the French army and was holding over
eighty miles of the line; and although the British high command was
keen to go on the offensive in any case, there is no doubt that the
Somme campaign helped to ease the pressure upon Verdun—just as
Passchendaele in 1917 took the German energies away from the
French part of the front while Pétain was desperately attempting to
rebuild his forces' morale after the mutinies, and waiting for the new
trucks, aircraft, and heavy artillery to do the work which massed infantry clearly could not. Finally, in the epic to-and-fro battles along the
western front between March and August 1918, France could rely not
only upon British and imperial divisions, but also upon increasing
numbers of American ones. And when Foch orchestrated his final
counteroffensive in September 1918, he could engage the 197 under-
strength German divisions with 102 French, 60 British Empire, 42
(double-sized) American, and 12 Belgian divisions.[215] Only with a *combination* of armies could the formidable Germans at last be driven
from French soil and the country be free again.

When the British entered the war in August 1914, it was with no
sense that they, too, would become dependent upon another Great
Power in order to secure ultimate victory. So far as can be deduced
from their prewar plans and preparations, the strategists had imagined

that while the Royal Navy was sweeping German merchantmen (and perhaps the High Seas Fleet) from the oceans, and while the German colonial empire was being seized by dominion and British Indian troops, a small but vital expeditionary force would be sent across the Channel to "plug" a gap between the French and Belgian armies and to hold the German offensive until such time as the Russian steam-roller and the French Plan XVII were driving deep into the Fatherland. The British, like all the other powers, were not prepared for a long war, although they had taken certain measures to avoid a sudden crisis in their delicate international credit and commercial networks. But un-like the others, they were also not prepared for large-scale operations on the continent of Europe.[216] It was therefore scarcely surprising that one to two years of intense preparation were needed before 1 million British troops stood ready in France, and that the explosion of govern-ment spending upon rifles, artillery, machine guns, aircraft, trucks, and ammunition merely revealed innumerable production deficien-cies which were only slowly corrected by Lloyd George's Ministry of Munitions.[217] Here again there were fantastic rises in output, as shown in Table 23.

Table 23. U.K. Munitions Production, 1914–1918[218]

	1914	1915	1916	1917	1918
Guns	91	3,390	4,314	5,137	8,039
Tanks	—	—	150	1,110	1,359
Aircraft	200	1,900	6,100	14,700	32,000
Machine guns	300	6,100	33,500	79,700	120,900

But that is scarcely surprising when one realizes that British defense expenditures rose from £91 million in 1913 to £1.956 billion in 1918, by which time it represented 80 percent of total government expendi-tures and 52 percent of the GNP.[219]

To give full details of the vast growth in the number of British and imperial divisions, squadrons of aircraft, and batteries of heavy artil-lery seems less important, therefore, than to point to the weaknesses which the First World War exposed in Britain's overall strategical position. The first was that while geography and the Grand Fleet's numerical superiority meant the Allies retained command of the sea in the *surface* conflict, the Royal Navy was quite unprepared to counter the unrestricted U-boat warfare which the Germans were implement-ing by early 1917. The second was that whereas the cluster of relatively cheap strategical weapons (blockade, colonial campaigns, amphibious operations) did not seem to be working against a foe with the wide-ranging resources of the Central Powers, the alternative strategy of direct military encounters with the German army also seemed incapa-ble of producing results—and was fearfully costly in manpower. By the time the Somme campaign whimpered to a close in November 1916, British casualties in that fighting had risen to over 400,000. Although this wiped out the finest of Britain's volunteers and shocked the politicians, it did not dampen Haig's confidence in ultimate victory. By the middle of 1917 he was preparing for yet a further offensive from Ypres northeastward to Passchendaele—a muddy nightmare which cost another 300,000 casualties and badly hurt morale throughout much of the army in France. It was, therefore, all too predictable that however much Generals Haig and Robertson protested, Lloyd George and the imperialist-minded War Cabinet were tempted to divert ever more British divisions to the Near East, where substantial territorial gains beckoned and losses were far fewer than would be incurred in storming well-held German trenches.[220]

Even before Passchendaele, however, Britain had assumed (despite this imperial campaigning) the leadership role in the struggle against Germany. France and Russia might still have larger armies in the field, but they were exhausted by Nivelle's costly assaults and by the German counterblow to the Brusilov offensive. This leadership role was even more pronounced at the economic level, where Britain functioned as the banker and loan-raiser on the world's credit markets, not only for itself but also by guaranteeing the monies borrowed by Russia, Italy, and even France—since none of the Allies could provide from their own gold or foreign-investment holdings anywhere near the sums required to pay the vast surge of imported munitions and raw materials from overseas. By April 1, 1917, indeed, inter-Allied war credits had risen to $4.3 billion, 88 percent of which was covered by the British government. Although this looked like a repetition of Britain's eighteenth-century role as "banker to the coalition," there was now one critical difference: the sheer size of the trade deficit with the United States, which was supplying billions of dollars' worth of munitions and foodstuffs to the Allies (but not, because of the naval blockade, to the Central Powers) yet required few goods in return. Neither the transfer of gold nor the sale of Britain's enormous dollar securities could close this gap; only borrowing on the New York and Chicago money markets, to pay the American munitions suppliers in dollars, would do the trick. This in turn meant that the Allies became ever more dependent upon U.S. financial aid to sustain their own war effort. In October 1916, the British Chancellor of the Exchequer was warning that "by next June, or earlier, the President of the American Republic would be in a position, if he wishes, to dictate his terms to us."[221] It was an altogether alarming position for "independent" Great Powers to be in.

But what of Germany? Its performance in the war had been staggering. As Professor Northedge points out, "with no considerable assistance from her allies, [it] had held the rest of the world at bay, had beaten Russia, had driven France, the military colossus of Europe for more than two centuries, to the end of her tether, and in 1917, had come within an ace of starving Britain into surrender."[222] Part of this was due to those advantages outlined above: good inner lines of communication, easily defensible positions in the west, and open space for mobile warfare against less efficient foes in the east. It was also due to the sheer fighting quality of the German forces, which possessed an array of intelligent, probing staff officers who readjusted to the new conditions of combat faster than those in any other army, and who by 1916 had rethought the nature of both defensive and offensive warfare.[223]

Finally, the German state could draw upon both a large population and a massive industrial base for the prosecution of "total war." Indeed, it actually mobilized more men than Russia—13.25 million to 13 million—a remarkable achievement in view of their respective overall populations; and always had more divisions in the field than Russia. Its own munitions production soared, under the watchful eye not only of the high command but of intelligent bureaucrat-businessmen such as Walther Rathenau, who set up cartels to allocate vital supplies and avoid bottlenecks. Adept chemists produced ersatz goods for those items (e.g., Chilean nitrates) cut off by the British naval blockade. The occupied lands of Luxembourg and northern France were exploited for their ores and coal, Belgian workers were drafted into German factories, Rumanian wheat and oil were systematically plundered following the 1916 invasion. Like Napoleon and Hitler, the German military leadership sought to make conquest pay.[224] By the first half of 1917, with Russia collapsing, France wilting, and Britain under the "counterblockade" of the U-boats, Germany seemed on the brink of victory. Despite all the rhetoric of "fighting to the bitter end," statesmen in London and Paris were going to be anxiously considering the possibilities of a compromise peace for the next twelve months until the tide turned.[225]

Yet behind this appearance of Teutonic military-industrial might, there lurked very considerable problems. These were not too evident before the summer of 1916, that is, while the German army stayed on the defensive in the west and made sweeping strikes in the east. But the campaigns of Verdun and the Somme were of a new order of magnitude, both in the firepower employed and the losses sustained; and German casualties on the western front, which had been around 850,000 in 1915, leaped to nearly 1.2 million in 1916. The Somme offensive in particular impressed the Germans, since it showed that the British were at last making an all-out commitment of national resources for victory in the field; and it led in turn to the so-called Hindenburg Program of August 1916, which proclaimed an enormous expansion in munitions production and a far tighter degree of controls over the German economy and society to meet the demands of total war. This combination of on the one hand an authoritarian regime exercising all sorts of powers over the population and on the other a great growth in government borrowing and printing of paper money rather than raising income and dividend taxes—which, in turn, produced high inflation—dealt a heavy blow to popular morale—an ingredient in grand strategy which Ludendorff was far less equipped to understand than, say, a politician like Lloyd George or Clemenceau.

Even as an economic measure, the Hindenburg Program had its problems. The announcement of quite fantastic production totals—doubling explosives output, trebling machine-gun output—led to all sorts of bottlenecks as German industry struggled to meet these demands. It required not only many additional workers, but also a massive infrastructural investment, from new blast furnaces to bridges over the Rhine, which further used up labor and resources. Within a short while, therefore, it became clear that the program could be achieved only if skilled workers were returned from military duty; accordingly, 1.2 million were released in September 1916, and a further 1.9 million in July 1917. Given the serious losses on the western front, and the still-considerable casualties in the east, such withdrawals meant that even Germany's large able-bodied male population was being stretched to its limits. In that respect, although Passchendaele was a catastrophe for the British army, it was also viewed as a disaster by Ludendorff, who saw another 400,000 of his troops incapacitated. By December 1917, the German army's manpower totals were consistently under the peak of 5.38 million men it had possessed six months earlier.[226]

The final twist in the Hindenburg Program was the chronic neglect of agriculture. Here, even more than in France or Russia, men and horses and fuel were taken from the land and directed toward the needs of the army or the munitions industry—an insane imbalance, since Germany could not (like France) compensate for such planning errors by obtaining foodstuffs from overseas to make up the difference. While agricultural production plummeted in Germany, food prices spiraled and people everywhere complained about the scarcity of food supplies. In one scholar's severe judgment, "by concentrating lopsidedly on producing munitions, the military managers of the German economy thus brought the country to the verge of starvation by the end of 1918."[227]

But that time was an epoch away from early 1917, when it was the Allies who were feeling the brunt of the war and when, indeed, Russia was collapsing in chaos and both France and Italy seemed not far from that fate. It is in this grand-strategical context, of each bloc being exhausted by the war but of Germany still possessing an overall military advantage, that one must place the high command's inept policies toward the United States in the first few months of 1917. That the

American polity was leaning toward the Allied side even before then was no great secret; despite occasional disagreements over the naval blockade, the general ideological sympathy for the Allied democracies and the increasing dependence of U.S. exporters upon the western European market had made Washington less than completely neutral toward Germany. But the announcement of the unrestricted U-boat campaign against merchant shipping and the revelations of the secret German offers to Mexico of an alliance (in the "Zimmermann Telegram") finally brought Wilson and the Congress to enter the war.[228]

The significance of the American entry into the conflict was not at all a military one, at least for twelve to fifteen months after April 1917, since its army was even less prepared for modern campaigning than any of the European forces had been in 1914. But its productive strength, boosted by the billions of dollars of Allied war orders, was unequaled. Its total industrial potential and its share of world manufacturing output was two and a half times that of Germany's now overstrained economy. It could launch merchant ships in their hundreds, a vital requirement in a year when the U-boats were sinking over 500,000 tons a month of British and Allied vessels. It could build destroyers in the astonishing time of three months. It produced half of the world's food exports, which could now be sent to France and Italy as well as to its traditional British market.

In terms of economic power, therefore, the entry of the United States into the war quite transformed the balances, and more than compensated for the collapse of Russia at this same time. As Table 24 (which should be compared with Table 22) demonstrates, the productive resources now arranged against the Central Powers were enormous.

Table 24. Industrial/Technological Comparisons with the United States but Without Russia

	U.K./U.S./France	Germany/Austria-Hungary
Percentages of world manufacturing production (1913)	51.7	19.2
Energy consumption (1913), million metric tons of coal equivalent	798.8	236.4
Steel production (1913) in million tons	44.1	20.2
Total industrial potential (U.K. in 1900=100)	472.6	178.4

Because of the "lag time" between turning this economic potential into military effectiveness, the immediate consequences of the American entry into the war were mixed. The United States could not, in the short time available, produce its own tanks, field artillery, and aircraft at anything like the numbers needed (and in fact it had to borrow from France and Britain for such heavier weaponry); but it could continue to pour out the small-arms munitions and other supplies upon which London, Paris, and Rome depended so much. And it could take over from the bankers the private credit arrangements to pay for all these goods, and transform them into intergovernmental debts. Over the longer term, moreover, the U.S. Army could be expanded into a vast force of millions of fresh, confident, well-fed troops, to be thrown into the European balance.[229] In the meanwhile, the British had to grind their way through the Passchendaele muds, the Russian army had disintegrated, German reinforcements had permitted the Central Powers to deal a devastating blow to Italy at Caporetto, and Ludendorff was withdrawing some of his forces from the east in order to launch a final strike at the weakened Anglo-French lines. Outside of Europe, it was true, the British were making important gains against Turkey in the Near East. But the capture of Jerusalem and Damascus would be poor compensation for the loss of France, if the Germans at last managed to do in the west what they had done everywhere else in Europe.

This was why the leaderships of all of the major belligerents saw the coming campaigns of 1918 as absolutely decisive to the war as a whole. Although Germany had to leave well over a million troops to occupy its new great empire of conquest in the east, which the Bolsheviks finally acknowledged in the Treaty of Brest-Litovsk (March 1918), Ludendorff had been switching forces westward at the rate of ten divisions a month since early November 1917. By the time the German war machine was poised to strike, in late March 1918, it had a superiority of almost thirty divisions over the Anglo-French forces, and many of its units had been trained by Bruchmüller and other staff officers in the new techniques of surprise "storm trooper" warfare. If they succeeded in punching a hole through the Allied lines and driving to Paris or the Channel, it would be the greatest military achievement in the war. But the risks also were horrendous, for Ludendorff was mobilizing the entire remaining resources of Germany for this single campaign; it was to be "all or nothing," a gamble of epic proportions. Behind the scenes, the German economy was weakening ominously. Its industrial output was down to 57 percent of the 1913 level. Agriculture was more neglected than ever, and poor weather contributed to the decline in output; the further rise in food prices increased domestic discontents. The overworked rolling stock was by now unable to move anything like the amount of raw materials from the eastern territories that had been planned. Of the 192 divisions Ludendorff deployed in the west, 56 were labeled "attack divisions," in its way a disguise for the fact that they would receive the lion's share of the diminishing stocks of equipment and ammunition.[230] It was a gamble which the high command believed had to succeed. But if the attack failed, German resources would be exhausted—and that just at the time when the Americans were at last capable of pouring nearly 300,000 troops a month into France, and the unrestricted U-boat campaign had been completely checked by the Allied convoys.

Ludendorff's early successes—crushing the outnumbered British Fifth Army, driving a wedge between the French and British forces, and advancing by early June 1918 to within thirty-seven miles of Paris in another one of his lunges—frightened the Allies into giving Foch supreme coordination of their Western Front forces, sending reinforcements from England, Italy, and the Near East, and again (privately) worrying about a compromise peace. Yet the fact was that the Germans *had* overextended themselves, and suffered the usual consequences of going from the defensive to the offensive. In the first two heavy blows against the British sector, for example, they had inflicted 240,000 British and 92,000 French casualties, but their own losses had risen to 348,000. By July, "the Germans lost about 973,000 men, and over a million more were listed as sick. By October there were only 2.5 million men in the west and the recruiting situation was desperate."[231] From mid-July onward, the Allies were superior, not simply in fresh fighting men, but even more so in artillery, tanks, and aircraft—allowing Foch to orchestrate a whole series of offensives by British Empire, American, and French armies so that the weakening German forces would be given no rest. At the same time, too, the Allies' military superiority and greater staying power was showing itself in impressive victories in Syria, Bulgaria, and Italy. All at once, in September/October 1918, the entire German-led bloc seemed to a panic-stricken Ludendorff to be collapsing, internal discontent and revolutions now interacting with the defeats at the front to produce surrender, chaos, and political upheaval.[232] Not only was the German military bid finished, therefore, but the Old Order in Europe was ruined as well.

In the light of the awful individual losses, suffering, and devastation which had occurred both in "the face of battle" and on the home fronts,[233] and of the way in which the First World War has been seen as a self-inflicted death blow to European civilization and influence in the world,[234] it may appear crudely materialistic to introduce another statistical table at this point (Table 25). Yet the fact is that these figures point to what has been argued above: that the advantages possessed by the Central Powers—good internal lines, the quality of the German army, the occupation and exploitation of many territories, the isolation and defeat of Russia—could not over the long run outweigh this massive disadvantage in sheer economic muscle, and the considerable disadvantage in the size of total mobilized forces. Just as Ludendorff's despair at running out of able-bodied troops by July 1918 was a reflection of the imbalance of forces, so the average *Frontsoldat's* amaze-

Table 25. War Expenditure and Total Mobilized Forces, 1914–1919[235]

	War Expenditure at 1913 Prices (billions of dollars)	Total Mobilized Forces (millions)
British Empire	23.0	9.5
France	9.3	8.2
Russia	5.4	13.0
Italy	3.2	5.6
United States	17.1	3.8
Other Allies*	− 0.3	2.6
Total Allies	57.7	40.7
Germany	19.9	13.25
Austria-Hungary	4.7	9.00
Bulgaria, Turkey	0.1	2.85
Total Central Powers	24.7	25.10

*Belgium, Rumania, Portugal, Greece, Serbia.

ment at how well provisioned were the Allied units which they overran in the spring of that year was an indication of the imbalance of production.[236]

While it would be quite wrong, then, to claim that the outcome of the First World War was predetermined, the evidence presented here suggests that the overall course of that conflict—the early stalemate between the two sides, the ineffectiveness of the Italian entry, the slow exhaustion of Russia, the decisiveness of the American intervention in keeping up the Allied pressures, and the eventual collapse of the Central Powers—correlates closely with the economic and industrial production and effectively mobilized forces available to each alliance during the different phases of the struggle. To be sure, generals still had to direct (or *mis*direct) their campaigns, troops still had to summon the individual moral courage to assault an enemy position, and sailors still had to endure the rigors of sea warfare; but the record indicates that such qualities and talents existed on both sides, and were not enjoyed in disproportionate measure by one of the coalitions. What *was* enjoyed by one side, particularly after 1917, was a marked superiority in productive forces. As in earlier, lengthy coalition wars, that factor eventually turned out to be decisive.

6
The Coming of a Bipolar World and the Crisis of the "Middle Powers": Part Two, 1919–1942

The Postwar International Order

The statesmen of the greater and lesser powers assembling in Paris at the beginning of 1919 to arrange a peace settlement were confronted with a list of problems both more extensive and more intractable than had been encountered by any of their predecessors in 1856, 1814–1815, and 1763. While many items on the agenda could be settled and incorporated into the Treaty of Versailles itself (June 28, 1919), the confusion prevailing in eastern Europe as rival ethnic groups jostled to establish "successor states," the civil war and interventions in Russia, and the Turkish nationalist reaction against the intended western division of Asia Minor meant that many matters were not fixed until 1920, and in some cases 1923. However, for the purposes of brevity, this group of agreements will be examined as a whole, rather than in the actual chronological order of their settlement.

The most striking change in Europe, measured in territorial-juridical terms, was the emergence of a cluster of nation-states—Poland, Czechoslovakia, Austria, Hungary, Yugoslavia, Finland, Estonia, Latvia, and Lithuania—in place of lands which were formerly part of the Habsburg, Romanov, and Hohenzollen empires. While the ethnically coherent Germany suffered far smaller territorial losses in eastern Europe than either Soviet Russia or the totally dissolved Austro-Hungarian Empire, its power was hurt in other ways: by the return of Alsace-Lorraine to France, and by border rectifications with Belgium and Denmark; by the Allied military occupation of the Rhineland, and the French economic exploitation of the Saarland; by the unprecedented "demilitarization" terms (e.g., minuscule army and coastal-defense navy, no air force, tanks, or submarines, abolition of Prussian General Staff); and by an enormous reparations bill. In addition, Germany also lost its extensive colonial empire to Britain, the self-governing dominions, and France—just as Turkey found its Near East territories turned into British and French mandates, distantly

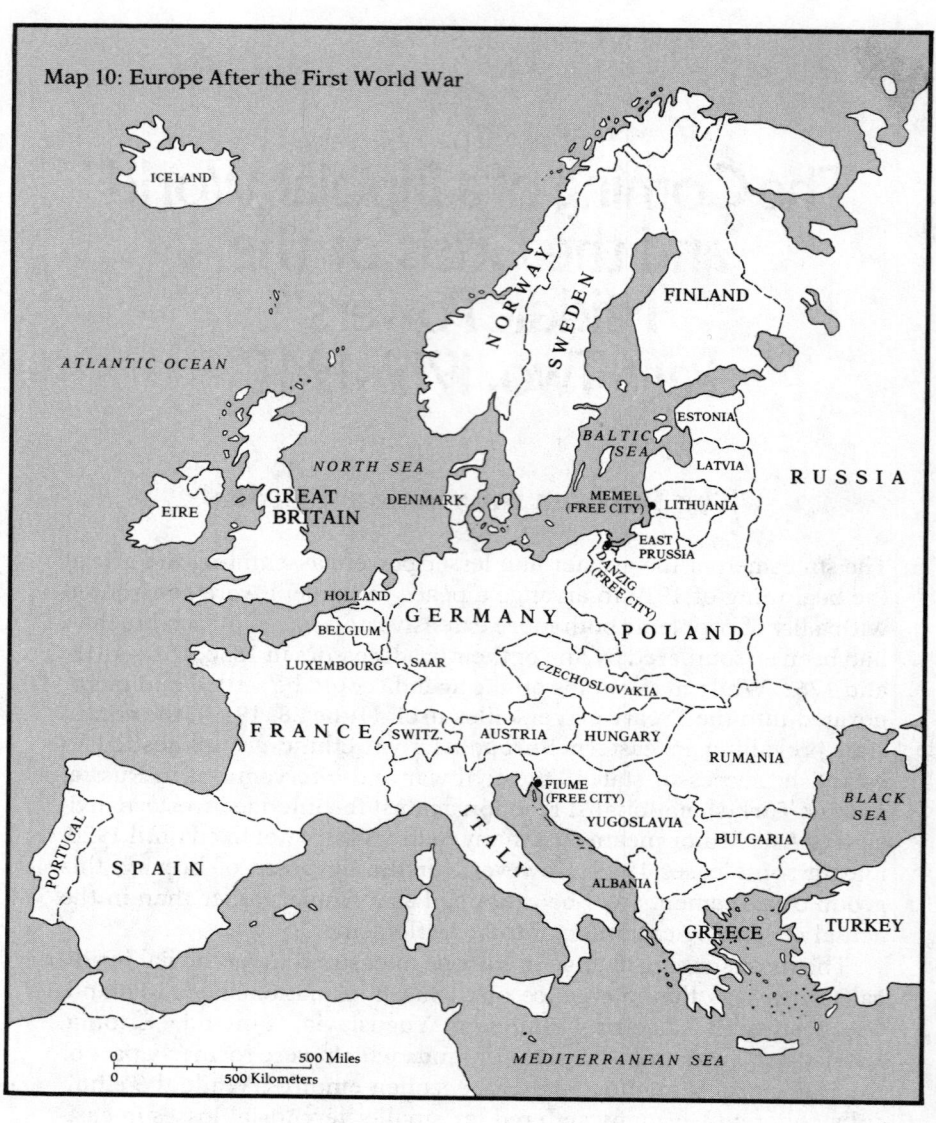

Map 10: Europe After the First World War

ICELAND

ATLANTIC OCEAN

NORWAY

SWEDEN

FINLAND

BALTIC SEA

ESTONIA

LATVIA

RUSSIA

NORTH SEA

EIRE

GREAT BRITAIN

DENMARK

MEMEL (FREE CITY)

LITHUANIA

EAST PRUSSIA

DANZIG (FREE CITY)

HOLLAND

BELGIUM

GERMANY

POLAND

LUXEMBOURG

SAAR

CZECHOSLOVAKIA

FRANCE

SWITZ.

AUSTRIA

HUNGARY

RUMANIA

BLACK SEA

FIUME (FREE CITY)

YUGOSLAVIA

BULGARIA

PORTUGAL

SPAIN

ITALY

ALBANIA

GREECE

TURKEY

MEDITERRANEAN SEA

500 Miles

500 Kilometers

supervised by the new League of Nations. In the Far East, Japan inherited the former German island groups north of the equator, although it returned Shantung to China in 1922. At the 1921–1922 Washington Conference, the powers recognized the territorial status quo in the Pacific and Far East, and agreed to restrict the size of their battle fleets according to relative formulae, thereby heading off an Anglo-American-Japanese naval race. In both the West and the East, therefore, the international system appeared to have been stabilized by the early 1920s—and what difficulties remained (or might arise in the future) could now be dealt with by the League of Nations, which met regularly at Geneva despite the surprise defection of the United States.[1]

The sudden American retreat into at least relative diplomatic isolationism after 1920 seemed yet another contradiction to those world-power trends which, as detailed above, had been under way since the 1890s. To the prophets of world politics in that earlier period, it was self-evident that the international scene was going to be increasingly influenced, if not dominated, by the three rising powers of Germany, Russia, and the United States. Instead, the first-named had been decisively defeated, the second had collapsed in revolution and then withdrawn into its Bolshevik-led isolation, and the third, although clearly the most powerful nation in the world by 1919, also preferred to retreat from the center of the diplomatic stage. In consequence, international affairs during the 1920s and beyond still seemed to focus either upon the actions of France and Britain, even though both countries had been badly hurt by the First World War, or upon the deliberations of the League, in which French and British statesmen were preeminent. Austria-Hungary was now gone. Italy, where the National Fascist Party under Mussolini was consolidating its hold after 1922, was relatively quiescent. Japan, too, appeared tranquil following the 1921–1922 Washington Conference decisions.

In a curious and (as will be seen) artificial way, therefore, it still seemed a Eurocentered world. The diplomatic histories of this period focus heavily upon France's "search for security" against a future German resurgence. Having lost a special Anglo-American military guarantee at the same time as the U.S. Senate rejected the Treaty of Versailles, the French sought to create a variety of substitutes: encouraging the formation of an "antirevisionist" bloc of states in eastern Europe (the so-called Little Entente of 1921); concluding individual alliances with Belgium (1920), Poland (1921), Czechoslovakia (1924), Rumania (1926), and Yugoslavia (1927); maintaining a very large army and air force to overawe the Germans and intervening—as in the 1923 Ruhr crisis—when Germany defaulted on the reparation payments; and endeavoring to persuade successive British administrations to provide a new military guarantee of France's borders, something which was achieved only indirectly in the multilateral

Locarno Treaty of 1925.[2] It was also a period of intense financial
diplomacy, since the interacting problem of German reparations and
Allied war debts bedeviled relations not only between the victors and
the vanquished, but also between the United States and its former
European allies.[3] The financial compromise of the Dawes Plan (1924)
eased much of this turbulence, and in turn prepared the ground for the
Locarno Treaty the following year; that was followed by Germany's
entry into the League and then the amended financial settlement of the
Young Plan (1929). By the late 1920s, indeed, with prosperity returning
to Europe, with the League apparently accepted as an important new
element in the international system, and with a plethora of states
solemnly agreeing (under the 1928 Pact of Paris) not to resort to war
to settle future disputes, the diplomatic stage seemed to have returned
to normal. Statesmen such as Stresemann, Briand, and Austen Chamberlain appeared, in their way, the latter-day equivalents of Metternich
and Bismarck, meeting at this or that European spa to settle the affairs
of the world.

Despite these superficial impressions, however, the underlying
structures of the post-1919 international system were significantly different from, and much more fragile than, those which influenced diplomacy a half-century earlier. In the first place, the population losses
and economic disruptions caused by four and a half years of "total"
war were immense. Around 8 million men were killed in actual
fighting, with another 7 million permanently disabled and a further 15
million "more or less seriously wounded"[4]—the vast majority of these
being in the prime of their productive life. In addition, Europe *excluding* Russia probably lost over 5 million civilian casualties through
what has been termed "war-induced causes"—"disease, famine and
privation consequent upon the war as well as those wrought by military conflict";[5] the Russian total, compounded by the heavy losses in
the civil war, was much larger. The wartime "birth deficits" (caused by
so many men being absent at the front, and the populations thereby not
renewing themselves at the normal prewar rate) were also extremely
high. Finally, even as the major battles ground to a halt, fighting and
massacres occurred during the postwar border conflicts in, for example, eastern Europe, Armenia, and Poland; and none of these war-
weakened regions escaped the dreadful influenza epidemic of
1918–1919, which carried off further millions. Thus, the final casualty
list for this extended period might have been as much as 60 million
people, with nearly half of these losses occurring in Russia, and with
France, Germany, and Italy also being badly hit. There is no known
way of measuring the personal anguish and the psychological shocks
involved in such a human catastrophe, but it is easy to see why the

participants—statesmen as well as peasants—were so deeply affected by it all.

The material costs of the war were also unprecedented and seemed, to those who viewed the devastated landscapes of northern France, Poland, and Serbia, even more shocking: hundreds of thousands of houses were destroyed, farms gutted, roads and railways and telegraph lines blown up, livestock slaughtered, forests pulverized, and vast tracts of land rendered unfit for farming because of unexploded shells and mines. When the shipping losses, the direct and indirect costs of mobilization, and the monies raised by the combatants are added to the list, the total charge becomes so huge as to be virtually incomprehensible: in fact, some $260 billion, which, according to one calculation, "represented about six and a half times the sum of all the national debt accumulated in the world from the end of the eighteenth century up to the eve of the First World War."[6] After decades of growth, world manufacturing production turned sharply down; in 1920 it was still 7 percent less than in 1913, agricultural production was about one-third below normal, and the volume of exports was only around half what it was in the prewar period. While the growth of the European economy as a whole had been retarded, perhaps as much as by eight years,* individual countries were much more severely affected. Predictably, Russia in the turmoil of 1920 recorded the lowest industrial output, equal to a mere 13 percent of the 1913 figure; but in Germany, France, Belgium, and much of eastern Europe, industrial output was at least 30 percent lower than before the conflict.[7]

If some societies were the more heavily affected by the war, then others of course escaped lightly—and many improved their position. For the fact was that modern war, and the industrial productivity generated by it, also had positive effects. In strictly economic and technological terms, these years had seen many advances: in automobile and truck production, in aviation, in oil refining and chemicals, in the electrical and dyestuff and alloy-steel industries, in refrigeration and canning, and in a whole host of other industries.[8] Naturally, it proved easier to develop and to benefit commercially from such advances if one's economy was far from the disruption of the front line; which is why the United States itself, but also Canada, Australia, South Africa, India, and parts of South America, found their economies stimulated by the industrial, raw-material, and foodstuffs demand of a Europe convulsed by a war of attrition. As in previous mercantilist conflicts, one country's loss was often another's gain—provided the

*That is to say, its output in 1929 totaled what it probably would have reached in 1921, had there been no war and had the pre-1913 growth rates continued.

**Table 26. World Indices of
Manufacturing Production, 1913–1925[9]**

	1913	1920	1925
World	100	93.6	121.6
Europe*	100	77.3	103.5
USSR	100	12.8	70.1
United States	100	122.2	148.0
Rest of World	100	109.5	138.1

*U.K., France, Belgium, Netherlands, Germany,
Denmark, Norway, Sweden, Finland, Switzerland,
Austria, Italy, Czechoslovakia, Hungary, Poland,
Rumania, Greece, and Spain.

latter avoided the costs of war, or was at least protected from the full blast of battle.

Such figures on world manufacturing production are very illuminating in this respect, since they record the extent to which Europe (and especially the USSR) were hurt by the war, while other regions gained substantially. To some degree, of course, the spread of industrialization from Europe to the Americas, Japan, India, and Australasia, and the increasing share of these latter territories in world trade, was simply the continuation of economic trends which had been in evidence since the late nineteenth century. Thus, according to one arcane calculation already mentioned earlier, the United States pre-1914 growth was such that it probably would have overtaken Europe in total output in the year 1925;[10] what the war did was to accelerate that event by a mere six years, to 1919. On the other hand, unlike the 1880–1913 changes, these particular shifts in the global economic balances were *not* taking place in peacetime over several decades and in accord with market forces. Instead, the agencies of war and blockade created their own peremptory demands and thus massively distorted the natural patterns of world production and trade. For example, shipbuilding capacity (especially in the United States) had been enormously increased in the middle of the war to counter the sinkings by U-boats; but after 1919–1920, there were excess berths across the globe. Again, the output of the steel industries of continental Europe had fallen during the war, whereas that of the United States and Britain had risen sharply; but when the European steel producers recovered, the excess capacity was horrific. This problem also affected an even greater sector of the economy—agriculture. During the war years, farm output in continental Europe had shriveled and Russia's prewar export trade in grain had disappeared, whereas there had been large increases in output in North and South America and in Australasia, whose farmers were the decided (if unpremeditating) beneficiaries of the archduke's death. But when European agriculture recovered by the late 1920s, producers across the world faced a fall-off in demand, and tumbling prices.[11] These sorts of structural distortions affected all regions, but were felt nowhere as severely as in east-central Europe, where the fragile "successor states" grappled with new boundaries, dislocated markets, and distorted communications. Making peace at Versailles and redrawing the map of Europe along (roughly) ethnic lines did not of itself guarantee a restoration of economic stability.

Finally, the financing of the war had caused economic—and later political—problems of unprecedented complexity. Very few of the belligerents (Britain and the United States were among the exceptions) had tried to pay for even part of the costs of the conflict by increasing taxes; instead most states relied almost entirely on borrowing, assuming that the defeated foe would be forced to meet the bill—as had happened to France in 1871. Public debts, now uncovered by gold, rose precipitously; paper money, pouring out of the state treasuries, sent prices soaring.[12] Given the economic devastation and territorial dislocations caused by the war, no European country was ready to follow the United States back onto the gold standard in 1919. Lax monetary and fiscal policies caused inflation to keep on increasing, with disastrous results in central and eastern Europe. Competitive depreciations of the national currency, carried out in a desperate attempt to boost exports, simply created more financial instability—as well as political rivalry. This was all compounded by the intractable related issues of intra-Allied loans and the victors' (especially France's) demand for substantial German reparations. All the European allies were in debt to Britain, and to a lesser extent to France; while those two powers were heavily in debt to the United States. With the Bolsheviks' repudiating Russia's massive borrowings of $3.6 billion, with the Americans asking for their money back, with France, Italy, and other countries refusing to pay off their debts until they had received reparations from Germany, and with the Germans declaring that they could not possibly pay the amounts demanded of them, the scene was set for years of bitter wrangling, which sharply widened the gap in political sympathies between western Europe and a disgruntled United States.[13]

If it was true that these quarrels seemed smoothed over by the Dawes Plan of 1924, the political and social consequences of this turbulence had been immense, especially during the German hyperinflation of the previous year. What was equally alarming, although less well understood at the time, was that the apparent financial and commercial stabilization of the world economy by the mid-1920s rested on far more precarious foundations than had existed prior to the First World War. Although the gold standard was being restored in most countries by then, the subtle (and almost self-balancing) pre-1914 mechanism of international trade and monetary flows based upon the City of London had not. London had, in fact, made desperate attempts to recover that role—including the 1925 fixing of the sterling convertibility rate at the prewar level of £1:$4.86, which badly hurt British exporters; and it also had resumed large-scale lending overseas. Nonetheless, the fact was that the center of world finance had naturally moved across the Atlantic between 1914 and 1919, as Europe's international debts increased and the United States became the world's greatest creditor nation. On the other hand, the quite different structure of the American economy—less dependent upon foreign commerce and much less integrated into the world economy, protectionist-inclined (especially in agriculture) rather than free-trading, lacking a full equivalent to the Bank of England, fluctuating much more wildly in its booms and busts, with politicians much more directly influenced by domestic lobbies—meant that the international financial and commercial system revolved around a volatile and flawed central point. There was now no real "lender of last resort," offering long-term loans for the infrastructural development of the world economy and stabilizing the temporary disjunctions in the international accounts.[14]

These structural inadequacies were concealed in the late 1920s, when vast amounts of dollars flowed out of the United States in short-term loans to European governments and municipalities, all willing to offer high interest rates in order to use such funds—not always wisely—both for development and to close the gap in their balance of payments. With short-term money being thus employed for long-term projects, with considerable amounts of investment (especially in central and eastern Europe) still going into agriculture and thus increasing the downward pressures on farm prices, with the costs of servicing these debts rising alarmingly and, since they could not be paid off by exports, being sustained only by further borrowings, the system was already breaking down in the summer of 1928, when the American domestic boom (and the Federal Reserve's reactive increase in interest rates) sharply curtailed the outflow of capital.

The ending of that boom in the "Wall Street crash" of October 1929 and the further reduction in American lending then instigated a chain reaction which appeared uncontrollable: the lack of ready credit reduced both investment and consumption; depressed demand among the industrialized countries hurt producers of foodstuffs and raw materials, who responded desperately by increasing supply and then witnessing the near-total collapse of prices—making it impossible for them in turn to purchase manufactured goods. Deflation, going off gold and devaluing the currency, restrictive measures on commerce and capital, and defaults upon international debts were the various expedients of the day; each one dealt a further blow to the global system of trade and credit. The archprotectionist Smoot-Hawley Tariff, passed (in the calculation of aiding American farmers) by the only country with a substantial trade surplus, made it even more difficult for other countries to earn dollars—and led to the inevitable reprisals, which devastated American exports. By the summer of 1932, industrial production in many countries was only half that of 1928, and world trade had shrunk by one-third. The value of European trade ($58 billion in 1928) was still down at $20.8 billion in 1935—a decline which in turn hit shipping, shipbuilding, insurance, and so on.[15]

Given the severity of this worldwide depression and the massive unemployment caused by it, there was no way international politics could escape from its dire effects. The fierce competition in manufactures, raw materials, and farm produce increased national resentments and impelled many a politician, aware of his constituents' discontents, into trying to make the foreigner pay; more extreme groups, especially of the right, took advantage of the economic dislocation to attack the entire liberal-capitalist system and to call for assertive "national" policies, backed if necessary by the sword. The more fragile democracies, in Weimar Germany especially but also in Spain, Rumania, and elsewhere, buckled under these politico-economic strains. The cautious conservatives who ruled Japan were edged out by nationalists and militarists. If the democracies of the West weathered these storms better, their statesmen were forced to concentrate upon domestic economic management, increasingly tinged with a beggar-thy-neighbor attitude. Neither the United States nor France, the main gold-surplus countries, were willing to bail out debtor states; indeed, France inclined more and more to use its financial strength to try to control German behavior (which merely intensified resentments on the other side of the Rhine) and to aid its own European diplomacy. Similarly, the "Hoover moratorium" on German reparations, which so infuriated the French, could not be separated from the issue of reductions in (and ultimately defaults on) war debts, which made the Americans bitter. Competitive devaluations in currency, and disagreements at the 1933 World Economic Conference about the dollar-sterling rate, completed this gloomy picture.

By that time, the cosmopolitan world order had dissolved into various rivaling subunits: a sterling block, based upon British trade patterns and enhanced by the "imperial preferences" of the 1932 Ottawa Conference: a gold block, led by France; a yen block, dependent upon Japan, in the Far East; a U.S.-led dollar block (after Roosevelt also went off gold); and, completely detached from these convulsions, a USSR steadily building "socialism in one country." The trend toward autarky was thus already strongly developed even before Adolf Hitler commenced his program of creating a self-sufficient, thousand-year Reich in which foreign trade was reduced to special deals and "barter" agreements. With France having repeatedly opposed the Anglo-Saxon powers over the treatment of German reparations, with Roosevelt claiming that the United States always lost out in deals with the British, and with Neville Chamberlain already convinced of his later remark that the American policy was all "words,"[16] the democracies were in no frame of mind to cooperate in handling the pressures building up for territorial charges in the flawed 1919 world order.

The Old World statesmen and foreign offices had always found it difficult either to understand or to deal with economic issues; but perhaps an even more disruptive feature, to those fondly looking back at the cabinet diplomacy of the nineteenth century, was the increasing influence of mass public opinion upon international affairs during the 1920s and 1930s. In some ways, of course, this was inevitable. Even before the First World War, political groups across Europe had been criticizing the arcane, secretive methods and elitist preconceptions of the "old diplomacy," and calling instead for a reformed system, where the affairs of state were open to the scrutiny of the people and their representatives.[17] These demands were greatly boosted by the 1914–1918 conflict, partly because the leaderships who demanded the total mobilization of society realized that society, in turn, would require compensations for its sacrifices and a say in the peace; partly because the war, fondly proclaimed by Allied propagandists as a struggle for democracy and national self-determination, did indeed smash the autocratic empires of east-central Europe; and partly because the powerful and appealing figure of Woodrow Wilson kept up the pressures for a new and enlightened world order even as Clemenceau and Lloyd George were proclaiming the need for total victory.[18]

But the problem with "public opinion" after 1919 was that many sections of it did *not* match that fond Gladstonian and Wilsonian vision of a liberal, educated, fair-minded populace, imbued with internationalist ideas, utilitarian assumptions, and respect for the rule of law. As Arno Mayer has shown, "the old diplomacy" which (it was widely claimed) had caused the World War was being challenged after 1917 not only by Wilsonian reformism, but also by the Bolsheviks' much more systematic criticism of the existing order—a criticism of considerable attraction to the organized working classes in *both* belligerent camps.[19] While this caused nimble politicians such as Lloyd George to invent their own "package" of progressive domestic and foreign policies, to neutralize Wilson's appeal and to check labor's drift toward socialism,[20] the impact upon more conservative and nationalist figures in the Allied camp was quite different. In their view, Wilsonian principles must be firmly rejected in the interests of national "security," which could only be measured in the hard cash of border adjustments, colonial acquisitions, and reparations; while Lenin's threat, which was much more frightening, had to be ruthlessly smashed, in its Bolshevik heartland and (especially) in the imitative soviets which sprang up in the West. The politics and diplomacy of the peacemaking,[21] in other words, was charged with background ideological and domestic-political elements to a degree unknown at the congresses of 1856 and 1878.

There was more. In the western democracies, the images of the First World War which prevailed by the late 1920s were of death, destruction, horror, waste, and the futility of it all. The "Carthaginian peace" of 1919, the lack of those benefits promised by wartime politicians in return for the people's sacrifices, the millions of maimed veterans and of war widows, the economic troubles of the 1920s, the loss of faith and the breakdown in Victorian social and personal relationships, were all blamed upon the folly of the July 1914 decisions.[22] But this widespread public recoil from fighting and militarism, mingled in many quarters with the hope that the League of Nations would render impossible any repetition of that disaster, was not shared by all of the war's participants—even if Anglo-American literature gives that impression.[23] To hundreds of thousands of former *Frontsoldaten* across the continent of Europe, disillusioned by the unemployment and inflation and boredom of the postwar bourgeois-dominated order, the conflict had represented something searing but positive: martial values, the camaraderie of warriors, the thrill of violence and action. To such groups, especially in the defeated nations of Germany and Hungary and in the bitterly dissatisfied victor nation of Italy, but also among the French right, the ideas of the new fascist movements—of order, discipline, and national glory, of the smashing of the Jews, Bolsheviks, intellectual decadents, and self-satisfied liberal middle classes—had great appeal. In their eyes (and in the eyes of their equivalents in Japan), it was struggle and force and heroism which were the enduring features of life, and the tenets of Wilsonian internationism which were false and outdated.[24]

What this meant was that international relations during the 1920s and 1930s continued to be complicated by ideology, and by the steady fissuring of world society into political blocs which only partly overlapped with the economic subdivisions mentioned earlier. On the one hand, there were the western democracies, especially in the English-speaking world, recoiling from the horror of the First World War, concentrating upon domestic (especially socioeconomic) issues, and massively reducing their defense establishments; and while the French leadership kept up a large army and air force out of fear of a revived Germany, it was evident that much of its public shared this hatred of war and desire for social reconstruction. On the other hand, there was the Soviet Union, isolated in so many ways from the global politico-economic system yet attracting admirers in the West because it offered, purportedly, a "new civilization" which *inter alia* escaped the Great Depression,[25] though the USSR was also widely detested. Finally, there were, at least by the 1930s, the fascistic "revisionist" states of Germany, Japan, and Italy, which were not only virulently anti-Bolshevik but also denounced the liberal-capitalist status quo that had been reestablished in 1919. All this made the conduct of foreign policy inordinately difficult for democratic statesmen, who possessed little grasp of either the fascist or the Bolshevik frame of mind, and yearned merely to return to that state of Edwardian "normalcy" which the war had so badly destroyed.

Compared with these problems, the post-1919 challenges to the Eurocentric world which were beginning to arise in the tropics were less threatening—but still important. Here, too, one can detect precedents prior to 1914, such as Arabi Pasha's revolt in Egypt, the young Turks' breakthrough after 1908, Tilak's attempts to radicalize the Indian Congress movement, and Sun Yat-sen's campaign against western dominance in China; by the same token, historians have noted how events such as the Japanese defeat of Russia in 1905 and the abortive Russian revolution of that same year fascinated and electrified protonationalist forces elsewhere in Asia and the Middle East.[26] Ironically, yet predictably, the more that colonialism penetrated underdeveloped societies, drew them into a global network of trade and finance, and brought them into contact with western ideas, the more this provoked an indigenous reaction; whether it came in the form of tribal unrest against restrictions upon their traditional patterns of life and trade or, more significantly, in the form of western-educated lawyers and intellectuals seeking to create mass parties and campaigning for national self-determination, the result was an increasing challenge to European colonial controls.

The First World War accelerated these trends in all sorts of ways. In the first place, the intensified economic exploitation of the raw materials in the tropics and the attempts to make the colonies contribute—both with manpower and with taxes—to the metropolitan powers' war effort inevitably caused questions to be asked about "compensation," just as it was doing among the working classes of Europe.[27] Furthermore, the campaigning in West, Southwest, and East Africa, in the Near East, and in the Pacific raised questions about the viability and permanence of colonial empires in general—a tendency reinforced by Allied propaganda about "national self-determination" and "democracy," and German counterpropaganda activities toward the Maghreb, Ireland, Egypt, and India. By 1919, while the European powers were establishing their League of Nations mandates—hiding their imperial interests behind ever more elaborate fig leaves, as A.J.P. Taylor once described it—the Pan African Congress had been meeting in Paris to put its point of view, the Wafd Party was being founded in Egypt, the May Fourth Movement was active in China, Kemal Ataturk was emerging as the founder of modern Turkey, the Destour party was reformulating its tactics in Tunisia, the Sarehat Islam had reached a membership of 2.5 million in Indonesia, and Gandhi was catalyzing the many different strands of opposition to British rule in India.[28]

More important still, this "revolt against the West" would no longer find the Great Powers united in the supposition that whatever their own differences, a great gulf lay between themselves and the less-developed peoples of the globe; this, too, was another large difference from the time of the Berlin West Africa Conference. Such unity had already been made redundant by the entry into the Great Power club of the Japanese, some of whose thinkers were beginning to articulate notions of an East Asian "co-prosperity sphere" as early as 1919.[29] And it was overtaken altogether by the coming of the two versions of the "new diplomacy" proposed by Lenin and Wilson—for whatever the political differences between those charismatic leaders, they had in common a dislike of the old European colonial order and a desire to transform it into something else. Neither of them, for a variety of reasons, could prevent the further extension of that colonial order under the League mandates; but their rhetoric and influence seeped across imperial demarcation zones and interacted with the mobilization of indigenous nationalists. This was evident in China by the late 1920s, where the old European order of treaty privileges, commercial penetration, and occasional gunboat actions was beginning to lose ground to competing alternative "orders" proposed by Russia, the United States, and Japan, and to wilt in the face of the resurgent Chinese nationalism.[30]

This did not mean that western colonialism was about to collapse. The sharp British response at Amritsar in 1919, the Dutch imprisonment of Sukarno and other Indonesian nationalist leaders and breaking-up of the trade unions in the late 1920s, the firm French reaction to Tonkinese unrest at the intense agricultural development of rice and rubber, all testified to the residual power of European armies and weaponry.[31] And the same could be said, of course, of Italy's belated imperial thrust into Abyssinia in the mid-1930s. Only the far larger shocks administered by the Second World War would really loosen these imperial controls. Nevertheless, this colonial unrest was of some importance to international relations in the 1920s and especially in the 1930s. First of all, it distracted the attention (and the resources) of certain of the Great Powers from their concern with the European balance of power. This was preeminently the case with Britain, whose leaders worried far more about Palestine, India, and Singapore than about the Sudetenland or Danzig—such priorities being reflected in their post-1919 "imperial" defense policy;[32] but involvements in Africa also affected France to the same degree, and of course quite distracted the Italian military. Furthermore, in certain instances the reemergence of extra-European and colonial issues was cutting right across the former 1914–1918 alliance structure. Not only did the question of imperialism cause Americans to be ever more distrustful of Anglo-French policies, but events such as the Italian invasion of Abyssinia and the Japanese aggression into mainland China divided Rome and

Tokyo from London and Paris by the 1930s—and offered possible partners to German revisionists. Here again, international affairs had become that bit more difficult to manage according to the prescriptions of the "old diplomacy."

The final major cause of postwar instability was the awkward fact that the "German question" had not been settled, but made more intractable and intense. The swift collapse of Germany in October 1918 when its armies still controlled Europe from Belgium to the Ukraine came as a great shock to nationalist, right-wing forces, who tended to blame "traitors within" for the humiliating surrender. When the terms of the Paris settlement brought even more humiliations, vast numbers of Germans denounced both the "slave treaty" and the Weimar-democratic politicians who had agreed to such terms. The reparations issue, and the related hyperinflation of 1923, filled the cup of German discontents. Very few were as extreme as the National Socialists, who appeared as a cranky demagogic fringe movement for much of the 1920s; but very few Germans were *not* revisionists, in one form or another. Reparations, the Polish corridor, restrictions on the armed forces, the separation of German-speaking regions from the Fatherland were not going to be tolerated forever. The only questions were how soon these restrictions could be abolished and to what extent diplomacy should be preferred to force in order to alter the status quo. In this respect, Hitler's coming to power in 1933 merely intensified the German drive for revisionism.[33]

The problem of settling Germany's "proper" place in Europe was compounded by the curious and unbalanced distribution of international power after the First World War. Despite its territorial losses, military restrictions, and economic instability, Germany after 1919 was still *potentially* an immensely strong Great Power. A more detailed analysis of its strengths and weaknesses will be given below, but it is worth noting here that Germany still possessed a much larger population than France and an iron-and-steel capacity which was around three times as big. Its internal communications network was intact, as were its chemical and electrical plants and its universities and technical institutes. "At the moment in 1919, Germany was down-and-out. The immediate problem was German weakness; but given a few years of 'normal' life, it would again become the problem of German strength."[34] Furthermore, as Taylor points out, the old balance of power on the European continent which had helped to restrain German expansionism was no more. "Russia had withdrawn; Austria-Hungary had vanished. Only France and Italy remained, both inferior in manpower and still more in economic resources, both exhausted by the war."[35] And, as time went on, first the United States and then Britain showed an increasing distaste for interventions in Europe, and an increasing disapproval of French efforts to keep Germany down.

Yet it was precisely this apprehension that France was *not* secure which drove Paris into seeking to prevent a revival of German power by all means possible: insisting on the full payment of reparations; maintaining its own large and costly armed forces; endeavoring to turn the League of Nations into an organization dedicated to preserving the status quo; and resisting all suggestions that Germany be admitted to "arm up" to France's level[36]—all of which, predictably, fueled German resentments and helped the agitations of the right-wing extremists.

The other device in France's battery of diplomatic and political weapons was its link with the eastern European "successor states." On the face of it, support for Poland, Czechoslovakia, and the other beneficiaries of the 1919–1921 settlements in that region was both a plausible and a promising strategy;[37] by it, German expansionism would be checked on each flank. In reality, the scheme was fraught with difficulties. Because of the geographical dispersion of the various populations under the former multinational empires, it had not been possible in 1919 to create a territorial settlement which was ethnically coherent; large groups of minorities therefore lived on the wrong side of every state's borders, offering a source not only of internal weakness but also of foreign resentments. In other words, Germany was not alone in desiring a revision of the Paris treaties; and even if France was eager to insist upon no changes in the status quo, it was aware that neither Britain nor the United States felt any great commitment to the hastily arranged and irregular boundaries in this region. As London made clear in 1925, there would be no Locarno-type guarantees in eastern Europe.[38]

The economic scene in eastern and central Europe made matters even worse, since the erection of customs and tariff barriers around these newly created countries increased regional rivalries and hindered general development. There were now twenty-seven separate currencies in Europe instead of fourteen as before the war, and an extra 12,500 miles of frontiers; many of the borders separated factories from their raw materials, ironworks from their coalfields, farms from their market. What was more, although French and British bankers and enterprises moved into these successor states after 1919, a much more "natural" trading partner for those nations was Germany, once it had recovered its own economic stability in the 1930s. Not only was it closer to, and better connected by road and rail with, the eastern European market, but it could readily absorb the area's agricultural surpluses in the way that farm-surplus France and imperial-preference Britain could not, offering in return for Hungarian wheat and Rumanian oil much-needed machinery and (later) armaments. Moreover, these countries, like Germany itself, had currency problems and thus found it easier to trade on a "barter" basis. Economically, therefore, Mitteleuropa could again steadily become a German-dominated zone.[39]

Many of the participants at the Paris negotiations of 1919 were aware of some (though obviously not all) of the problems mentioned above. However, they felt that, like Lloyd George, they could look to the newly created League of Nations "to remedy, to repair, and to redress. . . . [It] will be there as a Court of Appeal to readjust crudities, irregularities, injustices."[40] Surely any outstanding political or economic quarrel between states could now be settled by reasonable men meeting around a table in Geneva. That again seemed a plausible supposition to make in 1919, but it was to founder on hard reality. The United States would not join the League. The Soviet Union was treated as a pariah state and kept out of the League. So, too, were the defeated powers, at least for the first few years. When the revisionist states commenced their aggressions in the 1930s, they soon thereafter left the League.

Furthermore, because of the earlier disagreements between the French and British versions of what the League should be—a policeman or a conciliator—the body lacked enforcement powers and had no real machinery of collective security. Ironically, therefore, the League's actual contribution turned out to be not deterring aggressors, but confusing the democracies. It was immensely popular with war-wearied public opinion in the West, but its very creation then permitted many the argument that there was no need for national defense forces since the League would somehow prevent future wars. In consequence, the existence of the League caused cabinets and foreign ministers to wobble between the "old" and the "new" diplomacy, usually securing the benefits of neither, as the Manchurian and Abyssinian cases amply demonstrated.

In the light of all of the above difficulties, and of the overwhelming fact that Europe plunged into another great war only twenty years after signing the Treaty of Versailles, it is scarcely surprising that historians have seen this period as a "twenty years' truce" and portrayed it as a gloomy and fractured time—full of crises, deceits, brutalities, dishonor. But with book titles like *A Broken World, The Lost Peace,* and *The Twenty Years' Crisis* describing these entire two decades,[41] there is a danger that the great differences between the 1920s and the 1930s may be ignored. To repeat a remark made earlier, by the late 1920s, the Locarno and Kellogg-Briand (Pact of Paris) treaties, the settling of many Franco-German differences, the meetings of the League, and the general revival of prosperity seemed to indicate that the First World War was at last over as far as international relations were concerned. Within another year or two, however, the devastating financial and industrial collapse had shaken that harmony and had begun to interact with the challenges which the Japanese and German (and later Italian) nationalists would pose to the existing order. In a remarkably short space of time, the clouds of war returned. The system was under threat, in a fundamental way, just at a moment when the democracies were least prepared, psychologically and militarily, to meet it; and just as they were less coordinated than at any time since the 1919 settlement. Whatever the deficiencies and follies of any particular "appeaser" in the unhappy 1930s, therefore, it is as well to bear in mind the unprecedented complexities with which the statesmen of that decade had to grapple.

Before seeing how the international crises of this period unfolded into war, it is important once again to examine the particular strengths and weaknesses of each of the Great Powers, all of which had been affected not only by the 1914–1918 conflict but also by the economic and military developments of the interwar years. In this latter respect, Tables 12–18 above, showing the shifts in the productive balances between the powers, will be referred to again and again. Two further preliminary remarks about the economics of rearmament should be made at this point. The first concerns differential growth rates, which were much more marked during the 1930s than they had been, say, in the decade prior to 1914; the dislocation of the world economy into various blocs and the remarkably different ways in which national economic policy was pursued (from four-year plans and "new deals" to classic deflationary budgets) meant that output and wealth could be rising in one country while dramatically slowing down in another. Secondly, the interwar developments in military technology made the armed forces more dependent than ever upon the productive forces of their nations. Without a flourishing industrial base and, more important still, without a large, advanced scientific community which could be mobilized by the state in order to keep pace with new developments in weaponry, victory in another great war was inconceivable. If the future lay (to use Stalin's phrase) in the hands of the big battalions, they in turn increasingly rested upon modern technology and mass production.

The Challengers

The economic vulnerability of a Great Power, however active and ambitious its national leadership, is nowhere more clearly seen than in the case of Italy during the 1930s. On the face of it, Mussolini's fascist regime had brought the country from the hinterlands to the forefront of the diplomatic world. With Britain, it was one of the outside guarantors of the 1925 Locarno agreement; with Britain, France and Germany, it was also a signatory to the 1938 Munich settlement. Italy's claim to primacy in the Mediterranean had been asserted by the attack upon Corfu (1923), by intensifying the "pacification" of Libya, and by the very large intervention (of 50,000 Italian troops) in the Spanish Civil War. Between 1935 and 1937, Mussolini avenged the defeat of Adowa by his ruthless conquest of Abyssinia, boldly defying the League's sanctions and hostile western opinion. At other times, he supported the status quo, moving troops up to the Brenner in 1934 to deter Hitler from taking over Austria, and readily signing the anti-German accord at Stresa in 1935. His tirades against Bolshevism won him the admiration of many foreigners (Churchill included) in the 1920s, and he was wooed by all sides during the decade following— with Chamberlain traveling to Rome as late as January 1939 in an effort to stop Italy from drifting completely into the German camp.[42]

But diplomatic prominence was not the only measure of Italy's new greatness. This fascist state, with its elimination of factious party politics, its "corporatist" planning for the economy in the place of disputes between capital and labor, its commitment to government action, seemed to offer a new model to a disenchanted postwar European society—and one attractive to those who feared the alternative "model" being offered by the Bolsheviks. Because of Allied investments, industrialization had proceeded apace from 1915 to 1918, at least in those heavy industries related to arms production. Under Mussolini, the state committed itself to an ambitious modernization program, which ranged from draining the Pontine marshes, to the impressive development of hydroelectricity, to the improvements in the railway system. The electrochemical industry was furthered, and rayon and other artificial fibers were developed. Automobile production was increased, and the Italian aeronautical industry seemed to be among the most innovative in the world, its aircraft gaining a whole series of speed and altitude records.[43]

Military power, too, seemed to give good indications of Italy's rising status. Although he had not spent much on the armed services in the 1920s, Mussolini's belief in force and conquest and his rising desire to expand Italy's territories led to significant increases in defense spending during the 1930s. Indeed, a little over 10 percent of national income and as much as one-third of government income was devoted to the armed forces by the mid-1930s, which in absolute figures was more than was spent by Britain or France, and much more than the American totals. Smart new battleships were being laid down, to rival the French navy and the British Mediterranean Fleet, and to support Mussolini's claim that the Mediterranean was indeed *mare nostrum*. When Italy entered the war it possessed 113 submarines—"the largest submarine force in the world except perhaps that of the Soviet Union."[44] Even larger sums were being allocated to the air force, the Regia Aeronautica, in the years leading up to 1940, in keeping perhaps with early fascism's emphasis upon modernity, science, speed, and glamour. Both in Abyssinia and, even more, in Spain, the Italians demonstrated the uses of air power and convinced themselves—and many foreign observers—that they possessed the most advanced air force in the world. This buildup of the navy and the air force left fewer funds for the Italian army, but its thirty divisions were being substantially restructured in the late 1930s, and new tanks and artillery were being planned. Besides, Mussolini felt, there were the masses of fascist *squadristi* and trained bands, so that in another total war the nation might well possess the claimed "eight million bayonets." All this boded well for the creation of a second Roman Empire.

Alas for such dreams, fascist Italy was, in power-political terms, spectacularly weak. The key problem was that even "at the end of the First World War Italy, economically speaking, was a semideveloped country."[45] Its per capita income in 1920 was probably equal to that achieved by Britain and the United States in the early *nineteenth* century, and by France a few decades later. National income data concealed the fact that per capita income in the north was 20 percent above, in the south 30 percent below, the average; and the gap, if anything, was widening. Thanks to a continued flow of emigrants, Italy's population in the interwar years increased by only around 1 percent a year; since the gross domestic product grew by 2 percent a year, the average per capita rose by a mere 1 percent a year, which was not disastrous, but hardly an economic miracle. At the root of Italy's weakness was the continued reliance upon small-scale agriculture, which in 1920 accounted for 40 percent of GNP and absorbed 50 percent of the total working population.[46] It was a further sign of this economic backwardness that even as late as 1938 over half a family's expenditure went on food. Far from reducing these proportions, fascism, with its heavy emphasis upon the virtues of rural life, endeavored to support agriculture by a battery of measures, including protective tariffs, widespread land reclamation, and, finally, complete control of the wheat market. Important in the regime's calculations was the desire to reduce dependence upon foreign food producers and the strong wish to prevent a further drift of peasants into the towns, where they would boost the unemployment totals and add to the social problem. The consequence was a very heavy *under*employment in the countryside, with all of the corresponding features: low productivity, illiteracy, immense regional disparities.

Given the relatively backward nature of the Italian economy and the state's willingness to spend money both on armaments and on the preservation of village agriculture, it is not surprising that the amount of savings for entrepreneurial investment was low. If the First World War had already reduced the stock of domestic capital, the economic depression and the turn to protectionism were further blows. To be sure, companies boosted by government orders for aircraft or trucks could make a good profit, but it is unlikely that Italy's industrial development benefited (on the whole) from attempts at autarky; tariffs merely gave protection to inefficient producers, while the general neo-mercantilism of the age reduced the flow of foreign investments which had done much to stimulate Italian industrialization earlier. By 1938 Italy still possessed only 2.8 percent of world manufacturing production, produced 2.1 percent of its steel, 1.0 percent of its pig iron, 0.7 percent of its iron ore, and 0.1 percent of its coal, and consumed energy from modern sources at a rate far below that of any of the other Great Powers. Finally, in the light of Mussolini's evident eagerness to go to war against France, and sometimes even France and Britain combined, it is worth noting that Italy remained embarrassingly dependent upon imported fertilizer, coal, oil, scrap iron, rubber, copper, and other vital raw materials—80 percent of which had to come past Gibraltar or Suez, and much of which was carried in British ships. It was typical of the regime that no contingency plan had been prepared in the event of these imports ceasing, and that a policy of stockpiling such strategic materials was out of the question, since by the late 1930s Italy didn't even have the foreign currency to cover its current needs. This chronic currency shortage also helps to explain why the Italians also could not afford to pay for the German machine tools so vital for the production of the more modern aircraft, tanks, guns, and ships which were being developed in the years after 1935 or so.[47]

Economic backwardness also explains why, despite all the attention and resources which Mussolini's regime devoted to the armed forces, their actual performance and condition were poor—and getting worse. The navy was probably the best-equipped of the three services, but probably too weak to drive the Royal Navy out of the Mediterranean. It possessed no aircraft carriers—Mussolini had forbidden their construction—and was forced instead to rely upon the Regia Aeronautica, a poor arrangement given the lack of interservice cooperation. Its cruisers were fair-weather vessels, and its great array of submarines proved to be a heavy investment in obsolescence: "The boats lacked attack computers, their air-conditioning systems gave off poisonous gases when tubing ruptured under depth-charge attack, and they were relatively slow in diving, which proved embarrassing when enemy aircraft approached."[48] Similar signs of obsolescence could be seen in the Italian air force, which had shown itself capable of bombing (if not always hitting) Abyssinian tribesmen, and had then impressed many observers by its Spanish Civil War performances. But by the late 1930s the Fiat CR42 biplane was totally eclipsed by the newer British and German monoplanes; and even the bomber force suffered from having only light to medium bombers, with weak engines and stupendously ineffective bombs. Yet both the above services had secured increasing shares of the defense budget. The army, by contrast, saw its share drop from 58.2 percent in 1935–1936 to 44.5 percent in 1938–1939, and that at a time when it desperately needed modern tanks, artillery, trucks, and communications systems. The "main battle tank" of the Italian army, when it entered the Second World War, was the Fiat L.3, of three and a half tons, with no radio, little vision, and only two machine guns—this at a time when the latest German and French tank designs were close upon twenty tons and had much heavier weaponry.

Given the almost irremediable weaknesses which afflicted the Italian economy under fascism, it would be rash to suggest that it could ever have won a war against another proper Great Power; but its prospects were made the bleaker by the fact that its armed forces were the victims of early rearmament—and swift obsolescence. Since this was a common problem in the 1930s, affecting France and Russia to almost the same degree, it is important to go into it in a little more detail before returning to our specific analysis of Italy's weaknesses.

The key factor was the intense application of science and technology to military developments in this period, which was transforming weapon systems in all the services. Fighter aircraft, for example, were swiftly changing from maneuverable (but lightly armed and fabric-covered) biplanes which could do about 200 mph to "duraluminum monoplane aircraft laden with multiple heavy machine guns and cannon, cockpit armor and self-sealing fuel tanks"[49] which flew at up to 400 mph and required much more powerful engines. Bomber aircraft were changing—in those nations which could afford the move—from two-engined, shorter-range medium bombers to the massively expensive four-engined types capable of carrying large bomb loads and with a radius of over two thousand miles. Post–Washington Treaty battleships (e.g., of the *King George V, Bismarck,* and *North Carolina* sort), were much faster, better-armored, and equipped with far heavier antiaircraft defenses than their predecessors. The newer aircraft carriers were large, well-designed types, with a much greater striking power than the updated seaplane carriers and converted battle cruisers of the 1920s. Tank developers were rushing ahead with heavier, better-armed, and better-armored models which required far more powerful engines than those which had driven the light experimental prototypes of the pre-1935 years. Furthermore, all of these weapon systems were just beginning to be affected by the changes in electrical communications, by improvements in navigational devices and antisubmarine detection equipment, by early radar and improved radio equipment—which not only made the newer weapons so much more expensive, but also complicated the procurement process. Did one have enough of the new machine tools, gauges, and jigs to switch to these improved models? Could armaments works and electrical suppliers meet the rising

demand? Did they have enough spare plant, and trained engineers?
Dare one *stop* producing the tried but perhaps obsolescent older models while waiting for the newer types to be tested and then built?
Finally—and critically—how did these desperate rearmament efforts
relate to the state of the nation's economy, its access to overseas as well
as domestic resources, its ability to pay its way? These were, of course,
not new dilemmas—but they pressed upon the decision-makers of the
1930s with a far greater urgency than ever before.

It is in this technological-economic context (as well as in the diplomatic context) that the varying patterns of Great Power rearmament
in the 1930s can best be understood. There are many disparities in the
compilation of the actual annual totals of defense expenditures by
individual nations in this decade, but Table 27 can serve as a fair guide
to what was happening.

Table 27. Defense Expenditures of the Great Powers, 1930–1938[50]
(millions of current dollars)

	Japan	Italy	Germany	USSR	U.K.	France	U.S.
1930	218	266	162	722	512	498	699
1933	183	351	452	707	333	524	570
	(356)	(361)	(620)	(303)	(500)	(805)	(792)
	[387]						
1934	292	455	709	3479	540	707	803
	(384)	(427)	(914)	(980)	(558)	(731)	(708)
	[427]						
1935	300	966	1,607	5,517	646	867	806
	(900)	(966)	(2,025)	(1,607)	(671)	(849)	(933)
	[463]						
1936	313	1,149	2,332	2,933	892	995	932
	(440)	(1,252)	(3,266)	(2,903)	(911)	(980)	(1,119)
	[488]						
1937	940	1,235	3,298	3,446	1,245	890	1,032
	(1,621)	(1,015)	(4,769)	(3,430)	(1,283)	(862)	(1,079)
	[1,064]						
1938	1,740	746	7,415	5,429	1,863	919	1,131
	(2,489)	(818)	(5,807)	(4,527)	(1,915)	(1,014)	(1,131)
	[1,706]						

Seen in this comparative light, the Italian problem becomes clearer.
It had not been a great spender on armaments in absolute terms during
the first half of the 1930s, although even then it had needed to devote
a higher proportion of its national income to the armed services than
probably all other states except the USSR. But the extended Abyssinian
campaign, overlapped by the intervention in Spain, led to greatly increased expenditures between 1935 and 1937. Thus part of Italian
defense spending in those years was devoted to current operations, and
not to the buildup of the services or the armaments industry. On the
contrary, the Abyssinian and Spanish adventures gravely weakened

Italy, not only because of losses in the field, but also because the longer it fought, the more it needed to import—and pay for—vital strategic raw materials, causing the Bank of Italy's reserves to shrink to almost nothing by 1939. Unable to afford the machine tools and other equipment needed to modernize the air force and the army, the country was probably getting *weaker* in the two to three years prior to 1940. The army was not helped by its own reorganization, since the device of creating half again as many divisions by simply reducing each division from three to two regiments led to many officer promotions but to no real increase in efficiency. The air force, supported (if that is the right word) by an industry which was *less* productive than that of 1915–1918, claimed that it had over 8,500 planes; further investigations reduced that total to 454 bombers and 129 fighters, few of which would be regarded as first-rate in other air forces.[51] Without proper tanks or antiaircraft guns or fast fighters or decent bombs or aircraft carriers or radar or foreign currency or adequate logistics, Mussolini in 1940 threw his country into another Great Power war, on the assumption that it was already won. In fact, only a miracle, or the Germans, could prevent a debacle of epic proportions.

All of this emphasis upon weaponry and numbers does, of course, ignore the elements of leadership, quality of personnel, and national proclivity for combat; but the sad fact was that, far from compensating for Italy's matériel deficiencies, those elements merely added to its relative weakness. Despite superficial fascist indoctrination, nothing in Italian society and political culture had altered between 1900 and 1930 to make the army a more attractive career to talented, ambitious males; on the contrary, its collective inefficiency, lack of initiative, and concern for personal career prospects was stultifying—and amazed the German attachés and other military observers. The army was not the compliant tool of Mussolini; it could, and often did, obstruct his wishes, offering innumerable reasons why things could not be done. Its fate was to be thrust, often without prior consultation, into conflicts where something *had* to be done. Dominated by its cautious and inadequately trained senior officers, and lacking a backbone of experienced NCOs, the army's plight in the event of a Great Power war was hopeless; and the navy (except for the enterprising midget submarines) was little better off. If the officer corps and crews of the Regia Aeronautica were better educated and better trained, that would avail them little when they were still flying obsolescent aircraft, whose engines succumbed to the desert sands, whose bombs were hopeless, and whose firepower was pathetic. Perhaps it hardly needs saying that there was no chiefs of staff committee to coordinate plans between the services, or to discuss (let alone settle) defense priorities.

Finally, there was Mussolini himself, a strategical liability of the first order. He was not, it has been argued, the all-powerful leader on the lines of Hitler which he projected himself as being. King Victor Emmanuel III strove to preserve his prerogatives, and succeeded in keeping the loyalties of much of the bureaucracy and the officer corps. The papacy was also an independent, and rival, focus of authority for many Italians. Neither the great industrialists nor the recalcitrant peasantry were enthusiastic about the regime by the 1930s; and the National Fascist Party itself, or at least its regional bosses, seemed more concerned with the distribution of jobs than the pursuit of national glory.[52] But even had Mussolini's rule been absolute, Italy's position would be no better, given Il Duce's penchant for self-delusion, resort to bombast and bluster, congenital lying, inability to act and think effectively, and governmental incompetence.[53]

In 1939 and 1940, the western Allies frequently considered the pros and cons of having Italy fighting on Germany's side rather than remaining neutral. On the whole, the British chiefs of staff preferred Italy to be kept out of the war, so as to preserve peace in the Mediterranean and Near East; but there were powerful counterarguments, which seem in retrospect to have been correct.[54] Rarely in the history of human conflict has it been argued that the entry of an additional foe would hurt one's enemy more than oneself; but Mussolini's Italy was, in that way at least, unique.

The challenge to the status quo posed by Japan was also of a very individual sort, but needed to be taken much more seriously by the established Powers. In the world of the 1920s and 1930s, heavily colored by racist and cultural prejudices, many in the West tended to dismiss the Japanese as "little yellow men"; only during the devastating attacks upon Pearl Harbor, Malaya, and the Philippines was this crude stereotype of a myopic, stunted, unmechanical people revealed for the nonsense it was.[55] The Japanese navy trained hard, both for day and night fighting, and learned well; its attachés fed a continual stream of intelligence back to the planners and ship designers in Tokyo. Both the army and the naval air forces were also well trained, with a large stock of competent pilots and dedicated crewmen.[56] As for the army proper, its determined and hyperpatriotic officer corps stood at the head of a force imbued with the *bushido* spirit; they were formidable troops both in offensive and defensive warfare. The fanatical zeal which led to the assassination of (allegedly) weak ministers could easily be transformed into battlefield effectiveness. While other armies merely talked of fighting to the last man, Japanese soldiers took the phrase literally, and did so.

But what distinguished the Japanese from, say, Zulu warriors was that by this period the former possessed military-technical superiority as well as sheer bravery. The pre-1914 process of industrialization had been immensely boosted by the First World War, partly because of

Allied contracts for munitions and a strong demand for Japanese shipping, partly because its own exporters could step into Asian markets which the West could no longer supply.[57] Imports and exports tripled during the war, steel and cement production more than doubled, and great advances were made in chemical and electrical industries. As with the United States, Japan's foreign debts were liquidated during the war and it became a creditor. It also became a major shipbuilding nation, launching 650,000 tons in 1919 compared with a mere 85,000 tons in 1914. As the League of Nations *World Economic Survey* showed, the war had boosted its manufacturing production even more than that of the United States, and the continuation of that growth during the 1919–1938 period meant that it was second only to the Soviet Union in its overall rate of expansion (See Table 28).

Table 28. Annual Indices of Manufacturing Production, 1913–1938[58]
(1913 = 100)

	World	U.S.	Germany	U.K.	France	USSR	Italy	Japan
1913	100.0	100.0	100.0	100.0	100.0	100.0	100.0	100.0
1920	93.2	122.2	59.0	92.6	70.4	12.8	95.2	176.0
1921	81.1	98.0	74.7	55.1	61.4	23.3	98.4	167.1
1922	99.5	125.8	81.8	73.5	87.8	28.9	108.1	197.9
1923	104.5	141.4	55.4	79.1	95.2	35.4	119.3	206.4
1924	111.0	133.2	81.8	87.8	117.9	47.5	140.7	223.3
1925	120.7	148.0	94.9	86.3	114.3	70.2	156.8	221.8
1926	126.5	156.1	90.9	78.8	129.8	100.3	162.8	264.9
1927	134.5	154.5	122.1	96.0	115.6	114.5	161.2	270.0
1928	141.8	162.8	118.3	95.1	134.4	143.5	175.2	300.2
1929	153.3	180.8	117.3	100.3	142.7	181.4	181.0	324.0
1930	137.5	148.0	101.6	91.3	139.9	235.5	164.0	294.9
1931	122.5	121.6	85.1	82.4	122.6	293.9	145.1	288.1
1932	108.4	93.7	70.2	82.5	105.4	326.1	123.3	309.1
1933	121.7	111.8	79.4	83.3	119.8	363.2	133.2	360.7
1934	136.4	121.6	101.8	100.2	111.4	437.0	134.7	413.5
1935	154.5	140.3	116.7	107.9	109.1	533.7	162.2	457.8
1936	178.1	171.0	127.5	119.1	116.3	693.3	169.2	483.9
1937	195.8	185.8	138.1	127.8	123.8	772.2	194.5	551.0
1938	182.7	143.0	149.3	117.6	114.6	857.3	195.2	552.0

By 1938, in fact, Japan had not only become much stronger economically than Italy, but had also overtaken France in all of the indices of manufacturing and industrial production (see Tables 14–18 above). Had its military leaders not gone to war in China in 1937 and, more disastrously, in the Pacific in 1941, one is tempted to conclude that it would also have overtaken British output well before actually doing so, in the mid-1960s.

This is not to say that Japan had effortlessly overcome all of its economic problems, but merely that it was growing markedly stronger. Because of its primitive banking system, it had not found it easy to adjust to becoming a creditor nation during the First World War, and its handling of the money supply had caused great inflation—not to mention the "rice riots" of 1919.[59] As Europe resumed its peacetime production of textiles, merchant vessels, and other goods, Japan felt the pressure of renewed competition; the cost of its manufacturing, at this stage, was still generally higher than in the West. Furthermore, a heavy proportion of the Japanese population remained in small-plot agriculture, and these groups suffered not only from rising rice imports from Taiwan and Korea, but also from the collapse of the vital silk export trade when American demand fell away after 1930. Seeking to alleviate these miseries by imperial expansion was always a temptation for worried or ambitious Japanese politicians—the conquest of Manchuria, for example, meant economic benefits as well as military gains. On the other hand, when Japanese industry and commerce recovered during the 1930s, partly through rearmament and partly through the exploitation of captive East Asian markets, so its dependence upon imported raw materials grew (in this respect, at least, it was similar to Italy). As the Japanese steel industry expanded, it required larger amounts of pig iron and ore from China and Malaya. Domestic supplies of coal and copper were also inadequate for industry's requirements; but even that was less critical than the country's near-total reliance upon petroleum fuels of all sorts. Japan's quest for "economic security"[60]—a self-evident good in the eyes of its fervent nationalists and the military rulers—drove it ever forward, but with mixed results.

Despite—and, of course, in some ways because of—these economic difficulties, the finance ministry under Takahashi was willing to borrow recklessly in the early 1930s in order to allocate more to the armed services, whose share of government spending rose from 31 percent in 1931–1932 to 47 percent in 1936–1937;[61] when he finally took alarm at the economic consequences and sought to modify further increases, he was promptly assassinated by the militarists, and armaments expenditures spiraled upward. By the following year, the armed services were taking 70 percent of government expenditure and Japan was thus spending, in absolute terms, more than any of the far wealthier democracies. Thus the Japanese armed services were in a far better position than those of Italy by the late 1930s, and possibly also those of France and Britain. The Imperial Japanese Navy, legally restricted by the Washington Treaty to slightly over half the size of either the British or American navy, was in reality much more powerful than that. While the two leading naval powers economized during the 1920s and early 1930s, Japan built right up to the treaty limits—and, indeed, secretly went far beyond them. Its heavy cruisers, for example, displaced closer to 14,000 tons than the 8,000 tons required by the treaty. All of the Japanese major warships were fast and very heavily armed; its older battleships had been modernized, and by the late 1930s it was laying down the gigantic *Yamato*-class vessels, larger than anything else in the world. The most important element of all, although the battleship admirals didn't properly realize it, was Japan's powerful and efficient naval air service, with 3,000 aircraft and 3,500 pilots, which centered upon the ten carriers in the fleet but also included some deadly-efficient bomber and torpedo-carrying squadrons on land. Japanese torpedoes were of unequaled power and quality. Finally, the country also possessed the world's third-largest merchant marine, although (curiously) the navy itself virtually neglected antisubmarine warfare.[62]

Because of conscription, the Japanese army had ready access to manpower and could ingrain the recruits into its traditions of absolute obedience and mass maximum effort. While it had kept the size of the army limited in earlier years, its expansion program saw the 24 divisions and 54 air squadrons of 1937 grow to 51 active service divisions and 133 air squadrons by 1941. In addition, there were 10 depot divisions (for training), and a large number of independent brigade and garrison troops, probably equal to another 30 divisions. By the eve of war, therefore, Japan had an army of over 1 million men, backed by nearly 2 million trained reserves. It was not strong in tanks, for which neither the terrain nor the wooden bridges of much of East Asia were suitable, but it had good mobile artillery and was well trained for jungle work, river crossings, and amphibious landings. The army's 2,000 first-line aircraft (like the navy's) included the formidable Zero fighter, as fast and maneuverable as anything produced in Europe at the time.[63]

Japan's military effectiveness, therefore, was extremely high; but it was not free of weaknesses. Government decision-making in the 1930s was rendered erratic and, at times, incoherent by clashes between the various factions, by civil-military disputes, and by assassinations. In addition, there was the lack of proper coordination between the army and the navy—not a unique situation by any means, but the more dangerous in Japan's case since each service had a quite different enemy *and* area of operations in mind. While the navy anticipated a future war with either Britain or the United States, the army's eyes were fixed exclusively upon the Asian continent and the threat to Japanese interests there posed by the Soviet Union. Since the army was much more influential in Japanese politics and also dominated imperial general headquarters, its views generally prevailed. There was no effective opposition, from either the navy or the foreign office, although both were reluctant, when in 1937 the army insisted upon taking further action against China following the contrived Marco Polo Bridge incident. Despite a large-scale invasion of northern China from Manchurian soil, and landings along the Chinese coast, the Japanese army found it impossible to achieve a decisive victory. While losing great numbers of troops, Chiang Kai-shek kept up the struggle and moved even farther inland, pursued by Japanese striking columns and aircraft. The problem for Imperial General Headquarters was not so much the losses this campaigning involved—the army probably suffered only 70,000 casualties—but the stupendous costs of such inconclusive and extended warfare. By the end of 1937, there were over 700,000 Japanese troops in China, a number which steadily increased (though Willmott's figure of 1.5 million by 1938 seems far too high)[64] without ever managing to force the Chinese to surrender. The "China Incident," as Tokyo referred to it, was now costing $5 million a day and causing an even larger rise in defense spending. Rationing was introduced in 1938, as were a whole series of enactments which virtually put Japan onto a "total war" mobilization. The national debt spiraled upward at an alarming rate as the government borrowed more and more to pay for the enormous defense expenditures.[65]

What made this strategy even more difficult to sustain was Japan's shrinking stocks of foreign currency and raw materials, and her increasing dependence upon imports from the disapproving Americans, British, and Dutch. After her air forces had used up large amounts of fuel in the China campaigns, "factories were ordered to reduce their fuel by 37 percent, ships by 15 percent and automobiles by 65 percent."[66] This situation was the more intolerable to the Japanese since they believed that Chiang Kai-shek's forces were only able to keep up their resistance because of the flow of western supplies, via the Burma Road, French Indochina, or other routes. Logically, inexorably, the conviction grew that Japan would have to strike south, both to isolate China and to gain a firm grip upon the oil and other raw materials of Southeast Asia, the Dutch East Indies, and Borneo. This was, of course, the direction which the Japanese navy had always favored; yet even the army, despite its prior concern about the Soviet Union and its extensive operations in China, was forced slowly to admit that action was necessary to ensure Japan's economic security.

This led to the gravest problem of all. Given the armed strength which they had built up by the late 1930s, the Japanese could easily sweep the French out of Indochina and the Dutch out of the East Indies. Even the British Empire would have found it difficult to hold its own against Japan, as the strategic planners in Whitehall secretly admitted during the 1930s; and by the time war had broken out in Europe, a full British commitment to the Far East was impossible. It was quite another thing, however, for the Japanese to go to war against either Russia or the United States. In the prolonged and bloody border clashes with the Red Army around Nomonhan between May and August 1939, for example, Imperial General Headquarters was alarmed at the clear superiority of Soviet artillery and aircraft, and at the firepower of the much larger Russian tanks.[67] With the Kwantung (Manchuria) army possessing only half the number of divisions that the Russians had placed in Mongolia and Siberia, and with large forces increasingly bogged down in China, even the more extremist army officers recognized that war against the USSR had to be avoided—at least until the international circumstances were more favorable.

But if a northern war would expose Japan's limitations, would not a southern one also, if it ran the risk of bringing in the United States? And would the Roosevelt administration, which so strongly disapproved of the Japanese actions in China, stand idly by while Tokyo helped itself to the Dutch East Indies and Malaya, thereby escaping from American economic pressure? The "moral embargo" upon the export of aeronautical materials in June 1938, the abrogation of the American-Japanese trade treaty in the following year, and, most of all, the British-Dutch-U.S. ban of oil and iron-ore exports following the Japanese takeover of Indochina in July 1941 made it clear that "economic security" could be achieved only at the price of war with the United States. But the United States had nearly twice the population of Japan, and *seventeen* times the national income, produced five times as much steel, and seven times as much coal, and made eighty times as many motor vehicles each year. Its industrial potential, even in a poor year like 1938, was seven times larger than Japan's;[68] it might in other years be nine or ten times as large. Even granted the high level of Japanese patriotic fervor and the memory of its staggering successes against far larger opponents in 1895 (China) and 1905 (Russia), what it was now planning bordered on the incredible—and the absurd. Indeed, to such sober strategists as Admiral Yamamoto, an attack upon a country as powerful as the United States seemed folly, especially when it became clear that most of the Japanese army would remain in China; yet *not* to take on the United States after July 1941 would leave Japan exposed to western economic blackmail, which was also an intolerable notion. Unable to go back, the Japanese military leaders prepared to plunge forward.[69]

In the 1920s, Germany appeared to be by far the weakest and most troubled of those Great Powers which felt dissatisfied by the postwar territorial and economic arrangements. Shackled by the military provisions of the Versailles Treaty, burdened by the need to pay reparations, constrained strategically by the transfer of border regions to France and Poland, and convulsed internally by inflation, class tension, and the corresponding volatility and confusion of the electorate and the parties, Germany possessed nothing like the freedom of action in foreign affairs enjoyed by Italy and Japan. While things had vastly improved by the late 1920s in consequence of the general prosperity and of Stresemann's successes in enhancing Germany's position by diplomacy, the country still was a politically troubled "half-free" Great

Power when the financial and commercial crises of 1929–1933 devastated both its precarious economy and its much-disliked Weimar democracy.[70]

If the advent of Hitler transformed Germany's position in Europe within a matter of years, it is important to recall the points made earlier: that virtually every German was a "revisionist" to a greater or lesser degree and much of the early Nazi foreign-policy program represented a *continuity* with the past ambitions of German nationalists and the suppressed armed forces; that the 1919–1922 border settlements in east-central Europe were seen as unsatisfactory by many other nations and ethnic groups, who pressed for changes long before the Nazis seized power, and were willing to join Berlin in amending them; that Germany, despite its losses of territory, population, and raw materials, retained the industrial potential to be the greatest of the European powers; and that the international balances which were needed to contain a resurgence of German aggrandizement were now far more disparate, and much less coordinated, than prior to 1914. That Hitler soon achieved staggering successes in his scheme to improve Germany's diplomatic and military position is undoubted; but it is also clear that many existing circumstances favored his ruthless exploitation of opportunities.[71]

Hitler's "specialness," so far as the themes pursued in this book are concerned, lay in two areas. The first was the peculiarly intense and manic nature of the National Socialist Germany which he intended to create: a society racially "purified" by the elimination of Jews, gypsies, and any other allegedly non-Teutonic elements; a people whose minds and souls were given over to unquestioned support of the regime, which would thereby replace the older loyalties of class, church, region, and family; an economy mobilized and controlled for the purposes of expanding *Deutschtum* whenever or wherever the leader decreed that to be necessary, and against however many of the Great Powers; an ideology of force and struggle and hatred, which rejoiced in smashing foes and scorned the very idea of compromise.[72] Given the size and complexity of twentieth-century German society, it hardly needs remarking that this was an unreal vision: there were "limits to Hitler's power"[73] across the country; there were individuals, and interest groups, which supported him in 1932–1933, and even until 1938–1939, but with decreasing enthusiasm; and no doubt for all those who openly opposed the regime there were many others who developed a mentally internalized resistance. But despite such exceptions, there was also no question that the National Socialist regime was immensely popular and—even more important—absolutely unchallenged in respect to its disposition of national resources. With a political culture bent upon war and conquest and a political economy distorted to the extent that by 1938 52 percent of government expenditure and a massive 17 percent of gross national product was being poured into armaments, Germany had entered a different league from any of the other western European states. In the year of Munich, indeed, Germany was spending more upon weapons than Britain, France, and the United States combined. Insofar as the state apparatus could concentrate them, all German national energies were being mobilized for a renewed struggle.[74]

The second major feature of German rearmament was the frighteningly precarious state of the national economy as it heated up during this expansion. As has been noted above, both the Italian and the Japanese economies manifested similar problems by the late 1930s— and the same would happen to France and Britain when they sought to respond to the fantastic pace of arms increases. But in none of those countries was the buildup of the armed forces as sudden as in Germany. In January 1933 its army was, legally, supposed to be no more than 100,000 men, although well before Hitler's accession the military had secret plans to expand from a seven-division force to a twenty-one division force—just as it had privately prepared for the reestablishment of an air force, tank formations, and other elements banned by the Versailles Treaty. Hitler's general instruction of February 1933 to von Fritsch, "to create an army of the greatest possible strength,"[75] was simply taken by the planners to be the go-ahead to turn the earlier scheme into effect, free at last from financial and manpower restrictions. By 1935, however, conscription was announced and the army's ceiling raised to thirty-six divisions. The acquisition of Austrian units in 1938, the takeover of the Rhineland military police, the creation of armored divisions, and the reorganization of the Landwehr sent that figure ever higher. In the crisis period of late 1938, the army totaled forty-two active, eight reserve, and twenty-one Landwehr divisions; by the next summer, when the war began, the German field army's order of battle listed 103 divisions—a jump of thirty-two within one year.[76] The Luftwaffe's expansion was even greater and faster. German aircraft production of a mere thirty-six planes in 1932 rose to 1,938 in 1934 and 5,112 in 1936, and the service's twenty-six squadrons (July 1933 directive) rose to 302 squadrons, with over 4,000 front-line aircraft, at the outset of war.[77] If the navy was less impressive in size, then that was to a large degree due to the fact that (as Tirpitz earlier discovered) the creation of a powerful battle fleet took at least one to two decades. Nonetheless, by 1939 Admiral Raeder commanded a number of fast, modern warships, the navy had five times the number of personnel that it possessed in 1932, and it was spending twelve times as much as before Hitler came to power.[78] At sea, as well as on land and in the air, the German rearmament program was intent upon altering the balance of power as soon as possible.

While all this looked impressive from the outside, it was decidedly shaky within. The blows the German economy had received from the Versailles territorial arrangements, the great inflation of 1923, the payment of reparations, and the difficulty of reentering pre-1914 foreign markets meant that it was only in 1927–1928 that Germany's output equaled that achieved prior to the First World War. But this recovery was promptly ruined by the great economic crisis of the following few years, which hit Germany more severely than most other countries; by 1932, industrial production was only 58 percent that of 1928, exports and imports had been more than halved, the gross national product had fallen from 89 billion to 57 billion reichsmarks, and unemployment had swollen from 1.4 to 5.6 million people.[79] Much of Hitler's early popularity stemmed from the fact that the widespread programs of roadbuilding, electrification, and industrial investment greatly reduced the unemployment totals even before conscription did the rest.[80] By 1936, however, the economic recovery was being increasingly affected by the fantastic expenditure upon armaments. In the short term, this spending was yet another quasi-Keynesian government boost to capital investment and industrial growth. In the medium, let alone the long, term, the economic consequences were frightening. Probably only the U.S. economy could, without major difficulty, have withstood the strain placed upon it by this level of arms spending; the German economy certainly could not.

The first serious problem, little perceived by foreign observers at the time, was the quite chaotic structure of National Socialist decision-making, something which Hitler seems to have encouraged in order to retain ultimate authority. Despite the pronouncements of the Four-Year Plan, there was no coherent national program to relate the arms buildup to Germany's economic capacity and to allocate priorities between the services; Goering, nominally in charge of the plan, was a hopeless administrator. Instead, each branch pursued its own breakneck expansion, setting new (often preposterous) targets and then competing for the necessary allocations of capital investment and, especially, raw materials. To be sure, the situation would have been even more chaotic had the government not imposed strict controls upon labor, compelled private industry to reinvest its profits into manufactures approved of by the state and, through high taxation, deficit borrowing, checking wages and personal consumption, also forced an increasing amount of the national product into capital investment for the arms industry. But even when government expenditure soared to 33 percent of GNP by 1938 (and much "private" investment was by then really done at the state's request), there were insufficient resources to meet the overlapping and sometimes megalomaniacal demands of the armed services. The Z-Plan fleet being built for the German navy would have needed 6 million tons of fuel oil (equal to Germany's entire consumption in 1938); the Luftwaffe's plan to have 19,000 (!) front-line and reserve aircraft by 1942 would require "85 percent of the existing *world* production of oil."[81] In the meantime, each service struggled to get a larger share of skilled manpower, steel, ball bearings, petroleum, and other vital strategic materials.

Finally, this frantic arms buildup clashed with Germany's acute dependence upon imported raw materials. Rich only in coal, the Reich required vast amounts of iron ore, copper, bauxite, nickel, petroleum, rubber, and many other items upon which modern industry—and modern weapons systems—relied.[82] By contrast, the United States, the British Empire, and the Soviet Union were well endowed in all those respects. Before 1914, Germany had paid for such imports by its booming export of manufactures: in the 1930s, this was no longer possible, since German industry was now being redirected into the production of tanks, guns, and aircraft for the Wehrmacht's consumption. Furthermore, the costs of the First World War and of later reparations, together with the collapse in the traditional export trades, had drained Germany of virtually all foreign currency; in 1938, it possessed only 1 percent of the world's gold and financial reserves, compared with the United States' 54 percent and France's and Britain's 11 percent each.[83] Hence the strict regime of currency controls, barter arrangements, and other special "deals" instituted by Reich agencies in order to pay for vital imports without transferring gold or currency. Hence, too, the much proclaimed efforts to escape from such dependence by the production of synthetic substitutes (oil, fertilizer, etc.) under the Four-Year Plan. Each of these devices helped; none of them, or even all of them together, could balance the demands made by the arms buildup. This explains the recurrent crises within the German armaments industry, as the national stockpiles of raw materials were exhausted and funds ran out to pay for fresh supplies. In 1937, Raeder warned that the entire naval construction would have to be halted unless more materials were secured. And in January 1939, Hitler himself ordered massive reductions in allocations to the Wehrmacht of steel, copper, rubber, and other materials while the economy waged an "export battle" to raise foreign currency.[84]

There were three related consequences of the above for German power and policies. The first was that Germany was not as strong, militarily, by 1938–1939 as Hitler liked to boast and the western democracies feared. The field army, claiming a strength of 2.75 million men at the outset of war, contained a small number of mobile, well-armed divisions and a very long tail of underequipped reserve divisions; experienced officers and NCOs were almost overwhelmed by the need to train such a mass of raw soldiery. Munitions stocks were slim. Even the famed panzer units had fewer tanks than the Anglo-French totals at the onset of hostilities. The navy, which was planning for a war in the mid-1940s, described itself as "completely inadequately

armed for the great conflict with Britain"[85]—a fair summary in respect
to surface warships, even if the U-boats were going to help redress the
balance. As for the Luftwaffe, it was strong chiefly because its foes were
so chronically weak—but it always suffered from a lack of reserves and
supporting services. In the international crises of the late 1930s, it had
never been as powerful as its opponents had imagined—and both its
aircraft industry and its aircrews had found it very difficult to adjust
to the "second generation" of planes. For example, the number of
aircraft crews "fully operational" was far fewer than those defined as
"front-line" during the Munich crisis—and the very idea of bombing
London to a cinder was absurd.[86]

Still, it may be unwise to go all the way with recent revisionist
literature about Germany's unreadiness for war in 1939. At the end of
the day, military effectiveness is relative. Few, if any, armed services
claim that all their needs are satisfied; and the German weaknesses
have to be measured against those of their foes. When that is done, the
picture seems far more favorable to Berlin, especially because of the
efficiency of its armed services *in operational doctrine:* its army was
prepared to concentrate its tank forces, and then to allow them initiative on the battlefield, keeping in touch by radio; its air force, despite
tendencies toward "strategic" missions, was trained to give assistance
to the army's thrusts; its U-boat arm, though small, was flexible as to
tactics. All this was important compensation for, say, meager stocks of
rubber.[87]

This brings us to the second consequence. Because the German
armed forces had rearmed so rapidly that they severely strained the
economy, there was a massive temptation on Hitler's part to resort to
war in order to obviate such economic difficulties. As he well knew, the
acquisition of Austria brought with it not only another five divisions
of troops, some iron ore and oil fields, and a considerable metal industry, but also $200 million in gold and foreign-exchange reserves.[88] The
Sudetenland was less useful economically (though it did have coal
deposits), and by early 1939 the Reich's foreign currency position was
critical. It was scarcely surprising, therefore, that Hitler was greedily
eyeing the rest of Czechoslovakia and rushed to Prague in March 1939
to examine the booty once the occupation occurred. Apart from the
gold and currency assets held by the Czech national bank, the Germans
also seized large stocks of ores and metals, which were swiftly used to
aid German industry; while the large and profitable Czech arms industry could now be exploited to earn currency for Germany by selling (or
bartering) its products to clients in the Balkans. The aircraft, tanks,
and weapons of the substantial Czech army were also taken, partly to
equip new German divisions, and partly to be sold for foreign currency. All this, together with Czechoslovakia's industrial production,
was a great boost to German power in Europe, and permitted Hitler's

hectic (if somewhat hand-to-mouth) rearmament program to continue—until the next crisis. As Tim Mason has pointed out, "the only
'solution' open to this regime of the structural tensions and crises
produced by dictatorship and rearmament was more dictatorship and
rearmament.... A war for the plunder of manpower and materials lay
square in the dreadful logic of German economic development under
National Socialism."[89]

The third consequence—and problem—was this: just how far could
Germany maintain such a policy of conquest and plunder without
overextending itself? Once the initial German rearmament was under
way, and its armed services were equipped with modern weapons, the
pattern of overcoming weak neighbors and gaining fresh territories,
raw materials, and currency seemed self-fulfilling; by April/May 1939,
it was clear that Poland was the next stage. But even if that country
could be swiftly conquered, was Germany capable of facing France
and Britain—that is, engaging in a war which would be much more
challenging to a Greater German economy still heavily dependent
upon imported raw materials? The evidence suggests that while he was
willing to take the risk of fighting the western democracies in 1939,
Hitler hoped that they would once again back down and allow him
another limited war of plunder, against Poland alone; and this in turn
would help the German economy to prepare its first Great Power war,
somewhere in the mid-1940s.[90] Given the weakened economic and
strategic power of France and Britain, and the hesitancy of their political leaderships by 1939, even a premature struggle with those powers
may have seemed worth the risk—although if the military operations
were stalemated on the lines of the 1914–1918 war, Germany's initial
lead in modern armaments would probably be slowly eroded. Victory
for the Führer and his regime would, however, be much more problematical if the United States should lend its aid to the Allies; or if
operations were extended into Russia, where the sheer size of the
country implied lengthy, drawn-out fighting which placed a premium
on economic stamina.

On the other hand, since the Nazi regime lived upon conquest, and
Hitler was driven forward from one acquisition to the next, how and
where could a halt be called? The full logic of his megalomania implied
that no other state should be a challenge to Germany in Europe, and
possibly in the world. Only by this means would his foes be crushed,
the "Jewish problem" solved, and the Thousand-Year Reich established
on a firm footing.[91] Despite all the lines of continuity, the German
Führer was quite different from his Frederickian and Bismarckian
forebears in his fantastic schemes for world power and his ultimate
disregard for all the obstacles which stood in the way of this design.
Impelled as much by these manic, long-term ambitions as by the need

to escape from short-term crises, Hitler, like the Japanese, was committed to altering the international order as soon as possible.

France and Britain

The position of both France and Britain in the face of this gathering storm was one of acute and increasing difficulty. Although there were many important differences between them, both were liberal-capitalist democracies which had been badly hurt by the war, which were unable (despite their best efforts) to recover in any sustained way the rosy Edwardian political economy of their memories, which felt under large and growing pressure from the labor movement at home, and which possessed a public opinion eager to avoid another conflict and overwhelmingly concerned with domestic, "social" issues rather than foreign affairs. This is by no means to say that the diplomacy of London and Paris was identical; because of their quite different geographical-strategical positions, and the varying pressures brought to bear upon their respective governments, the two democracies frequently differed about how to handle the "German problem."[92] But while they quarreled as to the means, both were unanimous over the end; in the troubled post-1919 years, France and Britain were unquestionably status quo powers.

At the beginning of the 1930s, it was France which seemed the stronger and the more influential, at least on the all-important European scene. Throughout these years it possessed the second-largest army among the Great Powers (after the Soviet Union) and also the second-largest air force (again, the Russian totals were larger). Diplomatically, it was immensely influential, especially at Geneva and in eastern Europe. It had suffered severe economic turbulence in the years immediately following 1919, when the franc had to readjust to the awkward facts that it could no longer rely upon Anglo-American subsidies and that German reparations would be far less than expected. But Poincaré's 1926 stabilization of the currency found French industry in the middle of a remarkable boom; pig-iron production soared from 3.4 million tons in 1920 to 10.3 million tons in 1929, steel output from 3 to 9.7 million, automobiles from 40,000 to 254,000; while chemicals, dyestuffs, and electrical products had all escaped from the pre-war German domination. The favorable fixing of the franc helped French trade, and the Bank of France's large stockpile of gold gave it an influence throughout central and eastern Europe. Even when the "Great Crash" came, France seemed the least affected—partly because of its gold holdings and advantageously placed currency, partly because the French economy was much less dependent upon the international market than, say, Britain's.[93]

After 1933, however, the French economy began to collapse in a steady, systematic, frightening way. The vain attempts to avoid a devaluation of the franc when all of the other major trading countries had gone "off" gold meant that French exports became less and less competitive, and its foreign trade collapsed: "imports went down by 60 percent and exports by 70 percent."[94] After some years of paralysis, the 1935 decision to deflate heavily dealt a blow to the sagging French industrial sector, which was further hit when the 1936 Popular Front administration forced through a forty-hour working week and an increase in wages. That action, and the massive devaluation of the franc in October 1936, accelerated the already enormous flow of gold out of France, badly hurting its international credit. In the agriculture sector, which still employed half of the French nation, and whose yields were still the least efficient in western Europe, surplus production kept prices down and worsened the already low per capita income, a trend accelerated by the drift back to the villages of those losing their jobs in industry; the only (very dubious) benefit of this return to the land was that, as in Italy, it disguised the true level of unemployment. Housebuilding fell off dramatically. The newer industries, like automobiles, stagnated in France just as they were recovering elsewhere. In 1938, the franc was only 36 percent of its 1928 level, French industrial production was only 83 percent of that a decade earlier, steel output a mere 64 percent, building 61 percent. Perhaps the most awful figure—in view of the implications for French *power*—was that its national income in the year of Munich was 18 percent less than that in 1929;[95] and this in the face of a Germany which was fantastically more dangerous, and at a time when massive rearmament was vital.

It would be very easy, therefore, to explain the collapse of French military effectiveness in the 1930s solely in economic terms. Aided by the relative prosperity of the late 1920s, and worried about clandestine German rearmament, France had sharply increased her defense expenditures (especially upon the army) in the budget years 1929–1930 and 1930–1931. Alas, the false hopes placed in the Geneva disarmament talks, followed by the effects of the depression; both had their toll. By 1934, defense expenditures still represented the 4.3 percent of national income which they had done in 1930–1931, but the absolute sum was over 4 million francs less, since the economy was sinking so fast.[96] Although the Popular Front government of Léon Blum sought to reverse this decline in arms expenditures, it was not until 1937 that the 1930 defense estimates were exceeded—and most of that increase went into repairing the more obvious deficiencies in the field army, and into further fortifications. In these critical years, therefore, Germany bounded ahead, both economically and militarily:

France had fallen behind Britain and Germany in automobile production; it had slumped into fourth place in aircraft manufacturing, from first to fourth in less than a decade; its steel production had increased by a miserly 30 percent between 1932 and 1937, compared to the 300 percent increase enjoyed by German industry; its coal production showed a significant decline over the same five-year period, a development which is largely explained by the return of the Saar coal fields in early 1935 and the consequent increase in German production.[97]

With this swiftly weakening economy, and with the debt charges and the outlay for 1914–1918 war pensions composing *half* the total public expenditure, it was impossible for France to reequip its three armed forces satisfactorily even when, as in 1937 and 1938, it spent over 30 percent of its budget upon defense. Ironically, the ungrateful French navy was probably the best catered for, and possessed a well-balanced and modern fleet by 1939—which was of little help in stemming a German blow on land. Of all the services, the most badly affected was the French air force, which was continually starved of funds and for which a small-scale, scattered aeronautics industry eked out a living by producing a mere fifty or seventy planes a month between 1933 and 1937, about one-tenth of the German total. In 1937, for example, Germany built 5,606 aircraft, whereas France produced only 370 (or 743, depending upon the source one uses).[98] Only in 1938 did the government begin pouring money into the aircraft industry, thus producing all the inevitable bottlenecks which come with a too-sudden expansion, not to mention the design—and flying—difficulties caused by the move to newer, high-performance aircraft. The first eighty of the promising Dewoitine 520 fighters were accepted by the air force only in January-April 1940, for example, and its pilots were just beginning to practice flying the plane, when the Blitzkrieg struck.[99]

But behind these economic and production difficulties, most historians concede, lay deeper-seated social and political problems. Shocked by the losses of the Great War, depressed by repeated economic blows and disappointments, divided by class and ideological concerns which intensified as politicians struggled unsuccessfully with the problems of devaluation, deflation, the forty-hour work week, higher taxes, and rearmament, French society witnessed a severe collapse in public morale and cohesion as the 1930s advanced. Far from producing a *union sacrée,* the rise of fascism in Europe had caused—at least by the time of the Spanish Civil War—further divisions of French opinion, with the extreme right preferring (as the street chant went) Hitler to Blum, and with many among the left disliking both a rise in arms spending and the proposed abrogation of the forty-hour week. Such ideological clashes interacted with the volatility of the parties and the chronic instability of French interwar governments (twenty-four changes between 1930 and 1940) to give the impression of a society sometimes on the brink of civil war. At the very least, it was hardly capable of standing up to Hitler's bold moves and to Mussolini's distractions.[100]

As so often before in French politics, all this affected civil-military relations and the standing of the army in society.[101] But quite apart from the general atmosphere of suspicion and gloom in which France's leaders had to operate, there existed a whole array of specific weaknesses. No effective body existed, like the Committee of Imperial Defence or the Chiefs of Staff Sub-Committee in Great Britain, to bring together the military and the nonmilitary branches of government for strategic planning in a systematic way, or even to coordinate the views of the rival services. The leading figures in the army, Gamelin, Georges, Weygand, and (in the background) Pétain, were in their sixties and seventies, defensive-minded, cautious, uninterested in tactical innovations. While flatly rejecting de Gaulle's proposals for a smaller, modernized, tank army, they did not themselves grapple with alternative ways of using the newer weapons of war. The policy of combined arms was not practiced. Problems of battle control and communications (e.g., by radio) were ignored. The role of aircraft was downgraded. Although French intelligence provided lots of information about what the Germans were thinking, it was all ignored; there was open disbelief in the efficacy of using large-scale armored formations, as the Germans were doing in their maneuvers; and all the copies of translations of Guderian's *Achtung Panzer* sent to every garrison library in France remained unread.[102] What this meant was that even when French industry was galvanized into producing considerable numbers of tanks—many, like the SOMUA-35, of very good quality—there was no proper doctrine for their use.[103] Given such failures in command and training, it was going to be extraordinarily difficult for the French army to compensate for the country's sociopolitical malaise and economic decline if ever it came to another great war.

Nor could such weaknesses be overcome, as was the case prior to 1914, by successes in French diplomacy and an advantageous alliance strategy. On the contrary, as the 1930s unfolded, the contradictions in France's external policy became more open. The first of these had already been there, of course, in the irreconcilability of the post-Locarno adoption of the strategic defensive behind the Maginot Line, and the desire to stop German expansion in eastern Europe, if need be by going *forward* to aid France's continental allies as the treaties demanded. The German recovery of the Saarland in 1935 and Hitler's reoccupation of the demilitarized Rhineland zone made a French advance less possible, even had its army leaders been willing to contemplate offensive operations. But that was nothing to the blows which rained upon France's diplomatic and strategic position in 1936: the quarrel over the Abyssinian Crisis with Italy, turning the latter from a potential ally against Germany into a potential foe; the beginning of the Spanish Civil War, with its prospect of another fascist power being established in France's rear; and Belgium's withdrawal into neutrality, with its strategical implications. At the end of that calamitous year, France could no longer concentrate upon its northeast frontier alone; and the idea of its rushing into the Rhineland in order to help an eastern ally had become remote. At the time of the Munich crisis, therefore, many leading Frenchmen were petrified at the prospect of having to fulfill their obligation to Czechoslovakia.[104] Finally, once the Munich agreement had been signed, Paris found the USSR much more hostile to collaboration with the West, and unwilling any longer to take seriously the Franco-Russian pact of 1935.

In such gloomy diplomatic, military, and economic circumstances, it was scarcely surprising that French strategy essentially came to rest upon gaining full-scale British support in any future war with Germany. There were obvious economic reasons for this. France was heavily dependent upon imported coal (30 percent), copper (100 percent), oil (99 percent), rubber (100 percent), and other vital raw materials, much of which came from the British Empire and was carried by the British merchant fleet. If "total war" came, the sagging franc might again need the Bank of England's help to pay its way in the world; indeed, by 1936–1937, France already felt heavily dependent upon Anglo-American financial support.[105] Conversely, only with the Royal Navy's aid could Germany once more be cut off from overseas supplies. By the late 1930s, the assistance of the Royal Air Force was also required—as was the commitment of a fresh British expeditionary force. In all these respects, it has been argued, there was a long-term logic in the French policy of strategic passivism; assuming that any German strike on the west could be halted as in 1914, the superior resources of the Anglo-French empires would eventually prevail—and no doubt also compel the recovery of the Czech and Polish territories temporarily lost in the east.[106]

Yet it could hardly be said that this French strategy of "waiting for Britain" was an unqualified blessing. Obviously, it handed the initiative to Hitler, who after 1934 repeatedly showed that he knew how to take it. In addition, it tied France's hands (although there is considerable evidence that people like Bonnet and Gamelin preferred to be so constrained). Since 1919, the British had been urging the French to adopt a softer, more conciliatory policy toward Germany and strongly disliked what they perceived to be Gallic intransigence; and for years after Hitler's seizure of power, both Britain's government and its people exhibited little appreciation of France's security dilemma. More specifically, the British strongly disapproved of French military commitments to the "successor states" of eastern Europe, and when Anglo-French cooperation became unavoidable, they pressured Paris to repudiate its obligations. Even before the Czech crisis, Britain had

dislocated and undermined the old, hard-line French policy toward
Berlin—without, however, offering anything substantive in its place.
Only in the spring of 1939 did the two countries really come together
into a proper military alliance, and even then their mutual political
suspicions had not fully dissolved.[107] As we shall see below, it seems
fair to argue that Albion was not so much "perfidious" as it was myopic,
wishful-thinking, and obsessed with a score of domestic and imperial
problems; but that merely confirms the fact that it was a weak and
uncertain reed for French policy to rest upon if German expansionism
was to be contained.

Perhaps the greatest miscalculation of France was that Britain in
the late 1930s was as capable of helping check the German challenge
as it had been in 1914. Britain was still a considerable power, of course,
enjoying many strategical advantages and with a manufacturing output and industrial potential twice as large as France's; but its own
position, too, was less substantial and assured than it had been two
decades earlier. Psychologically, the British nation had been badly
scarred by the First World War and disenchanted by the fruitlessness
(so far as the populace could see it) of the "Carthaginian" peace which
followed. This public turnaway from militarism, continental involvements, and any concern for the balance of power coincided both with
the full advent of parliamentary democracy (through the 1918 and
1928 franchise extensions) and with the rise of the Labour Party. Even
more, perhaps, than in France, national politics in these decades
seemed to revolve around the "social" question—a fact reflected in the
small amount (10.5 percent) of public expenditure being devoted to the
armed forces by 1933 compared with the sums allocated the social
services (46.6 percent).[108] This was not a climate, Baldwin and Chamberlain frequently reminded their Cabinet colleagues, in which votes
could be gained by interfering in the intractable problems of east-
central Europe, whose boundaries were (in Whitehall's eyes) less than
sacred.

Even to those political groups and strategic planners who concerned themselves more with foreign affairs than with social issues or
electoral maneuvering, the post-1919 international scene suggested
caution and noncommitment. As soon as the war was over, the self-
governing dominions had pressed for a redefinition of their status.
When that had been effected, through the 1926 Balfour Declaration
and the 1931 Statute of Westminister, they had evolved into virtually
independent states, with (if they wished) separate foreign policies.
None of them was eager to fight over European issues; some, like Eire,
South Africa, and even Canada, were reluctant to fight over anything.
If Britain wished to maintain the image of imperial unity, it followed
that it could go to war only over an issue which would attract the
support of the dominions; and even when such separatism was

modified as the threat from Germany, Italy, and Japan increased, London remained aware of the important *extra*-European dimension to all its foreign-policy decisions.[109] More important still, in strictly military terms, were the "imperial-policing" activities in which the British army, and also the RAF, were engaged in India, Iraq, Egypt, Palestine, and elsewhere. For much of the interwar years, in fact, the British army found itself reverting to a Victorian role: the Russian threat to India was perceived as the greatest (if rather abstract) strategic danger; and keeping the natives quiet was the day-to-day operational activity.[110] Finally, this imperial strand in British grand strategy was powerfully reinforced by the Royal Navy's obsession with sending a "main fleet to Singapore" and with Whitehall's justifiable concern about defending its distant and vulnerable possessions against the Japanese.[111]

It was true that this strategical ambivalence of the British "Janus" was centuries old; but what was altogether more frightening was that it now had to be carried out with a much weakened industrial base. British manufacturing output had been sluggish in the 1920s, in part because of the return of sterling to the gold standard at too high a level. Although it did not suffer as dramatically as Germany and the United States, Britain's ailing economy was shaken to its roots by the worldwide slump after 1929. Textile production, which still provided 40 percent of British exports, was cut by two-thirds; coal, which provided another 10 percent of exports, dropped by one-fifth; shipbuilding was so badly hit that in 1933 production fell to 7 percent of its prewar figure; steel production fell by 45 percent in the three years 1929–1932 and pig-iron production by 53 percent. With international trade drying up and being replaced by currency blocs, Britain's share of global commerce continued in a downward trend, from 14.15 percent (1913) to 10.75 percent (1929) to 9.8 percent (1937). Moreover, the *invisible* earnings from shipping, insurance, and overseas investment, which for over a century had handsomely covered the *visible* trade gap, no longer could do so; by the early 1930s, Britain was living on its capital. The trauma of the 1931 crisis, involving the collapse of the Labour government and the decision to go off gold, made politicians all too aware of the country's economic vulnerability.[112]

To some degree, indeed, those leaders' apprehension may have been exaggerated. By 1934, the economy was slowly beginning to recover. While older industries in the north languished, newer ones—aircraft, automobiles, petrochemicals, electrical goods—were growing.[113] Trade within the "sterling block" provided a certain crutch to British exporters. The drop in food and raw materials prices aided the British consumer. But such palliatives were not sufficient to a Treasury worried about Britain's delicate credit abroad and about further runs on sterling. In their view, the overwhelming priority was for the country to pay its way in the world, which meant balancing the government's books, keeping taxes to a minimum, and controlling state spending. Even when the Manchurian crisis caused the government in 1932 to give up the famous Ten-Year Rule,* the Treasury was swift to insist that "this must not be taken to justify an expanding expenditure by the Defense Services without regard to the very serious financial and economic situation which still obtains."[114]

This combination of domestic-political and economic pressures ensured that, like France, Britain was cutting its defense expenditures during the early 1930s just when the dictator states were beginning to increase theirs. Not until 1936, following several years of studying the country's "defense deficiencies" and the twin shock of Hitler's open rearmament followed by the Abyssinian crisis, did British spending upon the armed services take its first substantial upward rise; but that year's allocation was less than Italy's and only one-third or one-quarter of Germany's. Even at that stage, Treasury controls and politicians' worries about domestic opinion prevented full-scale rearmament, which only really began in the crisis year of 1938. Well before that date, however, the armed services were warning of the impossibility of safeguarding "our trade, territory and vital interests against Germany, Italy and Japan at the same time," and urging the government "to reduce the number of our potential enemies and to gain the support of potential allies."[115] In other words, diplomacy—the diplomacy of appeasement—was required in order to defend this economically weakened, strategically overstretched empire from threats in the Far East, the Mediterranean, and Europe itself. In no foreign theater of war, the chiefs of staff felt, was Britain strong enough; and even that dismal fact was overshadowed by the alarming rise of the Luftwaffe, which made the inhabitants of the island state directly vulnerable for the first time to the military operations of an enemy.[116]

There is some evidence that the British chiefs of staff, too, were excessively gloomy about their country's prospects,[117] like the military professionals in virtually every other state; the First World War had made them cautious and pessimistic.[118] But there *was* no doubt that Britain had been overtaken in the air by Germany by 1936–1937, that its minuscule long-service army could do little on the continent of Europe, and that its navy would find it impossible to control European waters *and* to send a main fleet to Singapore. Perhaps even more perturbing to British decision-makers was that it was now extremely difficult to find those "potential allies" which the chiefs of staff demanded. The coalitions which Britain had woven together to counter Napoleon, the successful *ententes* and *rapprochements* which had been effected in the years after 1900, could no longer be found. Japan

---

*That is, the post-1919 directive that the armed services should frame their estimates on the assumption that they would not be engaged in a major war within the next ten years.

had drifted from being an ally to being a foe; the same had happened to Italy. Russia, the other "flank" power (to use Dehio's term)[119] which traditionally had joined Britain in opposing a continental hegemon, was now in diplomatic isolation and deeply suspicious of the western democracies. Almost as inscrutable and unpredictable, at least to frustrated Whitehall minds, was the policy of the United States in the early to middle 1930s; avoiding all diplomatic and military commitments, still unwilling to join the League, strongly opposed to the various British efforts to buy off the revisionist states (e.g., by admitting Japan's special place in East Asia, or offering special payments and exchange arrangements to Germany), and making it impossible—through the 1937 neutrality legislation—to borrow on the American markets in the way Britain had done to sustain its war effort between 1914 and 1917, the United States was persistently dislocating British grand strategy in the same, perhaps inadvertent, way that Britain was dislocating France's eastern European strategy.[120] This left, then, as potential allies only France itself, and the rest of the British Empire. France's diplomatic needs, however, drew Britain into commitments in Central Europe, which the dominions strongly opposed and which the whole structure of "imperial defense" was incapable of defending; on the other hand, the *extra*-European concerns of the empire took away the attention and resources required to contain the German threat. In consequence, the British during the 1930s found themselves engaged in a global diplomatic and strategical dilemma to which there was no satisfactory solution.[121]

This is not to deny that Baldwin, Chamberlain and their colleagues could have done more, or to claim that the determinants of British appeasement policy were such that all alternative policies proposed by Churchill and other critics were impracticable. There was a persistent willingness on the British government's part, despite all the counterevidence, to trust in "reasonable" approaches toward the Nazi regime. The emotional dislike of Communism was such that Russia's potential as a member of an antifascist coalition was always ignored or downgraded. Vulnerable eastern European states, like Czechoslovakia and Poland, were all too often regarded as nuisances, and the lack of sympathy for France's problems showed a fatal meanness of spirit. Germany's and Italy's power was consistently overrated, on the basis of slim evidence, whereas all British defense weaknesses were seized upon as a reason for inaction. Whitehall's views of the European balance of power were self-serving and short-term. Critics of the appeasement policy such as Churchill were systematically censored and neutralized, even as the government proclaimed that it could only follow (rather than give a lead to) public opinion.[122] For all the plausible, objectively valid grounds behind the British government's desire to avoid standing up to the dictator states, therefore, there is much in its ungenerous, narrow attitude that looks dubious, even at this distance in time.

On the other hand, any investigation of the economic and strategical realities ought also to admit that by the late 1930s, the basic problems affecting British grand strategy were not soluble merely by a change of attitude, or even of prime ministers. Indeed, the more Chamberlain was compelled—by Hitler's further aggressions, and by the outrage of British opinion—to abandon appeasement, the more the fundamental contradictions became evident. Though the chiefs of staff insisted upon massive increases in defense spending, the Treasury argued that such spending would be economically ruinous. Already in 1937, Britain, like France, was spending more of its GNP upon defense than either of those countries had done in the crisis years prior to 1914, but without any significant improvement in security—simply because of the far higher arms spending of the manically driven, overheated German state. But as British defense expenditures soared further—roughly, from 5.5 percent of GNP in 1937 to 8.5 percent in 1938, to 12.5 percent in 1939—its delicate economy also began to suffer. Even when money was released for arms increases, the inadequacy of British industrial plant and the critical shortage of skilled engineers slowed down the hoped-for production of aircraft, tanks, and ships; but this in turn compelled the services to place ever-larger orders for weapons, sheet steel, ball bearings, and other items with neutral countries such as Sweden and the United States, which further drained foreign-currency reserves and threatened the balance of payments. As the country's stocks of gold and dollars shrank, its international credit became shakier than ever. "If we were under the impression that we were as well able as in 1914 to conduct a long war," the Treasury coldly pointed out in response to the fresh rearmament measures of April 1939, "we were burying our head in the sand."[123] This was not a pleasant forecast for a power whose strategic planners assumed that they had no chance of winning a short war, but somehow hoped to prevail in a drawn-out conflict.

Equally serious contradictions were also surfacing in the military sphere on the eve of war. While Britain's 1939 decision to accept once again a formal "continental commitment" to France and its almost parallel decision to give the Mediterranean priority over Singapore in terms of naval deployments settled some long-standing strategical issues, they also left British interests in the Far East totally exposed to the next act of Japanese aggression. In a similarly contradictory way, Britain's swift guarantees to Poland in the spring of 1939, followed by further guarantees to Greece, Rumania, and Turkey, were signs of Whitehall's rediscovery of the importance of eastern Europe and the Balkans within the continental balance of power; but the fact was that the British armed forces had little prospect of defending those lands against determined German attack.

In sum, neither Chamberlain's stiffer policies toward Germany after March 1939 nor even his replacement by Churchill in May 1940 "solved" Britain's strategical and economic dilemmas; all they did was to redefine the problems. For an overstretched global empire at this late stage in its history—still controlling one-quarter of the globe but with only 9 to 10 percent of its manufacturing strength and "war potential"[124]—both appeasement and anti-appeasement brought disadvantages; there was only a choice of evils.[125] That the right choice was made in 1939, to stand up to Hitler's further act of aggression, is undoubted. But by that stage the balance of forces aligned against British interests in Europe and even more in the Far East had become so unfavorable that it was difficult to see how a clear-cut victory against fascism could be secured without the intervention of the neutral Great Powers. And that, too, would bring its problems.

The Offstage Superpowers

As noted above, one of the greatest difficulties which faced British and French decision-makers as they wrestled with the diplomatic and strategical challenges of the 1930s was the uncertainty which surrounded the stance of those two giant and somewhat detached Powers, Russia and the United States. Was it worth making further efforts to persuade them into an alliance against the fascist states, even if this involved substantial concessions to Moscow's and Washington's requirements, and provoked criticism at home? Which of these should be wooed more ardently, and in what respects? Would an open move, say, toward Russia merely provoke rather than deter a German or Japanese reaction? From the viewpoint of Berlin and Tokyo (less so of Rome), the attitude of Russia and the United States was equally important. Would these Powers remain aloof while Hitler reordered the boundaries of central Europe? How would they react to further Japanese expansion in China or operations against the old European empires in Southeast Asia? Would the United States give at least economic aid to the western democracies, as occurred between 1914 and 1917? And would the USSR be bought off, by economic and territorial deals? Finally, did those two enigmatic, introspective polities *really matter*? How strong were they, in fact? How important in the changing international order?

It was harder to attempt an answer to such questions in the case of a "closed" society like the Soviet Union. Nonetheless the outlines of Soviet economic growth and military power in that era now seem evident. The first and most obvious point was that Russia had been dreadfully reduced in strength, more than any of the other Great Powers, by the 1914–1918 conflict and then by the revolution and civil war. Its population had plummeted from 171 million in 1914 to 132 million in 1921. The loss of Poland, Finland, and the Baltic states removed many of the country's industrial plants, railways, and farms, and the prolonged fighting destroyed much that remained. The stupendous decline in manufacturing—down to 13 percent of its 1913 output by 1920—concealed the even greater collapse of certain key commodities: "thus only 1.6 percent of the prewar iron ore was being produced, 2.4 percent of the pig iron, 4.0 percent of the steel, and 5 percent of the cotton."[126] Foreign trade had disappeared altogether, the gross yield of crops was less than half the prewar figure, and per capita national income declined by more than 60 percent to a truly horrendous level. However, since the extreme severity of these falls was chiefly caused by the social and political chaos of the years 1917–1921, it followed that the establishment of Soviet rule (or indeed *any* rule) was bound to effect a recovery of sorts. The prewar and wartime development of Russian industry had bequeathed to the Bolsheviks an array of factories, railway works, and steel mills. There was a basic infrastructure of railways, roads, and telegraph lines. There were industrial workers who could return to the factories once the civil war was over. And there was an established pattern of agricultural production, and the sale of foodstuffs to the towns and cities, which could be restored once Lenin had decided (under the New Economic Policy of 1921) to abandon the fruitless attempts to "communize" the peasantry and instead to permit individual farming. By 1926, therefore, agricultural output had returned to its prewar level, followed two years later by industrial output. The war and revolution had cost Russia thirteen years of economic growth, but it now stood ready to resume its upward surge.

But that "surge" was unlikely to be swift enough—certainly not to the increasingly autocratic Stalin—while Russia labored under its traditional economic weaknesses. With no foreign investment available, capital had somehow to be raised from domestic sources to finance the development of large-scale industry *and* the creation of substantial armed forces in a hostile world. Given the elimination of a middle class, which could either have been encouraged to create capital or plundered for its existing wealth; given, too, the fact that 78 percent of Russian population (1926) remained in a bottom-heavy agricultural sector, which was still overwhelmingly in private hands, there seemed to Stalin only one way for the state to raise money and simultaneously increase the switch from farming to industry: that is, by the collectivization of agriculture, forcing the peasants into communes, destroying the kulaks, controlling the output from the land, and fixing both the wages paid to farm workers and the (far higher) prices of food for resale. In a frighteningly draconian way, the state thus interposed itself between rural producers and urban consumers, and extracted money from each to a degree that the czarist regime had never dared to do. This was accentuated by the deliberate price inflation, a variety of taxes and dues, and the pressures to show one's loyalty by buying state bonds. The overall result, represented in the crude macroeconomic statistics, was that the share of Russian GNP devoted to private consumption, which in other countries going through the "takeoff" to industrialization was around 80 percent, was driven down to the appalling level of 51 or 52 percent.[127]

There were two contrary, yet predictable economic consequences from this extraordinary attempt at a socialist "command economy." The first was the catastrophic decline in Soviet agricultural production, as kulaks (and others) resisted the forced collectivization and then were eliminated. The horrific preemptive slaughter of farm animals—"the number of horses fell from 33.5 million in 1928 to 16.6 million in 1935; and the number of cattle from 70.5 to 38.4 million"[128]—in turn produced a staggering decline in meat and grain outputs and in an already miserable standard of living, not to be recovered until Khrushchev's time. Esoteric calculations have been attempted as to the proportion of the national income which was later returned to agriculture in the form of tractors or electrification—as opposed to the amount siphoned off by collectivization and price controls[129]—but this is an arcane exercise for our purposes, since (for example) tractor factories, once established, were designed to be converted to the production of light tanks; peasants, of course, were not so useful in checking the Wehrmacht. What *was* incontrovertible was that for the moment, Soviet agricultural output collapsed. The casualties, especially during the 1933 famine, could be reckoned in millions of lives. When output began to recover in the late 1930s, it was expedited by hundreds of thousands of tractors, hordes of agricultural scientists, and armies of tightly controlled collectives. But the cost, in human terms, was immeasurable.

The second consequence was altogether brighter, at least for the purposes of Soviet economic-military power. Having driven private consumption's share of the GNP down to a level probably unmatched in modern history—and certainly far lower than, say, the Nazis could ever contemplate in Germany—the USSR was able to deploy the fantastic proportion of around 25 percent of GNP for industrial investment and still possess considerable sums for education, science, and the armed services. While the workplace of much of the Russian people was being transformed at a staggering rate, with the number employed in agriculture dropping from 71 percent to 51 percent in the twelve years 1928–1940, that population was also being educated at an unprecedented pace. This was vital at two levels, since Russia had always suffered—in comparison, say, with Germany or the United

States—from having a poorly trained and illiterate industrial work force, and in possessing only a minuscule number of engineers, scientists, and managers necessary for the higher direction and *steady improvement* of the manufacturing sector. With millions of workers now being trained, either in factory schools or in technical colleges, and then (slightly later) with a vast expansion in university numbers, the country was at last acquiring the trained cadres necessary for sustained growth; the number of graduate engineers in the "national economy" rose, for example, from 47,000 in 1928 to 289,900 in 1941.[130] Many of the figures touted by Soviet propagandists in this period were doubtless inflated and concealed various weak points, but the deliberate allocation of resources to growth was unquestionable. So, too, was the creation of enormous new power plants, steelworks, and factories beyond the Urals, invulnerable to attack from either the West or Japan.

The resulting upturn in manufacturing output and national income—even if one accepts the more cautious estimates—was something unprecedented in the history of industrialization. Because the actual volume and value of output in earlier years (e.g., 1913, let alone 1920) was so low, the percentage changes are almost meaningless— even if Table 28 above serves the useful point of showing how the USSR's manufacturing production was expanding during the Great Depression. However, if one examines only the period of the two Five-Year Plans (1928 to 1937), Russian national income rose from 24.4 to 96.3 billion rubles, coal output increased from 35.4 to 128 million tons and steel production from 4 to 17.7 million tons, electricity output rose sevenfold, machine-tool figures over twentyfold, and tractors nearly fortyfold.[131] By the late 1930s, indeed, Russia's industrial output had not only soared well past that of France, Japan, and Italy but had probably overtaken Britain's as well.[132]

Behind this impressive buildup, however, there still lurked many deficiencies. Although farm output slowly rose in the mid-1930s, Russian agriculture was now less capable than before of feeding the nation, let alone producing a surplus for export; and the yields per acre were still appallingly low. Despite fresh investment in railways, the communications system remained primitive and inadequate for the country's growing needs. In many industries there was a heavy dependence upon foreign firms and foreign expertise, especially from the United States. The "gigantism" of the plants and of the entire manufacturing processes made difficult any swift adjustments of the product mix or the introduction of new designs. There were inevitable bottlenecks, too, because the planned expansion of certain industries did not match the existing stocks of raw materials or skilled manpower. After 1937, the reorientation of the Soviet economy toward a massive armament program was bound to affect industrial continuity and to distort the earlier planning. Above all, there were the great purges.

Whatever the reasons for Stalin's manic, paranoid assault upon so many of his own people, the economic results were serious: "civil servants, managers, technicians, statisticians, even foremen"[133] were swept away into the camps, making Russia's shortage of trained personnel more acute than ever. While the terror no doubt drove many to demonstrate a Stakhanovite loyalty to the system, it also greatly inhibited innovation, experimentation, open discussion, and constructive criticism: "the simplest thing to do was to avoid responsibility, to seek approval from one's superior for any act, to obey mechanically any order received, regardless of local conditions."[134] It saved one's skin; but it did not help the growth of a complex economy.

Having been born out of a war, and feeling acutely threatened by potential enemies—Poland, Japan, Britain—the USSR devoted a large share of the state budget (12–16 percent) to defense expenditures for much of the 1920s. That share fell away during the early years of the first Five-Year Plan, by which time the regular Soviet armed forces had settled down to about 600,000 men, backed by a large but inefficient militia twice that size. The Manchurian crisis and Hitler's accession to power led to swift increases in the size of the army, to 940,000 in 1934 and 1.3 million in 1935. With the rise in industrial output and national income deriving from the Five-Year Plans, large numbers of tanks and aircraft were built. Innovative officers around Tukhachevsky were willing to study (if not fully accept) ideas from Douhet, Fuller, Liddell Hart, Guderian, and other western theorists of warfare, and by the early 1930s the USSR possessed not only a tank army but also a large paratroop force. While the Soviet navy remained small and ineffective, a large aircraft industry was created in the late 1920s, which for a while produced more planes each year than all the other powers combined (see Table 29).

Table 29. Aircraft Production of the Powers, 1932–1939[135]

	1932	1933	1934	1935	1936	1937	1938	1939
France	(600)	(600)	(600)	785	890	743	1,382	3,163
Germany	36	368	1,968	3,183	5,112	5,606	5,235	8,295
Italy	(500)	(500)	(750)	(1,000)	(1,000)	(1,500)	1,850	(2,000)
Japan	691	766	688	952	1,181	1,511	3,201	4,467
U.K.	445	633	740	1,140	1,877	2,153	2,827	7,940
United States	593	466	437	459	1,141	949	1,800	2,195
USSR	2,595	2,595	2,595	3,578	3,578	3,578	7,500	10,382

But these figures, too, concealed alarming weaknesses. The predictable corollary of Russian "gigantism" was an excessive emphasis upon quantity. Given the attributes of a command economy, this had resulted in the production of enormous numbers of aircraft and tanks by the early 1930s; by 1932, indeed, the USSR was producing over 3,000 tanks and over 2,500 aircraft—fantastically more than any other country in the world. Given the tremendous growth of the regular army after 1934, it must have been extraordinarily difficult to find sufficient highly trained officers and NCOs to supervise the tank battalions and air squadrons. It was even more difficult, in a country with a surplus of peasants and desperately short of skilled workers, to man a modern army and air force; despite the massive educational program, the country's chief weakness in the 1930s probably still lay in the poor training of many of its workers and soldiers. Furthermore, Russia, like France, was a victim of heavy investment in aircraft and tank types of the early 1930s. When the Spanish Civil War showed the limits, in speed, maneuverability, range, and toughness, of these first-generation weapons, the race to build faster aircraft and more powerful tanks was accelerated. But the Soviet arms industry, like a large vessel at sea, could not change course swiftly; and it seemed folly to stop production on existing types while newer models were being built and tested. (In this connection, it is interesting to note that "of the 24,000 Russian tanks operational in June 1941, only 967 were of a new design equivalent or superior to the German tanks of that time.")[136] On top of this, there came the purges. The decapitation of the Red Army—90 percent of all generals and 80 percent of all colonels suffered in Stalin's manic drive—not only had the overall effect of destroying so many trained officers, but had specific results which badly hurt the armed forces. By wiping out Tukhachevsky and the "modern warfare" enthusiasts, by eliminating those who studied German methods and British theories, the purges left the army in the hands of such politically safe but intellectually retarded figures as Voroshilov and Kuluk. One early result was the disbanding of the seven mechanized corps, a decision influenced by the argument that the Spanish Civil War had shown that tank formations could play no independent offensive role on the battlefield and that the vehicles should be distributed to rifle battalions in order to support the infantry. In much the same way it was decided that the TB-3 strategic bombers were of little use to the USSR.

With much of its air force obsolescent and its armored units disbanded, with the services cowed into blind obedience by the purges, Russia was much weaker at the end of the 1930s than it had been five or ten years earlier—and in the meantime both Germany and Japan had greatly increased their arms output and were becoming more aggressive. The post-1937 Five-Year Plan clearly involved an enormous arms buildup, equal to and in many areas—e.g., aircraft production—larger than Germany's own. But until that investment had translated itself into far larger and better-equipped armed forces, Stalin felt Russia to be passing through a "danger zone" at least as threatening as the years 1919–1922. These external circumstances help explain the various changes in Soviet diplomacy during the 1930s. Worried by the

Japanese aggression in Manchuria and perhaps even more by Hitler's Germany, Stalin faced the prospect of a potential two-front war in theaters thousands of miles apart (exactly the strategical dilemma which paralyzed British decision-makers). Yet his diplomatic tacking toward the West, which included Russia's 1934 entry into the League of Nations and the 1935 treaties with France and Czechoslovakia, did not bring the desired increase in collective security. Without a Polish agreement, there was really little Russia could do to aid France or Czechoslovakia—and vice versa. And the British frowned at these efforts to create a diplomatic "popular front" against Germany, which in part explains Stalin's caution during the Spanish Civil War; a triumphant socialist republic in Spain, Moscow feared, might drive Britain and France to the right, as well as embroil Russia in open conflict with Franco's supporters, Italy and Germany.

By 1938–1939, the external situation must have appeared more threatening than ever in Stalin's eyes (which makes his purges even more foolish and inexplicable). The Munich settlement not only seemed to confirm Hitler's ambitions in east-central Europe but— more worryingly—revealed that the West was not prepared to oppose them and might indeed prefer to divert German energies farther eastward. Since these two years also saw substantial border clashes between Soviet and Japanese armies in the Far East (necessitating the heavy reinforcement of the Russian divisions in Siberia), it was not surprising that Stalin, too, decided to follow an "appeasement" policy toward Berlin even if that meant sitting down with his ideological foe. Given the USSR's own political ambitions in eastern Europe, Moscow had far fewer reservations about a carving up of the independent states in that region, provided that its own share was substantial. The surprise Nazi-Soviet pact of August 1939 at least provided Russia with a buffer zone on its western border and more time for rearmament while the West fought Germany in consequence of Hitler's attack upon Poland. Feeding morsels to the crocodile (to use Churchill's phrase) seemed much better than being devoured by it.[137]

All this makes it inordinately difficult to measure Soviet power by the end of the 1930s, especially since statistics on "relative war potentials"[138] reflect neither internal morale nor quality of armed forces nor geographical position. Clearly, the Red Army no longer resembled that "formidable modern force of great weight with advanced equipment and exceptionally tough fighting men" (except in the latter respect) which Mackintosh described the 1936 army as being;[139] but how far it had lost ground was not clear. The 1939–1940 "Winter War" against Finland appeared to confirm its precipitous decline, yet the less-well-known 1939 clashes with Japan at Nomonhan showed a cleverly led, modern force in action.[140] It is also evident that Stalin was aghast at the devastating Blitzkrieg-style victories of the German army in 1940, and more than ever anxious not to provoke Hitler into a war. His other great and obvious worry was where Tokyo would decide to strike in the East—not that Japan was so mortal a foe, but the defense of Siberia was logistically very exhausting and would further weaken Russia's capacity against the German threat. The swift recall of Zhukov's armor, to join in the invasion of eastern Poland in September 1939, once a border truce in the east had been arranged with Japan, was illustrative of this precarious strategical juggling act.[141] On the other hand, by that time the damage inflicted upon the Red Army was being hastily repaired and its numbers increased (to 4,320,000 men by 1941), the entire Soviet economy was being deployed toward war production, massive new factories were being built in central Russia, and improved aircraft and tanks (including the formidable T-34) were being tested. The 16.5 percent of the budget allocated to defense spending in 1937 had jumped to 32.6 percent in 1940.[142] Like most of the other Great Powers in this period, therefore, the USSR was racing against time. More even than in 1931, Stalin needed to urge his fellow countrymen to close the productive gap with the West. "To slacken the tempo would mean falling behind. And those who fall behind get beaten. . . ." The Russia of the czars had suffered "continual beatings" because it had fallen behind in industrial productivity and military strength.[143] Under its even more autocratic and ruthless leader, the Soviet regime was determined to catch up fast. Whether Hitler would let it do so was impossible to say.

The relative power of the United States in world affairs during the interwar years was, curiously, in inverse ratio to that of both the USSR and Germany. That is to say, it was inordinately strong in the 1920s, but then declined more than any other of the Great Powers during the depressed 1930s, recovering only (and partially) at the very end of this period. The reason for its preeminence in the first of these decades has been made clear above. The United States was the only major country, apart from Japan, to benefit from the Great War. It became the world's greatest financial and creditor nation, in addition to its already being the largest producer of manufactures and foodstuffs. It had by far the largest stocks of gold. It had a domestic market so extensive that massive economies of scale could be practiced by giant firms and distributors, especially in the booming automobile industry. Its high standard of living and its ready availability of investment capital interacted in a mutually beneficial fashion to spur on further heavy investments in manufacturing industry, since consumer demand could absorb virtually all of the goods which increased productivity offered. In 1929, for example, the United States produced over 4.5 million motor vehicles, compared with France's 211,000, Britain's 182,000, and Germany's 117,000.[144] It was hardly surprising that there were fantastic leaps in the import of rubber, tin, petroleum, and other raw materials to feed this manufacturing boom; but exports, especially of cars, agricultural machinery, office equipment, and similar wares, also expanded throughout the 1920s, the entire process being aided by the swift growth of American overseas investments.[145] Yet even if this is well known, it still remains staggering to note that the United States in those years was producing "a larger output than that of the other six Great Powers *taken together*" and that "her overwhelming productive strength was further underlined by the fact that the gross value of manufactures produced per head of population in the United States was nearly twice as high as in Great Britain or Germany, and more than ten to eleven times as high as in the USSR or Italy."[146]

While it is also true, as the author of the above lines immediately notes, "that the United States' political influence in the world was in no respect commensurate with her extraordinary industrial strength,"[147] that may not have been so important in the 1920s. In the first place, the American people decidedly rejected a leading role in world politics, with all the diplomatic and military entanglements which such a posture would inevitably produce; provided American commercial interests were not deleteriously affected by the actions of other states, there was little cause to get involved in foreign events—especially those arising in eastern Europe or the Horn of Africa. Secondly, for all the *absolute* increases in American exports and imports, their place in its national economy was not large, simply because the country was so self-sufficient; in fact, "the proportion of manufactured goods exported in relation to their total production decreased from a little less than 10 percent in 1914 to a little under 8 percent in 1929," and the book value of foreign direct investments as a share of GNP remained unaltered[148]—which helps to explain why, despite a widespread acceptance of world-market ideas *in principle,* American economic policy was much more responsive to domestic needs. Except in respect to certain raw materials, the world outside was not that important to American prosperity. Finally, international affairs in the decade after 1919 did not suggest the existence of a major threat to American interests: the Europeans were still quarreling but much less so than in the early 1920s, Russia was isolated, Japan quiescent. Naval rivalry had been contained by the Washington treaties. In such circumstances, the United States could reduce its army to a very small size (about 140,000 regulars), although it did allow the creation of a reasonably large and modern air force, and the navy was permitted to develop its aircraft-carrier and heavy-cruiser programs.[149] While the generals and admirals predictably complained about receiving insufficient resources from Congress, and certain damaging measures were done to national security (like Stimson's 1929 decision to wind up the codebreaking service on the grounds that "gentlemen do not read each others mail"),[150] the fact was that this was a decade in which the United

States still could remain an economic giant but a military middle-weight. It was perhaps symptomatic of this period of tranquillity that the United States still did not possess a superior civil-military body for considering strategic issues, like the Committee of Imperial Defence in Britain or its own later National Security Council. What need was there for one when the American people had decisively rejected the ideas of war?

The leading role of the United States in bringing about the financial collapse of 1929 has been described above.[151] What is even more significant, for the purposes of measuring comparative national power, was that the subsequent depression and tariff wars hurt it much more than any other advanced economy. If this was partly due to the relatively uncontrolled and volatile nature of American capitalism, it was also affected by the fatal decision to opt for protectionism by the Smoot-Hawley tariffs of 1930. Despite the complaints by U.S. farmers and some industrial lobbies about unfair foreign competition, the country's industrial and agricultural productivity was such—as the surplus of exports over imports clearly showed—that a breakup of the open world trading order would hurt its exporters more than any others. "The nation's GNP had plummeted from $98.4 billion in 1929 to barely half that three years later. The value of manufactured goods in 1933 was less than one-quarter what it had been in 1929. Nearly fifteen million workers had lost their jobs and were without any means of support. . . . During this same period the value of American exports had decreased from $5.24 billion to $1.61 billion, a fall of 69 percent."[152] With other nations scuttling hastily into protective trading blocs, those American industries which did rely heavily upon exports were devastated. "Wheat exports, which had totaled $200 million ten years earlier, slumped to $5 million in 1932. Auto exports fell from $541 million in 1929 to $76 million in 1932."[153] World trade collapsed generally, but the U.S. share of foreign commerce contracted even faster, from 13.8 percent in 1929 to less than 10 percent in 1932. What was more, while certain other major powers steadily recovered output by the middle to late 1930s, the United States suffered a further severe economic convulsion in 1937 which lost much of the ground gained over the preceding five years. But because of what has been termed the "disarticulated world economy"[154]—that is, the drift toward trading blocs which were much more self-contained than in the 1920s—this second American slump did not hurt other countries so severely. The overall consequence was that in the year of the Munich crisis, the U.S. share of world manufacturing output was lower than at any time since around 1910 (see Table 30).

Because of the severity of this slump, and because of the declining share of foreign trade in the GNP, American policy under Hoover and especially under Roosevelt became even more introspective. In view of

**Table 30. Shares of World Manufacturing
Output, 1929–1938**[155]
(percent)

	1929	1932	1937	1938
United States	43.3	31.8	35.1	28.7
USSR	5.0	11.5	14.1	17.6
Germany	11.1	10.6	11.4	13.2
U.K.	9.4	10.9	9.4	9.2
France	6.6	6.9	4.5	4.5
Japan	2.5	3.5	3.5	3.8
Italy	3.3	3.1	2.7	2.9

the strength of isolationist opinion and Roosevelt's pressing set of problems at home, it could hardly be expected that he would give to international affairs the concentrated attention which both Cordell Hull and the State Department wished from him. Nevertheless, because of the crucial position which the United States continued to occupy in the world economy, there remains some substance in the criticism of "the occupation with domestic recovery" and the "desire for the appearance of immediate action and results [and] a national habit of policy formation that gave little sustained thought to the impact American programs might have on other nations."[156] The 1934 ban upon loans to any foreign government which had defaulted on its war debts, the 1935 arms embargo in the event of war, and the slightly later prohibition of loans to any belligerent power simply made the British and French more cautious than ever about standing up to the fascist states. The 1935 denunciations of Italy were accompanied by enormous increases in American petroleum supplies to Mussolini's regime, to the consternation of the British Admiralty. The various commercial restrictions upon Germany and Japan, in partial response to their aggression, "served to antagonize [both] without providing meaningful aid to the opponents of these nations. FDR's economic diplomacy created enemies without winning friends or supporting prospective allies."[157] Perhaps the most serious consequence—although the responsibility needs to be shared—was the mutual suspicions which arose between Whitehall and Washington precisely at a time when the dictator states were making their challenge.[158]

By 1937 and 1938, however, Roosevelt himself seems to have become more worried by the fascist threats, even if American public opinion and economic difficulties restrained him from taking the lead. His messages to Berlin and Tokyo became firmer, his encouragement of Britain and France somewhat warmer (even if that hardly helped those two democracies in the short term). By 1938, secret Anglo-American naval talks were taking place about how to deal with the twin challenges of Japan and Germany. The president's "quarantine" speech was an early sign that he would move toward economic discrimination against the dictator states. Above all, Roosevelt now pressed for large-scale increases in defense expenditures. As the figures in Table 26 above show, even in 1938 the United States was spending less on armaments than Britain or Japan, and only a fraction of the sums spent by Germany and the Soviet Union. Nonetheless, aircraft production virtually doubled between 1937 and 1938, and in the latter year Congress passed a "Navy Second to None" Act, allowing for a massive expansion in the fleet. By that time, too, tests were taking place on the prototype B-17 bomber, the Marines Corps was refining its doctrine of amphibious warfare, and the army (while not yet possessing a decent tank) was grappling with the problems of armored warfare and planning to mobilize a vast force.[159] When war broke out in Europe, none of the services was at all ready; but they were in better shape, relative to the demands of modern warfare, than they had been in 1914.

Even these rearmament measures scarcely disturbed an economy the size of the United States. The key fact about the American economy in the late 1930s was that it was greatly *underutilized*. Unemployment was around ten million in 1939, yet industrial productivity per man-hour had been vastly improved by investments in conveyor belts, electric motors (in place of steam engines), and better managerial techniques, although little of this showed through in *absolute* output figures because of the considerable reduction in work hours by the labor force. Given the depressed demand, which the 1937–1938 recession did not help, the various New Deal schemes were insufficient to stimulate the economy and take advantage of this underutilized productive capacity. In 1938, for example, the United States produced 26.4 million tons of steel, well ahead of Germany's 20.7 million, the USSR's 16.5 million, and Japan's 6.0 million; yet the steel industries of those latter three countries were working to full capacity, whereas *two-thirds* of American steel plants were idle. As it turned out, this underutilization was soon going to be changed by the enormous rearmament programs.[160] The 1940 authorization of a doubling (!) of the navy's combat fleet, the Army Air Corps' plan to create eighty-four groups with 7,800 combat aircraft, the establishment (through the Selective Service and Training Act) of an army of close to 1 million men—all had an effect upon an economy which was not, like those of Italy, France, and Britain, suffering from severe structural problems, but was merely underutilized because of the Depression. Precisely because the United States had an enormous spare capacity whereas other economies were overheating, perhaps the most significant statistics for understanding the outcome of the future struggle were not the 1938 figures of actual steel or industrial output, but those which attempt to measure national income (Table 31) and, however imprecise, "relative war potential" (Table 32). For in each case they remind us that if the United States had suffered disproportionately during the Great

Depression, it nonetheless remained (in Admiral Yamamoto's words) a sleeping giant.

Table 31. National Income of the Powers in 1937 and Percentage Spent on Defense[161]

	National Income (billions of dollars)	Percentage on Defense
United States	68	1.5
British Empire	22	5.7
France	10	9.1
Germany	17	23.5
Italy	6	14.5
USSR	19	26.4
Japan	4	28.2

Table 32. Relative War Potential of the Powers in 1937[162]

United States	41.7%
Germany	14.4%
USSR	14.0%
U.K.	10.2%
France	4.2%
Japan	3.5%
Italy	2.5%
(seven Powers 90.5%)	

The awakening of this giant after 1938, and especially after 1940, provides a final confirmation the crucial issue of *timing* in the arms races and strategical calculations of this era. Like Britain and the USSR a little earlier, the United States was now endeavoring to close the armaments gap which had been opened up by the prior and heavy defense spending of the fascist states. That it could outspend any other country, if the political will existed at home, was clear from the statistics: even as late as 1939, U.S. defense composed only 11.7 percent of total expenditures and a mere 1.6 percent of GNP[163]—percentages far, far less than in any of the other Great Powers. An increase in the defense-spending share of the American GNP to bring it close to the proportions devoted to armaments by the fascist states would automatically make the United States the most powerful military state in the world. There are, moreover, many indications that Berlin and Tokyo realized how such a development would constrict their opportunities for future expansion. In Hitler's case, the issue is complicated by his scorn for the United States as a degenerate, miscegenated power, but he also sensed that he dared not wait until the mid-1940s to resume his conquests, since the military balance would by then have decisively swung to the Anglo-French-American camp.[164] On the Japanese side, because the United States was taken more seriously, the calculations were more precise: thus, the Japanese navy estimated that whereas its warship strength would be a respectable 70 percent of the American navy in late 1941, "this would fall to 65 percent in 1942, to 50 percent in 1943, and to a disastrous 30 percent in 1944."[165] Like Germany, Japan also had a powerful strategical incentive to move soon if it was going to escape from its fate as a middleweight nation in a world increasingly overshadowed by the superpowers.

The Unfolding Crisis, 1931–1942

When the relative strengths and weaknesses of each of the Great Powers are viewed in their entirety, and also integrated into the economic and technological-military dynamics of the age, the course of international diplomacy during the 1930s becomes more comprehensible. This is not to imply that the *local* roots of the various crises—whether in Mukden, Ethiopia, or the Sudetenland—were completely irrelevant, or that there would have been no international problems if the Great Powers had been in harmony. But it is clear that when a regional crisis arose, the statesmen in each of the leading capitals were compelled to view such events in the light both of the larger diplomatic scene and, perhaps especially, of their pressing domestic problems. The British prime minister, MacDonald, put this nicely to his colleague Baldwin, after the 1931 Manchurian affair had interacted with the sterling crisis and the collapse of the second Labor government:

> We have all been so distracted by day to day troubles that we never had a chance of surveying the whole situation and hammering out a policy regarding it, but have had to live from agitation to agitation.[166]

It is a good reminder of the way politicians' concerns were often immediate and practical, rather than long-term and strategic. But even after the British government had recovered its breath, there is no sign that it contemplated a change in its circumspect policy toward Japan's conquest of Manchuria. Quite apart from the continued need to deal with economic problems, and the public's unrelenting dislike of entanglements in the Far East, British leaders were also aware of dominion pressures for peace and of the very rundown state of imperial defenses in a region where Japan enjoyed the strategical advantage. In any case, there were various Britons who approved of Tokyo's decision to deal with the irritating Chinese nationalists and many more who wanted to maintain good relations with Japan. Even when those sentiments waned, after further Japanese aggressions, the only way in which

Whitehall might be moved to stronger action would be in conjunction with the League and/or the other Great Powers.

But the League itself, however admirable its principles, had no effective means for preventing Japanese aggression in Manchuria other than the armed forces of its leading members. Thus its recourse to an investigative committee (the Lytton Commission) merely gave the Powers an excuse to delay action while at the same time Japan continued its conquest. Of the major states, Italy had no real interests in the Far East. Germany, although enjoying commercial and military ties with China, preferred to sit back and observe whether Japan's "revisionism" could offer a useful precedent in Europe. The Soviet Union *was* concerned about Japanese aggression, but was unlikely to be invited to cooperate with the other powers and had no intention of being pushed forward alone. The French, predictably, were caught in a dilemma: they had no wish to see precedents being set for altering existing territorial boundaries and flouting League resolutions; on the other hand, being increasingly worried about clandestine German rearmament and the need to maintain the status quo in Europe, the French were appalled at the idea of complications arising in the Far East which would direct attention, and possibly military resources, away from the German problem. While Paris publicly stood firm alongside League principles, it privately let Tokyo know that it understood Japan's problems in China.[167] By contrast, the U.S. government—at least as represented by Secretary of State Stimson—in no way condoned Japanese actions, rightly seeing in them a threat to the open-door world upon which, in theory, the American way of life was so dependent. But Stimson's high-principled condemnations attracted neither Hoover, who feared the consequent entanglements, nor the British government, which preferred trimming to crusading. The result was a Stimson-Hoover quarrel in their respective memoirs, and (more significant) a legacy of mistrust between Washington and London. All this offered a depressing and convincing example of what one scholar has termed "the limits of foreign policy."[168]

Whether or not the Japanese military's move into Manchuria in 1931 was carried out[169] without the home government's knowledge was less important than the fact that this action succeeded, and was expanded upon, without the West being able to do anything substantial. The larger consequences were that the League had been shown to be an ineffective instrument for preventing aggression, and that the three western democracies were incapable of united action. This was also evident in the contemporaneous discussion at Geneva concerning land and air disarmament; here, of course, the United States was missing, but the Anglo-French differences over how to respond to German demands for "equality" and the continued British evasion of any guarantee to ease France's fears meant that Hitler's new regime could walk out of the talks and denounce the existing treaties without fear of any retribution.[170]

The revival of a German threat by 1933 placed further strains upon Anglo-French-American diplomatic cooperation at a time when the World Economic Conference had broken down and the three democracies were erecting their own currency and trading blocs. Although France was the more directly threatened by Germany, it was Britain which felt that its freedom of maneuver had been more substantially impinged upon. By 1934 both the Cabinet and its Defence Requirements Committee conceded that while Japan was the more immediate danger, Germany was the greater long-term threat. But since it was not possible to be strong against both, it was important to achieve a reconciliation in one of those regions. Whereas some circles favored improving relations with Japan so as to be better able to stand up to Germany, the Foreign Office argued that an Anglo-Japanese understanding in the Far East would ruin London's delicate relations with the United States. On the other hand, it could be pointed out to those imperial and naval circles who wanted to give priority to strengthening British defenses in the Orient that it was impossible to turn one's back upon French concern over German revisionism and (after 1935) fatal to ignore the growing threat from the Luftwaffe. For the rest of the decade the decision-makers in Whitehall sought to escape from this strategical dilemma of facing potential enemies at opposite ends of the globe.[171]

In 1934 and 1935, however, such a dilemma seemed disturbing but not acute. If Hitler's regime was clearly an unpleasant one, he had shown himself surprisingly willing to negotiate a settlement with Poland; in any case, Germany was still considerably weaker in military terms than either France or Russia. Furthermore, the German effort to move into Austria following Dollfuss's assassination in 1934 had provoked Mussolini to deploy troops on the Brenner Pass as a warning. The prospect of Italy being associated with the status quo powers was especially comforting to France, which sought to bring an anti-German coalition together in the "Stresa Front" of April 1935. At almost the same time, Stalin indicated that he, too, wished to associate with the "peace-loving" states, and by 1935 the Soviet Union had not only joined the League of Nations but had instituted its security pacts with Paris and Prague. Although Hitler had made plain his opposition to an "eastern Locarno," it looked as if Germany was nicely contained on all sides. And in the Far East, Japan was quiet.[172]

By the second half of 1935, however, this encouraging scene was disintegrating fast without Hitler having lifted a finger. The differing Anglo-French perceptions of the "security problem" were already revealed in the British unease at France's renewed links with Russia on the one hand and the French dismay at the Anglo-German naval agreement of June 1935 on the other. Both measures had been taken unilaterally to gain extra security, France desiring to bring the USSR into the European balance, Britain eager to reconcile its naval needs in European waters and the Far East; but each step seemed to the other neighbor to give a wrong signal to Berlin.[173] Even so, such contradictions were damaging but not catastrophic, which could not be said of Mussolini's decision to invade Abyssinia following a series of local clashes and in vain pursuit of his own ambition to create a new Roman Empire. This, too, was a good example of a regional quarrel having extraordinarily broader ramifications. To the French, aghast at the idea of turning a new potential ally against Germany into a bitter foe, the whole Abyssinian episode was an unmitigated disaster: to allow a flagrant transgression of the League's principles was disturbing, as was Mussolini's muscle-flexing (for where might he strike next?); on the other hand, to drive Italy into the German camp would be an appalling act of folly in strictly *Realpolitik* terms—but the latter consideration was unlikely to sway the idealistic British.[174] Yet Whitehall's dilemma was at least as large, since it not only had to handle even greater public unease about Italy's blatant transgression of League principles, but also had to worry about what Japan might do in the Far East if the West was engaged in a Mediterranean imbroglio. Whereas France feared that quarreling with Italy would tempt Hitler into the Rhineland, Britain suspected that it would encourage Japan to expand farther into Asia, the more especially since, at that exact time, Tokyo was on the point of denouncing the naval treaties and going for an unrestricted fleet buildup.[175] In a larger sense, both were right; the difficulty, as usual, was in reconciling the immediate problem with the longer-term implication.

The French fears were proved correct first. The 1935 Anglo-French offer of a territorial readjustment in Northeastern Africa to Italy's favor (the Hoare-Laval Pact) had caused British public opinion in particular to explode in moral indignation. Yet while the London and Paris governments were torn between responding to that mood, and still in private facing the overwhelmingly plausible strategic and economic reasons why they should not go to war with Italy, Hitler chose to order a reoccupation of the demilitarized Rhineland (March 1936). In strictly military terms, that was not such a blow; it was highly unlikely by then that France could have launched an offensive strike against Germany, and quite impossible for the British to have done so.[176] But this further weakening of the Versailles settlement—and the total abandonment of the Locarno Treaty—raised the general issue of what was, or was not, an internationally acceptable way of altering the status quo. Because of the failure of its leading members to halt Mussolini's aggression in 1935–1936, the League was now pretty much discredited; it played little or no role, for example, either in the Spanish Civil War or in Japan's open assault upon China in 1937. If further changes in the existing territorial order were going to be checked, or at least controlled, that could only be done by determined moves against the "revisionist" states by the major "status quo" powers.

To none of the latter, however, did the threat to resort to arms seem a practical possibility. Indeed, just as the fascist countries were coming closer together (in November 1937 Germany and Japan signed their anti-Comintern pact, shortly after Mussolini had proclaimed the Rome-Berlin axis), their potential opponents were becoming even more introspective and disunited.[177] Despite American resentments at the Japanese invasion of China and the bombing of the U.S.S. *Panay*, 1937 was not a good year for Roosevelt to take decisive steps in overseas affairs even had he wished to: the economy had been hit by a renewed slump, and Congress was passing ever tighter neutrality legislation. Since all Roosevelt could offer was words of condemnation without any promise of action, his policies merely "tended to strengthen Anglo-French doubts about American reliability."[178] In a quite different way, Stalin also was concentrating upon domestic affairs, since his purges and show trials were then at their height. Although he cautiously extended aid to the Spanish republic in the Civil War, he was aware that many in the West disliked the "redshirts" even more than the "blackshirts," and that it would be highly dangerous to be pushed forward into an open conflict with the Axis. Japan's actions in the Far East, and the signing of the anti-Comintern pact, made him more cautious still.

Yet the Power worst affected of all in the years 1936–1937 was undoubtedly France. Not only was its economy sagging and its political scene so divided that some observers thought it close to civil war, but its own elaborate security system in Europe had been almost totally destroyed in a series of shattering blows. The German reoccupation of the Rhineland removed any lingering possibility that the French army could undertake offensive actions to put pressure upon Berlin; the country now seemed dangerously vulnerable to the Luftwaffe, just as the French air force was becoming obsolescent; the Abyssinian affair and the Rome-Berlin axis turned Italy from a potential ally into a most unpredictable and threatening foe; Belgium's retreat into isolation dislocated existing plans for the defense of France's northern frontiers, and there was no way (due to the cost) that the Maginot Line could be extended to close this gap; the Spanish Civil War raised the awful prospect of a fascist, pro-Axis state being created in France's rear; and in eastern Europe, Yugoslavia was tacking closer toward Italy and the Little Entente seemed moribund.[179]

In these gloomy, near-paralyzing circumstances, the role of Great Britain became of critical importance, as Neville Chamberlain (in May 1937) replaced Baldwin as prime minister. Concerned at his country's economic and strategical vulnerability and personally horrified at the prospect of war, Chamberlain was determined to head off any future crisis in Europe by making "positive" offers toward satisfying the dictators' grievances. Suspicious of the Soviet Union, disdainful of Roosevelt's "verbiage," impatient at what he felt was France's confused diplomacy of intransigence and passivity, and regarding the League as totally ineffective, the prime minister embarked upon his own strategy to secure lasting peace by appeasement. Even before then, London had been making noises to Berlin about commercial and colonial concessions; Chamberlain's contribution was to increase the pace by being willing to consider territorial changes in Europe itself. At the same time, and precisely because he saw in Germany the greatest danger, the prime minister was eager to improve relations with Italy in the hope of detaching that country from the Axis.[180] All this was bound to be controversial—it caused, *inter alia,* the resignation of Chamberlain's foreign secretary (Eden) early in 1938, criticism from the small but growing number of anti-appeasers at home, and increased suspicion in Washington and Moscow—but on the other hand it could well be argued that so many bold moves in the past history of diplomacy were also controversial. The real flaw in Chamberlain's strategy, understood by some in Europe but not by the majority, was that Hitler was fundamentally *unappeasable* and determined upon a future territorial order which small-scale adjustments alone could never satisfy.

If that conclusion became clear by 1939, and still more by 1940–1941, it was not evident either to the British or even the French government in the crisis year of 1938. The takeover of Austria in the spring of that year was an unpleasant instance of Hitler's fondness for unannounced moves, but could one really object to the principle of joining Germans with Germans? If anything, it merely intensified Chamberlain's conviction that the issue of the German-speaking minority in Czechoslovakia had to be settled before that crisis brought the Powers up to, and over, the brink of war. Admittedly, the question of the Sudetenland was a much more contentious one—Czechoslovakia, too, had rights to a sovereignty which had been internationally guaranteed, and the western Powers' desire to satisfy Hitler now seemed more influenced by negative selfish fears than by positive ideals—but the fact was that the Führer was the only leader at this time prepared to fight, and was indeed irritated that the prospect of smashing the Czechs was removed by the concessions he gained at the Munich conference. As ever, it took two to make a Great Power war; and in 1938 there was no willing opponent to Hitler.[181]

Because the political and public will for war was lacking in the west, it makes little sense here to enter into the long-lasting debate about what might have happened had Britain and France fought on Czechoslovakia's behalf, although it is worth noting that the military balance was not as favorable to Germany as the various apologists of appeasement suggested.[182] What is clear, however, is that that balance swung even more in Hitler's favor following the Munich settlement. The elimination of Czechoslovakia as a substantial middleweight European force by March 1939, the German acquisition of Czech armaments, factories, and raw materials, and Stalin's increasing suspicion of the West outweighed the factors working in favor of London and Paris such as the considerable increases in British arms output, the more intimate Anglo-French military cooperation, or the swing in British and dominion opinion in favor of standing up to Hitler. At the same time, Chamberlain failed (January 1939) to detach Italy from the Axis, or to deter it from its own aggressions in the Balkans—even if Mussolini, for urgent reasons of his own, would not fight immediately alongside his fellow dictator in a Great Power war against the western nations.

When Hitler began to apply pressure upon Poland in the late spring of 1939, therefore, the possibilities of avoiding a conflict were less than in the previous year—and the prospects of an Anglo-French victory should war break out were *much* less. Germany's annexation of the "rump" state of Czechoslovakia in March 1939 and Italy's move into Albania a month later had led the democracies, under mounting public pressure to "stop Hitler," to offer guarantees to Poland, Greece, Rumania, and Turkey, thus tying western Europe to the fate of eastern Europe to a degree which the British at least had never before contemplated. Yet Poland could not be directly assisted by the western countries, and any *indirect* assistance was going to be small in a period when the French army had assumed the strategic defensive and the British were concentrating so much of their resources upon improved aerial defenses at home. The only direct aid which could be given to Poland must come from the east, and if Chamberlain's government was unenthusiastic about agreements with Moscow, the Poles for their part were adamantly opposed to having the Red Army on their territory. Since Stalin's overwhelming concern was to buy time and avoid a war, and Hitler's need was to increase the pressure upon the western nations to abandon Poland, both dictators had a secular interest in doing a "deal" at Warsaw's expense, whatever their own ideological differences. The shock announcement of the Molotov-Ribbentrop pact (August 23, 1939) not only enhanced Germany's strategical position but also made a war over Poland virtually inevitable. This time "appeasement" was not an option open to London and Paris, even if the economic and military circumstances pointed (perhaps more than in the preceding years) to the avoidance of a Great Power conflict.[183]

The outbreak of the Second World War thus found Britain and France once again opposing Germany, and, as in 1914, a British expeditionary force was dispatched across the Channel while the Anglo-French navies imposed their maritime blockade.[184] In so many other respects, however, the strategical contours of this war were quite different from the previous one, and disadvantageous to the Allies. Not only was there no eastern front, but the political agreement between Berlin and Moscow to carve up Poland also led to commercial arrangements, so that an increasing flow of raw materials sent from Russia steadily obviated any effects which the blockade might have had upon the German economy. It was true that in the first year of the war, stocks of oil and other raw materials were still desperately low in Germany, but ersatz production, Swedish iron ore, and the growing supplies from Russia helped to bridge the gap. In addition, Allied inertia on the western front meant that there was little pressure upon German holdings of petroleum and ammunitions. Finally, there were no encumbrancing allies for Germany to prop up, like Austria-Hungary in the 1914–1918 war. Had Italy also joined in the conflict in September 1939, its own economic deficiencies might have posed an excessive strain upon the Reich's slender stocks and, arguably, dislocated the chances for the German westward strike in 1940. To be sure, Italy's participation would have complicated the Anglo-French position in the Mediterranean, but not perhaps by much, and Rome's neutrality made it a useful conduit for German trade—which is why many of the planners in Berlin hoped that Mussolini would remain on the sidelines.[185]

While the "phony war" did not put Germany's economic vulnerability to the test, it did allow Germany to perfect those elements of national strategy in which the Wehrmacht was so superior—that is, operational doctrine, combined arms, tactical air power, and decentralized offensive warfare. The Polish campaign in particular confirmed the efficacy of Blitzkrieg warfare, exposed a number of weaknesses (which could then be corrected), and strengthened German confidence in being able to overrun foes by rapid, surprise assaults and the proper concentration of aerial and armored power. This was again easily demonstrated in the swift overrunning of Denmark and the Netherlands, although geography made Norway both inaccessible to German panzer divisions and subject to the influence of British sea power, which is why that campaign was touch-and-go for a while until the Luftwaffe's dominance was established. But the best example of the superiority of German military doctrine and operational tactical ability came in the French campaign of May–June 1940, when the larger but less well organized Allied infantry and armored forces were torn apart by Guderian's clusters of tanks and motorized infantry. In all of these encounters, the attacker enjoyed a considerable air superiority. Unlike the 1914–1916 battles, therefore, in which neither side showed much skill in grappling with the newer condition of warfare, these 1940 campaigns revealed German advantages which seemed to obviate Germany's long-term economic vulnerability.[186]

What was more, by winning so decisively in 1939–1940 the German war machine greatly expanded its available sources of oil and raw materials. Not only could it (and did it!) plunder heavily from its defeated foes, but the elimination of France and Britain's obvious incapacity to launch a major military campaign also meant that there would be no serious drain upon the Wehrmacht's stocks through extensive campaigning. A land line had been made to Spanish raw materials, Swedish ores were now safe from Allied expeditions, and Russia, secretly appalled at Hitler's swift successes, was increasing its supplies. In these circumstances, Italy's entry into the war just as France was collapsing was not the economic embarrassment it might have been— and, indeed, distracted British resources away from Europe to the Near East, even if Italy's spectacularly unsuccessful campaigning showed how overrated it had been throughout the 1930s.[187]

Had the war continued simply with these three belligerents, it is difficult to say how long it might have gone on. The British Empire under Churchill was determined to continue the struggle and was mobilizing large numbers of men and stocks of munitions— outbuilding Germany both in aircraft and tank production in 1940, for example.[188] And while Britain's own holdings of gold and dollars were by then insufficient to pay for American supplies, Roosevelt was managing to undo the damaging neutrality legislation and to persuade Congress that it was in the country's own security interests to sustain Britain—by Lend-Lease, the "destroyers for bases" deal, convoy protection, and so on.[189] The overall result was to leave the two major combatants in the position of being unable to damage the other decisively. If the Battle of Britain had rendered impossible a German cross-Channel invasion, the imbalance of land forces made a British military entry into Europe quite out of the question. Bomber Command's raids upon Germany were good for British morale, but did little real damage at this stage. Despite occasional raids into the North Atlantic, the German surface fleet was in no position to take on the Royal Navy; on the other hand, the U-boat campaign was as threatening as ever, thanks to Doenitz's newer tactics and additional boats. In North Africa, Somalia, and Abyssinia, British Empire forces found it easy to take Italian-held positions, but extremely difficult to cope with the explosive form of warfare practiced by Rommel's Afrika Korps or by the German invading forces in Greece. The second year of what has been termed "the last European war" was, therefore, characterized by defensive victories and small-scale gains rather than by epic encounters and conquests.[190]

Inevitably, then, Hitler's fateful decision to invade Russia in June 1941 changed the entire dimensions of the conflict. Strategically, it meant that Germany now had to fight on several fronts and thus revert to its dilemma of 1914–1917—this being a particularly heavy strain for the Luftwaffe, which had its squadrons thinly spread between the west, the east, and the Mediterranean. It also ensured that the British Empire's position in the Middle East—which could surely have been over-run had Hitler dispatched there one-quarter of the troops and aircraft used for Operation Barbarossa—would remain, like the home islands, as a springboard for an enemy counteroffensive in the future. Most important of all, however, the sheer geographical extent and logistical demands of campaigning hundreds of miles deep into Russia under-mined the Wehrmacht's greatest advantage: its ability to launch shock attacks within limited confines, so as to overwhelm the enemy before its own supplies began to run out and its war machine slowed down. In contrast to the stupendous array of front-line strength assembled by Germany and its allies in June 1941, the supporting and follow-on resources were minimal, especially in the light of the poor road system; no thought had been given to winter warfare, since it was assumed that the struggle would be over within three months; German aircraft pro-duction in 1941 was significantly smaller than that of Britain or Russia, let alone the United States; the Wehrmacht had far fewer tanks than Russia; and the supplies of petroleum and ammunition were quickly run down in the extensive campaigning.[191] Even when the Wehrmacht was spectacularly successful in the field—and Stalin's inept deploy-ment orders in the face of the impending attack allowed the Germans to kill or capture three million Russians in the first four months of fighting—that did not of itself solve the problem. Russia could suffer appalling losses of men and equipment, and cede a million square miles of territory, and still not be defeated; the capture of Moscow, or perhaps even of Stalin himself, might not have forced a surrender, given the country's extraordinarily large reserves. In sum, this was a limitless war, and the Third Reich, for all its imposing successes and operational brilliance, was not properly equipped to fight it.

Whether Russia could have survived the German army at the gates of Moscow *and* a heavy attack by Japan upon Siberia in December 1941 is quite another matter, fascinating to speculate upon and impos-sible to answer. In signing both the Tripartite Pact (September 1940) with Germany and Italy and the later (April 1941) neutrality treaty with the Soviet Union, Japan had hoped to deter the USSR while con-centrating on its southern expansion; but many in Tokyo were tempted again to a war against Russia at the news of the German advance upon Moscow. If indeed the Japanese army had struck against its traditional foe in Asia instead of agreeing to the southern operations, it might still have been difficult for Roosevelt to persuade the American people to enter fully into such a war, and the assistance which the British could have given Russia in the Far East (had Churchill alone entered that conflict) would have been minimal. Instead of facing that dreadful two-front scenario, Stalin was able to switch his well-trained, winter-hardy divisions from Siberia in late 1941 to help blunt the German offensive and then to drive it back.[192] Seen from Tokyo's viewpoint, however, the decision to expand southward was utterly logical. The West's embargo on trade with Japan and freezing of its assets in July 1941 (following Tokyo's seizure of French Indochina) made both the army and the navy acutely aware that unless they gave in to American political demands *or* attempted to seize the oil and raw materials supplies of Southeast Asia, they would be economically ruined within a matter of months. From July 1941, therefore, a northern war against Russia became virtually impossible and southern operations virtually inevitable—but since the Americans were judged hardly likely to stand by while Japan helped itself to Borneo, Malaya, and the Dutch East Indies, their military installations in the western Pacific—and their fleet base at Pearl Harbor—also needed to be eliminated. Simply to keep up the momentum of their "China incident," the Japanese generals now found it necessary to support large-scale operations thousands of miles from home against targets they had scarcely heard of.[193]

December 1941 marked the second major turning point in a war which had now become global. The Russian counterattacks around Moscow in the same month confirmed that here, at least, the Blitzkrieg had failed. And if the stunning array of Japanese successes in the first six months of the Pacific war dealt heavy blows to the Allies, none of the territories lost (not even Singapore or the Philippines) was really vital in grand-strategical terms. What was much more important was that Japan's actions, and Hitler's gratuitous declaration of war upon the United States, at last brought into the conflict the most powerful country in the world. To be sure, industrial productivity alone could not ensure military effectiveness—and German operational skills in particular meant that simple man-to-man and dollar-to-dollar comparisons were foolish[194]—but the Grand Alliance, as Churchill fondly called it, was so superior in matériel terms to the Axis and its productive bases were so far away from the German and Japanese armed forces that it had the resources and the opportunity to build up an overwhelming military strength which none of the earlier opponents of fascist aggression could have hoped to possess. Within another year, in fact, de Tocqueville's forecast of 1835 concerning the emergence of a bipolar world was at last on the point of being realized.

STRATEGY & ECONOMICS TODAY & TOMORROW

7

Stability and Change in a Bipolar World, 1943-1980

At the news of the U.S. entry into the war, Winston Churchill openly rejoiced—and with good reason. As he later explained it, "Hitler's fate was sealed. Mussolini's fate was sealed. As for the Japanese, they would be ground to powder. All the rest was merely the proper application of overwhelming force."[1] Yet such confidence must have seemed wildly misplaced to more cautious minds on the Allied side during 1942 and until the first half of 1943. For six months after Pearl Harbor, Japanese forces had run rampant in the Pacific and Southeast Asia, overwhelming the European colonial empires, encircling China from the south, and threatening India, Australia, and Hawaii. In the Russo-German war, the Wehrmacht resumed its brutal offensives once the winter of 1941-1942 had passed and battled its way toward the Caucasus; at almost the same time, the far smaller German force under Rommel in North Africa had pushed to within fifty-five miles of Alexandria. The U-boat assault upon Allied convoys was proving deadlier than ever, with the highest losses of merchantmen occurring in the spring of 1943; yet the Anglo-American "counterblockade" of the German economy by means of strategic bombing was failing to achieve its purpose and was leading to severe casualties among the aircrews. If the fate of the Axis Powers *was* sealed after December 1941, there was little indication that they knew it.

"The Proper Application of Overwhelming Force"

Nevertheless, Churchill's basic assumption was correct. The conversion of the conflict from a European war to a truly global war may have complicated Britain's own strategical juggling act—as many historians have pointed out, the loss of Singapore was the result of the British concentration of aircraft and trained divisions in the Mediterranean theater[2]—but it totally altered the overall balance of forces once the newer belligerents were properly mobilized. In the meantime, the German and Japanese war machines could still continue their conquests; yet the further they extended themselves the less capable they were of meeting the counteroffensives which the Allies were steadily preparing.

The first of these came in the Pacific, where Nimitz's carrier-based aircraft had already blunted the Japanese drive into the Coral Sea (May 1942) and toward Midway (June 1942) and showed how vital naval air power was in the vast expanses of that ocean. By the end of the year, Japanese troops had been pulled out of Guadalcanal and Australian-American forces were pushing forward in New Guinea. When the counteroffensive through the central Pacific began late in 1943, the two powerful American battle fleets covering the Gilberts invasion were themselves protected by *four* fast-carrier task forces (twelve carriers) with overwhelming control of the air.[3] An even greater imbalance of force had permitted the British Empire divisions to crash through the German positions at El Alamein in October 1942 and to drive Rommel's units back toward Tunisia; when Montgomery ordered the attack, he had six times as many tanks as his opponent, three times as many troops, and almost complete command of the air. In the month following, Eisenhower's Anglo-American army of 100,000 men landed in French North Africa to begin a "pincer movement" from the west against the German-Italian forces, which would culminate in the latter's mass surrender in May 1943.[4] By that time, too, Doenitz had been compelled to withdraw his U-boat wolf packs from the North Atlantic, where they had suffered very heavy losses against Allied convoys now protected by very-long-range Liberators, escort carriers, and hunter-killer escort groups equipped with the latest radar and depth charges—and alerted by "Ultra" decrypts as to the U-boats' movements.[5] If it was to take longer for the Allies to achieve "command of the air" over Europe to complement their command of the sea, the solution was being swiftly developed in the form of the long-range Mustang fighter, which first accompanied the USAAF's bomber fleets in December 1943; within another few months, the Luftwaffe's capacity to defend the airspace above the Third Reich's soldiers, factories, and civilian population had been weakened beyond recovery.[6]

Even more ominous to the Wehrmacht high command was the changing balance of advantage along the eastern front. As early as August 1941, when many observers felt that Russia was in the process of being finished off as a Great Power, General Halder was gloomily confiding in the War Staff diary:

> We reckoned with about 200 enemy divisions. Now we have already counted 360 . . . not armed and equipped to our standards, and their

tactical leadership is often poor. But . . . if we smash a dozen of them, the Russians simply put up another dozen. . . . Time . . . favors them, as they are near their own resources, while we are moving farther and farther away from ours.[7]

In this sort of mass, reckless, brutalized fighting, the casualty figures were making even First World War totals seem modest. In the first five months of campaigning, the Germans claimed to have killed, wounded, or captured well over 3 million Russians.[8] Yet at that particular moment, when Stalin and the Stavka were planning the first counteroffensive around Moscow, the Red Army still had 4.2 million men in its field armies, and was numerically superior in tanks and aircraft.[9] To be sure, it could not match the professional expertise of the Germans either on land or in the air—even as late as 1944 the Russians were losing five or six men for every one German soldier[10]—and when the fearful winter of 1941–1942 passed, Hitler's war machine could again commence its offensive, this time toward Stalingrad and then disaster. After Stalingrad, in the summer of 1943, the Wehrmacht tried again, pulling together its armored forces to produce the fantastic total of seventeen panzer divisions for the encirclement of Kursk. Yet in what was to be by far the greatest tank battle of the Second World War, the Red Army countered with thirty-four armored divisions, some 4,000 vehicles to the German's 2,700. While the numbers of Soviet tanks had been reduced by over one-half within a week, they had smashed the greater part of Hitler's *Panzerarmee* in the process and were now ready for the unrelenting counteroffensive toward Berlin. At that point, news of the Allied landing in Italy provided Hitler with the excuse for withdrawing from what had been an unmitigated disaster, as well as confirming the extent to which the Reich's enemies were closing the ring.[11]

Was all this, then, merely the "proper application of overwhelming force"? Clearly, economic power was never the *only* influence upon military effectiveness, even in the mechanized, total war of 1939–1945; economics, to paraphrase Clausewitz, stood in about the same relationship to combat as the craft of the swordsmith to the art of fencing. And there were far too many examples of where the German and Japanese leadership made grievous political or strategical errors after 1941 which were to cost them dear. In the German case, this ranged from relatively small-scale decisions, like pouring reinforcements into North Africa in early 1943, just in time for them to be captured, to the appallingly stupid as well as criminal treatment of the Ukrainian and other non-Russian minorities in the USSR, who were happy to escape from the Stalinist embrace until checked by Nazi atrocities. It ran from the arrogance of assuming that the Enigma codes could never be broken to the ideological prejudice against employing German women in

munitions factories, whereas all Germany's foes willingly exploited
that largely untapped labor pool. It was compounded by rivalries
within the higher echelons of the army itself, which made it ineffective
in resisting Hitler's manic urge for overambitious offensives like Stalingrad and Kursk. Above all, there was what scholars refer to as the
"polycratic chaos" of rivaling ministries and subempires (the army, the
SS, the Gauleiter, the economics ministry), which prevented any coherent assessment and allocation of resources, let alone the hammering-
out of what elsewhere would be termed a "grand strategy." This was
not a serious way to run a war.[12]

While Japanese strategical mistakes were less egregious and counterproductive, they were nonetheless amazing. Because Japan was carrying out a "continental" strategy in which the army's influence
predominated, its operations in the Pacific and Southeast Asia had
been implemented with a minimum of force—only eleven divisions,
compared with the thirteen in Manchuria and the twenty-two in China.
Yet even when the American counteroffensive in the central Pacific
was under way, Japanese troop and aerial reinforcements to that region were far too tardy and far too small—especially as compared with
the resources allocated for the massive China offensives of 1943–1944.
Ironically, even when Nimitz's forces were closing upon Japan in early
1945, and its cities were being pulverized from the air, there were still
1 million soldiers in China and another 780,000 or so in Manchuria—
now incapable of being withdrawn because of the effectiveness of the
American submarine campaign.

Yet the Imperial Japanese Navy, too, needs to take its share of
the blame. The operational handling of key battles like Midway was
riddled with errors, but even when the aircraft carrier was proving
itself supreme in Pacific warfare, many Japanese admirals after
Yamamoto's death were wedded to the battleship and still looked for
the chance to fight a second Tsushima—as the 1944 Leyte Gulf operation and, even more symbolically, the one-way suicide trip of the
Yamato revealed. Japanese submarines, with their formidable
torpedoes, were utterly misused as scouts for the battle fleet or in
running supplies to beleaguered island garrisons, rather than being
deployed against the enemy's lines of communication. By contrast, the
navy failed to protect its own merchant marine, and was quite backward in developing convoy systems, antisubmarine techniques, escort
carriers, and hunter-killer groups, although Japan was even more dependent than Britain upon imported materials.[13] It was symptomatic
of this battle-fleet obsession that while the navy was allocating resources to the construction of giant *Yamato*-class vessels, it built *no*
destroyer escorts between 1941 and 1943—in contrast to the Americans' 331 ships.[14] Japan also completely lost the battle of intelligence,
codes, and decrypts.[15] All of this was about as helpful to the preserva-

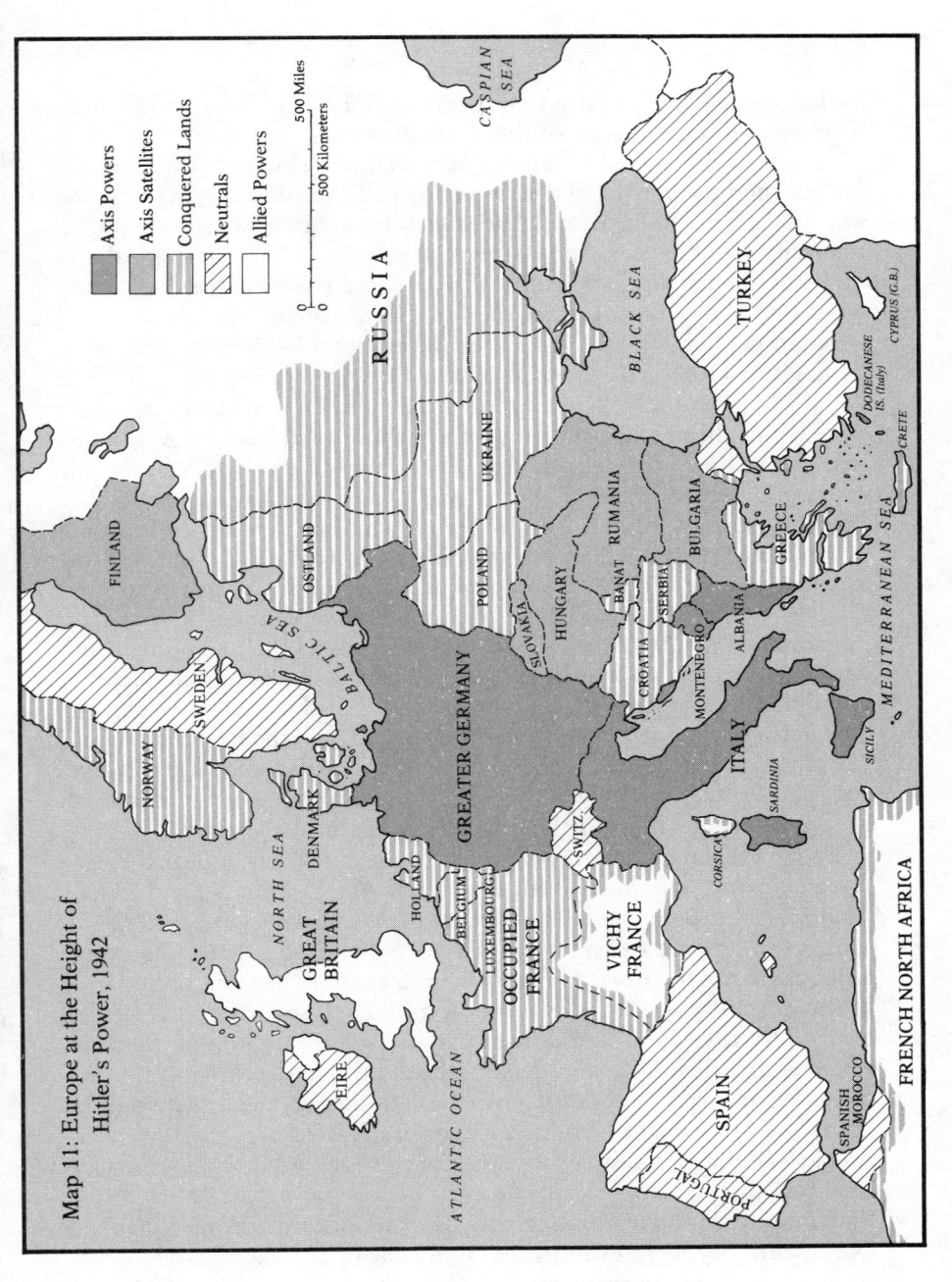

Map 11: Europe at the Height of Hitler's Power, 1942

Legend:
- Axis Powers
- Axis Satellites
- Conquered Lands
- Neutrals
- Allied Powers

500 Miles
500 Kilometers

RUSSIA

CASPIAN SEA

TURKEY

BLACK SEA

CYPRUS (G.B.)

DODECANESE IS. (Ital.)

CRETE

UKRAINE

BULGARIA

RUMANIA

GREECE

MEDITERRANEAN SEA

FINLAND

OSTLAND

POLAND

BANAT

SERBIA

ALBANIA

SICILY

SWEDEN

BALTIC SEA

SLOVAKIA

HUNGARY

CROATIA

MONTENEGRO

ITALY

SARDINIA

NORWAY

DENMARK

GREATER GERMANY

SWITZ.

CORSICA

NORTH SEA

GREAT BRITAIN

HOLLAND

BELGIUM

LUXEMBOURG

OCCUPIED FRANCE

VICHY FRANCE

ATLANTIC OCEAN

EIRE

SPAIN

PORTUGAL

SPANISH MOROCCO

FRENCH NORTH AFRICA

tion of a Greater East Asia Co-prosperity Sphere as German mistakes
were to the maintenance of the Thousand-Year Reich.

There is, obviously, no known way of "factoring out" those errors
(to use the economists' inelegant term) and thus discovering how the
Axis Powers might have fared had such follies been avoided. But unless
the Allies for their part had committed equally serious strategical and
political mistakes, it is difficult to see how their productive superiority
would not have prevailed in the long term. Obviously, a successful
German occupation of Moscow in December 1941 would have been
damaging to Russia's war effort (and to Stalin's regime); but would the
USSR's population have surrendered then and there when its only fate
would have been extermination—and when it still had large productive and military reserves thousands of miles to the east? Despite the
economic losses dealt by Operation Barbarossa—coal production
down by 57 percent, pig iron by 68 percent, and so on[16]—it is worth
noting that Russia produced 4,000 more aircraft than Germany in 1941
and 10,000 more in 1942, and this was for one front, as opposed to
Germany's three.[17] Given its increasing superiority in men, tanks, artillery, and planes, by the second year of the conflict the Red Army could
actually afford to sustain losses at a rate of five or six to one (albeit at
an appalling cost to its own troops) and still push forward against the
weakening Germans. By the beginning of 1945, on the Belorussian and
Ukrainian fronts alone, "Soviet superiority was both absolute and awesome, fivefold in manpower, fivefold in armor, over sevenfold in artillery and seventeen times the German strength in the air."[18]

Since the Anglo-American forces in France a few months earlier
were enjoying "an effective superiority of 20 to 1 in tanks and 25 to 1
in aircraft,"[19] the amazing fact is that the Germans did so well for so
long; even at the close of 1944, just as in September 1918, they were
still occupying territories far larger than the Reich's own boundaries
at the onset of war. To this question military historians have offered
a virtually unanimous response: that German operational doctrine,
emphasizing flexibility and decentralized decision-making at the *battlefield* level, proved far superior to the cautious, set-piece tactics of the
British, the bloody, full-frontal assaults of the Russians, and the enthusiastic but unprofessional forward rushes of the Americans; that German "combined-arms" experience was better than anybody else's; and
that the caliber and training of both the staff officers and the NCOs was
extraordinarily high, even in the final year of the war.

Yet our contemporary admiration for the German operational performance, which seems to be rising book by book,[20] ought not to
obscure the obvious fact that Berlin, like Tokyo, had overstretched
itself. In November 1943, General Jodl estimated that 3.9 million Germans (together with a mere 283,000 Axis-allied troops) were trying to
hold off 5.5 million Russians on the eastern front. A further 177,000

German troops were in Finland, while Norway and Denmark were garrisoned by 486,000 men. There were 1,370,000 occupation troops in France and Belgium. "Another 612,000 men were tied down in the Balkans, and there were 412,000 men in Italy. . . . Hitler's armies were scattered the length and breadth of Europe and were inferior in numbers and equipment on every front."[21] The same could be said of the Japanese divisions, spread thinly across the Far East from Burma to the Aleutian Islands.

Even in those campaigns which seemingly "changed the course of the war," one wonders whether an Axis victory rather than an Allied one would not merely have postponed the eventual outcome. Had, say, Nimitz lost more than one carrier at Midway, they would have been replaced, in that same year, by three new fleet carriers, three light fleet carriers, and fifteen escort carriers; in 1943, by five fleet carriers, six light fleet carriers, and twenty-five escort carriers; and in 1944, by nine fleet carriers and thirty-five escort carriers.[22] Similarly, in the critical years of the Battle of the Atlantic, the Allies lost 8.3 million tons of shipping overall in 1942 and 4 million tons in 1943, but those frightening totals were compensated for by Allied launchings of 7 million and 9 million tons of new merchant ships respectively. This was chiefly due to the fantastic explosion in American shipbuilding output, which by mid-1942 was already launching vessels faster than the U-boats could sink them—causing one notable authority to conclude, "In World War II, the German submarine campaign may have postponed, but did not affect the outcome."[23] On land, also—and the Second World War in Europe was preeminently a gunner's war and a tank crew's war—Germany's production of artillery pieces, self-propelled guns and tanks was considerably less than Russia's, let alone the combined Allied totals (see Table 33).

Table 33. Tank Production in 1944[24]

Germany	17,800
Russia	29,000
Britain	5,000
United States	17,500 (in 1943, 29,500)

But the most telling statistics of all relate to aircraft production (Table 34), for everyone could see that without command of the air it was impossible for armies and navies to operate effectively; *with* command of the air, one could not only achieve campaign victories, but also deal heavy blows at the foe's wartime economy.

Such figures, moreover, disguise the fact that the Anglo-American totals include a large number of heavy four-engined bombers, so that the Allied superiority is even more marked when the number of engines or the structure weight of the aircraft is compared with the Axis

Table 34. Aircraft Production of the Powers, 1939–1945[25]

	1939	1940	1941	1942	1943	1944	1945
United States	5,856	12,804	26,277	47,836	85,898	96,318	49,761
USSR	10,382	10,565	15,735	25,436	34,900	40,300	20,900
Britain	7,940	15,049	20,094	23,672	26,263	26,461	12,070
British Commonwealth	250	1,100	2,600	4,575	4,700	4,575	2,075
TOTAL ALLIES	24,178	39,518	64,706	101,519	151,761	167,654	84,806
Germany	8,295	10,247	11,776	15,409	24,807	39,807	7,540
Japan	4,467	4,768	5,088	8,861	16,693	28,180	11,066
Italy	1,800	1,800	2,400	2,400	1,600	—	—
TOTAL AXIS	14,562	16,815	19,264	26,670	43,100	67,987	18,606

totals.[26] Here was the ultimate reason why, despite extraordinary efforts by the Germans to retain command of the air,[27] their cities and factories and railway lines were increasingly devastated—as was, even more so, the almost totally unprotected Japanese homeland. Here, too, was the reason why Doenitz's U-boats had to keep below the surface; why Slim's Burma Army could reinforce Imphal; why American carriers could launch repeated attacks upon Japanese bases all over the western Pacific; and why Allied soldiers, whenever stopped by a stubborn German defense, could always call for aircraft to crush the enemy and get the offensive going again. On D-Day itself (June 6, 1944), it may be worth noting, the Germans could muster 319 aircraft against the Allies 12,837 in the west. To turn Clausewitz's phrase around, the art of fencing (like the art of war) indeed required skill and experience; but that would avail the fighter little if he ran out of stocks of swords. In the battle of the swordsmiths, the Allies were very clearly winning.

For the simple fact was that even after the expansion of the German and Japanese empires, the economic and productive forces ranged upon each side were *much more disproportionate* than in the First World War. According to the rough approximations which we have already seen,[28] the Greater Germany of 1938 had a share of the world's manufacturing output and a "relative war potential" which were both about equal to that of Britain and France combined. It was probably inferior to the total resources and war potential of the British and French *empires* combined; but those lands had not been mobilized to Germany's degree when war broke out, and, as discussed previously, the Allies were less than competent in the vital matter of operational expertise. Germany's acquisitions of territory in 1939 and (especially) in 1940 put it decisively ahead of the isolated and somewhat mauled Power which Churchill took control of. France's collapse and Italy's entry into the conflict therefore left the British Empire facing an agglomeration of military force which, in terms of war potential, was probably twice as strong; militarily, the Berlin-Rome Axis was unassailable on land, still inferior at sea, and about equal in the air—hence the British preference for fighting in North Africa rather than Europe. The German attack upon the USSR did not at first seem to change this balance, if only because of the disastrous casualties suffered by the Red Army, which were then compounded by the losses of Soviet territory and plant.

On the other hand, the decisive events of December 1941 entirely altered these balances: the Russian counterattack at Moscow showed that it would not fall to Blitzkrieg warfare; and the entry of Japan and the United States into what was now a global conflict brought together a "Grand Alliance" of enormous industrial-productive staying power. It could not *immediately* affect the course of the military campaigns, since Germany was still strong enough to renew its offensive in Russia during the summer of 1942, and Japan was enjoying its first six months of easy victories against the unprepared forces of the United States, the Dutch, and the British Empire. Yet all this could not obviate the fact that the Allies possessed *twice* the manufacturing strength (using the distorted 1938 figures, which downplay the U.S.' share), *three* times the "war potential," and *three* times the national income of the Axis powers, even when the French shares are added to Germany's total.[29] By 1942 and 1943, these figures of *potential* power were being exchanged into the hard currency of aircraft, guns, tanks, and ships; indeed, by 1943–1944 the United States alone was producing one ship a day and one aircraft every five minutes! What is more, the Allies were producing many newer *types* of weapons (Superfortresses, Mustangs, light fleet carriers), whereas the Axis powers could only produce advanced weapons (jet fighters, Type 23 U-boats) in relatively small quantities.

The best measure of this decisive shift in the balances comes from Wagenführ's figures for the armaments-production totals of the major combatants (see Table 35).

Table 35. Armaments Production of the Powers,
1940–1943[30]
(billions of 1944 dollars)

	1940	1941	1943
Britain	3.5	6.5	11.1
USSR	(5.0)	8.5	13.9
United States	(1.5)	4.5	37.5
Total of Allied *combatants*	3.5	19.5	62.5
Germany	6.0	6.0	13.8
Japan	(1.0)	2.0	4.5
Italy	0.75	1.0	—
Total of Axis *combatants*	6.75	9.0	18.3

Thus, in 1940 British armaments production was significantly behind Germany's but still growing fast, so that it was slightly superior by the following year—the last year in which the German economy was being operated at relative leisure. The twin military shocks of Stalingrad and North Africa, and Speer's assumption of the economics ministry, led to an enormous boost in German arms production by 1943;[31] and Japan, too, more than doubled its output. Even so, the increases in combined British and Soviet production during those two years equaled the rise in Axis output (G.B./USSR, $10 billion increase, 1941–1943; cf. Axis, $9.8 billion increase), and kept them still superior in total armaments production. But the most staggering change came with the *more than eightfold* rise in American arms output between 1941 and 1943, which meant that by the latter year the Allied total was over three times that of its foes—thereby finally realizing that imbalance in "war potential" and national income which had existed embryonically at the very beginning. No matter how cleverly the Wehrmacht mounted its tactical counterattacks on both the western and eastern fronts until almost the last months of the war, it was to be ultimately overwhelmed by the sheer mass of Allied firepower. By 1945, the thousands of Anglo-American bombers pounding the Reich each day and the hundreds of Red Army divisions poised to blast through to Berlin and Vienna were all different manifestations of the same blunt fact. Once again, in a protracted and full-scale coalition war, the countries with the deepest purse had prevailed in the end.

This was also true of Japan's own collapse in the Pacific war. It is now clear that the dropping of the atomic bombs in 1945 marked a watershed in the military history of the world, and one which throws into doubt the viability of mankind should a Great Power war with atomic weaponry ever be fought. Yet in the context of the 1945 campaigning, it was but one of a series of military tools which the United States then could employ to compel Japan to surrender. The successful American submarine campaign was threatening to starve Japan; the swarms of B-29 bombers were pounding its towns and cities to ashes (the Tokyo "fire raid" of March 9, 1945, caused approximately 185,000 casualties and destroyed 267,000 buildings); and the American planners and their allies were preparing for a massive invasion of the home islands. The mix of motives which, despite certain reservations, pushed toward the decision to drop the bomb—the wish to save Allied casualties, the desire to send a warning to Stalin, the need to justify the vast expenses of the atomic project—are still debated today;[32] but the point being made here is that it was the United States alone which at this time had the productive and technological resources not only to wage two large-scale conventional wars but also to invest the scientists, raw materials, and money (about $2 billion) in the development of a new weapon which might or might not work. The devastation inflicted upon Hiroshima, together with Berlin's fall into the hands of the Red

Army, not only symbolized the end of another war, it also marked the beginning of a new order in world affairs.

The New Strategic Landscape

The outlines of that new order were already being described by American military planners even as the conflict was at its height. As one of their policy papers expressed it:

> The successful termination of the war against our present enemies will find a world profoundly changed in respect of relative national military strengths, a change more comparable indeed with that occasioned by the fall of Rome than with any other change occurring during the succeeding fifteen hundred years. . . . After the defeat of Japan, the United States and the Soviet Union will be the only military powers of the first magnitude. This is due in each case to a combination of geographical position and extent, and vast munitioning potential.[33]

While historians might quibble at the claim that nothing of a comparable nature had occurred during the past fifteen hundred years, it was becoming clear that the global balance of power after the war would be totally different from that preceding it. Former Great Powers—France, Italy—were already eclipsed. The German bid for mastery in Europe was collapsing, as was Japan's bid in the Far East and Pacific. Britain, despite Churchill, was fading. The bipolar world, forecast so often in the nineteenth and early twentieth centuries, had at last arrived; the international order, in DePorte's words, now moved "from one system to another."[34] Only the United States and the USSR counted, so it seemed; and of the two, the American "superpower" was vastly superior.

Simply because much of the rest of the world was either exhausted by the war or still in a stage of colonial "underdevelopment," American power in 1945 was, for want of another term, *artificially* high, like, say, Britain's in 1815. Nonetheless, the actual dimensions of its might were unprecedented in absolute terms. Stimulated by the vast surge in war expenditures, the country's GNP measured in constant 1939 dollars rose from $88.6 billion (1939) to $135 billion (1945), and much higher ($220 billion) in current dollars. At last, the "slack" in the economy which the New Deal had failed to eradicate was fully taken up, and underutilized resources and manpower properly exploited: "During the war the size of the productive plant within the country grew by nearly 50 percent and the physical output of goods by more than 50 percent."[35] Indeed, in the years 1940 to 1944, industrial expansion in the United States rose at a faster pace—over 15 percent a year—than at any period before or since. Although the greater part of this growth was caused by war production (which soared from 2 percent of total output in 1939 to 40 percent in 1943), nonwar goods also increased, so that the civilian sector of the economy was not encroached upon as in the other combatant nations. Its standard of living was higher than any other country's, but so was its per capita productivity. Among the Great Powers, the United States was the only country which became richer—in fact, much richer—rather than poorer because of the war. At its conclusion, Washington possessed gold reserves of $20 billion, almost two-thirds of the world's total of $33 billion.[36] Again, ". . . more than half the total manufacturing production of the world took place within the U.S.A., which, in fact, turned out a third of the world production of goods of all types."[37] This also made it by far the greatest exporter of goods at the war's end, and even a few years later it supplied one-third of the world's exports. Because of the massive expansion of its shipbuilding facilities, it now owned half of the world supply of shipping. Economically, the world was its oyster.

This economic power was reflected in the military strength of the United States, which at the end of the war controlled 12.5 million service personnel, including 7.5 million overseas. Although this total was naturally going to shrink in peacetime (by 1948, the army's personnel was only one-ninth what it had been four years earlier), that merely reflected political choices, not real military potential. Given the early postwar assumptions about the limited overseas roles of the United States, a better indication of its strength lay in the tallies of its modern weaponry. By this stage, the U.S. Navy was unquestionably "second to none," its fleet of 1,200 major warships (centered upon dozens of aircraft carriers rather than battleships) now being considerably larger than the Royal Navy's, with no other significant maritime force existing. In both its carrier task forces and its Marine Corps divisions, the United States had amply demonstrated its capacity to project its power across the globe to any region accessible from the sea. Even more imposing was the American "command of the air"; the 2,000-plus heavy bombers which had pounded Hitler's Europe and the 1,000 ultra-long-range B-29s which had reduced many Japanese cities to ashes were to be supplemented by even more powerful jet-propelled strategic bombers like the B-36. Above all, the United States possessed a monopoly of atomic bombs, which promised to unleash a devastation upon any future enemy as horrific as that which had occurred at Hiroshima and Nagasaki.[38] As later analyses have pointed out, American military power may actually have been less than it seemed (there were very few A-bombs in stock, and dropping them had large political implications), and it was difficult to use it to influence the conduct of a country as distant, inscrutable, and suspicious as the USSR; but the image of ineffable superiority remained undisturbed until the Korean War, and was reinforced by the pleas of so many nations for American loans, weapons, and promises of military support.

Given the extraordinarily favorable economic and strategical position which the United States thus occupied, its post-1945 outward thrust could come as no surprise to those familiar with the history of international politics. With the traditional Great Powers fading away, it steadily moved into the vacuum which their going created; having become number one, it could no longer contain itself within its own shores, or even its own hemisphere. To be sure, the war itself had been the primary cause of this projection outward of American power and influence; because of it, for example, in 1945 it had sixty-nine divisions in Europe, twenty-six in Asia and the Pacific, and none in the continental United States.[39] Simply because it was politically committed to the reordering of Japan and Germany (and Austria), it was "over there"; and because it had campaigned via island groups in the Pacific, and into North Africa, Italy, and western Europe, it had forces in those territories also. There were, however, many Americans (especially among the troops) who expected that they would all be home within a short period of time, returning U.S. armed-forces deployments to their pre-1941 position. But while that idea alarmed the likes of Churchill and attracted isolationist Republicans, it proved impossible to turn the clock back. Like the British after 1815, the Americans in their turn found their informal influence in various lands hardening into something more formal—and more entangling; like the British, too, they found "new frontiers of insecurity" whenever they wanted to draw the line. The "Pax Americana" had come of age.[40]

The economic aspects of this new order were, at least, predictable enough. During the war, internationalists like Cordell Hull had argued, with some reason, that the global crisis of the 1930s had been in large part caused by a malfunctioning of the international economy: by protective tariffs, unfair economic competition, restricted access to raw materials, autarkic governmental policies. This eighteenth-century Enlightenment belief that "unhampered trade dovetails with peace"[41] was joined by the pressures exerted by export-oriented industries, which feared that a postwar slump might follow the decline in U.S. government spending unless new overseas markets were opened up to absorb the products of America's enhanced productivity. To this was added a determined, and perhaps excessive, advocacy by the military to ensure American control of (or unrestricted access to) strategically critical materials such as oil, rubber, and metal ores.[42] All this combined to make the United States committed to the creation of a new world order beneficial to the needs of western capitalism and, of course, to the most flourishing of the western capitalist states—though with the longer-term, Adam Smithian assurance that "the more efficient distribution of resources brought about by unimpeded trade would raise productivity all around and thus increase everybody's purchasing power."[43] Hence the package of international arrangements hammered out between 1942 and 1946—the setting-up of the International Monetary Fund, of the International Bank for Reconstruction and Development—and then the later General Agreement on Tariffs and Trade (GATT). Those countries wishing to secure some of the monies available for reconstruction and development under this new economic regime found themselves obliged to conform to American requirements on free convertibility of currencies and open competition (as the British did, despite their efforts to preserve imperial preference)[44]—or to stand clear of the entire system (as the Russians did, when they perceived how incompatible this was with socialist controls).

The practical flaws in such arrangements were, first, that the amount of money available was simply insufficient to deal with the devastation caused by six years of total war; and, secondly, that a laissez-faire system inevitably works to the advantage of the country in the most competitive position—in this case, the undamaged, hyper-productive United States—and to the detriment of those less well equipped to compete—nations devastated by war, with boundaries altered, masses of refugees, bombed-out housing, worn-out machinery, ruinous debts, lost markets. Only the later American perception of the twin dangers of widespread social discontent in Europe and growing Soviet influence, which stimulated the creation of the Marshall Plan, permitted funds to be released for the substantial industrial redevelopment of the "free world." By that time, however, the expansion of American economic influence was going hand in hand with the erection of an array of military-base and security treaties across the globe (below, pp. 389–90). Here, too, there are many parallels with the expansion of British bases and treaty relationships after 1815; but the most noticeable difference was that Britain, on the whole, was able to avoid the plethora of fixed and entangling alliances with other sovereign countries which the United States was now assuming. Almost all of these American commitments were, it is true, "a response to events"[45] as the Cold War unfolded; but regardless of the justification, the blunt fact was that they involved the United States in a degree of global overstretch totally at variance with its own earlier history.

Little of this seems to have worried the decision-makers of 1945, many of whom appear to have felt not only that this was the working out of "manifest destiny," but that they now had a golden opportunity to put right what the former Great Powers had managed to mess up. "American experience," exulted Henry Luce of *Life* magazine, "is the key to the future. . . . America must be the elder brother of nations in the brotherhood of man."[46] Not only China, in which extremely high hopes were placed, but all of the other countries of what was soon to be termed the Third World were encouraged to emulate American ideals of self-help, entrepreneurship, free trade, and democracy. "All these principles and policies are so beneficial and appealing to the sense of justice, of right and of the well-being of free peoples everywhere," Hull prophesized, "that in the course of a few years the entire international machinery should be working fairly satisfactorily."[47] Whoever was so purblind as not to appreciate that fact—whether old-fashioned British and Dutch imperialists, or leftward-tending European political parties, or the grim-faced Molotov—would be persuaded, by a mixture of sticks and carrots, in the right direction. As one American official put it, "It is now our turn to bat in Asia";[48] and, he might have added, nearly everywhere else as well.

The one area where American influence was highly unlikely to penetrate was that controlled by the Soviet Union, which in 1945 (and ever since) claimed to be the true victor of the fight against fascism. According to the Red Army's statistics, it had smashed a total of 506 German divisions; and of the 13.6 million German casualties and prisoners lost during the Second World War, 10 million met their fate on the eastern front.[49] Yet even before the Third Reich had collapsed, Stalin was switching dozens of divisions to the Far East, ready to unleash them upon Japan's denuded Kwantung Army in Manchuria when the time was ripe; which turned out to be, perhaps unsurprisingly, three days after Hiroshima. The extended campaign on the western front more than reversed the disastrous post-1917 slump in Russia's position in Europe; indeed, it actually restored it to something akin to that of the period 1814–1848, when its great army had been the gendarme of east-central Europe. Russian territorial boundaries expanded, in the north at the expense of Finland, in the center at the expense of Poland; and in the south, recovering Bessarabia, at the expense of Rumania. The Baltic states of Estonia, Latvia, and Lithuania were reincorporated into Russia. Part of East Prussia was taken, and a slice of eastern Czechoslovakia (Ruthenia, or Subcarpathian Ukraine) was also thoughtfully added, so that there was direct access to Hungary. To the west and southwest of this enhanced Russia lay a new *cordon sanitaire* of satellite states, Poland, East Germany, Czechoslovakia, Hungary, Rumania, Bulgaria, and (until they wriggled free) Yugoslavia and Albania. Between them and the West, the proverbial "iron curtain" was falling; behind that curtain, Communist party cadres and secret police were determining that the entire region would operate under principles totally at variance with Cordell Hull's hopes. The same was true in the Far East, where the swift occupation of Manchuria, North Korea, and Sakhalin not only avenged the war of 1904–1905, but allowed a link-up with Mao's Chinese Communists, who were also unlikely to swallow the gospel of laissez-faire capitalism.

But if this growth of Soviet influence looked imposing, its economic base had been badly hurt by the war—in contrast to the United States' undisturbed boom. Russia's population losses were appalling: 7.5 million in the armed forces; 6–8 million civilians killed by the Germans; plus the "indirect" war losses caused by the reduced food rations, forced labor, and vastly increased hours of work, so that "altogether probably some 20–25 million Soviet citizens died premature deaths between 1941 and 1945."[50] Since the casualties were mainly men, the consequent imbalance between the sexes greatly affected the country's demographic structure and caused a severe drop in the birthrate. The material damage done in the German-occupied parts of European Russia, the Ukraine, and Belorussia was so large as to be beyond normal imaginings:

> Of the 11.6 million horses in occupied territory, 7 million were killed or taken away, as were 20 out of 23 million pigs. 137,000 tractors, 49,000 grain combines and large numbers of cowsheds and other farm buildings were destroyed. Transport was hit by the destruction of 65,000 kilometers of railway track, loss of or damage to 15,800 locomotives, 428,000 goods wagons, 4,280 river boats, and half of all the railway bridges in the occupied territory. Almost 50 percent of all urban living space in this territory, 1.2 million houses, were destroyed, as well as 3.5 million houses in rural areas.
>
> Many towns lay in ruins. Thousands of villages were smashed. People lived in holes in the ground.[51]

It was scarcely surprising, therefore, that when the Russians moved into their "occupation zone" in Germany, they attempted to strip it of all movable assets, factory plant, rail lines, etc., as well as demanding compensations from other eastern European territories (Rumanian oil, Finnish timber, Polish coal).

It was true that the Soviet Union had outproduced Greater Germany in the armaments battle as well as outfighting it at the front; but it had done so by an incredibly single-minded concentration upon military-industrial production and by drastic decreases in every other sector—consumer goods, retail trade, and agricultural supplies (though the decline in food output was chiefly caused by German plunderings).[52] In essence, therefore, the Russia of 1945 was a military giant and, at the same time, economically poor, deprived, and unbalanced. With Lend-Lease cut off, and having rejected later American monies because of the political conditions attached to them, the Soviet Union reverted to its post-1928 program of enforced economic growth from its own resources—with the same strong emphasis upon producer goods (heavy industry, coal, electricity, cement) and transport to the detriment of consumer goods and agriculture, and with a natural reduction in military expenditures from their wartime levels. The result, after initial difficulties, was "a minor economic miracle"[53] so far as heavy industry was concerned, with output nearly doubling between 1945 and 1950. Obsessed by the need to rebuild the sinews of national power, the Stalinist regime had no problems in achieving that crude aim or in keeping the standard of living for most Russians down at pre-Revolution levels. Yet it also ought to be noted that, as with the post-1922 growth, much of the "recovery" of industrial production consisted of getting back to the *prewar* output; in the Ukraine, for example, metallurgical and electrical output around 1950 had reached, or just exceeded, the 1940 figures. Once again, because of war, Russia's economic growth had been choked back by a decade or so. More serious still, in the longer term, was the continued failure of the vital agricultural sector: with the emergency wartime incentive measures suppressed, and because of the totally inadequate (and misdirected) investment, farming wilted and food output slumped. Until his death, Stalin maintained his bitter vendetta against the peasantry's preference for private plots, thereby ensuring that the traditional low productivity and high inefficiency of Russian agriculture would continue.[54]

By contrast, Stalin was clearly intent upon maintaining a high level of military security in the postwar world. Given the need to rebuild the economy, it was not surprising that the enormous Red Army was reduced by two-thirds after 1945, to the still very substantial total of 175 divisions, supported by 25,000 front-line tanks and 19,000 aircraft. It still would remain, therefore, the largest defense establishment in the world—a fact justified (in Soviet eyes, at least) by its need to deter future aggressors and, more prosaically, to keep control of its newly acquired satellites in Europe as well as its conquests in the Far East. Although this was an enormous force, many of its divisions existed only in skeleton form, or were essentially garrison troops.[55] Moreover, the service ran the danger which had befallen the gigantic Russian army in the decades after 1815—increasing obsolescence, in the face of new military advances. This was to be combated not only by a substantial reorganization and modernization of the army's divisions,[56] but also by committing the economic and scientific resources of the Soviet state to the development of new weapon systems. By 1947–1948, the formidable MiG-15 jet fighter was going into service, and—in imitation of the Americans and British—a long-range strategic air force had been created. Captured German scientists and technicians were being used to develop a variety of guided missiles. Even during the war, resources had been allocated for the development of a Soviet A-bomb. And the Russian navy, which had been a mere ancillary arm in the struggle against Germany, was also being transformed, with the addition of new heavy cruisers and even more oceangoing submarines. Much of this weaponry was derivative and, by western standards, unsophisticated. What could not be doubted, however, was the Soviet determination not to be left behind.[57]

The third major element in the buttressing of Russian power was Stalin's renewed emphasis upon the internal discipline and absolute conformism of the late 1930s. Whether this was due to his increasing paranoia or a carefully calculated set of moves to reinforce his own dictatorial position—or a mixture of both—is hard to say; but the events spoke for themselves.[58] Anyone with foreign connections was suspect; returning prisoners-of-war were shot; the creation of the state of Israel, and thus an alternative source of Jewish loyalties, led to renewed anti-Semitic measures within Russia. The army leadership was cut down to size, with the respected Marshal Zhukov being removed as commander of the Soviet ground forces in 1946. Discipline within the Communist party itself, and admission to the same, was tightened; in 1948, the entire party leadership of Leningrad (which Stalin always disliked) was purged. Censorship was intensified, not only over literature and the creative arts, but also over the natural sciences, biology, linguistics. This overall "tightening" of the system naturally fitted in with the reasserted collectivization of agriculture mentioned earlier, and with the rise of Cold War tensions. It was also natural that a similar process of ideological stiffening and totalitarian controls should take place in the Soviet-dominated states of eastern Europe, where the elimination of rival parties, the holdings of show trials, the drive against individual rights and properties, became the order of the day. All this, and in particular the elimination of democracy in Poland and (in 1948) in Czechoslovakia, led to a considerable ebbing of western enthusiasm for the Soviet system. Again, it is unclear whether these measures were all carefully calculated—there was, and is, a crude logic in the Soviet elite's desire to isolate its satellites as well as its own people from the ideas and riches of the West—or whether it simply reflected Stalin's increasing paranoia as his end approached. Whatever the cause, there would be one massive stretch of territory totally immune from the influences of any "Pax Americana," and indeed offering an alternative to it.

This growth of the Soviet Empire appeared to confirm the geopolitical predictions of Mackinder and others that a gigantic military power would control the resources of the Eurasian "Heartland"; and that the further expansion of that state into the periphery or "Rimland" would need to be contested by the great maritime states if they were to preserve a global balance of power.[59] It would still be another few years before U.S. administrations, shaken by the Korean War, completely abandoned their earlier ideas of "One World" and replaced them with the image of an unrelenting superpower struggle across the international arena. Yet to a large extent this was implicit in the circumstances of 1945; the United States and the USSR were the only nations now capable, as de Tocqueville had once put it, of swaying the destinies of half the globe; and both had fallen prey to "globalist" thinking. "The USSR now is one of the mightiest countries of the world. One cannot decide now *any* serious problems of international relations without the USSR . . ." Molotov claimed in 1946,[60] an echo of the earlier American intimation to Moscow (when it seemed that Churchill and Stalin might come to a private agreement over eastern Europe) that "in this global war there is literally no question, political or military, in which the United States is not interested."[61] A serious clash of interests was inevitable.

But what of those former Great Powers, now merely middleweight countries, whose collapse was the obverse side of the rise of the superpowers? It needs to be said immediately that the defeated fascist states of Germany, Japan, and Italy were in a different category from that of Great Britain and, perhaps, of France also in the immediate post-1945 period. When the fighting ceased, the Allies went ahead with their plans to ensure that neither Germany nor Japan would ever again be a threat to the international order. This involved not only the long-term military occupation of both countries but, in the German case, its division into four occupation zones and then, later, into two separate German states. Japan was stripped of its overseas acquisitions (as was Italy in 1943), Germany of its European gains and of its older territories in the east (Silesia, East Prussia, etc.). The devastation caused by the strategic bombing, the overstraining of the transport system, the decline of the housing stock, and the lack of many raw materials and export markets was compounded by the Allied controls upon industry—and, in Germany, by the dismantling of industrial plant. German national income and output in 1946 was less than one-third that of 1938, a horrendous reduction.[62] In Japan, a similar economic regression had occurred; real national income in 1946 was only 57 percent that of 1934–1936 and real manufacturing wages were down to only 30 percent of the same; foreign trade was so minimal that even two years later, exports were only 8 percent and imports 18 percent of the 1934–1936 figure. Japan's shipping had been eliminated by the war, the number of cotton spindles cut from 12.2 million to 2 million, coal output halved, and so on.[63] Economically as well as militarily, their days as powerful nations seemed over.

Although Italy had switched sides in 1943, its economic fate was almost as grim. For two years, Allied forces had fought and bombed their way up the peninsula, severely adding to the damage caused by Mussolini's strategical extravagances. "In 1945 . . . Italy's gross national product had reverted to the 1911 level and had diminished by about 40 percent in real terms, as compared with 1938. The population, despite war losses, had increased largely as a result of repatriation from the colonies and the halt in emigration. The standard of living was alarmingly low, and but for international aid, especially from the United States, many Italians would have died of starvation."[64] Italian real wages were down to 26.7 percent of their 1913 value by 1945.[65] In fact, all of these countries were terribly dependent upon American aid during this period; and, as such, were little more than economic satellites.

It was difficult to tell the difference, in economic terms, between France and Germany. Four years of plundering by the Germans had been followed by months of large-scale fighting in 1944; "most waterways and harbors were blocked, most bridges destroyed, much of the railway system temporarily unusable."[66] Fohlen's indices of French imports and exports shows them plunging to virtually nothing by 1944–1945; France's national income by that time was only half that of 1938, itself a gloomy year.[67] France had no stocks of foreign currency, and the franc itself had not been accepted on the foreign exchanges; its value, when fixed at 50 to the dollar in 1944, was "purely fictitious,"[68] and within a year it had slid to 119 to the dollar; by 1949, when things seemed more stable, it was 420 to the dollar. French party politics, and in particular the role of the Communist party, obviously interacted with these purely economic problems of reconstruction, nationalization, and inflation.

On the other hand, the Free French had been members of the "Grand Alliance" against fascism and had fought in many of the major campaigns, as well as triumphing in their "civil" war against pro-Vichy forces in West Africa, the Levant, and Algeria. Given the German occupation of France and the division in French loyalties during the war, de Gaulle's organization was heavily dependent upon Anglo-American aid—which de Gaulle resented, even as he demanded more. Nonetheless, the British were eager to see France reestablished as a strong military Power in Europe as a check to Russia, rather than a collapsing Germany, and so France acquired many of the accouterments of Great Power status: an occupation zone in Germany, permanent membership in the UN Security Council, and so on. Although it could not regain its former mandates in Syria and Lebanon, it did seek to reassert itself in Indochina and in the protectorates of Tunisia and Morocco; and with its overseas departments and territories, it still possessed the second-largest colonial empire in the world and was determined to hang on to it.[69] To many outside observers, especially the Americans, this attempt to regain the trappings of first-class power status while so desperately weak economically—and so dependent upon American financial support—was nothing more than a *folie de grandeur*. And so, to a large extent, it was. Perhaps its chief consequence was to disguise, at least for some more years, the extent to which the strategical landscape of the globe had been altered by the war.

Although most Britons in 1945 would have felt indignant at the comparison, the continued appearance of their nation and empire as one of the Great Powers of the world also disguised the new strategical balances—as well as making it psychologically difficult for decision-makers in London to readjust to the politics of decline. The British Empire was the only major state which had fought through the Second World War from beginning to end. Under Churchill's leadership, it had been unquestionably one of the "Big Three." Its military performance, at sea, in the air, even on land, had been significantly better than in the First World War. By August 1945, all the possessions of the king-emperor—including Hong Kong—were back in British hands. British troops and airbases were sprawled across North Africa, Italy, Germany, Southeast Asia. Despite heavy losses, the Royal Navy possessed over 1,000 warships, nearly 3,000 minor war vessels, and nearly 5,500 landing craft. RAF Bomber Command was the second-largest strategic air force (by far) in the world. And yet, as Correlli Barnett has forcefully pointed out, "victory" was not

> synonymous with the preservation of British power. The defeat of Germany [and its allies] was only one factor, if a highly important factor, in such a preservation. For Germany might be defeated and yet British power still be brought to an end. What counted was not so much "victory" in itself, but the circumstances of the victory, and in particular the circumstances in which England found herself. . . .[70]

For the blunt fact was that in securing a victorious outcome to the war the British had severely overstrained themselves, running down their gold and dollar reserves, wearing out their domestic machinery, and (despite an extraordinary mobilization of their resources and population) becoming increasingly dependent upon American munitions, shipping, foodstuffs, and other supplies to stay in the fighting. While its need for such imports had risen year by year, its export trade had withered away—by 1944 it was a mere 31 percent of the 1938 figure. When the Labor government entered office in July 1945, one of the first documents it had to read was Keynes's hair-raising memorandum about the "financial Dunkirk" which the country was facing: its colossal trade gap, its weakened industrial base, its enormous overseas establishments, meant that American aid was desperately needed, to replace the cut-off Lend-Lease. Without that help, indeed, "a greater degree of austerity would be necessary than we have experienced at any time during the war. . . ."[71] Once again, as happened after the First World War, the goal of creating a home fit for heroes would have to be modified. But this time, it was impossible to believe that Britain was still at the center of the world politically.

Yet, the illusions of Great Power status lingered on, even among Labor ministers intent upon creating a "welfare state." The history of the next few years therefore involved an earnest British attempt to grapple with these irreconcilables—improving domestic standards of living, moving to a "mixed economy," closing the trade gap, and at the same time supporting a vastly extended array of overseas bases, in Germany, the Near East, and India, and maintaining large armed forces in the face of the worsening relations with Russia. As the detailed studies of the Attlee administration suggest,[72] it was remarkably successful in many respects: industrial productivity rose, the trade gap narrowed, social reforms were enacted, the European scene was stabilized. The Labor government also found it prudent to withdraw from India, to pull out of the chaos in Palestine, and to abandon the guarantees to Greece and Turkey, so that it was relieved of at least some of its more pressing overseas burdens. On the other hand, that economic recovery had itself depended upon the large loan Keynes had negotiated in Washington in 1945, upon the further massive support which came via Marshall Plan aid, and upon the still-devastated state of most of Britain's commercial rivals; it was, therefore, a delicate and conditional economic revival. Equally suspect, over the longer term, was the success of the British withdrawals of 1947. It certainly shed intolerable burdens; but that strategical "fancy footwork" was postulated on the assumption that in abandoning certain regions, Britain could relocate its bases to accord more with its real imperial interests—the Suez Canal rather than Palestine, Arabian oil rather than India. At this stage, there certainly was no intention in Whitehall of giving up the *rest* of the dependent empire, which in economic terms was more important to Britain than ever before.[73] Only further shocks and the rising costs of hanging on would later force another reappraisal of Britain's place in the world. In the meantime, however, it would remain an overextended but still powerful strategical entity, dependent upon the United States for security and yet also that country's most useful ally—and an important strategic collaborator—in a world dividing into two large power blocs.[74]

All the efforts of British and French governments to the contrary, however, there was no doubt about "the passing of the European age." While the U.S. GNP had surged by more than 50 percent in real terms during the war, Europe's as a whole (but minus the Soviet Union) had fallen by about 25 percent.[75] Europe's share of total world manufacturing output was lower than at any time since the early nineteenth century; even by 1953, when most of the war damage had been repaired, it possessed only 26 percent of the whole (compared with the United States' 44.7 percent).[76] Its population was now only about 15–16 percent of the total world population. In 1950 its per capita GNP was only about one-half of the United States'; moreover, the Soviet Union had by then significantly closed the gap, so that the total GNP of the powers was as shown in Table 36.

Table 36. Total GNP and per Capita GNP of the Powers in 1950[77]
(in 1964 dollars)

	Total GNP	Per Capita GNP
United States	381 billion	2,536
USSR	126	699
U.K.	71	1,393 (1951)
France	50	1,172
West Germany	48	1,001
Japan	32	382
Italy	29	626 (1951)

This eclipse of the European powers was reflected even more markedly in military personnel and expenditures. In 1950, for example, the United States spent $14.5 billion on defense and had 1.38 million military personnel, while the USSR spent slightly more ($15.5 billion) on its far larger armed forces of 4.3 million men. In both respects, the superpowers were far ahead of Britain ($2.3 billion; 680,000 personnel), France ($1.4 billion; 590,000 personnel), and Italy ($0.5 billion; 230,000 personnel), and of course Germany and Japan were still demilitarized. The Korean War tensions saw quite significant increases in the defense spending of the middleweight European powers in 1951, but they paled by comparison with the expenditures of the United States ($33.3 billion) and USSR ($20.1 billion). In that year alone, the defense expenditures of Britain, France, and Italy *combined* were less than one-fifth of the United States' and less than one third of the USSR's; and their *combined* military personnel was one-half of the United States' and one-third of Russia's.[78] In both relative economic strength and in military power, the European states seemed decidedly eclipsed.

Such an impression was, if anything, heightened by the coming of nuclear weapons and long-range delivery systems. It is clear from the record that many of the scientists working on the A-bomb were acutely aware that they were reaching toward a watershed in the entire history of warfare, weapon systems, and man's capacity for destruction; the successful test at Alamogordo on July 16, 1945, confirmed to the observers that "there had been brought into being something big and something new that would prove to be immeasurably more important than the discovery of electricity or any of the other great discoveries which have affected our existence." When the "strong, sustained, awesome roar which warned of doomsday"[79] was repeated in the actual carnage of Hiroshima and Nagasaki, there could be no further doubt of the weapon's power. Its creation left American decision-makers wrestling with the many practical consequences for the future. How did it affect conventional warfare? Should it be used immediately at the outset of war, or as a weapon of last resort? What were the implications, and potentialities, of developing bigger (H-bombs) and smaller (tactical) forms of nuclear weapons? Should the knowledge be shared with others?[80] It also undoubtedly gave a boost to the already existing Soviet development of nuclear weapons, since Stalin put his formidable security chief, Beria, in charge of the atomic program on the day after Hiroshima.[81] Although the Russians were clearly behind at this time, in the creation of both bombs and delivery systems, they caught up much faster than the Americans estimated they would. For some years after 1945, it seems fair to assume that the American nuclear advantage helped to "balance out" the Russian preponderance in conventional forces. But it was not long, certainly in the history of international relations, before Moscow began to catch up and thus to prove its own claim that the United States' monopoly of this weapon had been only a passing phase.[82]

The coming of atomic weapons transformed the "strategical landscape," since they gave to any state possessing them the capability of mass indiscriminate destruction, even of mankind itself. Much more narrowly, and immediately, the advent of this new level in weapons technology put increased pressure upon the traditional European states to catch up—or admit that they were indeed relegated to second-class status. Of course, in the case of Germany and Japan, and the economically and technologically weakened Italy, there was no prospect of joining the nuclear club. But to the government in London, even when Attlee replaced Churchill, it was inconceivable that the country should not possess those weapons, both as a deterrent and because they "were a manifestation of the scientific and technological superiority on which Britain's strength, so deficient if measured in sheer numbers of men, must depend."[83] They were seen, in other words, as a relatively *cheap* way of retaining independent Great Power influence—a calculation which, shortly afterward, appealed equally to the French.[84] Yet, however attractive that logic appeared to be, it was weakened by practical factors: that neither state would possess the weapons, and delivery systems, for some years; and that their nuclear arsenals would be minor compared with those of the superpowers, and might indeed be made obsolete by a further leap in technology. For all the ambitions of London and Paris (and, later on, China) to join the nuclear club, this striving during the early post-1945 decades was somewhat similar to the Austro-Hungarian and Italian efforts to possess their own *Dreadnought*-type battleships prior to 1914. It was, in other words, a reflection of weakness rather than strength.

The final element which seemed to emphasize that the world must now be viewed, strategically and politically, as bipolar rather than in its traditional multipolar form was the heightened role of *ideology*. To be sure, even in the age of classical nineteenth-century diplomacy, ideological factors had played a part in policy—as the actions of Metternich, Nicholas I, Bismarck, and Gladstone amply testified. This seemed much more the case in the interwar years, when a "radical right" and a "radical left" arose to challenge the prevailing assumptions of the "bourgeois-liberal center." Nonetheless, the complex dynamics of multipolar rivalries by the late 1930s (with British Tories like Churchill wanting an alliance with Communist Russia against Nazi Germany, and with liberal Americans wanting to support Anglo-French diplomacy in Europe but to dismantle the British and French empires outside Europe) made difficult all attempts to explain world affairs in ideological terms. During the war itself, moreover, differences on political and social principles could be subsumed under the overriding need to combat fascism. Stalin's suppression of the Communist International in 1943 and the West's admiration for the Russian resistance to Operation Barbarossa also seemed to blur earlier suspicions—especially in the United States, where *Life* magazine in 1943 airily claimed that the Russians "look like Americans, dress like Americans and think like Americans," and the *New York Times* a year later declared that "Marxian thinking in Soviet Russia is out."[85] Such sentiments, however naive, help to explain the widespread American reluctance to accept that the postwar world was not living up to their vision of international harmony—hence, for example, the pained and angry reactions of many to Churchill's famous "Iron Curtain" speech of March 1946.[86]

Yet, within another year or two, the ideological nature of what was now admitted to be the Cold War between Russia and the West was all too evident. The increasing signs that Russia would not permit parliamentary-type democracy in eastern Europe, the sheer size of the Russian armed forces, the civil war raging between Communists and their opponents in Greece, China, and elsewhere, and—last but by no means least—the growing fears of "the Red menace," spy rings, and internal subversion at home led to a massive swing in American sentiment, and one to which the Truman administration responded with alacrity. In his "Truman Doctrine" speech of March 1947, occasioned by the fear that Russia would enter into the power vacuum created by Britain's withdrawal of guarantees to Greece and Turkey, the president portrayed a world faced with a choice between two different sets of ideological principles:

One way of life is based upon the will of the majority, and is distinguished by free institutions, representative government, free elections, guarantees of individual liberty, freedom of speech and religion and freedom from political oppression. The second way of life is based upon the will of a minority forcibly imposed on the majority. It relies upon terror and oppression, a controlled press, framed elections and the suppression of personal freedom.[87]

It would be the policy of the United States, Truman continued, "to help free people to maintain their institutions and their integrity against aggressive movements that seek to impose upon them totalitarian regimes." Henceforward, international affairs would be presented, in even more emotional terms, as a Manichean struggle; in Eisenhower's words, "Forces of good and evil are massed and armed and opposed as rarely before in history. Freedom is pitted against slavery, lightness against dark."[88]

No doubt much of this rhetoric had a domestic purpose—and not just in the United States, but also in Britain, Italy, France, and wherever it was useful for conservative forces to invoke such language to discredit their rivals, or to attack their own governments for being "soft on Communism." What was also true was that it must have deepened Stalin's suspicions of the West, which was swiftly portrayed in the Soviet press as contesting the Russian "sphere of influence" in eastern Europe, surrounding the Soviet Union with new foes on all sides, establishing forward bases, supporting reactionary regimes against any Communist influences, and deliberately "packing" the United Nations. "The new course of American foreign policy," Moscow claimed, "meant a return to the old anti-Soviet course, designed to unloose war and forcibly to institute world domination by Britain and the United States."[89] This explanation, in turn, could help the Soviet regime to justify its crackdown upon internal dissidents, its tightening grip upon eastern Europe, its forced industrialization, its heavy spending upon armaments. Thus, the foreign and domestic requirements of the Cold War could feed off each other, mutually covered by an appeal to ideological principles. Liberalism and Communism, being both universal ideas, were "mutually exclusive";[90] this permitted each side to understand, and to portray, the whole world as an arena in which the ideological quarrel could not be separated from power-political advantage. One was either in the American-led bloc or the Soviet one. There was to be no middle way; in an age of Stalin and Joe McCarthy, it was imprudent to think that there could be. This was the new strategical reality, to which not merely the peoples of a divided Europe but also those in Asia, the Middle East, Africa, Latin America, and elsewhere would have to adjust.

The Cold War and the Third World

As it turned out, a large part of international politics over the following two decades *was* to concern itself with adjusting to that Soviet-American rivalry, and then with its partial rejection. In the beginning, the Cold War was centered upon remaking the boundaries of Europe. Underneath, therefore, it was still to do with the "German problem," since the resolution of that issue would in turn determine the amount of influence which the victorious Powers of 1945 would exert over Europe. The Russians had undoubtedly suffered more than any other country from German aggressions in the first half of the twentieth century, and, reinforced by Stalin's own paranoid demand for security, they were determined to permit no repetitions in the second half. Promoting the Communist world revolution was a secondary but not unconnected consideration, since Russia's strategic and political position was most likely to be enhanced if it could create other Marxist-led states which looked to Moscow for guidance. Such considerations, much more than any centuries-old drive toward warm-water ports, probably ordered the Soviet policy in the post-1945 world, even if it left open the detailed solution of the various issues. There was, in the first place, therefore, a determination to undo the territorial settlements of 1918–1922, with "roundings-off" for strategical purposes; as noted above, this meant the reassertion of Russian control over the Baltic states, the pushing westward of the Polish-Russian border, the elimination of East Prussia, and the acquisition of territories from Finland, Hungary, and Rumania. Little of this worried the West; indeed, much of it had been agreed to during the war. What was more perturbing was the Russian indications of how they intended to ensure that the formerly independent countries of east-central Europe would contain regimes "friendly to Moscow."

In this respect, the fate of Poland was a harbinger of what would occur elsewhere, although it was the more poignant because of Britain's 1939 decision to fight for that country's integrity, and because of the Polish contingents (and government in exile) which had operated in the West. The discovery of the mass grave of Polish officers at Katyn, the Russian disapproval of the Warsaw uprising, Stalin's insistence on altering Poland's boundaries, and the appearance of a pro-Moscow faction of Poles at Lublin made Churchill in particular suspicious of Russia's intentions; within another few years, with the installation of a puppet regime and the virtual elimination of any pro-western Poles from positions of power, those fears were realized.[91]

Moscow's handling of the Polish issue related to the "German problem" in all sorts of ways. Territorially, the westward adjustment of the boundaries not only reduced the size of German lands (as did the swallowing-up of East Prussia), it also gave the Poles an incentive to oppose any future German revision of the Oder-Neisse line. Strategically, the Russian insistence upon making Poland a secure "buffer zone" was intended to ensure that there could be no repetition of Germany's 1941 attack; it was logical, therefore, for Moscow to insist upon determining the fate of the German people as well. Politically, the support of the "Lublin" Poles was paralleled by the grooming of German Communists in exile to play a similar role when they returned to their homeland. Economically, Russia's exploitation of Poland and its eastern European neighbors was a foretaste of the stripping of German assets. When, however, it became obvious to Moscow that it would be impossible to win the German people's goodwill while systematically reducing them to penury, the asset-stripping ceased and Molotov's tone became much more encouraging. But those tactical shifts were of less importance than the obvious message that Russia intended to have a, if not *the*, major say in deciding Germany's future.[92]

Both in the Polish and the German cases, then, Russian policy was bound to clash with that of the West. Politically and economically the Americans, British, and French desired free-market ideas and democratic elections to be the norm throughout Europe (although London and Paris clearly wished the state to occupy a larger place than the laissez-faire Americans preferred). Strategically, the West was just as determined as Moscow to prevent any revival of German militarism, and the French especially were to worry about that until the mid-1950s; but none of them wanted to see the Wehrmacht's domination of Europe merely replaced by the Red Army's. And although both the French and the Italian governments after 1945 contained Communists, there was a deep mistrust of Marxist parties gaining real power anywhere—a feeling confirmed by the steady elimination of non-Communist parties in eastern Europe. Although there were still voices hoping for a reconciliation between Russia and the West, the fact was that their respective aims clashed in all manner of ways. If one side's program succeeded, the other would feel threatened; in that sense, at least, the Cold War seemed inevitable, until both sides agreed to compromise on their universalist assumptions.

For that reason, a step-by-step account of the escalation of the tensions is not necessary here;[93] it would have the same relevance to this analysis of the evolving dynamics of world power as would, say, a detailed account of Metternich's diplomacy in an earlier chapter. The chief features of the Cold War after 1945 are, however, worthy of examination, since they have continued to affect the conduct of international relations to this day.

The first of these was the intensification of the "split" between the two blocs in Europe. That this bifurcation had not occurred immediately in 1945 was understandable: the chief tasks then for the Allied occupation forces, and for the "successor" parties which emerged out of hiding and exile once the Germans had left, were pressing administrative ones—restoring communications and utilities, getting foodstuffs to the cities, housing the refugees, tracking down war criminals. Much of this led to a blurring of ideological positions: in the occupied zones of Germany, the Americans found themselves quarreling as much with the French as with the Russians; in national assemblies and cabinets being formed across Europe, Socialists sat alongside Communists in the east, Communists alongside Christian Democrats in the west. But by late 1946 and early 1947, the gap was widening and becoming more publicized: various plebiscites and regional elections in the German zones were showing "the political complexion of West Germany . . . beginning to differ markedly from that of East Germany";[94] the steady elimination of any non-Communist elements in Poland, Bulgaria, and Rumania was mirrored by the internal political crisis in France in April 1947, when the Communists were forced to resign from the government. A month after, the same happened in Italy. In Yugoslavia, Tito's political domination (in place of the Allied wartime agreements about shared power) was interpreted by the West as a further step in Moscow's planned advance. These disagreements, together with the Soviet Union's unwillingness to join the IMF and International Bank, especially disturbed those Americans who had hoped to preserve good relations with Moscow after the war.

It was only a modest leap in assumptions, therefore, for the West to suspect that Stalin also planned to acquire control in *western* and *southern* Europe when the circumstances were right and, indeed, to hurry those circumstances along. This was unlikely to occur by outright military force, although the increasing Russian pressure upon Turkey was worrying, and prompted Washington to station a naval task force in the eastern Mediterranean by 1946; rather, it might come about through the ability of Moscow's minions to take advantage of the continued economic dislocation and political rivalries caused by the war. The Greek Communist revolt was seen as one sign of this; the Communist-supported strikes in France another. The Russian bids to woo German public opinion were suspicious; so, too, if one really wanted to worry about things, was the strength of the Communists in northern Italy. Historians of each of those movements are nowadays more skeptical of how much they could have been controlled by a Moscow-conceived "master plan." The Greek Communists, Tito, and Mao Tse-tung cared most about their local foes, not a global Marxist order; and the leaders of Communist parties and trade unions in the West had to respond, first and foremost, to their followers' mood. On the other hand, a gain for Communism in any of those countries would undoubtedly have been welcome to Russia, provided it did not lead to a major war; and it is easy to understand why, at the time, Soviet experts like George Kennan were sympathetically heard when they argued the case for "containing" the Soviet Union.

Among all of the varied elements of the fast-evolving "strategy of containment,"[95] two stood out. The first, admitted by Kennan to be negative in nature although increasingly preferred by the military chiefs as offering more solid guarantees of stability, was to indicate to Moscow those regions of the globe which the United States "cannot permit . . . to fall into hands hostile to us."[96] Such states would, therefore, be given military support to build up their powers of resistance; and a Soviet attack on them would be regarded virtually as a *casus belli.* Much more positive, however, was the American recognition that resistance to Russian subversion was weakened because of "the profound exhaustion of physical plant and of spiritual vigor" caused by the Second World War.[97] The most crucial component of any long-term containment policy would therefore be a massive program of U.S. economic aid, to permit the rebuilding of the shattered industries, farms, and cities of Europe and Japan; for that would not only make the latter far less likely to be tempted by Communist doctrines of class struggle and revolution, it would also help to readjust the *power balances* in America's favor. If, to use Kennan's very plausible geopolitical argument, there were only "five centers of industrial and military power in the world which are important to us from the standpoint of national security"[98]—the United States itself, its rival the USSR, Great Britain, Germany and central Europe, and Japan—then it followed that by keeping the three last-named areas in the western camp and by building up their strength, there would be a resultant "correlation of forces" which would ensure that the Soviet Union was permanently inferior. Equally obvious, this strategy would be regarded with profound suspicion by Stalin's Russia, especially since it included the restoration of its two recent enemies, Germany and Japan.

Once again, therefore, an exact chronology of the various steps taken by each side during and after the "watershed year" of 1947 is less important than the general consequences. The U.S. replacement of the British guarantees to Greece and Turkey—symbolically, a transfer of responsibilities from the former global policeman to the rising one, and as much a part of London's logic as of Washington's[99]—was justified by Truman in terms of a "doctrine" which had no regional limitations. In the European context, however, the open American willingness "to help free peoples maintain their institutions" could be linked to the earnest discussions which were taking place about how to deal with the widespread economic distress, the food shortages, and the scarcity of coal which were afflicting the continent. The American administration's solution—the so-called Marshall Plan for massive aid "to place Europe on its feet economically"—was deliberately presented as an offering to *all* European nations, whether Communist or not. But whatever the attractions of receiving that aid may have been to Moscow, it did involve joint cooperation with western Europe, just at a time when the Soviet economy had returned to the most rigid forms of socialization and collectivization; and it took no genius to see that the *raison d'être* for the plan was to convince Europeans everywhere that private enterprise was better able to bring them prosperity than Communism. The result of Molotov's walkout from the Paris talks on the plan, and of the Russian pressure upon Poland and Czechoslovakia not to apply for aid, was that Europe became much more divided than before. In western Europe, boosted by the billions of dollars of American aid (especially to the larger states of Britain, France, Italy, and West Germany), economic growth shot ahead, integrated into a North Atlantic trading network. In eastern Europe, Communist controls were being tightened. The Cominform was set up in 1947, as a sort of reconstituted and only half-disguised Communist International. The pluralist regime in Prague was ended by a Communist coup in 1948. While Tito's Yugoslavia managed to escape from Stalin's claustrophobic embrace, other satellites found themselves subject to purges, and in 1949 they were forced to join Comecon (Council of Mutual Economic Assistance), which, far from being a Soviet Marshall Plan was "simply a new piece of machinery for milking the satellites."[100] Churchill may have been a little premature in his "Iron Curtain" description of 1946; two years later, his words seemed realized.

The intensification of East-West economic rivalries was complemented at the military level, and once again Germany was at the center of the dispute. In March 1947 the British and French had signed the Dunkirk Treaty, whereby each pledged all-out military support to the other signatory in the event of an attack by Germany (even though the Foreign Office in London held that contingency to be "rather academic" and was more concerned about western Europe's internal weaknesses). In March 1948 this pact was extended, by the Brussels Treaty, to include the Benelux countries. The latter agreement did not mention Germany by name, but it is fair to say that many politicians in western Europe (especially France) were still obsessed with the "German problem" at this time rather than the "Russian problem."[101] The antediluvian nature of their concerns was to be shaken up as 1948 unfolded. In the same month as the Brussels Treaty was signed, the Russians walked out of the Four-Power Control Council on Germany, claiming irreconcilable differences with the West over that country's economic and political future. Three months later, in an effort to end the black market and currency chaos in Germany, the three western control powers announced the creation of a new deutsche mark. The Russian response to this unilateral action was not only to ban the West German notes from their zone but to clamp down on movements in and out of Berlin, that island of western influence one hundred miles into their sphere.

If anything brought the extent of the antagonism close to home, it was the Berlin crisis of 1948–1949.[102] Already officials in Washington and London were discussing means whereby a grouping of the European states, the dominions, and the United States could stand together in the event of hostilities with Russia. While—as with the Marshall Plan—the Americans wished the Europeans to come forward first with schemes for military security, there was by this stage no doubt as to how seriously the United States took the Communist challenge. A full-blown "Red scare" at home complemented tougher actions abroad. In March 1948, Truman was even asking Congress to reinstate conscription, a request granted in the Selective Service Act of June of that year. All of these moves were boosted by the Soviet blockade of the land routes to Berlin. While the age of air power enabled the Americans and British to call Stalin's bluff by flying supplies into Berlin for the next eleven months, until the land access was restored, there had been many who argued for sending a military convoy to force its way to the city. It is difficult to believe that such an action would not have provoked a war; as it was, under a new treaty the United States moved a fleet of B-29 bombers to British airfields, a sign of their earnestness in the matter.

In these circumstances, even isolationist senators could be moved to support proposals for the creation of what was to be the North Atlantic Treaty Organization, with full American membership—and, indeed, with its chief strategical purpose being the provision of North American aid to the European states in the event of Russian aggression. In its early years, NATO reflected political concerns more than any exact military calculations, symbolizing as it did the historic shift in American diplomatic traditions as it took over from Britain as the leading western "flank" power, dedicated to maintaining the European equilibrium. In the view of the American and British governments, the chief task had been to tie the United States and Canada to the Brussels Pact signatories, and to extend the promise of mutual support to countries like Norway and Italy, which also felt insecure. On the day that the NATO treaty was signed, in fact, the U.S. Army had a mere 100,000 troops in Europe (compared with 3 million in 1945), and there existed only twelve divisions—seven French, two British, two American, one Belgian—in place to resist a Soviet push westward. Although the Russian forces at this period were nowhere near as large or capable as alarmist voices in the West claimed, the imbalance in each bloc's troop totals was disquieting; slightly later, those fears were increased by the thought that the Communists could sweep over the northern German plain as swiftly as they had crossed the Yalu during the Korean War. This meant that while the NATO strategy increasingly relied upon the "massive retaliation" of American long-range bombers to answer a Soviet invasion, there was a commitment to build up large conventional armed forces as well. In turn, this had the effect of tying all three of the western "flank" Powers—the United States, Canada, and Britain—to permanent military obligations on the continent of Europe to a degree which would have amazed their respective strategic planners in the 1930s.[103]

The NATO alliance did militarily what the Marshall plan had done economically; it deepened the 1945 division of Europe into two camps, with only traditional neutrals (Switzerland, Sweden), Franco's Spain, and certain special cases (Finland, Austria, Yugoslavia) in neither one nor the other. It was to be answered, in due course, by the Soviet-dominated Warsaw Pact. This deepening division, in turn, made the prospects for a reunification of Germany ever more remote. Despite French worries, the West German armed forces began to be built up within the NATO structure by the late 1950s—which was logical enough, if the West really wanted to narrow the gap in troop totals.[104] But that inevitably moved the USSR to develop an East German army, albeit under special controls. With each German state integrated into its respective military alliance, it became inevitable that both blocs would regard any future German attempt to become neutral with alarm and suspicion, as a blow to their own security. In Russia's case, this was reinforced, even after Stalin's death in 1953, by the conviction that any country which had become Communist should not be permitted to abandon that creed (the "Brezhnev Doctrine," to use later parlance). By October 1953, the U.S. National Security Council had privately accepted that the eastern European satellite states "could be freed only by general war or by the Russians themselves." As Bartlett cryptically notes, "Neither was possible."[105] In 1953, too, a rising in East Germany was swiftly put down. In 1956, alarmed at the Hungarian decision to withdraw from the Warsaw Pact, Russia moved its divisions back into that land and suppressed its independence. In 1961, in an admission of defeat, Khrushchev ordered the erection of the Berlin Wall to stem the flow of talent to the West. In 1968, the Czechs suffered the same fate as the Hungarians twelve years earlier, though the bloodshed was less. Each of these measures, taken by a Soviet leadership incapable (despite its official propaganda) of matching either the ideological or the economic appeal of the West, simply added to the division between the two blocs.[106]

The second main feature of the Cold War, its steady *lateral* escalation from Europe itself into the rest of the world, was hardly surprising. During much of the war itself, there had been an almost single-minded concentration of Russian energies upon dealing with the German threat; but that did not mean that Moscow had abandoned its political interest in the future of Turkey, Persia, and the Far East—

as was made plain in August 1945. It was therefore highly unlikely that Russia's quarrels with the West over European issues would be geographically limited to that continent, especially since the principles in dispute were of universal application—self-government versus national security, economic liberalism versus socialist planning, and so on. More important still, the war itself had caused immense social and political turbulence, from the Balkans to the East Indies; and even in countries not directly overrun by invading armies (for example, India, or Egypt), the mobilization of manpower, resources, and *ideas* had led to profound changes. Traditional social orders lay smashed, colonial regimes had been discredited, underground nationalist parties had flourished, and resistance movements had grown up, committed not only to military victory but also to political transformation.[107] There was, in other words, an immense degree of political turbulence in the world situation of 1945, which could be a threat to Great Powers eager to restore peacetime stability as soon as possible; but this could also be an opportunity for each of the superpowers, imbued with their universalist doctrines, to bid for support among the vast swathe of peoples emerging from the debris of the collapsed older order. During the war itself, the Allies had given aid to all manner of resistance movements struggling against their German and Japanese overlords, and it was natural for those groups to hope for a continuation of such aid after 1945, even while they engaged in jostling with rival contenders for power. That some of these partisan groups were Communist and others bitterly anti-Communist made it more difficult than ever for decision-makers in Moscow and Washington to separate these regional quarrels from their own global preoccupations. Greece and Yugoslavia had already demonstrated how a local, internal dispute could swiftly be given an international significance.

The first of the extra-European disputes between Russia and the West was very much a legacy of such *ad hoc* wartime arrangements; in 1941–1943 Iran had been placed under tripartite military protection, partly to ensure that it remained in the Allied camp, partly to ensure that none of the Allies gained undue economic influence with the Teheran regime.[108] When Moscow did not withdraw its garrison in early 1946, and instead seemed to be encouraging separatist, pro-Communist movements in the north, the traditional British objections to undue Russian influence in this part of the world were augmented, and then rather eclipsed, by the Truman administration's strong protests. The withdrawal of the Russian troops, soon followed by the Iranian army's suppression of the northern provinces and of the Tudeh (Communist) party itself, gave ample satisfaction in Washington, where it confirmed Truman's belief in the efficacy of "talking tough" to the Soviets. The case demonstrated, in Ulam's words, "the meaning of containment before the doctrine was actually enunciated,"[109] and psy-

chologically prepared Washington to react similarly against news of
Russian activities elsewhere. Thus, the continuing civil war in Greece,
Moscow's pressure upon the Turks for concessions at the Straits and
in the Kars border region, and the British government's 1947 declaration that it could no longer maintain its guarantees to those two nations triggered off a public American response (in the "Truman
Doctrine") which was already in embryonic form. As early as April
1946 the State Department was urging the need to give support to "the
United Kingdom and the *communications* of the British Commonwealth."[110] The growing acceptance of such views, and the way in
which Washington was beginning to link together the various crises
along the "northern tier" of those countries which blocked Russian
expansion into the eastern Mediterranean and Middle East, indicates
how swiftly the idealistic strands in American foreign policy were
being joined, if not altogether replaced by geopolitical calculation.

It was with this perception of the *global* advance of Communism
that the western Powers also viewed the changes occurring in the Far
East. In the case of the Dutch, who were soon to be ejected from their
"East Indies" by Sukarno's widely based nationalist movement, or the
French, quickly embroiled in an armed struggle with Ho Chi Minh's
Vietminh, or the British, soon engaged in counterinsurgency warfare
in Malaya, their response as old colonial powers might have been the
same even had no Communist existed east of Suez.[111] (On the other
hand, by the late 1940s it proved useful in gaining Washington's sympathies, and in France's case military aid also, to claim that the insurgents were master-minded by Moscow.) But the shock to the United
States of the "loss" of China was altogether more severe than these
challenges farther south. From the time of American missionary endeavors in the nineteenth century onward, enormous amounts of cultural and psychological (much less financial) capital had been invested
by the United States in that large and populous land; and this had been
blown up to even greater proportions by the press coverage of Chiang
Kai-shek's government during the war itself. In more than the religious
sense, the United States felt it had a "mission" in China.[112] And while
the professionals in the State Department and the military were increasingly aware of the Kuomintang's corruption and inefficiency,
their perceptions were not generally shared by public opinion, especially on the Republican right, which by the late 1940s was beginning
to see world politics in rigidly black-and-white terms.

The political turbulence and uncertainties which existed throughout the Orient in these years placed Washington in repeated dilemmas.
On the one hand, the American republic could not be seen to be the
supporter of corrupt Third World regimes or of decaying colonial
empires. On the other, it did not want the "forces of revolution" to
spread further, since that (it was claimed) would enhance Moscow's

influence. It was relatively easy to encourage the British to withdraw
from India in 1947, for it simply involved a transfer to a parliamentary,
democratic regime under Nehru. The same could be done in pressing
the Dutch to leave Indonesia by 1949, although Washington still worried about the growth of Communist insurgency there—as it did in the
Philippines (given independence in 1946). But elsewhere the "wobbling" was more in evidence. Instead of pushing ahead with the earlier
notions of a full-blown social transformation and demilitarization of
Japanese society, for example, Washington planners steadily moved
toward ideas of rebuilding the Japanese economy through the giant
firms *(zaibatsu),* and even toward encouraging the creation of Japan's
own armed forces—partly to ease the United States' economic and
military burdens, partly to ensure that Japan would be an anti-Communist bastion in Asia.[113]

This hardening of Washington's position by 1950 was the result of
two factors. The first was the increasing attacks upon the more flexible
"containment" policies of Truman and Acheson, not only by Republican critics and the fast-rising "red-baiter" Joe McCarthy, but also by
newer diehards within the administration itself, such as Louis Johnson, John Foster Dulles, Dean Rusk, and Paul Nitze—compelling Truman to act more assertively in order to protect his domestic political
flank. The second was the North Korean attack across the 38th parallel
in June 1950, which was swiftly interpreted by the United States as but
one part of an aggressive master plan orchestrated by Moscow. Together, these two factors gave the upper hand to those forces in Washington which desired a more active, and even belligerent, policy to stop
the rot. "We are losing Asia fast," wrote the influential journalist Stewart Alsop, invoking the homely imagery of a ten-pin bowling game. The
Kremlin was the hard-hitting, ambitious bowler.

> The head pin was China. It is down already. The two pins in the
> second row are Burma and Indochina. If they go, the three pins in
> the next row, Siam, Malaya, and Indonesia, are pretty sure to topple
> in their turn. And if all the rest of Asia goes, the resulting psychologi-
> cal, political and economic magnetism will almost certainly drag
> down the four pins of the fourth row, India, Pakistan, Japan and the
> Philippines.[114]

The consequences of this change of mind affected American policy
throughout East Asia. Its most obvious manifestation was the rapidly
escalating military support to South Korea—an unsavory and repres-
sive regime, which must share the blame for the conflict, but was at this
time seen as an innocent victim. The early U.S. air and naval support
was soon reinforced by army and marine divisions, which permitted
MacArthur to launch his impressive counterattack (Inchon) until the

northward advance of the United Nations forces in turn provoked
China's own intervention in October/November 1950. Denied the use
of A-bombs, the Americans were forced to conduct a campaign reminiscent of the trench warfare of 1914–1918.[115] By the time the cease-fire
was reached, in June 1953, the United States had spent about $50
billion to fight the war, had sent over 2 million servicemen to the war
zone, and had lost over 54,000 of them. While it had contained the
North, the United States had also created for itself a long-lasting and
substantial military commitment to the South from which it would be
difficult, if not impossible, to withdraw.

This fighting also led to significant changes in American policy
elsewhere in Asia. By 1949, many in the Truman administration had
given up support of Chiang Kai-shek in disgust, viewed the "rump"
government in Taiwan with contempt, and were thinking of following
the British in recognizing Mao's Communist regime. Within another
year, however, Taiwan was being supported and protected by the U.S.
fleet, and China itself was regarded as a bitter foe, against which (at
least in MacArthur's view) it would be necessary to use atomic weapons to counter its aggressions. In Indonesia, so important for its raw
materials and food supplies, the new government would be given aid
to fight the Communist insurgents; in Malaya, the British would be
encouraged to do the same; and in Indochina, while still pressing the
French to establish a more representative form of government, the
United States was now prepared to pour in arms and money to combat
the Vietminh.[116] No longer convinced that the moral and cultural appeal of American civilization was enough to prevent the spread of
communism, the United States turned increasingly to military-territorial guarantees, especially after Dulles became secretary of state.[117]
Even by August 1951 a treaty had reaffirmed U.S. air- and naval-base
rights to the Philippines and American commitments to the defense of
those islands. A few days later, Washington signed its tripartite security treaty with Australia and New Zealand. One week later, the peace
treaty with Japan was finally concluded, legally ending the Pacific war
and restoring full sovereignty to the Japanese state—but on the same
day a security pact was signed, keeping American forces both in the
home islands and in Okinawa. Washington's policy toward Communist
China remained unrelentingly hostile, and toward Taiwan increasingly supportive, even over such minor outposts as Quemoy and
Matsu.

The third major element in the Cold War was the increasing arms
race between the two blocs, along with the creation of supportive
military alliances. In terms of monies spent, the trend was by no means
an even one, as shown in Table 37.

The enormous surge in American defense expenditures for several
years after 1950 clearly reflected the costs of the Korean War, *and*

Table 37. Defense Expenditures of the Powers, 1948–1970[118]
(billions of dollars)

Date	U.S.	USSR	West Germany	France	U.K.	Italy	Japan	China
1948	10.9	13.1		0.9	3.4	0.4		
1949	13.5	13.4		1.2	3.1	0.5		2.0
1950	14.5	15.5		1.4	2.3	0.5		2.5
1951	33.3	20.1		2.1	3.2	0.7		3.0
1952	47.8	21.9		3.0	4.3	0.8		2.7
1953	49.6	25.5		3.4	4.5	0.7	0.3	2.5
1954	42.7	28.0		3.6	4.4	0.8	0.4	2.5
1955	40.5	29.5	1.7	2.9	4.3	0.8	0.4	2.5
1956	41.7	26.7	1.7	3.6	4.5	0.9	0.4	5.5
1957	44.5	27.6	2.1	3.6	4.3	0.9	0.4	6.2
1958	45.5	30.2	1.2	3.6	4.4	1.0	0.4	5.8
1959	46.6	34.4	2.6	3.6	4.4	1.0	0.4	6.6
1960	45.3	36.9	2.9	3.8	4.6	1.1	0.4	6.7
1961	47.8	43.6	3.1	4.1	4.7	1.2	0.4	7.9
1962	52.3	49.9	4.3	4.5	5.0	1.3	0.5	9.3
1963	52.2	54.7	4.9	4.6	5.2	1.6	0.4	10.6
1964	51.2	48.7	4.9	4.9	5.5	1.7	0.6	12.8
1965	51.8	62.3	5.0	5.1	5.8	1.9	0.8	13.7
1966	67.5	69.7	5.0	5.4	6.0	2.1	0.9	15.9
1967	75.4	80.9	5.3	5.8	6.3	2.2	1.0	16.3
1968	80.7	85.4	4.8	5.8	5.6	2.2	1.1	17.8
1969	81.4	89.8	5.3	5.7	5.4	2.2	1.3	20.2
1970	77.8	72.0	6.1	5.9	5.8	2.4	1.3	23.7

Washington's belief that it needed to rearm in a threatening world; the post-1953 decline was Eisenhower's attempt to control the "military-industrial complex" before it damaged both society and economy; the 1961–1962 increases reflected the Berlin Wall and Cuban missile crises; and the post-1965 jump in spending showed the increasing American commitment in Southeast Asia.[119] Although the Soviet figures are mere estimates and Moscow's policy was shrouded in mystery, it is probably fair to deduce that its own 1950–1955 buildup was caused by worries that war with the West would lead to devastating aerial attacks upon the Russian homeland unless its numbers of aircraft and missiles were greatly augmented; the 1955–1957 reductions reflect Khrushchev's *détente* diplomacy and efforts to release funds for consumer goods; and the very strong buildup after 1959–1960 reveals the worsening relations with the West, the humiliation over the Cuba crisis, and the determination to be strong in all services.[120] Communist China's more modest buildup was as much a reflection of its own economic growth as of anything else, but the 1960s defense increases suggest that Peking was willing to pay the price for its break with Moscow. As for the western European states, the figures in Table 37 show both Britain and France greatly increasing their defense expenditures at the time of the Korean War, and France's expenditures still rising until 1954 because of its embroilment in Indochina; but there-after both those powers, and West Germany, Italy, and Japan in their turn, permitted only modest increases (and an occasional decline) in defense spending. Apart from China's growth—and those figures also are very imprecise—the pattern of arms spending in the 1950s and 1960s still conveys the impression of a bipolar world.

Perhaps more significant than figures alone was the multilevel and multisided character of the arms race. Although shocked by the Russian achievement of manufacturing its own A-bomb in 1949, the United States believed that it could inflict far more damage upon the USSR in a nuclear exchange than the USSR could inflict on it. On the other hand, as the strongly ideological NSC-68 (National Security Council Memorandum 68, of January 1950) put it, it was imperative "to increase as rapidly as possible our general air, ground and sea strength and that of our allies to a point where we are militarily not so heavily dependent on atomic weapons."[121] Between 1950 and 1953, in fact, U.S. ground forces tripled in size, and although much of this was due to the calling-up of reserves to fight in Korea, there was also a determination to convert NATO from a set of general military obligations into an *on-the-ground* alliance—to forestall a Soviet overrunning of western Europe which both American and British planners feared likely at this time.[122] Although there was no real prospect of the fantastic total of ninety Allied divisions being created on the lines of the Lisbon Agreement of 1952, there was nonetheless a significant rise in military commitments to Europe—from one to five U.S. divisions by 1953, with Britain agreeing to station four divisions in Germany, so that a reasonable balance had been achieved by the mid-1950s, when the West German army was expanded to compensate for reductions made then by London and Paris. In addition, there were enormous increases in Allied expenditures upon their air forces, so that some 5,200 were available to NATO by 1953. While much less is known about the development of the Soviet army and air force in these years, it is clear that Zhukov was engaged upon significant reorganization once Stalin died—getting rid of masses of half-prepared troops, making units much more powerful, mobile, and compact, replacing artillery with missiles, and, in sum, giving them a much better capacity for offensive action than they had possessed in 1950–1951, when the West's fear of attack was greatest. At the same time, it is clear that Russia, too, was placing the greatest proportion of these budgetary increases upon defensive and offensive air power.[123]

A second and quite new area of the East-West arms race opened up at sea, although this was also in an irregular pattern. The U.S. Navy had finished the Pacific war trailing clouds of glory, because of the impressive performance of its fast-carrier task forces and its submarine fleet; and the Royal Navy also felt that it had had a "good war," and one much more decisively fought than the stalemated 1914–1918 conflict at sea.[124] But the coming of A-bombs (especially in the Bikini trials against a variety of warships) to be carried by long-range strategic bombers or missiles seemed to cast a cloud over the future of the traditional instruments of naval warfare and even over the aircraft carrier itself. In the post-1945 retrenchment of defense expenditures, and "rationalization" of the separate services into a unified defense ministry, both navies came under heavy pressure. They were rescued, at least to some extent, by the Korean War, which again saw amphibious landings, carrier-based air strikes, and the clever exploitation of western sea power. The U.S. Navy was also able to join the nuclear club with the creation of a new class of enormous carriers, possessing strike bombers equipped with atomic weapons, and, by the late 1950s, with the planned construction of nuclear-powered submarines capable of firing long-range ballistic missiles. The British, less able to afford modern carriers, nonetheless retained converted "commando" carriers for what were termed brushfire wars, and, like the French, also strove to create a submarine-based deterrent. If all western navies by 1965 contained fewer ships and men than in 1945, they certainly had a more powerful punch.[125]

But the greatest stimulus to the continued expenditure of these navies was the buildup of the Soviet fleet. During the Second World War itself, the Russian navy had achieved very little, despite its large submarine force, and most of its personnel had fought on land (or assisted at river crossings by the army). After 1945, Stalin permitted the construction of many more submarines, based upon superior German designs and probably to be employed in an extended coastal-defense role; but he also favored the creation of a larger surface navy, including battleships and aircraft carriers. This ambitious scheme was swiftly halted by Khrushchev, who saw no purpose in building large, expensive warships in an age of nuclear missiles; in this his views were identical to those of many politicians and air marshals in the West. What probably shook that assumption was the repeated examples of the use of surface sea power by Russia's most likely foes—the Anglo-French sea-based attack upon Suez in 1956, the landing of U.S. forces in Lebanon in 1958 (thus checking the Russian-backed Syrians), and especially the *cordon sanitaire* which American warships placed around Cuba in the tense confrontation of the missile crisis of 1962. The lesson which the Kremlin (urged on by the influential Admiral Gorschkov) drew from these incidents was that until Russia also possessed a powerful navy, it would continue to be at a serious disadvantage in the world-power stakes—a conclusion reinforced by the U.S. Navy's rapid move to Polaris-missile-carrying submarines in the early 1960s. The result was both a massive expansion in virtually all classes of vessels in the Red Navy—cruisers, destroyers, submarines of all types, hybrid aircraft-carriers—*and* a massive expansion in their deployment overseas, challenging western maritime predominance in, say, the Mediterranean or the Indian Ocean in a manner which Stalin had never attempted.[126]

This form of challenge could, however, be regarded in traditional terms, as was clear by the many comparisons which observers made between Admiral Gorschkov's buildup and Tirpitz's four decades earlier; and even if the Soviet Union appeared committed to a new "naval race," it would be decades (if at all) before it could match the massively expensive carrier task forces of the U.S. Navy. The really *revolutionary* aspect of the post-1945 arms race was occurring elsewhere, in the sphere of atomic weapons and long-range missiles to project them. Despite the horrific casualties caused at Hiroshima and Nagasaki, there still remained many who saw in atomic weapons "just another bomb" rather than a watershed in the history of man's capacity for destruction. Moreover, following the failure of the 1946 Baruch Plan to internationalize atomic-power developments, there was the comforting thought that the United States possessed a nuclear monopoly and that the Strategic Air Command's bombers compensated for (and deterred) the large Soviet superiority in ground forces;[127] the western European states in particular accepted that a Russian military invasion would be answered by American (and later British) airborne bombings with nuclear weapons.

Technological innovations, and Soviet advances especially, changed all that. Russia's successful explosion of an atomic device in 1949 (well before most western estimates had predicted) broke the American monopoly. More alarming still was the construction of long-range Russian bombers, especially of the Bison type, which by the mid-1950s not only were assumed to be capable of reaching the United States but also were (erroneously) supposed to exist in such large numbers that a "bomber gap" existed. While the resultant controversy signified both the difficulty of gaining hard evidence about Russian capabilities and the U.S. Air Force's tendency to exaggerate,[128] it was in fact only to be a few more years before the era of American invulnerability was over. In 1949 Washington had agreed to the production of a new "super" bomb (the H-bomb), of staggeringly larger destructive capacity. This seemed once again to promise to the United States a decisive advantage, and the early to middle 1950s witnessed, both in Foster Dulles's startling speeches and in the Air Force's own plans, a commitment to "massive retaliation" upon Russia or China in the event of the next war.[129] While this doctrine itself produced considerable private unease within both the Truman and Eisenhower administrations—leading to the buildup of conventional forces and tactical (i.e., "battlefield") nuclear weapons, as alternatives to unleashing Armageddon—the chief blow to that strategy came from the Russian side.

In 1953, Russia also tested an H-bomb, a mere nine months after the American test. Moreover, the Soviet government had devoted considerable resources to exploiting German wartime technology on rocketry. By 1955 the USSR was mass-producing a medium-range ballistic missile (the SS-3); by 1957 it had fired an intercontinental ballistic missile over a range of five thousand miles, using the same rocket engine which shot *Sputnik,* the earth's first artificial satellite, into orbit in October of the same year.

Shocked by these Russian advances, and by the implication that both U.S. cities and U.S. bomber forces might be vulnerable to a sudden Soviet strike, Washington committed massive resources to its own intercontinental ballistic missiles in order to close what was predictably termed "the missile gap."[130] But the nuclear arms race was not confined to such systems. From 1960 onward, each side was also swiftly developing the capacity to launch ballistic missiles from submarines; and by that time a whole variety of battlefield nuclear weapons, and shorter-range rockets, had been constructed. All this was attended by the intellectual wrestlings of both strategic planners and civilian analysts in their "think tanks" about how to manage the various stages of escalation in what was now a strategy of "flexible response." However clear the solutions proposed, none of this managed to escape from the awful problem that it was going to be difficult if not impossible to integrate nuclear weapons into the traditional ways of fighting conventional warfare (it was soon realized, for example, that the battlefield "nukes" would blow up most of Germany). Yet if recourse were had to launching high-yield H-bombs upon Russian and American soil, the mutual casualties and damage would be unprecedented. Locked in what Churchill called a mutual balance of terror, and unable to *dis*invent their weapons of mass destruction, Washington and Moscow threw more and more resources into the technology of nuclear warfare.[131] And while both Britain and France were pushing ahead with their own atomic bombs and delivery systems in the 1950s, it still seemed—by all contemporary measure of aircraft, missiles, and nuclear bombs themselves—that in this field, too, only the superpowers counted.

The final major element in this rivalry was the creation by both Russia and the West of alliances across the globe, and the competition to find new partners—or at least to prevent Third World countries from joining the other side. In the early years, this was overwhelmingly an American activity, flowing from its advantageous position in 1945, from the fact that it already had many garrisons and air bases outside the western hemisphere, and from the equally important fact that so many countries were looking to Washington for economic and sometimes military support. By contrast, the USSR was desperately needing to rebuild itself, its chief foreign concern was the stabilization of its own borders on terms favorable to Moscow, and it had neither the economic nor the military instruments of power to project itself farther afield. Despite territorial gains in the Baltic, northern Finland, and the Far East, Russia was still, relatively speaking, a landlocked superpower. Moreover, it now seems clear that Stalin's view of the world outside was one overwhelmingly charged with caution and suspicion—toward the West, which, he feared, would not tolerate open Communist gains (e.g., in Greece in 1947); and also toward those Communist leaders, such as Tito and Mao, who were certainly not "Soviet puppets."[132] The setting-up of the Cominform in 1947 and the strong propaganda about supporting revolutionaries abroad had echoes from the 1930s (and even more, from the 1918–1921 era); but in actual fact Moscow seems to have avoided foreign entanglements in this period.

Yet the view from Washington, as noted above, was that a master plan for world Communist domination was unfolding, step by step, and needed to be "contained." The proffered guarantees to Greece and Turkey in 1947 were the first sign of this change of course, and the 1949 NATO treaty was its most spectacular exemplar. With the further additions to NATO's membership in the 1950s, this meant that the United States was pledged "to the defense of most of Europe and even parts of the Near East—from Spitzbergen to the Berlin Wall and beyond to the Asian borders of Turkey."[133] But that was only the beginning of the American overstretch. The Rio Pact and the special arrangement with Canada meant that it was responsible for the defense of the entire western hemisphere. The ANZUS treaty created obligations in the southwestern Pacific. The confrontations in East Asia during the early 1950s had led to the signing of various bilateral treaties, whereby the United States was pledged to aid countries along the "rim"—Japan, South Korea, and Taiwan, as well as the Philippines. In 1954, this was buttressed further by the establishment of SEATO (the Southeast Asia Treaty Organization), whereby the United States joined Britain, France, Australia, New Zealand, the Philippines, Pakistan, and Thailand in promising mutual support to combat aggression in that vast region. In the Middle East, it was the chief sponsor of another regional grouping, the 1955 Baghdad Pact (later, the Central Treaty Organization, or CENTO), in which Britain, Turkey, Iraq, Iran, and Pakistan stood against subversion and attack. Elsewhere in the Middle East, the United States had evolved or was soon to evolve special agreements with Israel, Saudi Arabia, and Jordan, either because of the strong Jewish-American ties or in consequence of the 1957 "Eisenhower Doctrine," which proffered American aid to Arab states. Early in 1970, one observer noted,

> the United States had more than 1,000,000 soldiers in 30 countries, was a member of four regional defense alliances and an active

participant in a fifth, had mutual defense treaties with 42 nations, was a member of 53 international organizations, and was furnishing military or economic aid to nearly 100 nations across the face of the globe.[134]

This was an array of commitments about which Louis XIV or Palmerston would have felt a little nervous. Yet in a world which seemed to be swiftly shrinking in size and in which each part appeared to relate to another, these step-by-step pledges all had their logic. Where, in a bipolar system, could Washington draw the line—especially after it was claimed that its earlier definition that Korea was *not* vital had been an invitation to the Communist attack of the following year?[135] "This has become a very small planet," Dean Rusk argued in May 1965. "We have to be concerned with all of it—with all of its land, waters, atmosphere, and with surrounding space."[136]

If the projection of Soviet power and influence into the world outside was far less extensive, the years after Stalin's death nonetheless saw noteworthy advances. Khrushchev, it is clear, wanted the Soviet Union to be admired, even loved, rather than feared; he also wanted to redirect resources from the military to agricultural investment and consumer goods. His general foreign-policy ideas reflected his hope for a "thaw" in the Cold War. Overruling Molotov, he removed Soviet troops from Austria; he handed back the Porkkala naval base to Finland and Port Arthur to China; and he improved relations with Yugoslavia, arguing that there were "separate roads to socialism" (a position as upsetting to many of his Presidium colleagues as it was to Mao Tse-tung). Although 1955 saw the formal establishment of the Warsaw Pact, in response to West Germany's joining of NATO, Khrushchev was willing to open diplomatic relations with Bonn. He was also keen to improve relations with the United States, although his own volatility of manner and the by now chronic distrust with which Washington interpreted all Russian moves made a real *détente* impossible. In that same year, Khrushchev traveled to India, Burma, and Afghanistan. The Third World was from now on going to be taken seriously by the Soviet Union, just when more and more Afro-Asian states were gaining independence.[137]

Little of this was as complete or smooth-going a transformation as the ebullient Khrushchev would have liked. In April 1956, that instrument of Stalinist control the Cominform had been dissolved. Embarrassingly, two months later the Hungarian uprising—a "separate road" away from socialism—had to be put down with Stalinist resolve. Quarrels with China multiplied and, as will be discussed below, produced a deep cleft in the Communist world. *Détente* foundered on the rocks of the U-2 incident (1960), the Berlin Wall crisis (1961), and then the confrontation with the United States over Soviet missiles in Cuba

(1962). None of this, however, could turn back the Russian move toward world policy; the mere establishment of diplomatic relations with newly emergent countries and contact with their representatives at the United Nations made the growth of Soviet ties with the outside world inevitable. In addition, Khrushchev, eager to demonstrate the innate superiority of the Soviet system over capitalism, was bound to look for new friends abroad; his more pragmatic successors, after 1964, were interested in breaking the American cordon which had been placed around the USSR, *and* in checking Chinese influence. There were, moreover, many Third World countries eager to escape from what they termed "neocolonialism" and to institute a planned economy rather than a laissez-faire one—a preference which usually caused a cessation of western aid. All this fused to give Russian foreign policy a distinct "outward thrust."

This thrust began in a very decisive fashion in December 1953, by the signing of a trade agreement with India (neatly coinciding with Vice-President Nixon's visit to New Delhi), followed up by the 1955 offer to construct the Bhilai steel plant, and then by lots of military aid; this was a connection to the most important of the Third World powers, it simultaneously annoyed the Americans and the Chinese, and it punished Pakistan for its membership in the Baghdad Pact. Almost at the same time, in 1955–1956, the USSR and Czechoslovakia began giving aid to Egypt, replacing Washington in the funding of the Aswan Dam. Soviet loans also went to Iraq, Afghanistan, and North Yemen. Pronounced anti-imperialist states in Africa, such as Ghana, Mali, and Guinea, were also encouraged by Moscow. In 1960, the great breakthrough occurred in Latin America, when the USSR signed its first trade agreement with Castro's Cuba, then already becoming embroiled with an irritated United States. All this set a pattern which was not reversed by Khrushchev's fall. Having waged a strident propaganda campaign against imperialism, the USSR quite naturally offered "friendship treaties," trade credits, military advisers, and the rest to any newly decolonized nation. Russia could also benefit, in the Middle East, from the U.S. support of Israel (hence, for example, Moscow's increasing aid to Syria and Iraq as well as Egypt in the 1960s); it could gain kudos by offering military and economic assistance to North Vietnam; even in distant Latin America, it could proclaim its commitment to national-liberation movements. In this struggle for world influence, the USSR had now come a long way from Stalin's paranoid caution.[138]

But did this competition by Washington and Moscow for the affections of the rest of the globe, this mutual jostling for influence with the aid of treaties, credits, and weapons exports, mean that a bipolar world had indeed come into being, with everything significant in international affairs gravitating around the two opposing *Schwerpunkte* of the

United States and the USSR? From the viewpoint of a Dulles or a Molotov, that indeed was how the world was ordered. And yet, even as these two blocs competed across the globe, and in areas unknown to both in 1941, they were meeting up with a quite different trend. For a Third World was just at this time coming of age, and many of its members, having at last thrown off the controls of the traditional European empires, were in no mood to become mere satellites of a distant superpower, even if the latter could provide useful economic and military aid.

What was happening, in fact, was that one major trend in twentieth-century power politics, the rise of the superpowers, was beginning to interact with another, newer trend—the political fragmentation of the globe. In the Social Darwinistic and imperialistic atmosphere that had prevailed around 1900, it was easy to think that all power was being concentrated in fewer and fewer capitals of the world (see above, pp. 195–96) Yet the very arrogance and ambitiousness of western imperialism brought with it the seeds of its own destruction; the exaggerated nationalism of Cecil Rhodes, or the Panslavs, or the Austro-Hungarian military, provoked reactions among Boers, the Poles, the Serbs, the Finns; ideas of national self-determination, propagated to justify the unification of Germany and Italy, or the 1914 Allied decision to assist Belgium, seeped relentlessly eastward and southward, to Egypt, to India, to Indochina. Because the empires of Britain, France, Italy, and Japan had triumphed over the Central Powers in 1918 and had checked Wilson's ideas for a new world order in 1919, these stirrings of nationalism were only selectively encouraged: it was fine to grant self-determination to the peoples of eastern Europe, because they were European and thus regarded as "civilized"; but it was *not* fine to extend these principles to the Middle East, Africa, or Asia, where the imperialist powers extended their territories and held down independence movements. The shattering of those empires in the Far East after 1941, the mobilization of the economies and recruitment of the manpower of the other dependent territories as the war developed, the ideological influences of the Atlantic Charter, and the decline of Europe all combined to release the forces for change in what by the 1950s was being called the Third World.[139]

But it was described as a "third" world precisely because it insisted on its distinction both from the American- and the Russian-dominated blocs. This did not mean that the countries which met at the original Bandung conference in April 1955 were free of all ties and obligations to the superpowers—Turkey, China, Japan, and the Philippines, for example, were among those attending the conference for whom the term "nonaligned" would have been inappropriate.[140] On the other hand, they all pressed for increased decolonization, for the United Nations to focus upon issues other than the Cold War tensions, and for measures to change a world which was still economically dominated by white men. When the second major phase of decolonization occurred, in the late 1950s and early 1960s, the original members of the Third World movement could be joined by a large number of new recruits, smarting at the decades (or centuries) of foreign rule and grappling with the hard fact that independence had left them with a host of economic problems. Given the vast swelling of their numbers, they could now begin to dominate the United Nations General Assembly; originally a body of fifty (overwhelmingly European and Latin American) countries, the UN steadily changed into an organization of well over one hundred states with many new Afro-Asian members. This did not restrict the actions of the larger Powers that were permanent members of the Security Council and that possessed a veto—conditions insisted upon by a cautious Stalin. But it did mean that if either of the superpowers wished to appeal to "world opinion" (as the United States had done in getting the United Nations to aid South Korea in 1950), it had to gain the agreement of a body whose membership did not share the preoccupations of Washington and Moscow. Chiefly because the 1950s and 1960s were dominated by issues of decolonization, and by increasing calls to end "underdevelopment," causes which the Russians adroitly espoused, this Third World opinion had a distinctly anti-western flavor, from the Suez crisis of 1956 to the later issues of Vietnam, the Middle East wars, Latin America, and South Africa. Even at the formal summits of the nonaligned countries, the emphasis was increasingly placed upon anticolonialism; and the geographical sitings of those meetings (Belgrade in 1961, Cairo in 1964, and Lusaka in 1970) symbolized this shift away from Eurocentered issues. The agenda of world politics was no longer exclusively in the hands of those powers possessing the greatest military and economic muscle.[141]

The most prominent of the early advocates of nonalignment—Tito, Nasser, Nehru—symbolized this transformation. Yugoslavia was remarkable in breaking with Stalin (it was expelled from the Cominform as early as 1948) and yet maintaining its independence without a Russian invasion occurring. It was a policy firmly maintained after Stalin's death; not for nothing was the first nonaligned summit held in Belgrade.[142] Nasser had risen to fame throughout the Arab world after his 1956 clash with Britain, France, and Israel, was a fierce critic of western imperialism, and willingly accepted Soviet aid; yet he was not a puppet of Moscow—he "treated his home-grown communists badly and between 1959 and 1961 a vigorous anti-Soviet radio and press campaign was launched."[143] Pan-Arabism, and especially Muslim fundamentalism, were not natural partners for atheistic materialism, even if local Marxist intellectuals strove to produce a fusion of the two. As for India, long the symbolic leader of the "moderate" nonaligned states, the repeated infusions of Soviet economic and military aid, which rose to new heights following Sino-Indian and Pakistani-Indian clashes, did not stop Nehru from criticizing Russian actions elsewhere and being very suspicious of the Communist party of India. His condemnations of British policy at Suez was due to his dislike of *all* Great Power interventions abroad.

The very fact that so many new states were entering the international community in these years, and that Russia was eager to wean them away from the West without itself having much knowledge of local conditions, also meant that its diplomatic "gains" were frequently attended by "losses." The most spectacular example of this was China itself, which will be discussed further below; but there were many others. The 1958 change of regime in Iraq allowed Russia to pose as the friend of that Arab state and to offer it loans; four years later, a Ba'athist coup led to the bloody suppression of the Communist party there. Moscow's continued aid to India inevitably angered Pakistan; there was no way it could please the one without losing the other. In Burma, an early promising start foundered when that country banned *all* foreigners. In Indonesia, things were worse; after receiving masses of Russian and eastern-European aid, Sukarno's government had turned from Moscow to Peking by 1963. Two years later, the Indonesian army wiped out the Communist party with great ferocity. Sékou Touré in Guinea sent home the Russian ambassador in 1961 for involving himself in a local strike, and during the Cuban missile crisis he refused to let Soviet planes refuel at the airport they had specially extended at Conakry.[144] Russia's support of Lumumba in the Congo crisis of 1960 undermined his prospects, and his successor Mobutu closed down the Soviet embassy. The most spectacular instance of that sort of setback—and a major blow to Soviet influence—came in 1972, when Sadat ordered 21,000 Russian advisers out of Egypt.

The relationship between the Third World and the "first two worlds" was always, therefore, a complex and shifting one. There were, to be sure, countries which were persistently pro-Russian (Cuba, Angola) and others which were strongly pro-American (Taiwan, Israel), chiefly because they felt under threat from their neighbors. There were some which, following Tito's early lead, genuinely sought to be nonaligned. There were others which, while leaning toward one bloc because it offered them aid, strongly resisted undue dependence. And, finally, there were the frequent revolutions, civil wars, changes of regime, and border conflicts in the Third World which took Moscow and Washington by surprise. Local rivalries in Cyprus, in the Ogaden, along the India-Pakistan border, and in Kampuchea (Cambodia) embarrassed the superpowers, since each of the contending parties sought their aid. Like other Great Powers before them, both Russia and the United States had to grapple with the hard fact that their "universalist" message would not be automatically accepted by other societies and cultures.

The Fissuring of the Bipolar World

As the 1960s moved into the 1970s, there nevertheless remained good reasons why the Washington-Moscow relationship should continue to seem all-important in world affairs. Militarily, the USSR had drawn much closer to the United States, but both were still in a different league from everyone else. In 1974, for example, the United States was spending $85 billion and the USSR was spending $109 billion on defense, which was three to four times what was spent by China ($26 billion) and eight to ten times what was spent by the leading European states (U.K. $9.7 billion; France, $9.9 billion; West Germany, $13.7 billion);[145] and the American and Russian armed forces, of over 2 million and 3 million men, respectively, were much larger than those of the European states, and much better equipped than the 3 million men in the Chinese services. Both superpowers had over 5,000 combat aircraft, more than ten times the number possessed by the former Great Powers.[146] Their total tonnage in warships—the United States had 2.8 million tons, the USSR 2.1 million tons in 1974—was well ahead of Britain (370,000 tons), France (160,000 tons), Japan (180,000 tons), and China (150,000 tons).[147] But the greatest disparity lay in the numbers of nuclear delivery weapons, shown in Table 38.

Table 38. Nuclear Delivery Vehicles of the Powers, 1974[148]

	U.S.	USSR	Britain	France	China
Intercontinental ballistic missiles	1,054	1,575	—	—	—
Intermediate ballistic missiles	—	600	—	18	c. 80
Submarine-based ballistic missiles	656	720	64	48	—
Long-range bombers	437	140	—	—	—
Medium-range bombers	66	800	50	52	100

So capable had each superpower become of obliterating the other (and anyone else besides)—a state of affairs quickly named MAD, or Mutually Assured Destruction—that they began to evolve arrangements for controlling the nuclear arms race in various ways. There was, following the Cuban missile crisis, the installation of a "hot line" to allow each side to communicate in the event of another critical occasion; there was the nuclear test-ban treaty of 1963, also signed by the United Kingdom, which banned testing in the atmosphere, under water, and in outer space; there was the Strategic Arms Limitation Treaty (SALT I) of 1972, which set limits on the numbers of intercontinental ballistic missiles each side could possess and halted the Russian construction of an anti-ballistic-missile system; there was the extension of that agreement at Vladivostock in 1975, and, in the late 1970s, there were negotiations toward a SALT II treaty (signed in June 1979, but never ratified by the U.S. Senate). Yet these various measures of agreement, and the particular economic and domestic-political and foreign-policy motives which pushed each side into them, did not stop the arms race; if anything, the banning or limitation of one weapon system merely led to a transfer of resources to another area. From the late 1950s onward, the USSR steadily and inexorably increased its allocations to the armed forces; and while the pattern of American defense spending was distorted by its expensive war in Vietnam and then the public reaction against that venture, the long-term trend was also toward ever-higher totals. Every few years, newer weapon systems would be added: multiple warheads were fitted to each side's rockets; missile-carrying submarines augmented each side's navy; the nuclear stalemate in *strategic* missiles (provoking a European fear that the United States would not respond to a Soviet attack westward by unleashing long-range American missiles, since that could in turn provoke atomic strikes upon American cities) led to new types of medium-range or "theater" nuclear weapons, like the Pershing II and the cruise missiles being developed as answers to the Russian SS-20. The arms race and arms-control discussions of various sorts were obverse sides of the same coin; but each kept Washington and Moscow at the center of the stage.

In other fields, too, their rivalry appeared central. As mentioned earlier, one of the more notable features of the Soviet arms buildup since 1960 was the enormous expansion of its surface fleet—*physically*, as it constructed ever more powerful, missile-bearing destroyers and cruisers, then medium-sized helicopter carriers, then aircraft carriers;[149] and *geographically*, as the Soviet navy began to send more and more vessels into the Mediterranean and farther afield, to the Indian Ocean, West Africa, Indochina, and Cuba, where it was able to use an increasing number of bases. This last development reflected a very significant extension of American-Russian rivalries into the Third World, chiefly because of Moscow's further success in breaking into regions where foreign influence had hitherto been a western monopoly. The continued tension in the Middle East, and especially the Arab-Israeli wars of 1967 and 1973 (where American arms supplies to Israel were decisive), meant that various Arab states—Syria, Libya, Iraq—would remain looking to Moscow for assistance. The Marxist regimes of Southern Yemen and Somalia provided naval-base facilities to the Russian navy, giving it a new maritime presence in the Red Sea. But, as usual, breakthroughs were accompanied by setbacks: Moscow's apparent preference for Ethiopia led to the expulsion of Soviet personnel and ships from Somalia in 1977, just a few years after the same had happened in Egypt; and Russian advances in this area were countered by the growth of the American presence in Oman and Diego Garcia, naval-base rights in Kenya and Somalia, and increased arms shipments to Egypt, Saudia Arabia, and Pakistan. Farther to the south, however, the Soviet-Cuban military assistance to the MPLA forces in Angola, the frequent attempts of the Soviet-aided Libyan regime of Qaddafi to export revolution elsewhere, and the presence of Marxist governments in Ethiopia, Mozambique, Guinea, Congo, and other West African states suggested that Moscow was winning in the struggle for global influence. Its own military move into Afghanistan in 1979— the first such expansion (outside eastern Europe) since the Second World War—and Cuba's encouragement of leftist regimes in Nicaragua and Grenada furthered this impression that the American-Russian rivalry knew no limits, and provoked additional countermoves and increases in defense spending on Washington's part. By 1980, with a new Republican administration denouncing the Soviet Union as an "evil empire" against which massive defense forces and unbending policies were the only answer, little seemed to have changed since the days of John Foster Dulles.[150]

Yet, for all this focus upon the American-Russian relationship and its many ups and downs between 1960 and 1980, other trends had been at work to make the international power system much *less* bipolar than it had appeared to be in the earlier period. Not only had the Third World emerged to complicate matters, but significant fissures had occurred in what had earlier appeared to be the two monolithic blocs dominated by Moscow and Washington. The most decisive of these by far, with repercussions which are difficult to measure fully even at the present time, was the split between the USSR and Communist China. In retrospect, it may seem self-evident that even the allegedly "scientific" and "universalist" claims of Marxism would founder on the rocks of local circumstances, indigenous cultural strengths, and differing stages of economic development—after all, Lenin himself had had to make massive deviations from the original doctrine of dialectical materialism in order to secure the 1917 Revolution. And some foreign observers of Mao's Communist movement in the 1930s and 1940s were aware that he, at least, was not inclined to adhere slavishly to Stalin's dogmatic position toward the relative importance of workers and peasantry. They were also aware that Moscow, in its turn, had been less than wholehearted in its support of the Chinese Communist Party and had, even as late as 1946 and 1948, tried to balance it off against Chiang Kai-shek's Nationalists. This, in the USSR's view, would avoid the creation of "a vigorous new Communist regime established without the assistance of the Red Army in a country with almost three times the population of Russia [which] would inevitably become a competing pole of attraction within the world Communist movement."[151]

Nonetheless, the sheer extent of the split took most observers by surprise, and was for many years missed by a United States aroused by the fear of a global Communist conspiracy. Admittedly, the Korean War and the subsequent Chinese-American jockeying over Taiwan took attention from the lukewarm state of the Moscow-Peking axis, in which Stalin's relatively small amounts of aid to China were always tendered for a price which emphasized Russia's privileges in Mongolia and Manchuria. Although Mao was able to redress the balance in his 1954 negotiations with the Russians, his hostility to the United States over the offshore islands of Quemoy and Matsu and his more extreme adherence (at least at that time) to the belief in the inevitability of a clash with capitalism made him bitterly suspicious of Khrushchev's early *détente* policies. From Moscow's viewpoint, however, it seemed foolish in the late 1950s to provoke the Americans unnecessarily, especially when the latter had a clear nuclear advantage; it would also be a setback, diplomatically, to support China in its 1959 border clash with India, which was so important to Russia's Third World policy; and it would be highly unwise, given the Chinese proclivity to independent action, to aid their nuclear program without getting some controls over it—all of these being regarded as successive betrayals by Mao. By 1959, Khrushchev had canceled the atomic agreement with Peking and was proffering India far larger loans than had ever been given to China. In the following year, the "split" became open for all to see at the World Communist Parties' meeting in Moscow. By 1962–1963, things were worse still: Mao had denounced the Russians for giving in over Cuba, and then for signing the partial Nuclear Test Ban Treaty with the United States and Britain; the Russians had by then cut off all aid to China and its ally Albania and increased supplies to India; and the first of the Sino-Soviet border clashes occurred (although never as serious as those of 1969). More significant still was the news that in 1964 the Chinese had exploded their first atomic bomb and were hard at work on delivery systems.[152]

Strategically, this split was the single most important event since 1945. In September 1964, *Pravda* readers were shocked to see a report that Mao was not only claiming back the Asian territories which the Chinese Empire had lost to Russia in the nineteenth century, but also denouncing the USSR for its appropriations of the Kurile Islands, parts of Poland, East Prussia, and a section of Rumania. Russia, in Mao's view, had to be reduced in size—in respect to China's claims, by 1.5 million square kilometers![153] How much the opinionated Chinese leader had been carried away by his own rhetoric it is hard to say, but there was no doubt that all this—together with the border clashes and the development of Chinese atomic weapons—was thoroughly alarming to the Kremlin. Indeed, it is likely that at least some of the buildup of the Russian armed forces in the 1960s was due to this perceived new danger to the east as well as the need to respond to the Kennedy administration's defense increases. "The number of Soviet divisions deployed along the Chinese frontier was increased from fifteen in 1967 to twenty-one in 1969 and thirty in 1970"—this latter jump being caused by the serious clash at Damansky (or Chenpao) island in March 1969. "By 1972 forty-four Soviet divisions stood guard along the 4,500-mile border with China (compared to thirty-one divisions in Eastern Europe), while a quarter of the Soviet air force had been deployed from west to east."[154] With China now possessing a hydrogen bomb, there were hints that Moscow was considering a preemptive strike against the nuclear installation at Lop Nor—causing the United States to make its own contingency plans, since it felt that it could not allow Russia to obliterate China.[155] Washington had come a long way since its 1964 ponderings about joining the USSR in "preventative military action" to arrest China's development as a nuclear power![156]

This was hardly to say that Mao's China had emerged as a full-fledged third superpower. Economically, it had enormous problems—which were exacerbated by its leader's decision to initiate the "Cultural Revolution," with all its accompanying discontinuities and uncertainties. And while it might boast the largest army in the world, its people's militias were not likely to be a match for Soviet motor rifle divisions. China's navy was negligible compared with the expanding Russian fleet; its air force, though large, chiefly consisted of older planes; and its nuclear-delivery system was but in its infancy. Nonetheless, unless the USSR was prepared to run the risk of provoking the Americans and offending world opinion by launching a massive nuclear attack upon China, any fighting *at a lesser level* could quickly produce enormous casualties—which the Chinese seemed willing to accept, but Russian politicians in the Brezhnev era were less keen about. It was therefore not surprising that as Russo-Chinese relations worsened, Moscow should not only have shown interest in nuclear-arms-limitation talks with the West but also have quickened the pace of improving relations with countries like the Federal Republic of Germany, which under Willy Brandt seemed much more willing to foster *détente* than in Adenauer's days.

In the political and diplomatic arena, the Sino-Soviet split was even more embarrassing to the Kremlin. Although Khrushchev himself had been willing to tolerate "separate roads to socialism" (always provided those routes were not too divergent!), it was quite another thing for the USSR to be openly accused of having abandoned true Marxist principles; for its satellites and clients to be encouraged to throw off the Russian "yoke"; and for its diplomatic efforts in the Third World to be complicated by Peking's rival aid and propaganda—the more especially since Mao's brand of peasant-based Communism appeared often more appropriate than the Russian emphasis upon an industrial proletariat. This did not mean that the Soviet Empire in eastern Europe was in any real danger of following the Chinese lead—only the eccentric regime in Albania did so.[157] But it remained embarrassing to Moscow to be denounced by Peking for suppressing the Czech liberalization reforms in 1968, and again for its actions against Afghanistan in 1979. In the Third World, moreover, China was somewhat better placed to block Russian influence: it competed hard in North Yemen; it made much of its railway construction scheme in Tanzania; it criticized Moscow for failing to give sufficient support to the Vietminh and the Vietcong against the United States; and as it renewed relations with Japan, it warned Tokyo about a too-heavy economic collaboration with the Russians in Siberia. Once again, this was rarely an equal struggle—Russia could usually offer much more to Third World states in terms of credits and advanced arms, and could also project its influence by using Cuban and Libyan surrogates. But simply having to compete with a fellow Marxist state as well as with the United States was altogether more upsetting than the predictable, bipolar rivalries of two decades earlier.

In all sorts of ways, then, China's assertive and independent line made diplomatic relationships more complicated and baroque, especially in Asia. The Chinese had been stung by Moscow's wooing of India and even more by its dispatch of military supplies to New Delhi following Sino-Indian border clashes; not surprisingly, therefore, Peking gave support to Pakistan in its own clashes with India, and was strongly resentful of the Russian invasion of Afghanistan. China was further alienated by Moscow's support for North Vietnam's expansion in the late 1970s, by the latter's entry into Comecon, and by the increasing Russian naval presence in Vietnamese ports. When Vietnam invaded Cambodia in December 1978, China engaged itself in bloody and not very successful border clashes with its southern neighbor, which was in turn being heavily supplied with Russian weapons. By this stage, Moscow was even looking more favorably toward the Taiwan regime, and Peking was urging the United States to increase its naval forces in the Indian Ocean and western Pacific, to counter the Russian squadrons. A mere twenty years after China was criticizing the USSR for being too soft toward the West, it was pressing NATO to increase its defenses and warning both Japan and the Common Market against strengthening economic ties with Russia![158]

By comparison, the dislocations which occurred in the western camp from the early 1960s onward, caused chiefly by de Gaulle's campaign against American hegemony, were nowhere near as serious in the long term—although they certainly added to the impression that the two blocs were breaking up. With strong memories of the Second World War still in mind, de Gaulle seethed at the fact that he was treated as less than equal by the United States; he resented American policy during the Suez crisis in 1956, not to mention Dulles's habit of threatening a nuclear conflagration over issues like Quemoy. Although de Gaulle had more than enough to keep him busy for several years after 1958 as he sought to extricate France from Algeria, even at that time he criticized western Europe's subservience (as he saw it) to American interests. Like the British a decade earlier, he saw in nuclear weapons a chance to preserve Great Power status; when news of the first French atomic test of 1960 arrived, the general called out, "Hooray for France—since this morning she is stronger and prouder."[159] Determined to have France's nuclear deterrent totally independent, he angrily rejected Washington's offer of a Polaris missile system similar to Britain's because of the conditions the Kennedy administration attached to it. While this meant that France's own nuclear-weapons program would consume a far greater proportion of the total defense budget (perhaps as much as 30 percent) than it did elsewhere, de Gaulle and his successors felt the price was worth paying. At the same time, he began to pull France out of the NATO military structure, expelling that organization's HQ from Paris in 1966 and closing down all American bases on French soil. In parallel with this, he sought to improve France's relations with Moscow—where his actions were warmly applauded—and he ceaselessly proclaimed the need for Europe to stand on its own feet.[160]

De Gaulle's spectacular actions did not rest merely on Gallic rhetoric and cultural pride. Boosted by Marshall Plan aid and other American grants, and benefiting from Europe's general economic recovery after the late 1940s, the French economy had grown swiftly for almost two decades.[161] The colonial wars in Indochina (1950–1954) and Algeria (1956–1962) diverted French resources for a while, but not irremediably. Having negotiated very favorable terms for its national interests at the time of the formation of the European Economic Community in 1957, France was able to benefit from this larger market while restructuring its own agriculture and modernizing its industry. Although critical of Washington and firmly preventing British entry into the EEC, de Gaulle effected a dramatic reconciliation with Adenauer's Germany in 1963. And all the time he spoke of a need for Europe to stand on its own feet, to be free of superpower domination, to remember its glorious past and to cooperate—with France naturally showing the lead—in the pursuit of equally glorious destiny.[162] These were heady words, but they evoked a response on *both* sides of the Iron Curtain, and appealed to many who disliked both the Russian and American political cultures, not to mention their respective foreign policies.

By 1968, however, de Gaulle's own political career had been undermined by the students' and workers' revolt. The strains caused by modernization and the still relatively modest size of the French economy (3.5 percent of world manufacturing production in 1963)[163] meant that the country simply was not strong enough to play the influential role that the general had envisaged; and whatever the special agreements he proffered to the West Germans, the latter dared not abandon their tight links with the United States, upon which, in the final resort, Bonn politicians knew they heavily depended. Moreover, Russia's ruthless crushing of the Czech reforms in 1968 showed that the eastern superpower had no intention of letting the countries in its sphere evolve their own policies, let alone become part of a French-led, European-wide confederation.

Nonetheless, for all his hubris, de Gaulle had symbolized and accelerated trends which could not be stopped. Despite their military weaknesses compared with the United States and the USSR, the armed forces of the western European states were much larger and stronger, relatively speaking, than they had been in the post-1945 years; two of them had nuclear weapons and were developing delivery systems. Economically, as will be discussed in more detail below, the "recovery of Europe" had succeeded splendidly. What was more, despite Russia's 1968 invasion of Czechoslovakia, the era of the Cold War division of Europe into hermetically sealed blocs was being weakened. Willy Brandt's spectacular policy of reconciliation with Russia, with Poland and Czechoslovakia, and especially with the (at first very reluctant) East German regime between 1969 and 1973, chiefly on the basis of accepting the 1945 boundaries as permanent, inaugurated a period of blossoming East-West contacts. Western investments and technology flowed across the Iron Curtain, and this "economic *détente*" spilled over into cultural exchanges, the Helsinki Accords (of 1975) on human rights, and efforts to avert future military misunderstandings and to achieve mutual force reductions. To all this the superpowers, for their own good reasons, and with some inevitable reservations (especially on the Soviet side), gave their blessing. But perhaps the most significant fact had been the persistent pressures by the Europeans themselves to effect the *rapprochement;* even when relations cooled between Moscow and Washington, therefore, it was going to be extremely difficult in the future for either the USSR or the United States to halt this process.[164]

Of the two, the Americans were in a much better position than the Russians to adjust to the new, pluralistic international environment. Whatever de Gaulle's anti-American gestures, they were nowhere near the seriousness of Sino-Soviet border clashes, elimination of bilateral trade, ideological invective, and diplomatic jostling across the globe which, by 1969, were causing some observers to argue that a Russo-Chinese war was inevitable.[165] However much American administrations resented France's actions, they hardly needed to redeploy their armed forces because of such quarrels. In any case, NATO was still permitted to retain overflight rights and the fuel-oil pipeline which ran across France, and Paris kept up its special defense arrangements with West Germany—so that its troops, too, would be available if the Warsaw Pact forces struck westward. Finally, of course, it had been a fundamental axiom of American policy after 1945 that a strong and independent Europe (that is, independent from Russian domination) was in the United States' long-term interests and would help to reduce its defense burdens—even while admitting that such a Europe might also be an economic and perhaps a diplomatic competitor. It was for that reason that Washington had encouraged all moves toward European integration, and was urging Britain to join the EEC. By contrast, Russia might begin not only to feel insecure militarily if a powerful European confederation emerged in the West, but also to worry about the magnetic pull which such a body would exercise upon the Rumanians, Poles, and other satellite peoples. A policy of selective *détente* and economic cooperation with western Europe by Moscow was one thing, partly because it could bring technological and trading benefits, partly because it might draw the Europeans further away from the Americans, and partly because of the China challenge on Russia's Asian front. In the longer term, however, a prosperous, resurgent Europe which would overshadow the USSR in all respects except the military (and perhaps become strong in that area, too) could hardly be in Russia's best interests.[166]

Yet if, in retrospect, the United States was better placed to adjust to the changing patterns of world power, that was not obvious for many years after 1960. In the first place, there was a chronic dislike of "Asian Communism," with Mao's China replacing Khrushchev's Russia as the fomenter of world revolution in the eyes of many Americans. China's border war of 1962 with India, a country which Washington (like Moscow) wished to woo, confirmed the earlier aggressive image emanating from the clashes over Quemoy and Matsu; and *détente* between the United States and China was hardly conceivable in the early 1960s, when Mao's propaganda machine was denouncing the Russians for backing down over Cuba and for signing the limited nuclear-test-ban treaty with the West. Finally, between 1965 and 1968 China was in the convulsions of Mao's Cultural Revolution, which made the country appear chronically unstable as well as even more ideologically abhorrent to administrations in Washington. None of this pointed to "a situation in which much progress towards better relations with the United States was likely."[167]

Above all, of course, the United States in these years was itself increasingly convulsed by the problems emerging from the war in Vietnam. The North Vietnamese, and the Vietcong in the South, appeared to most Americans as but new manifestations of the creeping Asian Communism which had to be forcibly contained before it did even further damage; and since those revolutionary forces were being encouraged and supplied by China and Russia, both of the latter Powers (but perhaps especially the bitterly critical regime in Peking) could only be seen as part of a hostile Marxist coalition lined up against the "free world." Indeed, as the Johnson administration escalated its own buildup in Vietnam, decision-makers in Washington frequently worried about how far they could go *without* provoking the sort of Chinese intervention which had occurred in the Korean War.[168] From the Chinese government's standpoint, it must have been a matter of earnest debate throughout the 1960s about whether the growing clash with the Soviets to the north was as ominous as the ever-escalating American military and aerial operations to the south. Yet while in fact its own relationship with the ethnically different Vietnamese had traditionally been one of rivalry, and it was deeply suspicious of the amount of military hardware which Russia was giving to Hanoi, these tensions were invisible to most western eyes throughout the period of the Kennedy and Johnson administrations.

In so many ways, symbolic as well as practical, it would be difficult to exaggerate the impacts of the lengthy American campaign in Vietnam and other parts of Southeast Asia upon the international power system—or upon the national psyche of the American people themselves, most of whose perceptions of their country's role in the world still remain strongly influenced by that conflict, albeit in different ways. The fact that this was a war fought by an "open society"—and made the more open because of revelations like the Pentagon Papers, and by the daily television and press reportage of the carnage and apparent futility of it all; that this was the first war which the United States had unequivocally lost, that it confounded the victorious experiences of the Second World War and destroyed a whole array of reputations, from those of four-star generals to those of "brightest and best" intellectuals; that it coincided with, and in no small measure helped to cause, the fissuring of a consensus in American society about the nation's goals and priorities, was attended by inflation, unprecedented student protests and inner city disturbances, and was followed in turn by the Watergate crisis, which discredited the presidency itself for a time; that it seemed to many to stand in bitter and ironic contradiction to everything which the Founding Fathers had taught, and made the United States unpopular across most of the globe; and finally that the shamefaced and uncaring treatment of the GIs who came back from Vietnam would produce its own reaction a decade later and thus ensure that the memory of this conflict would continue to prey upon the public consciousness, in war memorials, books, television documentaries, and personal tragedies—all of this meant that the Vietnam War, although far smaller in terms of casualties, impacted upon the American people somewhat as had the First World War upon Europeans. The effects were seen, overwhelmingly, at the *personal* and *psychological* levels; more broadly, they were interpreted as a crisis in American civilization and in its constitutional arrangements. As such, they would continue to have significance quite independent of the strategical and Great Power dimensions of this conflict.

But the latter aspects are the most important ones for our survey, and require further mention here. To begin with, it provided a useful and sobering reminder that a vast superiority in military hardware and economic productivity will not always and automatically translate into military *effectiveness*. That does not undermine the thrust of the present book, which has stressed the importance of economics and technology in large-scale, protracted (and usually coalition) wars between the Great Powers when each combatant has been equally committed to victory. Economically, the United States may have been fifty to one hundred times more productive than North Vietnam; militarily, it possessed the firepower to (as some hawks urged) bomb the enemy back into the stone age—indeed, with nuclear weapons, it had the capacity to obliterate Southeast Asia altogether. But this was *not* a war in which those superiorities could be made properly effective. Fear of domestic opinion, and of world reaction, prevented the use of atomic weapons against a foe who could never be a *vital* threat to the United States itself. Worries about the American public's opposition to heavy casualties in a conflict whose legitimacy and efficacy came increasingly under question had similarly constrained the administration's use of the conventional methods of warfare; restrictions were placed on the bombing campaign; the Ho Chi Minh Trail through neutral Laos could not be occupied; Russian vessels bearing arms to Haiphong harbor could not be seized. It was important not to provoke the two major Communist states into joining the war. This essentially reduced the fighting to a series of small-scale encounters in jungles and paddy fields, terrain which blunted the advantages of American firepower and (helicopter-borne) mobility, and instead placed an emphasis upon jungle-warfare techniques and unit cohesion—which was much less of a problem for the crack forces than for the rapidly turning over contingents of draftees. Although Johnson followed Kennedy's lead in sending more and more troops to Vietnam (it peaked at 542,000, in 1969), it was never enough to meet General Westmoreland's demands; clinging to the view that this was still a limited conflict, the government refused to mobilize the reserves, or indeed to put the economy on a war footing.[169]

The difficulties of fighting the war on terms disadvantageous to the United States' real military strengths reflected a larger political problem—the discrepancy between means and ends (as Clausewitz might have put it). The North Vietnamese and the Vietcong were fighting for what they believed in very strongly; those who were not were undoubtedly subject to the discipline of a totalitarian, passionately nationalistic regime. The South Vietnamese governing system, by contrast, appeared corrupt, unpopular, and in a distinct minority, opposed by the Buddhist monks, unsupported by a frightened, exploited, and war-weary peasantry; those native units loyal to the regime and who often fought well were not sufficient to compensate for this inner corrosion. As the war escalated, more and more Americans questioned the efficacy of fighting for the regime in Saigon, and worried at the way in which all this was corrupting the American armed forces themselves— in the decline in morale, the rise in cynicism, indiscipline, drug-taking, prostitution, the increasing racial sneers at the "gooks," and atrocities in the field, not to mention the corrosion of the United States' own currency or of its larger strategic posture. Ho Chi Minh had declared that his forces were willing to lose men at the rate of ten to one—and when they were rash enough to emerge from the jungles to attack the cities, as in the 1968 Tet offensive, they often did; but, he continued, despite those losses they would still fight on. That sort of willpower was not evident in South Vietnam. Nor was American society itself, increasingly disturbed by the war's contradictions, willing to sacrifice everything for victory. While the latter feeling was quite understandable, given what was at stake for each side, the fact was that it proved impossible for an open democracy to wage a halfhearted war successfully. This was the fundamental contradiction, which neither McNamara's systems analysis nor the B-52 bombers based on Guam could alter.[170]

More than a decade after the fall of Saigon (April 1975), and with books upon all aspects of that conflict still flooding from the presses, it still remains difficult to assess clearly how it may have affected the U.S. position in the world. Viewed from a longer perspective, say, backward from the year 2000 or 2020, it might be seen as having produced a salutory shock to American global hubris (or to what Senator Fulbright called "the arrogance of power"), and thus compelled the country to think more deeply about its political and strategical priorities and to readjust more sensibly to a world already much changed since 1945—in other words, rather like the shock which the Russians received in the Crimean War, or the British received in the Boer War, producing in their turn beneficial reforms and reassessments.

At the time, however, the short-term effects of the war could not be other than deleterious. The vast boom in spending on the war, precisely at a time when domestic expenditures upon Johnson's "Great Society" were also leaping upward, badly affected the American economy in ways which will be examined below (pp. 434–35). Moreover, while the United States was pouring money into Vietnam, the USSR was devoting steadily larger sums to its nuclear forces—so that it achieved a rough strategic parity—and to its navy, which in these years emerged as a major force in global gunboat diplomacy; and this increasing imbalance was worsened by the American electorate's turn against military expenditures for most of the 1970s. In 1978, "national security expenditures" were only 5 percent of GNP, lower than they had been for thirty years.[171] Morale in the armed services plummeted, in consequence both of the war itself and of the postwar cuts. Shakeups in the CIA and other agencies, however necessary to check abuses, undoubtedly cramped their effectiveness. The American concentration upon Vietnam worried even sympathetic allies; its methods of fighting in support of a corrupt regime alienated public opinion, in western Europe as much as in the Third World, and was a major factor in what some writers have termed American "estrangement" from much of the rest of the planet.[172] It led to a neglect of American attention toward Latin America—and a tendency to replace Kennedy's hoped-for "Alliance for Progress" with military support for undemocratic regimes and with counterrevolutionary actions (like the 1965 intervention in the Dominican Republic). The—inevitably—open post-Vietnam War debate over the regions of the globe for which the United States would or *would not* fight in the future disturbed existing allies, doubtless encouraged its foes, and caused wobbling neutrals to consider re-insuring themselves with the other side. At the United Nations debates, the American delegate appeared increasingly beleaguered and isolated. Things had come a long way since Henry Luce's assertion that the United States would be the elder brother of nations in the brotherhood of man.[173]

The other power-political consequence of the Vietnam War was that it obscured, by perhaps as much as a decade, Washington's recognition of the extent of the Sino-Soviet split—and thus its chance to evolve a policy to handle it. It was therefore the more striking that this neglect should be put right so swiftly after the entry into the presidency of that bitter foe of Communism Richard Nixon, in January 1969. But Nixon possessed, to use Professor Gaddis's phrase, a "unique combination of ideological rigidity with political pragmatism"[174]—and the latter was especially manifest in his dealings with foreign Great Powers. Despite Nixon's dislike of domestic radicals and animosity toward, say, Allende's Chile for its socialist policies, the president claimed to be unideological when it came to global diplomacy. To him, there was no great contradiction between ordering a massive increase in the bombing of North Vietnam in 1972—to compel Hanoi to come closer to the American bargaining position for withdrawal from the South—and journeying to China to bury the hatchet with Mao Tse-tung in the same year. Even more significant was to be his choice of Henry Kissinger as his national security adviser (and later secretary of state). Kissinger's approach to world affairs was historicist and relativistic: events had to be seen in their larger context, and related to each other; Great Powers should be judged on what they did, not on their domestic ideology; an absolutist search for security was utopian, since that would make everyone else absolutely insecure—all that one could hope to achieve was relative security, based upon a reasonable balance of forces in world affairs, a mature recognition that the world scene would never be completely harmonious, and a willingness to bargain. Like the statesmen he had written about (Metternich, Castlereagh, Bismarck), Kissinger felt that "the beginning of wisdom in human as well as international affairs was knowing when to stop."[175] His aphorisms were Palmerstonian ("We have no permanent enemies") and Bismarckian ("The hostility between China and the Soviet Union served our purposes best if we maintained closer relations with each side than they did with each other"),[176] and were unlike anything in American diplomacy since Kennan. But Kissinger had a much greater chance to direct policy than his fellow admirer of nineteenth-century European statesmen ever possessed.[177]

Finally, Kissinger recognized the limitations upon American power, not only in the sense that the United States could not afford to fight a protracted war in the jungles of Southeast Asia *and* to maintain its other, more vital interests, but also because both he and Nixon could perceive that the world's balances were altering, and new forces were undermining the hitherto unchallenged domination of the two superpowers. The latter were still far ahead in terms of strictly military power, but in other respects the world had become more of a multipolar place: "In economic terms," he noted in 1973, "there are at least five major groupings. Politically, many more centers of influence have emerged. . . ." With echoes of (and amendments to) Kennan, he identified five important regions, the United States, the USSR, China, Japan, and western Europe; and unlike many in Washington and (perhaps) everyone in Moscow, he welcomed this change. A *concert* of large powers, balancing each other off and with no one dominating another, would be "a safer world and a better world" than a bipolar situation in which "a gain for one side appears as an absolute loss for the other."[178] Confident in his own abilities to defend American interests in such a pluralistic world, Kissinger was urging a fundamental reshaping of American diplomacy in the largest sense of that word.

The diplomatic revolution caused by the steady Sino-American *rapprochement* after 1971 had a profound effect on the "global correlation of forces." Although taken by surprise at Washington's move, Japan felt that it at last was able to establish relations with the People's Republic of China, which thus gave a further boost to its booming Asian trade. The Cold War in Asia, it appeared, was over—or perhaps it would be better to say that it had become more complicated: Pakistan, which had been a diplomatic conduit for secret messages between Washington and Peking, received the support of both those Powers during its clash with India in 1971; Moscow, predictably, gave strong support to New Delhi. In Europe, too, the balances had been altered. Alarmed by China's hostility and taken aback by Kissinger's diplomacy, the Kremlin deemed it prudent to conclude the SALT I treaty and to encourage the various other attempts to improve relations across the Iron Curtain. It also held back when, following its tense confrontation with the United States at the time of the 1973 Arab-Israeli war, Kissinger commenced his "shuttle diplomacy" to reconcile Egypt and Israel, effectively freezing Russia out of any meaningful role.

It is difficult to know how long Kissinger could have kept up his Bismarck-style juggling act had the Watergate scandal not swept Nixon from the White House in August 1974 and made so many Americans even more suspicious of their government. As it was, the secretary of state remained in his post during Ford's tenure of the presidency, but with increasingly less freedom for maneuver. Defense budget requisitions were frequently slashed by Congress. All further aid was cut off to South Vietnam, Cambodia, and Laos in February 1975, a few months before those states were overrun. The War Powers Act sharply pared the president's capacity to commit American troops overseas. Soviet-Cuban interventions in Angola could not, Congress had voted, be countered by sending CIA funds and weapons to the pro-western factions there. With the Republican right growing restive at this decline in American power abroad and blaming Kissinger for ceding away national interests (the Panama Canal) and old friends (Taiwan), the secretary of state's position was beginning to crumble even before Ford was swept out of power in the 1976 election.

As the United States grappled with serious socioeconomic problems throughout the 1970s and as different political groups tried to reconcile themselves to its reduced international position, it was perhaps inevitable that its external policies would be more erratic than was the case in placid times. Nonetheless, there were to be "swings" in policy over the next few years which were remarkable by any standards. Imbued with the most creditable of Gladstonian and Wilsonian beliefs about the need to create a "fairer" global order, Carter breezily entered an international system in which many of the other actors (especially in the world's "trouble spots") had no intention of conducting their policies according to Judeo-Christian principles. Given the Third World's discontent at the economic gap between rich and poor nations, which had been exacerbated by the 1973 oil crisis, there was prudence as well as magnanimity in his push for north-south cooperation, just as there was common sense in the terms of the renegotiated Panama Canal treaty, and in his refusal to equate every Latin American reformist movement with Marxism. Carter also took justified credit for "brokering" the 1978 Camp David agreement between Egypt and Israel—although he ought not to have been so surprised at the critical reaction of the other Arab nations, which in turn was to give Russia the opportunity to strengthen its ties with the more radical states in the Middle East. For all its worthy intentions, however, the Carter government foundered upon the rocks of a complex world which seemed increasingly unwilling to abide by American advice, and upon its own inconsistencies of policy (often caused by quarrels within the administration).[179] Authoritarian, right-wing regimes were berated and pressured across the globe for their human-rights violations, yet Washington continued to support President Mobutu of Zaire, King Hassan of Morocco, and the shah of Iran—at least until the latter's demise in 1979, which led to the hostages crisis, and in turn to the flawed attempt to rescue them.[180] In other parts of the globe, from Nicaragua to Angola, the administration found it difficult to discover democratic-liberal forces worthy of its support, yet hesitated to commit itself against Marxist revolutionaries. Carter also hoped to keep defense expenditures low, and appeared bewildered that *détente* with the USSR had halted neither that country's arms spending nor its actions in the Third World. When Russian troops invaded Afghanistan at the end of 1979, Washington, which was by then engaged in a large-scale defense buildup, withdrew the SALT II treaty, canceled grain sales to Moscow, and began to pursue—especially in Brzezinski's celebrated visits to China and Afghanistan—"balance-of-power" politics which the president had condemned only four years earlier.[181]

If the Carter administration had come into office with a set of simple recipes for a complex world, those of his successor in 1980 were no less simple—albeit drastically different. Suffused by an emotional reaction against all that had "gone wrong" with the United States over the preceding two decades, boosted by an electoral landslide much affected by the humiliation in Iran, charged by an ideological view of the world which at times seemed positively Manichaean, the Reagan government was intent upon steering the ship of state in quite new directions. *Détente* was out, since it merely provided a mask for Russian expansionism. The arms buildup would be increased, in all directions. Human rights were off the agenda; "authoritarian governments" were in favor. Amazingly, even the "China card" was suspect, because of the Republican right's support for Taiwan. As might have been expected, much of this simplemindedness also foundered on the complex realities of the world outside, not to mention the resistance of a Congress and public which liked their president's homely patriotism but suspected his Cold War policies. Interventions in Latin America, or in any place clad in jungles and thus reminiscent of Vietnam, were constantly blocked. The escalation of the nuclear arms race produced widespread unease, and pressure for renewed arms talks, especially when administration supporters talked of being able to "prevail" in a

nuclear confrontation with the Soviet Union. Authoritarian regimes in
the tropics collapsed, often made more unpopular by association with
the American government. The Europeans were bewildered at a logic
which forbade them to buy natural gas from the USSR, but permitted
American farmers to sell that country grain. In the Middle East, the
Reagan administration's inability to put pressure upon Mr. Begin's
Israel contradicted its strategy of lining up the Arab world in an anti-
Russian front. At the United Nations, the United States seemed more
isolated than ever; by 1984, it had withdrawn from UNESCO—a situation which would have amazed Franklin Roosevelt. By more than
doubling the defense budget in five years, the United States was certainly going to possess greater military hardware than it did in 1980;
but whether the Pentagon was receiving good value for its outpourings
was increasingly doubted, as was the question of whether it could
control its interservice rivalries.[182] The invasion of Grenada, trum-
peted as a great success, was in various *operational* aspects worryingly
close to a Gilbert and Sullivan farce. Last but not least, even sympathetic observers wondered if this administration could work out a
coherent grand strategy when so many of its members were quarreling
with one another (even after Haig's retirement as secretary of state),
when its chief appeared to give little attention to critical issues, and
when (with rare exceptions) it viewed the world outside through such
ethnocentric spectacles.[183]

Many of these issues will be returned to in the final chapter. The
point about listing the various troubles of the Carter and Reagan administrations *together* was that they had, taken as a whole, distracted
attention from the larger forces which were shaping global power
politics—and most particularly that shift from a bipolar to a multipolar world which Kissinger had much earlier detected and begun to
adjust to. (As will be seen below, the emergence of three additional
centers of political-cum-economic power—western Europe, China,
and Japan—did not mean that the latter were free of problems either;
but that is not the point here.) More important still, the American
concentration upon the burgeoning problems of Nicaragua, Iran, Angola, Libya, and so on was still tending to obscure the fact that the
country most affected by the transformations which were occurring in
global politics during the 1970s was probably the USSR itself—a consideration which deserves some further brief elaboration before this
section concludes.

That the USSR had enhanced its military strength in these years was
undoubted. Yet, as Professor Ulam points out, because of other developments, that simply meant that

the rulers of the Soviet Union were in a position to appreciate the
uncomfortable discovery made by so many Americans in the forties

and fifties: enhanced power does not automatically, especially in the
nuclear age, give a state greater security. From almost every point
of view, economically and militarily, in absolute and in relative
terms, the USSR under Brezhnev was much more powerful than it
had been under Stalin. And yet along with this greatly increased
strength came new international developments and foreign commitments that made the Soviet state more vulnerable to external
danger and the turbulence of world politics than it had been, say,
in 1952.[184]

Moreover, even in the closing years of the Carter administration the
United States had resumed a defense buildup which—continued at a
massive pace by the succeeding Reagan government—threatened to
restore U.S. military superiority in strategic nuclear weaponry, to enhance U.S. maritime supremacy, and to place a heavier emphasis than
ever before upon advanced technology. The annoyed Soviet reply that
they would not be outspent or outgunned could not disguise the awkward fact that this would place increased pressure upon an economy
which had significantly slowed down (pp. 429–32 below) and was not
well positioned to indulge in a high-technology race.[185] By the late
1970s, it was in the embarrassing position of needing to import large
amounts of foreign *grain*, not to mention technology. Its satellite empire in eastern Europe was, apart from the select Communist party
cadres, increasingly disaffected; the Polish discontents in particular
were a dreadful problem, and yet a repetition of the 1968 Czech invasion seemed to promise little relief. Far to the south, the threat of losing
its Afghan buffer state to foreign (probably Chinese) influences provoked the 1979 coup d'état, which not only turned out to be a military
quagmire but had a disastrous impact upon the Soviet Union's standing abroad.[186] Russian actions in Czechoslovakia, Poland, and Afghanistan had much reduced its appeal as a "model" to others, whether in
western Europe or in Africa. Muslim fundamentalism in the Middle
East was a disturbing phenomenon, which threatened (as in Iran) to
vent itself against local Communists as well as against pro-American
groupings. Above all, there was the relentless Chinese hostility, which,
thanks to the Afghan and Vietnam complications, seemed even more
marked at the end of the 1970s than it had at the beginning.[187] If any
of the two superpowers had "lost China," it was Russia. Finally, the
ethnocentricity and narrow suspiciousness of its aging rulers and the
obstructiveness of its domestic elites, the *nomenklatura,* toward
sweeping reforms were probably going to make a successful adjustment to the newer world balances even more difficult than for the
United States.

All this ought to have been of some consolation in Washington, and
acted as a guide to a more relaxed and sophisticated view of foreign-

policy problems, even when the latter were unexpected and unpleasant. On some issues, admittedly, such as modifying earlier support for Taiwan, the Reagan administration did become more pragmatic and conciliatory. Yet the language of the 1979–1980 election campaign was difficult to shake off, perhaps because it had not been mere rhetoric, but a fundamentalist view of the world order and of the United States' destined place in it. As had happened so often in the past, the holding of such sentiments always made it difficult for countries to deal with external affairs as they really were, rather than as they thought they should be.

The Changing Economic Balances, 1950 to 1980

In July 1971, Richard Nixon repeated his opinion to a group of news-media executives in Kansas City that there now existed five clusters of world economic power—western Europe, Japan, and China as well as the USSR and the United States. "These are the five that will determine the economic future and, *because economic power will be the key to other kinds of power,* the future of the world in other ways in the last third of this century."[188] Assuming that presidential remark upon the importance of economic power to be valid, it is necessary to get a deeper sense of the transformations which were occurring in the global economy since the early years of the Cold War; for although international trade and prosperity were to be subject to some unusual turbulences (especially in the 1970s), certain basic long-term trends can be detected which seemed likely to shape the state of world politics into the foreseeable future.

As with all of the earlier periods covered in this book, there can be no exactitude in the comparative economic statistics used here. If anything, the growth in the number of professional statisticians employed by governments and by international organizations and the development of much more sophisticated techniques since the days of Mulhall's *Dictionary of Statistics* have tended to show how difficult is the task of making proper comparisons. The reluctance of "closed" societies to publish their figures, differentiated national ways of measuring income and product, and fluctuating exchange rates (especially after the post-1971 decisions to abandon a gold-exchange standard and to adopt floating exchange rates) have all combined to cast doubt upon the correctness of any *one* series of economic data.[189] On the other hand, a *number* of statistical indications can be used, with a reasonable degree of confidence, to correlate with one another and to point to broad trends occurring over time.

The first, and by far the most important, feature has been what Bairoch rightly describes as "a totally unprecedented rate of growth in

world industrial output"[190] during the decades after the Second World
War. Between 1953 and 1975 that growth rate averaged a remarkable
6 percent a year overall (4 percent per capita), and even in the 1973–
1980 period the average increase was 2.4 percent a year, which was
very respectable by historical standards. Bairoch's own calculations of
the "production of world manufacturing industries"—essentially
confirmed by Rostow's figures on "world industrial production"[191]—
give some sense of this dizzy rise (see Table 39).

**Table 39. Production of World Manufacturing
Industries, 1830–1980[192]**
(1900 = 100)

	Total Production	Annual Growth Rate
1830	34.1	(0.8)
1860	41.8	0.7
1880	59.4	1.8
1900	100.0	2.6
1913	172.4	4.3
1928	250.8	2.5
1938	311.4	2.2
1953	567.7	4.1
1963	950.1	5.3
1973	1730.6	6.2
1980	3041.6	2.4

As Bairoch also points out, "The accumulated world industrial output between 1953 and 1973 was comparable in volume to that of the
entire century and a half which separated 1953 from 1800."[193] The
recovery of war-damaged economies, the development of new technologies, the continued drift from agriculture to industry, the harnessing of national resources within "planned economies," and the spread
of industrialization to the Third World all helped to effect this dramatic
change.

In an even more emphatic way, and for much the same reasons, the
volume of world trade also grew spectacularly after 1945, in contrast
to the distortions of the era of the two world wars:

**Table 40. Volume of World Trade,
1850–1971[194]**
(1913 = 100)

1850	10.1	1938	103
1896–1900	57.0	1948	103
1913	100.0	1953	142
1921–1925	82	1963	269
1930	113	1968	407
1931–1935	93	1971	520

What was more encouraging, as Ashworth points out, was that by 1957, for the first time ever world trade in manufactured goods exceeded those in primary produce, which itself was a consequence of the fact that the increase in the overall output of manufactures during these decades was considerably larger than the (very impressive) increases in agricultural goods and minerals (see Table 41).

**Table 41. Percentage Increases in World
Production, 1948–1968**[195]

	1948–1958	1958–1968
Agricultural goods	32%	30%
Minerals	40%	58%
Manufactures	60%	100%

To some extent, this disparity can be explained by the great increases in manufacturing and trade *among* the advanced industrial countries (especially those of the European Economic Community); but their rising demand for primary products and the beginnings of industrialization among an increasing number of Third World countries meant that the economies of most of the latter were also growing faster in these decades than at any time in the twentieth century.[196] Notwithstanding the damage which western imperialism did to many of the societies in other parts of the world, the exports and general economic growth of these societies do appear to have benefited most when the industrialized nations were in a period of expansion. Less-developed countries (LDCs), argues Foreman-Peck, grew rapidly in the nineteenth century when "open" economies like Britain's were expanding fast—just as they were the worst hit of all when the industrial world fell into depression in the 1930s. During the 1950s and 1960s, they once again experienced faster growth rates, because the developed countries were booming, raw-materials demand was rising, and industrialization was spreading.[197] After its nadir in 1953 (6.5 percent), Bairoch shows the Third World's share of world manufacturing production rising steadily, to 8.5 percent (1963), then 9.9 percent (1973), and then 12.0 percent (1980).[198] In the CIA's estimates, the less-developed countries' share of "gross world product" has also been increasing, from 11.1 percent (1960), to 12.3 percent (1970), to 14.8 percent (1980).[199]

Given the sheer number of people in the Third World, however, their share of world product was still disproportionately low—and their poverty horrifically manifest. The average GNP per capita in the industrialized countries was $10,660 in 1980, but only $1,580 per capita for the middle-income countries like Brazil, and a shocking $250 per capita for the very poorest Third World countries like Zaire.[200] For the fact was that while their proportion of world product and manufacturing output was arising *as a whole*, the gain was not shared in equal

proportion by all of the LDCs. Differences in wealth between some
countries in the tropics were large even as the colonialists withdrew—
just as they had been, in many cases, before the imperial era. They were
exacerbated by the uneven pattern of demand for the countries' products, by the varying levels of aid which each managed to secure, and
by the vicissitudes of climate, politics, tampering with the environment, and economic forces quite outside their control. Drought could
devastate a country for years. Civil wars, guerrilla activities, or the
forced resettlement of peasants could reduce agricultural output and
trade. Sinking world prices, say, of peanuts or tin could almost bring
a single-product economy to a halt. Soaring interest rates, or a rise in
the value of the U.S. dollar, could be body blows. A spiraling population growth, caused by western medical science's success in checking
disease, increased the pressure upon food stocks and threatened to
wipe out any gains in overall national income. On the other hand, there
were states which went through a "green revolution," with agricultural
output boosted by improved farming techniques and new strains of
plants. In addition, the massive earnings recorded by those countries
lucky enough to possess oil in the 1970s turned them into a different
economic category—although even these so-called OPEC-LDCs suffered as oil prices tumbled in the early 1980s. Finally, in one of the
most significant developments of all, there arose among Third World
countries a number of what Rosecrance terms "the trading states"—
South Korea, Taiwan, Singapore, and Malaysia, imitating Japan, West
Germany, and Switzerland in their entrepreneurship and commitment
to produce industrial manufactures for the global market.[201]

This disparity among less-developed nations points to the second
major feature of macroeconomic change over the past few decades—
the differential growth rates among the various nations of the globe,
which was as true of the larger, industrialized Powers as it was of the
smaller countries. Since this trend is the one which—on the record of
the preceding centuries—has ultimately had the greatest impact upon
the international power balances, it is worth examining in some detail
how it affected the major nations in these decades.

There can be no doubt that the economic transformation of Japan
after 1945 offered the most spectacular example of sustained modernization in these decades, outclassing almost all of the existing "advanced" countries as a commercial and technological competitor, and
providing a model for emulation by the other Asian "trading states."
To be sure, Japan had already distinguished itself almost a century
earlier by becoming the first Asian country to copy the West in both
economic and—fatefully for itself—military and imperialist terms. Although badly damaged by the 1937–1945 war, and cut off from its
traditional markets and suppliers, it possessed an industrial infrastructure which could be repaired and a talented, well-educated, and

socially cohesive population whose determination to improve themselves could now be channeled into peaceful commercial pursuits. For the few years after 1945, Japan was prostrate, an occupied territory, and dependent upon American aid. In 1950, the tide turned—ironically, to a large degree because of the heavy U.S. defense spending in the Korean War, which stimulated Japan's export-oriented companies. Toyota, for example, was in danger of foundering when it was rescued by the first of the U.S. Defense Department's orders for its trucks; and much the same happened to many other companies.[202]

There was, of course, much more to the "Japanese miracle" than the stimulant of American spending during the Korean War and, again, during the Vietnam War; and the effort to explain exactly how the country transformed itself, and how others can imitate its success, has turned into a miniature growth industry itself.[203] One major reason was its quite fanatical belief in achieving the highest levels of quality control, borrowing (and improving upon) sophisticated management techniques and production methods in the West. It benefited from the national commitment to vigorous, high-level standards of universal education, and from possessing vast numbers of engineers, of electronics and automobile buffs, and of small but entrepreneurial workshops as well as the giant *zaibatsu*. There was social ethos in favor of hard work, loyalty to the company, and the need to reconcile management-worker differences through a mixture of compromise and deference. The economy required enormous amounts of capital to achieve sustained growth, and it received just that—partly because there was so little expenditure upon defense by a "demilitarized" country sheltering under the American strategic umbrella, but perhaps even more because of fiscal and taxation policies which encouraged an unusually high degree of personal savings, which could then be used for investment purposes. Japan also benefited from the role played by MITI (its Ministry for International Trade and Industry) in "nursing new industries and technological developments while at the same time coordinating the orderly run-down of aging, decaying industries,"[204] all this in a manner totally different from the American laissez-faire approach.

Whatever the mix of explanations—and other experts upon Japan would point more strongly to cultural and sociological reasons, not to mention that indefinable "plus factor" of national self-confidence and willpower in a people whose time has come—there was no denying the extent of its economic success. Between 1950 and 1973 its gross domestic product grew at the fantastic average of 10.5 percent a year, far in excess of that of any other industrialized nation; and even the oil crisis in 1973–1974, with its profound blow to world expansion, did not prevent Japan's growth rates in subsequent years from staying almost twice as large as those of its major competitors. The range of manufactures in which Japan steadily became the dominant world producer was quite staggering—cameras, kitchen goods, electrical products, musical instruments, scooters, on and on the list goes. Japanese products challenged the Swiss watch industry, overshadowed the German optical industry, and devastated the British and American motorcycle industries. Within a decade, Japan's shipyards were producing over half of the world's tonnage of launchings. By the 1970s, its more modern steelworks were turning out as much as the American steel industry. The transformation of its automobile industry was even more dramatic—between 1960 and 1984 its share of world car production rose from 1 percent to 23 percent—and in consequence Japanese cars and trucks were being exported in their millions all over the world. Steadily, relentlessly, the country moved from low- to high-technology products—to computers, telecommunications, aerospace, robotics, and biotechnology. Steadily, relentlessly, its trade surpluses increased—turning it into a financial giant as well as an industrial one—and its share of world production and markets expanded. When the Allied occupation ended in 1952, Japan's "gross national product was little more than one-third that of France or the United Kingdom. By the late 1970s the Japanese GNP was as large as the United Kingdom's and France's *combined* and more than half the size of America's."[205] Within one generation, its share of the world's manufacturing output, and of GNP, had risen from around 2–3 percent to around 10 percent—and was not stopping. Only the USSR in the years after 1928 had achieved anything like that degree of growth, but Japan had done it far less painfully and in a much more impressive, broader-based way.

By comparison with Japan, *every* other large Power must seem economically sluggish. Nonetheless, when the People's Republic of China (PRC) began to assert itself in the years after its foundation in 1949, there were few observers who did not take it seriously. In part this may have reflected a traditional worry about the "Yellow Peril," since the sleeping giant in the East would clearly be a major force in world affairs just as soon as it had organized its 800 million population for national purposes. More important still was the very prominent, not to say aggressive, role which the PRC adopted toward foreign Powers almost since its inception, even if that may have been a nervous response to its perceived encirclement. The clashes with the United States over Korea and Quemoy and Matsu; the move into Tibet; the border struggles with India; the angry break with the USSR, and military confrontations in the disputed regions; the bloody encounter with North Vietnam; and the generally combative tone of Chinese propaganda (especially under Mao) as it criticized western imperialism and "Russian hegemonism" and urged on people's liberation movements across the globe made it a much more important, but also more incalculable, figure in world affairs than the discreet and subtle Japanese.[206] Simply because China possessed one-quarter of the world's population, its political lurches in one direction or another had to be taken seriously.

Nevertheless, measured on strictly economic criteria, the PRC seemed a classic case of economic backwardness. In 1953, for example, it was responsible for only 2.3 percent of world manufacturing production and had a "total industrial potential" equal only to 71 percent of Britain's in 1900![207] Its population, leaping upward by tens of millions of new mouths each year, consisted overwhelmingly of poor peasants whose per capita output was dreadfully low and rendered the state little in terms of "added value." The disruption caused by the warlords, the Japanese invasion, and then the civil war of the late 1940s was not stopped when the peasant communes took over from the landowners after 1949. Nevertheless, economic prospects were not entirely hopeless. China did possess a basic infrastructure of roads and light railways, its textile industry was substantial, its cities and ports were centers of entrepreneurial activity, and the Manchurian region in particular had been developed by the Japanese during the 1930s.[208] What the country required, if it was to enter the stage of industrial takeoff, was a long period of stability and massive infusions of capital. Both conditions were achieved to some degree—because of the dominance of the Communist Party, and the flow of Russian aid—as the 1950s evolved. The Five-Year Plan of 1953 consciously imitated those Stalinist priorities of developing heavy industry and of increasing steel, iron and coal production. By 1957, industrial output had doubled.[209] On the other hand, the amount of ready capital for industrial investment, whether raised internally or borrowed from Russia, was quite insufficient for a country of China's economic needs—and the Sino-Soviet split brought Russian financial and technical aid to an abrupt halt. In addition, Mao's fatuous decisions to achieve a "Great Leap Forward" by encouraging thousands of cottage-sized steelworks and his campaign for the "Cultural Revolution" (which led to the disgrace of technical experts, professional managers, and trained economists) slowed development considerably. Finally, throughout the 1950s and 1960s, the PRC's confrontationist diplomacy and its military clashes with almost all of its neighbors meant that far too large a proportion of the country's scarce resources had to be devoted to the armed forces.

The period of the Cultural Revolution was not *all* bad in economic terms; it did at least emphasize the importance of the rural areas, stimulating small-scale industries as well as improved farming techniques, and bringing basic medical and social care to the villages.[210] Nevertheless, significant increases in national product could come only from further industrialization, infrastructure improvements, and long-term investments—all of which were aided by the winding down of the Cultural Revolution and by the growth of trade with the United States, Japan, and other advanced economies. China's own coal and oil resources were being swiftly exploited, as were its stocks of many precious minerals. By 1980, its steel output of 37 million tons was well in excess of that of Britain or France, and its consumption of energy from modern sources was twice that of any of the leading European states.[211] By that date, too, its share of world manufacturing production had risen to 5.0 percent (from 3.9 percent in 1973), and was closing upon West Germany's.[212] This heady recent growth has not been unattended by problems, and the party leadership has had to readjust downward the targets for the country's "four moderniza-tions"; it is also worth repeating that when any of China's statistics of wealth or output are presented in per capita terms, its relative eco-nomic backwardness is again revealed. Yet, notwithstanding those deficiencies, it became clear over time that the Asian giant was at last on the move and determined to build an economic foundation ade-quate for its intended role as a Great Power.[213]

The fifth region of economic power identified by Nixon in his July 1971 speech had been "western Europe," which was of course more of a geographical expression than a unified assertive Power like China, the USSR, and the United States. Even the term itself meant different things to different people—it could be all of those countries outside the Russian-dominated sphere (and therefore include Scandinavia, Greece, and Turkey), or it could be the original (or enlarged) European Economic Community, which at least possessed an institutional frame-work, or it was often used as a shorthand for that cluster of formerly great states (Britain, France, Germany, Italy) which might need to be consulted, say, by the U.S. State Department before the latter initiated a new policy toward Russia or in the Middle East. Even that did not exhaust the possibilities of semantic confusion, since for much of this period the British regarded "Europe" as beginning on the other side of the English Channel; and there were, moreover, many committed European integrationists (not to mention German nationalists) who regarded the post-1945 division of the continent as a merely temporary condition, to be followed in the future by a joining of the countries of both sides into some larger union. Politically and constitutionally, therefore, it has been difficult to use the term "Europe" or even "west-ern Europe" as more than a figure of speech—or a vague cultural-geographical concept.[214]

At the economic level, however, there did seem to be a basic similarity in what was being experienced across Europe in these years. The most outstanding feature was the "sustained and high level of economic growth."[215] By 1949–1950, most countries were back to their prewar levels of output, and some (especially, of course, the wartime neutrals) were significantly ahead. But there then followed year after year of increased manufacturing output, of unprecedented levels of growth in exports, of a remarkable degree of full employment and historically high levels of disposable income as well as of investment capital. The result was to make Europe the fastest-growing region in the world, Japan excepted. "Between 1950 and 1970 European gross domestic product grew on average at about 5.5 percent per annum and 4.4 percent on a per capita basis, as against world average rates of 5.0 and 3.0 percent respectively. Industrial production rose even faster at 7.1 percent compared with a world rate of 5.9 percent. Thus by the latter date output per head in Europe was almost two and a half times greater than in 1950."[216] Interestingly enough, this growth was shared in all parts of the continent—in northwestern Europe's industrial core, in the Mediterranean lands, in eastern Europe; even the sluggish British economy grew faster during this period than it had for decades. Not surprisingly, Europe's relative place in the world economy, which had been declining since the turn of the century, soon began to expand. "During the period 1950 to 1970 her share of world output of goods and services (GDP) rose from 37 to 41 percent, while in the case of industrial production the increase was even greater, from 39 to 48 percent."[217] Both in 1960 and in 1970, the CIA figures were showing—admittedly on statistical evidence that can be disputed[218]—that the "European Community" possessed a larger share of gross world product than even the United States, and that it was twice as large as the Soviet Union's.

The reasons for Europe's economic recovery are, on reflection, not at all surprising. For too long, much of the continent had suffered from invasions, prolonged fighting and foreign occupation, bombings of towns, factories, roads, and railways, shortages of food and raw materials caused by blockade, the call-up of millions of men and killing off of millions of animals. Even before the fighting, Europe's "natural" economic development—that is, growth which evolved region by region, as new sources of energy and production revealed themselves, as new markets took off, as new technology spread—had been distorted by the actions of the nationalistically inclined *Machtstaat.*[219] Ever-higher tariff barriers had separated suppliers from their markets. Government subventions had kept inefficient firms and farmers protected from foreign competition. Increasingly large amounts of national income had been devoted to armaments spending rather than commercial enterprise. It was thus impossible to maximize Europe's economic growth in this "climate of blocks and autarky, of economic nationalism, and of gaining benefits by hurting others."[220] Now, after 1945, there were not only "new Europeans" like Monnet, Spaak, and Hallstein determined to create economic structures which would avoid the mistakes of the past, but there was also a helpful and beneficient United States, willing (through the Marshall Plan and other aid schemes) to finance Europe's recovery provided it was done as a cooperative venture.

Thus, a Europe whose economic potential had been distorted and underutilized by war and politics now had a chance to correct those deficiencies. There was a broad determination to "build anew" in both eastern and western parts of the continent, and a willingness to learn from the follies of the 1930s. State planning, whether of the Keynesian or socialistic variety, gave a concentrated thrust to this desire for social and economic improvement; the collapse (or discrediting) of older structures made innovation easier. The United States not only gave billions of dollars of Marshall Plan aid—"a shot in the arm at a critical time," as it was aptly described[221]—but also provided a defense umbrella under which the European states could shelter. (It was true that both Britain and France spent heavily on defense during the Korean War years and the period before their decolonizations—but they, and all their neighbors, would have had to devote much more of their scarce national resources to armaments had they not been protected by the United States.) Because there were fewer trade barriers, firms and individuals were able to flourish in a much larger market. This was especially so since trade *among* developed countries (in this case, the European states themselves) was always more profitable than trade elsewhere, simply because the mutual demand was greater. If the "foreign" trade of Europe rose faster than anything else in these decades, therefore, it was chiefly because much more buying and selling was going on among neighbors. In one generation after 1950, per capita income increased as much as it had during the century and a half prior to that date![222] The socioeconomic pace of this change was truly remarkable: the share of West Germany's working population engaged in agriculture, forestry and fishing dropped from 24.6 percent in 1950 to 7.5 percent in 1973, and in France it fell from 28.2 percent to 12.2 percent in the same period (and to 8.8 percent in 1980). Disposable incomes boomed as industrialization spread; in West Germany per capita income soared from $320 in 1949 to $9,131 in 1978, and in Italy it rose from $638 in 1960 to $5,142 in 1979. The number of automobiles per 1,000 of population rose from 6.3 in West Germany (1948) to 227 (1970), and in France from 37 to 252.[223] However one measured it, and despite continued regional disparities, the evidence of very real gains was clear.

This combination of general economic growth, together with wide variations in both the rate of change and its effects, can clearly be seen if one examines what happened in each of the former Great Powers. South of the Alps, there occurred what journalists hyperbolically termed "the Italian miracle," with the country's GNP in real terms rising nearly three times as fast after 1948 than it had during the interwar years; indeed, until 1963, when growth slowed, the Italian economy rose faster in these years than that of any other country except Japan and West Germany. Yet perhaps that, too, is not surprising in retrospect. It was always the least developed of the European "Big Four," which is another way of saying that its potential for growth had not been as fully exploited. Freed from the absurdities of fascist economic policies, and benefiting strongly from American aid, Italian manufacturers were able to utilize the country's lower wage costs and strong reputation in design to boost exports at an amazingly fast rate, especially within the Common Market. Hydroelectricity and cheaply imported oil compensated for the lack of indigenous coal supplies. Motor construction was a great stimulant. As local consumption levels boomed, FIAT, the domestic automobile producer, occupied an unchallenged position for many years in this home market, giving it a strong base for its export drive north of the Alps. Traditional manufactures, like shoes and fine clothes, were now joined by newer products; Italian refrigerators outsold any others in Europe by the 1960s. This was not, by any means, a story of unqualified success. The gap between north and south in Italy remained chronic. Social conditions, both in the inner cities and in the poorer rural areas, were far worse than in northern Europe. Governmental instability, a large "black economy," and a high public deficit, together with a higher than average inflation rate, affected the value of the lira and suggested that this economic recovery was a fragile one. Whenever European-wide comparisons of income, or industrialization, were made, Italy did not compare too well with its more advanced neighbors; when *growth* rates were compared, things looked much better. That is simply another way of saying that Italy had started from a long way behind.[224]

By contrast, Great Britain in 1945 was a long way ahead, at least among the larger European states; which may be part of the explanation for its relative economic decline during the four decades following. That is to say, since it (just like the United States) had not been so badly damaged by the war, its rate of growth was unlikely to be as high as in those countries recovering from years of military occupation and damage. Psychologically, too, as has been discussed above,[225] the fact that Britain was undefeated, that it was still one of the "Big Three" at Potsdam, and that it regained all of its worldwide empire made it difficult for people to see the need for drastic reforms in its own economic system. Far from producing newer structures, the war had preserved traditional institutions such as trade unions, the civil service, the ancient universities. Although the Labor administration of 1945–1951 pushed ahead with its plans for nationalization and for the creation of a "welfare state," a more fundamental restructuring of economic practices and of *attitudes* to work did not occur. Confident still in its special place in the world, Britain continued to rely upon captive colonial markets, struggled in vain to preserve the old parity for sterling, maintained extensive overseas garrisons (a great drain on the currency), declined to join in the early moves toward European unity, and spent more on defense than any of the other NATO powers apart from the United States itself.

The frailty of Britain's international and economic position was partially disguised in the early post-1945 period by the even greater weakness of other states, the prudent withdrawals from India and Palestine, the short-term surge in exports, and the maintenance of empire in the Middle East and Africa.[226] The humiliation at Suez in 1956 therefore came as a greater shock, since it revealed not only the weakness of sterling but also the blunt fact that Britain could not operate militarily in the Third World in the face of American disapproval. Nonetheless, it can be argued that the realities of decline were *still* disguised—in defense matters, by the post-1957 policy of relying upon the nuclear deterrent, which was far less expensive than large conventional forces yet suggested a continued Great Power status; and in economic matters, by the fact that Britain also shared in the general boom of the 1950s and 1960s. If its growth rates were about the lowest in Europe, they were nevertheless better than the expansion of previous decades and thus allowed Macmillan to claim to the British electors, "You've never had it so good!" Measured in terms of disposable income, or numbers of washing machines and automobiles, that claim was historically correct.

Measured against the much faster progress being made elsewhere, however, the country appeared to be suffering from what the Germans unkindly termed "the English disease"—a combination of militant trade unionism, poor management, "stop-go" policies by government, and negative cultural attitudes toward hard work and entrepreneurship. The new prosperity brought a massive surge in imports of better-designed European products and of cheaper Asian wares, in turn leading to balance-of-payments difficulties, sterling crises, and devaluations which helped to fuel inflation and thus higher wage demands. Price controls, legislation on wage increases, and fiscal deflation were employed at various times by British governments to check inflation and create the right circumstances for sustained growth. They rarely worked for long. The British automobile industry was steadily undermined by its foreign competitors, the once-booming shipbuilding industry grew to depend almost solely upon Admiralty orders, the producers of electrical goods and motorbikes found that they could no longer compete. Some companies (like ICI) were notable exceptions to this trend; the City of London's financial services held up well, and retailing remained strong—but the erosion of Britain's *industrial* base was remorseless. Joining the Common Market in 1971 did not provide the hoped-for panacea: it exposed the British market to even greater competition in manufactures, while tying Britain into the expensive farm-price policies of the EEC. North Sea oil also proved less than a godsend: it brought Britain massive foreign-currency earnings, but that so drove up the price of sterling that it hurt manufacturing exports.[227]

The economic statistics offer a measure of what Bairoch terms "the acceleration of the industrial decline of Great Britain."[228] Its share of world manufacturing production slipped from 8.6 percent in 1953 to 4.0 percent in 1980. Its share of world trade also fell away swiftly, from 19.8 percent (1955) to 8.7 percent (1976). Its gross national product, third-largest in the world in 1945, was overtaken by West Germany's, then by Japan's, then by France's. Its per capita disposable income was steadily overtaken by a host of smaller but richer European countries; by the late 1970s it was closer to those of Mediterranean states than to those of West Germany, France, or the Benelux countries.[229] To be sure, much of this decline in Britain's *shares* (whether of world trade or world GNP) was due to the fact that special technical and historical circumstances had given the country a disproportionately large amount of global wealth and commerce in earlier decades; now that those special circumstances had gone, and other countries were able to exploit their own potential for industrialization, it was natural that Britain's relative position should slip. Whether it should have slipped so much and so fast is another issue; whether it will slip further, relative to its European neighbors, is equally difficult to say. By the early 1980s, the decline seemed to be leveling off, leaving Britain still with the world's sixth-largest economy, and with very substantial armed forces. By comparison with Lloyd George's time, or even with Clement Attlee's in 1945, however, it was now just an ordinary, moderately large power, not a Great Power.

While the British economy was languishing in relative decline, West Germany was enjoying its *Wirtschaftswunder,* or "economic miracle." Once again, it is worth stressing how "natural," relatively speaking, this development was. Even in its truncated state, the Federal Republic possessed the most developed infrastructure in Europe, contained large internal resources (from coal to machine-tool plants), and had a highly educated population, perhaps especially strong in managers, engineers, and scientists, which was swollen by the emigration of talent from the east. For the past half-century or more, its economic powers had been distorted by the requirements of the German military machine. Now that the national energies could (as in Japan) be concentrated solely upon commercial success, the only question was the extent of the recovery. German big business, which had accommodated itself fairly easily to the Second Reich, to Weimar, and then to the Nazi period of rule, had to adjust to the new circumstances and pick up American management assumptions.[230] The big banks were once again able to play a large role in the direction of industry. The chemical and electrical industries soon reemerged to be the giants of European industry. Massively successful automobile companies, like Volkswagen and Mercedes, had their inevitable "multiplier effects" upon hundreds of small supplier firms. As exports boomed—Germany became second only to the United States in world export trade—increasing number of firms and local communities needed to bring in "guest workers" to meet the crying demand for unskilled labor. Once again, for the third time in a hundred years, the German economy was the powerhouse of Europe's economic growth.[231]

Statistically, then, the story seemed one of unbroken success. Even between 1948 and 1952, German industrial production rose by 110 percent and real GNP by 67 percent.[232] With the country having the highest gross investment levels in Europe, German firms benefited immensely from their ready access to capital. Steel output, virtually nonexistent in 1946, was soon the largest in Europe (over 34 million tons by 1960), and the same was true of most other industries. Year after year, the country had the largest growth in gross domestic product. Its GNP, a mere $32 billion in 1952, was the biggest in Europe (at $89 billion) by a decade later, and was over $600 billion by the late 1970s. Its per capita disposable income, a modest $1,186 in 1960 (when the United States' was $2,491), was an imposing $10,837 in 1979—ahead of the American average of $9,595.[233] Year after year, export surpluses were built up, with the deutsche mark needing frequent upward adjustment, and indeed becoming a sort of reserve currency. Although naturally worried at the competition posed by the even more efficient Japanese, the West Germans were undoubtedly the second most successful among the larger "trading states." This was the more impressive since the country had been separated from 40 percent of its territory and over 35 percent of its population; ironically, the German Democratic Republic was soon to show that it was the most productive and industrialized per capita of all of the eastern European states (including the USSR) despite the loss of millions of its talented labor force to the West. Had it been possible to return to the 1937 boundaries, a united Germany would once again have been far ahead of any economic rival in Europe and, indeed, perhaps not significantly behind the much larger USSR itself.

Precisely because Germany had been defeated and divided, and because its international status (and that of Berlin) continued to be regulated by the "treaty powers," this economic weight did not translate into political might. Feeling a natural responsibility toward Germans in the east, the Federal Republic was peculiarly sensitive to any warming or cooling in the NATO–Warsaw Pact relationship. It had the largest trade with eastern Europe and the USSR, yet it was obviously in the front line should another war occur. Soviet and (only slightly less) French alarm at any revival of "German militarism" meant that it could never become a nuclear Power. It felt guilty toward neighbors like the Poles and the Czechs, vulnerable toward Russia, heavily dependent upon the United States; it welcomed with gratitude the special Franco-German relationship offered by de Gaulle, but rarely felt able to use its economic muscle to control the more assertive policies of the French. Engaged in a profound intellectual confrontation with their own past, the West Germans were very happy to be seen as good team players, but *not* as decisive leaders in international affairs.[234]

This contrasted very markedly, then, with France's role in the post-war world or, more accurately, in the post-1958 world, when de Gaulle took over the helm of the state. As mentioned above (pp. 401-2), the economic progress which the planners around Monnet hoped to achieve after 1945 had been affected by colonial wars, party-political instability, and the weakness of the franc. Yet even at the time of the Indochinese and Algerian campaigns the French economy was growing fast. For the first time in many decades, its population was increasing, and thus fueling domestic demand. France was a rich, varied, but half-developed land, its economy stagnant since the early 1930s. Merely with the coming of peace, the infusion of American aid, the nationalization of utilities, and the stimulus of a larger market, growth was likely. Furthermore, France (like Italy) had a relatively low per capita level of industrialization, because of its small-town, agriculture-heavy economy, which meant that the increases in that regard were quite spectacular: from 95 in 1953, to 167 in 1963, to 259 in 1973 (relative to U.K. in 1900 = 100).[235] The annual rate of growth reached an average of 4.6 percent in the 1950s, and spurted to 5.8 percent in the 1960s, under the impetus of Common Market membership. The particular arrangements of the latter not only protected French agriculture from world-market prices, but gave it a large market within Europe. The general boom in the West aided the export of France's traditional high-added-value wares (clothes, shoes, wines, jewelry), which were now joined by aircraft and automobiles. Between 1949 and 1969, automobile production rose tenfold, aluminum sixfold, tractors and cement fourfold, iron and steel two and a half times.[236] The country had always been relatively rich, if underindustrialized; by the 1970s, it was a lot richer, and looked altogether more modern.

Nevertheless, France's growth was never as broadly based industrially as that of its neighbor across the Rhine, and President Pompidou's hopes that his country would soon overtake West Germany had little prospect of realization. With certain notable exceptions in the electrical, automobile, and aerospace industries, most French firms were still small and undercapitalized, and the prices of their products were too high compared with Germany's. Despite the "rationalization" of agriculture, many smallholdings remained—and were, in fact, sustained by the Common Market subvention policies; yet the pressures upon rural France, together with the social strain of industrial modernization (closing old steelworks, etc.) provoked outbursts of working-class discontent, of which the most famous were the 1968 riots. Poor in indigenous fuel supplies, France became heavily dependent upon imported oil, and (despite its ambitious nuclear-energy program) its balance of payments heavily fluctuated according to the world price of oil. Its trade deficit with West Germany steadily increased, and necessitated regular (if embarrassed) devaluations against the deutsche mark—which was probably a more reliable measure of France's economic standing than the wild fluctuations in the dollar-franc exchange rate. Even in periods of sustained economic growth, then, there was a certain precariousness to the French economy—which, in the event of shock, sent many prudent bourgeois across the Swiss frontier, bearing the family savings.

Yet France always had an impact upon affairs far larger than might be expected from a country with a mere 4 percent of the world GNP— and this was true not merely of the period of de Gaulle's presidency. It may have been due to sheer national-cultural assertiveness,[237] and that coinciding with a time when Anglo-American influences were waning, Russia was appearing more and more unattractive, and Germany was deferential. If western Europe *was* to have a leader and spokesman, France was a more obvious candidate than the isolationist British or the subdued Germans. Furthermore, successive French administrations quickly recognized that their country's modest real power could be buttressed by persuading the Common Market to adopt a particular line—on agricultural tariffs, high technology, overseas aid, cooperation at the United Nations, policy toward the Arab-Israeli conflict, and so on—which effectively harnessed what had become the world's largest trading bloc to positions favored by Paris. None of this restrained France from quite unilateral actions when the occasion seemed to merit it.

The fact that all four of these larger European states grew in wealth and output during these decades, together with their smaller neighbors, was not a guarantee of everlasting happiness. The early hopes toward ever-closer political and constitutional integration foundered upon the still-strong nationalism of its members, shown first of all by de Gaulle's France, and then by those states (Britain, Denmark, Greece) which had only later, and more warily, joined the EEC. Economic disputes, especially over the high cost of the farm-support policy, often paralyzed affairs in Brussels and Strasbourg. With neutral Eire a member, it was not possible to effect a common defense policy, which had to be left to NATO (from whose command structure the French had now absented themselves). The shock of the oil price rises in the 1970s seemed to hit Europe especially badly, and to take the steam out of the earlier optimism; despite widespread alarm, and considerable planning in Brussels, it seemed difficult to evolve high-technology policies to counter the Japanese and American challenges. Yet, notwithstanding these many difficulties, the sheer economic size of the EEC meant that the international landscape was now significantly different from that of 1945 or 1948. The EEC was by far the largest importer and exporter of the world's goods (although much of that was intra-European trade), and it contained, by 1983, by far the largest international currency and gold reserves; it manufactured more automobiles (34 percent) than either Japan (24 percent) or the United States (23 percent) and more cement than anyone else, and its crude-steel production was second only to that of the USSR.[238] With a total population in 1983 significantly larger than the United States' and almost exactly the same as Russia's—each having 272 million—the ten-member EEC had a substantially bigger GNP and share of world manufacturing production than the Soviet state, or the entire Comecon bloc. If politically and militarily the European Community was still immature, it was now a much more powerful presence in the global economic balances than in 1956.

Almost exactly the opposite could be said about the USSR, as it evolved from the 1950s to the 1980s. As has been described above (pp. 385–91), these were decades when the Soviet Union not only maintained a strong army, but also achieved nuclear-strategic parity with the United States, developed an oceangoing navy, and extended its influence in various parts of the world. Yet this persistent drive to achieve equality with the Americans on the global scene was not matched by parallel achievements at the economic level. Ironically (given Marx's stress upon the importance of the productive substructure in determining events), the country which claimed to be the world's original Communist state appeared to be suffering from increasing economic difficulties as time went on.

This is not to gainsay the quite impressive economic progress which was made in the USSR—and throughout the Soviet-dominated bloc—since Stalin's final years. In many respects, the region was even more transformed than western Europe during those few decades, although that may have been chiefly due to the fact that it was so much poorer and "underdeveloped" to begin with. At any event, measured in crude statistical terms, the gains were imposing. Russia's steel output, a mere 12.3 million tons in 1945, soared to 65.3 million tons in 1960, and to 148 million tons in 1980 (making the USSR the world's largest producer); electricity output rose from 43.2 million kilowatt-hours, to 292 million, to 1.294 billion, during the same periods; automobile production jumped from 74,000 units, to 524,000, to 2.2 million units; and this list of increases in products could be added to almost indefinitely.[239] Overall industrial output, averaging over 10 percent growth a year during the 1950s, increased from a notional 100 in 1953 to 421 in 1964,[240] which was a remarkable achievement—as were such obvious manifestations of Russian prowess as the Sputnik, space exploration, and military hardware. By the time of Khrushchev's political demise, the country had a far more prosperous, broader-based economy than under Stalin, and that absolute gain has steadily increased.

There were, however, two serious defects which began to overshadow these achievements. The first was the steady, long-term *decline* in the rate of growth, with industrial output each year since 1959 dropping from double-digit increases to a lower and lower figure, so that by the late 1970s it was down to 3–4 percent a year and still falling. In retrospect, this was a fairly natural development, since it has now become clear that the early, impressive annual increases were chiefly due to vast infusions of labor and capital. As the existing labor supply began to be fully utilized (and to compete with the requirements of the armed forces, and agriculture), the pace of growth could not help but fall back. As for capital investment, it was heavily directed into large-scale industry and defense-related production, which again emphasized quantitative rather than qualitative growth, and left many other sectors of the economy undercapitalized. Although the standard of living of the average Russian was improved by Khrushchev and his successors, nonetheless consumer demand could not (as in the West) stimulate growth in an economy in which personal consumption was being deliberately kept low in order to preserve national resources for heavy industry and the military. Above all, perhaps, there remained the chronic structural and climatic weaknesses affecting Soviet agriculture, the net output of which grew 4.8 percent a year in the 1950s but only 3 percent in the 1960s and 1.8 percent in the 1970s—despite all the attention and capital lavished upon it by anguished Soviet planners and their ministers.[241] Bearing in mind the size of the agricultural sector in the USSR, and the fact that its population rose by 84 million in the three decades after 1950, the overall increases in national product per capita were significantly less than the rates of *industrial* output, which were in themselves a somewhat "forced" achievement.

The second serious defect was, predictably enough, in terms of the Soviet Union's *relative* economic standing. During the 1950s and early 1960s, with its share both of world manufacturing output and of world trade increasing, Khrushchev's claim that the Marxist mode of production was superior and would one day "bury capitalism" seemed to have some plausibility to it. Since that time, however, the trend has become more worrying to the Kremlin. The European Community, led by its industrial half-giant West Germany, has become much wealthier and more productive than the USSR. The small island state of Japan grew so fast that its overtaking of Russia's total GNP became merely a matter of time. The United States, despite its own relative industrial decline, kept ahead in total output and wealth. The standard of living of the average Russian, and of his eastern-European confreres, did not close the gap with that in western Europe, toward which the peoples of the

Marxist economies looked with some envy. The newer technology, of computers, robotics, telecommunications, revealed the USSR and its satellites as poorly positioned to compete. And agriculture remained as weak as ever, in productive terms: in 1980, the American farm worker was producing enough food to supply sixty-five people, whereas his Russian equivalent turned out enough to feed only eight.[242] This, in turn, led to the embarrassing Soviet need to import increasing amounts of foodstuffs.

Many of Russia's own economic difficulties have been mirrored by those of its satellites, which also achieved high growth rates in the 1950s and early 1960s—though again from levels which were low compared with those of the West, and by following priorities which similarly emphasized centralized planning, heavy industry, and collectivization of agriculture.[243] While significant differences in prosperity and growth occurred among the eastern European states (and still do occur), the overall tendency was one of early expansion and then slowdown—leaving Marxist planners with a choice of difficult options. In Russia's case, additional farmland could be brought under cultivation, though the limits imposed by the winter ecology in the north and the deserts in the south restricted possibilities in that direction (and easily reminded many of how Khrushchev's confident exploitation of the "virgin lands" soon turned them into dustbowls);[244] similarly, more intensive exploitation of raw materials ran the danger of increasing inefficiencies in dealing with, say, oil stocks,[245] while extractive costs rose swiftly as soon as mining was extended into the permafrost region. More capital might be poured into industry and technology, but only at the cost of diverting resources either from defense—which has remained the number-one priority of the USSR, despite all the changes of leadership—or from consumer goods— slighting of which was seen to be highly unpopular (especially in eastern Europe) at a time when improved communications were making the West's relative prosperity even more obvious. Finally, Russia and its fellow Communist regimes could contemplate a series of reforms, not merely of the regular rooting-out-corruption and shaking-up-the-bureaucracy sort, but of the *system* itself, providing personal incentives, introducing a more realistic price mechanism, allowing increases in private farming, encouraging open discussion and entrepreneurship in dealing with the newer technologies, etc.; in other words, going for "creeping capitalism," such as the Hungarians were adroitly practicing in the 1970s. The difficulty of that strategy, as the Czech experiences of 1968 showed, was that "liberalization" measures threw into question the *dirigiste* Communist regime itself—and were therefore frowned upon by party ideologues and the military throughout the cautious Brezhnev era.[246] Reversing relative economic decline therefore had to be done carefully, which in turn made a striking success unlikely.

Perhaps the only consolation to decision-makers in the Kremlin was that their archrival, the United States, also appeared to be encountering economic difficulties from the 1960s onward and that it was swiftly losing the *relative* share of the world's wealth, production, and trade which it had possessed in 1945. Yet mention of that year is, of course, the most important fact in understanding the American relative decline. As argued above, the United States' favorable economic position at that point in history was both unprecedented and artificial. It was on top of the world partly because of its own productive spurt, but also because of the temporary weakness of other nations. That situation would alter, against the United States, with Europe's and Japan's recovery of prewar level of output; and it would alter still further with the general expansion of world manufacturing production (which rose more than threefold between 1953 and 1973), since it was inconceivable that the United States could maintain its one-half share of 1945 when new factories and industrial plant were being created all over the globe. By 1953, Bairoch calculates, the American percentage had fallen to 44.7 percent; by 1980 to 31.5 percent; and it was still falling.[247] For much the same reason, the CIA's economic indicators showed the United States' share of world GNP dropping from 25.9 percent in 1960 to 21.5 percent in 1980 (although the dollar's short-lived rise in the currency markets would see that share increase over the next few years).[248] The point was not that Americans were producing significantly less (except in industries generally declining in the western world), but that others were producing much more. Automobile production is perhaps the easiest way of illustrating the two trends which make up this story: in 1960, the United States manufactured 6.65 million automobiles, which was a massive 52 percent of the world output of 12.8 million such vehicles; by 1980, it was producing a mere 23 percent of the world output, but since the latter totaled 30 million units, the absolute American production had increased to 6.9 million units.

Yet despite that half-consoling thought—similar to the argument which the British used to half-console themselves seventy years earlier when their shares of world output began to be eroded—there was a worrying aspect to this development. The real question was not "Did the United States have to decline relatively?" but "Did it have to decline *so fast*?" For the fact was that even in the heyday of the Pax Americana, its competitive position was already being eroded by a disturbingly low average annual rate of growth of output per capita, especially as compared with previous decades (see Table 42).

Once again, it may be possible to argue that this was a historically "natural" development. As Michael Balfour remarks, for decades be-

**Table 42. Average Annual Rate of
Growth of Output per Capita,
1948–1962[249]**

	(1913–50)	1948–62
United States	(1.7)	1.6
U.K.	(1.3)	2.4
Belgium	(0.7)	2.2
France	(0.7)	3.4
Germany/FRG	(0.4)	6.8
Italy	(0.6)	5.6

fore 1950 the United States had increased its output faster than anyone else because it had been a major innovator in methods of standardization and mass production. As a result, it had "gone further than any other country to satisfy human needs and [was] already operating at a high level of efficiency (measured in terms of output per man per hour) so that the known possibilities for increasing output by better methods or better machinery were, in comparison with the rest of the world, smaller."[250] Yet while that was surely true, the United States was not helped by certain other secular trends which were occurring in its economy: fiscal and taxation policies encouraged high consumption, but a low personal savings rate; investment in R&D, except for military purposes, was slowly sinking compared with other countries; and defense expenditures themselves, as a proportion of national product, were larger than anywhere else in the western bloc of nations. In addition, an increasing proportion of the American population was moving from industry to services, that is, into low-productivity fields.[251]

Much of this was hidden during the 1950s and 1960s by the glamour developments of American high technology (especially in the air), by the high prosperity which triggered off consumer demand for flashy cars and color televisions, and by the evident flow of dollars from the United States to poorer parts of the world, as foreign aid, or as military spending, or as investment by banks and companies. It is instructive in this regard to recall the widespread alarm in the mid-1960s at what Servan-Schreiber called *le défi Americain*—the vast outward surge of U.S. investments into Europe (and, by extension, elsewhere), allegedly turning those countries into economic satellites; the awe, or hatred, with which giant multinationals like Exxon and General Motors were regarded; and, associated with these trends, the respect accorded to the sophisticated management techniques imbued by American business schools.[252] From a certain economic perspective, indeed, this transfer of U.S. investment and production was an indicator of economic strength and modernity; it took advantage of lower labor costs and ensured greater access in overseas markets. Over time, however, these capital flows eventually became so strong that they began to outweigh the surpluses which Americans earned on exports of manufactures, foodstuffs, and "invisible" services. Although this increasing payments deficit did see some gold draining out of the United States by the late 1950s, most foreign governments were content to hold more dollars (that being the leading reserve currency) rather than demand payment in gold.

As the 1960s unfolded, however, this cozy situation evaporated. Both Kennedy and (even more) Johnson were willing to increase American military expenditures overseas, and not just in Vietnam, although that conflict turned the flow of dollars exported into a flood. Both Kennedy and (even more) Johnson were committed to increases in domestic expenditures, a trend already detectable prior to 1960. Neither administration liked the political costs of raising taxes to pay for the inevitable inflation. The result was year after year of federal government deficits, soaring price rises, and increasing American industrial uncompetitiveness—in turn leading to larger balance-of-payments deficits, the choking back (by the Johnson administration) of foreign investments by U.S. firms, and then the latter's turn toward the new instrument of Eurodollars. In the same period, the U.S. share of world (non-Comecon) gold reserves shrank remorselessly, from 68 percent (1950) to a mere 27 percent (1973). With the entire international payments and money-flow system buckling under these interacting problems, and being further weakened by de Gaulle's angry counterattacks against what he regarded as America's "export of inflation," the Nixon administration found it had little choice but to end the dollar's link to gold in private markets, and then to float the dollar against other currencies. The Bretton Woods system, very much a creation of the days when the United States was financially supreme, collapsed when its leading pillar could bear the strains no more.[253]

The detailed story of the ups and downs of the dollar in the 1970s, when it was floating freely, are not for telling here; nor is the zigzag course of successive administrations' efforts to check inflation and to stimulate growth, always without causing too much pain politically. The higher-than-average inflation in the United States generally caused the dollar to weaken vis-à-vis the German and Japanese currencies in the 1970s; oil shocks, which hurt countries more dependent upon OPEC supplies (e.g., Japan, France), political turbulence in various parts of the world, and high American interest rates tended to push the dollar upward, as was the case by the early 1980s. Yet although these oscillations were important, and tended to add to global economic insecurities, they may be less significant for our purposes than the unrelenting longer-term trends, which were the decreasing productivity growth, which in the private sector fell from 2.4 percent (1965–1972), to 1.6 percent (1972–1977), to 0.2 percent (1977–1982);[254] the increasing federal deficits, which could be seen as giving a Keynesian-type "boost" to the economy, but at the cost of sucking in so much cash from abroad (attracted by the higher American interest rates) that it sent the dollar's price to artificially high levels and turned the country from a net lender to a net borrower; and the increasing difficulty American manufacturers found in competing with imported automobiles, electrical goods, kitchenware, and other manufactures. Not surprisingly, American per capita GNP, once the highest in the world, began to slip down the list.[255]

There were still consolations, to those who could see the American economy and its needs in larger terms than selected comparisons with Swiss incomes or Japanese productivity. As Calleo points out, post-1945 American policy did achieve some very basic and significant aims: domestic prosperity, as opposed to a 1930s-type slump; the containing of Soviet expansionism without war; the revival of the economies—and the democratic traditions—of western Europe, later joined by Japan to create "an increasingly integrated economic bloc," with "an imposing battery of multilateral institutions . . . to manage common economic as well as military affairs"; and, finally, "the transformation of the old colonial empires into independent states still closely integrated into a world economy."[256] In sum, it had maintained the liberal international order, upon which it, itself, increasingly depended; and while its share of world production and wealth had shrunk, perhaps faster than need have been the case, the redistribution of global economic balances still left an environment which was not too hostile to its own open-market and capitalist traditions. Finally, if it had seen its productive lead eroded by certain faster-growing economies, it had still maintained a very considerable superiority over the Soviet Union in almost all respects of true national power and—by clinging to its own entrepreneurial creed—remained open to the stimulus of managerial initiative and technological charge which its Marxist rival would have far greater difficulty in accepting.

A more detailed discussion of the implication of these economic movements must await the final chapter. It may, however, be useful to give in statistical form (see Table 43) the essence of the trends examined above, as they concern the global economic balances, namely the partial recovery of the share of world product in the hands of the less-developed countries; the remarkable growth of Japan and, to a lesser extent, of the People's Republic of China; the erosion of the European Economic Community's share even as it remained the largest economic bloc in the world; the stabilization, and then slow decline, of the USSR's share; and the much faster decline, but still far larger economic muscle, of the United States.

Indeed, by 1980, the final year in Table 43, the World Bank's figures of population, GNP per capita, and GNP itself, were very much point-

Table 43. Shares of Gross World Product, 1960–1980[257]
(percent)

	1960	1970	1980
Less-developed countries	11.1	12.3	14.8
Japan	4.5	7.7	9.0
China	3.1	3.4	4.5
European Economic Community	26.0	24.7	22.5
United States	25.9	23.0	21.5
Other developed countries	10.1	10.3	9.7
USSR	12.5	12.4	11.4
Other Communist countries	6.8	6.2	6.1

ing to a *multipolar* distribution of the global economic balances, as shown in Table 44.

Table 44. Population, GNP per Capita, and GNP in 1980[258]

	Population (millions)	GNP per Capita (dollars)	GNP (billions of dollars)
United States	228	11,360	2,590
USSR	265	4,550	1,205
Japan	117	9,890	1,157
EEC (12 states) of which	317	—	2,907
W. Germany	61	13,590	828
France	54	11,730	633
U.K.	56	7,920	443
Italy	57	6,480	369
West and East Germany together	78	—	950
China[259]	980	290 or 450	284 or 441

Finally, it might be useful to recall that these long-term shifts in the productive balances are of importance not so much for their own sake, but for their power-political implications. As Lenin himself noted in 1917–1918, it was the *uneven* economic growth rates of countries which led ineluctably to the rise of specific powers and the decline of others:

Half a century ago, Germany was a miserable, insignificant country, as far as its capitalist strength was concerned, compared with the strength of England at that time. Japan was similarly insignificant compared with Russia. Is it "conceivable" that in ten or twenty years' time the relative strength of the imperialist powers will have remained *un*changed? Absolutely inconceivable.[260]

And for all Lenin's own concentration upon the capitalist/imperialist states, the rule seems common to *all* national units, whatever their favored political economy, that uneven rates of economic growth would, sooner or later, lead to shifts in the world's political and military balances. This, certainly, has been the pattern observed in the four centuries of Great Power development prior to the present one. It therefore follows that the unusually rapid shifts in the centers of world production during the past two or three decades cannot avoid having repercussions upon the grand-strategical future of today's leading Powers, and rightly deserve the attention of one final chapter.

8
To the
Twenty-first Century

History and Speculation

A chapter with a title such as that above implies not merely a change in chronology but also, and much more significantly, a change in *methodology*. Even the very recent past is history, and although problems of bias and source make the historian of the previous decade "hard put to separate the ephemeral from the fundamental,"[1] he is still operating within the same academic discipline. But writings upon how the present may evolve into the future, even if they discuss trends which are already under way, can lay no claim to being historical truth. Not only do the raw materials change, from archivally based monographs to economic *forecasts* and political *projections*, but the validity of what is being written about can no longer be assumed. Even if there always were many methodological difficulties in dealing with "historical facts,"[2] past events like an archduke's assassination or a military defeat *did indeed occur*. Nothing one can say about the future has that certainty. Unforeseen happenings, sheer accidents, the halting of a trend, can ruin the most plausible of forecasts; if they do not, then the forecaster is merely lucky.

What follows, then, can only be provisional and conjectural, based upon a reasoned surmise of how present tendencies in global economics and strategy may work out—but with no guarantee that all (or any) of this will happen. The gyrations which have occurred in the international value of the dollar over the past few years and the post-1984 collapse in oil prices (with its differing implications, for Russia, for Japan, for OPEC) offer a good warning against drawing conclusions from economically based trends; and the world of politics and diplomacy has never been one which followed straight lines. Many a final chapter in works dealing with contemporary affairs has to be changed, only a few years later, in the wisdom of hindsight; it will be surprising if this present chapter survives unscathed.

Perhaps the best way to comprehend what lies ahead is to look *backward* briefly, at the rise and fall of the Great Powers over the past five centuries. The argument in this book has been that there exists a dynamic for change, driven chiefly by economic and technological developments, which then impact upon social structures, political systems, military power, and the position of individual states and empires. The speed of this global economic change has not been a uniform one, simply because the pace of technological innovation and economic growth is itself irregular, conditioned by the circumstance of the individual inventor and entrepreneur as well as by climate, disease, wars, geography, the social framework, and so on. In the same way, different regions and societies across the globe have experienced a faster *or* slower rate of growth, depending not only upon the shifting patterns of technology, production, and trade, but also upon their receptivity to the new modes of increasing output and wealth. As some areas of the world have risen, others have fallen behind—relatively or (sometimes) absolutely. None of this is surprising. Because of man's innate drive to improve his condition, the world has never stood still. And the intellectual breakthroughs from the time of the Renaissance onward, boosted by the coming of the "exact sciences" during the Enlightenment and Industrial Revolution, simply meant that the dynamics of change would be increasingly more powerful and self-sustaining than before.

The second major argument of this book has been that this uneven pace of economic growth has had crucial long-term impacts upon the relative military power and strategical position of the members of the states system. This again is unsurprising, and has been said many times before, although the emphasis and presentation of argument may have been different.[3] The world did not need to wait until Engels's time to learn that "nothing is more dependent on economic conditions than precisely the army and the navy."[4] It was as clear to a Renaissance prince as it is to the Pentagon today that military power rests upon adequate supplies of wealth, which in turn derive from a flourishing productive base, from healthy finances, and from superior technology. As the above narrative has shown, economic prosperity does not *always and immediately* translate into military effectiveness, for that depends upon many other factors, from geography and national morale to generalship and tactical competence. Nevertheless, the fact remains that all of the major shifts in the world's *military-power* balances have followed alterations in the *productive* balances; and further, that the rising and falling of the various empires and states in the international system has been confirmed by the outcomes of the major Great Power wars, where victory has always gone to the side with the greatest material resources.

While what follows is speculation rather than history, therefore, it is based upon the plausible assumption that these broad trends of the past five centuries are likely to continue. The international system, whether it is dominated for a time by six Great Powers or only two, remains anarchical—that is, there is no greater authority than the sovereign, egoistical nation-state.[5] In each particular period of time some of those states are growing or shrinking in their *relative* share of secular power. The world is no more likely to remain frozen in 1987 or 2000 than it was in 1870 or 1660. On the contrary, certain economists would argue that the very *structures* of international production and trade are changing faster than ever before: with agricultural and raw-materials products losing their relative value, with industrial "production" becoming uncoupled from industrial "employment," with knowledge-intensive goods becoming dominant in all advanced societies, and with world capital flows becoming increasingly detached from trade patterns.[6] All this, and the many new developments in science, are bound to influence international affairs. In sum, without the intervention of an act of God, or a disastrous nuclear conflagration, there will continue to be a dynamic of world power, essentially driven by technological and economic change. If the rosy forecasts of the impact of computers, robotics, biotechnology, and so on are correct—and if, in addition, forecasts of the success of a "green revolution" in parts of the Third World (with India and even China becoming regular net exporters of grain)[7] do turn out right—then the world *as a whole* could be a lot richer by the early twenty-first century. Even if technological progress is less dramatic, economic growth is likely to occur. Changing demographic patterns, with their impact upon demand, would ensure that, as would the more sophisticated exploitation of raw materials.

What is also clear is that this growth will be uneven—faster here, slower there, depending upon the conditions for change. It is this, more than anything else, which makes the prognoses that follow so provisional; for there is no guarantee that, for example, Japan's impressive economic expansion over the past four decades will continue during the next two; nor is it impossible for Russian growth rates, which have been declining since the 1960s, to increase again in the 1990s, given changes in that country's economic policy and mechanisms. On the evidence of existing trends, however, neither of those outcomes appears very likely. To put it another way, if it did happen that Japan stagnated and Russia boomed economically between now and the early twenty-first century, then that could only come about from changes in circumstances and policies far more drastic than it is reasonable to assume from the available evidence. Just because estimates of how the world will appear in fifteen or twenty-five years' time may go wrong does not mean that one should prefer implausible outcomes rather than sensible expectations based upon current broad developments.

It is reasonable to expect, for example, that one of the better-known "global trends" of today, the rise of the Pacific region, is likely to continue, simply because that development is so broad-based. It includes not only the economic powerhouse of Japan, but also that swiftly changing giant the People's Republic of China; not only the prosperous and established industrial states of Australia and New Zealand, but also the immensely successful Asian newly industrializing countries like Taiwan, South Korea, Hong Kong, and Singapore—as well as the larger Association of Southeast Asian Nations (ASEAN) lands of Malaysia, Indonesia, Thailand, and the Philippines; by extension, it also includes the Pacific states of the United States and provinces of Canada.[8] Economic growth in this vast area has been stimulated by a happy combination of factors: a spectacular rise in industrial productivity by export-oriented societies, in turn leading to great increases in foreign trade, shipping, and financial services; a marked move into the newer technologies as well as into cheaper, labor-intensive manufactures; and an immensely successful effort to increase agricultural output (especially grains and livestock) faster than total population growth. Each success has beneficially interacted with the others, to produce a rate of economic expansion which has far eclipsed that of the traditional western powers—as well as that of Comecon—in recent years.

In 1960, for example, the combined gross domestic product of the Asian-Pacific countries (i.e., excluding the United States) was a mere 7.8 percent of world GDP; by 1982, it had more than doubled, to 16.4 percent, and since then the area's growth rates have exceeded those of Europe, the United States, and the USSR by ever wider margins. It is very likely to contain over 20 percent of world GDP by the year 2000— the equal of Europe, or the United States; and that achievement will occur even on the basis of growth-rate differentials "much smaller" than those which have existed over the past quarter-century.[9] The dynamism of the Pacific basin has also been felt in the shifting economic balances within the United States itself during that same period. American trade with Asia and the Pacific was only 48 percent of that with Europe (OECD members) in 1960, but had risen to 122 percent of American-European trade by 1983—a change which has been accompanied by a redistribution of both population and income within the United States in the direction of the Pacific.[10] Despite a slowdown in, say, any *one* country's growth, or problems affecting a particular industry, it is evident that these trends are continuing as a whole. It is not surprising, therefore, that one economic expert has confidently predicted that the entire Pacific region, which now possesses 43 percent of the world's GNP, will enjoy a good 50 percent of it by the year 2000; and concludes, "The center of world economic gravity is shifting rapidly towards Asia and the Pacific, as the Pacific takes its place as one of the key centers of world economic power."[11] This sort of language has of course been heard frequently since the nineteenth century; but only with the massive growth of the region's commerce and productivity since 1960 has that forecast become a reality.

Similarly, it is also reasonable to assume that the next few decades will witness a continuation of a much less attractive but even broader trend: the spiraling cost of the arms race, which is fueled by the sheer expensiveness of newer weapon systems as well as by international rivalries. "One of the few constancies in history," it has been observed, "is that the scale of commitment on military spending has always risen."[12] And if that was true (granted some short-term fluctuations) for the wars and arms races of the eighteenth century, when weapons technology changed only slowly, it is much truer of the present century, when each new generation of aircraft, warships, and tanks is vastly more expensive than preceding ones, even when allowance is made for inflation. Edwardian statesmen, appalled that a pre-1914 battleship cost £2.5 million, would be staggered to learn that it now costs the British Admiralty £120 million and more for a replacement *frigate*! American legislators, who had willingly allocated funds for thousands of B-17 bombers in the late 1930s, now understandably wince at the Pentagon's estimate that the new B-1 bomber will cost over $200 billion for a mere one hundred planes. In all areas, the upward spiral is at work:

> Bombers cost two hundred times as much as they did in World War II. Fighters cost one hundred times or more than they did in World War II. Aircraft carriers are twenty times as expensive and battle tanks are fifteen times as expensive as in World War II. A Gato class submarine cost $5,500 per ton in World War II, compared with $1.6 million per ton for the Trident.[13]

Compounding these problems is the evidence that today's armaments industry is becoming increasingly divergent from commercial, free-market manufacturing. The former, usually concentrated in a few gigantic firms enjoying a special relationship with their own department of defense (whether in the United States, Britain, or France, or even more in the "command economy" of the USSR), is frequently protected from marketplace operations by the state's granting of exclusive contracts and cost-overrun guarantees, for products for which only it (and friendly states) will be the consumer. The latter, even in the case of giant companies like IBM and General Motors, has to struggle against cutthroat competition to win merely a *share* of the volatile internal and external markets in which quality, consumer taste, and price are vital variables. The former, driven by military men's desire to have the most advanced "state-of-the-art" weaponry so that their armed services may be able to fight in all possible (if sometimes highly implausible) battle scenarios, produces goods which are increasingly more expensive, more elaborate, and *much less numerous*. The latter, after initial heavy investment in the early prototypes of household goods or office computers, has its average unit costs pushed *downward*, because of market competition and large-scale production.[14] And while it may be true that the explosion in new technological and scientific developments since the late nineteenth century inevitably drove defense manufacturers into a relationship with governments which deviated from "free market" norms,[15] the present pace of this increase is an alarming one. The various proposals about "military reform" in the United States could perhaps prevent the result forecast by the cynics, that the entire Pentagon budget may be swallowed up on *one* aircraft by the year 2020; but even those efforts are unlikely to *reverse* the trend toward ever fewer weapons at ever higher cost.

While much of this is of course due to the growing and inescapable sophistication of weapons—like modern fighter aircraft, which may contain 100,000 separate parts—it is also caused by the continuing array of arms races on land, on and under the oceans, in the air, and in space. If the greatest of those rivalries is between NATO and the Warsaw Pact countries (which, thanks to the two superpowers, spend almost 80 percent of the world's investment in armaments, and possess 60–70 percent of its aircraft and ships), there are smaller yet still significant arms races—not to mention wars—in the Middle East, Africa, Latin America, and across Asia, from Iran to Korea. The consequence has been an explosion in Third World military expenditures, even by the poorest regimes, and large-scale increases in arms sales and transfers to those countries; by 1984, world arms imports of a colossal $35 billion had exceeded the world trade in grain ($33 billion). In the following year, it is also worth noting, world military expenditures had reached a total of about $940 billion, rather more than the entire income of the poorer half of this planet's population. What was more, that expenditure on weapons was rising faster than the global economy and most national economies were expanding. At the head were the United States and the USSR, each devoting well over $250 billion annually to defense and likely to push that total to over $300 billion in the near future. In most countries, spending on the armed forces was taking an increasing share of governmental budgets and of GNP, checked only (with very few exceptions of motive, as in Japan and Luxembourg) by economic weaknesses, shortage of hard currency, etc., rather than by a genuine commitment to reduce arms expenditures.[16] The "militarization of the world economy," as the Worldwatch Institute terms it, is now advancing faster than it has for a generation.[17]

These two trends—the uneven pattern of growth, with the global productive balances tilting toward the Pacific basin; and the spiraling costs of weapons and armed forces—are of course separate developments. Yet at the same time it is obvious that they are increasingly likely to interact and indeed are doing so already. Both of them are driven by the dynamic of technological and industrial change (even if individual arms races will have political and ideological motives as well). Both of them impinge heavily upon the national economy: the first by boosting wealth and productivity at a faster or slower pace, and by making certain societies more prosperous than others; the second by consuming national resources—measured not simply in terms of investment capital and raw materials, but also (and perhaps even more importantly) in the share of scientists, engineers, R&D personnel, engaged in defense-related production as opposed to commercial, export-oriented growth. Although it has been claimed that defense expenditures can have certain commercial economic spin-offs, it seems increasingly difficult to argue against the proposition that *excessive* arms spending will hurt economic growth.[18] The difficulties experienced by contemporary societies which are militarily top-heavy merely repeat those which, in their time, affected Philip II's Spain, Nicholas II's Russia, and Hitler's Germany. A large military establishment may, like a great monument, look imposing to the impressionable observer; but if it is not resting upon a firm foundation (in this case, a productive national economy), it runs the risk of a future collapse.

By extension, therefore, both of these trends have profound socioeconomic and political implications. Slow growth occurring in a particular country is likely to depress public morale, produce discontents, and exacerbate the discussion over national spending priorities; on the other hand, a fast pace of technological and industrial expansion will also have its consequences, especially upon a hitherto nonindustrialized society. Large-scale armaments spending, for its part, can benefit specific industries within the national economy; but it can also lead to a diversion of resources from other groups in society, and it can make that national economy less capable of handling the commercial challenges of other countries. Unless there is an enemy immediately at the gate, high defense spending in this century has nearly always provoked a "guns versus butter" controversy. Less publicly, but of even greater significance for our purposes, it has provoked a debate upon the proper relationship of economic strength to military power.[19]

Not for the first time in history, therefore, there looms today a tension between a nation's existence in an anarchic military-political world and its existence in a laissez-faire economic world; between on the one hand its search for strategic security, as represented by its investment in the latest weapon systems and in its large-scale diversion of national resources to the armed forces, and on the other hand its search for economic security, as represented by an enhanced national prosperity, which depends upon growth (which in turn flows from new methods of production and wealth creation), upon increased output, and upon flourishing internal and external demand—all of which may be damaged by excessive spending upon armaments. Precisely because a top-heavy military establishment may slow down the rate of economic growth and lead to a decline in the nation's share of world manufacturing output, and therefore wealth, and therefore *power*, the whole issue becomes one of the balancing the short-term security afforded by large defense forces against the longer-term security of rising production and income.

The tension between these conflicting aims is perhaps particularly acute in the late twentieth century because of the publicity given to the existence of various alternative "models" for emulation. On the one hand, there are the extremely successful "trading states"—chiefly in Asia, like Japan and Hong Kong, but also including Switzerland, Sweden, and Austria—which have taken advantage of the great growth in world production and in commercial interdependence since 1945, and whose external policy emphasizes peaceful, trading relations with other societies. In consequence, they have all sought to keep defense spending as low as is compatible with the preservation of national sovereignty, thereby freeing resources for high domestic consumption and capital investment. On the other hand, there are the various "militarized" economies—Vietnam in Southeast Asia, Iran and Iraq as they engage in their lengthy war, Israel and its jealous neighbors in the Near East, and the USSR itself—all of which allocate more (in some cases, much more) than 10 percent of their GNP to defense expenditures each year and, while firmly believing that such levels of spending are necessary to guarantee military security, manifestly suffer from that diversion of resources from productive, peaceful ends. Between the two poles of the merchant and the warrior states, so to speak, there lie most of the rest of the nations of this planet, not convinced that the world is a safe enough place to allow them to reduce arms expenditure to Japan's unusually low level, but also generally uneasy at the high economic and social costs of large-scale spending upon armaments, and aware that there is a certain trade-off between short-term military security and long-term economic security. For countries which have—again, in contrast to Japan—extensive overseas military obligations from which it would be difficult to escape, the problem is further compounded. Moreover, in many of the leading Powers the planners are acutely aware that they have to balance the spiraling cost of weaponry not only against productive investment but also against growing social requirements (especially as their overall population ages), which makes the allocation of spending priorities a more difficult task than ever.

The feat demanded of most if not all governing bodies as the world heads toward the twenty-first century is therefore a *threefold* one: simultaneously to provide military security (or some viable alternative security) for its national interests, *and* to satisfy the socioeconomic needs of its citizenry, *and* to ensure sustained growth, this last being essential both for the positive purposes of affording the required guns and butter at the present, and for the negative purpose of avoiding a relative economic decline which could hurt the people's military and economic security in the future. Achieving all three of those feats over a sustained period of time will be a very difficult task, given the uneven pace of technological and commercial change and the unpredictable fluctuations in international politics. Yet achieving the first two feats— or either one of them—without the third will inevitably lead to relative eclipse over the longer term, which has of course been the fate of all slower-growing societies that failed to adjust to the dynamics of world power. As one economist has soberly pointed out, "It is hard to imagine, but a country whose productivity growth lags 1 percent behind other countries over one century can turn, as England did, from the world's indisputed industrial leader into the mediocre economy it is today."[20]

Just how well (or badly) the leading nations seem placed to carry out this task is the focus of the rest of this chapter. It hardly needs emphasizing that since the varied demands of defense spending/military security, social/consumer needs, and investment for growth involve a triangular competition for resources, there is no absolutely perfect solution to this tension. Probably the best that can be achieved is that all three aims be kept in rough harmony, but just how that balance is reached will always be strongly influenced by national circumstances, not by some theoretical definition of equilibrium. A state surrounded by hostile neighbors will think it better to allocate more to military security than one whose citizens feel relatively unthreatened; a country rich in natural resources will find it easier to pay for guns and butter; a society determined upon economic growth in order to catch up to the others will have different priorities from one on the brink of war. Geography, politics, and culture will all ensure that one state's "solution" will never be exactly the same as another's. Nevertheless, the basic argument remains: without a rough balance between these competing demands of defense, consumption, and investment, a Great Power is unlikely to preserve its status for long.

China's Balancing Act

The competing claims of weapons modernization, the people's social requirements, and the need to channel all available resources into "productive" nonmilitary enterprises is nowhere more pressing than in the People's Republic of China (PRC), which is simultaneously the poorest of the major Powers and probably the least well placed strategically. Yet if the PRC suffers from certain chronic hardships, its present leadership seems to be evolving a grand strategy altogether more coherent and forward-looking than that which prevails in Moscow, Washington, or Tokyo, not to mention western Europe. And while the *material* constraints upon China are great, they are being ameliorated by an economic expansion which, *if it can be kept up,* promises to transform the country within a few decades.

The country's weaknesses are so well known as to require only a brief mention here. Diplomatically and strategically, Peking has regarded itself (with some justification) as being isolated and surrounded. If this was partly due to Mao's policies toward China's neighbors, it was also a consequence of the rivalry and ambitions of other powers in Asia during the preceding decades. The memories of Japan's earlier aggressions have not faded from the Chinese mind, and reinforce the caution with which the leadership in Peking regards that country's explosive growth in recent years. Despite the 1970s thaw in relations with Washington, the United States is also viewed with some suspicion—the more particularly under a Republican regime which seems overenthusiastic about constructing an anti-Russian bloc, which appears to nourish a lingering fondness for Taiwan, and which interferes too readily against Third World countries and revolutionary movements for Peking's liking. The future of Taiwan and the smaller offshore islands remains a thorny problem, and only half-submerged. The PRC's relations with India have stayed cool, being complicated by their respective ties to Pakistan and Russia. Notwithstanding recent "wooing" efforts by Moscow, China feels bound to see in the USSR its chief foreign danger—and not merely because of the masses of Russian divisions and aircraft deployed along the frontier, but also in consequence of the Russian invasion of Afghanistan and, more worryingly, in the military expansionism of the Soviet-supported Vietnamese state to the south. Somewhat like the Germans earlier in this century, therefore, the Chinese think deeply about "encirclement" even as they simultaneously strive to enhance their place in the global system of power.[21]

Moreover, this awkward, multilateral set of diplomatic tasks has to be managed by a country which is not very strong militarily or economically, when measured against its chief rivals. For all the size

of the Chinese Army in *numerical* terms, it remains woefully underequipped in modern instruments of warfare. Most of its tanks,
guns, aircraft, and warships are indigenous versions of Russian or
western models which China acquired years ago, and are certainly not
on a par with later, much more sophisticated types; a lack of hard
currency and an unwillingness to become too dependent upon other
nations have kept purchases of foreign arms to a minimum. Perhaps
even more worrying to Peking's leaders are the weaknesses in China's
combat effectiveness, due to the Maoist attacks upon professionalism
in the army and the preference for peasant militias—such utopian
solutions being of little assistance in the 1979 border war with Vietnam, whose battle-hardened and well-trained troops killed some
26,000 Chinese and wounded 37,000 others.[22] Economically, China
appears still further behind; even when amending its official per capita
GNP figures in a way which better accords with western concepts and
economic measurements,[23] the figure can hardly be more than a mere
$500, compared with well over $13,000 for many of the advanced
capitalist states and a respectable $5,000+ for the USSR. With its
population likely to rise from a billion people today to 1.2 or 1.3 billion
by the year 2000, the prospects of a major increase in personal income
may not be large; even in the next century the average Chinaman will
be poor, relative to the inhabitants of the established Powers. Furthermore, it hardly needs saying that the difficulties of governing such a
populous state, of reconciling the various factions (party, army,
bureaucrats, farmers), and of achieving growth without social and
ideological turbulence will test even the most flexible and intelligent
leadership. China's internal history for the past century does not offer
encouraging precedents for long-term strategies of development.

Nevertheless, the indications of reform and self-improvement in
China which have occurred over the past six to eight years are very
remarkable, and suggest that this period of Deng Xiaoping's leadership
may one day be seen in the way that historians view Colbert's France,
or the early stages of Frederick the Great's reign, or Japan in the
post–Meiji Restoration decades: that is, as a country straining to develop its power (in all senses of that word) by every pragmatic means,
balancing the desire to encourage enterprise and initiative and change
with an *étatiste* determination to direct events so that the national
goals are achieved as swiftly and smoothly as possible. Such a strategy
involves the ability to see how the separate aspects of government
policy relate to each other. It therefore involves a sophisticated balancing act, requiring careful judgments as to the speed at which these
transformations can safely occur, the amount of resources to be allocated to long-term as opposed to short-term needs, the coordination
of the state's internal and external requirements, and—last but not
least in a country which still has a "modified" Marxist system—the

ways by which ideology and practice can be reconciled. Although difficulties have occurred and new ones are likely to emerge in the future, the record so far is an impressive one.

It can be seen, for example, in the many ways in which the Chinese armed services are transforming themselves after the convulsions of the 1960s. The planned reduction of the People's Liberation Army (which includes the navy and air force) from 4.2 to 3 million personnel is, in fact, an enhancement of real strength, since far too many of them were merely support troops, used for railway-building and civic duties. Those remaining within the armed forces are likely to be of higher overall quality: new uniforms and the restoration of military ranks (abolished by Mao as being "bourgeois") are the outward sign of this; but they will be reinforced by replacing a largely volunteer army with conscription (to give the state access to high-quality personnel), by reorganizing the military regions and streamlining the staffs, and by improving officer training at the academies, which have also emerged from their period of Maoist disgrace.[24] Along with this will go a large-scale modernization of China's weaponry, which, although numerically substantial, suffers from considerable obsolescence. Its navy is being given an array of new vessels, from destroyers and escorts to fast-attack craft and even hovercraft; and it has built up a very substantial fleet of conventional submarines (107 in 1985), making it the third-largest such force in the world. Its tanks are now displaying laser rangefinders; its aircraft are becoming all-weather types, with modern radar. All this is attended by a willingness to experiment with large-scale maneuvers under modern battlefield conditions (one such 1981 maneuver involved six or seven Chinese armies backed by aircraft—which had been missing in the 1979 clash with Vietnam),[25] and to rethink the strategy of a "forward defense" along the frontiers with Russia in favor of counterattacks some way behind the long, exposed borders. The navy, too, is experimenting on a much larger scale: in 1980 an eighteen-vessel task force undertook an eight-thousand-nautical-mile mission in the South Pacific, in conjunction with China's latest intercontinental ballistic missile experiments. (Was this, one wonders, the first significant demonstration of Chinese sea power since Cheng Ho's cruises of the early fifteenth century? See pp. 6–7 above.)

More impressive still, for China's emergence as a Great Power militarily, has been the extraordinarily rapid development of its nuclear technology. Although the first Chinese tests occurred in Mao's time, he had publicly scorned nuclear weapons when preferring the merits of a "people's war"; the Deng leadership, by contrast, is intent upon taking China into the ranks of the *modern* military states as swiftly as possible. As early as 1980, China was testing ICBMs with a range of seven thousand nautical miles (which would encompass not only all of the USSR but also parts of the United States).[26] A year later, one of its rockets launched three space satellites, which is an indication of a multiple-warhead rocket technology. Most of China's nuclear forces are *land-based*, and medium-range rather than long-distance; but they are being joined by new ICBMs and, perhaps the most significant step of all (in terms of nuclear deterrence), by a fleet of missile-carrying submarines. Since 1982, China has been testing submarine-launched ballistic missiles and working on improvements of both range and accuracy. There are also reports of Chinese experimentation with tactical nuclear weapons. All this is backed up by large-scale atomic research, and by a refusal to have its nuclear weapons development "frozen" by international limitations agreements, since that would merely aid the existing Great Powers.

As against this evidence of military-technological prowess, it is also easy to point to continuing signs of weakness. There is always a significant time lag between producing an early prototype of a weapon and having large numbers of them, tried and tested, in the possession of the armed forces themselves; and this is particularly so with a country which is not rich in capital or scientific resources. Severe setbacks—including the possible explosion of a Chinese submarine while attempting to launch a missile; the cancellation or slowdown of weapons programs; the lack of expertise in metallic technology, advanced jet engines, and radar, navigation, and communications equipment—continue to hamper China's drive toward real military equality with the USSR and the United States. Its navy, despite the Pacific Ocean exercises, is far from being a "blue water" fleet, and its force of missile-bearing submarines will long remain behind those of the "Big Two," which are pouring funds into the development of gigantic types (*Ohio* class, *Alfa* class) that can dive deeper and run faster than any previous submarine.[27] Finally, the mention of finance is a reminder that as long as China is spending only one-eighth or thereabouts of the amount upon defense as the superpowers, there is no way it can achieve full parity; it cannot, therefore, plan to acquire *every* sort of weapon or to prepare for every conceivable threat.

Nonetheless, even China's existing military capability gives it an influence which is far more substantial than that existing some years ago. The improvements in training, organization, and equipment ought to place the PLA in a better position to meet regional rivals like Vietnam, Taiwan, and India than in the past two decades. Even the military balance vis-à-vis the Soviet Union may no longer be so disproportionately tilted in Moscow's favor. Should future disputes in Asia lead to a Sino-Russian war, the leadership in Moscow may find it politically difficult to consent to launching heavy nuclear strikes at China, both because of world reaction and because of the unpredictability of the American response; but if it did "go nuclear," there is less and less prospect of the Soviet armed forces being able to *guarantee* the destruction of China's growing land-based and (especially) sea-based missile systems before they can retaliate. On the other hand, if there is only conventional fighting, the Soviet dilemma remains acute. The fact that Moscow takes the possibility of war seriously can be gleamed from its deployment of around fifty divisions (including six or seven tank divisions) of Russian troops in its two military districts east of the Urals. And while it may be assumed that such forces can handle the seventy or more PLA divisions similarly stationed in the frontier area, their superiority may hardly be enough to ensure a striking victory—especially if the Chinese trade space for time in order to weaken the effects of a Soviet Blitzkrieg. To many observers, there now exists a "rough equivalence," a "balance of forces," in Central Asia[28]— and, if true, the strategical repercussions of that extend far beyond the immediate region of Mongolia.

But the most significant aspect of China's longer-term war-fighting power lies elsewhere: in the remarkably swift growth of its economy which has occurred during the past few decades and which seems likely to continue into the future. As was mentioned in the preceding chapter (see pp. 418–20), even before the Communists had firmly established their rule, China was a considerable manufacturing power— although that was disguised by the sheer size of the country, the fact that the vast majority of the population consisted of peasant farmers, and the disruptions of war and civil wars. The creation of a Marxist regime and the coming of domestic peace allowed production to shoot ahead, with the state actively encouraging both agricultural and industrial growth—although sometimes doing so (i.e., under Mao) by bizarre and counterproductive means. Writing in 1983–1984, one observer noted that "China has achieved annual growth rates in industry and agriculture since 1952 of around 10 percent and 3 percent respectively, and an overall growth of GNP of 5–6 percent per year."[29] If those figures do not match the achievements of such export-oriented Asian "trading states" as Singapore or Taiwan, they are impressive for a country as large and populous as China, and readily translate into an economic power of some size. By the late 1970s, according to one calculation, the Chinese industrial economy was as large as (if not larger than) those of the USSR and Japan in 1961.[30] Moreover, it is worth remarking once again that these *average* growth rates include the period of the so-called Great Leap Forward of 1958–1959; the break with Russia, and the withdrawal of Soviet funds, scientists, and blueprints in the early 1960s; and the turmoil of the Cultural Revolution, which not only distorted industrial planning but also undermined the entire educational and scientific system for nearly one generation. Had those events *not* occurred, Chinese growth would have been even faster overall—as may be gathered from the fact that over the past five years of Deng-led reforms, agriculture has averaged an 8 percent growth, and industry a spectacular 12 percent.[31]

To a very large degree, the agricultural sector remains both China's opportunity and its weak point. The East Asian methods of wet-rice cultivation are inordinately productive in yields per hectare, but are also extremely labor-intensive—which makes it difficult to effect a switch to, say, the large-scale, mechanized forms of agriculture used on the American prairies. Yet since agriculture forms over 30 percent of China's GDP and employs 70 percent of the population, decay (or merely a slowdown) in that sector will act as a drag upon the entire economy—as has clearly happened in the Soviet Union. This challenge is compounded by the population time bomb. Already China is attempting to feed a billion people on only 250 million acres of arable land (compared with the United States' 400 million acres of crops for its 230 million population);[32] can it possibly manage to feed another 200 million Chinese by the year 2000, without an increasing dependence upon imported food, which has both balance-of-payments and strategic costs? It is difficult to get a clear answer to that crucial question, in part because the experts point to different pieces of evidence. China's traditional export of foodstuffs slowly declined over the past three decades, and in 1980 it became, very briefly, a net *importer*.[33] On the other hand, the Chinese government is devoting massive scientific resources into achieving a "green revolution" on the Indian model, and Deng's encouragement of market-oriented reforms, together with large increases in agricultural purchase prices (without passing the cost on to the cities), have led to tremendous rises in food production over the past half-decade. Between 1979 and 1983—when much of the rest of the globe was suffering from economic depression—the 800 million Chinese in rural areas increased their incomes by about 70 percent, and their calorific intake was nearly as high as that of Brazilians or Malaysians. "In 1985, the Chinese produced 100 million more tons of grain than they did a decade earlier, one of the most productive surges ever recorded."[34] With the population increasing, and turning more and more to meat consumption (which requires yet more grain), the pressure to keep up this expansion in agricultural consumption will become more intense—and yet the acreage available remains restricted, and the growth in yields caused by the applications of fertilizer is bound to slow down. Nonetheless, the evidence suggests that China is managing to maintain this part of its elaborate balancing act with a considerable degree of success.

The future of China's drive toward industrialization is of even greater importance—but is a yet more delicate trick internally. It has been hampered not only by the lack of consumer purchasing power, but also by years of rather heavy-handed planning on the Russian and eastern European model. The "liberalization" measures of the past few years—getting state industries to respond to the commercial realities of quality, price, and market demand, encouraging the creation of privately run, small-scale enterprises, and allowing a great expansion in foreign trade[35]—have led to impressive rises in manufacturing output, but also to many problems. The creation of tens of thousands of private businesses has alarmed party ideologists, and the rise in prices (probably caused as much by the necessary adjustment to market costs as by the frequently denounced "racketeering" and "profiteering") has caused mutterings among urban workers, whose incomes have not risen as fast as either the farmers' or the entrepreneurs'. In addition, the foreign-trade boom quickly led to a sucking in of imported manufactures, and thus to a trade deficit. The statements made in 1986 by Prime Minister Zhao Ziyang that matters may have slipped somewhat "out of control" and that "consolidation" was needed for a while— together with the announced decrease in the hectic growth targets— are indications that internal and ideological problems remain.[36]

It is nevertheless remarkable that even the reduced growth rates are planned to be a very respectable 7.5 percent annually in future years (as opposed to the 10 percent rate since 1981). That itself would *double* China's GNP in less than ten years (a 10 percent rate would do the same in a mere seven years), yet for a number of reasons economic experts seem to feel that such a target can be achieved. In the first place, China's rate of savings and investment has been consistently in excess of 30 percent of GNP since 1970, and while that in turn brings problems (it reduces the proportion available for consumption, which is compensated for by price stability and income equality, which in turn get in the way of entrepreneurship), it also means that there are large funds available for productive investment. Secondly, there are huge opportunities for cost savings: China has been among the most profligate and extravagant countries in its consumption of energy (which caused declines in its quite considerable oil stocks), but its post-1978 energy reforms have substantially reduced the costs of one of industry's main "inputs" and thus freed money for investments elsewhere— or consumption.[37] Moreover, only now is China beginning to shake off the consequences of the Cultural Revolution. After more than a decade during which Chinese universities and research institutes were closed (or compelled to operate in a totally counterproductive way), it was predictable that it would take some time to catch up on the scientific and technological progress made elsewhere. "It is only against this background," it was remarked a few years ago,

> that one can understand the importance of the thousands of scientists who went to the United States and elsewhere in the West in the late 1970s for stays of one or two years and occasionally longer periods. . . . as early as 1985—and certainly by 1990—China will

have a cadre of many thousands of scientists and technicians familiar with the frontiers of their various fields. Tens of thousands more
trained at home as well as abroad will staff the institutes and enterprises that will implement the programs required to bring Chinese
industrial technology up to the best international standards, at least
in strategic areas of activity.[38]

In the same way, it could only be in the post-1978 period of encouraging (albeit selectively) foreign trade and investment in China that its
managers and entrepreneurs had the proper opportunity to pick and
choose from among the technological devices, patents, and production
facilities enthusiastically offered by western governments and companies which quite exaggerated the size of the Chinese market for such
items. Despite—or, rather, because of—the Peking government's desire
to control the level and contents of overseas trade, it is likely that
imports will be deliberately selected to boost economic growth.

The final and perhaps the most remarkable aspect of China's "dash
for growth" has been the very firm control upon defense spending, so
that the armed forces do not consume resources needed elsewhere. In
Deng's view, defense has to remain the fourth of China's much-vaunted
"four modernizations"—behind agriculture, industry, and science; and
although it is difficult to gain exact figures on Chinese defense spending
(chiefly because of different methods of calculation),[39] it seems clear
that the proportion of GNP allocated to the armed forces has been
tumbling for the past fifteen years—from perhaps 17.4 percent in 1971
(according to one source) to 7.5 percent in 1985.[40] This in its turn may
cause grumbling among the military and thus increase the internal
debate over economic priorities and policies; and it would clearly have
to be reversed if serious border clashes recurred in the north or the
south. Nonetheless, the fact that defense spending must take an inferior place is probably the most significant indication to date of
China's all-out commitment to economic growth, and stands in stark
contrast to both the Soviet obsession with "military security" and the
Reagan administration's commitment to pouring funds into the armed
services. As many experts have pointed out,[41] given China's existing
GNP and amount of national savings and investment within it, there
would be no real problem in spending much more than its current c.
$30 billion on defense. That it chooses not to do so reflects Peking's
belief that long-term security will be assured only when its present
output and wealth have been multiplied many times.

In sum: "The only events likely to stop this growth in its tracks
would be the outbreak of war with the Soviet Union or prolonged
political upheaval on the pattern of the Cultural Revolution. China's
management, energy, and agricultural problems are serious, but they
are the kinds of problems faced and overcome by all developing na-

tions during the growth process."[42] If that seems a remarkably rosy statement, it pales compared with *The Economist's* recent calculation that if China maintains an average 8 percent annual growth—which it calls "feasible"—it would soar past the British and Italian GNP totals well before 2000 and be vastly in excess of *any* European power by 2020.[43]

Chart 2. GDP Projections of China, India, and Certain Western European States, 1980–2020

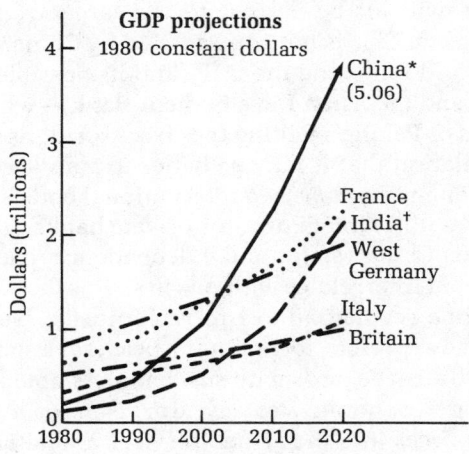

* Assuming 7 percent growth rate 1980-1985
  and 8 percent thereafter
† Assuming 5.5 percent growth rate 1980-1985
  and 7 percent thereafter
Other countries assuming average annual rates
  as in 1970-1982

Source: *The Economist*/IMF

The greatest mistake of all would be to assume that this sort of projection, with all the changeable factors that it rests upon, could ever work out with such exactitude. But the general point remains: China will have a very large GNP within a relatively short space of time, barring some major catastrophe; and while it will still be relatively poor in per capita terms, it will be decidedly richer than it is today.

Three further points are worth making about China's future impact upon the international scene. The first, and least important for our purposes, is that while the country's economic growth will boost its foreign trade, it is impossible to transform it into another West Germany or Japan. The sheer size of the domestic market of a continent-wide Power such as China, and of its population and raw-materials base, makes it highly unlikely that it would become as dependent upon

overseas commerce as one of the smaller, maritime "trading states."[44]
The extent of its labor-intensive agricultural sector and the regime's
determination not to become too reliant upon imported foodstuffs will
also be a drag upon foreign trade. What *is* likely is that China will
become an increasingly important producer of low-cost goods, like
textiles, which will help to pay for western—or even Russian—technology; but Peking is clearly determined *not* to become dependent upon
foreign capital, manufactures, or markets, or upon any one country or
supplier in particular. Acquiring foreign technology, tools, and production methods will all be subject to the larger requirements of
China's balancing act. This is not contradicted by China's recent membership in the World Bank and the IMF (and its possible future membership in GATT and the Asian Development Bank)—which are not so
much indications of Peking's joining the "free world" as they are of its
hard-nosed calculation that it may be better to gain access to foreign
markets, and to long-term loans, via international bodies than through
unilateral "deals" with a Great Power or private banks. In other words,
such moves protect China's status and independence. The second point
is separate from, but interrelates with, the first. It is that whereas in the
1960s Mao's regime seemed almost to relish in the frequent border
clashes, Peking now prefers to maintain peaceful relations with its
neighbors, even those it regards with suspicion. As noted above, peace
is central to Deng's economic strategy; war, even of a regional sort,
would divert resources into the armed services and alter the order of
priority among China's "four modernizations." It may also be the case,
as has been argued recently,[45] that China feels more relaxed about
relations with Moscow simply because its own military improvements
have created a rough equilibrium in central Asia. Having achieved a
"correlation of forces," or at least a decent defensive capacity, China
can concentrate more upon economic development.

Yet if its intentions are peaceable, China also emphasizes how determined it is to preserve its own complete independence, and how
much it disapproves of the two superpowers' military interventions
abroad. Even toward Japan the Chinese have kept a wary eye, restricting its share of the import/export trade and yet also warning Tokyo
not to get too heavily involved in developing Siberia.[46] Toward Washington and Moscow, China has been much more studied—and critical.
All of the Soviet suggestions for improving relations and even the
return of Soviet engineers and scientists to China in early 1986 have
not altered Peking's fundamental position: that a real improvement
cannot take place until Moscow makes concessions in some, if not all,
of the three outstanding issues—the Russian invasion of Afghanistan,
the Russian support of Vietnam, and the long-standing question of
central Asian boundaries and security.[47] On the other hand, U.S. policies in Latin America and the Middle East have come in for repeated

attack from Peking (as, to be sure, have similar Russian adventures in the tropics). Being economically one of the "less-developed countries" and inherently suspicious of the white races' domination of the globe makes China a natural critic of superpower intervention, even if it is not a formal member of the Third World movement and even if those criticisms are nowadays fairly mild compared to Mao's fulminations of the 1960s. And despite its earlier (and still powerful) hostility to Russian pretensions in Asia, the Chinese remain suspicious of the earnest American discussion of how and when to play the "China card."[48] In Peking's view, it may be necessary to incline toward Russia or (more frequently, since the Sino-Soviet quarrels) toward the United States, by measures including the joint monitoring of Russian nuclear testing and exchanging information over Afghanistan and Vietnam; but the ideal position is to be equidistant between the two, and to have them both wooing the Middle Kingdom.

To this extent, China's importance as a truly independent actor in the present (and future) international system is enhanced by what, for want of a better word, one might term its "style" of relating to the other Powers. This has been put so nicely by Jonathan Pollack that it is worth repeating *in extenso:*

> [W]eapons, economic strength, and power potential alone cannot explain the imputed significance of China in a global power equation. If its strategic significance is judged modest and its economic performance has been at best mixed, this cannot account for the considerable importance of China in the calculations of both Washington and Moscow, and the careful attention paid to it in other key world capitals. The answer lies in the fact that, notwithstanding its self-characterization as a threatened and aggrieved state, China has very shrewdly and even brazenly used its available political, economic, and military resources. Towards the superpowers, Peking's overall strategy has at various times comprised confrontation and armed conflict, partial accomodation, informal alignment, and a detachment bordering on disengagement, sometimes interposed with strident, angry rhetoric. As a result, China becomes all things to all nations, with many left uncertain and even anxious about its long-term intentions and directions.
>
> To be sure, such an indeterminate strategy has at times entailed substantial political and military risks. Yet the same strategy has lent considerable credibility to China's position as an emergent major power. China has often acted in defiance of the preferences or demands of both superpowers; at other times it has behaved far differently from what others expect. Despite its seeming vulnerability, China has not proven pliant and yielding toward either Moscow or Washington. . . . For all these reasons, China has assumed a singular international position, both as a participant in many of the central political and military conflicts in the post war era and as a

state that resists easy political or ideological categorization. . . . Indeed, in a certain sense China must be judged as a candidate superpower in its own right—not in imitation or emulation of either the Soviet Union or the United States, but as a reflection of Peking's unique position in global politics. In a long-term sense, China represents a political and strategic force too significant to be regarded as an adjunct to either Moscow or Washington or simply as an intermediate power.[49]

As a final point, it needs to be stressed again that although China is keeping a tight hold upon military expenditures at the moment, it has no intention of remaining a strategical "lightweight" in the future. On the contrary, the more that China pushes forward with its economic expansion in a Colbertian, *étatiste* fashion, the more that development will have power-political implications. This is the more likely when one recalls the attention China is giving to expanding its scientific/technological base, and the impressive achievements already made in rocketry and nuclear weapons when that base was so much smaller. Such a concern for enhancing the country's economic substructure at the expense of an immediate investment in weapons will hardly satisfy China's generals (who, like military groups everywhere, prefer short-term to long-term means of security). Yet as *The Economist* has nicely remarked:

> For [China's] military men with the patience to see the [economic] reforms through, there is a payoff. If Mr. Deng's plans for the economy as a whole are allowed to run their course, and the value of China's output quadruples, as planned, between 1980 and 2000 (admittedly big ifs), then 10 to 15 years down the line the civilian economy should have picked up enough steam to haul the military sector along more rapidly. That is when China's army, its neighbors and the big powers will really have something to think about.[50]

It is only a matter of time.

The Japanese Dilemma

The very fact that Peking is so purposeful about what is to happen in East Asia increases the pressures now bearing down upon Japan's (self-proclaimed) "omnidirectional peaceful diplomacy"—or what might more cynically be described as "being all things to all men."[51] The Japanese dilemma may perhaps be best summarized as follows:

Due to its immensely successful growth since 1945, the country enjoys a unique and very favorable position in the global economic and power-political order, yet that is also—the Japanese feel—an extremely delicate and vulnerable position, which could be badly deranged if international circumstances changed. The best thing that could happen from Tokyo's viewpoint, therefore, would be for the continuation of those factors which caused "the Japanese miracle" in the first place. But precisely because this is an anarchic world in which "dissatisfied" powers jostle alongside "satisfied" ones, and because the dynamic of technological and commercial change is driving so fast, the likelihood is that those favorable factors will diminish—or even disappear altogether. Given Japan's belief in the delicacy and vulnerability of its own position, it finds it hard openly to resist the pressures for change; instead, the latter must be slowed down, or deflected, by diplomatic compromise. Hence its constant advocacy of the peaceful solution to international problems, its alarm and embarrassment when it finds itself in a political crossfire between other countries, and its evident wish to be on good terms with everyone while it gets steadily richer.

The reasons for Japan's phenomenal economic success have already been discussed (see above, pp. 416–18). For over forty years the Japanese homeland has been protected by American nuclear and conventional forces, and its sea lanes by the U.S. Navy. Thus enabled to redirect its national energies from militaristic expansion and its resources from high defense spending, Japan has devoted itself to the pursuit of sustained economic growth, especially in export markets. This success could not have been achieved without its own people's commitment to entrepreneurship, quality control, and hard work, but it was also aided by certain special factors: the holding-down of the yen to an artificially low level for decade after decade in order to boost exports; the restrictions, both formal and informal, upon the purchase of imported foreign manufactures (although not, of course, of the vital raw materials which industry needed); and the existence of a liberal international trading order which placed few obstacles in the way of Japanese goods—and which was kept "open," despite the increasing burdens upon itself, by the United States. For the past quarter-century, therefore, Japan has been able to enjoy all of the advantages of evolving into a global economic giant, but without any of the political responsibilities and territorial disadvantages which have, historically, followed from such a growth. Little wonder that it prefers things to remain as they are.

Since the foundations of Japan's present success lie exclusively in the economic sphere, it is not surprising that this also is the field which worries Tokyo most. On the one hand (as will be discussed below), technological and economic growth offers fresh glittering prizes to the country whose political economy is best positioned for the coming twenty-first century; and only a few dispute the contention that Japan is in that favorable position.[52] On the other hand, its very success is already provoking a "scissors effect" reaction against its export-led expansion. The one "blade" of those scissors is the emulation of Japan by other ambitious Asian NICs (newly industrialized countries), such as South Korea, Singapore, Taiwan, Thailand, etc.—not to mention China itself at the lower end of the product scale (e.g., textiles).[53] All of these countries have far lower labor costs than Japan,* and are challenging strongly in fields in which the Japanese no longer enjoy decisive advantages—textiles, toys, domestic goods, shipbuilding, even (to a much less degree) steel and automobiles. This does not, of course, mean that Japan's production of ships, cars, trucks, and steel is doomed, but to the extent that it is increasingly necessary for them to move "up-market" (e.g., to higher-grade steels, or more sophisticated and larger-sized automobiles) they are withdrawing from the bottom end of a production spectrum where previously they were unchallenged; and one of the more important tasks of MITI (the Ministry for International Trade and Industry) is to plan the phasing out of industries which are no longer competitive—not only to make the decline less traumatic but also to arrange for the transfer of resources and personnel into other, more competitive sectors of the international economy.

The second, even more worrying blade of the scissors has been the increasingly hostile reaction of Americans and Europeans to the seemingly inexorable penetration of their domestic markets by Japanese products. Year after year, the populations of these prosperous markets have bought Japanese steel, machine tools, motorcycles, automobiles, and TV sets and other electrical goods. Year after year, Japan's trading surpluses with the EEC and the United States have widened. The European reaction has been the tougher one, ranging from import quotas to bureaucratic obstructionism (such as the French requirement that Japanese electrical goods be admitted only via an understaffed customs house in Poitiers).[54] Because of its own belief in an open world trading system, American administrations have hesitated to ban or otherwise restrict Japanese imports apart from dubious "voluntary" limits. But even the staunchest American advocates of laissez-faire have grown uneasy at a situation in which, essentially, the United States supplies Japan with foodstuffs and raw materials and receives Japanese manufactures in return—a sort of "colonial" or "underdevelopment" trading status it has not known for a century and a half. Moreover, the growing U.S. trade deficits with Japan—$62 billion in the fiscal year ending March 31, 1986—and the pressures from beleaguered American industries which have felt the brunt of this transpacific competition have increased Washington's demand for measures to reduce the imbalance—e.g., to encourage a rise in the exchange value of the yen, a substantial increase in American imports

*Which is why even Japanese firms are building factories there.

into Japan, and so on. As the western world drifts toward quasi-protec-
tionism, moreover, its tendency to put limits upon the *total* amount of
textiles or televisions imported implies that Japan will have to divide
that shrunken market with its Asian rivals.

It is scarcely surprising, therefore, that some Japanese spokesmen
deny that things are good, and point to an alarming conjunction of
threats to their present market shares and prosperity: the increasing
challenge by Asian NICs in so many industries; the restrictions upon
Japanese exports by western governments; the pressures to change
Japan's tax laws, divert monies from savings to consumption, and
ensure a large increase in imports; finally, the swift rise in the value
of the yen. All of these, it is claimed, could mean the end of Japan's
export-led boom, a decline in its payments surpluses, a slowing-down
in its growth rate (which has already been decelerating as its economy
becomes more "mature" and its potential for spectacular expansion
diminishes). In that connection, Japan worries that it is not only its
economy which is maturing: because of the age structure of its population, by 2010 it will have "the lowest ratio of working-age people (those
15 to 64 years old) among the leading industrial nations," which will
require high social security outlays and could lead to a loss of dynamism.[55] Moreover, all the attempts to get the Japanese consumer to
buy foreign-made manufactures (except those with a certain prestige,
like Mercedes cars) lead to domestic political controversy,[56] which
might in turn cause a possible breakdown in the consensus politics
which has been an integral part of Japan's sustained export-led expansion in the past.

Yet while it may be true that Japan's economic growth is slowing
down as it enters a more mature phase, and while it is certainly true
that other countries are unwilling to permit Japan to keep the economic advantages which aided its previous explosion of exports, there
nevertheless remain considerable substantive reasons why it is likely
to expand faster than the other *major* Powers in the future. In the first
place, as a country so incredibly dependent upon imported raw materials (99 percent of its oil, 92 percent of its iron, 100 percent of its
copper), it benefits enormously from the changing terms of trade
which have reduced the prices of so many ores, fuels, and foodstuffs;
the drop in world oil prices after 1980–1981, which saves Japan billions
of dollars of foreign currency each year, is only the most spectacular
of the falls in raw-materials and foodstuffs prices.[57] Furthermore,
while a rapid appreciation in the value of the yen is likely to cut some
of the country's exports overseas (depending always upon the elasticity
of demand), it also greatly reduces the cost of imports—and thus helps
industry to stay competitive and inflation to remain low. In addition,
the 1973 oil crisis stimulated the Japanese into searching for all sorts
of energy economies, which contribute to the still greater efficiency of

its industry; in the past decade alone, Japan has reduced its dependence on oil by 25 percent. In addition, that same crisis impelled Japan
into a sustained search for new sources of raw materials and a heavy
investment in such areas (somewhat akin to Britain's investments
overseas in the nineteenth century). None of this makes it *absolutely*
certain that Japan can rely upon a continued flow of low-priced raw
materials; but the auguries for that are good.

More significant still is the continued surge of Japanese industry
toward the most promising (and, ultimately, most profitable) sectors
of the economy for the early twenty-first century: that is, high technology. In other words, as Japan steadily pulls out of the production of
textiles, shipbuilding, basic steel—leaving them to countries with
lower labor costs—it clearly intends to be a (if not *the*) leading force
in those scientifically advanced manufactures which have a much
higher added value. Its achievements in the computing field are already so well known as to be legendary. Borrowing heavily from
American technology in the first instance, Japanese companies were
able to exploit all their native advantages (a protected home market,
MITI support, better quality control, a favorable yen-to-dollar ratio) as
well as—most probably—"dumping" at below-cost prices to drive most
American companies out of the production of semiconductors,
whether of the 16k RAM, the 64k RAM, or the later 256k RAM.[58]

Even more worrying to the American computer industry is the
evidence of Japan's determined move into two fresh (and much more
profitable) fields. The first is the production of advanced computers
themselves, particularly the sophisticated and extremely expensive
"fifth generation" supercomputers, which can work hundreds of times
faster than the largest existing machines and promise to give their
owners enormous benefits in everything from codebreaking to designing aircraft shapes. Already American experts are stunned by the speed
at which Japan has moved into this area, and at the amount of research
capital which MITI and large companies like Hitachi and Fujitsu are
pouring into it.[59] Yet the same is also happening in the field of computer *software*, where again American firms (and a few European
firms) were unchallenged until the early 1980s.[60] To be sure, the successful production both of supercomputers and of software is a much
larger task than making semiconductors, and will test Japan's designers to the utmost; and in the meantime both American and European
companies (the latter strongly supported by the in governments) are
preparing to meet the commercial challenge, while the U.S. Department of Defense will give its massive backing to ensuring that its
national firms remain ahead in the development of supercomputers.
Nonetheless, those bodies would be very sanguine to assume that
Japan can be permanently held off in these fields.

Since respected journals like *The Economist*, the *Wall Street Jour-*

nal, the *New York Times,* and many others frequently carry articles about Japan's move into further areas of high technology, it would be superfluous to repeat the details here. Mitsubishi's link-up with Westinghouse has been seen as evidence of Japan's increasing interest in the nuclear-power industry.[61] Biotechnology is also a large Japanese concern, especially with its implications for enhancing crop yields. So, too, is ceramics. The reports that the Japanese Aircraft Development Corporation has joined up with Boeing to produce a new generation of fuel-efficient aircraft for the 1990s—denounced by one American expert as a "Faustian bargain" whereby Japan will provide cheap finance and acquire U.S. technology and expertise[62]—may be even more significant for the future. But perhaps the most important (in terms of sheer output) will be the already impressive lead which Japan has in the field of industrial robots and its development of (experimental) entire factories virtually controlled by computers, lasers, and robots: the ultimate solution to the country's decreasing labor force! The latest figures show that "Japan continued to introduce about as many industrial robots as the rest of the world combined, several times the rate of introduction in the United States." Another survey indicates that the Japanese use their robots much more efficiently than Americans do.[63]

Behind all of these high-technology ventures are a cluster of broader, structural factors which continue to give Japan marked advantages over its chief rivals. The role of MITI as a sort of economic equivalent to the famous Prussian General Staff may have been exaggerated by foreigners,[64] but there seems little doubt that the broad direction which it gives to Japanese economic development by arranging research and funding for growth industries and a gentle euthanasia for declining ones has worked better to date than the uncoordinated laissez-faire approach of the United States. The second strength—one of the most important of all in explaining the rise and fall of particular firms and industries—is the large (and increasing) amount of money which is allocated to research and development in Japan. "The proportion of GNP devoted to R&D will virtually double this decade, rising from 2 percent of GNP in 1980 to an expected 3.5 percent by 1990. The United States has stabilized R&D expenses at about 2.7 percent of GNP. However, if military research is excluded, Japan is already devoting about as many man-hours to R&D as the United States and will soon be spending about as much for it. If present trends continue, Japan will take the lead in nonmilitary R&D spending by the early 1990s."[65] Even more interesting, perhaps, is the fact that a far higher proportion of Japanese R&D is paid for and done by industry itself than in Europe and the United States (where so much is done by governments or universities). In other words, it is aimed directly at the marketplace and is expected to pay its way quickly. "Pure" science is left to others, and tapped only when its commercial relevance becomes clear.

The third advantage is the very high level of national savings in Japan, which is especially marked compared with that in the United States. This is partly explained by the differences in tax systems, which in the United States have traditionally encouraged personal borrowing and consumer spending—and in Japan encourage private savings. On average, too, the individual in Japan has to save much more for his or her old age, since the pension schemes are usually less generous. What all this means is that Japanese banks and insurance companies are awash with funds and can provide industry with masses of low-interest capital. The share of GNP which is collected in Japan both as income tax *and* social security payments is much lower than in the other major capitalist-cum-"welfare state" societies, and the Japanese evidently intend to keep it that way, in order to free the money for investment capital.[66] Europeans who would like to imitate "the Japanese way" would first of all have to massively reduce their social welfare spending. Americans enamored of Japan's system would have to slash both defense and social expenditures, *and* to alter their taxation laws even more drastically than they have done so far.

The fourth strength is that Japanese firms have a virtually guaranteed home market in all except prestige and specialized manufactures—a situation no longer enjoyed by most American firms or (despite their protectionist efforts) by the majority of European companies. While much of this was aided by in-built bureaucratic practices and regulations designed to favor Japanese producers in their home market, even the abolition of such mercantilistic devices is unlikely to persuade Japan's consumers to "buy foreign," other than raw materials and basic foodstuffs; the high quality and familiarity of Japanese products, a strong cultural pride, and the complex structure of domestic distribution and sales will ensure that.

Finally, there is the very high quality of the Japanese work force— at least as measured by various mathematical and scientific aptitude tests—which is not only groomed in an intensely competitive public education system but also systematically trained by the companies themselves. Even fifteen-year-olds in Japan show a marked superiority in testable subjects (e.g., mathematics) over most of their western counterparts. In the higher reaches of learning, the balance is different: Japan has a dearth of Nobel Prize scientists, but it produces many more engineers than any western country (about 50 percent more than the United States itself). It also has nearly 700,000 R&D workers, which is more than Britain, France, and West Germany have combined.[67]

No statistically quantifiable assessment can be made of the combined effects of the above five factors, compared with conditions in other leading nations; but, taken together, they obviously give Japanese industry an immensely strong bedrock. So, too, does the docility and diligence of the Japanese work force and the harmony which seems to prevail in the industrial-relations system, where there are only company unions, a search for consensus, and virtually no strikes. There are, clearly, unattractive features here as well: longer hours of work, the all-pervading conformism to the company ethos (from the early-morning physical exercises onward), the absence of truly independent trade unions, the cramped housing conditions, the emphasis upon hierarchy and deference. Moreover, Japan also contains, outside the factory gates, a radicalized student body. Such facts, and other disturbing traits in Japanese society, have been commented on by many western observers[68]—some of whom appear to view the country with the same sort of horror and awe that continental Europeans manifested toward the "factory system" of early-nineteenth-century Britain. In other words, what is clearly a more effective arrangement of workers, and of society, in terms of *output* (and thus wealth creation) involves a disturbing challenge to traditional norms and individualist ways of behavior. And it is because the emulation of the Japanese industrial miracle would involve not merely the copying of this or that piece of technology or management but the imitation of much of the Japanese social system that observers such as David Halberstam argue, "This is America's newest and . . . most difficult challenge for the rest of the century . . . a much harder and more intense competition than . . . the political-military competition with the Soviet Union. . . ."[69]

As if these industrial strengths were not enough, they have been complemented by the amazingly swift emergence of Japan as the world's leading creditor nation, exporting tens of billions of dollars each year. This transformation, which has been under way since MITI's 1969 dismantling of export controls upon Japanese lending and its creation of financial inducements for overseas investments, is rooted in two basic causes. The first of these is the inordinately high level of personal savings in Japan—over 20 percent of Japanese wages are saved, so that by 1985 "the average total savings of Japanese households exceeded the average annual income for the first time"[70]— which has left financial institutions flush with funds that are increasingly invested abroad to gain a higher return. The second reason has been the unprecedentedly large trade surpluses occurring for Japan in recent years because of the explosion in its earnings from exports. Fearing that such surpluses would fuel domestic inflation (if returned home), the Japanese finance ministry has been encouraging the giant banks to invest vast sums overseas.[71] In 1983, the net outflow of Japanese capital was $17.7 billion; in 1984, it leaped to $49.7 billion; and in 1985, it leaped again, to $64.5 billion, turning Japan into the world's largest net creditor nation. By 1990, the director of the Institute for

International Economics forecasts, the rest of the world will owe Japan a staggering $500 billion; and by 1995, the Nomura Research Institute predicts, Japan's gross overseas assets will exceed $1 trillion.[72] Not surprisingly, Japanese banks and securities firms are rapidly becoming the largest and most successful in the world.[73]

The consequences of this vast surge in Japanese capital exports contain dangers as well as benefits for the world economy, and perhaps also for Japan itself. A considerable amount of these funds is invested into infrastructures around the globe (e.g., the English Channel tunnel) or into the opening of new iron-ore fields (e.g., in Brazil), which will benefit Tokyo indirectly or directly. Other monies are being channeled by Japanese companies and their balances into the creation of overseas subsidiaries (especially for production)—either to have Japanese goods manufactured in low-labor-cost countries so that they can remain competitive, or to place such plants within the territories of, say, EEC countries and the United States in order to obviate protectionist tariffs. The greater part of this capital flow has, however, gone into short-term bonds (especially U.S. Treasury bonds), which if ever recalled back to Japan in large amounts could unsettle the international financial system—just as in 1929—and place tremendous pressures upon U.S. dollars *and* the U.S. economy, since much of this money is going to finance the huge budget deficits incurred by the Reagan administration. On the whole, however, Tokyo is much more likely to keep recycling its surplus capital into new ventures overseas than to bring it home.

The rise of Japan in the past few years to be the world's leading net creditor nation—combined with the transformation of the United States from being the biggest lender to being the biggest borrower—has occurred so swiftly that it is still difficult to work out its full implications. Since "historically a creditor nation has led growth in each period of global economic expansion, and Japan's era is just arriving,"[74] it may well be that Tokyo's emergence as the leading world banker gives a further middle-to-long-term boost to international commerce and finance, following the earlier examples provided by the Netherlands, Britain, and the United States. What seems remarkable at this stage is that the surge in Japan's "invisible" financial role is occurring *before* there is any significant erosion of its immense "visible" industrial lead, as happened (for example) in the British case. Perhaps that may change, and swiftly, if the value of the yen soars too high and Japan experiences long-term "maturity" and slowdown in its manufacturing base and in its rate of productive growth. Yet even if this does happen—and there are reasons (as given above) to think that any decline of Japan as a manufacturing nation will be a slow process—one fact is clear: with the forecast amount of overseas assets in its hands by the year 2000, its current-account balances are bound to be handsomely supplemented by a vast flow of earnings from abroad. In all ways, therefore, Japan seems destined to get much richer.

Just how powerful, economically, will Japan be in the early twenty-first century? Barring large-scale war, or ecological disaster, or a return to a 1930s-style world slump and protectionism, the consensus answer seems to be: *much* more powerful. In computers, robotics, telecommunications, automobiles, trucks, and ships, and possibly also in biotechnology and even in aerospace, Japan will be either the leading or the second nation. In finance, it may by then be in a class of its own. Already it is reported that its per capita GNP has sailed past those of the United States and western Europe, giving it almost the highest standard of living on earth. What its share of world manufacturing output or of total world GNP will be is impossible to say. It is worth recalling that in 1951, Japan's total GNP was one-third of Britain's and one-twentieth (!) of the United States'; yet within three decades it had risen to be double Britain's and nearly half the United States'. To be sure, its rate of growth over those decades was unusually swift, because of special conditions. Yet according to many assessments,[75] the Japanese economy is still likely to expand about 1½ to 2 percent a year faster than the other large economies (except, of course, China) over the next several decades.* It is for that reason that scholars such as Herman Kahn and Ezra Vogel have argued that Japan will be "number one" economically in the early twenty-first century, and it is not surprising that many Japanese are fired by that very prospect. For a country which possesses only 3 percent of the world population and only 0.3 percent of its habitable land, it seems an almost unbelievable achievement; and but for the possibilities inherent in the new technology, one would be tempted to assume that Japan was already close to maximizing the potential of its people and land and that, like other relatively small peripheral or island states (Portugal, Venice, the Netherlands, even Britain in its time) it would one day be eclipsed by nations which had far larger resources and merely needed to copy its successful habits. For the foreseeable future, however, Japan's trajectory continues to rise upward.

No matter how one measures Japan's present and future economic strength, two facts are overriding. The first is that it is enormously

---

*Assuming that to be the case, it is still difficult for technical reasons to suggest what that means in exact figures. Many of the statistics commonly used (e.g., by the CIA) in international comparisons are based upon U.S. dollars and market exchange rates; thus the tumbling of the value of the dollar vis-à-vis the yen by nearly 40 percent in 1985–1986 could, by that reckoning, massively boost Japan's GNP total as compared with the United States' (and also as compared with the USSR's, since its GNP is often calculated in "geometric mean dollars").[76] Simply a rise in the yen from its present exchange value to 120 or even 100 to the dollar—which some economic experts think is its "true" rate[77]—would give Japan a total GNP close to the United States' and well in excess of Russia's. It is because of the problems caused by rapidly fluctuating exchange rates that some economists prefer to use "purchasing parity ratios," although that measurement also has its problems.

productive and prosperous, and getting much more so. The second is
that its *military* strength, and defense spending, bears no relation to
its place in the international economic order of things. It possesses a
reasonable-sized navy (including thirty-one destroyers and eighteen
frigates), a home-defense air force, and a modest army, but it is clearly
much less of a military power, relative to others, than it was in the
1930s, or even in the 1910s. More pertinent still for the debate upon
"burden-sharing"[78] is the fact that Japan allocates so relatively little for
defense. According to the figures in *The Military Balance,* in 1983
Japan spent $11.6 billion on defense, compared with $21–24 billion
spent by France, West Germany, and Britain, and a colossal $239
billion by the United States; per capita, therefore, the average Japanese
inhabitant had had to pay only $98 for defense that year, compared
with the average Briton's $439 and the average American's $1,023.[79]
Given its current prosperity, Japan seems to be getting off lightly from
the costs of defense—and in two related ways: the first is that it shelters
under the protection of others, namely, the United States; the second
is that its low defense outlays help it to keep down public spending and
thus provide more resources for the Japanese manufacturing effort
which is so hurting American and European competitors.[80]

Were Japan indeed to respond to the pressures of the U.S. government and of other western critics and to increase its defense spending
to the level allocated by the European NATO members—averaging
around 3–4 percent of GNP—the transformation would be dramatic
and would turn it (along with China) into the third-largest military
power in the world, with expenditures on defense of over $50 billion
a year. Nor is there any doubt, given Japan's technological and productive resources, that it could build, for example, carrier task forces for
its navy, or long-range missiles as a deterrent. That would certainly
benefit domestic firms like Mitsubishi, as well as providing a counter
to Soviet power in the Far East, thus rendering help to an overstretched
United States.

What is much more likely to happen, however, is that Tokyo will
endeavor to escape those external pressures, or at least to maintain
defense spending as low as it possibly can without provoking a rupture
with Washington. The chief reason has not been the purely symbolic
one of wishing to keep Japanese expenditures on defense within the
ceiling of 1 percent of GNP; by NATO definitions (i.e., by including
military pensions), it had already broken that barrier, and in any case,
it spent a considerably larger percentage of its GNP upon defense in
the early 1950s. Nor has it much to do with the conditions of the 1951
U.S.-Japan security treaty, which is the legal basis for the American
military presence in Japan, and which further encouraged Tokyo to
think of trade rather than strategic power; for the circumstances of the
1980s are now quite different from those of the Korean War. The real

reasons, in the view of the Japanese government, are the domestic and regional objections to a massive increase in its defense spending, and to a revision of the constitution, which forbids sending troops (or even selling arms) abroad. The memory of the militaristic excesses of the 1930s, of the wartime losses, and (especially) of the horrors of the A-bombs has ingrained upon the Japanese consciousness a dislike and suspicion of war and of the instruments of war which is at least as strong as western pacifism after the First World War; and while that may change in time, with the coming of a younger, more assertive generation, the prevailing opinion in the near future is much more likely to constrain the Tokyo government to keep increases in spending on the aptly named "self-defense forces" to modest levels.[81]

To these moral and ideological reasons there can be added economic ones. Among Japanese businessmen and politicians there is considerable opposition to increasing public spending (which, as mentioned above, is much lower in Japan than in any of the other OECD countries): to them, a doubling or trebling of defense expenditures must be paid for by either adding to the large public-sector deficit or raising taxes—and both are acutely disliked. Besides, it is argued, a large army and navy did not bring Japan "security," whether of the military or the economic sort, in the 1930s; and it is difficult to see at present how an increase in defense spending could prevent a possible cutoff of Arab oil—which is a far greater danger to Japan strategically than, say, the hypothetical nuclear winter, and explains Tokyo's desperate efforts to "lie low and say nothing" whenever there is a crisis in the Middle East. Is it not better, then, for Japan to abjure the use of force and to resolve all international disputes peacefully, as a cosmopolitan "trading state" should? Since modern war is so costly and is usually counterproductive, the Japanese feel that there is a lot of merit in their *zenhoi heiwa gaiko* ("omnidirectional peaceful diplomacy").

These feelings are no doubt reinforced by Tokyo's awareness that many of its neighbors would react with alarm to a large-scale buildup of Japanese military power. That would obviously be the response of the Russians—against whom, after all, the United States wants Japan to "burden-share" in defense matters, and who are still in dispute with Tokyo over the islands north of Hokkaido, and who probably feel that they have enough on their hands in the Far East with the expansion of Chinese power. But it would also be the response of those lands previously subjected to Japanese occupation—Korea, Taiwan, the Philippines, Malaysia, Indonesia—as well as Australia and New Zealand, all of which have reacted nervously to any signs of a revival of Japanese nationalism and *bushido* mentality, and which have encouraged Tokyo to "focus on productive nonmilitary ways to enhance Southeast Asian peace and security."[82] Above all, perhaps, there looms for Tokyo the difficulty of assuaging the suspicions of a touchy Peking, which still nurses memories of the Japanese atrocities of 1937–1945, and has also warned Japan not to get too heavily involved in developing Siberia (which in turn complicates the Tokyo-Moscow relationship) or to support Taiwan.

Even Japan's economic expansion (while bringing with it much-needed investments, plus some development aid and tourism) has left many of its neighbors suspicious, feeling that they are being sucked into a newer and more subtle version of the "Greater East Asia Co-Prosperity Sphere" once again—the more especially since Japan does not import very much (except raw materials) from those countries, yet sells a great deal of its own manufactures to them. Here, too, China has been the most outspoken, at first welcoming the late 1970s boom in Japanese trade and investments, then sharply curtailing them, partly because of its own balance-of-payments deficit, partly to avoid economic dependency upon any single foreign country which might take undue advantage of it; America's trade with China, Deng urged in 1979, "must come equal to Japan's,"[83] and thus prevent any possibility of a Japanese variant of "the imperialism of free trade."

All of these are, at the moment, merely straws in the wind, but they make politicians in Tokyo worry about how best to evolve a coherent external strategy for Japan as it moves toward the twenty-first century. There is no doubt that with its economic power expanding, it could become a second Venice—in the sense not just of extensive trading, but also of protecting its maritime sea lanes and of creating quasi-dependencies overseas; yet the internal and external objections to a strong Japan are such that not only will it avoid any move toward territorial acquisitions along old-fashioned imperialist lines, but it is also unlikely to increase its defense forces by very much. This latter conclusion, however, will increasingly irritate American circles who are pressing for "burden sharing" in the western Pacific. Ironically, therefore, Japan will be criticized if it does not substantially increase its spending upon arms, and it will be denounced if it does. Either way spells trouble to what has been nicely termed Japan's "maximal gain/minimum risk foreign policy."[84] This suggests, once again, a Japanese preference for as little change as possible in the military and political affairs of East Asia, even as the pace of economic growth quickens. That, too, compounds the dilemma, for even a non-Marxist would be puzzled to imagine how the profound economic transformation of Asia could avoid being attended by far-reaching changes in other spheres as well.

The deepest worries of the Japanese, therefore, are probably those which are rarely if ever discussed publicly—partly out of diplomatic discretion, partly to avoid bringing such developments about—and concern the future balance of power in East Asia itself. "Omnidirectional peaceful diplomacy" is all very well for the present, but how useful will it be if an overextended United States does withdraw from its Asian commitments, or finds it impossible to protect the flow of oil from Arabia to Yokohama? How useful if there is another Korean war? How useful if China begins to dominate the region? How useful if a declining and nervous USSR takes aggressive actions? There is, of course, no way of answering such hypothetical and alarming questions; yet even a mere "trading state" with small "self-defense forces" may one day find it unavoidable to provide some answers. As other nations have discovered in the past, commercial expertise and financial wealth sometimes no longer suffice in the anarchic world of international power politics.

The EEC—Potential and Problems

Of the five main concentrations of economic and military power in the world today, the only one that is not a sovereign nation-state is Europe—which at once defines the chief problem facing this region as it moves toward the emerging Great Power system of the early twenty-first century. Even if our consideration of the continent's future prospects excludes the Communist-controlled regimes in the east (as, for practical reasons, it must), we are still left with some states which are members of an economic-political organization (the EEC) but not of the chief military alliance (NATO), with others which adhere to the latter but not the former, and with important neutrals which are members of neither. Because of such anomalies, this section will focus upon the European Economic Community (and upon the policies of some of its leading members) rather than upon non-Communist Europe as a whole—for it is only in the EEC that an organization and structure exists, at least *potentially*, for a fifth world power.

But it is precisely because we are examining the EEC's *potential* rather than its present reality that the problem of guessing what it may be like in the year 2000 or 2020 is compounded. In some ways the situation is similar to that which, on a smaller scale, faced the members of the German Federation in the mid-nineteenth century.[85] A customs union existed which had proved to be so successful in stimulating trade and industry that it rapidly attracted new members, and it was clear that if that enlarged economic community was able to turn itself into a Power state it would be a major new actor in the international system—to which the established Great Powers would have to adjust accordingly. But so long as that transformation did not occur; so long as there were divisions among the members of the customs union about further economic integration and, still more, about political and military integration; so long as there were quarrels about which state should take the lead and disputes between the various parties and pressure groups about the benefits (or losses) accruing to them, then just so long would it stay divided, unable to realize its potential, and incapable of dealing as an equal with the other Great Powers. For all the differences of time and circumstance, the "German question" of the last century was a microcosm of the "European problem" of the present.

In its *potential,* the EEC clearly has the size, the wealth, and the productive capacity of a Great Power. With the adherence of Spain and Portugal, its twelve-member population now totals around 320 million—which is 50 million more than the USSR and almost half as big again as the U.S. population. Moreover, it is a highly trained population, with hundreds of universities and colleges across Europe and millions of scientists and engineers. While its average per capita income conceals great gulfs—say, between West German and Portuguese incomes—it is much richer on the whole than Russia, and some of its member states are richer per capita than the United States. As was pointed out earlier, it is by far the largest trading block in the world, although much of that is intra-European trade. Perhaps a better measure of its economic strength lies in its productive output, in automobiles, steel, cement, etc., which puts it ahead of the United States, Japan, and (except in steel) the USSR. Depending upon the annual statistics, and upon the wild swings in the value of the dollar relative to European currencies over the past six years, the total GNP of the EEC is about equal (1980, 1986) to that of the USA, or about two-thirds as big (1983–1984 figures). It is certainly far larger than Russia, Japan, or China in its share of world GNP or manufacturing output.

In military terms also, the European member states are far from negligible. Taking only the four largest countries (West Germany, France, Britain, Italy) into account, one finds their combined regular-army size to be over a million men, with a further 1.7 million in reserves[86]—a total which is of course smaller than the Russian and Chinese armies, but considerably larger than the U.S. Army. In addition, these four states possess hundreds of major surface warships and submarines and thousands of tanks, artillery, and aircraft. Finally, both France and Britain possess nuclear weapons, and delivery systems—sea-based and land-based. The implications and effectiveness of these military forces will be discussed below; the point being made here is simply that, *once combined,* the totals are very substantial. What is more, the spending upon these forces represents around 4 percent of the GNP, as a rough average. Were those countries, or, more significant still, the entire EEC, spending around 7 percent of total GNP on defense, as the United States is today, the sums allocated would be equal to hundreds of billions of dollars—that is, roughly the same amount as the two military superpowers spend.

And yet Europe's real power and effectiveness in the world is much less than the crude total of its economic and military strength would suggest—simply because of disunity. The armed forces, for example, not only suffer from a multitude of languages (a problem which the German Federation's members never had to face), but are equipped with many different weapons and have very marked differences in quality and training—between, say, the West German and the Greek armies, or the Royal Navy and the Spanish navy. Despite NATO's many attempts at standardization, one is still talking about a dozen armies, navies, and air forces of varying worth. But even those problems pale beside the obstacles at the *political* level, relating to the foreign and defense policy priorities of Europe. Ireland's traditional (and anachronistic) stance on neutrality prevents the EEC from discussing defense issues—although even if discussions occurred, they would probably soon founder upon Greek objections. Turkey, with its substantial army, is not a member of the EEC; and the Turkish and Greek armed forces often seem more worried about each other than about the Warsaw Pact. France's independent stance has (as will be seen below) military advantages and disadvantages; but it adds to the complications of consultation on defense and foreign-policy matters. Both Britain and France indulge in "out of area" operations and, indeed, still maintain an array of bases and troops overseas. For West Germany, the overriding defense issue—toward which *all* its forces are geared— is the security of its eastern frontier. Evolving a unified European policy toward, say, the Palestinian issue, or even toward the United States itself, is inordinately complex (and often fails), because of the differing interests and traditions of each of the member states.

In terms of economic integration, and of the constitutional and institutional arrangements that exist to implement decisions in the economic field, the EEC is obviously much further ahead; even so, as an "economic community," it is much more splintered than a sovereign state would ever be. Political ideology always affects economic policy and priorities. Coordination is difficult, if not impossible, when socialist regimes are in power in some of the member states and conservative parties are dominant in the others. Although the coordination of currencies is now more successful than it was, the occasional realignments which do take place (usually involving a revaluation of the German mark) are a reminder of the separate fiscal systems—and differentiated credit-worthiness—of the members. Despite proposals from the European Commission, there is as yet little progress toward a common European policy on a whole variety of issues, from full-scale airline deregulation to financial services. At too many of the common frontiers there are still customs posts, and lengthy checks, to the fury of the truck drivers. Even agriculture, the mainstay of the EEC's spending functions and one of the few economic sectors where there is a "common market," has proved to be a bone of contention.

And if it is indeed likely that world foodstuffs production will continue to expand, with India and other Asian countries increasingly entering the export markets, the pressure to reform the EEC's price-support system will build up, until the issue explodes into heated controversy again.

Finally, there is the persistent worry that after its postwar decades of economic growth and success, Europe is beginning to stagnate, and perhaps even to decline. The problems caused by the oil crisis of 1979—the steep rise in fuel prices, the pressure upon balance of payments, the general world depression in demand, output, and trade— seemed to hit the Europeans harder than many of the other major economies of the earth, as is indicated by Table 45.

Table 45. Growth in Real GNP, 1979–1983[87]
(percent)

	1979	1980	1981	1982	1983
United States	2.8	−0.3	2.6	−0.5	2.4
Canada	3.4	1.0	4.0	−4.2	3.0
Japan	5.1	4.9	4.0	3.2	3.0
China	7.0	5.2	3.0	7.4	9.0
EEC (ten)	3.5	1.1	−0.3	0.5	0.8

One of the chief concerns of the European states has been the effect of this slump upon employment levels—the number of people losing their jobs in western Europe in recent years has been much higher than at any time in the post-1945 era (for example, it leaped from 5.9 million to 10.2 million within the EEC between 1978 and 1982) and has shown little sign of coming down—which in turn swells the already extremely high level of social expenditures, leaving less for investment.[88] Nor has there been anything like the creation of new jobs on the scale which has occurred in the United States (chiefly in low-paying service industries) and Japan (in high technology and services) as the 1980s have unfolded. Whether one ascribes this to the lack of business incentives, high costs and immobility of the labor market, and bureaucratic over-regulation (as right-wingers tend to do), or to the failure of the state to plan and invest sufficiently (as the Left usually sees it), or to a fatal combination of both, the result is the same. More alarming still, to many commentators, have been the signs that Europe is falling behind its American and (especially) its Japanese competitors in the high-technology stakes of the future. Thus, the 1984–85 *Annual Economic Report* of the European Commission warned:

> The Community is now having to respond to the challenge of an emerging inferiority, by comparison with the United States and Japan, in industrial capacity in new and fast-growing technologies.

. . . The deteriorating world trade performance of the Community
in such fields as computers, micro-electronics, and equipment is
now generally recognized.[89]

Quite possibly, this picture of "Eurosclerosis" and "Europessimism"
has been painted too gloomily, for there are many other signs of European competitiveness—in quality automobiles, commercial and fighter
aircraft, satellites, chemicals, telecommunications systems, financial
services, etc. Nevertheless, the two most pressing issues remain in
doubt. Is the EEC, because of the sociopolitical diversity of its members, as capable as its overseas competitors of responding to swift and
large-scale shifts in employment patterns? Or is it designed more to
slow down the impact of economic changes upon uncompetitive sectors (agriculture, textiles, shipbuilding, coal, and steel), and, in being
so humane in the short term, disadvantaging itself in the longer term?
And is the EEC capable of mobilizing the scientific and investment
resources to remain a leading contender in the high-technology stakes,
when its own companies are nowhere near as big as the American and
Japanese giants, and when any "industrial strategy" has to be worked
out, not by the likes of MITI, but by *twelve* governments (plus the EEC
Commission), each exhibiting different concerns?

If one turned one's attention from the EEC as a whole to a brief
examination of the situation in which the leading *three* military/politi-
cal countries of Europe find themselves, the sense of "potential" being
threatened by "problems" is only reinforced. No state, arguably, manifests this ambivalence about the future more than the Federal Republic
of Germany, in large part because of its inheritance from the past and
the still "provisional" nature of the present structure of Europe.

Although many Germans fret about the economic prospects for
their country by the early twenty-first century, that can hardly be
regarded as the major concern (especially as compared with the economic difficulties facing other societies). While its total labor force is
only a little higher than Britain's or France's, its GNP is significantly
larger, reflecting an economy whose long-term productive growth has
been extremely impressive. It is the largest producer in the EEC of
steel, chemicals, electrical goods, automobiles, tractors, and (given
Britain's decline) even merchant ships and coal. Because of a remarkably low level both of inflation and of labor disputes, it has kept its
export prices competitive, despite the frequent upward valuations of
the deutsche mark—which are, after all, merely belated acknowledgments by other nations of West Germany's better economic performance. A heavy emphasis upon engineering and design in the German
management tradition (as opposed to the American emphasis upon
finance) has given it an international reputation for quality products.
Year after year, the German economy has notched up a surplus in its

PAUL KENNEDY

trade balances second only to Japan's. Its international reserves are larger than those of any other country in the world (except, presumably, those of Japan after the latter's recent surge), and the deutsche mark is often used by other nations as a reserve currency.

As against all this, one can point to those factors which give the Germans cause for *Angst*.[90] The EEC's agricultural price-support system, long a drain for the German taxpayer, redistributes resources from the most competitive to the least competitive sectors of the economy—and not just in the Federal Republic itself (where there are a surprisingly large number of small farms), but to the peasantry of southern Europe. This has obvious social value, but it is a burden proportionately much larger than the protection given to American and perhaps even to Japanese agriculture. The persistently high level of unemployment, a sign that the Federal Republic still has too large a proportion of its work force in older industries, is also a major drain upon the economy, keeping social-security payments at a very high proportion of GDP; and while unemployment among the youth can be alleviated by the impressively broad level of training and apprenticeships, and will also be eased by the rapid aging of the German population, this latter trend is perhaps regarded with the greatest unease of all. If it is clearly an exaggeration to believe that the German race will "die out," the steep decline in the birth rate will have obvious repercussions upon the German economy when an even larger share of the population consists of old-age pensioners. Along with this demographic fear goes the much less tangible worry that the "successor generation" will not want to work as earnestly as those who rebuilt Germany from the wartime ashes, and that with higher wage costs and far shorter working weeks than the Japanese, even German productivity growth will not keep up with the challenge from the Pacific basin.

Even so, none of those problems are insuperable, provided the Germans can maintain their "package" of low inflation, quality goods, high investment in new technology, superior design and salesmanship, and labor peace. (At the very least, one can say that if the problems named above affect the German economy, how much more will they hurt the economies of most of its less competitive neighbors!) What is much more difficult to forecast is whether the extraordinarily complex and quite unique contours of the "German question" as they have existed since the late 1940s will continue unchanged into the twenty-first century: that is, whether there will continue to be two "Germanies," separated by hostile alliances, despite the growing intimacy between them; whether the NATO alliance (of which the Federal Republic is such a central part) can defend the German lands without destroying them, should East-West relations worsen into hostilities; and whether, in the event of a diminution in American power and a reduction of its forces in Europe, Germany and its major EEC/NATO

partners can provide an adequate substitute for the U.S. strategic umbrella which has served so well for the past forty years. None of these
interrelated issues are crying out for an immediate solution, but all of
them are giving thoughtful observers grounds for concern.

The "German-German" relationship will probably seem, at this
time, the most hypothetical of the cluster. As has been made clear in
the preceding chapters, the proper place of the German people within
the European states system has troubled statesmen for at least the past
century and a half.[91] If all those speaking the German tongue are
brought together as one nation-state—as has been the European norm
for nearly two centuries—the resultant concentration of population
and industrial might would always make Germany the economic
power center of west-central Europe. That itself need not *necessarily*
turn it into the dominant military-territorial force in Europe as well,
in the way that the imperialism of both the Wilhelmine and (even
more) the Nazi eras led to a German bid for hegemony. In a bipolar
world which, militarily, is still dominated by Washington and Moscow,
in an age when major Great Power aggressions run the risk of triggering a nuclear war, and with a post-1945 "de-Nazified" generation of
German politicians running affairs in Bonn and East Berlin, the notion
of any future Germanic bid for "mastery in Europe" seems anachronistic. Even were it attempted, the balance of European (let alone global)
power would prevail against it. In abstract terms, therefore, there is
surely nothing wrong *and a lot that is right* with permitting the 62
million "West" Germans and 17 million "East" Germans to reunite,
particularly when each population increasingly perceives that it has
more in common with the other than with its superpower guardian.

Yet the tragic fact is that however logical that solution is in one
sense—and however much the two German peoples are showing signs
(despite the ideological gulf) of their common inheritance and culture—the present political realities speak against it, even if it took the
form of a loose Germanic federation on the nineteenth-century model,
as has been ingeniously suggested.[92] For the blunt fact is that East
Germany serves as a strategical barrier for the Soviet control over the
buffer states of eastern Europe (not to say the jump-off position for a
move to the west); and since the men in the Kremlin still think in terms
of imperialist *Realpolitik,* letting the German Democratic Republic
gravitate toward (and into) the Federal Republic would be regarded as
a major blow. As one authority has recently pointed out, based on
present forces alone, a unified Germany could field over 660,000 regular troops plus 1.5 million paramilitary and reservists. The USSR could
not view with equanimity a unified German nation with an army of 2
million on its western flank.[93] On the other hand, it seems difficult to
see why a *peacefully* united Germany should want to maintain armed
forces of that size, forces which reflect present Cold War tensions. It

is also difficult to believe that despite its heavy-handed emphasis upon the lessons of the Second World War, even the Soviet leadership accepts its own propaganda about German revanchism and neo-Nazism (which has been an increasingly difficult position to maintain since Willy Brandt's period of office). But what is also clear is that Moscow has a congenital dislike of withdrawing from *anywhere,* and also worries deeply about the political consequences of a reunited Germany. Not only would it be a formidable economic Power in its own right—with a total GNP dangerously close to the USSR's own, at least in formal dollar-equivalent terms—but it also would act as a trading magnet for all of its eastern European neighbors. Even more fundamental a point: how could Russia withdraw from East Germany without provoking the question of a similar withdrawal from Czechoslovakia, Hungary, and Poland—leaving as the USSR's western frontier the dubious Polish/Ukrainian borderline, which is temptingly close for the fifty million Ukrainians?

What remains, therefore, is a state of suspended animation. Intra-German trade relations are likely to grow (clouded only by the occasional tension between the superpowers); each German state is likely to become relatively more productive and richer than its neighbors; each will swear loyalty to its supranational military (NATO/Warsaw Pact) and economic (EEC/Comecon) organizations while making special arrangements with its Germanic sister state. It is impossible to forecast how Bonn would react should the Soviet Union itself be shaken and upset from within—and should that coincide with serious unrest in the German Democratic Republic. It is also impossible to forecast how the "East" Germans would react if there was to be a Warsaw-Pact offensive westward. Certainly, the special Soviet "control" arrangements over the Democratic Republic's army, and the shadowing of every one of its divisions by a Russian motor-rifle division, suggest that even the grim men in the Kremlin worry about setting German against German—as well they should.

But the more concrete and immediate problem which the Federal Republic faces—and has faced since its existence—has been to discover a viable defense policy in the event of a war in Europe. From the beginning (see pp. 378–79), the apprehension that a vastly superior Red Army could strike westward without much hindrance led both the Germans and their fellow Europeans to rely upon the U.S. nuclear deterrent as their chief security. Ever since the USSR acquired the capacity to hit the American homeland with its own ICBMs, however, that strategy has been in doubt—would Washington really begin a nuclear interchange in response to a Russian conventional attack on the northern German plain?—even if it has never been officially abandoned. This is also true of the related question of whether the United States would unleash strategic nuclear attacks against the Soviet Union (again, inviting reprisals upon its own cities) if the Russians contented themselves with firing short- or *intermediate*-range missiles (SS-20s) solely at European targets. There has been, to be sure, no lack of proposals for creating a "credible deterrent" to meet such contingencies: installing Pershing II and various forms of cruise-missile systems to counter the Russian SS-20s; producing an enhanced-radiation (or "neutron") bomb, intended to kill off invading Warsaw Pact troops without damage to buildings and infrastructure; and—in the French case—reliance upon a Paris-controlled deterrent force as an alternative to an uncertain American defense system. All of these, however, have their own attendant problems;[94] and, quite apart from the political reactions which they provoke, each of them points to the uniquely contradictory nature of nuclear weapon systems—that having recourse to them is more than likely to lead to the destruction of that which one wishes to defend.

It is scarcely surprising, therefore, that while successive West German administrations have paid lip service to the value of NATO's nuclear-deterrence strategy, and have foresworn the acquisition of nuclear weapons for themselves, they have been to the fore in the creation of a strong *conventional* defense system. As it is, the Bundeswehr has not only the largest of the NATO armies in Europe (335,000 troops, with 645,000 trained reserves)[95] but also one of extremely high quality and with good equipment; provided it did not lose command of the air, it would give an impressive account of itself. On the other hand, the steeply declining birthrate makes it increasingly difficult to maintain the Bundeswehr at full strength, while the government's desire to keep defense spending down to 3.5 to 4 percent of GNP means that it will be difficult for the armed services to procure as much new equipment as they need.[96] At the end of the day, such weakness can be overcome—just as the deficiencies in the less-well-equipped Allied armies stationed in West Germany could be overcome, given the political will. However, this still leaves the Germans facing the uncomfortable (for some, intolerable) dilemma that any outbreak of large-scale hostilities in central Europe would lead to incalculable bloodshed and material loss on their territory.

It is not surprising, therefore, that since at least the time of Willy Brandt's chancellorship the government in Bonn has been to the fore in its pursuit of *détente* in Europe—and not merely with its German sister state, but also with eastern European nations and with the USSR itself, in an endeavor to calm their traditional fears of a too-strong Germany; and that it, more than all its NATO partners, has partaken in and financed East-West trade in the Cobdenite belief that economic interdependence makes war more difficult (and also no doubt because West German banks and industries are so favorably placed to take advantage of that commerce). This does not imply a move into "neu-

tralism" for the two Germanies—as is sometimes proposed by left-wing
Social Democrats and the Green Party—for that would depend upon
securing Moscow's consent to East German neutralism as well, which
is highly unlikely. What it does mean is that West Germany sees its
security problem concentrated almost exclusively in Europe and shuns
any "out-of-area" capability—let alone the occasional extra-European
actions in which the French and British still indulge. By extension,
therefore, it dislikes being forced to take a position on the (in its view)
distracting and distant issues in the Near East and farther afield, and
that in turn leads it into disagreements with a U.S. government which
feels that the preservation of western security cannot be so neatly
limited to central Europe. In its relationship to Moscow and East Berlin on the one hand and to non-European issues on the other, West
Germany finds it difficult if not impossible to conduct a merely bilateral diplomacy; it must, instead, have regard for the reactions of Washington (and, often, of Paris). That, too, is a price which has to be paid
for its awkward and unique position in the international power system.[97]

If the Federal Republic finds the economic challenges less intracti-
ble than foreign- and defense-policy problems, the same cannot be said
for the United Kingdom. It, too, is the legatee of a historical past—and,
of course, of a geographical position—which strongly influences its
policy toward the world outside. But, as we have seen in earlier chapters, it is also the country among the former Great Powers whose
economy and society have found it hardest to adjust to the shifting
patterns of technology and manufacturing in the post-1945 decades
(and in many respects in the decades before). The most devastating
impact of the global changes has been upon manufacturing, a sector
which once earned Britain the title "workshop of the world." It is true
that among many of the advanced economies of the world, manufacturing's share of output and employment has been steadily shrinking
while other sectors (e.g., services) have grown; but in Britain's case the
fall has been much more precipitous. Not only has its proportion of
world manufacturing output continued its remorseless decline *relatively*, but it has also decreased *absolutely*. More shocking still has
been the abrupt switch in the place of manufactures in Britain's foreign trade. While it may be difficult to prove *The Economist*'s tart
observation that "since 1983, Britain's trade balance on manufactures
has been in deficit for the first time since the Romans invaded Britain,"
it is a fact that even in the late 1950s exports of manufactures were
three times as big as imports.[98] Now that surplus has gone. What is
more, the decline in employment occurs not only in older industries
but also in the "sunrise" high-technology firms.[99]

If the fall in Britain's manufacturing competitiveness is a century-
old tale,[100] it has clearly been accelerated by the discovery of North Sea

oil, which while producing earnings to cover the visible trade gap has also had the effect of turning sterling into a "petrocurrency," sending its value to unrealistically high levels for a while and making many of its exports uncompetitive. Even when the oil runs out, causing sterling to decline further, it is not at all clear that that would *ipso facto* lead to a revival in manufacturing: plant has been scrapped, foreign markets lost (perhaps permanently), and international competitiveness eroded by higher than average rises in unit labor costs. Britain's shift into services is somewhat more promising, but it nonetheless remains as true here as in the United States that many services (from window cleaning to fast food) neither earn foreign currency nor are particularly productive. Even in the expanding, high-earning fields of international banking, investment, commodity dealing, and so on, it seems clear that the competition is, if anything, more intense—and in the past thirty years "Britain's share of world trade in services has fallen from 18 percent to 7 percent."[101] As banking and finance become a global business, increasingly dominated by those (chiefly American and Japanese) firms with massive capital resources in New York *and* London *and* Tokyo, the British share may diminish further. Finally, future developments in telecommunications and office equipment are already suggesting that white-collar jobs may soon follow the path already trodden by blue-collar workers in the West.

None of this, one hopes, portends a cataclysm. A general growth in world output and trade would help to keep the British economy afloat, even if its share of the whole gently declined and its per capita GNP was steadily being overtaken by many more nations, from Italy to Singapore. The decline could intensify, if a change of government led to large increases in social spending (rather than productive investment), higher taxation levels, a drop in business confidence, and a flight from sterling; it might slow down, with a government which adopted a less strict monetary policy, evolved a coherent "industrial strategy," and cooperated with fellow Europeans in marketable (and nonprestige) ventures. It also may be true, as one economist maintains,[102] that British manufacturing is now altogether leaner, fitter, and more competitive, having undergone an "industrial renaissance." But the auguries for a spectacular turnaround are not good; the relative immobility and lack of training in the labor market, the high unit costs, and the comparative smallness of even the largest British manufacturing firms are very considerable handicaps. The output of engineers and scientists is still dismally low. Above all, there is the poor level of investment in R&D: for every $1 spent in Britain on R&D in the early 1980s, $1.50 was spent in Germany, $3 in Japan, and $8 in the United States—yet 50 percent of that British R&D was devoted to nonproductive defense activities, compared with Germany's 9 percent and Japan's minuscule amount.[103] By contrast with its chief rivals (except the

United States), British R&D is both much less related to industry's needs and much less paid for by industry itself.

The large proportion devoted to defense-related R&D brings us onto the other horn of the British dilemma. If it was an unambitious, obscure, isolated, pacific state, its slow industrial anemia would be a pity—but irrelevant to the international power system. Yet the fact is that, although much shrunken from its Victorian heyday, Britain still remains—or claims to be—one of the leading "midsized" Powers of the globe. Its defense budget is the third- or fourth-largest (depending upon how one measures China's total), its navy the fourth-largest, its air force the fourth-largest[104]—all of which, it might be thought, is significantly out of proportion to its geographical size (a mere 245,000 square kilometers), its population (56 million) and its modest, declining share of world GNP (3.38 percent in 1983). Furthermore, despite its imperial sunset, it still has very extensive strategical commitments abroad: not only in the 65,000 troops and airmen in Germany as its contribution to NATO's Central Front, but also in garrisons and naval bases across the globe—Belize, Cyprus, Gibraltar, Hong Kong, the Falklands, Brunei, the Indian Ocean. Despite all the premature announcements, it is still not one with Nineveh and Tyre.[105]

This divergence between Britain's shrunken economic state and its overextended strategical posture is probably more extreme than that affecting any other of the larger Powers, except Russia itself. It therefore finds itself particularly vulnerable to the fact that weapon prices are rising 6 to 10 percent faster than inflation, and that every new weapon system is three to five times costlier than that which it is intended to replace. It is made the more vulnerable in consequence of domestic-political constraints upon defense spending; while Conservative administrations feel it necessary to contain arms spending in order to reduce the deficit, any alternative regime would feel inclined to chop defense expenditures in absolute terms. Quite apart from this political dilemma, however, there looms for Britain a fundamental and (soon) unavoidable choice: *either* to cut allocations to all of the armed services, placing each of them in a less than effective state; *or* to cut some of the nation's defense commitments.

Yet as soon as that proposition is stated, the obstacles emerge. Command of the air is taken to be axiomatic (hence the RAF's superior budget), even while the cost of new Euro-fighters is spiraling out of sight. By far the greatest British overseas commitment is to Germany and Berlin (almost $4 billion), but even now those 55,000 troops, 600 tanks, and 3,000 other armored vehicles are, despite high morale, underprovisioned. However, any reduction in the size of the BAOR (British Army on the Rhine) or fancy-footwork scheme to keep half the troops in British rather than German garrisons is likely to trigger off such *political* repercussions—from German grief, to Belgian emulation, to American annoyance—that it could be totally counterproductive. A second alternative is to reduce the size of the surface fleet—the Ministry of Defence solution of 1981, until the Falklands crisis upset that scheme.[106] But while such an alternative probably has the most advocates in Whitehall's corridors of power, it looks ill-timed in the face of Russia's rising naval challenge and the increasing American emphasis upon NATO having an "out-of-area" thrust. (And it is certainly a contradiction for the advocates of enhancing NATO's conventional forces in Europe to agree to reductions in the alliance's second-largest fleet of Atlantic escorts.) A more possible candidate for "cuts" would be Britain's expensive and (while emotionally understandable) vastly overextended commitments in the Falkland Islands: but even that retrenchment would probably only postpone a longer decision for several years. Finally, there is the investment in the very expensive Trident submarine-based ballistic-missile system, the costs of which seem to rise month by month.[107] Given the Conservative government's enthusiasm for an advanced and "independent" deterrent system—not to mention the way in which the Trident boats may actually be altering the overall nuclear balance (see below, p. 506)—that decision is only likely with a radical change of administration in Britain, which in turn might throw more than future defense policy into question.

At the end of the day, however, the awkward choice is there. As the *Sunday Times* has put it, "Unless something is done soon, this country's defense policy will increasingly consist of trying to do the same job with less money, which can only be bad for Britain and NATO."[108] This leaves the politicians (of *any* party) with the alternative of reducing certain commitments, and enduring the consequences thereof; or of increasing defense expenditures still further—and Britain spends proportionately more (5.5 percent of GNP) than any other European NATO partner except Greece—and thereby reducing its own investment in productive growth and its long-term prospects for an economic recovery. As with most decaying Powers, there is only a choice of hard options.

The same dilemma confronts Britain's neighbor across the Channel, even if that has been concealed by the lack of sustained domestic questioning of France's defense policy, and by a significantly better (if still flawed) economic performance since the 1950s. At the end of the day, Paris, like London, has to grapple with the problem of being only a "midsized" Power with extensive national interests and overseas commitments, the defense of which is coming under steadily increased pressure from escalating weapon costs.[109] While its population is the same as Britain's, its total GNP and its per capita GNP are larger. The French produce more cars and more steel than the British and have a very large aerospace industry. Unlike Britain, France remains heavily

dependent upon imported oil; on the other hand, it still runs a considerable surplus in agricultural goods, which are heavily subsidized by
the EEC. In a number of significant high-technology fields—telecommunications, space satellites, aircraft, nuclear power—the French
have shown a strong commitment to keeping abreast with worldwide
competition. If France's economy was badly dented by the Socialist
administration's dash for growth in the early 1980s (just when all its
major trading partners were retrenching fiscally), the stricter policies
which followed seem to have reduced inflation, cut the trade gap, and
stabilized the franc, all of which ought to allow for a resumption in
French economic growth.

But whenever France's economic structure and prospects are compared with those of its powerful neighbor across the Rhine—or with
Japan's—the precariousness shows through. While France is still spectacularly adroit in exporting fighter aircraft, wines, and grain, it "remains relatively weak in selling run-of-the-mill manufactured goods
abroad."[110] Too many of its customers have been unstable Third World
countries that order lavish projects like dams or Mirages and then have
difficulty paying for them; by contrast, the "import penetration" of
industrial goods, automobiles, and electrical appliances into France
indicates broad fields where it is not competitive. Its trade deficit with
West Germany grows year by year and, since French prices always rise
faster than those in Germany, will in all probability lead to further
devaluations of the franc. The northern landscape of France is still
scarred with decaying industries—coal, iron, steel, shipbuilding—and
much of its automobile industry is also feeling the strain. And while
the new technologies seem full of promise, neither can they absorb
France's many unemployed nor are they receiving the levels of investment necessary to keep pace with German, Japanese, and American
technologies. More worrying still for a country as economically (and,
of perhaps greater import, psychologically) attached to agriculture is
the looming crisis of global overproduction of grains, dairy produce,
fruit, wine, etc.—with its increasing strain upon French and EEC budgets if farm-support prices are maintained and its threat of social
unrest if prices are cut. Until a few years ago, Paris could rely upon
Community funds to aid in restructuring agriculture; now, most of that
cash is likely to go to the peasants of Spain, Portugal, and Greece. All
this may leave France without the capital resources necessary for a
much larger R&D effort and for sustained, high-tech-based growth
over the next two decades.

It is in this larger context, of fixing priorities for France's future,
that one needs to view the debate over national defense policy. In many
ways, there is much that is impressive about French strategy, and
military actions, in recent times. Recognizing (and assertively voicing)
the increasing doubts about the credibility of the American strategic

nuclear deterrent, France has provided itself with its own "triad" of delivery systems for use in the event of Soviet aggression. By keeping in its own hands every aspect of its nuclear deterrent (from production to targeting), and by insisting that its entire force of missiles will be loosed at Russia if deterrence fails, Paris feels it has a more certain way of holding the Kremlin in check. At the same time, it has maintained one of the largest land armies and has a substantial garrison in south-western Germany and a commitment to come to the Federal Republic's aid; while being outside the NATO command structure, and thus able to proffer an independent "European" voice on strategic issues, it has not dislocated the military need for reinforcing the Central Front in the event of a Russian attack. The French have also maintained an extra-European role and—by means of occasional military interventions overseas, the presence of their garrisons and advisers in Third World countries, and their successful arms-sales policy—offered an alternative influence (and source of supply) to either the USSR or the United States. If this has sometimes irritated Washington—and if French nuclear testing in the South Pacific has rightly annoyed the countries of that region—then Moscow in its turn can hardly be comforted by the various and sometimes unpredictable displays of Gallic independence. Furthermore, since both the right and the left in France support the idea of the nation's playing a distinct role abroad, French claims and actions for that purpose do not provoke the domestic criticism which would occur in virtually all other Western societies. All this had led foreign observers (and, of course, Frenchmen themselves) to describe their policy as logical, hard-nosed, realistic, and so on.

Yet the policy itself is not without its problems—as some French commentators are beginning openly to admit[111]—and must cause the historically minded to recall the gap which existed between the theory and the reality of France's defense policy prior to 1914 and 1939. In the first place, there is a great deal of truth in the cold observation that all of France's posturings of independence have taken place behind the American shield and guarantee to western Europe, both conventional and nuclear. A Gaullist policy of assertiveness was only possible, Raymond Aron pointed out, because for the first time in this century France was not in the front line.[112] But what if that security disappears? That is, what if the American nuclear deterrent is admitted to be noncredible? What if the United States, over time, steadily pulls back its troops, tanks, and aircraft from Europe? Under certain circumstances, both of those eventualities might be seen as welcome. Yet, as the French themselves admit, they can hardly appear so in the light of Moscow's recent policies: steadily building up its own nuclear *and* European-based conventional forces to excessive levels, keeping a tight hold upon its eastern European satellites, and launching "peace offensives" designed perhaps particularly to wean the West German public out of the NATO alliance and into neutralism. Many of the signs of what has been termed France's "New Atlanticism"[113]—a stiffer tone toward the Soviet Union, criticism of neutralist tendencies among the German Social Democrats, the Franco-German agreement for the forward deployment in Germany (possibly with tactical nuclear weapons) of the Force d'Action Rapide, the closer links with NATO[114]—are obvious consequences of French concern about the future. Until Moscow changes, Paris is bound to worry that the USSR might move *into* western Europe when (or even before) the United States has moved *out*.

But if that threat became more likely, what could France do about it in *practical* terms? Naturally, it could increase its conventional forces still further, moving toward the creation of an enhanced Franco-German army strong enough to hold off a Russian assault even if U.S. forces were diminished (or even absent). In the view of people like Helmut Schmidt,[115] this is the logical extension not only of the Paris-Bonn *entente* but also of international trends (e.g., the weakening of American capacities). There are all sorts of political and organizational difficulties in the way of such a scheme—ranging from the possible attitude of a future left-of-center German administration, to questions of command, language and deployment, to the touchy issue of French tactical nuclear weapons[116]—but in any event such a strategy is likely to founder upon one insuperable reef: lack of money. France is currently spending about 4.2 percent of its GNP upon defense (compared with the United States' 7.4 percent and Britain's 5.5 percent), but given the delicate state of the French economy, that percentage cannot be increased by very much. Moreover, France's independence in atomic-weapons development means that its nuclear strategic forces absorb up to 30 percent of the defense budget, far more than elsewhere. What is left is not enough for the AMX battle tank, advanced aircraft, the new nuclear-powered aircraft carrier, "smart" battlefield weapons, and so on. While certain increases in the French armed forces may be likely, that could not possibly satisfy all requirements.[117] Just as in Britain's case, therefore, the French are being faced with the awkward choice of either eliminating some weapon systems (and roles) entirely or forcing economies upon all of them.

Equally worrying are the doubts being raised about France's nuclear deterrent, both at the technical and the (related) strategical level. Parts of the triad of French nuclear weaponry—the land-based missiles, and especially the aircraft—suffer from deterioration over time and even their costly upgrading and modernization may not keep pace with newer weapons technology.[118] This problem may become particularly acute if significant breakthroughs occur in American Strategic Defense Initiative (SDI) technology, and if the Russians in their turn develop a much larger system of ballistic-missile defense. Nothing is more disturbing, from the French viewpoint, than the two superpowers enhancing their potential invulnerability while Europe remains exposed. As against this, there is the significant buildup of the French submarine-launched ballistic-missile system (discussed below, p. 506). However, the general principle remains: advanced technology could render useless existing types of weaponry, and certainly will make the cost of any replacements much more expensive. In any case, the French are caught in the same trap of credibility as all of the other nuclear Powers. If Paris thinks it increasingly unlikely that the United States would risk a strategic nuclear exchange with the USSR because the German frontier had been invaded, how likely is its own promise to "go nuclear" on behalf of the Federal Republic? (The West Germans hardly believe it.) Even the Gaullist tradition of defending the "sanctuary" of France by firing off all its missiles at Russia hangs upon the unproven assumption that the French people prefer obliteration to a possible (or likely) defeat by conventional means. "Tearing an arm off the Russian bear" has always sounded like a good phrase, until it is remembered that one will certainly be devoured by the bear; and that Russia's own antimissile defenses may limit the damage it will suffer. Obviously, the official posture of French nuclear strategy is not going to be altered soon, if at all. But it is worth wondering how realistic it is, should the East-West balance worsen and the United States weaken.[119]

France's problem, then, is that so many demands are pressing upon its own modest national resources. Given demographic and structural-economic trends, the high share of national income consumed by social security is likely to continue, and probably increase. Large funds may soon be needed for the agricultural sector. At the same time, the modernization of the armed forces requires substantial amounts of money. Yet all of these have to be balanced against—and take away from—the pressing need for vastly enlarged investment in R&D and in advanced industrial processes. If it cannot allocate the monies necessary for the last-named purpose, it will over time put into jeopardy the prospects of affording defense, social security, and all the rest. Obviously this dilemma is not France's alone, although it is the French above all who have argued for a distinctively "European" position on international economic and defense issues—and who therefore most clearly articulate European concerns. For this reason, too, it is Paris which has usually taken the lead in initiating new policies—deepening Franco-German military ties, producing European Airbuses and satellites, and so on. Many of these schemes have met with skepticism among France's neighbors at this Gallic fondness for bureaucratic planning and prestige endeavors, or with the suspicion that French companies are likely to be awarded the lion's share of Euro-funded projects. Other schemes, however, have already proved their worth or seem to hold a rich promise.

Europe's "problems" are, of course, more than those considered here: they include aging populations and aging industries, ethnic discontents in the inner cities, the gap between the prosperous north and the poorer south, the political/linguistic tensions in Belgium, Ulster, and northern Spain. Pessimistic observers also occasionally allude to the possibility of a "Finlandization" of certain European states (Denmark, West Germany), which would then become dependent upon Moscow. Since that development could only follow from a leftward political shift in the countries concerned, it is difficult to estimate its likelihood. As it is, if one considers Europe—as represented chiefly by the EEC—as a *power-political* unit in the global system, the most important issues it faces are clearly those discussed above: how to evolve a common defense policy for the coming century which will be viable even in what may be an era of significant change in the international power balances; and how to remain competitive against the very formidable economic challenges posed by new technology and new commercial competitors. In the case of the other four regions and societies examined in this chapter, it is possible to suggest what changes are likely to occur over time in their present position: that Japan and China will probably see their status in the world enhanced, and that the USSR and even the United States will see theirs eroded. But Europe remains an enigma. If the European Community can really act together, it may well improve its position in the world, both militarily and economically. If it does not—which, given human nature, is the more plausible outcome—its relative decline seems destined to continue.

The Soviet Union and Its "Contradictions"

The word "contradiction" in Marxist terminology is a very specific one, and refers to the tensions which (it is argued) inherently exist within the capitalist system of production and will inevitably cause its demise.[120] It may therefore seem deliberately ironic to employ the same expression to describe the position in which the Soviet Union, the world's first Communist state, now finds itself. Nevertheless, as will be described below, in a number of absolutely critical areas there seems to be opening up an ever-widening gap between the aims of the Soviet state and the methods employed to reach them. It proclaims the need for enhanced agricultural and industrial output, yet hobbles that possibility by collectivization and by heavy-handed planning. It asserts the overriding importance of world peace, yet its own massive arms buildup and its link with "revolutionary" states (together with its revolutionary heritage) serve to increase international tensions. It claims to require absolute security along its extensive borders, yet its hitherto unyielding policy toward its neighbors' own security concerns worsens

THE RISE AND FALL OF THE GREAT POWERS

Moscow's relations—with western and eastern Europe, with Middle East peoples, with China and Japan—and in turn makes the Russians feel "encircled" and *less* secure. Its philosophy asserts the ongoing dialectical process of change in world affairs, driven by technology and new means of production, and inevitably causing all sorts of political and social transformations; and yet its own autocratic and bureaucratic habits, the privileges which cushion the party elites, the restrictions upon the free interchange of knowledge, and the lack of a personal-incentive system make it horribly ill-equipped to handle the explosive but subtle high-tech future which is already emerging in Japan and California. Above all, while its party leaders frequently insist that the USSR will never again accept a position of military inferiority, and even more frequently urge the nation to increase production, it has clearly found it difficult to reconcile those two aims; and, in particular, to check a Russian tradition of devoting too high a share of national resources to the armed forces—with deleterious consequences for its ability to compete with other societies commercially. Perhaps there are other ways of labeling all these problems, but it does not seem inappropriate to term them "contradictions."

Given the emphasis in Marxian philosophy upon the *material* basis of existence, it may seem doubly ironic that the chief difficulties facing the USSR today are located in its economic substructure; and yet the evidence gleaned by western experts—not to mention the increasingly open acknowledgments by the Soviet leadership itself—leave no doubt that that is so. It would be interesting to know how Khrushchev, who in the 1950s confidently forecast that the USSR would overtake the United States economically and "bury" capitalism, would have felt about Mr. Gorbachev's 1986 admissions to the 27th Communist Party Congress:

> Difficulties began to build up in the economy in the 1970s, with the rates of economic growth declining visibly. As a result, the targets for economic development set in the Communist Party program, and even the lower targets of the 9th and 10th 5-year plans were not attained. Neither did we manage to carry out the social program charted for this period. A lag ensued in the material base of science and education, health protection, culture and everyday services.
>
> Though efforts have been made of late, we have not succeeded in fully remedying the situation. There are serious lags in engineering, the oil and coal industries, the electrical engineering industry, in ferrous metals and chemicals in capital construction. Neither have the targets been met for the main indicators of efficiency and the improvement of the people's standard of living.
>
> Acceleration of the country's socio-economic development is the

key to all our problems; immediate and long-term, economic and
social, political and ideological, internal and external.[121]

To which it might be remarked that the final statement could have been
made by *any* government in the world, and that the mere recognition
of economic problems is no guarantee that they will be solved.

The most critical area of weakness in the economy during the entire
history of the Soviet Union has been agriculture, which is the more
amazing when it is recalled that a century ago Russia was one of the
two largest grain exporters in the world. Yet since the early 1970s it has
needed to import tens of millions of tons of wheat and corn each year.
If world food-production trends continue, Russia (and certain other
socialist economies of eastern Europe) will share with parts of Africa
and the Near East the dubious distinction of being the only countries
which have changed from being net food *exporters* to *importers* on a
large-scale and sustained way over recent years.[122] In Russia's case,
this embarrassing stagnation in agricultural output has not been for
want of attention or effort; since Stalin's death, every Soviet leader has
pressed for increases in food production, in order to meet consumer
demand and to fulfill the promised rises in the Russian standard of
living. It would be wrong to assume that such rises have not occurred—
clearly, the average Russian is much better off now than in 1953, when
his situation was desperate. But what is much more depressing is that
after some decades of drawing closer to the West, his standard of living
is falling behind again—despite all the resources which the state commits toward agriculture, which swallows up nearly 30 percent of total
investment (cf. 5 percent in the United States) and employs over 20
percent of the labor force (cf. 3 percent in the United States). Merely
in order to maintain standards of living, the USSR is compelled to
invest approximately $78 billion in agriculture each year, *and* to subsi-
dize food prices by a further $50 billion—despite which it seems "to be
moving further and further away from being the exporter it once
was"[123] and instead needs to pour out further billions of hard currency
to import grain and meats to make up its own shortfalls in agricultural
output.

There are, it is true, certain *natural* reasons for the precariousness
of Soviet agriculture, and for the fact that its productivity is about
one-seventh that of American farming. Although the USSR is often
regarded as geographically rather similar to the United States—both
being continent-wide, northern-hemisphere states—it actually lies
much farther to the north: the Ukraine is on the same latitude as
southern Canada. Not only does this make it difficult to grow corn, but
even the Soviet wheat-growing regions endure far colder winters—and
are subject to more frequent droughts—than states like Kansas and
Oklahoma. The four years 1979–1982 were particularly bad in that

respect, and so embarrassed the government that it stopped giving details of agricultural output (although its average import of 35 million tons of grain each year provided a clue!). Even the "good" year of 1983 did not make the USSR self-sufficient—and it was followed in turn by yet another disastrous year of cold and drought.[124] Moreover, any attempt to increase production by extending the wheat acreage into the "virgin lands" is always constricted by frosts in the north and the arid conditions in the south.

Nevertheless, no outside observers are convinced that it is climate alone which has depressed Soviet agricultural output.[125] By far the biggest problems are simply caused by the "socialization" of agriculture. To keep the Russian populace happy, food prices are held artificially low through subsidies, so that "meat costing the state $4 a pound to produce sells for 80 cents a pound"[126]—which, for example, makes it cheaper for peasants to buy and feed bread and potatoes to their livestock than to use unprocessed grain. The vast amounts of state investment in agriculture are thrown at large-scale projects (dams, drainage) rather than at individual barns or up-to-date small tractors that an ordinary peasant might want. Decisions as to planting, investment, and so on are taken not by those who work the fields but by managers and bureaucrats. The denial of responsibility and initiative to the individual peasants is probably the single greatest reason for disappointing yields, chronic inefficiencies, and enormous wastage— although the wastage is clearly affected also by the inadequate storage facilities and lack of year-round roads, which causes "approximately 20 percent of the grain, fruit and vegetable harvest, and as much as 50 percent of the potato crop [to perish] because of poor storage, transportation and distribution."[127] What could be done if the system were altered in its fundamentals—that is, a massive change away from collectivization towards individual peasant-run farming—is indicated by the fact that the existing private plots produce around 25 percent of Russia's total crop output, yet occupy a mere 4 percent of the country's arable land.[128]

Yet whatever the noises about "reform" from the highest levels, the indications are that the Soviet Union is not contemplating following Mr. Deng's large-scale agricultural changes to anything like the extent of China's "liberalization" (see above), even when it is clear that Russian output is falling far behind that of its adventurous neighbor.[129]

Although the Kremlin is unlikely to explain openly why it prefers the present system of collectivized agriculture despite its manifest inefficiencies, two reasons for this inflexibility stand out. The first is that a massive extension of private plots, the creation of many more private markets, and increases in the prices paid for agricultural produce would imply significant rises in the peasantry's share of national income—to the detriment of the resentful urban population and, per-

Chart 3. Grain Production in the Soviet Union and China, 1950–1984

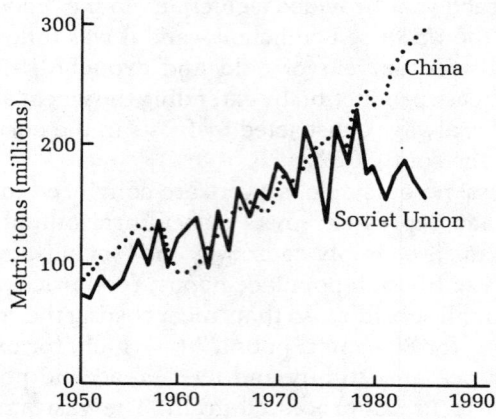

Source: Brown et. al. / U.S. Department of Agriculture

haps, of industrial investment. It would mean, in other words, the final triumph of Bukharin's policies (which favored agricultural incentives) and the demise of Stalin's prejudices.[130] Secondly, it would mean a decline in the powers of the bureaucrats and managers who run Soviet agriculture, and thus have implications for all of the other spheres of decision-making. While it is surely true that "individual farmers making day-to-day decisions in response to market signals, changing weather, and the conditions of their crops have a combined intelligence far exceeding that of a centralized bureaucracy, however well designed and competently staffed,"[131] what might that imply for the future of the "centralized bureaucracy"? If it *is* correct that there is a consistent, embarrassing relationship between "socialism and national food deficits,"[132] then that can hardly have escaped the Politburo's attention. But from its own perspective, it may seem better—safer, certainly—to maintain "socialist" (i.e., collectivized) farming even if that implies rising food imports, rather than to admit the failure of the Communist system and to remove the existing controls upon so large a segment of society.

By the same token, it is also difficult for the USSR to amend its industrial sector. To some observers, that may hardly seem necessary, given the remarkable achievements of the Soviet economy since 1945 and the fact that it outproduces the United States in, for example, machine tools, steel, cement, fertilizers, oil, and so on.[133] Yet there are many signs that Soviet industry, too, is stagnating and that the period of relatively easy expansion—caused by fixing ambitious output targets, and then devoting masses of finance and manpower to meeting those figures—is coming to a close. Part of this is due to increasing labor and energy shortages, which are discussed separately below. Equally important, however, are the repeated signs that manufacturing suffers from an excess of bureaucratic planning, from being too concentrated upon heavy industry, and from being unable to respond either to consumer choice or to the need to alter products to meet new demands or markets. Producing masses of cement is not necessarily a good thing, if the excessive investment in it has taken resources from a more needy sector; if the actual cement-production process has been very wasteful of energy; if the final product has to be transported long distances across the country, thus placing further strains upon the overworked railway system; and if the cement itself has to be distributed among the thousands of building projects which Soviet planners authorized but have never been able to complete.[134] The same remarks might be made about the enormous Soviet steel industry, much of the output of which seems to be wasted—causing some scholars to marvel at the "paradox of industrial plenty in the midst of consumer poverty."[135] There are, to be sure, efficient sectors in Soviet industry (usually related to defense, which can command large resources and *must* compete with the West), but the overall system suffers from concentrating upon production without much concern for market prices and consumer demand. Since Soviet factories cannot go out of business, as in the West, they also lack the ultimate stimulus to produce efficiently. However many tinkerings there are to assist industrial growth at a faster rate, it is difficult to believe that they will produce a sustained breakthrough if the existing system of a "planned economy" remains.

Yet if today's levels of Soviet industrial efficiency are scarcely tolerable (or, judging from the harsher tone of the government, increasingly intolerable), the system is likely to be even more damaged by three further pressures bearing down upon it. The first of these concerns energy supplies. It has become increasingly obvious that the great expansion in Soviet industrial output since the 1940s heavily depended upon plentiful supplies of coal, oil and natural gas, almost without regard to cost. In consequence, the "energy waste" and "steel waste" in both the USSR and its chief satellites is extraordinary, compared with western Europe, as shown in Table 46.

In Russia's case, this misuse of "inputs" may have seemed tolerable

Table 46. Kilos of Coal Equivalent and Steel Used to Produce $1,000 of GDP in 1979–1980[136]

	Coal	Steel		Coal	Steel
Russia	1,490	135	Britain	820	38
East Germany	1,356	88	West Germany	565	52
Czechoslovakia	1,290	132	France	502	42
Hungary	1,058	88	Switzerland	371	26

when its energy supplies were so plentiful and (relatively) easily accessible; but the awful fact is that this is no longer the case. It may have been that the CIA's famous 1977 forecast that Soviet oil production would soon peak, and then rapidly decline, *was* premature; nonetheless, Russian oil output did drop a little in 1984 and 1985, for the first time since the Second World War.[137] More alarming still is the fact that the remaining (and very considerable) stocks of oil—and of natural gas—are to be found at much deeper levels or in regions, like western Siberia, badly affected by permafrost. Over the past decade, as Gorbachev reported in 1985, the cost of extracting an additional ton of Soviet oil had risen by 70 percent and this problem was, if anything, intensifying.[138] Hence, to a large degree, the very extensive commitment by Russia to building up its nuclear-power output as swiftly as possible, thus doubling its share of electricity production (from 10 percent to 20 percent) by 1990. It is too soon to know how far the disaster at the Chernobyl plant will hurt those plans—the four reactors at Chernobyl produced one-seventh of the total Russian nuclear-generated electricity, so that their shutdown implied an increased use of other fuel stocks—but what is obvious is that it will both increase costs (because of additional safety measures) and reduce the pace of the planned development of the industry.[139] Finally, there is the awkward fact that the energy sector already absorbs so much capital—about 30 percent of all industrial investment—and that amount is bound to rise sharply. It seems difficult to believe the recent report that "a simple continuation of recent investment trends in oil, coal and electric power, combined with the targeted investment increase for natural gas, will absorb virtually the *entire* available increase in capital resources for Soviet industry over the period 1981–5,"[140] simply because the implications elsewhere are too severe. Nevertheless, the overall pattern is clear: merely to keep the economy growing at a modest pace, the energy sector will require an increased share of the GNP.[141]

Equally problematic, from the viewpoint of the Russian leadership, is the challenge posed in the high-technology areas of robotics, supercomputers, lasers, optics, telecommunications, and so on, where the USSR is in danger of increasingly falling behind the West. In the narrower, strictly military sense, there is the threat that "smart" battlefield weapons and advanced detection systems could neutralize Russia's *quantitative* advantages in military hardware: thus, supercomputers might be able to decrypt Russian codes, to locate submarines under the ocean's surface, to handle a fast-moving battle scene, and—last but not least—to protect American nuclear bases (as implied in President Reagan's "Star Wars" program); while sophisticated radar, laser, and guidance-control technology might allow western aircraft and artillery/rocket forces to locate and destroy enemy planes and tanks with impunity—as Israel regularly does to Syrian (Soviet-equipped) weapon-systems. Merely to keep up with these advanced technologies requires ever-larger allocations of scientific and engineering resources to Russia's defense-related sector.[142]

In the civilian field, the problem is even greater. Given the limitations which are being reached in such classic "inputs" as labor and capital investment, high technology is rightly perceived as being vital for increasing Russian output. To give but one example, the large-scale use of computers could greatly reduce wastage in the discovery, production, and distribution of energy supplies. But the adoption of this new technology not only implies heavy investments (taken from where?), it also challenges the intensely secretive, bureaucratic, and centralized Soviet system. Computers, word processors, telecommunications, being knowledge-intensive industries, can best be exploited by a society which possesses a technology-trained population that is encouraged to experiment freely and to exchange new ideas and hypotheses in the widest possible way. This works well in California and Japan, but threatens to loosen the Russian state's monopoly of information. If, even today, senior scientists and scholars in the Soviet Union are forbidden to use copying machines personally (the copying departments are staffed by the KGB), then it is hard to see how the country could move toward the widespread use of word processors, interactive computers, electronic mail, etc. without a substantial loosening of police controls and censorship.[143] As in agriculture, therefore, the regime's commitment to "modernization" and its willingness to allocate additional resources of money and manpower are vitiated by an economic substructure and a political ideology which are basic obstacles to change.

By comparison, then, the increasing reliance of the Soviet Union upon imported technologies and machinery—whether legally traded goods, or stolen from the West—is a less fundamental if still serious problem. The extent of the industrial and scientific espionage (whether for military or commercial purposes) can obviously not be quantified, but seems to be yet another indication of Russia's worry that it is falling behind.[144] The more regular trade—importing western technology (and also eastern-European manufactures) in exchange for Russian raw materials—is a traditional way in which the country seeks to "close the gap"; it was done in the 1890–1914 period, and again in the 1920s. In that sense, all that has changed is the more modern nature of the product: oil-drilling machinery, rolled steel, pipe, computers, machine tools, equipment for the chemical/plastics industry, etc. What must be much more worrying to Soviet planners is the accumulating evidence that the imported technology takes longer to set up, and is used much less efficiently than in the West.[145] The second problem is the availability of hard currency for the purchase of such technology. Traditionally, this could be circumvented by importing manufactured goods from fellow Comecon countries (thus involving no loss of hard currency), but the latter's products have increasingly failed to keep up with those from the West, even if they still have to be accepted to prevent a collapse of their eastern-European economies.[146] And while Russia has normally paid for a large proportion of western imports through the barter or direct sale of surplus oil, its prospects (and those of eastern Europe) may be shrinking because of the uncertainties in oil prices, its own growing energy needs, and the general change in the terms of trade for raw materials as manufacturing processes become more sophisticated.[147] At the same time as Russian earnings from oil and other raw materials (except, presumably, gas) shrink, the payments for a variety of imports remain high—all of which presumably reduces the sums available for investment.

The third major cause for concern about Russia's future economic growth lies in demographics. The position here is so gloomy that one scholar began his recent survey "Population and Labor Force" with the following blunt statement:

> On any basis, short-term or long-term, the prospects for the development of Soviet population and manpower resources until the end of the century are quite dismal. From the reduction in the country's birthrate to the incredible increase in the death rates beyond all reasonable past projections; from the decrease in the supply of new entrants to the labor force, compounded by its unequal regional distribution, to the relative ageing of the population, not much hope lies before the Soviet government in these trends.[148]

While all of these elements are serious—and interacting—the most shocking trend has been the steady deterioration in both life expectancy and infant mortality rates since the 1970s and perhaps earlier. Because of a slow erosion in hospital and general health care, poor standards of sanitation and public hygiene, and the fantastic levels of alcoholism, death rates in the Soviet Union have increased, especially among the working males: "Today, the average Soviet man can expect to live for only about 60 years, six years less than in the mid-1960s."[149] Equally shocking has been the rise in infant mortality—the only industrialized country where this has occurred—to a point where infant deaths are, comparatively, over three times the U.S. rate, despite the enormous numbers of Soviet doctors. Yet if the Russian population is dying off faster than before, its birthrates are slowing down sharply. Because (presumably) of urbanization, higher female participation in the work force, poor housing conditions, and other disincentives, the crude overall birthrate has been steadily dropping, more particularly among the *Russian* population of the country. The consequences of all these trends is that the male Russian population of the country is scarcely increasing at all.

The implications of all this have been disturbing Russia's leaders for some time, and are obviously behind the exhortations to increase family size, the stricter campaign against alcoholism, and the efforts to persuade older workers to remain in the factories. The first is that the country clearly requires a larger proportion of resources to be devoted to health care and social security, especially as the percentage of older population increases: in this the USSR is no different from other industrialized countries (except in its increased death rates), but this again raises the issue of spending priorities. Secondly, there are the implications for both Soviet industry and the armed services, given the drastic fall-off in the rate of growth of the labor force: according to projections, between 1980 and 1990 the labor force will enjoy a net increase of "only 5,990,000 persons, whereas during the preceding ten years the estimated increase in the labor force was 24,217,000."[150] To leave the military's problems until later, this trend reminds us again that a large part of the growth in Russian industrial output in the 1950s to the 1970s was due to an enhanced labor force, rather than increases in efficiency; from now on economic expansion can no longer rely upon a fast-increasing work force in manufacturing. To a considerable extent, of course, this difficulty could be overcome if more able-bodied males were released from agriculture; but the problem there is that an excessive number of youths in the Slavic areas have already left the communes for the city, whereas the surplus which does exist in the non-Slavic republics is more poorly educated, often has little knowledge of the Russian language, and would require an immense investment in training for industry. This brings us to the final trend which makes Moscow planners uneasy: that since the fertility rates in central Asian republics like Uzbekistan are three times larger than among the Slavic and Baltic peoples, a major shift in the long-term population balances is under way. In consequence, the Russian population's share is expected to decline from 52 percent in 1980 to only 48 percent by 2000.[151] For the first time in the history of the USSR, Russians will not be in the majority.

This catalog of difficulties may seem too gloomy to certain commentators. Military-related production in the USSR is often impressive and is constantly driven to improve itself because of the dynamic of the arms-race itself.[152] As one historian (admittedly writing in 1981)[153] points out, the picture cannot be seen as altogether negative, especially if one looks at Soviet economic achievements over the past half-century; and it has been a habit among western observers to exaggerate Russia's strengths in one period and its weaknesses in the next. Nevertheless, however much the USSR has improved itself since Lenin's time, the awkward facts are that it has not caught up with the West and, indeed, that the gap in real standards of living seems to have been widening since the later years of the Brezhnev regime; that it is being overtaken, by all measures of per capita output and industrial efficiency, by Japan and certain other Asian countries; and that its slow-down in rate of growth, its aging population, and its difficulties with climate, energy stocks, and agriculture cast a dark shadow over the claims and exhortations of the Soviet leadership.

It is in this context, then, that Gorbachev's belief that "acceleration of the country's socioeconomic development is the key to all our problems" becomes the more understandable. And yet, quite apart from natural difficulties (permafrost, etc.), two main *political* obstacles stand in the way of producing a "leap forward" on the Chinese model. The first is the entrenched position of the party officials, bureaucrats, and other members of the elite, who enjoy a large array of privileges (depending upon rank) which cushion them from the hardships of everyday life in the Soviet Union, and who monopolize power and influence. To decentralize the planning and pricing system, to free the peasants from communal controls, to allow managers of factories a greater freedom of action, to offer incentives for individual enterprise rather than party loyalty, to close outdated plants, to refuse to accept shoddy products, and to allow a far freer circulation of information would be seen by those in power as dire threats to their own position. Exhortations, more flexible planning, enhanced investments in this or that sector, and disciplinary drives against alcoholism or corrupt management are one thing; but all proposed changes, Soviet party officials have stressed, have to take place "within the framework of scientific socialism" and without "any shifts toward a market economy or private enterprise."[154] In the opinion of one recent visitor, "the Soviet Union needs its inefficiencies to remain Soviet";[155] if that is so, all Mr. Gorbachev's urgings about the need for a "profound transformation" of the system are unlikely to make much impact upon the long-term growth rates.

The second political obstacle lies in the very significant share of GNP devoted by the USSR to defense. How best to calculate the totals and how that measures with western defense spending has exercised many analysts; the CIA's 1975 announcement that the ruble prices of Soviet weaponry were twice as high as previously estimated—and that Russia was probably spending 11–13 percent of GNP upon defense rather than 6–8 percent—led to all sorts of misinterpretations of what that meant.[156] But the exact figures (which may not even be available to Soviet planners) are less significant than the fact that although the growth in armaments spending slowed down after 1976, the Kremlin appears to have allocated around twice as much of the country's product to this area as has the USA, even under Reagan's arms buildup; and this in turn means that the Soviet armed forces have siphoned off vast

stocks of trained manpower, scientists, machinery, and capital investment which could have been devoted to the civilian economy. This
does *not* mean, according to certain economic forecasts, that a large
reduction in defense expenditures would quickly lead to a great surge
in Russia's growth rates, simply because of the fact that it would take
a long time before, say, a T-72 tank-assembly factory could be retooled
to do something else.[157] On the other hand, if the arms race with NATO
over the rest of this century drove up the share of Russian defense
spending from 14 to 17 percent or more of GNP by the year 2000, a
larger and larger amount of equipment such as machine-building and
metalworking tools would be consumed by the military, crowding out
the share of investment capital going to the rest of industry. Yet, while
economists believe that "this will represent a tremendous problem for
Soviet decision-makers,"[158] all the indications are that defense expenditures *will* rise faster than GNP growth—and have the consequent
effect upon prosperity and consumption.

   Like every other one of the large Powers, therefore, the USSR has
to make a choice in its allocations of national resources between (1)
the requirements of the military—in this case, with their built-in ability
to articulate Russia's security needs; and (2) the increasing desire of
the Russian populace for consumer goods and better living and working conditions, not to mention improved social services to check the
high death and sickness rates; and (3) the needs of both agriculture and
industry for fresh capital investment, in order to modernize the economy, increase output, keep abreast of the advances of others, and in
the longer term satisfy both the defense and the social requirements
of the country.[159] As elsewhere, this involves difficult choices by the
decision-makers concerned; yet one has the sense that however large
and pressing are the needs both of the Russian consumer and of "modernizing" the economy, the traditional obsession by Moscow with military security means that the fundamental choice has already been
made. Unless the Gorbachev regime really manages to transform
things, guns will always come before butter and, if need be, before
economic growth as well. This, as much as any other characteristic,
makes Russia basically different from Japan and western Europe, and
even from China and the United States.

   Historically, then, the Kremlin today follows the tradition of the
Romanov czars, and of Stalin himself, in its desire to have armed
forces equal to (and, if preferable, larger than) those of any other
Power. There is no doubt that at the present time, the military strength
of the USSR is extremely imposing. To try to offer a realistic figure for
annual totals of current Soviet defense expenditures would probably
be a deception: on the one hand, Moscow's *official* figures are absurdly
low, concealing large amounts of defense-related spending under
other headings ("science," the space programs, internal security, civil

defense, and construction); on the other hand, western estimates of the real total are complicated by the artificial dollar-ruble exchange rate, limited understanding of Soviet budgetary procedures, the difficulties in, say, the CIA's effort to put a "dollar cost" on a Russian-made weapon or manpower costs, and institutional/ideological biases. The result is an array of "guestimates," which one can choose according to one's fancy.[160] What is not in question, however, is the massive modernization which has occurred in all branches of the Soviet armed forces, both nuclear and conventional, on land and sea and in the air. Whether one considers the rapid growth of Russian land- and sea-based strategic missile systems, the thousands of aircraft and tens of thousands of main battle tanks, the extraordinary developments in the surface navy and in the submarine fleet, the specialist activities (airborne and amphibious warfare units, chemical warfare, intelligence and "disinformation" activities), the end result is impressive. It may or may not have cost as much in real terms as the Pentagon's own allocations; but it undoubtedly gives the USSR a range of military capabilities which only the rival American superpower possesses. This is *not* a twentieth-century military Potemkin village, ready to collapse at the first serious testing.[161]

On the other hand, the Soviet war machine also has its own weaknesses and problems, and certainly ought not to be presented as an omnipotent force, able to execute with consummate efficiency all of the possible military operations which the Kremlin might require of it. Since the dilemmas which face the strategy-makers of the *other* large Powers of the globe are also being pointed out in this chapter, it is only proper to draw attention to the great variety of difficulties confronting Russia's military-political leadership—without, however, jumping to the opposite conclusion that the Soviet Union is therefore unlikely to "survive" for very long.[162]

Some of the difficulties facing Russian military decision-makers over the middle to longer term derive directly from the economic and demographic problems of the Soviet state which have been outlined above. The first is in technology. Since Peter the Great's time—to repeat a point made in the previous chapters of this book—Russia has always enjoyed its greatest military advantage vis-à-vis the West when the pace of weapons technology has slowed down enough to allow a standardization of equipment and thus of fighting units and tactics—whether that be the eighteenth-century infantry column or the mid-twentieth-century armored division. Whenever an upward spiral in weapons technology has placed an emphasis upon quality rather than quantity, however, the Russian advantage has diminished. And while it is clearly true that Russia has substantially closed the technological gap with the West which existed in czarist times, and that its military enjoys unrivaled access to the scientific and productive resources of a state-run economy, there nonetheless is evidence of significant lag times[163] in a large number of technological processes. One of the two clearest signs of this is the unease with which the Soviet Union has watched its weaponry being repeatedly outclassed by American hardware in the surrogate battles which have taken place in the Middle East and elsewhere over the past few decades. Admittedly, the quality of North Korean, Egyptian, Syrian, and Libyan pilots and tank crews was never of the highest, but even if it had been, there are grounds to doubt if they could have prevailed against American weapons with far superior avionics, radar equipment, miniaturized guidance systems, and so on. It has probably been in response to this that western experts on the Soviet military report a constant effort to upgrade quality[164] and to produce—a few years later—"mirror images" of U.S. weapon systems. But this in turn draws Soviet planners into the same vortex which threatens western defense programs: more sophisticated equipment leads to much longer building times, larger maintenance schedules, heavier (usually) and vastly more expensive (always) hardware, and a decline in production numbers. This is not a comforting trend for a Power which has traditionally relied upon large numbers of weapons to carry out its various and disparate strategical tasks.

The second sign of Soviet unease about technological obsolescence relates to the so-called Strategic Defense Initiative (SDI) of the Reagan administration. It seems difficult at this stage to believe that it would really make the United States completely invulnerable to nuclear attack (for example, it can do nothing against low-flying "cruise" missiles), but the protection it may give to American missile sites and airbases and the added strain upon the Soviet defense budget of producing many more rockets and warheads to swamp the SDI system with sheer numbers can hardly be welcome to the Kremlin. More worrying still, perhaps, are the implications for high-tech *conventional* warfare. One commentator has pointed out:

> A defense that can protect against 99 percent of the Soviet nuclear arsenal may be judged as not good enough, given the destructive potential of the weapons that could survive. . . . [But if] the United States could achieve a technological superiority that would assure destruction of much of the Soviet Union's conventionally armed aircraft, tanks, and ships, the Soviet numerical advantage would be less threatening. Technology judged less than ideal for SDI may be perfectly applicable for nonnuclear combat.[165]

This, in turn, compels a much larger Russian investment into the advanced technologies of lasers, optics, supercomputers, guidance systems, and navigation: in other words, as one Russian spokesman has put it, there will be "a whole new arms race at a much higher technological level."[166] Judging from the 1984 warnings of Marshal Ogarkov, then chief of military staff, about the awful consequences of Russia's failing to match western technology, the Red Army seems less than confident that it could win that sort of race.

At the other end of the spectrum, there lies a potential demographic threat to Russia's traditional advantage in *quantity*, that is, in manpower. As noted above, this is the result of two trends: the overall decline in total USSR birthrate, and the rising share of births in the non-Russian regions. If this is leading to difficulties in the allocation of manpower between agriculture and industry, then it is even more of a long-term problem for military recruitment. In round terms, there ought not to be a problem in taking 1.3 to 1.5 million recruits each year from the 2.1 million males available; but an increasing proportion comes from the Asiatic youth of Turkestan, many of whom are not well versed in the Russian language, have a far lower level of mechanical (let alone electronic) competence, and are sometimes strongly influenced by Islam. All of the studies of the ethnic composition of the Soviet armed forces reveal that the officer corps and NCOs are overwhelmingly Slavic—as are the rocket forces, the air force, the navy, and the technical forces.[167] So, too, unsurprisingly, are the Category I (first-class) divisions of the Red Army. By contrast, the Category II and (especially) Category III divisions and most of service and transport units are manned by non-Slavs, which raises an interesting question about the effectiveness of these "follow-on" divisions in a conventional war against NATO, if the Category I divisions required substantial reinforcement. Labeling this bias "racialistic" and (Great Russian) "nationalistic," as many western commentators do, is less significant in strictly military terms than the fact that a considerable portion of available Soviet manpower is regarded as unreliable and inefficient by the general staff—which is probably a true judgment, given the reports of Muslim fundamentalism throughout southern Russia and the bewilderment of those troops at, say, having to invade Afghanistan.

In other words, like the Austro-Hungarian Empire eighty years ago or, for that matter, the *Czarist* Empire eighty years ago—the Russian leadership faces a "nationality problem"[168] undimmed by the ideology of Marxism. To be sure, the control apparatus now is altogether more formidable than that existing prior to 1914, and one ought perhaps to take with a pinch of salt claims that, for example, the Ukraine is a "hotbed" of disaffection.[169] Nevertheless, long memories about how Ukrainians welcomed the German invaders in 1941, reports of discontent in the Baltic provinces, the forcible (and successful) Georgian protests at the 1978 attempt to make Russian the equal-first language in that republic; above all, perhaps, the straddling across the Sino-Soviet border of millions of Kazakhs and Uighers, and the existence of 48 million Muslims north of the unstable borders with Turkey, Iran, and Afghanistan: these facts seem to prey upon the minds of the Russian leadership and to add to their insecurities. More specifically, they provoke an increasing concern about where to place the shrinking numbers of the more "reliable" Slavic youth. Should they be directed into the armed forces, to the Category I divisions and other prestige services, even if fewer and fewer of them are available for industry and agriculture, both of which desperately need infusions of trained and loyal recruits? Or should the non-Slavic population form a growing proportion of the Red Army, despite the risks to military efficiency, in order to release Russians and fellow Slavs for civilian purposes?[170] Since the Soviet tradition is one of "safety first," probably the former tendency will prevail; but far from solving the dilemma, that merely reflects a choice between evils.

If the economic components of what Soviet strategists term "the correlation of forces"[171] is a cause for concern among the Politburo, those same leaders can hardly draw much encouragement from the more strictly *military* aspects of the fast-changing global balance of power. However imposing and alarming the Soviet military machine appears to outside observers, it is nonetheless worth measuring those forces against the array of strategical tasks which the Soviet military may be called upon to carry out.

In undertaking such an exercise, it is useful to separate a consideration of conventional warfare from that which may involve nuclear weapons. For obvious reasons, *the* item in the military balances which has attracted most attention and the most concern is the armory of strategic nuclear weapons in the hands of the Great Powers, and especially of the United States and the USSR, both of which possess the capacity to devastate the globe. For the record, it may be worth reproducing the 1986 "count" of their strategic nuclear warheads by the International Institute of Strategic Studies (see Table 47).

Table 47. Estimated Strategic Nuclear Warheads[172]

	U.S.	USSR
ICBM-borne warheads	2,118	6,420
SLBM-borne warheads	5,536	2,787+
Aircraft-borne warheads	2,520	680
Totals	10,174	9,987+

Precisely how one reacts to such figures depends upon one's interests. To those concerned with numbers alone, or with the possible misrepresentation of numbers, there will be a keen checking of the subtotals and a reminder of the fact that additional large stocks of *tactical* nuclear weapons are also held by each superpower.[173] To a very considerable number of nonofficial commentators, and to many

of the public at large, the sheer extent and destructive capacity of the
nuclear weaponry held in these two arsenals is an indication of political incapacity or mental sickness, which threatens all daily life on
this planet and should be abolished or greatly reduced as soon as
possible.[174] On the other hand, there is that whole cluster of commentators—in think tanks and universities, as well as in defense
departments—who have accepted the possibility that nuclear weapons
might indeed be *used,* as part of a national strategy; and who therefore
devote their intellectual energies to an intensive study of the respective
weapon systems, of escalation strategies and war-gaming, of the pros
and cons of arms control and verification agreements, of "throw-
weights," "footprints," and "equivalent megatonnages," targeting policies, and "second-strike" scenarios.[175]

How to deal with "the nuclear problem"[176] within a five-century
survey such as this obviously presents a major difficulty. Is it not the
case that the existence of nuclear weapons—or, rather, the possibility
of their mass deployment—has made redundant any consideration of
war, of strategy, of economics, from a traditional viewpoint? In the
event of an all-out exchange of strategic nuclear weapons, would not
estimates of their impact on the "shifting power balances" in world
affairs be irrelevant to everyone in the northern hemisphere (and perhaps to everyone in the southern hemisphere as well)? Did not the
traditional pattern—of Great Power rivalries turning from time to time
into open warfare—finally come to an end in 1945?

There is, obviously, no way of answering such questions with certainty. Yet there are indications that today's Great Powers may be
returning to more traditional assumptions about the use of force despite—in many ways, *because of*—the existence of nuclear weapons. In
the first place, there appears to be now—and probably has been for
some years—an essential balance in nuclear armaments between the
two superpowers. For all the debate about "windows of opportunity"
and the possibilities of one side or the other having a "first-strike
capability," it is clear that neither Washington nor Moscow possesses
any guarantee that it could obliterate its rival without the likelihood
of also suffering devastation; and the coming of a "Star Wars" technology will not significantly alter that fact. In particular, the possession
by each side of a great number of *submarine*-launched ballistic missiles, located in underwater craft which are difficult to detect,[177] makes
it inconceivable for either side to assume that it could knock out its
enemy's nuclear-weapons capacity all at once. This fact, more than—or
at least as much as—fears of a "nuclear winter" will stay the hand of
decision-makers, unless they are dragged down by some accidentally
induced escalation. It therefore follows that each side is locked into a
nuclear stalemate from which it cannot retreat—it being practically
impossible either to disinvent nuclear technology or for one (or both)

superpowers to give up possession of the weapons—and from which it cannot gain real advantage—since each power's new system is countered or imitated by the other, and since it is too risky actually to use the weapons themselves.

In other words, the vast nuclear armories of each superpower will continue to exist, but (barring an accidental "triggering") they are in all likelihood unusable, because they contradict the ancient assumption that in war, as in most other things, there ought to be a balance between means and ends. In a nuclear war, by contrast, the risk is run of inflicting and incurring such damage to mankind that no political, ideological, or economic purpose would be served by it. Although masses of brainpower are devoted to evolving a "nuclear-war-fighting strategy," it is difficult to contest Jervis's observation that "a rational strategy for the employment of nuclear weapons is a contradiction in terms."[178] Once the first missile is unleashed, there would be an end to the "mutual hostage" position into which each side has been locked ever since the United States lost its nuclear monopoly. The results then might be so cataclysmic that no rational political leadership is likely to take the first step across the threshold. Unless there is an inadvertent nuclear war—which is, because of human error or technical malfunction, always possible[179]—each side is likely to be deterred from "going nuclear." If a clash does occur, both the political and the military leaderships will endeavor to "contain" it at the level of conventional fighting.

This does not address what may be a far more serious problem for the two rival superpowers over the next twenty years and beyond: that of nuclear proliferation into countries in the more volatile parts of the world—the Near East, the Indian subcontinent, South Africa, possibly Latin America.[180] Since the states concerned are not part of the Great Power system, the awful possibility of their resorting to nuclear weapons in some regional clash is not considered here: on the whole it seems fair to conclude that the United States and the USSR have a shared interest in halting nuclear proliferation, since it makes global politics more complicated than ever before. If anything, the trend toward proliferation may cause the superpowers to appreciate what they have in common.

In a quite different league—from Moscow's viewpoint, certainly—are the fast-expanding nuclear armories of China, Britain, and France. Until a few years ago, it was commonly assumed that all three of those nations were merely marginal factors in the nuclear balance, and that their nuclear strategy was not at all "credible," since they could only inflict (in all three cases) limited damage upon the USSR in exchange for their own atomic obliteration. But the indications are that that assumption may soon require modification. The most alarming tendency—again, from Moscow's viewpoint—is the increasing nuclear capacity of the People's Republic of China, about which it has been concerned for the past twenty-five years.[181] If the PRC can develop not only a more sophisticated land-based ICBM system but also—as seems its intention—a long-range, submarine-based ballistic-missile system, and if Sino-Soviet disputes are not settled to mutual satisfaction, then the USSR faces the possibility of a future armed clash along the borders which might escalate into a nuclear interchange with its Chinese neighbor. As things are at present, the devastation of the PRC would be immense; but Moscow cannot exclude the possibility that at least a certain number (and, the 1990s, a larger number) of Chinese nuclear missiles would hit the Soviet Union.

More worrying technically, although perhaps less alarming politically, is the buildup of the British and French nuclear delivery and warhead capacities. Until recently, the "deterrent" effect of both of these Powers' strategic weapon systems appeared dubious. In the rather implausible event of their being involved in a nuclear interchange with the USSR, and with the United States neutral (which is, after all, the justification for the British and French systems), it was difficult to see them risking national suicide when they could only inflict partial damage upon Russia from their own modest delivery systems. In the next few years, however, the devastation which each of those midsized Powers could do to the USSR will be multiplied many times, because of the vast enhancement of their submarine-launched ballistic-missile systems. For example, Britain's acquisition of submarines carrying the Trident II missile system—derided by *The Economist* as "the Rolls Royce of nuclear missiles"[182] because of its high cost and excessive striking power—will give that country a nearly invulnerable deterrent force which could destroy more than 350 Soviet targets, instead of the present sixteen-plus targets. In rather the same way, France's new submarine *L'Inflexible,* with the longer-range, multiwarhead M-4 missile, is probably capable of attacking ninety-six Soviet targets—"more than all of France's five earlier nuclear submarines combined"[183]—and when the other boats have been reequipped with the same M-4 missile, France's strategic warheads will have increased *fivefold,* allowing it also to be theoretically capable of hitting hundreds of Russian targets from thousands of miles away.

What this means in real terms it is, of course, impossible to forecast. In Britain itself many prominent figures have found the idea that their country would *independently* use its nuclear weapons against Russia to be, literally, "incredible";[184] and such critics are unlikely to be swayed by the counterargument that the country's own suicide would at least be attended by inflicting much heavier damage upon the USSR than was possible hitherto. In France, too, public opinion—and some strategic commentators—find its declared deterrent policy to be scarcely credible.[185] On the other hand, it seems fair to assume that

Russian military planners, who take nuclear-war-fighting possibilities very seriously indeed, must find these recent developments disturbing. Not only will they face *four* countries—instead of the United States alone—with the potential to inflict heavy (perhaps extraordinarily heavy) damage upon the Soviet heartland, but they must consider what the *subsequent* world military balances would look like if Russia was involved in a nuclear interchange with one of these Powers (say, China) while the others were neutral observers of such mutually inflicted devastation. Hence the Soviets' repeated insistence that in any overall Strategic Arms Limitation Treaty with the United States the Anglo-French systems have to be taken into account, *and* that the USSR must have a certain margin of nuclear force to take care of China. All this, it seems reasonable to suggest, makes nuclear weapons an ever more dubious instrument of *rational* military policy from the Kremlin's viewpoint.

If, however, this leaves conventional weapons as the chief measure of Soviet military power—and the chief tool for securing the political aims of the Soviet state—it is difficult to believe that Russian planners can feel much more assured at the present state of the international military balance. This may seem a bold statement to make in view of the very extensive publicity which has been given to the far larger totals of Soviet aircraft, tanks, artillery, and infantry divisions in assessments of the U.S.-USSR "military balance"—not to mention the frequent assertion that NATO forces, unable to hold their own in a large-scale conventional war in Europe, would be compelled to "go nuclear" within a matter of days. Yet an increasing number of the most recent academic studies of the "balance" are now suggesting that that is precisely what exists—namely, a situation in which "there still appears to be insufficient overall strength on *either* side to guarantee victory."[186] To reach this conclusion involves both very detailed comparative analyses (e.g., of the composition of the U.S. as opposed to Russian tank divisions) and considerations of certain larger and intangible factors (e.g., the role of China, the reliability of the Warsaw Pact), and only a summary of these arguments can be provided here. If, however, this evidence is even roughly correct, it also cannot be very comforting to Soviet planners.

The first and most obvious point to be made is that any analysis of the *conventional* balance of forces needs to measure the rival alliances as a whole, especially in their European context. As soon as that is done, it becomes evident that the non-American parts of NATO are much more significant than the non-Russian parts of the Warsaw Pact. Indeed, as the 1985 British Defence White Paper made pains to point out, "European countries were providing the major part of the ready [NATO] forces stationed in Europe: 90 percent of the manpower, 85 percent of the tanks, 95 percent of the artillery and 80 percent of the combat aircraft; and over 70 percent of the major warships in Atlantic and European waters. . . . The full mobilized strength of European forces was nearly 7 million men as against 3.5 million for the United States."[187] It is, of course, also true that the United States has deployed 250,000 men *in situ* in Germany, that the army divisions and air squadrons which it plans to pour across the Atlantic in the event of a European war would be critical reinforcements, and that NATO as a whole depends upon the American nuclear deterrent and upon American sea power. But the point is that the North Atlantic Alliance is much more evenly balanced between, as it were, the twin pillars of the "arch," than is the Warsaw Pact, which is top-heavy and skewed toward Moscow. It is also worth noting that America's NATO allies spend six times more on defense than Russia's Warsaw Pact allies; indeed, Britain, France, and West Germany *each* spend more than the non-Russian Warsaw Pact countries together.[188]

If, then, the strength of the two alliances is measured as a whole, and without the curious omissions and provisos which have characterized some of the more alarmist western assessments,* a picture emerges of strategical parity in most respects; and even where the Warsaw Pact has the edge in numbers, that does not look decisive. For example, each alliance appears to have roughly similar "total ground forces in Europe"; they also have similar "total ground forces" and "total ground force reserves."[189] In the *roundest* sense of all, the Warsaw Pact's 13.9 million men (6.4 million "main forces" and 7.5 million reserves) is not vastly greater than NATO's 11.9 million men (5 million "main forces" and 6.8 million reserves), the more especially since a large proportion of the Warsaw Pact total consists of Category III units and reserve forces of the Red Army. Even on the critically important Central Front, where NATO forces are most seriously outnumbered by the masses of Russian armored and motor-rifle divisions, the Warsaw Pact's advantage is not a very comforting one—especially when it is recalled how difficult it would be to conduct fast, offensive, "maneuver warfare" in the crowded terrain of northern Germany and when it is realized how many of Russia's 52,000 "main battle tanks" are the obsolescent T-54s—which would simply clog up the roads. Provided NATO has sufficient reserves of ammunition, fuel, replacement weaponry, etc., it certainly seems to be in a much better position to blunt a Soviet conventional offensive than it was in the 1950s.[190]

In addition, there is the incalculable element of the integrity and cohesion of the respective military alliances. That NATO has many weaknesses is undeniable: from the frequent transatlantic disputes

---

*It is, for example, all too easy to show the Warsaw Pact as massively superior by including, say, all of Russia's armed forces (even those deployed against China), and by excluding, say, France's.

over "burden sharing" to the tricky issue of intergovernmental consultation in the event of pressure to launch nuclear missiles. Neutralist and anti-NATO sentiment, detectable in left-of-center parties from West Germany and Britain to Spain and Greece, is also a cause of periodic concern.[191] And if there were to be, at some future time, a "Finlandization" of any of the states lying along the Warsaw Pact's western boundary (especially, of course, West Germany itself), then that would be a massive strategical gain to the USSR as well as providing economic relief. Yet even if such a scenario is possible *in theory*, that can hardly compare with the worries which Moscow must presently entertain about the reliability of its "empire" in eastern Europe. The broad-based popularity of the Solidarity movement in Poland, the evident East German wishes to improve relations with Bonn, the "creeping capitalism" of the Hungarians, the economic woes which are affecting not merely Poland and Rumania but all of eastern Europe, pose extraordinarily difficult problems for the Soviet leadership. They are not issues which can be readily solved by the use of the Red Army; nor, however, does it appear that fresh doses of "scientific socialism" would provide an answer satisfactory to the eastern Europeans. Despite the Kremlin's recent rhetoric about the modernization and reexamination of Marxist economic and social policies, it is difficult to see Russia relinquishing its many controls over eastern Europe. Yet these varied signs of political discontent and economic distress must call ever more into question the reliability of the *non-Russian* armies in the Warsaw Pact.[192] The Polish armed forces, for example, can hardly be reckoned an addition to the pact's strength; if anything, the reverse is true, since they—and the critically important Polish road and rail lines—would need close Red Army supervision in wartime.[193] Similarly, it is difficult to imagine the Czech and Hungarian armies enthusiastically rushing forward to assault NATO positions upon Moscow's orders. Even the attitudes of East German forces, probably the most effective and modernized of Russia's allies, may be affected by the order to attack westward. It is true that the great bulk (four-fifths) of the Warsaw Pact's forces are Russians, and that Soviet divisions would be the real spearhead in any conventional war with the West; but it will be a considerable task for Red Army commanders both to conduct such a war and to keep an eye upon the million or more eastern European soldiers, most of them not very efficient and some of them not very reliable.[194] The possibility (however remote) that NATO may even seek to respond to a Warsaw Pact offensive by mounting its own counteroffensive, into, say, Czechoslovakia,[195] can only increase an unease which is probably as much political as it is military.

Since the early 1960s, moreover, Russian planners have had to juggle with an even more horrifying problem: the possibility that they might be involved in a large-scale conflict with NATO *and* with China.

If this occurred at the same time, then the prospects of switching reinforcements from one front or to another would be severely limited, if not impossible; but even if the war was being fought only on one front, the Kremlin might well fear to redeploy divisions from a region which, while technically neutral, had large armed forces of a potential foe arrayed along the border. As it is, the USSR is compelled to keep about fifty divisions and 13,000 tanks ready for the eventuality of a Sino-Soviet clash; and although the Russian forces are more modern and mobile than the Chinese, it is hard to envisage how they could ensure a total victory—not to mention a prolonged occupation—against an army four times as large.[196] All this necessarily assumes that the war would remain a conventional one (which, given some Russian hints about how they would crush China, may be a totally flawed assumption); but if there *is* a Russo-Chinese nuclear exchange, Soviet planners would then have to wonder whether their country might be left in a position of inferiority vis-à-vis the still neutral, yet very critical, West. In the same way, a Soviet Union badly hurt by either nuclear or large-scale conventional fighting against NATO must worry about how to handle Chinese pressures if it had been reduced to a "broken-backed" status.[197]

Although China is (apart from NATO) the most serious concern for Soviet planners simply because of its size, it is not difficult to imagine Soviet worries about the entire Asian "flank." In the largest geopolitical sense, it looks as if the age-old tendency of Muscovite/Russian policy, steady territorial expansion across Asia, has come to a halt. The re-emergence of China, the independence (and growing strength) of India, the economic recovery of Japan—not to mention the assertiveness of many smaller Asian states—has surely put to rest the nineteenth-century fear of a Russia gradually taking control of the entire continent. (The very idea nowadays would make the Soviet general staff blanch with alarm!) To be sure, this would still not prevent Moscow from making marginal gains, as in Afghanistan; but the duration of that conflict and the hostility it has provoked elsewhere in the region merely confirm that any further extensions of Russian territory would be at an incalculable military and political cost. By contrast with the self-confident Russian announcements of its "Asian mission" a century ago, the rulers in the Kremlin now have to worry about Muslim fundamentalism seeping across its southern borders from the Middle East, about the Chinese threat, and about complications in Afghanistan, Korea, and Vietnam. Whatever the number of divisions positioned in Asia, it can probably never seem enough to give "security" along such a vast periphery, especially since the Trans-Siberian Railway is still terribly vulnerable to disruption by an enemy rocket strike, which in turn would have dire implications for the Soviet forces in the Far East.[198]

Given the traditional concern of the Russian regime for the safety of the homeland, it is scarcely surprising that Soviet capacities both at sea and in the overseas world are, relatively speaking, much less significant. This is not to deny the very impressive expansion of the Red Navy over the past quarter-century, and the great variety of new and more powerful submarines, surface vessels, and even experimental aircraft carriers which are being laid down. Nor is it to deny the large expansion of the Soviet merchant marine and fishing fleets, and their significant strategical roles.[199] But there is as yet nothing in the USSR's naval armory which has the striking power of the U.S. Navy's fifteen carrier task forces. Moreover, once the comparison is between the fleets of the two *alliances* rather than the two superpowers, the sizable contributions of the non-American NATO navies makes an immense difference.

Table 48. NATO and Warsaw Pact Naval Strengths[200]

	Warsaw Pact			Nato		
	Non-Soviet	USSR	Total	Total	U.S.	Non-U.S.
Nuclear submarines	—	105	105	97	85	12
Diesel submarines	6	168	174	137	5	132
Major surface warships	3	184	187	376	149	227
Naval aircraft	52	755	807	2533	2250	283

"Even if China is excluded, the Western Allies have twice as many major surface combatants and three times as much naval air power as the Warsaw Pact, and practically as many submarines," as shown in Table 48. If one adds to this the fact that many more of the Warsaw Pact's large surface warships and submarines are over twenty years old, that its capacity to detect enemy submarines is more limited, and that 75 percent of the Red Navy's personnel are conscripts (in contrast to the West's long-service professionals), it is difficult to see how the USSR would be in a position to bid for "command of the sea" in the near future.[201]

Finally, if indeed the real purpose of the newer and larger surface warships of the Soviet navy is to form an "ocean bastion" in, say, the Barents Sea to protect its nuclear-missile submarines from Allied attack—that is, if the Russian fleet is being chiefly designed to guard the country's *strategic deterrent* as it moves offshore[202]—then this clearly gives it little surplus force (apart from its older submarines) to interdict NATO's maritime lines of communication. By extension, therefore, there would be little prospect of the USSR's being able to render help to its scattered overseas bases and troop deployments in the event of a major conflict with the West. As it is, despite all of the publicity given to Russia's penetration of the Third World, it has very few forces stationed overseas (i.e., outside eastern Europe and Afghanistan), and its only major overseas bases are in Vietnam, Ethiopia, South Yemen, and Cuba, all of which require large amounts of direct financial aid, which seems to be being increasingly resented in Russia itself. It may be that the USSR, having recognized the vulnerability of its Trans-Siberian Railway in the event of a war in which China is involved, is systematically attempting to create a sea line of communication (SLOC), via the Indian Ocean, to its Far East territories. As things are at the moment, however, that route must still appear a very precarious one. Not only are the USSR's spheres of influence not comparable with the far larger array of American (plus British and French) bases, troops, and overseas fleets stationed across the globe, but the few Russian positions which do exist, being exposed, are very vulnerable to western pressures in wartime. If China, Japan, and certain smaller pro-western countries are brought into the equation, the picture looks even more unbalanced. To be sure, the forcible exclusion of the Soviet Union from the Third World would not be a great blow economically— since its trade, investments and loans in those lands are minuscule compared with those of the West[203]—but that is simply another reflection of its being *less* than a global Power.

Although all of this may seem to be overstating the odds which are stacked against the Soviet Union, it is worth noting that its own planners clearly do think about "worst-case" analyses; and also that its arms-control negotiators always resist any idea of having a mere *equality* of forces with the United States, arguing instead that Russia needs a "margin" to ensure its security against China and to take account of its eight-thousand-mile border. To any reasonable outside observer, the USSR already has more than enough forces to guarantee its security, and Moscow's insistence upon building ever-newer weapon systems simply induces insecurity in everyone else. To the decision-makers in the Kremlin, heirs to a militaristic and often paranoid tradition of statecraft, Russia appears surrounded by crumbling frontiers—in eastern Europe, along the "northern tier" of the Middle East, and in its lengthy shared border with China; yet having pushed out so many Russian divisions and air squadrons to stabilize those frontiers has not produced the hoped-for invulnerability. Pulling back from eastern Europe or making border concessions to China is also feared, however, not only because of the local consequences but because it may be seen as an indication of Moscow's loss of willpower. And at the same time as the Kremlin wrestles with these traditional problems of ensuring *territorial* security for the country's extensive landward border, it must also try to keep up with the United States in rocketry, satellite-based weapons, space exploration, and so on. Thus, the USSR—or, better, the Marxist system of the USSR—is being tested both quantitatively and qualitatively in the world power stakes; and it does not like the odds.

But those odds (or "correlation of forces") would obviously be better if the economy were healthier, which brings us back to Russia's long-term problem. Economics matters to the Soviet military, not merely because they are Marxist, and not only because it pays for their weapons and wages, but also because they understand its importance for the outcome of a lengthy, Great Power, coalition war. It *might* be true, the *Soviet Military Encyclopedia* conceded in 1979, that a global coalition war would be short, especially if nuclear weapons were used. "However, taking into account the great military and economic potentials of possible coalitions of belligerent states, it is not excluded that it might be protracted also."[204] But if such a war is "protracted," the emphasis will again be upon economic staying power, as it was in the great coalition wars of the past. With that assumption in mind, it cannot be comforting to the Soviet leadership to reflect that the USSR possesses only 12 or 13 percent of the world's GNP (or about 17 percent, if one dares to include the Warsaw Pact satellites as *plus* factors); and that it is not only far behind both the United States and western Europe in the size of its GNP, but it is also being overtaken by Japan and may—if long-term growth rates continue as they are—even find itself being approached by China in the next thirty years. If that seems an extraordinary claim, it is worth recalling the cold observation by *The Economist* that in 1913 "Imperial Russia had a real product per man-hour 3½ times greater than Japan's [but it] has spent its nigh 70 socialist years slipping relatively backwards, to maybe a quarter of Japan's rate now."[205] However one assesses the military strength of the USSR at the moment, therefore, the prospect of its being only the fourth or fifth among the great productive centers of the world by the early twenty-first century cannot but worry the Soviet leadership, simply because of the implications for long-term Russian power.

This does *not* mean that the USSR is close to collapse, any more than it should be viewed as a country of almost supernatural strength. It *does* mean that it is facing awkward choices. As one Russian expert has expressed it, "The policy of guns, butter, and growth—the political cornerstone of the Brezhnev era—is no longer possible . . . even under the more optimistic scenarios . . . the Soviet Union will face an economic crunch far more severe than anything it encountered in the 1960s and 1970s."[206] It is to be expected that the efforts and exhortations to improve the Russian economy will intensify. But since it is highly unlikely that even an energetic regime in Moscow would either abandon "scientific socialism" in order to boost the economy or drastically cut the burdens of defense expenditures and thereby affect the military core of the Soviet state, the prospects of an escape from the contradictions which the USSR faces are not good. Without its massive military power, it counts for little in the world; *with* its massive military power, it makes others feel insecure and hurts its own economic prospects. It is a grim dilemma.[207]

This can hardly be an unalloyed pleasure for the West, however, since there is nothing in the character or tradition of the Russian state to suggest that it could ever accept imperial decline gracefully. Indeed, historically, *none* of the overextended, multinational empires which have been dealt with in this survey—the Ottoman, the Spanish, the Napoleonic, the British—ever retreated to their own ethnic base until they had been defeated in a Great Power war, or (as with Britain after 1945) were so weakened by war that an imperial withdrawal was politically unavoidable. Those who rejoice at the present-day difficulties of the Soviet Union and who look forward to the collapse of that empire might wish to recall that such transformations normally occur at very great cost, and not always in a predictable fashion.

The United States: The Problem of Number One in Relative Decline

It is worth bearing in mind the Soviet Union's difficulties when one turns to analyze the present and the future circumstances of the United States, because of two important distinctions. The first is that while it can be argued that the American share of world power has been declining *relatively* faster than Russia's over the past few decades, its problems are probably nowhere near as great as those of its Soviet rival. Moreover, its *absolute* strength (especially in industrial and technological fields) is still much larger than that of the USSR. The second is that the very unstructured, laissez-faire nature of American society (while not without its weaknesses) probably gives it a better chance of readjusting to changing circumstances than a rigid and *dirigiste* power would have. But that in turn depends upon the existence of a national leadership which can understand the larger processes at work in the world today, and is aware of both the strong and the weak points of the U.S. position as it seeks to adjust to the changing global environment.

Although the United States is at present still in a class of its own economically and perhaps even militarily, it cannot avoid confronting the two great tests which challenge the *longevity* of every major power that occupies the "number one" position in world affairs: whether, in the military/strategical realm, it can preserve a reasonable balance between the nation's perceived defense requirements and the means it possesses to maintain those commitments; and whether, as an intimately related point, it can preserve the technological and economic bases of its power from relative erosion in the face of the ever-shifting patterns of global production. This test of American abilities will be the greater because it, like Imperial Spain around 1600 or the British Empire around 1900, is the inheritor of a vast array of strategical commitments which had been made decades earlier, when the nation's political, economic, and military capacity to influence world affairs seemed so much more assured. In consequence, the United States now runs the risk, so familiar to historians of the rise and fall of previous Great Powers, of what might roughly be called "imperial overstretch": that is to say, decision-makers in Washington must face the awkward and enduring fact that the sum total of the United States' global interests and obligations is nowadays far larger than the country's power to defend them all simultaneously.

Unlike those earlier Powers that grappled with the problem of strategical overextension, the United States also confronts the possibility of nuclear annihilation—a fact which, many people feel, has changed the entire nature of international power politics. If indeed a large-scale nuclear exchange were to occur, then any consideration of the United States' "prospects" becomes so problematical as to make it pointless—even if it also is the case that the American position (because of its defensive systems, and geographical extent) is probably more favorable than, say, France's or Japan's in such a conflict. On the other hand, the history of the post-1945 arms race so far suggests that nuclear weapons, while mutually threatening to East and West, also seem to be mutually unusable—which is the chief reason why the Powers continue to increase expenditures upon their *conventional* forces. If, however, the possibility exists of the major states someday becoming involved in a nonnuclear war (whether merely regional or on a larger scale), then the similarity of strategical circumstances between the United States today and imperial Spain or Edwardian Britain in their day is clearly much more appropriate. In each case, the declining number-one power faced threats, not so much to the security of its own homeland (in the United States' case, the prospect of being conquered by an invading army is remote), but to the nation's interests abroad—interests so widespread that it would be difficult to defend them all at once, and yet almost equally difficult to abandon any of them without running further risks.

Each of those interests abroad, it is fair to remark, was undertaken by the United States for what seemed very plausible (often very pressing) reasons at the time, and in most instances the reason for the American presence has not diminished; in certain parts of the globe, U.S. interests may now appear larger to decision-makers in Washington than they were a few decades ago.

That, it can be argued, is certainly true of American obligations in the Middle East. Here is a region, from Morocco in the west to Afghanistan in the east, where the United States faces a number of conflicts and problems whose mere listing (as one observer put it) "leaves one breathless."[208] It is an area which contains so much of the world's surplus oil supply; which seems so susceptible (at least on the map) to Soviet penetration; toward which a powerfully organized domestic lobby presses for unflinching support for an isolated but militarily efficient Israel; in which Arab states of a generally pro-western inclination (Egypt, Saudi Arabia, Jordan, the Gulf emirates) are under pressure from their own Islamic fundamentalists as well as from external threats such as Libya; and in which all the Arab states, whatever their own rivalries, oppose Israel's policy toward the Palestinians. This makes the region very important to the United States, but at the same time bewilderingly resistant to any simple policy option. It is, in addition, the region in the world which, at least in some parts of it, seems most frequently to resort to war. Finally, it contains the only territory—Afghanistan—which the Soviet Union is attempting to conquer by means of armed force. It is hardly surprising, therefore, that the Middle East has been viewed as requiring constant American attention, whether of a military or a diplomatic kind. Yet the memory of the 1979 debacle in Iran and of the ill-fated Lebanon venture of 1983, the diplomatic complexities of the antagonisms (how to assist Saudi Arabia without alarming Israel), and the unpopularity of the United States among the Arab masses all make it extremely difficult for an American government to conduct a coherent, long-term policy in the Middle East.

In Latin America, too, there are seen to be growing challenges to the United States' national interests. If a major international debt crisis is to occur anywhere in the world, dealing a heavy blow to the global credit system and especially to U.S. banks, it is likely to begin in this region. As it is, Latin America's economic problems have not only lowered the credit rating of many eminent American banking houses, but they have also contributed to a substantial decline in U.S. manufacturing exports to that region. Here, as in East Asia, the threat that the advanced, prosperous countries of the world will steadily increase tariffs against imported, low-labor-cost manufactures, and be ever less generous in their overseas-aid programs, is a cause for deep concern. All this is compounded by the fact that, economically and socially, Latin America has been changing remarkably swiftly over the past few decades;[209] at the same time, its demographic explosion is pressing ever harder upon the available resources, and upon the older conservative governing structures, in a considerable number of states. This has led to broad-based movements for social and constitutional reforms, or even for outright "revolution"—the latter being influenced by the present radical regimes in Cuba and Nicaragua. In turn, these movements have produced a conservative backlash, with reactionary governments proclaiming the need to eradicate all signs of domestic

Communism, and appealing to the United States for help to achieve that goal. These social and political fissures often compel the United States to choose between its desire to enhance democratic rights in Latin America and its wish to defeat Marxism. It also forces Washington to consider whether it can achieve its own purposes by political and economic means alone, or whether it may have to resort to military action (as in the case of Grenada).

By far the most worrying situation of all, however, lies just to the south of the United States, and makes the Polish "crisis" for the USSR seem small by comparison. There is simply no equivalent in the world for the present state of Mexican–United States relations. Mexico is on the verge of economic bankruptcy and default, its internal economic crisis forces hundreds of thousands to drift illegally to the north each year, its most profitable trade with the United States is swiftly becoming a brutally managed flow of hard drugs, and the border for all this sort of traffic is still extraordinarily permeable.[210]

If the challenges to American interests in East Asia are farther away, that does not diminish the significance of this vast area today. The largest share of the world's population lives there; a large and increasing proportion of American trade is with countries on the "Pacific rim"; two of the world's future Great Powers, China and Japan, are located there; the Soviet Union, directly and (through Vietnam) indirectly, is also there. So are those Asian newly industrializing countries, delicate quasi-democracies which on the one hand have embraced the capitalist laissez-faire ethos with a vengeance, and on the other are undercutting American manufacturing in everything from textiles to electronics. It is in East Asia, too, that a substantial number of American military obligations exist, usually as creations of the early Cold War.

Even a mere listing of those obligations cannot fail to suggest the extraordinarily wide-ranging nature of American interests in this region. A few years ago, the U.S. Defense Department attempted a brief summary of American interests in East Asia, but its very succinctness pointed, paradoxically, to the almost limitless extent of those strategical commitments:

> The importance to the United States of the security of East Asia and the Pacific is demonstrated by the bilateral treaties with Japan, Korea, and the Philippines; the Manila Pact, which adds Thailand to our treaty partners; and our treaty with Australia and New Zealand—the ANZUS Treaty. It is further enhanced by the deployment of land and air forces in Korea and Japan, and the forward deployment of the Seventh Fleet in the Western Pacific. Our foremost regional objectives, in conjunction with our regional friends and allies, are:

—To maintain the security of our essential sea lanes and of the United States' interests in the region; to maintain the capability to fulfill our treaty commitments in the Pacific and East Asia; to prevent the Soviet Union, North Korea, and Vietnam from interfering in the affairs of others; to build a durable strategic relationship with the People's Republic of China; and to support the stability and independence of friendly countries.[211]

Moreover, this carefully selected prose inevitably conceals a considerable number of extremely delicate political and strategic issues: how to build a good relationship with the PRC without abandoning Taiwan; how to "support the stability and independence of friendly countries" while trying to control the flood of their exports to the American market; how to make the Japanese assume a larger share of the defense of the western Pacific without alarming its various neighbors; how to maintain U.S. bases in, for example, the Philippines without provoking local resentments; how to reduce the American military presence in South Korea without sending the wrong "signal" to the North . . .

Larger still, at least as measured by military deployments, is the American stake in western Europe—the defense of which is, more than anything else, the strategic rationale of the American army and of much of the air force and the navy. According to some arcane calculations, in fact, 50 or 60 percent of American general-purpose forces are allocated to NATO, an organization in which (critics repeatedly point out) the other members contribute a significantly lower share of their GNP to defense spending even though Europe's total population and income are now larger than the USA's own.[212] This is not the place to rehearse the various European counterarguments in the "burden-sharing" debate (such as the social cost which countries like France and West Germany pay in maintaining conscription), or to develop the point that if western Europe was "Finlandized" the USA would probably spend even more on defense than at the moment.[213] From an American strategical perspective, the unavoidable fact is that this region has always seemed more vulnerable to Russian pressure than, say, Japan—partly because it is *not* an island, and partly because on the other side of the European land frontier the USSR has concentrated the largest proportion of its land and air forces, significantly greater than what may be reasonably needed for internal-security purposes. This still may not give Russia the military capacity to overrun western Europe (see pp. 507–9), but it is not a situation in which it would be prudent to withdraw substantial U.S. ground and air forces unilaterally. Even the outside possibility that the world's largest concentration of manufacturing production *might* fall into the Soviet orbit is enough to convince the Pentagon that "the security of western

Europe is particularly vital to the security of the United States."[214]

Yet however logical the American commitment to Europe may be strategically, that fact itself is no guarantee against certain military and political complications which have led to transatlantic discord. Although the NATO alliance brings the United States and western Europe close together at one level, the EEC itself is, like Japan, a rival in economic terms, especially in the shrinking markets for agricultural products. More significantly, while *official* European policy has always been to stress the importance of being under the American "nuclear umbrella," a broad-based unease exists among the general publics at the implications of siting U.S. weapons (cruise missiles, Pershing IIs, Trident-bearing submarines—let alone neutron bombs) on European soil. But if, to return to an earlier point, both superpowers would try to avoid "going nuclear" in the event of a major clash, that still leaves considerable problems in guaranteeing the defense of western Europe by *conventional* means. In the first place, that is a very expensive proposition. Secondly, even if one accepts the evidence which is beginning to suggest that the Warsaw Pact's land and air forces could in fact be held in check, such an argument is predicated upon a certain enhancement of NATO's current strength. From that perspective, nothing could be more upsetting than proposals to reduce or withdraw U.S. forces in Europe—however pressing that might be for economic reasons or for the purpose of buttressing American deployments elsewhere in the world. Yet carrying out a grand strategy which is both global and flexible is extremely difficult when so large a portion of the American armed forces are committed to one particular region.

In view of the above, it is not surprising that the circles most concerned about the discrepancy between American commitments and American power are the armed services themselves, simply because they would be the first to suffer if strategical weaknesses were exposed in the harsh test of war. Hence the frequent warnings by the Pentagon against being forced to carry out a global logistical juggling act, switching forces from one "hot spot" to another as new troubles emerge. If this was particularly acute in late 1983, when additional U.S. deployments in Central America, Grenada, Chad, and the Lebanon caused the former chairman of the Joint Chiefs of Staff to proclaim that the "mismatch" between American forces and strategy "is greater now than ever before,"[215] the problem had been implicit for years beforehand. Interestingly, such warnings about the American armed forces being "at full stretch" are attended by maps of "Major U.S. Military Deployment Around the World"[216] which, to historians, look extraordinarily similar to the chain of fleet bases and garrisons possessed by that former world power, Great Britain, at the height of its strategic overstretch.[217]

On the other hand, it is hardly likely that the United States would

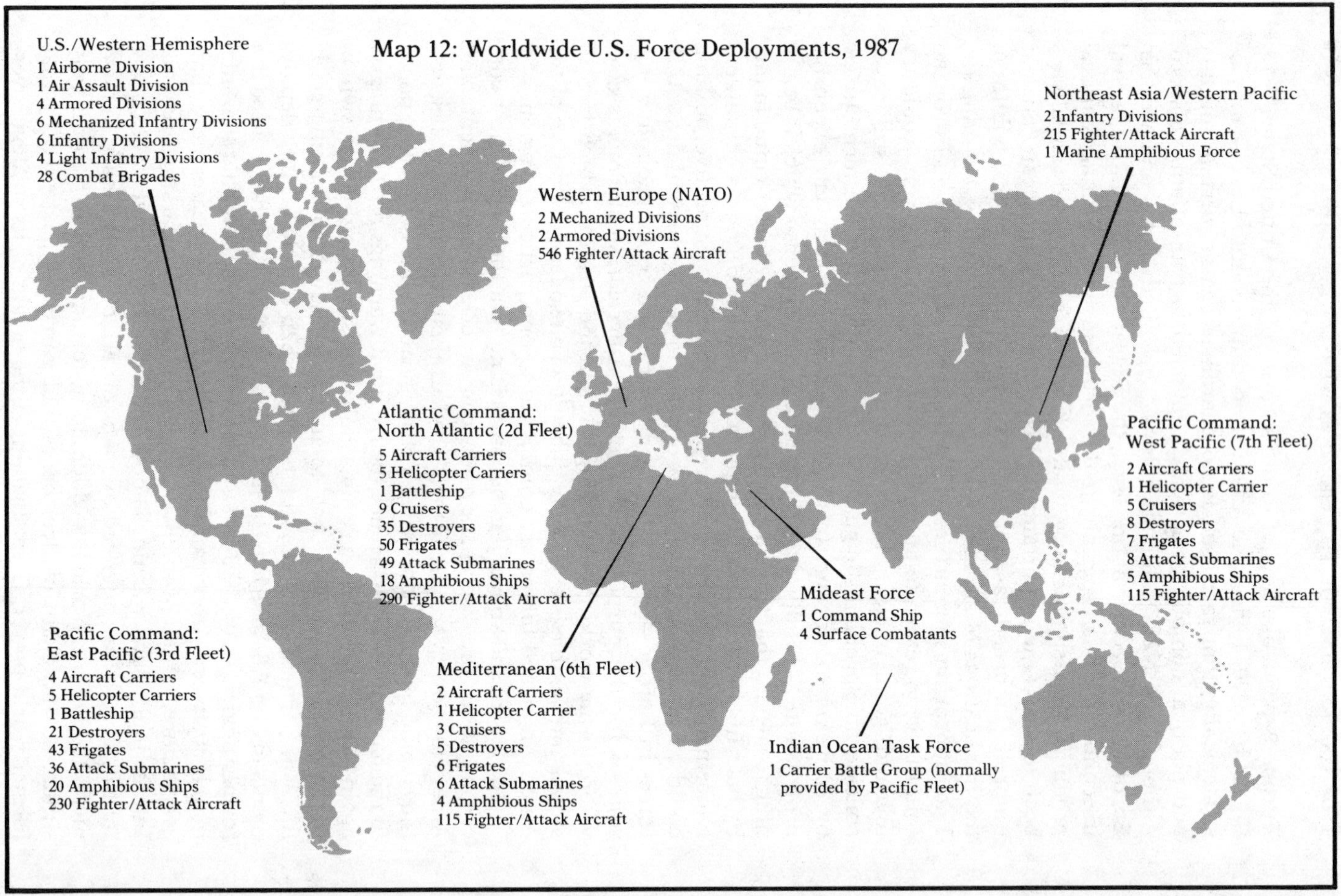

Map 12: Worldwide U.S. Force Deployments, 1987

U.S./Western Hemisphere
1 Airborne Division
1 Air Assault Division
4 Armored Divisions
6 Mechanized Infantry Divisions
4 Infantry Divisions
4 Light Infantry Divisions
28 Combat Brigades

Northeast Asia/Western Pacific
2 Infantry Divisions
215 Fighter/Attack Aircraft
1 Marine Amphibious Force

Pacific Command:
West Pacific (7th Fleet)
2 Aircraft Carriers
1 Helicopter Carrier
5 Cruisers
8 Destroyers
7 Frigates
8 Attack Submarines
5 Amphibious Ships
115 Fighter/Attack Aircraft

Western Europe (NATO)
2 Mechanized Divisions
2 Armored Divisions
546 Fighter/Attack Aircraft

Atlantic Command:
North Atlantic (2d Fleet)
5 Aircraft Carriers
5 Helicopter Carriers
1 Battleship
9 Cruisers
35 Destroyers
50 Frigates
49 Attack Submarines
18 Amphibious Ships
290 Fighter/Attack Aircraft

Mideast Force
1 Command Ship
4 Surface Combatants

Indian Ocean Task Force
1 Carrier Battle Group (normally
provided by Pacific Fleet)

Mediterranean (6th Fleet)
2 Aircraft Carriers
1 Helicopter Carrier
3 Cruisers
5 Destroyers
6 Frigates
6 Attack Submarines
4 Amphibious Ships
115 Fighter/Attack Aircraft

Pacific Command:
East Pacific (3rd Fleet)
4 Aircraft Carriers
5 Helicopter Carriers
1 Battleship
21 Destroyers
43 Frigates
36 Attack Submarines
20 Amphibious Ships
230 Fighter/Attack Aircraft

Source: American Defense Annual, 1987–1988

be called upon to defend *all* of its overseas interests simultaneously
and without the aid of a significant number of allies—the NATO members in western Europe, Israel in the Middle East, and, in the Pacific,
Japan, Australia, possibly China. Nor are all the regional trends
becoming unfavorable to the United States in defense terms; for example, while aggression by the unpredictable North Korean regime is
always possible, that would hardly be welcomed by Peking nowadays—and, in addition, South Korea itself has grown to possess over
twice the population and four times the GNP of North Korea. In the
same way, while the expansion of Russian forces in the Far East is
alarming to Washington, that is considerably balanced off by the growing threat posed by the PRC to Russia's land and sea lines of communication with the Orient. The recent, sober admission by the U.S. defense
secretary that "we can never afford to buy the capabilities sufficient to
meet all of our commitments with one hundred percent confidence"[218]
is surely true; but it may be less worrying than at first appears if it is
also recalled that the total of potential anti-Soviet resources in the
world (United States, western Europe, Japan, PRC, Australasia) is far
greater than the total of resources lined up on Russia's side.

Despite such consolations, the fundamental grand-strategical dilemma remains: the United States today has roughly the same massive
array of military obligations across the globe as it had a quarter-century ago, when its shares of world GNP, manufacturing production,
military spending, and armed forces personnel were so much larger
than they are now.[219] Even in 1985, forty years after its triumphs of the
Second World War and over a decade after its pull-out from Vietnam,
the United States had 520,000 members of its armed forces abroad
(including 65,000 afloat).[220] That total is, incidentally, substantially
more than the overseas deployments in peacetime of the military and
naval forces of the British Empire at the height of its power. Nevertheless, in the strongly expressed opinion of the Joint Chiefs of Staff, and
of many civilian experts,[221] it is simply not enough. Despite a near-
trebling of the American defense budget since the late 1970s, there has
occurred a "mere 5 percent increase in the numerical size of the armed
forces on active duty."[222] As the British and French military found in
their time, a nation with extensive overseas obligations will always
have a more difficult "manpower problem" than a state which keeps its
armed forces solely for home defense; and a politically liberal and
economically laissez-faire society—aware of the unpopularity of conscription—will have a greater problem than most.[223]

Possibly this concern about the gap between American interests
and capabilities in the world would be less acute had there not been
so much doubt expressed—since at least the time of the Vietnam War—
about the *efficiency* of the system itself. Since those doubts have been
repeatedly aired in other studies, they will only be summarized here;

this is not a further essay on the hot topic of "defense reform."[224] One major area of contention, for example, has been the degree of interservice rivalry, which is of course common to most armed forces but seems more deeply entrenched in the American system—possibly because of the relatively modest powers of the chairman of the Joint Chiefs of Staff, possibly because so much more energy appears to be devoted to procurement as opposed to strategical and operational issues. In peacetime, this might merely be dismissed as an extreme example of "bureaucratic politics"; but in actual wartime operations— say, in the emergency dispatch of the Rapid Deployment Joint Task Force, which contains elements from all four services—a lack of proper coordination could be fatal.

In the area of military procurement itself, allegations of "waste, fraud and abuse"[225] have been commonplace. The various scandals over horrendously expensive, *under*performing weapons which have caught the public's attention in recent years have plausible explanations: the lack of proper competitive bidding and of market forces in the "military-industrial complex," and the tendency toward "gold-plated" weapon systems, not to mention the striving for large profits. It is difficult, however, to separate those deficiencies in the procurement process from what is clearly a more fundamental happening: the intensification of the impacts which new technological advances make upon the art of war. Given that it is in the high-technology field that the USSR usually appears most vulnerable—which suggests that American *quality* in weaponry can be employed to counter the superior Russian *quantity* of, say, tanks and aircraft—there is an obvious attraction in what Caspar Weinberger termed "competitive strategies" when ordering new armaments.[226] Nevertheless, the fact that the Reagan administration in its first term spent over 75 percent more on new aircraft than the Carter regime but acquired only 9 percent more planes points to *the* appalling military-procurement problem of the late twentieth century: given the technologically driven tendency toward spending more and more money upon fewer and fewer weapon systems, would the United States and its allies really have enough sophisticated and highly expensive aircraft and tanks in reserve after the early stages of a ferociously fought conventional war? Does the U.S. Navy possess enough attack submarines, or frigates, if heavy losses were incurred in the early stages of a *third* Battle of the Atlantic? If not, the results would be grim; for it is clear that today's complex weaponry simply cannot be replaced in the short times which were achieved during the Second World War.

This dilemma is accentuated by two other elements in the complicated calculus of evolving an effective American defense policy. The first is the issue of budgetary constraints. Unless external circumstances became much more threatening, it would be a remarkable act of political persuasion to get national defense expenditures raised much above, say, 7.5 percent of GNP—the more especially since the size of the federal deficit (see below, pp. 527–28) points to the need to balance governmental spending as the first priority of state. But if there is a slowing-down or even a halt in the increase in defense spending, coinciding with the continuous upward spiral in weapons costs, then the problem facing the Pentagon will become much more acute.

The second factor is the sheer variety of military contingencies that a global superpower like the United States has to plan for—all of which, in their way, place differing demands upon the armed forces and the weaponry they are likely to employ. This again is not without precedent in the history of the Great Powers; the British army was frequently placed under strain by having to plan to fight on the North-west Frontier of India *or* in Belgium. But even that challenge pales beside the task facing today's "number one." If the critical issue for the United States is preserving a nuclear deterrent against the Soviet Union, at *all* levels of escalation, then money will inevitably be poured into such weapons as the MX missile, the B-1 and "Stealth" bombers, Pershing IIs, cruise missiles, and Trident-bearing submarines. If a large-scale conventional war against the Warsaw Pact is the most probable scenario, then the funds presumably need to go in quite different directions: tactical aircraft, main battle tanks, large carriers, frigates, attack submarines, and logistical services. If it is likely that the United States and the USSR will avoid a direct clash, but that both will become more active in the Third World, then the weapons mix changes again: small arms, helicopters, light carriers, an enhanced role for the U.S. Marine Corps become the chief items on the list. Already it is clear that a large part of the controversy over "defense reform" stems from differing assumptions about the *type* of war the United States might be called upon to fight. But what if those in authority make the wrong assumption?

A further major concern about the efficiency of the system, and one voiced even by strong supporters of the campaign to "restore" American power,[227] is whether the present decision-making structure permits a proper grand strategy to be carried out. This would not merely imply achieving a greater coherence in military policies, so that there is less argument about "maritime strategy" versus "coalition warfare,"[228] but would also involve effecting a synthesis of the United States' long-term political, economic, and strategical interests, in place of the bureaucratic infighting which seems to have characterized so much of Washington's policymaking. A much-quoted example of this is the all-too-frequent *public* dispute about how and where the United States should employ its armed forces abroad to enhance or defend its national interests—with the State Department wanting clear and firm responses made to those who threaten such interests, but the Defense

Department being unwilling (especially after the Lebanon debacle) to get involved overseas except under special conditions.[229] But there also have been, and by contrast, examples of the Pentagon's preference for taking unilateral decisions in the arms race with Russia (e.g., SDI program, abandoning SALT II) without consulting major allies, which leaves problems for the State Department. There have been uncertainties attending the role played by the National Security Council, and more especially individual national security advisers. There have been incoherencies of policy in the Middle East, partly because of the intractibility of, say, the Palestine issue, but also because the United States' strategical interest in supporting the conservative, pro-Western Arab states against Russian penetration in that area has often foundered upon the well-organized opposition of its own pro-Israel lobby. There have been interdepartmental disputes about the use of economic tools—from boycotts on trade and embargoes on technology transfer to foreign-aid grants and weapons sales and grain sales—in support of American diplomatic interests, which affect policies toward the Third World, South Africa, Russia, Poland, the EEC, and so on, and which have sometimes been uncoordinated and contradictory. No sensible person would maintain that the many foreign-policy problems afflicting the globe each possess an obvious and ready "solution"; on the other hand, the preservation of long-term American interests is certainly not helped when the decision-making system is attended by frequent disagreements within.

All this has led to questions by gloomier critics about the overall political culture in which Washington decision-makers have to operate. This is far too large and complex a matter to be explored in depth here. But it has been increasingly suggested that a country needing to reformulate its grand strategy in the light of the larger, uncontrollable changes taking place in world affairs may not be well served by an electoral system which seems to paralyze foreign-policy decision-making every two years. It may not be helped by the extraordinary pressures applied by lobbyists, political action committees, and other interest groups, all of which, by definition, are prejudiced in respect to this or that policy change; nor by an inherent "simplification" of vital but complex international and strategical issues through a mass media whose time and space for such things are limited, and whose *raison d'être* is chiefly to make money and secure audiences, and only secondarily to inform. It may also not be helped by the still-powerful "escapist" urges in the American social culture, which may be understandable in terms of the nation's "frontier" past but is a hindrance to coming to terms with today's more complex, integrated world and with *other* cultures and ideologies. Finally, the country may not always be assisted by its division of constitutional and decision-making powers, deliberately created when it was geographically and strategically isolated from the rest of the world two centuries ago, and possessed a decent degree of time to come to an agreement on the few issues which actually concerned "foreign" policy, but which may be harder to operate when it has become a global superpower, often called upon to make swift decisions vis-à-vis countries which enjoy far fewer constraints. No single one of these presents an insuperable obstacle to the execution of a coherent, long-term American grand strategy; their cumulative and interacting effect is, however, to make it much more difficult than otherwise to carry out needed changes of policy if that seems to hurt special interests and occurs in an election year. It may therefore be here, in the cultural and domestic-political realms, that the evolution of an effective overall American policy to meet the twenty-first century will be subjected to the greatest test.

The final question about the proper relationship of "means and ends" in the defense of American global interests relates to the economic challenges bearing down upon the country, which, because they are so various, threaten to place immense strains upon decision-making in national policy. The extraordinary breadth and complexity of the American economy makes it difficult to summarize what is happening to all parts of it—especially in a period when it is sending out such contradictory signals.[230] Nonetheless, the features which were described in the preceding chapter (pp. 432–35) still prevail.

The first of these is the country's relative industrial decline, as measured against world production, not only in older manufactures such as textiles, iron and steel, shipbuilding, and basic chemicals, but also—although it is far less easy to judge the final outcome of this level of industrial-technological combat—in global shares of robotics, aerospace, automobiles, machine tools, and computers. Both of these pose immense problems: in traditional and basic manufacturing, the gap in wage scales between the United States and newly industrializing countries is probably such that no "efficiency measures" will close it; but to lose out in the competition in future technologies, if that indeed should occur, would be even more disastrous. In late 1986, for example, a congressional study reported that the U.S. trade surplus in high-technology goods had plunged from $27 billion in 1980 to a mere $4 billion in 1985, and was swiftly heading into a deficit.[231]

The second, and in many ways less expected, sector of decline is agriculture. Only a decade ago, experts in that subject were predicting a frightening global imbalance between feeding requirements and farming output.[232] But such a scenario of famine and disaster stimulated two powerful responses. The first was a massive investment into American farming from the 1970s onward, fueled by the prospect of ever-larger overseas food sales; the second was the enormous (western-world-funded) investigation into scientific means of increasing Third World crop outputs, which has been so successful as to turn growing numbers of such countries into food *exporters,* and thus competitors of the United States. These two trends are separate from, but have coincided with, the transformation of the EEC into a major producer of agricultural surpluses, because of its price-support system. In consequence, experts now refer to a "world awash in food," [233] which in turn leads to sharp declines in agricultural prices and in American food exports—and drives many farmers out of business.

It is not surprising, therefore, that these economic problems have led to a surge in protectionist sentiment throughout many sectors of the American economy, and among businessmen, unions, farmers, and their congressmen. As with the "tariff reform" agitation in Edwardian Britain,[234] the advocates of increased protection complain of unfair foreign practices, of "dumping" below-cost manufactures on the American market, and of enormous subsidies to foreign farmers—which, they maintain, can only be answered by U.S. administrations abandoning their laissez-faire policy on trade and instituting tough countermeasures. Many of those individual complaints (e.g., of Japan shipping below-cost silicon chips to the American market) have been valid. More broadly, however, the surge in protectionist sentiment is also a reflection of the erosion of the previously unchallenged U.S. manufacturing supremacy. Like mid-Victorian Britons, Americans after 1945 favored free trade and open competition, not just because they held that global commerce and prosperity would be boosted in the process, but also because they knew that they were most likely to benefit from the abandonment of protectionism. Forty years later, with that confidence ebbing, there is a predictable shift of opinion in favor of protecting the domestic market and the domestic producer. And, just as in that earlier British case, defenders of the existing system point out that enhanced tariffs might not only make domestic products *less* competitive internationally, but that there also could be various external repercussions—a global tariff war, blows against American exports, the undermining of the currencies of certain newly industrializing countries, and a return to the economic crisis of the 1930s.

Along with these difficulties affecting American manufacturing and agriculture there are unprecedented turbulences in the nation's finances. The uncompetitiveness of U.S. industrial products abroad and the declining sales of agricultural exports have together produced staggering deficits in visible trade—$160 billion in the twelve months to May 1986—but what is more alarming is that such a gap can no longer be covered by American earnings on "invisibles," which is the traditional recourse of a mature economy (e.g., Great Britain before 1914). On the contrary, the only way the United States can pay its way in the world is by importing ever-larger sums of capital, which has transformed it from being the world's largest creditor to the world's largest debtor nation *in the space of a few years.*

Compounding this problem—in the view of many critics, *causing* this problem[235]—have been the budgetary policies of the U.S. government itself. Even in the 1960s, there was a tendency for Washington to rely upon deficit finance, rather than additional taxes, to pay for the increasing cost of defense and social programs. But the decisions taken by the Reagan administration in the early 1980s—i.e., large-scale increases in defense expenditures, plus considerable decreases in taxation, but *without* significant reductions in federal spending elsewhere—have produced extraordinary rises in the deficit, and consequently in the national debt, as shown in Table 49.

Table 49. U.S. Federal Deficit, Debt, and
Interest, 1980–1985[236]
(billions of dollars)

	Deficit	Debt	Interest on Debt
1980	59.6	914.3	52.5
1983	195.4	1,381.9	87.8
1985	202.8	1,823.1	129.0

The continuation of such trends, alarmed voices have pointed out, would push the U.S. national debt to around $13 *trillion* by the year 2000 (fourteen times that of 1980), and the interest payments on such debt to $1.5 *trillion* (twenty-nine times that of 1980).[237] In fact, a lowering of interest rates could bring down those estimates,[238] but the overall trend is still very unhealthy. Even if federal deficits could be reduced to a "mere" $100 billion annually, the compounding of national debt and interest payments by the early twenty-first century will still cause quite unprecedented totals of money to be diverted in that direction. Historically, the only other example which comes to mind of a Great Power so increasing its indebtedness in *peacetime* is France in the 1780s, where the fiscal crisis contributed to the domestic political crisis.

These American trade and federal deficits are now interacting with a new phenomenon in the world economy—what is perhaps best described as the "dislocation" of international capital movements from the trade in goods and services. Because of the growing integration of the world economy, the volume of trade both in manufactures and in financial services is much larger than ever before, and together may amount to some $3 trillion a year; but that is now eclipsed by the stupendous level of capital flows pouring through the world's money markets, with the London-based Eurodollar market alone having a volume "at least 25 times that of world trade."[239] While this trend was fueled by events in the 1970s (the move from fixed to floating exchange rates, the surplus funds flowing from OPEC countries), it has also been stimulated by the U.S. deficits, since the only way the federal government has been able to cover the yawning gap between its expenditures and its receipts has been to suck into the country tremendous amounts of liquid funds from Europe and (especially) Japan—turning the United States, as mentioned above, into the world's largest debtor country by far.[240] It is, in fact, difficult to imagine how the American economy could have got by *without* the inflow of foreign funds in the early 1980s, even if that had the awkward consequence of sending up the exchange value of the dollar, and further hurting U.S. agricultural and manufacturing exports. But that in turn raises the troubling question about what might happen if those massive and volatile funds were pulled out of the dollar, causing its value to drop precipitously.

The trends have, in turn, produced explanations which suggest that alarmist voices are exaggerating the gravity of what is happening to the U.S. economy and failing to note the "naturalness" of most of these developments. For example, the midwestern farm belt would be much less badly off had not so many individuals bought land at inflated prices and excessive interest rates in the late 1970s. Again, the move from manufacturing into services is an understandable one, which is occurring in all advanced countries; and it is also worth recalling that U.S. manufacturing *output* has been rising in absolute terms, even if employment (especially blue-collar employment) in manufacturing industry has been falling—but that again is a "natural" trend, as the world increasingly moves from material-based to knowledge-based production. Similarly, there is nothing wrong in the metamorphosis of American financial institutions into *world* financial institutions, with a triple base in Tokyo, London, and New York, to handle (and profit from) the great volume of capital flows; that can only boost the nation's earnings from services. Even the large annual federal deficits and the mounting national debt are sometimes described as being not too serious, after allowance is made for inflation; and there exists in some quarters a belief that the economy will "grow its way out" of these deficits, or that measures will be taken by the politicians to close the gap, whether by increasing taxes or cutting spending or a combination of both. A too-hasty attempt to slash the deficit, it is pointed out, could well trigger off a major recession.

Even more reassuring are said to be the positive signs of growth in the American economy. Because of the boom in the services sector, the United States has been creating jobs over the past decade faster than at any time in its peacetime history—and certainly a lot faster than in western Europe. As a related point, its far greater degree of labor mobility eases such transformations in the job market. Furthermore, the enormous American commitment in high technology—not just in California, but in New England, Virginia, Arizona, and many other parts of the land—promises ever greater outputs of production, and thus of national wealth (as well as ensuring a strategical edge over the USSR). Indeed, it is precisely because of the opportunities that exist in the American economy that it continues to attract millions of immigrants, and to stimulate thousands of new entrepreneurs; while the floods of capital which pour into the country can be tapped for further investment, especially into R&D. Finally, if the shifts in the global terms of trade are indeed leading to lower prices for foodstuffs and raw materials, that ought to benefit an economy which still imports enormous amounts of oil, metal ores, and so on (even if it hurts particular American producers, like farmers and oilmen).

Many of these individual points may be valid. Since the American economy is so large and variegated, some sectors and regions are likely to be growing at the same time as others are in decline—and to characterize the whole with sweeping generalizations about "crisis" or "boom" is therefore inappropriate. Given the decline in raw-materials prices, the ebbing of the dollar's unsustainably high exchange value of early 1985, the general fall in interest rates—and the impact of all three trends upon inflation and upon business confidence—it is not surprising to find some professional economists being optimistic about the future.[241]

Nevertheless, from the viewpoint of American grand strategy, and of the economic foundation upon which an effective, long-term strategy needs to rest, the picture is much less rosy. In the first place, given the worldwide array of military liabilities which the United States has assumed since 1945, its capacity to carry those burdens is obviously less than it was several decades ago, when its share of global manufacturing and GNP was much larger, its agriculture was not in crisis, its balance of payments was far healthier, the government budget was also in balance, and it was not so heavily in debt to the rest of the world. In that larger sense, there is something in the analogy which is made by certain political scientists between the United States' position today and that of previous "declining hegemons."[242]

Here again, it is instructive to note the uncanny similarities between the growing mood of anxiety among thoughtful circles in the United States today and that which pervaded all political parties in Edwardian Britain and led to what has been termed the "national efficiency" movement: that is, a broad-based debate within the nation's decision-making, business, and educational elites over the various measures which could reverse what was seen to be a growing uncompetitiveness as compared with other advanced societies. In terms of commercial expertise, levels of training and education, efficiency of production, standards of income and (among the less well-off) of living, health, and housing, the "number-one" power of 1900 seemed to be losing its position, with dire implications for the country's long-term *strategic* position; hence the fact that the calls for "renewal" and "reorganization" came at least as much from the Right as from the Left.[243] Such campaigns usually do lead to reforms, here and there; but their very existence is, ironically, a confirmation of decline, in that such an agitation simply would not have been necessary a few decades earlier, when the nation's lead was unquestioned. A strong man, the writer G. K. Chesterton sardonically observed, does not worry about his bodily efficiency; only when he weakens does he begin to talk about health.[244] In the same way, when a Great Power is strong and unchallenged, it will be much less likely to debate its capacity to meet its obligations than when it is relatively weaker.

More narrowly, there could be serious implications for American grand strategy if its industrial base continued to shrink. Were there ever to be a large-scale future war which remained conventional (because of the belligerents' mutual fear of triggering a nuclear holocaust), then one is bound to wonder what the impact upon U.S. productive capacities would be after years of decline in certain key industries, the erosion of blue-collar employment, and so on. In this connection, one is reminded of Hewins's alarmed cry in 1904 about the impact of British industrial decay upon *that* country's power:[245]

> Suppose an industry which is threatened [by foreign competition] is one which lies at the very root of your system of National defence, where are you then? You could not get on without an iron industry, a great Engineering trade, because in modern warfare you would not have the means of producing, and maintaining in a state of efficiency, your fleets and armies.

It is hard to imagine that the decline in American industrial capacity could be so severe: its manufacturing base is simply that much broader than Edwardian Britain's was; and—an important point—the "defense-related industries" have not only been sustained by repeated Pentagon orders, but have paralleled the shift from materials-intensive into knowledge-intensive (high-technology) manufacturing, which over the longer term will also reduce the West's reliance upon critical raw materials. Even so, the very high proportion of, say, semiconductors which are assembled in foreign countries and then shipped to the United States,[246] or—to think of a product as far removed from semiconductors as possible—the erosion of the American shipping and shipbuilding industry, or the closing down of so many American mines and oilfields—such trends cannot but be damaging in the event of another long-lasting, Great Power, coalition war. If, moreover, historical precedents are of any validity at all, the most critical constraint upon any "surge" in wartime production has usually been in the area of skilled craftsmen[247]—which, once again, causes one to wonder about the massive long-term decline in American blue-collar (i.e., usually skilled-craftsmen) employment.

A quite different problem, but one equally important for the sus-

taining of a proper grand strategy, concerns the impact of slow economic growth upon the American social/political consensus. To a
degree which amazes most Europeans, the United States in the twentieth century has managed to avoid ostensible "class" politics. This is
due, one imagines, to the facts that so many of its immigrants were
fleeing from socially rigid circumstances elsewhere; that the sheer size
of the country allowed those who were disillusioned with their economic position to "escape" to the West, and simultaneously made the
organization of labor much more difficult than in, say, France or Britain; and that those same geographical dimensions, and the entrepreneurial opportunities within them, encouraged the development of
a largely unreconstructed form of laissez-faire capitalism which has
dominated the political culture of the nation (despite occasional counterattacks from the left). In consequence, the "earnings gap" between
rich and poor in the United States is significantly larger than in any
other advanced industrial society; and, by the same token, state expenditures upon social services form a lower share of GNP than in comparable countries (except Japan, which appears to have a much stronger
family-based form of support for the poor and the aged).

This lack of "class" politics despite the obvious socioeconomic disparities has obviously been helped by the fact that the United States'
overall growth since the 1930s offered the prospect of individual better-
ment to a majority of the population; and by the more disturbing fact
that the poorest *one-third* of American society has not been "mobilized" to become regular voters. But given the differentiated birthrate
between the white ethnic groups on the one hand and the black and
Hispanic groups on the other—not to mention the changing flow of
immigrants into the United States, and given also the economic metamorphosis which is leading to the loss of millions of relatively high-
earning jobs in manufacturing, and the creation of millions of poorly
paid jobs in services, it may be unwise to assume that the prevailing
norms of the American political economy (low government expenditures, low taxes on the rich) would be maintained if the nation entered
a period of sustained economic difficulty caused by a plunging dollar
and slow growth. What this also suggests is that an American polity
which responds to external challenges by increasing defense expenditures, and reacts to the budgetary crisis by slashing the existing social
expenditures, may run the risk of provoking an eventual political backlash. As with all of the other Powers surveyed in this chapter, there are
no easy answers in dealing with the constant three-way tension between defense, consumption, and investment in settling national priorities.

This brings us, inevitably, to the delicate relationship between slow
economic growth and high defense spending. The debate upon "the
economics of defense spending" is a highly controversial one, and—

bearing in mind the size and variety of the American economy, the stimulus which can come from large government contracts, and the technical spin-offs from weapons research—the evidence does not point simply in one direction.[248] But what is significant for our purposes is the comparative dimension. Even if (as is often pointed out) defense expenditures formed 10 percent of GNP under Eisenhower and 9 percent under Kennedy, the United States' relative share of global production and wealth was at that time around *twice* what it is today; and, more particularly, the American economy was not then facing the challenges to either its traditional or its high-technology manufactures. Moreover, if the United States at present continues to devote 7 percent or more of its GNP to defense spending while its major economic rivals, especially Japan, allocate a far smaller proportion, then *ipso facto* the latter have potentially more funds "free" for civilian investment; if the United States continues to invest a massive amount of its R&D activities into military-related production while the Japanese and West Germans concentrate upon commercial R&D; and if the Pentagon's spending drains off the majority of the country's scientists and engineers from the design and production of goods for the world market while similar personnel in other countries are primarily engaged in bringing out better products for the civilian consumer, then it seems inevitable that the American share of world manufacturing will steadily decline, and also likely that its economic growth rates will be slower than in those countries dedicated to the marketplace and less eager to channel resources into defense.[249]

It is almost superfluous to say that these tendencies place the United States on the horns of a most acute dilemma over the longer term. Simply because it is *the* global superpower, with far more extensive military commitments than a regional Power like Japan or West Germany, it requires much larger defense forces—in just the same way as imperial Spain felt it needed a far larger army than its contemporaries and Victorian Britain insisted upon a much bigger navy than any other country. Furthermore, since the USSR is seen to be the major military threat to American interests across the globe and is clearly devoting a far greater proportion of *its* GNP to defense, American decision-makers are inevitably worried about "losing" the arms race with Russia. Yet the more sensible among these decision-makers can also perceive that the burden of armaments is debilitating the Soviet economy; and that if the two superpowers continue to allocate ever-larger shares of their national wealth into the unproductive field of armaments, the critical question might soon be: "Whose economy will decline *fastest*, relative to such expanding states as Japan, China, etc.?" A low investment in armaments may, for a globally overstretched Power like the United States, leave it feeling vulnerable everywhere; but a very heavy investment in armaments, while bringing greater security in the short term, may so erode the commercial competitiveness of the American economy that the nation will be *less* secure in the long term.[250]

Here, too, the historical precedents are not encouraging. For it has been a common dilemma facing previous "number-one" countries that even as their relative economic strength is ebbing, the growing foreign challenges to their position have compelled them to allocate more and more of their resources into the military sector, which in turn squeezes out productive investment and, over time, leads to the downward spiral of slower growth, heavier taxes, deepening domestic splits over spending priorities, and a weakening capacity to bear the burdens of defense.[251] If this, indeed, is the pattern of history, one is tempted to paraphrase Shaw's deadly serious quip and say: "Rome fell; Babylon fell; Scarsdale's turn will come."[252]

In the largest sense of all, therefore, the only answer to the question increasingly debated by the public of whether the United States can preserve its existing position is "no"—for it simply has not been given to any one society to remain *permanently* ahead of all the others, because that would imply a freezing of the differentiated pattern of growth rates, technological advance, and military developments which has existed since time immemorial. On the other hand, this reference to historical precedents does *not* imply that the United States is destined to shrink to the relative obscurity of former leading Powers such as Spain or the Netherlands, or to disintegrate like the Roman and Austro-Hungarian empires; it is simply too large to do the former, and presumably too homogeneous to do the latter. Even the British analogy, much favored in the current political-science literature, is not a good one if it ignores the differences in *scale*. This can be put another way: the geographical size, population, and natural resources of the British Isles would suggest that it ought to possess roughly 3 or 4 percent of the world's wealth and power, *all other things being equal;* but it is precisely because all other things are *never* equal that a peculiar set of historical and technological circumstances permitted the British Isles to expand to possess, say, 25 percent of the world's wealth and power in its prime; and since those favorable circumstances have disappeared, all that it has been doing is returning down to its more "natural" size. In the same way, it may be argued that the geographical extent, population, and natural resources of the United States suggest that it ought to possess perhaps 16 or 18 percent of the world's wealth and power, but because of historical and technical circumstances favorable to it, that share rose to 40 percent or more by 1945; and what we are witnessing at the moment is the early decades of the ebbing away from that extraordinarily high figure to a more "natural" share. That decline is being masked by the country's enormous military capabilities at present, and also by its success in "internationalizing" American capitalism and culture.[253] Yet even when it declines to occupy its "natural" share of the world's wealth and power, a long time into the future, the United States will still be a very significant Power in a multipolar world, simply because of its size.

The task facing American statesmen over the next decades, therefore, is to recognize that broad trends are under way, and that there is a need to "manage" affairs so that the *relative* erosion of the United States' position takes place slowly and smoothly, and is not accelerated by policies which bring merely short-term advantage but longer-term disadvantage. This involves, from the president's office downward, an appreciation that technological and therefore socioeconomic change is occurring in the world faster than ever before; that the international community is much more politically and culturally diverse than has been assumed, and is defiant of simplistic remedies offered either by Washington or Moscow to its problems; that the economic and productive power balances are no longer as favorably tilted in the United States' direction as in 1945; and that, even in the military realm, there are signs of a certain redistribution of the balances, away from a bipolar to more of a multipolar system, in which the conglomeration of American economic-cum-military strength is likely to remain larger than that possessed by any one of the others individually, but will not be as disproportionate as in the decades which immediately followed the Second World War. This, in itself, is not a bad thing if one recalls Kissinger's observations about the disadvantages of carrying out policies in what is always seen to be a bipolar world (see pp. 407–8); and it may seem still less of a bad thing when it is recognized how much more Russia may be affected by the changing dynamics of world power. In all of the discussions about the erosion of American leadership, it needs to be repeated again and again that the decline referred to is relative not absolute, and is therefore perfectly natural; and that the only serious threat to the real interests of the United States can come from a failure to adjust sensibly to the newer world order.

Given the considerable array of strengths still possessed by the United States, it ought not *in theory* to be beyond the talents of successive administrations to arrange the diplomacy and strategy of this readjustment so that it can, in Walter Lippmann's classic phrase, bring "into balance . . . the nation's commitments and the nation's power."[254] Although there is no obvious, single "successor state" which can take over America's global burdens in the way that the United States assumed Britain's role in the 1940s, it is nonetheless also true that the country has fewer problems than an imperial Spain besieged by enemies on all fronts, or a Netherlands being squeezed between France and England, or a British Empire facing a bevy of challengers. The tests before the United States as it heads toward the twenty-first century are certainly daunting, perhaps especially in the economic sphere; but the nation's resources remain considerable, *if* they can be properly organized, and *if* there is a judicious recognition of both the limitations and the opportunities of American power.

Viewed from one perspective, it can hardly be said that the dilemmas facing the United States are unique. Which country in the world, one it tempted to ask, is *not* encountering problems in evolving a viable military policy, or in choosing between guns and butter and investment? From another perspective, however, the American position is a very special one. For all its economic and perhaps military decline, it remains, in Pierre Hassner's words, "the decisive actor in every type of balance and issue."[255] Because it has so much power for good or evil, because it is the linchpin of the western alliance system and the center of the existing global economy, what it does, *or does not do,* is so much more important than what any of the other Powers decides to do.

Epilogue

After a five-hundred-year survey of the rise and fall of the Great Powers within the international system, there is a case for concluding with a substantial final section on *theory* and *methodology*, in which the author would engage the proliferating theories upon "war and the cycle of relative power,"[1] "global wars, public debts, and the long cycle,"[2] "the size and duration of empires,"[3] and the various other attempts[4] by political scientists to make some sense of the whole and—usually—to suggest implications for the future. But this is not a work of political science, even if it hopes to have offered a large body of detailed facts and commentaries to those scholars in that discipline who are investigating the larger patterns of war and change in the international order.

This section will also not attempt to offer a conclusive summary of where we stand now, for that would contradict one of the chief messages of this book, which is that the international system is subject to constant changes, not only those caused by the day-to-day actions of statesmen and the ebb and flow of political and military events, but also those caused by the deeper transformations in the foundations of world power, which in time make their way through to the surface.

Nevertheless, it is proper to offer a few general observations before closing this study. It has been argued throughout the book that so far as the international system is concerned, wealth and power, or economic strength and military strength, are always relative and should be seen as such. Since they are relative, and since all societies are subject to the inexorable tendency to change, then the international balances can *never* be still, and it is a folly of statesmanship to assume that they ever would be. Given the anarchic and competitive nature of rivalries between nations, the history of international affairs over the past five centuries has all too frequently been a history of warfare, or at least of preparation for warfare—both of which consume resources which societies might use for other "goods," whether public or private. Whatever the stage of economic and scientific development reached, each century has therefore witnessed a debate about the extent to which national wealth ought to be used for military purposes. It has also recorded a debate about how best to enhance national prosperity, not only because of the individual benefits which increased wealth brings, but also because of the recognition that economic growth, productivity, flourishing finances, will all affect a Great Power's relative prospects if another international conflict occurs. Indeed, the outcome of all of the major, lengthy wars among the Great Powers which have been surveyed here repeatedly points to the crucial influences of productive economic forces—both during the struggle itself, and during those periods *between* wars when differentiated growth rates cause the various Powers to become relatively stronger or weaker. To a large degree, the outcome of the great coalition wars of the period 1500–1945 confirms the shifts which have been taking place, over a longer period, at the economic level. The new territorial order established at the end of each war thus reflects the redistribution of power which has been taking place within the international system. The coming of peace, however, does not stop this process of continual change; and the differentiated pace of economic growth among the Great Powers ensures that they will go on, rising and falling, relative to each other.

Whether the existence of "rising" and "falling" Powers in an anarchical world order must always lead to war is not certain. Most of the historical literature assumed that "war" and "the Great Power system" go hand in hand. Mackinder, one of the founding fathers of neomercantilist and geopolitical thought, held that "the great wars of history . . . are the outcome, direct or indirect, of the unequal growth of nations."[5] But did this pattern cease in 1945? It may indeed be the case that the advent of nuclear weapons, with their built-in threat to turn any exchange of fire into mutual devastation, has finally checked the habit of resorting to armed conflict in response to secular shifts in the Great Power balances, leaving only indirect, small-scale, "surrogate" wars. However, it might also be the case that the mutual apprehensions of nuclear weapons merely ensure that future conflicts, if they occur between the Great Powers, would remain conventional—although even they would be dreadfully bloody affairs, given modern battlefield weaponry.

Obviously, no one knows the answer to such critical questions. Those who assume that mankind would not be so foolish as to become involved in another ruinously expensive Great Power war perhaps need reminding that that belief was also widely held for much of the nineteenth century; and, indeed, Norman Angell's book *The Great Illusion*, which became an international bestseller with its argument that war would be economically disastrous to both victors and vanquished, appeared as late as 1910, as the European general staffs were quietly finalizing their war plans.

Whatever the likelihood of nuclear or conventional clashes between the major states, it is clear that important transformations in the balances *are* occurring, and will continue, probably at a faster pace than before. What is more, they are occurring at the two separate but interacting levels of economic production and strategic power. Unless the trends of the past two decades alter (but why should they?), the *pattern* of world politics looks roughly as follows:

First, there will be a shift, both in shares of total world product and total world military spending, from the five largest concentrations of strength to many more nations; but that will be a gradual process, and no other state is likely to join the present "pentarchy" of the United States, the USSR, China, Japan, and the EEC in the near future.

Secondly, the global productive balances between these five have already begun to tilt in certain directions: away from Russia and the United States, away also from the EEC, to Japan and China. This does not make for a *balanced* five-sided arrangement in economic terms, for the United States and the EEC have roughly the same productive and trading muscle (though the former gains immensely by being a military state); the USSR and Japan are also roughly equal (though Japan is growing the faster), with each having only around two-thirds of the productive power of the previous two; and the PRC is still a long way behind, but growing fastest of all.

Thirdly, in military terms there still exists a bipolar world, in that only the United States and the USSR have the capacity to ensure each other's destruction—and the destruction of any other country. Nevertheless, that bipolarity may be being slowly eroded, both at the *nuclear* level, either because such weapons are unusable under most circumstances, or because China, France, and Britain are each acquiring massive additions to their own nuclear arsenals; and at the *conventional* level, because of the steady buildup of Chinese strength, plus the growing realization that a West German–French (with, possibly, British and Italian) agglomeration of land, sea, and air forces would be an extremely large combination of power, if those nations really could work together effectively. For domestic-political reasons, that is not likely to happen in the near future; but the very fact that such a potential exists places a further uncertainty over the "bipolar" system, at least at the conventional level. By contrast, no one is at present suggesting that Japan will transform itself into a great military Power; yet all acquainted with the pattern of "war and change in world politics" would find it unsurprising if, one day, a different political leadership in Tokyo decided to turn its economic strength into a larger degree of military strength.

If Japan did decide to become a more active military presence in world affairs, it would presumably be because it felt it could no longer preserve its interests by acting simply as a "trading state";[6] in strengthening its armed forces, it would therefore be hoping to enhance its power and influence internationally to an extent that could not be achieved by nonmilitary measures. Yet the history of the past five hundred years of international rivalry demonstrates that military "security" alone is never enough. It may, over the shorter term, deter or defeat rival states (and that, for most political leaders and their publics, is perfectly satisfactory). But if, by such victories, the nation overextends itself geographically and strategically; if, even at a less imperial level, it chooses to devote a large proportion of its total income to "protection," leaving less for "productive investment," it is likely to find its economic output slowing down, with dire implications for its long-term capacity to maintain both its citizens' consumption demands and its international position.[7] Already this is happening in the case of the USSR, the United States, and Britain; and it is significant that both China and West Germany are struggling to avoid an excessive investment in military spending, both suspecting that it would affect their long-term growth prospects.

We therefore return to the conundrum which has exercised strategists and economists and political leaders from classical times onward. To be a Great Power—by definition, a state capable of holding its own against any other nation[8]—demands a flourishing economic base. In List's words, "War or the very possibility of war makes the establishment of a manufacturing power an indispensable requirement for a nation of the first rank. . . ."[9] Yet by going to war, or by devoting a large share of the nation's "manufacturing power" to expenditures upon "unproductive" armaments, one runs the risk of eroding the national economic base, especially vis-à-vis states which are concentrating a greater share of their income upon productive investment for long-term growth.

All of this was fully recognized by the classical writers on political economy. Those who followed Adam Smith's preferences inclined to keep defense expenditures low; those sympathetic to List's notion of *Nationaloekonomie* wanted to see the state possess greater instruments of force. All of them, if they were honest, admitted that it was really a matter of choice, and a difficult choice at that.[10] Ideally, of course, "profit" and "power" should go hand in hand. Far too often, however, statesmen found themselves confronted with the usual dilemma: between buying military security, at a time of real or perceived danger, which then became a burden upon the national economy; or keeping defense expenditures low, but finding one's interests sometimes threatened by the actions of other states.[11]

The present large Powers in the international system are thus compelled to grapple with the twin challenges which have confronted all their predecessors: first, with the uneven pattern of economic growth, which causes some of them to become wealthier (and, usually, stronger), relative to others; and second, with the competitive and occasionally dangerous scene abroad, which forces them to choose between a more immediate military security and a longer-term economic security. *No* general rule will provide the decision-makers of the time with a universally applicable course of action. If they neglect to provide adequate military defenses, they may be unable to respond if a rival Power takes advantage of them; if they spend too much on armaments—or, more usually, upon maintaining at growing cost the military obligations they had assumed in a previous period—they are likely to overstrain themselves, like an old man attempting to work beyond his natural strength. None of this is made easier by the "law of the increasing cost of war."[12] Even if, to take the most often cited example, one actually can prevent the entire U.S. Air Force budget from being consumed by the production of a *single* aircraft in the year 2020, the cost escalation of modern weaponry is an alarming tendency for all governments—and their taxpayers.

Each of today's large Powers—the United States, the USSR, China, Japan, and (putatively) the EEC—is therefore left grappling with the age-old dilemmas of rise and fall, with the shifting pace of productive growth, with technological innovation, with changes in the international scene, with the spiraling cost of weapons, with alterations in the power balances. Those are not developments which can be controlled by any one state, or individual. To paraphrase Bismarck's famous remark, all of these Powers are traveling on "the stream of Time," which they can "neither create nor direct," but upon which they can "steer with more or less skill and experience."[13] How they emerge from that voyage depends, to a large degree, upon the wisdom of the governments in Washington, Moscow, Tokyo, Peking, and the various European capitals. The above analysis has tried to suggest what the prospects are likely to be for each of those polities and, in consequence, for the Great Power system as a whole. But that still leaves an awful lot depending upon the "skill and experience" with which they manage to sail on "the stream of Time."

Notes

CHAPTER ONE
The Rise of the Western World

1. W. H. McNeill, *A World History* (London, 1979 edn.), p. 295; idem, *The Rise of the West* (Chicago, 1967), p. 565; J. M. Roberts, *The Pelican History of the World* (Harmondsworth, Mdssx., 1980), p. 519; G. Barraclough (ed.), *The Times Atlas of World History* (London, 1978), p. 153.

2. For surveys of international relations in Europe around 1500, see *The New Cambridge Modern History* (hereafter *NCMH*), vol. 1, *The Renaissance 1493–1520*, ed. G. R. Potter (Cambridge, 1961), espec. chs. 7–14; vol. 2, *The Reformation 1520–1529*, ed. G. R. Elton (Cambridge, 1958), chs. 10–11 and 16; G. R. Elton, *Reformation Europe 1517–1559* (London, 1963), ch. 2; G. Mattingly, *Renaissance Diplomacy* (Harmondsworth, Mddsx., 1965), pp. 115ff.

3. There are succinct accounts of Ming China in McNeill, *Rise of the West,* pp. 524–34; and Roberts, *History of the World,* pp. 424–44. For more detail, C. O. Hucker, *China's Imperial Past* (Stanford, Calif., 1975), pp. 303ff; J. A. Harrison, *The Chinese Empire* (New York, 1972); W. Eberhard, *A History of China* (2nd edn., London, 1960), pp. 232–70; M. Elvin, *The Pattern of the Chinese Past* (London, 1973).

4. Y. Shiba, *Commerce and Society in Sung China* (Ann Arbor, Mich., 1970); J. Needham, *The Development of Iron and Steel Technology in China* (London, 1958); L.-S. Yang, *Money and Credit in China* (Cambridge, Mass., 1952); and espec. W. H. McNeill, *The Pursuit of Power: Technology, Armed Forces and Society Since 1000 A.D.* (Chicago, 1983), ch. 2.

5. The great source (in English) for the above is J. Needham, *Science and Civilization in China,* vol. 4, pt. 3, *Civil Engineering and Nautics* (Cambridge, 1971), espec. pp. 379–536; but see also Lo Jung-pang, "The Emergence of China as a Sea Power During the Late Sung and Early Yuan Periods," *Far Eastern Quarterly,* vol. 14 (1955), pp. 489–503; C. G. Reynolds, *Command of the Sea: The History and Strategy of Maritime Empires* (New York, 1974), pp. 98–104.

6. For what follows, see McNeill, *World History,* pp. 254–55; Needham, *Science and Civilization in China,* vol. 4, pt. 3, pp. 524ff; R. Dawson, *Imperial China* (London, 1972), pp. 230ff; Lo Jung-pang, "The Decline of the Early Ming Navy," *Orient Extremus,* vol. 5 (1958), pp. 149–68; and Ho Ping-Ti, "Economic and Institutional Factors in the Decline of the Chinese Empire," in C. C. Cipolla (ed.), *The Economic Decline of Empires* (London, 1970), pp. 274–76, although in general the picture given is less gloomy than other accounts. See also the careful comparisons in J. Needham, *The Grand Titration: Science and Society*

in East and West (London, 1969), passim; and in E. L. Jones, *The European Miracle: Environments, Economies and Geopolitics in the History of Europe and Asia* (Cambridge, 1981).

7. Jones, *European Miracle*, ch. 9; F. Braudel, *The Mediterranean and the Mediterranean World in the Age of Philip II*, 2 vols. (London, 1972), vol. 2, pp. 661ff; P. Wittek, *The Rise of the Ottoman Empire* (London, 1938); H. Inalcik, *The Ottoman Empire: The Classical Age 1300–1600* (New York, 1973); M. A. Cook (ed.), *A History of the Ottoman Empire to 1730* (Cambridge, 1976); M.G.S. Hodgson, *The Venture of Islam*, vols. 2 and 3 (Chicago/London, 1924); C. M. Kortepeter, *Ottoman Imperialism During the Reformation* (London, 1973).

8. A. C. Hess, "The Evolution of the Ottoman Seaborne Empire in the Age of the Oceanic Discoveries, 1453–1525," *American Historical Review*, vol. 75, no. 7 (December 1970), pp. 1892–1919; Braudel, *Mediterranean*, vol. 2, pp. 918ff; Reynolds, *Command of the Sea*, pp. 112ff; and the comments in J. F. Guilmartin, *Gunpowder and Galleys: Changing Technology and Mediterranean Warfare at Sea in the Sixteenth Century* (Cambridge, 1974).

9. Jones, *European Miracle*, pp. 176ff; Cook (ed.), *History of the Ottoman Empire*, espec. pp. 103ff; B. Lewis, "Some Reflections on the Decline of the Ottoman Empire," in Cipolla (ed.), *Economic Decline of Empires*, pp. 215–34; H.A.R. Gibbs and H. Bowen, *Islamic Society and the West*, vol. 1, 2 pts. (London, 1950 and 1957), pt. 1, pp. 273ff.; pt. 2, pp. 1–37. See also H. Inalcik, *The Ottoman Empire: Conquest, Organization and Economy: Collected Studies* (London, 1978), chs. 10–13.

10. Jones, *European Miracle*, p. 182.

11. For the gloomy side, see ibid., ch. 10; Roberts, *History of the World*, pp. 415–23; W. H. Moreland, *From Akbar to Aurangzeb: A Study in Indian Economic History* (London, 1923); M. D. Morris, "Values as an Obstacle to Economic Growth in South Asia," *Journal of Economic History*, vol. 27 (1967), pp. 588–607. For a brighter presentation, A. J. Qaisar, *The Indian Response to European Technology and Culture, A.D. 1498–1707* (Delhi, India, 1982), passim; and, for a slightly later period, C. A. Bayley, *Rulers, Townsmen and Bazaars* (Cambridge, 1983).

12. McNeill, *Rise of the West*, pp. 645–49; Jones, *European Miracle*, pp. 157–59; R. Bendix, *Kings or People: Power and the Mandate to Rule* (Berkeley/Los Angeles, 1978), pp. 431ff; G. B. Sansom, *The Western World and Japan* (London, 1950), pp. 3–208; idem, *A History of Japan*, vols. 2–3 (London, 1961 and 1964); C. R. Boxer, *The Christian Century in Japan 1549–1650* (Berkeley, 1951); J. W. Hall, *Government and Local Power in Japan* (Princeton, 1966); D. M. Brown, "The Impact of Firearms on Japanese Warfare," *Far Eastern Quarterly*, vol. 7 (1947), pp. 236–45; R. P. Toby, *State and Diplomacy in Early Modern Japan* (Princeton, N.J., 1984).

13. McNeill, *World History*, pp. 328–43; Bendix, *Kings or People*, pp. 491ff; I. Wallerstein, *The Modern World System*, vol. 1, *Capitalist Agriculture and the Origins of the European World-Economy in the Sixteenth Century* (New York/London, 1974), pp. 301–24; G. Vernadsky, *The Tsardom of Muscovy 1547–1682* (New Haven, Conn., 1969); R. H. Fisher, *The Russian Fur Trade 1550–1700* (Berkeley, Calif., 1943); M. Florinsky, *Russia: A Short History* (New York, 1964), chs. 3–9; R. J. Kerner, *The Urge to the Sea* (New York, 1971 reprint); T. Szamuely, *The Russian Traditions* (London, 1974); L. Kochan and R. Abraham, *The Making of Modern Russia* (Harmondsworth, Mddsx., 2nd edn., 1983), chs. 3–6.

14. See Roberts, *History of the World*, p. 585: "So little was Russia known even in the [seventeenth] century that a French king could write to the Tsar, not knowing that the prince whom he addressed had been dead for ten years." Note

also the condescending remarks of English traders in Russia in Kochan and Abraham, *Making of Modern Russia,* pp. 56–57.

15. This is the title, of course, of E. L. Jones's impressive book. It, and the important work by W. H. McNeill, *The Pursuit of Power,* have strongly influenced my argument in the following paragraphs. See also McNeill, *Rise of the West,* passim; Wallerstein, *Modern World System;* D. C. North and R. P. Thomas, *The Rise of the Western World* (Cambridge, 1973); J. H. Parry, *The Establishment of the European Hegemony 1415–1715* (3rd edn., New York, 1966); S. Viljoen, *Economic Systems in World History* (London, 1974), passim; P. Chaunu, *European Expansion in the Later Middle Ages* (Amsterdam, 1979).

16. H. C. Darby, "The Face of Europe on the Eve of the Great Discoveries," in *NCMH,* vol. 1, pp. 20–49; N. J. G. Pounds and S. S. Ball, "Core-Areas and the Development of the European States System," *Annals of the Association of American Geographers,* vol. 54 (1964), pp. 24–40; R. G. Wesson, *State Systems: International Relations, Politics and Culture* (New York, 1978), p. 111; Jones, *European Miracle,* ch. 7.

17. N. J. G. Pounds, *An Historical Geography of Europe 1500–1840* (Cambridge, 1979), ch. 1; C. Cipolla, *Before the Industrial Revolution: European Society and Economy 1000–1700* (2nd edn., London, 1980), passim; C. Cipolla (ed.), *The Fontana Economic History of Europe,* vol. 1, *The Middle Ages* (London, 1972), ch. 7; E. Samhaber, *Merchants Make History* (London, 1963), pp. 130ff.; Wallerstein, *Modern World System,* vol. 1, pp. 42ff.; Braudel, *Mediterranean,* vol. 1, pp. 188–224.

18. Roberts, *History of the World,* pp. 505–6; J. H. Parry, *The Age of Reconnaissance* (2nd edn., London, 1966), pp. 60ff.

19. Quoted in Jones, *European Miracle,* p. 235.

20. McNeill, *Pursuit of Power,* ch. 3; J. U. Nef, *War and Human Progress* (New York, 1968 edn.), ch. 2; R. A. Preston, S. F. Wise, and H. O. Werner, *Men in Arms* (London, 1962), ch. 7; C. Cipolla, *Guns and Sails in the Early Phase of European Expansion 1400–1700* (London, 1965), passim; and R. Bean, "War and the Birth of the Nation State," *Journal of Economic History,* vol. 33 (1973), pp. 203–21.

21. One is bound to put quotation marks around the word "national," since so many men in the French army were mercenaries: see V. G. Kiernan, "Foreign Mercenaries and Absolute Monarchy," *Past and Present,* vol. 11 (1957), p. 72. For the general comments above, see McNeill, *Pursuit of Power,* ch. 3; H. Thomas, *History of the World* (New York, 1979 edn.), ch. 24; M. E. Mallet, *Mercenaries and Their Masters: Warfare in Renaissance Italy* (London, 1976); and J. R. Hale, "Armies, Navies and the Art of War," *NCMH,* vol. 2, espec. pp. 486ff; idem, *War and Society in Renaissance Europe 1450–1620* (London, 1985), ch. 2.

22. Cipolla, *Guns and Sails,* passim; Nef, *War and Human Progress,* pp. 46ff.

23. C. Duffy, *Siege Warfare: The Fortress in the Early Modern World 1494–1660* (London, 1979), chs. 1–2; McNeill, *Pursuit of Power,* ch. 3; Wesson, *State Systems,* pp. 112ff; Braudel, *Mediterranean,* vol. 2., pp. 845ff; J. R. Hale, "The Early Development of the Bastion: An Italian Chronology c. 1450—c.1534," in Hale et al. (eds.), *Europe in the Later Middle Ages* (London, 1965), pp. 466–94.

24. For what follows, see Parry, *Age of Reconnaissance,* ch. VII; Reynolds, *Command of the Sea,* pp. 106ff; P. Padfield, *Guns at Sea* (London, 1973), pt. 1; G. V. Scammell, *The World Encompassed: The First European Maritime Empires, c. 800–1650* (Berkeley, Calif., 1981), which places the fifteenth-century voyages in the broader sweep of European expansionism.

25. Jones, *European Miracle,* p. 80. The importance of "efficient economic organi-

zation" is also repeatedly stressed in North and Thomas, *Rise of the Western World*, p. 1 and passim.

26. This is the thrust of Guilmartin's excellent study, *Gunpowder and Galleys*, passim.

27. For the Portuguese experience, see Parry, *Age of Reconnaissance;* P. Padfield, *Tide of Empires: Decisive Naval Campaigns in the Rise of the West*, vol. 1, *1481–1654* (London, 1979), ch. 2; C. R. Boxer, *The Portuguese Seaborne Empire 1415–1825* (London, 1969); V. Magalhaes-Godinho, *L'économie de l'Empire Portugais aux XVᵉ et XVIᵉ siècles* (Paris, 1969); B. W. Diffie and C. D. Winius, *Foundations of the Portuguese Empire 1415–1580* (Minneapolis, 1977); Wallerstein, *Modern World System*, p. 325ff; Braudel, *Mediterranean*, vol. 2, pp. 1174–76; Scammell, *World Encompassed*, ch. 5.

28. P. M. Kennedy, *The Rise and Fall of British Naval Mastery* (London/New York, 1976), p. 18.

29. Padfield, *Tide of Empires*, vol. 1, p. 49.

30. Whether the Portuguese government itself benefited so much is more doubtful: see M. Newitt, "Plunder and the Rewards of Office in the Portuguese Empire," in M. Duffy (ed.), *The Military Revolution and the State 1500–1800* (Exeter Studies in History, Exeter, 1980), pp. 10–28;. and W. Reinhard, *Geschichte der europäischen Expansion*, vol. 1 (Stuttgart, 1983), ch. 3 and 5.

31. Wallerstein, *Modern World System*, p. 170; C. H. Haring, *The Spanish Empire in America* (New York, 1947); Parry, *Spanish Seaborne Empire*, passim; Scammell, *World Encompassed*, ch. 6; C. Gibson, *Spain in America* (New York, 1966).

32. Wallerstein, *Modern World System*. See also Jones, *European Miracle*, ch. 4; Parry, *Age of Reconnaissance*, pt. 3; Roberts, *History of the World*, pp. 600ff; *Cambridge Economic History of Europe*, vol. 4, *The Economy of Expanding Europe in the Sixteenth and Seventeenth Centuries* (Cambridge, 1967), passim. A sensible warning against *anticipating* a real "world system" is contained in R. A. Dodgshon, "A Spatial Perspective," *Peasant Studies*, vol. 6, no. 1 (January 1977), pp. 8–19.

33. For the beginnings of this challenge to the Iberian trading monopoly overseas, see *NCMH*, vol. 1, ch. 16, and vol. 3, ch. 17; Padfield, *Tide of Empires*, ch. 4; Scammell, *World Encompassed*, ch. 7 and 9.

34. K. Mendelsohn, *Science and Western Domination* (London, 1976), passim; Nef, *War and Human Progress*, ch. 3; Elton, *Reformation Europe*, pp. 292ff; McNeill, *Rise of the West*, pp. 592–98; Cipolla (ed.), *Fontana Economic History of Europe*, vol. 2, ch. 3; A. Wolf, *A History of Science, Technology and Philosophy in the Sixteenth and Seventeenth Centuries* (New York, 1935).

35. Jones, *European Miracle*, pp. 170–71 and passim; and cf. A. G. Frank, *World Accumulation 1492–1789* (New York/London, 1978), pp. 137ff.

36. See again Mendelssohn, *Science and Western Domination*, which stresses the importance of scientific observation and prediction; and McNeill, *Rise of the West*, pp. 593–99.

CHAPTER TWO
The Habsburg Bid for Mastery, 1519–1659

1. C. Oman, *A History of the Art of War in the Sixteenth Century* (London, 1937), p. 3. For the earlier wars, see idem, *A History of the Art of War in the Middle Ages*, 2 vols. (London, 1924).

2. See the warning about this in G. R. Elton, *Reformation Europe 1517–1559* (London, 1963), pp. 305ff.

3. Ibid., p. 35.
4. R. A. Stradling, *Europe and the Decline of Spain: A Study of the Spanish System, 1580–1720* (London/Boston, 1981), p. 44.
5. For example, Gattinara's declaration to Charles V that "God has set you on the path towards a world monarchy," quoted in *NCMH*, vol. 2, pp. 301ff.; and the quotations in H. Kamen, *Spain 1469–1714* (London, 1983), p. 67.
6. Oman, *War in the Sixteenth Century*, p. 5. This book remains the best *military* narrative for this period. Useful succinct accounts of these 140 years are in the three relevant volumes of *Fontana History of Europe*: G. R. Elton, *Reformation Europe 1517–1559* (London, 1963); J. H. Elliott, *Europe Divided 1559–1598* (London, 1968); and G. Parker, *Europe in Crisis 1598–1648* (London, 1979). See also *NCMH*, vols. 2–5; and H. G. Koenigsberger, *The Habsburgs and Europe 1516–1660* (Ithaca/London, 1971).
7. *NCMH*, vol. 2, ch. 11 and 17.
8. V. S. Mamatey, *Rise of the Habsburg Empire 1526–1815* (Huntingdon, N.Y., 1978 edn.), p. 9.
9. Details in Oman, *War in the Sixteenth Century*, pp. 703ff; Braudel, *Mediterranean World*, vol. 2, pp. 904–1237.
10. H. C. Koenigsberger, "Western Europe and the Power of Spain," in *NCMH*, vol. 3, pp. 234–318; G. Parker, *Spain and the Netherlands 1559–1659* (London, 1979), passim; C. Wilson, *The Transformation of Europe 1558–1648* (London, 1976), chs. 8–9.
11. The international nature of the rivalry is well covered in Parker, "The Dutch Revolt and the Polarization of International Politics," in *Spain and the Netherlands*, pp. 74ff; and, for a more economic/social interpretation, J. V. Polisensky, *The Thirty Years War* (London, 1971), espec. ch. 4.
12. C. V. Wedgewood, *The Thirty Years War* (London, 1964 edn.), chs. 3–6.
13. Parker, *Europe in Crisis*, p. 252; J. H. Elliott, *The Count-Duke of Olivares* (New Haven, Conn., 1986), p. 495.
14. Parker, *Spain and the Netherlands*, pp. 54–77; C. R. Boxer, *The Dutch Seaborne Empire 1600–1800* (London, 1972), pp. 25–26.
15. For the final years of conflict, see Stradling, *Europe and the Decline of Spain*, chs. 2–4; J. Stoye, *Europe Unfolding 1648–1688* (London, 1969), chs. 3–4.
16. Apart from specific works cited in the notes below, this section has been much influenced by a number of excellent studies of Spanish imperial power, namely: J. H. Elliott, *Imperial Spain 1469–1716* (Harmondsworth, Mddsx., 1970); J. Lynch, *Spain Under the Habsburgs*, 2 vols. (Oxford, 1964 and 1969); Stradling, *Europe and the Decline of Spain*, passim. Also used were two older works, R. Trevor Davies, *The Golden Century of Spain 1501–1621* (London, 1937); and B. Chudoba, *Spain and the Empire 1519–1643* (New York, 1969 edn.). Finally, there is John Elliott's thoughtful article, reproduced in Cipolla (ed.), *Economic Decline of Empires*, as "The Decline of Spain," pp. 168–95.
17. Koenigsberger, *Habsburgs and Europe*, p. xi.
18. R. Ehrenberg, *Das Zeitalter der Fugger: Geldkapital und Creditverkehr im 16. Jahrhundert*, 2 vols. (Jena, 1896); E. Samhaber, *Merchants Make History* (London, 1963), ch. 8; and see the broad recent survey by G. Parker, "The Emergence of Modern Finance in Europe 1500–1730," in Cipolla (ed.), *Fontana Economic History of Europe*, vol. 2, pp. 527–89.
19. *NCMH*, vol. 1, ch. 7; R. A. Kann, *A History of the Habsburg Empire 1526–1918* (Berkeley/Los Angeles/London, 1974), chs. 1–2.
20. Lynch, *Spain Under the Habsburgs*, vol. 1, p. 77.
21. M. Roberts, "The Military Revolution, 1560–1660," in Roberts, *Essays in Swedish History* (London, 1967), pp. 195–225; G. Parker, " 'The Military Revolution,

1560–1660'—a Myth?" in Parker, *Spain and the Netherlands*, pp. 86–105; M. van Creveld, *Supplying War: Logistics from Wallenstein to Patton* (Cambridge, 1977), pp. 5–6; J. R. Hale, "Armies, Navies, and the Art of War," in *NCMH*, vol. 2, pp. 481–509, and vol. 3, pp. 171–208; McNeill, *Pursuit of Power*, ch. 4; R. Bean, "War and the Birth of the Nation State," *Journal of Economic History*, vol. 33 (1973), pp. 203–21.

22. G. Parker, *The Army of Flanders and the Spanish Road 1567–1659: The Logistics of Spanish Victory and Defeat in the Low Countries War* (Cambridge, 1972), p. 6.

23. I.A.A. Thompson, *War and Government in Habsburg Spain 1560–1620* (London, 1976), p. 16; more generally, see Reynolds, *Command of the Sea*, chs. 4–6.

24. Lynch, *Spain Under the Habsburgs*, vol. 1, pp. 53–58.

25. Ibid., p. 128. See also Parker, *Army of Flanders and the Spanish Road*, ch. 6.

26. Braudel, *Mediterranean World*, vol. 2, p. 841; and, for a full breakdown, Parker, "Lepanto (1571): the Costs of Victory," in *Spain and the Netherlands*, pp. 122–34.

27. *NCMH*, vol. 3, pp. 275ff.; Parker, "Why Did the Dutch Revolt Last So Long?", and "Mutiny and Discontent in the Spanish Army of Flanders 1572–1607," in *Spain and the Netherlands*, pp. 45–64, 106–21.

28. Thompson, *War and Government in Habsburg Spain*, ch. 3.

29. Ibid., pp. 36ff, 89ff; Lynch, *Spain Under the Habsburgs*, vol. 2, pp. 30ff.

30. For further details, see J. Regla, "Spain and Her Empire," in *NCMH*, vol. 5, pp. 319–83; Lynch, *Spain Under the Habsburgs*, vol. 2, chs. 4–5; Elliott, *Imperial Spain*, ch. 10; Stradling, *Europe and the Decline of Spain*, chs. 3–5; but see also Kamen, *Spain 1469–1714*, arguing for a later "recovery."

31. See the interesting remarks of Braudel about the disadvantages facing the two "overlarge" empires of Spain and Islam, in *Mediterranean World*, vol. 2, pp. 701–03.

32. The fluctuations of Spanish effort from one theater to another are nicely charted in Parker, "Spain, Her Enemies and the Revolt of the Netherlands, 1559–1648," in *Spain and the Netherlands*, pp. 17–42.

33. Lynch, *Spain Under the Habsburgs*, vol. 1, p. 347.

34. Ibid., vol. 2, p. 70.

35. E. Heischmann, *Die Anfänge des stehenden Heeres in Oesterreich* (Vienna, 1925).

36. *NCMH*, vol. 5, chs. 18 and 20; Kann, *History of the Habsburg Empire*.

37. See the excellent analysis of the war in the Netherlands in Duffy, *Siege Warfare*, ch. 4.

38. Parker, *Spain and the Netherlands*, pp. 185, 188.

39. Idem, *Army of Flanders and the Spanish Road*, pp. 50ff.

40. *NCMH*, vol. 3, p. 308.

41. Cited in Parker, *Europe in Crisis*, p. 238.

42. Ibid., p. 239.

43. For what follows, see Kamen, *Spain 1469–1714*, pp. 81ff, 161ff, 214ff; H. G. Koenigsberger, "The Empire of Charles V in Europe," in *NCMH*, vol. 2, pp. 301–33; and the extended version in Koenigsberger, *Habsburgs and Europe*, passim.

44. H. G. Koenigsberger, *The Government of Sicily Under Philip II* (London, 1951), passim.

45. Idem, *The Habsburgs and Europe*, passim; and see also the excellent new study by D. Stella, *Crisis and Continuity: The Economy of Spanish Lombardy in the Seventeenth Century* (Cambridge, Mass., 1979).

46. Parker, *Spain and the Netherlands*, pp. 21–22.

47. *NCMH,* vol. 1, pp. 450ff, and vol. 2, pp. 320ff; Elliott, *Imperial Spain,* chs. 5 and 8; Lynch, *Spain Under the Habsburgs,* vol. 1, pp. 53ff and passim, and vol. 2, pp. 3ff.

48. For what follows, see Cipolla, *Before the Industrial Revolution,* pp. 250ff; J. V. Vives, "The Decline of Spain in the Seventeenth Century," in Cipolla (ed.), *Economic Decline of Empires,* pp. 121–67, Davies, *Golden Century of Spain,* chs. 3 and 8; Wallerstein, *Modern World System,* vol. 1, pp. 191ff; as well as the books by Elliott and Lynch.

49. Cipolla, *Guns and Sails,* p. 33; Thompson, *War and Government in Habsburg Spain,* p. 25.

50. D. Maland, *Europe in the Seventeenth Century* (London, 1966), p. 214; Lynch, *Spain Under the Habsburgs,* vol. 2, pp. 139ff. But this Spanish policy of tolerating trade with their Dutch enemies was often reversed, as is made clear in Israel's article, note 82 below.

51. Thompson, *War and Government in Habsburg Spain,* p. i; Parker, *Europe in Crisis,* pp. 71–75; more generally, Hale, *War and Society in Renaissance Europe,* chs. 8–9.

52. Parker, *Spain and the Netherlands,* p. 96.

53. *NCMH,* vol. 2, p. 472.

54. Ibid., vol. 1, ch. 10; and espec. M. Wolfe, *The Fiscal System of Renaissance France* (New Haven/London, 1972), chs. 2–3.

55. Oman, *War in the Sixteenth Century,* pp. 393–536, gives the military details of the French wars. For the politics, see J.H.M. Salmon, *Society in Crisis: France in the Sixteenth Century* (London, 1975), passim; and R. Briggs, *Early Modern France 1560–1715* (Oxford, 1977), ch. 1.

56. Nef, *War and Human Progress,* pp. 103ff; Wolfe, *Fiscal System of Renaissance France,* ch. 8; Salmon, *Society in Crisis,* pp. 301ff; E. J. Hamilton, "Origin and Growth of National Debt in Western Europe," *American Economic Review,* vol. 37, no. 2 (1947), pp. 119–20.

57. *NCMH,* vol. 3, pp. 314–17; Wolfe, *Fiscal System of Renaissance France,* ch. 8; Salmon, *Society in Crisis,* ch. 12; Briggs, *Early Modern France,* pp. 80ff; Parker, *Europe in Crisis,* pp. 119–22.

58. Parker, *Europe in Crisis,* pp. 17ff, 246ff; J. B. Wolf, *Toward a European Balance of Power 1620–1715* (Chicago, 1970), pp. 17–19.

59. A. Guery, "Les finances de la monarchie Française," *Annales,* vol. 33, no. 2 (1978), pp. 216–39, espec. pp. 228–30, 236. The similarity of the strains upon both France and Spain is well argued in J. H. Elliott, *Richelieu and Olivares* (Cambridge, 1984), especially chs. 3 and 5–6; and in M. S. Kimmell, "War, State Finance, and Revolution," in P. McGowan and C. W. Kegley (eds.), *Foreign Policy and the Modern World-System* (Beverly Hills, Calif., 1983), pp. 89–124.

60. E. H. Jenkins, *A History of the French Navy* (London, 1973), ch. 4; Briggs, *Early Modern France,* pp. 128–44; Parker, *Europe in Crisis,* pp. 276ff.

61. R. Stradling, "Catastrophe and Recovery: The Defeat of Spain 1639–43," *History,* vol. 64, no. 211 (June 1979), pp. 205–19.

62. On English economic history in this period, see Cipolla, *Before the Industrial Revolution,* pp. 276–96; D. C. Coleman, *The Economy of England 1450–1750* (Oxford, 1977); B. Murphy, *A History of the British Economy* (London, 1973), pt. 1, ch. 4; C. Hill, *Reformation to Industrial Revolution* (Harmondsworth, Mddsx. 1969); R. Davis, *English Overseas Trade 1500–1700* (London, 1973). Among the more prominent political surveys are G. R. Elton, *England Under the Tudors* (London, 1955); D. M. Loades, *Politics and the Nation 1450–1660* (London, 1974), pp. 118ff; and P. Williams, *The Tudor Regime* (Oxford, 1979), espec. chs. 2 and 9. On the crown's finances, see the older work F. C. Dietz,

English Public Finance 1485–1641, vol. 1, *English Government Finance 1485–1558* (London, 1964 edn.).

63. Nef, *War and Human Progress*, pp. 10–12, 71–73, 87–88.

64. C. Barnett, *Britain and Her Army 1509–1970: A Military, Political and Social Survey* (London, 1970), ch. 1; Oman, *War in the Sixteenth Century*, pp. 285ff; G. J. Millar, *Tudor Mercenaries and Auxiliaries 1485–1547* (Charlottesville, Va., 1980). For the later period, see C. G. Cruikshank, *Elizabeth's Army* (2nd edn., Oxford, 1966).

65. Williams, *Tudor Regime*, pp. 64ff; Dietz, *English Government Finance*, chs. 7–14; Hill, *Reformation to Industrial Revolution*, ch. 6; P. S. Crowson, *Tudor Foreign Policy* (London, 1973), ch. 25.

66. K. R. Andrews, *Elizabethan Privateering* (Cambridge, 1964); indem, *Trade, Plunder and Settlement* (Cambridge, 1983); Padfield, *Tide of Empires*, vol. 1, pp. 120ff; D. B. Quinn and A. N. Ryan, *England's Sea Empire, 1550–1642* (London, 1983), ch. 5; Scammell, *World Encompassed*, pp. 465ff.

67. As quoted in Kennedy, *British Naval Mastery*, p. 28. See also M. Howard, "The British Way in Warfare" (Neale Lecture, London, 1975); Barnett, *Britain and Her Army*, pp. 25ff, 51ff; R. B. Wernham, "Elizabethan War Aims and Strategy," in *Elizabethan Government and Society*, ed. S. T. Bindoff, J. Hurstfield, and C. H. Williams (London, 1961), pp. 340–68. See also the two general surveys by Wernham, *Before the Armada: The Growth of English Foreign Policy 1485–1588* (London, 1966), and *The Making of Elizabethan Foreign Policy 1588–1603* (Berkeley/Los Angeles/London, 1980).

68. For these figures, see F. C. Dietz, "The Exchequer in Elizabeth's Reign," *Smith College Studies in History*, vol. 8, no. 2 (January 1923); idem, *English Public Finance 1485–1641*, vol. 2, *1558–1641*, chs. 2–5; W. R. Scott, *The Constitution and Finance of English, Scottish and Irish Joint Stock Companies to 1720*, 3 vols. (Cambridge, 1912), vol. 3, pp. 485–544.

69. Loades, *Politics and the Nation*, pp. 301ff; R. Ashton, *The Crown and the Money Market 1603–1640* (Oxford, 1960), passim, espec. chs. 2 and 7.

70. R. Ashton, *The English Civil War: Conservatism and Revolution 1603–1649* (London, 1979); C. Hill, *The Century of Revolution 1603–1714* (Edinburgh, 1961), pt. 1; C. Russell (ed.), *The Origins of the English Civil War* (London, 1973); L. Stone, *The Causes of the English Revolution 1529–1642* (London, 1972); Loades, *Politics and the Nation*, pp. 327ff.

71. Kennedy, *British Naval Mastery*, pp. 44ff; Barnett, *Britain and Her Army*, pp. 90ff; Hill, *Reformation to Industrial Revolution*, pp. 155ff; J. R. Jones, *Britain and the World 1649–1815* (London, 1980), pp. 51ff. See also two important German studies: B. Martin, "Aussenhandel und Aussenpolitik Englands unter Cromwell," *Historische Zeitschrift*, vol. 218, no. 3 (June 1974), pp. 571–92; and H. C. Junge, *Flottenpolitik und Revolution: Die Entstehung der englischen Seemacht während der Herrschaft Cromwells* (Stuttgart, 1980).

72. M. Ashley, *Financial and Commercial Policy Under the Cromwellian Protectorate* (London, 1962 edn.), p. 48.

73. C. Hill, *Century of Revolution*, p. 161.

74. North and Thomas, *Rise of the Western World*, pp. 118, 150, and passim.

75. What follows relies heavily upon the writings of Michael Roberts, not only his classic *Gustavus Adolphus*, 2 vols. (London, 1958), but also his broader surveys: *Essays in Swedish History* (London, 1967); *Gustavus Adolphus and the Rise of Sweden* (London, 1973); (ed.), *Sweden's Age of Greatness, 1632–1718* (London, 1973); and *The Swedish Imperial Experience 1560–1718* (Cambridge, 1979).

76. Cipolla, *Guns and Sails*, pp. 52ff; Roberts, *Gustavus Adolphus*, vol. 2, pp. 107ff;

Wallerstein, *Modern World System*, vol. 2, pp. 203ff; and E. F. Heckscher, *An Economic History of Sweden* (Cambridge, Mass., 1963), ch. 4, espec. pp. 101ff.

77. There is a brief summary of the reforms in Roberts, *Gustavus Adolphus and the Rise of Sweden*, chs. 6–7; full details in idem, *Gustavus Adolphus*, vol. 2, pp. 63–304.

78. See F. Redlich, "Contributions in the Thirty Years War," *Economic History Review*, 2nd series, vol. 12 (1959), pp. 247–54, as well as his larger work, *The German Military Enterpriser and His Work Force*, 2 vols. (Wiesbaden, 1964). M. Ritter, "Das Kontributionssystem Wallensteins," *Historische Zeitschrift*, vol. 90 (1902), and A. Ernstberger, *Hans de Witte: Finanzmann Wallensteins* (Wiesbaden, 1954), have further details. For Sweden, see Roberts, *Gustavus Adolphus and the Rise of Sweden*, ch. 8; and S. Lundkvist, "Svensk krigsfinansiering 1630–1635," *Historisk tidskrift*, 1966, pp. 377–421, with a German summary.

79. Roberts, "Charles XI," in *Essays in Swedish History*, p. 233.

80. Idem, *Swedish Imperial Experience*, pp. 132–37.

81. Ibid., p. 51.

82. G. Parker, *The Dutch Revolt* (London, 1977), supersedes all other accounts of the sixteenth-century phase of the "Eighty Years War." For the later struggle, see the important article by J. I. Israel, "A Conflict of Empires: Spain and the Netherlands, 1618–1648," *Past and Present*, no. 76 (1977), pp. 34–74; and idem, *The Dutch Republic and the Hispanic World, 1606–1661* (Oxford, 1982).

83. G. Gash, *Renaissance Armies 1480–1650* (Cambridge, 1975), p. 106.

84. C. Wilson, *The Dutch Republic and the Civilization of the Seventeenth Century* (London, 1968), p. 31. See also Wallerstein, *Modern World System*, vol. 1, pp. 199ff; vol. 2, ch. 2.

85. Quoted from Parker, *Dutch Revolt*, p. 249; Reynolds, *Command of the Sea*, pp. 158ff; Boxer, *Dutch Seaborne Empire*, passim; Padfield, *Tide of Empires*, vol. 1, ch. 5; Scammell, *World Encompassed*, ch. 7.

86. On this "shift" from the Mediterranean to the Atlantic world, see Cipolla, *Before the Industrial Revolution*, ch. 10; Braudel, *Mediterranean World*, vol. 2; Wallerstein, *Modern World System*, vols. 1 and 2; and R. T. Rapp, "The Unmaking of the Mediterranean Trade Hegemony," *Journal of Economic History*, vol. 35 (1975), pp. 499–525, with some useful reservations about what was happening.

87. On the losses caused to the United Provinces by the war, see Parker, "War and Economic Change," passim, and Israel, "Conflict of Empires," passim. On Amsterdam's financial role, and official debts, see Parker, "Emergence of Modern Finance in Europe," pp. 549ff, 573ff; V. Barbour, *Capitalism in Amsterdam in the Seventeenth Century* (Baltimore, 1950), passim; André-E. Sayous, "Le rôle d'Amsterdam dans l'histoire du capitalisme commercial et financier," *Revue Historique*, vol. 183, no. 2 (October–December 1938), pp. 242–80.

88. Bean, "War and the Birth of the Nation State," passim. See also S. E. Finer, "State and Nation-Building in Europe: The Role of the Military," in C. Tilly (ed.), *The Formation of National States in Western Europe* (Princeton, 1975), pp. 84–163.

89. *NCMH*, vol. 3, ch. 16; Wesson, *State Systems*, pp. 121ff; O. Ranum (ed.), *National Consciousness, History and Political Culture in Early-Modern Europe* (Baltimore/London, 1975); and E. D. Marcu, *Sixteenth Century Nationalism* (New York, 1976). This was also seen in the "national" economic theories of the time: see G. H. McCormick, "Strategic Considerations in the Development of Economic Thought," pp. 4–8, in G. H. McCormick and R. E. Bissess (eds.), *Strategic Dimensions of Economic Behavior* (New York, 1984).

90. Among the more general interpretations and syntheses, see Tilly (ed.), *Formation of National States in Western Europe*, passim; Bendix, *Kings or People*, pp.

247ff; Wallerstein, *Modern World System,* vol. 1, ch. 3; V. G. Kiernan, "State and Nation in Western Europe," *Past and Present,* vol. 31 (1965), pp. 20–38; J. H. Shennan, *The Origins of the Modern European State 1450–1725* (London, 1974); H. Lubasz (ed.), *The Development of the Modern State* (New York, 1964).
91. Cited in Creveld, *Supplying War,* p. 17.
92. Ibid., pp. 13–17.
93. See again Elliott, *Richelieu and Olivares,* ch. 6.

CHAPTER THREE
Finance, Geography, and the Winning of Wars, 1660–1815

1. For basic political narratives of this period, see D. McKay and H. M. Scott, *The Rise of the Great Powers 1648–1815* (London, 1983), an excellent survey; *NCMH,* vols. 5–9; W. Doyle, *The Old European Order 1660–1800* (Oxford, 1978); E. N. Williams, *The Ancien Regime in Europe 1648–1789* (Harmondsworth, Mddsx., 1979 edn.). Europe in the outside world is treated in J. H. Parry, *Trade and Dominion: The European Overseas Empire in the Eighteenth Century* (London, 1971); G. Williams, *The Expansion of Europe in the Eighteenth Century* (London, 1966). For cartographical representations of these trends, see G. Barraclough (ed.), *Times Atlas of World History,* pp. 192ff.
2. On military and naval developments generally, see Nef, *War and Human Progress,* pt. 2; Ropp, *War in the Modern World,* chs. 1–4; Preston, Wise, and Werner, *Men in Arms,* chs. 9–12; McNeill, *Pursuit of Power,* chs. 4–6; H. Strachan, *European Armies and the Conduct of War* (London/Boston, 1983), chs. 1–4; J. Childs, *Armies and Warfare in Europe 1648–1789* (Manchester, 1982). On navies, see Reynolds, *Command of the Sea,* chs. 6–9; Kennedy, *Rise and Fall of British Naval Mastery,* chs. 3–5; Padfield, *Tide of Empires,* vol. 2.
3. On these developments, see, in addition to the references in note 2 above, A. Corvisier, *Armies and Societies in Europe 1494–1789* (Bloomington, 1979), espec. pt. 2; Howard, *War in European History,* ch. 4; van Creveld, *Supplying War,* pp. 10ff; C. Tilly (ed.), *The Formation of National States in Western Europe* (Princeton, N.J., 1975), espec. S. E. Finer's essay "State-and-Nation-Building in Europe: The Role of the Military," pp. 84–163.
4. G. Parker, "Emergence of Modern Finance in Europe," passim; Tilly (ed.), *Formation of National States in Western Europe,* chs. 3–4; F. Braudel, *The Wheels of Commerce,* vol. 2 of *Civilization and Capitalism, 15th–18th Centuries* (London, 1982); H. van der Wee, "Monetary, Credit and Banking Systems," in E. R. Rich and C. H. Wilson (eds.), *The Cambridge Economic History of Europe,* vol. 5 (Cambridge, 1977), pp. 290–392; P.G.M. Dickson and J. Sperling, "War Finance, 1689–1714," in *NCMH,* vol. 6, ch. 9. Note also K. A. Rasler and W. R. Thompson, "Global Wars, Public Debts, and the Long Cycle," *World Politics,* vol. 35 (1983), pp. 489–516; and C. Webber and A. Wildavsky, *A History of Taxation and Expenditure in the Western World* (New York, 1986), pp. 250ff.
5. The term refers, of course, to the title of P.G.M. Dickson's excellent book *The Financial Revolution in England: A Study in the Development of Public Credit 1688–1756* (London, 1967).
6. This endless debate is covered in W. Sombart, *Krieg und Kapitalismus* (Munich, 1913); Nef, *War and Human Progress;* and many later books and articles. See the useful introduction and bibliography in J. M. Winter (ed.), *War and Economic Development* (Cambridge, 1975).
7. Parker, "Emergence of Modern Finance," passim; Wallerstein, *Modern World System,* vol. 2, pp. 57ff; C. H. Wilson, *Anglo-Dutch Commerce and Finance in*

the Eighteenth Century (Cambridge, 1966 reprint); V. Barbour, *Capitalism in Amsterdam in the Seventeenth Century* (Baltimore, 1950), espec. ch. 6. Above all, see now J. C. Riley, *International Government Finance and the Amsterdam Capital Market 1740–1815* (Cambridge, 1980).

8. See the discussion on this in Wilson, "Decline of the Netherlands," in *Economic History and the Historian: Collected Essays* (London, 1969), pp. 22–47; and idem, *Anglo-Dutch Commerce and Finance;* as well as the references in note 23 below.

9. Riley, *International Government Finance*, chs. 6–7.

10. For general comparisons of the French and British economies, financial policies, and fiscal systems, see Wallerstein, *Modern World System*, vol. 2, chs. 3 and 6; P. Mathias and P. O'Brien, "Taxation in Britain and France, 1715–1810," *Journal of European Economic History*, vol. 5, no. 3 (Winter 1976), pp. 601–49; F. Crouzet, "L'Angleterre et France au XVIIIe siècle: essai d'analyse comparée de deux croissances économiques," *Annales*, vol. 21 (1966), pp. 254–91; McNeill, *Pursuit of Power*, espec. ch. 6; N.F.R. Crafts, "Industrial Revolution in England and France: Some Thoughts on the Question: 'Why was England First?' " *Economic History Review*, 2nd series, vol. 30 (1977), pp. 429–41. There is a brief synopsis in P. Kriedte, *Peasants, Landlords and Merchant Capitalists: Europe and the World Economy, 1500–1800* (Leamington Spa, 1983), pp. 115ff.

11. Mathias and O'Brien, "Taxation in Britain and France," passim; and for the earlier period, see again Dickson and Sperling, "War Finance 1689–1714," passim. There is, however, nothing quite like R. Braun's penetrating comparative essay "Taxation, Sociopolitical Structure, and State-Building," in Tilly (ed.), *Formation of National States in Western Europe*, pp. 243–327.

12. Dickson, *Financial Revolution in England*, p. 198. For the institutional story, see J. H. Clapham, *The Bank of England*, vol. 1, *1694–1797* (Cambridge, 1944); and H. Roseveare, *The Treasury: The Evolution of a British Institution* (London/New York, 1969); and compare with the much less satisfactory (and irregular) situation prior to 1688: C. D. Chandaman, *The English Public Revenue 1660–1688* (Oxford, 1975).

13. Riley, *International Government Finance*, chs. 4 and 6; Wilson, *Anglo-Dutch Commerce and Finance*, passim; A. C. Carter, "Dutch Foreign Investment, 1738–1800," *Economica*, n.s., vol. 20 (November 1953), pp. 322–40. The role of Dutch finance in Britain's growth is also stressed (and perhaps exaggerated) in Wallerstein, *Modern World System*, vol. 2, pp. 279ff; but note also the interesting arguments in L. Neal, "Interpreting Power and Profit in Economic History: A Case Study of the Seven Years War," *Journal of Economic History*, vol. 37 (1977), pp. 34–35.

14. Dickson, *Financial Revolution in England*, p. 9, which is the source for Table 2.

15. Bishop Berkeley's quotation is from ibid., p. 15. For McNeill's argument about the "feedback loop," see *Pursuit of Power*, pp. 178, 206ff.

16. The most useful study here is J. F. Bosher, *French Finances, 1770–1795* (Cambridge, 1970); but see also the articles by Dickson and Sperling, "War Finance," and Mathias and O'Brien, "Taxation in Britain and France," as well as the references in Chapter 2 above to the writings of Bonney, Dent, and Guery. See also the older work R. Mousnier, "L'evolution des finances publiques en France et en Angleterre pendant les guerres de la Ligue d'Augsburg et de la Succession d'Espagne," *Revue Historique*, vol. 44, no. 205 (1951), pp. 1–23.

17. Bosher, *French Finances 1770–1795*, p. 20. This argument is summarized in Bosher's article "French Administration and Public Finance in their European Setting," *NCMH*, vol. 8, ch. 20. For calculations of the amount of taxes siphoned

off into private hands, see Mathias and O'Brien, "Taxation in Britain and France," pp. 643–46.

18. The direct quotations come from J. G. Clark, *La Rochelle and the Atlantic Economy During the Eighteenth Century* (Baltimore/London, 1981), pp. 23, 226; and see in particular chs. 1 and 7, as well as the conclusion. That story can be compared with the British experience, as recounted in R. Davis, *The Rise of the Atlantic Economies* (London, 1975); W. E. Minchinton (ed.), *The Growth of English Overseas Trade in the Seventeenth and Eighteenth Centuries* (London, 1969); A. Calder, *Revolutionary Empire: The Rise of the English-Speaking Empires from the Fifteenth Century to the 1780s* (London, 1981), bks. 2–3; as well as a host of specialized books upon individual ports and trades.

19. See the illuminating detail in the chapters "Finances" and "Supply and Equipment" in L. Kennet, *The French Armies in the Seven Years War: A Study in Military Organization and Administration* (Durham, N.C., 1967). For the navy's weaknesses, particularly with respect to provisions and timber, see P. W. Bamford, *Forests and French Sea Power 1660–1789* (Toronto, 1956), passim; and Jenkins, *History of the French Navy*, ch. 8; and the remarkable analysis by J. F. Bosher, "Financing the French Navy in the Seven Years War: *Beaujon, Goossens et compagnie* in 1759," to be published in *U.S. Naval Institute Proceedings.* For a British comparison, see D. A. Baugh, *British Naval Administration in the Age of Walpole* (Princeton, 1965), passim.

20. For these comparative statistics, see Bosher, *French Finances 1770–1795*, pp. 23–24. This can be supplemented by R. D. Harris, "French Finances and the American War, 1777–1783," *Journal of Modern History*, vol. 46, no. 2 (1976), pp. 233–58; G. Ardent, "Financial Policy and Economic Infrastructure of Modern States and Nations," in Tilly (ed.), *Formation of National States in Western Europe*, pp. 217ff; Hamilton, "Origin and Growth of the National Debt in Western Europe," pp. 122–24. The place of taxation in the French crisis of the late 1780s is delineated in Doyle, *The Old European Order*, pp. 313–20; and *NCMH*, vol. 8, chs. 20–21. For Pitt's reforms, see J. Ehrman, *The Younger Pitt*, 2 vols. to date (London, 1969 and 1983), vol. 1, pp. 239ff; and J.E.D. Binney, *British Public Finance and Administration, 1774–1792* (Oxford, 1958), passim.

21. There is no prospect of giving a satisfactory (let alone an exhaustive) list of references to the war finance of these other states. In general, see Tilly (ed.), *Formation of National States in Western Europe*, chs. 3–4; *NCMH*, vol. 6, pp. 20ff, 284ff; and C. Moraze, "Finance et despotisme, essai sur les despotes eclaires," *Annales*, vol. 3 (1948), pp. 279–96. For Prussia, see the brief remarks in *NCMH*, vol. 7, pp. 296ff, and vol. 8, pp. 7ff, 565ff; and C. Duffy, *The Army of Frederick the Great* (Newton Abbott, 1974), ch. 8. For the Habsburg Empire, see idem, *The Army of Maria Theresa: The Armed Forces of Imperial Austria, 1740–1780* (London, 1977), ch. 10. Even in Russia's case, where conscription operated and the resources of the country were ransacked for military purposes, the earlier self-sufficiency in cash and kind had been replaced by an increasing recourse to foreign loans and paper money by the final decade of the eighteenth century; see idem, *Russia's Military Way to the West: Origins and Nature of Russian Military Power 1700–1800* (London, 1981), pp. 36–38, 179–180.

22. Jones, *Britain and Europe in the Seventeenth Century*, ch. 5; Kennedy, *Rise and Fall of British Naval Mastery*, pp. 50ff.

23. J. G. Stork-Penning, "The Ordeal of the States: Some Remarks on Dutch Politics During the War of the Spanish Succession," *Acta Historiae Neerlandica*, vol. 2 (1967), pp. 107–41; C. R. Boxer, "The Dutch Economic Decline," in Cipolla (ed.), *Economic Decline of Empires;* Wilson, "Taxation and the Decline of Empires:

An Unfashionable Theme," in *Economic History and the Historian*, pp. 114–27; Wolf, *Toward a European Balance of Power*, ch. 7. See also the synopsis in C. P. Kindleberger, "Commercial Expansion and the Industrial Revolution," *Journal of European Economic History*, vol. 4, no. 3 (Winter 1975), pp. 620ff.

24. A. C. Carter, *The Dutch Republic in Europe in the Seven Years War* (London, 1971), especially ch. 7; and, more generally, idem, *Neutrality or Commitment: the Evolution of Dutch Foreign Policy (1667–1795)* (London, 1975), an excellent survey.

25. Carter, *Neutrality or Commitment*, pp. 89ff; and the relevant chapters in E. H. Kossmann, *The Low Countries 1780–1940* (Oxford, 1978).

26. Figures from Doyle, *Old European Order*, p. 242. For France under Louis XIV, see *NCMH*, vols. 5–6; A. de St. Leger and P. Sagnac, *La Prepondérance française, Louis XIV, 1661–1715* (Paris, 1935); R. M. Hatton (ed.), *Louis XIV and Europe* (London, 1976); P. Goubert, *Louis XIV and Twenty Million Frenchmen* (London, 1970); and J. B. Wolf, *Louis XIV* (London, 1968).

27. For excellent analyses of the military-geopolitical problems facing the rulers in Vienna during this period, see K. A. Roider, *Austria's Eastern Question 1700–1790* (Princeton, N.J., 1982); and C. W. Ingrao, "Habsburg Strategy and Geopolitics during the Eighteenth Century," in G. E. Rothenberg, B. K. Kiraly, and P. F. Sugar (eds.), *East Central European Society and War in the Pre-Revolutionary Eighteenth Century* (New York, 1982), pp. 49–96. See also the running commentary in D. Mackay, *Prince Eugene of Savoy* (London, 1977).

28. O. Hufton, *Europe: Privilege and Protest 1730–1789* (London, 1980), p. 155. See also *NCMH*, vol. 8, ch. 10; Kann, *History of the Habsburg Empire*, chs. 3 and 5; and, more generally, E. Wangermann, *The Austrian Achievement* (New York, 1973); and V. S. Mamatey, *Rise of the Habsburg Empire 1526–1815* (New York, 1971). See also the very useful comments in Duffy, *Army of Maria Theresa*, passim.

29. Hufton, *Europe: Privilege and Protest*, ch. 7; Williams, *Ancien Regime in Europe*, chs. 13–16; Wallerstein, *Modern World System*, vol. 2, pp. 225ff; F. L. Carsten, *The Origins of Prussia* (Oxford, 1954), passim; H. Rosenberg, *Bureaucracy, Aristocracy and Autocracy: The Prussian Experience 1660–1815* (Cambridge, Mass., 1958). There is also a good survey of the Prussian reforms and system in *NCMH*, vol. 7, ch. 13.

30. G. Craig, *The Politics of the Prussian Army 1640–1945* (Oxford, 1955), pp. 22ff; Duffy, *Army of Frederick the Great*, passim; T. N. Dupuy, *A Genius for War: The German Army and General Staff, 1807–1945* (Englewood Cliffs, N.J., 1977), pp. 17ff; P. Paret, *Yorck and the Era of Prussian Reform* (Princeton, N.J., 1961), passim.

31. For a brief but very useful analysis, see P. Dukes, *The Emergence of the Super-Powers: A Short Comparative History of the USA and the USSR* (London, 1970), chs. 1–2.

32. Quoted from P. Bairoch, "International Industrialization Levels from 1750 to 1980," *Journal of European Economic History*, vol. 11, no. 2 (Spring 1982), p. 291. See also L. H. Gipson, *The Coming of the Revolution 1763–1775* (New York, 1962), pp. 13–18; R. M. Robertson, *History of the American Economy* (3rd edn., New York, 1973), p. 64.

33. *NCMH*, vol. 7, ch. 14, and vol. 8, ch. 11; Kochan and Abraham, *Making of Modern Russia*, chs. 7–9; Duffy, *Russia's Military Way to the West*, passim; P. Dukes, *The Making of Russian Absolutism 1613–1801* (London, 1982), passim; M. Falkus, *The Industrialization of Russia 1700–1914* (London, 1972), chs. 2–3; M. Raeff, *Imperial Russia 1682–1825* (New York, 1971), passim; and the many

comments on Russia's rise in M. S. Anderson, *Europe in the Eighteenth Century* (London, 1961), espec. ch. 9.

34. A. de Tocqueville, *Democracy in America*, 2 vols. (New York, 1945 edn.), p. 452; and see also the prognostications reported in Dukes, *Emergence of the Super-Powers*, chs. 1–3; H. Gollwitzer, *Geschichte des weltpolitischen Denkens*, 2 vols. (Göttingen, 1972, 1982), vol. 1, pp. 403ff; and the commentary in W. Woodruff, *America's Impact on the World: A Study of the Role of the United States in the World Economy 1750–1970* (New York, 1973).

35. A. T. Mahan, *The Influence of Sea Power upon History 1660–1783* (London, 1965 edn.), p. 29.

36. On which see Kennedy, *The Rise and Fall of the British Naval Mastery*, introduction and chs. 3–5; M. Howard, *The British Way in Warfare* (Neale Lecture, University of London, 1974), passim; Jones, *Britain and the World*, chs. 1–2 and passim.

37. D. E. C. Eversley, "The Home Market and Economic Growth in England 1750–1780," in E. L. Jones and G. E. Mingay (eds.), *Land, Labour and Population of the Industrial Revolution* (London, 1967), pp. 206–59; F. Crouzet, "Toward an Export Economy: British Exports During the Industrial Revolution," *Explorations in Economic History*, vol. 17 (1980), pp. 48–93; P. J. Cain and A. G. Hopkins, "The Political Economy of British Expansion Overseas, 1750–1914," *Economic History Review*, 2nd series, vol. 33, no. 4 (1980), pp. 463–90.

38. Quoted in H. Richmond, *Statesmen and Sea Power* (Oxford, 1946), p. 111; and see further details of this strategical debate in R. Pares, "American versus Continental Warfare 1739–63," *English Historical Review*, vol. 51, no. 103 (1936), pp. 429–65; Wallerstein, *Modern World-System*, vol. 2, pp. 246ff; G. Niedhart, *Handel und Krieg in der britischen Weltpolitik 1738–1763* (Munich, 1979), pp. 64ff.

39. L. Dehio, *The Precarious Balance* (London, 1963), p. 118.

40. These figures—all *approximations*—come from a variety of sources, including Cipolla, *Before the Industrial Revolution*, p. 4; A. Armengaud, "Population in Europe 1700–1914," in C. M. Cipolla (ed.), *Fontana Economic History of Europe*, vol. 3 (1976), pp. 22–76; *NCMH*, vol. 8, p. 714; B. R. Mitchell, *European Historical Statistics, 1750–1970* (London, 1975), pt. A; W. Woodruff, *Impact of Western Man: A Study of Europe's Role in the World Economy 1750–1960* (New York, 1967), p. 104.

41. Corvisier, *Armies and Societies in Europe 1494–1789*, p. 113, gives different figures from Childs, *Armies and Warfare in Europe 1648–1789*, p. 42—and both differ on occasions from data given in specific works on national armies or individual wars.

42. These figures are taken from Anderson, *Europe in the Eighteenth Century*, pp. 144–45, with somewhat different ones given in L. W. Cowie, *Eighteenth-Century Europe* (London, 1963), pp. 141–42. Again, amendments have been made in the light of what seems to be a more authoritative source: thus, the 1779 figures come from J. Dull, *The French Navy and American Independence* (Princeton, N.J., 1975), appendix F; and the 1790 totals from O. von Pivka, *Navies of the Napoleonic Era* (Newton Abbott, 1980), p. 30 (but cf. *NCMH*, vol. 8, p. 190).

43. See pp. 135–37 below.

44. For what follows, see McKay and Scott, *Rise of the Great Powers*, pp. 14ff; Stoye, *Europe Unfolding 1648–1688*, ch. 9; Wolf, *Toward a European Balance of Power*, passim; idem, *The Emergence of the Great Powers 1685–1715* (New York, 1951), chs. 1–7; *NCMH*, vol. 5, ch. 9; St. Leger and Sagnac, *La Préponderance française*, passim; and Hatton (ed.), *Louis XIV and Europe*, passim.

45. L. Andre, *Michel Le Tellier et Louvois* (Paris, 1943 edn.); C. Jones, "The Military

Revolution and the Professionalization of the French Army under the Ancien Régime," in M. Duffy (ed.), *The Military Revolution and the State 1500–1800* (Exeter Studies in History, no. 1, Exeter, 1980), pp. 29–48; Jenkins, *History of the French Navy*, ch. 5.

46. Jones, *Britain and the World*, pp. 100–110; idem, *Country and Court 1658–1714* (London, 1978), pp. 106ff; Padfield, *Tide of Empires*, vol. 2, ch. 4.

47. McKay and Scott, *Rise of the Great Powers*, pp. 34ff; Hatton (ed.), *Louis XIV and Europe*, passim.

48. *NCMH*, vol. 6, ch. 7; Wolf, *Toward a European Balance of Power*, ch. 4; McKay and Scott, *Rise of the Great Powers*, pp. 43–50.

49. G. Symcox, *The Crisis of French Seapower 1689–1697* (The Hague, 1974), passim; Jenkins, *History of the French Navy*, pp. 69–88; Padfield, *Tide of Empires*, vol. 2, ch. 5.

50. For these remarks, see Symcox, *Crisis of French Seapower*, passim; Kennedy, *Rise and Fall of British Naval Mastery*, pp. 76–80; G. N. Clarke, *The Dutch Alliance and the War Against French Trade 1688–1697* (New York, 1971 edn.), passim; D. G. Chandler, "Fluctuations in the Strength of Forces in English Pay sent to Flanders During the Nine Years War, 1688–1697," *War and Society*, vol. 1, no. 2 (September 1983), pp. 1–20; S. B. Baxter, *William III and the Defense of European Liberty 1650–1702* (Westport, Conn., 1976 reprint), pp. 288ff.

51. McKay and Scott, *Rise of the Great Powers*, pp. 54–63; Wolf, *Toward a European Balance of Power*, ch. 7; *NCMH*, vol. 6, ch. 12.

52. For military events, and tactics, in this war, see G. Chandler, *The Art of Warfare in the Age of Marlborough* (London, 1976); Barnett, *Britain and Her Army*, pp. 152ff; McKay, *Prince Eugene of Savoy*, pp. 58ff.

53. Mahan, *Influence of Sea Power upon History*, ch. 5; Kennedy, *Rise and Fall of British Naval Mastery*, pp. 82–88; Padfield, *Tide of Empires*, vol. 2, pp. 156ff; Jones, *Britain and Europe in the Seventeenth Century*, ch. 7; *NCMH*, vol. 6, chs. 11–13, 15.

54. For the Peace of Utrecht, see McKay and Scott, *Rise of the Great Powers*, pp. 63–66; *NCMH*, vol. 6, ch. 14. On the *Asiento* concession, see G. J. Walker, *Spanish Politics and Imperial Trade, 1700–1789* (Bloomington, 1979), ch. 4.

55. J. W. Stoye, *The Siege of Vienna* (London, 1964); T. M. Barker, *Double Eagle and Crescent* (Albany, N.Y., 1967); McKay, *Prince Eugene of Savoy*, chs. 3 and 5; *NCMH*, vol. 6, ch. 19. For characteristics of military warfare in eastern Europe, see B. K. Kiraly and G. E. Rotherberg (eds.), *War and Society in Eastern Europe*, vol. 1 (New York, 1979), espec. pp. 1–33, 361ff.

56. For Charles XII, see R. M. Hatton, *Charles XII of Sweden* (London, 1968), and her ch. 20(i) in *NCMH*, vol. 6, as well as the comments in Roberts, *Swedish Imperial Experience*. For Peter, see M. S. Anderson, *Peter the Great* (London, 1978); R. Wittram, *Peter I: Czar und Kaiser*, 2 vols. (Göttingen, 1964); B. H. Sumner, *Peter the Great and the Emergence of Russia* (London, 1940); *NCMH*, vol. 6, chs. 20(i) and 21.

57. McKay and Scott, *Rise of the Great Powers*, p. 92.

58. Dehio, *Precarious Balance*, p. 102.

59. McKay and Scott, *Rise of the Great Powers*, ch. 4.

60. *NCMH*, vol. 7, ch. 9. For the policies of the individual powers, see A. M. Wilson, *French Foreign Policy During the Administration of Cardinal Fleury* (Cambridge, Mass., 1936); P. Langford, *The Eighteenth Century, 1688–1815: British Foreign Policy* (London, 1976), pp. 71ff; Kann, *History of the Habsburg Empire*, pp. 90ff.

61. Padfield, *Tide of Empires*, vol. 2, pp. 194ff; R. Pares, *War and Trade in the West Indies 1739–1763* (Oxford, 1936); M. Savelle, *Empires to Nations: Expansion in*

America, 1713–1824 (Minneapolis, 1974), ch. 6; Walker, *Spanish Politics and Imperial Trade,* espec. pt. 3; W. L. Dorn, *Competition for Empire 1740–1763* (New York, 1940). For the War of Austrian Succession, see *NCMH,* vol. 7, ch. 17.

62. Dorn, *Competition for Empire,* passim; Pares, *War and Trade,* passim; idem, "American versus Continental Warfare," passim; *NCMH,* vol. 7, chs. 20 and 22; Padfield, *Tide of Empires,* vol. 2, pp. 224ff; Saville, *Empires to Nations,* pp. 135ff; C. M. Andrews, "Anglo-French Commercial Rivalry, 1700–1750," *American Historical Review,* vol. 20 (1915), pp. 539–56, 761–80; P.L.R. Higonnet, "The Origins of the Seven Years War," *Journal of Modern History,* vol. 40 (1968), pp. 57–90.

63. See again Carter, *Dutch Republic in the Seven Years War,* passim; Walker, *Spanish Politics and Imperial Trade.*

64. On the Seven Years War generally, see *NCMH,* vol. 7, ch. 20; McKay and Scott, *Rise of the Great Powers,* pp. 192–200. British policy is covered in Niedhart, *Handel und Krieg in der britischen Weltpolitik,* pp. 121–38; Jones, *Britain and the World,* pp. 207ff; B. Tunstall, *William Pitt, Earl of Chatham* (London, 1938); J. S. Corbett, *England in the Seven Years War: A Study in Combined Strategy,* 2 vols. (London, 1907); R. Savory, *His Britannic Majesty's Army in Germany During the Seven Years War* (Oxford, 1966). The lackluster French effort is nicely described in Kennett, *French Armies in the Seven Years War;* the improved Austrian performance in Duffy, *Army of Maria Theresa.* Russia's early role is described in H. H. Kaplan, *Russia and the Outbreak of the Seven Years War* (Berkeley, Calif., 1968); and Duffy, *Russia's Military Way to the West,* pp. 92ff. Succinct accounts of Prussia's performance are in Duffy, *Army of Frederick the Great;* and J. Kunisch, *Das Mirakel des Hauses Brandenburg* (Munich, 1978), with useful comparisons.

65. Cited in Kennedy, *Rise and Fall of British Naval Mastery,* p. 106; and see also Pares, "American versus Continental Warfare," passim. On Pitt's difficulties in the ministry of 1757–1762, see R. Middleton, *The Bells of Victory* (Cambridge, 1985).

66. Quoted in H. Rosinski, "The Role of Sea Power in the Global Warfare of the Future," *Brassey's Naval Annual* (1947), p. 103. For French financial weaknesses during the Seven Years War, see again Kennett, *French Armies in the Seven Years War,* and Bosher, "Financing the French Navy in the Seven Years War," passim.

67. For the above, see McKay and Scott, *Rise of the Great Powers,* pp. 253–58; *NCMH,* vol. 8, pp. 254ff; J. F. Ramsay, *Anglo-French Relations 1763–70: A Study of Choiseul's Foreign Policy* (Berkeley, Calif., 1939); H. M. Scott, "The Importance of Bourbon Naval Reconstruction to the Strategy of Choiseul after the Seven Years War," *International History Review,* vol. 1 (1979), pp. 17–35; R. Abarca, "Classical Diplomacy and Bourbon 'Revanche' Strategy, 1763–1770," *Review of Politics,* vol. 32 (1970), pp. 313–37; M. Roberts, *Splendid Isolation 1763–1780* (Stenton Lecture, Reading, 1970).

68. For what follows, see I. R. Christie, *Wars and Revolutions: Britain 1760–1815* (London, 1982), chs. 4–6; P. Mackesy, *The War for America 1775–1783* (London, 1964); B. Donoughue, *British Politics and the American Revolution* (London, 1964); G. S. Brown, *The American Secretary: The Colonial Policy of Lord George Germain 1775–1778* (Ann Arbor, Mich., 1963); *NCMH,* vol. 8, chs. 15–19; and the useful collection of essays in D. Higginbotham (ed.), *Reconsiderations on the Revolutionary War* (Westport, Conn., 1978). There is a good survey of the newer literature in H. M. Scott, "British Foreign Policy in the Age of the American Revolution," *International History Review,* vol. 6 (1984), pp. 113–25.

69. D. Syrett, *Shipping and the American War 1775–83* (London, 1970), p. 243 and passim. See also N. Baker, *Government and Contractors: The British Treasury and War Supplies 1775–1783* (London, 1971); R. A. Bowler, *Logistics and the Failure of the British Army in America 1775–1783* (Princeton, N.J., 1975); E. E. Curtis, *The Organization of the British Army in the American Revolution* (Menston, Yorkshire, 1972 reprint). For the American side, see the excellent survey D. Higginbotham, *The War of American Independence* (Bloomington, Ind., 1977 ed.).

70. Barnett, *Britain and Her Army*, p. 225.

71. Figures are from Kennedy, *Rise and Fall of British Naval Mastery*, p. 111. See also the excellent work by Dull, *French Navy and American Independence;* and A. T. Patterson, *The Other Armada: The Franco-Spanish Attempt to Invade Britain in 1779* (Manchester, 1960). For the diplomatic aspects, see I. de Madariaga, *Britain, Russia and the Armed Neutrality of 1780* (London, 1962); S. F. Bemis, *The Diplomacy of the American Revolution* (New York, 1935); and Higginbotham, *The War of American Independence*, ch. 10; most recently, Dull, *A Diplomatic History of the American Revolution* (New Haven, Conn., 1985).

72. For what follows, see McKay and Scott, *Rise of the Great Powers*, ch. 8; *NCMH*, vol. 8, chs. 9 and 12; I. de Madariaga, *Russia in the Age of Catherine the Great* (London, 1981).

73. Ehrman, *Younger Pitt*, vol. 1, pp. 516–71, and vol. 2, pp. 42ff; Jones, *Britain and the World*, pp. 252ff; Binney, *British Public Finance and Administration;* and, for comparisons with France's economy in the 1780s, see again Crouzet, "Angleterre et France"; Mathias and O'Brien, "Taxation in Britain and France, 1715–1810"; and Nef, *War and Human Progress*, pp. 282ff.

74. For the military reforms, see *NCMH*, vol. 8, pp. 190ff, and vol. 9, ch. 3; McNeill, *Pursuit of Power*, pp. 158ff; Strachan, *European Armies and the Conduct of War*, pp. 25ff; R. S. Quimby, *The Background of Napoleonic Warfare* (New York, 1957); D. Bien, "The Army in the French Enlightenment: Reform, Reaction and Revolution," *Past and Present*, no. 85 (1979), pp. 68–98; and G. Rothenberg, *The Art of Warfare in the Age of Napoleon* (Bloomington, Ind., 1978). For the early stages of the campaigning, see M. Glover, *The Napoleonic Wars: An Illustrated History 1792–1815* (New York, 1979); S. T. Ross, *Quest for Victory: French Military Strategy 1792–1799* (London/New York, 1973), chs. 1–4; G. Rothenberg, *Napoleon's Great Adversaries: The Archduke Charles and the Austrian Army 1792–1814* (London, 1982), ch. 2.

75. British policy and strategy is covered in Jones, *Britain and the World*, pp. 259ff; Ehrman, *Younger Pitt*, vol. 2, pts. 4–5; Christie, *Wars and Revolutions*, pp. 215–326; J. M. Sherwig, *Guineas and Gunpowder: British Foreign Aid in the Wars with France 1793–1815* (Cambridge, Mass., 1969), chs. 1–4; M. Duffy, "British Policy in the War Against Revolutionary France," in C. Jones (ed.), *Britain and Revolutionary France: Conflict, Subversion and Propaganda* (Exeter Studies in History, no. 5, Exeter, 1983); D. Geggus, "The Cost of Pitt's Caribbean Campaigns, 1793–1798," *Historical Journal*, vol. 26, no. 2 (1983), pp. 691–706.

76. Quoted in Glover, *Napoleonic Wars*, p. 50. For Napoleon as strategist and commander, see D. G. Chandler, *The Campaigns of Napoleon* (New York, 1966); C. Barnett, *Napoleon* (London, 1978); Rothenberg, *Art of Warfare in the Age of Napoleon;* and the running commentary in G. Lefevre, *Napoleon*, 2 vols. (London/New York, 1969).

77. See A. B. Rodger, *The War of the Second Coalition, 1798–1801* (Oxford, 1964); P. Mackesy, *Statesmen at War: The Strategy of Overthrow, 1798–1799* (London, 1974); the controversial comments in E. Ingram, *Commitment to Empire:*

Prophecies of the Great Game in Asia, 1797–1800 (Oxford, 1981); Sherwig, *Guineas and Gunpowder*, chs. 6–7; Rothenberg, *Napoleon's Great Adversaries*, ch. 3. For the French side, see Ross, *Quest for Victory*, chs. 5–12; and idem, *European Diplomatic History 1789–1815: France Against Europe* (Malabar, Fla., 1981 reprint), ch. 6. The Russian intervention is covered in A. A. Lobanov-Rostovsky, *Russia and Europe 1789–1825* (Durham, N.C., 1947), pp. 43–64; and Duffy, *Russia's Military Way to the West*, pp. 208ff.

78. Jones, *Britain and the World*, pp. 272–80; C. Emsley, *British Society and the French Wars 1793–1815* (London, 1979), chs. 4–5; Lefevre, *Napoleon*, vol. 1, chs. 5 and 7; Glover, *Napoleonic Wars*, pp. 83–84. See also the comments in E. L. Presseisen, *Amiens and Munich: Comparisons in Appeasement* (The Hague, 1978).

79. Lefevre, *Napoleon*, vol. 1, chs. 7 and 9; Ross, *European Diplomatic History*, ch. 8; Chandler, *Campaigns of Napoleon*, pt. 7; Glover, *Napoleonic Wars*, ch. 3; Rothenberg, *Napoleon's Great Adversaries*, ch. 5; Sherwig, *Guineas and Gunpowder*, chs. 7–8; Jones, *Britain and the World*, pp. 281–87; Marcus, *Naval History of England*, vol. 2, pp. 221–302.

80. For what follows, see Jones, *Britain and the World*, pp. 289ff; F. Crouzet, *L'Economie britannique et le Blocus Continental 1806–1813*, 2 vols. (Paris, 1958); idem, "Wars, Blockade, and Economic Change in Europe 1792–1815," *Journal of Economic History*, vol. 24 (1964), pp. 567–88; Kennedy, *Rise and Fall of British Naval Mastery*, pp. 143–45; *NCMH*, vol. 9, pp. 326ff; E. F. Heckscher, *The Continental System* (Oxford, 1922). For the debate over the impact of the 1793–1815 struggle upon the British economy, see, in addition, Emsley, *British Society and the French Wars*, chs. 7–8; J. E. Cookson, "Political Arithmetic and War 1793–1815," *War and Society*, vol. 1, no. 2 (1983), pp. 37–60; G. Hueckel, "War and the British Economy, 1793–1815: A General Equilibrium Analysis," *Explorations in Economic History*, vol. 10, no. 4 (Summer, 1973), pp. 365–96; P. Deane, "War and Industrialisation," in Winter (ed.), *War and Economic Development*, pp. 91–102; J. L. Anderson, "Aspects of the Effects on the British Economy of the War Against France, 1793–1815," *Australian Economic History Review*, vol. 12 (1972), pp. 1–20.

81. See Table 2, above. For British war finances, see N. J. Silberling, "Financial and Monetary Policy of Great Britain During the Napoleonic Wars," *Quarterly Journal of Economics*, vol. 38 (1923–24), pp. 214–33; E. B. Schumpeter, "English Prices and Public Finance, 1660–1822," *Review of Economic Statistics*, vol. 20 (1938), pp. 21–37; A. Hope-Jones, *Income Tax in the Napoleonic Wars* (Cambridge, 1939); P. O'Brien, *British Financial and Fiscal Policy in the Wars Against France, 1793–1815* (Oxford, 1984).

82. L. Bergeron, *France Under Napoleon* (Princeton, N.J., 1981), pp. 37ff, 159ff; G. Brunn, *Europe and the French Imperium, 1799–1815* (New York, 1938), chs. 4–5; S. B. Clough, *France: A History of National Economics 1789–1939* (New York, 1939), chs. 2–3; Lefevre, *Napoleon*, vol. 2, chs. 1–4; C. Trebilcock, *The Industrialization of the Continental Powers 1780–1914* (London, 1981), pp. 125ff.

83. Bergeron, *France Under Napoleon*, pp. 167ff, 184ff; Crouzet, "Wars, Blockade, and Economic Change," passim.

84. Bergeron, *France Under Napoleon*, pp. 37ff; Lefevre, *Napoleon*, vol. 2, pp. 171ff; Clough, *France*, chs. 2–3.

85. For what follows, see Bergeron, *France Under Napoleon*, pp. 40–41; Lefevre, *Napoleon*, vol. 2, p. 291; McNeill, *Pursuit of Power*, pp. 198ff; Brunn, *Europe and the French Imperium*, pp. 73–75, 110ff; E. J. Hobsbawm, *The Age of Revolution 1789–1848* (London, 1962), p. 97; G. Rudé, *Revolutionary Europe 1783–*

1815 (London, 1964), ch. 13 and espec. pp. 274–75; S. Schama, "The Exigencies of War and the Politics of Taxation in the Netherlands 1795–1810," in Winter (ed.), *War and Economic Development,* pp. 111, 117, 128.

86. Quoted in Glover, *Napoleonic Wars,* p. 129; and compare with Guibert's remarkable pre-Revolution forecast of a people "who, knowing how to make war cheaply and live on the spoils of victory, was not obliged to lay down its arms for reasons of finance"—as cited in *NCMH,* vol. 8, p. 217; and with Spenser Wilkinson's remarks, quoted in Tilly (ed.), *Formation of National States in Western Europe,* pp. 147–48, 152.

87. Glover, *Napoleonic Wars,* pp. 140–41; Jones, *Britain and the World,* pp. 22, 317; Sherwig, *Guineas and Gunpowder,* chs. 9–10.

88. Figures from Glover, *Napoleonic Wars,* p. 152; see also Chandler, *Campaigns of Napoleon,* p. 734. For the Austrian army's campaigning—and recuperation— see Rothenberg, *Napoleon's Great Adversaries,* pp. 123ff.

89. For the Peninsular War, see the relevant parts of Glover, *Campaigns of Napoleon:* J. Weller, *Wellington in the Peninsula* (London, 1962); R. Glover, *Peninsular Preparation: The Reform of the British Army, 1795–1809* (Cambridge, 1963); M. Glover, *The Peninsular War, 1807–1814: A Concise History* (Newton Abbott, 1974); Sherwig, *Guineas and Gunpowder,* pp. 198ff. The French side is covered in J. Thiry, *La Guerre d'Espagne* (Paris, 1966); Ross, *European Diplomatic History,* pp. 276ff; G. H. Lovett, *Napoleon and the Birth of Modern Spain,* 2 vols. (New York, 1965). The importance of the Spanish contribution is rightly stressed in D. Gates, *The Spanish Ulcer: A History of the Peninsula War* (London, 1986).

90. Brunn, *Europe and the French Imperium,* ch. 8; Rudé, *Revolutionary Europe,* chs. 13–14; Lefevre, *Napoleon,* vol. 2, chs. 7–8; J. Godechet, B. F. Hyslop, and D. L. Dowd, *The Napoleonic Era in Europe* (New York, 1971), espec. ch. 8; G. Best, *War and Society in Revolutionary Europe, 1770–1870* (London, 1982), chs. 11–13; R. J. Rath, *The Fall of the Napoleonic Kingdom of Italy* (New York, 1941), chs. 1–2.

91. Crouzet, "Wars, Blockade and Economic Change," passim; Glover, *Napoleonic Wars,* chs. 4–5; O. Connelly, *Napoleon's Satellite Kingdoms* (New York, 1965), passim. For Russian policy, see Chandler, *Campaign of Napoleon,* pp. 739ff; *NCMH,* vol. 9, pp. 512ff; Lobanov-Rostovsky, *Russia in Europe, 1789–1825,* passim; and, earlier, H. Ragsdale, *Détente in the Napoleonic Era: Bonaparte and the Russians* (Lawrence, Kansas, 1980).

92. Chandler, *Campaigns of Napoleon,* pts. 13–14; Glover, *Napoleonic Wars,* pp. 160ff; Ross, *European Diplomatic History,* pp. 310ff; A. Palmer, *Napoleon in Russia* (New York, 1967); C. Duffy, *Borodino and the War of 1812* (London, 1973); Lefevre, *Napoleon,* vol. 2, ch. 9; G. Blond, *La Grande Armée 1804/1815* (Paris, 1979).

93. Glover, *Napoleonic Wars,* p. 193; Sherwig, *Guineas and Gunpowder,* chs. 12– 13, espec. pp. 287–88; Rothenberg, *Napoleon's Great Adversaries,* pp. 178ff.

94. Which is perhaps why it is almost completely ignored in so many of the standard military and diplomatic histories of this period. For details, see E. B. Potter (ed.), *Sea Power: A Naval History,* 2nd edn. (Annapolis, Md., 1981), ch. 10, and bibliography on p. 392; B. Perkins, *Prologue to War: England and the United States 1805–1812* (Berkeley, Calif., 1961); A. T. Mahan, *Sea Power in Its Relations to the War of 1812,* 2 vols. (London, 1905); Marcus, *Naval History of England,* vol. 2, ch. 16.

95. Ingram, *Commitment to Empire,* passim; G. J. Adler, "Britain and the Defence of India—The Origins of the Problem, 1798–1815," *Journal of Asian History,* vol. 6 (1972), pp. 14–44.

96. Chandler, *Campaigns of Napoleon*, pt. 17; Glover, *Napoleonic Wars*, pp. 212ff; Lefevre, *Napoleon*, vol. 2, ch. 10; Blond, *La Grand Armée*, ch. 16; H. Lachouque, *Waterloo* (Paris, 1972); U. Pericoli and M. Glover, *1815: The Armies at Waterloo* (London, 1973).

97. For details on the 1814–1815 settlements, see Sherwig, *Guineas and Gunpowder*, ch. 14; *NCMH*, vol. 9, ch. 24; E. V. Gulick, *Europe's Classical Balance of Power* (New York, 1967 edn.), passim; C. K. Webster, *The Foreign Policy of Castlereagh, 1812–1815: Britain and the Reconstruction of Europe* (London, 1931); H. G. Nicolson, *The Congress of Vienna* (London/New York, 1946); D. Dakin, "The Congress of Vienna, 1814–15, and Its Antecedents," in A. Sked (ed.), *Europe's Balance of Power 1815–1848* (London, 1979).

98. Gulick, *Europe's Classical Balance of Power*, p. 304. See also the comments in H. Kissinger, *A World Restored: Metternich, Castlereagh and the Problems of Peace 1812–1822* (Boston, 1957).

99. For a succinct coverage of the extensive literature, see P. J. Marshall, "British Expansion in India in the Eighteenth Century: An Historical Revision," *History*, vol. 60 (1975), pp. 28–43; as well as the remarks in Ingram, *Commitment to Empire*.

100. See Braudel, *Wheels of Commerce*, pp. 403ff, for a useful discussion of the importance of long-distance trade. For the specifically British context, I have benefited from reading Patrick O'Brien's paper "The Impact of the Revolutionary and Napoleonic Wars, 1793–1815, on the Long Run Growth of the British Economy" (Davis Center Paper, 1983).

101. This literature is covered in Crouzet, "Toward an Export Economy," passim; Cain and Hopkins, "The Political Economy of British Expansion Overseas, 1750–1914," passim; R. Davis, *The Industrial Revolution and British Overseas Trade* (Leicester, 1979); N.F.R. Crafts, "British Economic Growth, 1700–1831: A Review of the Evidence," *Economic History Review*, 2nd series, vol. 36 (1983), pp. 177–99.

102. The phrase is used in F. Crouzet, *The Victorian Economy* (London, 1982), p. 1.

103. Glover, *Napoleonic Wars*, pp. 182–83.

104. Quoted in Marcus, *Naval History of England*, vol. 2, p. 501.

CHAPTER FOUR
Industrialization and the Shifting Global Balances, 1815–1885

1. S. Pollard, *Peaceful Conquest: The Industrialization of Europe 1760–1970* (Oxford, 1981), passim. For good treatments of the Industrial Revolution in the West on a *country-by-country* basis, see T. Kemp, *Industrialization in Nineteenth-Century Europe* (London, 1969); W. O. Henderson, *The Industrial Revolution on the Continent: Germany, France, Russia 1800–1914* (London, 1967 edn.); C. Trebilcock, *The Industrialization of the Continental Powers 1780–1914* (London, 1981); C. M. Cipolla (ed.), *Fontana Economic History of Europe*, vol. 3, *The Industrial Revolution* (London, 1973); A. S. Milward and S. B. Saul, *The Economic Development of Continental Europe 1780–1870* (London, 1973).

2. C. M. Cipolla, "Introduction," in Cipolla (ed.), *Industrial Revolution*, p. 7.

3. D. Landes, *The Unbound Prometheus: Technological Change and Industrial Development in Western Europe from 1750 to the Present* (Cambridge, 1969), p. 41.

4. Ibid.

5. Braudel, *Civilization and Capitalism*, vol. 1, pp. 42ff.

6. For details, see McNeill, *Pursuit of Power,* pp. 185ff; G. Rudé, *Paris and London in the Eighteenth Century: Studies in Popular Protest* (New York, 1971), passim.

7. T. S. Ashton, *The Industrial Revolution 1760–1830* (Oxford, 1968 edn.), p. 129. For other excellent studies of British economic change in this period, see Mathias, *First Industrial Nation,* passim; Hobsbawm, *Industry and Empire,* chs. 2–4 and 6; and Crouzet, *Victorian Economy,* pt. 1, from where the population and GNP figures given in the preceding paragraph come.

8. Landes, *Unbound Prometheus,* pp. 97–98.

9. Ashton, *Industrial Revolution,* p. 129.

10. Mathias, *First Industrial Nation,* p. 5.

11. Bairoch, "International Industrialization Levels from 1750 to 1980," pp. 296 and 294 respectively. In the "Methodological Appendix" to this important essay, Bairoch discusses how he reaches these figures. Bairoch's assumptions are by no means uncontested, however: see A. Maddison, "A Comparison of Levels of GDP per Capita in Developed and Developing Countries, 1700–1980," *Journal of Economic History,* vol. 43 (1983), pp. 27–41.

12. Bairoch, "International Industrialization Levels," pp. 290ff; Crouzet, *Victorian Economy,* Introduction.

13. Woodruff, *Impact of Western Man,* passim; D. Fieldhouse, *The Colonial Empires: A Comparative Survey from the Eighteenth Century* (London, 1966), pt. 2; idem, *Economics and Empire 1830–1916* (London, 1973), passim.

14. On which see V. Kiernan, *European Empires from Conquest to Collapse, 1815–1960* (London, 1982); Strachen, *European Armies and the Conduct of War,* ch. 6.

15. Figures from Fieldhouse, *Colonial Empires,* p. 178.

16. This has now been very well covered in D. R. Headrich, *The Tools of Empire: Technology and European Imperialism in the Nineteenth Century* (Oxford, 1981), ch. 2 and passim.

17. E. Hobsbawm, *The Age of Capital 1848–1875* (London, 1975), ch. 7.

18. Bairoch, "International Industrialization Levels," p. 291. For a new study which stresses (and perhaps *over*stresses) the relative slowness of British economic expansion in these decades, see N.F.R. Crafts, *British Economic Growth During the Industrial Revolution* (Oxford, 1985).

19. Crouzet, *Victorian Economy,* pp. 4–5.

20. Quoted in R. Hyam, *Britain's Imperial Century 1815–1914* (London, 1975), p. 47. For further details, see B. Porter, *The Lion's Share: A Short History of British Imperialism 1850–1970* (London, 1976), passim; Cain and Hopkins, "The Political Economy of British Expansion Overseas, 1750–1914," passim; Crouzet, "Towards an Export Economy," passim; J. B. Williams, *British Commercial Policy and Trade Expansion 1750–1850* (Oxford, 1972), passim.

21. P. Bairoch, "Europe's Gross National Product: 1800–1975," *Journal of European Economic History,* vol. 5, no. 2 (Fall 1976), p. 282. And see Table 10 below.

22. D. French, *British Economic and Strategic Planning, 1905–1915* (London, 1982), ch. 1, "Nineteenth-Century Political Economy and the Problem of War," is a good introduction to these ideas.

23. See H. Strachan, *Wellington's Legacy: The Reform of the British Army, 1830–54* (Manchester, 1984).

24. These seem reasonable assumptions, based upon the crude figures of British GNP and government expenditures available in A. T. Peacock and J. Wiseman, *The Growth of Public Expenditure in the United Kingdon* (London, 1967 edn.); and P. Flora (ed.), *State, Economy and Society in Western Europe 1875–1975,* vol. 1 (Frankfurt/London, 1983), especially pt. 4, p. 441.

25. Figures taken from the "Correlates of War" print-out data made available

through the Inter-University Consortium for Political and Social Research at the University of Michigan.

26. C. Lloyd, *The Nation and the Navy* (London, 1961), p. 223.
27. For details, see Kennedy, *Rise and Fall of British Naval Mastery*, ch. 6; and espec. C. J. Bartlett, *Great Britain and Sea Power 1815–1853* (Oxford, 1963), passim. For some regional manifestations: G. S. Graham, *Great Britain in the Indian Ocean: A Study of Maritime Enterprise 1810–1850* (Oxford, 1967); B. Gough, *The Royal Navy and the North West Coast of America 1810–1914* (Vancouver, 1971); G. Fox, *British Admirals and Chinese Pirates 1832–1869* (London, 1940).
28. A.G.L. Shaw (ed.), *Great Britain and the Colonies 1815–1865* (London, 1970), p. 2. Also important here are Hyam, *Britain's Imperial Century*, passim; Porter, *Lion's Share*, passim; J. Gallagher and R. Robinson, "The Imperialism of Free Trade," *Economic History Review*, 2nd series, vol. 6, no. 1 (1953), pp. 1–15.
29. For British assumptions, see B. Porter, *Britain, Europe and the World, 1850–1982: Delusions of Grandeur* (London/Boston, 1983), ch. 1; B. J. Wendt, "Freihandel und Friedenssicherung: Zur Bedeutung des Cobden-Vertrags von 1860 zwischen England und Frankreich," *Vierteljahresschrift fur Sozial- und Wirtschafts-geschichte*, vol. 61 (1974), pp. 29ff. For the economic details, see Cain and Hopkins, "Political Economy of British Expansion Overseas," passim; L. H. Jenks, *Migration of British Capital to 1875* (London, 1963 edn.); Crouzet, *Victorian Economy*, chs. 10–11 and passim; Mathias, *First Industrial Nation*, ch. 11; A. H. Imlah, *Economic Elements in the "Pax Britannica"* (Cambridge, Mass., 1958). The complementarity in the trading/payments relationships is nicely covered in S. B. Saul, *Studies in British Overseas Trade 1870–1914* (Liverpool, 1960); and J. Foreman-Peck, *A History of the World Economy: International Economic Relations since 1850* (Brighton, Sussex, 1983), espec. chs. 1–6.
30. For this argument, see Kennedy, *Rise and Fall of British Naval Mastery*, ch. 7.
31. F. Crouzet, "Towards an Export Economy," p. 70.
32. Porter, *Britain, Europe and the World*, chs. 1–2. For the strategical implications of Britain's increasing reliance upon "service" industries, see P. Kennedy, *Strategy and Diplomacy, 1860–1945: Eight Essays* (London/Boston, 1983), ch. 3; French, *British Economic and Strategic Planning*, passim.
33. Quoted in Higham, *Britain's Imperial Century*, p. 49.
34. See pp. 131–33 above.
35. Kemp, *Industrialization in Nineteenth-century Europe*, chs. 2–3; Pollard, *Peaceful Conquest*, chs. 2–3; T. Hamerow, *Restoration, Revolution, Reaction: Economics and Politics in Germany* (Princeton, N.J., 1958).
36. J. Droz, *Europe Between Revolutions 1815–1848* (London, 1967), p. 18.
37. D. Thomson, *Europe Since Napoleon* (Harmondsworth, Mddsx., 1966 edn.), p. 111; and see also Best, *War and Society in Revolutionary Europe*, pt. 3; A. Sked, "Metternich's Enemies or the Threat from Below," in Sked (ed.), *Europe's Balance of Power 1815–1848* (London, 1979), ch. 8.
38. F. R. Bridge and R. Bullen, *The Great Powers and the European States System 1815–1914* (London, 1980), chs. 2–3; Craig, *Politics of the Prussian Army*, pp. 65ff.; R. Albrecht-Carrié, *A Diplomatic History of Europe Since the Congress of Vienna* (London, 1965 edn.), chs. 1 and 3–4. The best study of Prussian and German-state affairs in this period is now T. Nipperdey, *Deutsche Geschichte 1800–1866* (Munich, 1983).
39. D. Showalter, *Railroads and Rifles: Soldiers, Technology and the Unification of Germany* (Hamden, Conn., 1975), passim; Dupuy, *Genius for War*, chs. 4–6; *NCMH*, vol. 10, *The Zenith of European Power 1830–70*, chs. 12 and 19; L. H.

Addington, *The Patterns of War Since the Eighteenth Century* (Bloomington, Ind., 1984), pp. 39ff.

40. See again Mamatey, *Rise of the Habsburg Empire 1526–1815*, passim; Kann, *A History of the Habsburg Empire*, chs. 3 and 5.

41. A. Sked, "The Metternich System, 1815–48," in Sked (ed.), *Europe's Balance of Power 1815–1848*, ch. 5; Bridge and Bullen, *Great Powers and the European States System*, passim; Albrecht-Carrié, *Diplomatic History*, chs. 3–4; P. W. Schroeder, "World War I as a Galloping Gertie," *Journal of Modern History*, vol. 44 (1972), pp. 319–45—which echoes some of the remarks in his *Austria, Britain and the Crimean War: The Destruction of the European Concert* (Ithaca, N.Y., 1972).

42. Quoted in C. McEvedy, *The Penguin Atlas of Recent History* (Harmondsworth, Mddsx., 1982), p. 8; see also Droz, *Europe Between Revolutions*, pp. 170ff.

43. G. Rothenberg, *The Army of Francis Joseph* (West Lafayette, Ind., 1976), pp. xi, 61. See also A. Sked, *The Survival of the Habsburg Empire: Radetzky, The Imperial Army and the Class War, 1848* (London, 1979), pt. 1.

44. D. F. Good, *The Economic Rise of the Habsburg Empire, 1750–1914* (Berkeley, Calif., 1984) is best here.

45. Rothenberg, *Army of Francis Joseph*, p. 9; and J. Niemeyer, *Das oesterreichische Militärwesen im Umbruch* (Osnabruck, 1979), pp. 43–45.

46. See Rothenberg, *Army of Francis Joseph*, pp. 10, 41, 46, 58, for financial allocations; and G. A. Craig, "Command and Staff Problems in the Austrian Army, 1740–1866," in M. Howard (ed.), *The Theory and Practice of War* (London, 1965), pp. 43–67, for institutional difficulties.

47. Rothenberg, *Army of Francis Joseph*, p. 19; Kann, *History of the Habsburg Empire*, ch. 6; A. Sked, "The Metternich System," in *Europe's Balance of Power 1815–1848*, passim.

48. For a succinct survey, see R. Bullen, "France and Europe, 1815–48: The Problems of Defeat and Recovery," in Sked (ed.), *Survival of the Habsburg Empire*, pp. 122–44. For economic histories, see again Clough, *France; A History of National Economics*, passim; F. Caron, *An Economic History of Modern France* (New York, 1979), pt. 1; T. Kemp, *Economic Forces in French History* (London, 1971), chs. 6–8, 10.

49. Bullen, "France and Europe, 1815–48," pp. 125–26.

50. Ibid.

51. McNeill, *Pursuit of Power*, p. 213, fn. 57.

52. As quoted in Milward and Saul, *Economic Development of Continental Europe 1780–1870*, pp. 307–9. See also Clough, *France*, pp. 41ff; Trebilcock, *Industrialization of the Continental Powers 1780–1914*, pp. 130ff; Kemp, *Economic Forces in French History*, pp. 106ff.

53. Calculated from the figures produced in Table 10 of Bairoch, "International Industrialization Levels from 1750 to 1980," p. 296. See also the figures offered in R. E. Cameron, "Economic Growth and Stagnation in France 1815–1914," *Journal of Modern History*, vol. 30 (1958), pp. 1–13.

54. For these arguments, see Caron, *Economic History of Modern France*, espec. ch. 1. The study by P. O'Brien and C. Keydor, *Economic Growth in Britain and France 1780–1914* (London, 1978), is also a useful corrective to the older literature; but since it is not concerned with what they describe as "the mercantilist jargon of 'national power'" (p. 176), its implications are not so important for our analysis. For a critique of O'Brien and Keydor's handling of comparative statistics, see V. Hentschel, "Produktion, Wachstum und Produktivität in England, Frankreich und Deutschland von der Mitte des 19. Jahrhundert bis zum

Ersten Weltkrieg," *Vierteljahresschrift fur Sozial- und Wirtschaftsgeschichte*, vol. 68 (1981), pp. 457–510.

55. R. Cameron, *France and the Economic Development of Europe 1800–1914* (Princeton, N.J. 1961); Trebilcock, *Industrialization of the Continental Powers*, pp. 176ff; A. Rowley, *Evolution économique de la France de milieu du xixe siècle à 1914* (Paris, 1982), pp. 413ff.

56. McNeill, *Pursuit of Power*, pp. 226ff. French tactical and strategical (as well as technical) innovations are nicely compared in C. E. Hamilton, "The Royal Navy, *La Royale*, and the Militarization of Naval Warfare, 1840–1870," *Journal of Strategic Studies*, vol. 6 (1983), pp. 182–212.

57. In Padfield's definition: see *Tide of Empires*, vol. 1, foreword; and see again Bullen, "France and Europe," passim. France's colonial endeavors are briefly covered in Fieldhouse, *Colonial Empires*, ch. 13.

58. This was Palmerston's phrase of April 1848: see *NCMH*, vol. 10, p. 260. For general surveys of Russia's international position after 1815, see Bridge and Bullen, *Great Powers and the European States System*, passim; Lobanov-Rostovsky, *Russia and Europe 1789–1825*, passim; R. W. Seton-Watson, *The Russian Empire 1801–1917* (Oxford, 1967), ch. 9.

59. See the discussion in M. E. Falkus, *The Industrialization of Russia 1700–1914* (London, 1972), ch. 4; W. C. Blackwell, *The Beginnings of Russian Industrialization, 1800–1860* (Princeton, N.J., 1968); and idem, *The Industrialization of Russia: An Historical Perspective* (New York, 1970), chs. 1–2.

60. Bairoch, "Europe's Gross National Product, 1800–1975," Table 4, p. 281.

61. Ibid., Table 6, p. 286.

62. Kochan and Abraham, *Making of Modern Russia*, p. 164.

63. Ibid., chs. 9–10; Trebilcock, *Industrialization of the Continental Powers*, ch. 4; Falkus, *Industrialization of Russia*, chs. 4–5; Dukes, *Emergence of the Super-Powers*, chs. 3–4.

64. J. S. Curtiss, *The Russian Army Under Nicholas I, 1825–1855* (Durham, N.C., 1965), passim; Best, *War and Society in Revolutionary Europe*, ch. 18; Seton-Watson, *Russian Empire*, pp. 289ff; J. Keep, "The Military Style of the Romanov Rulers," *War and Society*, vol. 1, no. 2 (1983), pp. 61–84. For the Anglo-Russian rivalry, see D. Gillard, *The Struggle for Asia 1828–1961* (London, 1977); E. Ingram, *The Beginning of the Great Game in Asia 1828–1834* (Oxford, 1979); Ingram (ed.), "The Great Game in Asia," *International History Review*, vol. 2, no. 2 (April 1980), special issue.

65. Curtiss, *Russian Army Under Nicholas I*, pp. 310–11.

66. By far the best study is J. S. Curtiss, *Russia's Crimean War* (Durham, N.C., 1979); but see also A. Seaton, *The Crimean War: A Russian Chronicle* (London, 1977), passim; idem, *The Russian Army of the Crimea* (Reading, Berkshire, 1973).

67. D. W. Mitchell, *A History of Russian and Soviet Sea Power* (New York, 1974), ch. 8.

68. For these details, see Curtiss, *Russia's Crimean War*, passim; Seaton, *Crimean War*, passim; Seton-Watson, *Russian Empire*, pp. 319ff; Blackwell, *Beginnings of Industrialization in Russia*, pp. 183ff; and the very good summary in W. Baumgart, *The Peace of Paris, 1856* (Santa Barbara, Calif., 1981), pp. 68–80, from where the quotation comes.

69. Baumgart, *Peace of Paris*, pp. 72–74; Seton-Watson, *Russian Empire*, p. 248; W. Pintner, "Inflation in Russia During the Crimean War Period," *American Slavic and East European Review*, vol. 18 (1959), pp. 85-87.

70. Baumgart, *Peace of Paris*, pp. 25–31.

71. Ibid., pp. 31ff.; Barnett, *Britain and Her Army*, pp. 283–91; E. M. Spiers, *The*

Army and Society 1815–1914 (London, 1980), ch. 4; J.A.S. Grenville, *Europe Reshaped 1848–1878* (London, 1976), ch. 10.

72. O. Anderson, *A Liberal State at War* (London, 1967), passim.
73. Figures taken from the "Correlates of War" print-out data, made available through the Inter-University Consortium for Political and Social Research at the University of Michigan.
74. See again MacDonagh, *Liberal State at War*, and compare with Schroeder, *Austria, Britain and the Crimean War*, Baumgart, *The Peace of Paris*, and N. Rich, *Why the Crimean War?: A Cautionary Tale* (Hanover, N.H., 1985), pp. 157ff, which concentrate much more upon Palmerston's belligerent *tone*.
75. Quoted in D.C.B. Lieven, *Russia and the Origins of the First World War* (London, 1983), p. 21. See also D. Beyrau, *Militär und Gesellschaft im vorrevolutionären Russland* (Göttingen, 1984).
76. W. E. Mosse, *Alexander II and the Modernization of Russia* (New York, 1962 edn.), passim; Kochan and Abraham, *Making of Modern Russia*, ch. 10; Seton-Watson, *Russian Empire*, pt. 4; Falkus, *Industrialization of Russia 1700–1914*, ch. 5; Blackwell, *Industrialization of Russia*, ch. 2.
77. See again Dukes, *Emergence of the Super-Powers*, chs. 3–4; Gollwitzer, *Geschichte des weltpolitischen Denkens*, vol. 1, chs. 3–4.
78. Covered in K. Bourne, *Britain and the Balance of Power in North America 1815–1908* (London, 1967).
79. "Correlates of War" print-out data; for the railway mileages, see W. W. Rostow, *The World Economy, History and Prospect* (Austin, Texas, 1978), p. 152. See also W. H. Becker and S. F. Wells, Jr. (eds.), *Economics and World Power: An Assessment of American Diplomacy Since 1789* (New York, 1984), pp. 56ff.
80. The literature upon the American Civil War is staggeringly large. I found most useful H. Hattaway and A. Jones, *How the North Won: A Military History of the Civil War* (Urbana, Ill., 1983); P. J. Parish, *The American Civil War* (New York, 1975); A. R. Millett and P. Maslowski, *For the Common Defense: A Military History of the United States of America* (New York, 1984), chs. 6–7; R. F. Weigley, *History of the United States Army* (Bloomington, Ind., 1984 edn.), chs. 10–11; Ropp, *War in the Modern World*, pp. 175–194; Addington, *Patterns of War*, pp. 62–82.
81. Millett and Maslowski, *For the Common Defense*, p. 155.
82. R. F. Weigley, *The American Way of War: A History of the United States Military Strategy and Policy* (Bloomington, Ind., 1977 edn.); Millett and Maslowski, *For the Common Defense*, passim.
83. For brief details of that position, see K. Bourne, *Victorian Foreign Policy 1830–1902* (Oxford, 1970), pp. 90–96; and, in much more detail, E. D. Adams, *Great Britain and the American Civil War*, 2 vols. (London, 1925).
84. J. Luvaas, *The Military Legacy of the Civil War: The European Inheritance* (Chicago, 1959), passim.
85. For post–Crimean War diplomacy in Europe, see Bridge and Bullen, *Great Powers and the European State System*, pp. 88ff; Albrecht-Carrié, *Diplomatic History*, pp. 94ff; W. E. Mosse, *The Rise and Fall of the Crimean System 1855–71* (London, 1963); NCMH, vol. 10, ch. 10, pp. 268ff; A. J. P. Taylor, *The Struggle for Mastery in Europe 1848–1918* (Oxford, 1954), pp. 83ff.
86. Rothenberg, *Army of Francis Joseph*, pp. 52ff.
87. McNeill, *Pursuit of Power*, ch. 7; C. Harvie, *War and Society in the 19th Century*, block 4, unit 10 of *War and Society* (The Open University, Bletchley, 1973); Strachan, *European Armies*, ch. 8; Ropp, *War in the Modern World*, ch. 6; Showalter, *Railroads and Rifles*, passim; NCMH, vol. 10, ch. 12; M. Glover, *Warfare from Waterloo to Mons* (London, 1980), pts. 2–3.

88. For Prussian military developments, see again Dupuy, *Genius for War*, pp. 75ff; Showalter, *Railroads and Rifles*, passim; Strachan, *European Armies*, pp. 98ff. For the mistakes made in 1866, see M. van Creveld, *Command in War* (Cambridge, Mass., 1985), ch. 4; G. A. Craig, *The Battle of Koeniggratz* (London, 1965), passim. The Austrian side is summarized in Rothenberg, *Army of Francis Joseph*, pp. 66ff.

89. See again van Creveld, *Command in War*, pp. 140ff; M. Howard, *The Franco-Prussian War* (London, 1981 edn.), passim.

90. For military details, see Craig, *Koeniggratz*, passim; for the diplomatic and political background, O. Pflanze, *Bismarck and the Development of Germany: The Period of Unification 1815–1871* (Princeton, N.J., 1963), chs. 13–15.

91. Howard, *Franco-Prussian War*, offers outstanding coverage of these events. For French military weaknesses, see also R. Holmes, *The Road to Sedan: The French Army, 1866–70* (London, 1984).

92. Howard, *Franco-Prussian War*, p. 1; and Holmes, *Road to Sedan*, passim, for the French side.

93. The raw figures are available in Flora, *State, Economy and Society in Western Europe 1815–1975*, vol. 1; and in B. R. Mitchell, *European Historical Statistics 1750–1975* (2nd edn., New York, 1981), e.g., coal figures on p. 381, etc. For comparative analyses of the two nations' economies, see again Trebilcock, *Industrialization of the Continental Powers*, chs. 2–3; Kemp, *Industrialization in Nineteenth-Century Europe*, chs. 3–4; Landes, *Unbound Prometheus*, ch. 4.

94. The diplomacy of the Franco-Prussian War is covered in Taylor, *Struggle for Mastery in Europe*, pp. 201–17; W. E. Mosse, *The European Powers and the German Question 1848–1870* (Cambridge, 1958); E. Kolb (ed.), *Europa und die Reichsgründung (Historische Zeitschrift, Beiheft 6, Munich, 1980)*, passim; Bridge and Bullen, *Great Powers and the European States System*, pp. 108ff.

95. On which see A. Mitchell, *The German Influence in France After 1870: The Formation of the French Republic* (Chapel Hill, N.C., 1979); and idem, *Victors and Vanquished: The German Influence on Army and Church in France after 1870* (Chapel Hill, N.C., 1984).

96. See the revealing figures in Taylor, *Struggle for Mastery in Europe*, pp. xxiv–xxvi (and the remark on p. xxiii, fn. 4); also D. Mack Smith, *Italy: A Modern History* (Ann Arbor, Mich., 1959); and C. J. Lowe and F. Marzari, *Italian Foreign Policy 1870–1940* (London, 1975).

97. To use the terms employed by P. W. Schroeder, "The Lost Intermediaries: The Impact of 1870 on the European System," *International History Review*, vol. 6 (1984), p. 14.

98. On the implications of which, see ibid., passim.

99. Taylor, *Struggle for Mastery in Europe*, pp. 218ff; Bridge and Bullen, *Great Powers and the European State System*, pp. 112ff; W. L. Langer, *European Alliances and Alignments 1871–1890* (New York, 1950 edn.), passim; Grenville, *Europe Reshaped 1848–1878*, ch. 18. British policy is well covered in K. Hildebrand, "Grossbritannien und die deutsche Reichsgründung," in Kolb (ed.), *Europa und die Reichsgründung*, pp. 37ff.

100. For a good discussion, see A. Hillgruber, *Bismarcks Aussenpolitik* (Freiburg, 1972), briefly summarized in idem, *Die gescheiterte Grossmacht: Eine Skizze des Deutschen Reiches 1871–1945* (Düsseldorf, 1980), pp. 17–30.

101. A. Hillgruber, "Die 'Krieg-in-Sicht'-Krise 1875," in E. Schulin (ed.), *Gedenkschrift Martin Göhring, Studien zur europäischen Geschichte* (Wiesbaden, 1968), pp. 239–53; P. Kennedy, *The Rise of the Anglo-German Antagonism, 1860–1914* (London/Boston, 1980), pp. 29–31.

102. Hillgruber, *Die gescheiterte Grossmacht*, pp. 30ff.; and for stimulating discus-

sions of the longer-term issues, see D. Calleo, *The German Problem Reconsidered: Germany and the World Order, 1870 to the Present* (New York/Cambridge, 1978), espec. chs. 2–4; W. D. Gruner, *Die deutsche Frage: Ein Problem der europäischen Geschichte seit 1800* (Munich, 1985), passim; K. Hildebrand, "Staatskunst oder Systemzwang? Die 'Deutsche Frage' als Problem der Weltpolitik," *Historische Zeitschrift*, no. 228 (1979).

103. Taylor, *Struggle for Mastery in Europe*, pp. 228ff; Langer, *European Alliances and Alignments*, chs. 3–5; B. Jelavich, *The Great Powers, the Ottoman Empire, and the Straits Question 1870–1887* (Bloomington, Ind., 1973).

104. Quoted in Seton-Watson, *Russian Empire*, p. 455. For the naval side, see Mitchell, *A History of Russian and Soviet Sea Power*, pp. 184–90. More generally, see B. H. Sumner, *Russia and the Balkans 1870–1880* (London, 1937).

105. See the essays by Beyrau (on Russia) and Rumpler (on Austria-Hungary) in Kolb (ed.), *Europa und die Reichsgründung*; Taylor, *Struggle for Mastery in Europe*, ch. 12; Langer, *European Alliances and Alignments*, chs. 6–7; W. Windelband, *Bismarck und die europäischen Grossmächte 1878–85* (Essen, 1940); B. Waller, *Bismarck at the Crossroads* (London, 1974).

106. Taylor, *Struggle for Mastery in Europe*, ch. 13; Langer, *European Alliances and Alignments*, chs. 7–9; *NCMH*, vol. 11, chs. 20–22.

107. Kennedy, *Rise and Fall of British Naval Mastery*, pp. 189–90.

CHAPTER FIVE
The Coming of a Bipolar World and the Crisis of the "Middle Powers": Part One, 1885–1918

1. For full details, see S. E. Crowe, *The Berlin West African Conference 1884–1885* (Westport, Conn., 1970 reprint). For the general background, see again Langer, *European Alliances and Alignments*, ch. 9; *NCMH*, vol. 11, chs. 20–22; and the various chapters in E. A. Benians et al. (eds.), *The Cambridge History of the British Empire*, vol. 3, *The Empire-Commonwealth 1870–1919* (Cambridge, 1959).

2. See generally D. M. Pletcher, "Economic Growth and Diplomatic Adjustment, 1861–1898," in W. H. Becker and S. F. Wells (eds.), *Economics and World Power: An Assessment of American Diplomacy Since 1789* (New York, 1984), pp. 119–71; M. Plesur, *America's Outward Thrust: Approaches to Foreign Affairs 1865–1890* (DeKalb, Ill., 1971), pp. 151ff; W. A. Williams, *The Roots of the Modern American Empire* (New York, 1969), p. 262.

3. Crowe, *Berlin West Africa Conference*, p. 220.

4. G. F. Hudson, *The Far East in World Affairs* (2nd ed., London, 1939), p. 74.

5. This general story can be followed in G. Barraclough, *An Introduction to Contemporary History* (Harmondsworth, Mddsx., 1967), chs. 3–4; A. de Porte, *Europe Between the Super Powers* (New Haven/London, 1979) chs. 1–5; *NCMH*, vol. 12, *The Shifting Balance of World Forces, 1898–1965*, passim; W. R. Keylor, *The Twentieth-Century World: An International History* (Oxford, 1984), pt. 1; J. Bartlett, *The Global Conflict, 1880–1970: The International Rivalry of the Great Powers* (London, 1984), chs. 1–9; F. H. Hinsley, *Power and the Pursuit of Peace* (Cambridge, 1967), pp. 300ff.

6. Barraclough, *Contemporary History*, ch. 3; F. Fischer, *War of Illusions: German Policies from 1911 to 1914* (London, 1975), ch. 3; Kennedy, *Rise and Fall of British Naval Mastery*, ch. 7.

7. J.A.S. Grenville, *Lord Salisbury and Foreign Policy: The Close of the Nineteenth Century, 1895–1902* (London, 1964), pp. 165–66; and more generally, W. L.

Langer, *The Diplomacy of Imperialism 1890–1902* (2nd ed., New York, 1965), ch. 3 and p. 505.

8. Fischer, *War of Illusions*, pp. 36ff.
9. Ibid., p. 35.
10. Cited in P. Kennedy, *Strategy and Diplomacy 1860–1965: Eight Essays* (London, 1983), pp. 157–58.
11. H. Gollwitzer, *Geschichte des weltpolitischen Denkens*, vol. 2, *Zeitalter des Imperialismus und Weltkriege* (Göttingen, 1982), p. 198.
12. P. Kennedy, *The Rise of the Anglo-German Antagonism, 1860–1914* (London/Boston, 1980), chs. 16–17.
13. Idem, *Strategy and Diplomacy*, p. 46; Keylor, *Twentieth-Century World*, pp. 27ff.
14. Amery comment, on H. J. Mackinder, "The Geographical Pivot of History," *Geographical Journal*, vol. 23, no. 6 (April 1904), p. 441.
15. Thucydides, *The Peleponnesian War* (Harmondsworth, Mddsx., 1954), p. 49. For a discussion of this view, see R. Gilpin, *War and Change in World Politics* (Cambridge, 1981).
16. Landes, *Unbound Prometheus*, p. 259.
17. Figures taken from the "Correlates of War" print-out data made available through the Inter-University Consortium for Political and Social Research at the University of Michigan.
18. C. E. Black et al., *The Modernization of Japan and Russia: A Comparative Study* (New York, 1975), pp. 6–7; and, for the now classic account, W. W. Rostow, *The Process of Economic Growth* (2nd edn., Oxford, 1960).
19. Ibid.
20. Figures from Bairoch, "International Industrialization Levels from 1750 to 1980," pp. 294, 302.
21. "Correlates of War" print-out data.
22. Ibid.
23. Bairoch, "International Industrialization Levels," pp. 292, 299.
24. Ibid., pp. 296, 304.
25. C. Barnett, *The Collapse of British Power* (London/New York, 1972), p. xi.
26. Wright, *Study of War*, pp. 670–71.
27. Ibid. The 1890 total for the United States is given as only 40,000 by Wright, which is clearly a mistake.
28. See pp. 188–89 above.
29. See Table 14 above. Italian history generally in this period is covered in D. Mack Smith, *Italy, A Modern History* (Ann Arbor, 1969), pp. 101ff; C. Seton Watson, *Italy from Liberalism to Fascism* (London, 1967), pp. 129–412. It is noticeable that there is no "Italy" section in the *New Cambridge Modern History*, vol. 11, *1870–98*, and only a few pages, 482–87, in vol. 12, *1898–1945*.
30. Kemp, *Industrialization in Nineteenth-Century Europe*, ch. 6.
31. See the references in A. Tamborra, "The Rise of Italian Industry and the Balkans," *Journal of European Economic History*, vol. 3, no. 1 (1974), pp. 87–120. Other useful studies are G. Mori, "The Genesis of Italian Industrialization," *Journal of European Economic History*, vol. 4, no. 1 (Spring 1975), pp. 79–94; idem, "The Process of Industrialization in Italy: Some Suggestions, Problems and Questions," *Journal of European Economic History*, vol. 8, no. 1 (Spring 1979), pp. 60–82; Trebilcock, *Industrialization of the Continental Powers 1780–1914*, ch. 5; Pollard, *Peaceful Conquest*, pp. 229–32; Seton-Watson, *Italy from Liberalism to Fascism*, pp. 284ff; S. B. Clough, *The Economic History of Modern Italy, 1830–1914* (New York, 1964); L. Cafagua, "The Industrial Revolution in

Italy 1830–1914," in C. Cipolla (ed.), *Fontana Economic History of Europe*, vol. 4, pt. 1, *The Emergence of Industrial Societies*, pp. 287–325.

32. A. S. Milward and S. B. Saul, *The Development of the Economies of Continental Europe 1850–1914* (Cambridge, Mass., 1977), pp. 253ff; J. S. Cohen, "Financing Industrialization in Italy, 1894–1914: The Partial Transformation of a Late-Comer," *Journal of Economic History*, vol. 27 (1967), pp. 363–82; V. Castronovo, "The Italian Takeoff: A Critical Re-examination of the Problem," *Journal of Italian History*, vol. 1 (1978), pp. 492–510.

33. R.J.B. Bosworth, *Italy, the Least of the Great Powers: Italian Foreign Policy Before the First World War* (Cambridge, 1979), p. 4.

34. See the interesting (and thoroughly depressing) collection of articles on "Italian Military Efficiency" in *Journal of Strategic Studies*, vol. 5, no. 2 (1982), pp. 248ff; J. Gooch, "Italy Before 1915: The Quandary of the Vulnerable," in E. R. May (ed.), *Knowing One's Enemies: Intelligence Assessment Before the Two World Wars* (Princeton, N.J., 1984), pp. 205ff; J. Whittam, *The Politics of the Italian Army 1861–1918* (London, 1977), passim; and idem, "War Aims and Strategy: The Italian Government and High Command 1914–1919," in B. Hunt and A. Preston (eds.), *War Aims and Strategic Policy in the Great War* (London, 1977), pp. 85–104.

35. P. Halpern, *The Mediterranean Naval Situation, 1908–1914* (Cambridge, Mass., 1971), ch. 7; A. J. Marder, *The Anatomy of British Sea Power* (Hamden, Conn., 1964 reprint), pp. 174–75.

36. Bosworth, *Italy, the Least of the Great Powers*, passim. See also idem, *Italy and the Approach of the First World War* (London, 1983); Lowe and Marzari, *Italian Foreign Policy, 1870–1940*, passim.

37. P. Kennedy, "The First World War and the International Power System," in S. E. Miller (ed.), *Military Strategy and the Origins of the First World War* (Princeton, N.J., 1985), p. 15.

38. W. R. Keylor, *The Twentieth-Century World*, pp. 14–15. For other general accounts, see *NCMH*, vol. 12, ch. 12; I. Nish, *Japan's Foreign Policy, 1869–1942* (London, 1978); R. Storry, *Japan and the Decline of the West in Asia 1894–1943* (London, 1979).

39. The political and economic modernization of Japan is briefly covered in R. Storry, *A History of Modern Japan* (Harmondsworth, Mddsx., 1982 edn.), ch. 5; and in much more detail in W. H. Beasley, *The Meiji Restoration* (Stanford, Calif., 1972); E. H. Norman, *Japan's Emergence as a Modern State* (New York, 1940); T. Smith, *Political Change and Industrial Development in Japan: Government Enterprise 1868–1880* (Stanford, Calif., 1955).

40. The economic aspects of Japanese modernization can be followed in G. S. Allen, *A Short Economic History of Japan* (London, 1981 edn.), chs. 2–5; L. Klein and K. Ohkawa (eds.), *Economic Growth: The Japanese Experience Since the Meiji Era* (Holmwood, Ill., 1968); Rostow, *World Economy*, pp. 416–25; K. Ohkawa and H. Rosovsky, *Japanese Economic Growth* (Stanford, Calif., 1973).

41. E. B. Potter (ed.), *Sea Power: A Naval History* (Annapolis, Md., 1981), pp. 166–168; Glover, *Warfare from Waterloo to Mons*, pp. 181–84.

42. Quoted in Storry, *Japan and the Decline of the West in Asia*, p. 30.

43. On which see now I. Nish, *The Origin of the Russo-Japanese War* (London, 1985), passim. The conflict itself is best described in J. N. Westwood, *Russia Against Japan, 1904–5: A New Look at the Russo-Japanese War* (London, 1986), and is also covered in Storry, *Japan and the Decline of the West in Asia*, chs. 4–5; S. Okamoto, *The Japanese Oligarchy and the Russo-Japanese War* (New York, 1970); J. A. White, *The Diplomacy of the Russo-Japanese War* (Princeton, N.J., 1964). The war at sea is briefly covered in Potter (ed.), *Sea Power*, pp.

168ff, and P. Padfield, *The Battleship Era* (London, 1972), pp. 167ff; on land, P. Walden, *The Short Victorious War: A History of the Russo-Japanese War, 1904–5* (New York, 1974).

44. See A. J. Sherman, "German-Jewish Bankers in World Politics: The Financing of the Russo-Japanese War," *Leo Baeck Institute Yearbook*, vol. 28 (1983), pp. 59–73.

45. Cited in Kennedy, *Rise of the Anglo-German Antagonism*, p. 464.

46. For general accounts of Germany's economic growth, see Fisher, *War of Illusions*, pt. 1; Calleo, *The German Problem Reconsidered*, ch. 4; N. Stone, *Europe Transformed 1878–1916* (London, 1983), pp. 159ff; W. G. Hoffmann, *Das Wachstum der Deutschen Wirtschaft seit der Mitte des 19. Jahrhunderts*, (Berlin, 1965); W. O. Henderson, *The Rise of German Industrial Power, 1834–1914*, (Berkeley/Los Angeles, 1972), pt. 3; M. Kitchen, *The Political Economy of Germany 1815–1914* (London, 1978).

47. I took this figure from p. 2 of John Gooch's paper "Italy During the First World War," for the forthcoming first volume of *Military Effectiveness*, eds. A. Millett and W. Murray.

48. See the figures in Calleo, *German Problem Reconsidered*, pp. 66, 68.

49. Quoted in J. Steinberg, "The Copenhagen Complex," *Journal of Contemporary History*, vol. 1, pt. 3 (1966), p. 26.

50. Langer, *Diplomacy of Imperialism*, p. 96; and see again Gollwitzer, *Geschichte des weltpolitischen Denkens*, vol. 2, pp. 83–252; idem, *Europe in the Age of Imperialism* (London, 1969), passim; W. Baumgart, *Imperialism: The Idea and Reality of British and French Colonial Expansion 1880–1914* (Oxford, 1982), pt. 3.

51. For these quotations, see respectively, Kennedy, *Rise of the Anglo-German Antagonism*, p. 311; J. C. Röhl, "A Document of 1892 on Germany, Prussia, and Poland," *Historical Journal*, vol. 7 (1964), pp. 144ff; Fisher, *War of Illusions*, ch. 3.

52. I take this term from H.-U. Wehler, *Bismarck und der Imperialismus* (Cologne, 1969), pt. 3, pp. 112ff.

53. See the assessments in A. J. Marder, *From the Dreadnought to Scapa Flow: The Royal Navy in the Fisher Period*, vol. 1, *The Road to War 1904–1914* (London, 1961), ch. 13; Kennedy, *Rise and Fall of British Naval Mastery*, chs. 8–9.

54. Kennedy, *Strategy and Diplomacy*, p. 160.

55. B. F. Schulte, *Die deutsche Armee* (Düsseldorf, 1977); V. R. Berghahn, *Germany and the Approach of War in 1914* (London/New York, 1974), chs. 1 and 6. For good examples of the many fatuous underestimations of German military power (especially as compared with Russia and France), see P. Towle, "The European Balance of Power in 1914," *Army Quarterly and Defense Journal*, vol. 104 (1974), pp. 333–62.

56. All of these figures from Wright, *Study of War*, pp. 670–71.

57. J. K. Tanenbaum, "French Estimates of Germany's Operational War Plans," in May (ed.), *Knowing One's Enemies*, p. 162.

58. Calleo, *German Problem Reconsidered*, introduction.

59. Kennedy, *Rise of the Anglo-German Antagonism*, p. 311.

60. See again Gilpin, *War and Change in World Politics*, passim.

61. For compelling evidence of this, see the articles in J.G.C. Röhl and N. Sombart (eds.), *Kaiser Wilhelm II: New Interpretations* (Cambridge, 1982).

62. Quoted in G. A. Craig, *Germany 1866–1965* (Oxford, 1978), p. 336. There is good evidence of this confusion of purpose in I. N. Lambi, *The Navy and German Power Politics 1862–1914* (London/Boston, 1984).

63. Fisher, *War of Illusions,* passim; Berghahn, *Germany and the Approach of War,* passim.

64. This is explored further in P. Kennedy (ed.), *The War Plans of the Great Powers 1880–1914* (London/Boston 1979), introduction.

65. Calleo, *German Problem Reconsidered,* p. 5.

66. Quoted in Kennedy, *Strategy and Diplomacy,* p. 157.

67. See the charts for France, Great Britain, and Austria-Hungary's "Relative Power" in C. F. Doran and W. Parsons, "War and the Cycle of Relative Power," *American Political Science Review,* vol. 74 (1980), p. 956.

68. Taylor, *Struggle for Mastery in Europe,* p. xxviii.

69. There is a brief coverage in Kann, *History of the Habsburg Empire,* pp. 461ff; a good survey in Milward and Saul, *Development of the Economies of Continental Europe 1850–1914,* pp. 271ff; and a more sophisticated analysis, comparing the empire with Italy and Spain, in Trebilcock, *Industrialization of the Continental Powers,* ch. 5.

70. Bairoch, "Europe's Gross National Product 1800–1975," p. 287.

71. L. L. Farrar, *Arrogance and Anxiety: The Ambivalence of German Powers 1849–1914* (Iowa City, Iowa, 1981), ch. 3, fns. 9 and 18. Farrar calculates "power" by multiplying population and manufacturing production. The early section of this present chapter should indicate that power is a much more complex phenomenon.

72. For comparative growth rates, see Good, *The Economic Rise of the Habsburg Empire 1750–1914,* p. 239; for industrial potential, see Table 17 above.

73. Figures from Good, *Economic Rise of the Habsburg Empire,* p. 150.

74. For what follows, see the brilliant description in Stone, *Europe Transformed,* pp. 303ff; Kann, *History of the Habsburg Empire,* ch. 8; C. A. MacArtney, *The Habsburg Empire 1790–1918* (London, 1969), chs. 14–17; A. J. May, *The Habsburg Monarchy 1862–1916* (Cambridge, Mass., 1960), pp. 343ff.

75. Rothenberg, *Army of Francis Joseph,* ch. 9; Langer, *Diplomacy of Imperialism,* pp. 596–98; and espec. C. Andrew, *Théophile Delcassé and the Making of the Entente Cordiale* (London, 1968), pp. 127ff.

76. Quoted in Stone, *Europe Transformed,* pp. 316–17; see also Rothenberg, *Army of Francis Joseph,* p. 106.

77. Wright, *Study of War,* pp. 670–71, columns 10–12; also useful is Rothenberg, *Army of Francis Joseph,* pp. 125–26, 148, 160, 172.

78. For the state of the Austro-Hungarian navy, see Halpern, *Mediterannean Naval Situation,* ch. 6. The state of the army prior to 1914 is covered in Rothenberg's excellent *Army of Francis Joseph,* chs. 9–12; N. Stone, "Moltke and Conrad: Relations between the Austro-Hungarian and German General Staffs 1909–1914," in Kennedy (ed.), *War Plans of the Great Powers 1880–1914,* pp. 222ff; idem, *The Eastern Front 1914–1917* (London, 1975), ch. 4; idem, "Austria-Hungary," in May (ed.), *Knowing One's Enemies,* pp. 37ff.

79. Rothenberg, *Army of Francis Joseph,* p. 159, also pp. 152, 163.

80. Ibid., p. 159. And see also Stone, "Moltke and Conrad," in Kennedy (ed.), *War Plans of the Great Powers.*

81. Stone, "Austria-Hungary," p. 52.

82. See here P. W. Schroeder's powerful and elegant plea that the Great Powers (Britain especially) should have preserved the Austro-Hungarian Empire in order to save the status quo: "World War I as a Galloping Gertie," *Journal of Modern History,* vol. 44, no.3 (1972), pp. 319–45. It is not unlike pleading that after 1945 the United States and USSR should have tried to preserve the British Empire in order to avoid subsequent instability in the Third World.

83. For French foreign policy, see the older work E. M. Carroll, *French Public*

Opinion and Foreign Affairs 1880–1914 (London, 1931); G. F. Kennan, *The Decline of Bismarck's European Order: Franco-Russian Relations 1875–1890* (Princeton, N.J., 1979); Andrew, *Théophile Delcassé and the Making of the Entente Cordiale;* J.F.V. Keiger, *France and the Origins of the First World War* (London, 1983).

84. There is no comprehensive history of French defense policy in this period; but there are useful details in D. Porch, *The March to the Marne: The French Army 1871–1914* (Cambridge, 1981); P.-M. de la Gorce, *The French Army: A Military Political History* (New York, 1963), chs. 1–5; R. D. Challenor, *The French Theory of the Nation in Arms 1866–1939* (New York, 1955); as well as the references in notes 88–89 below.

85. Marder, *Anatomy of British Sea Power,* pp. 71–3, 86–7, 107–9, 124ff; and the references in Kennedy, *Rise of the Anglo-German Antagonism,* ch. 11, fn. 27.

86. French colonialism and the French colonial empire are covered in A. S. Kanya-Forstner, *The Conquest of the Western Sudan: A Study in French Military Imperialism* (Cambridge, 1969); R. Betts, *Tricouleur: The French Empire* (London, 1978): H. Brunschwig, *French Colonialism, 1871–1916: Myths and Realities* (London, 1966); R. Girardet, *L'idée coloniale en France de 1871 à 1962* (Paris, 1972); J. Ganiage, *L'expansion coloniale de la France sous la Troisième République 1871–1914* (Paris, 1968).

87. For a good summary of this argument, see A. S. Kanya-Forstner, "French Expansion in Africa: The Mythical Theory," in R. Owen and R. Sutcliffe (eds.), *Studies in the Theory of Imperialism* (London, 1972), pp. 285ff.

88. French naval policy is covered briefly in Jenkins, *History of the French Navy,* pp. 303ff; Williamson, *Politics of Grand Strategy,* pp. 227ff; Halpern, *Mediterranean Naval Situation,* pp. 47ff; and T. Ropp, *The Development of a Modern Navy: French Naval Policy 1871–1904* (Annapolis, Md., 1987), passim.

89. This may also explain why so many historians have tended to focus upon civil-military relations in France rather than military policy *per se.* For examples, in addition to the works listed in note 84 above, see R. Girardet, *La société militaire dans la France contemporaine* (Paris, 1953); G. Krumeich, *Armaments and Politics in France on the Eve of the First World War* (Leamington Spa, 1986).

90. For what follows, see Milward and Saul, *Development of the Economies of Continental Europe 1850–1914,* ch. 2; Kemp, *Industrialization in Nineteenth-Century Europe,* ch. 3; idem, *Economic Forces in French History,* ch. 9; Trebilcock, *Industrialization of the Continental Powers,* ch. 3 (an excellent and sophisticated survey); Rowley, *Evolution économique de la France du Milieu du XIXe siècle à 1914,* passim; Caron, *Economic History of Modern France,* pt. 1; J. H. Clapham, *The Economic Development of France and Germany, 1815–1914* (Cambridge, 1948); R. Price, *The Economic Modernization of France* (London, 1975).

91. Kemp, *Industrialization in Nineteenth-Century Europe,* pp. 71–72.

92. The literature upon French banking and overseas investment is enormous; for a brief summary, see Kindleberger, *Financial History of Western Europe,* pp. 225ff; Trebilcock, *Industrialization of the Continental Powers,* pp. 173ff; R. Cameron, *France and the Economic Development of Europe* (Princeton, 1961), passim. The Russian loans and Franco-Russian diplomacy are covered in R. Girault, *Emprunts russes et investisements français en Russie, 1887–1914* (Paris, 1973); and Krumeich, *Armaments and Politics in France,* ch. 6.

93. Trebilcock, *Industrialization of the Continental Powers,* p. 182.

94. Ibid., p. 158.

95. Bairoch, "Europe's Gross National Product," p. 281; idem, "International In-

dustrialization Levels," p. 297; Wright, *Study of War*, pp. 670–71. See also the careful comparisons in V. Hentschel, "Produktion, Wachstum and Productivität in England, Frankreich and Deutschland von der Mitte des 19. Jahrhunderts bis zum Ersten Weltkrieg," *Vierteljahresschrift fur Sozial- und Wirtschaftsgeschichte*, vol. 68 (1981), pp. 457–510. All this quite contradicts Stone, *Europe Transformed*, p. 282.

96. See the overwhelming evidence in Mitchell, *Victors and Vanquished*, chs. 1–5, espec. pp. 109–11.

97. Porch, *March to the Marne*, p. 227.

98. For repeated examples of these sort of claims, see E. Weber, *The Nationalist Revival in France, 1905–1916* (Berkeley, Calif., 1959); H. Contamine, *La Revanche, 1871–1914* (Paris, 1957); Krumeich, *Armament and Politics in France*, passim.

99. Ibid. See also Williamson, *Politics of Grand Strategy*, chs. 5 and 8; B. H. Liddell Hart, "French Military Ideas Before the First World War," in M. Gilbert (ed.), *A Century of Conflict, 1850–1950* (London, 1966), pp. 133–48.

100. For what follows, see Andrew, *Théophile Delcassé and the Making of the Entente Cordiale*, passim; Keiger, *France and the Origins of the First World War*, chs. 1 and 4.

101. J. J. Becker, *1914: Comment les Français sont entrés dans la guerre* (Paris, 1977); J. Joll, *The Origins of the First World War* (London/New York, 1984), ch. 8.

102. J. Remak, "1914—The Third Balkan War: Origins Reconsidered," reprinted in Koch (ed.), *Origins of the First World War*, pp. 89–90.

103. The phrase used first in R. Robinson and J. Gallagher, with A. Denny, *Africa and the Victorian: The Official Mind of Imperialism* (2nd edn., London, 1981). For a discussion of this term, and their other ideas, see P. Kennedy, "Continuity and Discontinuity in British Imperialism 1815–1914," in C. C. Eldridge (ed.), *British Imperialism in the Nineteenth Century* (London, 1984), pp. 20–38.

104. See again Bourne, *Britain and the Balance of Power in North America*, passim. For the settlement of these differences, and other aspects of the relationship, see B. Perkins, *The Great Rapprochement* (New York, 1969).

105. Gillard, *Struggle for Asia*, passim; F. Kazemzadeh, *Russian and Britain in Persia, 1864–1914* (New Haven, Conn., 1968); E. Hölzle, *Die Selbstentmachtung Europas*, pp. 85ff.

106. L. K. Young, *British Policy in China 1895–1902* (Oxford, 1970); P. Lowe, *Britain in the Far East: A Survey from 1819 to the Present* (London, 1981) chs. 3–4.

107. Hobsbawm, *Industry and Empire*, p. 150. See also P. J. Cain, *Economic Foundations of British Overseas Expansion 1815–1914* (London, 1980), ch. 9; W. G. Hynes, *The Economics of Empire: Britain, Africa and the New Imperialism, 1870–95* (London, 1979), passim; Cain and Hopkins, "Political Economy of British Expansion Overseas," pp. 485ff.

108. For details, see the early chapters of Grenville, *Lord Salisbury and Foreign Policy*.

109. Marder, *Anatomy of British Sea Power*, passim; Kennedy, *Rise and Fall of British Naval Mastery*, chs. 7–8; and J. Gooch, *The Plans of War: The General Staff and British Military Strategy c. 1900–1916* (London, 1974), cover naval and military planning.

110. In consequence, the literature is enormous and grows each year. Hobsbawm, *Industry and Empire*, pp. 136–53, 172–85; Landes, *Unbound Prometheus*, pp. 326–58; and Mathias, *First Industrial Nation*, pp. 243–52, 306–34, 365–426, are still very instructive. Crouzet, *Victorian Economy*, pp. 371ff, is a succinct new survey.

111. Cited in Kennedy, *Rise of the Anglo-German Antagonism,* p. 315.
112. Quoted in N. Mansergh, *The Commonwealth Experience* (London, 1969), p. 134.
113. Kennedy, *Rise of the Anglo-German Antagonism,* p. 307, and passim, for similar quotations.
114. Quotation in G. R. Searle, *The Quest for National Efficiency 1899–1914* (Oxford, 1971), p. 5, with a wealth of further detail on this mood.
115. Porter, *Lion's Share,* pp. 353–54.
116. Taylor, *Struggle for Mastery in Europe,* p. xxix; Peacock and Wiseman, *Growth of Public Expenditure in the United Kingdom,* p. 166; Kennedy, *Rise of the Anglo-German Antagonism,* ch. 17.
117. Figures from W. Woodruff, "The Emergence of an Industrial Economy 1700–1914," in Cipolla (ed.), *Fontana Economic History of Europe,* vol. 4, pt. 2, *The Emergence of Industrial Societies,* p. 707.
118. On which theme see Porter's excellent *Britian, Europe and the World,* passim.
119. Kennedy, *Rise and Fall of British Naval Mastery,* pp. 195ff.
120. Mansergh, *Commonwealth Experience,* ch. 5; D. C. Gordon, *The Dominion Partnership in Imperial Defense 1870–1914* (Baltimore, Md., 1965).
121. On which see J. Ehrman, *Cabinet Government and War 1890–1940* (Cambridge, 1958); F. A. Johnson, *Defense by Committee* (London, 1960).
122. See note 102 above.
123. Superbly analyzed in M. Howard, *The Continental Commitment* (London, 1972), passim.
124. French, *British Economic and Strategic Planning,* passim; Kennedy, "Strategy versus Finance in Twentieth-Century Britain," in *Strategy and Diplomacy,* pp. 89–106; and the stimulating treatment in Porter, *Britain, Europe and the World,* ch. 3.
125. Cited in Fischer, *War of Illusions,* p. 402.
126. The words are those of Buchanan, British ambassador to Russia, as quoted in K. Wilson, "British Power in the European Balance, 1906–1914," in D. Dilks (ed.), *Retreat from Power: Studies in Britain's Foreign Policy in the Twentieth Century,* 2 vols. (London, 1981), vol. 1, p. 39.
127. Which are, respectively, the rough subtitle and the main title of R. Ropponen, *Die Kraft Russlands: Wie beurteilte die politische und militarische Führung der europäischen Grossmächte in der Zeit von 1905 bis 1914 die Kraft Russlands?* (Helsinki, 1968), an extraordinarily rich compilation.
128. The following section on the Russian economy prior to 1914 is based upon G. Grossman, "The Industrialization of Russia and the Soviet Union," in Cipolla (ed.), *Fontana Economic History of Europe,* vol. 4, pt. 2, pp. 486ff; R. Munting, *The Economic Development of the USSR* (London, 1982), ch. 1; O. Crisp, *Studies in the Russian Economy Before 1914* (London, 1976), espec. ch. 1, "The Pattern of Industrialization in Russia, 1700–1914"; Seton-Watson, *Russian Empire,* pp. 506ff, 647ff; Blackwell, *Industrialization of Russia,* ch. 2; M. E. Falkus, *Industrialization of Russia 1700–1914,* chs. 7–9; Milward and Saul, *Development of the Economies of Continental Europe,* pp. 365–423; the comparisons in Black (ed.), *Modernization of Japan and Russia,* passim; and the many statistics in the older work of M. S. Miller, *The Economic Development of Russia, 1905–1914* (London, 1926).
129. Crisp, "Pattern of Industrialization," pp. 40–41.
130. Munting, *Economic Development,* p. 34; Girault, *Emprunts russes et Investisements français en Russie,* passim; and J. P. Machay, *Pioneer for Profit: Foreign Entrepreneurs and Russian Industrialization* (Chicago/London, 1970), passim. For indigenous entrepreneurs, see R. Portal, "Muscovite Industrialists: The

Cotton Sector 1861–1914," in W. L. Blackwell (ed.), *Russian Economic Development from Peter the Great to Stalin* (New York, 1974), pp. 161–96.

131. Munting, *Economic Development*, p. 31. More generally, A. Gershrenkon, *Economic Backwardness in Historical Perspective* (Cambridge, Mass., 1962); M. Falkus, "Aspects of Foreign Investment in Tsarist Russia," *Journal of European Economic History*, vol. 8, no. 1 (Spring 1979), pp. 14–16. For the latest, very sophisticated (but therefore very complex) diagnosis, see P. Gatrell, *The Tsarist Economy, 1850–1917* (London, 1986), passim.

132. See Tables 14–18 above; and A. Nove's excellent comparative statistics in *An Economic History of the USSR* (Harmondsworth, Mddsx., 1969), pp. 14–15.

133. Munting, *Economic Development*, pp. 27; Trebilcock, *Industrialization of the Continental Power*, pp. 216ff, 247ff.

134. Grossman, "Industrialization of Russia and the Soviet Union," p. 489.

135. Ibid., p. 486.

136. Lieven, *Russia and the Origins of the First World War*, p. 4. Chs. 1 and 5 of Lieven's book are compelling in this respect, as is T. H. von Laue, *Sergei Witte and the Industrialization of Russia* (New York, 1963).

137. Lieven, *Russia and the Origins of the First World War*, p. 13; H. Rogge, *Russia in the Age of Modernization and Revolution 1881–1917* (London, 1983), pp. 77ff; Falkus, "Aspects of Foreign Investment," p. 10.

138. Stone, *Europe Transformed*, pp. 257ff, is especially good here. See also Seton-Watson, *Russian Empire*, pp. 541ff; Milward and Saul, *Development of the Economies of Continental Europe*, pp. 397ff; J.H.L. Keep, "Russia," in *NCMH*, vol. 9, p. 369.

139. Stone, *Europe Transformed*, pp. 212–13. See also Blackwell, *Industrialization of Russia*, pp. 32ff.

140. Stone, *Europe Transformed*, p. 244.

141. Seton-Watson, *Russian Empire*, pp. 485ff, 607ff, 643ff; Rogge, *Russia in the Age of Modernization and Revolution*, ch. 9. For the army's dislike of internal-police roles, see J. Bushnell, *Mutiny and Repression: Russian Soldiers in the Revolution of 1905–1906* (Bloomington, Ind., 1985), pp. 32ff.

142. Lieven, *Russia and the Origins of the First World War*, ch. 5; Joll, *Origins of the First World War*, pp. 102ff.

143. See Tables 14–18 above.

144. K. Neilson, "Watching the 'Steamroller': British Observers and the Russian Army before 1914," *Journal of Strategic Studies*, vol. 8, no. 2 (June 1985), p. 213.

145. And not surprising, since the War Office's "Military Reports" on foreign countries covered "geography, topography, ethnography, defences, trade, resources, communications, political condition, etc."—see T. G. Ferguson, *British Military Intelligence, 1870–1914* (Frederick, Md., 1984), p. 223.

146. O. Crisp, quoted in Lieven, *Russia and the Origins of the First World War*, p. 9; and see the details in J. Bushnell, "Peasants in Uniform: The Tsarist Army as a Peasant Society," *Journal of Social History*, vol. 13 (1980), pp. 565–76. See also A. K. Wildman, *The End of the Russian Imperial Army* (Princeton, 1980), chs. 1–2.

147. The quotation is from Fuller, "The Russian Empire," in May (ed.), *Knowing One's Enemies*, p. 114, and passim. Also important here is J. Bushnell, "The Tsarist Officer Corps, 1881–1914: Customs, Duties, Inefficiencies," *American Historical Review*, vol. 86 (1981), pp. 753–80; P. Kenez, "Russian Officer Corps Before the Revolution: The Military Mind," *Russian Review*, vol. 31 (1972), pp. 226–36. Bushnell's study *Mutiny and Repression* contains further eye-opening details, as does W. C. Fuller, *Civil-Military Conflict in Imperial Russia 1881–1914* (Princeton, N.J., 1985).

148. Fuller, "Russian Empire," passim; A. K. Wildman, *End of the Russian Imperial Army*, chs. 1–2; W. B. Lincoln, *Passage Through Armageddon: The Russians in the War and Revolution 1914–1918* (New York, 1986), pp. 52ff.

149. Lieven, *Russia and the Origins of the First World War*, pp. 149–50; Stone, *Eastern Front*, p. 134 (from where the quotation comes).

150. The confusions of prewar Russian planning are covered in Stone, *Eastern Front*, pp. 30ff; Lieven, *Russia and the Origins of the First World War*, ch. 5; L.C.F. Turner, "The Russian Mobilization in 1914," rev. version, in Kennedy, *War Plans of the Great Powers*, pp. 252–62; Fuller, "Russian Empire," pp. 111ff.

151. Mitchell, *History of Russian and Soviet Sea Power*, p. 279.

152. Doran and Parsons, "War and the Cycle of Relative Power," p. 956.

153. D. M. Pletcher, "1861–1898: Economic Growth and Diplomatic Adjustments," in W. H. Becker and S. F. Wells (eds.), *Economics and World Power: An Assessment of American Diplomacy Since 1789* (New York, 1984), p. 120. For other surveys of this growth, see M. L. Eysenbach, *American Manufactured Exports 1897–1914: A Study of Growth and Comparative Advantage* (New York, 1976); H. G. Vatter, *The Drive to Industrial Maturity: The U. S. Economy, 1860–1914* (Westport, Conn., 1975 edn.).

154. Stone, *Europe Transformed*, pp. 211ff; cf. R. M. Robertson, *History of American Economy* (New York, 1975 edn.), ch. 13.

155. Barraclough, *Introduction to Contemporary History*, p. 51.

156. Taken from Q. Wright, *Study of War*, pp. 670–71, with my calculations on per capita income.

157. See Tables 15–16 above—but cf. Taylor, *Struggle for Mastery in Europe*, p. xxx.

158. Farrar, *Arrogance and Anxiety*, p. 39, fn. 168.

159. Ibid.; D. H. Aldcroft, *From Versailles to Wall Street: The International Economy in the 1920s* (Berkeley/Los Angeles, 1977), p. 98, Table 4.

160. Keylor, *Twentieth-Century World*, p. 39; cf. Crouzet, *Victorian Economy*, p. 342, fn. 153.

161. Woodruff, *America's Impact on the World*, p. 161.

162. W. LaFeber, *The New Empire: An Interpretation of American Expansion 1860–1898* (Ithaca, N.Y., 1963); W. A. Williams, *The Roots of the Modern American Empire* (New York, 1969). For more general surveys of American foreign policy, see T. A. Bailey, *A Diplomatic History of the American People* (New York, 1974, edn.); R. D. Schulzinger, *American Diplomacy in the Twentieth Century* (New York/Oxford, 1984), chs. 2–3.

163. Pletcher, "1861–1898," pp. 124ff; T. McCormick, *China Market: America's Quest for Informal Empire* (Chicago, 1967); D. G. Munro, *Intervention and Dollar Diplomacy in the Caribbean 1900–1921* (Princeton, N.J., 1964); E. R. May, *Imperial Democracy: The Emergence of America as a Great Power* (New York, 1961), pp. 5–6; Perkins, *Great Rapprochment*, pp. 122ff.

164. For a critical analysis, see M. de Cecco, *Money and Empire: The International Gold Standard 1890–1914* (Oxford, 1974), pp. 110–126; for the 1907 crisis, see J. H. Clapham, *The Economic History of Modern Britain*, 3 vols. (Cambridge, 1938), vol. 3, pp. 55ff.

165. The literature upon the motives and actions of American imperialism between 1895 and 1914 is colossal. Apart from the references in notes 162 and 163 above, see also R. Dallek, *The American Style of Foreign Policy* (New York, 1983), chs. 1–3; E. R. May, *American Imperialism: A Speculative Essay* (New York, 1968); G. F. Linderman, *The Mirror of War: American Society and the Spanish-American War* (Ann Arbor, Mich., 1974); Howard K. Beale, *Theodore Roosevelt and the Rise of America to World Power* (New York, 1962 edn.).

166. Dallek, *American Style of Foreign Policy*, p. 23

167. Beale, *Theodore Roosevelt and the Rise of America to World Power*, passim; Dallek, *American Style of Foreign Policy*, ch. 2; Schulzinger, *American Diplomacy in the Twentieth Century*, pp. 24–38.

168. See especially the criticisms in G. F. Kennan, *American Diplomacy* (Chicago, 1984 edn.), chs. 1–3; and Dallek, *American Style of Foreign Policy*, passim.

169. U.S. naval growth and naval policy in this period are now very well covered. Apart from Potter (ed.), *Sea Power*, chs. 15 and 17–18, see K. J. Hagan (ed.), *In Peace and War: Interpretations of American Naval History, 1775–1978* (Westport, Conn., 1978), chs. 9–10; W. R. Braisted, *The United States Navy in the Pacific*, 2 vols. (Austin, Texas, 1958 and 1971); and the older works H. and M. Sprout, *The Rise of American Naval Power, 1776–1918* (Princeton, N.J., 1946 edn.), and W. Mills, *Arms and Men* (New York, 1956), ch. 2.

170. Apart from Braisted's important works, see R. D. Challenor, *Admirals, Generals and American Foreign Policy 1898–1914* (Princeton, N.J., 1973); J.A.S. Grenville and G. B. Young, *Politics, Strategy and American Diplomacy: Studies in Foreign Policy, 1873–1917* (New Haven, Conn., 1966).

171. Challenor, *Admirals, Generals, and American Foreign Policy*, passim; H. H. Herwig, *Politics of Frustration: The United States in German Naval Planning, 1889–1941* (New York, 1976). For the improvement in Anglo-American relations, see C. S. Campbell, *From Revolution to Rapprochement: The United States and Great Britain, 1783–1900* (New York, 1974), chs. 13–14.

172. Millet and Maslowski, *For the Common Defense*, chs. 9–10. For further details, see D. F. Trask, *The War with Spain in 1898* (New York, 1981); and G. A. Cosmas, *An Army for Empire: The United States Army in the Spanish-American War* (Columbia, Missouri, 1971). Also useful on the change of attitudes is J. L. Abrahamson, *America Arms for a New Century* (New York, 1981); R. Weigley, *History of the United States Army*, chs. 13–14.

173. See again Tables 14–20 above.

174. F. Gilbert, *The End of the European Era, 1890 to the Present* (3rd edn., New York, 1984), p. 110. For detailed analyses of these decades, see Taylor, *Struggle for Mastery in Europe*, pp. 325ff; Bridge and Bullen, *Great Powers and the European States System*, chs. 6–8; Albrecht-Carrié, *Diplomatic History of Europe Since the Congress of Vienna*, pp. 207ff; Bartlett, *Global Conflict*, chs. 2–3.

175. B. Waller, *Bismarck at the Crossroads: The Reorientation of German Foreign Policy After the Congress of Berlin 1878–1880* (London, 1974), p. 195. See also Taylor, *Struggle for Mastery*, pp. 258ff; and Kennan, *Decline of Bismarck's European Order*, pp. 73ff.

176. Kennan, *Decline of Bismarck's European Order*, passim; and idem, *The Fateful Alliance: France, Russia, and the Coming of the First World War* (New York, 1984), passim. The German side is well covered in N. Rich, *Friedrich von Holstein*, 2 vols. (Cambridge, 1965), vol. 1, passim.

177. The argument that the European scene was "stabilized" in the 1890s, permitting the turn toward colonial issues, is best covered in W. L. Langer, *The Diplomacy of Imperialism 1890–1902* (New York, 1951 edn.), passim.

178. Langer's phrase: see ibid., ch. 13; and, more generally, Padfield, *Battleship Era*, ch. 14.

179. On this transformation, see again Perkins, *Great Rapprochement*, passim; Campbell, *From Revolution to Rapprochement*, ch. 14.

180. The standard work here is I. H. Nish, *The Anglo-Japanese Alliance* (London, 1966); but see also C. J. Lowe, *The Reluctant Imperialists: British Foreign Policy 1878–1902*, 2 vols. (London, 1967), vol. 1, ch. 10.

181. Taylor, *Struggle for Mastery in Europe*, ch. 18; Andrew, *Delcassé and the Mak-*

ing of the Entente Cordiale, passim; Albrecht-Carrié, *Diplomatic History*, pp. 232ff. See also the comments in M. Behnen, *Rüstung-Bündnis-Sicherheit* (Tübingen, 1985).

182. This is best covered in Andrew, *Delcassé*, passim; and G. L. Monger, *The End of Isolation; British Foreign Policy 1900–1907* (London, 1963).

183. O. J. Hale, *Germany and the Diplomatic Revolution 1904–1906* (Philadelphia, Pa., 1931); Kennedy, *Rise of the Anglo-German Antagonism*, ch. 14.

184. Kennedy, *Rise of the Anglo-German Antagonism*, pp. 268ff; further details in B. Vogel, *Deutsche Russlandpolitik, 1900–1906* (Düsseldorf, 1973).

185. The complicated events are covered in the works by Taylor, Monger, Andrew, Rich, and Kennedy, cited above. See also H. Raulff, *Zwischen Machtpolitik und Imperialismus: Die deutsche Frankreichpolitik 1904–5* (Düsseldorf, 1976); and Lambi's excellent *Navy and German Power Politics 1862–1914*, ch. 13.

186. Taylor, *Struggle for Mastery*, ch. 19; Z. Steiner, *Britain and the Origins of the First World War* (London, 1977), ch. 2 et seq. For the Russian response to the 1909 humiliation, see Lieven, *Russia and the Origin of the First World War*, pp. 36ff.

187. Steiner, *Britain and the Origins of the First World War*, pp. 200ff; Williamson, *Politics of Grand Strategy*, passim, espec. ch. 7.

188. The most detailed study of these events is L. Albertini, *The Origin of the War of 1914*, 3 vols. (London, 1952–57); but there are good succinct accounts in L.C.F. Turner, *Origins of the First World War* (London, 1970); J. Joll, *Origins of the First World War*, chs. 2–3; and Langhorne, *Collapse of the Concert of Europe*, chs. 6–7.

189. The literature upon pre-1914 war plans is immense; for surveys, see P.M. Kennedy (ed.), *The War Plans of the Great Powers 1880–1914* (London/Boston, 1979); S. E. Miller (ed.), *Military Strategy and the Origins of the First World War* (Princeton, N.J., 1985); J. Snyder, *The Ideology of the Offensive* (Ithaca, N.Y., 1984).

190. Strachan, *European Armies and the Conduct of War*, ch. 9; B. E. Schmitt and H. C. Vedeler, *The World in the Crucible 1914–1919* (New York, 1984), pp. 62ff.

191. Kennedy, *Rise and Fall of British Naval Mastery*, ch. 9.

192. For this argument, see L. L. Farrar, *The Short-War Illusion* (Santa Barbara, Calif., 1973), passim.

193. On which see, briefly, Schulzinger, *American Diplomacy in the Twentieth Century*, pp. 62ff; and, in more detail, D. M. Smith, *The Great Departure: The United States and World War I, 1914–1920* (New York, 1965); P. Devlin, *Too Proud to Fight: Woodrow Wilson's Neutrality* (New York, 1975); E. R. May, *The World War and American Isolation* (Chicago, 1966 edn.); A. S. Link, *Wilson*, 5 vols. to date (Princeton, N.J., 1947–65), vols. 3–5.

194. Bosworth, *Italy, the Least of the Great Powers*, is best here.

195. On which distractions, see P. Guinn, *British Strategy and Politics, 1914–1918* (Oxford, 1965); Beloff, *Imperial Sunset*, vol. 1, ch. 5; and D. French, *British Strategy and War Aims 1914–1916* (London/Boston, 1986), passim.

196. Rothenberg, *Army of Francis Joseph*, chs. 12–14, is an excellent analysis of Austro-Hungarian military policy—including both strengths and weaknesses—during the war.

197. For this argument, see Steiner, *Britain and the Origins of the First World War*, ch. 9; Kennedy, *Rise of the Anglo-German Antagonism*, pp. 458ff.

198. For a more extended argument on these lines, see Kennedy, *British Naval Mastery*, ch. 9.

199. Ibid.

200. Strachen, *European Armies and the Conduct of War*, ch. 9; and see also the

excellent analysis of the problem in S. Bidwell and D. Graham, *Fire-Power: British Army Weapons and Theories of War, 1904–1945* (London, 1982), chs. 4–8. For a succinct survey, see B. Bond, "The First World War," in *NCMH.*, vol. 12, ch. 7.

201. For excellent examples, see Stone, *Eastern Front*, p. 265 and passim.

202. Van Creveld, *Supplying War*, ch. 4, is convincing here. See also the critique in G. Ritter, *The Schlieffen Plan* (New York, 1958), and in L.C.F. Turner, "The Significance of the Schlieffen Plan," in Kennedy (ed.), *War Plans of the Great Powers*, pp. 199–221.

203. For further details, see Stone, *Eastern Front*, chs. 3–8; Schmitt and Vedeler, *World in the Crucible*, chs. 4–5; B. H. Liddell Hart, *History of the First World War* (London, 1970 edn.), chs. 4–5; Lincoln, *Passage Through Armageddon*, chs. 2–4.

204. Schmitt and Vedeler, *World in the Crucible*, ch. 6; J. L. Stokesbury, *A Short History of World War I* (New York, 1981), chs. 11–12.

205. See, for example, Stone on Russia, in *Eastern Front*, ch. 9; Barnett on Britain, in *Collapse of British Power*, pp. 113ff; McNeill on France, in *Pursuit of Power*, pp. 318ff.

206. Apart from McNeill's excellent general survey, see also G. Hardach, *The First World War 1914–1918* (London, 1977), espec. chs. 4 and 6; and A. Marwick, *War and Social Change in the Twentieth Century* (London, 1974), chs. 2–3.

207. See again Rothenberg, *Army of Francis Joseph*, chs. 12–14; for the internal problems, Kann, *History of the Habsburg Empire*, ch. 9; A. J. May, *The Passing of the Habsburg Monarchy, 1914–1918*, 2 vols. (Philadelphia, Pa., 1966), passim.

208. See especially the paper by J. Gooch, "Italy During the First World War," in the forthcoming collection A. Millett and W. Murray (eds.), *Military Effectiveness*.

209. J.A.S. Grenville, *A World History of the Twentieth Century 1900–1945* (London, 1980), vol. 1, pp. 218–19.

210. Stone, *Eastern Front*, passim, has excellent details (even if his case for Russia's industrial successes begs certain questions). See also Seton-Watson, *Russian Empire*, pp. 698ff; and D. R. Jones, "Imperial Russia's Armed Forces at War, 1914–1918: An Analysis of Combat Effectiveness," in Millett and Murray (eds.), *Military Effectiveness*. The role of the Moscow industrialists and their quarrels with the ministries is detailed in L. H. Siegelbaum, *The Politics of Industrial Mobilization in Russia, 1914–1917* (New York, 1984); and there is further massive detail in A. L. Sidorov, *The Economic Position of Russia During the First World War* (Moscow, 1973 trans.). The czar's own efforts are examined in D. R. Jones, "Nicholas II and the Supreme Command," *Sbornik*, vol. 11 (1985), pp. 47–83.

211. Schmitt and Vedeler, *World in the Crucible*, pp. 188–99. This quotation is from N. Golovine, *Russian Army in the World War* (New Haven, 1932), p. 281. For the casualty numbers, and the discontents at the "second-category" call-up, see Wildman, *End of the Russian Imperial Army*, ch. 3; and the nice survey in Lincoln, *Passage Through Armageddon*, passim.

212. G. Pedrocini, *Les mutineries de 1917* (Paris, 1967), is the best of a number of studies on this crisis.

213. McNeill, *Pursuit of Power*, p. 322, with a good synthesis of the literature. See also Hardach, *First World War*, pp. 86ff, 131ff.

214. See the older work M. Ange-Laribé, *L'agriculture pendant la guerre* (Paris, 1925), as well as the coverage in Hardach and McNeill.

215. Figures from Stokesbury, *Short History of World War I*, p. 289.

216. Kennedy, "Great Britain Before 1914," in May (ed.), *Knowing One's Enemies*, pp. 172–204; French, *British Economic and Strategic Planning*, passim.

217. See again Barnett, *Collapse of British Power*, pp. 113ff; Hardach, *First World War*, pp. 77ff; McNeill, *Pursuit of Power*, pp. 325ff; R.J.Q. Adams, *Arms and the Wizard: Lloyd George and the Ministry of Munitions, 1915* (London, 1978), passim.
218. Figures from Hardach, *First World War*, p. 87.
219. Kennedy, *Realities Behind Diplomacy*, p. 146, with the figures drawn from tables in Peacock and Wiseman, *Growth of Public Expenditure in the United Kingdom*.
220. Bond, "First World War," passim in *NCMH*, vol. 12; Guinn, *British Strategy and Politics*, passim: Schmitt and Vedeler, *World in the Crucible*, chs. 6–8; D. R. Woodward, *Lloyd George and the Generals* (Newark, N.J., 1983).
221. Quoted in Beloff, *Imperial Sunset*, vol. 1, p. 255. For full details, see now K. Burk, *Britain, America and the Sinews of War 1914–1918* (London/Boston, 1985).
222. F. S. Northedge, *The Troubled Giant: Britain Among the Great Powers* (London, 1966), p. 623.
223. Well covered in T. Lupfer, "The Dynamics of Doctrine: The Changes in German Tactical Doctrine During the First World War," *Leavenworth Papers*, no. 4 (Fort Leavenworth, Kans., 1981); and Van Creveld, *Command in War*, pp. 168ff.
224. Hardach, *First World War*, pp. 55ff; G. Feldman, *Army, Industry and Labor in Germany 1914–1918* (Princeton, N.J., 1966).
225. See the nervous consideration of this in Beloff, *Imperial Sunset*, pp. 239ff, 246ff, 271.
226. Hardach, *The First World War*, pp. 63ff; McNeill, *The Pursuit of Power*, pp. 338ff; Bond, "The First World War," pp. 198–99, in *NCMH*, vol. 12.
227. Full details are in A. Skalweit, *Die Deutsche Kriegsnährungswirtschaft* (Berlin, 1927), with a summary in Hardach, *First World War*, pp. 112ff. For the impact of the war upon the German people, see J. Kocka, *Facing Total War: German Society 1914–1918* (Leamington Spa, Warwick, 1984), chs. 2 and 4; McNeill, *Pursuit of Power*, p. 340, for the quotation.
228. See the references in note 193 above. For a historiographical summary, see D. M. Smith, "National Interest and American Intervention, 1917: An Historical Appraisal," *Journal of American History*, vol. 52 (1965), pp. 5–24.
229. The American contribution is ably summarized in Millett and Maslowski, *For the Common Defense*, ch. 11; Weigley, *History of the United States Army*, ch. 16; T. K. Nenninger, "American Military Effectiveness in World War I," in Millett and Murray (eds.), *Military Effectiveness* (forthcoming).
230. Strachan, *European Armies and the Conduct of War*, p. 148. See also the useful details in Ritter, *The Sword and the Scepter*, 4 vols. (London, 1975), vol. 4, pp. 119ff, 229ff.
231. Bond, "First World War," *NCMH*, vol. 12, p. 199, which provides these figures; Schmitt and Vedeler, *World in the Crucible*, p. 261. For detailed studies of the 1918 campaigning, see J. Toland, *No Man's Land: The Story of 1918* (London, 1980); H. Essame, *The Battle for Europe, 1918* (New York, 1972); B. Pitt, *1918—The Last Act* (New York, 1962).
232. For details, see Schmitt and Vedeler, *World in the Crucible*, p. 255ff, 376ff; A. J. Ryder, *The German Revolution of 1918* (Cambridge, 1967), passim.
233. J. Keegan, *The Face of Battle* (Harmondsworth, Mddsx., 1978), passim; J. Williams, *The Home Fronts: Britain, France and Germany, 1914–1918* (London, 1972); A. Marwick, *The Deluge—British Society in the First World War* (London, 1965); idem, *War and Social Change in the Twentieth Century*, chs. 2–3.
234. This theme runs through Kennan's books; for example, see *Decline of Bis-*

marck's European Order, p. 3. In a similar vein is Hölzle, *Die Selbstentmach-tung Europas.* For surveys of the psychological-cultural impact, referring to the more detailed literature, see Schmitt and Vedeler, *World in the Crucible,* pp. 476ff, and J. Joll, *Europe Since 1870* (London, 1973), espec. ch. 11.

235. War expenditure figures from Hardach, *First World War,* p. 153; total mobilized forces from Barraclough (ed.), *Atlas of World History,* p. 252.

236. See the anecdotes in M. Middlebrook, *The Kaiser's Battle: 21 March 1918* (London, 1978).

CHAPTER SIX
The Coming of a Bipolar World and the Crisis of the "Middle Powers": Part Two, 1919–1942

1. For the 1919–1923 settlements, see the general treatments in *NCMH,* vol. 12, ch. 8; Albrecht-Carrié, *Diplomatic History of Europe,* pp. 360ff; G. Ross, *The Great Powers and the Decline of the European States System 1914–1945* (London, 1983), ch. 3; R. J. Sontag, *A Broken World, 1919–1939* (New York, 1971), chs. 1 and 4; M. L. Dockrill and J. D. Goold, *Peace Without Promise: Britain and the Peace Conferences 1919–23* (London, 1981), passim; S. Marks, *The Illusion of Peace: International Relations in Europe 1918–1933* (London, 1976), ch. 1.

2. Ross, *Great Powers,* ch. 4; Marks, *Illusion of Peace,* ch. 3; A.J.P. Taylor, *The Origins of the Second World War* (Harmondsworth, Mddsx., 1964 edn.), ch. 3; J. Jacobsen, *Locarno Diplomacy: Germany and the West 1925–1929* (Princeton, N.J., 1972); and G. Grun, "Locarno, Ideal and Reality," *International Affairs,* vol. 31 (1955), pp. 477–85, are best here.

3. The literature upon reparations and war debts has now turned into a flood. Among the more important recent works are M. Trachtenberg, *Reparation in World Politics: France and European Diplomacy 1916–1923* (New York, 1980); W. A. McDougall, *France's Rhineland Diplomacy 1914–1924* (Princeton, N.J., 1978); H. Rupieper, *The Cuno Government and Reparations, 1922–1923* (London, 1979); S. A. Shuker, *The End of French Predominance in Europe: The Financial Crisis of 1924 and the Adoption of the Dawes Plan* (Chapel Hill, N.C., 1976); D. P. Silverman, *Reconstructing Europe After the Great War* (Cambridge, Mass., 1982). Marks, *Illusion of Peace,* ch. 2, is also useful, and there is a good summary in Kindleberger, *Financial History of Western Europe,* pt. 4.

4. D. H. Aldcroft, *From Versailles to Wall Street, 1919–1929* (London, 1977), p. 13. This is a good summary of all of the post-1919 studies (often sponsored by the Carnegie Foundation) on "the costs of the war," as well as the more recent literature.

5. Aldcroft, *From Versailles to Wall Street,* p. 14.

6. Aldcroft, *The European Economy 1914–1980* (London, 1978), p. 19.

7. Aldcroft, *From Versailles to Wall Street,* pp. 34–35, 98ff.

8. Rostow, *World Economy,* pp. 194–200, has a good summary; but see also Kenwood and Lougheed, *Growth of the International Economy,* ch. 11; A. S. Milward, *The Economic Effects of the World Wars in Britain* (London, 1970), passim; Landes, *Unbound Prometheus,* ch. 6.

9. I. Svennilson, *Growth and Stagnation in the European Economy,* (Geneva, 1954), pp. 204–05.

10. Farrar, *Arrogance and Anxiety,* p. 39, fn. 17.

11. Aldcroft, *From Versailles to Wall Street,* ch. 1 and pp. 99–101: Kenwood and Lougheed, *Growth of the International Economy,* pp. 176ff. For details of the

collapse in American farm prices after 1919, see Robertson, *History of the American Economy*, p. 515.

12. For a good summary, see Hardach, *First World War*, ch. 6; also Aldcroft, *From Versailles to Wall Street*, pp. 30ff.

13. See the references in note 3 above; and Aldcroft, *From Versailles to Wall Street*, ch. 4.

14. See here the essays in Rowland (ed.), *Balance of Power or Hegemony: The Inter-War Monetary System;* C. P. Kindleberger, *The World in Depression 1929–1939* (California, 1973), passim, but especially chs. 1 and 4; A. Fishlow, "Lessons from the Past: Capital Markets During the 19th Century and the Interwar Period," *International Organization*, vol. 39, no. 3 (1985), especially pp. 415–27. There is also a very good analysis in Kennedy, *Over Here*, pp. 334–47.

15. For an analysis of these events, see Aldcroft, *From Versailles to Wall Street*, chs. 7–11; Kindleberger, *World in Depression*, chs. 3–9; idem, *Financial History of Western Europe*, ch. 20.

16. Kindleberger, *World in Depression*, p. 231; Rowland, "Preparing the American Ascendancy: The Transfer of Economic Power from Britain to the United States, 1933–1944," in Rowland (ed.), *Balance of Power or Hegemony*, pp. 198ff. For Chamberlain's quote, see D. Reynolds, *The Creation of the Anglo-American Alliance, 1937–61* (London, 1981), p. 16 and passim; also C. A. MacDonald, *The United States, Britain and Appeasement 1936–1939* (London, 1980).

17. A.J.P. Taylor, *The Trouble-Makers: Dissent over Foreign Policy, 1789–1939* (London, 1969 edn.), chs. 4–6; Z. S. Steiner, *The Foreign Office and Foreign Policy 1898–1914* (Cambridge, 1969), passim; G. A. Craig and A. L. George, *Force and Statecraft: Diplomatic Problems of Our Time* (Oxford, 1983), ch. 5.

18. See, for example, L. Martin, *Peace Without Victory—Woodrow Wilson and the English Liberals* (New York, 1973 edn.); Taylor, *Trouble-Makers*, ch. 5.

19. A. J. Mayer, *Political Origins of the New Diplomacy* (New York, 1970 edn.), passim; S. R. Grabaud, *British Labour and the Russian Revolution 1917–1924* (Cambridge, Mass., 1956); F. S. Northedge and A. Wells, *Britain and Soviet Communism: The Impact of a Revolution* (London, 1982), ch. 8.

20. G. Schmidt, "Wozu noch politische Geschichte?" *Aus Politik und Zeitgeschichte*, B17/75 (April 1975), pp. 32ff.

21. Mayer, *Politics and Diplomacy of Peacemaking: Containment and Counter-Revolution at Versailles 1918–1919* (London, 1968); Joll, *Europe Since 1870*, ch. 9, "Revolution and Counter-Revolution." There is also good detail upon these fears of revolution in C. S. Maier, *Recasting Bourgeois Europe* (Princeton, N.J., 1975), espec. ch. 1.

22. Joll, *Europe Since 1870*, chs. 9–12; Sontag, *Broken World*, pp. 24ff.

23. Schmitt and Vedeler, *World in the Crucible*, pp. 476ff; B. Bengonzi, *Heroes' Twilight* (New York, 1966); P. Fussell, *The Great War and Modern Memory* (New York, 1975); cf. Barnett, *Collapse of British Power*, pp. 426ff.

24. See again Joll, *Europe Since 1870*, pp. 262ff; Gollwitzer, *Geschichte des Weltpolitischen Denkens*, vol. 2, pp. 538ff.; A. Hamilton, *The Appeal of Fascism* (London, 1971): P. Hayes, *Fascism* (London, 1973), passim; R.A.L. Waite, *Vanguard of Nazism: The Free Corps Movement in Postwar Germany* (Cambridge, Mass., 1952), passim; J. Diehl, *Paramilitary Politics in Weimar Germany* (Bloomington, Ind., 1977).

25. D. Caute, *The Fellow Travellers* (London, 1973); Northedge and Wells, *Britain and Soviet Communism*, chs. 6–8.

26. For what follows, see the excellent analysis in Barraclough, *Introduction to Contemporary History*, ch. 6, "The Revolt Against the West"; and the maps in Barraclough (ed.), *Atlas of World History*, pp. 248, 260–61. See also Gollwitzer,

Geschichte des weltpolitischen Denkens, vol. 2, pp. 575ff; *NCMH,* vol. 12, chs. 10–12; H. Bull and A. Watson, *The Expansion of International Society* (Oxford, 1984), espec. pt. 3; R. F. Holland, *European Decolonization 1918–1981* (London, 1985), ch. 1; H. Griml, *Decolonization: The British, French, Dutch, and Belgian Empires 1919–1963* (London, 1978) chs. 1–3.

27. For a good example on the British side, see B. R. Tomlinson, *The Political Economy of the Raj 1914–1947* (Cambridge, 1979), passim; more generally, Tomlinson, "The Contraction of England: National Decline and the Loss of Empire," *Journal of Imperial and Commonwealth History,* vol. 11 (1982), pp. 58–72; Thornton, *Imperial Idea and its Enemies,* chs. 4–6; Beloff, *Imperial Sunset,* vol. 1, ch. 6.

28. Barraclough, *Introduction to Contemporary History,* pp. 156–58.

29. Storry, *Japan and the Decline of the West in Asia,* pp. 107ff; Grenville, *World History of the Twentieth Century,* pp. 117ff; Keylor, *Twentieth-Century World,* pp. 229ff; Gollwitzer, *Geschichte des weltpolitischen Denkens,* vol. 2, pp. 575ff.

30. A. Iriye, *After Imperialism: The Search for a New Order in the Far East 1921–1931* (New York, 1978 edn.), passim.

31. Kiernan, *European Empires from Conquest to Collapse,* ch. 13; *NCMH,* vol. 12, pp. 319, 324–25; C. M. Andrew and A. S. Kanya-Forstner, *The Climax of French Imperial Expansion 1914–1924* (Stanford, Calif., 1981), p. 246.

32. Howard, *Continental Commitment,* pp. 56ff; B. Bond, *British Military Policy Between the Two World Wars* (Oxford, 1980), chs. 1, 3–4.

33. For discussions of this "continuity" in German policy after 1919, see the general treatments in Calleo, *German Problem Reconsidered,* passim; Gruner, *Die deutsche Frage,* pp. 126ff; Hillgruber, *Germany and the Two World Wars,* passim. See also two important new works: G. Stoakes, *Hitler and the Quest for World Dominion: Nazi Ideology and Foreign Policy in the 1920s* (Leamington Spa, Warwickshire, 1986); M. Lee and W. Michalka, *German Foreign Policy 1917–1933: Continuity or Break?* (Leamington Spa, Warwickshire, 1987).

34. Taylor, *Origins of the Second World War,* p. 48.

35. Ibid. For other surveys of the post-1919 "balance," see DePorte, *Europe Between the Super-Powers,* ch. 3; Thomson, *Europe Since Napoleon,* pp. 622ff.; Ross, *Great Powers and the Decline of the European States System,* chs. 3–6.

36. E. M. Bennett, *German Rearmament and the West, 1932–1933* (Princeton, N.J., 1979), pp. 92ff, is best here.

37. P. Wandycz, *France and Her Eastern Allies 1919–25* (Minneapolis, Minn., 1962), passim; and the classic older work A. Wolfers, *Britain and France Between Two Wars* (New York, 1966 edn.), especially ch. 8. Later French efforts to contain Germany in eastern Europe are explored in L. Radice, *Prelude to Appeasement, East Central European Diplomacy in the early 1930s* (New York, 1981), chs. 3–4.

38. W. N. Medlicott, *British Foreign Policy Since Versailles, 1919–1963* (London, 1968), pp. 61–63; Ross, *Great Powers,* p. 57; A. Orde, *Britain and International Security 1920–1926* (London, 1978), passim. For the continuity of this policy, see P. W. Schroeder, "Munich and the British Tradition," *Historical Journal,* vol. 19 (1976), pp. 223–43.

39. A. Teichova, *An Economic Background to Munich* (Cambridge, 1974) passim; D. Kaiser, *Economic Diplomacy and the Origins of the Second World War* (Princeton, N.J., 1980), passim; B. J. Wendt, "England und der deutsche 'Drang nach Südosten,' " in I. Geiss and B. J. Wendt (eds.), *Deutschland in der Weltpolitik des 19. und 20. Jahrhunderts* (Düsseldorf, 1973), pp. 483–512.

40. Quoted in Northedge, *Troubled Giant,* p. 220. There is a good and succinct survey of the League's activities in *NCMH,* vol. 12, ch. 9; and in Ross, *Great Powers,* ch. 7.

41. E. H. Carr, *The Twenty Years Crisis 1919–1939* (London, 1939); Sontag, *Broken World*, passim; A. Adamthwaite, *The Lost Peace: International Relations in Europe 1918–1939* (London, 1980), passim.

42. D. Mack Smith, *Mussolini: A Biography* (New York, 1982) is a good portrayal of the man, though less so of Italian politics and economy under him. For those aspects, see M. Knox, *Mussolini Unleashed 1939–1941* (Cambridge, 1982), ch. 1; J. Whittam, "The Italian General Staff and the Coming of the Second World War," in A. Preston (ed.), *General Staffs and Diplomacy Before the Second World War* (London, 1978), pp. 77–97; A. Raspin, "Wirtschaftliche und politische Aspekte der italienischen Aufrüstung Anfang der dreissiger Jahre bis 1940," in F. Forstmeier and H. E. Volkmann (eds.), *Wirtschaft und Rüstung am Vorabend des Zweiten Weltkrieges* (Düsseldorf, 1975), pp. 202–21; B. R. Sullivan, "The Italian Armed Forces, 1918–1940," in Millett and Murray (eds.), *Military Effectiveness*, vol. 2 (forthcoming).

43. S. Ricossa, "Italy," in Cipolla (ed.), *Fontana Economic History of Europe*, vol. 6, no. 1, pp. 272ff; R. Higham, *Air Power: A Concise History* (Manhattan, Kan., 1984 edn.), p. 48; J. W. Thompson, *Italian Civil and Military Aircraft 1930–1945* (Fallbrook, Calif., 1963).

44. Knox, *Mussolini Unleashed*, p. 20.

45. Quoted from Ricossa, "Italy," p. 266; see also, Knox, *Mussolini Unleashed*, pp. 30–31, 43.

46. Ricossa, "Italy," p. 270.

47. Knox, *Mussolini Unleashed*, ch. 1; Mack Smith, *Mussolini's Roman Empire*, ch. 13; Raspin, "Wirtschaftliche und Politische Aspekte," passim; W. Murray, *The Change in the European Balance of Power, 1938–1939* (Princeton, N.J., 1984), pp. 110ff.

48. Knox, *Mussolini Unleashed*, p. 48.

49. Ibid., p. 73. More generally, see McNeill, *Pursuit of Power*, pp. 350ff; W. Murray, "German Air Power and the Munich Crisis," in B. Bond and I. Roy (eds.), *War and Society*, vol. 1 (1976), pp. 107–18.

50. The figures with neither parentheses nor brackets come from Hillman, "Comparative Strength of the Powers," in A. J. Toynbee and F. T. Ashton-Gwatkin (eds.), *The World in 1939* (London, 1952), Table VI, p. 454, with currency conversions at the exchange rates he gives in the footnote. The figures in parentheses come from the "Correlates of War" print-out. One suspects that currency changes are responsible for some of the discrepancies, as are different national accounting practices. In Japan's case the matter is further complicated by the distinctions made between regular and "extraordinary" defense spending, and between "forces in homeland" and "others" (e.g., China War). The figures in brackets are from K. Ohkawa and M. Shinohara (eds.), *Patterns of Japanese Economic Development* (New Haven, Conn., 1979), and do *not* include "others."

51. Mack Smith, *Mussolini's Roman Empire*, pp. 177–78.

52. Knox, *Mussolini Unleashed*, pp. 9–16; idem, "Conquest, Foreign and Domestic, in Fascist Italy and Nazi Germany", *Journal of Modern History*, vol. 56 (1986), pp. 1–57.

53. On this, Mack Smith, *Mussolini*, is overwhelming.

54. See below, pp. 340–41.

55. These racial/cultural attitudes are nicely covered in Thorne, *The Issue of War: States, Societies, and the Far Eastern Conflict of 1941–1945* (London, 1985), passim. See also Storry, *Japan and the Decline of the West in Asia*, passim.

56. Howarth, *Fighting Ships of the Rising Sun*, pp. 199ff.

57. Allen, *Short Economic History of Modern Japan*, pp. 100ff.

58. League of Nations, *World Economic Survey* (Geneva, 1945), Table III, p. 134.
59. Allen, *Economic History*, pp. 101–13; Storry, *Japan and the Decline of the West in Asia*, p. 115.
60. On this important theme, see espec. J. B. Crowley, *Japan's Quest for Autonomy: National Security and Foreign Policy 1930–1958* (Princeton, N.J., 1966), passim; M. A. Barnhart, "Japan's Economic Security and the Origins of the Pacific War," *Journal of Strategic Studies*, vol. 4, no. 2 (1981), pp. 105–24; J. W. Morley (ed.), *Dilemmas of Growth in Prewar Japan* (Princeton, N.J., 1971).
61. Allen, *Economic History of Modern Japan*, p. 141.
62. Howarth, *Fighting Ships of the Rising Sun*, pt. 4; H. P. Willmott, *Empires in the Balance* (Annapolis, Md., 1982), ch. 3; A. J. Marder, *Old Friends, New Enemies: The Royal Navy and the Imperial Japanese Navy* (Oxford, 1981), ch. 11; S. E. Pelz, *Race to Pearl Harbor* (Cambridge, Mass., 1974), espec. pts. 1 and 5; C. Bateson, *The War with Japan* (East Lansing, Mich., 1968), ch. 2.
63. Willmott, *Empires in the Balance*, pp. 89ff; R. H. Spector, *Eagle Against the Sun: The American War with Japan* (New York, 1985), chs. 2 and 4; S. Hayashi with A. Coox, *Kogun: The Japanese Army in the Pacific War* (Westport, Conn., 1978 reprint), ch. 1.
64. Willmott, *Empires in the Balance*, p. 55; P. M. Kennedy, "Japan's Strategic Decisions, 1939–45," in Kennedy, *Strategy and Diplomacy 1870–1945*, pp. 182ff; C. Boyd, "Military Organizational Effectiveness: Imperial Japanese Armed Forces Between the World Wars," in Millett and Murray (eds.), *Military Effectiveness*, vol. 2. Pelz, *Race to Pearl Harbor*, ch. 12, is very good on the army-navy quarrels. The China War itself is covered in F. Dorn, *The Sino-Japanese War 1937–1941* (New York, 1974).
65. Barnhart, "Japan's Economic Security," pp. 112–16.
66. Barnhart, "Japan's Economic Security," p. 114, from where the quote comes. See also B. Martin, "Aggressionspolitik als Mobilisierungsfaktor: Der militärische und wirtschaftliche Imperialismus Japans 1931 bis 1941," in F. Forstmeier and H.-E. Volkmann (eds.), *Wirtschaft und Rüstung am Vorabend des Zweiten Weltkrieges* (Düsseldorf, 1975), pp. 234–35.
67. Hayashi and Coox, *Kogun*, pp. 14–17; M. A. Barnhart, "Japanese Intelligence Before the Second World War," in May (ed.), *Knowing One's Enemies*, pp. 435–37; and espec. A. Coox, *Nomonhan*, 2 vols. (Stanford, Calif., 1985), passim.
68. Wright, *Study of War*, p. 672; Overy, *Air War*, p. 151; Bairoch, "World Industrialization Levels," p. 299.
69. For the decision itself, see Willmott, *Empires in the Balance*, ch. 3; Hayashi and Coox, *Kogun*, pp. 19ff; Barnhart, "Japan's Economic Security," pp. 116ff; I. Nobutaka (ed.), *Japan's Decision for War* (Stanford, Calif., 1967), passim; Spector, *Eagle Against the Sun*, ch. 4; R. J. Butow, *Tojo and the Coming of War* (Princeton, N.J., 1961).
70. For general surveys, see Craig, *Germany 1866–1945*, pp. 396ff; A. J. Nicholls, *Weimar and the Rise of Hitler* (London, 1979 edn.), passim. For summaries of the massive historiography, and hotly contested debates upon Germany in the Nazi era, see I. Kershaw, *The Nazi Dictatorship* (London, 1985); and K. Hildebrand, *The Third Reich* (London/Boston, 1984).
71. Taylor, *Origins of the Second World War*, passim; J. Hiden, *Germany and Europe 1919–1939* (London, 1977), espec. ch. 7; F. Fischer, *Bündnis der Eliten* (Düsseldorf, 1979). For details of the "continuity" among the armed forces, see G. Schreiber, *Revisionismus und Weltmachtstreben* (Stuttgart, 1978), passim; J. Dülffer, *Weimar, Hitler und die Marine: Reichspolitik und Flottenbau 1920–1939* (Düsseldorf, 1973); M. Geyer, *Aufrüstung oder Sicherheit* (Wiesbaden, 1980). Also important for what follows is *Das Deutsche Reich und der Zweite*

Weltkrieg, vol. 1, *Ursachen und Voraussetzungen der deutschen Kriegspolitik*, eds. W. Deist et al. (Stuttgart, 1979).

72. A. Bullock, *Hitler: A Study in Tyranny* (London, 1962 edn.); A. Hillgruber, *Germany and the Two World Wars* (Cambridge, Mass., 1981), espec. chs. 5 and 8; N. Rich, *Hitler's War Aims*, 2 vols. (London, 1973–74); G. Weinberg, *The Foreign Policy of Hitler's Germany*, 2 vols. (Chicago, 1970 and 1980); and the literature in M. Hauner, "A Racial Revolution?" *Journal of Contemporary History*, vol. 19 (1984), pp. 669–87; Calleo, *The German Problem Reconsidered*, pp. 85–95; Gruner, *Die deutsche Frage*, pp. 145ff; A. Kuhn, *Hitlers aussenpolitisches Programm* (Stuttgart, 1970); E. Jackel, *Hitler's Weltanschauung* (Middletown, Conn., 1982).

73. The term comes from E. N. Petersen, *The Limits of Hitler's Power* (Princeton, N.J., 1969); but see also Craig, *Germany 1860–1945*, ch. 17; Kershaw, *Nazi Dictatorship*, chs. 4 and 7; Hildebrand, *Third Reich*, pp. 83ff, 152ff; also I. Kershaw, *Popular Opinion and Political Dissent in the Third Reich: Bavaria 1933–1945* (Oxford, 1983).

74. Murray, *Change in the European Balance of Power*, pp. 20–21; Hillman, "Comparative Strength of the Great Powers," p. 454.

75. Quoted in A. Seaton, *The German Army 1933–45* (London, 1982), p. 55. See also Craig, *Politics of the Prussian Army*, pp. 397ff.

76. Seaton, *German Army 1933–45*, chs. 3–4, covers this breakneck expansion, as does W. Deist, *The Wehrmacht and German Rearmament* (London, 1981), chs. 3 and 6, with references to the extensive further literature.

77. For more details, see Deist, *Wehrmacht*, ch. 4; Overy, *Air War*, p. 21; W. Murray, *Luftwaffe* (Baltimore, Md., 1985), ch. 1; E. L. Homze, *Arming the Luftwaffe* (Lincoln, Neb., 1976); K.-H. Volker, *Die deutsche Luftwaffe 1933–1939* (Stuttgart, 1967).

78. Deist, *Wehrmacht*, p. 81; with much more detail in Dülffer, *Weimar, Hitler und die Marine*, passim; and M. Salewski, *Die deutsche Seekriegsleitung 1935–1945*, 3 vols. (Frankfurt, 1970–75).

79. R. J. Overy, *The Nazi Economic Recovery 1932–1938* (London, 1932), pp. 19ff.

80. Ibid., pp. 28ff. Overy's brief work contains full references to further studies on the German economy under the Nazis.

81. Deist, *Wehrmacht*, pp. 89–91 and passim; A. S. Milward, *The German Economy at War* (London, 1965), pp. 17–24.

82. Murray, *Change in the European Balance of Power*, pp. 4ff, is the best summary here; but see also Hillmann, "Comparative Strength of the Powers," pp. 368ff.

83. Murray, *Balance of Power*, p. 15.

84. Ibid., pp. 15–16. See also the important chapter by H.-E. Volkmann, "Die NS-Wirtschaft in Vorbereitung des Krieges," in Deist, et al., *Ursachen und Voraussetzungen der deutschen Kriegspolitik*, espec. pp. 349ff.

85. Deist, *Wehrmacht*, p. 90; Seaton, *German Army*, pp. 93–96.

86. Quoted in Murray, *Luftwaffe*, p. 20; idem., "German Air Power and the Munich Crisis," in Bond and Roy (eds.), *War and Society*, vol. 1, passim; Deist, *Wehrmacht*, pp. 66–69.

87. B. R. Posen, *The Sources of Military Doctrine: France, Britain and Germany Between the World Wars* (Ithaca, N.Y., 1984), passim; W. Murray, "German Army Doctrine, 1918–1939, and the Post-1945 Theory of Blitzkrieg Strategy," in C. Fink et al. (eds.), *German Nationalism and the European Response 1890–1945* (Chapel Hill, N.C., 1985), pp. 71–94; Dupuy, *Genius for War*, ch. 15.

88. Murray, *Balance of Power*, pp. 150–51; and Volkmann, "Die NS-Wirtschaft in Vorbereitung des Krieges," pp. 323ff. Details of the relationship between Germany's economic difficulties and Hitler's "forward" policy are in B. A. Carroll,

Design for Total War: Arms and Economics in the Third Reich (The Hague, 1968); T. W. Mason, "Innere Krise und Angriffskrieg 1938/39," in Forstmeier and Volkmann (eds.), *Wirtschaft und Rüstung am Vorabend des zweiten Weltkrieges,* pp. 158–88; J. Dulffer, "Der Beginn des Krieges 1939," *Geschichte und Gesellschaft,* vol. 2 (1976), pp. 443–70.

89. T. W. Mason, "Some Origins of the Second World War," p. 125, in E. M. Robertson (ed.), *The Origins of the Second World War* (London, 1971); idem, "Innere Krise und Angriffskrieg 1938/39," passim. Murray, *Balance of Power,* pp. 290ff, details the 1938 and 1939 plunder.

90. R. J. Overy, "Hitler's War and the German Economy: A Reinterpretation," *Economic History Review,* 2nd series, vol. 35 (1982), pp. 272–91, is important here.

91. Hillgruber, *Germany and the Two World Wars,* passim; Deist, *Wehrmacht,* ch. 7; Murray, *Luftwaffe,* pp. 81ff; M. Hauner, "Did Hitler Want a World Dominion?" *Journal of Contemporary History,* vol. 13, pp. 15–32; J. Thies, *Architekt der Weltherrschaft: Die "Endziele" Hitlers* (Düsseldorf, 1976), passim; and see the historiographical discussion in Kershaw, *Nazi Dictatorship,* ch. 6.

92. On which see the two older works A. Wolfers, *Britain and France Between the Wars* (New York, 1940); and W. M. Jordan, *Britain, France and the German Problem* (London, 1943); as well as the essays in N. Waites (ed.), *Troubled Neighbours: Franco-British Relations in the Twentieth Century* (London, 1971); and N. Rostow, *Anglo-French Relations 1934–1936* (London, 1984), passim.

93. C. Fohlen, "France," in Cipolla (ed.), *Fontana Economic History of Europe,* vol. 6, no. 1, pp. 80–86; T. Kemp, *The French Economy 1913–39: The History of a Decline* (New York, 1972), chs. 5–7; G. Ziebura, "Determinanten der Aussenpolitik Frankreichs 1932–1939," in K. Rohe (ed.), *Die Westmächte und das Dritte Reich 1933–1939* (Paderborn, 1982), pp. 136ff. There are lots of details (also prejudiced commentary) in A. Sauvy, *Histoire économique de la France entre les deux guerres,* 2 vols. (Paris, 1965–67); and more balance in *Histoire économique et sociale de la France,* vol. 4, pt. 2, *1914–1950,* eds. F. Braudel and E. Labrousse (Paris, 1980).

94. Fohlen, "France," p. 88.

95. Ibid., pp. 86–91; Landes, *Unbound Prometheus,* pp. 388ff; Kemp, *French Economy 1913–39,* chs. 8–12 (with very good details); Caron, *Economic History of Modern France,* pp. 258ff.

96. The best source here is R. Frankenstein, *Le Prix du réarmement français 1935–1939* (Paris, 1939), passim, but p. 303 for the spending totals. The national-income figure is taken from A. Adamthwaite, *France and the Coming of the Second World War* (London, 1977), p. 164. See also B. A. Lee, "Strategy, Arms and the Collapse of France 1939–1940," in R.T.B. Langhorne (ed.), *Diplomacy and Intelligence During the Second World War* (Cambridge, 1985), pp. 63ff.

97. R. J. Young, *In Command of France: French Foreign Policy and Military Planning 1933–1940* (Cambridge, Mass., 1978), ch. 1; see also the essays in *Les Relations franco-allemandes 1933–1939* (Paris, 1976).

98. Frankenstein, *Le Prix du réarmement français,* p. 317; idem, "The Decline of France, and French Appeasement Policies 1936–9," in Mommsen and Kettenacker (eds.) *Fascist Challenge and the Policy of Appeasement,* p. 238; Overy, *Air War,* p. 21. The relatively generous treatment of the navy—and that service's ingratitude—is detailed in R. Chalmers Hood, *Royal Republicans: The French Naval Dynasties Between the World Wars* (Baton Rouge, La., 1985).

99. Frankenstein, *Le Prix des réarmement français,* p. 319; Murray, *Change in the European Balance of Power,* pp. 107–8. The navy's strength by then is assessed

in P. Masson, "La Marine française en 1939–40," *Revue historique des armées*, No. 4 (1979), pp. 57–77.

100. No attempt will be made here to cover all the literature upon French politics and society in the 1930s and its relationship to the 1940 "strange defeat." There are important surveys in J. B. Duroselle, *La Décadence 1932–1939* (Paris, 1979); R. Hohne, "Innere Desintegration und äusserer Machtzerfall: Die französische Politik in den Jahren 1933–36," in Rohe (ed.), *Die Westmächte und das Dritte Reich*, pp. 157ff; H. Dubief, *Le Déclin de la IIIe République 1929–1938* (Paris, 1976); J. Joll (ed.), *The Decline of the Third Republic* (New York, 1959). There is also a useful summary in J. C. Cairns, "Some Recent Historians and the 'Strange Defeat' of 1940," *Journal of Modern History*, vol. 46 (1974), pp. 60–85.

101. For details, see A. Horne, *The French Army and Politics 1870–1970* (London, 1984), ch. 3; P.C.F. Bankwitz, *Maxime Weygand and Civil-Military Relations in Modern France* (Cambridge, Mass., 1967); the more technical details in Frankenstein, *Le Prix du réarmement français*, and H. Dutailly, *Les Problèmes de l'Armée de terre française 1933–1939* (Paris, 1980); and the more cautionary comments in R. A. Doughty, "The French Armed Forces, 1918–1940," in Millett and Murray (eds.), *Military Effectiveness*, vol. 2.

102. Adamthwaite, *France and the Coming of the Second World War*, p. 166; Gorce, *French Army: A Military-Political History*, pp. 270ff; Young, "French Military Intelligence and Nazi Germany," in May (ed.), *Knowing One's Enemies*, pp. 271–309.

103. Posen, *Sources of Military Doctrine*, ch. 4; Doughty, "French Armed Forces, 1918–1940," passim; Murray, *Change in the European Balance of Power*, pp. 97ff; L. Mysyrowicz, *Autopsie d'une Défaite; Origines de l'effondrement militaire français de 1940* (Lausanne, 1973). But the most thorough analysis is now R. A. Doughty, *The Seeds of Disaster: The Development of French Army Doctrine 1919–1939* (Hamden, Conn., 1985).

104. French diplomacy in these critical years is best covered in Adamthwaite, *France and the Coming of the Second World War*, passim; Duroselle, *La Décadence*, passim; and P. Wandycz, *The Twilight of the French Eastern Alliances, 1926–1936* (forthcoming).

105. See R. Girault, "The Impact of the Economic Situation on the Foreign Policy of France, 1936–9," in Mommsen and Kettenacker (eds.), *Fascist Challenge and the Policy of Appeasement*, pp. 209–26.

106. In particular, see Young, "La Guerre de Longue Durée: Some Reflections on French Strategy and Diplomacy in the 1930s," in Preston (ed.), *General Staffs and Diplomacy Before the Second World War*, pp. 41–64; and Posen, *Sources of Military Doctrine*, pp. 112ff, 127ff. For full diplomatic details, see Adamthwaite, *France and the Coming of the Second World War*, especially pt 3; the contributions to *Les Relations Franco-Britanniques 1935–39* (Paris, 1975); and Young, *In Command of France*, chs. 8–9.

107. Apart from the details in Adamthwaite's and Young's books, see also Barnett, *Collapse of British Power;* Howard, *Continental Commitment;* and last but not least, J. C. Cairns, "A Nation of Shopkeepers in Search of a Suitable France," *American Historical Review*, vol. 79 (1974), pp. 710–43.

108. Figures from Kennedy, *Realities Behind Diplomacy*, p. 240. It is impossible to list even one-tenth of the studies upon British "appeasement" policies in the 1930s; but there are very useful summative essays in Mommsen and Kettenacker (eds.), *Fascist Challenge and the Power of Appeasement*, chs. 6–13 and 19–25; and massive detail (and an enormous bibliography) in G. Schmidt, *England in der Krise: Grundzüge und Grundlagen der britischen Appeasement-Politik, 1930–1937* (Opladen, 1981).

109. See especially R. Ovendale, *Appeasement and the English-Speaking World* (Cardiff, 1975), as well as his ch. 23 in Mommsen and Ketternacker (eds.), *Fascist Challenge;* R. F. Holland, *Britain and the Commonwealth Alliance, 1918–1939* (London, 1981).

110. B. Bond, *British Military Policy Between Two World Wars* (Oxford, 1980), espec. chs. 1 and 4, is best here.

111. R. Meyers, "British Imperial Interests and the Policy of Appeasement," and W. R. Louis, "The Road to Singapore: British Imperialism in the Far East 1932–1942," both in Mommsen and Kettenacher (eds.), *Fascist Challenge;* A. J. Marder, *Old Friends, New Enemies: The Royal Navy and the Imperial Japanese Navy* (Oxford, 1981); L. R. Pratt, *East of Malta, West of Suez: Britain's Mediterranean Crisis* (London, 1975); S. W. Roskill, *Naval Policy Between the Wars,* vol. 2 (London, 1976).

112. Kennedy, *British Naval Mastery,* ch. 10. For details of the policy implications, see the varying assessments in G. C. Peden, *British Rearmament and the Treasury 1932–1939* (Edinburgh, 1979); R. P. Shay, *British Rearmament in the Thirties: Politics and Profits* (Princeton, N.J., 1977); Barnett, *Collapse of British Power,* ch. 5; and N. H. Gibbs, *Grand Strategy,* vol. 1 (London, 1976), passim.

113. For the economic recovery and newer industries, see Pollard, *Development of the British Economy,* ch. 3; H. W. Richardson, *Economic Recovery in Britain, 1932–1939* (London, 1967); B.W.E. Alford, *Depression and Recovery? British Economic Growth 1918–1939* (London, 1972).

114. Cited in Howard, *Continental Commitment,* p. 99. For fuller details, see Peden, *British Rearmament and the Treasury,* chs. 3–4; see also R. Meyers, *Britische Sicherheitspolitik 1934–1938* (Düsseldorf, 1976); and Gibbs, *Grand Strategy,* vol. 1, ch. 4.

115. Howard, *Continental Commitment,* pp. 120–21.

116. Details in U. Bialer, *The Shadow of the Bomber: The Fear of Air Attack and British Politics 1932–1939* (London, 1980); M. Smith, *British Air Strategy Between the Wars* (Oxford, 1984), espec. pt. 2.

117. For this argument, see especially Barnett, *Collapse of British Power,* and Murray, *Change in the European Balance of Power.*

118. D. C. Watt, *Too Serious a Business: European Armed Forces and the Approach of the Second World War* (London, 1975), is the key work here.

119. See again Dehio, *Precarious Balance.* For good surveys of the British Cabinet's awareness of the country's strategical dilemmas, see Barnett, *Collapse of British Power;* Howard, *The Continental Commitment;* Posen, *Sources of Military Doctrine,* ch. 5; D. Dilks, "The Unnecessary War? Military Advice and Foreign Policy in Great Britain 1931–1939," in Preston (ed.), *General Staffs and Diplomacy Before the Second World War,* pp. 98–132; and G. Schmidt's thoughtful essay in Rohe (ed.), *Die Westmächte und das Dritte Reich,* pp. 29–56.

120. Schmidt, in Rohe (ed.), *Die Westmächte,* pp. 46ff; C. A. MacDonald, *United States, Britain and Appeasement, 1936–1939,* passim.

121. Schmidt, *England in der Krise,* ch. 1, is best here; but see also the above-named works by Howard, Bond, Barnett, Dilks, Gibbs, and Meyers; and the good summary in G. Niedhart, "Appeasement: Die Britische Antwort auf die Krise des Weltreichs und des internationalen Systems vor dem Zweiten Weltkrieg," *Historische Zeitschrift,* vol. 226 (1978), pp. 68–88.

122. Barnett, *Collapse of British Power,* passim; Murray, *Change in the European Balance of Power,* passim; Kennedy, *Realities Behind Diplomacy,* pp. 290ff; A. Adamthwaite, "The British Government and the Media, 1937–1938," *Journal of Contemporary History,* vol. 18 (1983), pp. 281–97.

123. Cited in Barnett, *Collapse of British Power,* p. 564.

124. Hillmann, "Comparative Strength of the Great Powers," in Toynbee (ed.), *World in March 1939*, pp. 439, 446.
125. For more details of this argument, see Kennedy, "Strategy versus Finance in Twentieth-Century Britain," in *Strategy and Diplomacy*, pp. 100–6; and for an even more deterministic view, Porter, *Britain, Europe and the World*, pp. 86ff, 95ff.
126. Figures from Pollard, *Peaceful Conquest*, p. 294; but see also Munting, *Economic Development of the USSR*, pp. 45ff; Nove, *Economic History of Russia*, chs. 6–10; and the interesting discussion in Grossman, "The Industrialization of Russia and the Soviet Union," in Cipolla (ed.), *Fontana Economic History of Europe*, vol. 4, pt. 2, pp. 501ff.
127. S. H. Cohn, *Economic Development in the Soviet Union* (Lexington, Mass., 1970), pp. 70–71; F. D. Holzmann, "Financing Soviet Economic Development," in Blackwell (ed.), *Russian Economic Development from Peter the Great to Stalin*, pp. 259–76; Kochan and Abraham, *Making of Modern Russia*, pp. 361ff. See also M. Lewin, *Russian Peasants and Soviet Power* (Evanston, Ill., 1968).
128. W. A. Lewis, *Economic Survey 1919–1939* (London, 1949), p. 131; Nove, *Economic History*, ch. 7; Munting, *Economic Development of the USSR*, p. 99; H. J. Ellison, "The Decision to Collectivize Agriculture," in Blackwell (ed.), *Russian Economic Development from Peter the Great to Stalin*, pp. 241–55.
129. On which see Munting, *Economic Development of the USSR*, pp. 106ff.
130. Nove, *Economic History*, p. 232; Lewis, *Economic Survey*, p. 133; M. McCauley, *The Soviet Union Since 1917* (London, 1981), pp. 85–87.
131. Munting, *Economic Development of the Soviet Union*, p. 93; Nove, *Economic History*, pp. 187ff; Blackwell, *Industrialization of Russia*, pp. 132ff; Lewis, *Economic Survey*, p. 125.
132. See Hillmann, "Comparative Strength of the Great Powers," in Toynbee (ed.), *World in March 1939*, pp. 439, 446; Black et al., *Modernization of Japan and Russia*, pp. 195–97; S. H. Cohn, "The Soviet Economy: Performance and Growth," in Blackwell (ed.), *Russian Economic Development from Peter the Great to Stalin*, pp. 321–51.
133. Nove, *Economic History*, p. 236. For further details, see Kochan and Abraham, *Making of Modern Russia*, pp. 382ff; R. Conquest, *The Great Terror* (London, 1968).
134. Nove, *Economic History*, p. 236.
135. Figures from Overy, *Air War*, p. 21. The Italian figures for the years 1932–37 (not available in Overy) were provided by my colleague Brian Sullivan, but are only rough estimates; the same is true of the 1932–34 French figures, generally thought to be about 50 a month—see Young, *In Command of France*, p. 164. Relative neglect of the navy is covered in Mitchell, *History of Russia and Soviet Sea Power*, ch. 17.
136. McNeill, *Pursuit of Power*, p. 350, fn. 77. For the subsequent comments on Soviet military development generally, see J. Erickson, *The Soviet High Command, 1918–1941* (London, 1962), passim; E. F. Ziemke, "The Soviet Armed Forces in the Interwar Period," in Millett and Murray (eds.), *Military Effectiveness*, vol. 1; B. H. Liddell Hart (ed.), *The Red Army* (New York, 1956), chs. 3–9. Russian defense expenditures are detailed in Nove, *Economic History*, pp. 227–28; and Munting, *Economic Development of the USSR*, p. 114.
137. Ulam, *Expansion and Coexistence*, chs. 5–6; J. Haslam, *The Soviet Union and the Struggle for Collective Security in Europe 1933–39* (New York, 1984); and J. Hochmann, *The Soviet Union and the Failure of Collective Security 1934–1938* (Ithaca, N.Y., 1984), are best here.
138. Hillmann, "Comparative Strength of the Great Powers," p. 446.

139. M. Mackintosh, "The Red Army 1920–36," in Liddell Hart (ed.), *Red Army*, p. 63.

140. Erickson, *Soviet High Command*, pp. 532ff, 542ff; K. Dittmar and G. J. Antonov, "The Red Army in the Finnish War," in Liddell Hart (ed.), *Red Army*, pp. 79–92. Above all, Coox, *Nomonhan*, passim.

141. Erickson's works—*The Soviet High Command; The Road to Stalingrad*, early chapters; and "Threat Identification and Strategic Appraisal by the Soviet Union, 1930–1941," in May (ed.), *Knowing One's Enemies*, pp. 375–423—are best here. For diplomatic background, see W. Carr, *Poland to Pearl Harbor* (London, 1985), chs. 3–4.

142. Figures from Nove, *Economic History*, p. 228.

143. Quoted in Munting, *Economic Development of the USSR*, p. 86; see also Ziemke, "Soviet Armed Forces," passim, for the frantic preparations in 1939–1941.

144. Rostow, *World Economy*, p. 210.

145. See the excellent analysis in M. P. Leffler, "Expansionist Impulses and Domestic Constraints, 1921–1932," in Becker and Wells (eds.), *Economics and World Power*, pp. 246–48.

146. Hillmann, "Comparative Strength of the Great Powers," in Toynbee (ed.), *World in March 1939*, pp. 421–22.

147. Ibid., p. 422.

148. Leffler, "Expansionist Impulses and Domestic Constraints," in Becker and Wells (eds.), *Economics and World Power*, p. 258.

149. For a good, succinct survey of American defense policy between the wars, see Millett and Maslowski, *For the Common Defense*, ch. 12.

150. H. Yardley, *The American Black Chamber* (New York, 1931), pp. 262–63.

151. See above, pp. 281–82.

152. R. M. Hathaway, "Economic Diplomacy in a Time of Crisis," in Becker and Wells (eds.), *Economics and World Power*, pp. 277–78.

153. L. Silk, "Protectionist Mood: Mounting Pressure," *New York Times*, Sept. 17, 1985, p. D1; Robertson, *History of the American Economy*, pp. 516ff.

154. Kindleberger, *World in Depression*, ch. 12 and pp. 280–87.

155. Table from Hillman, "Comparative Strength of the Great Powers," in Toynbee (ed.), *World in March 1939*, p. 439.

156. Hathaway, "Economic Diplomacy in a Time of Crisis," in Becker and Wells (eds.), *Economics and World Power*, p. 285.

157. Ibid., pp. 309, 312. For a brief survey, Schulzinger, *America Diplomacy in the Twentieth Century*, pp. 147ff.

158. This is well covered in MacDonald, *United States, Britain and Appeasement 1936–1939*, passim; and Carr, *Poland to Pearl Harbor*, ch. 1. See also D. Reynolds, *Creation of the Anglo-American Alliance 1937–1941*, chs. 1-2; A. Offner, *American Appeasement. United States Foreign Policy and Germany 1933–1938* (Cambridge, Mass., 1969); and N. Graebner, *America as a World Power* (Wilmington, Del., 1984), ch. 2.

159. Millett and Maslowski, *For the Common Defense*, pp. 386ff; Mills, *Arms and Men*, pp. 237ff; J. A. Iseley and P. A. Crowl, *The U. S. Marines and Amphibious War* (Princeton, N.J., 1945); M. H. Gillie, *Forging the Thunderbolt* (Harrisburg, Pa., 1947); M. S. Watson, *Chief of Staff: Pre-War Plans and Preparations* (Washington, D.C., 1950); J. Major, "The Navy Plans for War, 1937–1941," in Hagan (ed.), *In Peace and War*, pp. 237ff; Weighley, *History of the United States Army*, pp. 416ff.

160. Robertson, *History of the American Economy*, pp. 709ff. The steel statistics

come from Hillmann, "Comparative Strength of the Great Powers," in Toynbee (ed.), *World in March 1939,* p. 443 and fn.

161. Figures from Wright, *Study of War,* p. 672.

162. Figures from Hillmann, "Comparative Strength of the Great Powers," in Toynbee (ed.), *World in March 1939,* p. 446.

163. M. S. Kendrick, *A Century and a Half of Federal Expenditures* (New York, 1955), p. 12.

164. The extensive literature upon Hitler's views of the United States are conveniently summarized in Herwig, *Politics of Frustration,* pp. 179ff. See also the commentaries in Weinberg, *Foreign Policy of Hitler's Germany,* vols. 1–2; idem, *World in the Balance* (New Hampshire/London, 1981) pp. 53–136.

165. Cited in Willmott, *Empires in the Balance,* p. 62; see also Pelz, *Race to Pearl Harbor,* pp. 217–18, 224.

166. Cited in Thorne, *Limits of Foreign Policy,* p. 90—a book which makes superfluous all previous studies of the Manchurian crisis.

167. Ibid., pp. 148ff, 231ff.

168. Ibid., passim; Crowley, *Japan's Quest for Autonomy,* pp. 161ff; A. Rappaport, *Henry L. Stimson and Japan, 1931–1933* (Chicago, 1963); Schulzinger, *American Diplomacy,* pp. 148ff.

169. Crowley, *Japan's Quest for Autonomy,* ch. 2; Storry, *History of Modern Japan,* pp. 186ff.

170. Bennett, *German Rearmament and the West,* is best here.

171. See above, pp. 315–20; and Howard, *The Continental Commitment,* ch. 5. The 1934 arguments for and against an Anglo-Japanese understanding are nicely covered in W. R. Louis, "The Road to Singapore: British Imperialism in the Far East 1932–42," in Mommsen and Kettenacker (eds.), *Fascist Challenge and the Policy of Appeasement,* pp. 359ff.

172. Ross, *The Great Powers and the Decline of the European States System,* pp. 85–87; Ulam, *Expansion and Coexistence,* ch. 5.

173. This is now most fully covered in Rostow, *Anglo-French Relations 1934–36,* espec. ch. 5; but see also Taylor, *Origins of the Second World War,* ch. 5; Ross, *Great Powers,* pp. 90ff. The Anglo-German naval agreement is treated in E. Haraszti, *Treaty-Breakers or "Realpolitiker"? The Anglo-German Naval Agreement of June 1935* (Boppard, 1974).

174. F. Hardie, *The Abyssinian Crisis* (London, 1974), passim; A. J. Marder, "The Royal Navy in the Italo-Ethiopian War 1935–36," *American Historical Review,* vol. 75 (1970), pp. 1327–56; R.A.C. Parker, "Great Britain, France and the Ethiopian Crisis 1935–1936," *English Historical Review,* vol. 89 (1974), pp. 293–32; Mack Smith, *Mussolini's Roman Empire,* ch. 5; F. D. Laurens, *France and the Italio-Ethiopian Crisis, 1935–6* (The Hague, 1967); G. Baer, *Test Case: Italy, Ethiopia, and the League of Nations* (Stanford, Calif., 1976).

175. Pelz, *Road to Pearl Harbor,* pt. 4.

176. Now covered in J. T. Emmerson, *The Rhineland Crisis* (London, 1977), and E. Haraszti, *The Invaders: Hitler Occupies the Rhineland* (Budapest, 1983). See also Rostow, *Anglo-French Relations 1934–36,* pp. 233ff.

177. See again Rohe (ed.), *Die Westmächte und das Dritte Reich,* passim.

178. Ross, *Great Powers,* p. 98; see also MacDonald, *The United States, Great Britain, and Appeasement,* passim.

179. See above, pp. 313–14.

180. Although we still await the second volume of D. Dilks's authoritative biography, the literature upon Chamberlain and "appeasement" is already enormous. For surveys, see the relevant chapters in Mommsen and Kettenacker (eds.), *Fascist Challenge and the Policy of Appeasement; K. Middlemas, *Diplomacy of*

Illusion: The British Government and Germany 1937–39 (London, 1972); M. Cowling, *The Impact of Hitler: British Politics and British Policies 1933–1940*, passim; Barnett, *Collapse of British Power*, ch. 5. Also very important is M. Gilbert, *Winston Churchill*, vol. 5, *1922–1939* (London, 1976).

181. By far the most comprehensive analysis is now T. Taylor, *Munich: The Price of Peace* (New York, 1979); but see also A.J.P. Taylor, *Origins of the Second World War*, ch. 8; Middlemas, *Diplomacy of Illusion*, pp. 211ff; Weinberg, *Foreign Policy of Hitler's Germany*, vol. 2, chs. 10–11; K. Robbins, *Munich, 1938* (London, 1968).

182. W. Murray, "Munich, 1938; The Military Confrontation," *Journal of Strategic Studies*, vol. 2 (1979), pp. 282–302; Barnett, *Collapse of British Power*, pp. 505ff; Kennedy, *Realities Behind Diplomacy*, pp. 291–93.

183. The unfolding of events in 1939 is covered in Murray, *Change in the European Balance of Power*, chs. 8–10; Taylor, *Origins of the Second World War*, chs. 9–11; S. Aster, *1939: The Making of the Second World War* (London, 1973); Weinberg, *Foreign Policy of Hitler's Germany*, vol. 2, pp. 465ff; Barnett, *Collapse of British Power*, pp. 554ff; H. Graml (ed.), *Summer 1939: Die Grossmächte und der europäische Krieg* (Stuttgart, 1979); D. Kaiser, *Economic Diplomacy and the Origins of the Second World War*, pp. 263ff.

184. For the overall strategical dimension in 1939–1940, see Kennedy, *Rise and Fall of British Naval Mastery*, pp. 300ff; Murray, *Change in the European Balance of Power*, pp. 310ff; B. H. Liddell Hart, *History of the Second World War* (London, 1970), pp. 16ff; *Grand Strategy*, vols. 1 (Gibbs) and 2 (Butler).

185. Murray, *Change in the European Balance of Power*, pp. 314–21; cf. Pratt, *East of Malta, West of Suez*, ch. 6; Gibbs, *Grand Strategy*, pp. 664ff; G. Schreiber et al., *Der Mittelmeerraum und Südosteuropa*, vol. 3 of *Das Deutsche Reich und der Zweite Weltkrieg* (Stuttgart, 1984), ch. 1.

186. K. A. Maier et al., *Die Errichtung des Hegemonie auf dem europäischen Continent*, vol. 2 of *Das Deutsche Reich und der Zweite Weltkrieg* (Stuttgart, 1979), passim; Murray, *Change in the European Balance of Power*, ch. 10; idem, *Luftwaffe*, ch. 2; Overy, *Air War*, pp. 26–30; Posen, *Sources of Military Doctrine*, ch. 3; J. A. Gunsberg, *Divided and Conquered: The French High Command and the Defeat of the West, 1940* (Westport, Conn., 1979). For a good analysis of the reasons for the Allied inertia and the German decision to attack, see also J. Mearsheimer, *Conventional Deterrence* (Ithaca, N.Y., 1983), chs. 3–4.

187. Knox, *Mussolini Unleashed*, is best on those repeated Italian disasters; but see also Schreiber et al., *Mittelmeerraum*, pts. 2–3 and 5. For a more sympathetic account of Italy's weaknesses, see J. L. Sadkovich, "Minerals, Weapons and Warfare: Italy's Failure in World War II," accepted for *Storia contemporanea*.

188. Overy, *Air War*, p. 28; Kennedy, *Rise and Fall of British Naval Mastery*, p. 309.

189. Carr, *Poland to Pearl Harbor*, pp. 99ff; Reynolds, *Creation of the Anglo-American Alliance*, pp. 108ff. See also J. Leutze, *Bargaining for Supremacy: Anglo-American Naval Relations 1937–1941* (Chapel Hill, N.C., 1977).

190. J. Lukacs, *The Last European War, September 1939/December 1941* (London, 1977); H. Baldwin, *The Crucial Years 1939–41* (New York, 1976); Carr, *Poland to Pearl Harbor*, passim. For the German side, A. Hillgruber, *Hitler's Strategie: Politik und Kriegsführung 1940–41* (Frankfurt, 1965).

191. Van Creveld, *Supplying War*, ch. 5; Murray, *Luftwaffe*, chs. 3–4; Milward, *German Economy at War*, pp. 39ff. For full details of the early campaigning, see H. Boog et al., *Der Angriff auf die Sowjetunion*, vol. 4 of *Das Deutsche Reich und der Zweite Weltkrieg* (Stuttgart, 1983); and A. Clark, *Barbarossa: The Russo-German Conflict 1941–1945* (London, 1965), pp. 71–216. For the Russian

side, Erickson, *Road to Stalingrad,* passim; A. Seaton, *The Russo-German War 1941–45* (London, 1971).

192. Erickson, *Stalingrad,* pp. 237ff; Carr, *From Poland to Pearl Harbor,* pp. 150ff.
193. Willmott, *Empires in the Balance,* pp. 68ff, is best here; but see also J. Morley (ed.), *The Fateful Choice: Japan's Advance into Southeast Asia, 1939–1941* (New York, 1980).
194. Dupuy, *Genius for War,* appendix E.

CHAPTER SEVEN
Stability and Change in a Bipolar World, 1943–1980

1. Quoted in Spector, *Eagle Against the Sun,* p. 123.
2. For a brief summary, Liddell Hart, *History of the Second World War,* pp. 230–33; J. Neidpath, *The Singapore Naval Base and the Defense of Britain's Eastern Empire 1919–41* (Oxford, 1981), ch. 8; Barclay, *Empire Is Marching,* chs. 8–9.
3. Spector, *Eagle Against the Sun,* chs. 8–12; Liddell Hart, *History of the Second World War,* chs. 23 and 29.
4. Liddell Hart, *History of the Second World War,* chs. 20–22, and 25.
5. Ibid., ch. 24; S. W. Roskill, *The War at Sea,* 3 vols. (London, 1954–1961); F. H. Hinsley et al., *British Intelligence in the Second World War,* vol. 2 (London, 1981), ch. 26.
6. By far the best survey now is Murray, *Luftwaffe,* chs. 5–7; but see also N. Frankland, *The Bomber Offensive Against Germany* (London, 1965).
7. Quoted in Ropp, *War in the Modern World,* p. 336.
8. Ibid., p. 334. For much fuller details, see Erickson, *Road to Stalingrad,* passim; idem, *The Road to Berlin* (London, 1983), passim; E. F. Ziemke, *Stalingrad to Berlin: The German Defeat in the East 1942–1945* (Washington, D.C., 1968); Clark, *Barbarossa,* passim; and Seaton, *Russo-German War 1941–45,* passim.
9. Erickson, *Road to Stalingrad,* p. 272.
10. Dupuy, *Genius for War,* p. 343.
11. Clark, *Barbarossa,* chs. 17–18; Erickson, *Road to Berlin,* ch. 4.
12. These rivalries come out clearly in Clark, *Barbarossa,* passim; and are covered in more detail in Milward, *German Economy at War,* espec. ch. 6; Speer's own *Inside the Third Reich* (New York, 1982 edn.), pts. 2–3; Seaton, *German Army, 1933–45,* chs. 9–11; Hildebrand, *Third Reich,* pp. 49ff.
13. Kennedy, "Japanese Strategic Decisions, 1939–45," in *Strategy and Diplomacy,* pp. 181–95; C. G. Reynolds, "Imperial Japan's Continental Strategy," *U.S. Naval Institute Proceedings,* vol. 109 (August 1983), pp. 65–71; Spector, *Eagle Against the Sun,* passim; and the excellent survey by A. Coox, "The Effectiveness of the Japanese Military Establishment in World War II," in Millett and Murray (eds.), *Military Effectiveness,* vol. 3.
14. Willmott, *Empires in the Balance,* p. 89.
15. R. Lewin, *The American Magic: Codes, Cyphers and the Defeat of Japan* (New York, 1982), is the best synthesis.
16. Clark, *Barbarossa,* p. 228; Erickson, *Road to Stalingrad,* ch. 6. For Soviet war production, see Nove, *Economic History of the USSR.,* ch. 10; Munting, *Economic Development of the USSR,* ch. 5; A. Milward, *War, Economy and Society 1939–1945* (Berkeley, Calif., 1979), pp. 94ff.
17. See Table 34 below; and Overy, *Air War,* pp. 49ff.
18. Erickson, *Road to Berlin,* p. 447. See also the figures in Liddell Hart (ed.), *Red Army,* ch. 13.

19. Liddell Hart, *History of the Second World War*, p. 559.
20. For this trend, see such works as Dupuy, *Genius for War*, passim; M. van Creveld, *Fighting Power: German and U.S. Army Performance, 1939–1945* (Westport, Conn., 1982), passim; M. Hastings, *Overlord: D-Day and the Battle for Normandy* (London, 1984), pp. 14, 370, and passim.
21. Ropp, *War in the Modern World*, p. 342. For details of the Japanese "overstretch," see Hayashi and Coox, *Kogun*. More generally, see the similar argument in A. J. Levine, "Was World War II a Near-Run Thing?" *Journal of Strategic Studies*, vol. 8, no. 1 (March 1985), pp. 38–63.
22. Figures from Willmott, *Empires in the Balance*, p. 98.
23. Ropp, *War in the Modern World*, p. 328, quoting from S. E. Morison, *History of United States Naval Operations*, vol. 10, *The Atlantic Battle Won* (Boston, 1956), p. 64. For further details, see Roskill, *The War at Sea*, 3 vols., passim; Liddell Hart, *History of the Second World War*, ch. 24; Potter (ed.), *Sea Power*, ch. 24; Levine, "Was World War II a Near-Run Thing?" pp. 46ff.
24. For comparisons, see Kennedy, *Rise and Fall of British Naval Mastery*, pp. 309–10; Seaton, *German Army 1933–45*, p. 239 (Seaton includes self-propelled guns with these tank totals).
25. Overy, *Air War*, p. 150. Overy's figures for Italian production in the first half of the war are much less than those given in Table XVIII of James J. Sadkovich's article "Minerals, Weapons and Warfare: Italy's Failure in World War II," *Storia contemporanea* (forthcoming).
26. Overy, *Air War*, p. 150.
27. Murray, *Luftwaffe*, chs. 6–7.
28. See Tables 30 and 32 above.
29. Hillman, "Comparative Strength of the Powers," in Toynbee (ed.), *World in March 1939*, pp. 439, 446; Wright, *Study of War*, p. 672. See also R. W. Goldsmith, "The Power of Victory: Munitions Output in World War II," *Military Affairs*, vol. 10 (Spring 1946), pp. 69–80.
30. Figures from R. Wagenführ, *Die deutsche Industrie im Kriege 1939–1945* (Berlin, 1963), pp. 34, 87. The Italian figures are my own very rough "guestimates," based upon the size of its economy relative to those of the other Powers. For further comparisons, see F. Forstmeier and H. E. Volkmann (eds.), *Kriegswirtschaft und Rüstung 1939–1945* (Düsseldorf, 1977).
31. Milward, *German Economy at War*, pp. 72ff; Wagenführ, *Die deutsche Industrie in Kriege*, ch. 3; and for more general comparisons, Aldcroft, *European Economy 1914–1980*, pp. 124ff.
32. Spector, *Eagle Against the Sun*, ch. 23; L. Giovannetti and F. Freed, *The Decision to Drop the Bomb* (London, 1967), passim; H. Feis, *The Atomic Bomb and the End of World War II* (Princeton, N.J., 1966 edn.), passim; G. Alperowitz, *Atomic Diplomacy: Hiroshima and Potsdam* (London, 1966); M. J. Sherwin, *A World Destroyed: The Atomic Bomb and the Grand Alliance* (New York, 1975).
33. Cited in M. Matloff, *Strategic Planning for Coalition Warfare, 1943–1944* (Washington, D.C., 1959), pp. 523–24.
34. DePorte, *Europe Between the Superpowers*, ch. 4.
35. W. Ashworth, *A Short History of the International Economy Since 1850* (London, 1975), p. 268. See also the figures in Milward, *War, Economy and Society 1939–1945*, p. 63.
36. Rowland (ed.), *Balance of Power or Hegemony*, p. 220.
37. Ashworth, *Short History of the International Economy Since 1850*, p. 268.
38. Apart from the early chapters of L. Freedman, *The Evolution of Nuclear Strategy* (London, 1981), see also D. A. Rosenberg, "The Origins of Overkill: Nuclear Weapons and American Strategy, 1945–1960," *International Security*, vol. 7,

no. 4 (Spring 1983); M. Mandelbaum, *The Nuclear Question: The United States and Nuclear Weapons 1946–1976* (New York, 1979).

39. Figures from W. P. Mako, *U.S. Ground Forces and the Defense of Central Europe* (Washington, D.C., 1983), p. 8.

40. R. Steel, *Pax Americana* (New York, 1977), ch. 2. For the parallels with Britain after 1815, see above, pp. 151–58; and T. Smith, *The Pattern of Imperialism: The United States, Great Britain and the Late-Industrializing World Since 1815* (Cambridge, 1981), pp. 182ff.

41. M. Balfour, *The Adversaries: America, Russia, and the Open World, 1941–62* (London, 1981), p. 14.

42. G. Kolko, *The Politics of War 1943–1945* (New York, 1968), passim; Becker and Wells (eds.), *Economics and World Power*, chs. 6–7; R. Keohane, "State Power and Industry Influence: American Foreign Oil Policy in the 1940s," *International Organization*, vol. 36 (Winter 1982), pp. 165–83; A. E. Eckes, *The United States and the Global Struggle for Minerals* (Austin, Texas, 1979).

43. Balfour, *Adversaries*, p. 15.

44. On which see R. N. Gardner, *Sterling-Dollar Diplomacy* (New York, 1969), passim.

45. The phrase used in Steel, *Pax Americana*, p. 10.

46. Quoted by R. Dallek, "The Postwar World: Made in the USA," in S. J. Ungar (ed.), *Estrangement: America and the World* (New York, 1985), p. 32.

47. Cited in J. W. Spanier, *American Foreign Policy Since World War II* (London, 1972 edn.), p. 26. See also R. A. Divine, *Second Chance: The Triumph of Internationalism in America During World War II* (New York, 1971), passim.

48. Thorne, *Issue of War*, p. 206. See also M. P. Leffler's recent writings: "The American Conception of National Security and the Beginnings of the Cold War, 1945–48," *American Historical Review*, vol. 89 (1984), pp. 349–81; and his Lehrman Institute paper "Security and Containment Before Kennan: The Identification of American Interests at the End of World War II," passim.

49. Erickson, *Road to Berlin*, p. ix.

50. G. Hosking, *A History of the Soviet Union* (London, 1985), p. 296.

51. Nove, *Economic History of the USSR*, p. 285.

52. See the figures in Munting, *Economic Development of the USSR*, p. 118.

53. McCauley, *Soviet Union Since 1917*, p. 138. For further details, see Nove, *Economic History of the USSR*, pp. 140–42.

54. McCauley, *Soviet Union Since 1917*, pp. 140–42.

55. For details, see M. A. Evangelista, "Stalin's Postwar Army Reappraised," *International Security*, vol. 7, no. 3 (1982–83), pp. 110–38.

56. Mackintosh, *Juggernaut: A History of the Soviet Armed Forces*, pp. 272–73.

57. Ibid. See also the relevant chapters in Liddell Hart (ed.), *The Red Army*, pt. 2; D. Holloway, *The Soviet Union and the Arms Race* (New Haven, Conn., 1983), pp. 15ff; Mitchell, *History of Russian and Soviet Sea Power*, pp. 469ff.

58. Hosking, *History of the Soviet Union*, ch. 11, is best here. See also McCauley, *Soviet Union Since 1917*, ch. 5; Nove, *Economic History*, pp. 266ff; Ulam, *Expansion and Coexistence*, pp. 467ff.

59. Spanier, *American Foreign Policy Since World War II*, p. 3; G. Challiand and J.-P. Rageau, *Strategic Atlas: A Comparative Geopolitics of the World's Powers* (New York, 1985), pp. 18ff; J. L. Gaddis, *Strategies of Containment* (New York, 1982), pp. 57ff; and the comments in A. K. Henrikson, "America's Changing Place in the World: From 'Periphery' to 'Center'?" in J. Gottman (ed.), *Center and Periphery* (Beverly Hills, Calif., 1980), pp. 73–100.

60. Ulam, *Expansion and Coexistence*, p. 405.

61. Cited in H. Feis, *Churchill-Roosevelt-Stalin* (Princeton, N.J., 1967), p. 462.

62. Landes, *Unbound Prometheus*, p. 488, fn. 1.

63. Allen, *Short Economic History of Modern Japan*, pp. 187ff, and the relevant tables in appendix B.

64. Ricossa, "Italy 1920–1970," in Cipolla (ed.), *Fontana Economic History of Europe*, vol. 6, pt. 1, p. 240.

65. Ibid., p. 316.

66. Wright, *Ordeal of Total War*, p. 264.

67. Fohlen, "France 1920–1970," in Cipolla (ed.), *Fontana Economic History of Europe*, vol. 6, pt. 1, pp. 92, 109.

68. Ibid., p. 100.

69. De Gaulle's attitude toward the Anglo-Saxon powers is superbly brought out in F. Kersaudy, *Churchill and de Gaulle* (London, 1981), as well as in de Gaulle's own *Memoires de Guerre*, 3 vols. (Paris, 1954–59). For French colonial policy during and after the war, see L. von Albertini, *Decolonization* (New York, 1971 edn.), pp. 358ff; and—with British comparisons—Smith, *Pattern of Imperialism*, ch. 3.

70. Barnett, *Collapse of British Power*, pp. 587–88; and, in a similar tone, Porter, *Britain, Europe and the World 1850–1982*, pp. 111ff.

71. Cited in Kennedy, *Realities Behind Diplomacy*, p. 318, with further details of Britain's economic position. See also Hobsbawm, *Industry and Empire*, pp. 356ff; Barnett, *The Audit of War* (London, 1986), passim.

72. The best of these is K. O. Morgan, *Labour in Power 1945–1951* (Oxford, 1984), passim, and also appendices 3–5. But see also the relevant chapters in K. Harris, *Attlee* (London, 1982), and A. Bullock, *Ernest Bevin: Foreign Secretary* (Oxford, 1983). Economic policy is detailed in A. Cairncross, *Years of Recovery: British Economic Policy 1945–51* (London, 1985), and summarized in D. H. Aldcroft, *The British Economy*, vol. 1 (London, 1986), ch. 8.

73. See especially H. M. Sachar, *Europe Leaves the Middle East 1936–1954* (London, 1972); W. R. Louis, *The British Empire in the Middle East, 1945–1951* (Oxford, 1984); and H. Rahman, "British Post-Second World War Military Planning for the Middle East," *Journal of Strategic Studies*, vol. 5, no. 4 (December 1982), pp. 511–30, for details of the enhanced importance of the region. The post-1945 economic value of the empire is summarized in Porter, *Lion's Share*, pp. 319ff.

74. On this cooperation, see T. H. Anderson, *The United States, Great Britain and the Cold War, 1944–1947* (Columbia, Mo., 1981), for early interchanges; J. Baylis, *Anglo-American Defense Relations 1939–1980* (London, 1981), for a general assessment; and Bartlett, *Global Conflict*, pp. 269ff.

75. See the details in Bairoch, "Europe's Gross National Product, 1800–1975," pp. 291–92.

76. See Bairoch, "International Industrialization Levels," p. 304, cf. p. 296.

77. The per capita GNP figures for 1950 are taken from S. H. Cohn, *Economic Development in the Soviet Union* (Lexington, Mass., 1970), appendix C, Table C-1. To obtain the national GNP figures, I multiplied by the population size given in "The Correlates of War" print-out.

78. "Correlates of War" print-out data.

79. Quotations from Sherwin, *World Destroyed*, p. 314.

80. On which see Freedman, *Evolution of Nuclear Strategy*, passim; and the very useful survey in A. L. Friedberg, "A History of U. S. Strategic 'Doctrine,' 1945–1980," *Journal of Strategic Studies*, vol. 3, no. 3 (December 1983), pp. 40ff. For some early published examples of these ponderings, see B. Brody, *The Absolute Weapon* (New York, 1946); idem, *Strategy in the Nuclear Age* (Princeton, N.J., 1959); H. Kahn, *On Thermonuclear War* (Princeton, N.J., 1960); J. Slessor,

Strategy for the West (London, 1954); P.M.S. Blackett, *Fear, War, and the Bomb* (New York, 1948).

81. Holloway, *Soviet Union and the Arms Race*, ch. 2; J. Prados, *The Soviet Estimate: U.S. Intelligence Analysis and Russian Military Strength* (New York, 1982), pp. 17ff; R. L. Garthoff, *Soviet Strategy in the Nuclear Age* (New York, 1958), passim; H. S. Dinerstein, *War and the Soviet Union* (London, 1962 edn.), especially chs. 1–6.

82. Prados, *Soviet Estimate*, pp. 17–18; Freedman, *Evolution of Nuclear Strategy*, ch. 5 et seq.; T. B. Larson, *Soviet-American Rivalry* (New York, 1978), pp. 178ff.

83. M. Growing, *Independence and Deterrence: Britain and Atomic Energy 1945–1952*, 2 vols. (London, 1974), vol. 1, p. 184. See also L. Freedman, *Britain and Nuclear Weapons* (London, 1980); A. Pierce, *Nuclear Politics: The British Experience with an Independent Strategic Nuclear Force, 1939–1970* (London, 1972); and J. Groom, *British Thinking About Nuclear Weapons* (London, 1974).

84. See below, p. 401; and Freedman, *Evolution of Nuclear Strategy*, ch. 21; W. Kohl, *French Nuclear Diplomacy* (Princeton, N.J., 1971), passim, with fuller references.

85. Dallek, *American Style of Foreign Policy*, p. 130.

86. Ibid., p. 152.

87. Quoted in Balfour, *Adversaries*, p. 71. For the changes in American policy and opinion, see also Anderson, *United States, Great Britain, and the Cold War, 1944–1947*, chs. 6–7; J. L. Gaddis, *The United States and the Origins of the Cold War, 1941–1947* (New York, 1972); and B. R. Kuniholm, *The Origins of the Cold War in the Near East* (Princeton, N.J., 1980), passim.

88. Dallek, *American Style of Foreign Policy*, p. 170.

89. Ulam, *Expansion and Coexistence*, p. 437.

90. G. Lichtheim, *Europe in the Twentieth Century* (London, 1972), p. 351.

91. Balfour, *Adversaries*, pp. 8ff; and for fuller details, L. E. Davis, *The Cold War Begins: Soviet-American Conflict over Eastern Europe* (Princeton, N.J., 1974); Feis, *Churchill-Roosevelt-Stalin*, passim; B. Dovrig, *The Myth of Liberation* (Baltimore, Md., 1973); A. Polonsky, *The Great Powers and the Polish Question 1941–1945* (London, 1976); V. Rothwell, *Britain and the Cold War 1941–47* (London, 1982), espec. ch. 3; R. Douglas, *From War to Cold War 1942–1948* (London, 1981), passim.

92. Ulam, *Expansion and Coexistence*, chs. 7–9; T. Wolfe, *Soviet Power and Europe, 1945–1970* (Baltimore, Md., 1970); M. McCauley (ed.), *Communist Power in Europe, 1944–1949* (London, 1977); W. Taubman, *Stalin's American Policy: From Entente to Detente to Cold War* (New York, 1982), passim.

93. Nor is it proposed to give a full bibliography of the enormous literature upon the Cold War. Balfour, *Adversaries;* Larson, *Soviet-American Rivalry;* Ulam, *Expansion and Coexistence;* and Bartlett, *Global Conflict*, chs. 10–11, all provide surveys with references to the further literature. See also note 87 above.

94. Balfour, *Adversaries*, p. 94; M. Balfour and J. Mair, *Four-Power Control in Germany and Austria 1945–1946* (London, 1956); Rothwell, *Britain and the Cold War*, ch. 6. See also the very important collection J. Foschepoth (ed.), *Kalter Krieg und deutsche Frage* (Göttingen, 1985), espec. pt. 3.

95. A reference to Gaddis's excellent survey, *Strategies of Containment*.

96. Ibid., p. 30.

97. Ibid., p. 31.

98. Ibid., p. 30.

99. Anderson, *United States, Great Britain and the Cold War*, passim; Bullock, *Ernest Bevin: Foreign Secretary*, espec. ch. 10; Kuniholm, *Origins of the Cold War in the Near East*, passim; Keylor, *Twentieth-Century World*, pp. 270–71.

100. Apart from Ulam's book, see also the references in note 92 above; and M. D. Shulman, *Stalin's Foreign Policy Reappraised* (New York, 1969); M. Kaser, *Comecon* (London, 1967); J. K. Hoensch, *Sowjetische Osteuropa-Politik 1945–1974* (Düsseldorf, 1977).

101. See the references in R. Poidevin, "Die Neuorientierung der französischen Deutschlandpolitik in 1948/9," in Foschepoth (ed.), *Kalter Krieg und deutsche Frage;* J. W. Young, *Britain, France and the Unity of Europe 1945–51* (Leicester, 1984), especially ch. 5; Douglas, *From War to Cold War,* pp. 167ff; and, for British ambivalences, see S. Greenwood, "Return to Dunkirk: The Origins of the Anglo-French Treaty of March 1947," *Journal of Strategic Studies,* vol. 6, no. 4 (December 1983), pp. 49–65.

102. Bullock, *Bevin,* pp. 571ff; W. P. Davison, *The Berlin Blockade* (Princeton, N.J., 1958); the relevant chapters in R. Morgan, *The United States and West Germany 1945–73* (London, 1974); J. H. Backer, *Winds of History: The German Years of Lucius DuBignon Clay* (New York, 1983), ch. 10; M. Bell, "Die Blockade Berlins-Konfrontation der Allierten in Deutschland," in Foschepoth (ed.), *Kalter Krieg und deutsche Frage,* pp. 217ff.

103. Evangelista, "Stalin's Postwar Army Reconsidered," passim; W. LaFeber, *America, Russia, and the Cold War 1945–1975* (New York, 1976), pp. 83ff; Lord Ismay, *NATO—the First Five Years, 1949–1954* (Utrecht, 1954); Gaddis, *Strategies of Containment,* pp. 72ff; A. K. Henrikson, "The Creation of the North Atlantic Alliance, 1948–1952," *Naval War College Review,* vol. 32, no. 3 (May/June 1980), pp. 4–39; L. S. Kaplan, *The United States and NATO: The Formative Years* (Lexington, Ky., 1984), passim.

104. On which see A. Grosser, *West Germany from Defeat to Rearmament* (London, 1955); R. McGeehan, *The German Rearmament Question* (Urbana, Ill., 1971); D. Lerner and R. Aron, *France Defeats EDC* (New York, 1957); DePorte, *Europe Between the Superpowers,* pp. 158ff; and T. Schwarz, "The Case of German Rearmament: Alliance Crisis in the 'Golden Age,'" *Fletcher Forum* (Summer 1984), pp. 295–309.

105. Bartlett, *Global Conflict,* p. 312.

106. Ulam, *Expansion and Coexistence,* pp. 544ff; D. J. Dallin, *Soviet Foreign Policy After Stalin* (Philadelphia, Pa., 1961); R. A. Remington, *The Warsaw Pact* (Cambridge, Mass., 1971).

107. On which see again Kolko, *Politics of War,* passim; and Thorne, *Issue of War.*

108. Kolko, *Politics of War,* pp. 298ff; Kuniholm, *Origins of the Cold War in the Near East,* passim; Louis, *British Empire in the Middle East,* pp. 53ff.

109. Ulam, *Expansion and Coexistence,* p. 428; and see also Anderson, *United States, Great Britain and the Cold War,* pp. 103ff.

110. Cited in Bartlett, *Global Conflict,* p. 261 (my emphasis); and see again the works by Anderson, Louis, and Kuniholm above.

111. Griml, *Decolonization,* pp. 183ff, is a good summary; also, Kiernan, *European Empires from Conquest to Collapse,* pp. 210ff; Holland, *European Decolonization 1918–1981,* pp. 86ff.

112. M. Heald and L. S. Kaplan, *Culture and Diplomacy: The American Experience* (Westport, Conn., 1977), chs. 5 and 8; P. A. Varg, *Missionaries, Chinese, and Diplomats . . . 1890–1952* (Princeton, N.J., 1952); A. Iriye, *Across the Pacific* (New York, 1967); and, more specifically, B. W. Tuchman, *Stilwell and the American Experience in China* (New York, 1971); H. Feis, *The China Tangle* (Princeton, N.J., 1953), passim; N. B. Tucker, *Patterns in the Dust: Chinese-American Relations and the Recognition Controversy 1949–50* (New York, 1983).

113. M. Schaller, *The American Occupation of Japan: The Origins of the Cold War*

in Asia (New York, 1985), which places U.S. policy toward Japan in a much wider East Asian and Cold War context; and W. S. Borden, *The Pacific Alliance* (Madison, Wis., 1984), passim.

114. Cited in Schaller, *American Occupation of Japan*, p. 232; see also Smith, *The Pattern of Imperialism*, pp. 193–94. American policy in the region is well covered in W. W. Stueck, *The Road to Confrontation* (Chapel Hill, N.C., 1981); R. M. Blum, *Drawing the Line: The Origin of American Containment Policy in East Asia* (New York, 1982); B. Cumings, *The Origins of the Korean War* (Princeton, N.J., 1981); N. Yonosuke and A. Iriye (eds.), *The Origins of the Cold War in Asia* (New York, 1977). See also R. Dingman, "Strategic Planning and the Policy Process: American Plans for War in East Asia, 1945–50," *Naval War College Review*, vol. 32, no. 6 (1979), pp. 4–21.

115. There is a succinct account of the Korean War in Millett and Maslowski, *For the Common Defense*, pp. 484ff; and much more detail in D. Rees, *Korea: The Limited War* (New York, 1966); F. H. Heller, (ed.), *The Korean War: A 25-Year Perspective* (Kansas, 1977); as well as the U. S. official histories.

116. N. A. Graebner, *America as a World Power* (Wilmington, Del., 1984), ch. 7, "Global Containment: The Truman Years"; Tucker, *Patterns in the Dust*, passim; D. Borg and W. Heinrichs (eds.), *Uncertain Years: Chinese-American Relations, 1947–50* (New York, 1980), passim; Schaller, *American Occupation of Japan*, chs. 11–15; E. M. Irving, *The First Indochina War: French and American Policy, 1945–1954* (London, 1975).

117. For the stiffer mood, see Gaddis, *Strategies of Containment*, chs. 5–6. See also the thoughtful piece by R. Jervis, "The Impact of the Korean War on the Cold War," *Journal of Conflict Resolution*, vol. 24, no. 4 (December 1980), pp. 563–92.

118. "Correlates of War" print-out data.

119. See also the chart in R. W. DeGrasse, *Military Expansion, Economic Decline* (Armonk, NY, 1983), p. 119.

120. Holloway, *Soviet Union and the Arms Race*, pp. 43, 115ff. It is, of course, impossible to obtain reliable Soviet spending figures, and the "explicit" defense-expenditure share of the budget is much too low; see F. D. Holzman, *Financial Checks on Soviet Defense Expenditures* (Lexington, Mass., 1975), passim.

121. Cited in Gaddis, *Strategies of Containment*, p. 100. See also S. F. Wells, "Sounding the Tocsin: NSC-68 and the Soviet Threat," *International Security*, vol. 4 (Fall 1979), pp. 116–38, and Paul Nitze's reply, "The Development of NSC-68," *International Security*, Spring 1980, pp. 159–69; Paul Y. Hammond, "NSC-68: Prologue to Rearmament," in W. R. Schilling et al., *Strategy, Politics, and Defense Budgets* (New York, 1962), pp. 267–378.

122. See Bartlett, *Global Conflict*, pp. 303ff; and the details on NATO's build-up in Ismay, *NATO*, passim; T. P. Ireland, *Creating the Entangling Alliance* (London, 1981); and Kaplan, *United States and NATO*, pp. 143ff.

123. Mackintosh, *Juggernaut*, pp. 292ff; the various essays in Liddell Hart (ed.), *Red Army*, pt. 2; Wolfe, *Soviet Power and Europe*, passim; A. Lee, *The Soviet Air Force* (London, 1961); R. Kilmarx, *A History of Soviet Air Power* (London, 1962).

124. Reynolds, *Command of the Sea*, pp. 530–43; Kennedy, *Rise and Fall of British Naval Mastery*, ch. 11.

125. Reynolds, *Command of the Sea*, pp. 545ff; Hagan (ed.), *In Peace and War: Interpretations of American Naval History 1775–1978*, chs. 15–16; Potter (ed.), *Sea Power*, chs. 31–32; J. Woods (pseud.), "The Royal Navy Since World War II," *U.S. Naval Institute Proceedings*, vol. 108, no. 3 (March 1982), pp. 82ff.

126. Mitchell, *History of Russian and Soviet Sea Power*, chs. 21–22, covers the post-1945 buildup. See also N. Polmar, *Soviet Naval Developments, 1982* (4th edn., Annapolis, Md., 1981), pp. 3–13; R. W. Herrick, *Soviet Naval Strategy* (Annapolis, Md., 1968); L. L. Whetton, "The Mediterranean Threat," *Survival*, no. 8 (August 1980), pp. 252–58; G. Jukes, "The Indian Ocean in Soviet Naval Policy," *Adelphi Papers*, no. 87 (May 1972). Very important in this connection are the works of M. MccGwire, *Soviet Naval Developments* (New York, 1973), *Soviet Naval Policy* (New York, 1975), and *Soviet Naval Influence* (New York, 1977), summarized in idem, "The Rationale for the Development of Soviet Seapower," in J. Baylis and G. Segal (eds.), *Soviet Strategy* (London, 1981), pp. 210ff.

127. On which see G. Herken, *The Winning Weapon: The Atomic Bomb in the Cold War 1945–1950* (New York, 1980); Freedman, *Evolution of Nuclear Strategy*, pp. 38ff; but see also H. R. Borowski, *A Hollow Threat: Strategic Air Power and Containment before Korea* (Westport, Conn., 1982). For implications and comparisons, M. Mandelbaum, *The Nuclear Revolution: International Politics Before and After Hiroshima* (New York, 1981).

128. Prados, *Soviet Estimate*, ch. 4, is best here.

129. Gaddis, *Strategies of Containment*, chs. 4–5, gives the overall context. See also D. A. Rosenberg, "American Atomic Strategy and the Hydrogen Bomb Decision," *Journal of American History*, vol. 66 (June 1979), pp. 62–87; idem, " 'A Smoking Radiating Ruin at the End of Two Hours': Documents on American Plans for Nuclear War with the Soviet Union, 1954–55," *International Security*, vol. 6, no. 3 (Winter 1981–82), pp. 3–38; Freedman, *Evolution of Nuclear Strategy*, ch. 6; Weigley, *The American Way of War*, ch. 17.

130. Prados, *Soviet Estimate*, chs. 5–8; also E. Bottome, *The Missile Gap* (Rutherford, N.J., 1971), passim.

131. Freedman, *Evolution of Nuclear Strategy*, pp. 175ff; Friedberg, "A History of the U.S. Strategic 'Doctrine,' 1945 to 1980," pp. 41ff. Also very useful is John Gaddis, "The Origins of Self-Deterrence: The United States and the Non-Use of Nuclear Weapons, 1945–1958" (ms.). The strategic thinkers are discussed in G. Herken, *Counsels of War* (New York, 1985), and F. Kaplan, *The Wizards of Armageddon* (New York, 1983).

132. R. V. Daniels, *Russia, The Roots of Confrontation* (Cambridge, Mass., 1985), p. 234; McCauley, *The Soviet Union Since 1917*, pp. 155ff; Ulam, *Expansion and Coexistence*, chs. 9–10.

133. Steele, *Pax Americana*, p. 9; and, in more detail, R. E. Osgood, *NATO: The Entangling Alliance* (Chicago, Ill., 1962), passim; DePorte, *Europe Between the Superpowers*, pp. 115ff; Kaplan, *United States and NATO*.

134. Steele, *Pax Americana*, p. 134. See also R. Aron, *The Imperial Republic* (London, 1975); D. Horowitz, *The Free World Colossus* (New York, 1971 edn.); Schulzinger, *American Diplomacy in the Twentieth Century*, chs. 11–12.

135. Keylor, *Twentieth-Century World*, p. 375; J. L. Gaddis, "The Strategic Perspective: The Rise and Fall of the 'Defensive Perimeter' Concept," in Borg and Heinrichs (eds.), *Uncertain Years*, pp. 61–118; and—with some very good quotations—Schaller, *The American Occupation of Japan*, pp. 279ff.

136. Quoted in Woodruff, *America's Impact on the World*, p. 65.

137. Ulam, *Expansion and Coexistence*, pp. 539ff; McCauley, *Soviet Union Since 1917*, pp. 198ff; Daniels, *Russia: The Roots of Confrontation*, pp. 333ff.

138. The literature on this topic is now overwhelming. Among the more important studies are G. Jukes, *The Soviet Union in Asia* (Berkeley, Calif., 1973); H. D. Cohn, *Soviet Policy Toward Black Africa* (New York, 1972); R. H. Donaldson, *Soviet Policy Toward India* (Cambridge, Mass., 1974); R. Kanet (ed.), *The Soviet*

Union and the Developing Nations (Baltimore, Md., 1974); E. Taborsky, *Communist Penetration of the Third World* (New York, 1963).

139. P. Lyon, "The Emergence of the Third World," in H. Bull and A. Watson (eds.), *The Expansion of International Society* (Oxford, 1984), pp. 229ff, as well as the other essays in sec. 3; Barraclough, *Introduction to Contemporary History,* ch. 6; R. Emerson, *From Empire to Nation: The Rise to Self-Assertion of Asian and African Peoples* (Cambridge, Mass., 1962), passim.

140. Lyon, "Emergence of the Third World," in Bull and Watson (eds.), *Expansion of International Society,* p. 229; idem, *Neutralism* (Leicester, 1963); G. H. Jansen, *Afro-Asia and Non-Alignment* (London, 1966).

141. Apart from the works in note 139 above, see also L. S. Stavrianos, *Global Rift: The Third World Comes of Age* (New York, 1981); R. A. Mortimer, *The Third World Coalition in International Politics* (New York, 1980); R. L. Rothstein, *The Weak in the World of the Strong: The Developing Countries in the International System* (New York, 1977); idem, *The Third World and U.S. Foreign Policy* (Boulder, Colo., 1981).

142. Balfour, *Adversaries,* pp. 157ff; Ulam, *Expansion and Coexistence,* pp. 461ff; D. Rusinov, *The Yugoslav Experiment, 1948–1974* (London, 1977); Lyon, "Emergence of the Third World," passim.

143. McCauley, *Soviet Union Since 1917,* p. 204. More generally, see the references in note 138 above, and R. C. Horn, *The Soviet Union and India: The Limits of Influence* (New York, 1981); R. H. Donaldson (ed.), *The Soviet Union in the Third World: Successes and Failures* (Boulder, Colo., 1981); M. H. Haykal, *The Sphinx and the Commissar: The Rise and Fall of Soviet Influence in the Middle East* (London, 1978); K. Dawisha, *Soviet Foreign Policy Towards Egypt* (London, 1979), passim.

144. McCauley, *Soviet Union Since 1917,* p. 210; Donaldson (ed.), *Soviet Union in the Third World: Successes and Failures,* passim; A. Dawisha and K. Dawisha (eds.), *The Soviet Union in the Middle East* (New York, 1982).

145. "Correlates of War" print-out data, which is more reliable than *Military Balance* (see following note) figures for the early 1970s.

146. *The Military Balance 1974–75* (London, 1974), pp. 7, 10; cf. pp. 19, 22.

147. H. Pemsel, *Atlas of Naval Warfare* (London, 1977), p. 159.

148. *Military Balance 1974–75,* pp. 75–77; for China, pp. 48–49.

149. See the references in note 126 above.

150. For Soviet-American relations in the 1970s, see Keylor, *Twentieth-Century World,* pp. 364ff, 405ff; Schulzinger, *American Diplomacy in the Twentieth Century,* pp. 299ff; S. Hoffman, *Primacy or World Order* (New York, 1978), passim; Lawson, *Soviet-American Rivalry,* passim; McCauley, *Soviet Union Since 1917,* pp. 238ff; Daniels, *Russia: The Roots of Confrontation,* pp. 321ff, and the full bibliography on pp. 394–96. Above all, there is now R. L. Garthoff, *Détente and Confrontation: American-Soviet Relations from Nixon to Reagan* (Washington, D.C., 1985), with enormous detail.

151. Keylor, *Twentieth-Century World,* p. 371.

152. For what follows see R. C. Thornton, *The Bear and the Dragon* (New York, 1972); R. C. North, *Moscow and the Chinese Communists* (Stanford, Calif. 1953); R. R. Simmons, *The Strained Alliance* (New York, 1975); G. Ginsburgs and C. F. Pinkele, *The Sino-Soviet Territorial Dispute, 1949–64* (New York, 1978); D. Floyd, *Mao Against Khrushchev* (New York, 1964); A. D. Low, *The Sino-Soviet Dispute* (Rutherford, N.J., 1976); and a good brief summary in Bartlett, *Global Conflict,* pp. 325ff.

153. Ulam, *Expansion and Coexistence,* p. 693; O. E. Clubb, *China and Russia: The "Great Game"* (New York, 1971), passim, gives more details, as does J. Camil-

leri, *Chinese Foreign Policy: The Maoist Era and Its Aftermath* (Seattle, Wash., 1980).

154. Keylor, *Twentieth-Century World*, p. 398.
155. H. Kissinger, *The White House Years* (Boston, 1979), pp. 172ff; and the important analysis in D. L. Strode, "Arms Control and Sino-Soviet Relations," *Orbis*, vol. 28, no. 1 (Spring 1984), pp. 163–88.
156. Gaddis, *Strategies of Containment*, p. 210, fn.
157. W. E. Griffith (ed.), *Communism in Europe: Continuity, Change and the Sino-Soviet Dispute*, 2 vols. (Cambridge, Mass., 1964–66); J. G. Whelan, *World Communism, 1967–1969: Soviet Attempts to Reestablish Control* (Library of Congress, Legislative Reference Service, Washington, D.C., 1970); Z. Brzezinski, *The Soviet Bloc: Unity and Conflict* (Cambridge, Mass., 1967 edn.).
158. See the nice, brief survey by C. Bell, "China and the International Order," in Bull and Watson (ed.), *Expansion of International Society*, ch. 17; more detailed in M. B. Yahuda, *China's Role in World Affairs* (New York, 1978).
159. Cited in W. L. Kohl, *French Nuclear Diplomacy* (Princeton, N.J., 1971), p. 103. See also W. Mendl, *Deterrence and Persuasion: French Nuclear Armament in the Context of National Policy, 1945–1969* (London, 1970); M. M. Harrison, *Reluctant Ally: France and Atlantic Security* (Baltimore, Md., 1981); and espec. E. Kolodziej, *French International Policy Under de Gaulle and Pompidou: The Politics of Grandeur* (Ithaca, N.Y., 1974).
160. Kolodziej, *French International Policy*, passim; A. Grosser, *The Western Alliance: European-American Relations since 1945* (London, 1980), pp. 183ff, 209ff.
161. See below, pp. 427–28.
162. There is a succinct survey of de Gaulle's policies in De Porte, *Europe Between the Superpowers*, pp. 229ff; and Keylor, *Twentieth-Century World*, pp. 346ff.
163. Bairoch, "International Industrialization Levels," p. 304.
164. Keylor, *Twentieth-Century World*, pp. 354ff, 408ff; A. Bronke and D. Novak (eds.), *The Communist States in the Era of Detente, 1971–1977* (Oakville, Ont., 1979); R. L. Tokes, *Euro-Communism and Détente* (New York, 1978); G. B. Ginsburgs and A. Z. Rubinstein (eds.), *Soviet Foreign Policy Towards Western Europe* (New York, 1978); L. L. Whetten, *Germany's Ostpolitik* (London, 1971); and W. E. Griffith, *The Ostpolitik of the Federal Republic of Germany* (Cambridge, Mass., 1978), cover the German aspects.
165. H. Salisbury, *The Coming War Between Russia and China* (London, 1969), passim.
166. Some of these concerns are discussed in E. Morton and G. Segal (eds.), *Soviet Strategy Toward Western Europe* (London, 1984).
167. Bartlett, *Global Conflict*, p. 355. See also G. Segal, *The Great Power Triangle* (London, 1982); R. Sutter, *China Watch: Toward Sino-American Reconciliation* (Baltimore, Md., 1978), passim; and the essays in R. H. Solomon (ed.), *The China Factor: Sino-American Relations and the Global Scene* (New York, 1981), and G. Segal (ed.), *The China Factor: Peking and the Superpowers* (London, 1982), espec. B. Garrett, "The United States and the Great Power Triangle," pp. 76–104.
168. Gaddis, *Strategies of Containment*, pp. 249–50, 259.
169. A. Kendrick, *The Wound Within: America in the Vietnam Years, 1945–1974* (Boston, 1974); T. Powers, *The War at Home: Vietnam and the American People, 1964–1968* (New York, 1973); F. Fitzgerald, *Fire in the Lake: The Vietnamese and the Americans in Vietnam* (Boston, 1972); W. O'Neill, *Coming Apart* (New York, 1971); R. J. Lifton, *Home from the War: Vietnam Veterans* (New York, 1973); L. Baskir and P. Strauss, *Chance and Circumstance: The War, The Draft, and the Vietnam Generation* (New York, 1978); and G. Kolko,

Vietnam: Anatomy of a War, 1940–1975 (New York, 1986), are among some of the welter of good books on these themes.

170. Again, the literature on the American strategy and conduct of the war is already overwhelming. Millett and Maslowski, *For the Common Defense*, ch. 17, is a good summary. H. G. Summers, *On Strategy: A Critical Analysis of the Vietnam War* (New York, 1972) examines the war through Clausewitzian spectacles. B. Palmer, *The 25-Year War: America's Military Role in Vietnam* (New York, 1984), espec. pt. 2, "Assessment"; S. Karnow, *Vietnam: A History* (New York, 1984); G. C. Herring, *America's Longest War: The United States and Vietnam, 1950–1975* (New York, 1979), are all important.

171. Figures from Gaddis, *Strategies of Containment*, p. 359; see also Millett and Maslowski, *For the Common Defense*, pp. 565ff.

172. See again Ungar (ed.), *Estrangement: America and the World*, passim; but especially G. Hodgson, "Disorder Within, Disorder Without."

173. This may be seen, *inter alia*, in the titles of many American studies on the international system and the United States' place in it. Apart from Ungar (ed.), *Estrangement*, see also K. A. Oye et al. (eds.), *Eagle Entangled: U.S. Foreign Policy in a Complex World* (New York, 1979); R. D. Keohane, *After Hegemony* (Princeton, N.J., 1974); J. Kwitny, *Endless Enemies* (New York, 1984); and the important earlier work S. Hoffman, *Gulliver's Troubles* (New York, 1968).

174. Gaddis, *Strategies of Containment*, p. 275. And see again the references in note 167 above, and the very useful survey in Garthoff, *Détente and Confrontation*, pp. 24ff.

175. Gaddis, *Strategies of Containment*, p. 179. See also Kissinger's own *White House Years*; and H. Starr, *Henry Kissinger: Perceptions of International Politics* (Lexington, Ky., 1982), passim. Dallek, *American Style of Foreign Policy*, ch. 9, is much more critical.

176. Gaddis, *Strategies of Containment*, pp. 284, 297.

177. Compare Kennan, *Decline of Bismarck's European Order*, with Kissinger, "The White Revolutionary: Reflections on Bismarck," *Daedelus*, vol. 97 (Summer 1968), pp. 888–924.

178. Gaddis, *Strategies of Containment*, pp. 280–82; and, in more detail, two fine studies: C. Bell, *The Diplomacy of Détente: The Kissinger Era* (New York, 1977); and R. S. Litwak, *Détente and the Nixon Doctrine: American Foreign Policy and the Pursuit of Stability, 1969–1975* (Cambridge, 1984).

179. Apart from the (often contradictory) memoirs of Carter, his secretary of state, Vance, and his national security adviser, Brzezinski, see the coverage in Garthoff, *Détente and Confrontation*, pp. 563ff; and, much more briefly, Ambrose, *Rise to Globalism*, ch. 15; Schulzinger, *American Diplomacy*, pp. 316ff; and John Gaddis's final thoughts in the "Epilogue" to *Strategies of Containment*. Above all, see G. Smith, *Morality, Reason and Power: American Diplomacy in the Carter Years* (New York, 1986), passim, but espec. pp. 241ff.

180. B. Rubin, *Paved with Good Intentions: The United States and Iran* (New York, 1980), passim; G. Sick, *All Fall Down: America's Tragic Encounter with Iran* (New York, 1985); and Smith, *Morality, Reason and Power*, ch. 9, are best here.

181. Garthoff, *Détente and Confrontation*, chs. 26–27, is best here.

182. See, *inter alia*, J. S. Gansler, *The Defense Industry* (Cambridge, Mass., 1980), passim; J. Fallows, *National Defense* (New York, 1981), especially ch. 3; R. W. DeGrasse, *Military Expansion, Economic Decline* (Armonk, N.Y., 1983); J. Coates and M. Kilian, *Heavy Losses* (New York, 1985 edn.), passim.

183. See the biting comments in Schulzinger, *American Diplomacy*, pp. 339ff; S. Talbott, *Deadly Gambits: The Reagan Administration and the Stalemate in Nuclear Arms Control* (New York, 1984), with revealing details; Haig's own

memoir, *Caveat* (New York, 1984); E. Luttwak, *The Pentagon and the Art of War* (New York, 1985).

184. Ulam, *Dangerous Relations: The Soviet Union in World Politics 1970–1982* (New York, 1983), p. 39.

185. D. Holloway, *The Soviet Union and the Arms Race* (New Haven, 1984, 2nd ed.), pp. 134ff; and the more technical analysis is A. Bergson, "Technological Progress," in Bergson and H. S. Levine (eds.), *The Soviet Economy: Toward the Years 2000* (London, 1983), pp. 34–78.

186. Garthoff, *Détente and Confrontation,* pp. 887ff, is excellent here. See also H. S. Bradsher, *Afghanistan and the Soviet Union* (Durham, N.C., 1983), passim; and T. T. Hammond, *Red Flag over Afghanistan* (Boulder, Colo., 1984), passim.

187. Garthoff, *Détente and Confrontation,* pp. 982ff. See also the works cited in note 167 above, as well as B. Garrett, "China Policy and the Constraints of Triangular Logic," in K. A. Oye et al. (eds.), *Eagle Defiant: United States Foreign Policy in the 1980s* (Boston, 1983), espec. pp. 245ff.

188. Gaddis, *Strategies of Containment,* p. 280 (my emphasis).

189. This is most critically the case, of course, in respect to *Russian* data: see F. D. Holzmann, "Soviet Military Spending: Assessing the Numbers Game," *International Security,* vol. 6, no. 4 (Spring 1982), pp. 78–101, which is a good introduction to this subject.

190. Bairoch, "International Industrialization Levels," p. 276.

191. Rostow, *World Economy,* p. 662. (The chief difference is that Rostow uses a 1913 = 100 baseline, whereas Bairoch has chosen 1900.)

192. Bairoch, "International Industrialization Levels," p. 273.

193. Ibid., p. 276.

194. From Rostow, *World Economy,* p. 669.

195. Ashworth, *Short History of the International Economy,* pp. 287–88.

196. Ibid., p. 289; and the more detailed discussion in Bairoch, *The Economic Development of the Third World Since 1900* (Berkeley, Calif., 1975), passim.

197. Foreman-Peck, *History of the World Economy,* p. 376.

198. Bairoch, "International Industrialization Levels," p. 304.

199. See the table in Oye et al. (eds.), *Eagle Defiant,* p. 8.

200. G. Blackburn, *The West and the World Since 1945* (New York, 1985), p. 96; and Bairoch, *Economic Development,* passim, with a good bibliography on pp. 250–52.

201. R. Rosecrance, *The Rise of the Trading State* (New York, 1985), espec. ch. 7; and M. Smith et al., *Asia's New Industrial World* (New York, 1985).

202. See Schaller, *American Occupation of Japan,* p. 289.

203. Of which perhaps the most important study has been E. F. Vogel, *Japan as Number One: Lessons for America* (New York, 1980 edn.).

204. Smith et al., p. 18; C. Johnson, *MITI and the Japanese Miracle* (Stanford, Calif., 1982), passim.

205. Vogel, *Japan as Number One,* pp. 9–10 (my emphasis). Allen, *A Short Economic History of Modern Japan,* pt. 2, is very valuable here. The automobile statistics come from *The Economist,* November 2, 1985, p. 111.

206. Most of the writings upon China after 1945 seem to have focused upon Mao or upon cultural/ideological issues, rather than its external policy: but there is Bell, "China and the International Order," in Bull and Watson (eds.), *The Expansion of International Society,* pp. 255–67; H. Harding (ed.), *China's Foreign Relations in the 1980s* (New Haven, Conn., 1984), espec. chs. 1 and 5–6; A. D. Barnett, *China and the Major Powers in East Asia* (Washington, D.C., 1977); M. Yahuda, *China's Role in World Affairs* (New York, 1978); P. Van Ness, *Revolution and Chinese Foreign Policy* (Berkeley, Calif., 1971); and R. H. Sol-

omon (ed.), *The China Factor: Sino-American Relations and the Global Scene* (Englewood Cliffs, N.J., 1981), with some very useful chapters.

207. Bairoch, "International Industrialization Levels," pp. 299, 302.
208. Rostow, *World Economy*, pp. 525ff; and D. H. Perkins (ed.), *China's Modern Economy in Historical Perspective* (Stanford, Calif., 1975), passim.
209. Blackburn, *West and the World Since 1945*, p. 77.
210. Ibid.; and Bairoch, *Economic Development of the Third World*, pp. 188ff, 201ff, which comments approvingly on the attention the Chinese gave to agriculture.
211. "Correlates of War" print-out data for 1980.
212. Bairoch, "International Industrialization Levels," p. 304.
213. D. H. Perkins, "The International Consequences of China's Economic Development," in Solomon (ed.), *China Factor*, pp. 114–136, is important here.
214. Some of Europe's dilemmas are discussed in DePorte, *Europe Between the Superpowers*, passim; J. R. Wegs, *Europe Since 1945* (New York, 1984, 2nd edn.), espec. chs. 8–15; S. Holt, *The Common Market: The Conflict of Theory and Practice* (London, 1967).
215. Aldcroft, *European Economy 1914–1980*, p. 161.
216. Ibid.; and see also Landes, *Unbound Prometheus*, ch. 7; Pollard, *Peaceful Conquest*, ch. 9; Maddison, "Economic Policy and Performance in Europe 1913–1970," in Cipolla (ed.), *Fontana Economic History of Europe*, vol. 5, pt. 2, pp. 476ff. For the early period, there are detailed studies: M. M. Postan, *An Economic History of Western Europe, 1945–1964* (London, 1967); and A. S. Milward, *The Reconstruction of Western Europe, 1945–1951* (London, 1984).
217. Aldcroft, *European Economy*, pp. 161–62.
218. Oye et al. (eds.), *Eagle Defiant*, p. 8, and notes in Table 1-1.
219. For this argument, see again Pollard, *Peaceful Conquest*, passim.
220. Ibid., p. 305
221. Ibid., p. 171.
222. Aldcroft, *European Economy*, p. 161.
223. See the data in Wegs, *Europe Since 1945*, ch. 9; A. S. Deaton, "The Structure of Demand 1920–1970," in Cipolla (ed.), *Fontana Economic History of Europe*, vol. 5, pt. 1.
224. Ricossa, "Italy, 1920–1970," in Cipolla (ed.), *Fontana Economic History of Europe*, vol. 6, pt. 1, pp. 290ff; G. Scimone, "The Italian Miracle," in J. Hennessy et al., *Economic "Miracles"* (London, 1964); G. H. Hildebrand, *Growth and Structure in the Economy of Modern Italy* (Cambridge, Mass., 1965).
225. See above, pp. 367–68.
226. Porter, *Britain, Europe and the World*, ch. 5; Kennedy, *Realities behind Diplomacy*, chs. 7–8.
227. The literature on Britain's post-1945 relative economic decline is enormous. See, *inter alia*, Gamble, *Britain in Decline*, passim; Kirby, *Decline of British Economic Power Since 1870*, ch. 5; F. Blackaby (ed.), *De-industrialization* (London, 1979), passim; W. Beckerman (ed.), *Slow Growth in Britain: Causes and Consequences* (Oxford, 1979); J. Eatwell, *Whatever Happened to Britain?* (London, 1982), passim.
228. Bairoch, "International Industrialization Levels," p. 303.
229. Wegs, *Europe Since 1945*, p. 161. The figures for world manufacturing production are from Bairoch, those for shares of world trade from Kirby, *Decline*, p. 149, table 15.
230. V. Berghahn, *Unternehmer und Politik in der Bundesrepublik* (Frankfurt, 1985), passim; K. Hardach, *The Political Economy of Germany in the Twentieth Century* (Berkeley, Calif., 1980), pp. 140ff.
231. For fuller details, Hardach, *Political Economy of Germany*, pp. 178ff; L. Er-

hard's satisfied account, *The Economics of Success* (Princeton, N.J., 1963), passim; Hardach, "Germany 1914–1970," in Cipolla (ed.), *Fontana Economic History of Europe*, vol 6., pt. 1, pp. 217ff; Landes, *Unbound Prometheus*, pp. 502ff, 531ff; Balfour, *Adversaries*, pp. 122ff.

232. Hardach, "Germany 1914–1970," in Cipolla (ed.), *Fontana Economic History of Europe*, vol. 6, pt. 1, p. 221.

233. Wegs, *Europe Since 1945*, p. 161.

234. The Federal Republic's diplomatic and security concerns, and the attitude of other Powers to them, are examined in DePorte, *Europe Between the Superpowers*, pp. 1180ff; C. M. Kelleher, *Germany and the Politics of Nuclear Weapons* (New York, 1975); W. F. Hanrieden, *West German Foreign Policy 1949–1963* (Stanford, Calif., 1967); Willis, *France, Germany and the New Europe*, passim; Calleo, *The German Problem Reconsidered*, pp. 161ff; P. Windsor, *German Reunification* (London, 1969), passim; Kaiser, *German Foreign Policy in Transition*, passim; Gruner, *Die deutsche Frage*, pp. 176ff.

235. Bairoch, "International Industrialization Levels," p. 302.

236. Fohlen, "France 1920–1970," in Cipolla (ed.), *Fontana Economic History of Europe*, vol. 6, pt. 1, pp. 100ff; E. Malinraud, *La Croissance française* (Paris, 1972), passim; M. Parodi, *L'économie et la société française de 1945 à 1970* (Paris, 1971); Caron, *Economic History of Modern France*, pp. 182ff; R. F. Kuisel, *Capitalism and the State in Modern France* (Cambridge, 1981), chs. 7–9; and Kindleberger, "The Postwar Resurgence of the French Economy," in S. Hoffman (ed.), *In Search of France* (Cambridge, Mass., 1963).

237. See again Kolodziej, *French International Policy Under de Gaulle and Pompidou: The Politics of Grandeur.*

238. See the statistics in the CIA's *Handbook of Economic Statistics, 1984*, pp. 16ff.

239. See, for example, Hosking, *History of the Soviet Union*, appendix C ("Selected Indices of Industrial and Agricultural Production"), p. 483; Munting, *Economic Development of the USSR*, p. 133; Nove, *Economic History of the USSR*, pp. 340, 387; J. P. Nettl, *The Soviet Achievement* (London, 1967), ch. 6.

240. Munting, *Economic Development of the USSR*, p. 133.

241. The problems of Soviet agriculture have been the focus of massive attention in the scholarly literature; see, in particular, the useful essays 4 and 5 in Bergson and Levine (eds.), *Soviet Economy: Toward the Year 2000*; D. M. Schooner, "Soviet Agricultural Policies," in *Soviet Economy in a Time of Change* (Washington, D.C., 1979; Papers, Joint Economic Committee, U.S. Congress), pp. 87–115; and Munting, *Economic Development of the USSR*, pp. 142ff, 160ff.

242. CIA, *Handbook of Economic Statistics, 1984*, p. 27.

243. Cipolla (ed.), *Fontana Economic History of Europe*, vol. 5, pt. 2, pp. 476ff, and vol. 6, pt. 2, pp. 593ff; N. Spulber, *The State and Economic Development in Eastern Europe* (New York, 1966), passim; Kaser, *Comecon*, passim; and an excellent summary in Aldcroft, *European Economy 1914–1980*, ch. 6.

244. Nove, *Economic History*, pp. 330ff, 363ff; Bergson and Levine (eds.), *Soviet Economy: Toward the Year 2000*, p. 148.

245. Details in M. I. Goldman, *The Enigma of Soviet Petroleum* (London/Boston, 1980), which has a rosier view of the future of Russian oil production than the CIA, but acknowledges the problem of waste.

246. Much of this will be discussed again in the final chapter, but see Bergson and Levine (eds.), *Soviet Economy: Toward the Year 2000*, espec. pp. 402ff; H. S. Rowen, "Living with a Sick Bear," *National Interest*, no. 2 (Winter 1985–86), pp. 14–26; M. I. Goldman, *USSR in Crisis: The Failure of an Economic System* (New York, 1983); P. Dibb, *The Soviet Union: The Incomplete Super-power*

(London, 1985), ch. 3; T. J. Colton, *The Dilemma of Reform in the Soviet Union* (New York, 1984), passim. For eastern Europe's problems, see the "Cracks in the Soviet Empire?" issue of *International Security*, vol. 6, no. 3 (Winter 1981–82).

247. Bairoch, "International Industrialization Levels," p. 304.

248. See Table 43 below; and cf. CIA, *Handbook of Economic Statistics, 1984*, p. 4—which (being computed in U.S. dollars) will presumably have quite altered figures for 1987, because of the decline in the value of the American currency.

249. Balfour, *Adversaries*, p. 204.

250. Ibid., p. 193.

251. L. Thurow, "America Among Equals," in Ungar (ed.), *Estrangement*, pp. 159–78; idem, *The Zero-Sum Game* (New York, 1980), passim, but espec. chs. 1 and 4; DeGrasse, *Military Expansion, Economic Decline*, espec. ch. 2.

252. See, in particular, Grosser, *Western Alliance*, pp. 217ff; J. J. Servan-Schreiber, *The American Challenge* (Harmondsworth, Middlesex, 1969 edn.), espec. pt. 2; R. Barnet, *Global Reach* (New York, 1974), passim; S. Rolfe, *The International Corporation* (Paris, 1969); as well as Woodruff, *America's Impact on the World*, ch. 4.

253. Becker and Wells (ed.), *Economics and World Power*, chs. 7–8; D. Calleo, *The Imperious Economy* (Cambridge, Mass., 1982), passim; J. Gowa, *Closing the Gold Window: Domestic Politics and the End of Bretton Woods* (Ithaca, N.Y., 1983); G. Epstein, "The Triple Debt Crisis," *World Policy Journal*, vol. 2, no. 4 (Fall 1985), pp. 628ff; *Economist*, October 5, 1985, "Monetary Reform" Survey, p. 11.

254. Thurow, "America Among Equals," in Ungar (ed.), *Estrangement*, p. 163.

255. Idem, *Zero-Sum Society*, pp. 3–4. (The U.S. figures presumably looked better with the dollar's rise, 1983–1985, and worsened again with the currency's post-1985 decline.)

256. Calleo, "Since 1961: American Power in a New World," in Becker and Wells (eds.), *Economics and World Power*, pp. 391–93.

257. Oye et al. (eds), *Eagle Defiant*, p. 8 (with a note about the sources used).

258. I have taken the population and GNP per capita figures from Chaliand and Gageau, *Strategic Atlas*, pp. 214–20, which bases its figures on the World Bank's *Report on World Development, 1982*. The total GNP is my extrapolation.

259. Given the assertion by Perkins, in Solomon (ed.), *China Factor*, pp. 118–119, that China's per capita GNP in 1979 was more likely between $400 and $500 than the official conversion figure of $266, I have included a calculation for 1980 based on $450 per capita.

260. Cited in Gilpin, *War and Change in World Politics*, pp. 76–77.

CHAPTER EIGHT
To the Twenty-first Century

1. Keylor, *Twentieth-Century World*, p. 405.

2. The classic statement here is E. H. Carr, *What Is History?* (Harmondsworth, Mddsx., 1964), ch. 1, "The Historian and his Facts"; but see also D. Thomson, *The Aims of History* (London, 1969), ch. 4.

3. See, *inter alia*, Gilpin, *War and Change in World Politics*; G. Modelski, "The Long Cycle of Global Politics and the Nation-State," *Comparative Studies in Society and History*, vol. 20 (April 1978), pp. 214–35; Rasler and Thompson, "Global Wars, Public Debts, and the Long Cycle," passim; McNeill, *Pursuit of Power*, passim; Rosecrance, *Action and Reaction in World Politics*, passim.

4. As in the well-known quotation in *Herr Eugen Dühring's Revolution in Science* (London, 1936), p. 188.
5. The political-science literature here is overwhelming. For a sampling, see M. Wight, *Power Politics* (Harmondsworth, Mddsx., 1979); K. Waltz, *Man, the State and War* (New York, 1959); H. Bull, *The Anarchical Society* (New York, 1977).
6. See, for example, P. F. Drucker, "The Changed World Economy," *Foreign Affairs,* vol. 64, no. 4 (Spring 1986), pp. 768–91—a remarkable article. See also the figures given in "Beyond Factory Robots," *Economist,* July 5, 1986, p. 61.
7. Drucker, "Changed World Economy," pp. 771–72; "China and India," *Economist,* Dec. 21, 1985, pp. 66–67.
8. Again, the literature on this theme is immense. For good general introductions, see S. B. Linder, *The Pacific Century* (Stanford, Calif., 1986); J. W. Morley (ed.), *The Pacific Basin* (New York, 1986); M. Smith et al., *Asia's New Industrial World* (London, 1985); K. E. Calder, "The Making of a Trans-Pacific Economy," *World Policy Journal,* vol. 2, no. 4 (Fall 1985), pp. 593–623.
9. Linder, *Pacific Century,* pp. 13–14.
10. Ibid., pp. 6, 15.
11. P. Drysdale, "The Pacific Basin and Its Economic Vitality," in Morley (ed.), *Pacific Basin,* p. 11.
12. Mathias, *First Industrial Nation,* p. 44.
13. M. Kaldor, *The Baroque Arsenal* (London, 1982), p. 18. For further examples—from a quite different source—see F. Cooper, "Affordable Defense: In Search of a Strategy," *Journal of the Royal United Services Institute for Defense Studies,* vol. 130, no. 4 (December 1985), p. 4. Also very useful is the special survey "Defense Technology," *Economist,* May 21, 1983.
14. The key work here (by an in-house expert) is J. S. Gansler, *The Defense Industry* (Cambridge, Mass., 1980).
15. On which see McNeill, *Pursuit of Power,* passim; and Kaldor, *Baroque Arsenal,* passim.
16. *The Military Balance 1985–86,* pp. 170–73; and the SIPRI (Stockholm International Peace Research Institute) publication *The Arms Race and Arms Control* (London, 1982), especially chs. 2–3.
17. L. Brown et al., *State of the World, 1986* (New York, 1986), p. 196.
18. "Excessive" is, of course, a haphazard term; for if a country feels under acute pressure from foreign foes (e.g., Israel), it seems inappropriate to employ that term. On the other hand, the historical record suggests that if a particular nation is allocating *over the long term* more than 10 percent (and in some cases—when it is structurally weak—more than 5 percent) of GNP to armaments, that is likely to limit its growth rate.
19. For some examples of this, see Cipolla (ed.), *Economic Decline of Empires,* passim; Kennedy, *Strategy and Diplomacy,* ch. 3; F. Lewis, "Military Spending Questioned," *New York Times,* Nov. 11, 1986, pp. D1, D5.
20. Reported in "The Elusive Boom in Productivity," *New York Times,* April 8, 1984, business section, pp. 1, 26. See also "Richer Than You," *Economist,* Oct. 25, 1986, pp. 13–14.
21. See T. Fingar (ed.), *China's Quest for Independence* (Boulder, Colo., 1980), passim; G. Segal and W. Tow (eds.), *Chinese Defense Policy* (London, 1984); Chaliand and Rageau, *Strategic Atlas,* p. 143; and the important essays in R. H. Solomon (ed.), *The China Factor: Sino-American Relations and the Global Scene* (Englewood Cliffs, N. J., 1981); and J. Camilleri, *Chinese Foreign Policy: The Maoist Era and Its Aftermath* (Seattle, Wash., 1980).
22. G. Segal, *Defending China* (London, 1985), covers in detail the decline in

Chinese combat effectiveness; see also H. W. Jencks, *From Missiles to Muskets: Politics and Professionalism in the Chinese Army 1945–1981* (Boulder, Colo., 1982).

23. See D. H. Perkins, "The International Consequences of China's Economic Development," in Solomon (ed.), *China Factor*, p. 118.

24. See the important article "A New Long March in China," *Economist*, Jan. 25, 1986, pp. 29–31; J. T. Dreyer, "China's Military Modernization," *Orbis*, vol. 27, no. 4 (Winter 1984), pp. 1011–26; *Military Balance 1985–1986*, pp. 111–15; M. Y. M. Kan, "Deng's Quest for Military Modernization and National Security," in *Mainland China's Modernization: Its Prospects and Problems* (Berkeley, Calif., 1982), pp. 227–44.

25. Dreyer, "China's Military Modernization," p. 1017.

26. Ibid., p. 1016. See also J. D. Pollack, "China as a Nuclear Power," in W. H. Overholt (ed.), *Asia's Nuclear Future* (Boulder, Colo., 1977), passim.

27. For a brief survey of these weaknesses, see again Dreyer, "China's Military Modernization," pp. 1017ff. On submarine developments, see *New York Times*, April 1, 1986, pp. C1, C3.

28. "As China Grows Strong," *Economist*, Jan. 25, 1986, p. 11; and espec. G. Segal, "Defense Culture and Sino-Soviet Relations," *Journal of Strategic Studies*, vol. 8, no. 2 (June 1985), pp. 180–98, with fuller references.

29. B. Reynolds, "China in the International Economy," in H. Harding (ed.), *China's Foreign Relations in the 1980s* (New Haven, Conn., 1984), p. 75.

30. D. H. Perkins, "The International Consequences of China's Economic Development," in Solomon (ed.), *China Factor*, pp. 115–16; and for more detail, Perkins (ed.), *China's Modern Economy in Historical Perspective* (Stanford, Calif., 1975), passim; and A. D. Barnett, *China's Economy in Global Perspective* (Washington, D.C., 1981), passim.

31. *New York Times*, March 27, 1986, p. A14; Rostow, *World Economy*, pp. 532ff.

32. Perkins, "International Consequences," in Solomon (ed.), *China Factor*, p. 128.

33. Reynolds, "China in the International Economy," in Harding (ed.), *China's Foreign Relations in the 1980s*, p. 87.

34. Quoted in Brown et al., *State of the World, 1986*, p. 19; and see also, "China and India: Two Billion People Discover the Joys of the Market," *Economist*, Dec. 21, 1985, pp. 66–67.

35. "China and India"; and see the amazing eyewitness details of the recent transformation in O. Schell, *To Get Rich Is Glorious: China in the 80s* (New York, 1985).

36. *New York Times*, March 27, 1986, p. A14; and, more generally, K. Lieberthal, "Domestic Politics and Foreign Policy," in Harding (ed.), *China's Foreign Relations in the 1980s*, pp. 58ff. See also the CIA report "China: Economic Performance in 1985" (Washington, D.C., 1986); and, finally, the extremely intelligent article by A. D. Barnett, "Ten Years After Mao," *Foreign Affairs*, vol. 65, no. 1 (Fall 1986), pp. 37–65.

37. See again the important article "China and India," *Economist*, Dec. 21, 1985, pp. 65–70, espec. p. 68; and *Ramses*, 1982, *The State of the World Economy* (Cambridge, Mass., 1982), pp. 286–87.

38. Perkins, "International Consequences," pp. 130–31.

39. *Military Balance 1985–86*, p. 112; Perkins, "The International Consequences . . .", in Solomon (ed.), *China Factor*, p. 132.

40. See the table in Brown et al., *State of the World, 1986*, p. 207.

41. Perkins, "International Consequences," in Solomon (ed.), *China Factor*, pp. 132–33; *Economist*, Jan. 25, 1986, p. 29.

42. Perkins, "International Consequences," in Solomon (ed.), *China Factor*, p. 120.

43. This projection assumes that "the four largest economies in Western Europe grow in 1985–2000 at the same pace as they did in 1970–82" (which the paper admits may be too pessimistic): "China and India," p. 69.
44. *Ramses*, 1982, p. 285; the figures in Morley (ed.), *Pacific Basin*, p. 13; Reynolds, "China in the International Economy," pp. 73–74. By comparison, see again Rosecrance, *Rise of the Trading State*, passim.
45. See again Segal, "Defense Culture and Sino-Soviet Relations," passim.
46. But note R. Taylor, *The Sino-Japanese Axis* (New York, 1985).
47. "Russia and China," *Economist*, March 29, 1986, pp. 34–35. This does not, however, make it automatically a member of an "anti-Soviet united front," as is argued in C. D. McFetridge, "Some Implications of China's Emergence as a Great Power," *Journal of the Royal United Services Institute for Defense Studies*, vol. 128, no. 3 (September 1983), p. 43.
48. On which see J. G. Stoessinger, *Nations in Darkness: China, Russia and America* (New York, 1978), passim; Solomon (ed.), *China Factor*, passim; Segal (ed.), *China Factor*, passim; and Harding (ed.), *China's Foreign Relations in the 1980s*, passim, espec. ch. 6.
49. Pollack, "China and the Global Strategic Balance," in Harding (ed.), *China's Foreign Relations in the 1980s*, pp. 173–74.
50. "A New Long March in China," *Economist*, Jan. 25, 1986, p. 31.
51. For this policy, see in particular E. A. Olsen, *U.S.-Japan Strategic Reciprocity: A Neo-Internationalist View* (Stanford, Calif., 1985), passim; the remarks on Japan in R. A. Scalapino, "China and Northeast Asia," in Solomon (ed.), *China Factor*, pp. 193ff.; Scalapino (ed.), *The Foreign Policy of Modern Japan* (Berkeley, Calif., 1977); T. J. Pempel, "Japanese Foreign Economic Policy," ch. 5 of P. J. Katzenstein (ed.), *Between Power and Plenty: Foreign Economic Policies of Advanced Industrial States* (Madison, Wis., 1978).
52. This is perhaps best argued in Vogel, *Japan as Number One;* but see also his article "Pax Nipponica?" *Foreign Affairs*, vol. 64, no. 4 (Spring 1986), pp. 752–67; and H. Kahn, *The Emerging Japanese Superstate* (London, 1971). For a contrary argument, see "High Technology: Clash of the Titans," *Economist*, Aug. 23, 1986, pp. 318ff, which points to the U.S. advantages.
53. See again Smith et al., *Asia's New Industrial World;* and Linder, *Pacific Century*, passim.
54. For what follows, see Linder, *Pacific Century*, pp. 107ff; E. Wilkinson, *Misunderstanding: Europe versus Japan* (Tokyo, 1981); "Is It Too Late to Stop the Slide to Protectionism?" *Times* (London), Jan. 14, 1982, p. 15; Olsen, *U.S.-Japan Strategic Reciprocity*, ch. 4.
55. "Japan Frets About Tomorrow," *New York Times*, April 30, 1986, pp. D1–D2.
56. "Obstacles to Change in Japan," *New York Times*, April 29, 1986, p. D1.
57. See the figures in the *CIA Handbook of Economic Statistics, 1984*, pp. 50–54; the weekly *Economist* index on commodity prices; and Drucker, "Changed World Economy," passim.
58. See the useful summary in R. B. Reich, "Japan in the Chips," *New York Review of Books*, July 5, 1985; and "Silicon Valley Has a Big Chip About Japan," *Economist*, March 20, 1986, pp. 63–64.
59. "Big Japanese Gain in Computers Seen," *New York Times*, Feb. 13, 1984, pp. A1, A19; "Will Japan Leapfrog America on Superfast Computers?" *Economist*, March 6, 1982, p. 95.
60. "Japan Sets Next Target," *Sunday Times* (London), Nov. 29, 1981.
61. "Westinghouse/Mitsubishi," *Economist*, Feb. 6, 1982, p. 65.
62. R. B. Reich, "A Faustian Bargain with the Japanese," *New York Times*, April

6, 1986, business section, p. 2; "Japanese All Set for Take-off," *Times* (London), Nov. 11, 1981; Smith et al., *Asia's New Industrial World,* pp. 21–24.

63. The quotation is from Vogel, "Pax Nipponica," p. 753. More generally, see "Japanese Technology," *Times* (London), June 14, 1983, "Special Report," pp. i–viii. The more successful Japanese exploitation of robotics technology is outlined in B. J. Feder, "New Challenge in Automation," *New York Times,* Oct. 30, 1986, p. D2.

64. "Reconsider Japan," *Economist,* April 26, 1986, pp. 19–22; but see again Johnson, *MITI and the Japanese Miracle;* Vogel, *Japan as Number One,* pp. 70ff.

65. Vogel, "Pax Nipponica," p. 754.

66. See the tables in *Economist,* July 9, 1983, "Japan Survey" section, p. 7; and Pempel, "Japanese Foreign Economic Policy," pp. 171–72.

67. *Economist,* April 26, 1986, p. 22; Vogel, "Pax Nipponica," p. 753; idem, *Japan as Number One,* ch. 7; Smith et al., *Asia's New Industrial World,* pp. 13ff.

68. For example, S. Kamata, *Japan in the Passing Lane* (New York, 1984); J. Taylor, *Shadows of the Rising Sun: A Critical View of the "Japanese Miracle"* (New York, 1984); "There Can be Clouds Too," *Economist,* July 9, 1983, "Japan Survey."

69. D. Halberstam, "Can We Rise to the Japanese Challenge?" *Parade,* Oct. 9, 1983, pp. 4–5; and the even more alarming piece by T. H. White, "The Danger from Japan," *New York Times Magazine,* July 28, 1985.

70. "The New Global Top Banker: Tokyo and Its Mighty Money," *New York Times,* April 27, 1986, pp. 1, 16.

71. F. Marsh, *Japanese Overseas Investment* (Economist Intelligence Unit, London, 1983); *Times* (London), April 22, 1983.

72. For these figures and forecasts, see "Japan Investing Enormous Sums of Cash Abroad," *New York Times,* March 11, 1986, pp. A1, D12; "The New Global Top Banker," *New York Times,* April 27, 1986, pp. 1, 16.

73. "Japan's Investment Bankers Head for the Big Wide World," *Economist,* April 19, 1986, pp. 91–94; D. Burstein, "When the Yen Leaves the Sky It May Capture the Earth," *New York Times,* Sept. 3, 1986, p. A27.

74. "New Global Top Banker," p. 1.

75. See the table in Linder, *Pacific Century,* p. 12, quoting the *Japan in the Year 2000* study.

76. See CIA, *Handbook of Economic Statistics, 1984,* p. 33, fn. b.

77. "The Yen Also Rises," *New York Times,* March 5, 1986, p. D2.

78. See again the very pertinent study by Olsen, *U.S.-Japan Strategic Reciprocity,* passim.

79. See the figures in *Military Balance 1985–86,* pp. 170–72.

80. Olsen, *U.S.-Japan Strategic Reciprocity,* passim; Z. Brzezinski, "Japan Should Increase Spending for Defense," *New Haven Register,* Aug. 16, 1985, "Forum," p. 15.

81. There is a good flavor of the Japanese antiwar movement in Storry, *History of Modern Japan,* ch. 11. See also *Economist,* Aug. 16, 1985, pp. 21–22.

82. Olsen, *U.S.-Japan Strategic Reciprocity,* p. 149.

83. See the discussion in Reynolds, "China in the International Economy," in Harding (ed.), *China's Foreign Relations in the 1980s,* ch. 3 (and espec., p. 86, from where the quotation comes); Scalapino, "China and Northeast Asia," in Solomon (ed.), *China Factor,* espec. pp. 193ff. On the other hand, see Taylor, *Sino-Japanese Axis,* passim.

84. Scalapino, "China and Northeast Asia," p. 200. See also the comments on Japanese external policy in "Japan Survey," *Economist,* Dec. 7, 1985, pp. 10ff.

85. See again Gruner, *Die deutsche Frage,* espec. ch. 4.

86. I take these totals from *The Military Balance 1985–86*, pp. 40–43, 46–54.
87. CIA, *Handbook of Economic Statistics, 1984*, p. 37.
88. The unemployment figures were taken from *The Economist Diary, 1984*, p. 44. For the rising social expenditures, see the OECD report of March 1985, *Social Expenditures 1960–1990*.
89. Quoted in Linder, *Pacific Century*, p. 108.
90. See the review article, "Down to Earth: A Survey of the West German Economy," *Economist*, Feb. 4, 1984.
91. Calleo, *German Problem Reconsidered*, and Gruner, *Die Deutsche Frage*, are best here; but see also DePorte, *Europe Between the Superpowers*, pp. 180ff.
92. W. Gruner, "Der Deutsche Bund—Modell fur eine Zwischenlösung?" *Politik und Kultur*, vol. 9 (1982), no. 5.
93. P. Dibb, *The Soviet Union: The Incomplete Superpower* (London, 1986), pp. 43–44.
94. The literature on European defense and nuclear weapons is enormous. I have relied upon A. J. Pierre (ed.), *Nuclear Weapons in Europe* (New York, 1984); the debate provoked by M. Bundy et al., "Nuclear Weapons and the Atlantic Alliance," *Foreign Affairs*, vol. 6, no. 4 (Spring 1982), pp. 753–68; and by *Strengthening Conventional Deterrence in Europe: Proposals for the 1980s* (New York, 1983); J. D. Steinbrunner and L. V. Segal (eds.), *Alliance Security: NATO and the No-First-Use Question* (Washington, D.C., 1983); G. Prins (ed.), *The Nuclear Crisis Reader* (New York, 1984).
95. *Military Balance 1985–86*, p. 49.
96. "West German Defense: Early Warnings," *Economist*, June 29, 1985, p. 46.
97. See again the good discussion in Calleo, *German Problem Reconsidered*, chs. 8–9; and J. Dean, "Directions in Inner-German Relations," *Orbis*, vol. 29, no. 3 (Fall 1985), pp. 609–32; and G. F. Treverton, *Making the Alliance Work: The United States and Europe* (Ithaca, N.Y., 1985), passim.
98. "When the Oil Runs Out," *Economist*, Oct. 19, 1985, p. 65; "After the Oil Years," *Economist*, March 6, 1985, p. 57.
99. "Manufacturing," *Economist*, Sept. 28, 1985, p. 57.
100. See again Gamble, *Britain in Decline;* Kirby, *Decline of British Economic Power Since 1870;* Eatwell, *Whatever Happened to Britain;* and S. Pollard, *The Wasting of the British Economy* (London, 1982).
101. "After the Oil Years," *Economist*, March 6, 1986, p. 57.
102. A. Waters, *Britain's Industrial Renaissance* (London, 1986)—Waters having been, of course, Mrs. Thatcher's economic adviser.
103. "Scientists' Lament," *Economist*, Jan. 18, 1986, p. 16.
104. See again the statistics in *Military Balance 1985–86*.
105. The share of world GNP is calculated from CIA, *Handbook of Economic Statistics, 1984*, p. 32. For a devastating attack upon this attempt to maintain an overextended defense posture, see A. Barnett, "The Dangerous Dream," *New Statesman*, June 17, 1983, pp. 9–11. Less critical, but equally sobering, is "Yes, But How Do We Pay for It?" *Times* (London), June 15, 1983.
106. "Navy Wins War of the Frigates," *The Sunday Times* (London), Oct. 17, 1982; C. Wain, "The Navy's Future", *The Listener*, Aug. 19, 1982.
107. See *The Economist*'s frequent assaults upon it for that reason: e.g., "Trident: Bad Money After Bad," Nov. 3, 1984, p. 34; "Not Trident," Feb. 9, 1985, p. 16. The government's rationale for Trident is in *Statement on the Defense Estimates, 1985*, vol. 1 (Cmnd. 9430-1).
108. "Message to the New Defense Secretary: Think Small," *Sunday Times* (London), Jan. 12, 1986, p. 16; see also "Defense Budget Costs Go over the Top," *Daily Telegraph*, Dec. 10, 1985. There are excellent surveys of the problem—

and various proposals to deal with it—in J. Baylis (ed.), *Alternative Approaches to British Defense Policy* (London, 1983), passim.

109. For French defense policy, see generally M. M. Harrison, *The Reluctant Ally: France and Atlantic Security* (Baltimore, Md., 1981); R. F. Laird, *France, the Soviet Union, and the Nuclear Weapons Issue* (Boulder, Col., 1985); and D. S. Yost, *France's Deterrent Posture* (Adelphi Papers, nos. 194 and 195).

110. "France" survey, *Economist*, Feb. 9, 1985, p. 8.

111. See, in particular, the work by P. Lellouche, *L'avenir de la guerre* (Paris, 1985), nicely discussed in D. S. Yost, "Radical Change in French Defense Policy," *Survival*, vol. 28 (Jan./Feb., 1986), pp. 53–68; R. F. Laird, "The French Strategic Dilemma," *Orbis*, vol. 28, no. 2 (Summer 1984), pp. 307–28.

112. R. S. Rudney, "Mitterand's New Atlanticism: Evolving French Attitudes toward NATO," *Orbis*, vol. 28, no. 1 (Spring 1984), p. 99, citing Aron.

113. Ibid., passim.

114. "Chirac Is Pledged to Stick with NATO and Bonn," *New York Times*, April 6, 1986, "The Week in Review" section p. 2.

115. H. Schmidt, *A Grand Strategy for the West* (New Haven, Conn., 1985), pp. 41–43, 55–57. See also J. P. Pigasse, *Le bouclier d'Europe* (Paris, 1982).

116. See the discussion in Yost, "Radical change in French defense policy?"; as well as idem, *France and Conventional Defense in Central Europe* (Boulder, Colo., 1985).

117. "The French are Ready to Cross the Rhine," *Economist*, July 13, 1985, pp. 43–44; "French Defence: Count on Us," *Economist*, Oct. 25, 1986, pp. 50–51.

118. P. Stares, "The Modernization of the French Strategic Nuclear Force," *Journal of the Royal United Services Institute*, vol. 125, no. 4 (December 1980), p. 37.

119. See again Laird, "French Strategic Dilemma," passim; and P. Lellouche, "France and the Euromissiles," *Foreign Affairs*, Winter 1983–84, pp. 318–34.

120. See the analysis in L. Kolakowski, *Main Currents of Marxism*, vol. 1, *The Founders* (Oxford, 1981 edn.), ch. 13, "The Contradictions of Capital"; and Engels's discussion of contradictions in "Socialism: Utopian and Scientific," in *The Essential Left* (London, 1960), pp. 130ff.

121. "Excerpts from Gorbachev's Speech to the Party," *New York Times*, Feb. 26, 1986. See also "Making Mr. Gorbachev Frown," *Economist*, March 8, 1986, p. 67; S. Bialer, "The Harsh Decade: Soviet Policies in the 1980s," *Foreign Affairs*, vol. 59, no. 5 (Summer 1981), pp. 999–1020.

122. Brown et al., *State of the World, 1986*, pp. 14–19; "Focus: Food," *Economist*, April 12, 1986, p. 107.

123. M. I. Goldman, *USSR in Crisis: The Failure of an Economic System* (New York, 1983), p. 86. For further analyses, see Bergson and Levine (eds.), *Soviet Economy: Toward the Year 2000*, chs. 4–5. How swiftly (relatively) the USSR's position has been worsened can be seen by rereading the rosier assessment of the gap between it and the United States being closed by the year 2000 in Larson's very sober *Soviet-American Rivalry* (written in 1976–77?), p. 272.

124. As reported in "Soviet Is Facing Sixth Poor Harvest in a Row," *New York Times*, Aug. 28, 1985, pp. A1, D17. More generally, R. E. M. Mellor, *The Soviet Union and Its Geographical Problems* (London, 1982); Larson, *Soviet-American Rivalry*, pp. 17ff.

125. For what follows, see Hosking, *History of the Soviet Union*, pp. 392ff; J. R. Millar, "The Prospects for Soviet Agriculture," in M. Bornstein (ed.), *The Soviet Economy: Continuity and Change* (Boulder, Colo., 1981), pp. 273–91 (more optimistic than most); Goldman, *USSR in Crisis*, ch. 3.

126. "The Soviet Economy," *New York Times*, March 15, 1985, pp. A1, A6.

127. Goldman, *USSR in Crisis*, p. 81.

128. Ibid., p. 83; and the remarks in Nove, *Economic History of the USSR*, pp. 362ff.

129. Reprinted from Brown et al., *State of the World*, 1986, p. 18.

130. See again Goldman, *USSR in Crisis*, pp. 70–71; and, more broadly, R. W. Tucker, "Swollen State, Spent Society: Stalin's Legacy to Brezhnev's Russia," *Foreign Affairs*, vol. 60, no. 2 (Winter 1981–82), pp. 415ff.

131. Brown et al., *State of the World, 1986*, p. 18.

132. Ibid., p. 11.

133. See the comparative figures in CIA, *Handbook of Economic Statistics, 1984*, pp. 28–30.

134. Goldman, *USSR in Crisis*, p. 40, has some remarkable figures on that inefficiency. See also the extremely thoughtful piece by J. S. Berliner, "Planning and Management," in Bergson and Levine (eds.), *Soviet Economy: Toward the Year 2000*, pp. 350–89.

135. The phrase comes from Daniels, *Russia: The Roots of Confrontation*, p. 289.

136. Taken from "Inputs Misused," *Economist*, July 6, 1985, p. 12, which (itself employing the words "used to produce *even an alleged* $1,000-worth of GDP") clearly suspects that the *real* figures could be worse.

137. This is best discussed in M. I. Goldman, *The Enigma of Soviet Petroleum: Half-Full or Half-Empty* (London, 1980), passim; but see also L. Silk, "Soviet Oil Troubles," *New York Times*, June 5, 1985, p. D2.

138. "Russia Drills Less Oil, OPEC Keeps It Cheap," *Economist*, June 8, 1985, p. 65.

139. *Economist*, May 3, 1986, pp. 55–57; more generally, see R. W. Campbell, "Energy," in Bergson and Levine (eds.), *Soviet Economy: Toward the Year 2000*, pp. 191ff.

140. Dibb, *Soviet Union: The Incomplete Superpower*, p. 93.

141. Campbell, "Energy," pp. 213–14, in Bergson and Levine (eds.), *Soviet Economy: Toward the Year 2000*; see also L. Dienes, "An Energy Crunch Ahead in the Soviet Union?" in Bornstein (ed.), *Soviet Economy*, pp. 313–43.

142. See below, pp. 500–502.

143. Goldman, "A Low-Tech Economy at Home," *New York Times*, Feb. 19, 1984, business section, p. 2; and the interesting details in R. Amann and J. Cooper (eds.), *Industrial Innovation in the Soviet Union* (New Haven, Conn., 1982).

144. "Losing Battle," *Wall Street Journal*, July 25, 1984.

145. Apart from Goldman, *USSR in Crisis*, p. 131, see R. Amann et al. (eds.), *The Technological Level of Soviet Industry* (New Haven, Conn., 1977).

146. Goldman, *USSR in Crisis*, ch. 6; "Shadows over Comecon," *Economist*, May 29, 1982, pp. 84–85; Comecon Survey, *Economist*, April 20, 1985. pp. 3–18.

147. See again Drucker, "Changed World Economy," passim; "Oil's Decline Seen Curbing Soviet Plans," *New York Times*, March 10, 1986; "East European Trade," *Economist*, Oct. 26, 1985, p. 119. The implications for eastern Europe are also analyzed in T. Gustafson, "Energy and the Soviet Union," *International Security*, vol. 6, no. 3 (Winter 1981–82), pp. 65–89.

148. M. Feshbach, "Population and Labor Force," in Bergson and Levine (eds.), *Soviet Economy: Toward the Year 2000*, p. 79. See also Goldman, *USSR in Crisis*, pp. 100ff; and T. J. Colton, *The Dilemma of Reform in the Soviet Union* (New York, 1984), pp. 15ff.

149. "Sick Men of Europe," *Economist*, March 22, 1986, p. 53.

150. Dibb, *Soviet Union: The Incomplete Superpower*, pp. 92–93.

151. Feshbach, "Population and Labor Force," in Bergson and Levine (eds.), *Soviet Economy: Toward the Year 2000*, passim.

152. See the argument in J. W. Kiser, "How the Arms Race Really Helps Moscow," *Foreign Policy*, no. 60 (Fall 1985), pp. 40–51.

153. Munting, *Economic Development of the USSR*, p. 208.

154. "Gorbachev's Plans: Westerners See a Lot of Zeal, but Little Basic Change," *New York Times,* Feb. 23, 1986, p. 16; "Russia Under Gorbachev," *Economist,* Nov. 16, 1985, p. 21.

155. "The Soviet Economy," *New York Times,* March 15, 1985, pp. A1, A6, quoting Leonard Silk; Colton, *Dilemma of Reform in the Soviet Union,* ch. 3; Daniels, *Russia: The Roots of Confrontation,* pp. 273ff; J. F. Hough and M. Fainsod, *How the Soviet Union Is Governed* (Cambridge, Mass., 1979).

156. This is best covered by F. D. Holzman's articles "Are the Soviets Really Outspending the U.S. on Defense?" *International Security,* vol. 4, no. 4 (Spring 1980), pp. 86–104, and "Soviet Military Spending: Assessing the Numbers Game," *International Security,* vol. 6, no. 4 (Spring 1982), pp. 78–101; as well as idem, *Financial Checks on Soviet Defense Expenditures* (Lexington, Mass., 1975). See also Holloway, *Soviet Union and the Arms Race,* pp. 114ff; Dibb, *Soviet Union: The Incomplete Superpower,* pp. 80ff.

157. This point is made both by Colton, *Dilemma of Reform in the Soviet Union,* p. 91; and Bond and Levine, "An Overview," in Bergson and Levine (eds.), *Soviet Economy: Toward the Year 2000,* pp. 19–21.

158. Ibid., p. 20, the source of this quotation; see also; "Can Andropov Control His Generals?" *Economist,* Aug. 6, 1983, pp. 33–35.

159. L. H. Gelb, "A Common Desire for Guns and Butter," *New York Times,* Nov. 10, 1985, "The Week in Review" section, p. 2.

160. See the table in Holloway, *Soviet Union and the Arms Race,* p. 114; and the discussion in *Military Balance 1985–86,* pp. 17–20; Holzman, "Soviet Military Spending," passim; W. T. Lee, *The Estimation of Soviet Defense Expenditures 1955–75* (New York, 1977), passim; G. Adams, "Moscow's Military Costs," *New York Times,* Jan. 10, 1984, p. A23.

161. For details, one can consult the somewhat bloodcurdling annual publication of the U.S. Defense Department *Soviet Military Power,* and the Committee on the Present Danger's *Can America Catch Up?*—views contested by such critics as T. Gervasi, *The Myth of Soviet Military Supremacy* (New York, 1986), and A. Cockburn, *The Threat: Inside the Soviet Military Machine* (New York, 1984 edn.). For details presented nonpolemically, see the annual *Military Balance,* and the annual report by SIPRI (Stockholm International Peace Research Institute). A good general work is J. Steele, *Soviet Power* (New York, 1984), but see also Dibb, *Soviet Union: The Incomplete Superpower;* and Holloway, *Soviet Union and the Arms Race,* as well as the references following.

162. A. Amalrik, *Will the Soviet Union Survive Until 1984?* (New York, 1970). See also M. Garder, *L'Agonie du régime en Russie sovietique* (Paris, 1966), and the subsequent debate in the journal *Problems of Communism;* and Colton, *Dilemma of Reform in the Soviet Union,* passim.

163. See the comparative tables in Bergson, "Technological Progress," in Bergson and Levine (eds.), *Soviet Economy: Toward the Year 2000,* pp. 51ff; Rostow, *World Economy,* p. 434; Holloway, *Soviet Union and the Arms Race,* pp. 134ff.

164. "Soviet Arms: Their Quality Is Upgraded," *New York Times,* Feb. 12, 1984; Cockburn, *The Threat,* pp. 455–56.

165. Alex Gliksman, "Behind Moscow's Fear of 'Star Wars,'" *New York Times,* Feb. 13, 1986.

166. Quoted in Flora Lewis, "Soviet SDI Fears," *New York Times,* March 6, 1986, p. A27.

167. Dibb, *Soviet Union: The Incomplete Superpower,* pp. 51ff; J. Kazokins, "Nationality in the Soviet Army," *Journal of the Royal United Services Institute for Defense Studies,* vol. 130, no. 4 (December 1985), pp. 27–34. For a rosier pic-

ture, E. Jones, "Manning the Soviet Military," *International Security,* vol. 7, no. 1 (Summer 1982), pp. 105–31.

168. On which see Dibb, Soviet Union: *The Incomplete Superpower,* pp. 44ff, "The Nationality Problem"; Hosking, *History of the Soviet Union,* ch. 14; Daniels, *Russia, The Roots of Confrontation,* pp. 315ff; as well as the more detailed studies, like H. Carrere d'Encausse, *Decline of an Empire* (New York, 1979); M. Rywkin, *Moscow's Muslim Challenge* (New York, 1982); A. Bennigsen and M. Broxup, *The Islamic Threat to the Soviet State* (London, 1983); and S. E. Wimbush (ed.), *Soviet Nationalities in Strategic Perspective* (New York, 1985).

169. J. Anderson, "Ukraine a Hotbed of Dissent, Nationalism" (syndicated article), *New Haven Register,* June 13, 1985; but see also P. T. Potichny (ed.), *The Ukraine in the Seventies* (Oakville, Ont., 1982); Hosking, *History of the Soviet Union,* pp. 432ff.

170. Apart from Kazokins, "Nationality in the Soviet Army," passim, see the eye-opening details in Cockburn, *Threat,* pp. 74ff; E. Jones, "Minorities in the Soviet Armed Forces," *Comparative Strategy,* vol. 3, no. 4 (1982), pp. 285–318; and the Rand Corporation studies S. Curran and D. Ponomoreff, *Managing the Ethnic Factor in the Russian and Soviet Armed Forces: An Historical Overview* (Santa Monica, Calif., 1982); and E. Brunner, Jr., *Soviet Demographic Trends and the Ethnic Composition of Draft Age Males, 1980–1985* (Santa Monica, Calif., 1981).

171. On which term see, for example, the coverage in D. Leebaert (ed.), *Soviet Military Thinking* (London, 1981), espec. the essays in pt. 1; J. Baylis and G. Segal (eds.), *Soviet Strategy* (London, 1981), espec. essays 4 and 5.

172. *Military Balance 1985–86,* p. 180.

173. For example, Gervasi, *Myth of Soviet Military Supremacy,* passim, but espec. pp. 116–18.

174. For examples: J. Schell, *The Fate of the Earth* (New York, 1982); H. Caldicott, *Nuclear Madness* (Brookline, Mass., 1979); E. P. Thompson, *Zero Option* (London, 1982).

175. There is a good brief survey of these strategic ideas in E. Bottome, *The Balance of Terror* (Boston, Mass., 1986 edn.), chs. 4–7 (and a glossary of terms, pp. 243–54); A. W. Garfinkle, *The Politics of the Nuclear Freeze* (Philadelphia, Pa., 1984); and T. Powers, *Thinking About Nuclear Weapons* (New York, 1983).

176. Of the vast array of studies on this problem, I prefer M. Mandelbaum, *The Nuclear Future* (Ithaca, N.Y., 1983); R. Jervis, *The Illogic of American Nuclear Strategy* (Ithaca, N.Y., 1984); and S. Zuckerman, *Nuclear Illusion and Reality* (London, 1982). Also useful is S. M. Keeny and W.K.H. Panofsky, "MAD vs. NUTS: the Mutual Hostage Relationship of the Superpowers," *Foreign Affairs,* vol. 60, no. 2 (Winter 1981–82), pp. 287–304.

177. See again "In Battle of Wits, Submarines Evade Advanced Efforts at Detection," *New York Times,* April 1, 1986, p. C1; and the comments in McGwire, "Rationale for the Development of Soviet Seapower," passim, on the difficulties the USSR has had with integrating American SLBMs into its strategic planning.

178. The quote is from Jervis, *Illogic of American Nuclear Strategy.* For an example of "war-fighting" writers, see C. Gray, "Nuclear Strategy: A Case for a Theory of Victory," *International Security,* vol. 4 (Summer 1979), pp. 54–87.

179. See especially P. Bracken, *The Command and Control of Nuclear Weapons* (New Haven, Conn., 1983); also N. Calder, *Nuclear Nightmares* (Harmondsworth, Mddsx., 1981).

180. On which theme, see in particular J. C. Snyder and S. F. Wells (eds.), *Limiting Nuclear Proliferation* (Cambridge, Mass., 1985); Mandelbaum, *Nuclear Future,* ch. 3; G. Quester (ed.), *Nuclear Proliferation: Breaking the Chain* (Madison,

Wis., 1981). By contrast, K. N. Waltz, "Toward Nuclear Peace," Wilson Center, International Security Studies Program, Working Paper no. 16.

181. D. L. Strode, "Arms Control and Sino-Soviet Relations," *Orbis*, vol. 28, no. 1 (Spring 1984), espec. p. 168ff.

182. *The Economist*, 9 February, 1985, "Not Trident," p. 16. See also, Gervasi, *The Myth of Soviet Military Supremacy*, p. 171.

183. "France Tests Longer-Range Sub Missile," *New York Times*, March 6, 1986, p. A3. See also the table outlining the buildup of French nuclear warheads in *New York Times*, April 6, 1986, "The Week in Review" section, p. 2.

184. For example, "Powell Derides Nuclear 'Last Resort,' " *Times* (London), June 1, 1983, p. 4; Lord Carver, "Why Britain Should Reject Trident," *Sunday Times* (London), Feb. 21, 1982.

185. See again Yost, "Radical Change in French Defense Policy?"

186. Dibb, *Soviet Union: The Incomplete Superpower*, p. 161. By contrast, see Gervasi, *Myth of Soviet Military Supremacy*, ch. 26, which argues that NATO numbers are in fact superior. Also important are the *International Security* essays edited by S. E. Miller, *Conventional Forces and American Defense Policy* (Princeton, N. J., 1986).

187. *Statement on the Defense Estimates, 1985*, vol. 1 (Cmnd 9430), summarized in *Survey of Current Affairs*, vol. 15, no. 6 (June 1985), p. 179.

188. As pointed out by F. D. Holzman, "What Defense-Spending Gap?" *New York Times*, March 4, 1986.

189. See Dibb, *Soviet Union: The Incomplete Superpower*, p. 162; *Military Balance 1985–86*, pp. 186–87; R. L. Fischer, *Defending the Central Front: The Balance of Forces* (Adelphi Papers, no. 127, London, 1976).

190. This is a tricky (and highly disputed) topic. For the optimists' view—with which, for what it is worth, this author agrees—see J. Mearsheimer, "Why the Soviets Can't Win Quickly in Central Europe," pp. 121–57, and B. R. Posen, "Measuring the European Conventional Balance," pp. 79–120, both in Miller (ed.), *Conventional Forces and American Defense Policy*. See also Steele, *Soviet Power*, pp. 76ff; and C. N. Donnelly, "Tactical Problems Facing the Soviet Army: Recent Debates in the Soviet Military Press," *International Defense Review*, vol. 11, no. 9 (1978), pp. 1405–12. More sobering assessments are provided by R. A. Mason, "Military Strategy," in E. Moreton and G. Segal (eds.), *Soviet Strategy Toward Western Europe* (London, 1984), pp. 175–202; P. A. Peterson and J. G. Hines, "The Conventional Offensive in Soviet Theater Strategy," *Orbis*, vol. 27, no. 3 (Fall 1983), pp. 695–739; and—calling attention to the possibility of Soviet use of dual-purpose missiles (i.e., tactical nuclear missiles)—D. M. Gormley, "A New Dimension to Soviet Theater Strategy," *Orbis*, vol. 29, no. 3 (Fall 1985), pp. 537–69. There is a good recent survey, "NATO's Central Front," in *Economist*, Aug. 30, 1986.

191. This is now best treated in Treverton, *Making the Alliance Work*, passim; but see also J. Joffe, "European-American Relations: The Enduring Crisis," *Foreign Affairs*, vol. 59 (Spring 1981).

192. V. Bunce, "The Empire Strikes Back: The Evolution of the Eastern Bloc from a Soviet Asset to a Soviet Liability," *International Organization*, vol. 39, no. 1 (Winter 1985), pp. 13–28. See also the articles on "Cracks in the Soviet Empire?" in *International Security*, vol. 6, no. 3 (Winter 1981–82); D. R. Herspring and I. Volgyes, "Political Reliability in the Eastern European Warsaw Pact Armies," *Armed Forces and Society*, vol. 6, no. 2 (Winter 1980), pp. 270–96; A. R. Johnson et al., *East European Military Establishments: The Warsaw Pact Northern Tier* (New York, 1982).

193. D. A. Andelman, "Contempt and Crisis in Poland," *International Security,* vol. 6, no. 3 (Winter 1981–82), pp. 90–104.

194. Herspring and Volgyes, "Political Reliability," passim; B. S. Lambeth, "Uncertainties for the Soviet War Planner," in Miller (ed.), *Conventional Forces and American Defense Policy,* pp. 181–82; W. E. Griffith, "Superpower Problems in Europe: A Comparative Assessment," *Orbis,* vol. 29, no. 4 (Winter 1986), pp. 748–49.

195. See the controversial proposal of S. P. Huntington, "Conventional Deterrence and Conventional Retaliation in Europe," in Miller (ed.), *Conventional Forces and American Defense Policy,* pp. 251–75. And for a wide-ranging consideration of all these issues, see E. R. Alterman, "Central Europe: Misperceived Threats and Unforeseen Dangers," *World Policy Journal,* vol. 2, no. 4 (Fall 1985), pp. 681–709.

196. See the discussion in Dibb, *Soviet Union: The Incomplete Superpower,* pp. 165–66; Segal, *Defending China,* passim; idem, "Defense Culture and Sino-Soviet Relations," passim; and pp. 449–51 above.

197. Dibb, *Soviet Union: The Incomplete Superpower,* pp. 147ff; Segal, "The China Factor," in Moreton and Segal (eds.), *Soviet Strategy Towards Western Europe,* pp. 154–59; Strode, "Arms Control and Sino-Soviet Relations," passim.

198. See Steele, *Soviet Power,* ch. 8, "Asian Anxieties"; also T. B. Millar, "Asia in the Global Balance," in D. H. McMillen (ed.), *Asian Perspectives on International Security* (London, 1984); Segal (ed.), *The Soviet Union in East Asia* (Boulder, Colo., 1983); M. Hauner, "The Soviet Geostrategic Dilemma" (ms. article for Foreign Policy Research Institute).

199. See again McGwire, "Rationale for the Development of Soviet Seapower," in Baylis and Segal (eds.), *Soviet Strategy,* pp. 210–54; Polmar, *Soviet Naval Developments,* passim.

200. Figures from Dibb, *Soviet Union: The Incomplete Superpower,* p. 172.

201. The quotation is from ibid., p. 171; but see also Steele, *Soviet Power,* pp. 33–36; and Cockburn, *Threat,* ch. 15.

202. McGwire, "The Rationale," pp. 226ff; Dibb, *Soviet Union: The Incomplete Superpower,* pp. 167–74.

203. See the comparative statistics in Smith, *Pattern of Imperialism,* p. 215; the argument in Steele, *Soviet Power,* chs. 9–12; F. Fukuyama, "Gorbachev and the Third World," *Foreign Affairs,* vol. 64, no. 4 (Spring 1986), pp. 715–31; K. Menon, *Soviet Power and the Third World* (New York, 1985).

204. Quoted in Dibb, *Soviet Union: The Incomplete Superpower,* p. 160. Note also, N. Eberstadt, " 'Danger' to the Soviet," *New York Times,* Sept. 26, 1983, p. A21, which argues how weak the USSR's influence would be if nuclear weapons did not exist.

205. "If Gorbachev Dares," *Economist,* July 6, 1985.

206. Quotations from Bialer, "Politics and Priorities," in Bergson and Levine (eds.), *Soviet Economy: Toward the Year 2000,* pp. 403, 405.

207. For considerations of Russia's problems and future, see H. S. Rosen, "Living with a Sick Bear," *National Interest,* no. 2 (Winter 1985–86), pp. 14–26; Garthoff, *Détente and Confrontation,* chs. 29–30; Colton, *Dilemma of Reform in the Soviet Union,* passim; Goldman, *USSR in Crisis,* ch. 7; Dibb, *Soviet Union: The Incomplete Superpower,* ch. 8; and the entire issue of *Orbis,* vol. 30, no. 2 (Summer 1986).

208. B. Rubin, "The Reagan Administration and the Middle East," in Oye et al., (eds.), *Eagle Defiant,* p. 367—a good survey. See also H. Saunders, *The Middle East Problem in the 1980s* (Washington, D.C., 1981). For particular problems, see P. Jabber, "Egypt's Crisis, America's Dilemma," *Foreign Affairs,* vol. 64, no.

5 (Summer 1986), pp. 960–80; and R. W. Tucker, "The Arms Balance and the Persian Gulf," in *The Purposes of American Power* (New York, 1981), ch. 4.

209. A. F. Lowenthal, "Ronald Reagan and Latin America: Coping with Hegemony in Decline," in Oye et al. (eds.), *Eagle Defiant*, pp. 311ff; R. Bonachea, "The United States and Central America," in Kaplan, *Global Power*, pp. 209–41; P. A. Armella et al. (eds.), *Financial Policies and the World Capital Markets: The Place of Latin American Countries* (Chicago, Ill., 1983).

210. "An Economy Struggles to Break Its Fall," *New York Times*, June 8, 1986, p. E3; "Hard Times in Mexico Cause Concern in U.S.," *New York Times*, Oct. 19, 1986, pp. 1, 20.

211. *Report of the Secretary of Defense Caspar W. Weinberger to the Congress, on Fiscal Year 1984 Budget* (Washington, D.C., 1983), p. 17.

212. "NATO: Burdens Shared," *Economist*, Aug. 4, 1984, p. 3. See also the discussion of this in Calleo, *Imperious Economy*, pp. 169–71, and in fns. 16–17 on pp. 256–57; E. Conine, "Do the Interests of the U.S. Really Cover the World?" (syndicated column), *New Haven Register*, Feb. 7, 1985, p. 11; M. Kahler, "The United States and Western Europe," in Oye et al. (eds.), *Eagle Defiant*, ch. 9; and, especially, Treverton, *Making the Alliance Work*, passim.

213. There are useful discussions in Mako, *U.S. Ground Forces and the Defense of Central Europe*, passim; Treverton, *Making the Alliance Work*, passim; L. Sullivan, "A New Approach to Burden-Sharing," *Foreign Policy*, no. 60 (Fall 1985), pp. 91ff; K. Knorr, "Burden-Sharing in NATO: Aspects of U.S. Policy," *Orbis*, vol. 29, no. 3 (Fall 1985), pp. 517–36.

214. *Report of the Secretary of Defense . . . Fiscal Year 1984*, p. 17.

215. "Military Forces Stretched Thin, Army Chief Says," *New York Times*, Aug. 10, 1983, pp. A1, A3.

216. "U.S. Forces: Need Arising for More Troops, Ships and Planes," *New York Times*, Oct. 26, 1983, p. A16 (with map).

217. See, for example, the map in the endpapers of Barnett, *Collapse of British Power*, and of Marder, *Anatomy of British Sea Power*.

218. C. W. Weinberger, "U.S. Defense Strategy," *Foreign Affairs*, vol. 64, no. 4 (Spring 1986), p. 678. In this connection, see also B. R. Posen and S. Van Evera, "Defense Policy and the Reagan Administration: Departure from Containment," in Miller (ed.) *Conventional Forces and American Defense Policy*, pp. 19–61.

219. For the statistical evidence of this, see Oye et al. (eds.), *Eagle Defiant*, ch. 1; Bairoch, "International Industrialization Levels from 1750 to 1980," passim. For other measurements, see A. Bergeson and C. Sahoo, "Evidence of the Decline of American Hegemony in World Production," *Review*, vol. 8, no. 4 (Spring 1985), pp. 595–611; and S. D. Krasner, "United States Commercial and Monetary Policy," in Katzenstein (ed.), *Between Power and Plenty*, pp. 58–59, 68–69.

220. *Military Balance 1985–86*, p. 13.

221. For a good example, see E. A. Cohen, "When Policy Outstrips Power—American Strategy and Statecraft," *Public Interest*, no. 75 (Spring 1984), pp. 3–19.

222. Luttwak, *Pentagon and the Art of War*, p. 256.

223. See especially E. A. Cohen, *Citizens and Soldiers: The Dilemma of Military Service* (Ithaca, N.Y., 1985), chs. 7–9; and Canby's interesting remarks on the European experience, in "Military Reform and the Art of War," Wilson Center, International Security Studies Program, working paper no. 41, pp. 8ff.

224. For a sampling, see G. Hart with W. S. Lind, *America Can Win* (Bethesda, Md., 1986); Kaufman, *Reasonable Defense*, passim; Luttwak, *Pentagon and the Art of War*, passim; J. Record, "Reagan's Strategy Gap," *New Republic*, Oct. 29,

1984, pp. 17–21; J. Fallows, *National Defense* (New York, 1981); idem, "The Spend-Up," *Atlantic,* July 1986, pp. 27–31; Gansler, *Defense Industry,* passim; S. L. Canby, "Military Reform and the Art of War," passim; "Forum: Military Reform and Defense Planning," *Orbis,* vol. 27, no. 2 (Summer 1983), pp. 245–300. Also very important in this connection is the powerful exposé of A. T. Hadley, *The Straw Giant: Triumph and Failure: America's Armed Forces* (New York, 1986).

225. Kaufman, *Reasonable Defense,* p. 35; "Bungling the Military Build-Up," *New York Times,* Jan. 27, 1985, business section, pp. 1, 8; Gansler, *Defense Industry,* passim; Fallows, "The Spend-Up," passim; but see also Luttwak, *Pentagon and the Art of War,* ch. 5, for interesting correctives.

226. Weinberger, "U.S. Defense Strategy," p. 694; but see the doubts expressed in Record, "Reagan's Strategy Gap"; Fallows, "The Spend-Up"; and Canby, "Military Reform and the Art of War;" as well as the reasoned defense of high-technology weapons by K. N. Lewis in the *Orbis* forum "Military Reform."

227. Among which I would include Luttwak, *Pentagon and the Art of War;* Canby, "Military Reform and the Art of War"; and Cohen, "When Policy Outstrips Power."

228. See, for example, R. W. Komer, *Maritime Strategy or Coalition Defense?* (Cambridge, Mass., 1984), passim, and the debate in 1986 in journals such as *International Security* upon the Reagan administration's "maritime strategy."

229. Recently spelled out again in Weinberger, "U.S. Defense Strategy," pp. 684ff. See also "Schultz-Weinberger Discord," *New York Times,* Dec. 11, 1984, pp. A1, A12.

230. See, for example, L. C. Thurow, "Losing the Economic Race," *New York Review of Books,* Sept. 27, 1984, pp. 29–31; cf. W. D. Nordhaus, "On the Eve of a Historic Economic Boom," *New York Times,* April 6, 1986, which followed shortly after P. G. Petersen's article in the same paper, "When the Economic Valium Wears Off."

231. S. M. Bodner, "Our Trade Gap Is Really a Standard of Living Gap," *New York Times,* May 6, 1986 (letters); and "Why America Cannot Pay its Way," *Economist,* July 13, 1985, p. 69, both cover the problems facing traditional industries. For the debate upon future technologies, see "High Technology: Clash of the Titans," *Economist,* Aug. 23, 1986. For the congressional study, see "A Disturbing New Deficit," *Time,* Nov. 3, 1986, p. 56.

232. For example, while *The Global 2000 Report to the President* (Washington, D.C., 1980), vol. 1, pp. 18–19, referred to absolute increases in world grain production, it forecast increasing deficits in China, South Asia, and western Europe.

233. "Farmers' Slipping Share of the Market," *New York Times,* May 26, 1986; "Farm Imports Rise as Exports Plunge," *New York Times,* April 20, 1986; "Elephant-High Farm Debts," *Economist,* Sept. 14, 1985, p. 17.

234. For a good brief survey, see P. Cain, "Political Economy in Edwardian England: The Tariff-Reform Controversy," in A. O'Day (ed.), *The Edwardian Age,* (London, 1979), pp. 34–59.

235. Petersen, "When the Economic Valium Wears Off," passim; F. Rohatyn, "The Debtor Economy: A Proposal," *New York Review of Books,* Nov. 8, 1984, pp. 16–21; J. Chace, *Solvency, the Price of Survival* (New York, 1981), chs. 1–2.

236. *President's Private Sector Survey on Cost Control,* report, as reprinted in "Of Debt. Deficits, and the Death of a Republic" (Figgie International advertisement), *New York Times,* April 20, 1986, p. F9. This advertisement misprints the 1985 total of interest as $179 billion; it is in fact $129 billion.

237. Ibid.

238. "Cost of Paying Interest Eases Dramatically for U.S.," *New York Times*, Dec. 28, 1986, pp. 1, 24.
239. The quotation is from Drucker, "Changed World Economy," p. 782. See also M. Shubik and P. Bracken, "Strategic Purpose and the International Economy," in McCormick and Bissell (eds.), *Strategic Dimensions of Economic Behaviour*, p. 212.
240. Drucker, "Changed World Economy," passim; S. Marriss, *Deficits and the Dollar: The World Economy at Risk* (Washington, D.C., 1985); and the comments in "As America Diets, Allies Must Eat" (lead article), *New York Times*, Jan. 17, 1986; "A Nation Hooked on Foreign Funds," *New York Times*, Nov. 18, 1984, business section, pp. 1, 24; "U.S. as Debtor: A Threat to World Trade," *New York Times*, Sept. 22, 1985, business section, p. 3.
241. See again Nordhaus, "On the Eve of a Historic Economic Boom"; the uncharacteristically rosy argument in "America Manufactures Still," *Economist*, April 19, 1986, p. 81; and L. Silk, "Can the U.S. Remain No. 1?" *New York Times*, Aug. 10, 1984, p. D2 (a question, incidentally, which would not have been asked ten to twenty years ago).
242. Rasler and Thompson, "Global Wars, Public Debts, and the Long Cycle," passim; Gilpin, *War and Change in World Politics*, passim.
243. This is best described in G. R. Searle, *The Quest for National Efficiency: A Study in British Politics and British Political Thought, 1899–1914* (Oxford, 1971).
244. Quoted in ibid., p. 101.
245. See above, p. 228–29.
246. See the Brookings study by J. Grunwald and K. Flamm, *The Global Factory: Foreign Assembly in International Trade* (Washington, D.C., 1985); and P. Seabury, "International Policy and National Defense," *Journal of Contemporary Studies*, Spring 1983.
247. See, for example, the British experience in the late 1930s, as detailed in Gibbs, *Grand Strategy*, vol. 1, p. 311.
248. Gansler, *Defense Industry*, pp. 12ff; and especially R. W. DeGrasse, *Military Expansion, Economic Decline* (Armonk, N.Y., 1985 edn.); G. Adama, *The Iron Triangle* (New York, 1981); Thurow, "How to Wreck the Economy," *New York Review of Books*, May 14, 1981, pp. 3–8; Kaufmann, *A Reasonable Defense*, pp. 33–34; more generally, G. Kennedy, *Defense Economics* (London, 1983), espec. ch. 8; S. Chan, "The Impact of Defense Spending on Economic Performance: A Survey of Evidence and Problems," *Orbis*, vol. 29, no. 2 (Summer 1985), pp. 403ff; B. Russett, "Defense Expenditures and National Well-Being," *American Political Science Review*, vol. 76, no. 4 (December 1982), pp. 767–77.
249. Kaldor, *Baroque Arsenal*, passim; DeGrasse, *Military Expansion, Economic Decline*, passim; Thurow, "How to Wreck the Economy," passim; Chace, *Solvency*, ch. 2; E. Rothschild, "The American Arms Boom," in E. P. Thompson and D. Smith (eds.), *Protest and Survive* (Harmondsworth, Mddsx., 1980), pp. 170ff; Rosecrance, *Rise of the Trading State*, chs. 6 and 10.
250. E. Rothschild, "The Costs of Reaganism," *New York Review of Books*, March 15, 1984, pp. 14–17.
251. See again Cipolla, *Economic Decline of Empires;* and Rasler and Thompson, "Global Wars, Public Debts, and the Long Cycle," passim.
252. The quip is from *Misalliance* (1909), and in the original reads "Hindhead's turn will come." As Hobsbawm notes, in *Industry and Empire*, p. 193, this was an obvious jibe at the stockbroker townships south of London, prospering while other parts of the economy were coming under pressure.
253. See above, p. 357. Also useful in this connection is B. Russett, "America's

Continuing Strengths," *International Organization,* vol. 39, no. 2 (Spring 1985), pp. 207–31.
254. W. Lippman, *U.S. Foreign Policy: Shield of the Republic* (Boston, Mass., 1943), pp. 7–8; and see again Cohen, "When Policy Outstrips Power"; and the conclusions in E. Bottome, *The Balance of Terror* (Boston, Mass., 1986 edn.), pp. 235–42.
255. P. Hassner, "Europe and the Contradictions in American Policy," in R. Rosecrance (ed.), *America as an Ordinary Power* (Ithaca, N.Y., 1976), pp. 60–86. See also Helmut Schmidt's insistence, in *Grand Strategy for the West*, p. 147, that "the leadership role can only be assumed by the United States."

EPILOGUE

1. See again Doran and Parsons, "War and the Cycle of Relative Power," passim; G. Modelski, "Wars and the Great Power System," passim; idem, "The Long Cycle of Global Politics and the Nation-State," passim. See also J. Levy, *War in the Modern Great Power System* (Lexington, Ky., 1983).
2. Rasler and Thompson, "Global Wars, Public Debts, and the Long Cycle," passim.
3. L. E. Davis and R. A. Huttenback, "The Cost of Empire," in R. L. Ransom et al. (eds.), *Exploration in the New Economic History* (New York, 1982), pp. 41–69; R. Taagepera, "Size and Duration of Empires: Systematics of Size," *Social Science Research*, vol. 7 (1978), pp. 108–27; idem, "Growth Curves of Empires," *General Systems*, vol. 13 (1968), pp. 171–75.
4. I am thinking here of the various scholars influenced by Wallerstein's "world-system" ideas. For example, A. Bergesen, "Cycles of War in the Reproduction of the World Economy," in P. M. Johnson and W. R. Thompson (eds.), *Rhythms in Politics and Economics* (New York, 1985); E. Friedman (ed.), *Ascent and Decline in the World-System* (Beverly Hills, Calif., 1982); Bergesen (ed.), *Studies in the Modern World-System* (New York, 1980); McGowan and Kegley (eds.), *Foreign Policy and the Modern World-System*, passim.
5. Gilpin, *War and Change in World Politics*, p. 93.
6. Rosecrance, *Rise of the Trading State*, passim.
7. Gilpin, *War and Change in World Politics*, pp. 158–59, has a very good discussion of this point.
8. See the analysis in Wight, *Power Politics*, ch. 3.
9. Quoted by McCormick, on p. 19 of his article "Strategic Considerations in the Development of Economic Thought," in McCormick and Bissell (eds.), *Strategic Dimensions of Economic Behavior.*
10. Ibid.
11. Kennedy, "Strategy versus Finance in Twentieth Century Britain"; and also J. H. Maurer, "Economics, Strategy, and War in Historical Perspective," in McCormick and Bissell (eds.), *Strategic Dimensions of Economic Behavior*, pp. 59–83.
12. Gilpin's term; see *War and Change in World Politics*, p. 162.
13. Cited in Pflanze, *Bismarck and the Development of Germany*, p. 17.

Bibliography

Abarca, R. "Classical Diplomacy and Bourbon 'Revanche' Strategy, 1763–1770," *Review of Politics* 32 (1970).

Abrahamson, J.L. *America Arms for a New Century*. New York, 1981.

Adama, G. *The Iron Triangle*. New York, 1981.

Adams, E.D. *Great Britain and the American Civil War*, 2 vols. London, 1925.

Adams, R.J.Q. *Arms and the Wizard: Lloyd George and the Ministry of Munitions, 1915*. London, 1978.

Adamthwaite, A. *France and the Coming of the Second World War 1936–1939*. Cambridge, 1977.

———, "The British Government and the Media, 1937–1938," *Journal of Contemporary History* 18 (1983).

———. *The Lost Peace: International Relations in Europe 1918–1939*. London, 1980.

Addington, L.H. *The Patterns of War Since the Eighteenth Century*. Bloomington, Ind., 1984.

Adler, G.J., "Britain and the Defence of India—the Origins of the Problem, 1798–1815," *Journal of Asian History* 6 (1972).

Albertini, L. *The Origin of the War of 1914*, 3 vols. London, 1952–57.

Albertini, R. von. *Decolonization*. New York, 1971 edn.

Albrecht-Carrié, R. *A Diplomatic History of Europe Since the Congress of Vienna*. London, 1965 edn.

Aldcroft, D.H. *The British Economy*, vol. 1. London, 1986.

———. *From Versailles to Wall Street: The International Economy in the 1920s*. Berkeley, Calif., 1977.

———. *The European Economy, 1914–1980*.

Alford, B.W.E. *Depression and Recovery: British Economic Growth 1918–1939*. London, 1972.

Allen, G.S. *A Short Economic History of Japan*. London, 1981 edn.

Alperowitz, G. *Atomic Diplomacy: Hiroshima and Potsdam*. London, 1966.

Alterman, E.R., "Central Europe: Misperceived Threats and Unforeseen Dangers," *World Policy Journal* 2 (1985).

Amalrik, A. *Will the Soviet Union Survive until 1984?* New York, 1970.

Amann, R., and J. Cooper, eds. *Industrial Innovation in the Soviet Union*. New Haven, Conn., 1982.

———, et al., eds. *The Technological Level of Soviet Industry*. New Haven, Conn., 1977.

Ambrose, S. *Rise to Globalism: American Foreign Policy Since 1938*. 4th edn., New York, 1985.

Andelman, D.A., "Contempt and Crisis in Poland," *International Security* 6 (1981–2).

Anderson, J.L., "Aspects of the Effects on the British Economy of the War Against France, 1793–1815," *Australian Economic History Review* 12 (1972).

Anderson, M.S. *Europe in the Eighteenth Century*. London, 1961.

———. *Peter the Great*. London, 1978.

Anderson, O. *A Liberal State at War*. London, 1967.

Anderson, T.H. *The United States, Great Britain and the Cold War, 1944–1947*. Columbia, Mo., 1981.

André, L. *Michel le Tellier et Louvois*. Paris, 1943 edn.

Andrew, C.M., and A.S. Kanya-Forstner. *The Climax of French Imperial Expansion 1914–1924*. Stanford, Calif., 1981.

———. *Théophile Delcassé and the Making of the Entente Cordiale*. London, 1968.

Andrews, C.M., "Anglo-French Commercial Rivalry 1700–1750," *American Historical Review* 20 (1915).

Andrews, K.R. *Elizabethan Privateering*. Cambridge, 1964.

———. *Trade, Plunder and Settlement*. Cambridge, 1983.

Ange-Laribe, M. *L'agriculture pendant la guerre*. Paris, 1925.

Armella, P.A., et al., eds. *Financial Policies and the World Capital Markets: The Place of Latin American Countries*. Chicago, 1983.

Aron, R. *The Imperial Republic*. London, 1975.

Ashley, M. *Financial and Commercial Policy under the Cromwellian Protectorate*. London, 1962 edn.

Ashton, R. *The Crown and the Money Market 1603–1640*. Oxford, 1960.

Ashton, T.S. *The Industrial Revolution 1760–1830*. Oxford, 1968 edn.

Ashworth, W. *A Short History of the International Economy Since 1850*. London, 1975.

Aster, S. *1939: The Making of the Second World War*. London, 1973.

Backer, J.H. *Winds of History: The German Years of Lucius DuBignon Clay*. New York, 1983.

Baer, G. *Test Case: Italy, Ethiopia, and the League of Nations*. Stanford, Calif., 1976.

Bailey, T.A. *A Diplomatic History of the American People*. New York, 1974 edn.

Bairoch, P., "International Industrialization Levels from 1750 to 1980," *Journal of European Economic History* 11 (1982).

———, "Europe's Gross National Product: 1800–1975," *Journal of European Economic History* 5 (1976).

———. *The Economic Development of the Third World Since 1900*. Berkeley, Calif., 1975.

Baker, N. *Government and Contractors: The British Treasury and War Supplies 1775–1783*. London, 1971.

Baldwin, H. *The Crucial Years 1939–41*. New York, 1976.

Balfour, M. *The Adversaries: America, Russia, and the Open World, 1941–1962*. London, 1981.

———, and J. Mair. *Four-Power Control in Germany and Austria 1945–1946*. London, 1956.

Bamford, P.W. *Forests and French Sea Power 1660–1780*. Toronto, 1956.

Bankwitz, P.C.F. *Maxime Weygand and Civil-Military Relations in Modern France*. Cambridge, Mass., 1967.

Barbour, V. *Capitalism in Amsterdam in the Seventeenth Century*. Baltimore, 1950.

Barclay, G. *The Empire Is Marching: A Study of the Military Effort of the British Empire*. London, 1976.

Barker, T.M. *Double Eagle and Crescent*. Albany, N.Y., 1967.

Barnet, R. *Global Reach*. New York, 1974.

Barnett, A.D. *China and the Major Powers in East Asia*. Washington, D.C., 1977.

———. *China's Economy in Global Perspective*. Washington, D.C., 1981.

——, "Ten Years After Mao," *Foreign Affairs* 65 (1986).

Barnett, C. *Britain and Her Army 1509–1970: A Military, Political and Social Survey.* London, 1970.

——. *Napoleon.* London, 1978.

——. *The Audit of War.* London, 1986.

——. *The Collapse of British Power.* London, 1972.

Barnhart, M.A., "Japan's Economic Security and the Origins of the Pacific War," *The Journal of Strategic Studies* 4 (1981).

Barraclough, G., ed. *The Times Atlas of World History.* London, 1978.

——. *An Introduction to Contemporary History.* Harmondsworth, Mddsx., 1967.

Bartlett, C.J. *Great Britain and Sea Power 1815–1853.* Oxford, 1963.

——. *The Global Conflict, 1880–1970: The International Rivalry of the Great Powers.* London, 1984.

Baskir, L., and P. Strauss. *Chance and Circumstance: The War, the Draft, and the Vietnam Generation.* New York, 1978.

Bateson, C. *The War with Japan.* East Lansing, Mich., 1968.

Baugh, D.A. *British Naval Administration in the Age of Walpole.* Princeton, N.J., 1965.

Baumgart, W. *Imperialism: The Idea and Reality of British and French Colonial Expansion.* Oxford, 1982.

——. *The Peace of Paris, 1856.* Santa Barbara, Calif., 1981.

Baxter, S.B. *William III and the Defense of European Liberty 1650–1702.* Westport, Conn., 1976 reprint.

Bayley, C.A. *Rulers, Townsmen and Bazaars.* Cambridge, 1983.

Baylis, J., ed. *Alternative Approaches to British Defense Policy.* London, 1983.

——, and G. Segal, eds. *Soviet Strategy.* London, 1981.

——. *Anglo-American Defense Relations 1939–1980.* London, 1981.

Beale, H.K. *Theodore Roosevelt and the Rise of America to World Power.* New York, 1962 edn.

Bean, R., "War and the Birth of the Nation State," *Journal of Economic History* 33 (1973).

Beasley, W.H. *The Meiji Restoration.* Stanford, Calif., 1972.

Becker, J.J. *1914: Comment les Français sont entrés dans la guerre.* Paris, 1977.

Becker, W.H., and S. F. Wells, Jr., eds. *Economics and World Power: An Assessment of American Diplomacy Since 1789.* New York, 1984.

Beckerman, W., ed. *Slow Growth in Britain: Causes and Consequences.* Oxford, 1979.

Behnen, M. *Rüstung-Bündnis-Sicherheit.* Tübingen, 1985.

Bell, C. *The Diplomacy of Détente: The Kissinger Era.* New York, 1977.

Beloff, M. *Imperial Sunset,* vol. i, *Britain's Liberal Empire.* London, 1969.

Bemis, S.F. *The Diplomacy of the American Revolution.* New York, 1935.

Bendix, R. *Kings or People: Power and the Mandate to Rule.* Berkeley, Calif., 1978.

Bengonzi, B. *Heroes' Twilight.* New York, 1966.

Benians, E.A., ed. *The Cambridge History of the British Empire,* vol. iii, *The Empire-Commonwealth 1870–1919.* Cambridge, 1959.

Bennett, E.M. *German Rearmament and the West, 1932–33.* Princeton, N.J., 1979.

Bennigson, A., and M. Broxup. *The Islamic Threat to the Soviet State.* London, 1983.

Bergeron, L. *France under Napoleon.* Princeton, N.J., 1981.

Bergeson, A., ed. *Studies in the Modern World-System.* New York, 1980.

——, and C. Sahoo, "Evidence of the Decline of American Hegemony in World Production," *Review* 8 (1985).

Berghahn, V.R. *Germany and the Approach of War in 1914.* London, 1974.

——. *Unternehmer und Politik in der Bundesrepublik.* Frankfurt, 1985.

Bergson, A., and H. S. Levine, eds. *The Soviet Economy: Toward the Year 2000.* London, 1983.

Best, G. *War and Society in Revolutionary Europe, 1770–1870.* London, 1982.

Betts, R. *Tricouleur: The French Colonial Empire.* London, 1978.

Beyrau, D. *Militär und Gesellschaft im vorrevolutionären Russland.* Göttingen, 1984.

Bialer, S., "The Harsh Decade: Soviet Policies in the 1980s," *Foreign Affairs* 59 (1981).

Bialer, U. *The Shadow of the Bomber: The Fear of Air Attack and British Politics 1932–1939.* London, 1980.

Bidwell, S., and D. Graham. *Fire-Power: British Army Weapons and Theories of War, 1904–1945.* London, 1982.

Bien, D., "The Army in the French Enlightenment: Reform, Reaction and Revolution," *Past and Present* 85 (1979).

Bindoff, S.T., J. Hurstfield, and C.H. Williams, eds. *Elizabethan Government and Society.* London, 1961.

Binney, J.E.D. *British Public Finance and Administration 1774–1792.* Oxford, 1958.

Black, C.E., et al. *The Modernization of Japan and Russia: A Comparative Study.* New York, 1975.

Blackaby, F., ed. *De-industrialization.* London, 1979.

Blackburn, G. *The West and the World Since 1945.* New York, 1985.

Blackett, P.M.S. *Fear, War, and the Bomb.* New York, 1948.

Blackwell, W.L. *The Beginnings of Russian Industrialization, 1800–1860.* Princeton, N.J., 1968.

————. *The Industrialization of Russia: An Historical Perspective.* New York, 1970.

————, ed. *Russian Economic Development from Peter the Great to Stalin.* New York, 1974.

Blond, G. *La Grande Armée 1804/1815.* Paris, 1979.

Blum, R.M. *Drawing the Line: The Origin of American Containment Policy in East Asia.* New York, 1982.

Bond, B. *British Military Policy Between Two World Wars.* Oxford, 1980.

————, "The First World War," *New Cambridge Modern History,* vol. 12 (rev. edn.). Cambridge, 1968.

Boog, H., et al., eds. *Das Deutsche Reich und der Zweite Weltkrieg,* vol. 4, *Der Angriff auf die Sowjetunion.* Stuttgart, 1983.

Borden, W.S. *The Pacific Alliance.* Madison, Wi., 1984.

Borg, D., and W. Heinrichs, eds. *Uncertain Years: Chinese-American Relations, 1947–1950.* New York, 1980.

Bornstein, M., ed. *The Soviet Economy: Continuity and Change.* Boulder, Col., 1981.

Borowski, H.R. *A Hollow Threat: Strategic Air Power and Containment Before Korea.* Westport, Conn., 1982.

Bosher, J.F., "Financing the French Navy in the Seven Years War: Beaujou, Goossens et compagnie in 1759," *U.S. Naval Institute Proceedings,* forthcoming.

————, "French Administration and Public Finance in Their European Setting," *New Cambridge Modern History,* vol. viii. Cambridge, 1965.

————. *French Finances 1770–1795.* Cambridge, 1975.

Bosworth, J.R.B. *Italy and the Approach of the First World War.* London, 1983.

————. *Italy, the Least of the Great Powers: Italian Foreign Policy Before the First World War.* Cambridge, 1979.

Bottome, E. *The Balance of Terror.* Boston, 1986 edn.

————. *The Missile Gap.* Rutherford, N.J., 1971.

Bourne, K. *Britain and the Balance of Power in North America 1815–1908.* London, 1967.

————. *Victorian Foreign Policy 1830–1902.* Oxford, 1970.

Bowler, A. *Logistics and the Failure of the British Army in the America 1775–1783.* Princeton, N.J., 1975.

Boxer, C.R. *The Christian Century in Japan 1549–1650.* Berkeley, Calif., 1951.

———. *The Dutch Seaborne Empire 1600–1800.* London, 1972.

———. *The Portuguese Seaborne Empire 1415–1825.* London, 1969.

Bracken, P. *The Command and Control of Nuclear Weapons.* New Haven, Conn., 1983.

Bradsher, H.S. *Afghanistan and the Soviet Union.* Durham, N.C., 1983.

Braisted, W.R. *The United States Navy in the Pacific,* 2 vols. Austin, Tex., 1958, 1971.

Braudel, F. *The Mediterranean and the Mediterranean World in the Age of Philip II,* 2 vols. London, 1972.

———, and E. Labrousse, eds. *Histoire économique et sociale de la France,* vol. iv. Paris, 1980.

———. *Civilization and Capitalism, 15th–18th Centuries,* 3 vols. London, 1981–84.

Bridge, F.R., and R. Bullen. *The Great Powers and the European States System 1815–1914.* London, 1980.

Briggs, R. *Early Modern France 1560–1715.* Oxford, 1977.

Brodie, B. *Strategy in the Nuclear Age.* Princeton, N.J., 1959.

———. *The Absolute Weapon.* New York, 1946.

Bronke, A., and D. Novak, eds. *The Communist States in the Era of Détente, 1971–1977.* Oakville, Ont., 1979.

Brown, D.M., "The Impact of Firearms on Japanese Warfare," *Far Eastern Quarterly* 7 (1947).

Brown, G.S. *The American Secretary: The Colonial Policy of Lord George Germain 1775–1778.* Ann Arbor, Mich., 1963.

Brown, L., et al. *State of the World, 1986.* New York, 1986.

Brunn, G. *Europe and the French Imperium, 1799–1815.* New York, 1938.

Brunner, E., Jr. *Soviet Demographic Trends and the Ethnic Composition of Draft Age Males, 1980–1995.* Santa Monica, Calif., 1981.

Brunschwig, H. *French Colonialism, 1871–1916: Myths and Realities.* London, 1966.

Brzezinski, Z. *The Soviet Bloc: Unity and Conflict.* Cambridge, Mass., 1967 edn.

Bull, H. *The Anarchical Society.* New York, 1977.

———, and A. Watson, eds. *The Expansion of International Society.* Oxford, 1984.

Bullock, A. *Ernest Bevin, Foreign Secretary.* Oxford, 1983.

———. *Hitler: A Study in Tyranny.* London, 1962 edn.

Bunce, V., "The Empire Strikes Back: The Evolution of the Eastern Bloc from a Soviet Asset to a Soviet Liability," *International Organization* 39 (1985).

Bundy, M., et al., "Nuclear Weapons and the Atlantic Alliance," *Foreign Affairs* 62 (1982).

Burk, K. *Britain, America and the Sinews of War 1914–1918.* London, 1985.

Bushnell, J. *Mutiny and Repression: Russian Soldiers in the Revolution of 1905–1906.* Bloomington, Ind., 1985.

———, "Peasants in Uniform: The Tsarist Army as a Peasant Society," *Journal of Social History* 13 (1980).

———, "The Tsarist Officer Corps, 1881–1915: Customs, Duties, Inefficiencies," *American Historical Review* 86 (1981).

Butler, J.R.M. *Grand Strategy,* vol. ii. London, 1957.

Butow, R.J. *Tojo and the Coming of War.* Princeton, N.J., 1961.

Cain, P.J.. *Economic Foundations of British Overseas Expansion 1815–1914.* London, 1980.

———, and A.G. Hopkins, "The Political Economy of British Expansion Overseas, 1750–1914," *Economic History Review* 33 (1980).

Cairncross, A. *Years of Recovery: British Economic Policy 1945–51.* London, 1985.

Cairns, J.C., "A Nation of Shopkeepers in Search of a Suitable France," *American Historical Review* 79 (1974).

———, "Some Recent Historians and the 'Strange Defeat' of 1940," *Journal of Modern History* 46 (1974).

Calder, A. *Revolutionary Empire: The Rise of the English-Speaking Empires from the Fifteenth Century to the 1780's.* London, 1981.

Calder, K.E., "The Making of a Trans-Pacific Economy," *World Policy Journal* 2 (1985).

Calder, N. *Nuclear Nightmares.* Harmondsworth, Mddsx., 1981.

Caldicott, H. *Nuclear Madness.* Brookline, Mass., 1979.

Calleo, D. *The German Problem Reconsidered: Germany and the World Order, 1870 to the Present.* New York, 1978.

———. *The Imperious Economy.* Cambridge, Mass., 1982.

Cameron, R.E., "Economic Growth and Stagnation in France 1815–1914," *Journal of Modern History* 30 (1958).

———. *France and the Economic Development of Europe 1800–1914.* Princeton, N.J., 1961.

Camilleri, J. *Chinese Foreign Policy: The Maoist Era and Its Aftermath.* Seattle, 1980.

Campbell, C.S. *From Revolution to Rapprochement: The United States and Great Britain, 1783–1900.* New York, 1974.

Canby, S.L., "Military Reform and the Art of War," Wilson Center, International Security Studies Program, working paper 41. Washington, D.C., 1982.

Caron, F. *An Economic History of Modern France.* New York, 1979.

Carr, E.H. *The Twenty Years Crisis 1919–1939.* London, 1939.

———. *What Is History?* Harmondsworth, Mddsx., 1964.

Carr, W. *Poland to Pearl Harbor.* London, 1985.

Carrere d'Encausse, H. *Decline of an Empire.* New York, 1979.

Carroll, B.A. *Design for Total War: Arms and Economics in the Third Reich.* The Hague, 1968.

Carroll, E.M. *French Public Opinion and Foreign Affairs 1880–1914.* London, 1931.

Carsten, F.L. *The Origins of Prussia.* Oxford, 1954.

Carter, A.C., "Dutch Foreign Investment, 1738–1800," *Economica* 20 (1953).

———. *Neutrality or Commitment: The Evolution of Dutch Foreign Policy (1667–1795).* London, 1975.

———. *The Dutch Republic in the Seven Years War.* London, 1971.

Castronovo, V., "The Italian Takeoff: A Critical Re-examination of the Problem," *Journal of Italian History* 1 (1978).

Caute, D. *The Fellow Travellers.* London, 1973.

Cecco, M. de. *Money and Empire: The International Gold Standard 1890–1914.* Oxford, 1974.

Central Intelligence Agency, "China: Economic Performance in 1985." Washington, D.C., 1986.

———. *Handbook of Economic Statistics,* Washington, D.C., 1984.

Chace, J. *Solvency, the Price of Survival.* New York, 1981.

Challenor, R.D. *Admirals, Generals and American Foreign Policy 1898–1914.* Princeton, N.J., 1973.

———. *The French Theory of the Nation in Arms 1866–1939.* New York, 1955.

Challiand, G., and J.-P. Rageau. *Strategic Atlas: A Comparative Geopolitics of the World's Powers.* New York, 1985.

Chalmers Hood, R. *Royal Republicans: The French Naval Dynasties Between the World Wars.* Baton Rouge, La., 1985.

Chan, S., "The Impact of Defense Spending on Economic Performance: A Survey of Evidence and Problems," *Orbis* 29 (1985).

Chandaman, C.D. *The English Public Revenue 1660–1688.* Oxford, 1975.

Chandler, D.G., "Fluctuation in the Strength of Forces in English Pay Sent to Flanders During the Nine Years War, 1688–1697," *War and Society* 1 (1983).

——. *The Art of Warfare in the Age of Marlborough.* London, 1976.

——. *The Campaigns of Napoleon.* New York, 1966.

Chaunu, P. *European Expansion in the Later Middle Ages.* Amsterdam, 1979.

Childs, J. *Armies and Warfare in Europe 1648–1789.* Manchester, 1982.

Christie, I.R. *Wars and Revolutions: Britain 1760–1815.* London, 1982.

Chudoba, B. *Spain and the Empire 1519–1643.* New York, 1969 edn.

Cipolla, C., ed. *The Economic Decline of Empires.* London, 1970.

——. *The Fontana Economic History of Europe,* 6 vols. London, 1972–76.

——. *Before the Industrial Revolution: European Society and Economy 1000–1700,* 2nd edn. London, 1980.

——. *Guns and Sails in the Early Phase of European Expansion 1400–1700.* London, 1965.

Clapham, J.H. *The Bank of England,* vol. i, *1694–1797.* Cambridge, 1944.

——. *The Economic Development of France and Germany, 1815–1914.* Cambridge, 1948.

——. *The Economic History of Modern Britain,* 3 vols. Cambridge, 1938.

Clark, A. *Barbarossa: The Russo-German Conflict 1941–1945.* London, 1965.

Clark, J.G. *La Rochelle and the Atlantic Economy During the Eighteenth Century.* Baltimore, 1981.

Clarke, G.N. *The Dutch Alliance and the War Against French Trade 1688–1697.* New York, 1971 edn.

Clough, S.B. *France: A History of National Economics 1789–1939.* New York, 1939.

——. *The Economic History of Modern Italy, 1830–1914.* New York, 1964.

Clubb, O.E. *China and Russia: The "Great Game."* New York, 1971.

Coates, J., and M. Kilian. *Heavy Losses.* New York, 1985 edn.

Cockburn, A. *The Threat: Inside the Soviet Military Machine.* New York, 1984 edn.

Cohen, E.A. *Citizens and Soldiers: The Dilemma of Military Service.* Ithaca, N.Y., 1985.

——, "When Policy Outstrips Power—American Strategy and Statecraft," *The Public Interest* 75 (1984).

Cohen, J.S., "Financing Industrialization in Italy, 1898–1914: The Partial Transformation of a Latecomer," *Journal of Economic History* 27 (1967).

Cohn, H.D. *Soviet Policy Toward Black Africa.* New York, 1972.

Cohn, S.H. *Economic Development in the Soviet Union.* Lexington, Mass., 1970.

Coleman, D.C. *The Economic History of England 1450–1750.* Oxford, 1977.

Colton, T.J. *The Dilemma of Reform in the Soviet Union.* New York, 1984.

Connelly, O. *Napoleon's Satellite Kingdoms.* New York, 1965.

Conquest, R. *The Great Terror.* London, 1968.

Contamine, H. *La Revanche, 1871–1914.* Paris, 1957.

Cook, M.A., ed. *A History of the Ottoman Empire to 1730.* Cambridge, 1976.

Cookson, J.E., "Political Arithmetic and War 1793–1815," *War and Society* 1 (1983).

Cooper, F., "Affordable Defense: In Search of a Strategy," *Journal of the Royal United Services Institute for Defence Studies* 130 (1985).

Coox, A. *Nomonhan,* 2 vols. Stanford, Calif., 1985.

Corbett, J.S. *England in the Seven Years War: A Study in Combined Strategy,* 2 vols. London, 1907.

Corvisier, A. *Armies and Societies in Europe 1494–1789.* Bloomington, Ind., 1979.

Cosmas, G.A. *An Army for Empire: The United States Army in the Spanish-American War.* Columbia, Mo., 1971.

Cowie, L.W. *Eighteenth-Century Europe.* London, 1963.

Cowling, M. *The Impact of Hitler: British Politics and British Policies 1933–1940.* Cambridge, 1975.

Crafts, N.F.R. *British Economic Growth During the Industrial Revolution.* Oxford, 1985.

———, "British Economic Growth, 1700–1831: A Review of the Evidence," *Economic History Review* 36 (1983).

———, "Industrial Revolution in England and France: Some Thoughts on the Question: 'Why Was England First?'" *Economic History Review* 30 (1977).

Craig, G.A. *Germany 1866–1965.* Oxford, 1978.

———. *The Battle of Koeniggratz.* London, 1965.

———. *The Politics of the Prussian Army 1640–1945.* Oxford, 1955.

———, and A. G. George. *Force and Statecraft: Diplomatic Problems of Our Time.* Oxford, 1983.

Creveld, M. van. *Command in War.* Cambridge, Mass., 1985.

———. *Fighting Power: German and U.S. Army Performance, 1939–1945.* Westport, Conn., 1982.

———. *Supplying War: Logistics from Wallenstein to Patton.* Cambridge, 1977.

Crisp, O. *Studies in the Russian Economy Before 1914.* London, 1976.

Crouzet, F., "L'Angleterre et France au XVIIIe siècle: essai d'analyse comparée de deux croissances économiques," *Annales* 21 (1966).

———. *L'Economie britannique et le Blocus Continental 1806–1813,* 2 vols. Paris, 1958.

———. *The Victorian Economy.* London, 1982.

———, "Toward an Export Economy: British Exports During the Industrial Revolution," *Explorations in Economic History* 17 (1980).

———, "Wars, Blockade and Economic Change in Europe, 1792–1815," *Journal of Economic History* 24 (1964).

Crowe, S.E. *The Berlin West African Conference 1884–1885.* Westport, Conn., 1970 reprint.

Crowley, J.B. *Japan's Quest for Autonomy: National Security and Foreign Policy 1930–1958.* Princeton, N.J., 1966.

Crowson, P.S. *Tudor Foreign Policy.* London, 1973.

Cruikshank, C.G. *Elizabeth's Army.* 2nd edn., Oxford, 1966.

Cumings, B. *The Origins of the Korean War.* Princeton, N.J., 1981.

Curran, S., and D. Ponomoreff. *Managing the Ethnic Factor in the Russian and Soviet Armed Forces: An Historical Overview.* Santa Monica, Calif., 1982.

Curtis, E.E. *The Organization of the British Army in the American Revolution.* Menston, Yorkshire, 1972 reprint.

Curtiss, J.S. *Russia's Crimean War.* Durham, N.C., 1979.

———. *The Russian Army Under Nicholas I, 1825–1855.* Durham, N.C., 1965.

Dallek, R. *The American Style of Foreign Policy.* New York, 1983.

Dallin, D.J. *Soviet Foreign Policy After Stalin.* Philadelphia, 1961.

Daniels, R.V. *Russia, The Roots of Confrontation.* Cambridge, Mass., 1985.

Darby, H.C., "The Face of Europe on the Eve of the Great Discoveries," *New Cambridge Modern History,* vol. i. Cambridge, 1961.

Davies, R.T. *The Golden Century of Spain 1501–1621.* London, 1937.

Davis, L.E. *The Cold War Begins: Soviet-American Conflict over Eastern Europe.* Princeton, N.J., 1974.

Davis, R. *English Overseas Trade 1500–1700.* London, 1973.

———. *The Industrial Revolution and British Overseas Trade.* Leicester, 1979.

———. *The Rise of the Atlantic Economies.* London, 1975.

Davison, W.P. *The Berlin Blockade.* Princeton, N.J., 1958.

Dawisha, A., and K. Dawisha, eds. *The Soviet Union in the Middle East.* New York, 1982.

Dawisha, K. *Soviet Foreign Policy Towards Egypt.* London, 1979.

Dawson, R. *Imperial China.* London, 1972.

Dean, J., "Directions in Inner-German Relations," *Orbis* 29 (1985).

DeGrasse, R.W. *Military Expansion, Economic Decline.* Armonk, N.Y., 1983.

Dehio, L. *The Precarious Balance.* London, 1963.

Deist, W. *The Wehrmacht and German Rearmament.* London, 1981.

———, et al., eds. *Das Deutsche Reich und der Zweite Weltkrieg,* vol. 1, *Ursachen und Voraussetzungen der deutschen Kriegspolitik.* Stuttgart, 1979.

De Gaulle, C. *Mémoires de Guerre,* 3 vols., Paris, 1954–59.

DePorte, A. *Europe Between the Superpowers.* New Haven, Conn., 1979.

de St. Leger, A., and P. Sagnac. *Lá Préponderance française, Louis XIV, 1661–1715.* Paris, 1935.

Devlin, P. *Too Proud to Fight: Woodrow Wilson's Neutrality,* New York, 1975.

Dibb, P. *The Soviet Union: The Incomplete Super-power.* London, 1985.

Dickson, P.G.M. *The Financial Revolution in England: A Study in the Development of Public Credit 1688–1756.* London, 1967.

———, and J. Sperling, "War Finance, 1689–1714," *New Cambridge Modern History,* vol. vi. Cambridge, 1970.

Diehl, J. *Paramilitary Politics in Weimar Germany.* Bloomington, Ind., 1977.

Dietz, F.C. *English Public Finance 1485–1641,* 2 vols. London, 1964 edn.

———, "The Exchequer in Elizabeth's Reign," *Smith College Studies in History* 8 (1923).

Diffie, B.W., and C. D. Winius. *Foundations of the Portuguese Empire 1415–1580.* Minneapolis, 1977.

Dilks, D., ed. *Retreat from Power: Studies in Britain's Foreign Policy in the Twentieth Century,* 2 vols. London, 1981.

Dinerstein, H.S. *War and the Soviet Union.* London, 1962 edn.

Dingman, R., "Strategic Planning and the Policy Process: American Plans for War in East Asia, 1945–50," *Naval War College Review* 32 (1979).

Divine, R.A. *Second Chance: The Triumph of Internationalism in America During World War II.* New York, 1971.

Dockrill, M.L., and J. D. Goold. *Peace Without Promise: Britain and the Peace Conferences 1919–1923.* London, 1981.

Dodgshon, R.A., "A Spatial Perspective," *Peasant Studies* 6 (1977).

Donaldson, R.H., ed. *The Soviet Union in the Third World: Successes and Failures.* Boulder, Col., 1981.

———. *Soviet Policy Toward India.* Cambridge, Mass., 1974.

Donnelly, C.N., "Tactical Problems Facing the Soviet Army: Recent Debates in the Soviet Military Press," *International Defense Review* 11 (1978).

Donoughue, B. *British Politics and the American Revolution.* London, 1964.

Doran, C.F., and W. Parsons, "War and the Cycle of Relative Power," *American Political Science Review* 74 (1980).

Dorn, F. *The Sino-Japanese War 1937–1941.* New York, 1974.

Dorn, W.L. *Competition for Empire 1740–1763.* New York, 1940.

Doughty, R.A. *The Seeds of Disaster: The Development of French Army Doctrine 1919–1939.* Hamden, Conn., 1985.

Douglas, R. *From War to Cold War 1942–1948.* London, 1981.

Dovrig, B. *The Myth of Liberation.* Baltimore, Md., 1973.

Doyle, W. *The Old European Order 1660–1800.* Oxford, 1978.

Dreyer, J.T., "China's Military Modernization," *Orbis* 27 (1984).

Droz, J. *Europe Between Revolutions 1815–1848.* London, 1967.

Drucker, P.F., "The Changed World Economy," *Foreign Affairs* 64 (1986).

Dubief, H. *Le Declin de la IIIᵉ République 1929–1938.* Paris, 1976.

Duffy, C. *Borodino and the War of 1812.* London, 1973.

———. *Russia's Military Way to the West: Origins and Nature of Russian Military Power 1700–1800.* London, 1981.

———. *Siege Warfare: The Fortress in the Early Modern World 1494–1660.* London, 1979.

———. *The Army of Frederick the Great.* Newton Abbott, 1974.

———. *The Army of Maria Theresa: The Armed Forces of Imperial Austria 1740–1780.* London, 1977.

Duffy, M., ed. *The Military Revolution and the State 1500–1800.* Exeter, 1980.

Dukes, P. *The Emergence of the Super-Powers: A Short Comparative History of the USA and the USSR.* London, 1970.

———. *The Making of Russian Absolutism 1613–1801.* London, 1982.

Dülffer, J., "Der Beginn des Krieges 1939," *Geschichte und Gesellschaft* 2 (1976).

———. *Weimar, Hitler und die Marine: Reichspolitik und Flottenbau 1920–1939.* Düsseldorf, 1973.

Dull, J. *A Diplomatic History of the American Revolution.* New Haven, Conn., 1985.

———. *The French Navy and American Independence.* Princeton, N.J., 1975.

Dupuy, N. *A Genius for War: The German Army and General Staff, 1807–1945.* Englewood Cliffs, N.J., 1977.

Duroselle, J.B. *La Décadence 1932–1939.* Paris, 1979.

Dutailly, H. *Les Problèmes de l'Armée de terre française 1933–1939.* Paris, 1980.

Eatwell, J. *Whatever Happened to Britain?* London, 1982.

Eberhard, W. *A History of China,* 2nd edn. London, 1960.

Eckes, A.E. *The United States and the Global Struggle for Minerals.* Austin, Tex., 1979.

Ehrenberg, R. *Das Zeitalter der Fugger: Geldkapital und Creditverkehr im 16. Jahrhundert,* 2 vols. Jena, 1896.

Ehrman, J. *Cabinet Government and War 1890–1940.* Cambridge, 1958.

———. *The Younger Pitt,* 2 vols. London, 1969, 1983.

Eldridge, C.C., ed. *British Imperialism in the Nineteenth Century.* London, 1984.

Elliott, J.H. *Europe Divided 1559–1598.* London, 1968.

———. *Imperial Spain 1469–1716.* Harmondsworth, Mddsx., 1970.

———. *Richelieu and Olivares.* Cambridge, 1984.

———. *The Count-Duke of Olivares.* New Haven, Conn., 1986.

Elton, G.R., ed. *The New Cambridge Modern History,* vol. ii, *The Reformation 1520–1559.* Cambridge, 1958.

———. *England Under the Tudors.* London, 1955.

———. *Reformation Europe 1517–1559.* London, 1963.

Elvin, M. *The Pattern of the Chinese Past.* London, 1963.

Emerson, R. *From Empire to Nation: The Rise to Self-Assertion of Asian and African Peoples.* Cambridge, Mass., 1962.

Emmerson, J.T. *The Rhineland Crisis.* London, 1977.

Emsley, C. *British Society and the French Wars 1793–1815.* London, 1979.

Engels, F. *Herr Eugen Dühring's Revolution in Science.* London, 1936 edn.

———, "Socialism: Utopian and Scientific," in *The Essential Left.* London, 1960.

Epstein, G., "The Triple Debt Crisis," *World Policy Journal* 2 (1985).

Erhard, L. *The Economics of Success.* Princeton, N.J., 1963.

Erickson, J. *The Road to Berlin.* London, 1983.

———. *The Road to Stalingrad.* London, 1975.

———. *The Soviet High Command, 1918–1941.* London, 1962.

Ernstberger, A. *Hans de Witte: Finanzmann Wallensteins.* Wiesbaden, 1954.

Essame, H. *The Battle for Europe, 1918.* New York, 1972.

Evangelista, M.A., "Stalin's Postwar Army Reappraised," *International Security* 7 (1982–3).

Eysenbach, M.L. *American Manufactured Exports 1897–1914: A Study of Growth and Comparative Advantage.* New York, 1976.

Falkus, M. *The Industrialization of Russia 1700–1914.* London, 1972.

———, "Aspects of Foreign Investment in Tsarist Russia," *Journal of European Economic History* 8 (1979).

Fallows, J. *National Defense.* New York, 1981.

Farrar, L.L. *Arrogance and Anxiety: The Ambivalence of German Power 1849–1914.* Iowa City, Ia., 1981.

———. *The Short War Illusion.* Santa Barbara, Calif., 1973.

Feis, H. *Churchill-Roosevelt-Stalin.* Princeton, N.J., 1967.

———. *The Atomic Bomb and the End of World War II.* Princeton, N.J., 1966 edn.

———. *The China Tangle.* Princeton, N.J., 1953.

Feldman, G. *Army, Industry and Labor in Germany 1914–1918.* Princeton, N.J., 1966.

Ferguson, T.G. *British Military Intelligence 1870–1914.* Frederick, Md., 1984.

Fieldhouse, D. *Economics and Empire 1830–1914.* London, 1973.

———. *The Colonial Empires: A Comparative Study from the Eighteenth Century.* London, 1966.

Fingar, T., ed. *China's Quest for Independence.* Boulder, Col., 1980.

Fink, C.L., et al., eds. *German Nationalism and the European Response 1890–1945.* Chapel Hill, N.C., 1985.

Fischer, E. *The Passing of the European Age.* Cambridge, Mass., 1943.

Fischer, F. *Bündnis der Eliten.* Düsseldorf, 1979.

———. *War of Illusions: German Policies from 1911 to 1914.* London, 1975.

Fischer, R.L., "Defending the Central Front: The Balance of Forces," *Adelphi Papers* 127 (1976).

Fisher, R.H. *The Russian Fur Trade 1550–1700.* Berkeley, Calif., 1943.

Fishlow, A., "Lessons from the Past: Capital Markets During the 19th Century and the Interwar Period," *International Organization* 39 (1985).

Fitzgerald, F. *Fire in the Lake: The Vietnamese and the Americans in Vietnam.* Boston, 1972.

Flora, P., ed. *State, Economy and Society in Western Europe 1875–1975,* vol. i. Frankfurt, 1983.

Florinsky, M. *Russia: A Short History.* New York, 1964.

Floyd, D. *Mao Against Khrushchev.* New York, 1964.

Foreman-Peck, J. *A History of the World Economy: International Economic Relations Since 1850.* Brighton, Sussex, 1983.

Forstmeier, F., and H. E. Volkmann, eds. *Kriegswirtschaft und Rüstung 1939–1945.* Düsseldorf, 1977.

———. *Wirtschaft und Rüstung am Vorabend des Zweiten Weltkrieges.* Düsseldorf, 1975.

Foschepoth, J., ed. *Kalter Krieg und deutsche Frage.* Göttingen, 1985.

Fox, G. *British Admirals and the Chinese Pirates 1832–1869.* London, 1940.

Frank, A.G. *World Accumulation 1492–1789.* New York, 1978.

Frankenstein, R. *Le Prix du réarmement français 1935–1939.* Paris, 1939.

Frankland, N. *The Bomber Offensive Against Germany.* London, 1965.

Freedman, L. *Britain and Nuclear Weapons.* London, 1980.

———. *The Evolution of Nuclear Strategy.* London, 1981.

French, D. *British Economic and Strategic Planning, 1905–1915.* London, 1982.

———. *British Strategy and War Aims 1914–1916.* London, 1986.

Friedberg, A.L., "A History of US Strategic 'Doctrine,' 1945–1980," *Journal of Strategic Studies* 3 (1983).

Friedman, E., ed. *Ascent and Decline in the World-System.* Beverly Hills, Calif., 1982.

Fukuyama, F., "Gorbachev and the Third World," *Foreign Affairs* 64 (1986).

Fuller, W.C. *Civil-Military Conflict in Imperial Russia 1881–1914.* Princeton, N.J., 1985.

Fussell, P. *The Great War and Modern Memory.* New York, 1975.

Gaddis, J.L. *Strategies of Containment.* New York, 1982.

——, "The Origins of Self-Deterrence: The United States and the Non-Use of Nuclear Weapons, 1954–1958," forthcoming.

——. *The United States and the Origins of the Cold War, 1941–1947.* New York, 1972.

Gallagher, J., and R. Robinson, "The Imperialism of Free Trade," *Economic History Review* 6 (1953).

Gansler, J.S. *The Defense Industry.* Cambridge, Mass., 1980.

Garder, M. *L'Agonie du régime en Russie soviétique.* Paris, 1966.

Gardner, R.N. *Sterling-Dollar Diplomacy.* New York, 1969.

Garfinkle, A.W. *The Politics of the Nuclear Freeze.* Philadelphia, 1984.

Garthoff, R.L. *Détente and Confrontation: American-Soviet Relations from Nixon to Reagan.* Washington, D.C., 1985.

——. *Soviet Strategy in the Nuclear Age.* New York, 1958.

Gash, G. *Renaissance Armies 1480–1650.* Cambridge, 1975.

Gates, D. *The Spanish Ulcer: A History of the Peninsula War.* London, 1986.

Gatrell, P. *The Tsarist Economy, 1850–1917.* London, 1983.

Geggus, D., "The Cost of Pitt's Caribbean Campaigns, 1793–1798," *Historical Journal* 26 (1983).

Geiss, I., and B. J. Wendt, eds. *Deutschland in der Weltpolitik des 19. und 20. Jahrhunderts.* Düsseldorf, 1973.

Gershrenkon, A. *Economic Backwardness in Historical Perspective.* Cambridge, Mass., 1962.

Gervasi, T. *The Myth of Soviet Military Supremacy.* New York, 1986.

Geyer, M. *Aufrüstung oder Sicherheit.* Wiesbaden, 1980.

Gibbs, H.A.R., and H. Bowen. *Islamic Society and the West,* 2 vols. London, 1950, 1957.

Gibbs, N.H. *Grand Strategy,* vol. i. London, 1976.

Gibson, C. *Spain in America.* New York, 1966.

Gilbert, F. *The End of the European Era, 1890 to the Present,* 3rd edn. New York, 1984.

Gilbert, M., ed. *A Century of Conflict, 1850–1950.* London, 1966.

——. *Winston Churchill,* vol. v, *1922–1939.* London, 1976.

Gillard, D. *The Struggle for Asia 1828–1961.* London, 1977.

Gillie, M.H. *Forging the Thunderbolt.* Harrisburg, Penn., 1947.

Gilpin, R. *War and Change in World Politics.* Cambridge, 1981.

Ginsburgs, G., and C. F. Pinkele. *The Sino-Soviet Territorial Dispute, 1949–64.* New York, 1978.

——, and A. Z. Rubinstein, eds. *Soviet Foreign Policy Towards Western Europe.* New York, 1978.

Giovannetti, L., and F. Freed. *The Decision to Drop the Bomb.* London, 1967.

Gipson, L.H. *The Coming of the Revolution 1763–1775.* New York, 1962.

Girardet, R. *La société militaire dans la France contemporaine.* Paris, 1953.

——. *L'idée coloniale de la France sous la Troisième République 1871–1914.* Paris, 1968.

Girault, R. *Emprunts russes et investisements français en Russie, 1887–1914.* Paris, 1973.

Global 2000 Report to the President, The. Washington, D.C., 1980.

Glover, M. *The Napoleonic Wars: An Illustrated History 1792–1815.* New York, 1979.

———. *The Peninsular War, 1807–1814: A Concise History.* Newton Abbott, 1974.

———. *Warfare from Waterloo to Mons.* London, 1980.

Glover, R. *Peninsular Preparation: The Reform of the British Army, 1795–1809.* Cambridge, 1963.

Godechet, J., B. F. Hyslop, and D. L. Dowd. *The Napoleonic Era in Europe.* New York, 1971.

Goldman, M.I. *The Enigma of Soviet Petroleum: Half-Full or Half-Empty?* London, 1980.

———. *USSR in Crisis: The Failure of an Economic System.* New York, 1983.

Goldsmith, R.W., "The Power of Victory: Munitions Output in World War II," *Military Affairs* 10 (1946).

Gollwitzer, H. *Europe in the Age of Imperialism.* London, 1969.

———. *Geschichte des weltpolitischen Denkens,* 2 vols. Göttingen, 1972, 1982.

Golovine, N. *Russian Army in the World War.* New Haven, Conn., 1932.

Gooch, J. *The Plans of War: The General Staff and British Military Strategy c. 1900–1916.* London, 1974.

Good, D.F. *The Economic Rise of the Habsburg Empire, 1750–1914.* Berkeley, Calif., 1984.

Gorce, P.-M. de la. *The French Army: A Military Political History.* New York, 1963.

Gordon, D.C. *The Dominion Partnership in Imperial Defense 1870–1914.* Baltimore, Md., 1965.

Gormley, D.M., "A New Dimension to Soviet Theater Strategy," *Orbis* 29 (1985).

Gottman, J., ed. *Center and Periphery.* Beverly Hills, Calif., 1980.

Goubert, P. *Louis XIV and Twenty Million Frenchmen.* London, 1970.

Gough, B. *The Royal Navy and the North West Coast of America 1810–1914.* Vancouver, 1971.

Gowa, J. *Closing the Gold Window: Domestic Politics and the End of Bretton Woods.* Ithaca, N.Y., 1983.

Grabaud, S.R. *British Labour and the Russian Revolution 1917–1924.* Cambridge, Mass., 1956.

Graebner, N.A. *America as a World Power.* Wilmington, Del., 1984.

Graham, G.S. *Great Britain in the Indian Ocean: A Study of Maritime Enterprise 1810–1850.* Oxford, 1967.

Graml, H., ed. *Sommer 1939, Die Grossmächte und der europäische Krieg.* Stuttgart, 1979.

Gray, C., "Nuclear Strategy: A Case for a Theory of Victory," *International Security* 4 (1979).

Greenwood, S., "Return to Dunkirk: The Origins of the Anglo-French Treaty of March 1947," *Journal of Strategic Studies* 6 (1983).

Grenville, J.A.S., and G. B. Young. *Politics, Strategy and American Diplomacy: Studies in Foreign Policy, 1873–1917.* New Haven, Conn., 1966.

———. *A World History of the Twentieth Century 1900–1945.* London, 1980.

———. *Europe Reshaped 1848–1878.* London, 1976.

———. *Lord Salisbury and Foreign Policy: The Close of the Nineteenth Century, 1895–1902.* London, 1964.

Griffith, W.E., ed. *Communism in Europe: Continuity, Change and the Sino-Soviet Dispute,* 2 vols. Cambridge, Mass., 1964–66.

———, "Superpower Problems in Europe: A Comparative Assessment," *Orbis* 29 (1986).

———. *The Ostpolitik of the Federal Republic of Germany.* Cambridge, Mass., 1978.
Groom, J. *British Thinking About Nuclear Weapons.* London, 1974.
Grosser, A. *The Western Alliance: European-American Relations Since 1945.* London, 1980.
———. *West Germany from Defeat to Rearmament.* London, 1955.
Growing, M. *Independence and Deterrence: Britain and Atomic Energy 1945–1952,* 2 vols. London, 1974.
Grün, G., "Locarno, Ideal and Reality," *International Affairs* 31 (1955).
Gruner, W., "Der Deutsche Bund—Modell für eine Zwischenlösung?" *Politik und Kultur* 9 (1982).
———. *Die deutsche Frage: Ein Problem der europäischen Geschichte seit 1800.* Munich, 1985.
Grunwald, J., and K. Flamm. *The Global Factory: Foreign Assembly in International Trade.* Washington, D.C., 1985.
Guéry, A., "Les finances de la monarchie française," *Annales* 33 (1978).
Guilmartin, J.F. *Gunpowder and Galleys: Changing Technology and Mediterranean Warfare at Sea in the Sixteenth Century.* Cambridge, 1974.
Guinn, P. *British Strategy and Politics, 1914–1918.* Oxford, 1965.
Gulick, E.V. *Europe's Classical Balance of Power.* New York, 1967 edn.
Gunsberg, J.A. *Divided and Conquered: The French High Command and the Defeat of the West, 1940.* Westport, Conn., 1979.
Gustafson, T., "Energy and the Soviet Union," *International Security* 6 (1981–82).
Hadley, A.T. *The Straw Giant: Triumph and Failure: America's Armed Forces.* New York, 1986.
Hagan, K.J., ed. *In Peace and War: Interpretations of American Naval History, 1775–1978.* Westport, Conn., 1978.
Haig, A. *Caveat.* New York, 1984.
Hale, J.R., ed. *Europe in the Later Middle Ages.* London, 1965.
———, "Armies, Navies and the Art of War," *New Cambridge Modern History,* vol. ii. Cambridge, 1958.
———. *War and Society in Renaissance Europe 1450–1620.* London, 1985.
Hale, O.J. *Germany and the Diplomatic Revolution 1904–1906.* Philadelphia, 1931.
Hall, J.W. *Government and Local Power in Japan.* Princeton, N.J., 1966.
Halpern, P. *The Mediterranean Naval Situation, 1908–1914.* Cambridge, Mass., 1971.
Hamerow, T. *Restoration, Revolution, Reaction: Economics and Politics in Germany.* Princeton, N.J., 1958.
Hamilton, A. *The Appeal of Fascism.* London, 1971.
Hamilton, C.E., "The Royal Navy, *La Royale* and the Militarization of Naval Warfare, 1840–1870," *Journal of Strategic Studies* 6 (1983).
Hamilton, E.J., "Origin and Growth of National Debt in Western Europe," *American Economic Review* 37 (1947).
Hammond, T.T. *Red Flag over Afghanistan.* Boulder, Col., 1984.
Hanrieder, W.F. *West German Foreign Policy 1949–1963.* Stanford, Calif., 1967.
Haraszti, E. *The Invaders: Hitler Occupies the Rhineland.* Budapest, 1983.
———. *Treaty-Breakers or 'Realpolitiker'? The Anglo-German Naval Agreement of June 1935.* Boppard, 1974.
Hardach, G. *The First World War 1914–1918.* London, 1977.
Hardach, K. *The Political Economy of Germany in the Twentieth Century.* Berkeley, Calif., 1980.
Hardie, F. *The Abyssinian Crisis.* London, 1974.
Harding, H., ed. *China's Foreign Relations in the 1980s.* New Haven, Conn., 1984.
Haring, C.H. *The Spanish Empire in America.* New York, 1947.
Harris, K. *Attlee.* London, 1982.

Harris, R.D., "French Finances and the American War, 1777–1783," *Journal of Modern History* 46 (1976).

Harrison, J.A. *The Chinese Empire.* New York, 1972.

Harrison, M.M. *Reluctant Ally: France and Atlantic Security.* Baltimore, 1981.

Hart, G., and W. S. Lind. *America Can Win.* Bethesda, Md., 1986.

Harvie, C. *War and Society in the 19th Century.* Bletchley, 1973.

Haslam, J. *The Soviet Union and the Struggle for Collective Security in Europe 1933–39.* New York, 1984.

Hastings, M. *Overlord: D-Day and the Battle for Normandy.* London, 1984.

Hattaway, H., and A. Jones. *How the North Won: A Military History of the Civil War.* Urbana, Ill., 1983.

Hatton, R.M., ed. *Louis XIV and Europe.* London, 1976.

———. *Charles XII of Sweden.* London, 1968.

Hauner, M., "A Racial Revolution," *Journal of Contemporary History* 19 (1984).

———, "Did Hitler Want a World Dominion?," *Journal of Contemporary History* 13 (1968).

———, "The Soviet Geostrategic Dilemma," Foreign Policy Research Institute, forthcoming.

Hayashi, S., and A. Coox. *Kogun: The Japanese Army in the Pacific War.* Westport, Conn., 1978 reprint.

Hayes, P. *Fascism.* London, 1973.

Haykal, M.H. *The Sphinx and the Commissar: The Rise and Fall of Soviet Influence in the Middle East.* London, 1978.

Headrich, D.R. *The Tools of Empire: Technology and European Imperialism in the Nineteenth Century.* Oxford, 1981.

Heald, M., and L. S. Kaplan. *Culture and Diplomacy: The American Experience.* Westport, Conn., 1977.

Hecksher, E.F. *An Economic History of Sweden.* Cambridge, Mass., 1963.

———. *The Continental System.* Oxford, 1922.

Heischmann, E. *Die Anfänge des stehenden Heeres in Oesterreich.* Vienna, 1925.

Heller, F.H., ed. *The Korean War: A 25-Year Perspective.* Lawrence, Kan., 1977.

Henderson, W.O. *The Industrial Revolution on the Continent: Germany, France, Russia 1800–1914.* London, 1967 edn.

———. *The Rise of German Industrial Power, 1834–1914.* Berkeley, Calif., 1972.

Hennessy, J., et al. *Economic "Miracles."* London, 1964.

Henrickson, A.K., "The Creation of the North Atlantic Alliance, 1948–1952," *Naval War College Review* 32 (1980).

Hentschel, V., "Produktion, Wachstum und Produktivität in England, Frankreich und Deutschland von der Mitte des 19. Jahrhunderts bis zum Ersten Weltkrieg," *Vierteljahresschrift für Sozial- und Wirtschaftsgeschichte* 68 (1981).

Herken, G. *Counsels of War.* New York, 1985.

———. *The Winning Weapon: The Atomic Bomb in the Cold War 1945–1950.* New York, 1980.

Herrick, R.W. *Soviet Naval Strategy.* Annapolis, Md., 1968.

Herring, G. *America's Longest War: The United States and Vietnam, 1950–1975.* New York, 1979.

Herspring, D.R., and I. Volgyes, "Political Reliability in the Eastern European Warsaw Pact Armies," *Armed Forces and Society* 6 (1980).

Herwig, H.H. *Politics of Frustration: The United States in German Naval Planning, 1889–1941.* New York, 1976.

Hess, A.C., "The Evolution of the Ottoman Seaborne Empire in the Age of Oceanic Discoveries, 1453–1525," *American Historical Review* 75 (1970).

Hiden, J. *Germany and Europe 1919–1939.* London, 1977.

Higginbotham, D., ed. *Reconsiderations on the Revolutionary War.* Westport, Conn., 1978.

———. *The War of American Independence.* Bloomington, Ind., 1977 edn.

Higham, R. *Air Power: A Concise History.* Manhattan, Kan., 1984 edn.

Higonnet, P.L.R., "The Origins of the Seven Years War," *Journal of Modern History* 40 (1968).

Hildebrand, G.H. *Growth and Structure in the Economy of Modern Italy.* Cambridge, Mass., 1965.

Hildebrand, K., "Staatskunst oder Systemzwang? Die 'Deutsche Frage' als Problem der Weltpolitik," *Historische Zeitschrift* 228 (1979).

———. *The Third Reich.* London, 1984.

Hill, C. *Reformation to Industrial Revolution.* Harmondsworth, Mddsx., 1969.

———. *The Century of Revolution 1603–1714.* Edinburgh, 1961.

Hillgruber, A. *Bismarcks Aussenpolitik.* Freiburg, 1972.

———. *Die gescheiterte Grossmacht: Eine Skizze des Deutschen Reiches 1871–1945.* Düsseldorf, 1980.

———. *Germany and the Two World Wars.* Cambridge, Mass., 1981.

———. *Hitlers Strategie: Politik und Kriegsführung 1940–41.* Frankfurt, 1965.

Hinsley, F.H., et al. *British Intelligence in the Second World War,* vol. ii. London, 1981.

———. *Power and the Pursuit of Peace.* Cambridge, 1967.

Hobsbawm, E.J. *The Age of Capital 1848–1875.* London, 1975.

———. *Industry and Empire.* Harmondsworth, Mddsx., 1969.

———. *The Age of Revolution 1789–1848.* London, 1962.

Hochmann, J. *The Soviet Union and the Failure of Collective Security 1934–1938.* Ithaca, N.Y., 1984.

Hodgson, M.G.S. *The Venture of Islam.* Chicago, 1924.

Hoensch, J.K. *Sowjetische Osteuropa-Politik 1945–1974.* Düsseldorf, 1977.

Hoffman, S., ed. *In Search of France.* Cambridge, Mass., 1963.

———. *Gulliver's Troubles.* New York, 1968.

———. *Primacy or World Order?* New York, 1978.

Hoffmann, W.G. *Das Wachstum der deutschen Wirtschaft seit der Mitte des 19. Jahrhunderts.* Berlin, 1965.

Holland, R.F. *Britain and the Commonwealth Alliance, 1918–1939.* London, 1981.

———. *European Decolonization: The British, French, Dutch, and Belgian Empires 1919–1963.* London, 1978.

Holloway, D. *The Soviet Union and the Arms Race,* 2nd edn. New Haven, Conn., 1984.

Holmes, R. *The Road to Sedan: The French Army, 1866–1870.* London, 1984.

Holt, S. *The Common Market: The Conflict of Theory and Practice.* London, 1967.

Holzle, E. *Die Selbstentmachtung Europas.* Göttingen, 1975.

Holzman, F.D., "Are the Soviets Really Outspending the US on Defense?," *International Security* 4 (1980).

———. *Financial Checks on Soviet Defense Expenditures.* Lexington, Mass., 1975.

———, "Soviet Military Spending; Assessing the Numbers Game," *International Security* 6 (1982).

Homze, E.L. *Arming the Luftwaffe.* Lincoln, Neb., 1976.

Hope-Jones, A. *Income Tax in the Napoleonic Wars.* Cambridge, 1939.

Horn, R.C. *The Soviet Union and India. The Limits of Influence.* New York, 1981.

Horne, A. *The French Army and Politics 1870–1970.* London, 1984.

Horowitz, D. *The Free World Colossus.* New York, 1971 edn.

Hosking, G. *A History of the Soviet Union.* London, 1985.

Hough, J.F., and M. Fainsod. *How the Soviet Union Is Governed.* Cambridge, Mass., 1979.

Howard, M. ed. *The Theory and Practice of War.* London, 1965.

———. *The British Way in Warfare.* Neale Lecture, London, 1975.

———. *The Continental Commitment.* London, 1972.

———. *The Franco-Prussian War.* London, 1981 edn.

Howarth, S. *The Fighting Ships of the Rising Sun: The Drama of the Imperial Japanese Navy 1895–1945.* New York, 1983.

Hucker, C.O. *China's Imperial Past.* Stanford, Calif., 1975.

Hudson, G.F. *The Far East in World Affairs,* 2nd edn. London, 1939.

Hueckel, G., "War and the British Economy, 1793–1815: A General Equilibrium Analysis," *Explorations in Economic History* 10 (1972).

Hufton, O. *Europe: Privilege and Protest 1730–1789.* London, 1980.

Hunt, B., and A. Preston, eds. *War Aims and Strategic Policy in the Great War.* London, 1977.

Hyam, R. *Britain's Imperial Century 1815–1914.* London, 1975.

Hynes, W.G. *The Economics of Empire: Britain, Africa and the New Imperialism, 1870–95.* London, 1979.

Imlah, A.H. *Economic Elements in the "Pax Britannica."* Cambridge, Mass., 1958.

Inalcik, H. *The Ottoman Empire: Conquest, Organization and Economy: Collected Studies.* London, 1978.

———. *The Ottoman Empire: The Classical Age 1300–1600.* New York, 1973.

Ingram, E., ed., "The Great Game in Asia," *The International History Review* 2 (1980).

———. *Commitment to Empire: Prophecies of the Great Game in Asia, 1797–1800.* Oxford, 1981.

———. *The Beginning of the Great Game in Asia 1828–1834.* Oxford, 1979.

Ireland, T.P. *Creating the Entangling Alliance.* London, 1981.

Iriye, A. *Across the Pacific.* New York, 1967.

———. *After Imperialism: The Search for a New Order in the Far East 1921–1931.* New York, 1978 edn.

Irving, E.M. *The First Indochina War: French and American Policy, 1945–1954.* London, 1975.

Iseley, J.A., and P. A. Crowl. *The U.S. Marines and Amphibious War.* Princeton, N.J., 1945.

Ismay, Lord. *NATO—The First Five Years, 1949–1954.* Utrecht, 1954.

Israel, J.I., "A Conflict of Empires: Spain and the Netherlands, 1618–1648," *Past and Present* 76 (1977).

———. *The Dutch Republic and the Hispanic World, 1606–1661.* Oxford, 1982.

Jabber, P., "Egypt's Crisis, America's Dilemma," *Foreign Affairs* 64 (1986).

Jackel, E. *Hitler's Weltanschauung.* Middletown, Conn., 1982.

Jacobsen, J. *Locarno Diplomacy: Germany and the West 1925–1929.* Princeton, N.J., 1972.

Jansen, G.H. *Afro-Asia and Non-Alignment.* London, 1966.

Jelavich, B. *The Great Powers, the Ottoman Empire, and the Straits Question 1870–1887.* Bloomington, Ind., 1973.

Jencks, H.W. *From Missiles to Muskets: Politics and Professionalism in the Chinese Army 1945–1981.* Boulder, Col., 1982.

Jenkins, E.H. *A History of the French Navy.* London, 1973.

Jenks, L.H. *Migration of British Capital to 1875.* London, 1963 edn.

Jervis, R. *The Illogic of American Nuclear Strategy.* Ithaca, N.Y., 1984.

———, "The Impact of the Korean War on the Cold War," *Journal of Conflict Resolution* 24 (1980).

Joffe, J., "European-American Relations: The Enduring Crisis," *Foreign Affairs* 59 (1981).

Johnson, A.R., et al. *East European Military Establishments: The Warsaw Pact Northern Tier.* New York, 1982.

Johnson, C. *MITI and the Japanese Miracle: The Growth of Industrial Policy 1925–1975.* Stanford, Calif., 1982.

Johnson, F.A. *Defense by Committee.* London, 1960.

Johnson, P.M., and W. R. Thompson, eds. *Rhythms in Politics and Economics.* New York, 1985.

Joll, J., ed. *The Decline of the Third Republic.* New York, 1959.

———. *Europe Since 1870.* London, 1973.

———. *The Origins of the First World War.* London, 1984.

Jones, C., ed. *Britain and Revolutionary France: Conflict, Subversion and Propaganda.* Exeter, 1983.

Jones, D.R., "Nicholas II and the Supreme Command," *Sbornik* 11 (1985).

Jones, E., "Manning the Soviet Military," *International Security* 7 (1982).

———, "Minorities in the Soviet Armed Forces," *Comparative Strategy* 3 (1982).

Jones, E.L., and G. E. Mingay, eds. *Land, Labour and Population of the Industrial Revolution.* London, 1967.

———. *The European Miracle: Environments, Economies and Geopolitics in the History of Europe and Asia.* Cambridge, 1981.

Jones, J.R. *Britain and the World 1649–1815.* London, 1980.

———. *Country and Court 1658–1714.* London, 1978.

Jordan, W.M. *Britain, France and the German Problem.* London, 1943.

Jukes, G., "The Indian Ocean in Soviet Naval Policy," *Adelphi Papers* 87 (1972).

———. *The Soviet Union in Asia.* Berkeley, Calif., 1973.

Junge, C. *Flottenpolitik und Revolution: Die Entstehung der englischen Seemacht während der Herrschaft Cromwells.* Stuttgart, 1980.

Kahn, H. *On Thermonuclear War.* Princeton, N.J., 1960.

———. *The Emerging Japanese Superstate.* London, 1971.

Kaiser, D. *Economic Diplomacy and the Origins of the Second World War.* Princeton, N.J., 1980.

Kaldor, M. *The Baroque Arsenal.* London, 1982.

Kamata, S. *Japan in the Passing Lane.* New York, 1984.

Kamen, H. *Spain 1469–1714.* London, 1983.

Kan, M.Y.M. *Mainland China's Modernization: Its Prospects and Problems.* Berkeley, Calif., 1982.

Kanet, R., ed. *The Soviet Union and the Developing Nations.* Baltimore, 1974.

Kann, R.A. *A History of the Habsburg Empire 1526–1918.* Berkeley, Calif., 1974.

Kanya-Forstner, A.S. *The Conquest of the Western Sudan: A Study in French Military Imperialism.* Cambridge, 1969.

Kaplan, F. *The Wizards of Armageddon.* New York, 1983.

Kaplan, H. *Russia and the Outbreak of the Seven Years War.* Berkeley, Calif., 1968.

Kaplan, L.S. *The United States and NATO: The Formative Years.* Lexington, Ky., 1984.

Karnow, S. *Vietnam: A History.* New York, 1984.

Kaser, M. *Comecon.* London, 1967.

Katzenstein, P.J., ed. *Between Power and Plenty: Foreign Economic Policies of Advanced Industrial States.* Madison, Wi., 1978.

Kazemzadeh, F. *Russia and Britain in Persia 1864–1914.* New Haven, Conn., 1968.

Kazokins, J., "Nationality in the Soviet Army," *Journal of the Royal United Services Institute for Defense Studies* 130 (1985).

Keegan, J. *The Face of Battle.* Harmondsworth, Mddsx., 1978.

Keeny, S.M., and W.K.H. Panofsky, "MAD vs. NUTS: The Mutual Hostage Relationship of the Superpowers," *Foreign Affairs* 60 (1981–82).

Keep, J.H.L., "The Military Style of the Romanov Rulers," *War and Society* 1 (1983).

———, "Russia," *New Cambridge Modern History,* vol. xi. Cambridge, 1962.

Keiger, J.F.V. *France and the Origins of the First World War.* London, 1983.

Kelleher, C.M. *Germany and the Politics of Nuclear Weapons.* New York, 1975.

Kemp, T. *Economic Forces in French History.* London, 1971.

———. *Industrialization in Nineteenth-Century Europe.* London, 1969.

———. *The French Economy 1913–39: The History of a Decline.* New York, 1972.

Kendrick, A. *The Wound Within: America in the Vietnam Years, 1945–1974.* Boston, 1974.

Kendrick, M.S. *A Century and a Half of Federal Expenditures.* New York, 1955.

Kenez, P., "Russian Officer Corps Before the Revolution: The Military Mind," *Russian Review* 31 (1972).

Kennan, G.F. *The Decline of Bismarck's European Order: Franco-Russian Relations 1875–1890.* Princeton, N.J., 1979.

———. *American Diplomacy.* Chicago, 1984 edn.

———. *The Fateful Alliance: France, Russia, and the Coming of the First World War.* New York, 1984.

Kennedy, D. *Over Here: The First World War and American Society.* Oxford, 1980.

Kennedy, G. *Defense Economics.* London, 1983.

Kennedy, P.M., ed. *The War Plans of the Great Powers 1880–1914.* London, 1979.

———. *Strategy and Diplomacy, 1860–1945: Eight Essays.* London, 1983.

———. *The Realities Behind Diplomacy.* London, 1981.

———. *The Rise and Fall of British Naval Mastery.* London, 1976.

———. *The Rise of the Anglo-German Antagonism, 1860–1914.* London, 1980.

Kennet, L. *The French Armies in the Seven Years War: A Study in Military Organization and Administration.* Durham, N.C., 1967.

Keohane, R.O., "State Power and Industry Influence: American Foreign Oil Policy in the 1940s," *International Organization* 36 (1982).

———. *After Hegemony.* Princeton, N.J., 1974.

Kerner, R.J. *The Urge to the Sea.* New York, 1971 reprint.

Kersaudy, F. *Churchill and De Gaulle.* London, 1981.

Kershaw, I. *Popular Opinion and Political Dissent in the Third Reich: Bavaria 1933–1945.* Oxford, 1983.

———. *The Nazi Dictatorship.* London, 1985.

Keylor, W.R. *The Twentieth-Century World: An International History.* Oxford, 1984.

Kiernan, V.G. *European Empires from Conquest to Collapse, 1815–1960.* London, 1982.

———, "Foreign Mercenaries and Absolute Monarchy," *Past and Present* 11 (1957).

———, "State and Nation in Western Europe," *Past and Present* 31 (1965).

Kilmarx, R. *A History of Soviet Air Power.* London, 1962.

Kindleberger, C.P. *A Financial History of Western Europe.* London, 1984.

———, "Commercial Expansion and the Industrial Revolution," *Journal of European Economic History* 4 (1975).

———. *The World in Depression 1929–1939.* Berkeley, Calif., 1973.

Kiraly, B.K., and G. E. Rothenberg, eds. *War and Society in Eastern Europe,* vol. i. New York, 1979.

Kiser, J.W., "How the Arms Race Really Helps Moscow," *Foreign Policy* 60 (1985).

Kissinger, H. *A World Restored: Metternich, Castlereagh and the Problems of Peace 1812–1822.* Boston, 1957.

———. *The White House Years.* Boston, 1979.

———. "The White Revolutionary: Reflections on Bismarck," *Daedelus* 97 (1968).

Kitchen, M. *The Political Economy of Germany 1815–1914.* London, 1978.

Klein, L., and K. Ohkawa, eds. *Economic Growth: The Japanese Experience Since the Meiji Era.* Holmwood, Ill., 1968.

Knorr, K., "Burden-Sharing in NATO: Aspects of US Policy," *Orbis* 29 (1985).

Knox, M., "Conquest, Foreign and Domestic, in Fascist Italy and Nazi Germany," *Journal of Modern History* 56 (1986).

———. *Mussolini Unleashed 1939–1941.* Cambridge, 1982.

Koch, H.W., ed. *The Origins of the First World War.* London, 1982.

Kochan, L., and R. Abraham. *The Making of Modern Russia.* Harmondsworth, Mddsx., 1983 edn.

Kocka, J. *Facing Total War: German Society 1914–1918.* Leamington Spa, 1984.

Koenigsberger, H.G., "The Empire of Charles V in Europe," *New Cambridge Modern History,* vol. ii. Cambridge, 1958.

———, "Western Europe and the Power of Spain," *New Cambridge Modern History,* vol. 3. Cambridge, 1968.

———. *The Government of Sicily Under Philip II.* London, 1951.

———. *The Habsburgs and Europe 1516–1660.* Ithaca, N.Y., 1971.

Kohl, W.L. *French Nuclear Diplomacy.* Princeton, N.J., 1971.

Kolakowski, L. *Main Currents of Marxism,* vol. i, *The Founders.* Oxford, 1981 edn.

Kolb, E. ed. "Europa und die Reichsgründung," *Historische Zeitschrift,* Beiheft 6. Munich, 1980.

Kolko, G. *The Politics of War 1943–1945.* New York, 1968.

———. *Vietnam: Anatomy of a War, 1940–1975.* New York, 1986.

Kolodziej, E. *French International Policy Under De Gaulle and Pompidou: The Politics of Grandeur.* Ithaca, N.Y., 1974.

Komer, R.W. *Maritime Strategy or Coalition Defense?* Cambridge, Mass., 1984.

Kortepeter, C.M. *Ottoman Imperialism During the Reformation.* London, 1973.

Kriedte, P. *Peasants, Landlords and Merchant Capitalists: Europe and the World Economy, 1500–1800.* Leamington Spa, 1983.

Krumeich, G. *Armaments and Politics in France on the Eve of the First World War.* Leamington Spa, 1986.

Kuhn, A. *Hitlers aussenpolitisches Programm.* Stuttgart, 1970.

Kuisel, R.F. *Capitalism and the State in Modern France.* Cambridge, 1981.

Kuniholm, B.R. *The Origins of the Cold War in the Near East.* Princeton, N.J., 1980.

Kunisch, J. *Das Mirakel des Hauses Brandenburg.* Munich, 1978.

Kwitny, J. *Endless Enemies.* New York, 1984.

Lachouque, H. *Waterloo.* Paris, 1972.

LaFeber, W. *America, Russia, and the Cold War 1945–1975.* New York, 1976.

———. *The New Empire: An Interpretation of American Expansion 1860–1898.* Ithaca, N.Y., 1963.

Laird, R.F. *France, the Soviet Union, and the Nuclear Weapons Issue.* Boulder, Col., 1986.

———, "The French Strategic Dilemma," *Orbis* 28 (1984).

Lambi, I.N. *The Navy and German Power Politics 1862–1914.* London, 1984.

Landes, D. *The Unbound Prometheus: Technological Change and Industrial Development in Western Europe from 1750 to the Present.* Cambridge, 1969.

Langer, W.L. *European Alliances and Alignments 1871–1890.* New York, 1950 edn.

———. *The Diplomacy of Imperialism 1890–1902,* 2nd edn. New York, 1965.

Langford, P. *The Eighteenth Century 1688–1815: British Foreign Policy.* London, 1976.

Langhorne, R.T.B., ed. *Diplomacy and Intelligence During the Second World War.* Cambridge, 1985

Larson, T.B. *Soviet-American Rivalry.* New York, 1978.

Laue, T.H. von. *Sergei Witte and the Industrialization of Russia.* New York, 1963.

Laurens, F.D. *France and the Italo-Ethiopian Crisis, 1935–6.* The Hague, 1967.

League of Nations. *World Economic Survey.* Geneva, 1945.

Lee, A. *The Soviet Air Force.* London, 1961.

Lee, M., and W. Michalka. *German Foreign Policy 1917–1933: Continuity or Break?* Leamington Spa, 1987.

Lee, W.T. *The Estimation of Soviet Defense Expenditures 1955–75.* New York, 1977.

Leebaert, D., ed. *Soviet Military Thinking.* London, 1981.

Lefebvre, G. *Napoleon,* 2 vols. London, 1969.

Leffler, M.P., "Security and Containment Before Kennan: The Identification of American Interests at the End of World War II," Lehrman Institute Paper, forthcoming.

——, "The American Conception of National Security and the Beginnings of the Cold War, 1945–48," *American Historical Review* 89 (1984).

Lellouche, P. *L'avenir de la guerre.* Paris, 1985.

——, "France and the Euromissiles," *Foreign Affairs* 62 (1983–84).

Lerner, D., and R. Aron. *France Defeats EDC.* New York, 1957.

Leutze, J. *Bargaining for Supremacy: Anglo-American Naval Relations 1937–1941.* Chapel Hill, N.C., 1977.

Levine, A.J., "Was World War II a Near-Run Thing?," *Journal of Strategic Studies* 8 (1985).

Levy, J. *War in the Modern Great Power System.* Lexington, Ky., 1983.

Lewin, M. *Russian Peasants and Soviet Power.* Evanston, Ill., 1968.

Lewin, R. *The American Magic: Codes, Ciphers and the Defeat of Japan.* New York, 1982.

Lewis, W.A. *Economic Survey 1919–1939.* London, 1949.

Lichtheim, G. *Europe in the Twentieth Century.* London, 1972.

Liddell Hart, B.H., ed. *The Red Army.* New York, 1956.

——. *History of the First World War.* London, 1970 edn.

——. *History of the Second World War.* London, 1970.

Lieven, D.C.B. *Russia and the Origins of the First World War.* London, 1983.

Lifton, R.J. *Home from the War: Vietnam Veterans.* New York, 1973.

Lincoln, W.B. *Passage Through Armageddon: The Russians in the War and Revolution 1914–1918.* New York, 1986.

Linder, S.B. *The Pacific Century.* Stanford, Calif., 1986.

Linderman, G.F. *The Mirror of War: American Society and the Spanish-American War.* Ann Arbor, Mich., 1974.

Link, A.S. *Wilson,* 5 vols. Princeton, N.J., 1947–65.

Lippmann, W. *U.S. Foreign Policy: Shield of the Republic.* Boston, 1943.

Litwak, R.S. *Détente and the Nixon Doctrine: American Foreign Policy and the Pursuit of Stability, 1969–1975.* Cambridge, 1984.

Lloyd, C. *The Nation and the Navy.* London, 1961.

Loades, D.M. *Politics and the Nation 1450–1660.* London, 1974.

Lobonov-Rostovsky, A.A. *Russia and Europe 1789–1825.* Durham, N.C., 1947.

Lo Jung-pang, "The Decline of the Early Ming Navy," *Orient Extremus* 5 (1958).

——, "The Emergence of China as a Sea Power During the Late Sung and Early Yuan Periods," *Far Eastern Quarterly* 14 (1955).

Louis, W.R. *The British Empire in the Middle East, 1945–1951.* Oxford, 1984.

Lovett, G.H. *Napoleon and the Birth of Modern Spain,* 2 vols. New York, 1965.

Low, A.D. *The Sino-Soviet Dispute.* Rutherford, N.J., 1976.

Lowe, C.J., and F. Marzari. *Italian Foreign Policy 1870–1940.* London, 1975.

Lowe, P. *Britain in the Far East: A Survey from 1819 to the Present.* London, 1981.

Lubasz, H., ed. *The Development of the Modern State.* New York, 1964.

Lukacs, J. *The Last European War, September 1939/December 1941.* London, 1977.

Lundkvist, S., "Svensk krigsfinansiering 1630–1635" (with German summary), *Historisk tidskrift* (1966).

Lupfer, T., "The Dynamics of Doctrine: The Changes in German Tactical Doctrine During the First World War," *Leavenworth Papers* 4. Leavenworth, Kan., 1981.

Luttwak, E. *The Pentagon and the Art of War.* New York, 1985.

Luvaas, J. *The Military Legacy of the Civil War: The European Inheritance.* Chicago, 1959.

Lynch, J. *Spain Under the Habsburgs,* 2 vols. Oxford, 1964, 1969.

Lyon, P. *Neutralism.* Leicester, 1963.

Macartney, C.A. *The Habsburg Empire 1790–1918.* London, 1969.

McCauley, M., ed. *Communist Power in Europe, 1944–1949.* London, 1977.

———. *The Soviet Union Since 1917.* London, 1981.

McCormick, T. *China Market: America's Quest for Informal Empire.* Chicago, 1967.

MacDonald, C.A. *The United States, Britain and Appeasement 1936–1939.* London, 1980.

McDougall, W.A. *France's Rhineland Diplomacy 1914–1924.* Princeton, N.J., 1978.

McEvedy, C. *The Penguin Atlas of Recent History.* Harmondsworth, Mddsx., 1982.

McFetridge, C.D., "Some Implications of China's Emergence as a Great Power," *Journal of the Royal United Services Institute for Defence Studies* 128 (1983).

McGeehan, R. *The German Rearmament Question.* Urbana, Ill., 1971.

McGowan, P., and C. W. Kegley, eds. *Foreign Policy and the Modern World-System.* Beverly Hills, Calif., 1983.

Machay, J.P. *Pioneer for Profit: Foreign Entrepreneurs and Russian Industrialization.* Chicago, 1970.

Mack Smith, D. *Italy: A Modern History.* Ann Arbor, Mich., 1959.

———. *Mussolini's Roman Empire.* London, 1976.

———. *Mussolini: A Biography.* New York, 1982.

Mackay, D. *Prince Eugene of Savoy.* London, 1977.

MacKay, D., and H. M. Scott. *The Rise of the Great Powers 1648–1815.* London, 1983.

Mackesy, P. *Statesman at War: The Strategy of Overthrow, 1798–1799.* London, 1974.

———. *The War for America 1775–1783.* London, 1964.

Mackinder, H.J., "The Geographical Pivot of History," *Geographical Journal* 23 (1904).

Mackintosh, M. *Juggernaut: A History of the Soviet Armed Forces.* New York, 1967.

McMillen, D.H., ed. *Asian Perspectives on International Security.* London, 1984.

McNeill, W.H. *A World History.* London, 1979 edn.

———. *The Pursuit of Power: Technology, Armed Forces and Society Since 1000 A.D.* Chicago, 1983.

———. *The Rise of the West.* Chicago, 1967.

Madariaga, I. de. *Britain, Russia and the Armed Neutrality of 1780.* London, 1962.

———. *Russia in the Age of Catherine the Great.* London, 1981.

Maddison, A., "A Comparison of Levels of GDP per Capita in Developed and Developing Countries, 1700–1980," *Journal of Economic History* 43 (1983).

Magalhaes-Godinho, V. *L'économie de l'Empire Portugais aux XVe et XVIe siècles.* Paris, 1969.

Mahan, A.T. *Sea Power in Its Relations to the War of 1812,* 2 vols. London, 1905.

———. *The Influence of Sea Power upon History 1660–1783.* London, 1965 edn.

Maier, C.S. *Recasting Bourgeois Europe.* Princeton, N.J., 1975.

Maier, K.A., et al., eds. *Das Deutsche Reich und der Zweite Weltkrieg,* vol. 2, *Die Errichtung der Hegemonie auf dem europäischen Kontinent.* Stuttgart, 1979.

Mako, W.P. *U.S. Ground Forces and the Defense of Central Europe.* Washington, D.C., 1983.

Maland, D. *Europe in the Seventeenth Century.* London, 1966.

Malinraud, E. *La Croissance française.* Paris, 1972.

Mallet, M.E. *Mercenaries and Their Masters: Warfare in Renaissance Italy.* London, 1976.

Mamatey, V.S. *Rise of the Habsburg Empire 1526–1815.* Huntingdon, N.Y., 1978 edn.

Mandelbaum, M. *The Nuclear Future.* Ithaca, N.Y., 1983.

———. *The Nuclear Question: The United States and Nuclear Weapons 1946–1976.* New York, 1979.

———. *The Nuclear Revolution: International Politics Before and After Hiroshima.* New York, 1981.

Mansergh, N. *The Commonwealth Experience.* London, 1969.

Marder, A.J. *From the Dreadnought to Scapa Flow: The Royal Navy in the Fisher Period,* vol. i, *The Road to War, 1904–1914.* London, 1961.

———. *Old Friends, New Enemies: The Royal Navy and the Imperial Japanese Navy.* Oxford, 1981.

———. *The Anatomy of British Sea Power.* Hamden, Conn., 1964 reprint.

———, "The Royal Navy in the Italo-Ethiopian War 1935–36," *American Historical Review* 75 (1970).

Marks, S. *The Illusion of Peace: International Relations in Europe 1918–1933.* London, 1976.

Marriss, S. *Deficits and the Dollar: The World Economy at Risk.* Washington, D.C., 1985.

Marsh, F. *Japanese Overseas Investment.* London, 1983.

Marshall, P.J., "British Expansion in India in the Eighteenth Century: An Historical Revision," *History* 60 (1975).

Martin, B., "Aussenhandel und Aussenpolitik Englands unter Cromwell," *Historische Zeitschrift* 218 (1974).

Martin, L. *Peace Without Victory—Woodrow Wilson and the English Liberals.* New York, 1973 edn.

Marwick, A. *The Deluge—British Society in the First World War.* London, 1965.

———. *War and Social Change in the Twentieth Century.* London, 1974.

Masson, P., "La Marine française en 1939–40," *Revue historique des armées* 4 (1979).

Mathias, P. *The First Industrial Nation: An Economic History of Britain 1700–1914.* London, 1969.

———, and P. O'Brien. "Taxation in Britain and France, 1715–1810," *Journal of European Economic History* 5 (1976).

Matloff, M. *Strategic Planning for Coalition Warfare, 1943–1944.* Washington, D.C., 1959.

Mattingly, G. *Renaissance Diplomacy.* Harmondsworth, Mddsx., 1965.

May, A.J. *The Habsburg Monarchy 1862–1916.* Cambridge, Mass., 1960.

———. *The Passing of the Habsburg Monarchy, 1914–1918,* 2 vols. Philadelphia, 1966.

May, E.R., ed. *Knowing One's Enemies: Intelligence Assessment Before the Two World Wars.* Princeton, N.J., 1984.

———. *American Imperialism: A Speculative Essay.* New York, 1968.

———. *Imperial Democracy: The Emergence of America as a Great Power.* New York, 1961.

———. *The World War and American Isolation.* Chicago, 1966 edn.

Mayer, A.J. *Political Origins of the New Diplomacy.* New York, 1970 edn.

———. *Politics and Diplomacy of Peacemaking: Containment and Counterrevolution at Versailles 1918–1919.* London, 1968.

MccGwire, M. *Soviet Naval Developments*. New York, 1973.
———. *Soviet Naval Influence*. New York, 1977.
———. *Soviet Naval Policy*. New York, 1975.
Mearsheimer, J. *Conventional Deterrence*. Ithaca, N.Y., 1983.
Medlicott, W.N. *British Foreign Policy Since Versailles, 1919–1963*. London, 1968.
Mellor, R.E.M. *The Soviet Union and Its Geographical Problems*. London, 1982.
Mendelsohn, K. *Science and Western Domination*. London, 1976.
Mendl, W. *Deterrence and Persuasion: French Nuclear Armament in the Context of National Policy, 1945–1969*. London, 1970.
Menon, K. *Soviet Power and the Third World*. New York, 1985.
Meyers, R. *Britische Sicherheitspolitik 1934–1938*. Düsseldorf, 1976.
Middlebrook, M. *The Kaiser's Battle: 21 March 1918*. London, 1978.
Middlemas, K. *Diplomacy of Illusion: The British Government and Germany 1937–39*. London, 1972.
Middleton, R. *The Bells of Victory*. Cambridge, 1985.
Military Balance, The. International Institute of Strategic Studies. London, annual.
Millar, G.J. *Tudor Mercenaries and Auxiliaries 1485–1547*. Charlottesville, Va., 1980.
Miller, M.S. *The Economic Development of Russia, 1905–1914*. London, 1926.
Miller, S.E., ed. *Military Strategy and the Origins of the First World War*. Princeton, N.J., 1985.
———, ed. *Conventional Forces and American Defense Policy*. Princeton, N.J., 1986.
Millett, A.R., and W. Murray, eds. *Military Effectiveness*. Forthcoming.
———, and P. Maslowski. *For the Common Defense: A Military History of the United States of America*. New York, 1984.
Mills, W. *Arms and Men*. New York, 1956.
Milward, A.S. *The Economic Effects of the World Wars in Britain*. London, 1970.
———. *The German Economy at War*. London, 1965.
———. *The Reconstruction of Western Europe, 1945–1951*. London, 1984.
———. *War, Economy and Society 1939–1945*. Berkeley, Calif., 1979.
———, and S. B. Saul. *The Development of the Economies of Continental Europe 1850–1914*. Cambridge, Mass., 1977.
———. *The Economic Development of Continental Europe 1780–1870*. London, 1973.
Minchinton, W.E., ed. *The Growth of English Overseas Trade in the Seventeenth and Eighteenth Centuries*. London, 1969.
Mitchell, A. *The German Influence in France after 1870: The Formation of the French Republic*. Chapel Hill, N.C., 1979.
———. *Victors and Vanquished: The German Influence on Army and Church in France after 1870*. Chapel Hill, N.C., 1984.
Mitchell, B.R. *European Historical Statistics 1750–1970*. London, 1975.
Mitchell, D.W. *A History of Russian and Soviet Sea Power*. New York, 1974.
Modelski, G., "The Long Cycle of Global Politics and the Nation-State," *Comparative Studies in Society and History* 20 (1978).
Mommsen, W.J., and L. Kettenacker, eds. *The Fascist Challenge and the Policy of Appeasement*. London, 1983.
Monger, G.L. *The End of Isolation: British Foreign Policy 1900–1907*. London, 1963.
Morazé, C., "Finance et despotisme, essai sur les despotes éclairés," *Annales* 3 (1948).
Moreland, W.H. *From Akbar to Aurangzeb: A Study in Indian Economic History*. London, 1923.
Moreton, E., and G. Segal, eds. *Soviet Strategy Toward Western Europe*. London, 1984.
Morgan, K.O. *Labour in Power 1945–1951*. Oxford, 1984.

Morgan, R. *The United States and West Germany 1945–1973.* London, 1974.

Mori, G., "The Genesis of Italian Industrialization," *Journal of European Economic History* 4 (1975).

———, "The Process of Industrialization in Italy: Some Suggestions, Problems and Questions," *Journal of European Economic History* 8 (1979).

Morison, S.E. *History of the United States Naval Operations,* vol. x, *The Atlantic Battle Won.* Boston, Mass., 1956.

Morley, J.W., ed. *Dilemmas of Growth in Prewar Japan.* Princeton, N.J., 1971.

———, ed. *The Fateful Choice: Japan's Advance into Southeast Asia, 1939–1941.* New York, 1980.

———, ed. *The Pacific Basin.* New York, 1986.

Morris, M.D., "Values as an Obstacle to Growth in South Asia," *Journal of Economic History* 27 (1967).

Mortimer, R.A. *The Third World Coalition in International Politics.* New York, 1980.

Morton, E., and G. Segal, eds. *Soviet Strategy Toward Western Europe.* London, 1984.

Mosse, W.E. *Alexander II and the Modernization of Russia.* New York, 1962 edn.

———. *The European Powers and the German Question 1848–1870.* Cambridge, 1958.

———. *The Rise and Fall of the Crimean System 1855–1871.* London, 1963.

Mousnier, R., "L'Evolution des finances publiques en France et en Angleterre pendant les guerres de la Ligue d'Augsbourg et de la Succession d'Espagne," *Revue Historique* 44 (1951).

Mowat, C.L., ed. *New Cambridge Modern History,* vol. xii (rev. ed.), *The Shifting Balance of World Forces.* Cambridge, 1968.

Munro, D.G. *Intervention and Dollar Diplomacy in the Caribbean 1900–1921.* Princeton, N.J., 1964.

Munting, R. *The Economic Development of the USSR.* London, 1982.

Murphy, B. *A History of the British Economy.* London, 1973.

Murray, W., "German Air Power and the Munich Crisis," *War and Society* 1 (1976).

———. *Luftwaffe.* Baltimore, Md., 1985.

———, "Munich, 1938: The Military Confrontation," *Journal of Strategic Studies* 2 (1979).

———. *The Change in the European Balance of Power, 1938–1939.* Princeton, N.J., 1984.

Mysyrowicz, L. *Autopsie d'une Defaite: Origines de l'effrondrement militaire français de 1940.* Lausanne, 1973.

Neal, L., "Interpreting Power and Profit in Economic History: A Case Study of the Seven Years War," *Journal of Economic History* 37 (1977).

Needham, J. *Science and Civilization in China,* vol. iv, *Civil Engineering and Nautics.* Cambridge, 1971.

———. *The Development of Iron and Steel Technology in China.* London, 1958.

———. *The Grand Titration. Science and Society in East and West.* London, 1969.

Nef, J.U. *War and Human Progress.* New York, 1968.

Neidpath, J. *The Singapore Naval Base and the Defense of Britain's Eastern Empire 1919–1941.* Oxford, 1981.

Neilson, K., "Watching the 'Steamroller': British Observers and the Russian Army Before 1914." *Journal of Strategic Studies* 8 (1985).

Nettl, J.P. *The Soviet Achievement.* London, 1967.

Nicholls, A.J. *Weimar and the Rise of Hitler.* London, 1979 edn.

Nicolson, H.G. *The Congress of Vienna.* London, 1946.

Niedhart, G., "Appeasement: Die britische Antwort auf die Krise des Weltreichs und des internationalen Systems vor dem zweiten Weltkrieg," *Historische Zeitschrift* 226 (1978).

———. *Handel und Krieg in der britischen Weltpolitik 1738–1763.* Munich, 1979.

Niemeyer, J. *Das österreichische Militärwesen im Umbruch.* Osnabrück, 1979.

Nipperdey, T. *Deutsche Geschichte 1800–1866.* Munich, 1983.

Nish, I. *Japan's Foreign Policy, 1869–1942.* London, 1978.

———. *The Anglo-Japanese Alliance.* London, 1966.

———. *The Origins of the Russo-Japanese War.* London, 1985.

Nitze, P., "The Development of NSC-68," *International Security* 5 (1980).

Nobutaka, I, ed. *Japan's Decision for War.* Stanford, Calif., 1967.

Norman, E.H. *Japan's Emergence as a Modern State.* New York, 1940.

North, D.C., and R. P. Thomas. *The Rise of the Western World.* Cambridge, 1973.

North, R.C. *Moscow and the Chinese Communists.* Stanford, Calif., 1953.

Northedge, F.S., and A. Wells. *Britain and Soviet Communism: The Impact of a Revolution.* London, 1982.

———. *The Troubled Giant: Britain Among the Great Powers.* London, 1966.

Nove, A. *An Economic History of the USSR.* Harmondsworth, Mddsx., 1969.

O'Brien, P. *British Financial and Fiscal Policy in the Wars Against France, 1793–1815.* Oxford, 1984.

———, and C. Keydor. *Economic Growth in Britain and France 1780–1914.* London, 1978.

O'Day, A., ed. *The Edwardian Age.* London, 1979.

Offner, A. *American Appeasement, United States Foreign Policy and Germany 1933– 1938.* Cambridge, Mass., 1969.

Ohkawa, K., and H. Rosovsky. *Japanese Economic Growth.* Stanford, Calif., 1973.

———, and M. Shinohara, eds. *Patterns of Japanese Economic Development.* New Haven, Conn., 1979.

Okamoto, S. *The Japanese Oligarchy and the Russo-Japanese War.* New York, 1970.

Olsen, E.A. *U.S.-Japan Strategic Reciprocity: A Neo-Internationalist View.* Stanford, Calif., 1985.

Oman, C. *A History of the Art of War in the Middle Ages,* 2 vols. London, 1924.

———. *A History of the Art of War in the Sixteenth Century.* London, 1937.

O'Neill, W. *Coming Apart.* New York, 1971.

Orde, A. *Britain and International Security 1920–1926.* London, 1978.

Osgood, R.E. *NATO: The Entangling Alliance.* Chicago, 1962.

Ovendale, R. *Appeasement and the English-Speaking World.* Cardiff, 1975.

Overholt, W.H., ed. *Asia's Nuclear Future.* Boulder, Col., 1977.

Overy, R.J., "Hitler's War and the German Economy: A Reinterpretation," *Economic History Review* 35 (1982).

———. *The Air War, 1939–1945.* New York, 1980.

———. *The Nazi Economic Recovery 1932–1938.* London, 1982.

Owen, R., and R. Sutcliffe, eds. *Studies in the Theory of Imperialism.* London, 1972.

Oye, K.A., et al., eds. *Eagle Defiant: United States Foreign Policy in the 1980s.* Boston, 1983.

———, et al., eds. *Eagle Entangled: U.S. Foreign Policy in a Complex World.* New York, 1979.

Padfield, P. *Guns at Sea.* London, 1973.

———. *The Battleship Era.* London, 1972.

———. *Tide of Empires: Decisive Naval Campaigns in the Rise of the West,* 2 vols. London, 1979, 1982.

Palmer, A. *Napoleon in Russia.* New York, 1967.

Palmer, B. *The 25-Year War: America's Military Role in Vietnam.* New York, 1984.

Pares, R., "American versus Continental Warfare 1739–1763," *English Historical Review* 51 (1936).

——. *War and Trade in the West Indies 1739–1763*. Oxford, 1936.

Paret, P. *Yorck and the Era of Prussian Reform*. Princeton, N.J., 1961.

Parish, P.J. *The American Civil War*. New York, 1975.

Parker, G. *Europe in Crisis 1598–1648*. London, 1979.

——. *Spain and the Netherlands 1559–1659*. London, 1979.

——. *The Army of Flanders and the Spanish Road 1567–1659: The Logistics of Spanish Victory and Defeat in the Low Countries War*. Cambridge, 1972.

——. *The Dutch Revolt*. London, 1977.

Parker, R.A.C., "Great Britain, France and the Ethiopian Crisis 1935–1936," *English Historical Review* 89 (1974).

Parodi, M. *L'économie et la société française de 1945 a 1970*. Paris, 1971.

Parry, J.H. *The Age of Reconnaissance*, 2nd edn. London, 1966.

——. *The Establishment of the European Hegemony 1415–1715*, 3rd edn. New York, 1966.

——. *Trade and Dominion: The European Overseas Empire in the Eighteenth Century*. London, 1971.

Patterson, A.T. *The Other Armada: The Franco-Spanish Attempt to Invade Britain in 1779*. Manchester, 1960.

Peacock, A.T., and J. Wiseman. *The Growth of Public Expenditure in the United Kingdom*. London, 1967 edn.

Peden, G.C. *British Rearmament and the Treasury 1932–1939*. Edinburgh, 1979.

Pedroncini, G. *Les mutineries de 1917*. Paris, 1967.

Pelz, S.E. *Race to Pearl Harbor*. Cambridge, Mass., 1974.

Pemsel, H. *Atlas of Naval Warfare*. London, 1977.

Pericoli, U., and M. Glover. *1815: The Armies at Waterloo*. London, 1973.

Perkins, B. *Prologue to War: England and the United States 1805–1812*. Berkeley, Calif., 1961.

——. *The Great Rapprochement*. New York, 1969.

Perkins, D.H., ed. *China's Modern Economy in Historical Perspective*. Stanford, Calif., 1975.

Petersen, E.N. *The Limits of Hitler's Power*. Princeton, N.J., 1969.

Petersen, P.A., and J. G. Hines, "The Conventional Offensive in Soviet Theater Strategy," *Orbis* 27 (1983).

Pflanze, O. *Bismarck and the Development of Germany: The Period of Unification 1815–1871*. Princeton, N.J., 1963.

Pierre, A.J. *Nuclear Politics: The British Experience with an Independent Strategic Nuclear Force, 1939–1970*. London, 1972.

——, ed. *Nuclear Weapons in Europe*. New York, 1984.

Pigasse, J.P. *Le bouclier d'Europe*. Paris, 1982.

Pintner, W., "Inflation in Russia During the Crimean War Period," *American Slavic and East European Review* 18 (1959).

Pitt, B. *1918—The Last Act*. New York, 1962.

Pivka, O. von. *Navies of the Napoleonic Era*. Newton Abbott, 1980.

Plesur, M. *America's Outward Thrust: Approaches to Foreign Affairs 1865–1890*. DeKalb, Ill., 1971.

Polisensky, J.V. *The Thirty Years War*. London, 1971.

Pollard, S. *Peaceful Conquest: The Industrialization of Europe 1760–1970*. Oxford, 1981.

——. *The Wasting of the British Economy*. London, 1982.

Polmar, N. *Soviet Naval Developments, 1982*, 4th edn. Annapolis, Md., 1981.

Polonsky, A. *The Great Powers and the Polish Question 1941–1945*. London, 1976.

Porch, D. *The March to the Marne: The French Army 1871–1914.* Cambridge, 1981.
Porter, B. *Britain, Europe and the World, 1850–1982: Delusions of Grandeur.* London, 1983.
———. *The Lion's Share: A Short History of British Imperialism 1850–1970.* London, 1976.
Posen, B.R. *The Sources of Military Doctrine: France, Britain and Germany Between the World Wars.* Ithaca, N.Y., 1984.
Postan, M.M. *An Economic History of Western Europe, 1945–1964.* London, 1967.
Potichny, P.T., ed. *The Ukraine in the Seventies.* Oakville, Ont., 1982.
Potter, E.B., ed. *Sea Power: A Naval History.* Annapolis, Md., 1981.
Potter, G.R., ed. *The New Cambridge Modern History,* vol i, *The Renaissance 1493–1520.* Cambridge, 1961.
Pounds, N.J.G. *An Historical Geography of Europe 1500–1840.* Cambridge, 1979.
———, and S. S. Ball, "Core Areas and the Development of the European States System," *Annals of the Association of American Geographers* 54 (1964).
Powers, T. *The War at Home: Vietnam and the American People, 1964–1968.* New York, 1973.
———. *Thinking About Nuclear Weapons.* New York, 1983.
Prados, J. *The Soviet Estimate: U.S. Intelligence Analysis and Russian Military Strength.* New York, 1982.
Pratt, L.R. *East of Malta, West of Suez: Britain's Mediterranean Crisis.* London, 1975.
Presseisen, E.L. *Amiens and Munich: Comparisons in Appeasement.* The Hague, 1978.
Preston, A., ed. *General Staffs and Diplomacy Before the Second World War.* London, 1978.
Preston, R.A., S. F. Wise, and H. O. Werner. *Men in Arms.* London, 1962.
Price, R. *The Economic Modernization of France.* London, 1975.
Prins, G, ed. *The Nuclear Crisis Reader.* New York, 1984.
Qaisar, A.J. *The Indian Response to European Technology and Culture, A.D. 1498–1707.* Delhi, 1982.
Quester, G. *Nuclear Proliferation: Breaking the Chain.* Madison, Wi., 1981.
Quimby, R.S. *The Background of Napoleonic Warfare.* New York, 1957.
Quinn, D.B., and A. N. Ryan. *England's Sea Empire, 1550–1642.* London, 1983.
Radice, L. *Prelude to Appeasement: East Central European Diplomacy in the Early 1930s.* New York, 1981.
Raeff, M. *Imperial Russia 1682–1825.* New York, 1971.
Ragsdale, H. *Détente in the Napoleonic Era: Bonaparte and the Russians.* Lawrence, Kan., 1980.
Rahman, H., "British Post-Second World War Military Planning for the Middle East," *Journal of Strategic Studies* 5 (1982).
Ramsay, J.F. *Anglo-French Relations 1763–70: A Study of Choiseul's Foreign Policy.* Berkeley, Calif., 1939.
Ransom, R.L., et al., eds. *Explorations in the New Economic History.* New York, 1982.
Ranum, O., ed. *National Consciousness, History and Political Culture in Early Modern Europe.* Baltimore, 1975.
Rapp, R.T., "The Unmaking of the Mediterranean Trade Hegemony," *Journal of Economic History* 35 (1975).
Rappaport, A. *Henry L. Stimson and Japan, 1931–1933.* Chicago, 1963.
Rasler, K.A., and W. R. Thompson, "Global Wars, Public Debts, and the Long Cycle," *World Politics* 35 (1983).
Rath, R.J. *The Fall of the Napoleonic Kingdom of Italy.* New York, 1941.

Raulff, H. *Zwischen Machtpolitik und Imperialismus: Die deutsche Frankreichpolitik 1904–5.* Düsseldorf, 1976.

Reamington, R.A. *The Warsaw Pact.* Cambridge, Mass., 1971.

Redlich, F. "Contributions in the Thirty Years War," *Economic History Review* 12 (1959).

———. *The German Military Enterpriser and His Work Force,* 2 vols. Wiesbaden, 1964.

Rees, D. *Korea: The Limited War.* New York, 1966.

Regla, J., "Spain and Her Empire," *New Cambridge Modern History,* vol. v. Cambridge, 1961.

Reinhard, W. *Geschichte der europäischen Expansion,* vol. i. Stuttgart, 1983.

Les Relations franco-allemandes 1933–1939. Paris, 1976.

Les Relations franco-britanniques 1935–39. Paris, 1975.

Reynolds, C.G. *Command of the Sea: The History and Strategy of Maritime Empires.* New York, 1974.

———, "Imperial Japan's Continental Strategy," *U.S. Naval Institute Proceedings* 109 (1983).

Reynolds, D. *The Creation of the Anglo-American Alliance, 1937–1961.* London, 1981.

Rich, N. *Friedrich von Holstein,* 2 vols. Cambridge, 1965.

———. *Hitler's War Aims,* 2 vols. London, 1973–74.

———. *Why the Crimean War?: A Cautionary Tale.* Hanover, N.H., 1985.

Richardson, H.W. *Economic Recovery in Britain, 1932–1939.* London, 1967.

Richmond, H. *Statesmen and Sea Power.* Oxford, 1946.

Riley, J.C. *International Government Finance and the Amsterdam Capital Market 1740–1815.* Cambridge, 1980.

Ritter, G. *The Schlieffen Plan.* New York, 1958.

———. *The Sword and the Scepter,* 4 vols. London, 1975.

Ritter, M., "Das Kontributionssystem Wallensteins," *Historische Zeitschrift* 90 (1902).

Robbins, K. *Munich, 1938.* London, 1968.

Roberts, J.M. *The Pelican History of the World.* Harmondsworth, Mddsx., 1980.

Roberts, M. *Essays in Swedish History.* London, 1967.

———. *Gustavus Adolphus and the Rise of Sweden.* London, 1973.

———. *Gustavus Adolphus,* 2 vols. London, 1958.

———. *Splendid Isolation 1763–1780.* Stenton Lecture, Reading, 1970.

———. *The Swedish Imperial Experience 1560–1718.* Cambridge, 1979.

Robertson, E.M., ed. *The Origins of the Second World War.* London, 1971.

Robertson, R.M. *History of American Economy.* New York, 1975 edn.

Robinson, R., J. Gallagher, and A. Denny. *Africa and the Victorians: The Official Mind of Imperialism,* 2nd edn. London, 1982.

Rodger, A.B. *The War of the Second Coalition, 1798–1801.* Oxford, 1964.

Rogge, H. *Russia in the Age of Modernization and Revolution 1881–1917.* London, 1983.

Rohe, K., ed. *Die Westmächte und das Dritte Reich 1933–1939.* Paderborn, 1982.

Röhl, J.C.G., "A Document of 1892 on Germany, Prussia, and Poland," *Historical Journal* 7 (1964).

———, and N. Sombart, eds. *Kaiser Wilhelm II: New Interpretations.* Cambridge, 1982.

Roider, K.A. *Austria's Eastern Question 1700–1790.* Princeton, N.J., 1982.

Rolfe, S. *The International Corporation.* Paris, 1969.

Ropp, T. *The Development of a Modern Navy: French Naval Policy 1871–1904.* Annapolis, Md., 1987.

————. *War in the Modern World.* Durham, N.C., 1959.

Ropponen, R. *Die Kraft Russlands: Wie beurteilte die politische und militärische Führung der europäischen Grossmächte in der Zeit von 1905 bis 1914 die Kraft Russlands?* Helsinki, 1968.

Rosecrance, R., ed. *America as an Ordinary Power,* Ithaca, N.Y., 1976.

————. *The Rise of the Trading State.* New York, 1985.

Rosenberg, D.A., "A Smoking Radiating Ruin at the End of Two Hours: Documents on American Plans for Nuclear War with the Soviet Union, 1954–55," *International Security* 6 (1981–82).

————, "American Atomic Strategy and the Hydrogen Bomb Decision," *Journal of American History* 66 (1979).

————, "The Origins of Overkill: Nuclear Weapons and American Strategy, 1945–1960," *International Security* 7 (1983).

Rosenberg, H. *Bureaucracy, Aristocracy and Autocracy: The Prussian Experience 1660–1815.* Cambridge, Mass., 1958.

Roseveare, H. *The Treasury: The Evolution of a British Institution.* London, 1969.

Rosinski, H., "The Role of Sea Power in the Global Warfare of the Future," *Brassey's Naval Annual* (1947).

Roskill, S.W. *Naval Policy Between the Wars,* vol. ii. London, 1976.

————. *The War at Sea,* 3 vols. London, 1954–61.

Ross, G. *The Great Powers and the Decline of the European States System 1914–1945.* London, 1983.

Ross, S.T. *European Diplomatic History 1789–1815: France Against Europe.* Malabar, Fla., 1981 reprint.

————. *Quest for Victory: French Military Strategy 1792–1799.* London, 1973.

Rostow, N. *Anglo-French Relations 1934–1936.* London, 1984.

Rostow, W.W. *The Process of Economic Growth,* 2nd edn. Oxford, 1960.

————. *The World Economy: History and Prospect.* Austin, Tex., 1978.

Rothenberg, G.E., B. K. Kiraly, and P. F. Sugar, eds. *East Central European Society and War in the Pre-Revolutionary Eighteenth Century.* New York, 1982.

————. *Napoleon's Great Adversaries: The Archduke Charles and the Austrian Army 1792–1814.* London, 1982.

————. *The Army of Francis Joseph.* West Lafayette, Ind., 1976.

————. *The Art of Warfare in the Age of Napoleon.* Bloomington, Ind., 1978.

Rothstein, R.L. *The Third World and U.S. Foreign Policy.* Boulder, Col., 1981.

————. *The Weak in the World of the Strong: The Developing Countries in the International System.* New York, 1977.

Rothwell, V. *Britain and the Cold War 1941–47.* London, 1982.

Rowen, H.S., "Living with a Sick Bear," *The National Interest* 2 (1985–86).

Rowland, B.M., ed. *Balance of Power or Hegemony: The Inter-War Monetary System.* New York, 1976.

Rowley, A. *Evolution économique de la France de milieu du XIXe siècle à 1914.* Paris, 1982.

Rubin, B. *Paved with Good Intentions: The United States and Iran.* New York, 1980.

Rudé, G. *Paris and London in the Eighteenth Century: Studies in Popular Protest.* New York, 1971.

————. *Revolutionary Europe 1783–1815.* London, 1964.

Rudney, R.S., "Mitterrand's New Atlanticism: Evolving French Attitudes Toward NATO," *Orbis* 28 (1984).

Rupieper, H. *The Cuno Government and Reparations, 1922–1923.* London, 1979.

Rusinov, D. *The Yugoslav Experiment, 1948–1974.* London, 1977.

Russell, C., ed. *The Origins of the English Civil War.* London, 1973.

Russett, B., "America's Continuing Strengths," *International Organization* 39 (1985).

————, "Defense Expenditures and National Well-being," *American Political Science Review* 76 (1982).

Ryder, A.J. *The German Revolution of 1918.* Cambridge, 1967.

Rywkin, M. *Moscow's Muslim Challenge.* New York, 1982.

Sachar, H.M. *Europe Leaves the Middle East 1936–1954.* London, 1972.

Sadkovich, J.J., "Minerals, Weapons and Warfare: Italy's Failure in World War II," *Storia contemporanea,* forthcoming.

Salewski, M. *Die deutsche Seekriegsleitung 1935–1945,* 3 vols. Frankfurt, 1970–75.

Salisbury, H. *The Coming War Between Russia and China.* London, 1969.

Salmon, J.M.H. *Society in Crisis: France in the Sixteenth Century.* London, 1975.

Samhaber, E. *Merchants Make History.* London, 1963.

Sansom, G.B. *A History of Japan,* 3 vols. London, 1958–66.

————. *The Western World and Japan.* London, 1950.

Saul, S.B. *Studies in British Overseas Trade 1870–1914.* Liverpool, 1960.

Saunders, H. *The Middle East Problem in the 1980s.* Washington, D.C., 1981.

Sauvy, A. *Histoire économique de la France entre les deux guerres,* 2 vols. Paris, 1965–67.

Savelle, M. *Empires to Nations: Expansion in America, 1713–1824.* Minneapolis, 1974.

Savory, R. *His Britannic Majesty's Army in Germany During the Seven Years War.* Oxford, 1966.

Sayous, A., "Le role d'Amsterdam dans l'histoire du capitalisme commercial et financier," *Revue Historique* 183 (1938).

Scalapino, R.A., ed. *The Foreign Policy of Modern Japan.* Berkeley, Calif., 1977.

Scammell, G.V. *The World Encompassed: The First European Maritime Empires, c. 800–1650.* Berkeley, Calif., 1981.

Schaller, M. *The American Occupation of Japan: The Origins of the Cold War in Asia.* New York, 1985.

Schell, J. *The Fate of the Earth.* New York, 1982.

Schell, O. *To Get Rich Is Glorious: China in the 80s.* New York, 1985.

Schilling, W.R., et al. *Strategy, Politics, and Defense Budgets.* New York, 1962.

Schmidt, G. *England in der Krise: Grundzüge und Grundlagen der britischen Appeasement-Politik, 1930–1937.* Opladen, 1981.

————, "Wozu noch politische Geschichte?," *Aus Politik und Zeitgeschichte* B17 (1975).

Schmidt, H. *A Grand Strategy for the West.* New Haven, Conn., 1985.

Schmitt, B.E., and H. C. Vedeler. *The World in the Crucible 1914–1919.* New York, 1984.

Schooner, D.M. *Soviet Economy in a Time of Change.* Washington, D.C., 1979.

Schreiber, G., et al., eds. *Das Deutsche Reich und der Zweite Weltkrieg,* vol. iii, *Der Mittelmeerraum und Südosteuropa.* Stuttgart, 1984.

————. *Revisionismus und Weltmachtstreben.* Stuttgart, 1978.

Schroeder, P.W. *Austria, Britain and the Crimean War: The Destruction of the European Concert.* Ithaca, N.Y., 1972.

————, "Munich and the British Tradition," *Historical Journal* (1976).

————, "The Lost Intermediaries: The Impact of 1870 on the European System," *International History Review* 6 (1984).

————, "World War I as a Galloping Gertie," *Journal of Modern History* 44 (1972).

Schulin, E., ed. *Gedenkschrift Martin Göhring: Studien zur europäischen Geschichte.* Wiesbaden, 1968.

Schulte, B.F. *Die deutsche Armee.* Düsseldorf, 1977.

Schulzinger, R.D. *American Diplomacy in the Twentieth Century.* New York, 1984.

Schumpeter, E.B., "English Prices and Public Finance, 1660–1822," *Review of Economic Statistics* 20 (1938).

Schwartz, T., "The Case of German Rearmament: Alliance Crisis in the 'Golden Age,'" *The Fletcher Forum* (1984).

Scott, H.M., "British Foreign Policy in the Age of the American Revolution," *International History Review* 6 (1984).

———, "The Importance of Bourbon Naval Reconstruction to the Strategy of Choiseul after the Seven Years War," *International History Review* 1 (1979).

Scott, W.R. *The Constitution and Finance of English, Scottish and Irish Joint Stock Companies to 1720*, 3 vols. Cambridge, 1912.

Seabury, P., "International Policy and National Defense," *Journal of Contemporary Studies* (1983).

Searle, G.R. *The Quest for National Efficiency: A Study in British Politics and British Political Thought, 1899–1914*. Oxford, 1971.

Seaton, A. *The Crimean War: A Russian Chronicle*. London, 1977.

———. *The German Army 1933–1945*. London, 1982.

———. *The Russian Army of the Crimea*. Reading, Berkshire, 1973.

———. *The Russo-German War 1941–45*. London, 1971.

Segal, G., ed. *The China Factor: Peking and the Superpowers*. London, 1982.

———. *The Soviet Union in East Asia*. Boulder, Col., 1983.

———, and W. Tow, eds. *Chinese Defense Policy*. London, 1984.

———. *Defending China*. London, 1985.

———, "Defense Culture and Sino-Soviet Relations," *Journal of Strategic History* 8 (1985).

———. *The Great Power Triangle*. London, 1982.

Servan-Schreiber, J.J. *The American Challenge*. Harmondsworth, Mddsx., 1969 edn.

Seton-Watson, C. *Italy from Liberalism to Fascism*. London, 1967.

Seton-Watson, R.W. *The Russian Empire 1801–1917*. Oxford, 1967.

Shaw, A.G.L., ed. *Great Britain and the Colonies 1815–1865*. London, 1970.

Shay, R.P. *British Rearmament in the Thirties: Politics and Profits*. Princeton, N.J., 1977.

Shennan, J.H. *The Origins of the Modern European State 1450–1725*. London, 1974.

Sherman, A.J., "German-Jewish Bankers in World Politics: The Financing of the Russo-Japanese War," *Leo Baeck Institute Yearbook* 28 (1983).

Sherwig, J.M. *Guineas and Gunpowder: British Foreign Aid in the Wars with France 1793–1815*. Cambridge, Mass., 1969.

Sherwin, M.J. *A World Destroyed: The Atomic Bomb and the Grand Alliance*. New York, 1975.

Shiba, Y. *Commerce and Society in Sung China*. Ann Arbor, Mich., 1970.

Showalter, D. *Railroads and Rifles: Soldiers, Technology and the Unification of Germany*. Hamden, Conn., 1975.

Shuker, S.A. *The End of French Predominance in Europe: The Financial Crisis of 1924 and the Adoption of the Dawes Plan*. Chapel Hill, N.C., 1976.

Shulman, M.D. *Stalin's Foreign Policy Reappraised*. New York, 1969.

Sick, G. *All Fall Down: America's Tragic Encounter with Iran*. New York, 1985.

Sidorov, A.L. *The Economic Position of Russia During the First World War*. Moscow, 1973.

Siegelbaum, L.H. *The Politics of Industrial Mobilization in Russia, 1914–1917*. New York, 1984.

Silberling, N.J., "Financial and Monetary Policy of Great Britain During the Napoleonic Wars," *Quarterly Journal of Economics* 38 (1923–24).

Silverman, D.P. *Reconstructing Europe After the Great War*. Cambridge, Mass., 1982.

Simmons, R.R. *The Strained Alliance*. New York, 1975.

Skalweit, A. *Die deutsche Kriegsnährungswirtschaft*. Berlin, 1927.

Sked, A., ed. *Europe's Balance of Power 1815–1848*. London, 1979.

——. *The Survival of the Habsburg Empire: Radetsky, the Imperial Army and the Class War, 1848*. London, 1979.

Slessor, J. *Strategy for the West*. London, 1954.

Smith, D.M., "National Interest and American Intervention, 1917: An Historical Appraisal," *Journal of American History* 52 (1965).

——. *The Great Departure: The United States and World War I, 1914–1920*. New York, 1965.

Smith, G. *Morality, Reason and Power: American Diplomacy in the Carter Years*. New York, 1986.

Smith, M., et al. *Asia's New Industrial World*. London, 1985.

——. *British Air Strategy Between the Wars*. Oxford, 1984.

Smith, T. *Political Change and Modern Development in Japan: Government Enterprise 1868–1880*. Stanford, Calif., 1955.

——. *The Pattern of Imperialism: The United States, Great Britain and the Late-Industrializing World Since 1815*. Cambridge, 1981.

Snyder, J. *The Ideology of the Offensive*. Ithaca, N.Y., 1984.

Snyder, J.C., and S. F. Wells, eds. *Limiting Nuclear Proliferation*. Cambridge, Mass., 1985.

Solomon, R.H., ed. *The China Factor: Sino-American Relations and the Global Scene*. Englewood Cliffs, N.J., 1981.

Sombart, W. *Krieg und Kapitalismus*. Munich, 1913.

Sontag, R.J. *A Broken World, 1919–1939*. New York, 1971.

Spanier, J.W. *American Foreign Policy Since World War II*. London, 1972 edn.

Spector, R.H. *Eagle Against the Sun: The American War with Japan*. New York, 1985.

Speer, A. *Inside the Third Reich*. New York, 1982 edn.

Spiers, E.M. *The Army and Society 1815–1914*. London, 1980.

Sprout, H., and M. Sprout. *The Rise of American Naval Power, 1776–1918*. Princeton, N.J., 1946 edn.

Spulber, N. *The State and Economic Development in Eastern Europe*. New York, 1966.

Stares, P., "The Modernization of the French Strategic Nuclear Force," *Journal of the Royal United Services Institute for Defence Studies* 125 (1980).

Starr, H. *Henry Kissinger: Perceptions of International Politics*. Lexington, Ky., 1982.

State of the World Economy, The. Cambridge, Mass., 1982.

Stavrianos, L.S. *Global Rift: The Third World Comes of Age*. New York, 1981.

Steel, R. *Pax Americana*. New York, 1977.

Steele, J. *Soviet Power*. New York, 1984.

Steinberg, J., "The Copenhagen Complex," *Journal of Contemporary History* 1 (1966).

Steinbrunner, D.D., and L. V. Segal, eds. *Alliance Security: NATO and the No-First-Use Question*. Washington, D.C., 1983.

Steiner, Z.S. *Britain and the Origins of the First World War*. London, 1977.

——. *The Foreign Office and Foreign Policy 1898–1914*. Cambridge, 1969.

Stella, D. *Crisis and Continuity: The Economy of Spanish Lombardy in the Seventeenth Century*. Cambridge, Mass., 1979.

Stoakes, G. *Hitler and the Quest for World Dominion: Nazi Ideology and Foreign Policy in the 1920s*. Leamington Spa, 1986.

Stockholm International Peace Research Institute. *The Arms Race and Arms Control*. London, 1982.

Stoessinger, J.G. *Nations in Darkness: China, Russia and America.* New York, 1978.
Stokesbury, J.L. *A Short History of World War I.* New York, 1981.
Stone, L. *The Causes of the English Revolution 1529–1642.* London, 1972.
Stone, N. *Europe Transformed 1878–1919.* London, 1983.
———. *The Eastern Front 1914–1917.* London, 1975.
Stork-Penning, J.G., "The Ordeal of the States: Some Remarks on Dutch Politics During the War of the Spanish Succession," *Acta Historiae Neerlandica* 2 (1967).
Storry, R. *A History of Modern Japan.* Harmondsworth, Mddsx., 1982 edn.
———. *Japan and the Decline of the West in Asia 1894–1943.* London, 1979.
Stoye, J.W. *Europe Unfolding 1648–1688.* London, 1969.
———. *The Siege of Vienna.* London, 1964.
Strachan, H. *European Armies and the Conduct of War.* London, 1983.
———. *Wellington's Legacy: The Reform of the British Army, 1830–1854.* Manchester, 1984.
Stradling, R.A., "Catastrophe and Recovery: The Defeat of Spain 1639–43," *History* 64 (1979).
———. *Europe and the Decline of Spain: A Study of the Spanish System, 1580–1720.* London, 1981.
Strengthening Conventional Deterrence in Europe: Proposals for the 1980s. New York, 1983.
Strode, D.L., "Arms Control and Sino-Soviet Relations," *Orbis* 28 (1984).
Stueck, W.W. *The Road to Confrontation.* Chapel Hill, N.C., 1981.
Sullivan, L., "A New Approach to Burden-Sharing," *Foreign Policy* 60 (1985).
Summers, H.G. *On Strategy: A Critical Analysis of the Vietnam War.* New York, 1972.
Sumner, B.H. *Peter the Great and the Emergence of Russia.* London, 1940.
———. *Russia and the Balkans 1870–1880.* London, 1937.
Sutter, R. *China Watch: Toward Sino-American Reconciliation.* Baltimore, 1978.
Svennilson, I. *Growth and Stagnation in the European Economy.* Geneva, 1954.
Symcox, G. *The Crisis of French Sea Power 1689–1697.* The Hague, 1974.
Syrett, D. *Shipping and the American War 1775–83.* London, 1970.
Szamuely, T. *The Russian Traditions,* London, 1974.
Taagepera, R., "Growth Curves of Empires," *General Systems* 13 (1968).
———, "Size and Duration of Empires: Systematics of Size," *Social Science Research* 7 (1978).
Taborsky, E. *Communist Penetration of the Third World.* New York, 1963.
Talbott, S. *Deadly Gambits: The Reagan Administration and the Stalemate in Nuclear Arms Control.* New York, 1984.
Tamborra, A., "The Rise of Italian Industry and the Balkans," *Journal of European Economic History* 3 (1974).
Taubman, W. *Stalin's American Policy: From Entente to Détente to Cold War.* New York, 1982.
Taylor, A.J.P. *The Origins of the Second World War.* Harmondsworth, Mddsx., 1964 edn.
———. *The Struggle for Mastery in Europe 1848–1918.* Oxford, 1954.
———. *The Trouble-Makers: Dissent over Foreign Policy, 1789–1939.* London, 1969 edn.
Taylor, J. *Shadows of the Rising Sun: A Critical View of the "Japanese Miracle."* New York, 1984.
Taylor, R. *The Sino-Japanese Axis.* New York, 1985.
Taylor, T. *Munich: The Price of Peace.* New York, 1979.
Teichova, A. *An Economic Background to Munich.* Cambridge, 1974.
Thies, J. *Architekt der Weltherrschaft: Die "Endziele" Hitlers.* Düsseldorf, 1976.

Thiry, J. *La Guerre d'Espagne.* Paris, 1966.

Thomas, H. *History of the World.* New York, 1979 edn.

Thompson, E.P. *Zero Option.* London, 1982.

——, and D. Smith, eds. *Protest and Survive.* Harmondsworth, Mddsx., 1980.

Thompson, I.A.A. *War and Government in Habsburg Spain 1560–1620.* London, 1976.

Thompson, J.W. *Italian Civil and Military Aircraft 1930–1935.* Fallbrook, Calif., 1963.

Thomson, D. *Europe Since Napoleon.* Harmondsworth, Mddsx., 1966 edn.

——. *The Aims of History.* London, 1969.

Thorne, C. *The Issue of War: States, Societies, and the Far Eastern Conflict of 1941–1945.* London, 1985.

——. *The Limits of Foreign Policy: The West, the League and the Far Eastern Crisis of 1931–1933.* London, 1972.

Thornton, A.P. *The Imperial Idea and Its Enemies.* London, 1966.

Thornton, R.C. *The Bear and the Dragon.* New York, 1972.

Thucydides. *The Peleponnesian War.* Harmondsworth, Mddsx., 1954 edn.

Thurow, L. *The Zero-Sum Society.* New York, 1980.

Tilly, C., ed. *The Formation of the National States in Western Europe.* Princeton, N.J., 1975.

Toby, R.P. *State and Diplomacy in Early Modern Japan.* Princeton, N.J., 1984.

Tocqueville, A. de. *Democracy in America,* 2 vols. New York, 1945 edn.

Tokes, R.L. *Euro-Communism and Détente.* New York, 1978.

Toland, J. *No Man's Land: The Story of 1918.* London, 1980.

Tomlinson, B.R., "The Contraction of England: National Decline and the Loss of Empire," *Journal of Imperial and Commonwealth History* 11 (1982).

——. *The Political Economy of the Raj 1914–1947.* Cambridge, 1979.

Towle, P., "The European Balance of Power in 1914," *Army Quarterly and Defense Journal* 104 (1974).

Toynbee, A.J., and F. T. Ashton-Gwatkin, eds. *The World in 1939.* London, 1952.

Trachtenberg, M. *Reparation in World Politics: France and European Diplomacy 1916–1923.* New York, 1980.

Trask, D.F. *The War with Spain in 1898.* New York, 1981.

Trebilcock, C. *The Industrialization of the Continental Powers 1780–1914.* London, 1981.

Treverton, G.F. *Making the Alliance Work: The United States and Europe.* Ithaca, N.Y., 1985.

Tuchman, B.W. *Stilwell and the American Experience in China.* New York, 1971.

Tucker, N.B. *Patterns in the Dust: Chinese-American Relations and the Recognition Controversy 1949–50.* New York, 1983.

Tucker, R.W., "Swollen State, Spent Society: Stalin's Legacy to Brezhnev's Russia," *Foreign Affairs* 60 (1981–82).

——. *The Purposes of American Power.* New York, 1981.

Tunstall, B. *William Pitt, Earl of Chatham.* London, 1938.

Turner, L.C.F. *Origins of the First World War.* London, 1970.

Ulam, A. *Dangerous Relations: The Soviet Union in World Politics 1970–1982.* New York, 1983.

——. *Expansion and Coexistence: The History of Soviet Foreign Policy 1917–1973.* New York, 1974.

Ungar, S.J., ed. *Estrangement: America and the World.* New York, 1985.

van der Wee, H., "Monetary, Credit and Banking Systems," *The Cambridge Economic History of Europe,* vol. v. Cambridge, 1977.

Van Ness, P. *Revolution and Chinese Foreign Policy.* Berkeley, Calif., 1971.

Varg, P.A. *Missionaries, Chinese, and Diplomats... 1890–1952.* Princeton, N.J., 1952.

Vatter, H.G. *The Drive to Industrial Maturity: The U.S. Economy, 1860–1914.* Westport, Conn., 1975 edn.

Vernadsky, G. *The Tsardom of Muscovy, 1547–1682.* New Haven, Conn., 1969.

Viljoen, S. *Economic Systems in World History.* London, 1974.

Vogel, B. *Deutsche Russlandpolitik, 1900–1906.* Düsseldorf, 1973.

Vogel, E.F. *Japan as Number One: Lessons for America.* New York, 1980 edn.

———, "Pax Nipponica?," *Foreign Affairs* 64 (1986).

Volcker, K.-H. *Die deutsche Luftwaffe 1933–1939.* Stuttgart, 1967.

Wagenfuhr, R. *Die deutsche Industrie im Kriege 1939–1945.* Berlin, 1963.

Waite, R.A.L. *Vanguard of Nazism: The Free Corps Movement in Postwar Germany.* Cambridge, Mass., 1952.

Waites, N., ed. *Troubled Neighbours: Franco-British Relations in the Twentieth Century.* London, 1971.

Walden, P. *The Short Victorious War: A History of the Russo-Japanese War, 1904–5.* New York, 1974.

Walker, G.J. *Spanish Politics and Imperial Trade 1700–1789.* Bloomington, Ind., 1979.

Waller, B. *Bismarck at the Crossroads: The Reorientation of German Foreign Policy After the Congress of Berlin 1878–1880.* London, 1974.

Wallerstein, I. *The Modern World System,* 2 vols. to date. London, 1974, 1980.

Waltz, K. *Man, the State and War.* New York, 1959.

Waltz, K.N., "Toward Nuclear Peace," Wilson Center, International Security Studies, Working Paper 16.

Wandycz, P. *France and Her Eastern Allies 1919–1925.* Minneapolis, 1962.

———. *The Twilight of the French Eastern Alliances, 1926–1936,* forthcoming.

Wangermann, E. *The Austrian Achievement.* New York, 1973.

Waters, A. *Britain's Industrial Renaissance.* London, 1986.

Watson, M.S. *Chief of Staff: Pre-War Plans and Preparations.* Washington, D.C., 1950.

Watt, D.C. *Too Serious a Business: European Armed Forces and the Approach of the Second World War.* London, 1975.

Webber, C., and A. Wildavsky. *A History of Taxation and Expenditure in the Western World.* New York, 1986.

Weber, E. *The Nationalist Revival in France, 1905–1916.* Berkeley, Calif., 1959.

Webster, C.K. *The Foreign Policy of Castlereagh, 1812–1815: Britain and the Reconstruction of Europe.* London, 1931.

Wedgewood, C.V. *The Thirty Years War.* London, 1964 edn.

Wegs, J.R. *Europe Since 1945,* 2nd edn. New York, 1984.

Wehler, H.-U. *Bismarck und der Imperialismus.* Cologne, 1969.

Weigley, R.F. *History of the United States Army.* Bloomington, Ind., 1984 edn.

———. *The American Way of War: A History of the United States Military Strategy and Policy.* Bloomington, Ind., 1977 edn.

Weinberg, G. *The Foreign Policy of Hitler's Germany,* 2 vols. Chicago, 1970, 1980.

Weinberger, C. *Report of the Secretary of Defense Caspar W. Weinberger to the Congress on Fiscal Year 1984 Budget.* Washington, D.C., 1983.

———, "U.S. Defense Strategy," *Foreign Affairs* 64 (1986).

Weller, J. *Wellington in the Peninsula.* London, 1962.

Wells, S.F., "Sounding the Tocsin: NSC-68 and the Soviet Threat," *International Security* 4 (1979).

Wendt, B.J., "Freihandel und Friedenssicherung: Zur Bedeutung des Cobden-Vertrags von 1860 zwischen England und Frankreich," *Vierteljahresschrift für Sozial- und Wirtschaftsgeschichte* 61 (1974).

Wernham, R.B. *Before the Armada: The Growth of English Foreign Policy 1485–1588.* London, 1966.

——. *The Making of Elizabethan Foreign Policy 1588–1603.* Berkeley, Calif., 1980.

Wesson, R.G. *State Systems: International Relations: Politics and Culture.* New York, 1978.

Westwood, J.N. *Russia Against Japan, 1904–5: A New Look at the Russo-Japanese War.* London, 1986.

Whelan, J.G. *World Communism, 1967–1969: Soviet Attempts to Reestablish Control.* Washington, D.C., 1970.

Whetten, L.L. *Germany's Ostpolitik.* London, 1971.

——, "The Mediterranean Threat," *Survival* 8 (1980).

White, J.A. *The Diplomacy of the Russo-Japanese War.* Princeton, N.J., 1964.

Whittam, J. *The Politics of the Italian Army 1861–1918.* London, 1977.

Wight, M. *Power Politics.* Harmondsworth, Mddsx., 1979.

Wildman, A.K. *The End of the Russian Imperial Army.* Princeton, N.J., 1980.

Wilkinson, E. *Misunderstanding: Europe versus Japan.* Tokyo, 1981.

Williams, E.N. *The Ancien Régime in Europe 1648–1789.* Harmondsworth, Mddsx., 1979 edn.

Williams, G. *The Expansion of Europe in the Eighteenth Century.* London, 1966.

Williams, J. *The Home Fronts: Britain, France and Germany, 1914–1918.* London, 1972.

Williams, J.B. *British Commercial Policy and Trade Expansion 1750–1850.* Oxford, 1972.

Williams, P. *The Tudor Regime.* Oxford, 1979.

Williams, W.A. *The Roots of the Modern American Empire.* New York, 1969.

Willmott, H.P. *Empires in the Balance.* Annapolis, Md., 1982.

Wilson, A.M. *French Foreign Policy During the Administration of Cardinal Fleury.* Cambridge, Mass., 1936.

Wilson, C.H., ed. *Economic History and the Historian: Collected Essays.* London, 1969.

——. *Anglo-Dutch Commerce and Finance in the Eighteenth Century.* Cambridge, 1966 reprint.

——. *The Dutch Republic and the Civilization of the Seventeenth Century.* London, 1968.

——. *The Transformation of Europe 1558–1648.* London, 1976.

Wimbush, W.E., ed. *Soviet Nationalities in Strategic Perspective.* New York, 1985.

Windelband, W. *Bismarck und die europäischen Grossmächte 1878–85.* Essen, 1940.

Windsor, P. *German Reunification.* London, 1969.

Winter, J.M., ed. *War and Economic Development.* Cambridge, 1975.

Wittek, P. *The Rise of the Ottoman Empire.* London, 1938.

Wittram, R. *Peter I. Czar und Kaiser,* 2 vols. Göttingen, 1964.

Wolf, A. *A History of Science, Technology and Philosophy in the Sixteenth and Seventeenth Centuries.* New York, 1935.

Wolf, J.B. *Louis XIV.* London, 1968.

——. *The Emergence of the Great Powers 1685–1715.* New York, 1951.

——. *Toward a European Balance of Power 1620–1715.* Chicago, 1970.

Wolfe, M. *The Fiscal System of Renaissance France.* New Haven, Conn., 1972.

Wolfe, T. *Soviet Power and Europe, 1945–1970.* Baltimore, Md., 1970.

Wolfers, A. *Britain and France Between Two Wars.* New York, 1966 edn.

Woodruff, W. *America's Impact on the World: A Study of the Role of the United States in the World Economy 1750–1970.* New York, 1973.

——. *Impact of Western Man: A Study of Europe's Role in the World Economy 1750–1960.* New York, 1967.

Woods, J. (pseudonym), "The Royal Navy Since World War II," *U.S. Naval Institute Proceedings* 108 (1982).

Woodward, D.R. *Lloyd George and the Generals.* Newark, N.J., 1983.

Wright, G. *The Ordeal of Total War, 1939–1945.* New York, 1968.

Wright, Q. *A Study of War.* Chicago, 1942.

Yahuda, M.B. *China's Role in World Affairs.* New York, 1978.

Yang, L.-S. *Money and Credit in China.* Cambridge, Mass., 1952.

Yardley, H. *The American Black Chamber.* New York, 1931.

Yonosuke, N., and A. Iriye, eds. *The Origins of the Cold War in Asia.* New York, 1977.

Yost, D.S. *France and Conventional Defense in Central Europe.* Boulder, Col., 1985.

———, "France's Deterrent Posture," *Adelphi Papers* 194 and 195 (1985).

Young, J.W. *Britain, France and the Unity of Europe 1945–51.* Leicester, 1984.

Young, L.K. *British Policy in China 1895–1902.* Oxford, 1970.

Young, R.J. *In Command of France: French Foreign Policy and Military Planning 1933–1940.* Cambridge, Mass., 1978.

Ziemke, E.F. *Stalingrad to Berlin: The German Defeat in the East 1942–1945.* Washington, D.C., 1968.

Zuckerman, S. *Nuclear Illusion and Reality.* London, 1982.

Index

About the Author

PAUL KENNEDY was born in the north of England, at Wallsend-on-Tyne, in 1945. He attended the University of Newcastle, where he graduated with first class honors in history, and received his doctorate from Oxford.

Professor Kennedy has researched and lectured at a variety of places in Europe and North America. He is a Fellow of the Royal Historical Society, a former Visiting Fellow of the Institute for Advanced Study at Princeton, and of the Alexander von Humboldt Foundation in West Germany. In 1983 Kennedy moved to Yale to become the J. Richardson Dilworth Professor of History, with a focus on modern strategic and international affairs. A frequent reviewer for and contributor to *The New York Times, The New Republic, The Washington Post, The Atlantic* and *The Economist,* Paul Kennedy lives in Hamden, Connecticut, with his wife, Catherine, and their three sons.